Diseases of the Breast

Diseases of the Breast

Edited by

JAY R. HARRIS, MD

Professor of Radiation Oncology
Harvard Medical School
Clinical and Educational Director
Joint Center for Radiation Therapy
Department of Radiation Oncology
Beth Israel Hospital
Dana-Farber Cancer Institute
Boston, Massachusetts

MARC E. LIPPMAN, MD

Professor of Medicine and Pharmacology
Georgetown University Medical School
Director, Vincent T. Lombardi Cancer Research Center
Washington, DC

MONICA MORROW, MD

Associate Professor of Surgery
Northwestern University Medical School
Director, Lynn Sage Comprehensive Breast Program
Northwestern Memorial Hospital
Chicago, Illinois

SAMUEL HELLMAN, MD

A.N. Pritzker Distinguished Service Professor
Department of Radiation and Cellular Oncology
The University of Chicago
Chicago, Illinois

With 101 additional contributors

Lippincott - Raven
P U B L I S H E R S
Philadelphia • New York

Developmental Editor: Eileen Wolfberg
Associate Managing Editor: Grace R. Caputo
Production Manager: Caren Erlichman
Senior Production Coordinator: Kevin P. Johnson
Senior Design Coordinator: Kathy Kelley-Luedtke
Indexer: Maria Coughlin
Compositor: Tapsco, Inc.
Printer/Binder: Quebecor/Kingsport

Library of Congress Cataloging-in-Publication Data

Diseases of the breast/edited by Jay R. Harris . . . [et al.]; with 101 contributors.
    p. cm.
   Includes bibliographical references and index.
   ISBN 0-397-51470-0 (alk. paper)
   1. Breast—Cancer. 2. Breast—Diseases.   I. Harris, Jay R.
   [DNLM: 1. Breast Neoplasms. 2. Breast—pathology. 3. Breast—
physiopathology. WP 870 D611 1996]
RC280.B8D49 1996
618.1′9—dc20
DNLM/DLC
for Library of Congress   95-4853
                                                   CIP

The material contained in this volume was submitted as previously unpublished
material, except in the instances in which credit has been given to the source from
which some of the illustrative material was derived.

Great care has been taken to maintain the accuracy of the information contained
in the volume. However, neither Lippincott-Raven Publishers nor the editors can
be held responsible for errors or for any consequences arising from the use of the
information herein.

The authors and publisher have exerted every effort to ensure that drug selection
and dosage set forth in this text are in accord with current recommendations and
practice at the time of publication. However, in view of ongoing research, changes
in government regulation, and the constant flow of information relating to drug
therapy and drug reactions, the reader is urged to check the package insert for each
drug for any change in indications and dosage and for added warnings and
precautions. This is particularly important when the recommended agent is a new or
infrequently employed drug.

Materials appearing in this book prepared by individuals as part of their official
duties as U.S. Government employees are not covered by the above-mentioned
copyright.

9 8 7 6 5 4 3

CONTRIBUTORS

ALAN D. AARON, MD
Assistant Professor of Orthopaedics
Georgetown University Hospital
Washington, DC

DORIT D. ADLER, MD
Associate Professor of Radiology
Associate Director, Division of Breast Imaging
University of Michigan Medical Center
Ann Arbor, Michigan

MADELINE M. BARNICLE, RN, MSN, OCN
Oncology Clinical Specialist
Rush Cancer Institute
Rush-Presbyterian–St Luke's Medical Center
Chicago, Illinois

LESLIE BERNSTEIN, PhD
Professor
University of Southern California School of Medicine
Department of Preventive Medicine
Kenneth Norris Jr. Comprehensive Cancer Center
Los Angeles, California

JOHN BOSTWICK III, MD
Professor and Chairman
Department of Plastic Surgery
Division of Plastic and Reconstructive Surgery
Emory University School of Medicine
The Emory Clinic
Atlanta, Georgia

GLENN D. BRAUNSTEIN, MD
Professor of Medicine
University of California, Los Angeles, UCLA School
    of Medicine
Chairman, Department of Medicine
Cedars-Sinai Medical Center
Los Angeles, California

R. JAMES BRENNER, MD, JD
Associate Clinical Professor
University of California, Los Angeles, UCLA School
    of Medicine
Director, Breast Imaging Services
Joyce Eisenberg Keefer Breast Center
John Wayne Cancer Institute
Saint John's Hospital and Health Center
Director, Tower Breast Imaging Center
Los Angeles, California

LOUISE A. BRINTON, PhD
Chief, Environmental Studies Section
Environmental Epidemiology Branch
National Cancer Institute
Bethesda, Maryland

NILS BRÜNNER, MD, PhD
Finsen Laboratory
Copenhagen, Denmark

FRANÇOIS CAMPANA, MD
Chief, Brachytherapy Unit
Radiotherapy Department
Institut Curie
Paris, France

NATHAN I. CHERNY, MBBS, FRACP
Pain and Palliative Medicine Physician
Department of Internal Medicine
Shaare Zedek Medical Center
Jerusalem, Israel

GARY M. CLARK, PhD
Professor of Medicine
Division of Medical Oncology
University of Texas Health Science Center
    at San Antonio
San Antonio, Texas

ROBERT CLARKE, PhD
Associate Professor of Physiology and Biophysics
Georgetown University Medical Center
Vincent T. Lombardi Cancer Research Center
Washington, DC

CATHY COLEMAN, RN, OCN
Vice President, Breast Center Development
Comprehensive Cancer Centers
Salick Health Care
Los Angeles, California

STEVEN E. COME, MD
Associate Professor of Medicine
Harvard Medical School
Director, Hematology-Oncology Units
Beth Israel Hospital
Boston, Massachusetts

JAMES L. CONNOLLY, MD
Associate Professor of Pathology
Harvard Medical School
Director of Anatomic Pathology
Beth Israel Hospital
Boston, Massachusetts

SUSAN S. DEVESA, PhD
Chief, Descriptive Studies Section
Biostatistics Branch
Environmental Epidemiology Branch
National Institutes of Health
National Cancer Institute
Bethesda, Maryland

ROBERT B. DICKSON, PhD
Professor of Cell Biology and Pharmacology
Associate Director of Basic Science
Vincent T. Lombardi Cancer Research Center
Georgetown University Medical School
Washington, DC

KAREN HASSEY DOW, RN, RPhD, FAAN
Associate Professor
School of Nursing
University of Central Florida
Orlando, Florida

ROSEMARY B. DUDA, MD
Assistant Professor
Harvard Medical School
Chief, Division of Surgical Oncology
Beth Israel Hospital
Attending Physician
Dana Farber Cancer Institute
Boston, Massachusetts

TIMOTHY J. EBERLEIN, MD
Professor of Surgery
Harvard Medical School
Director, Biologic Cancer Therapy Program
Director, Division of Surgical Oncology
    Department of Surgery

Brigham and Women's Hospital
Surgical Director, Breast Evaluation Center
Dana-Farber Cancer Institute
Boston, Massachusetts

W. PHIL EVANS III, MD
Medical Director
Susan G. Komen Breast Center
Baylor University Medical Center
Dallas, Texas

KATHLEEN M. FOLEY, MD
Professor of Neurology, Neuroscience, and Clinical
    Pharmacology
Cornell University Medical Center
Chief, Pain Service
Department of Neurology
Memorial Sloan-Kettering Cancer Center
New York, New York

BRUNO D. FORNAGE, MD
Professor of Radiology
Department of Diagnostic Radiology
University of Texas M.D. Anderson Cancer Center
Houston, Texas

ROGER S. FOSTER, JR., MD
Wadley Glenn Professor of Surgery
Emory University School of Medicine
Chief of Surgical Services
Crawford Long Hospital of Emory University
Atlanta, Georgia

ALAIN FOURQUET, MD
Chief of Service
Radiotherapy Department
Institut Curie
Paris, France

RONNIE J. FREILICH, MD, BS, FRACP, MD
Neuro-Oncology Fellow
Memorial Sloan-Kettering Cancer Center
New York, New York

SUZANNE A.W. FUQUA, PhD
Division of Medical Oncology
Department of Medicine
University of Texas Health Science Center
    at San Antonio
San Antonio, Texas

MICHELE A. GADD, MD
Massachusetts General Hospital Cancer Center
Comprehensive Breast Health Center
Harvard Medical School
Boston, Massachusetts

JUDY E. GARBER, MD
Assistant Professor of Medicine
Harvard Medical School
Dana-Farber Cancer Institute
Boston, Massachusetts

REBECCA GELMAN, PhD
Associate Professor of Biostatistics
Harvard Medical School
Harvard School of Public Health
Dana-Farber Cancer Institute
Boston, Massachusetts

LYNN H. GERBER, MD
Chief, Department of Rehabilitation Medicine
Clinical Center
National Institutes of Health
Bethesda, Maryland

TERESA GILEWSKI, MD
Assistant Professor of Medicine
Cornell University Medical Center
Assistant Attending Physician
Memorial Sloan-Kettering Cancer Center
New York, New York

J. PETER GLASS, MD
Associate Professor of Medicine
Division of Neurology
Duke University Medical Center
Durham, North Carolina

JAY R. HARRIS, MD
Professor of Radiation Oncology
Harvard Medical School
Clinical and Educational Director
Joint Center of Radiation Therapy
Department of Radiation Oncology
Beth Israel Hospital
Dana-Farber Cancer Institute
Boston, Massachusetts

DANIEL F. HAYES, MD
Assistant Professor of Medicine
Harvard Medical School
Medical Director, Breast Evaluation Center
Dana-Farber Cancer Institute
Boston, Massachusetts

SAMUEL HELLMAN, MD
A.N. Pritzker Distinguished Service Professor
Department of Radiation and Cellular Oncology
The University of Chicago
Chicago, Illinois

BRIAN E. HENDERSON, MD
Department of Preventive Medicine
University of Southern California School of Medicine
Kenneth Norris Jr. Comprehensive Cancer Center
La Jolla, California

SUSAN FLAMM HONIG, MD
Associate Professor of Medicine
Director, Breast Cancer Consultation Group
Division of Hematology/Oncology
Vincent T. Lombardi Cancer Research Center
Washington, DC

GABRIEL N. HORTOBAGYI, MD
Professor of Medicine
Chairman, Department of Breast and Gynecologic
   Medical Oncology
University of Texas M.D. Anderson Cancer Center
Houston, Texas

MARY JANE HOULIHAN, MD
Instructor in Surgery
Harvard Medical School
Senior Associate in Surgery
Beth Israel Hospital
Boston, Massachusetts

DAVID J. HUNTER, MD
Associate Professor of Epidemiology
Harvard Medical School
Department of Medicine
Brigham and Women's Hospital
Boston, Massachusetts

CLAUDINE ISAACS, MD, FRCPC
Instructor in Medicine
Vincent T. Lombardi Cancer Research Center
Georgetown University Medical Center
Washington, DC

LORI JARDINES, MD
Assistant Professor
Director of Breast Surgery
Department of Surgery
Medical College of Pennsylvania
Philadelphia, Pennsylvania

L. CANDICE JENNINGS, MD
Instructor in Orthopaedic Surgery
Harvard Medical School
Assistant, Orthopaedic Surgery
Massachusetts General Hospital
Boston, Massachusetts

V. CRAIG JORDAN, PhD, DSc
Professor of Molecular Pharmacology and Biological
   Chemistry
Department of Pharmacology
Professor of Cancer Pharmacology
Director of the Breast Cancer Research Program
Associate Director for Cancer Prevention and Control
Robert H. Lurie Cancer Center
Northwestern University Medical School
Chicago, Illinois

WILLIAM KAPLAN, MD†
Associate Professor of Radiology
Harvard Medical School
Chief Oncologist, Nuclear Medicine
Dana-Farber Cancer Institute
Boston, Massachusetts

JON F. KERNER, PhD
Associate Director for Cancer Prevention and Control
Vincent T. Lombardi Cancer Research Center
Georgetown University Medical Center
Washington, DC

V. SUZANNE KLIMBERG, MD
Chief, Breast Service
Arkansas Cancer Research Center
University of Arkansas for Medical Sciences
Little Rock, Arkansas

DANIEL B. KOPANS, MD
Associate Professor of Radiology
Director of Breast Imaging
Massachusetts General Hospital
Boston, Massachusetts

DONALD R. LAUB, MD
Clinical Associate Professor of Surgery
Stanford University School of Medicine
Stanford, California

GAIL S. LEBOVIC, MA, MD
Attending Surgeon
Stanford University Hospital
Stanford, California

FABIO LEONESSA, MD
Research Instructor
Department of Physiology and Biophysics
Vincent T. Lombardi Cancer Research Center
Georgetown University Medical Center
Washington, DC

ROBERT LERNER, MD
Clinical Professor of Surgery
State University of New York Health Science Center
    at Brooklyn College of Medicine
Brooklyn, New York

MARC E. LIPPMAN, MD
Professor of Medicine and Pharmacology
Director, Vincent T. Lombardi Cancer Research Center
Georgetown University Medical School
Washington, DC

GREG J. MACKAY, MD
Department of Plastic Surgery
Division of Plastic and Reconstructive Surgery
Emory University School of Medicine
Atlanta, Georgia

COLETTE M. MAGNANT, MD, FACS
Assistant Professor of Surgery
Director, Trauma Services
Surgical Director, Multidisciplinary Breast Program
Georgetown University Medical Center
Georgetown University School of Medicine
Washington, DC

DAVID MALKIN, MD
Assistant Professor
Division of Oncology
Department of Pediatrics
The Hospital for Sick Children
University of Toronto
Toronto, Ontario, Canada

MARY JANE MASSIE, MD
Professor of Clinical Psychiatry
Cornell University Medical College
Attending Psychiatrist, Psychiatry Service
Director, Barbara White Fishman Breast Cancer
    Counseling Service
Memorial Sloan-Kettering Cancer Center
New York, New York

BERYL McCORMICK, MD
Associate Professor of Radiation Oncology in Medicine
Cornell University Medical College
Associate Attending Physician
New York Hospital
Memorial Sloan-Kettering Cancer Center
New York, New York

MARSHA D. McNEESE, MD
Associate Professor
Department of Radiotherapy
University of Texas M.D. Anderson Cancer Center
Houston, Texas

STEVEN S. MENTZER, MD
Associate Professor of Surgery
Division of Thoracic Surgery
Director of Lung Transplant Program
Brigham and Women's Hospital
Boston, Massachusetts

MALCOLM S. MITCHELL, MD
Professor of Medicine
USCD Cancer Center
Director, Center for Biological Therapy
    and Melanoma Research
University of California, San Diego, School of Medicine
La Jolla, California

MICHAEL P. MOORE, MD, PhD
Assistant Clinical Professor
Columbia Presbyterian Medical Center
New York, New York

† Deceased

MONICA MORROW, MD
Associate Professor of Surgery
Northwestern University Medical School
Director, Lynn Sage Comprehensive Breast Program
Northwestern Memorial Hospital
Chicago, Illinois

LARRY NORTON, MD
Professor of Medicine
Chief, Breast Cancer Medicine Service
Cornell University Medical Center
Memorial Sloan-Kettering Cancer Center
New York, New York

C. KENT OSBORNE, MD
Professor of Medicine
Interim Chief, Division of Medical Oncology
University of Texas Health Science Center
San Antonio, Texas

MICHAEL P. OSBORNE, MD
Director and Chief Executive Officer
Strang Cancer Prevention Center
New York, New York

JANET ROSE OSUCH, MD
Associate Professor of Surgery
Michigan State University College of Human Medicine
East Lansing, Michigan

WILLIAM P. PETERS, MD
President, Michigan Cancer Foundation
Director, Meyer L. Prentis Comprehensive
    Cancer Center
Detroit, Michigan

JEANNE A. PETREK, MD
Associate Professor Surgery
Cornell University Medical College
Associate Attending Surgeon
Breast Service
Memorial Sloan-Kettering Cancer Center
New York, New York

PETER M. RAVDIN, MD, PhD
Associate Professor of Medical Oncology
Division of Medical Oncology
University of Texas Health Science Center
San Antonio, Texas

ABRAM RECHT, MD
Associate Professor of Radiation Oncology
Harvard Medical School
Radiation Oncologist
Joint Center for Radiation Therapy
Deputy Section Chief

Department of Radiation Oncology
Beth Israel Hospital
Breast Evaluation Center
Dana-Farber Cancer Institute
Boston, Massachusetts

BARBARA K. RIMER, DrPH
Professor of Community and Family Medicine
Director, Cancer Prevention, Detection
    and Control Research
Duke University School of Medicine
Durham, North Carolina

ANNE DE LA ROCHEFORDIÈRE, MD
Senior Radiation Oncologist
Radiotherapy Department
Institut Curie
Paris, France

LISA R. ROGERS, DO
Associate Professor of Neurology
Wayne State University School of Medicine
Detroit, Michigan

PETER PAUL ROSEN, MD
Professor of Pathology
Cornell University Medical College
Attending Pathologist and Member
Memorial Sloan-Kettering Cancer Center
New York, New York

JULIA H. ROWLAND, PhD
Assistant Professor of Psychiatry
Director, Psycho-Oncology Program
Vincent T. Lombardi Cancer Research Center
Georgetown University Medical Center
Washington, DC

NORMAN L. SADOWSKY, MD
Clinical Professor of Radiology
Tufts University School of Medicine
Director, Faulkner-Sagoff Centre for Breast Health Care
Faulkner Hospital
Boston, Massachusetts

BRUNO SALVADORI, MD
Director, Surgical Oncology
National Cancer Institute
Milan, Italy

LOWELL E. SCHNIPPER, MD
Theodore W. and Evelyn G. Gerenson Associate
    Professor of Medicine
Harvard Medical School
Chief, Oncology Division
Beth Israel Hospital
Boston, Massachusetts

STUART J. SCHNITT, MD
Associate Professor of Pathology
Harvard Medical School
Associate Director of Surgical Pathology
Beth Israel Hospital
Boston, Massachusetts

LAWRENCE N. SHULMAN, MD
Assistant Professor of Medicine
Harvard Medical School
Clinical Director
Hematology–Oncology Division
Brigham and Women's Hospital
Boston, Massachusetts

S. EVA SINGLETARY, MD
Associate Professor of Surgery
Chief of Surgical Breast Services
Department of Surgical Oncology
University of Texas M.D. Anderson Cancer Center
Houston, Texas

BARBARA L. SMITH, MD, PhD
Assistant Professor
Harvard Medical School
Director, Comprehensive Breast Health Center
Massachusetts General Hospital
Boston, Massachusetts

DEMPSEY S. SPRINGFIELD, MD
Associate Professor of Orthopaedic Surgery
Harvard Medical School
Visiting Orthopaedic Surgeon
Massachusetts General Hospital
Boston, Massachusetts

PATRICIA S. STEEG, PhD
Chief
Women's Cancers Section
Laboratory of Pathology
National Cancer Institute
Bethesda, Maryland

DAVID J. SUGARBAKER, MD
Associate Professor of Surgery
Harvard Medical School
Chief, Division of Thoracic Surgery
Brigham and Women's Hospital
Boston, Massachusetts

MARK S. TALAMONTI, MD
Assistant Professor of Surgery
Northwestern University Medical School
Chicago, Illinois

KENNETH K. TANABE, MD
Assistant Professor of Surgery
Harvard Medical School
Division of Surgical Oncology
Department of Surgery
Massachusetts General Hospital
Boston, Massachusetts

RICHARD L. THERIAULT, DO, FACP
Associate Professor of Medicine
Department of Breast and Gynecologic Medical
    Oncology
University of Texas M.D. Anderson Cancer Center
Houston, Texas

ERIK W. THOMPSON, PhD
Assistant Professor of Cell Biology
Georgetown University Medical School
Washington, DC

ANN D. THOR, PhD
Associate Professor of Pathology
University of Vermont College of Medicine
Burlington, Vermont
Clinical Associate Professor
Massachusetts General Hospital
Boston, Massachusetts

BRUCE J. TROCK, PhD
Director of Molecular Epidemiology
Vincent T. Lombardi Cancer Research Center
Georgetown University Medical Center
Washington, DC

RENA VASSILOPOULOU-SELLIN, MD
Section of Endocrinology
University of Texas M.D. Anderson Cancer Center
Houston, Texas

UMBERTO VERONESI, MD
Scientific Director
European Institute of Oncology
Milano, Italy

VICTOR G. VOGEL, MD, MHS, FACP
Associate Professor of Medicine and Epidemiology
Chief, Section of Clinical Cancer Prevention
Division of Cancer Prevention
University of Texas M.D. Anderson Cancer Center
Houston, Texas

RICHARD L. WAHL, MD
Professor of Internal Medicine and Radiology
Director of Nuclear Imaging
Departments of Radiology and Internal Medicine
University of Michigan Medical Center
Ann Arbor, Michigan

RAYMOND P. WARRELL, JR., MD
Professor of Medicine
Cornell University Medical College
Member
Memorial Sloan-Kettering Cancer Center
New York, New York

BARBARA L. WEBER, MD
Associate Professor of Medicine and Genetics
Director, Breast Cancer Program
University of Pennsylvania Cancer Center
Hematology–Oncology Division
Department of Medicine
Hospital of the University of Pennsylvania
Philadelphia, Pennsylvania

ANTON WELLSTEIN, MD, PhD
Professor of Pharmacology and Medicine
Georgetown University Medical Center
Vincent T. Lombardi Cancer Research Center
Washington, DC

WALTER C. WILLETT, MD
Frederick John Stare Professor of Epidemiology
     and Nutrition
Chairman, Nutrition Department
Harvard School of Public Health
Boston, Massachusetts

DAVID P. WINCHESTER, MD, FACS
Chairman
Department of Surgery
Evanston Hospital
Evanston, Illinois

JANET WOLTER, MD
Professor of Medicine
Section of Medical Oncology
Rush-Presbyterian–St Luke's Medical Center
Rush University
Rush Cancer Institute
Chicago, Illinois

DAVID W. YANDELL, ScD
Associate Professor of Pathology
Department of Pathology
University of Vermont College of Medicine
Burlington, Vermont

PREFACE

Interest in and knowledge about breast diseases, especially breast cancer, have increased greatly in recent years. A number of factors have contributed to this, the foremost of which are the high occurrence of breast cancer in westernized countries and the dramatic upswing in this incidence during the past few decades. Clinical investigators have also helped define various benign diseases of the breast and have described their management and relation to subsequent breast cancer development. Moreover, clinical trials performed throughout the world have contributed considerable information about the early detection and management of breast cancer using surgery, radiation therapy, and systemic therapies, including chemotherapy and hormonal interventions. Finally, rapid advances in the understanding of the molecular biology and genetics of both normal tissues and cancers have raised optimism that new, more specific methods can be developed to identify a woman's risk for breast cancer, to prevent or at least detect the disease at an earlier stage, and, failing this, to cure it with minimal toxicity. Ultimately a source of hope, these factors have nevertheless caused considerable anxiety in the population, as well as provided a proliferation of information important for clinicians dealing with diseases that strike the breast.

Diseases of the Breast is intended as a single-source compilation of the new knowledge on breast diseases presented in a form accessible to practicing clinicians. Although it is widely recognized that multidisciplinary interaction and information sharing are essential to effective clinical management of diseases of the breast, new developments are rapidly demonstrating that clinicians also need to be knowledgeable about advances in basic science. A prominent example of how advances in basic science can rapidly enter the clinical arena is the discovery of the first genetic mutations at specific loci shown to be associated with a high risk of breast cancer. Clinicians are now faced with patient questions about the nature and meaning of such testing as well as its risks and benefits. We believe that other advances in basic science will quickly be reflected in clinical practice.

For *Diseases of the Breast,* we invited a large, diverse, and distinguished group of experts to summarize the current knowledge about breast diseases, including clinical features, management, and underlying biologic and epidemiologic factors. In assembling these contributions, we have tried to make the book comprehensive and timely, as well as accessible to practicing clinicians. We believe that this book will also be an aid to basic and translational scientists concerned about a breast cancer problem by providing clinical information that can help focus their energies and talents. We hope that *Diseases of the Breast* will be a useful resource for both clinicians and scientists and will foster the understanding and communication necessary to provide optimal patient care and to rapidly achieve advances in managing diseases of the breast, especially breast cancer.

Jay R. Harris, MD
Marc E. Lippman, MD
Monica Morrow, MD
Samuel Hellman, MD

CONTENTS

1 *Breast Development and Anatomy* 1
MICHAEL P. OSBORNE

2 *Biochemical Control of Breast Development* 15
ROBERT B. DICKSON

3 *Benign Disorders* 27

3.1 *Pathology of Benign Breast Disorders* 27
STUART J. SCHNITT · JAMES L. CONNOLLY

3.2 *Papillary Lesions* 42
MICHELE A. GADD

3.3 *Fibroadenoma and Hamartoma* 45
MARY JANE HOULIHAN

3.4 *Duct Ectasia, Periductal Mastitis, and Infections* 49
KENNETH K. TANABE

3.5 *Gynecomastia* 54
GLENN D. BRAUNSTEIN

3.6 *Fat Necrosis, Hematoma, and Trauma* 61
COLETTE M. MAGNANT

4 *Clinical Evaluation* 67

4.1 *Physical Examination of the Breast* 67
MONICA MORROW

4.2 *Imaging Analysis of Breast Lesions* 71
DANIEL B. KOPANS

4.3 *New Methods for Breast Cancer Imaging* 84
DORIT D. ADLER · RICHARD L. WAHL

5 *Management of Common Breast Disorders* 99

5.1 *Etiology and Management of Breast Pain* 99
V. SUZANNE KLIMBERG

5.2 *Nipple Discharge* 106
DAVID P. WINCHESTER

5.3 *Abnormalities on Physical Examination* 110
JANET ROSE OSUCH

5.4 *The Abnormal Mammogram* 114
MARK S. TALAMONTI · MONICA MORROW

5.5 *Abnormalities of the Breast in Pregnancy and Lactation* 122
JEANNE A. PETREK

5.6 *Medicolegal Aspects of Breast Cancer Evaluation and Treatment* 125
R. JAMES BRENNER

6 *Biopsy Techniques* 133

6.1 *Techniques for Diagnosis of Palpable Breast Masses* 133
ROGER S. FOSTER, JR.

6.2 *Preoperative Imaging-Guided Needle Localization and Biopsy of Nonpalpable Breast Lesions* 139
DANIEL B. KOPANS · BARBARA L. SMITH

6.3 *Stereotactic Core Breast Biopsy* 144
W. PHIL EVANS III

6.4 *Ultrasound-Guided Percutaneous Needle Biopsy of Nonpalpable Breast Masses* 152
BRUNO D. FORNAGE

**7 Etiology and Pathogenesis
of Breast Cancer** 159

EPIDEMIOLOGIC FACTORS

7.1 *Incidence, Demographics,
and Environmental Factors* 159
LOUISE A. BRINTON · SUSAN S. DEVESA

7.2 *Familial Breast Cancer* 168
BARBARA L. WEBER · JUDY E. GARBER

7.3 *Endogenous and Exogenous
Hormonal Factors* 185
BRIAN E. HENDERSON · LESLIE BERNSTEIN

7.4 *Dietary Factors* 201
DAVID J. HUNTER · WALTER C. WILLETT

7.5 *Molecular Epidemiology* 213
BRUCE J. TROCK

BIOLOGIC FACTORS

7.6 *Oncogenes and Suppressor Genes* 221
ROBERT B. DICKSON · MARC E. LIPPMAN

7.7 *Animal Models of Breast Cancer* 235
ROBERT CLARKE

7.8 *In Vitro Models of Breast Cancer* 245
ROBERT CLARKE · FABIO LEONESSA
NILS BRÜNNER · ERIK W. THOMPSON

7.9 *Estrogen and Progesterone Receptors
and Breast Cancer* 261
SUZANNE A.W. FUQUA

7.10 *Autocrine and Paracrine Factors
in the Normal and the Neoplastic
Breast* 272
ROBERT B. DICKSON · MARC E. LIPPMAN

7.11 *Control of Invasion and Metastasis* 284
PATRICIA S. STEEG

7.12 *Control of Angiogenesis* 293
ANTON WELLSTEIN

7.13 *Immunology and Immunotherapy
of Breast Cancer* 298
MALCOLM S. MITCHELL

8 Breast Cancer Screening 307
BARBARA K. RIMER

**9 Management of the High-Risk and the
Concerned Patient** 323
JUDY E. GARBER · BARBARA L. SMITH

10 Prevention of Breast Cancer 335

10.1 *Biologic Considerations in Breast Cancer
Prevention* 335
V. CRAIG JORDAN

10.2 *Clinical Considerations in Breast Cancer
Prevention* 341
VICTOR G. VOGEL

11 In Situ Carcinomas 355

11.1 *Ductal Carcinoma in Situ* 355
MONICA MORROW · STUART J. SCHNITT
JAY R. HARRIS

11.2 *Lobular Carcinoma in Situ* 369
MONICA MORROW · STUART J. SCHNITT

12 Natural History of Breast Cancer 375
JAY R. HARRIS · SAMUEL HELLMAN

13 Invasive Mammary Carcinoma 393
PAUL PETER ROSEN

**14 Molecular Pathology of Breast
Carcinoma** 445
ANN D. THOR · DAVID W. YANDELL

15 Staging of Breast Carcinoma 457
JAY R. HARRIS

16 Prognostic and Predictive Factors 461
GARY M. CLARK

**17 Treatment of Early-Stage
Breast Cancer** 487

17.1 *Local Management of Invasive
Breast Cancer* 487
JAY R. HARRIS · MONICA MORROW

17.2 *Adjuvant Systemic Therapy of Primary
Breast Cancer* 548
C. KENT OSBORNE · GARY M. CLARK
PETER M. RAVDIN

17.3 *Breast Conservation Trials From
the Milan National Cancer
Institute* 579
UMBERTO VERONESI · BRUNO SALVADORI

**18 Treatment of Locally Advanced
and Inflammatory Breast Cancer** 585
GABRIEL N. HORTOBAGYI
S. EVA SINGLETARY · MARSHA D. McNEESE

19 Breast Reconstruction 601

19.1 *Reconstructive Breast Surgery* 601
GREG J. MACKAY · JOHN BOSTWICK III

19.2 *Silicone Autoimmune Disease* 620
GAIL S. LEBOVIC · DONALD R. LAUB

**20 Evaluation of Patients After
Primary Therapy** 629
DANIEL F. HAYES · WILLIAM KAPLAN

**21 Local–Regional Recurrence After
Mastectomy or Breast-Conserving
Therapy** 649
ABRAM RECHT · DANIEL F. HAYES
TIMOTHY J. EBERLEIN · NORMAN L. SADOWSKY

22 Treatment of Metastatic Disease 669

22.1 Hormonal Therapy
and Chemotherapy 669
SUSAN FLAMM HONIG

22.2 High-Dose Chemotherapy
for Breast Cancer 735
WILLIAM P. PETERS

22.3 Biologic Therapy of Breast Cancer 743
MARC E. LIPPMAN

22.4 Cytokinetics and Breast Cancer
Chemotherapy 751
TERESA GILEWSKI · LARRY NORTON

23 Specific Sites and Emergencies 769

23.1 Brain Metastases in Patients
With Breast Cancer 769
J. PETER GLASS · KATHLEEN M. FOLEY

23.2 Epidural Metastasis 779
RONNIE J. FREILICH · KATHLEEN M. FOLEY

23.3 Leptomeningeal Metastasis 789
LISA R. ROGERS · KATHLEEN M. FOLEY

23.4 Brachial Plexopathy in Patients
With Breast Cancer 796
NATHAN I. CHERNY · KATHLEEN M. FOLEY

23.5 Ocular Metastases From
Breast Cancer 808
BERYL McCORMICK

23.6 Local Treatment
of Bone Metastases 811
ALAN D. AARON · L. CANDICE JENNINGS
DEMPSEY S. SPRINGFIELD

23.7 Medical Treatment
of Bone Metastases 819
RICHARD L. THERIAULT

23.8 Lymphatic Spread
of Breast Cancer 827
CLAUDINE ISAACS

23.9 Malignant Effusions 833
LAWRENCE N. SHULMAN · DAVID J. SUGARBAKER

23.10 Hypercalcemia 840
RAYMOND P. WARRELL, JR.

23.11 Bone Marrow Metastases 847
STEVEN E. COME · LOWELL E. SCHNIPPER

23.12 Management of Discrete Pulmonary
Nodules 853
STEVEN S. MENTZER · DAVID J. SUGARBAKER

24 Special Therapeutic Problems 859

24.1 Male Breast Cancer 859
MICHAEL P. MOORE

24.2 Phyllodes Tumors 863
JEANNE A. PETREK

24.3 Paget Disease 870
ROSEMARY B. DUDA

24.4 Other Cancers in the Breast 876
LORI JARDINES

24.5 Breast Cancer and Pregnancy 883
JEANNE A. PETREK

24.6 Occult Primary Cancer With
Axillary Metastases 892
ALAIN FOURQUET · ANNE DE LA ROCHEFORDIÈRE
FRANÇOIS CAMPANA

24.7 Lymphedema 896
JEANNE A. PETREK · ROBERT LERNER

24.8 Managing Menopausal Symptoms 903
RENA VASSILOPOULOU-SELLIN

24.9 Breast Cancer in Underserved
Minorities 910
JON F. KERNER

**25 Patient Rehabilitation
and Support** 919

25.1 Psychologic Reactions to Breast Cancer
Diagnosis, Treatment,
and Survival 919
JULIA H. ROWLAND · MARY JANE MASSIE

25.2 Rehabilitation Management for Women
With Breast Cancer: Maximizing
Functional Outcomes 939
LYNN H. GERBER

25.3 Support Programs 948
JANET WOLTER

25.4 Nursing Care in Patient Management
and Quality of Life 951
KAREN HASSEY DOW · MADELINE M. BARNICLE

**26 Organizing a Comprehensive
Breast Center** 963
CATHY COLEMAN · GAIL S. LEBOVIC

**27 Basic Tools for Advancing Knowledge
in Breast Cancer** 971

27.1 Techniques in Molecular Biology 971
DAVID MALKIN

27.2 Techniques in the Interpretation
of Clinical Trials 986
REBECCA GELMAN

Index 1007

Diseases of the Breast

Diseases of the Breast, edited by Jay R. Harris,
Marc E. Lippman, Monica Morrow, and Samuel Hellman.
Lippincott-Raven Publishers, Philadelphia, © 1996.

Breast Development and Anatomy

MICHAEL P. OSBORNE

The breasts, or mammary glands, of mammals are important for the survival of the newborn and thus of the species. Nursing of the young in the animal kingdom has many physiologic advantages for the mother, such as aiding postpartum uterine involution, as well as for the neonate in terms of the transfer of immunity and bonding. In humans, social influences have reduced the prevalence of breastfeeding of neonates and may have interfered with its physiologic role. It has become increasingly apparent that the advantages of nursing are substantial for both mother and child.

An understanding of the morphology and physiology of the breast and the many endocrine interrelationships of both is essential to the study of the pathophysiology of the breast and the management of benign, preneoplastic, and neoplastic disorders.

Embryology

During the fifth week of human fetal development, the ectodermal primitive milk streak, or "galactic band," develops from axilla to groin on the embryonic trunk.[1] In the region of the thorax, the band develops to form a mammary ridge, whereas the remaining galactic band regresses. Incomplete regression or dispersion of the primitive galactic band leads to accessory mammary tissues, found in 2% to 6% of women.

At 7 to 8 weeks of gestation, a thickening occurs in the mammary anlage (milk hill stage), followed by invagination into the chest wall mesenchyme (disk stage) and tridimensional growth (globular stage). Further invasion of the chest wall mesenchyme results in a flattening of the ridge (cone stage) at 10 to 14 weeks of gestation. Between 12 and 16 weeks, mesenchymal cells differentiate into the smooth muscle of the nipple and areola. Epithelial buds develop (budding stage) and then branch to form 15 to 25 strips of epithelium (branching stage) at 16 weeks; these strips represent the future secretory alveoli.[2] The secondary mammary anlage then develops, with differentiation of hair follicle, sebaceous gland, and sweat gland elements, but only the sweat glands develop fully at this time. Phylogenetically, the breast parenchyma is believed to develop from sweat gland tissue. In addition, special apocrine glands develop to form the Montgomery glands around the nipple. The developments described thus far are independent of hormonal influences.

During the third trimester of pregnancy, placental sex hormones enter the fetal circulation and induce canalization of the branched epithelial tissues (canalization stage).[3,4] This process continues from the 20th to the 32nd week of gestation. At about term, 15 to 25 mammary ducts are formed, with coalescence of duct and sebaceous glands near the epidermis. Parenchymal differentiation occurs at 32 to 40 weeks with the development of lobular–alveolar structures that contain colostrum (end-vesicle stage). A fourfold increase in mammary gland mass occurs at this time, and the nipple–areolar complex develops and becomes pigmented. In the neonate, the stimulated mammary tissue secretes colostral milk (sometimes called witch's milk), which can be expressed from the nipple for 4 to 7 days postpartum in most neonates of either sex. In the newborn, colostral secretion declines over a 3- to 4-week period, owing to involution of the breast after withdrawal of placental hormones. During early childhood, the end vesicles become further canalized and develop into ductal structures by additional growth and branching.

Molecular Biology of Mammary Gland Development

Normal development of the mammalian breast depends on a combination of systemic mammotrophic hormones as well as local cell–cell interactions.[5,6] The local cellular interactions appear to be mediated by a variety of growth factors, some of which belong to the epidermal growth factor (EGF), transforming growth factor β (TGF-β), fibroblast growth factor (FGF), and *Wnt* gene families.[7–11] Some of these growth regulators have been shown to affect mammary cell growth and differentiation in experimental systems,[10–16] whereas their differential expression in the developing breast suggests that they may act in concert with systemic hormones during normal glandular development.[7–11] Systemic hormonal alterations also combine with local cellular effects to promote involution of the mammary gland following lactation.[17]

TGF-α, a member of the EGF family, may play a role in both ductal growth and alveolar development of the mammary gland. Ectopic expression of TGF-α causes significant alterations in mammary epithelial growth and differentiation in transgenic mice and other systems,[12–14] and the in vivo localization of TGF-α to actively growing end buds of the mouse mammary gland is consistent with a role in normal ductal development.[7,8] In addition, the changing temporal and spatial expression pattern of TGF-α in the breast during pregnancy suggests that it may function in mediating lobuloalveolar development.[8] TGF-α is up-regulated in both mammary ductal epithelium and stromal fibroblasts during rat and human pregnancy.[8] It is therefore possible that TGF-α functions as an autocrine or paracrine intermediate in directing hormonally induced mammary morphogenesis.[7,8,12]

Studies of the growth factors FGF-1 and FGF-2 in the mouse have suggested that they function in promoting mammary ductal development during sexual maturity.[9] At the onset of ovarian function, FGF-1 expression is up-regulated in ductal epithelium and may provide an autocrine growth stimulus for the proliferating breast. In contrast, FGF-2 is expressed in the mammary stroma where it may act indirectly as a ductal morphogen through its influence on extracellular matrix composition. Both FGF-1 and FGF-2 are well known angiogenic factors and may also contribute to early breast development by stimulating neovascularization during ductal growth.[9]

The principal members of the TGF-β family, TGF-β1, -β2 and -β3 appear to be involved in ductal morphogenesis of the virgin mouse mammary gland and in regulating the onset of lactation.[10] TGF-β may govern early ductal development by maintaining an open ductal branching pattern required for subsequent alveolar development.[10] Maintenance of this ductal architecture requires suppression of lateral bud growth, and TGF-β inhibits ductal growth both in vitro and in transgenic mice, possibly through its effects on extracellular matrix deposition.[10,15] In addition, the TGF-β family may play a role in inhibition of lactation. TGF-β expression levels are down-regulated during lactation, and milk production is impaired in TGF-β transgenic mice.[10,16]

Several members of the *Wnt* gene family of secreted glycoproteins are expressed in the developing mouse mammary gland and may play a role in its normal development.[18,19] The first characterized member of this family, *Wnt*-1, was initially identified as an oncogene in mouse mammary tumor virus (MMTV)-induced mammary tumors and induces mammary hyperplasia when expressed in the mammary glands of transgenic mice.[11] Although *Wnt*-1 is not expressed during normal mammary development, at least 6 other members of the *Wnt* family are differentially expressed in the mouse mammary gland during early development, pregnancy, and lactation.[18,19] Because some of these genes can mimic the effects of *Wnt*-1 in mammary cell lines, it seems likely that they influence growth or differentiation in vivo.[11,20] The spatial expression patterns of these *Wnt* genes have not yet been reported, with the exception of *Wnt*-2. That expression of this gene during early mammary development has been localized to the growing epithelial end buds suggests that it may be involved in early ductal morphogenesis.[19]

The postlactational breast requires a combination of lactogenic hormone deprivation, as well as local signals, to undergo glandular involution.[17] The process of involution is characterized by apoptotic cell death and tissue remodeling.[21] Certain gene products associated with apoptosis are up-regulated during mammary involution; however, the factors that trigger the cell death pathway have not been clearly defined.[17] Local extracellular proteases involved in tissue remodeling are up-regulated during breast regression, and this may result in part from the action of TGF-β1 in the postlactational gland.[17]

The regulated expression of locally acting growth factors in the developing breast acts in combination with circulating hormones to control mammary growth, differentiation, and regression. Further investigation of the function of ligands in vivo will undoubtedly have importance for the understanding of both breast development and mammary tumorigenesis.

Abnormal Breast Development

CONGENITAL ABNORMALITIES

The most frequently observed abnormality seen in both sexes is an accessory nipple (polythelia). Ectopic nipple tissue may be mistaken for a pigmented nevus, and it may occur at any point along the milk streak from the axilla to the groin. Rarely, accessory true mammary glands develop. These are most often located in the axilla (polymastia). During pregnancy and lactation, an accessory breast may swell; occasionally, if it has an associated nipple, the accessory breast may function.

Hypoplasia is the underdevelopment of the breast; congenital absence of a breast is termed *amastia*. When breast tissue is lacking but a nipple is present, the condition is termed *amazia*. A wide range of breast abnormalities have been described and may be classified as follows[22,23]:

- Unilateral hypoplasia, contralateral normal
- Bilateral hypoplasia with asymmetry
- Unilateral hyperplasia, contralateral normal
- Bilateral hyperplasia with asymmetry
- Unilateral hypoplasia, contralateral hyperplasia
- Unilateral hypoplasia of breast, thorax, and pectoral muscles (Poland syndrome)

Most of these abnormalities are not severe. The severest deformity, amastia or marked breast hypoplasia, is associated with hypoplasia of the pectoral muscle in 90% of cases,[24] but the reverse does not apply. Ninety-two percent of women with pectoral muscle abnormalities have a normal breast.[25] Congenital abnormalities of the pectoral muscle are usually manifested by the lack of the lower third of the muscle and an associated deformity of the ipsilateral rib cage. The association among absence of the pectoral muscle, chest wall deformity, and breast abnormalities was first recognized by Poland in 1841. The original description, however, did not note the concomitant abnormalities of the hand (synbrachydactyly, with hypoplasia of the middle phalanges and central skin webbing),[26] and considerable controversy has evolved concerning the validity of the eponym for this congenital syndrome.[27,28]

ACQUIRED ABNORMALITIES

The most common—and avoidable—cause of amazia is iatrogenic. Injudicious biopsy of a precociously developing breast results in excision of most of the breast bud and subsequent marked deformity during puberty. The use of radiation therapy in prepubertal females to treat either hemangioma of the breast or intrathoracic disease may also result in amazia. Traumatic injury of the developing breast, such as that resulting from a severe cutaneous burn, with subsequent contracture, may also result in deformity.

Normal Breast Development During Puberty

Puberty in girls begins at the age of 10 to 12 years as a result of the influence of hypothalamic gonadotropin-releasing hormones secreted into the hypothalamic–pituitary portal venous system. The basophilic cells of the anterior pituitary release follicle-stimulating hormone (FSH) and luteinizing hormone (LH). FSH causes the primordial ovarian follicles to mature into graafian follicles, which secrete estrogens, primarily in the form of 17β-estradiol. These hormones induce the growth and maturation of the breasts and genital organs.[29] During the first 1 to 2 years after menarche, hypothalamic–adenohypophyseal function is unbalanced because the maturation of the primordial ovarian follicles does not result in ovulation or a luteal phase. Therefore, ovarian estrogen synthesis predominates over luteal progesterone synthesis. The physiologic effect of estrogens on the maturing breast is to stimulate longitudinal ductal growth of ductal epithelium. Terminal ductules also form buds that precede further breast lobules. Simultaneously, periductal connective tissues increase in volume and elasticity, with enhanced vascularity and fat deposition. These initial changes are induced by estrogens synthesized in immature ovarian follicles, which are anovulatory; subsequently, mature follicles ovulate, and the corpus luteum releases progesterone. The relative role of these hormones is not clear. In experi-

mental studies, estrogens alone induce a pronounced ductular increase, whereas progesterone alone does not. The two hormones together produce full ductular–lobular–alveolar development of mammary tissues.[29] The marked individual variation in development of the breast makes it impossible to categorize histologic changes on the basis of age.[3,4] Breast development by age has been described by external morphologic changes. The evolution of the breast from childhood to maturity has been divided into five phases by Tanner,[30] as shown in Table 1-1.

Morphology

THE ADULT BREAST

The adult breast lies between the second and sixth ribs in the vertical axis and between the sternal edge and the midaxillary line in the horizontal axis (Fig. 1-1). The average breast measures 10 to 12 cm in diameter, and its average thickness centrally is 5 to 7 cm. Breast tissue also projects into the axilla as the axillary tail of Spence. The contour of the breast varies but is usually domelike, with

TABLE 1-1
Phases of Breast Development

PHASE I	
Age: puberty	Preadolescent elevation of the nipple with no palpable glandular tissue or areolar pigmentation
PHASE II	
Age: 11.1 ± 1.1 y	Presence of glandular tissue in the subareolar region. The nipple and breast project as a single mound from the chest wall.
PHASE III	
Age: 12.2 ± 1.09 y	Increase in the amount of readily palpable glandular tissue with enlargement of the breast and increased diameter and pigmentation of the areola. The contour of the breast and nipple remains in a single plane.
PHASE IV	
Age: 13.1 ± 1.15 y	Enlargement of the areola and increased areolar pigmentation. The nipple and areola form a secondary mound above the level of the breast.
PHASE V	
Age: 15.3 ± 1.7 y	Final adolescent development of a smooth contour with no projection of the areola and nipple

(After Tanner JM. Wachstun und Reifung des Menschen. Stuttgart, Georg Thieme Verlag, 1962)

FIGURE 1-1   Normal anatomy of the breast and pectoralis major muscle.

1. Perforating branches from internal mammary artery and vein
2. Pectoral branches from thoracoacromial artery and vein
3. External mammary branch from lateral thoracic artery and vein
4. Branches from subscapular and thoracodorsal arteries and veins
5. Lateral branches of third, fourth, and fifth intercostal arteries and veins
6. Internal mammary artery and veins
7. Sternocostal head of pectoralis major muscle
8. Clavicular head of pectoralis major muscle
9. Axillary artery and vein
10. Cephalic vein
11. Axillary sheath
12. Latissimus dorsi muscle
13. Serratus anterior muscle
14. External abdominal oblique muscle

a conical configuration in the nulliparous woman and pendulous in the parous woman. The breast comprises three major structures: skin, subcutaneous tissue, and breast tissue, with the last comprising both parenchyma and stroma. The parenchyma is divided into 15 to 20 segments that converge at the nipple in a radial arrangement. The collecting ducts draining each segment are 2 mm in diameter, with subareolar lactiferous sinuses 5 to 8 mm in diameter. Between 5 and 10 major collecting milk ducts open at the nipple.

The nomenclature of the duct system is varied. The branching system may be named in a logical fashion, starting with the collecting ducts in the nipple and extending to the ducts draining each alveolus, as shown in Table 1-2.

Each duct drains a lobe made up of 20 to 40 lobules. Each lobule consists of 10 to 100 alveoli or tubulosaccular secretory units. The microanatomy has been described in detail by Parks.[31] The stroma and subcutaneous tissues of the breast contain fat, connective tissue, blood vessels, nerves, and lymphatics.

The skin of the breast is thin and contains hair follicles,

TABLE 1-2
Nomenclature of the Breast Epithelial System

MAJOR DUCTS

Collecting ducts

Lactiferous sinuses

Segmental ducts

Subsegmental ducts

TERMINAL DUCT–LOBULAR UNIT

Terminal ducts

    Extralobular

    Intralobular

Lobules

Alveoli

sebaceous glands, and eccrine sweat glands. The nipple, which is located over the fourth intercostal space in the nonpendulous breast, contains abundant sensory nerve endings, including Ruffini-like bodies and end-bulbs of Krause. Moreover, sebaceous and apocrine sweat glands are present, but no hair follicles. The areola is circular and pigmented, measuring 15 to 60 mm in diameter. The Morgagni tubercles, located near the periphery of the areola, are elevations formed by the openings of the ducts of the Montgomery glands. The Montgomery glands are large, sebaceous glands capable of secreting milk; they represent an intermediate stage between sweat and mammary glands. Fascial tissues envelop the breast. The superficial pectoral fascia envelops the breast and is continuous with the superficial abdominal fascia of Camper. The undersurface of the breast lies on the deep pectoral fascia, covering the pectoralis major and anterior serratus muscles. Connecting these two fascial layers are fibrous bands (Cooper suspensory ligaments) that represent the "natural" means of support of the breast.

BLOOD SUPPLY OF THE BREAST

The principal blood supply to the breast is derived from the internal mammary and lateral thoracic arteries. Approximately 60% of the breast, mainly the medial and central parts, is supplied by the anterior perforating branches of the internal mammary artery. About 30% of the breast, mainly the upper, outer quadrant, is supplied by the lateral thoracic artery. The pectoral branch of the thoracoacromial artery; the lateral branches of the third, fourth, and fifth intercostal arteries; and the subscapular and thoracodorsal arteries all make minor contributions to the blood supply.

LYMPHATIC DRAINAGE OF THE BREAST

Lymph Vessels

The subepithelial or papillary plexus of the lymphatics of the breast are confluent with the subepithelial lymphatics over the surface of the body. These valveless lymphatic vessels communicate with subdermal lymphatic vessels and merge with the Sappey subareolar plexus. The subareolar plexus receives lymphatic vessels from the nipple and areola and communicates by way of vertical lymphatic vessels equivalent to those connecting the subepithelial and subdermal plexus elsewhere.[32] Lymph flows unidirectionally from the superficial to deep plexus and from the subareolar plexus through the lymphatic vessels of the lactiferous duct to the perilobular and deep subcutaneous plexus. The periductal lymphatic vessels lie just outside the myoepithelial layer of the duct wall.[33]

Flow from the deep subcutaneous and intramammary lymphatic vessels moves centrifugally toward the axillary and internal mammary lymph nodes. Injection studies with radiolabeled colloid[34] have demonstrated the physiology of lymph flow and have countered the old hypothesis of centripetal flow toward the Sappey subareolar plexus. About 3% of the lymph from the breast is estimated to flow to the internal mammary chain, whereas 97% flows to the axillary nodes.[35] Drainage of lymph to the internal mammary chain may be observed following injection of any quadrant of the breast.

Axillary Lymph Nodes

The topographic anatomy of the axillary lymph nodes has been studied as the major route of regional spread in primary mammary carcinoma. The anatomic arrangement of the axillary lymph nodes has been subject to many different classifications. The most detailed studies are those of Pickren, which show the pathologic anatomy of tumor spread.[36] Axillary lymph nodes may be grouped as the apical or subclavicular nodes, lying medial to the pectoralis minor muscle, and the axillary vein lymph nodes, grouped along the axillary vein from the pectoralis minor muscle to the lateral limit of the axilla; the interpectoral (Rotter) nodes, lying between the pectoralis major and minor muscles along the lateral pectoral nerve; the scapular group, comprising the nodes lying along the subscapular vessels; and the central nodes, lying beneath the lateral border of the pectoralis major muscle and below the pectoralis minor muscle (Fig. 1-2). Other groups can be identified, such as the external mammary nodes lying over the axillary tail and the paramammary nodes located in the subcutaneous fat over the upper, outer quadrant of the breast.

An alternative method of delineating metastatic spread, for the purposes of determining pathologic anatomy and metastatic progression, is to divide the axillary lymph nodes into arbitrary levels.[37] Level I lymph nodes lie lateral to the lateral border of the pectoralis minor muscle, level II nodes lie behind the pectoralis minor muscle, and level III nodes are located medial to the medial border of the pectoralis minor muscle (Fig. 1-3). These levels can be determined accurately only by marking them at the time of surgery with tags.

INTERNAL MAMMARY LYMPH NODES. The internal mammary nodes lie in the intercostal spaces in the parasternal region. The nodes lie close to the internal mammary vessels in extrapleural fat and are distributed in the inter-

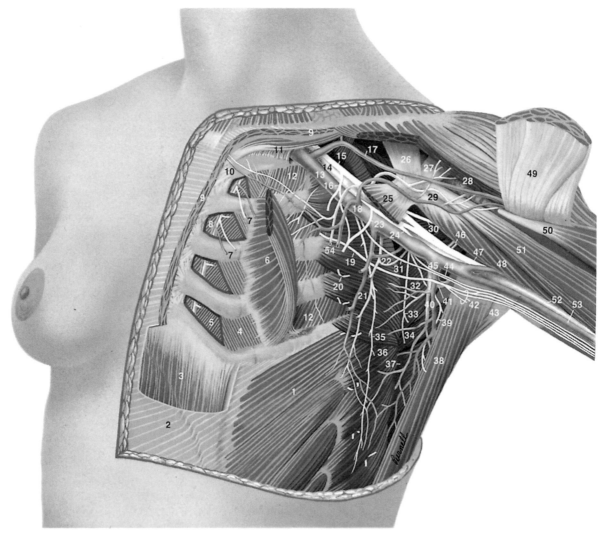

FIGURE 1-2 Chest wall muscles and vascular anatomy.

1. External abdominal oblique muscle
2. Rectus sheath
3. Rectus abdominis muscle
4. Internal intercostal muscle
5. Transverse thoracic muscle
6. Pectoralis minor muscle
7. Perforating branches from internal mammary artery and vein
8. Internal mammary artery and vein
9. Cut edge of pectoralis major muscle
10. Sternoclavicular branch of thoracoacromial artery and vein
11. Subclavius muscle and Halsted ligament
12. External intercostal muscle
13. Axillary vein
14. Axillary artery
15. Lateral cord of brachial plexus
16. Lateral pectoral nerve (from the lateral cord)
17. Cephalic vein
18. Thoracoacromial vein
19. Intercostobrachial nerve
20. Lateral cutaneous nerves
21. Lateral thoracic artery and vein
22. Scapular branches of lateral thoracic artery and vein
23. Medial pectoral nerve (from medial cord)
24. Ulnar nerve
25. Pectoralis minor muscle
26. Coracoclavicular ligament
27. Coracoacromial ligament
28. Cut edge of deltoid muscle
29. Acromial and humeral branches of thoracoacromial artery and vein
30. Musculocutaneous nerve
31. Medial cutaneous nerve of arm
32. Subscapularis muscle
33. Lower subscapular nerve
34. Teres major muscle
35. Long thoracic nerve
36. Serratus anterior muscle
37. Latissimus dorsi muscle
38. Latissimus dorsi muscle
39. Thoracodorsal nerve
40. Thoracodorsal artery and vein
41. Scapular circumflex artery and vein
42. Branching of intercostobrachial nerve
43. Teres major muscle
44. Medial cutaneous nerve of forearm
45. Subscapular artery and vein
46. Posterior humeral circumflex artery and vein
47. Median nerve
48. Coracobrachialis muscle
49. Pectoralis major muscle
50. Biceps brachii muscle, long head
51. Biceps brachii muscle, short head
52. Brachial artery
53. Basilic vein
54. Pectoral branch of thoracoacromial artery and vein

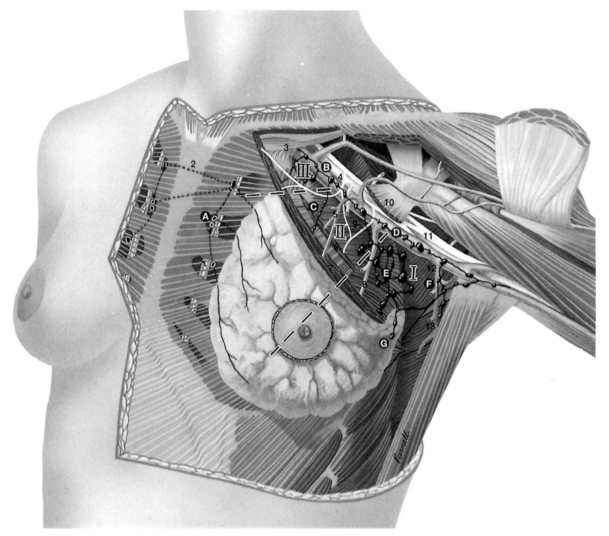

FIGURE 1-3 The lymphatic drainage of the breast showing lymph node groups and levels.

 1. Internal mammary artery and vein
 2. Substernal cross drainage to contralateral internal
    mammary lymphatic chain
 3. Subclavius muscle and Halsted ligament
 4. Lateral pectoral nerve (from the lateral cord)
 5. Pectoral branch from thoracoacromial vein
 6. Pectoralis minor muscle
 7. Pectoralis major muscle
 8. Lateral thoracic vein
 9. Medial pectoral nerve (from the medial cord)
10. Pectoralis minor muscle
11. Median nerve
12. Subscapular vein
13. Thoracodorsal vein

A. Internal mammary lymph nodes
B. Apical lymph nodes
C. Interpectoral (Rotter) lymph nodes
D. Axillary vein lymph nodes
E. Central lymph nodes
F. Scapular lymph nodes
G. External mammary lymph nodes
Level I lymph nodes: lateral to lateral border of pecto-
    ralis minor muscle
Level II lymph nodes: behind pectoralis minor muscle
Level III lymph nodes: medial to medial border of
    pectoralis minor muscle

costal spaces, as shown in Figure 1-3. From the second intercostal space downward, the internal mammary nodes are separated from the pleura by a thin layer of fascia in the same plane as the transverse thoracic muscle. The number of lymph nodes described in the internal mammary chain varies. The nodes lie medial to the internal mammary vessels in the first and second intercostal spaces in 88% and 76% of cases, respectively, whereas they lie lateral to the vessels in the third intercostal space in 79% of cases. The prevalence of nodes in each intercostal space is as follows: first space, 97%; second space, 98%; third space, 82%, fourth space, 9%; fifth space, 12%; and sixth space, 62%.[38] The pathologic anatomy of this route of lymphatic drainage in the spread of breast disease has been described by Handley and Thackray[39] and Urban and Marjani.[40]

In the presence of nodal metastases, obstruction of the physiologic routes of lymphatic flow may occur, and alternative pathways may then become important. The alternative routes that have been described are deep, substernal, cross drainage to the contralateral internal mammary chain[41,42]; superficial presternal crossover, lateral intercostal, and mediastinal drainage[43]; and spread through the rectus abdominis muscle sheath to the subdiaphragmatic and subperitoneal plexus (the Gerota pathway). This last route allows the direct spread of tumor to the liver and retroperitoneal lymph nodes. Substernal crossover is demonstrable by isotope imaging of the lymph nodes[44] and may be of significance in early breast cancer.[44]

MUSCULAR AND NEURAL ANATOMY

The important muscles in the region of the breast are the pectoralis major and minor, serratus anterior, and latissimus dorsi muscles, as well as the aponeurosis of the external oblique and rectus abdominis muscles (see Fig. 1-2).

The pectoralis minor muscle arises from the outer aspect of the third, fourth, and fifth ribs and is inserted into the medial border of the upper surface of the coracoid process of the scapula. The muscle is usually prefixed, rather than postfixed, and is innervated by the medial pectoral nerve, which arises mainly from the medial cord of the brachial plexus (G-8, T-1 segmental origin) and descends posteriorly to the muscle crossing the axillary vein anteriorly. The nerve enters the interpectoral space, passing through the muscle itself in 62% of cases and around the lateral border as a single branch in 38% of cases.[45] Varying numbers of branches passing through the muscle provide motor supply to the lateral part of the pectoralis major muscle. The terms *medial* and *lateral pectoral nerves* are confusing: the standard terminology refers to their brachial plexus origin, rather than their anatomic positions. Changes in terminology have been proposed but have not yet been generally accepted. The arrangement of these nerves is of particular importance in performing the modified radical (Patey) mastectomy.

The serratus anterior muscle stabilizes the scapula on the chest wall. The muscle arises by a series of digitations from the upper eight ribs laterally; its origin from the first rib is in the posterior triangle of the neck. At its origin from the fifth, sixth, seventh, and eighth ribs, it interdigitates with the origin of the external oblique muscle. The muscle inserts into the vertebral border of the scapula on its costal surface and is supplied by the long thoracic nerve of Bell (the nerve to the serratus anterior muscle). The origin of this important nerve is the posterior aspect of the C-5, C-6, and C-7 roots of the brachial plexus. It passes posteriorly to the axillary vessels, emerging on the chest wall high in the medial part of the subscapular fossa. The nerve lies superficial to the deep fascia overlying the anterior serratus muscle and marks the posterior limit of dissection of the deep fascia. Preservation of the nerve to the serratus anterior muscle as it passes downward is essential to avoid "winging" of the scapula and loss of shoulder power.

The latissimus dorsi muscle, the largest muscle in the body, is characterized by a wide origin from the spinous processes and supraspinous ligaments of the seventh thoracic vertebra downward, including all the lumbar and sacral vertebrae. The muscle inserts, by a narrow tendon forming the posterior axillary fold, into a 2.5-cm insertion in the bicipital groove of the humerus. As the muscle spirals around the teres major muscle, the surfaces of the muscle become reversed to the point of insertion. The muscle is supplied by the thoracodorsal nerve (the nerve to the latissimus dorsi muscle), which arises from the posterior cord of the brachial plexus, with segmental origin from C-6, C-7, and C-8. The nerve passes behind the axillary vessels, approaches the subscapular vessels from the medial side, and then crosses anterior to these vessels to enter the medial surface of the muscle. The nerve passes through the axilla and is intimately involved in the scapular group of lymph nodes. Resection of the nerve does not result in any important cosmetic or functional defect; nevertheless, it should be preserved when possible.

An important landmark in the apex of the axilla is the origin of the subclavius muscle, which arises from the costochondral junction of the first rib. At the tendinous part of the lower border of this muscle, two layers of the clavipectoral fascia fuse together to form a well-developed band, the costocoracoid ligament, which stretches from the coracoid process to the first costochondral junction (the Halsted ligament). At this point, the axillary vessels (the vein being anterior to the artery) enter the thorax, passing over the first rib and beneath the clavicle. Many unnamed small branches of the axillary vein pass to its lower border from the axilla. Near the apex, a small artery, the highest thoracic artery, arises from the axillary artery and lies on the first and second ribs.

Muscular Abnormalities

Congenital absence of the sternocostal head of the pectoralis major muscle and its associated abnormalities are described earlier in this chapter. In 5% of cadavers, a sternalis muscle may be found lying longitudinally between the sternal insertion of the sternocleidomastoid muscle and the rectus abdominis muscle. The pectoralis minor muscle is inserted into the head of the humerus as well as the coracoid process of the scapula in 15% of cases. Part of the tendon then passes between the two parts of the coracoacromial ligament to insert into the coracohumeral ligament. Rarely, the axillopectoral muscle arises as a separate part of the latissimus dorsi muscle and crosses the base of the axilla superficially, then passes deep to the pectoralis major muscle to join its insertion or to continue to the coracoid process (the Langer axillary arch). This anatomic arrangement may cause compression of the axillary vessels[46] and difficulty in orientation during axillary dissection.

TABLE 1-3
Characteristics of Human Breast Lobules

Lobule Type	Lobule Area (mm²)	Component Structures	Component Area ($\times 10^{-2}$/mm²)	Number of Components/Lobule	Number of Components/mm²	Number Cells/ Area Section
I	0.048 ± 0.0444	Alveolar bud	0.232 ± 0.090	11.20 ± 6.34	253.8 ± 50.17	32.43 ± 14.07
II	0.060 ± 0.026	Ductule	0.167 ± 0.035	47.0 ± 11.70	682.4 ± 169.0	13.14 ± 4.79
III	0.129 ± 0.049	Ductule	0.125 ± 0.029	81.0 ± 16.6	560.4 ± 25.0	11.0 ± 2.0
IV	0.250 ± 0.060	Acini	0.120 ± 0.050	180.0 ± 20.8	720.0 ± 150.0	10.0 ± 2.3

(After Russo J, Russo IH. Development of human mammary gland. In: Neville MC, Daniel CW, eds. The mammary gland. New York, Plenum, 1987:67)

MICROANATOMY OF BREAST DEVELOPMENT

The developing breast at puberty has been described in detail by Russo and Russo[47] as growing and dividing ducts that form club-shaped terminal end buds (TEBs). Growing TEBs form new branches, twigs, and small ductules termed *alveolar buds*. Alveolar buds subsequently differentiate into the terminal structure of the resting breast named the "acines" by German pathologists or the "ductule" by Dawson.[3] The term *alveolus* is best applied to the resting secretory unit and *acines* to the fully developed secretory unit of pregnancy and lactation.[47]

Lobules develop during the first few years after menarche. The alveolar buds cluster around a terminal duct and form type I (virginal) lobules, comprising about 11 alveolar buds lined by 2 layers of epithelium. Full differentiation of the mammary gland proceeds through puberty, takes many years, and may not be fully completed if interrupted by pregnancies.

Detailed microanatomic studies of the breast have shown the presence of three distinct types of lobules.[47] Type I lobules, previously described, are the first generation of lobules that develop just after the menarche. The transition to type II and type III gradually results from continued sprouting of new alveolar buds. The characteristics of the four lobular types are described in Tables 1-3 and 1-4.

MICROSCOPIC ANATOMY OF THE ADULT BREAST

In the immature breast, the ducts and alveoli are lined by a two-layer epithelium consisting of a basal cuboidal layer and a flattened surface layer. In the presence of estrogens at puberty and subsequently, this epithelium proliferates, becoming multilayered (Fig. 1-4*A*). Three alveolar cell types have been observed: superficial (luminal) A cells, basal B cells (chief cells), and myoepithelial cells.

Superficial, or luminal, A cells are dark, basophilic-staining cells that are rich in ribosomes. Superficial cells undergo intercellular dehiscence, with swelling of the mitochondria, and become grouped, forming buds within the lumen. Basal B cells, or chief cells, are the major cell type in mammary epithelium. They are clear, with an ovoid nucleus without nucleoli. Where the basal cells are

in contact with the lumen, microvilli occur on the cell membrane. Intracytoplasmic filaments are similar to those in myoepithelial cells, suggesting their differentiation toward that cell type. Myoepithelial cells are located around alveoli and small excretory milk ducts between the inner aspect of the basement membrane and the tunica propria. Myoepithelial cells are arranged in a branching, starlike fashion. The sarcoplasm contains filaments 50 to 80 nm in diameter; these myofilaments are inserted by hemidesmosomes into the basal membrane. These cells are not innervated but are stimulated by the steroid hormones prolactin and oxytocin.

Physiology

MICROSCOPY, MORPHOLOGY, AND THE MENSTRUAL CYCLE

Histologic changes in the normal breast have been identified in relation to the endocrine variations of the menstrual cycle.[48] Normal menstrual cycle–dependent histologic

TABLE 1-4
Proliferative Activity of Human Breast Terminal Duct—Lobular Unit Components as Measured by DNA-Labeling Index

Structure	Index
Terminal end-bud	15.8 ± 5.2
Type I lobule	5.5 ± 0.5
Type II lobule	0.9 ± 1.2
Type III lobule	0.25 ± 0.3
Terminal duct	1.2 ± 0.5

(After Russo J, Russo IH. Development of human mammary gland. In: Neville MC, Daniel CW, eds. The mammary gland. New York, Plenum, 1987:67)

FIGURE 1-4 **A.** One normal, inactive lobule from the breast of a 35-year-old woman. Alveolar cells are small and the lumina are inconspicuous. Much of the lobular space is occupied by capillaries and stroma. (Hematoxylin–eosin stain; ×40.) **B.** Portions of three adjacent, lactating lobules from the breast of a 25-year-old woman who was 3 weeks postpartum. There is cytoplasmic vacuolization of the alveolar cells, which have proliferated, leading to marked enlargement of the lobule. (Hematoxylin–eosin stain; ×40.)

changes in both stroma and epithelium have been observed and are summarized in Table 1-5.

Cyclic changes in the sex steroid hormone levels during the menstrual cycle profoundly influence breast morphology. Under the influence of FSH and LH during the follicular phase of the menstrual cycle, increasing levels of estrogen secreted by the ovarian graafian follicles stimulate breast epithelial proliferation. During this proliferative phase, the epithelium exhibits sprouting, with increased cellular mitoses, RNA synthesis, increased nuclear density, enlargement of the nucleolus, and changes in other intercellular organelles. In particular, the Golgi apparatus, ribosomes, and mitochondria increase in size or number. During the follicular phase, at the time of maximal estrogen synthesis and secretion in midcycle, ovulation occurs. A second peak occurs in the midluteal phase, when luteal progesterone synthesis is maximal. Similarly, progestogens induce changes in the mammary epithelium during the luteal phase of the ovulatory cycles. Mammary ducts dilate, and the alveolar epithelial cells differentiate into secretory cells, with a partly monolayer arrangement. The combination of these sex steroid hormones and other hormones results in the formation of lipid droplets in the alveolar cells and some intraluminal secretion. The changes in breast epithelium in response to hormones are mediated through either intracellular steroid receptors or membrane-bound peptide receptors. The presence of steroid receptors for estrogen and progestogens in the cytosol of normal mammary epithelium has been demonstrated.[49] It is through the binding of these hormones to specific receptors that the molecular changes, with their observed morphologic effects, are induced as physiologic changes. Similarly, membrane receptors are present to mediate the actions of prolactin. Increases in endogenous estrogen may also exert a histamine-like effect on the mammary microcircula-

tion,[50] resulting in an increased, maximal blood flow 3 to 4 days premenstrually, with an average increase in breast volume of 15 to 30 cm³.[4] Premenstrual breast fullness is attributable to increasing interlobular edema and enhanced ductular–acinar proliferation under the influence of estrogens and progestogens. With the onset of menstruation, following a rapid decline in the circulating levels of sex steroid hormones, secretory activity of the epithelium regresses.

Postmenstrually, tissue edema is reduced, and regression of the epithelium ceases as a new cycle begins with concomitant rises in estrogen levels. Minimum breast volume is observed 5 to 7 days after menstruation. That cyclic variations in DNA synthesis occur during the menstrual cycle has been shown by tritiated thymidine incorporation into the nuclei of short-term cultured normal breast tissue. Increased DNA synthesis occurs during the luteal phase,[51–54] and decreased DNA synthesis occurs during the follicular phase.[51,52] Cyclic cell deletion (apoptosis) occurs 3 days after the peak of mitoses to maintain a balance of cell proliferation and cell death[53,54]; however, a progression of cell population over each ovulatory cycle permits continued development of the budding structure to the age of 35.[4,29]

BREAST CHANGES DURING PREGNANCY

During pregnancy, marked ductular, lobular, and alveolar growth occurs as a result of the influence of luteal and placental sex steroids, placental lactogen, prolactin, and chorionic gonadotropin (see Fig. 1-4B). In experimental studies, these effects are observed when estrogen and progesterone cause a release of prolactin by reducing the hypothalamic release of prolactin-inhibiting factor (PIF).[55] Prolactin in humans is also released progressively during

TABLE 1-5
Morphologic Criteria for Phase Assignment

Phase Secretion	Days	Stroma	Lumen	Epithelium			
				Cell Types	Orientation of Epithelial Cells	Mitoses	Active
I Proliferative	3–7	Dense, cellular	Tight	Single, predominant pale eosinophilic cell	No stratification apparent	Present average 4/ 10 HPF	None
II Follicular	8–14	Dense, cellular, collagenous	Defined	1. Luminal columnar basophilic cell 2. Intermediate pale cell 3. Basal clear cell with hyperchromatic nucleus (myoepithelial)	Radial around lumen	Rare	None
III Luteal	15–20	Loose, broken	Open with some secretion	1. Luminal basophilic cell 2. Intermediate pale cell 3. Prominent vacuolization of basal clear cell (myoepithelial)	Radial around lumen	Absent	None
IV Secretory	21–27	Loose, edematous	Open with secretion	1. Luminal basophilic cell 2. Intermediate pale cell 3. Prominent vacuolization of basal clear cell (myoepithelium)	Radial around lumen	Absent	Active apocrine secretion from luminal cell
V Menstrual	28–2	Dense, cellular	Distended with secretion	1. Luminal basophilic cell with scant cytoplasm	Radial around lumen	Absent	Rare

HPF, high-power field.

(After Vogel PM, et al. The correlation of histologic changes in the human breast with menstrual cycle. Am J Pathol 1981;104:23)

pregnancy and probably stimulates epithelial growth and secretion.[56,57] Prolactin increases slowly during the first half of pregnancy; during the second and third trimesters, blood levels of prolactin are three to five times higher than normal, and mammary epithelium initiates protein synthesis.

In the first 3 to 4 weeks of pregnancy, marked ductular sprouting occurs with some branching, and lobular formation occurs under estrogenic influence. At 5 to 8 weeks, breast enlargement is significant, with dilatation of the superficial veins, heaviness, and increasing pigmentation of the nipple–areolar complex. In the second trimester, lobular formation exceeds ductular sprouting under progestogenic influence. The alveoli contain colostrum but no fat, which is secreted under the influence of prolactin. From the second half of pregnancy onward, increasing breast size results not from mammary epithelial proliferation but from increasing dilatation of the alveoli with colostrum, as well as from hypertrophy of myoepithelial cells, connective tissue, and fat. If these processes are interrupted by early delivery, lactation may be adequate from 16 weeks of pregnancy onward.

At the beginning of the second trimester, the mammary alveoli, but not the milk ducts, lose the superficial layer of A cells. Before this, as in the nonpregnant woman, the two-layer structure is maintained. In the second and third trimesters, this monolayer differentiates into a colostrum–cell layer and accumulates eosinophilic cells, plasma cells, and leukocytes around the alveoli. As pregnancy continues, colostrum, composed of desquamated epithelial cells, accumulates. Aggregations of lymphocytes, round cells, and desquamated phagocytic alveolar cells (foam cells) may be found in colostrum; these are termed the Donné corpuscles.

LACTATION

After parturition, an immediate withdrawal of placental lactogen and sex steroid hormones occurs. During pregnancy, these hormones antagonize the effect of prolactin on mammary epithelium. Concomitant to the abrupt removal of the placental hormones, luteal production of the sex steroid hormones also ceases. A nadir is reached on the fourth to fifth day postpartum; at this time, the secretion of PIF from the hypothalamus into the hypothalamoadenohypophyseal portal system decreases. This reduction in PIF secretion allows the transmembrane secretion of prolactin by pituitary lactotrophs. Sex steroid hormones are not necessary for successful lactation, and physiologic increases, such as may occur with postpartum ovulatory cycles, do not inhibit it.

Prolactin, in the presence of growth hormone, insulin, and cortisol, converts the mammary epithelial cells from a presecretory to a secretory state. During the first 4 or 5 days after birth, the breasts enlarge, owing to the accumulation of secretions in the alveoli and ducts. The initial secretion is of colostrum, a thin, serous fluid that is, at first, sticky and yellow. Colostrum contains lactoglobulin, which is identical to blood immunoglobulins. The importance of these immunoglobulins is unknown; many maternal antibodies cross the placenta, transferring passive immunity to the fetus in utero. Fatty acids, such as decadienoic acid, phospholipids, fat-soluble vitamins, and lactalbumin, in colostrum have considerable nutritional value. Following colostrum secretion, transitional milk and then mature milk are elaborated.

Mechanisms of Milk Synthesis and Secretion

The effects of prolactin are mediated through membrane receptors in the mammary epithelial cells. The release of prolactin is maintained and stimulated by suckling, as is the release of corticotropin (adrenocorticotropic hormone; ACTH). The mammary cells are cuboidal, depending on the degree of intracellular accumulation of secretions. The DNA and RNA of the nuclei increase, and abundant mitochondria, ribosomes, and rough endoplasmic reticulum, with a prominent Golgi apparatus, are apparent in the epithelial cells. Complex protein, mild fat, and lactose synthetic pathways are activated, as are water–ion transport mechanisms. These processes are initiated by the activation of hormone-specific membrane receptors. Changes in cyclic adenosine monophosphate (cAMP) stimulate milk synthesis through the induction of messenger and transfer RNA. Prolactin stimulates cAMP-induced protein kinase activity, resulting in the phosphorylation of milk proteins. Polymerase activity and cellular transcription are enhanced.[29]

Large fat vacuoles develop and move toward the apex of the cell. At the same time, the nucleus also moves toward the apex. As the water intake of the cell increases, longitudinal cellular striations may be observed. Ultimately, the vacuoles pass from the cell along with part of the cell membrane and cytoplasm; the apical cell membrane reconstitutes as secretion takes place.

Enhanced activity occurs during suckling. Fat is secreted chiefly through an apocrine mechanism, lactose is secreted through a merocrine mechanism, and the secretion of proteins occurs as a result of a combination of mechanisms. Ions enter the milk by diffusion and active transport. Relatively little holocrine secretion is thought to take place. The end result of secretion and subsequent intraductal dilution of extracellular fluid is milk, comprising a suspension of proteins—casein, α-lactalbumin, and β-lactoglobulin—and fat in a lactose–mineral solution. The white appearance of milk is due to emulsified lipids and calcium caseinate, whereas the yellow color of butterfat is due to the presence of carotenoids.

Mechanisms of Milk Ejection

The removal of milk by suckling is aided by active ejection. Sensory nerve endings in the nipple–areolar complex are activated by tactile stimuli. Impulses pass by way of sensory nerves through the dorsal roots to the spinal cord. In the spinal cord, impulses are relayed through the dorsal, lateral, and ventral spinothalamic tracts to the mesencephalon and lateral hypothalamus. Inhibition of PIF secretion permits the unimpeded secretion of prolactin from the anterior pituitary. Simultaneously, through a different pathway in the paraventricular nucleus, the synthesis of oxytocin occurs. Oxytocin is released from the posterior pituitary neurovesicles by impulses traveling along the neurosecretory fibers of the hypothalamoneurohypophyseal tract. Oxytocin released into the systemic circulation acts on the myoepithelial cells, which contract and eject milk from the alveoli into the lactiferous ducts and sinuses. This phenomenon is specific to oxytocin, and changes in intramammary ductal pressures of 20 to 25 mmHg may be observed in relation to peak blood levels. Oxytocin also acts on the uterus and cervix to promote involution. This effect may be stimulated by cervical dilatation and by vaginal stretching through the ascending afferent neural pathways (Ferguson reflex).

Complex neuroendocrine interactions determine normal lactation. An appreciation of these mechanisms is essential to the understanding of abnormalities and to the treatment of problems of lactation.[29]

Menopause

Declining ovarian function in late premenopause through the menopause leads to regression of epithelial structures and stroma. The duct system remains, but the lobules shrink and collapse. The last structures to appear with sexual maturity are the first ones to regress.[29]

References

1. Hamilton NJ, Boyd JD, Mossman HW. Human embryology. Cambridge, Heffer, 1968:428.
2. Hughes ESR. Development of mammary gland. Ann R Coll Surg Engl 1950;6:99.
3. Dawson EK. A histological study of the normal mamma in relation to tumour growth. I. Early development to maturity. Edinb Med J 1934;41:653.
4. Dabelow A. Milchdruse. In: Bargman W (ed): Handbuch der Mikroskopishen Anatomie des Menschen, vol 3, part 3. Berlin, Springer-Verlag, 1957.
5. Daniel CW, Silberstein GB. Postnatal development of the rodent mammary gland. In: Neville MC, Daniel CW, eds. The mammary gland: development, regulation, and function. New York, Plenum, 1987:3.
6. Vonderhaar BK. Regulation of development of the normal mammary gland by hormones and growth factors. In: Lippman ME, Dickson RB, eds. Breast cancer: cellular and molecular biology. Boston, Kluwer, 1988:251.
7. Snedeker SM, Brown CF, DiAugustine RP. Expression and functional properties of transforming growth factor alpha and epidermal growth factor during mouse mammary gland ductal morphogenesis. Proc Natl Acad Sci USA 1991;88:2760.
8. Liscia DS, Merlo G, Ciardiello F, et al. Transforming growth factor-alpha messenger RNA localization in the developing adult rat and human mammary gland by in situ hybridization. Dev Biol 1990;140:123.
9. Coleman-Krnacik S, Rosen JM. Differential temporal and spatial gene expression of fibroblast growth factor family members during mouse mammary gland development. Mol Endocrinol 1994;8:218.
10. Robinson SD, Silberstein GB, Roberts AB, et al. Regulated expression and growth inhibitory effects of transforming factor-α isoforms in mouse mammary gland development. Development 1991;113:867.
11. Nusse R, Varmus HE. *Wnt* genes. Cell 1992;69:1073.
12. Coleman S, Silberstein GB, Daniel CW: Ductal morphogenesis in the mouse mammary gland: evidence supporting a role for epidermal growth factor. Dev Biol 1988;127:304.
13. Vonderhaar BK. Local effects of EGF, α-TGF, and EGF-like growth factors on lobuloalveolar development of the mouse mammary gland in vivo. J Cell Physiol 1987;132:581.
14. Matsui Y, Halter SA, Holt JT, Hogan BL, Cofey RJ. Development of mammary hyperplasia and neoplasia in MMTV-TGF alpha transgenic mice. Cell 1990;61:1147.
15. Pierce DF Jr, Johnson MD, Matsui Y, et al. Inhibition of mammary duct development but not alveolar outgrowth during pregnancy in transgenic mice expressing active TGF-beta 1. Genes Dev 1993;7:2308.
16. Jhappan C, Geiser AG, Kordon EC, et al. Targetting expression of a transforming growth factor α1 transgene to the pregnant mammary gland inhibits alveolar development and lactation. EMBO J 1993;12:1835.
17. Strange R, Feng L, Saurer S, et al. Apoptotic cell death and tissue remodelling during mouse mammary gland involution. Development 1992;115:49.
18. Gavin BJ, McMahon AP. Differential regulation of the *Wnt* gene family during pregnancy and lactation suggests a role in postnatal development of the mammary gland. Mol Cell Biol 1992;12:2418.
19. Buhler TA, Dale TC, Kieback C, et al. Localization and quantification of *Wnt*-2 gene expression in mouse mammary development. Dev Biol 1993;155:87.
20. Blasband A, Schryver B, Papkoff J. The biochemical properties and transforming potential of human *Wnt*-2 are similar to *Wnt*-1. Oncogene 1992;7:153.
21. Pitelka DR. The mammary gland. In: Weiss L, ed. Cell and tissue biology. Baltimore, Urban & Schwarzenberg, 1988:877.
22. Maliniac JW: Breast deformities and their origin. New York, Grune & Stratton, 1950:163.
23. Simon BE, Hoffman S, Kahn S. Treatment of asymmetry of the breasts. Clin Plast Surg 1975;2:375.
24. Trier WC. Complete breast absence. Plast Reconstr Surg 1965;36:430.
25. Pers M. Aplasias of the anterior thoracic wall, the pectoral muscle, and the breast. Scand J Plast Reconstr Surg 1968;2:125.
26. Beals RK, Crawford S. Congenital absence of the pectoral muscles. Clin Orthop 1976;119:166.
27. McDowell F. On the propagation, perpetuation and parroting of erroneous eponyms such as "Poland's syndrome." Plast Reconstr Surg 1977;59:561.
28. Ravitch MM. Poland's syndrome: a study of an eponym. Plast Reconstr Surg 1977;59:508.
29. Vorherr H. The breast: morphology, physiology and lactation. New York, Academic, 1974.
30. Tanner JM. Wachstun und Reifung des Menschen. Stuttgart, Georg Thieme Verlag, 1962.
31. Parks AG. The micro-anatomy of the breast. Ann R Coll Surg Engl 1959;25:235.
32. Spratt JS, Shieber W, Dillard B. Anatomy and surgical technique of groin dissection. St Louis, CV Mosby, 1965.
33. Bonsor GM, Dossett JA, Jull JW. Human and experimental breast cancer. Springfield, Charles C Thomas, 1961.
34. Turner-Warwick RT. The lymphatics of the breast. Br J Surg 1959;46:574.
35. Hultborn KA, Larsen LG, Raghnult I: The lymph drainage from the breast to the axillary and parasternal lymph nodes: studied with the aid of colloidal Au^{198}. Acta Radiol 1955;43:52.
36. Pickren JW. Lymph node metastases in carcinoma of the female mammary gland. Bull Roswell Park Mem Inst 1956;1:79.
37. Berg JW. The significance of axillary node levels in the study of breast carcinoma. Cancer 1955;8:776.
38. Stibbe EP. The internal mammary lymphatic glands. J Anat 1918;52:257.
39. Handley RS, Thackray AC. Invasion of internal mammary lymph nodes in carcinoma of the breast. Br Med J 1954;1:161.
40. Urban JA, Marjani MA. Significance of internal mammary lymph node metastases in breast cancer. Am J Roentgenol 1971;111:130.
41. Rouviere H. Anatomie des lymphatiques de l'homme. Paris, Masson, 1932.
42. Ege GN. Internal mammary lymphoscintigraphy. Radiology 1975;118:101.
43. Thomas JM, Redding WH, Sloane JP. The spread of breast cancer: importance of the intrathoracic lymphatic route and its relevance to treatment. Br J Cancer 1979;40:540.
44. Osborne MP, Jeyasingh K, Jewkes RF, et al. The preoperative detection of internal mammary lymph node metastases in breast cancer. Br J Surg 1979;66:813.
45. Moosman DA. Anatomy of the pectoral nerves and their preservation in modified mastectomy. Am J Surg 1980;139:883.
46. Boontje AH. Axillary vein entrapment. Br J Surg 1979;66:331.
47. Russo J, Russo IH. Development of human mammary gland. In: Neville MC, Daniel CW, eds. The mammary gland. New York, Plenum, 1987:67.
48. Vogel PM, Georgiade NG, Fetter BF, et al. The correlation of histologic changes in the human breast with the menstrual cycle. Am J Pathol 1981;104:23.
49. Wittliff JL, Lewko WM, Park DC, et al. Hormones, receptors and breast cancer. In: McGuire WL, ed. Steroid binding proteins of

mammary tissues and their clinical significance in breast cancer, vol 10. New York, Raven, 1978:327.

50. Zeppa R. Vascular response of the breast to estrogen. J Clin Endocrinol Metab 1969;29:695.

51. Masters JRW, Drife JO, Scarisbrick JJ. Cyclic variations of DNA synthesis in human breast epithelium. JNCI 1977;58:1263–1265.

52. Meyer SJ. Cell proliferation in normal breast ducts, fibroadenomas and other ductal hyperplasia as measured by tritiated thymidine: effects of menstrual phase, age and oral contraceptive hormones. Hum Pathol 1977;8:67–81.

53. Anderson TJ, Ferguson DJP, Raab GM. Cell turnover in the "resting" human breast: influence of parity, contraceptive pill, age and laterality. Br J Cancer 1982;46:376–382.

54. Ferguson DJP, Anderson TJ: Morphological evaluation of cell turnover in relation to the menstrual cycle in the "resting" human breast. Br J Cancer 1981;44:177–181.

55. MacLeod RM, Abad A, Eidson LI. In vivo effect of sex hormones on the in vitro synthesis of prolactin and growth hormone in normal and pituitary tumor–bearing rats. Endocrinology 1969;84:1475.

56. Tyson JE, Hwang P, Guyda H, et al. Studies of prolactin secretion in human pregnancy. Am J Obstet Gynecol 1972;113:14.

57. Turkington RW. Multiple hormonal interactions: the mammary gland. In: Litwack G, ed. Biochemical actions of hormones. New York, Academic, 1972:55.

2

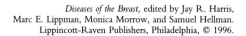

Diseases of the Breast, edited by Jay R. Harris,
Marc E. Lippman, Monica Morrow, and Samuel Hellman.
Lippincott-Raven Publishers, Philadelphia, © 1996.

Biochemical Control of Breast Development

ROBERT B. DICKSON

Hormone Action

Development of the normal breast, mammary carcinogenesis, and progression of breast cancer are regulated by hormonal factors. The endocrine steroids, peptides, and other molecules produced by the glandular tissue of the ovaries, pituitary, endocrine pancreas, thyroid, and adrenal cortex are the best defined of these factors. Following their initial interaction with their cognate nuclear or cell-surface receptors, these hormones govern multiple aspects of cellular function. On a more local level of control, normal and malignant mammary tissues synthesize additional hormone-like substances. One class of these local factors is known as the *paracrine hormones;* these are factors synthesized and released by one cell type to modulate the function of neighboring mammary cells of the same or different type. A second class is known as the *juxtacrine factors.* Juxtacrine growth factors are growth regulatory molecules that remain exposed on the surface of a cell after their synthesis and modulate adjacent cells by contacting their receptors. A third class of local factors is known as the *autocrine (or intracrine) hormones.* These soluble molecules, synthesized by one cell type, act back on the same cell type through surface or intracellular receptors, respectively.

Following their synthesis, polypeptide factors may be routed to multiple destinations, depending in part on features of their primary sequence. An initial point of regulation of growth-factor function occurs during translation of its mRNA to protein. If a signal sequence is encoded by the gene for a growth factor, then the factor is routed in the endoplasmic reticulum to a secretory pathway. There may be additional mechanisms for secretory routing of factors, such as adherence of the factor to other proteins undergoing contemporary synthesis. Some growth factors may also undergo disulfide-linked homodimeric or heterodimeric formation during their synthesis. During passage

of a growth factor to the cell surface, carbohydrate additions (*O*- and *N*-glycosylation, glycosaminoglycan addition), proteolytic cleavages, sulfation, phosphorylation, and esterification with lipids may also occur. Some growth factors are immediately secreted after synthesis, whereas others remain on the cell surface as transmembrane molecules after their synthesis. After secretion, growth factors may adhere to extracellular matrix molecules, they may interact with receptors on nearby cells, or they may enter the general circulation and exert distant effects. If a growth factor is not routed for secretion or to the cell surface, it is initially synthesized and released into the cell cytoplasm. From the cytoplasm, it can accumulate in the nucleus if it has a nuclear transfer signal and a nuclear cognate–binding protein. Alternatively, the factor may remain in the cytoplasm, awaiting cell death for its release into the local environment.

A central, organizing principle of endocrine hormone action in the breast has emerged from studies indicating that systemic hormones regulate local production of growth factors in the gland. The interaction of growth factors with other hormone-induced gene products regulates glandular function and sometimes the dysfunction of cancer.[1,2] A corresponding hierarchy of endocrine-growth factor regulation also appears to exist for other endocrine-regulated glandular tissues (endometrium and prostate gland) and their associated cancers[3,4] (see Fig. 2-1).

Although polypeptide growth factors are among the most widely studied local hormonal modulators, phospholipid degradation products, such as lysophospholipids, prostaglandins, fatty acids, and other molecular classes, may serve such functions as well. Polypeptide growth factors act primarily through cell-surface receptors, most of which function as homodimeric or heterodimeric tyrosine or serine–threonine protein kinases to add phosphate groups to protein substrates and to trigger cascades of intracellular kinases and phosphatases. Other routes of peptide hor-

Hierarchy of Modulators of Breast Development

FIGURE 2-1 Heirarchy of modulators of breast development. cAMP, cyclic adenosine monophosphate; CSF, colony-stimulating factor; EGF, epidermal growth factor; FGF, fibroblast growth factor; GF, growth factor; IGF, insulin-like growth factor; Jak–STAT, Janus kinase–signal transducers and activators of transcription; MAP, mitogen-activated protein; PI3K, phosphatidylinositol-3-kinase; PKC, protein kinase C; PLC-γ, phospholipase C γ; PLD, phospholipase D; TGF-β, transforming growth factor β; TPA, tissue plasminogen activator; UPA, urinary-type plasminogen activator.

mone action include additional signal transduction mechanisms, such as cyclic adenosine monophosphate (cAMP), Ca^{2+} influx, lipid turnover (phospholipase C or D, phosphatidyl-3-inositol kinase) or protein kinase C. Signal transduction ultimately results in altered transcription of genes, altered stability of mRNA, regulation of protein synthesis, and modification of protein stability, function, and localization. Cellular properties under the control of growth factors include cell division, differentiation, motility, glandular compartmentalization, and death. The three principal differentiated cell types of the mammary gland (stromal fibroblasts, myoepithelial, and epithelial cells) communicate by paracrine factors. Autocrine mechanisms

may also exist, particularly for epithelial cells.[5] Endothelial and immune inflammatory cells also play important local regulatory roles.

Hormonal Control of Mammary Development, Growth, and Differentiation

The initial development of the mammary gland involves both a prepubertal interaction between an epithelial rudiment at the nipple and the underlying fatty stroma and a

Stage by Stage Action of Regulatory Factors on Mammary Epithelium

Epithelial rudiment

(+) Transplacental maternal
    hormones of pregnancy   Unknown local factors
(−) Fetal testosterone

Ductal penetration into fat pad

(+) Estrogen and growth   (+?) TGF-α, amphiregulin;
    hormone   (−?) TGF-β
                               (+) IGF-1

Ductal elongation and branching following puberty

(+) Prolactin, insulin   (+) IGF-1
Growth hormone   (+?) TGF-α, amphiregulin
Glucocorticoids   (−?) TGF-β
Estrogen, progesterone   (+?) FGF

Lobuloalveolar differentiation

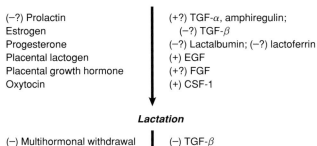

(−?) Prolactin   (+?) TGF-α, amphiregulin;
Estrogen   (−?) TGF-β
Progesterone   (−?) Lactalbumin; (−?) lactoferrin
Placental lactogen   (+) EGF
Placental growth hormone   (+?) FGF
Oxytocin   (+) CSF-1

Lactation

(−) Multihormonal withdrawal   (−) TGF-β

Postlactational apoptosis and glandular involution

FIGURE 2-2 Stage-by-stage action of regulatory factors on mammary epithelium. CSF, colony-stimulating factor; EGF, epidermal growth factor; FGF, fibroblast growth factor; IGF, insulin-like growth factor; TGF, transforming growth factor.

response to maternal hormones of pregnancy and lactation. In the female, estrogens interact with the primordial epithelial–stromal unit to promote ductal development and penetration into the fat (Fig. 2-2). This stromal inductive effect may be partially mimicked in a rodent model by mammary epithelial transplantation into the stroma of the embryologically related salivary gland. In the developing male, androgens interact with the epithelial–stromal unit to induce destruction of the epithelial rudiment. The exact nature of the local stromal–epithelial inductive factors for both sexes is not known.

During pubertal development, ductal elongation and branching occur. Based on studies with rodents, these processes appear to be under positive regulation by ovarian estrogen and pituitary growth hormone. An additional, important endocrine hormone is oxytocin, which induces myoepithelial proliferation and differentiation.[6] Growth hormone may mediate its effects through local production

of insulin-like growth factor I (IGF-I).[7] The agricultural use of growth hormone to enhance bovine lactational productivity is an area of current public controversy because of the possibility of slightly increased levels of hormones in milk. The most important local regulators of estrogen in the mammary gland are not yet fully established, but likely candidates include members of the epidermal growth factor family (EGF, TGF-α, and amphiregulin) and the transforming growth factor β family (TGF-β1, TGF-β2, TGF-β3).[5]

The final stage of development, known as *lobuloalveolar differentiation,* occurs during pregnancy. Lobuloalveolar development is regulated by many endocrine hormones, some of which are of placental origin: prolactin; growth hormone and its local mediator, IGF-1; insulin; glucocorticoids; estrogen; and progesterone.[5,7–8] During completion of lobuloalveolar growth, the gland becomes competent to carry out lactation. Among the hormones of lactation, growth hormone may again play a central role because, in transgenic mouse models, the growth hormone gene can influence the gland to attain its full lactational competence in the absence of pregnancy itself.[2] The final, irreversible, terminal differentiation of the epithelium produces secretory cells characterized by their ability to synthesize and secrete milk proteins, such as casein, and lipids.[8,9] As synthesis of milk products is induced, direct negative regulatory effects of lactogenic hormones, such as prolactin,[10] and milk proteins, such as lactoferrin,[11] on local growth factor pathways and on epithelial proliferation may occur. Secretion of milk is regulated by pituitary oxytocin, released in response to neural pathways and activated by suckling. The initial mammary secretory product, colostrum, and milk itself are rich sources of polypeptide growth factors and growth factor–binding proteins. These regulatory molecules, in turn, may be important both in mammary growth and differentiation and in control of neonatal development, metabolism and endocrine function.[6,12]

EGF and TGF-α, which is a structural and functional homologue of EGF, can produce similar biologic effects in mouse mammary explants and cultured human and mouse mammary epithelial cell lines.[13–15] The production and roles of these factors in normal and malignant mammary proliferation and differentiation have been emerging in the past few years. TGF-α mRNA has been detected in mammary epithelium by in situ hybridization during the proliferative, lobuloalveolar development stage of rodent and human pregnancy.[16] Some growth factors may also exert an endocrine function. Although this function has been recognized for many years for the IGF factors, it may also be true of other growth factors. In this regard, circulating, mouse salivary gland–derived EGF appears to be necessary for spontaneous mammary tumor formation in the mouse model as well as for growth of the tumors once they are formed.[17,18]

A significant amount of research has characterized the tissue location of various polypeptide growth factor classes during the stages of mammary development. A detailed study in the mouse observed TGF-α mRNA transcripts to the growing epithelial cell—cap layer of the growing terminal and buds in virgin and pregnant states. TGF-α expression was not detected in lactation. In contrast, EGF mRNA transcripts were localized to inner cell layers of the end buds and to ductal luminal cells of virgin, pregnant, and lactating glands.[19] The mRNA for the EGF-related growth factor, amphiregulin, was expressed in stromal cells, luminal epithelial cells, myoepithelial cells of branching ducts, and epithelial cap cells in virgin and pregnant mice.[20] These EGF family growth factors are thus likely to function as regulators of all stages of mammary growth and as potentially critical components of milk. Other stimulatory factors, such as the fibroblast growth factors FGF-1 and FGF-4, have been localized to ductal luminal cells. In contrast, FGF-2 and FGF-7 were expressed in stromal cells of the virgin mouse gland.[21] In the human gland, FGF-1 and FGF-2 and FGF receptors have been localized to both myoepithelial and epithelial cells.[22]

Finally, growth-inhibitory, differentiation-inducing TGF-β (three isoforms) family members are all produced in mammary epithelial cells. This growth factor family, like some FGF and EGF family members, binds heparin and is deposited into the extracellular matrix following secretion. Production of TGF-β increases during midpregnancy and lactation; it is thought eventually to suppress lactation, as well as ductal budding.[23,24] Growth factor regulation of the mammary gland almost certainly depends on a finely controlled balance between action of stimulatory and inhibitory factors at the local level. In mouse and human mammary epithelial cells in culture, EGF, IGF, and FGF family members are clearly stimulatory, whereas TGF-β family members are inhibitory of proliferation. Growth factor pellet implantation studies in the mouse mammary gland have largely confirmed these in vitro results in vivo.[25,26]

A final consideration of regulatory factors in mammary development involves the vascular endothelium and infiltrating immune cells. The growing vascular endothelial cells may provide additional growth factors to the developing gland, although this area has not yet been studied. In one study, in mice genetically deficient in the growth factor colony-stimulating factor 1 (CSF-1), the development of the mammary gland was incomplete; lobuloalveolar development was premature, and a failure, not in milk protein synthesis, but in its secretion, was noted. The natural source of CSF-1 in the breast is unknown, but a strong candidate is macrophages,[27] which also secrete EGF.[28]

In rodent models, an additional series of genes termed the *WNT family* clearly plays a vital role in gland development and tumorigenesis. Some of these genes appear to have growth factor—like function; they are differentially expressed in pregnancy and lactation, and they are transcriptionally activated as oncogenes in mouse mammary tumor virus (MMTV)—induced cancer.[7]

After weaning, withdrawal of the terminally differentiated luminal epithelial cells of the lactating gland from the steroid hormones and growth factors of pregnancy results in their programmed death, a process termed *apoptosis*.[29,30]

This process is characterized by an influx of Ca^{2+}, activation of an internucleosomal nuclease, and activation of tissue transglutaminase. Cells degrade their DNA in an adenosine triphosphate (ATP)-dependent fashion, the tissue undergoes autoproteolytic destruction and shrinkage, and differentiated function is lost. Detailed biochemical studies also implicate the cytokine—growth factor signal transduction enzyme protein kinase C in the process, in addition to several other gene products, such as the growth factor TGF-β, a mitochondrial suppressor of the process termed Bcl-2, the transcription factor oncogene termed c-myc, the tumor-suppressor gene p53, and additional proteins TRPM-2 and Fas/APO-1.[30] During this glandular involution, myoepithelial cells may play an assisting role with their increased synthesis of collagenolytic enzymes.[5]

A similar, but less marked, cyclicity also occurs in the proliferation and development of the mammary gland in women under regulation of the menstrual cycle. Proliferation of mammary epithelial cells is maximal in the luteal phase of the cycle, as progesterone, in the presence of estrogen, rises to a peak. This is followed by a synchronous wave of epithelial apoptosis on cessation of proliferation. This type of pattern may also exist in the shorter estrous cycles of rodents. The cyclic processes of proliferation and apoptosis in the mammary gland are 180 degrees out of phase with corresponding events in the endometrium, where mitoses are primarily in the follicular phase. Thus, although progesterone is a hormone that opposes the actions of estrogen on proliferation in the endometrium, the opposite is true in the breast.[31,32]

Depending on the various developmental stages, different types of ovary-controlled, hormonally dependent proliferative processes occur in the mammary gland. During puberty, estrogen-dependent growth may occur by expansion of a stem cell population (termed *cap cells* in the rodent) within the invading, terminal ramifications of the ductal network. These cells may give rise both to epithelial and myoepithelial cells of the gland. During the subsequent, normal reproductive cycles of pregnancy and lactation, an estrogen- and progesterone-dependent growth process may depend on expansion of a more differentiated multipotent population within the ducts and their terminal alveoli.[33] Each of these distinct, hormone-dependent proliferative processes depends on a proper epithelial—mesenchymal interaction allowing most local influences, including paracrine growth factors, to act. Although most cellular and molecular studies on breast development, proliferation, differentiation, and carcinogenesis have focused on epithelial cells, some research has included characterization of different mammary stromal cell types and their roles.[34]

Basement Membrane

A critically important feature of mammary differentiation is the organizational influence exerted by the basement membrane. Contact with this structure polarizes epithelial cells, organizes their secretory function, and contributes to regulation of genes important for mammary differentiation.[35] This structure is a complex, lattice-like scaffolding that is synthesized and assembled at the interface of epithelium and its underlying stroma. Its principal constituents include collagen IV, laminin, fibronectin, and heparan sulfate proteoglycans. The basement membrane is undoubtedly a plastic structure, undergoing cyclic assembly and destruction (*remodeling*). Proteolytic enzymes of multiple classes capable of degrading the basement membrane have been identified in stromal fibroblasts, blood vessels, and myoepithelial cells. A good example is the collagenase enzyme MMP-2. The basally located, myoepithelial cells appear to present high levels of this enzyme on their surfaces.[36] As discussed later in this chapter, breast cancer is characterized by progressive loss of controls of basement membrane and of hormones on proliferation and on epithelial differentiation (a process termed *epithelial–mesenchymal transition*), by genomic instability (mutations, deletions, amplifications, and chromosomal rearrangements), by alteration in nuclear matrix structure and function, and by loss of normal tissue organization and compartmentalization (*metastasis*).[36,37]

Steroid Action

As introduced earlier, estrogen and progesterone are well-established steroid endocrine regulators of mammary growth and differentiation. The two hormones appear to work together to promote mammary epithelial growth, differentiation, and survival. Whereas both steroids are commonly thought to be primarily important between the years of puberty and menopause, local aromatization of adrenal androgens provides additional estrogens in the postmenopausal years. Both estrogen and progesterone act through their nuclear receptors to modulate transcription of target genes. Genes encoding the receptors for each are members of a large superfamily of transcription-modulating factors. Whereas the estrogen receptor is thought to be a homodimer, the progesterone receptor is a heterodimeric protein. Research on each system has defined additional, alternately spliced variants, thought to be encoded by a single gene for each receptor. The biologic roles of these additional variant receptor subunits are under investigation. Each steroid receptor dimer is also associated with other proteins, including heat shock proteins, and associates with its cognate palindromic DNA elements on ligand binding. DNA interaction of steroid receptors occurs through zinc finger structures of the receptors and promotes formation of a stable initiation complex to promote transcription of responsive genes.[38,39]

Other studies suggest that the signal transduction pathways induced by growth factors and hormones may directly or indirectly regulate steroid receptor function. In the rat uterus, cAMP and IGF-1 appear to be able to modulate the estrogen receptor, presumably through phosphorylation; transcription of estrogen-responsive genes is induced.[40] cAMP and IGF-1 are also known to modulate estrogen receptor function in breast cancer cells. After treatment of cells with these molecules, the antiestrogen tamoxifen behaves as a more highly estrogenic compound.[41] Similar alterations in the antagonistic response of the progesterone receptor pathway to the antiprogestin mifepristone (RU 486) have been reported after cAMP stimulation.[42] The steroids are also well known for their ability to modulate directly the expression of nuclear protooncogenes downstream of growth factor pathways.[43] These findings provide multiple mechanisms to support a role for growth factors in the progressive expression of a more malignant phenotype and escape from normal hormonal control.

Peptide Hormone Action

At least four major pathways of polypeptide hormone action have been defined for mammary epithelial cells. The best-known pathway is that principally used by the tyrosine kinase receptors (EGF, FGF, and IGF-insulin families). Each factor acts through a homodimeric or heterodimeric cell-surface receptor to trigger receptor tyrosine autophosphorylation and transphosphorylation of a variety of substrate proteins in the cytoplasm. Several proteins, such as GRB-2, SOS, and IRS-1 bind to the tyrosine phosphorylated residues on the receptor through domains termed SH-2 domains. Another protein, termed Ras, then binds to help anchor the developing complex in the membrane. A cascade of subsequent, serine–threonine phosphorylations of Raf-1 kinase, mitogen-activated protein (MAP) kinase kinase, MAP kinase, and transcription factors and regulation of cell-cycle kinases completes the cascade.[44] A second pathway is triggered by TGF-β family members when they bind to their heterodimeric receptors and trigger a serine–threonine kinase activity. Although the details of the pathway are not clear, cell-cycle kinases (described later) and their inhibitors are then modulated.[45] Third, prolactin, growth hormone, and some cytokines act by interaction of their receptors with a member of the cytoplasmic JAK tyrosine kinase family. This kinase triggers transcription of genes through the action of a transcription factor of the STAT family.[46] Finally, growth factors and inflammatory cytokines (such as tumor necrosis factor [TNF]) stimulate phospholipase C, PI3-kinase, and protein kinase C (PKC) in cells, leading to serine–threonine phosphorylations of multiple metabolic determinants.[47,48]

This brief summary of signal transduction is highly simplified. In particular, the potential for diverse heterodimerization partners within many of the receptor families presents a vast potential for signal modulation.

Regulation of Genes Encoding Milk Proteins

The principal function of the terminal differentiation state of the mammary gland is the apocrine secretion of milk. Milk consists of lipids, nutrient proteins, growth factors, and many other biologically active molecules.[49] Among the best-studied milk proteins are casein, lactalbumin, and the whey acidic protein. Many of the genes encoding these proteins contain a consensus sequence in their promoters termed the *milk box*, in addition to other regulatory sequences. Use of cell lines and transgenic animals has facilitated study of the detailed regulation of these genes and the nature of their mammary-specific expression.[50,51]

Further research has established the nature of the transcription factor that activates milk protein synthesis in response to prolactin. This factor, termed Mgf, is a member of the STAT family of transcription factors. The regulation of expression of the casein gene depends on a balance between its activation by Mgf and its repression by another factor, termed *YY1*. In addition, a novel mechanism of gene regulation has been observed for β-casein. The mRNA of β-casein binds and sequesters a single-stranded nucleic acid–binding protein whose role is to inhibit gene expression.[52–54]

Mammary Epithelial Cell Cycle

The collection of endocrine, autocrine, and paracrine regulators of mammary epithelial proliferation is funneled to a common pathway, the cell cycle. This ultimate regulatory pathway consists of a series of proteins known as the cyclin-dependent kinases (CDKs), their activating subunits, which are the cyclins, and their inhibitory subunits, the CDK inhibitors. As noted earlier, the principal proliferative cell type in the gland is the epithelial cell; indeed, most of the cancers of the breast are of epithelial origin.

The early G_1 phase of the cell cycle is regulated by the cyclin D family, CDK2, CDK4, and CDK5. G_1-S is regulated by cyclin E-CDK2. S is driven by cyclin A-CDK2 and G_2M by cyclin B/A-CDC-2. Most of the stimulatory growth factor pathways seem to up-regulate cyclin D family members, whereas TGF-β inhibits CDK4 and induces at least one CDK inhibitor. Other oncogenes and suppressor genes, described in Chapter 7.6, have additional functions to dysregulate the cell-cycle proteins.[27,55,56]

Defective Regulation of Breast Epithelial Growth in Cancer

The basis for our understanding of ovarian endocrine influences on the malignant mammary gland may be traced back to the late 1800s.[57] More recent studies have specifically identified ovarian estrogens and progesterone as the principal ovarian effectors. Studies of rodent models of carcinogen-induced and spontaneous mammary cancer have demonstrated that both progestins and estrogens are able to support initial tumor formation and early tumor growth.[58–60] More recent studies have also implicated growth factors. Experiments with transgenic mice have demonstrated overexpression of several growth factors and their receptors, including those of the EGF class, as strong risk factors for mammary cancer.[61] In rodent models, early stages in spontaneous mammary neoplasia are also sensitive to growth factor stimulation,[62] whereas the most malignant metastatic stages are characterized by overproduction of growth factors and insensitivity to their exogenous supplementation.[1]

Numerous studies since the 1950s have shown that administration of sustained doses of estrogens or progestins can lead to development of malignant mammary tumors in specific rodent strains.[58,63] Estrogens and progestins may interact in both normal and malignant rodent and human breast, based on the requirement of estrogen, acting through its receptor to induce expression of progesterone receptor. Thus, both hormones working together may regulate other genes, such as growth factors and cell cycle–associated genes.[64] Both estrogenic and progestational components of the oral contraceptives are considered potential risk factors in breast cancer,[28,31,65] although most women taking these drugs do not appear to have a significantly increased risk of breast cancer.[28] Other established risk factors for breast cancer are known to include family history, patient history, a prolonged reproductively competent phase of life, late pregnancy, and excessive consumption of alcohol. Certain additional, controversial, putative risk factors include a high-fat diet and cigarette smoking.[66,67] The mechanisms of these risk factors are not known, but they most likely include prolonged hormonal stimulation of proliferation, DNA damage, dysregulated growth factor secretion and action, and disregulated cell cycle–associated genes. A long-standing observation has been that early pregnancy is protective, perhaps through induction of glandular differentiation.[28]

Estrogen and progesterone receptors have been localized by immunohistochemical study to a luminal subpopulation of ductal and lobular epithelial cells in women and rodents. These receptors are absent from epithelial cells of the terminal end buds, the most proliferative regions of the gland. Whether epithelial cells containing steroid receptors serve a precursor role in breast cancer is not known, although sex steroids are considered to be requirements for most breast cancers in women.[68,69] Indeed, approximately one third of breast cancers are hormonally responsive when they become metastatic. Although a large fraction of breast tumors may be able to respond directly to sex steroids, a body of literature strongly supports an indirect role of stromal fibroblasts (and possibly other cell types) to modulate positively steroidal growth regulation. Mechanisms of this effect are thought to involve stromal cytochrome P-450–mediated metabolism systems. These aromatize adrenal androgens (such as androstenedione) to estrogens, particularly in postmenopausal women. Moreover, growth factors produced by the cancer, including those under hormonal control, are thought to induce the P-450 enzymes responsible for local estrogen production.[70] In analogy with normal gland growth noted earlier, growth of breast tumor cells in vitro in response to estrogen is also markedly enhanced in vitro by coculture with fibroblasts, suggesting paracrine cooperation in the hormonal response.[34,71] The biochemical nature of this paracrine control remains uncertain, although the growth factor IGF-II appears to be a strong candidate.[72] Hormone responsivity of breast cancer is important for its treatment.[73]

Estrogen and progesterone receptor–negative breast cancers differ in multiple respects from their steroid receptor–positive counterparts. These differences appear to include higher proliferative and invasive rates in vivo and in vitro, altered expression of certain growth factor receptors (high levels of EGF and erbB-2 receptors but low IGF-I receptors), elevated expression of phases I and II enzymes of drug metabolism, more aberrant nuclear morphology, increased invasiveness, and loss of certain indicators of epithelial differentiation. These differences may indicate at least two distinct stages of differentiation or two different biologic types of breast cancer.[5] Perhaps also relevant is the observation that essentially all breast adenocarcinomas are characterized by expression of ductal luminal keratins.[74] These observations may support an argument that breast cancers may be derived from a luminal or luminal-committed, estrogen receptor– and progesterone receptor–positive stage of differentiation. Later malignant progression could encompass phenotypic dedifferentiation from this luminal lineage. Malignant progression involves multiple genetic and phenotypic changes. Important chromosomal regions containing common defects in breast cancer include the following loci: rearrangements with common breakpoints at 1p13 and 1q21, deletions on 1p (14–21), rearrangements on 6p, 7p, 11q (22–23), and 16q, and chromosomal imbalances of 8p, 13q, and 17p.

Biochemical Regulation of Tissue Compartmentalization

As described earlier in this chapter, the mammary epithelium has a homotypic affinity for itself and is capable of inducing production of a basement membrane, where it forms an interface with an adjacent stromal compartment. The basement membrane exerts a further influence to promote epithelial differentiation and sequestration. Proper compartmentalization of the breast thus requires cell–cell interactions and cell–substrate interactions. Both serve to regulate proper structure and differentiated function. Both types of adhesion may send intracellular signals in addition to their direct contribution to maintenance of tissue architecture.[33,75] Both homotypic adhesion of epithelial cells and heterotypic adhesion of epithelial to myoepithelial cells may be critical. In addition, the epithelial–mesenchymal interface is strongly inductive of basement membrane formation. Finally, vascular endothelium and immune cells must be able to penetrate the tissue space and maintain sufficient plasticity to respond to the variable metabolic states of tissue growth, milk production, and tissue death.[76]

The principal cell–cell adhesion molecule in the mammary epithelium is the calcium-dependent E-cadherin, also termed *uvomorulin* or *L-CAM*. This molecule is proposed as a tumor-suppressor gene in the breast.[77] Cell–cell adhesion restricts motility[78] and promotes differentiation.[79] A second important interaction is that of cell–substratum. This type of interaction is mediated by the heterodimeric RGD–consensus–binding transmembrane integrin class of surface molecules, as well as several nonintegrin molecules. Most integrins bind more than one ligand (collagen, fibronectin, laminin, fibrinogen, thrombospondin, and vitronectin), and a few ($\alpha_2\beta_1$, $\alpha_5\beta_1$, and $\alpha_3\beta_1$) may participate in cell–cell adhesion as well as cell–substrate adhesion.

Defective Regulation of Tissue Compartmentalization in Cancer

In addition to dysregulated proliferation, at least two other cellular processes seem to occur during malignant progression of breast cancer: loss of differentiated properties and loss of proper tissue compartmentalization (metastasis). Loss of cell–cell attachment, altered cell–substratum attachment, and altered cytoskeletal organization seem to play a role in loss of differentiation. The same three influences, plus cell locomotion, proteolysis, survival, and proliferation at distant sites,[80] contribute to metastasis.

As noted previously, the major cell–cell adhesion molecule thought to be involved in mammary epithelial differentiation is E-cadherin. Loss of expression of E-cadherin is associated with a more motile, fibroblastic morphology in breast cancer, with increased invasiveness, and with metastasis.[81] One subset of breast cancer cells is negative for expression of E-cadherin, expresses the mesenchymal intermediate filament vimentin (along with epithelial keratins), and expresses an even more strongly motile and invasive phenotype.[81,82] These characteristics are indicative of an epithelial mesenchymal transition (EMT) and are associated with poor histologic grade in clinical breast cancer.[83] The EMT process is known to occur frequently in other contexts during embryogenesis.[78] Loss of expression of $\alpha_2\beta_1$, $\alpha_3\beta_1$, $\alpha_5\beta_1$, and $\alpha_6\beta_1$, also a proposed tumor suppressor,[84] and increased expression of a 67-kd nonintegrin laminin binding protein are also associated with loss of differentiation in breast cancer.[75]

Other studies have suggested that loss of expression of the estrogen and progesterone receptors may be associated with an EMT process in breast cancer.[82] The overall mechanism for induction of the EMT remains unknown, but it seems to be associated with primary defects in arrangement of desmosomal and cytoskeletal proteins.[85] PKC expression may be a likely regulator; it seems to increase during malignant progression and chemotherapy resistance. A primary substrate of PKC is an actin filament cross-linking protein thought to be involved in motility.[86–88] PKC also mediates induction of the genes encoding multiple matrix-degrading proteases by means of AP-1 promoter interactions, cell–substrate adhesion through NF-kB promoter interactions, and breast cancer cell invasiveness.[89–93] Because retinoids are known to antagonize AP-1 regulated genes through RAR and RXR receptors, these lipid-soluble hormone-like substances may have antimetastatic potential.[94] In addition, the drug, bryostatin-1, appears to be a relatively nontoxic anti-PKC drug with therapeutic potential.[91,95–97]

Attachment of cells to a matrix substratum is thus critical both for differentiation[84] and for metastasis.[80] Other studies noted earlier implicated down-regulation of certain of the heterodimeric integrin class of attachment molecules as necessary for metastasis.[98,99] Cell–substratum adhesion itself may signal the cell through a tyrosine kinase termed FAK (focal adhesion kinase). This kinase is up-regulated in invasive breast cancer.[100] Finally, additional adhesion events may come into play in metastasis: expression of the vascular angiogenesis-associated integrin $\alpha_v\beta_3$, function of nonintegrin I-CAM-1, and function of the platelet–tumor cell adhesion integrin $\alpha_{IIb}\beta_3$ in embolus formation.[75,101] Moreover, additional adhesion molecules are involved in the final metastatic stages of tumor extravasation after vascular embolus trapping: E-selectin, V-CAM-1, and CD44.[75]

Metastases are initially marked by local invasion of the cancer across the basement membrane to the stromal area. This transition is thought to depend on abnormal tissue remodeling (local proteolysis) and tumor cell motility. Two collagen IV–selective degrading enzymes, 92-kd (MMP-9) and 72-kd (MMP-2) gelatinase, are under intense current scrutiny in this respect.[102] Plasmin production (from the tumor cell–secreted plasminogen activator urokinase, UPA), cathepsin D, a novel 80-kd broad-substrate matrix-degrading metalloproteinase, cathepsin B, and cathepsin L are potentially important.[102–105] UPA and MMPs (including a specialized MMP, MT-MMP, that activates others) are the most widely studied enzymes for development of potential antimetastatic therapy.[106–108] UPA and its inhibitor, PAI-1, are now considered to be strong indicators of poor prognosis in breast cancer; they are primarily secreted by stromal cells adjacent to invasive breast cancer. MMPs may also be synthesized by stromal cells in the area of the tumor.[109]

Summary and Future Prospects

This chapter attempts to review the multifactoral nature of breast development (see Fig. 2-1). Endocrine hormones are positioned at the top of a complex regulatory heirarchy. They deliver important modulatory signals to the local tissue. Adhesion molecules and growth factors are extremely important influences on local tissue function. Each of these two classes of regulators also delivers signals into the cell. Signal transduction from growth factors is now recognized to be diverse and complex; signals from adhesion molecules are only at the beginning of their understanding. Finally, endocrine and local influences exert their ultimate effects on cell growth, tissue remodeling, and milk production. Consideration of each of these topics is essential to the understanding of dysregulated tissue function in breast cancer. Indeed, the cancer genes known as oncogenes arise from normal regulators of these multiple pathways as the function of tumor-suppressor genes is lost.

References

1. Dickson RB, Lippman ME. Estrogenic regulation of growth and polypeptide growth factor secretion in human breast carcinoma. Endocr Rev 1987;8:29.
2. Suchard M, Landers JP, Sandhu NP, et al. Steroid hormone regulation of nuclear proto-oncogenes. Endocr Rev 1993;14:659.
3. Murphy LJ. Growth factors and steroid hormone action in endometrial cancer. J Steril Biochem Mol Biol 1994;48:419.
4. Bahgal I, Bailey J, Hitzmann K, et al. Epidermal growth factor-dependent stimulation of amphiregulin expression in androgen-stimulated human prostate cancer cells. Mol Biol Cell 1994;5:339.
5. Dickson RB, Lippman ME. Growth regulation of normal and malignant breast epithelium. In: Bland KI, Copeland EM, eds. The breast. Philadelphia, WB Saunders, 1991:363.
6. Bano M, Kidwell WR, Dickson RB. MDGF-1: a multifunctional growth factor in human milk and human breast cancer. In: Dickson RB, Lippman ME, eds. Mammary tumorigenesis and malignant progression. Boston, Kluwer, 1994:193.
7. Ruan W, Newman CB, Kleinberg DL. Intact and amino-terminally shortened forms of insulin-like growth factor I induce mammary gland differentiation and development. Proc Natl Acad Sci USA 1992;89:10872.
8. Sakakura T. Mammary embryogenesis. In: Neville MC, Daniel CW, eds. The mammary gland. New York, Plenum, 1987:37.
9. Russo J, Russo I. Development of the human mammary gland. In: Neville MC, Daniel CW, eds. The mammary gland. New York, Plenum, 1987:67.
10. Fenton SE, Sheffield LG. Prolactin inhibits epidermal growth factor (EGF)-stimulated signaling events in mouse mammary epithelial cells by altering EGF receptor function. Mol Biol Cell 1993;4:773.
11. Bezault J, Bhimani R, Wiprovnick J, et al. Human lactoferrin inhibits growth of solid tumors and development of experimental metastases in mice. Cancer Res 1994;54:2310.
12. Salomon DS, Kidwell WR. Tumor associated growth factors in malignant rodent and human mammary epithelial cells. In: Lippman ME, Dickson RB, eds. Breast cancer: cellular and molecular biology. Boston, Kluwer, 1988:363.
13. Vonderhaar BK. Regulation of development of the normal mammary gland by hormones and growth factors. In: Lippman ME, Dickson RB, eds. Breast cancer: cellular and molecular biology. Boston, Kluwer, 1988:251.
14. Stampfer MR. Isolation and growth of human mammary epithelial cells. J Tissue Cult Meth 1985;9:107.
15. Salomon DS, Perroteau I, Kidwell WR, et al. Loss of growth responsiveness to epidermal growth factor and enhanced production of alpha-transforming growth factors in *ras*-transformed mouse mammary epithelial cells. J Cell Physiol 1987;130:397.
16. Liscia DS, Merlo G, Ciardiello F, et al. Transforming growth factor-α messenger RNA localization in the developing adult rat and human mammary gland by in situ hybridization. Dev Biol 1990;140:123.
17. Oka T, Tsutsumi O, Kurachi H, et al. The role of epidermal

growth factor in normal and neoplastic growth of mouse mammary epithelial cells. In: Lippman ME, Dickson RB, eds. Breast cancer: cellular and molecular biology. Boston, Kluwer, 1988:343.

18. Kurachi H, Okamoto S, Oka T. Evidence for the involvement of the submandibular gland epidermal growth factor in mouse mammary tumorigenesis. Proc Natl Acad Sci USA 1985;81:5940.

19. Snedeker SM, Brown CF, DiAugustine RP. Expression and functional properties of transforming growth factor α and epidermal growth factor during mouse mammary gland ductal morphogenesis. Proc Natl Acad Sci USA 1991;88:276.

20. Kenney NJ, Huang R-P, Johnson G, et al. Detection and location of amphiregulin and cripto-1 expression in the developing mouse mammary gland. FASEB J 1995 (in press).

21. Coleman-Krnacik S, Rosen JM. Differential temporal and spatial gene expression of fibroblast growth factor family members during mouse mammary gland development. Mol Endocrinol 1994;8:218.

22. Coombes RC, Gomm JJ, Lugmani YA, et al. Acidic and basic FGF and their receptors in normal and malignant breast cells. (Abstract). Proc Am Assoc Cancer Res 1994.

23. Jhappan C, Geiser AG, Kordon EC, et al. Targeting expression of a transforming growth factor β1 transgene to the pregnant mammary gland inhibits alveolar development and lactation. EMBO 1993;12:1835.

24. Wooster R, Neuhausen SL, Mangion J, et al. Localization of a breast cancer susceptibility gene, BRCA2, to chromosome 13q12-13. Science 1994;265:2088.

25. Daniel C, Silberstein GB. Local effects of growth factors. In: Lippman ME, Dickson RB, eds. Regulatory mechanisms in breast cancer. Boston, Kluwer, 1990:79.

26. Dickson RB. Growth factors as local regulators of normal and malignant human mammary epithelium. In: Schonberg D, ed. Growth factors and reproduction. New York, Springer-Verlag, 1991:129.

27. Pines J. Arresting developments in cell-cycle control. TIBS 1994; 19:143.

28. Committee on the Relationship Between Oral Contraceptives and Breast Cancer. Oral contraceptives and breast cancer. Washington DC, National Academy Press, 1991:1.

29. Strange R, Li F, Suarer S, Burkhardt A, et al. Apoptic cell death and tissue remodelling during mouse mammary gland involution. Development 1992;115:49.

30. Collins MKL, Perkins GR, Gemma R-T, et al. Growth factors as survival factors: regulation of apoptosis. Bioessays 1994;16:133.

31. Anderson TJ, Battersby S, Macintyre CCA. Proliferative and secretory activity in human breast during natural and artificial menstrual cycles. Am J Pathol 1988;130:193.

32. Longacre TA, Bartow SA. A correlative morphologic study of human breast and endometrium in the menstrual cycle. Am J Surg Pathol 1986;10:382.

33. Daniel CW, Silberstein GB. Developmental biology of the mammary gland. In: Neville MC, Daniel CW, eds. The mammary gland. New York, Plenum, 1987:3.

34. Haslam SZ. Stromal–epithelial interactions in normal and neoplastic mammary gland. In: Lippman ME, Dickson RB, eds. Regulatory mechanisms in breast cancer. Boston, Kluwer, 1990:401.

35. Streuli CH, Bailey N, Bissell MJ. Control of mammary epithelial differentiation: basement membrane induces tissue-specific gene expression in the absence of cell–cell interaction and morphological polarity. J Cell Biol 1991;115:1383.

36. Monteagudo C, Merino MJ, San-Juan J, et al. Immunohistochemical distribution of type IV collagenase in normal, benign, and malignant breast tissue. Am J Pathol 1990;136:585.

37. Khanuja PS, Lehr JE, Soule HD, et al. Nuclear matrix proteins in normal and breast cancer cells. Cancer Res 1993;53:3394.

38. Green S, Chambon P. The estrogen receptor: from perception to mechanism. In: Parker MG, ed. Nuclear hormone receptors. London, Academic, 1991:15.

39. Read LD, Katzenellenbogen BS. Characterization and regulation of estrogen and progesterone receptors in breast cancer. In: Dickson RB, Lippman ME, eds. Genes, oncogenes, and hormones. Boston, Kluwer, 1992:277.

40. Aronica SM, Katzenellenbogen BS. Stimulation of estrogen receptor-mediated transcription and alteration in the phosphorylation state of the rat uterine estrogen receptor by estrogen, cyclic adenosine monophosphate, and insulin-like growth factor-1. Mol Endocrinol 1993;7:743.

41. Fujimoto N, Katzenellenbogen BS. Alteration in the agonist/antagonist balance of antiestrogens by activation of protein kinase: a signaling pathway in breast cancer cells: antiestrogen selectivity and promoter dependence. Mol Endocrinol 1994;8:296.

42. Nordeen SK, Bona BJ, Moyer ML. Latent agonist activity of the steroid antagonist, RU486, is unmasked in cells treated with activators of protein kinase A. Mol Endocrinol 1993;7:731.

43. Kahn SA, Stancel GM, eds. Protooncogenes and growth factors in steroid hormone-induced growth and differentiation. Ann Arbor, CRC, 1993:1.

44. Hall A. A biochemical function for ras: at last. Science 1994; 244:1413.

45. Yan Z, Winnwer S, Friedman E. Two different signal transduction pathways can be activated by FGFβ_1 in epithelial cells. J Biol Chem 1994;269:13231.

46. Darnell JE, Kerr IM, Storb GR. Jak-STAT pathways and transcriptional activation in response to INFs and other extracellular signalling pathways. Science 1994;264:1415.

47. Mangelsdorf-Soderquist A, Todderud G, Carpenter G. Elevated membrane association of phospholipase c-γ 1 in MDA-468 mammary tumor cells. Cancer Res 1992;52:4526.

48. Soltoff SP, Carraway KL, Priget SA, et al. ErbB$_3$ is involved in activating phosphatidyl-inositol-3-kinase by epidermal growth factor. Mol Cell Biol 1994;14:3550.

49. Grosvenor CE, Picciano MF, Baumrucker CR. Hormones and growth factors in milk. Endocr Rev 1992;14:720.

50. Greenberg NM, Wolfe J, Rosen JM. Casein gene expression: from transfection to transgenics. In: Dickson RB, Lippman ME, eds. Genes, oncogenes, and hormones. Boston, Kluwer, 1991:379.

51. McKnight RA, Burdon T, Pursel VG, et al. The whey acidic protein. In: Dickson RB, Lippman ME, eds. Genes, oncogenes, and hormones. Boston, Kluwer, 1991:399.

52. Wakao H, Gouilleux F, Groner B. Mammary gland factor (Mgf) is a novel member of the cytokine regulated transcription factor gene family and confers the prolactin response. EMBO J 1994;13:2182.

53. Happ B, Groner B. The activated mammary gland specific nuclear factor (Mgf) enhances *in vitro* transcription of the beta-casein gene promoter. J Steroid Biochem 1993;47:21.

54. Altiok S, Groner B. β-casein mRNA sequesters a single-stranded nucleic acid-binding protein which negatively regulates the β-casein gene promoter. Mol Cell Biol 1994;14:6004.

55. Sutherland RL, Watts CKW, Musgrove EA. Cyclin gene expression and growth control in normal and neoplastic breast epithelium. J Steroid Biochem Mol Biol 1993;47:99.

56. Muller R, Mumberg D, Lucibello L. Signals and genes in the control of cell cycle progression. Biochem Biophys Acta 1993; 1155:151.

57. Beatson GT. On the treatment of inoperable cases of carcinoma of the mamma: suggestion for a new method of treatment, with illustrative cases. Lancet 1896;2:104.

58. Welsch CW. Host factors affecting the growth of carcinogen-

induced rat mammary carcinomas: a review and tribute to Charles Brenton Huggins. Cancer Res 1985;45:3415.

59. Jabara AG, Toyne PH, Harcourt AG. Effects of time and duration of progesterone administration on mammary tumors induced by DMBA in Sprague Dawley rats. Br J Cancer 1973;27:63.

60. Robinson SP, Jordan VC. Reversal of the antitumor effects of tamoxifen by progesterone in the DMBA-induced rat mammary carcinoma model. Cancer Res 1987;47:5386.

61. Dickson RB, Gottardis MM, Merlino GT. Molecular insights into breast cancer from transgenic mouse models. Bioessays 1991; 13:591.

62. Medina D, Kittrell FS, Oborn CJ, et al. Growth factor dependency and gene expression in preoeplastic mouse mammary epithelial cells. Cancer Res 1993;53:668.

63. Molinolo AA, Lanari C, Charreau EH, et al. Mouse mammary tumors induced by medroxy progesterone acetate: immunohistochemistry and hormonal receptors. J Natl Cancer Inst 1987; 79:1341.

64. Clarke CL, Sutherland RL. Progestin regulation of cellular proliferation. Endocr Rev 1990;11:266.

65. McCarty KS. Proliferative stimuli in the normal breast: estrogens or progestins. Hum Pathol 1989;20:1137.

66. Willett WC, Hunter DJ, Stampfer MJ, et al. Dietary fat and fiber in relation to risk of breast cancer. JAMA 1992;268:2037.

67. Calle E, Miracle-McMahill HL, Thun MJ, et al. Cigarette smoking and risk of fatal breast cancer. Am J Epidemiol 1994;139:1001.

68. Daniel CW, Silberstein GA, Strickland P. Direct action of 17β estradiol in mouse mammary ducts analyzed by sustained release implants and steroid autoradiography. Cancer Res 1987;47:6052.

69. Dulbecco R. Experimental studies in mammary development and cancer: relevance to human cancer. Adv Oncol 1990;5:3.

70. Simpson ER, Merrill JC, Hollub AJ, et al. Regulation of estrogen biosynthesis by human adipose cells. Endocr Rev 1984;10:136.

71. Donjacour AA, Cunha GR. Stromal regulation of epithelial function. In: Lippman ME, Dickson RB, eds. Regulatory mechanisms in breast cancer. Boston, Kluwer, 1990:335.

72. Cullen KJ, Lippman ME. Stromal-epithelial interactions in breast cancer. In: Lippman ME, Dickson RB, eds. Genes, oncogenes and hormones. Boston, Kluwer, 1992:413.

73. Early Breast Cancer Trialists' Collaborative Group: Systemic treatment of early breast cancer by hormonal, cytotoxic, and immune therapy. Lancet 1992;339:1.

74. Taylor-Papadimitriou J, Lane EB. Keratin expression in the mammary gland. In: Neville MC, Daniel CW, eds. The mammary gland. New York, Plenum, 1987:181.

75. Maemura M, Dickson RB. Are cellular adhesion molecules involved in the metastasis of breast cancer? Breast Cancer Res Treat 1994 (in press).

76. Luscinskas, FW, Lawler J. Integrins as dynamic regulators of vascular function. FASEB J 1994;8:929.

77. Vleminck K, Vakaet L Jr, Mareel M, et al. Genetic manipulation of E-cadherin expression of epithelial tumor cells reveals an invasion suppressor role. Cell 1991;66:107.

78. Boyer B, Tucker GC, Thiery JP, et al. Alternative patterns of mitogenesis and cell scattering induced by acidic FGF and a function of cell density in a rat bladder carcinoma cell line. Cell Regulat 1990;1:975.

79. Strange R, Li F, Friis RR, et al. Mammary epithelial differentiation *in vitro*: minimum requirements for a functional response to hormonal stimulation. Cell Growth Differ 1991;2:549.

80. Liotta LA, Steeg PS, Stetler-Stevenson WG. Cancer metastasis and angiogenesis: an imbalance of positive and negative regulation. Cell 1991;64:327.

81. Sommers CL, Thompson EW, Torri JA, et al. Cell adhesion molecule uvomorulin expression in human breast cancer cell lines: relationship to morphology and invasive capacities. Cell Growth Differ 1991;2:365.

82. Thompson EW, Paik S, Brunner N, et al. Association of increased basement membrane–invasiveness with absence of estrogen receptor and expression of vimentin in human breast cancer cell lines. J Cell Physiol 1992;150:534.

83. Gamallo C, Palacios J, Suarez A, et al. Correlation of E-cadherin expression with differentiation grade and histological type in breast carcinoma. Am J Pathol 1993;142:987.

84. Sager R, Anisowicz A, Neveu M, et al. Identification by differential display of alpha 6 integrin as a candidate tumor suppressor gene. FASEB J 1993;7:964.

85. Boyer B, Tucker GC, Valles AM, et al. Rearrangements of desmosomal and cytoskeletal proteins during the transition from epithelial to fibroblastoid organization in cultured rat bladder carcinoma cells. J Cell Biol 1989;109:1495.

86. Lee SA, Karaszkiewicz JW, Anderson WB. Elevated level of nuclear protein kinase C in multidrug-resistant MCF-7 human breast carcinoma cells. Cancer Res 1992;52:3750.

87. O'Brian CA, Vogel VG, Singletary SE, et al. Elevated protein kinase C expression in human breast tumor biopsies relative to normal breast tissue. Cancer Res 1989;49:3215.

88. Hartwig JH, Thelen M, Rosen A, et al. MARCKS in an actin filament crosslinking protein regulated by protein kinase C and calcium–calmodulin. Nature 1992;356:618.

89. Isakov N, Gopas J, Priel E, et al. Effect of protein kinase C–activating tumor promoters on metastases formation by fibrosarcoma cells. Invasion Metastasis 1991;11:14.

90. Eck SL, Perkins ND, Carr DP, et al. Inhibition of phorbol ester-induced cellular adhesion by competitive binding of NF-kB in vivo. Mol Cell Biol 1993;13:6530.

91. Johnson MD, Torri J, Lippman ME, et al. Regulation of the invasiveness of the human breast cancer cell line MCF-7 by agents that act through protein kinase C. Proceedings of the Keystone Symposium on Breast and Prostate Cancer II, Lake Tahoe, 1994.

92. Birkedal-Hansen H, Moore WGI, Bodden MK, et al. Matrix metalloproteinases: a review. Crit Rev Oral Biol Med 1993;4:197.

93. Olson EN, Burgess R, Staudinger J. Protein kinase C as transducers of nuclear signals. Cell Growth Differ 1993;4:699.

94. Salbert G, Fanjul F, Piedrafita J, et al. Retinoic acid receptors and retinoid X receptor-α down-regulate the transforming growth factor-β_1 promoter by antagonizing AP-1 activity. Mol Endocrinol 1993;7:1347.

95. Dumont JA, Jones Jr WD, Bitonti AJ. Inhibition of experimental metastasis and cell adhesion of B16F1 melanoma cells by inhibitors of protein kinase C. Cancer Res 1992;52:1195.

96. Hornung RL, Pearson JW, Beckwith M, et al. Preclinical evaluation of bryostatin as an anticancer agent against several murine tumor cell lines: *in vitro* versus *in vivo* activity. Cancer Res 1992;52:101.

97. Kennedy MJ, Prestigiacomo LJ, Tyler G, et al. Differential effects of bryostatin 1 and phorbol ester on human breast cancer cell lines. Cancer Res 1992;52:1278.

98. Schwartz MA, Ingber DT. Integrating with integrins. Mol Biol Cell 1994;5:389.

99. Hynes RO. Integrins: a family of cell surface receptors. Cell 1987;48:549.

100. Weiner TM, Liu ET, Craven RJ, et al. Expression of focal adhesion kinase gene and invasion cancer. Lancet 1993;342:1024.

101. Sympson CJ, Talhouk RS, Alexander CM, et al. Targeted expression of stromelysin-1 in mammary gland provides evidence for a role of proteinases in branching morphogenesis and the require-

ment for an intact basement membrane for tissue-specific gene expression. J Cell Biol 1994;125:681.

102. Goldberg GI, Eisen AZ. Extracellular matrix metalloproteinase in tumor invasion and metastases. In: Lippman ME, Dickson RB, eds. Regulatory mechanisms in breast cancer. Boston, Kluwer, 1991:421.

103. Rochefort H, Augereau P, Capony F, et al. The 52k cathepsin D of breast cancer: structure, regulation, function, and clinical value. In: Lippman ME, Dickson RB, eds. Breast cancer: cellular and molecular biology. Boston, Kluwer, 1988:207.

104. Sloan BF. Cathepsin B and cystatins: evidence for a role in cancer progression. Semin Cancer Biol 1990;1:137.

105. Kane SE, Gottesman MM. The role of cathepsin L in malignant transformation. Semin Cancer Biol 1990;1:127.

106. Crowley CW, Cohen RL, Lucas BK, et al. Prevention of metastasis by inhibition of the urokinase receptor. Proc Natl Acad Sci USA 1993;90:5021.

107. Stack MS, Gray RD, Pizzo SV. Modulation of murine B16F10 melanoma plasminogen activator production by a synthetic peptide derived from the laminin A chain. Cancer Res 1993; 53:1998.

108. Sato H, Takino T, Okada Y, et al. A matrix metalloproteinase expressed on the surface of invasive tumor cells. Nature 1994;370:61.

109. Basset P, Bellocq JP, Wolf C, et al. A novel metalloproteinase gene specifically expressed in stromal cells of breast cancer. Nature 1990;348:699.

3

Benign Disorders

Diseases of the Breast, edited by Jay R. Harris,
Marc E. Lippman, Monica Morrow, and Samuel Hellman.
Lippincott-Raven Publishers, Philadelphia, © 1996.

3.1
Pathology of Benign Breast Disorders
Stuart J. Schnitt ▪ James L. Connolly

Benign breast disorders are a heterogeneous group of lesions that clinically and radiographically span the entire spectrum of breast abnormalities. Some benign lesions have findings on physical examination or imaging studies that are similar to those of breast cancer, necessitating a biopsy or an excision to make this distinction.

Once a breast lesion has been shown to be benign on pathologic examination, the most important clinical consideration is the risk of subsequent breast cancer associated with that lesion. For many years, physicians have known that some benign breast lesions are more closely associated with breast cancer than others. Two types of studies have evaluated this relationship. In the first type, the prevalence of benign alterations in breasts with cancer were compared with the prevalence of these conditions in breasts without cancer.[1,2] Although these studies demonstrated that some benign lesions are more common in cancer-containing breasts, the histologic coexistence of certain benign breast lesions with breast cancer is not sufficient to establish that those benign lesions impart an increased cancer risk.

More recent studies evaluated the subsequent risk of developing breast cancer in patients who have had a benign breast biopsy and for whom long-term follow-up is available.[3–12] In these studies, the benign biopsies were reviewed, and the type of benign lesions present were recorded and were related to the risk of breast cancer. In some of these studies, it was also possible to observe the interaction of histologic findings with other factors such as family history of breast cancer, time since biopsy, and menopausal status in determining cancer risk. The results

of these studies have provided important information regarding the risk of breast cancer associated with benign breast lesions, and this information is useful in patient management, counseling, and follow-up. These studies have further indicated that terms such as *fibrocystic disease, chronic cystic mastitis,* and *mammary dysplasia* are not clinically meaningful because they encompass a heterogeneous group of processes, some physiologic and some pathologic, with widely varying cancer risks.[2,13,14]

Foremost among the follow-up studies evaluating benign breast disease and cancer risk is the retrospective cohort study of Dupont, Page, Rogers, and coworkers.[4,15] In this study, the slides of benign breast biopsies from over 3000 women in Nashville were reviewed, and the histologic lesions present were categorized, using strictly defined criteria, into one of three categories: nonproliferative lesions, proliferative lesions without atypia, and atypical hyperplasias.[4,15,16] The risk of developing breast cancer was then determined for each of these groups. This system provides a pragmatic, clinically relevant approach to benign breast lesions and has been supported by a consensus conference of the College of American Pathologists.[17] As discussed later in this chapter, the findings of the Nashville group have now largely been confirmed by other investigators.

Nonproliferative Lesions

Nonproliferative lesions, as defined by Dupont and Page,[4] include cysts, papillary apocrine change, epithelial-related calcifications, and mild hyperplasia of the usual type. *Cysts* are fluid-filled, round to ovoid structures that vary in size from microscopic to grossly evident (Fig. 3.1-1). *Gross cysts,* as defined by Haagensen,[18] are those large enough to produce palpable masses. Cysts are derived from the terminal duct lobular unit. The epithelium usually consists of two layers: an inner (luminal) epithelial layer and an outer myoepithelial layer. In some cysts, the epithelium is markedly attenuated or absent; in others, the lining epithelium shows apocrine metaplasia, characterized by granular eosinophilic cytoplasm and apical cytoplasmic protrusions (snouts). *Papillary apocrine change* is characterized by a proliferation of ductal epithelial cells in which all cells show the foregoing apocrine features. *Epithelial-related calcifications* are frequently observed in breast tissue and may be seen in normal ducts and lobules or in virtually any pathologic condition in the breast. Moreover, calcifications may also be seen in the breast stroma as well as in

blood vessel walls. *Mild hyperplasia of the usual type* is defined as an increase in the number of epithelial cells within a duct that is more than two, but not more than four, epithelial cells in depth. In this type of hyperplasia, the epithelial cells do not cross the lumen of the involved space.

In the study of Dupont and Page,[4] 70% of the biopsy specimens showed nonproliferative lesions. The risk of subsequent breast cancer among these patients was not increased, compared with that of women who have had no breast biopsy (relative risk [RR], 0.89), even in patients with a family history of breast cancer (in a mother, sister, or daughter). The only group of patients in the nonproliferative category with an increased risk of developing breast cancer was that with gross cysts and a family history of breast cancer. The RR with gross cysts alone was 1.5, but it was 3 in patients with gross cysts and positive family

FIGURE 3.1-1 A. This fibrotic breast tissue contains grossly apparent cysts. The cysts are often blue in the fresh state; hence, their designation as blue dome cysts. **B.** Photomicrograph showing breast tissue containing a cyst that is surrounded by fibrous stroma and is lined by a flattened layer of epithelial cells.

histories.[4] Although Dupont and Page initially included fibroadenomas among the nonproliferative lesions, the results of a more recent study by these investigators indicated a higher relative risk for breast cancer among patients with fibroadenoma than in patients with other nonproliferative lesions (see Fibroadenomas).

Proliferative Lesions Without Atypia

Included in the group of proliferative lesions without atypia are *moderate or florid hyperplasias of the usual type, intraductal papillomas,* and *sclerosing adenosis.*[4,19] Moderate or florid hyperplasias of the usual type are intraductal epithelial proliferations more than four epithelial cells in depth. They are characterized by a tendency to bridge and often distend the involved space. The proliferation may have a solid, fenestrated, or papillary architecture. If spaces remain within the duct lumen, they are irregular and variable in shape. The cells comprising this type of proliferation are cytologically benign and variable in size, shape, and orientation. Often, one can discern two distinct cell populations: epithelial cells and myoepithelial cells. A fibrovascular stroma is sometimes present (Fig. 3.1-2). *Intraductal papillomas* are discussed later in this chapter. *Sclerosing adenosis* is most often an incidental microscopic finding, but it may manifest as a palpable mass (the so-called adenosis tumor). Microscopically, these lesions consist of a proliferation of glandular (acinar) structures and stroma in a lobulocentric configuration. Particularly in the center of such lesions, the stroma may compress and distort the glandular elements, producing a pattern that may mimic infiltrating carcinoma (Fig. 3.1-3). In some cases, the epithelial cells in sclerosing adenosis show prominent apocrine features (apocrine adenosis). Many examples of sclerosing adenosis

are associated with calcifications that may, in turn, be seen on mammograms.

In the series of Dupont and Page,[4,19] proliferative lesions without atypia were seen in 26% of biopsies, and such lesions were associated with a mildly elevated risk for the subsequent development of breast cancer (RR, 1.6). This risk was only slightly higher in women with proliferative lesions and positive family histories (RR, 2.1).

Atypical Hyperplasia

Atypical hyperplasias are proliferative lesions of the breast that possess some of the features of carcinoma in situ,[4,15,16] and these lesions are categorized as either ductal or lobular in type. *Atypical ductal hyperplasias* are lesions that have some of the architectural and cytologic features of ductal carcinoma in situ, such as nuclear monomorphism, regular cell placement, and round regular spaces, in at least part of the involved space (Fig. 3.1-4). Similarly, *atypical lobular hyperplasias* are characterized by changes similar to those of lobular carcinoma in situ, but they lack the complete criteria for that diagnosis (Fig. 3.1-5). In addition to involving lobular units, cells of atypical lobular hyperplasia may also involve ducts.[20]

In the study of Dupont and Page,[4] patients with atypical hyperplasia had a substantially increased risk of developing breast cancer. In that study, atypical hyperplasia (of either ductal or lobular type) was identified in only 4% of the biopsy specimens, but the risk of breast cancer for patients with atypical hyperplasia was 4.4 times that of the general population. Further, among patients with atypical hyperplasia and family histories of breast cancer, the relative risk of subsequent breast cancer was 8.9, approaching that of patients with carcinoma in situ.[4,15] Patients whose biopsy

FIGURE 3.1-2 Florid intraductal hyperplasia is characterized by a proliferation of cytologically benign epithelial cells that fill and distend the duct. The nuclei vary in size, shape, and orientation. The spaces within the duct are also variable in size and contour.

FIGURE 3.1-3 Sclerosing adenosis. **A.** Low-power photomicrograph demonstrating a lobulocentric proliferation of stromal and epithelial elements. **B.** High-power examination revealing epithelial cells entrapped in a fibrotic stroma. The cells are cytologically benign, but the pattern simulates that of invasive carcinoma.

specimens showed atypical lobular hyperplasia involving both lobules and ducts had a higher relative risk of developing cancer (RR, 6.8) than those with either atypical lobular hyperplasia alone (RR, 4.3) or only ductal involvement by atypical lobular hyperplasia cells (RR, 2.1).[20]

Certain considerations are important in interpreting the results of studies such as that of Dupont and Page. First, an understanding of the difference between relative risk and absolute risk is necessary to counsel individual patients properly. This distinction is discussed in Chapter 9. Furthermore, the risk of developing breast cancer in the study of Dupont and Page was not constant over the follow-up period; it was highest in the first 10 years after the benign breast biopsy. The relative risk for women with atypical hyperplasia was 9.8 during the first 10 years, and it fell to 3.6 after 10 years.[21] Finally, whether the combined effects of histology and family history on cancer risk in women with atypical hyperplasia represent a true interaction or

simply the presence of two separate risk factors is not yet clear.

Given the apparent clinical importance of the diagnosis of atypical hyperplasia, the ability of pathologists accurately and reproducibly to distinguish this lesion from florid hyperplasia without atypia, on the one hand, and from noncomedo (well-differentiated or low-grade) ductal carcinoma in situ, on the other hand, is a matter of legitimate concern. This problem was addressed in several studies.[22-24] In one of these studies, conducted by Rosai,[22] five highly respected breast pathologists were asked to apply the criteria they used in their daily practice to categorize a series of proliferative breast lesions. Under these conditions, not a single case occurred in which all five pathologists arrived at the same diagnosis, and in only 18% of the cases did four of the five pathologists agree. The results of another study suggest that, with standardization of histologic criteria among pathologists, interobserver

FIGURE 3.1-4 Atypical ductal hyperplasia. Near the center of this space is a proliferation of relatively uniform epithelial cells with monomorphic, round nuclei. This proliferation involves only a portion of the space, however. In other areas, the proliferating epithelial cells maintain their orientation to one another. Thus, this lesion has some of the features of noncomedo ductal carcinoma in situ and is best categorized as atypical ductal hyperplasia.

variability in the diagnosis of proliferative breast lesions can be reduced. In that study,[23] six experienced breast pathologists were instructed to use the same diagnostic criteria (ie, those of Page and coworkers) for categorizing a series of proliferative breast lesions. Complete agreement among all six pathologists was observed in 58% of the cases, and all but one pathologist arrived at the same diagnosis in 71%. The results of these studies indicate that, although the use of standardized histologic criteria improves inter-observer concordance in the diagnosis of these lesions,

even under these circumstances some proliferative lesions defy reproducible categorization.

Some authors have suggested that quantitative criteria should also be used to aid in the distinction between atypical ductal hyperplasia and ductal carcinoma in situ. For example, Page and coworkers[15] require that all the features of ductal carcinoma in situ be uniformly present throughout at least two separate spaces before ductal carcinoma in situ is diagnosed. Lesions that have the qualitative features of noncomedo ductal carcinoma in situ that do not fulfill this quantitative criterion are categorized as atypical hyperplasias. Tavassoli and Norris[6] suggested that the risk of breast cancer associated with small foci of noncomedo ductal carcinoma in situ (ie, less than 2 mm) is similar to that associated with atypical ductal hyperplasia; therefore, they classify lesions that fulfill the qualitative criteria for noncomedo ductal carcinoma in situ but that are less than 2 mm in size as atypical ductal hyperplasias. Although the identification of biologic or genetic markers that may be useful to distinguish atypical ductal hyperplasia from ductal carcinoma in situ is an area of active investigation, no such markers exist at this time, and this distinction must be made on the basis of routine histologic evaluation.

The results of several other follow-up studies in which the participating pathologists used the diagnostic criteria of Dupont, Page, and Rogers have been published.[7,8,11] These results are summarized in Tables 3.1-1 and 3.1-2. The risk estimates observed in these studies are consistent and suggest that this system of classifying benign breast lesions can, in fact, be applied to different populations of patients by different pathologists. These studies have also provided new information regarding benign breast disease and breast cancer risk. For example, in both the Nurse's Health Study and the Breast Cancer Detection Demonstration Project (BCDDP) study, breast cancer risk in women with atypical hyperplasia was influenced by meno-

FIGURE 3.1-5 Atypical lobular hyperplasia. The acini contain a proliferation of small, uniform cells, which are discohesive in some areas; however, the involved acinar structures are not distended by this proliferation. Because this lesion has some features of lobular carcinoma in situ, it is most appropriately categorized as atypical lobular hyperplasia.

TABLE 3.1-1
Relative Risk of Breast Cancer According to Histologic Category of Benign Breast Disease in Studies Using the Criteria of Dupont, Page, and Rogers[4,15,16]

Study	Study Design	Nonproliferative	Proliferative Without Atypia*	Atypical Hyperplasia*
Nashville[4]	Retrospective cohort	1	1.9 (1.6–2.3)	5.3 (3.1–8.8)
Nurse's Health Study[8]	Case-control	1	1.6 (1.0–2.5)	3.7 (2.1–6.8)
BCDDP[11]	Case-control	1	1.3 (0.77–2.2)	4.3 (1.7–11.0)
Florence, Italy[7]	Case-control	1	1.3 (0.5–3.5)	13.0 (4.1–41.7)

BCDDP, Breast Cancer Detection Demonstration Project.

* Numbers in parentheses are 95% confidence intervals for relative risks.

pausal status. In the Nurse's Health Study,[8] the relative risk of developing breast cancer was 5.9 among premenopausal women with atypical hyperplasia, compared with 2.3 for postmenopausal women with atypical hyperplasia. In the BCDDP study,[11] the relative risk for women with atypical hyperplasia was 12 for premenopausal patients and 3.3 for postmenopausal patients. Menopausal status did not have a significant effect on breast cancer risk for patients with proliferative disease without atypia in either of these studies. These results suggest that the hormonal milieu modifies breast cancer risk in women with atypical hyperplasia. These studies have also demonstrated that the risk of breast cancer in patients with atypical hyperplasia (of both ductal and lobular types) is approximately equal in both breasts.[7,25] This finding suggests that atypical hyperplasia is best considered a marker of increased risk rather than a precursor lesion. Moreover, with the increasing use of mammographic screening, atypical hyperplasias are diagnosed more frequently than in the past. For example, when a biopsy is performed because of a palpable mass, atypical hyperplasia is seen in only about 2% to 4% of cases.[4,26] In contrast, atypical hyperplasia was identified in 12% to 17% of biopsies performed because of the presence of mammographic microcalcifications.[27,28]

Some follow-up studies evaluating benign breast disease and breast cancer risk have used diagnostic criteria other than those of the Nashville group for categorizing benign breast lesions.[3,5,9,10,12] In general, the breast cancer risk in the highest-risk groups in these studies is not as great as in the studies that have used the combined histologic and cytologic criteria outlined by Dupont, Page, and Rogers.

In summary, the results of these follow-up studies indicate that the majority of women who have a benign breast biopsy are not at increased risk of developing breast cancer. A substantially increased breast cancer risk is seen only in the small percentage of patients whose benign breast biopsies show atypical hyperplasia using strictly defined histologic and cytologic criteria, particularly when accompanied by a family history of breast cancer.

OTHER BENIGN LESIONS
Fibroadenomas

On gross examination, fibroadenomas are pseudoencapsulated and are sharply delimited from the surrounding breast tissue. They are usually spheric or ovoid but may be multilobulated. When cut, the tumor bulges above the level of

TABLE 3.1-2
*Effect of Family History of Breast Cancer on Relative Risk of Breast Cancer**

Study	Proliferative Disease Without Atypia†		Atypical Hyperlasia†	
	No FH	FH	No FH	FH
Nashville[4]	1.9 (1.2–3.0)	2.7 (1.4–5.3)	4.3 (2.4–7.8)	8.4 (2.6–27)
Nurse's Health Study[8]	1.3 (0.8–2.2)	4.5 (1.1–18.4)	3.7 (1.9–7.0)	7.3 (1.1–50.1)
BCDDP[11]	1.7 (0.9–3.2)	2.6 (1.0–6.4)	4.2 (1.4–12.0)	22.0 (2.4–203)

FH, family history of breast cancer in mother, sister, or daughter; BCDDP, Breast Cancer Detection Demonstration Project.

* Relative risks compared with women with nonproliferative lesions.

† Numbers in parentheses are 95% confidence intervals for relative risks.

the surrounding breast tissue. The cut surface is most typically gray-white, and small, punctate, yellow-to-pink soft areas and slitlike spaces are commonly observed. Occasionally, the tumor has a gelatinous, mucoid consistency.

Microscopically, fibroadenomas have both epithelial and stromal components. The histologic pattern depends on which of these components predominates. In general, the epithelial component consists of well-defined, glandlike, and ductlike spaces lined by cuboidal or columnar cells with uniform nuclei. Varying degrees of epithelial hyperplasia are frequently observed. The stromal component consists of connective tissue that has a variable content of acid mucopolysaccharides and collagen (Fig. 3.1-6). In older lesions and in postmenopausal patients, the stroma may become hyalinized, calcified, or even ossified (ancient fibroadenoma). On rare occasions, mature adipose tissue or smooth muscle comprises a portion of the stroma.[29,30] Fibroadenomas may undergo partial, subtotal, or total infarction. Pregnancy and lactation are the most common predisposing factors. A relative vascular insufficiency in the face of increased metabolic activity in the breast has been postulated to underlie this phenomenon.[29] Variants of fibroadenomas include juvenile fibroadenomas[31–34] and giant fibroadenomas,[29,33] as discussed in Chapter 3.3. Carcinoma involving fibroadenomas and the risk of subsequent carcinoma associated with fibroadenomas are also discussed in Chapter 3.3.

Adenoma

Adenomas of the breast are well-circumscribed tumors composed of benign epithelial elements with sparse, inconspicuous stroma.[35] The last feature differentiates these lesions from fibroadenomas, in which the stroma is an integral part of the tumor. For practical purposes, adenomas may be divided into two major groups: tubular adenomas and lactating adenomas.

TUBULAR ADENOMAS. These occur in young women as well-defined, freely movable nodules that clinically resemble fibroadenomas.[35] Gross examination reveals a well-circumscribed, tan-yellow, firm tumor. On microscopic examination, tubular adenomas are separated from the adjacent breast tissue by a pseudocapsule and are composed of a proliferation of uniform, small, tubular structures with a scant amount of intervening stroma. The tubules are composed of an inner epithelial layer and an outer myoepithelial layer, and they resemble normal breast acini at both light microscopic and ultrastructural levels. In some cases, this pattern is admixed with that of a fibroadenoma, suggesting a relationship between the two tumors.

LACTATING ADENOMAS (NODULAR LACTATIONAL HYPERPLASIA). These occur as one or more freely movable masses during pregnancy or in the postpartum period.[35] They are grossly well circumscribed and lobulated, and on cut section they appear tan and softer than tubular adenomas. On microscopic examination, these lesions have lobulated borders and are composed of glands lined by cuboidal cells with secretory activity, identical to the lactational changes normally observed in breast tissue during pregnancy and the puerperium. Although some authors believe that these lesions are the result of lactational changes superimposed on a preexisting tubular adenoma, others have suggested that they represent new lesions and are merely nodular foci of hyperplasia in the lactating breast.

In a review of 42 breast adenomas that demonstrated lactational changes, O'Hara and Page[36] observed an overlapping spectrum of morphologic features in fibroadenomas with lactational changes and in lactating and tubular adenomas. These authors suggested that all these lesions may have a common pathogenesis.

Rarely, adenomatous tumors resembling dermal sweat-gland neoplasms are observed as primary lesions in the breast parenchyma (eg, clear cell hidradenoma and eccrine spirade-

FIGURE 3.1-6 In this fibroadenoma, the tumor is well circumscribed and is separated from the adjacent breast tissue by a rim of dense collagen. Both glandular and stromal elements are apparent.

noma)[29,35] or nipple (eg, syringomatous adenoma).[37,38] Pleomorphic adenomas, histologically identical to those seen in the salivary glands, have also been described in the breast.[29]

Adenomas of the Nipple

Adenoma of the nipple has been described by a variety of names, including florid papillomatosis of the nipple ducts,[39] subareolar duct papillomatosis,[29] papillary adenoma of the nipple,[40] and erosive adenomatosis of the nipple.[41] It is not a true adenoma of the breast as defined by Hertel and associates[35] because of its prominent stromal component.

On macroscopic examination, some adenomas of the nipple appear as solid, gray-tan, poorly demarcated tumors in the nipple and subareolar region; in other cases, no gross lesion is evident. Microscopically, the dominant feature is a proliferation of small, glandlike structures. Solid and papillary proliferation of ductal epithelium is also usually evident; however, the papillary pattern may be inconspicuous or totally absent. In advanced lesions, glandular epithelium extends onto the surface of the nipple, a phenomenon that results in the clinically evident reddish, granular appearance. Squamous epithelium frequently extends into the superficial regions of the involved ducts, sometimes with the formation of keratinaceous cysts. The lesions usually show considerable stromal fibrosis. This connective tissue may distort and entrap the epithelial elements, resulting in a pattern mimicking invasive carcinoma. The lesion is distinguishable from carcinoma by the preservation of a double layer of epithelium in the proliferating glands (an inner epithelial layer and an outer myoepithelial layer), minimal nuclear atypicality, the absence of necrosis, and the overall low-power configuration.

A few cases of carcinoma associated with adenomas of the nipple have been reported.[42–44] In most cases, however, the lesion is entirely benign. Reports of recurrence most likely represent cases in which the initial resection failed to remove the lesion completely.

Intraductal Papillomas

A variety of lesions in the breast are characterized by a papillary configuration grossly or microscopically (Fig. 3.1-7). These include solitary intraductal papillomas, multiple (peripheral) papillomas, and papillomatosis. *Solitary intraductal papillomas* are lesions of the larger ducts. *Multiple (peripheral) papillomas* arise in the terminal duct–lobular units and are less uniformly recognized. Although some authors include these in the category of papillomatosis, others recognize a clinicopathologic entity characterized clinically by an indistinct mass with or without nipple discharge and pathologically by multiple small, but grossly evident, papillary lesions.[18] *Papillomatosis* is a term used to describe microscopic foci of intraductal hyperplasia with a papillary architecture and is therefore included by Dupont and Page in the category of proliferative lesions without atypia.[4] One variant, juvenile papillomatosis (swiss cheese disease), is a distinct clinicopathologic entity that occurs most commonly in adolescents and young

women.[45–49] These lesions are considered in detail in Chapter 3.2.

Microglandular Adenosis

Microglandular adenosis (MGA) is an uncommon lesion that may be identified as an incidental finding in breast tissue excised for a variety of other lesions, or it may appear as a palpable mass. Most women in whom this lesion has been reported are older than 40 years of age, but patients as young as 28 years and as old as 82 years have been reported to have MGA. On gross examination, MGA is generally described as an ill-defined area of firm, rubbery tissue, usually 3 to 4 cm in diameter. The importance of this lesion is that it may be mistaken for a well-differentiated (tubular) carcinoma on histologic examination. Microscopically, the lesion of MGA is characterized by a poorly circumscribed, haphazard proliferation of small, round glands in the breast stroma and adipose tissue. Unlike sclerosing adenosis, MGA does not have a lobulocentric, organoid configuration. The glands are composed of a single layer of cuboidal epithelial cells with clear to slightly eosinophilic cytoplasm and small, regular nuclei. The cells stain strongly for S100 protein, and the glands are surrounded by basement membrane material.[50–52] Eosinophilic secretions are frequently present within the glandular lumina. The stroma is typically composed of dense, relatively acellular collagen, which usually demarcates the lesion from the adjacent parenchyma. In some areas, the stroma is minimal, and the proliferating glands lie exposed in adipose tissue (Fig. 3.1-8).

The relation between MGA and cancer has been addressed in several studies. Simultaneous or subsequent carcinoma was reported in 4 of the 13 patients originally reported by Rosen,[53] in 1 of the 11 patients described by Tavassoli and Norris,[54] and in none of the 6 patients reported by Clement and Azzopardi.[55] Rosenblum and coworkers described 7 cases of MGA associated with carcinoma.[56] More recently, James and associates[51] noted carcinoma arising in or in conjunction with MGA in 14 of 60 cases (23%). Thus, in some cases, MGA may be associated with carcinoma. The recommended approach to the management of patients with MGA is complete, local excision of the lesion and careful follow-up.

Radial Scars

Radial scars[57] have been described in the literature by a variety of names, including sclerosing papillary proliferation,[58] nonencapsulated sclerosing lesion,[59] and indurative mastopathy.[60] Their importance lies in that they may simulate carcinoma on mammographic, gross, and microscopic examinations.

Radial scars are most frequently incidental findings in breast tissue excised because of another abnormality. They may also be detected by mammography, as soft tissue densities with irregular, serrated edges, similar in appearance to carcinomas. They are often multiple, with as many as 31 lesions observed in a single breast.[61] These lesions are typically less than 1 cm in diameter and, on gross examina-

FIGURE 3.1-7 Intraductal papilloma. **A.** Low-power photomicrograph demonstrating the papillary lesion within a dilated duct. **B.** Higher-power view demonstrating that the papillae are composed of central fibrovascular cores covered by two layers of cells, a myoepithelial layer (lying closer to the cores) and an epithelial layer (lying closer to the duct lumen).

tion, are irregular, gray white, and indurated with central retraction—an appearance identical to that of scirrhous carcinoma. Similar lesions of greater size (larger than 1 cm) have been termed *complex sclerosing lesions.*[62]

Microscopically, these lesions have a stellate configuration and consist of a central, fibroelastotic core containing entrapped glandular elements. Radiating from this core are ducts with varying degrees of epithelial hyperplasia and papillomatosis. Ducts at the periphery may be dilated cystically. Sclerosing adenosis and apocrine metaplasia frequently accompany the lesion. The surrounding breast tissue typically shows varying degrees of intraductal hyperplasia and adenosis. The entrapped glands in the center of the lesion may be confused with the glands of tubular carcinoma. The low-power configuration of the lesion permits the correct diagnosis.

The significance of radial scars with regard to the subsequent development of carcinoma is controversial. Some authors have argued that these lesions may represent incip-

ient tubular carcinoma[58] or a stage in the development of many invasive breast cancers.[63] An autopsy study demonstrated that these lesions are significantly more common in breasts of cancer patients than in noncancerous breasts[61]; however, this evidence is clearly not sufficient to prove that these lesions are precancerous. Follow-up studies have failed to show an increased incidence of breast cancer in patients who have had a radial scar excised.[57,60] Available evidence suggests that the premalignant potential of these lesions is the same as that of their constituent parts.[61,64] Local excision is the treatment of choice.

Granular Cell Tumors

Granular cell tumors are uncommonly found in the breast but, when present, simulate carcinoma on clinical, mammographic, and pathologic examination.[65,66] Patients present with a palpable mass that may be associated with skin retraction or fixation to skeletal muscles of the chest wall.

FIGURE 3.1-8 A. Microglandular adenosis is characterized by a proliferation of small, glandular structures composed of a single layer of epithelial cells. The cells have clear to eosinophilic cytoplasm. The glands are round, and many contain eosinophilic material within their lumina. (Compare this lesion with that found in cases of tubular carcinoma.) **B.** Well-differentiated, infiltrating, ductal (tubular) carcinoma is composed of well-formed glands, many of which are ovoid and have tapering ends. The epithelial cells that constitute the tubules show minimal nuclear atypicality; apocrine snouts are apparent at the luminal aspect of the cells.

The similarity of granular cell tumors to carcinoma is also evident on mammographic examination, on which they resemble scirrhous carcinoma. Gross examination of the lesion reveals a firm tumor that is gray-white to tan and that may be gritty when cut with a knife, similar to the macroscopic appearance of many carcinomas. Microscopically, these lesions are identical to granular cell tumors in other sites, consisting of a poorly circumscribed proliferation of clusters of cells in which the most characteristic feature is prominent granularity of the cytoplasm. On electron microscopic examination, these granules correspond to secondary lysosomes.

Granular cell tumors are almost invariably benign and are adequately treated by wide local excision. Rare cases of malignant granular cell tumors have been reported in both the breast and extramammary sites.

Granular cell tumors were initially considered to be myogenic in origin (hence their earlier designation as granular cell myoblastomas), but more recent ultrastructural and immunohistochemical evidence supports a neurogenic origin for these tumors.[66,67]

Fibromatosis

Fibromatosis of the breast is analogous to fibromatosis in other sites (eg, desmoid tumors of the abdominal wall) and is characterized by a locally invasive, nonencapsulated proliferation of well-differentiated spindle cells.[68–73] These tumors have the capacity to recur locally if inadequately excised, but they do not metastasize. Patients typically present with a palpable mass that is sometimes associated with skin retraction or fixation to the underlying pectoral muscle. On mammography, these lesions are indistinguishable from carcinomas. Gross pathologic examination reveals an ill-defined, firm, gray-white lesion. Microscopically, fibromatoses consist of interlacing bundles of spindle-shaped cells surrounded by collagen. The cells show minimal to no cytologic atypism, and mitoses are only infrequently encountered. The proliferation tends to surround and entrap preexisting ducts and lobules without destroying them. The edges of the lesion infiltrate irregularly into the adjacent parenchyma. On electron microscopic examination, some tumor cells have the ultrastructural features of fibroblasts, whereas others appear to be myofibroblasts.

The proper treatment for these lesions consists of wide local excision. Although metastases have not been reported, lesions may recur locally. Zayid and Dehmis[74] described an exceptional case in which a patient treated with mastectomy subsequently developed multiple tumor recurrences in the chest wall that ultimately resulted in her death.

A few reported cases of fibromatosis of the breast have been associated with Gardner syndrome.[70] Another case occurred in a patient with familial multicentric fibromatosis.[74]

Miscellaneous Benign Tumors and Tumor-Like Lesions

Lipomas consist of encapsulated nodules of mature adipose tissue. Although true lipomas occur in the breast, many lesions designated *lipoma* probably represent foci of fatty breast tissue without a true capsule. *Adenolipoma* is a term applied to a benign fatty tumor of the breast containing entrapped lobular epithelial elements[29]; however, the distinction between this lesion and breast tissue with prominent stromal adipose tissue is often unclear.

Benign vascular lesions of the breast parenchyma are relatively uncommon and most often represent incidental microscopic findings. In a series of 550 mastectomy specimens from patients with breast carcinoma, the incidence of benign hemangiomas was 1.2%.[75] Benign vascular lesions of the breast may be divided into four major categories: *perilobular hemangiomas, angiomatoses, venous hemangiomas,* and *hemangiomas involving the mammary subcutaneous tissue.*[76-79] The major significance of these lesions is that they must be distinguished from angiosarcomas.[80] Benign angiomatous lesions are almost always microscopic in size and lack interanastomosing channels, endothelial proliferation, and atypia. Complete excision is recommended for all vascular lesions of the breast. *Pseudoangiomatous hyperplasia of the mammary stroma* is a benign stromal proliferation that simulates a vascular lesion.[81,82] The lesion is often seen as an incidental microscopic finding, but it may occur as a palpable mass. Microscopic examination reveals a densely fibrotic stroma containing complex interanastomosing spaces, some of which have spindle-shaped cells at their margins simulating endothelial cells. Ultrastructural examinations have demonstrated that the spaces appear to be due to separation and disruption of collagen fibers, however, and the associated spindle cells are fibroblasts. The significance of this lesion is that it must be distinguished from angiosarcoma.

Chondromatous lesions of the breast are uncommon. Although chondromatous changes are most often seen in breast carcinomas and sarcomas, chondroid metaplasia may readily be seen in fibroadenomas and intraductal papillomas. A few cases of *chondrolipoma* have also been reported,[83,84] as has a single case of *choristoma* containing cartilage.[85]

Leiomyomas of the breast are most often seen in the areolar region and rarely occur in the breast parenchyma.[29]

The histologic characteristics are the same as those of leiomyomas in other tissue.

Neurofibromas and *neurilemomas (schwannomas)* are benign nerve sheath tumors. These lesions are most frequently seen in the breast in patients with neurofibromatosis and are most common in the areolar area.[18]

Adenomyoepitheliomas are uncommon lesions composed of a combination of epithelial and myoepithelial elements. These lesions appear as palpable masses and are adequately treated by complete local excision.[86-89] Lesions composed exclusively of myoepithelial cells (*myoepitheliomas*) have also been described.[89,90]

Ductal adenomas are circumscribed nodules composed of glandular structures within a fibrotic stroma. Many of these lesions appear to represent extensively sclerotic intraductal papillomas.[91,92]

Mucocele-like lesions are characterized by cystic accumulations of mucus within the breast stroma.[93,94] The mucoid character of these lesions is usually evident on gross examination. Microscopically, the epithelium lining these cysts may assume a variety of histologic appearances including flat cuboidal epithelium, papillary hyperplasia, atypical ductal hyperplasia, and ductal carcinoma in situ. These lesions must be completely excised and carefully examined histologically, to rule out the possibility of invasive mucinous carcinoma.

Collagenous spherulosis is a lesion detected incidentally during microscopic examination of breast tissue removed because of another abnormality. It is characterized by a fenestrated proliferation of epithelial and myoepithelial cells and intraluminal spherules composed of variable amounts of basement membrane–like material and collagen. This lesion is important to recognize because it must be distinguished from adenoid cystic carcinoma and intraductal signet ring cell carcinoma.[95]

Inflammatory and Reactive Disorders

MAMMARY DUCT ECTASIA (PERIDUCTAL MASTITIS)

Mammary duct ectasia occurs primarily in perimenopausal and postmenopausal women and is characterized by dilatation of the subareolar ducts.[18] Considerable controversy exists regarding the most appropriate name for this condition: some authors consider ductal dilatation to be the primary event, whereas others consider the ectatic ducts to be the consequence of prior periductal inflammation.

Duct ectasia is a frequent pathologic finding in breast tissue obtained at autopsy and in surgically excised material. It has been observed on microscopic examination in 30% to 40% of women older than 50 years. Clinically evident disease, however, occurs much less frequently.[96] Details regarding the clinical presentation of patients with duct ectasia are presented in Chapter 3.4.

A wide spectrum of pathologic changes is observed in this condition. Cut section of the gross specimen often reveals dilated, thick-walled ducts that contain pasty, yellow-brown secretions. The intervening stroma may be

FIGURE 3.1-9   Fat necrosis. The fatty breast tissue is infiltrated by histiocytes containing foamy cytoplasm.

fibrotic. On microscopic examination, some specimens show prominent inspissation of lipid-rich material within ducts, accompanied by periductal inflammation. Rupture or leakage of these ducts results in release of this material into the adjacent stroma, with subsequent inflammation and fat necrosis (Fig. 3.1-9). Plasma cells may be a prominent component of the periductal and stroma inflammatory infiltrate. Many cases previously designated as plasma cell mastitis probably represent a stage in the evolution of duct ectasia. In other cases, the histologic picture is dominated by periductal fibrosis and ductal dilatation with minimal inflammation.

As alluded to earlier, the pathogenesis of this condition has not been fully established. Available evidence suggests, however, that the primary event is periductal inflammation, and duct ectasia is the ultimate outcome of this disorder. In support of this premise, Dixon and associates[96]

observed that inflammation around nondilated ducts predominates in younger patients with this condition, whereas duct dilatation and nipple retraction are more common in older patients. Thus, the postulated sequence of events in the evolution of this disease is that periductal inflammation leads to periductal fibrosis, which subsequently results in ductal dilatation. The cause of the initial inflammatory response remains obscure, however.

REACTIONS TO FOREIGN MATERIAL

Foreign body–type granulomatous inflammation has been described following injection within the breast of a variety of substances, including paraffin and silicone. Clinically, these lesions generally appear as firm nodules that may be tender.[97]

Various tissue reactions have been reported in associa-

FIGURE 3.1-10   Radiation effects. This terminal duct–lobular unit contains scattered, enlarged, epithelial cells with large, diffusely hyperchromatic nuclei (*arrows*). Cellular polarity is maintained, and no evidence of epithelial cell proliferation is present.

tion with mammary implants.[98,99] One of these is the formation of a fibrous capsule in the surrounding tissue. In 10% to 40% of patients, contracture of this capsule results in breast tightness or firmness and deformation of the implant necessitating either capsulotomy or removal of the implant and the surrounding capsule. Histologic examination of the capsular tissue shows varying degrees of fibrosis, chronic inflammation, fat necrosis, granulation tissue, fibrin deposition, and histiocytes and foreign body giant cells, often with demonstrable silicone and, in some cases in which it has been used as part of the implant shell, polyurethane. In some cases, the capsule surrounding breast implants develops a cellular lining that histologically, immunohistochemically, and ultrastructurally resembles either normal synovium or synovium with papillary hyperplasia (proliferative synovitis) and has physiologic properties similar to those of synovium.[100–104] This change has been variably described as pseudoepithelialization, synovial metaplasia, or capsular synovial hyperplasia. Factors associated with development of synovial-type metaplasia in this setting are not known. Some investigators have suggested that this condition is a consequence of mechanical forces (eg, micromotion and friction) between the implant and the surrounding tissue.

PATHOLOGIC CHANGES ASSOCIATED WITH RADIATION THERAPY FOR CARCINOMA

Breast-conserving surgery, followed by radiation therapy, is becoming an increasingly common treatment for patients with early-stage breast cancer. The effects of therapeutic doses of ionizing radiation on the skin of the breast have been well described and are identical to the radiation-induced alterations in skin overlying any irradiated site.[105]

Fat necrosis may occur in the breast following local excision and radiotherapy for carcinoma. These lesions may be indistinguishable from carcinoma by clinical and radiographic examination, requiring complete histologic examination for accurate diagnosis.[106] The most characteristic pathologic finding in breast tissue excised following primary radiotherapy for carcinoma is epithelial cell atypicality in the terminal duct–lobular unit (TDLU), usually associated with varying degrees of lobular sclerosis and atrophy[107] (Fig. 3.1-10). These changes may be distinguished from carcinoma involving the TDLU by the preservation of polarity and cohesion and by the absence of cellular proliferation and distention of the involved TDLU in areas of radiation-induced change. Similar epithelial changes have been described in patients treated with chemotherapy before tumor excision.[108] Less frequently, epithelial atypia in large (extralobular) ducts, atypical fibroblasts in the stroma, and radiation-related vascular changes may be observed. Stromal fibrosis, a characteristic effect of radiation in other organs, is so variable among both irradiated patients and non-irradiated control subjects that it is not, by itself, a reliable marker for radiation-induced injury in the breast.

SARCOIDOSIS

Involvement of the breast by sarcoidosis is rare, but when present, may clinically simulate a neoplasm.[109–111] Histologically, the lesions consist of typical, noncaseating granulomas with varying numbers of giant cells present in the interlobular and intralobular connective tissue. A diagnosis of sarcoidosis should be made only after other causes of granulomatous inflammation, such as mycobacterial, fungal, and parasitic infections or reactions to foreign materials, have been excluded. Sarcoidosis should also be distinguished from *granulomatous mastitis,* a lesion in which granulomas are associated with microabscesses and that may respond to corticosteroid therapy.[112–115]

DIABETIC MASTOPATHY

Patients with insulin-dependent diabetes occasionally develop palpable breast masses that, on histologic examination, show a characteristic constellation of features.[116,117] These include dense, keloid-like fibrosis, lymphocytic infiltrates in association with ducts and lobules (lymphocytic ductitis and lobulitis), lymphocytic vasculitis, and epithelioid fibroblasts in the stroma. Although the pathogenesis of this lesion is unknown, it may represent an autoimmune reaction.

References

1. Page DL, Dupont WD. Anatomic indicators (histologic and cytologic) of increased breast cancer risk. Breast Cancer Res Treat 1993;28:157.
2. Love SM, Gelman RS, Silen W. Fibrocystic "disease" of the breast: a nondisease? N Engl J Med 1982;307:1010.
3. Kodlin D, Winger EE, Morganstern NL, et al. Chronic mastopathy and breast cancer: a follow-up study. Cancer 1977;39:2603.
4. Dupont WD, Page DL. Risk factors for breast cancer in women with proliferative breast disease. N Engl J Med 1985;312:146.
5. Carter CL, Cook DK, Micozzi MS, et al. A prospective study of the development of breast cancer in 16,692 women with benign breast disease. Am J Epidemiol 1988;128:467.
6. Tavassoli FA, Norris HF. A comparison of long-term follow-up for atypical intraductal hyperplasia and intraductal hyperplasia of the breast. Cancer 1990;65:518.
7. Palli D, Del Turco MR, Simoncini R, et al. Benign breast disease and breast cancer: a case-control study in a cohort in Italy. Int J Cancer 1991;47:703.
8. London SJ, Connolly JL, Schnitt SJ, et al. A prospective study of benign breast disease and the risk of breast cancer. JAMA 1992;267:941.
9. Krieger N, Hiatt RA. Risk of breast cancer after benign breast diseases: variation by histologic type, degree of atypia, age at biopsy and length of follow-up. Am J Epidemiol 1992;135:619.
10. McDivitt RW, Stevens JA, Lee NC, et al. Histologic types of benign breast disease and the risk of breast cancer. Cancer 1992;69:1408.
11. Dupont WD, Parl FF, Hartmann WH, et al. Breast cancer risk associated with proliferative breast disease and atypical hyperplasia. Cancer 1993;71:1258.
12. Bodian CA, Perzin KH, Lattes R, et al. Prognostic significance of benign proliferative breast disease. Cancer 1993;71:3896.

13. Hutter RVP. Goodbye to "fibrocystic disease." N Engl J Med 1985;312:179.

14. Hughes LE, Mansel RE, Webster DJT. Aberrations of normal development and involution (ANDI): a new perspective on pathogenesis and nomenclature of benign breast disorders. Lancet 1987;2:1316.

15. Page DL, Dupont WD, Rogers LW, et al. Atypical hyperplastic lesions of the female breast: a long-term follow-up study. Cancer 1985;55:2698.

16. Page DL, Rogers LW. Combined histologic and cytologic criteria for the diagnosis of mammary atypical ductal hyperplasia. Hum Pathol 1992;23:1095.

17. Consensus Meeting. Is "fibrocystic disease" of the breast precancerous? Arch Pathol Lab Med 1986;110:171.

18. Haagensen CD. Diseases of the breast, ed 3. Philadelphia, WB Saunders, 1986.

19. Jensen RA, Page DL, Dupont WD, et al. Invasive breast cancer risk in women with sclerosing adenosis. Cancer 1989;64:1977.

20. Page DL, Dupont WD, Rogers LW. Ductal involvement by cells of atypical lobular hyperplasia: a long-term follow-up study of cancer risk. Hum Pathol 1988;19:201.

21. Dupont WD, Page DL. Relative risk of breast cancer varies with time since diagnosis of atypical hyperplasia. Hum Pathol 1989;20:723.

22. Rosai J. Borderline epithelial lesions of the breast. Am J Surg Pathol 1991;15:209.

23. Schnitt SJ, Connolly JL, Tavassoli FA, et al. Interobserver reproducibility in the diagnosis of ductal proliferative breast lesions using standardized criteria. Am J Surg Pathol 1992;16:1133.

24. Bodian CA, Perzin KH, Lattes R, et al. Reproducibility and validity of pathologic classifications of benign breast disease and implications for clinical applications. Cancer 1993;71:3908.

25. Connolly JL, Schnitt SJ, London S, et al. Both atypical lobular hyperplasia (ALH) and atypical ductal hyperplasia (ADH) predict for bilateral breast cancer risk. Lab Invest 1992;66:13A.

26. Schnitt SJ, Wang HH. Histologic sampling of grossly benign breast biopsies. How much is enough? Am J Surg Pathol 1989;13:505.

27. Owings DV, Hann L, Schnitt SJ. How thoroughly should needle localization breast biopsies be sampled for microscopic examination? A prospective mammographic–pathologic correlative study. Am J Surg Pathol 1990;14:578.

28. Rubin E, Visscher DW, Alexander RW, et al. Proliferative disease and atypia in biopsies performed for nonpalpable lesions detected mammographically. Cancer 1988;61:2077.

29. Azzopardi JG. Problems in breast pathology. Philadelphia, WB Saunders, 1976.

30. Goodman ZD, Taxy JB. Fibroadenomas of the breast with prominent smooth muscle. Am J Surg Pathol 1981;5:99.

31. Oberman HA. Breast lesions in the adolescent female. In: Sommers SC, Rosen PP, eds. Pathology annual, part 1. Norwalk, CT, Appleton-Century-Crofts, 1979.

32. Nambiar R, Kutty K. Giant fibroadenoma (cytosarcoma phyllodes) in adolescent females: a clinicopathologic study. Br J Surg 1974;61:113.

33. Ashikari R, Farrow JH, O'Hara J. Fibroadenomas in the breast of juveniles. Surg Gynecol Obstet 1971;132:259.

34. Mies C, Rosen PP. Juvenile fibroadenomas with atypical epithelial hyperplasia. Am J Surg Pathol 1987;11:184.

35. Hertel BF, Zaloudek C, Kempson RL. Breast adenomas. 1976;Cancer 37:2891.

36. O'Hara MF, Page DL. Adenomas of the breast and ectopic breast under lactational influences. Hum Pathol 1985;16:707.

37. Rosen PP. Syringomatous adenoma of the nipple. Am J Surg Pathol 1983;7:739.

38. Jones MW, Norris HJ, Snyder RC. Infiltrating syringomatous adenoma of the nipple: a clinical and pathological study of 11 cases. Am J Surg Pathol 1989;13:197.

39. Jones DB. Florid papillomatosis of the nipple ducts. Cancer 1955;8:315.

40. Perzin KH, Lattes R. Papillary adenoma of the nipple (florid papillomatosis, adenoma, adenomatosis): a clinicopathologic study. Cancer 1972;29:996.

41. Smith EJ, Kron SD, Gross PR. Erosive adenomatosis of the nipple. Arch Dermatol 1970;102:330.

42. Gudjonsdottir A, Hagerstrand I, Ostberg G. Adenoma of the nipple with carcinomatous development. Acta Pathol Microbiol Scand [A] 1971;79:676.

43. Bhagavan BS, Patchevsky AS, Koss LG. Florid subareolar duct papillomatosis (nipple adenoma) and mammary carcinoma: report of three cases. Hum Pathol 1973;4:289.

44. Rosen PP, Caicco JA. Florid papillomatosis of the nipple: a study of 51 patients, including nine with mammary carcinoma. Am J Surg Pathol 1986;102:87.

45. Rosen PP, Cantrell B, Mullen DL, et al. Juvenile papillomatosis (Swiss cheese disease) of the breast. Am J Surg Pathol 1980;4:3.

46. Rosen PP, Lyngholm B, Kinne DW, et al. Juvenile papillomatosis and family history of breast carcinoma. Cancer 1982;49:2591.

47. Rosen PP, Holmes G, Lesser ML, et al. Juvenile papillomatosis and breast carcinoma. Cancer 1985;55:1345.

48. Bazzochi F, Santini D, Martinelli G, et al. Juvenile papillomatosis (epitheliosis) of the breast: a clinical pathological study of 13 cases. Am J Clin Pathol 1986;86:745.

49. Rosen PP, Kimmel M. Juvenile papillomatosis of the breast: a follow-up study of 41 patients having biopsies before 1979. Am J Clin Pathol 1990;93:599–603.

50. Diaz NM, McDivitt RW, Wick MR. Microglandular adenosis of the breast: an immunohistochemical comparison with tubular carcinoma. Arch Pathol Lab Med 1991;115:578.

51. James BA, Cranor ML, Rosen PP. Carcinoma of the breast arising in microglandular adenosis. Am J Clin Pathol 1993;100:507.

52. Tavassoli FA, Bratthauer GL. Immunohistochemical profile and differential diagnosis of microglandular adenosis. Mod Pathol 1993;6:318.

53. Rosen PP. Microglandular adenosis: a benign lesion simulating invasive mammary carcinoma. Am J Surg Pathol 1983;7:137.

54. Tavassoli FA, Norris HJ. Microglandular adenosis of the breast: a clinicopathologic study of 11 cases with ultrastructural observations. Am J Surg Pathol 1983;7:731.

55. Clement PB, Azzopardi JG. Microglandular adenosis of the breast: a lesion simulating tubular carcinoma. Histopathology 1983;7:169.

56. Rosenblum MK, Purrazzella R, Rosen PP. Is microglandular adenosis a precancerous disease? A study of carcinoma arising in microglandular adenosis. Lab Invest 1985;52:57A.

57. Andersen JA, Gram JB. Radial scar in the female breast: a long-term follow-up study of 32 cases. Cancer 1984;53:2557.

58. Fenoglio C, Lattes R. Sclerosing papillary proliferations in the female breast: a benign lesion often mistaken for carcinoma. Cancer 1974;33:691.

59. Fisher ER, Palekar AS, Kotwal N, et al. A nonencapsulated sclerosing lesion of the breast. Am J Clin Pathol 1979;71:240.

60. Rickert RR, Kalisher L, Hutter RVP. Indurative mastopathy: a benign sclerosing lesion of breast with elastosis which may simulate carcinoma. Cancer 1981;47:561.

61. Wellings SR, Alpers CE. Subgross pathologic features and incidence of radial scars in the breast. Hum Pathol 1984;15:475.

62. Page DL, Anderson TJ. Diagnostic histopathology of the breast. Edinburgh, Churchill Livingstone, 1987.

63. Linell F, Ljungberg O, Andersson I. Breast carcinoma: aspects of early stages, progression and related problems. Acta Pathol Microbiol Scand [A] 1980;272(Suppl):14.

64. Nielsen M, Christensen L, Andersen J. Radial scars in women with breast cancer. Cancer 1987;59:1019.

65. DeMay RM, Kay S. Granular cell tumors of the breast. In: Sommers SC, Rosen PP, eds. Pathology annual, part 1. Norwalk, CT, Appleton-Century-Crofts, 1984.

66. Damiani S, Koerner FC, Dickersin GR, Cook MG, Eusebi V. Granular cell tumor of the breast. Virchows Arch Pathol Anat Histopathol [A] 1992;420:219–226.

67. Ingram DL, Mossler JA, Snowhite J, et al. Granular cell tumors of the breast: steroid receptor analysis and localization of carcinoembryonic antigen, myoglobin and S100 protein. Arch Pathol Lab Med 1984;108:897.

68. Gump FE, Sternschein MJ, Wolff M. Fibromatosis of the breast. Surg Gynecol Obstet 1981;153:57.

69. Ali M, Fayemi AO, Braun EV, et al. Fibromatosis of the breast. Am J Surg Pathol 1979;3:501.

70. Rosen Y, Sozos CP, Gardner B. Fibromatosis of the breast. Cancer 1978;41:1409.

71. Hanna WM, Jambrosic J, Fish E. Aggressive fibromatosis of the breast. Arch Pathol Lab Med 1985;109:260.

72. Wargotz ES, Norris HJ, Austin RM, et al. Fibromatosis of the breast: a clinical and pathological study of 28 cases. Am J Surg Pathol 1987;11:38.

73. Rosen PP, Ernsberger D. Mammary fibromatosis: a benign spindle-cell tumor with significant risk for local recurrence. Cancer 1989;63:1363.

74. Zayid I, Dehmis C. Familial multicentric fibromatosis-desmoids. Cancer 1969;24:786.

75. Rosen PP, Ridolfi RL. The perilobular hemangioma: a benign microscopic vascular lesion of the breast. Am J Clin Pathol 1977;68:21.

76. Jozefczyk MA, Rosen PP. Vascular tumors of the breast. II. Perilobular hemangiomas and hemangiomas. Am J Surg Pathol 1985;9:491.

77. Rosen PP. Vascular tumors of the breast. III. Angiomatosis. Am J Surg Pathol 1985;9:652.

78. Rosen PP. Vascular tumors of the breast. IV. The venous hemangioma. Am J Surg Pathol 1985;9:659.

79. Rosen PP. Vascular tumors of the breast. V. Nonparenchymal hemangiomas of mammary subcutaneous tissues. Am J Surg Pathol 1985;9:723.

80. Donnell RM, Rosen PP, Lieberman PH, et al. Angiosarcoma and other vascular tumors of the breast: pathologic analysis as a guide to prognosis. Am J Surg Pathol 1981;5:629.

81. Vuitch MF, Rosen PP, Erlandson RA. Pseudoangiomatous hyperplasia of mammary stroma. Hum Pathol 1986;17:185.

82. Ibrahim RE, Sciotto CG, Weidner N. Pseudoangiomatous hyperplasia of mammary stroma: some observations regarding its clinicopathologic spectrum. Cancer 1989;63:1154.

83. Kaplan L, Walts A. Benign chondrolipomatous tumor of the human female breast. Arch Pathol Lab Med 1977;101:149.

84. Marsh WL, Lucas JG, Olsen J. Chondrolipomas of the breast. Arch Pathol Lab Med 1989;113:369.

85. Metcalf JS, Ellis B. Choristoma of the breast. Hum Pathol 1985;16:739.

86. Cohen MB, Fisher PE. Schwann cell tumors of the breast and mammary region. Surg Pathol 1991;4:47.

87. Rosen PP. Adenomyoepithelioma of the breast. Hum Pathol 1987;18:1232.

88. Young RH, Clement PB. Adenomyoepithelioma of the breast: a report of three cases and review of the literature. Am J Clin Pathol 1988;89:308.

89. Tavassoli FA. Myoepithelial lesions of the breast: myoepitheliosis, adenomyoepithelioma, and myoepithelial carcinoma. Am J Surg Pathol 1991;15:554.

90. Erlandson RA, Rosen PP. Infiltrating myoepithelioma of the breast. Am J Surg Pathol 1982;6:795.

91. Azzopardi JG, Salm P. Ductal adenoma of the breast: a lesion which can mimic carcinoma. J Pathol 1984;144:15.

92. Lammie GA, Millis RR. Ductal adenoma of the breast: a review of 15 cases. Hum Pathol 1989;20:903.

93. Rosen PP. Mucocele-like tumors of the breast. Am J Surg Pathol 1986;10:464.

94. Ro J, Sneige N, Sahin AA, et al. Mucocele-like tumor of the breast associated with a typical ductal hyperplasia or mucinous carcinoma: a clinicopathologic study of seven cases. Arch Pathol Lab Med 1991;115:137.

95. Clement PB, Young RH, Azzopardi JG. Collagenous spherulosis of the breast. Am J Surg Pathol 1987;11:411.

96. Dixon JM, Anderson TJ, Lumsden AB, et al. Mammary duct ectasia. Br J Surg 1983;70:601.

97. Symmers W. The breasts. In: Symmers W. Systematic pathology. Edinburgh, Churchill Livingstone, 1978.

98. Sanchez-Guerrero J, Schur PH, Sergent JS, et al. Silicone breast implants and rheumatic disease: clinical, immunologic, and epidemiologic studies. Arthritis Rheum 1994;37:158.

99. Bridges AJ, Vasey FB. Silicone breast implants: history, safety and potential complications. Arch Intern Med 1993;153:2638.

100. Chase DR, Oberg KC, Chase RL, et al. Pseudoepithelialization of breast implant capsules. Int J Surg Pathol 1994;1:151.

101. Raso DS, Crymes LW, Metcalf JS. Histological assessment of fifty breast capsules from smooth and textured augmentation and reconstruction mammoplasty prostheses with emphasis on the role of synovial metaplasia. Mod Pathol 1994;7:310.

102. del Rosario AD, Bui HY, Singh J, et al. The synovial metaplasia of breast implant capsules: a light and electron microscopic study (Abstract) Lab Invest 1994;70:14A.

103. Hameed M, Erlandson R, Rosen P. Capsular synovial hyperplasia around mammary implants similar to detritic synovitis: a morphologic and immunohistochemical study of 15 cases. Am J Surg Pathol 1995;19:433.

104. Emery JA, Hardt NS, Caffee H, et al. Breast implant capsules share synovial transporting capabilities. (Abstract) Lab Invest 1994;70:15A.

105. Fajardo LJ. Pathology of radiation injury. New York, Masson Publishing, 1982.

106. Clarke D, Curtin JL, Martinez A, et al. Fat necrosis of the breast simulating recurrent carcinoma after primary radiotherapy in the management of early stage breast carcinoma. Cancer 1983;52:442.

107. Schnitt SJ, Connolly JL, Harris JR, et al. Radiation-induced changes in the breast. Hum Pathol 1984;15:545.

108. Kennedy SM, Merino MJ, Swain S, Lippman ME. The effects of hormonal and chemotherapy on tumoral and nonneoplastic breast tissue. Hum Pathol 1990;21:192.

109. Gansler TS, Wheeler JE. Mammary sarcoidosis: two cases and literature review. Arch Pathol Lab Med 1984;108:673.

110. Ross MJ, Merino MJ. Sarcoidosis of the breast. Hum Pathol 1985;16:185.

111. Fitzgibbons PL, Smiley DF, Kern WH. Sarcoidosis presenting initially as breast mass: report of two cases. Hum Pathol 1985;16:851.

112. Kessler E, Wolloch Y. Granulomatous mastitis: a lesion clinically simulating carcinoma. Am J Clin Pathol 1972;58:642.

113. Dettertogh DA, Rossof AH, Harris AA, et al. Prednisone management of granulomatous mastitis. N Engl J Med 1980;303:799.

114. Fletcher A, Magrath IM, Riddell RH, et al. Granulomatous mastitis: a report of seven cases. J Clin Pathol 1982;35:941.

115. Kessler EI, Katzav JA. Lobular granulomatous mastitis. Surg Pathol 1990;3:115.

116. Tomaszewski JE, Brooks JSJ, Hicks D, et al. Diabetic mastopathy: a distinctive clinicopathologic entity. Hum Pathol 1992;23:780.

117. Seidman JD, Schnapper LA, Phillips LE. Mastopathy in insulin-requiring diabetes mellitus. Hum Pathol 1994;25:819.

3.2

Papillary Lesions

MICHELE A. GADD

Isolated papillary lesions of the breast are relatively rare, accounting for less than 10% of all benign lesions removed at breast biopsy.[1-4] As a group, benign papillary lesions include a variety of subtypes based on a combination of clinical and pathologic characteristics. These include solitary and multiple papillomas, papillomatosis, papillomatosis of the nipple, and juvenile papillomatosis. Although each of these lesions can present as an isolated form of benign breast disease, papillary lesions tend to occur in settings in which additional manifestations of benign breast pathology are present.

Most of what is known about papillary lesions is based on series reviewed before 1980. No direct link between breast carcinoma and benign papillary lesions has been made, but certain subtypes are associated with an increased risk of concurrent or subsequent breast carcinoma. Because many of these early series failed to critically separate the various forms of papillary disease, the rates of recurrence and risk of subsequent carcinoma after treatment for some subtypes may be inflated. Benign papillary lesions of the breast are similar histologically, they all grow slowly, and the recommended treatment is uniformly complete local excision. The unique features of these lesions are derived from their location within the breast and the extent of parenchymal involvement.

Solitary Intraductal Papillomas

The most frequently encountered benign papillary lesion is a solitary intraductal papilloma arising from a single major collecting duct located in the subareolar region of the breast.[5] Solitary intraductal papillomas tend to present in perimenopausal women between 35 and 55 years of age. No associations between family history or other previously identified risk factors for breast carcinoma have been identified.

Most lesions are less than 0.5 cm in diameter and rarely are palpable, but intraductal papillomas ranging from 3 to 10 cm in diameter have been reported.[5,6] The location of an intermittent mass often correlates with the area of nipple discharge identified by compression at physical examination, referred to as the *trigger point*.[1] The incidence of unilateral nipple discharge, either bloody or serous, ranges from 50% to 90% and is more likely to be present in centrally located lesions.[7-10] In a review of 91 patients with spontaneous nipple discharge alone, 56 (61%) were found to have intraductal papillomas and 5 (6%) had carcinomas. In 69 patients with discharge and masses, the incidences of papilloma and carcinoma were similar.[11] The presence of nipple discharge alone should therefore indi-

cate the possibility of an underlying solitary intraductal papilloma.

Asymptomatic intraductal papillomas can be detected mammographically by the presence of a mass or calcifications.[1] The similarities between the clinical presentations of benign papillary lesions and of papillary carcinomas make differentiating the two a challenge. Cytomorphologic studies have failed to accurately distinguish benign papillary breast lesions from malignant lesions based on the extent of cellularity and the presence of single cells.[12,13] Therefore, surgical biopsy is necessary in all cases to determine whether malignancy is present.

Local recurrence rates vary from 3% to 12%, which undoubtedly reflects the adequacy of initial excision.[4,14] The recommended treatment for solitary intraductal papillomas is local excision of the dilated duct.[3,15] A ductogram can be useful in localizing the affected duct if it is not obvious on clinical examination or mammography. For relatively peripheral papillomas, a probe can be placed for surgical localization to limit the dissection. If the involved duct is not identified by a complete evaluation, total duct excision is recommended.

The natural history of a solitary intraductal papilloma is one of an isolated benign lesion associated with little risk of subsequent carcinoma (Table 3.2-1). Although earlier reports suggested that the incidence of subsequent carcinoma was high enough to warrant mastectomy, a more careful evaluation of these series reveals only a slightly increased risk relative to the general population. There is no clear explanation for the inordinately high incidence of subsequent carcinoma in the series of Buhl-Jorgensen and colleagues.[16] Because many of these lesions were removed by biopsy, a closely associated incidental carcinoma may have been missed.[16] Ciatto and associates[17] reported a relative risk of 3.33 of developing an ipsilateral breast cancer 1 to 8 years after treatment for a papilloma. This report and others support long-term follow-up in patients who have been treated for a solitary intraductal papilloma.

Multiple Peripheral Papillomas

Multiple peripheral papillomas occur much less frequently than solitary papillomas and are characterized by distinctly different clinical and pathologic features[5] (Table 3.2-2). Multiple papillomas tend to occur in groups of peripheral ducts, which together form a palpable mass and are rarely associated with nipple discharge. In nearly 15% of patients, these lesions are bilateral. Typical mammographic findings include round, oval, or slightly lobulated well-circumscribed nodules with or without associated calcifications.[1]

TABLE 3.2-1
*Risk of Development of Carcinoma
After Having Solitary Intraductal Papilloma*

Investigators	Cases (N)	Follow-Up (y)		Subsequent Cancer
		Range	Median	
Shie, 1942[14]	27	3–8	4	0
Estes & Phillips, 1949[7]	34	1–14	5	0
Haagenson et al, 1951[6]	76	4–21	10	0
Lewison & Lyons, 1952[4]	23	1–25	11	0
Snyder & Chaffin, 1954[3]	30	5–16	8	0
Hendrick, 1957[8]	207	5–18		1% CL
Moore et al, 1961[9]	125	1–21		3% IP
Kraus & Neubecker, 1962[10]	19	8–14		0
Buhl-Jorgenson et al, 1968[16]	51	6–16		7% IP, 9% CL
Kodlin et al, 1977[2]	80	1–25	7	5%
Ciatto et al, 1991[17]	225	2–14	7	4% IP

IP, ipsilateral carcinoma; CL, contralateral carcinoma.

Local recurrence rates after resection are as high as 24%.[15] Cardenosa and Eklund[1] reported that 43% of patients with multiple peripheral papillomas had associated atypical ductal hyperplasia, which also has been considered a risk factor for breast carcinoma. Therefore, it is necessary to evaluate the mammogram and biopsy specimen carefully for additional breast abnormalities that may increase the risk of subsequent carcinoma development.

Several authors[5,18,19] have reported that subsequent ipsilateral breast carcinoma develops in 10% to 33% of patients with multiple peripheral papillomas. The anatomic relation between peripheral papillomas and a concurrent carcinoma was studied by Ohuchi and coworkers[20] using a three-dimensional reconstructive approach. They demonstrated that carcinomas with multifocal origins in the terminal ductal lobular units were connected to peripherally located papillomas. Similarly, Murad and associates[21] reported malignant changes in association with multiple papillomas in 29% of patients. These observations and the reported risk of subsequent carcinoma suggest that multiple peripheral papillomas may be precursors of early breast carcinoma.

Despite this long-term risk, current treatment recommendations include complete local excision to reduce the frequency of local recurrence and close lifelong follow-up so that any subsequent carcinoma can be detected in its early stage.

Papillomatosis

Papillomatosis (epitheliosis) is a microscopic papillary proliferation of the ductal epithelial cells that tends to extend into the lumen of smaller ductules and that, unlike the solitary and multiple papillomas, has little to no fibrovascular stalk.[5] This process usually involves ducts scattered irregularly throughout the breast and is less likely to be focally extensive. Consequently, it is rarely associated with a mass and is difficult to detect. If central sclerosis occurs within the ducts, the resulting distortion often makes it difficult to distinguish between papillomatosis and carcinoma.

Papillomatosis appears to be a common component of benign epithelial hyperplasia.[22,23] Compared with other papillary subtypes, papillomatosis is most frequently associ-

TABLE 3.2-2
Characteristic Features of Papillary Lesions of the Breast

Parameter	Solitary Intraductal Papilloma	Multiple Peripheral Papilloma	Juvenile Papillomatosis
Age	41 y	48 y	23 y
Palpable mass	57%	98%	95%+
Size	<0.5 mm	>2 cm	2.5 cm
Location			
Central	92%	26%	
Peripheral	8%	74%	95%+
Bilaterality	4%	14%	4%
Nipple discharge	76%	20%	15%
Recurrence	5%	25%	15%
Subsequent carcinoma	5%	25%	4%

ated with additional elements of fibrocystic disease. In Dupont and Page's 1985 review of benign proliferative breast lesions,[22] women with proliferative lesions but without atypical hyperplasia were reported to be at 1.9 times the risk of developing cancer as women without proliferative lesions, whereas women with atypical hyperplasia were at 5.3 times the risk of cancer as women without proliferative lesions. Similarly, the increased risk of cancer ranged from 2.1 to 3.9 in a review by Bodian and coworkers[23] of patients with proliferative changes and varying degrees of epithelial atypia. The presence of papillomatosis alone does not appear to predispose a patient to the development of subsequent breast carcinoma. The treatment of papillomatosis and subsequent surveillance schedule should therefore be determined by the presence of associated breast abnormalities.

Papillary Lesions of the Nipple

Papillary lesions of the nipple, referred to as *florid papillomatosis*, tend to assume one or more of three distinct morphologic growth patterns, as described by Rosen and Caicco.[24] These patterns include sclerosing papillomatosis, papillomatosis adenosis, and adenosis. A nipple papilloma initially presents as a bulge just beneath the nipple and enlarges slowly over months to years before causing symptoms. Left untreated, many papillomas eventually break through the nipple surface. Patients present with nipple erosions, ulcerations, or masses, and often have serous or bloody discharge.[25,26] Because of this constellation of symptoms, it is often a challenge to differentiate papilloma of the nipple from Paget disease or eczematous dermatitis. An alternative form of nipple papillomatosis is characterized by a lesion within the nipple that is diffusely infiltrating.[5]

Papillary lesions of the nipple are extremely rare. Most patients present between the ages of 40 and 50 years. These lesions are not associated with a positive family history or other risk factors for breast carcinoma. In Rosen and Caicco's 1986 series,[24] 2 of 51 patients were men, both of whom demonstrated a concurrent carcinoma arising within the nipple lesion. In 7 of 49 (12%) women with papillary lesions of the nipple, concurrent carcinomas were discovered. Results of a review by Perzin and Lattes[26] of 65 patients with papillary lesions of the nipple revealed that 13 (20%) had concurrent carcinomas. When patients with concurrent carcinomas are excluded from these reviews, the risk of recurrence after local excision and the risk of subsequent carcinoma are approximately 4%.[24,26] Therefore, complete excision of the papillary lesion is sufficient. The coexistence of a concurrent carcinoma warrants a thorough examination of both breasts at the time of diagnosis.

Juvenile Papillomatosis

Juvenile papillomatosis was originally described by Rosen and colleagues in 1980[27] and again in 1985[28] after the establishment of the Juvenile Papillomatosis Registry. Juvenile papillomatosis generally occurs in women between the ages of 10 and 44 years; the average age is 23 years. Patients usually present with localized upper outer quadrant masses 2 to 3 cm in diameter and no associated discharge (see Table 3.2-2). The lesions are typically small and multicystic. Microscopically, they consist of a constellation of changes characteristic of fibrocystic disease, including apocrine metaplasia, duct stasis, sclerosing adenosis, and varying degrees of epithelial atypia.

Based on a review of the patients and families in the Juvenile Papillomatosis Registry, the incidence appears to be increased in women with positive family histories. In Rosen and colleague's review of 180 patients, 12 (7%) had first-degree relatives with breast cancer, and 38 of 80 (48%) had one or more second-degree relatives with breast cancer. A subsequent report by Bazzocchi and associates[29] of 13 patients with juvenile papillomatosis revealed positive family histories in 4 (33%) patients.

Among the patients in the Papillomatosis Registry, recurrent juvenile papillomatosis was identified in 25 (14%) patients. Seven (4%) patients presented with concurrent carcinomas, and only 2 had carcinoma 8 to 9 years after treatment. In the series of Bazzocchi and coworkers, a coexisting carcinoma was present in 15% of patients. Although the numbers are small, there was a correlation between the development of carcinoma, positive family history, and increased age (27 years) at diagnosis. The overall long-term risks of carcinoma remain uncertain as a result of the still-inadequate length of follow-up in these Registry patients. The recommended treatment is conservative surgery with lifelong follow-up. It is imperative that complete excision of the lesion be performed to prevent recurrence.

Summary

Papillary lesions of the breast occur alone or in conjunction with additional manifestations of benign breast disease. Therefore, both breasts should be carefully evaluated to rule out the presence of concurrent lesions. The treatment for an isolated papillary lesion is complete local excision. However, when deciding on a treatment plan, the coexisting pathology should be taken into consideration. After treatment, a surveillance schedule should be discussed, taking into consideration the differences in the malignant potential of these lesions.

References

1. Cardenosa G, Eklund G. Benign papillary neoplasms of the breast: mammographic findings. Radiology 1991;181:751.
2. Kodlin D, Winger E, Morgenstein N, et al. Chronic mastopathy and breast cancer: a follow-up study. Cancer 1977;39:2603.
3. Snyder W, Chaffin L. Main duct papilloma of the breast. Arch Surg 1954;70:680.

4. Lewison E, Lyons J. Relationship between benign disease and cancer. Arch Surg 1952;66:949.
5. Haagensen C. Diseases of the breast, ed 3. Philadelphia, WB Saunders, 1986.
6. Haagensen C, Stout A, Phillips J. The papillary neoplasms of the breast. I. Benign intraductal papilloma. Ann Surg 1951;133:18.
7. Estes A, Phillips C. Papilloma of lacteal duct. Surg Gynecol Obstet 1949;89:345.
8. Hendrick J. Intraductal papilloma of the breast. Surg Gynecol Obstet 1957;105:215.
9. Moore S, Pearce J, Ring E. Intraductal papilloma of the breast. Surg Gynecol Oncol 1961;112:153.
10. Kraus F, Neubecker R. The differential diagnosis of papillary tumors of the breast. Cancer 1962;15:444.
11. Gulay H, Bora S, Kilicturgay S, et al. Management of nipple discharge. J Am Coll Surg 1994;178:471.
12. Jeffrey P, Ljung B-M. Benign and malignant papillary lesions of the breast. Am J Clin Pathol 1994;101:500.
13. Dawson A, Mulford D. Benign versus malignant papillary neoplasms of the breast. Acta Cytol 1994;38:23.
14. Shie E. On the prognosis of the papilloma of the lactiferous ducts. Acta Chir Scand 1942;87:417.
15. Haagensen C, Bodian C, Haagensen D. Breast carcinoma: risk and detection. Philadelphia, WB Saunders, 1981.
16. Buhl-Jorgensen S, Fischermann K, Johanson H, et al. Cancer risk in intraductal papilloma and papillomatosis. Surg Gynecol Obstet 1968;127:1307.
17. Ciatto S, Andreoli C, Cirillo A, et al. The risk of breast cancer subsequent to histologic diagnosis of benign intraductal papilloma follow-up study of 339 cases. Tumori 1991;77:41.
18. Carter D. Intraductal papillary tumors of the breast. Cancer 1977;39:1689.
19. Kilgore A, Fleming R, Ramos M. The incidence of cancer with nipple discharge and the risk of cancer in the presence of papillary disease of the breast. Surg Gynecol Obstet 1953;96:649.
20. Ohuchi N, Abe R, Kasai M. Possible cancerous change of intraductal papillomas of the breast: a 3-D reconstruction study of 25 cases. Cancer 1984;54:605.
21. Murad T, Contesso G, Mouriesse H. Papillary tumors of the large lactiferous ducts. Cancer 1981;48:122.
22. Dupont W, Page D. Risk factors for breast cancer in women with proliferative breast disease. N Engl J Med 1985;312:146.
23. Bodian C, Perzin K, Lattes R, et al. Prognostic significance of benign proliferative breast disease. Cancer 1993;71:3896.
24. Rosen P, Caicco J. Florid papillomatosis of the nipple: a study of 51 patients, including nine with mammary carcinoma. Am J Surg Pathol 1986;10:87.
25. Brownstein M, Phelps R, Magnin P. Papillary adenoma of the nipple: analysis of fifteen new cases. J Am Acad Dermatol 1985;12:707.
26. Perzin K, Lattes R. Papillary adenoma of the nipple (florid papillomatosis, adenoma, adenomatosis). Cancer 1972;29:996.
27. Rosen P, Cantrell B, Mullen D, et al. Juvenile papillomatosis (Swiss cheese disease) of the breast. Am J Surg Pathol 1980;4:3.
28. Rosen P, Holmes G, Lesser M, et al. Juvenile papillomatosis and breast cancer. Cancer 1985;55:1345.
29. Bazzocchi F, Santini D, Martinelli G, et al. Juvenile papillomatosis (epitheliosis) of the breast: a clinical and pathologic study of 13 cases. Am J Clin Pathol 1986;86:745.

3.3

Fibroadenoma and Hamartoma

MARY JANE HOULIHAN

Fibroadenoma

A fibroadenoma may present on a mammogram as either a palpable mass or as a nodular density. The palpable mass is classically well defined, rubbery in texture, and mobile. Mammographically, a fibroadenoma usually appears as a well-circumscribed nodule that may or may not contain coarse calcifications.

Fibroadenomas present most frequently in patients between the ages of 20 to 50 years. A history of premenstrual breast pain and a family history of breast cancer are associated with an increased tendency toward the development of a fibroadenoma; oral contraceptives containing 50 μg of ethinyl estradiol seem to be protective.[1] Fibroadenomas rarely present in the male breast.[2] These lesions usually present as a solitary mass but may present as multiple lesions in 10% to 15% of cases.[3,4] No race-associated differences in frequency or age at presentation have been identified.[4,5] The exact prevalence of fibroadenoma is unknown; however, a 1951 autopsy series of 225 women showed that 8% of women under 40 years of age and 10% of women over 40 years of age had nonpalpable fibroadenomas.[6]

ETIOLOGY

Once thought to be benign noeplasms, fibroadenomas are now believed to represent a hyperplastic process that involves a single terminal ductal–lobular unit and its surrounding connective tissue.[7,8] As the lesion enlarges, adjacent ductal–lobular units are incorporated by the exuberant overgrowth of the connective tissue. Immunohistochemical and electron microscopic studies indicate that the cell of origin may be a fibroblast.[9] Surrounding tissues are not invaded but compressed. Fibroadenomas are considered to be an aberration of normal development.[10] The epithelial elements of a fibroadenoma are similar in appearance to the normal cells in other terminal ductal–lobular units as shown by light and electron microscopy,[11] whereas the connective tissue elements differ in appearance compared with other stroma. Cytogenetic studies of fibroadenoma cells have shown no abnormalities of the epithelial units but have shown occasional abnormal chromosomes in some of the stromal cells.[12] Clonal analysis of fibroadenomas has shown both their epithelial and stromal cell components to be polyclonal, suggesting a hyperplastic rather than a neoplastic process.[13] Although most consider fibroadenomas to represent a hyperplastic process, Koerner and O'Connell[14] have postulated that fibroadenomas are in fact neoplastic nodules for a number of reasons: (1) the lesions represent a focal proliferative process; (2) chromosomal abnormalities are observed in some of the cells that compose a fibroadenoma; and (3) human adenovirus 9, when injected into rats, causes a breast lesion similar both morphologically and functionally to a fibroadenoma.

The exact cause of fibroadenomas is unknown but is believed to be due to a hormonal imbalance. Martin and colleagues[15] and Sitruk-Ware and associates[16] have noted lower circulating levels of progesterone in women with fibroadenomas compared with controls; estrogen levels, however, remained unchanged.

HORMONAL INFLUENCE

Fibroadenomas have estrogen and progesterone receptors, the levels of which vary during the menstrual cycle.[17] The estrogen receptor is located on the epithelial cells.[18] Estrogen receptor protein levels are greater in patients with greater epithelial cell proliferation, and lower estrogen receptor values are associated with greater stromal proliferation.[15]

Because fibroadenomas contain the same elements as normal breast tissue, their response to hormonal changes is similar. These lesions tend to enlarge during pregnancy, to lactate, and to become smaller after weaning.[19] Fibroadenomas also involute like normal fibroglandular breast tissue after menopause. In postmenopausal patients receiving hormone replacement therapy with estrogen alone, fibroadenomas may increase in size relative to the surrounding breast parenchyma.[20,21] On the other hand, neither fibroadenoma frequency[22] nor rate of growth[23] is affected by oral contraceptives.

CANCER WITHIN A FIBROADENOMA

In more than 160 cases, fibroadenomas have been associated with carcinomas, including lobular carcinoma in situ (lobular neoplasia), infiltrating lobular and ductal carcinomas, and intraductal carcinomas.[24,25,26] The carcinoma is usually discovered as an incidental finding when a fibroadenoma is removed from a woman in her early to midforties, although these lesions have been reported in women ranging in age from the late teens into the seventies. No clinical or mammographic features are diagnostic of carcinoma within a fibroadenoma. In more than half of cases, the lesion identified has been lobular carcinoma in situ (lobular neoplasia). Intraductal carcinoma was identified in 20% of cases, infiltrating ductal carcinoma in another 20%, and infiltrating lobular carcinoma in 10%. Management of these lesions should be similar to that of carcinoma in other parts of the breast, that is, the tumor size and histopathologic characteristics should determine subsequent local therapy and the need for adjuvant therapy. Because lobular carcinoma in situ is a marker for increased risk, not a cancer or precancerous lesion, no further local treatment is indicated. Women with this lesion should, however, be carefully monitored.

FIBROADENOMA AND THE SUBSEQUENT RISK OF BREAST CANCER

Whether the fibroadenoma is a marker for significant increased subsequent risk for breast cancer remains uncertain. Historically, it had been widely accepted that fibroadenomas did not confer an increased subsequent cancer risk. In two early studies, only 1 patient in 317 subsequently developed cancer.[27,28]

Since 1980, four population-based, retrospective cohort studies have shown a small but definite increased risk for breast cancer development (relative risk, 1.3 to 1.9).[29,30,31,32] Unlike other benign breast lesions, such as atypical hyperplasia in which the breast cancer risk decreases over time, the risk associated with fibroadenomas appears to be persistent. This odds ratio (less than 2) is of scientific interest but should have little impact on clinical management.

Of interest is a recent report by DuPont and coworkers,[33] which described certain histologic and cytologic patterns of fibroadenomas associated with increased breast cancer risk. In a case-control study, patients with complex fibroadenomas—defined as fibroadenomas with cysts greater than 3 mm in diameter, sclerosing adenosis, epithelial calcifications, or papillary changes—had an increased relative risk of 3.1. Proliferative disease in the surrounding tissue was more common adjacent to complex compared with noncomplex fibroadenoma ($P = .002$). Patients with proliferative disease adjacent to a fibroadenoma and with family histories of breast cancer had a risk of 3.87. These observations are the first to show that various histologic subtypes of fibroadenomas may be important indicators of subsequent breast cancer risk. Because fibroadenomas consist of the same elements in the breast and are under the same environmental influences as the breast, it is not surprising that lesions that confer increased risk in the breast tissue also confer increased risk within a fibroadenoma. It is surprising, however, that some lesions of little or no consequence in the breast parenchyma seem to incur greater risk when found within a fibroadenoma and that this risk persists without decreasing over time. No major changes should be undertaken in the clinical treatment of women with histories of fibroadenoma until the observations of DuPont and associates are reproduced in other study populations. Until then, pathologists should begin to better define the histology of fibroadenomas and of the surrounding parenchyma.

MANAGEMENT

Fibroadenomas usually appear as solitary 1- to 2-cm lesions detected by the woman herself. The more characteristic the presentation, the more likely that the tissue diagnosis will be a fibroadenoma. In other words, a 1- to 2-cm, solitary, firm, rubbery, nontender, well-circumscribed mass discovered in a woman under 30 years of age is probably a fibroadenoma. The fewer of these features present, the greater the likelihood that a lesion is something other than a fibroadenoma. For example, lesions larger than 5 cm may be either benign or malignant phylloides tumors or a fibroadenoma variant, such as giant fibroadenoma or juvenile fibroadenoma.

The natural history of fibroadenomas varies. Because these lesions are thought to be an aberration of natural development, they may grow, regress, or remain unchanged as the hormonal environment changes. Haagensen[3] observed that most fibroadenomas stop growing when they reach 2 to 3 cm in diameter.

Because fibroadenomas are benign lesions, one may argue that their removal is not indicated. A diagnosis based on clinical examination alone, however, is not absolute, given that the clinical diagnosis of a fibroadenoma at biopsy is inaccurate 27% to 50% of the time.[34,35] The safest clinical course is to obtain a tissue diagnosis of all solid dominant masses. Excisional biopsy remains the procedure of choice and may be done as an outpatient procedure while the patient is under local anesthesia. The excisional biopsy should be done through an incision directly overlying the mass and following one of the natural skin lines, the Langer line. The dissection should proceed directly to the mass through the subcutaneous tissue and normal fibroglandular breast tissue. Either a clamp or a traction suture may be placed through the mass. The mass should be excised without removal of more than a few millimeters of surrounding normal breast parenchyma. The subcutaneous tissue should then be reapproximated and the skin closed with either an absorbable or nonabsorbable subcuticular stitch. Alternative tissue sampling methods may be considered in women under 25 years of age or in patients with multiple fibroadenomas. When using alternative techniques such as aspiration cytology or core needle biopsy, their limitations should be recognized. Aspiration cytology is useful for differentiating fibroadenomas from carcinomas[36] and phylloides tumors,[37] but differentiating fibroadenomas from other benign lesions is more difficult.[4] Because fibroadenomas and normal breast tissue consist of the same cellular components, adequate sampling of the mass in question is important when performing an aspiration cytology. Core needle biopsy, particularly of nonpalpable lesions, is an increasingly accepted biopsy option.[38] Adequate tissue sampling should be achieved to obtain a diagnosis with core biopsies. Unlike palpable, solid lesions for which a tissue diagnosis is warranted, nonpalpable, benign-appearing lesions may be followed using periodic mammographic surveillance without obtaining a tissue diagnosis.[39]

MULTIPLE FIBROADENOMAS

In 10% to 15% of patients, multiple fibroadenomas are present either at the time of initial presentation or over an extended period. Rather than performing excisional biopsies of all masses (which leaves a woman with multiple breast scars) clinicians should consider one of two management options. One is to excise one of the masses for tissue diagnosis and follow the remainder of the masses with regular breast examinations and radiologic studies. The second is to perform core-needle biopsies of all palpable masses and to confirm that the nonpalpable masses have ultrasound characteristics consistent with those of fibroadenomas. With either of these options, excisional biopsy is advisable for any mass for which the diagnosis is questioned.

FIBROADENOMA VARIANTS

Fibroadenoma variants include giant fibroadenoma and juvenile fibroadenoma. Giant fibroadenomas are masses larger than 5 cm[4] and are usually found in the breasts of pregnant or lactating women. If possible, excision should be delayed until after pregnancy. As the hormonal milieu changes after birth, these lesions frequently shrink.

Juvenile fibroadenomas occur in adolescent females. These lesions usually occur around the time of puberty and are marked by a rapidly growing mass that causes a distortion of the overlying skin with prominent veins and asymmetry of the breasts (see Fig. 4.1-2). The differential diagnosis includes phylloides tumor, fibrosarcoma of the breast, or virginal hypertrophy.

Juvenile fibroadenomas account for 0.5% to 2% of all fibroadenomas.[4,40] These lesions are benign and do not undergo malignant transformation. Management is excision of the mass, which may be difficult due to its size.[41] General anesthesia or intravenous sedation should be considered in these patients. Various approaches to excision of these lesions, including a lateral or inframammary fold incision, have been advocated in an effort to preserve the central breast bud; however, a direct surgical approach seems to be as reasonable. An incision should be placed directly over the mass along one of the natural skin lines. The mass should be excised, sparing the normal surrounding breast tissue.[42] Further breast development is usually normal and symmetric.[43]

Hamartomas

Hamartomas, also known as fibroadenolipomas, are uncommon breast lesions. Only 16 were identified in 10,000 mammograms during a 9-year period.[44] Hamartomas are well-circumscribed, mobile masses. Mammographically, these lesions consist of fibroglandular tissue admixed with fat and surrounded by a capsule of connective tissue.[45] The halo of connective tissue surrounding the lesions differentiates these masses from fibroadenomas. The classic mammographic appearance of hamartomas, however, may be less common than previously reported. Twelve of 17 mammograms of patients with biopsy-proven hamartomas did not have the classic appearance.[46] Because these lesions can be diagnosed mammographically, biopsy of a classic hamartoma is not indicated. If the mass in question lacks the classic features of a hamartoma, however, it should be removed by enucleation.

References

1. Sitruk-Ware R, Thalabard JC, Benotmane A, et al. Risk factors for breast fibroadenoma in young women. Contraception 1989;40:251.

2. Ansah-Boateng Y, Tavasoli FA. Fibroadenoma and cystosarcoma phylloides of the male breast. Mod Pathol 1992;5:114.

3. Haagensen CD. Diseases of the breast, ed 3. Philadelphia, WB Saunders, 1986:267.

4. Dent DM, Cant PF. Fibroadenoma. World J Surg 1989;13:706.

5. Bartow SA, Pathak DR, Black WC, et al. Prevalence of benign, atypical and malignant lesions in populations at different risk for breast cancer. Cancer 1987;60:2751.

6. Franz VK, Pickren JW, Melcher AW, et al. Incidence of chronic cystic disease in so-called "normal breasts:" a study based on 225 post-mortem examinations. Cancer 1951;40:762.

7. Demetrakopoulous NJ. Three dimensional reconstruction of a human mammary fibroadenoma. Q Bull Northwest Univ Med School 1958;32:221.

8. Azzopardi J. Problems in breast pathology. Major Prob Pathol 1979;11:39.

9. Reddick RL, Shin TK, Sawhney D, et al. Stromal proliferations of the breast: an ultrastructural and immunohistochemical evaluation of cystosarcoma phylloides, juvenile fibroadenoma. Hum Pathol 1987;18:45.

10. Hughes LE, Mansel RE, Webster DJT. Aberrations of normal development and involution (ANDI): a new perspective on pathogenesis and nomenclature of benign breast disorders. Lancet 1987;2:1316.

11. Archer F, Omar M. The fine structure of fibro-adenoma of the human breast. J Pathol 1969;99:113.

12. Fletcher JA, Pinkus GS, Weidner N, et al. Lineage restricted clonality in biphasic solid tumors. Am J Pathol 1991;138:1199.

13. Noguchi S, Motomura K, Inaji H, et al. Clonal analysis of fibroadenoma and phylloides tumor of the breast. Cancer Res 1993;53:4071.

14. Koerner FC, O'Connell JX. Fibroadenoma: morphological observations and theory of pathogenesis. Pathol Annu 1994;29 Pt 1:1.

15. Martin PM, Kutten F, Serment H, et al. Progesterone receptors in breast fibroadenomas. J Steroid Biochem 1979;11:1295.

16. Sitruk-Ware R, Sterkers N, Mauvais-Jarvis P. Benign breast disease. I. Hormonal investigation. Obstet Gynecol 1979;53:457.

17. Kutten F, Fournier S, Durand JC, et al. Estradiol and progesterone receptors in human breast fibroadenomas. J Clin Endocrinol Metab 1981;52:1225.

18. Balakrishnan A, Yang J, Beattie CW, et al. Estrogen receptor in dissociated and cultured human breast fibroadenoma epithelial cells. Cancer Lett 1987;34:233.

19. Moran, CS. Fibroadenoma of the breast during pregnancy and lactation. Arch Surg 1935;31:688.

20. Cyrlak D, Wong CH. Mammographic changes in post-menopausal women undergoing hormonal replacement therapy. Am J Roentgenol 1993;161:1177.

21. Meyer JE, Freena TN, Polger M, et al. Enlarging occult fibroadenomas. Radiology 1992;183:639.

22. Fechner RE. Fibroadenomas in patients receiving oral contraceptives: a clinical and pathologic study. Am J Clin Pathol 1970;53:857.

23. Wilkenson S, Anderson TJ, Rifkind E, et al. Fibroadenoma of the breast: a follow-up of conservative management. Br J Surg 1989;76:390.

24. Fukuda M, Nagao K, Nishimura R, et al. Carcinoma arising in a fibroadenoma of the breast: a case report and review of the literature. Jpn J Surg 1989;19:593.

25. Pick PW, Iossifides IA. Occurrence of breast carcinoma within a fibroadenoma: a review. Arch Pathol Lab Med 1984;108:590.

26. Oyyello L, Gump FE. The management of patients with carcinomas in fibroadenomatous tumors of the breast. Surg Gynecol Obstet 1985;160:99.

27. Oliver RL, Major RC. Cyclomastopathy: a physio-pathological conception of some benign breast tumors, with an analysis of four hundred cases. Am J Cancer 1934;21:1.

28. Semb C. Pathologico-anatomical and clinical investigations of fibroadenomatosis cystica mammae and its relation to other pathological conditions in the mamma, especially cancer. Acta Chir Scand 1928;(Suppl 10)64:1.

29. DuPont WD, Page DL. Risk factors for breast cancer in women with proliferative breast disease. N Engl J Med 1985;312:146.

30. London SJ, Connolly JL, Schnitt SJ, et al. A prospective study of benign breast disease and the risk of breast cancer. JAMA 1992;267:941.

31. DuPont WE, Parl FF, Hartman WH, et al. Breast cancer associated with proliferative breast disease and atypical hyperplasia. Cancer 1993;71:125.

32. McDivitt RW, Stevens JA, Lee NC, et al. Histologic types of benign breast disease and the risk for breast cancer: the Cancer and Steroid Hormone Study Group. Cancer 1992;69:1408.

33. DuPont WD, Page DL, Parl FF, et al. Long-term risk of breast cancer in women with fibroadenoma. N Engl J Med 1994;331:10.

34. Cant PJ, Madden MV, Close PM, et al. Case for conservative management of selected fibro-adenomas of the breast. Br J Surg 1987;74:857.

35. Wilkinson S, Anderson TJ, Rifkind E, et al. Fibroadenoma of the breast: a follow-up of conservative management. Br J Surg 1989;76:390.

36. Bottles K, Chan JS, Holly EA, et al. Cytologic criteria for fibroadenoma: a step-wise logistic regression analysis. Am J Clin Pathol 1988;89:707.

37. Simi U, Moretti D, Iaconni P, et al. Fine needle aspiration cytopathology of phylloides tumor: differential diagnosis with fibroadenoma. Acta Cytol 1988;32:63.

38. Parker SH, Tovin JD, Jobe WE, et al. Non-palpable lesions: stereotactic automated large core biopsies. Radiology 1991;180:403.

39. Sickles EA. Non-palpable, circumscribed, non–calcified solid breast masses: likelihood of malignancy based on lesion size and age of patient. Radiology 1994;192:439.

40. Mies C, Rosen PP. Juvenile fibroadenoma with atypical epithelium. Am J Surg Pathol 1987;11:184.

41. Davis C Jr, Patel V. Surgical problems in the management of giant fibroadenoma of the breast. Am J Obstet Gynecol 1985;152:1010.

42. Rouanet P, Givron O, Rouanet G, et al. Giant fibroadenoma of the breast: reconstruction of the breast after resection using the dermal vault technique. Ann Chir Plastic Esthetics 1991;36:200.

43. Block GE, Zlatnick PA. Giant fibroadenoma of the breast. Arch Surg 1960;80:665.

44. Hessler C, Schnyder P, Ozzello L. Hamartoma of the breast: diagnostic observation of 16 cases. Radiology 1978;126:95.

45. Kopans DB. Breast imaging. Philadelphia, JB Lippincott, 1989:260.

46. Helvie MA, Adler DD, Rebner M, et al. Breast hamartomas: variable mammographic appearance. Radiology 1989;170:417.

3.4

Duct Ectasia, Periductal Mastitis, and Infections

KENNETH K. TANABE

Mammary Duct Ectasia and Periductal Mastitis

Mammary duct ectasia and periductal mastitis represent an entity known by several other names, including mastitis obliterans,[1] varicocele tumor,[2] plasma cell mastitis,[3] comedomastitis,[4] periductal mastitis,[5] and secretory disease of the breast.[6] The variety of names given to this pathologic entity reflects several of its histopathologic characteristics. The predominant cell in the periductal inflammation is the plasma cell.[3] *Duct ectasia* is a term that refers to the dilated ducts that are filled with plugs of keratin and stagnant secretions. *Periductal mastitis* refers to the inflammatory process frequently identified around these ducts. Burkett[7] is credited with the first written description of this entity in 1850, labeling it a "morbid condition of the lactiferous ducts."

The reported incidence of mammary duct ectasia ranges from 5.5% to 25%, depending on the defining criteria used and patients studied.[5,8–11] Some degree of duct dilatation normally occurs with aging.[12] The incidence of duct ectasia and periductal mastitis is probably overestimated in some reports through inclusion of patients with histologic changes that are part of the normal processes of aging and ductal involution.[11] The peak incidence of duct ectasia and periductal mastitis in most series occurs in women between 40 and 49 years of age,[11] although it has been observed in women between 30 and 90 years of age and also in men.[13,14]

ETIOLOGY AND PATHOGENESIS

Pregnancy and breastfeeding are no longer considered important in the etiology of duct ectasia and periductal mastitis.[15] It remains to be resolved whether duct dilatation is the initiating event that leads to periductal mastitis or whether periductal mastitis is the initiating event that leads to duct wall damage and subsequent duct dilatation. Haagensen[16] proposed that duct dilatation and distention lead to atrophy of the duct epithelium. He suggested that this process is followed by loss of integrity of the duct wall and extravasation of irritating lipid material, which then causes an inflammatory reaction. This hypothesis accounts for the common coexistence of duct ectasia and periductal mastitis. In this proposed mechanism, duct obstruction leads to duct dilatation. Squamous metaplasia of the ductal epithelium with subsequent plugging of the duct by keratin scales may be a source of duct obstruction.[17–19] Nipple inversion has also been proposed as a source of duct obstruction.[20,21]

An alternate mechanism of development of duct ectasia and periductal mastitis has been forwarded by Dixon and colleagues,[11,15] who reviewed patients with mammary duct ectasia and noted that younger patients with this condition frequently had severe periductal inflammation located adjacent to nondilated ducts. In contrast, older patients with this disease more commonly had duct dilatation as the predominant histologic finding, with minimal adjacent periductal inflammation. These findings suggest that duct ectasia may be the result of periductal mastitis rather than the initiating event. In this model, periductal inflammation and fibrosis are causes of nipple retraction and inversion rather than consequences of it.

Infection by anaerobes and other bacteria may also play a role in the pathogenesis of this disease in some patients. A high percentage of patients with duct ectasia have bacteria in their nipple discharges.[22] Furthermore, broad-spectrum antibiotics appear to be successful in treating the periareolar inflammation associated with this condition;[23] however, excised specimens containing duct ectasia and periductal mastitis are sterile in some patients.[24–26] Therefore, the exact role of bacteria in the early pathogenesis of mammary duct ectasia and periductal mastitis remains unclear. Nonetheless, the presence of these bacteria in some patients appears to have significant ramifications. The wound infection rate after breast biopsies containing duct ectasia and periductal mastitis is 10.2%, compared with 2% after biopsies showing no evidence of this condition.[27] Furthermore, the organisms recovered from these postoperative infections are similar to those isolated from the nipple discharge of patients with duct ectasia or periductal mastitis.[22] These bacteria may also play a role in the subsequent development of nonpuerperal breast abscesses (see below). Another potential mechanism in the pathogenesis of duct ectasia and periductal mastitis may be autoimmunity; a histologic pattern resembling duct ectasia and periductal mastitis is seen in mice experimentally immunized with autologous mammary tissue.[28]

CLINICAL FEATURES

Mammary duct ectasia and periductal mastitis may present as breast pain, a breast mass, nipple discharge, nipple retraction, a nonpuerperal breast abscess, or a mammary fistula.[11,29,31] The pain is commonly subareolar and noncyclical.[15] It may be present alone or together with other symptoms. The nipple discharge varies in color from cream to green, and it may contain occult blood. The discharge can be unilateral or bilateral and frequently emanates from multiple ducts. Mammary duct ectasia and periductal mastitis account for 3% to 12% of benign breast lumps, and the signs and symptoms at presentation reflect the age of the patient.[11,27,30] Nipple retraction and noninflammatory masses occur more commonly in older women, whereas pain and nonpuerperal abscesses occur more commonly in younger women. These data are somewhat speculative because younger patients whose symptoms are limited to breast pain rarely undergo biopsy, and clinicopathologic correlation is therefore rarely obtained. Of women undergoing operation for pathology ultimately shown to be duct ectasia, 45% have nipple discharge, 32% have nipple inversion, 47% have a mass, and 12% have an abscess.[11,27,30]

Mammograms obtained from patients with duct ectasia or periductal mastitis frequently show tubular dilated ducts.[32] Calcifications may be present in the lumen and walls of the dilated ducts. Intense periductal mastitis may mammographically simulate carcinoma. Although patients with mammary duct ectasia and nipple discharge frequently have characteristic findings noted on galactography, carcinoma can coexist with mammary duct ectasia. Therefore, galactography cannot reliably exclude the presence of a carcinoma.

TREATMENT

The treatment of patients with mammary duct ectasia or periductal mastitis varies with clinical presentation. Patients who present with a mass must undergo biopsy to exclude a diagnosis of carcinoma. Patients with persistent, bloody, or cytologically suspicious nipple discharge should undergo duct excision for diagnostic purposes, even if galactographic findings are consistent with duct ectasia. Management of patients with nipple discharge or breast pain is discussed in Chapters 5.2 and 5.1, respectively. Duct ectasia and periductal mastitis can also give rise to nonpuerperal breast abscesses and fistulas, the management of which is described later.

Mammary Fistulas

Mammary fistulas, also known as Zuska disease,[33] squamous metaplasia of the lactiferous ducts,[34] and mammillary fistula,[20] represent a rare complication of duct ectasia and periductal mastitis. Despite their association with duct ectasia and periductal mastitis, their underlying pathology and etiology remain unclear. Zuska and colleagues[33] noted that the fistulas are frequently lined by squamous epithelium and concluded that fistulas represent dilated lactiferous ducts. Lambert and coworkers[35] reported the common association of mammary fistulas with chronic inflammation; however, they were able to identify a communication between the fistula and a lactiferous duct in only 10.5% of cases. The role of bacteria in the pathogenesis of this condition remains unclear; however, staphylococci and anaerobes are commonly isolated from mammary fistulas.[17] Nipple inversion has been postulated to be important in the etiology of mammary fistulas.[19] In contrast, Passaro and colleagues[17] identified nipple inversion in only

6 of 51 patients with mammary fistulas. It is reasonable to assume that mammary fistulas represent one clinical manifestation of underlying duct ectasia and periductal mastitis.

Patients with mammary fistulas frequently present with chronic, intermittent nipple discharge,[17,33,35] which may be associated with a swelling or mass at the border of the areola and skin. The average duration of symptoms has been reported to be over 3 years.[17]

Zuska and colleagues[33] have noted the parallels between management of anal fistulas and mammary fistulas. Simple incision and drainage frequently results in recurrences. Masupialization, wedge excision of a portion of areola, and excision of the abscess have also been suggested as treatment approaches.[26,36] Successful elimination of this disease, however, requires complete excision of the diseased lactiferous ducts including the terminal portion of the involved duct in the nipple. Failure to remove the terminal portion of the diseased duct may lead to disease recurrence.[17] The wound may be packed open and allowed to close by secondary intention, or it may be loosely closed over a drain with absorbable sutures.

Nonpuerperal Breast Abscesses and Fistulas

Nonpuerperal breast abscesses are now far more common than puerperal breast abscesses. In a recent review, only 8.5% of breast abscesses were in the puerperium, and only 3% of these were lactating at the time of presentation.[37] Both men and women can be affected.[38] Subareolar nonpuerperal breast abscesses appear to be a distinct clinical entity and to have a more aggressive natural history than peripheral breast abscesses.[39] Compared with patients with subareolar abscesses, patients with peripheral abscesses more often have conditions such as diabetes, steroid therapy, or other infected skin lesions that predispose them to infections.[38]

ETIOLOGY AND PATHOGENESIS

Patients with duct ectasia or periductal mastitis may be at higher risk for the development of breast abscesses. It remains unclear whether the presence of periductal mastitis or the presence of obstructed, secretion-filled ducts is more important in the development of breast abscesses. Although nipple inversion may provide a portal of entry for pathogenic bacteria, Ekland and Zeigler[38] found nipple inversion in only 9% of patients with their first subareolar abscess and in 19% of patients with a recurrent abscess. Only a minority of patients have nipple inversion that precedes the development of a breast abscess, and other mechanisms of bacterial seeding may be important. Furthermore, nipple inversion may even be a result of mastitis, with its attendant thickening and shortening of ducts due to chronic inflammation.[40]

Organisms cultured from nonpuerperal breast abscesses

differ from those cultured from puerperal abscesses. Staphylococci and α-hemolytic streptococci are the most common aerobic and facultative organisms recovered from nonpuerperal breast abscesses.[37–39,41] A variety of gram-positive and gram-negative anaerobic bacteria are also frequently recovered from nonpuerperal breast abscesses. It has been suggested that routine cultures frequently overlook the involvement of these anaerobic bacteria in this clinical entity.[42]

CLINICAL PRESENTATION

Patients with nonpuerperal breast abscesses most commonly present with localized tenderness, fluctuance, erythema, and induration.[38] Systemic signs of infection, including fever and leukocytosis, may be present. Patients with a breast abscess occurring as a complication of duct ectasia or periductal mastitis may present with a breast mass associated with overlying induration and erythema. These clinical signs resemble those seen in patients with inflammatory breast carcinoma; however, most patients with inflammatory breast carcinoma do not have any associated duct ectasia or periductal mastitis.

TREATMENT

Patients with peripheral nonpuerperal breast abscesses must be distinguished from those with subareolar nonpuerperal abscess, because the latter condition frequently recurs after simple incision and drainage.[37] Subareolar breast abscesses tend to be indolent, chronic, and recurrent in nature. Watt-Boolsen and colleagues[43] reported the recurrence rate for nonpuerperal subareolar abscesses to be 38% after simple incision and drainage. In that series, 10 of 11 recurrences were fistulas that developed within the surgical incision. Other authors have reported similar recurrence rates after incision and drainage.[37,44,45] It is generally believed that the underlying pathology (ie, damaged, obstructed ducts and accumulated debris) remains after incision and drainage, eventually resulting in recurrence of infection and abscess formation.

Several authors have concluded that excision of affected tissue in the treatment of subareolar breast abscesses leads to a lower recurrence rate than does simple incision and drainage. The acute phase of this treatment approach involves incision and drainage of the abscess, together with administration of broad-spectrum antibiotics. A portion of the abscess cavity wall should be excised and examined for the presence of carcinoma.[38,39,42] The wound should be irrigated copiously, and dressings should be changed frequently over the next few days. After resolution of the acute inflammatory process, the major duct system beneath the areola should be excised using a circumareolar incision.[37,38,46] During this procedure, a fine probe is inserted into the cavity to identify any sinus tracts that communicate with the nipple. Any identified sinus tracts are completely excised, as is a wedge of the nipple. The wound may either be left open and allowed to close by secondary intention, or it may be loosely approximated over a small drain if the edges are clean. This approach provides an excellent cosmetic result with a minimal risk for recurrence.

Women who become pregnant after major duct excision are able to lactate only in the breast that did not undergo operation. Although some engorgement of the operated breast may occur, galactoceles are extraordinarily rare.[47,48]

Puerperal Mastitis and Abscess

Cellulitis that develops in the lactating breast is commonly termed puerperal mastitis or lactational mastitis.[49–51] Two patterns of occurrence have been noted: epidemic and sporadic.

Epidemic puerperal mastitis is a hospital-acquired infection seen in nursing mothers. The most commonly isolated pathogen is *Staphylococcus aureus*, which can be recovered from both nipple aspirates and the suckling neonate.[49–51] It is commonly believed that the infant may transmit this pathogen to the mother's breast and vice versa. Heavy seeding of multiple ducts generally occurs, thereby resulting in inflammation of several nonadjacent areas of the breast.[52] Involved segments are typically red, warm, tender, and painful.[53] Because the infant harbors the pathogen, adequate treatment of the mother involves weaning the suckling infant. Failure to break the cycle may result in recurring infections or worsening of the initial episode. Progression of this pathologic process may result in abscess formation, with or without development of a fistula.[54] Administration of antibiotics to treat *S aureus* infection along with manual compression, warmth, and pumping of the affected breast represent the most effective regimen for epidemic puerperal mastitis. This entity has become rare, probably as a result of shortened hospital stays, improved hygiene, and prompt recognition and treatment.

In contrast to epidemic puerperal mastitis, sporadic disease frequently involves a single region of the breast, as defined by the underlying duct anatomy. Leary[55] has reported the incidence of mastitis in the puerperal period to be 1%, a figure far lower than that of Fulton,[56] who reported a 9% incidence in the puerperal period. As with the epidemic form of the disease, *S aureus* appears to be the most commonly isolated pathogen in sporadic puerperal mastitis.[39,52] An irritated or cracked nipple is frequently associated with this infection and may provide a portal of entry for the bacteria.[12] These nipple problems are more prevalent during the early weeks of nursing, as is sporadic puerperal mastitis. Patients typically present within the first few weeks of nursing with a segment of one breast that is red, warm, and tender. The underlying infection typically occurs in the periductal tissue, and purulent material may not be present in the ductal system.[52] Generalized signs of infection such as fevers, chills, and leukocytosis are commonly present.

Thomsen and associates[57] described a method to distinguish women with puerperal mastitis from those with milk stasis or noninfectious inflammation—two other conditions that have similar clinical presentations. Their diagnostic approach relies on a leukocyte count of the breast milk and a quantitative culture of bacteria in the milk. Patients with plugged ducts causing milk stasis have fewer than 10^6 white blood cells (WBCs)/mL of breast milk and fewer than 10^3 bacteria/mL of breast milk. Women with noninfectious breast inflammation have more than 10^6 WBCs/mL but fewer than 10^3 bacteria/mL of breast milk. Women with puerperal mastitis will have more than 10^6 WBCs/mL and over 10^3 bacteria/mL of breast milk. Although Thomsen and colleagues suggested that antibiotics be administered only to patients with elevated WBC and bacterial counts, I believe antibiotics should be empirically administered to any patient with florid mastitis.

Unlike in epidemic puerperal mastitis, the suckling infant is not believed to be the source of bacterial seeding in women with sporadic puerperal mastitis.[39,52] Therefore, although weaning was once thought to be the mainstay of treatment, this approach is no longer recommended. Weaning may lead to breast engorgement and milk stasis, which may actually promote the development of puerperal mastitis. This concept is supported by the observation that many episodes of mastitis follow periods of missed feedings or attempts at weaning.[52] In the experience of Thomsen and coworkers,[57] emptying the breast as part of treatment for puerperal mastitis significantly improved the outcome. Other investigators have also reported that emptying of the breast shortens the duration of symptoms.[52,58] Consequently, women who have sporadic puerperal mastitis are now treated with appropriate antibiotics and encouraged to continue breastfeeding or breast pumping. The infant does not require any specific antibiotic therapy, and no adverse factors affect an infant who continues to breast feed.[39,52] Warmth and manual pressure to the involved areas may also speed resolution of the process.

Patients who do not immediately seek medical attention for treatment of puerperal mastitis or those whose disease progresses despite treatment may develop a breast abscess.[54] Diagnosis of a breast abscess is usually not difficult; sufferers commonly present with worsening local symptoms, fluctuance, and systemic manifestations. Fluctuance, however, may occasionally be difficult to detect, and any patient who does not immediately respond to antibiotic administration and emptying of the breast should undergo breast sonography to detect a deep-seated abscess. Patients in whom abscesses are identified should immediately undergo exploration with incision and adequate abscess drainage. General anesthesia is frequently necessary for this procedure. Care must be taken to break up all loculations within the abscess. Biopsy of the cavity wall should be done to check for the presence of an associated carcinoma.[38,39,42] The wound should be copiously irrigated and closed loosely over a drain.[39] Broad-spectrum antibiotics should be administered because polymicrobial infection is common.[39,52] Unlike subareolar nonpuerperal breast abscesses, these abscesses heal rapidly with appropriate treatment, and recurrence or the subsequent development of fistulas after simple incision and drainage is rare.[39]

Uncommon Breast Infections

Tuberculosis, actinomycosis, blastomycosis, sporotrichosis, syphilis, and candidal intertrigo are very rare causes of breast infections. In contrast to developing countries, developed countries have an extremely low incidence of tuberculous mastitis.[59] The reported incidence in India ranges from 1% to 4.5% of breast problems requiring operation.[59-61] Women, especially those in their reproductive years, appear to be at the highest risk for mammary tuberculosis.[62] McKeown and Wilkinson[63] described five histologically distinct variants of tuberculous mastitis: acute miliary tubercular mastitis, nodular tuberculous mastitis, disseminated tuberculous mastitis, sclerosing tuberculous mastitis, and tuberculous mastitis obliterans. The most common symptom is a painful, solitary mass,[64] which may be fixated to the overlying skin. Axillary lymph nodes may also be palpably enlarged. The diagnosis is difficult to make preoperatively and is most commonly made at the time of specimen analysis. The optimal treatment involves excision of the mass plus administration of antituberculous medications.

Although cervicofacial actinomycosis is the most common presentation for patients infected with *Actinomyces israelii*, primary and secondary infection of the breast may occur.[65] The clinical presentation may mimic inflammatory breast carcinoma, and the diagnosis is usually made postoperatively. Abscess drainage and débridement of devitalized tissue, combined with high-dose tetracycline therapy, is the treatment of choice.[66] Mastectomy is indicated only when all nonviable tissue must be removed.

Blastomycosis[67] and sporotrichosis[68] of the breast are rare and result either from primary infection of the breast or from extension of pulmonary disease through the chest wall. Axillary lymph nodes may be enlarged, and the correct diagnosis is rarely suspected before abscess drainage. Histologic analysis of the abscess wall with special fungal stains, fungal cultures of the abscess contents, and special serological tests confirm the diagnosis. Administration of amphotericin B is the treatment of choice; however, saturated potassium iodide may be sufficient therapy for cutaneous sporotrichosis.

Primary syphilis of the breast is a sexually transmitted disease. Identification of *Treponema pallidum* by dark-field examination of samples from the primary chancre confirms the diagnosis. This chancre usually begins to heal spontaneously within 2 to 6 weeks, and the patient then develops secondary syphilis. Patients with secondary syphilis may present with gummas of the breast.[59] The treatment of primary and secondary syphilis is high-dose penicillin.

Cutaneous candidal intertrigo of the inframammary fold may present with a lesion characterized by weeping, damp scales, and surrounding erythema.[70] The clinical diagnosis can be confirmed by identification of filaments or budding cells in scraped material. Treatment of this condition requires improved aeration of the affected area, decreased maceration, and application of topical antifungal agents such as nystatin.

Finally, suppurative mastitis may occur in neonates and

infants.[71] Nipple discharge should be collected for Gram stain, cell count, and bacterial culture. These studies will allow distinction between this entity and physiologic neonatal mastitis that develops in response to transplacental passage of maternal hormones. Physiologic neonatal mastitis resolves spontaneously soon after birth. Suppurative neonatal mastitis should be treated with incision and drainage combined with appropriate antibiotics. Breast tissue should not be resected because this may result in subsequent agenesis or abnormal breast development.

References

1. Ingier A. Ueber obliterierende Mastitis. Virchows Arch 1909; 198:338.
2. Bloodgood JC. The clinical picture of dilated ducts beneath the nipple frequently to be palpated as a doughy wormlike mass: the varicocoele of the breast. Surg Gynecol Obstet 1923;36:486.
3. Adair FR. Plasma cell mastitis, a lesion simulating mammary carcinoma: a clinical and pathological study with a report of ten cases. Arch Surg 1933;29:735.
4. Tice GI, Dockerty MB, Harrington SW. Comedomastitis: a clinical and pathological study of data in 172 cases. Surg Gynecol Obstet 1948;87:525.
5. Foote FW, Stewart FW. Comparative studies of cancerous versus noncancerous breasts. Ann Surg 1945;121:6.
6. Ingleby H, Gershon-Cohen J. Comparative anatomy, pathology and roentgenology of the breast. Philadelphia, University of Pennsylvania, 1960:472.
7. Birkett J. The diseases of the breast. London, Longman, 1850:64.
8. Frantz VK, Pickren JW, Melcher GW, Auchincloss JH. Incidence of chronic cystic disease in so-called "normal breasts;" a study based on 225 postmortem examinations. Cancer 1951;47:762.
9. Geschickter CF. Diseases of the breast. Philadelphia, JB Lippincott, 1948.
10. Sandison AT, Walker JC. Inflammatory mastitis, mammary duct ectasia and mammillary fistula. Br J Surg 1962;50:57.
11. Dixon JM. Periductal mastitis/duct ectasia. World J Surg 1989;13:715.
12. Haagenson CD. Diseases of the breast, ed 3. Philadelphia, WB Saunders, 1986.
13. Mansel RE, Morgan WP. Duct ectasia in the male. Br J Surg 1979;66:660.
14. Webster DJT. Benign disorders of the male breast. Br J Surg 1989;13:726.
15. Dixon JM, Anderson TJ, Lumsden AB, et al. Mammary duct ectasia. Br J Surg 1983;70:601.
16. Haagensen CD. Mammary-duct ectasia: a disease that may simulate carcinoma. Cancer 1951;4:749.
17. Passaro ME, Broughan TA, Sebek BA, et al. Lactiferous fistula. J Am Coll Surg 1994;178:29.
18. Habif DV, Perzin KH, Lipton R, et al. Subareolar abscess associated with squamous metaplasia of the lactiferous ducts. Am J Surg 1970;119:523.
19. Powell BC, Maull KI, Sachatello C. Recurrent subareolar abscess of the breast and squamous metaplasia of the lactiferous ducts: a clinical syndrome. South Med J 1977;70:935.
20. Atkins JJB. Mammillary fistula. Br Med J 1955;2:1473.
21. Caswell HT, Urnett WE. Chronic recurrent breast abscess secondary to inversion of the nipple. Surg Gynecol Obstet 1956;102:439.
22. Bundred NJ, Dixon JMJ, Lumsden AB, et al. Are the lesions of duct ectasia sterile? Br J Surg 1985;72:844.
23. Dixon JM, Lee ECG, Greenhall MJ. Treatment of periareolar inflammation associated with periductal mastitis using metronidazole and flucloxacillin: a preliminary report. Br J Clin Pract 1988;42:78.
24. Aitken RJ, Hood J, Going JJ, et al. Bacteriology of mammary duct ectasia. Br J Surg 1988;75:1040.
25. Ewing M. Stagnation in the main ducts of the breast. J R Coll Surg Edinb 1963;8:134.
26. Kilgore AR, Fleming R. Recurring lesions in the areolar area. Calif Med 1952;77:190.
27. Dixon JM, Chetty U, Forrest APM. Wound infection after breast biopsy. Br J Surg 1988;75:918.
28. Davies JD. Histological study of mammae in oestrogenized rats after mammary isoimmunization. Br J Exp Pathol 1972;53:406.
29. Walker JC, Sandison AT. Mammary duct ectasia: a clinical study. Br J Surg 1964;51:350.
30. Thomas WG, Williamson RCN, Davies JC, et al. The clinical syndrome of mammary duct ectasia. Br J Surg 1982;69:423.
31. Devitt JE. Benign breast disease in the postmenopausal woman. World J Surg 1989;13:731.
32. Asch T, Frey C. Radiographic appearance of mammary duct ectasia. N Engl J Med 1962;266:86.
33. Zuska JJ, Cirle G, Ayres WW. Fistulas of lactiferous ducts. Am J Surg 1951;81:312.
34. Sebek BA. Periareolar abscess associated with squamous metaplasia of lactiferous ducts (Zuska's disease). Lab Invest 1988;58:83.
35. Lambert ME, Betts CD, Sellwood RA. Mammillary fistula. Br J Surg 1986;73:367.
36. Patey DH, Thackray AC. Pathology and treatment of mammary-duct fistula. Lancet 1958;2:871.
37. Scholefield JJ, Duncan JL, Rogers K. Review of a hospital experience of breast abscesses. Br J Surg 1987;74:469.
38. Ekland DA, Zeigler MG. Abscess in the nonlactating breast. Arch Surg 1973;107:398.
39. Benson EA. Management of breast abscesses. World J Surg 1989;13:753.
40. Rees BI, Gravelle IH, Hughes LE. Nipple retraction in duct ectasia. Br J Surg 1977;64:577.
41. Brook I. Microbiology of non-puerperal breast abscesses. J Infect Dis 1988;157:377.
42. Walker AP, Edmiston CE, Krepel CJ, et al. A prospective study of the microflora of nonpuerperal breast abscess. Arch Surg 1988;107:908.
43. Watt-Boolsen S, Rasmussen NR, Blichert-Toft M. Primary periareolar abscess in the nonlactating breast: risk of recurrence. Am J Surg 1987;153:571.
44. Leach RD, Phillips I, Eykyn SJ, et al. Anaerobic subareolar breast abscess. Lancet 1979;2:35.
45. Bates T, Down RHL, Tant DR, et al. The current treatment of breast abscesses in hospital and in general practice. Practioner 1973;211:541.
46. Maier WP, Berger A, Derrick BM. Periareolar abscess in the nonlactating breast. Am J Surg 1982;144:359.
47. Hadfield GH. Further experience of the operation for the excision of the major system of the breast. Br J Surg 1968;55:530.
48. Urban JA. Non-lactational nipple discharge. Cancer J Clin 1978;28:131.
49. Ravenholt RT, Wright P, Mulhern M. Epidemiology and prevention of nursery-derived staphylococcal disease. N Engl J Med 1957;257:789.
50. Colbeck JC. An extensive outbreak of staphylococcal infections in maternity units: use of bacteriophage typing in investigation and control. Can Med Assoc J 1949;61:557.
51. Sherman AJ. Report of an outbreak at Philadelphia General Hospital. Obstet Gynecol 1956;7:268.
52. Niebyl JR, Spence MR, Parmley TH. Sporadic (nonepidemic) puerperal mastitis. J Reprod Med 1978;20:97.
53. Soltau DHK, Hatcher GW. Some observations on the aetiology of breast abscess in the puerperium. Br Med J 1970;1:1603.

54. Gibbard GF. Sporadic and epidemic puerperal breast infections. Am J Obstet Gynecol 1953;65:1038.

55. Leary JWG. Acute puerperal mastitis: a view. Calif Med 1948;68:147.

56. Fulton AA. Incidence of puerperal and lactational mastitis in an industrial town of some 43,900 inhabitants. Br Med J 1945;1:693.

57. Thomsen AC, Hansen KB, Moller BR. Leukocyte counts and microbiologic cultivation in the diagnosis of puerperal mastitis. Am J Obstet Gynecol 1983;146:938.

58. Marshall BR, Hepper JK, Zirbel CC. Sporadic puerperal mastitis: an infection that need not interrupt lactation. JAMA 1975;233:1377.

59. Goldman KP. Tuberculosis of the breast. Tubercle 1978;59:41.

60. Webster CS. Tuberculosis of the breast. Am J Surg 1939;45:557.

61. Azzopardi JF. Problems in breast pathology. Philadelphia, WB Saunders, 1979:399.

62. Morgan M. Tuberculosis of the breast. Surg Gynecol Obstet 1931;53:593.

63. McKeown KC, Wilkinson KW. Tuberculous disease of the breast. Br J Surg 1952;39:420.

64. Dharkar RS, Kanhere MH, Vaishy ND, et al. Tuberculosis of the breast. J Indian Med Assoc 1968;50:207.

65. Lloyd-Davies JA. Primary actinomycosis of the breast. Br J Surg 1951;38:378.

66. Braude AI. Actinomycosis. In: Braude AI, ed. Medical microbiology and infectious diseases. Philadelphia, WB Saunders, 1981:846.

67. Braude AI. North American blastomycosis. In: Braude AI, ed. Medical microbiology and infectious diseases. Philadelphia, WB Saunders, 1981:989.

68. Braude AI. Sporotrichosis. In: Braude AI, ed. Medical microbiology and infectious diseases. Philadelphia, WB Saunders, 1981:1573.

69. Adair FE. Gumma of the breast: its differential diagnosis from carcinoma. Ann Surg 1924;79:44.

70. Edwards JJE. Moniliasis of the skin. In: Braude AI, ed. Medical microbiology and infectious diseases. Philadelphia, WB Saunders, 1981:1582.

71. Burry VF, Beezley M. Infant mastitis due to gram-negative organisms. Am J Dis Child 1972;124:736.

3.5

Gynecomastia

GLENN D. BRAUNSTEIN

Benign proliferation of the glandular tissue of the male breast constitutes the histologic hallmark of gynecomastia, which, if great enough, appears clinically as palpable or visual enlargement of the breast. This condition is exceedingly common and may be a sign of a serious underlying pathologic condition, may cause physical or emotional discomfort, or may be confused with other breast problems, most significantly carcinoma.

Prevalence

Breast glandular proliferation commonly occurs in infancy, during puberty, and in older age. It has been estimated that between 60% and 90% of infants exhibit the transient development of palpable breast tissue due to estrogenic stimulation from the maternal–placental–fetal unit. This stimulus for breast growth ceases as the estrogens are cleared from the neonatal circulation and the breast tissue gradually regresses over a 2- to 3-week period. Although population studies have shown that the prevalence of pubertal gynecomastia varies widely, most have indicated that 30% to 60% of pubertal boys exhibit gynecomastia, which generally begins between 10 and 12 years of age, with the highest prevalence between 13 and 14 years of age corresponding to Tanner stage III or IV of pubertal development, followed by involution that is generally complete by ages 16 to 17 years.[1-9] The percentage of adult males exhibiting gynecomastia increases with advancing age, with the highest prevalence being found in the 50- to 80-year age range (Fig. 3.5-1). The prevalence of the condition in men ranges between 24% and 65%, the differences between series being accounted for by the defining criteria and by the population studied.[10-16]

Pathogenesis

No inherent differences appear to exist in the hormonal responsiveness of the male or female breast glandular tissue.[9,17] It is the hormonal milieu, the duration and intensity of stimulation, and the individual's breast tissue sensitivity that determine the type and degree of glandular proliferation. Under the influence of estrogens, the ducts elongate and branch, the ductal epithelium becomes hyperplastic, the periductal fibroblasts proliferate, and the vascularity increases. This histologic picture is found early in the course of gynecomastia and is often referred to as the *florid* stage. Acinar development is not seen in males, because it requires the presence of progesterone in concentrations found during the luteal phase of the menstrual cycle.[18] Androgens exert an antiestrogen effect on rodent breast cancer models and the human MCF-7 breast cancer cell line and are thought to antagonize at least some of the effects of estrogens in normal breast tissue.[19] Accordingly, gynecomastia is generally considered to represent an imbalance between the breast stimulatory effects of estrogen and the inhibitory effects of androgens. In fact, alterations in the estrogen/androgen ratio have been found in many of the conditions associated with gynecomastia. Such alterations can occur through a variety of mechanisms (Table 3.5-1).

In men, the testes secrete 95% of the testosterone, 15% of the estradiol, and less than 5% of the estrone produced

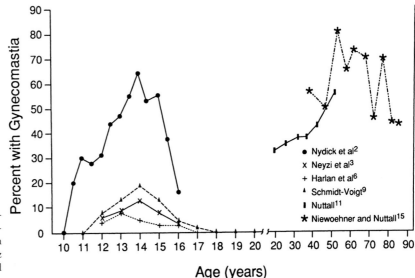

FIGURE 3.5-1 Prevalence of gynecomastia at various chronologic ages. Data were derived from multiple population studies.[2,3,6,9,11,15] (Adapted from Braunstein GD. Pubertal gynecomastia. In: Lifshitz F, ed. Pediatric endocrinology. New York, Marcel Dekker, 1995 [in press]).

daily. Most of the circulating estrogens are derived from the extraglandular conversion of estrogen precursors by extragonadal tissues including the liver, skin, fat, muscle, bone, and kidney. These tissues contain the aromatase enzyme that converts testosterone to estradiol and androstenedione, an androgen primarily secreted by the adrenal glands, to estrone. Estradiol and estrone are interconverted in extragonadal tissues through the activity of the 17-ketosteroid reductase enzyme. This enzyme is also responsible for the interconversion of testosterone and androstenedione. When androgens and estrogens enter the circulation, either from the direct secretion from gonadal tissues or from the sites of extragonadal metabolism, most are bound to sex hormone–binding globulin (SHBG), a protein derived primarily from the liver and one which has a greater affinity for androgens than for estrogens. The non-SHBG sex hormones circulate either in the free or unbound state or are weakly bound to albumin. These free or weakly bound fractions are able to cross the plasma membrane of target cells and are bound to cytoplasmic steroid receptors. In some target tissues, testosterone is converted to dihydrotestosterone through the action of the 5α-reductase enzyme. Both testosterone and dihydrotestosterone bind to the same androgen receptor and are translocated into the nucleus. Each also binds to the hormone-responsive element of the appropriate genes, resulting in the initiation of transcription and hormone action. A similar sequence of events occurs after the binding of estradiol or estrone to the cytoplasmic estrogen receptor.[18]

From a pathophysiologic standpoint, an imbalance between estrogen and androgen concentrations or effects can occur due to abnormalities at several levels (see Table 3.5-1). Overproduction of estrogens from testicular or adrenal neoplasms, or enhanced extraglandular conversion of estrogen precursors to estrogens may elevate the total estrogen concentration. Such extraglandular conversion may occur directly in the breast tissue. Indeed, increased

aromatization of androgens to estrogens has been noted in pubic skin fibroblasts from some patients with idiopathic gynecomastia.[20] Elevations of the absolute quantity of circulating free estrogens may occur if estrogen metabolism is slowed or if SHBG-bound estrogens are displaced from the protein. Conversely, decreased secretion of androgens from the testes—due to primary defects in the testes or secondary to loss of tonic stimulation by pituitary gonadotropins, enhanced metabolic degradation of androgens, or increased binding of androgens to SHBG—results in decreases in free androgens that could antagonize the effect of estrogens on the breast glandular tissue. As noted previously, androgen and estrogen balance depend not only on the amount and availability of free androgens and estrogens, but also on their ability to act at the target tissue level. Thus, defects in the androgen receptor or displacement of androgens from their receptors by drugs with antiandrogenic effects (eg, spironolactone) result in decreased androgen action and, hence, decreased estrogen antagonism at the breast glandular cell level. Finally, the inherent sensitivity of an individual's breast tissue to estrogen or androgen action may predispose some persons to develop gynecomastia even in the presence of apparently normal concentrations of estrogens and androgens.

Associated Conditions

Tables 3.5-2 and 3.5-3 list the various conditions that have been associated with gynecomastia. Although the list is relatively long, almost two thirds of the patients have either pubertal gynecomastia (approximately 25%), drug-induced gynecomastia (10% to 20%), or no underlying abnormality detected (idiopathic gynecomastia; approximately 25%). Most of the remainder will have cirrhosis or malnutrition (8%), primary hypogonadism (8%), testicular tumors (3%), secondary hypogonadism (2%), hyperthy-

TABLE 3.5-1
Pathophysiologic Mechanisms for Gynecomastia

ABSOLUTE INCREASE IN FREE ESTROGENS

Direct secretion from:

    Maternal–placental–fetal unit

    Testes

    Adrenal glands

Extraglandular aromatization of precursors

Displacement from sex hormone–binding globulin

Decreased metabolism

Exogenous estrogen administration

DECREASED ENDOGENOUS FREE ANDROGENS

Decreased secretion

Increased metabolism

Increased binding to sex hormone–binding globulin

**RELATIVE INCREASE IN FREE ESTROGEN/
FREE ANDROGEN RATIO**

ANDROGEN INSENSITIVITY

Congenital defects in androgen receptor structure and function

Displacement of androgens from androgen receptor

OTHER

Estrogen-like effect of drugs

Possible enhanced sensitivity of breast tissue

(Braunstein GD. Gynecomastia. N Engl J Med 1993;328:490)

roidism (1.5%), or renal disease (1%).[21] For most pathologic conditions, alterations in the balance between estrogen and androgen levels or action occur through several of the pathophysiologic mechanisms outlined in Table 3.5-1. One of the best examples is the gynecomastia associated with spironolactone. This aldosterone antagonist inhibits the testicular biosynthesis of testosterone, enhances the conversion of testosterone to the less potent androgen androstenedione, increases the aromatization of testosterone to estradiol, displaces testosterone from SHBG (leading to an increase in its metabolic clearance rate), and binds to the androgen receptors in target tissues, thereby acting as an antiandrogen.[22] For an in-depth discussion of the pathophysiology of gynecomastia associated with each of the conditions listed in Tables 3.5-2 and 3.5-3, the reader is referred to several reviews.[13,17,18,21,23,24]

Evaluation

Most patients with gynecomastia are asymptomatic, with the condition detected during a physical examination. Patients with recent onset of gynecomastia due to drugs or one of the pathologic conditions noted in Tables 3.5-2

and 3.5-3, however, may present with breast or nipple pain and tenderness. Approximately 10% to 15% of patients recall a history of breast trauma just before or at the time of discovery of the breast enlargement.[17,25] It is unclear whether breast trauma itself causes gynecomastia. It is likely that, in many patients with an antecedent history of trauma, the breast irritation from the trauma actually led to the discovery of pre-existing gynecomastia. Although half of patients have clinically apparent bilateral gynecomastia, histologic studies have shown that virtually all patients have bilateral involvement.[14] This discrepancy may be explained by assynchronous growth of the two breasts and differences in the amount of breast glandular and stromal proliferation.

Gynecomastia must be differentiated from other conditions that cause breast enlargement. Although neurofibromas, dermoid cysts, lipomas, hematomas, and lymphangiomas may enlarge portions of the breast, these abnormalities are usually easily distinguished from gynecomastia on historical or clinical grounds. The two conditions that are most important to differentiate are pseudogynecomastia and breast carcinoma. *Pseudogynecomastia* refers to enlargement of the breasts due to fat deposition rather than to glandular proliferation. Patients with this condition often have generalized obesity and do not complain of breast pain or tenderness. Additionally, the breast

TABLE 3.5-2
Conditions Associated With Gynecomastia

PHYSIOLOGIC

Neonatal

Pubertal

Involutional

PATHOLOGIC

Neoplasms

    Testicular (germ cell, Leydig cell, Sertoli cell, sex cord)

    Adrenal (adenoma or carcinoma)

    Ectopic production of human chorionic gonadotropin

Primary gonadal failure

Secondary hypogonadism

Enzymatic defects of testosterone production★

Androgen-insensitivity syndromes★

True hermaphroditism★

Liver disease

Starvation, especially during the recovery phase

Renal disease and dialysis

Hyperthyroidism

Excessive extraglandular aromatase activity

Drugs (see Table 3.5-3)

Idiopathic

★ These conditions are usually associated with ambiguity of genitalia or deficient virilization.

(Braunstein GD. Gynecomastia. N Engl J Med 1993;328:490)

TABLE 3.5-3
Drugs Associated With Gynecomastia

HORMONES

Androgens and anabolic steroids★

Chorionic gonadotropin★

Estrogens and estrogen agonists★

ANTIANDROGENS OR INHIBITORS OF ANDROGEN SYNTHESIS

Cyproterone★

Flutamide★

ANTIBIOTICS

Isoniazid

Ketoconazole★

ANTIULCER MEDICATIONS

Cimetidine★

Ranitidine

Omprazole

CANCER CHEMOTHERAPEUTIC AGENTS

Alkylating agents★

CARDIOVASCULAR DRUGS

Amiodarone

Captopril

Digitoxin★

Diltiazem

Enalapril

Methyldopa

Nifedipine

Reserpine

Spironolactone★

Verapamil

PSYCHOACTIVE AGENTS

Diazepam

Haloperidol

Phenothiazine

Tricyclic antidepressants

DRUGS OF ABUSE

Alcohol

Amphetamines

Heroin

Marijuana

OTHER

Phenytoin

Penicillamine

★ A strong relation has been established. Other relations have been proposed on the basis of epidemiologic studies or challenge–rechallenge studies of individual patients or small groups of patients.

(Braunstein GD. Gynecomastia. N Engl J Med 1993;328:490)

examination should allow the correct diagnosis. The breasts are best examined while the patient is lying on his back with his hands behind his head. The examiner places his or her thumb on one side of the breast and the second finger on the other side. The fingers are then gradually brought together without applying more than superficial pressure to the skin. Patients with gynecomastia have a rubbery or firm disk of tissue that extends concentrically out from the nipple and that either is easily palpated or offers some resistance to the apposition of the fingers, whereas those with pseudogynecomastia exhibit no such mound of tissue, and no resistance is felt as the fingers are brought together.

Differentiation of gynecomastia from breast carcinoma usually can be accomplished through careful physical examination. Carcinoma of the breast in men is usually eccentric in location and unilateral (rather than subareolar and bilateral) and is hard or firm, whereas gynecomastia tends to be rubbery to firm in texture. Patients with carcinoma may also exhibit skin dimpling and nipple retraction, are more likely to have a nipple discharge (60%) than are patients with gynecomastia (2%), and may present with axillary lymphadenopathy.[25] If the two conditions cannot be differentiated on clinical grounds, then mammography, fine-needle aspiration for cytologic examination, or open biopsy should be done. With the exception of the Klinefelter syndrome (XXY genotype), no well-established data indicate that gynecomastia predisposes to the development of carcinoma. Patients with the Klinefelter syndrome do have a 16-fold higher risk of developing breast carcinoma than do men without the syndrome.[26]

After a clinical diagnosis of gynecomastia has been made several etiologies should be investigated through a thorough history and physical examination. A careful history of medication use is essential, specifically regarding ingestion of the drugs listed in Table 3.5-3. A history of liver or renal disease, especially if the patient has been receiving hemodialysis for the latter, may point to the underlying etiology. A history of weight loss, tachycardia, tremulousness, diaphoresis, heat intolerance, and hyperdefecation, with or without the presence of a goiter, raises the possibility of hyperthyroidism. The patient should be evaluated for the signs and symptoms of hypogonadism including loss of libido, impotence, decreased strength, and testicular atrophy. A careful examination for abdominal masses, which may be present in nearly half the patients with adrenocortical carcinoma, and a meticulous examination for testicular masses is an essential part of the evaluation.

The next step depends on the results of the clinical evaluation. If any of the drugs listed in Table 3.5-3 have been ingested, they should be discontinued and the patient re-examined in 1 month. If the drug was the inciting agent, then a decrease in breast pain and tenderness should occur during that time. If the patient is of pubertal age and has an otherwise normal general physical and testicular examination, he probably has transient or persistent pubertal gynecomastia. Re-examination at 6-month intervals should determine whether the condition is transient or persistent. At this time, medical or surgical therapy should be considered. If during routine clinical examination an adult is found to have asymptomatic gynecomastia without the presence of underlying disease, the patient should have biochemical assessments of liver, kidney, and thyroid function. In a patient with normal results, no further tests are necessary, but the patient should be reevaluated in 6 months. Conversely, if the gynecomastia is of recent onset or if the patient complains of pain or tenderness, additional studies including measurements of serum concentrations of human chorionic gonadotropin, estradiol, testosterone, and luteinizing hormone should be done.

The algorithm outlined in Figure 3.5-2 can be used to discern the underlying abnormality, if any, responsible for the breast enlargement.[21] An elevated level of human chorionic gonadotropin in the serum indicates the presence of a testicular or nongonadal germ cell tumor or, rarely, a nontrophoblastic neoplasm that secretes the hormone ectopically. A testicular ultrasound should be done, and, if no testicular mass is found, a chest radiograph and abdominal computed tomographic scan or magnetic resonance imaging study should be done in an effort to localize an extragonadal human chorionic gonadotropin-producing tumor. Most nontrophoblastic tumors that secrete the hormone are bronchogenic, gastric, renal cell, or hepatic carcinomas. An elevated serum concentration of luteinizing hormone associated with a low testosterone level is indicative of primary hypogonadism, whereas a low testosterone level and a low or normal luteinizing hormone level suggests secondary hypogonadism due to a hypothalamic or pituitary abnormality. Serum prolactin

concentration should be determined in this situation to rule out a prolactin-secreting pituitary adenoma, which can cause hypogonadotropic hypogonadism. Elevated serum concentrations of luteinizing hormone and testosterone are found with hyperthyroidism as well as in patients with various forms of androgen resistance due to androgen receptor disorders. Thyroid function tests can distinguish between these conditions. If an elevated serum estradiol level is found along with a normal or suppressed concentration of luteinizing hormone, a testicular ultrasound is indicated to rule out a Leydig cell, Sertoli cell, or sex cord testicular tumor. If the ultrasound is normal, a computed tomographic scan or magnetic resonance imaging scan of the adrenal glands should be done to detect an estrogen-secreting adrenal neoplasm. If both the testes and adrenal glands appear normal, the increased estradiol level is probably due to enhanced extraglandular aromatization of estrogen precursors to estrogens. In this situation, estrone levels are often relatively higher than estradiol concentrations. Finally, if all of these endocrine measurements are normal, the patient is considered to have idiopathic gynecomastia.

Prevention

Two situations exist in which gynecomastia may be prevented. The first is in patients who require a medication. Avoidance of the drugs listed in Table 3.5-3 decreases the

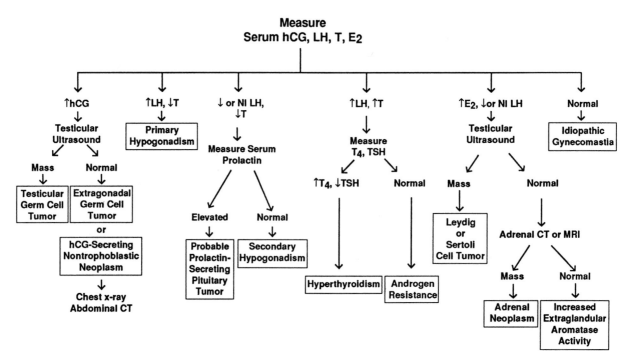

FIGURE 3.5-2 Algorithim providing interpretation of serum hormone levels and recommendations for further evaluation of patients with gynecomastia. hCG, human chorionic gonadotropin; LH, luteinizing hormone; T, testosterone; E2, estradiol; CT, computed tomography; T4, thyroxine; TSH, thyroid-stimulating hormone; MRI, magnetic resonance imaging. (Braunstein GD. Gynecomastia. N Engl J Med 1993;328:490)

risk for drug-induced breast stimulation. Also, not all the therapeutic agents within the drug groups listed in the table cause gynecomastia to the same extent. For example, when considering the use of a calcium-channel blocker in an older man, the clinician should remember that nifedipine has been associated with the highest frequency of gynecomastia, followed by verapamil, with diltiazem having the lowest association.[23,27] Similarly, the incidence of gynecomastia in patients receiving H_2-receptor or parietal cell proton-pump blockers is highest with cimetidine, then ranitidine, and least with omeprazole.[23,28] The second area of prevention occurs among patients with prostate cancer who are about to receive estrogens. Numerous studies have shown that prophylactic administration of low-dose radiation (900 rad) greatly reduces the appearance of gynecomastia.[29]

Treatment

Discontinuation of the offending drug or correction of the underlying condition that altered the estrogen–androgen balance results in regression of gynecomastia in recent-onset breast growth. As noted previously, histologic studies of the breast tissue from men with gynecomastia have shown a marked duct epithelial cell proliferation, inflammatory cell infiltration, increase in stromal fibroblasts, and enhanced vascularity early in the course of the disorder. It is during this proliferative, or florid, stage that patients may complain of breast pain and tenderness. This stage persists for a variable period, but usually lasts less than a year and is followed by spontaneous resolution or enters an inactive stage. There is a reduction in the epithelial proliferation, dilation of the ducts, and hyalinization and fibrosis of the stroma.[10,14,30] The inactive stage is usually asymptomatic. This histologic picture predominates in men whose gynecomastia is detected during a routine physical examination. When considering therapeutic approaches, it is important to appreciate that, after the inactive stage is reached, the gynecomastia is unlikely to spontaneously regress and is also unlikely to respond to medical therapies. Another important factor to consider is that most gynecomastia regresses spontaneously. Indeed, a large proportion of boys develop pubertal gynecomastia, but very few exhibit persistent breast glandular enlargement. Similarly, in a group of patients with gynecomastia from various causes, 85% of untreated patients had spontaneous improvement.[25] This finding emphasizes the difficulties in assessing the response to any medical intervention.

The indications for therapy are severe pain, tenderness, or embarrassment sufficient to interfere with the patient's normal daily activities. Surgical removal of the breast glandular and stromal tissue has been the mainstay of interventional therapy. Subcutaneous mastectomy through a periaerolar incision with contouring of the breast by suction-assisted lipectomy to remove the subglandular adipose tissue is the current surgical procedure of choice.[31] This technique should be used as primary therapy in patients with long-standing gynecomastia and as definitive therapy in patients who fail to respond to a series of medical therapies.

Three types of medical therapy—androgens, antiestrogens, and aromatase inhibitors—have been tested in patients with gynecomastia. Because this condition has a high frequency of spontaneous regression, the decision of when to treat is often difficult. It is also difficult to assess the utility of most medications that have been tried given the small sample sizes and nonblinded, uncontrolled designs of most studies. Nevertheless, with the exception of early pubertal gynecomastia, which has been present for less than 3 months, I recommend a trial of medical therapy for patients with moderate to severe symptoms.

Testosterone administration has not been shown to be more effective than placebo and carries the risk of exacerbating the condition by being aromatized to estradiol.[25] Dihydrotestosterone, a nonaromatizable androgen, given either by injection or percutaneously has been followed by a reduction in breast volume in 75% of patients, with complete resolution in approximately one quarter.[32] Responders had a decrease in breast tenderness within 1 to 2 weeks, without side effects. The androgenic progestogen danazol has also been tried in uncontrolled trials and a single placebo-controlled study, the latter showing a complete resolution in 23% of patients receiving danazol and only a 12% response in those given placebo.[33] Although the investigators believed that this drug was safe and well tolerated, other studies using danazol to treat other conditions have noted side effects including edema, weight gain, acne, nausea, and muscle cramps.

The two antiestrogens that have been tested are clomiphene citrate and tamoxifen. Response rates of 36% to 95% have been reported for clomiphene citrate, but two of the three systematic studies indicated that less than half of patients had a decrease in breast volume of 20% or more or were satisfied with the results.[34,35,36] No side effects were noted by the investigators when the drug was used in doses of 50 to 100 mg/d orally. In other settings, the drug has been associated with gastrointestinal distress and visual problems. Tamoxifen, given in doses of 10 mg orally twice a day, has been studied in two randomized, double-blind studies in a combined total of 16 patients.[37,38] This therapy was associated with an statistically significant reduction in pain and breast size, although neither study reported complete remissions. A complete response was reported in 80% of patients studied in an uncontrolled trial.[39] None of the studies has reported any side effects from tamoxifen given in these doses, and, in view of its safety, I usually recommend a 3-month trial of the drug for patients with painful gynecomastia.

The aromatase inhibitor testolactone has been given to a small number of patients with pubertal gynecomastia for up to 6 months at a dose of 450 mg/d orally without side effects.[40] The authors of this uncontrolled study reported a decrease in breast size after 2 months of therapy. Thus, insufficient data currently exist to recommend this drug as a first-line agent. On theoretical grounds, however, this medication appears to be beneficial in patients whose gynecomastia is primarily the result of enhanced extraglandular aromatization of estrogen precursors.

References

1. Jung FT, Shafton AL. Mastitis, mazoplasia, mastalgia, and gynecomastia in normal adolescent males. Ill Med J 1938;73:115.

2. Nydick M, Bustos J, Dale JH Jr, et al. Gynecomastia in adolescent boys. JAMA 1961;178:449.

3. Neyzi O, Alp H, Yalcindag A, et al. Sexual maturation in Turkish boys. Ann Hum Biol 1975;2:251.

4. Lee PA. The relationship of concentrations of serum hormones to pubertal gynecomastia. J Pediatr 1975;86:212.

5. Fara GM, DelCorvo G, Bernuzzi S, et al. Epidemic of breast enlargement in an Italian school. Lancet 1979;2:295.

6. Harlan WR, Grillo GP, Cornoni-Huntley J, et al. Secondary sex characteristics of boys 12 to 17 years of age: the U.S. Health Examination Survey. J Pediatr 1979;95:293.

7. Moore DC, Schlaepfer LV, Paunier L, et al. Hormonal changes during puberty. V. Transient pubertal gynecomastia: abnormal androgen–estrogen ratios. J Clin Endocrinol Metab 1984;58:492.

8. Biro FM, Lucky AW, Huster GA, et al. Hormonal studies and physical maturation in adolescent gynecomastia. J Pediatr 1990;116:450.

9. Schmidt-Voigt J. Brustdruenschwellungen bei mannlichen Jugendlichen des Pubertatsalters (Pubertatsmakromastie). Z Kinderheilkd 1941;62:590.

10. Williams MJ. Gynecomastia: its incidence, recognition and host characterization in 447 autopsy cases. Am J Med 1963;34:103.

11. Nuttall FQ. Gynecomastia as a physical finding in normal men. J Clin Endocrinol Metab 1979;48:338.

12. Ley SB, Mozaffarian GA, Leonard JM, et al. Palpable breast tissue versus gynecomastia as a normal physical finding. Clin Res 1980;28:24A.

13. Carlson HE. Gynecomastia. N Engl J Med 1980;303:795.

14. Andersen JA, Gram JB. Male breast at autopsy. APMIS 1982;90:191.

15. Niewoehner CB, Nuttall FQ. Gynecomastia in a hospitalized male population. Am J Med 1984;77:633.

16. Murray NP, Daly MJ. Gynaecomastia and heart failure: adverse drug reaction or disease process? J Clin Pharm Therap 1991;16:275.

17. Hall PF. Gynaecomastia. Glebe, Australasian Medical Publishing Company, 1959.

18. Wilson JD, Aiman J, MacDonald PC. The pathogenesis of gynecomastia. Adv Intern Med 1980;29:1.

19. Rochefort H, Garcia M. The estrogenic and antiestrogenic activities of androgens in female target tissues. Pharmacol Ther 1984;23:193.

20. Bulard J, Mowszowicz I, Schaison G. Increased aromatase activity in pubic skin fibroblasts from patients with isolated gynecomastia. J Clin Endocrinol Metab 1987;64:618.

21. Braunstein GD. Gynecomastia. N Engl J Med 1993;328:490.

22. Rose LI, Underwood RH, Newmark SR, et al. Pathophysiology of spironolactone-induced gynecomastia. Ann Intern Med 1977;87:398.

23. Thompson DF, Carter JR. Drug-induced gynecomastia. Pharmacotherapy 1993;13:37.

24. Braunstein GD. Pubertal gynecomastia. In: Lifshitz F, ed. Pediatric endocrinology. New York, Marcel Dekker, 1995 (in press).

25. Treves N. Gynecomastia: the origins of mammary swelling in the male: an analysis of 406 patients with breast hypertrophy, 525 with testicular tumors, and 13 with adrenal neoplasms. Cancer 58;11:1083.

26. Fentiman IS. Male breast cancer. In: Detection and treatment of early breast cancer. Philadelphia, JB Lippincott, 1990;207.

27. Tanner LA, Bosco LA. Gynecomastia associated with calcium channel blocker therapy. Arch Intern Med 1988;148:379:27.

28. Lindquist M, Edwards IR. Endocrine adverse effects of omeprazole. BMJ 1992;305:451.

29. Waterfall NB, Glaser MG. A study of the effects of radiation on prevention of gynaecomastia due to oestrogen therapy. Clin Oncol (R Coll Radiol) 1979;5:257.

30. Nicolis GL, Modlinger RS, Gabrilove JL. A study of the histopathology of human gynecomastia. J Clin Endocrinol Metab 1971;32:173.

31. Young VL, Brown DM, Young AE. Gynecomastia. Mod Med 1991;88:153.

32. Kuhn J–M, Roca R, Laudat M–H, et al. Studies on the treatment of idiopathic gynaecomastia with percutaneous dihydrotestosterone. Clin Endocrinol (Oxf) 1983;19:513.

33. Jones DJ, Davison DJ, Holt SD, et al. A comparison of danazol and placebo in the treatment of adult idiopathic gynaecomastia: results of a prospective study in 55 patients. Ann R Coll Surg Engl 1990;72:296.

34. Stepanas AV, Burnet RB, Harding PE. Clomiphene in the treatment of pubertal–adolescent gynecomastia: a preliminary report. J Pediatr 1977;90:651.

35. Plourde PV, Kulin HE, Santner SJ. Clomiphene in the treatment of adolescent gynecomastia: clinical and endocrine studies. Am J Dis Child 1983;137:1080.

36. LeRoith D, Sobel R, Glick SM. The effect of clomiphene citrate on pubertal gynaecomastia. Acta Endocrinol (Copenh) 1980;95:177.

37. Parker LN, Gray DR, Lai MK, et al. Treatment of gynecomastia with tamoxifen: a double-blind crossover study. Metabolism 1986;35:705.

38. McDermott MT, Hofeldt FD, Kidd GS. Tamoxifen therapy for painful idiopathic gynecomastia. South Med J 1990;83:1283.

39. Alagaratnam TT. Idiopathic gynecomastia treated with tamoxifen: a preliminary report. Clin Ther 1987;9:483.

40. Zachmann M, Eiholzer U, Muritano M, et al. Treatment of pubertal gynaecomastia with testolactone. Acta Endocrinol (Copenh) (Suppl) 1986;279:218.

3.6

Fat Necrosis, Hematoma, and Trauma

COLETTE M. MAGNANT

Breast Trauma and Hematoma

Trauma to the breast has been overlooked in most trauma texts because it is not a threat to life or limb. The actual presence of significant breast trauma often serves as a marker for more serious thoracic injuries, including pulmonary contusions, pneumothorax, hemopneumothorax, flail chest, and blunt cardiac injuries. Breast injuries include physical findings of ecchymoses, erythema, and edema, as well as soft tissue disruption from missile and stab wounds. Most breast trauma is mild and self-limiting; it rarely requires definitive therapy in isolation.

In addition to obvious penetrating injuries such as stab and missile wounds, blunt mechanisms are common in causes in the limited literature on traumatic injuries to the breast. Motor vehicle crashes account for nearly 60% of all traumatic injuries in the United States and are believed to cause most cases of breast trauma as well. In deceleration mechanisms over 55 miles per hour, the increased use of seat restraints with a three-point design (lap belt and shoulder harness) often creates force sufficient to cause fractured clavicle and ribs as well as mesenteric and splenic injuries. Direct chest wall trauma to the driver from impact with the steering wheel and dash also may lead to soft tissue injuries of the breast in addition to more serious cardiothoracic trauma.[1] Other blunt mechanisms, such as direct blows from assaults, falls, and other vehicular mechanisms, have not been reported.

Seat belt injuries causing subcutaneous rupture of the breast have been reported.[2,3] The mechanism of injury is thought to be compression of the soft tissue of the breast between the shoulder harness and bony thorax as the torso decelerates, combined with shearing of the soft tissues due to rotation of the trunk[3] (Fig. 3.6-1). In severe cases, the breast tissue can actually be divided in two at the line of impact of the shoulder harness. The resulting ecchymosis and pain usually resolve spontaneously, although widespread fat necrosis with subsequent deformity of the breast may require cosmetic surgery. Rupture of implants or of the fibrous capsule surrounding the implants has been reported in women who have undergone augmentation mammaplasty[4] or implant reconstruction who have suffered even mild blunt trauma. Removal and replacement of the implant is important, especially with silicone gel implants, to prevent future silicone granuloma formation.

Breast hematoma is the most common sequela of minor trauma to the breast.[5] These patients present with tender masses, usually with overlying ecchymosis early in the postinjury course. If patients fail to present in the acute period and the clinical signs of trauma are absent with palpable breast masses, careful evaluation and follow-up with biopsy is essential, since 9% to 20% of women with breast cancer have histories of antecedent trauma.[6]

Breast hematoma can occur secondary to surgical intervention, including fine-needle aspiration, stereotactic core biopsy, and excisional biopsy. Sickles and colleagues[7] reviewed 80 women who had undergone fine-needle aspiration of 94 breast masses and who then underwent mammography within 1 month. Seventeen benign lesions demonstrated poorly defined, irregular margins suggestive of malignancy, and all occurred when aspiration preceded mammography by less than 2 weeks. Their recommendation is to obtain a mammogram before performing aspiration or to delay mammography until 2 weeks after aspiration to prevent this difficulty in diagnosis.[7,8]

The incidence of postoperative hematoma after excisional breast biopsy ranges from 0.5% to 4%, depending on the series.[9–12] Common causes include inadequate hemostasis, altered platelet function secondary to ingestion of nonsteroidal antiinflammatory agents or salicylate-containing compounds, and, less frequently, bleeding disorders. Hematomas can make subsequent physical exami-

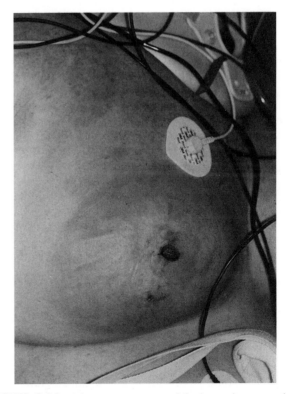

FIGURE 3.6-1 Subcutaneous rupture of the breast due to seat belt injury in a multiply injured trauma patient.

nation and mammographic evaluation difficult, especially after a needle localization biopsy, in which the presence of a residual mass or calcification may be obscured by the hematoma at the 3- to 6-month follow-up mammogram. Drainage of the biopsy cavity[13] and pressure dressings[14] have been shown to be of no value in the prevention of hematomas. Meticulous attention to hemostasis is important in preventing this complication.

The clinical management of breast hematomas is aimed at relief of symptoms. A patient presenting with an enlarging hematoma within hours of surgery should be returned to the operating room for evacuation of the hematoma and cauterization or ligation of the bleeding vessel. When the patient presents more than 24 hours after surgery, analgesics and support with a brassiere usually make her more comfortable. Once the hematoma has liquefied, as evidenced by fluctuance under the incision, aspiration may give some relief as well. Hematomas under pressure may drain spontaneously through the incision 1 or 2 weeks after surgery. When this occurs, the remainder of the hematoma can be expressed through a small opening in the incision, and the opening is allowed to heal secondarily. Primary incision and evacuation of a hematoma usually are not necessary unless the hematoma becomes secondarily infected.

The difficulty in interpreting the physical examination and mammogram of a patient with a postoperative hematoma is especially important in patients who elect to undergo lumpectomy and radiation therapy for treatment of their breast cancer.[15] Hematomas can make the breast difficult to inspect, and a recurrence of the carcinoma may go unnoticed. The hematoma may also become infected or liquefy and drain through the incision. If this occurs, the definitive surgery or radiation treatment for the breast cancer may be delayed.

Spontaneous hemorrhage into a breast cancer or cyst is rare but can occur. Cytologic evaluation of the fluid is often negative for cancer cells in this setting. If a breast mass does not completely resolve after aspiration of bloody fluid, excisional biopsy is important to rule out a malignancy.

Mondor Disease of the Breast

Mondor disease of the breast is an uncommon condition first reported in 1869 by Fagge[16] and later discussed in detail in 1939 by Mondor[17] as superficial thrombophlebitis of the lateral thoracic or superior thoracoepigastric veins. Mondor disease usually presents as a tender subcutaneous cord in the breast sometimes associated with dimpling of the overlying skin but without systemic signs of infection (Fig. 3.6-2). Its causes include benign conditions such as trauma to the breast, infections, breast surgery, excessive physical strain, and rheumatoid arthritis. Associated carcinoma has been reported in 5% to 12.7% of cases.[18,19] Mammography should be performed to rule out an underlying malignancy.[20] Mondor disease has been found to be associated with breast conservation surgery and radiation therapy

as a treatment for carcinoma of the breast.[21] The process is usually self-limiting and resolves spontaneously in 2 to 10 weeks. Local application of heat and nonsteroidal anti-inflammatory agents can give some relief of symptoms.

Fat Necrosis

Fat necrosis of the breast is a benign condition that can mimic breast carcinoma. In 1920, Lee and Adair[26] first reported on two patients thought to have breast carcinoma for which they underwent radical mastectomy; on histologic review of the specimen, they were found to have fat necrosis. Hadfield's subsequent series in 1929[27] reported on 45 women with fat necrosis of whom 12 (26%) underwent nontherapeutic mastectomy for the mistaken diagnosis of breast carcinoma. Adair and Munzer[28] reported on 110 cases of fat necrosis in 1947.

The cause of fat necrosis was originally considered to be blunt trauma to the breast. A history of antecedent trauma was reported in 14 (32%) of 44 patients in Haagensen's[29] series, 41 (37%) of 110 women in Adair and Munzer's series,[28] and 3 (40%) of 7 patients in Meyer and colleagues' series.[30] The actual incidence of prior trauma is probably higher than reported, since the breasts are prone to injury because of their vulnerable position and soft tissue composition, but many patients may not remember a minor traumatic incident. Surgical trauma secondary to biopsy and reduction mammaplasty[31] can also lead to fat necrosis. Infection, duct ectasia[32] with subsequent duct erosion, and extrusion of irritative intraductal debris into the surrounding fat, and injection of foreign materials such as paraffin, silicone, and narcotics into the breast[33–35] have also caused fat necrosis. Conservative treatment of breast carcinoma with lumpectomy and radiation therapy may also result in fat necrosis.[36]

Autologous fat transplantation using the liposuction technique to fill in irregular contours and small soft tissue defects in the breast has led to fat necrosis secondary to poor blood supply of the injected fat. Hartrampf and Bennett[37] argue against injection of autologous fat for cosmetic and reconstructive purposes, since it may lead to fat necrosis and can mimic carcinoma.

Many patients who undergo modified radical mastectomy for carcinoma now choose transverse rectus abdominis muscle (TRAM) flap reconstruction for the defect.[38] The lack of circulation in the medial and lateral tips of the TRAM flap increases the likelihood of fat necrosis in these areas.[38,39] These patients typically present with firm, painless masses that may simulate carcinoma on physical examination. Subsequent mammography and biopsy must be performed to rule out malignancy.

The predominant clinical findings in patients with fat necrosis are single or multiple firm, round, or irregular masses, which can be associated with overlying skin tethering or thickening. Masses are usually painless and immobile, raising the specter of carcinoma. Fat necrosis usually presents in the superficial tissue of the breast, which can cause dimpling of the overlying skin. Although fat necrosis

FIGURE 3.6-2 Mondor disease of the breast. **A.** Previous biopy incision. **B.** Subcutaneous cord characteristic of Mondor disease.

can occur anywhere in the breast, a central location in the subareolar area is most common.[5] Surgical biopsy is usually necessary to make the diagnosis.

The classic mammographic findings associated with fat necrosis include dystrophic calcifications and lipid cysts that may or may not be calcified (Fig. 3.6-3). Other radiographic features, such as spiculated densities, often with overlying skin thickening or retraction and branching, rodlike or angular calcifications, can be indistinguishable from carcinoma.[40] The only reliable finding is lipid cysts. Fine-needle aspiration, stereotactic core biopsy, or needle localization and excisional biopsy are mandatory to rule out carcinoma (Fig. 3.6-4).

Patients who present soon after trauma with physical sequelae such as ecchymosis and painful masses in the breast can be safely observed. Breast masses may initially increase in size and later become smaller as the acute inflammatory process resolves.[5] If patients present later with painless masses and histories of trauma that cannot be substantiated, the diagnosis of fat necrosis must be established by biopsy.

Warfarin-Induced Breast Necrosis

An unusual type of breast necrosis was first reported by Flood and associates in 1943.[41] The patient presented with massive necrosis of the breast caused by therapy with the oral anticoagulant warfarin. Kipen[42] reported on two subsequent cases in 1961 and established the link with the drug. Since the original report, 29 cases of massive necrosis of the breast have been reported. The necrosis typically

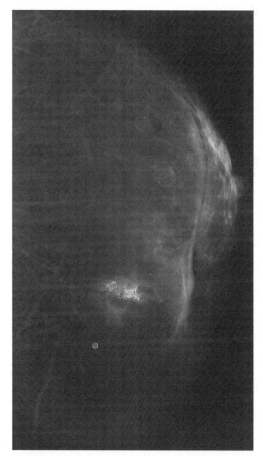

FIGURE 3.6-3 Mammogram showing dystrophic calcifications of the breast and calcified and noncalcified lipid cysts characteristic of fat necrosis.

FIGURE 3.6-4 Low-power photomicrograph of fat necrosis characterized by degeneration of adipocytes with surrounding lymphoplasmacytic infiltrates and fibrosis. Central cleared-out spaces of remaining uninvolved fat are visible.

occurs 3 to 5 days after initiation of warfarin therapy. The prothrombin time is usually in the therapeutic range.

The cause of warfarin-associated necrosis is not well understood, and proposed mechanisms include direct vascular toxicity of warfarin, altered hormonal balance, and disseminated intravascular coagulation. A deficiency of protein C has been demonstrated in some patients with warfarin-induced necrosis.[43,44] Protein C is a naturally circulating anticoagulant that cleaves activated factors V and VIII, destroying their procoagulant activity. A deficiency of protein C results in recurrent thrombotic episodes, which may be responsible for the massive tissue necrosis. Warfarin-induced breast necrosis is self-limited and fails to respond to a variety of treatments, including steroids, vasodilators, vitamin K, dextran, hypothermia, and sympathetic nerve blocks.[45] Wide débridement or simple mastectomy, which may require skin graft or myocutaneous flap closure, is the only effective treatment.

References

1. Cogbill TH, Landercasper J. Injury to the chest wall. In: Moore EE, Mattox KL, Feliciano DV, eds. Trauma, ed 2. Norwalk, CT, Appleton & Lange, 1991:327.
2. Eastwood D. Subcutaneous rupture of the breast: a seat belt injury. Br J Surg 1972;59:491.
3. Dawes R, Smallwood J, Taylor I. Seat belt injury to the female breast. Br J Surg 1986;73:106.
4. Bellon A, Cowley R, Hoopes J. Blunt chest trauma: evaluation of the augmented breast. J Trauma 1980;20:982.
5. Morrow M. Breast trauma, hematoma, and fat necrosis. In: Harris JR, Hellman S, Henderson IC, et al, eds. Breast diseases, ed 2. Philadelphia, JB Lippincott, 1991:43.
6. Donegan W, Spratt J. Cancer of the breast, ed 3. Philadelphia, WB Saunders, 1988:64.
7. Sickles EA, Klein DL, Goodson WH, et al. Mammography after needle aspiration of palpable breast masses. Am J Surg 1983;145:395.
8. Klein DL, Sickles EA. Effects of needle aspiration on the mammographic appearance of the breast: a guide to the proper timing of the mammography examination. Radiology 1982;145:44.
9. Landercasper J, Gundersen S, Sungersen A, et al. Needle localization and biopsy of nonpalpable lesions of the breast. Surg Gynecol Obstet 1987;164:399.
10. Ostrow LB, DuBois JJ, Hoefer RA Jr, et al. Needle-localized biopsy of occult breast lesions. South Med J 1987;80:29.
11. Homer M, Smith T, Marchant D. Outpatient needle localization and biopsy for nonpalpable lesions. JAMA 1984;252:2452.
12. Kaelin CM, Smith TJ, Homer MJ, et al. Safety, accuracy, and diagnostic yield of needle localization biopsy of the breast performed using local anesthesia. J Am Coll Surg 1994;179:267.
13. Warren HW, Griffith CD, McLean L, et al. Should breast biopsy cavities be drained? Ann R Coll Surg 1994;76:39.
14. Johnstone AJ, Thompson AM, Charles M, et al. Wound compression pads are of no value after local anaesthetic breast biopsy. Ann R Coll Surg Engl 1991;73:303.
15. Orford JE, Ingram DM, Kaard AO, et al. Scar formation after breast-conserving surgery for cancer: Sir Charles Gairdner Hospital Breast Cancer Group. Br J Surg 1993;80:1003.
16. Fagge CH. Remarks on certain cutaneous affections. Guy's Hospital Report 1869–70;15:302.
17. Mondor H. Tronculite sous-sutane subaigue de la paroi thoracique anterolaterale. Mem Acad Chir Paris 1939;65:1271.
18. Farrow JH. Thrombophlebitis of the superficial veins of the breast and anterior chest wall. Surg Gynecol Obstet 1955;101:63.
19. Catania S, Zurrida S, Veronesi P, et al. Mondor's disease in breast cancer. Cancer 1992;69:2267.
20. Tabar L, Dean P. Mondor's disease: clinical, mammographic and pathologic features. Breast 1981;7:17.
21. Magnant CM, Sznyter L, Potter J, et al. Mondor's disease presenting in post-radiation breast cancer patients. (Abstract) Breast Cancer Res Treat 1992;23:156.
22. Hershman M, Archer M. Mondor's disease and breast cancer. Br J Clin Pract 1987;41:979.
23. Halkier E, Bodker A. Mondor's disease: a review of five cases. Acta Chir Scand 1983;149:333.
24. Chiedozi L, Aghahowa J. Mondor's disease associated with breast cancer. Surgery 1987;103:438.

25. Green R, Dowden R. Mondor's disease in plastic surgery patients. Ann Plast Surg 1988;20:231.

26. Lee B, Adair F. Traumatic fat necrosis of the female breast and its differentiation from carcinoma. Ann Surg 1920;37:189.

27. Hadfield G. Fat necrosis of the breast. Br J Surg 1929;17:673.

28. Adair F, Munzer J. Fat necrosis of the female breast. Am J Surg 1947;74:117.

29. Haagensen C. Traumatic fat necrosis in the breast. In: Haagensen CD, ed. Diseases of the breast, ed 3. Philadelphia, WB Saunders, 1986:369.

30. Meyer J, Silverman P, Gandbhir L. Fat necrosis of the breast. Arch Surg 1978;113:801.

31. Barber C, Libshitz H. Bilateral fat necrosis of the breast following reduction mammoplasty. Am J Roentgenol 1977;128:508.

32. Paulus D. Benign diseases of the breast. Radiol Clin North Am 1983;21:38.

33. Schwartz G. Benign neoplasms and "inflammations" of the breast. Clin Obstet Gynecol 1982;25:373.

34. Aonobe H, Sato Y, Suzuki Y. Bilateral fat necrosis of the breast: report of a case. Acta Med Okayama 1980;34:343.

35. Blair NP. Misdiagnosis of bilateral breast cancer. (Letter) Can J Surg 1992;35:345.

36. Rostom A, El-Sayed M. Fat necrosis of the breast: an unusual complication of lumpectomy and radiotherapy in breast cancer. Clin Radiol 1987;38:31.

37. Hartrampf CR Jr, Bennett GK. Autologous fat from liposuction for breast augmentation. (Letter) Plast Reconstruct Surg 1987;80:646.

38. Hartrampf CR, Scheflan M, Black PW. Breast reconstruction with a transverse abdominal island flap. Plast Reconstruct Surg 1982; 69:216.

39. Hartrampf CR Jr, Bennett GK. Autogenous tissue reconstruction in the mastectomy patient: a critical review of 300 patients. Ann Surg 1987;205:508.

40. Bassett L, Gold R, Cove H. Mammographic spectrum of traumatic fat necrosis: the fallibility of "pathognomonic" signs of carcinoma. Am J Roentgenol 1978;130:119.

41. Flood E, Redish M, Rociek S, et al. Thrombophlebitis migrans disseminata: report of a case in which gangrene of a breast occurred. NY State J Med 1943;43:1121.

42. Kipen C. Gangrene of the breast: a complication of anticoagulant therapy. N Engl J Med 1961;265:638.

43. McGehee WG, Klotz TA, Epstein DJ, et al. Coumarin necrosis associated with hereditary protein C deficiency. Ann Intern Med 1984;100:59.

44. Rose VL, Kwaan HC, Williamson K, et al. Protein C antigen deficiency and warfarin necrosis. Am J Clin Pathol 1986;86:653.

45. Kagan R, Glassford H. Coumadin-induced breast necrosis. Am Surg 1981;47:509.

4

Clinical Evaluation

Diseases of the Breast, edited by Jay R. Harris,
Marc E. Lippman, Monica Morrow, and Samuel Hellman.
Lippincott-Raven Publishers, Philadelphia, © 1996.

4.1
Physical Examination of the Breast
MONICA MORROW

Obtaining a careful history is the initial step in a breast examination. Regardless of the presenting complaint, baseline information regarding menstrual status and breast cancer risk factors should be obtained. The basic elements of a breast history are listed in Table 4.1-1. In premenopausal women, the date of the last menstrual period and the regularity of the cycle are useful in evaluating breast

TABLE 4.1-1
Components of the Medical History of a Breast Problem

ALL WOMEN

Age at menarche
Number of pregnancies
Number of live births
Age at first birth
Family history of breast cancer including affected relative, age of onset, and presence of bilateral disease
History of breast biopsies (and histologic diagnosis if available)

PREMENOPAUSAL WOMEN

Date of last menstrual period
Length and regularity of cycles
Use of oral contraceptives

POSTMENOPAUSAL WOMEN

Date of menopause
Use of hormone replacement therapy

nodularity, pain, and cysts. Postmenopausal women should be questioned about use of hormone replacement therapy, given that many benign breast problems are uncommon after menopause in the absence of exogenous hormones. Specific information about the patient's presenting complaint is then elicited. A breast lump is the most common clinical breast problem causing women to seek treatment and remains the most common presentation of breast carcinoma. Haagensen[1] observed that 65% of 2198 breast cancer cases identified before the use of screening mammography presented as breast masses. Breast pain, a change in the size and shape of the breast, nipple discharge, and changes in the appearance of the skin are infrequent symptoms of carcinoma. The evaluation and management of these conditions is described in Chapter 5. In general, the duration of symptoms, their persistence over time, and their fluctuation with the menstrual cycle should be assessed.

Technique of Breast Examination

A woman must be disrobed from the waist up for a complete breast examination. Although attention to modesty is appropriate and a gown or drape should be provided, inspection is an important part of the examination, and subtle abnormalities are best appreciated by comparing the appearance of both breasts. Breast examination should be done with the patient in both the sitting and supine positions, and care should be taken at all times to be gentle.

The steps of a breast examination are illustrated in Figure 4.1-1.

The breasts should initially be inspected while the patient is in the sitting position with her arms relaxed (see Figure 4.1-1*A*). A comparison of breast size and shape should be made. If a size discrepancy is noted, its chronicity should be determined. Many women's breasts are not identical in size, and the finding of small size discrepancies is rarely a sign of malignancy. Differences in breast size that are of recent onset or progressive in nature, however, may be due to both benign and malignant tumors and require further evaluation (Fig. 4.1-2). Alterations in breast shape, in the absence of previous surgery, are of more concern. Superficially located tumors may cause bulges in the breast contour or retraction of the overlying skin. The skin retraction seen with superficial tumors may be due

FIGURE 4.1-1 Inspection of the patient in the upright position with arms relaxed (**A**) and pectoral muscles contracted (**B**) **C.** Palpation of the axillary nodes. The patient's ipsilateral arm is supported to relax the pectoral muscle. **D.** Palpation of the breast in the upright position. **E.** Palpation of the breast in the supine position. The breast is stabilized with one hand.

FIGURE 4.1-2 Marked breast asymmetry due to a benign breast tumor.

to direct extension of tumor or fibrosis. Tumors deep within the substance of the breast that involve the fibrous septae (Cooper ligaments) may also cause retraction. Retraction is not itself a prognostic factor except when due to the direct extension of tumor into the skin, and for this reason it is not a part of the clinical staging of breast cancer.[2] Although retraction is often a sign of malignancy, benign lesions of the breast such as granular cell tumors[3] and fat necrosis[4] also cause retraction. Other benign causes of retraction include surgical biopsy and thrombophlebitis of the thoracoepigatric vein (Mondor disease) (Fig. 4.1-3).

The skin of the breast and the nipples should also be carefully inspected. Edema of the skin of the breast (peau d'orange), when present, is usually extensive and readily apparent. Localized edema is frequently most prominent in the lower half of the breast and periareolar region and is most noticeable when the patient's arms are raised. Although breast edema usually occurs due to obstruction of the dermal lymphatics with tumor cells, it may also be caused by extensive axillary lymph node involvement related to metastatic tumor, primary diseases of the axillary nodes, or axillary dissection. Some degree of breast edema is very common after irradiation of the breast and should not be considered abnormal in this circumstance. Erythema is another sign of pathology that is evident on inspection. Erythema may be due to cellulitis or abscess in the breast, but a diagnosis of inflammatory carcinoma should always be considered. The erythema of inflammatory carcinoma usually involves the entire breast and is distinguished from the inflammation due to infection by the absence of breast tenderness and fever. A small percentage of large-breasted women will have mild, dependent erythema of the most pendulous portion of the breast, a condition which resolves when the patient lies down and which is of no concern.

Examination of the nipples should include inspection for symmetry, retraction, and changes in the character of

the skin. The new onset of nipple retraction should be regarded with a high index of suspicion, except when it occurs immediately after cessation of breast feeding. Ulceration and eczematous changes of the nipple may be the first signs of Paget disease. (This condition is discussed in detail in Chapter 24.3.) The initial nipple abnormality may be limited in extent, but, if untreated, it progresses to involve the entire nipple.

After inspection with the arms relaxed, the patient should be asked to raise her arms to allow a more complete inspection of the lower half of the breasts (see Fig. 4.1-4*A* and *B*). Inspection is completed with the patient contracting her pectoral muscles by pressing her hands against her hips (see Fig. 4.1-1*B*). This maneuver often highlights subtle areas of retraction not readily apparent with the arms relaxed.

The next step in the examination is palpation of the regional nodes. Examination of the axillary and supraclavicular nodes is done optimally with the patient upright. The right axilla is examined with the physician's left hand while supporting the patient's flexed right arm (see Fig. 4.1-1*C*). This position allows relaxation of the pectoral muscle and access to the axillary space and is reversed to examine the left axilla. If lymph nodes are palpable, their size and character (soft, firm, tender) should be noted, as well as whether they are single, multiple, or matted together. An assessment of whether the nodes are mobile or fixed should also be made. Based on this information, the physician can assess whether the nodes are clinically suspicious. Many women have palpable axillary nodes secondary to hangnails, minor abrasions of the arm, or folliculitis of the axilla, and nodes that are small (1 cm or less), soft, and mobile (especially if bilateral) should not be regarded with a high level of suspicion. In contrast, palpable

FIGURE 4.1-3 Breast retraction due to thrombophlebitis of the thoracoepigastric vein (Mondor disease). The characteristic pattern of lateral retraction superior to the nipple and crossing to the midline below the nipple is seen.

FIGURE 4.1-4 **A.** Patient with her arms at her sides. Breasts appear normal. **B.** With arms raised, retraction in right inferior breast is readily apparent.

supraclavicular adenopathy is uncommon and is an indication for further evaluation.

After completion of the nodal evaluation, palpation of the breasts should be done with the patient erect. Examination of the breast tissue in this position allows detection of lesions that might be obscured with the patient supine, such as those in the tail of the breast. The breast should be gently supported with one hand while examination is done with the flat portions of the fingers (see Fig. 4.1-1*D*). Pinching breast tissue between two fingers always results in the perception of a mass and is a common error of inexperienced examiners and women attempting self-examination.

The breast examination is completed with the patient in the supine position and the ipsilateral arm raised above the head (see Fig. 4.1-1*E*). In patients with extremely large breasts, it may be necessary to place a folded towel or a small pillow beneath the ipsilateral shoulder to elevate the breast, but this is not routinely necessary. The breast tissue is then systematically examined. Whether the examination is done using a radial search pattern or concentric circular pattern is unimportant, provided that the entire breast is examined. The examination should extend superiorly to the clavicle, inferiorly to the lower rib cage, medially to the sternal border, and laterally to the mid-axillary line. Examination is done with one hand while the other hand stabilizes the breast. The amount of pressure needed to examine the breast tissue varies but should not cause the patient discomfort.

One of the most difficult aspects of breast examination results from the nodular irregular texture of normal breasts in premenopausal women. Normal breasts tend to be most nodular in the upper outer quadrants where the glandular tissue is concentrated, in the inframammary ridge area,

and in the subareolar region. The characteristics that distinguish a dominant breast mass include the absence of other abnormalities of a similar character, density that differs from the surrounding breast tissue, and three dimensions. Generalized lumpiness is not a pathologic finding. Comparing the breasts is often helpful in determining whether a questionable area requires further evaluation. If the patient notices a mass not evident to the examiner, she should be asked to indicate the area of concern. The location of the perceived abnormality and the character of the breast tissue in the region should be described in the medical record. If uncertainty remains regarding the significance of an area of nodular breast tissue in a premenopausal woman, a repeat examination at a different time during the menstrual cycle may clarify the issue. If a dominant mass is identified it should be measured, and its location, mobility, and character should all be described in the medical record. The identification of a dominant mass is an indication for further evaluation. The steps in the evaluation of a palpable mass are described in Chapter 5.3.

References

1. Haagensen CD. Diseases of the breast. Philadelphia, WB Saunders, 1986:502.
2. American Joint Committee on Cancer. Manual for staging of cancer, ed 3. Philadelphia, JB Lippincott, 1988:145.
3. Gold DA, Hermann G, Schwartz IS, et al. Granular cell tumor of the breast. Breast Dis 1989;2:211.
4. Adair F, Munzer J. Fat necrosis of the female breast. Am J Surg 1947;74:117.
5. Tabar L, Dean P. Mondor's disease: clinical, mammographic and pathologic features. Breast 1981;7:17.

4.2
Imaging Analysis of Breast Lesions
DANIEL B. KOPANS

High-Quality Screening at Reduced Cost

The use of mammography to screen asymptomatic women 40 years of age and over for early detection of breast cancer has been shown to reduce mortality rates by 20% to 30%.[1] Mammography is the only technique with proven efficacy for breast cancer screening.

In an era of diminishing health care resources, cost is a major concern for the initiation of any type of screening. For the benefits of screening to be available to *all* women, the cost of mammography must be reduced. Because the quality of the mammographic image is directly related to early detection of cancers, however, cost reduction must not result in reduced image quality.

An efficient approach to screening can maintain quality and reduce cost. As has been shown in Europe and the United States, costs can be reduced by separating screening from the more costly evaluation of women who have a clinically evident problem or a problem detected by mammographic screening (diagnosis).[2,3] The screening mammogram is created at a center dedicated to breast cancer screening (or in a mobile facility), the quality of the study is ensured by expertly trained technologists, and the patient leaves. Using this approach, four women can be screened per hour. To enhance the radiologist's productivity, the screening studies are interpreted later in batches. This approach is similar to that used for cervical cancer screening, and, although the psychologic implications differ, mammography is the Pap test for the breast. One disadvantage of batch interpretation is that the patient does not receive an immediate report. This is more than offset by the reduced expense from efficient screening and the added advantage that reading mammograms on an alternator, in batches, permits double reading.

Double Reading

As has been shown in the interpretation of chest radiographs and other images, the perception of an abnormality is complicated by the psychovisual phenomenon that guarantees that significant abnormalities, visible in retrospect, are periodically overlooked by even the most experienced observer.[4] The failure to perceive an abnormality differs between observers. Errors can be reduced by having more than one reader. Mammographic interpretation is no exception. Double reading has been shown to improve the breast cancer detection rate by 5% to 15%.[5-7] Unless performed efficiently, double reading increases the cost of screening because both reviewers must be paid. A surprising amount of time is wasted handling films. Removing films from their envelope, organizing them on viewboxes, replacing them in their folders, and doing paperwork can account for several minutes for each case. This time expenditure can amount to an hour or more (depending on the number of films reviewed) not directly involved in film interpretation. If this work is duplicated by each radiologist, the time and cost become prohibitive. Further, although a psychologic benefit is derived from having the radiologist on site to provide the patient with a review and summary of her mammogram, this approach does not represent the best use of resources. The value of mammography lies in early detection of breast cancers. It is well known that mammography cannot be used to exclude breast cancer; therefore, having the radiologist reassure the patient that a study result is negative has no real value. Resources would be better directed toward increasing the ability to detect early lesions through double reading. This goal is best accomplished by delaying the interpretation and mounting mammograms on an alternator (multiviewer) in batches, thus permitting multiple review with little increase in cost.

In our experience, double reading increased the breast cancer detection rate by 7%. Using this approach, the first reader reviews films that were preloaded methodically on a multiviewer and completes all the paperwork involved in film interpretation. A second reader then concentrates completely on film review and does a second reading in a fraction of the time required by the first reader. In our study of 5900 screening mammograms, 39 cancers were identified. The methodical reader detected 8 more cancers than did the rapid reader, but the rapid reader detected an additional 3 cancers that were not appreciated by the methodical reader. Through efficient organization, and a slight delay (24 hours) for the patient in receiving her report, the false-negative rate can be reduced with virtually no increase in cost.

Screening Versus Diagnosis

The value of mammography for screening is well established. Although it is frequently used to evaluate women with signs or symptoms of breast cancer, the use of mammography as a diagnostic procedure is less efficacious. In 1979, Moskowitz[8] first emphasized the difference between detection (screening) and diagnosis. *Detection* is the process of finding breast abnormalities that may be cancer. *Diagnosis* is the process of determining which of the abnormalities actually is cancer. Understanding this distinction is critical for the proper use of mammography and other breast imaging techniques.

Mammography is unsurpassed in enabling the detection of anomalies in the breast, many of which represent early breast cancer but is less valuable when used as a diagnostic method of differentiating benign from malignant lesions. Radiologists have a fairly complete understanding of the underlying histopathologic changes that account for some of the mammographic findings; however, many benign and malignant lesions share similar morphologic characteristics when viewed mammographically. The differentiation is often insufficient to obviate the need for a tissue diagnosis.

Because tissue diagnosis (breast biopsy) is relatively safe and the consequences of early breast cancer detection critical, the accuracy of a noninvasive diagnostic study used instead of biopsy should be extremely high. Thus far, no imaging technologies are sufficiently accurate to obviate the need for a biopsy when a lesion is deemed suspicious by mammography.

As with any test, the likelihood that a given finding represents malignancy is a statistical probability. Many morphologic criteria are generally accepted as having a very high probability of malignancy. For example, a spiculated mass (Fig. 4.2-1) is virtually certain to indicate a malignant process if the patient has not had previous breast surgery to explain the finding. Nevertheless, benign, idiopathic lesions such as a radial scar (Fig. 4.2-2) occasionally have the same appearance. A tissue diagnosis is the only way to be certain. Other lesions, such as the solitary round or oval circumscribed mass (Fig. 4.2-3), have such a low probability of malignancy that many would argue that a tissue diagnosis is not justified and that monitoring the lesion at short intervals to assess its stability and permit early intervention should it change is a more reasonable approach.[9] Other findings are always due to benign processes and are associated with cancer only coincidentally.

Morphologic criteria have been established to assist in diagnosis. Before the instigation of an invasive procedure, it is important to analyze and categorize breast anomalies so that appropriate action can be taken. Mammography and ultrasound should be used to maximize the diagnosis of early cancers and to reduce the need for biopsy of benign lesions whenever possible.

Intervention Thresholds

As with many medical procedures, screening and the earlier detection of breast cancer represent a combination of science and art. The vagaries of perception and the importance of double reading have already been discussed, but an additional factor helps to determine the success of a screening program. This element is the threshold at which the radiologist recommends intervention. Breast cancer presents in various ways on a mammogram. Several of these overlap with the presentation of benign lesions, and many of these lesions have a very low probability of malignancy (less than 5%). Legitimate disagreement exists as to how aggressively these low-probability lesions should be treated. The influence of intervention threshold was shown in a study involving 10 radiologists who were asked to review a series of 150 mammographic studies without the knowledge that they included 27 cancer cases.[10] Almost one third of the cancers were borderline lesions. The radiologist who had the highest true-positive rate also had the highest false-positive rate (a low threshold for intervention), whereas the radiologist who had the lowest false-positive rate had the lowest false-negative rate (a high threshold for intervention).[11]

In an effort to reduce screening costs, great pressure exists to reduce the number of false-positive interpretations of mammograms, particularly the number of biopsies that prove to be for benign reasons. The ratio of the true-positive biopsy results to the total number of biopsies represents the positive predictive value. Given that the features of breast cancer overlap the features of many benign processes, a high true-positive rate can only be achieved at the expense of a high false-negative rate.[12] The only way to attain a high positive predictive value (a higher cancer-to-benign ratio) is for the radiologist to allow cancers with borderline morphology to pass through the screen.[13] This approach may be acceptable to reduce the induced costs of screening (patient anxiety and the cost of

FIGURE 4.2-1 Typical appearance of a spiculated cancer.

FIGURE 4.2-2 This spiculated lesion could be a malignancy but proved to be a benign radial scar.

biopsies, both traumatic and economic),[14] but it may reduce the ability of the screen to reduce mortality.[15,16]

Positive Predictive Value of a Mammographically Initiated Biopsy

Mammography is an excellent method for finding early-stage cancers, but no absolute criteria distinguish malignant from benign lesions. Lesions that are round or ovoid and that have sharply defined margins are statistically more likely to be benign,[17] but some cancers have similar shapes and margins.[18] Even the classic spiculated margin, a finding that is almost invariably due to malignancy, can occasionally be caused by a benign lesion such as a radial scar or an area of fat necrosis.[19,20] The microcalcifications that are associated with cancer are frequently indistinguishable morphologically from those produced by benign processes.[21] Ultrasound may be used to differentiate cysts from solid masses, but a cytologic or tissue diagnosis is frequently the only way to confidently distinguish a benign from a malignant lesion.

As the use of mammographic screening has increased, attention has been focused on the number of biopsies being done for what prove to be benign findings. As with any screening test, the sensitivity of the test can only increase at the expense of a higher false-positive rate. The false-positive rate is also a function of the probability of cancer in the population. Thus, the older a woman is, the greater the positive predictive value for a biopsy prompted by mammography.

The appropriate positive predictive value for biopsied lesions has been debated. By definition, the positive pre-

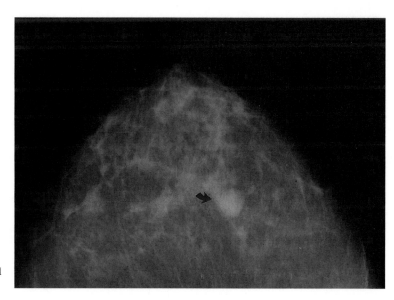

FIGURE 4.2-3 A solitary circumscribed mass that proved to be a cyst.

dictive value for a biopsy is the ratio of the number of biopsies showing cancer to the number of biopsies done to diagnose those lesions. The positive predictive value, however, must be evaluated in the context of the sensitivity of detection and the size and stage of the cancers diagnosed.[22] Because the features of breast cancer overlap the features of many benign processes, a high true-positive rate can only be achieved at the expense of a high false-negative rate.[23] The only way to attain a high positive predictive value (a higher cancer-to-benign ratio) is for the radiologist to allow cancers with borderline morphology to pass through the screen.[24] This approach may be acceptable to reduce the induced costs of screening (patient anxiety and the cost of biopsies, both traumatic and economic).[25] The optimal threshold for intervention has yet to be determined. A high threshold for intervention results in missing early cancers. The maintenance of a low threshold for intervention may result in fewer cancers per biopsy (more biopsies with benign results) but permits the diagnosis of cancers at a point in their growth when at least half of the invasive lesions are less than 1 cm in diameter and when 20% to 30% of the cancers are still intraductal. Higher positive predictive values can be achieved but only at the expense of early detection.

The detection of invasive lesions less than 1 cm in diameter is important. Rosen and colleagues[26] showed improved survival for stage I cancers that are under 1 cm when compared to stage I cancers 1.1 to 1.9 cm.[26] Other data also suggest the importance of detecting cancers 1 cm or smaller.[27] These thresholds can be achieved, but they require active investigation of lesions while they are still small and may not have the characteristic appearance of cancer. Most published series of needle-localized breast biopsies find malignancy in 20% to 35% of specimens.[28–30] The use of imaging-guided fine-needle aspiration biopsy for cellular (cytologic) evaluation[31] or core needle biopsy for histologic[32,33] evaluation of these lesions, if performed accurately, can reduce the need for excisional biopsy, but, as a result of sampling errors, the diagnosis of some cancers may be delayed.[34]

Many biopsies for benign abnormalities can be avoided by monitoring the lesions classified by the radiologist as probably benign using short-interval follow-up to establish the stability of benign lesions and to detect expeditiously any change among the few that prove to be benign.[35] This approach is the same that the clinician uses for palpable lesions that are probably benign but that he or she wishes to monitor for several months.

Monitoring Results: The Breast Imaging Audit

The best method to determine the success of a screening program is an audit that evaluates the cancer detection rate and the types of cancers detected. The Mammography Quality Standards Act, passed by Congress and administered by the Food and Drug Administration, became effective in October 1994. As part of the requirement for licensure, mammography facilities are required to monitor the results of their breast cancer detection programs. Sickles and associates[36] described in detail an audit of a screening practice. Each facility should monitor, among other parameters, the number of women screened, the number recalled for additional evaluation, the number recommended for biopsy, the positive predictive value of the biopsies, and the number, size, and stage of cancers detected. Many of these factors vary with the population being screened and with the prior probability of cancer in a particular population, so no absolute figures exist for these data. In our practice, in which we screen women beginning at 40 years of age, we recall approximately 7% of women for additional evaluation after their first screen (prevalence). This figure decreases to less than 4% on subsequent screens. Approximately 2% to 3% of women are recommended for a biopsy based on their first mammogram. This figure decreases to 1% to 2% on subsequent screens. We detect approximately 8 cancers per 1000 women in the first screen and 2 to 3 per 1000 in subsequent screens. Approximately 30% of the cancers detected are ductal carcinoma in situ (DCIS). Among the invasive cancers, about 50% are 1 cm or smaller, and less than 20% of the women diagnosed with breast cancer have positive axillary lymph nodes. These figures are not necessarily optimal, but, by evaluating the results of a screening effort, thresholds can be adjusted to improve the success of the program.

The optimal threshold for intervention has yet to be determined. A high threshold for intervention results in missing early cancers. The maintenance of a low threshold for intervention may result in fewer cancers per biopsy (more biopsies with benign results) but permits the diagnosis of cancers at a point in their growth when at least 50% of the invasive lesions are less than 1 cm in diameter and when 20% to 30% of the cancers are still intraductal. Higher positive predictive values can be achieved, but only at the expense of early detection.

Mammography

The primary role of mammography is to screen women with no symptoms to detect breast cancer at a smaller size and earlier stage than the woman's self-examination or her doctor's routine evaluation might ordinarily achieve. This has been shown to reduce or delay breast cancer mortality.[37–40]

Mammography is also used to evaluate women with palpable abnormalities; however, its utility in this setting is limited.[41] The mammogram may reinforce the diagnosis of cancer and help to avoid overlooking a malignancy.[42] Rarely, the mammogram may show a clearly benign lesion, and a biopsy can be avoided (Fig. 4.2-4), but, because some palpable cancers are invisible mammographically, the study cannot be used to exclude cancer. If the clinical examination raises concern, *a negative mammographic result should not delay further investigation.*

FIGURE 4.2-4 This calcified fibroadenoma requires no further evaluation.

It is best to think of mammography primarily as a screening study. Management of a clinically apparent lesion must ultimately be determined by the clinical evaluation. Even among women with symptoms, mammography is used primarily for screening. Because mammography cannot be used to exclude breast cancer, and because the mammographic findings are frequently not specific in women with symptoms, its primary value for these women is to survey the remainder of the ipsilateral breast and to screen the contralateral breast to detect clinically occult cancer.[43]

Ultrasound

Ultrasound technology has evolved over many years. Original hopes that ultrasound could be an effective screening technique did not survive scientific scrutiny. Rigorous evaluation of whole-breast ultrasound proved both that ultrasound was incapable of detecting early-stage cancers with any reliability and that scanning the breast with ultrasound raised concern for suspicious areas that never proved to be malignant.[44]

Ultrasound instrumentation has improved significantly,

but it remains to be shown scientifically that improved imaging has any significant effect on the sensitivity or specificity of the technique.

For many years, investigators have hoped that the ultrasound measurement of blood flow using the Doppler effect would increase the ability of the technique to differentiate benign from malignant lesions. Because many breast cancers appear to have a substantial neovasculature (at the microscopic level), and because most benign lesions do not have increased blood flow, the rationale for Doppler imaging appears to be sound. Unfortunately, the clinical results have not been particularly convincing. Many cancers can be shown to have increased blood flow, particularly at their periphery. High-velocity flow seems to be almost only found in breast cancers.[45] Although preliminary reports suggested a high sensitivity and specificity for Doppler,[46] other studies were not as successful, suggesting poor discrimination between normal and cancerous tissues.[47] The most optimistic report concluded that "color Doppler signal in a lesion otherwise thought to be benign should prompt a biopsy, while the absence of signals in an indeterminate lesion is reassuring."[48] The clinical application of this determination is not particularly useful. It might provide an approach to lesions that are thought to be benign as additional reassurance, but, depending on the lesions placed in this category, the use of Doppler imaging would only add to the cost of care, given that these lesions would otherwise be untreated. Indeterminate lesions would still require cytologic or histologic confirmation.

Because benign lesions may exhibit increased flow and, more importantly, because a significant number of cancers (particularly those less than 1 cm in diameter) do not exhibit evidence of abnormal flow,[49,50] Doppler is not yet reliable for distinguishing benign from malignant lesions. Given the safety and accuracy of breast biopsy and the overlap of benign and malignant characteristics with Doppler imaging, it is difficult to rely on Doppler analysis. At this time, Doppler is not a clinically useful test for the evaluation of breast lesions.

Although continued investigation and development of ultrasound is strongly urged, it is likely that the sonographic characteristics of normal and abnormal breast tissues are such that the modality itself will never have greater use than cyst-solid differentiation and as a guide for selected interventional procedures.[51-53]

ULTRASOUND AND PALPABLE MASSES

The routine use of ultrasound in the evaluation of palpable masses remains controversial. If a palpable mass is shown ultrasonographically to be a cyst (Fig. 4.2-5), no reason exists to aspirate it. If ultrasonographic evidence of a cyst averts any further intervention, then its use to evaluate palpable lesions is efficacious. Some physicians, however, argue that a palpable cyst interferes with the clinical evaluation of the tissue under it and choose to aspirate these lesions. Other palpable cysts are aspirated because they are uncomfortable, or even painful, and still others are aspirated because the patient prefers not to have a lump. Aspiration has the advantage that the problem is simultaneously

FIGURE 4.2-5 A lesion that is round or oval with sharp anterior and posterior walls, no internal echoes, and enhanced posterior echoes is a benign cyst and requires no further intervention.

diagnosed and eliminated. If a lesion is to be aspirated, despite ultrasonographic evidence that it is a cyst, then the ultrasound will have been superfluous. In general, we only use ultrasound on palpable masses that have resisted aspiration but are still believed to be cysts. Occasionally, a cyst may have a thick wall or be sufficiently mobile as to defy clinically guided aspiration. Ultrasonographic evidence that these lesions are indeed cysts can avoid an excisional biopsy.

Because ultrasound may be an expensive and unnecessarily redundant procedure in the evaluation of palpable masses, the technique is primarily valuable for the analysis of lesions that are not palpable but are detected by mammography—principally solitary masses that approach 1 cm in size or larger. Sonographic analysis should be confined to cyst-solid differentiation, given that the differentiation of a benign solid mass from a malignant lesion is not reliably accurate.

Analyzing Lesions Detected by Mammography

Mammographic analysis should be systematic and proceed following the simple sequence:

Find it.
Is it real?
Where is it?
What is it?
What should be done about it?

FIND IT

The ability to detect early cancers is related to the quality of the mammogram. Cancers cannot be detected if the tissues in which they grow are not imaged because of poor positioning or because the film is improperly exposed or processed. High-quality mammography is required. As noted, double reading should be encouraged.

If previous mammograms are available, they should be compared with the present mammogram study to identify changes. New masses or indeterminate calcifications should be carefully evaluated because the breast is relatively stable on mammograms from year to year. Because changes may be slow to evolve and difficult to appreciate from one year to the next, it is best to compare the current study to one from at least two years previous.

IS IT REAL?

Most findings that may elicit concern on a screening study prove on follow-up imaging to be a benign superimposition of normal structures. Thus, before significant concern is raised, the radiologist should determine that a perceived abnormality is, in fact, three-dimensionally real. Numerous methods have been developed to accomplish this,[54] including repositioning of the breast and magnification mammography.

WHERE IS IT?

When a lesion has been found and confirmed as three-dimensionally real, its location in the breast should be established if further evaluation is indicated. This can be accomplished using altered mammographic positions,[55] ultrasound,[56] or computed tomography.[57]

WHAT IS IT?

The first major step in mammographic analysis is to determine whether the detected change can be categorized as a benign finding. If its morphology clearly indicates a benign structure, further evaluation is unnecessary. If it is not clearly benign, analysis should proceed.

After an anomaly has been detected, the interpreter should, in every instance, have specific reasons for rendering a specific interpretation. Thresholds and guidelines should be defined so that analysis is based not on subjective assessment, but on objective criteria. For example, it is not sufficient to say, "I think these are benign calcifications." One must be able to explain why they are categorized as such, for example, because they are smooth, round, larger than 1 mm, and have lucent centers. These benign characteristics support the interpretation.

The radiologist should report the type of breast tissues evident by mammography, ranging from the breast that appears to be almost entirely fat, to the breast that contains some fibroglandular densities, to the breast that is heterogeneously dense, to the breast that is extremely dense.

The American College of Radiology Reporting and Data System (BIRADS) has been designed to provide a dictionary of terminology and a report organization that ends in a decision-oriented final assessment of a mammogram.[58] This approach should be used and defines five assessment categories for grouping findings:

1. A negative mammogram. There is no abnormality to report.
2. A benign finding—negative. This indicates the presence of a lesion, such as a calcifying fibroadenoma, that the radiologist wishes to document so that a less experienced observer will not mistake it as a significant abnormality, while indicating that the overall mammogram shows no evidence of cancer.
3. A finding that is probably benign, but short interval follow-up is recommended. This assessment is directly comparable to the clinical situation where the clinician palpates an abnormality, believes that it is a benign change, but wishes to evaluate it over several months to confirm its regression or stability.
4. An abnormality that is indeterminate, but the risk for cancer is measurable, and a biopsy should be considered. This category is incompletely defined and may contain lesions that have a probability of malignancy from 2% to 5% (the solitary circumscribed mass) to as high as perhaps 40% to 50%. If the radiologist has sufficient data to permit accurate figures, the use of probabilities may be helpful for the patient and her physician.
5. A lesion that has the morphologic appearance indicating that it is likely to be breast cancer and needs to be biopsied.

The first, second, and last categories are fairly straightforward. Benign changes require no further evaluation. Changes suggesting malignancy require intervention. No data other than anecdotal reports indicate that the high-probability lesion requires additional evaluation other than a tissue diagnosis. Some suggest that, in cases in which conservation therapy (lumpectomy and radiation therapy) is to be used, additional evaluation in high-probability lesions may involve magnification views in an attempt to better define the extent of a lesion[59] or to search for multifocality.

Within the indeterminate category, additional evaluation using special views (especially magnification) may be useful to better refine the morphologic characteristics of the lesion and to develop probabilities for a specific type of lesion.

Mammographic Appearance of Breast Cancer

Breast cancer usually presents as one or a combination of the following:

- A mass
- Associated calcifications
- Architectural distortion
- Asymmetry (of architecture, tissue density, or duct dilatation)
- Skin or nipple changes

Skin thickening or retraction and nipple retraction or inversion are generally changes found in association with later-stage cancers and are usually evident on clinical inspection. Mammography should be done to emphasize the analysis of the breast tissues. High-contrast mammograms maximize the perception of breast cancer, and images should be obtained to permit assessment of the breast parenchyma, with imaging of the skin and nipples being of secondary importance.

ANALYZING CALCIFICATIONS

Analysis of calcifications includes an evaluation of their location, size, number, morphology, and distribution.

Location

The major determination is whether calcifications are truly intramammary or in the skin. This aspect may seem trivial, yet numerous women have had unnecessary surgery in attempts to remove calcifications that were in fact benign skin deposits.[60] It is not difficult to appreciate the fact that most skin calcifications project over the breast in two views, given that only thin portions of the skin are actually seen in tangent on two-view mammography. Tangential views of the skin containing the calcifications confirm the location of these particles.

Size

Breast cancers rarely produce calcifications larger than 1 mm, and most calcifications associated with breast cancer are under 0.5 mm in diameter.

Number

The use of a threshold number to categorize suspicious groupings of calcifications has caused much discussion. A figure of five per cubic centimeter has been derived from general experience and from a large series published by Egan and associates[61] in which the probability of malignancy was zero when fewer than five calcific particles were present in a volume of tissue. Obviously, this phenomenon is observational and not a fact of nature. Some cancers undoubtedly indicate their presence by forming fewer than five calcifications, but the statistical probability of malignancy increases with the number of calcifications. One must always consider the morphology and distribution of the calcifications when assessing their significance.

Morphology

Morphology is the most important element in the analysis of calcifications. The shapes of the particles and the heterogeneity of the shapes and sizes are frequently valuable in determining the likely cause of the deposits. A better understanding of the microscopic histologic and pathologic environment in which calcifications form also helps us to understand the morphologic changes seen on mam-

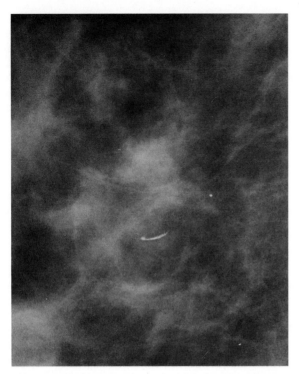

FIGURE 4.2-6 Calcifications, termed *milk of calcium,* that sink to the dependent portion of a cyst are a clear indication of a benign process.

mography.[62] Calcifications that can be categorized as the result of benign processes need no further evaluation.

Calcifications that form in the acinar structures of the lobule are virtually always benign. Probably due to the mold in which they form (the dilated acini), these calcifications are often smooth and round. Solid or lucent-centered spheres are almost always due to benign processes. Sedimented calcium that settles to the bottom of cysts formed by dilated acini are also benign forms of calcium deposits. The appearance of crescent-shaped calci-

fications that are concave on the horizontal beam lateral view (Fig. 4.2-6) can secure a benign mammographic diagnosis.[63]

Other lucent-centered calcifications include those that may form around the benign debris that can accumulate in ducts. Skin calcifications may also appear as lucent-centered calcifications.

Solid rod-shaped calcifications (Fig. 4.2-7), as well as lucent-centered, tubular forms, are usually due to calcifications within or around normal or ectatic ducts.[64] These forms of benign secretory calcification are almost always larger than 0.5 mm in diameter and can rarely be confused with malignant calcifications.

Very thin deposits associated with the rim of breast cysts are another form of calcification that should not elicit concern. These eggshell calcifications are only serendipitously associated with breast cancer. Thicker spherical deposits are usually due to fat necrosis (Fig. 4.2-8).

Vascular calcifications with their distinctive parallel-track appearance have such typical morphologic characteristics that they can be ignored.

The initial assessment of calcifications is made to determine whether they conform to these well-established benign morphologic presentations. If the characteristics of the calcifications are such that they cannot be reliably attributed to benign processes, additional evaluation is indicated. Magnification mammography is the primary technique used to further analyze calcifications. A clearer appreciation of the morphology and distribution of the calcifications is afforded by magnification, and this technique is used to ultimately decide, using objective criteria, whether a biopsy is needed to establish a firm diagnosis.

Calcifications that vary in size (most smaller than 0.5 mm) and shape are a cause for concern (Fig. 4.2-9). Calcifications due to breast cancer are either due to cellular secretion or to the calcification of necrotic cancer cells. Virtually all calcifications that form in breast cancers (including invasive lesions) form in the intraductal portion of the cancer. Although the multiplying cells can expand

FIGURE 4.2-7 These rod-shaped calcifications are benign secretory deposits.

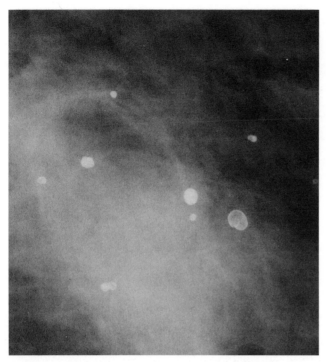

FIGURE 4.2-8 The spherical calcifications of fat necrosis.

the duct, the necrosis usually occurs irregularly in the duct's center. One study suggests that this process occurs when the tumor diameter enlarges beyond 180 μm.[65] The cells in the center become hypoxic as their distance from their blood supply increases, and eventually the center of the tumor becomes necrotic. Because this irregular process occurs at the center of the intraductal cancer, the calcifications formed are very small and irregular. Although these calcifications have been termed *casting,* they are actually the result of irregular patterns of tissue necrosis within cancers in a duct. Their distribution, however, is guided by the course of the duct and yields a very distinctive linear, branching (Fig. 4.2-10) pattern. This pattern of calcium distribution is known as comedonecrosis. In other cancers, the secretion of calcification into the cribriform spaces generated by some cancers probably accounts for the less characteristic patterns of calcium deposition.

Distribution

CLUSTERED. Many cancer calcifications form in nonspecific patterns. These calcifications are the most difficult to accurately analyze and are the cause of most benign biopsies. Heterogeneous calcifications whose pattern of distribution can only be termed *clustered* and cannot be accurately classified as benign may be caused by adenosis, peripheral duct papillomas, hyperplasia, and other benign breast conditions. Unfortunately, cancer can also produce these clusters of calcifications, and biopsy is needed to establish an accurate diagnosis.

SEGMENTAL. This distribution is thought to represent calcifications within a single duct network. A lobe or segment of the breast is defined by the major duct opening on the nipple and its branches spreading into the breast and terminating in its lobules. Many believe that breast cancer is a process that is initially confined to a single duct network. True multicentric cancer (involving multiple duct networks) is unusual, whereas multifocality (cancer at multiple sites within one duct network) appears to be relatively common.[66] Calcifications whose distribution suggests a duct network are of concern.

REGIONAL OR DIFFUSELY SCATTERED CALCIFICATIONS. Calcifications that appear to be randomly distributed throughout large volumes or throughout the breast are almost always benign. Although breast cancer can be extensive, such cases are unusual, and diffusely scattered calcifications are almost always due to benign processes.

ANALYZING MASSES

Masses should be evaluated based on their size, shape, margins, location and attenuation on radiographic evaluation.

Size

The size of a cancer at the time of diagnosis is a significant prognostic indicator.[67] Although the traditional staging of breast cancer uses 2 cm as the cutoff for stage I infiltrating cancers, even within stage I lesions a significant difference exists in prognosis that improves with the diminishing tumor diameter.[68] Many years ago, Gallagher and Martin[69] showed the benefit of finding infiltrating cancers 5 mm or smaller. This goal is desirable but difficult to achieve,

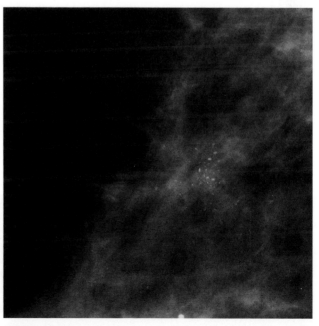

FIGURE 4.2-9 Heterogeneous calcifications of breast cancer.

FIGURE 4.2-10 The typical calcifications of a comedocarcinoma.

even with mammography. Several studies have looked at 1 cm as a threshold and have shown that finding infiltrating cancers smaller than 1 cm has a survival benefit that is almost as high as that achieved using a 5-mm threshold.[70–72] This goal is achievable. Since 1978, 57% of the infiltrating lesions detected by our screen have been under 1 cm. Certainly for spiculated and ill-defined masses, no size threshold should exist, and a biopsy should be recommended at any size for these lesions. For the most likely benign circumscribed mass, however, a threshold for investigation (ultrasound, aspiration, or biopsy) should be considered for solitary lesions approaching 1 cm in diameter.

Shape

Masses can be divided into round, oval, lobulated, and irregular shapes (Fig. 4.2-11). The probability of malignancy increases with these variations, depending on the appearance of lesion margins. An area of architectural distortion not associated with a mass in an area without prior surgery is frequently due to an underlying malignancy.

MARGINS. The interface between a lesion and the surrounding tissue is one of the most important factors in determining the significance of a mass (Fig. 4.2-12). Circumscribed masses whose margins form a sharp, abrupt transition with the surrounding tissue are almost always benign (Fig. 4.2-13). The halo of apparent lucency that can surround these masses is an optical illusion of the Mach effect[73] caused by the retina's appreciation of this abrupt transition between structures. Magnification mammography with increased resolution can increase the confidence of circumscription or show a less well-defined margin that should increase concern.

The microlobulated margin reflects the irregular surface that can be produced by a breast cancer. The irregular protrusions that form at a tumor's edge can form short undulations at the surface of the lesion when viewed mammographically.

An obscured margin occurs when the normal surrounding tissue hides the true edge of the lesion. The interpreter must decide whether a lesion's margin is obscured or truly infiltrative. The latter finding raises the level of concern.

Most breast cancers have an irregular interface as they invade the surrounding tissue. This produces the truly ill-defined margin that should raise concern. The probability of malignancy is high in lesions with ill-defined margins, although benign masses including cysts and fibroadenomas may have similar margins.

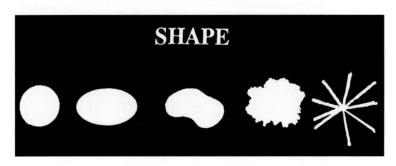

FIGURE 4.2-11 Round, oval, lobulated, irregular, and spiculated architectural distortion define the mammographic appearances of lesions.

FIGURE 4.2-12 The margins of a mass may be well circumscribed, obscured, microlobulated, ill-defined, or spiculated.

The classic breast cancer has a spiculated margin because of fibrous projections extending from the main tumor mass. Careful microscopic analysis of these projections shows associated cancer cells, although, by convention, the diameter of a cancer is measured across the tumor mass and excludes the spicules. Spiculated masses (or areas of architectural distortion that appear spiculated) should always undergo biopsy unless the distortion can be directly attributed to previous surgery. The analysis of breast lesions is thus aided by the presence of some historical information. Knowledge of previous surgery, the site of the incision, and, in particular, the site from which tissue was removed are important for the interpretation of both masses and calcifications. Architectural distortion is not uncommon during the first year after any form of breast surgery, but this distortion should resolve in almost all cases within 12 to 18 months.[74] Complete healing may be delayed if the breast has been irradiated. Postsurgical fat necrosis can produce calcifications that can be confusing.[75]

Sclerosing duct hyperplasia (radial scar) may produce spicules, and its likelihood can be suggested from morphologic criteria, but a biopsy is still required to make a safe diagnosis.[76]

Location

Location is primarily useful when the morphology of a mass suggests an intramammary lymph node. These findings are extremely common and are recognizably visible in about 5% of mammograms. Typically, these are reniform masses smaller than 1 cm with a lucent notch (Fig. 4.2-14) that occur at the edge of the breast tissue in the outer portions of the breast. They may be found as far as three quarters of the distance from the chest wall to the nipple.

X-Ray Attenuation

Lesions that truly contain fat (not those that merely appear to have or trap fat) are never malignant. The oil cyst form of fat necrosis that contains gelatinized fat defined by a thin capsule is characteristic. Lipomas and high-fat–content galactoceles present no diagnostic dilemma and are always benign. Similarly mixed-density hamartomas are always benign.

Most breast cancers have a higher radiographic attenuation than an equal volume of fibroglandular tissue, probably due to the dense fibrosis associated with these lesions. Many cancers are isodense, and some, such as colloid cancers, are less attenuating, thus giving this characteristic a less than perfect correlation. Benign lesions can also have

FIGURE 4.2-13 This cyst has a well-circumscribed margin.

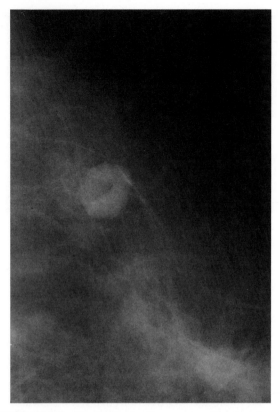

FIGURE 4.2-14   A typical benign intramammary lymph node.

higher attenuation. Cysts containing blood are frequently dense for their size.

OTHER FINDINGS

Other features involved in the assessment of a mass include skin and nipple changes and associated calcifications. Skin changes are occasionally useful, although they are usually equally or more evident on clinical evaluation. Skin thickening or nipple changes are often late findings in breast cancer. Only rarely are skin changes the predominant finding in an early breast cancer.

Pleomorphic calcifications that are under 0.5 mm found in association with a mass are of concern, as they would be if no mass were present. The presence of large (bigger than 0.5 mm) calcifications in a mass make it more likely to be a benign lesion such as an involuting fibroadenoma or papilloma.

Adjunctive Assessment

To arrive at a final assessment additional techniques beyond the standard two-view mammogram are useful. Magnification mammography results in an absolute increase in resolving capability. The morphology and number of calcifications are better appreciated using magnifi-

cation. The margins of masses are seen with greater clarity, and this feature may aid in the assessment of these lesions. One should use magnification carefully. The focal spot must be sufficiently small to permit the amount of magnification desired without the creation of geometric unsharpness. The use of the spot compression device to better spread overlapping structures can be combined with magnification, but the operator should recognize that spot compression may squeeze a true lesion out of the field of view, and, if a suspicious lesion seems to disappear with spot compression, this possibility should be considered. For as yet unexplained reasons, true architectural distortion may not be as evident on magnification. I therefore prefer to use spot compression without magnification as the first step in evaluating an area of architectural distortion. Other special views can be used to better visualize questionable lesions by rolling the breast[77] or angling the tube.

The use of ultrasound has already been discussed. I use ultrasound primarily in the assessment of mammographically detected nonpalpable lesions to differentiate cystic from solid masses. If ultrasound is to be relied on, strict criteria must be observed to safely diagnose a cyst. The margins should be well defined with sharply defined anterior and posterior walls. There should be *no* internal echoes, and posterior acoustic enhancement must be present. If any of these criteria are questionable, aspiration to confirm a cyst is prudent.

References

1. Fletcher SW, Black W, Harris R, et al. Report of the International Workshop on Screening for Breast Cancer. J Natl Cancer Inst 1993;85:1644.
2. Sickles EA, Weber WN, Galvin HB, et al. Mammographic screening: how to operate successfully at low cost. Radiology 1986;160:95.
3. Bird RE, McLelland R. How to initiate and operate a low-cost screening mammography center. Radiology 1986;161:43.
4. Revesz G, Kundel HL. Psychophysical studies of detection errors in chest radiology. Radiology 1977;123:559.
5. Bird RE. Professional quality assurance for mammographic screening programs. Radiology 1990;177:587.
6. Tabar L, Fagerberg G, Duffy S, et al. Update of the Swedish two-county program of mammographic screening for breast cancer. Radiol Clin North Am 1992;30:187.
7. Thurfjell EL, Lernevall KA, Taube AAS. Benefit of independent double reading in a population-based mammography screening program. Radiology 1994;191:241.
8. Moskowitz M. Screening is not diagnosis. Radiology 1979;133:265.
9. Sickles EA. Periodic mammographic follow-up of probably benign lesions: results of 3184 consecutive cases. Radiology 1991;179:463.
10. Elmore JG, Wells CK, Lee CH, et al. Variability in radiologists' interpretations of mammograms. N Engl J Med 1994;331:1493.
11. Kopans DB. The accuracy of mammographic interpretation. N Engl J Med 1994;331:1521.
12. D'Orsi CJ. To follow or not to follow, that is the question. Radiology 1992;184:306.
13. Kopans DB. Mammography screening for breast cancer. Cancer 1993;72:1809.
14. Sickles EA. Periodic mammographic follow-up of probably benign lesions: results of 3184 consecutive cases. Radiology 1981;179:463.

15. Peer PG, Holland R, Jan HCL. Age-specific effectiveness of Nijmegen population-based breast cancer-screening program: assessment of early indicators of screening effectiveness. J Natl Cancer Inst 1994;86:436.

16. Kopans DB. Efficacy of screening mammography for women in their forties. J Natl Cancer Inst 1994;86:1721.

17. Moskowitz M. The predictive value of certain mammographic signs in screening for breast cancer. Cancer 1983;51:1007.

18. Sickles EA. Nonpalpable, circumscribed, noncalcified solid breast masses: likelihood of malignancy based on lesion size and age of patient. Radiology 1994;192:439.

19. Cohen MI, Matthies HJ, Mintzer RA, et al. Indurative mastopathy: a cause of false-positive mammograms. Radiology 1985;155:69.

20. Bassett LW, Gold RH, Cove HC. Mammographic spectrum of traumatic fat necrosis: the fallibility of "pathognomonic" signs of carcinoma. AJR 1978;130:119.

21. Rouanet P, Lamarque JL, Naja A, et al. Isolated clustered microcalcifications: diagnostic value of mammography: series of 400 cases with surgical verification. Radiology 1994;190:479.

22. Kopans DB. The positive predictive value of mammography. AJR 1992;158:521.

23. D'Orsi CJ. To follow or not to follow, that is the question. Radiology 1992;184:306.

24. Kopans DB. Mammography screening for breast cancer. Cancer 1993;72:1809.

25. Sickles EA. Periodic mammographic follow-up of probably benign lesions: results of 3184 consecutive cases. Radiology 1981;179:463.

26. Rosen PP, Groshen S, Saigo PE, et al. A long-term follow-up study of survival in stage I (T1 N0 M0) and stage II (T1 N1 M0) breast carcinoma. J Clin Oncol 1989;7:355.

27. Tabar L, Fagerberg G, Day N, et al. Breast cancer treatment and natural history: new insights from results of screening. Lancet 1992;339:412.

28. Gisvold JJ, Martin JK. Prebiopsy localization of nonpalpable breast lesions. AJR 1984;143:477.

29. Meyer JE, Kopans DB, Stomper PC, et al. Occult breast abnormalities: percutaneous preoperative needle localization. Radiology 1984;150:335.

30. Rosenberg AL, Schwartz GF, Feig SA, et al. Clinically occult breast lesions: localization and significance. Radiology 1987;162:167.

31. Azevado E, Svane G, Auer G. Stereotactic fine-needle biopsy in 2594 mammographically detected non-palpable lesions. Lancet 1989;1:1033.

32. Parker SH, Lovin JD, Jobe WE, et al. Nonpalpable breast lesions: stereotactic automated large-core biopsies. Radiology 1991;180:403.

33. Elvecrog EL, Lechner MC, Nelson MT. Nonpalpable breast lesions: correlation of stereotaxic large-core needle biopsy and surgical biopsy results. Radiology 1993;188:453.

34. Kopans DB. Review of stereotaxic large-core needle biopsy and surgical biopsy results in nonpalpable breast lesions. Radiology 1993;189:665.

35. Sickles EA. Periodic mammographic follow-up of probably benign lesions: results of 3184 consecutive cases. Radiology 1981;179:463.

36. Sickles EA, Ominsky SH, Sollitto RA, et al. Medical audit of a rapid-throughput mammography screening practice: methodology and results of 27,114 examinations. Radiology 1990;175:323.

37. Shapiro S, Venet W, Strax P, et al. Periodic screening for breast cancer: the health insurance plan project and its sequelae, 1963–1986. Baltimore, Johns Hopkins University, 1988.

38. Tabar L, Gad A, Holmberg LH, et al. Reduction in mortality from breast cancer after mass screening with mammography. Lancet 1985;13:829.

39. Morrison AS, Brisson J, Khalid N. Breast cancer incidence and mortality in the breast cancer detection demonstration project. J Natl Cancer Inst 1988;80:17.

40. Tabar L, Gad A, Holmberg L, et al. Significant reduction in advanced breast cancer, results of the first seven years of mammography screening in Kopparberg, Sweden. Diagn Imag Clin Med 1985;54:158.

41. Kopans DB. Breast imaging and the "standard of care" for the "symptomatic" patient. Radiology 1993;187:608.

42. Meyer JE, Kopans DB. Analysis of mammographically obvious breast carcinomas with benign results on initial biopsy. Surg Gynecol Obstet 1981;153:570.

43. Kopans DB, Meyer JE, Cohen AM, et al. Palpable breast masses: the importance of preoperative mammography. JAMA 1981;246:2819.

44. Kopans DB, Meyer JE, Lindfors KK. Whole breast ultrasound imaging: four-year follow up. Radiology 1985;157:505.

45. Cosgrove DO, Bamber JC, Davey JB, et al. Color Doppler signals from breast tumors. Radiology 1990;176:175.

46. Schoenberger SG, Sutherland CM, Robinson AE. Breast neoplasms: duplex sonographic imaging as an adjunct in diagnosis. Radiology 1988;168:665.

47. Adler DD, Carlson PL, Rubin JM, et al. Doppler ultrasound color flow imaging in the study of breast cancer: preliminary findings. Ultrasound Med Biol 1990;16:553.

48. Cosgrove DO, Kedar RP, Bamber JC, et al. Breast diseases: color doppler US in differential diagnosis. Radiology 1993;189:99.

49. Dock W. Duplex sonography of mammary tumors: a prospective study of 75 patients. J Ultrasound Med 1993;2:79.

50. Dixon JM, Walsh J, Paterson D, et al. Colour doppler ultrasonography studies of benign and malignant breast lesions. Br J Surg 1992;79:259.

51. Bassett LW, Kimme-Smith C. Breast sonography. AJR 1991;156:449.

52. Jackson VP. The role of US in breast imaging. Radiology 1990;177:305.

53. Fornage BD, Faroux MJ, Simatos A. Breast masses: US-guided fine-needle aspiration biopsy. Radiology 1987;162:409.

54. Sickles EA. Practical solutions to common mammographic problems: tailoring the examination. AJR 1988;151:31.

55. Swann CA, Kopans DB, McCarthy KA, et al. Localization of occult breast lesions: practical solutions to problems of triangulation. Radiology 1987;163:577.

56. Kopans DB, Meyer JE, Lindfors KK, et al. Breast sonography to guide aspiration of cysts and preoperative localization of occult breast lesions. AJR 1984;144:489.

57. Kopans DB, Meyer JE. Computed tomography guided localization of clinically occult breast carcinoma: the "N" skin guide. Radiology 1982;145:211.

58. D'Orsi CJ, Kopans DB. Mammographic feature analysis. Semin Roentgenol 1993;28:204.

59. Sadowsky NL, Semine A, Harris JR. Breast imaging: a critical aspect of breast conserving treatment. Cancer 1990;65:2113.

60. Kopans DB, Meyer JE, Homer MJ, et al. Dermal deposits mistaken for breast calcifications. Radiology 1983;149:592.

61. Egan RL, McSweeney MB, Sewell CW. Intrammary calcifications without an associated mass in benign and malignant diseases. Radiology 1980;137:1.

62. Kopans DB. Breast imaging. Philadelphia, JB Lippincott, 1989.

63. Sickles EA, Abele JS. Milk of calcium within tiny benign breast cysts. Radiology 1981;141:655.

64. Levitan LH, Witten DM, Harrison EG. Calcification in breast disease: mammographic–pathologic correlation. Radiology 1964;92:29.

65. Mayr NA, Staples JJ, Robinson RA, et al. Morphometric studies in intraductal breast carcinoma using computerized image analysis. Cancer 1991;67:2805.

66. Holland R, Hendriks JHCL, Verbeck ALM, et al. Extent, distribution, and mammographic/histological correlations of breast ductal carcinoma in situ. Lancet 1990;335:519.

67. Carter CL, Allen C, Henson DE. Relation of tumor size, lymph node status, and survival in 24,740 breast cancer cases. Cancer 1989;63:181.

68. Rosen PP, Groshen PE, Kinne DW, et al. A long-term follow-up study of survival in stage I (T1,N0,M0) and stage II (T1,N1,M0) breast carcinoma. J Clin Oncol 1989;7:355.

69. Gallagher HS, Martin JE. Early phases in the development of breast cancer. Cancer 1969;24:1170.

70. Fisher B, Slack NH, Bross IDJ, et al. Cancer of the breast: size of neoplasm and prognosis. Cancer 1969;24:1071.

71. Tabar L, Duffy SW, Krusemo UB. Detection method, tumour size and node metastases in breast cancers diagnosed during a trial of breast cancer screening. Eur J Cancer Clin Oncol 1987;23:959.

72. Rosner D, Lane WW. Node-negative minimal invasive breast cancer patients are not candidates for routine systemic adjuvant therapy. Cancer 1990;66:199.

73. Swann CA, Kopans DB, Koerner FC, et al. The halo sign and malignant breast lesions. AJR 1987;149:1145.

74. Sickles EA, Herzog KA. Mammography of the postsurgical breast. AJR 1981;136:585.

75. Bassett LW, Gold RH, Cove HC. Mammographic spectrum of traumatic fat necrosis: the fallibility of "pathognomonic" signs of carcinoma. AJR 1978;130:119.

76. Mitnick JS, Vazquez MF, Harris MN, et al. Differentiation of radial scar from scirrhous carcinoma of the breast: mammographic–pathologic correlation. Radiology 1989;173:697.

77. Swann CA, Kopans DB, McCarthy KA, et al. Practical solutions to problems of triangulation and preoperative localization of breast lesions. Radiology 1987;163:577.

4.3

New Methods for Breast Cancer Imaging

DORIT D. ADLER ▪ RICHARD L. WAHL

Mammography currently represents the best imaging modality for the early detection and diagnosis of breast cancer. Although numerous advances and improvements in mammography have occurred within the last decades and have greatly improved image quality, the technique is not without shortcomings resulting in limitations in the sensitivity and specificity of this breast imaging modality. Multiple areas of research have therefore been sought not only to improve film–screen mammography, but also to consider entirely new techniques in the study of breast cancer.

Although this review is not intended to include all methods currently under investigation, those chosen for discussion represent areas in which major efforts have provided data suggesting exciting future applications. These include magnetic resonance imaging (MRI), digital mammography, computer-aided diagnosis (CAD), positron emission tomography (PET), single-photon emission imaging, and computed tomography (SPECT).

Magnetic Resonance Imaging of the Breast

The breast was one of the earliest sites studied with MRI.[1-5] It became apparent, however, that no major advantages existed over conventional breast imaging methods as a result of the overlap in relaxation times between benign and malignant tissues. Interest in breast MRI waned until the introduction of MRI contrast agents, specifically gadolinium diethylenetriaminepentaacetic acid (Gd-DTPA). Within the last decade, numerous reports have been published addressing the potential role of contrast enhanced MRI in the detection and diagnosis of breast cancer.[6-15] Ongoing changes and improvements in MRI technology have resulted in the application of a large number of pulse sequences and acquisition methods.

The basic premise behind the value of contrast enhanced MRI is analogous to the concept of contrast-enhanced computed tomography (CT). Beyond approximately 2 mm in size, tumors must create neovascularity, resulting in marked further growth as well as the potential to invade and metastasize.[16,17] This so-called angiogenesis results in regions of hypervascularity, occurring predominantly at the periphery of the tumor and creating beds for pooling of contrast agents. Although angiogenesis is a critical feature in the growth of malignant tumors, it is not unique to the malignant neoplasms inasmuch as angiogenic benign tumors exist, and the hypervascularity associated with benign conditions such as inflammatory lesions likely accounts for some of the overlap in enhancement characteristics. Gadolinium is known to distribute in the extracellular space and to accumulate in tissues with expanded interstitial spaces as well as those with increased vascularity. Breast cancers have been shown to have increased capillary permeability as well as an enlarged interstitial space.[18]

Although the morphologic features of a lesion may provide some clue to its cause, the data on contrast-enhanced MRI of the breast have addressed various aspects of the enhancement behavior of breast lesions and tissues including the amount, speed, and shape of enhancement.[9,11,12,19-23] In response to these considerations, certain technologic features must be met for breast MRI, including the need for high resolution and rapid acquisition.

Three-dimensional (3D) MRI has many advantages over conventional two-dimensional (2D) techniques. 3D imaging is optimally suited for thin-slice studies because no gaps occur between slices and 3D has a much lower practical limit on slice thickness than 2D. This allows the detection of small enhancing lesions that might otherwise be missed if large-slice thicknesses were utilized. Many slices can be obtained in a short time for later image reformation in any plane. 3D pulse sequences favor short repetition times, and the overall use of more projections improves the signal/noise ratio by the square root of the number of slices.[13,24] Among the fast-scan sequences that have gained popularity in breast MRI are gradient-recalled acquisition in a steady state, fast imaging with steady precession, fast adiabatic trajectory in steady state, and fast low-angle shot.[8,9,22] These fast imaging sequences have a much higher sensitivity for Gd-DTPA when compared with the previously used spin echo sequences. Fat-suppression methods have also been utilized so that enhancing breast lesions that would appear bright on the MRI image would not be obscured by the otherwise bright surrounding fatty tissue.[13,14,25–27] Another method for elimination of fat signals involves subtraction of the entire set of precontrast images from the postcontrast set.[22,23]

Certain potential roles for MRI in the study of breast cancer have been identified. These include increasing sensitivity and specificity of breast cancer detection as compared with mammography,[8] identifying recurrences in women treated by lumpectomy and radiation therapy,[28,29] and monitoring response to chemotherapy.[26,30]

The potential role for MRI in identifying cancers not detected by conventional imaging methods has created great interest (Fig. 4.3-1). Proper identification of multifocal and multicentric carcinoma so that appropriate treatment choices are selected is critical in patient management. In this role, MRI should have no false-negatives, and technical requirements are rigorous. These requirements include high resolution (approximately 1 mm in all dimensions), fat suppression, and rapid acquisition.[8] Specialized sequences have been developed to fulfill this role, although many of them are not yet commercially available.[8,31]

Most published reports have shown that with contrast-enhanced MRI, breast cancers enhance with gadolinium[9–12,22,23,29,32–34] (Fig. 4.3-2). Cancers missed on this basis have been attributed to problems with technique or interpretation.[22] Insufficient doses of contrast and size of carcinoma smaller than the slice thickness have also resulted in some false-negative results.[34] If there is an absence of signal enhancement, carcinoma larger than the slice thickness can be excluded with a high degree of confidence. Preliminary data suggest that certain histologic types of cancer such as invasive lobular carcinoma may enhance weakly or not at all.[23,34] In limited nonrandomized studies that have focused primarily on problem cases, the sensitivity of breast MRI has ranged between 88% and 100%,[22,23,29,31] with 100% sensitivity reported in patients with recurrent carcinoma following radiation therapy.[22,29] As mentioned, however, the presence of contrast enhancement can result from either malignant or benign lesions. Because of this potential for false-positive diagnoses, the clinical utility of MRI for increasing the sensitivity of breast cancer detection cannot be realistically met without the availability of MRI-guided biopsy.[8]

Another potential role for breast MRI is in improving specificity of breast cancer detection, particularly when compared with mammography. A strong criticism of mammography has been the generation of large numbers of biopsies that prove benign. In this capacity, MRI need only display lesions seen on mammography. Therefore, there should be no false-negative results while minimizing false-positives inasmuch as the MRI is performed to decrease the number of false-positive biopsies generated by mammography. Technologic requirements for this role are much less stringent and more readily available than those required for increasing sensitivity. The true false-negative rate for breast MRI is currently unknown, however, because all reported series have been based on biopsy results of suspicious lesions. A more accurate estimate

FIGURE 4.3-1 A 68-year-old woman presented with an axillary mass that showed metastatic adenocarcinoma at biopsy. Mammogram (*not shown*) demonstrated no suspicious findings. Sagittal MR images before (**A**) and after (**B**) contrast administration demonstrate a large, irregularly marginated, enhancing mass in the inferior aspect of the breast (*arrows*). Histologic study showed invasive ductal carcinoma. (Harms SE, Flamig DP, Hesley KL, et al. MR imaging of the breast with rotating delivery of excitation off resonance: clinical experience with pathologic correlation. Radiology 1993;187:493)

FIGURE 4.3-2 A 35-year-old woman noted a thickening in her left breast. **A.** Craniocaudal view from mammogram shows dense tissue and an area of architectural distortion (*arrows*) corresponding to the palpable finding. **B.** Coronal MR images before (*top*) and after (*bottom*) contrast administration shows a large area of abnormal contrast enhancement in the left lower outer quadrant (*arrows*). Histologic study showed invasive ductal carcinoma.

would require comparison of MRI results with serial sectioning of mastectomy specimens.[8] The specificity of MRI for breast cancer reported in certain series has been variable, with most results approximately 30% to 40%,[22,31] although some reports have achieved specificity as high as 97%.[22] One of the competitors for this MRI role is core needle biopsy, which provides histologic results. If this method is not employed, however, MRI could be used potentially to decrease the number of false-positive biopsies, a role achieved in many European centers.[8]

As previously mentioned, enhancement patterns have been studied in an attempt to differentiate benign and malignant tumors. The signal intensity of benign and malignant lesions is thought to be determined primarily by water content and fibrotic cells. Similar signal patterns may

therefore result from either benign or malignant lesions if both have high water content, high cellular content, or marked fibrosis.[22] In 1989, Kaiser and associates[9] reported that, in a small group of patients who had dynamic studies in which a section with a suspicious finding was imaged every 60 seconds for 10 minutes after contrast administration, all cancers showed rapid enhancement that essentially plateaued at 2 minutes, whereas benign lesions had a much lower increase in enhancement to 8 minutes, and by 20 to 30 minutes there was overlap between benign and malignant lesions. Stack and colleagues[11] found a significant difference between malignant tumors, which showed a steep increase in enhancement during the first 60 seconds after contrast administration followed by a smaller and more gradual increase, and benign lesions, which demonstrated a smaller overall increase in intensity at relatively slow rates. Dynamic MRI studies showed early contrast enhancement simultaneous with vascular enhancement 1 minute 34 seconds after contrast enhancement in 61 of 64 nonpalpable breast cancers reported by Gilles and associates.[23] Despite this 95% sensitivity, enhancement of benign lesions resulted in 53% specificity in the same series. These results suggest that early signal intensity measurements obtained immediately after gadolinium administration would provide better differentiation of benign from malignant disease. Other experts, however, have discontinued dynamic studies because some malignant tumors were found to enhance slowly, with a peak beyond 5 minutes.[22] As previously noted, some malignant tumors enhance poorly or not at all.[23,34]

The shape of enhancement has also been studied to provide an additional potential clue to the cause of a lesion.[22] Most carcinomas have been described as having focal, irregularly shaped enhancement, or enhancement along a duct, although diffuse enhancement, also seen in benign conditions, has similarly limited this type of analysis. Optimization of the dosage of contrast agent is also being addressed. Heywang-Kobrunner and colleagues[34] reported that conspicuity of malignant lesions was much improved using a higher dose of 0.16 mmol gadopentetate dimeglumine per kilogram of body weight compared with the more common dose of 0.1 mmol/kg. This included three small malignant foci visible only with the higher dose. No adverse reactions occurred, although the incremental cost of contrast agents is a disadvantage. In addition, no data for techniques other than the one used in this single series are currently available.

Among other applications of MRI in the breast cancer patient are the potential to identify residual or recurrent tumor and the ability to monitor treatment (Figs. 4.3-3 and 4.3-4). Studies have shown that postoperative scars older than 6 months do not enhance after contrast administration.[35] Recurrent tumor has been documented to en-

FIGURE 4.3-3 A 55-year-old woman has been treated for invasive ductal carcinoma of the right breast 6 years earlier. **A.** Mammogram shows increased density in the upper (*arrows*) and lower (*arrowhead*) breast. **B.** Dynamic MR image obtained 1 minute 34 seconds after contrast injection shows enhancement of several nodules in the breast and subcutaneous tissue (*arrows*). The scar tissue (*arrowheads*) does not enhance. Histologic study revealed multifocal invasive ductal carcinoma with cutaneous involvement. (Gilles R, Guinebretiere JM, Shapeero LG, et al. Assessment of breast cancer recurrence with contrast-enhanced subtraction MR imaging: preliminary results in 26 patients. Radiology 1993;188:473)

FIGURE 4.3-4 Invasive ductal carcinoma. Increased density in the retroareolar region and a small mass in the upper breast were seen on the mammogram (*not shown*). **A.** Diffuse enhancement of the retroareolar area (*left-pointing arrow*) with thickened enhancing skin (*right-pointing arrows*) is seen in the MR images following contrast administration. The mass seen on the mammogram also enhanced (not shown). **B.** Following chemotherapy, one sees marked reduction in the degree of postcontrast enhancement and skin thickening, although mild enhancement persists in the inferior aspect of the breast (*arrow*). (Harms SE, Flamig DP, Hesley KL, et al. MR imaging of the breast with rotating delivery of excitation off resonance: clinical experience with pathologic correlation. Radiology 1993;187:493)

hance. The additional use of a dynamic MRI subtraction study after gadolinium injection has allowed recurrent tumor to be differentiated from scarring and glandular tissue.[28] This method has also been shown useful in assessing residual tumor following chemotherapy.[30]

The field of breast MRI is evolving. Although exciting preliminary results have been obtained in the potential role of MRI in the earlier detection and diagnosis of breast cancer, striking factors have surfaced. Few patients have been reported in the English scientific journals.[22,23] Among results that appear most promising, the methods used are not universally available. Dose-comparison studies for a broad range of pulse sequences will be needed to identify optimal doses of contrast agent weighed against potential disadvantages. Lack of biopsy confirmation, particularly by MRI-directed methods, is a significant problem.[36] How does one confirm that a suspicious area seen on MRI has

truly been sampled? Even with radiographically guided localization methods, a certain percentage of lesions are not successfully removed at surgery.[37] How then can one rely on methods for which no guidance is available[9] and for which specimen MRI cannot be performed?

Even groups with the greatest experience disagree on which are the best methods.[22] There does, however, appear to be consensus that breast MRI as it currently exists should be confined to certain difficult clinical cases and that decisions for clinical management must be made in conjunction with mammographic and clinical information. Contrast-enhanced breast MRI should not be used as an isolated modality. As described by Heywang-Kobrunner,[22] existing problems for breast MRI include the lack of agreement on the optimal technique, the lack of agreement on interpretation guidelines, and the uncertain place of MRI in the diagnostic workup of the woman with a breast problem. Data for MRI of in situ carcinomas are extremely limited. Multiinstitutional trials are being designed and initiated both in the United States and elsewhere, to address many of these issues.[22]

Digital Mammography

Most experts agree that the next major strides in mammography will occur in the field of digital mammography.[37a] Marked improvements have already occurred in mammography as a result of improvements in design of dedicated mammographic units, development of new film–screen combinations, changes in breast positioning, and film processing. Although these areas continue to serve as foci for research, some inherent features of the mammographic film–screen system cannot be modified. Basic to this method is that film is performing multiple functions: it serves as the image acquisition detector as well as the means of displaying and storing the information. This combination of tasks results in compromises. Limitations exist in the range of radiographic exposures that can be recorded on film, and restrictions in the contrast that can be displayed may not allow more subtle lesions to be visualized. At high frequencies, noise in the imaging system is due to film graininess. If the tasks of image acquisition, display, and storage could be separated, each function could be optimized. Digital technology provides this opportunity.

Digital technology presents many potential advantages over conventional mammography.[38] Digital systems have a wide dynamic range, enabling a large field of exposure data to be handled. A wider range of tissue contrast can be seen, and subtle contrast differences can be amplified. A consistent response to radiation significantly reduces the need for repeat examinations secondary to exposure error. Computerized image processing techniques can be used and altered when the information is displayed, allowing enhancement of various image features. Image storage is much more efficient using high-quality computerized methods such as optical disks. Computerized applications also introduce the opportunity to utilize teleradiology, allowing image transmission to distant sites. In addition, computerized programs to aid in detection and diagnosis can be applied, as described in the next section of this chapter.

Digital detectors can be considered under the two broad categories of area detectors and scanned beam detectors.[38,39] In the latter, long acquisition times are involved because image acquisition occurs in a sequential fashion. Among area detectors, demagnification cameras have already found limited clinical utility in commercially available stereotaxic biopsy units. Utilizing this approach, a large-area phosphor is coupled to a small-area detector such as a charge coupled device using lenses or fiberoptic tapers. Current designs, however, offer only limited fields of view of approximately 5×5 cm^2. Other area detectors utilize photostimulable phosphors, amorphous selenium, or amorphous silicon.

Most reported series have used conventional mammograms that are then digitized, usually by means of high-resolution optical scanners.[40–43] Although many of the applications of digital technology can subsequently be applied, the quality of the digital image remains limited by the quality of the original information on the film. In addition, the time and cost to produce the conventional image have not been salvaged.

Among the strengths of conventional mammography are the excellent spatial resolution provided by film–screen combinations that can resolve on the order of 15 to 20 lp/mm. The requirements of a system with high spatial resolution and high contrast sensitivity have been among the challenges in developing a digital mammography system. The digital image is composed of a 2D matrix with numeric values corresponding to a picture element (pixel). The value of each pixel for a corresponding area in the breast is proportional to the amount of radiation passing through that area of tissue. Spatial resolution partly depends on pixel size, with improved resolution inversely proportional to that size. Practical limitations exist in the development of small pixel sizes, however, including cost and detector design.

Most studies to date have reported a spatial resolution of 0.1 mm per pixel for digital mammographic units corresponding to approximately 5 lp/mm,[40–42,44] focusing primarily on the ability of observers to detect lesions, especially calcifications, rather than classifying them. Classification would require more detailed information, to assess morphologic features. Investigators have postulated that, using image processing methods, the digital limitations in spatial resolution would be compensated, allowing detection comparable to that reported with conventional mammography.

An early study by Chan and associates[40] found that using a pixel size of 0.1 mm resulted in lower detection of microcalcifications than on conventional images. Karssemeijer and colleagues[41] found no change in detectability of small objects that would be representative of microcalcifications with digitization, whereas detectability was improved for low contrast objects. In the more challenging task of characterization of microcalcifications, this group similarly found no significant change with digitization compared with conventional studies. Oestmann and colleagues[44] tested the performance of a digitally acquired mammography system and also reported equivalent detectability of malignant microcalcifications using conventional images and digital images with 5 lp/mm resolution, although fewer individual calcifications could be resolved with the digital system.

Nab and associates[42] reported no difference in detectability of both microcalcifications and masses using a digital system with 0.1 mm per pixel spatial resolution, compared with the analogue images. The digital mammograms were viewed on a high-resolution monitor, and observers could manipulate contrast by adjusting window width and level. This might in part explain the improved results compared with those of Chan and colleagues,[40] in which hard copies of the digitized images used by the observers did not allow for interactive contrast manipulation.

Results of such early work employing digital mammography are particularly encouraging considering the foregoing study limitations. Many studies have involved few cases.[40,43–45] Some have had limited numbers of observers,[42–44] whereas others have included large numbers,[40,41] sometimes with a wide range of experience in interpreting mammograms.[40,41,45] In a study by Kimme-Smith and associates[45] in which microcalcifications were viewed on matched contact and microfocal spot magnification images and television-digitized enhanced images, inexperienced breast radiologists had more misdiagnoses with the TV-enhanced images. This finding might suggest that any one system may not provide uniform results, depending on observer experience. Some studies have included training sets of digitized mammograms,[41,42,44] whereas others have not.[40,43,45] Familiarization with this method is apparently needed because images may be different from those to which the radiologist is accustomed.[41]

Most existing studies have not approached a true clinical setting and have offered only single views,[41–43] including a disproportionate number of abnormalities, or have limited the time of film reading.[40] As stressed by Kimme-Smith and associates,[45] studies of digitally enhanced mammograms need to consider not only lesion detectability, but the ability to form diagnostic conclusions from such images. Although observers may subjectively prefer enhanced images, it remains to be shown that diagnostic accuracy would be improved.

The benefit of digital mammographic systems in interventional procedures has already been demonstrated in one reported series. Dershaw and colleagues[46] were able to decrease the time of needle-localization procedures by 50% without diminishing accuracy of the localization or the number of needle passes required. No significant increase in the number of images obtained was noted, and overall, an approximately 50% reduction in radiation dose was achieved. Despite these advantages, 17% of the procedures attempted could not be completed with the digital units, largely as a result of the small field of view (5 × 5 cm), the difficulty in imaging near the chest wall or axilla, and an inability to visualize some fine calcifications and soft tissue masses.

A pilot study to compare detectability of lesions on teleradiology-transmitted mammograms resulted in no significant differences for detection of masses or calcifications compared with conventional mammograms, although skin and nipple abnormalities were better detected by conventional methods[47] (Fig. 4.3-5). Although this early work also does not simulate the typical clinical setting, it suggests an important application of digital technology, particularly to facilitate consultation and to provide mammographic services at distant and underserved sites.

Although detector design represents a major challenge in development of digital technology, an appropriate display system must also be produced to meet the requirements of higher spatial resolution, greater brightness, and increased contrast compared with conventional television display systems.[39] The importance of developing digital mammography has been recognized and is pursued extensively, including collaborative efforts among federal and

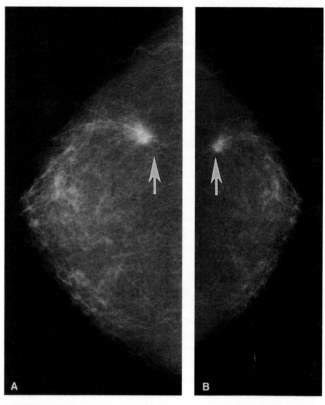

FIGURE 4.3-5 Craniocaudal views of a 1-cm spiculated carcinoma (*arrows*). Conventional screen-film (**A**) and teleradiology (**B**) images. (Fajardo LL, Yoshino MT, Seeley GW, et al. Detection of breast abnormalities on teleradiology transmitted mammograms. Invest Radiol 1990; 25:1111)

federally supported laboratories, academic institutions, and private industry.[15,39,48]

Computer-Aided Diagnosis

In approximately 15% to 20% of patients with breast cancer, the tumor is not seen on mammography. In some instances, missed detection may result from the subtle nature of the lesion. Observer factors such as distraction, fatigue, or oversight are also known to play a role. The area of CAD presents an exciting application and extension of digital technology. Computers can consistently scan all parts of an image without becoming tired or distracted.

CAD represents a computerized analysis of the radiographic information used by the radiologist as a "second opinion." The radiologist still decides the significance of the findings and makes appropriate recommendations. The goals of CAD are to improve mammographic sensitivity by increasing detection of potentially significant lesions and to improve specificity by reducing false-positive interpretations, ultimately reducing false-positive breast biopsies.

The two major areas of CAD in mammography fall

under the categories of detection and classification methods. These have been primarily directed toward study of microcalcifications and masses. Every subset of CAD has its own special set of requirements; for example, classification schemes require greater spatial resolution than detection schemes, and calcification detection necessitates finer digitization than does mass detection.

Numerous investigators have addressed these different applications, which are summarized in detail elsewhere.[49–51] In brief, Winsberg and associates[52] first described a method comparing density patterns in different areas of the same and opposite breast. Spiesberger[53] initially demonstrated the use of computers to detect microcalcifications. Although early research was limited by the state of computerized technology at the time, the plethora of recent publications in this area attests to the renewed interest resulting from advances in digital computer technology and the increased use of mammography.[50,54]

Chan and coworkers[55,56] reported on the feasibility of applying a specialized preprocessing step known as the *difference image approach* for the detection of microcalcification clusters (Fig. 4.3-6A). In this technique, a signal-suppressed image is subtracted from a signal-enhanced image to remove structured background (see Fig. 4.3-6B). Signal extraction methods based on size, contrast, number, and clustering of signals are applied to isolate calcification clusters from remaining background noise. A final digital image identifying the suspicious computer-detected areas using circles or arrows can then be provided to the radiologist (see Fig. 4.3-6C). Although this preliminary study achieved an 82% true-positive detection accuracy with one false-positive detection per image, later work demonstrated that sensitivity for detection could be increased to 94%, with two false-positive detections per image for subtle microcalcification clusters that may be missed by radiologists (Chan et al, presented at the American Association of Physics meeting, July 1991). False-positive results have been reduced by 60% with an artificial neural network (ANN) trained to recognize microcalcifications.[57] Many other methods to detect calcifications have also been described.[58–60] Most CAD programs can be operated in a range of sensitivity with a trade-off in specificity. The appropriate operating point in clinical practice has yet to be determined, based on the patient population and other considerations.

Detection of masses has been approached in various ways. Giger and Yin and their colleagues developed an image-processing technique using multiple subtraction images to enhance asymmetries between both breasts to detect subtle masses.[61,62] This bilateral subtraction method was reported to be better for initial detection of mammographic masses than for a single-image processing method.[63] Potential masses are identified based on optical densities, geometric patterns, and asymmetries between both breasts, with feature extraction techniques applied to decrease false-positive detections. Computerized methods have also used selected texture features to detect masses.[64]

Different approaches to image processing and feature analysis for detection of spiculation have been reported.[60,65] Kegelmeyer and associates[66] developed a method for analyzing local edge orientation to identify spicules, with every pixel in the image analyzed by the computer. The edge information was subsequently merged by the computer with local texture measures to eliminate false-positive detections with the algorithm alone achieving 100% sensitivity and 82% specificity (Fig. 4.3-7).

Other computerized applications have included techniques to classify mammograms as fatty or dense, based on the hypothesis that breasts that are automatically identified as dense, and potentially more difficult to interpret, could be examined by more experienced radiologists.[67] Giger and colleagues[68] developed a method to classify masses whereby border information is extracted to quantify the degree of spiculation. A preliminary study using texture features to distinguish between masses and normal breast parenchyma has demonstrated the feasibility of using such a classification scheme (Petrosian et al, unpublished data).

Nishikawa and colleagues[69] used ANN for decision making in mammography. ANN simulates human problem solving by learning from repeated presentation of examples. Using human extracted features, these investigators reported that ANN correctly classified all malignant cases (100% sensitivity), with 41% false-positive results, comparing favorably with radiologists, who achieved 89% sensitivity and 60% false-positive results for the same cases. Cheng and associates have shown the feasibility of training an ANN classifier to detect mass regions using texture features (unpublished data). Getty and Wu and their associates[70,71] reported that features merged by human observers can be merged by computers to arrive at a correct diagnosis.

In 1990, Chan and coworkers[72] showed that CAD significantly improved radiologists' accuracy in detecting clustered microcalcifications in a receiver operating characteristic study. This improvement occurred in experienced as well as in less expert mammographers. The investigators also analyzed the effect of the computer's false-positive rate on radiologists' accuracy in cluster identification. It appeared that, when the computer detected subtle calcifications also seen by the radiologist, the observer's confidence level increased. When the computer failed to detect more subtle clusters that were also likely missed by the radiologist, however, the radiologist might have been falsely reassured and prematurely stopped the search. Kegelmeyer and associates[66] found a statistically significant increase in radiologists' screening efficacy using a computerized method for detecting spiculated breast lesions. The algorithm increased the sensitivity of the average radiologists participating in the study by nearly 10% without decreasing average specificity. Subjectively, observers valued the computer for confirming a negative impression.

Astley and colleagues[60] studied factors affecting radiologists' perception of microcalcifications and the effects of cues on detection performance. Although these investigators also found that the detection performance of the observers was significantly higher with prompts than without, the observers required significantly longer to examine prompted than unprompted images.

FIGURE 4.3-6 **A.** General scheme for the automated detection of clustered microcalcifications on mammograms. **B.** Difference image. **C.** A single suspicious calcification cluster was isolated by the computer from remaining background noise (*not shown*). The computer-detected area is superimposed on the original mammogram. The scheme has correctly identified the malignant calcifications.

Giger and associates[73] used CAD schemes with a six-monitor view station as well as a single monitor system (Fig. 4.3-8). The six-monitor view station has been optimized for rapid retrieval and display of images including zoom and roam capabilities. Screen buttons allow the user to select cases, manipulate gray scale, and use CAD results.

Images can be viewed initially without CAD to allow an unassisted impression to be formed. To achieve the same goal, a delay mode has been adapted to a single monitor system.

CAD is still at a developmental stage. Even so, existing data suggest a promising and important role for this tech-

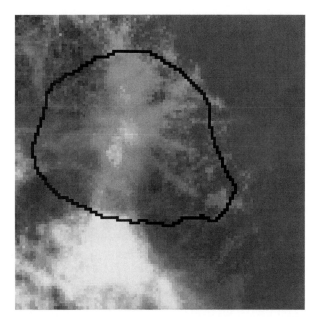

FIGURE 4.3-7 Computer detection scheme has correctly outlined a malignant mass. (Kegelmeyer WP, Pruneda JM, Bourland PD, et al. Computer-aided mammographic screening for spiculated lesions. Radiology 1994;191:331)

be challenging with current methods. PET may address these questions.

As do all nuclear medicine tests, PET shows physiologic changes in addition to localizing the process spatially, and it does so more quantitatively than other nuclear medicine procedures. Despite resolution superior to that of PET, standard anatomic methods such as CT and MRI remain limited in their capability to characterize masses as viable tumor or scar, in determining whether mildly enlarged lymph nodes represent tumor or a benign process, and in detecting small cancer foci less than 1 cm in diameter. Similarly, CT and MRI have not generally been successful in predicting whether cancers will respond to therapy. PET may answer some of these difficult diagnostic problems by supplying a quantitative metabolic characterization of tissues. The fusion (ie, 3D coregistration of data sets) of PET metabolic images and CT or MRI anatomy into "anatometabolic" images additionally provides a unique method for displaying complex anatomic and physiologic information in a single image.[75]

Initially, PET imaging studies in patients with breast cancer used carbon-11 (^{11}C)-labeled tracers to determine blood flow to the tumor or oxygen extraction or utilization by tumors.[76] An alternative radiopharmaceutical for PET has been ^{18}F–fluoro-17-β-estradiol, with specificity

nique in the future of breast imaging. Currently, different methods cannot be compared because various data bases comprising different cases and varying difficulty of cases are used.[54,74] One cannot automatically assume that a computerized scheme that has achieved a high sensitivity with one data base will achieve similar results with different data or in a true patient population. It is also unlikely that widespread application of CAD will be achieved until whole-breast direct digital systems become available, obviating the time and expense to digitize conventional mammograms. Because CAD is not used independently, however, its application need not await a perfect technique. It will likely be clinically useful before that stage, particularly if computer-detected lesions differ from those detected by the radiologist.

Positron Emission Tomography

Despite the progress noted previously, detecting breast cancer in younger women with mammographically dense breasts or in the surgically altered breast remains a challenge, as does determining which breast lesions require biopsy. Mammography is less sensitive in dense breasts and has a relatively low specificity. Once breast cancer is identified by conventional techniques, the only reliable method for determining whether tumor has disseminated to regional lymph nodes has been surgical removal and pathologic examination of the axillary nodes. Similarly, detecting and characterizing metastatic foci of tumor involvement in some soft tissues and bone can sometimes

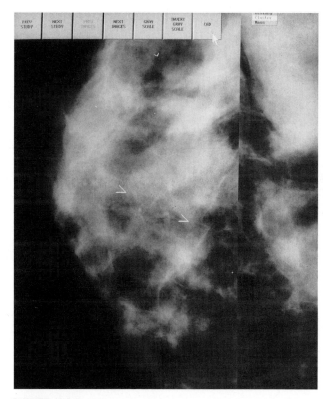

FIGURE 4.3-8 Computer-aided diagnosis (CAD) has detected a small cluster of microcalcifications in the midportion of the right breast. After use of the zoom feature, the calcifications are better visualized. Arrowheads indicate CAD output. (Giger ML, Doi K, MacMahon H, et al. An "intelligent" workstation for computer-aided diagnosis. Radiographics 1993;13:647)

for the estrogen receptors expressed on many breast cancers.[77] PET showed uptake of the radiotracer in the primary breast mass and the axillary nodes in 93% of estrogen receptor–positive tumors, and radiotracer uptake correlated positively with levels of estrogen receptors.[76] Imaging estrogen receptor–negative tumors was generally unsuccessful. This tracer approach is associated with moderate hepatic uptake of the tracer, which limits the utility of scans of the upper part of the abdomen.

Cancers generally have altered metabolism compared with normal tissues, which potentially can be detected using specific metabolic tracers labeled with positron emitters. The tracer most commonly applied for PET of tumors has been one that shows the excessive glycolysis of the tumor cell. Breast cancers have been shown to overexpress the glucose transport molecule GLUT1, which may contribute to increased glucose accumulation.[78] Fluorode-oxyglucose (FDG) is a structural analogue of glucose. In the absence of an inflammatory process, high FDG uptake into a tumor is most consistent with the presence of viable tumor cells.

Increased transport and utilization of several amino acids is also common in cancers. L-[methyl-^{11}C]-methionine PET has been used in the imaging of breast cancer. Initial data indicate that ^{11}C-methionine PET can be used to image large primary breast cancers, but it has limited value in imaging small lesions or lesions in the liver because of the high background uptake.[79]

The feasibility of imaging breast cancer using PET with FDG was demonstrated in several patients in 1989.[80,81] Subsequently, the feasibility of imaging primary, regional, and systemic metastases of breast cancer using FDG PET was shown in a larger series of patients in whom 25 of 25 known cancer foci (breast, regional lymph node, soft tissue, and bone) were detected. Of interest was the detection of primary tumors in several women with radiographically dense breasts. Feasibility studies have demonstrated that PET can show primary breast cancers in women with silicone breast implants.[82] Preliminary studies of FDG PET in staging for the presence or absence of axillary nodal metastases suggest significant promise for noninvasive staging of the axillary nodes[83–86] (Fig. 4.3-9). False-negative results have been reported, however, and fewer foci are seen on PET scans than on histologic examination. Other nodal groups such as internal mammary or supraclavicular

FIGURE 4.3-9 A. Axial PET scan demonstrates intense fluorodeoxyglucose (FDG) uptake (*arrows*) in the right breast, which is involved with inflammatory carcinoma. **B.** Intense FDG uptake seen in right axillary lymph node metastases (*arrows*).

nodes can also be imaged. This noninvasive staging application of PET warrants prospective trials to estimate carefully the accuracy of noninvasive staging and thus to assess whether the number of diagnostic lymph node dissections performed can be reduced.

Initial reports of PET imaging of primary breast carcinomas are encouraging, but this field is in its developmental stages. Most published studies have examined breast masses larger than 1 cm in diameter, in which sensitivity for cancer detection is nearly 100%. The accuracy of PET in characterizing smaller breast cancers has yet to be defined.[82,86] In breast masses larger than 1 cm, increased FDG uptake has been seen in cancers, whereas less FDG uptake has generally been seen in benign lesions. Indeed, preliminary reports suggest a greater than 90% accuracy in such characterization of mass lesions.[86] More study needs to be done to determine the accuracy of the FDG PET method, including its accuracy in detecting and characterizing small primary tumors, before the clinical utility of the method can be firmly defined. The resolution of PET scanners is improving, and machine performance characteristics and the technical approach to the study may affect accuracy. With higher-resolution scanning, PET may be expected to have increased applicability to detection and assessment of small primary lesions. In addition, correcting uptake for lesion size has become possible, probably allowing for enhanced accuracy in assessing small lesions.[86]

An important consideration in PET tumor imaging is that the axial field of view of the PET camera is generally limited (15 cm or less). This limitation can be overcome by obtaining multiple scanning levels, but the number of levels that can be imaged is limited by the half-life of the tracer and its time to optimal tumor targeting.[85] This is particularly a problem for ^{11}C-labeled compounds, the half-life of which is 20 minutes.

For true quantitation of tracer uptake, transmission images are generally obtained to measure body thickness. Detailed imaging of a region of the body is recommended for the assessment of regional disease. Whole-body imaging, without attenuation, may be most appropriate to screen for metastatic disease, although its quantitative ability and, possibly, its sensitivity are less[83,85] (Fig. 4.3-10).

Interpretation of PET images is generally a form of "hotspot" imaging for most PET tracers. Simple quantification of images can be done by measuring tumor–nontumor uptake ratios using a digital computer or by determining the *standardized uptake value,* which reflects the uptake of the tracer in tumor or normal tissues.[87] Generally, the higher the standard uptake value, the more likely it is that malignant tumor is present. Accurately determining this value for small tumors is challenging, however, because of the limits of scanner resolution.

The quantitative features of PET suggest that it has a potentially important role as a noninvasive method of assessing tumor response to therapy. Tumors that have responded to a variety of treatments generally have much lower FDG or other tracer uptake than they did at the outset of therapy. Successful radiotherapy or chemotherapy is usually associated with a decline in tracer uptake compared with baseline pretreatment levels.

A prospective evaluation of PET during breast cancer

FIGURE 4.3-10 Whole-body posterior presentation of fluorodeoxyglucose (FDG) uptake shows small foci of FDG uptake (*arrows*). Normal FDG uptake is seen in the heart, bladder, and kidneys.

chemohormonal therapy showed that, in women treated with a multiagent regimen, the tumor FDG uptake declined rapidly and significantly, just 8 days after treatment was initiated. Further declines in tumor FDG uptake were apparent at 21, 42, and 63 days of treatment in the patients who went on to complete or partial responses assessed 6 months later, whereas no significant decline in FDG uptake was seen in the nonresponding patients when examined 63 days after initiation of treatment. This preliminary study also showed that the tumor metabolic changes preceded changes in tumor size.[88] These findings suggest that PET may have an important role as a noninvasive early indicator of treatment efficacy, and thus may have a possible role in planning chemotherapy.

Single-Photon Emission Imaging and Single-Photon Emission Computed Tomography

A disadvantage of PET imaging is the high cost of PET scanners and short half-life and, thus, the limited availability of cyclotron-produced radiopharmaceuticals. Although

PET scanner prices have continued to decline, and FDG is becoming more widely available, nuclear medicine imaging of breast lesions and cancers would be much more accessible to patients if more standard radiolabels (single-photon emitters) could be used for imaging. Standard nuclear medicine examinations such as the radionuclide bone scan performed with technetium-99m (^{99m}Tc)-diphosphonates are routinely used in the staging of high-risk tumors and in the follow-up of patients with such lesions. These single-photon studies are more commonly performed using the SPECT approach, which can help in detecting and locating small foci of cancer in bone. Because bone scans image the reaction of bones to tumor and not the tumor itself, this represents a limitation of the method.

SPECT scanning is also applied to hepatic imaging. In patients with hepatic lesions identified on CT or ultrasound, labeled red blood cell imaging can be particularly helpful in lesion characterization. Increased red blood cell uptake is essentially diagnostic of hemangioma, and for lesions larger than 1.5 cm in diameter, the technique is highly sensitive.

Single-photon imaging is routinely used to assess cardiac function (ejection fraction) both before and during chemotherapy. SPECT has also been applied to this method of imaging. Radiolabeled monoclonal antibodies reactive with breast cancer have been shown to localize and to allow imaging of many primary and metastatic tumor foci.[89,90] Absolute tumor accumulation of the antibodies relative to background levels and relatively long periods from tracer injection until imaging are limitations of the antibody approach, although it remains under intensive study. Smaller antibody fragments or peptides reacting with breast cancer and labeled with ^{99m}Tc possibly may be applied in this setting.

Two tracers previously used most extensively for cardiac imaging have been used for breast imaging. Thallium-201 (^{201}Tl), a radiopharmaceutical that reflects tumor blood flow and viable tumor cell number, has been reported to separate malignant from benign primary breast lesions more than 1.5 cm in diameter reasonably well.[91] Some benign lesions, however, do accumulate ^{201}Tl, and a positive ^{201}Tl study must be viewed as suggestive but not diagnostic of cancer. There has also been limited but rapidly expanding experience with the ^{99m}Tc-labeled organonitrile, ^{99m}Tc-sestamibi. This agent accumulates in many primary breast cancers to a greater extent than in normal breast, probably because of the active mitochondrial accumulation of the agent. Experience with this agent is limited, but it suggests a high negative predictive value for the test.[92,93] With both ^{201}Tl and ^{99m}Tc-sestamibi, planar and SPECT imaging can be done, but high-resolution planar imaging of the breasts has mainly been performed. Larger prospective trials with ^{201}Tl and ^{99m}Tc-sestamibi will be necessary to determine their role in evaluating primary breast lesions. The role of these agents in evaluating metastatic disease is not well defined but is probably less than for FDG, because studies in animal models have shown superior targeting of FDG than of ^{201}Tl to breast cancer. If ^{201}Tl, ^{99m}Tc-sestamibi, or FDG PET can help to segregate breast lesions into low– and high–cancer risk groups, the number of biopsies performed possibly can be reduced.

In summary, several metabolic and physiologic imaging methods that use nuclear medicine techniques are showing promise in breast cancer imaging. Before widespread clinical application can be expected, the precise role of these techniques will need to be defined through controlled prospective trials comparing metabolic imaging with other, more standard methods or with biopsy data and ultimately with patient outcome. Already, however, these methods are increasingly used to help solve selected problems in the management of known or suspected breast cancer, and single-photon imaging of bone, hemangioma, and cardiac blood pool is routine. Clearly, many breast cancers have altered metabolism compared with normal breast tissue and benign lesions. Exploitation of these metabolic differences in imaging should add specificity to anatomic imaging techniques and may, in some cases, replace them.

ACKNOWLEDGMENTS

The authors are grateful for the assistance of H.P. Chan and T. Chenevert and for illustrations provided by L. Fajardo, M. Giger, R. Gilles, S. Harms, W.P. Kegelmeyer, and W. Pierce. Dr. Wahl's work was funded in part by NIH grant no. CA 52880.

References

1. Bovee VM, Creyghton JH, Getreuer KW, et al. NMR relaxation and images of human breast tumors in vitro. Phil Trans R Soc Lond (Biol) 1980;289.
2. Mansfield P, Morris PG, Ordidge R. Carcinoma of the breast imaged by NMR. Br J Radiol 1979;52:242.
3. El Yousef SJ, Alfidi RJ, Duchesneau RH, et al. Initial experience with nuclear magnetic resonance (NMR) imaging of the human breast. J Comput Assist Tomogr 1983;7:215.
4. El Yousef SJ, Duchesneau RH, Alfidi RJ, et al. Magnetic resonance imaging of the breast: work-in-progress. Radiology 1984;150:761.
5. Stelling CB, Wang PC, Lieber A, et al. Prototype coil for magnetic resonance imaging of the female breast: work in progress. Radiology 1985;154:457.
6. Heywang SH, Hahn D, Schmid H, et al. MR imaging of the breast using gadolinium-DTPA. J Comput Assist Tomogr 1986;10:199.
7. Hachiya J, Seki T, Okada M, et al. MR imaging of the breast with Gd-DTPA enhancement: comparison with mammography and ultrasonography. Radiat Med 1991;9:232.
8. Harms SE, Flamig DP. MR imaging of the breast. J Magn Reson Imaging 1993;3:277.
9. Kaiser WA, Zeitler E. MR imaging of the breast: fast imaging sequences with and without Gd-DTPA. Radiology 1989;170:681.
10. Heywang SH, Wolf A, Pruss E, et al. MR imaging of the breast with Gd-DTPA: use and limitations. Radiology 1989;171:95.
11. Stack JP, Redmond OM, Codd MB, et al. Breast disease: tissue characterization with Gd-DTPA enhancement profiles. Radiology 1990;174:491.
12. Kaiser WA, Zeitler E. MR imaging of the breast: fast imaging sequences with and without Gd-DTPA: preliminary observations. Radiology 1989;170:681.

13. Pierce WB, Harms SE, Flamig DP, et al. Three-dimensional gadolinium-enhanced MR imaging of the breast: pulse sequence with fat suppression and magnetization transfer contrast. Radiology 1991;181:757.

14. Rubens DTO, Herman S, Chacko AK, et al. Gadopentate dimeglumine-enhanced chemical-shift MR imaging of the breast. AJR 1991;157:267.

15. Adler DD, Wahl RL. New methods for imaging the breast: techniques, findings, and potential. AJR 1995;164:19.

16. Jensen HM, Chen J, De Vault MR, et al. Angiogenesis induced by "normal" human breast tissue: a probable marker for precancer. Science 1982;218:293.

17. Blood CH, Zetter BR. Tumor interactions with the vasculature: angiogenesis and tumor metastasis. Biochim Biophys Acta 1990;1032:89.

18. Revel D, Brasch R, Paajanen H, et al. Gd-DTPA contrast enhancement and tissue differentiation in MR imaging of experimental breast carcinoma. Radiology 1986;158:319.

19. Haase A, Frahm J, Matthaei D, et al. FLASH imaging: rapid NMR imaging using low flip angle pulses. J Magn Reson Imaging 1986;67:258.

20. Frahm J, Haase A, Matthaei D. Rapid three-dimensional NMR imaging using the FLASH technique. J Comput Assist Tomogr 1986;10:363.

21. Orel SG, Schnall MD, LiVolsi VA, et al. Suspicious breast lesions: MR imaging with radiologic–pathologic correlation. Radiology 1994;190:485.

22. Heywang-Kobrunner SH. Contrast-enhanced magnetic resonance imaging of the breast. Invest Radiol 1994;29:94.

23. Gilles R, Guinebretiere JM, Lucidarme O, et al. Nonpalpable breast tumors: diagnosis with contrast-enhanced subtraction dynamic MR imaging. Radiology 1994;191:625.

24. Harms SE, Flamig DP, Griffey RH. Three-dimensional imaging. In: Higgins CB, Hricak H, Helms CA, eds. Magnetic resonance imaging of the body, ed 2. New York, Raven, 1992;199.

25. Flamig DP, Pierce WB, Harms SE, et al. Magnetization transfer contrast in fat-suppressed steady-state three-dimensional MR images. Magn Reson Med 1992;26:122.

26. Harms SE, Flamig DP, Hesley KL, et al. Fat-suppressed three-dimensional MR imaging of the breast. Radiographics 1993;13:247.

27. Merchant TE, Thelissen GRP, Kievit HC, et al. Breast disease evaluation with fat-suppressed magnetic resonance imaging. Magn Reson Imaging 1992;10:335.

28. Gilles R, Guinebretiere JM, Shapeero LG, et al. Assessment of breast cancer recurrence with contrast-enhanced subtraction MR imaging: preliminary results in 26 patients. Radiology 1993;188:473.

29. Lewis-Jones HG, Whitehouse GH, Leinster SJ. The role of magnetic resonance imaging in the assessment of local recurrent breast cancer. Clin Radiol 1991;43:197.

30. Gilles R, Guinebretiere JM, Toussaint C, et al. Locally advanced breast cancer: contrast-enhanced subtraction MR imaging of response to preoperative chemotherapy. Radiology 1994;191:633.

31. Harms SE, Flamig DP, Hesley KL, et al. MR imaging of the breast with rotating delivery of excitation off resonance: clinical experience with pathologic correlation. Radiology 1993;187:493.

32. Harms SE, Flamig DP, Helsey KL, et al. Magnetic resonance imaging of the breast. Magn Reson Q 1992;8:139.

33. Heywang SH, Wolf A, Pruss E, et al. MR imaging of the breast with Gd-DTPA: use and limitations. Radiology 1989;171:95.

34. Heywang-Kobrunner SH, Haustein J, Pohl C, et al. Contrast-enhanced MR imaging of the breast: comparison of two different doses of gadopentate dimeglumine. Radiology 1994;181:639.

35. Heywang SH, Hilbertz T, Beck R, et al. Gd-DTPA enhanced MR imaging of the breast in patients with postoperative scarring and silicon implants. J Comput Assist Tomogr 1990;14:348.

36. Hussman K, Reuslo R, Phillips JJ, et al. MR mammographic localization: work in progress. Radiology 1993;189:915.

37. Norton LW, Zelyman BE, Pearlman NW. Accuracy and cost of needle localization breast biopsy. Arch Surg 1988;123:947.

37a. Kopans D, Pleves D. Breast imaging: state-of-the art and technologies of the future. Presented at the National Cancer Institutes Consensus Conference. September, 1991.

38. Yaffe MJ. Digital mammography. In: Haus AG, Yaffe MJ, eds. Syllabus: a categorical course on the technical aspects of breast imaging: clinical aspects of breast cancer and mammography. Oak Brook, IL, Radiological Society of North America, 1993;271.

39. Winfield D, Silbiger M, Brown GS, et al. Technology transfer in digital mammography: report of the Joint National Cancer Institute. National Aeronautics and Space Administration Workshop, May 19–20, 1993. Invest Radiol 1994;29:507.

40. Chan HP, Vyborny CJ, MacMahon H, et al. Digital mammography ROC studies of the effects of pixel size and unsharp-mask filtering on the detection of subtle microcalcifications. Invest Radiol 1987;22:581.

41. Karssemeijer N, Frieling JTM, Hendriks JHCL. Spatial resolution in digital mammography. Invest Radiol 1993;28:413.

42. Nab HW, Karssemeijer N, Van Erving LJTHO, et al. Comparison of digital and conventional mammography: a ROC study of 270 mammograms. Med Inform 1992;17:125.

43. Kimme-Smith C, Bassett LW, Gold RH, et al. Digital mammography: a comparison of two digitization methods. Invest Radiol 1989;24:869.

44. Oestmann JW, Kopans DB, Hall DA, et al. A comparison of digitized storage phosphors and conventional mammography in the detection of malignant microcalcifications. Invest Radiol 1988;23:725.

45. Kimme-Smith C, Gold RH, Bassett LW, et al. Diagnosis of breast calcifications: comparison of contact, magnified, and television-enhanced images. AJR 1989;153:963.

46. Dershaw DD, Fleischman RC, Liberman L, et al. Use of digital mammography in needle localization procedures. AJR 1993;161:559.

47. Fajardo LL, Yoshino MT, Seeley GW, et al. Detection of breast abnormalities on teleradiology transmitted mammograms. Invest Radiol 1990;25:1111.

48. Shtern F. Digital mammography and related technologies: a perspective from the National Cancer Institute. Radiology 1992;183:629.

49. Giger ML. Computer-aided diagnosis. In: Haus AG, Yaffe MJ, eds. Syllabus: a categorical course on the technical aspects of breast imaging: clinical aspects of breast cancer and mammography. Oak Brook, IL, Radiological Society of North America, 1993;283.

50. Vyborny CJ, Giger ML. Computer vision and artificial intelligence in mammography. AJR 1994;162:699.

51. Vyborny C. Can computers help radiologists read mammograms? Radiology 1994;191:315.

52. Winsberg F, Elkin M, Macy J, et al. Detection of radiographic abnormalities in mammograms by means of optical scanning and computer analysis. Radiology 1967;89:211.

53. Spiesberger W. Mammogram inspection by computer. IEEE Trans Biomed Eng 1979;26:213.

54. Acharya RS, Goldgof DB, eds. Biomedical image processing and biomedical visualization. Proc SPIE 1993;1905:442, 690.

55. Chan HP, Doi K, Galhotra S, et al. Image feature analysis and computer-aided diagnosis in digital radiography. 1. Automated detection of microcalcifications in mammography. Med Phys 1987;14:538.

56. Chan HP, Doi K, Vyborny CJ, et al. Computer-aided detection of microcalcifications in mammograms: methodology and preliminary clinical study. Invest Radiol 1988;23:664.

57. Chan HP, Lo SC, Helvie MA, et al. Recognition of mammographic microcalcifications with artificial neural network. (Abstract) Radiology 1993;189:318.

58. Fam BW, Olson SL, Winter PF, et al. Algorithm for the detection of

five clustered calcifications on film mammograms. Radiology 1988; 169:333.

59. Davies DH, Dance DR. Automatic computer detection of clustered calcifications in digital mammograms. Phys Med Biol 1990;35:111.

60. Astley S, Hutt I, Adamson S, et al. Automation in mammography: computer vision and human perception. Proc SPIE 1993;1905:716.

61. Giger ML, Yin FF, Doi K, et al. Investigation of methods for the computerized detection and analysis of mammographic masses. Proc SPIE 1990;1233:183.

62. Yin FF, Giger ML, Doi K, et al. Computerized detection of masses in digital mammograms: analysis of bilateral subtraction images. Med Phys 1991;18:955.

63. Yin FF, Giger ML, Vyborny CJ, et al. Comparison of bilateral-subtraction and single-image processing techniques in the computerized detection of mammographic masses. Invest Radiol 1993;28:473.

64. Petrosian AA, Chan HP, Helvie MA, et al. Computer-aided diagnosis in mammography: detection of masses by texture analysis. Med Phys 1993;20:880.

65. Ng SL, Bischof WF. Automated detection and classification of breast tumors. Comp Biomed Res 1992;25:218.

66. Kegelmeyer WP, Pruneda JM, Bourland PD, et al. Computer-aided mammographic screening for spiculated lesions. Radiology 1994;191:331.

67. Hajnal S, Taylor P, Dilhuydy MH, et al. Classifying mammograms by density: rationale and preliminary results. Proc SPIE 1993;1905:478.

68. Giger ML, Yin FF, Doi K, et al. Investigation of methods for the computerized detection and analysis of mammographic masses. Proc SPIE 1990;1233:183.

69. Nishikawa RM, Giger ML, Doi K, et al. Computer-aided detection and diagnosis of masses and clustered microcalcifications from digital mammograms. Proc SPIE 1993;1905:422.

70. Getty DJ, Pickett RM, D'Orsi CJ, et al. Enhanced interpretation of diagnostic images. Invest Radiol 1988;23:240.

71. Wu Y, Giger ML, Doi K, et al. Artificial neural networks in mammography: application to decision making in the diagnosis of breast cancer. Radiology 1993;187:81.

72. Chan HP, Doi K, Vyborny CJ, et al. Improvement in radiologists' detection of clustered microcalcifications on mammograms: the potential of computer-aided diagnosis. Invest Radiol 1990;25:1102.

73. Giger ML, Doi K, MacMahon H, et al. An "intelligent" workstation for computer-aided diagnosis. Radiographics 1993;13:647.

74. Nishikawa RM, Giger ML, Doi K, et al. Effect of case selection on the performance of computer-aided detection schemes. Med Phys 1994;21:265.

75. Wahl RL, Quint LE, Cieslak RD, et al. "Anatometabolic" tumor imaging: fusion of FDG PET with CT or MRI to localize foci of increased activity. J Nucl Med 1993;34:1190.

76. Beaney RP, Lammertsma AA, Jones T, et al. Positron emission tomography for in-vivo measurement of regional blood flow, oxygen utilization, and blood volume in patients with breast carcinoma. Lancet 1984;1:131.

77. Mintun MA, Welch MJ, Siegel BA, et al. Breast cancer: PET imaging of estrogen receptors. Radiology 1988;169:45.

78. Brown RS, Wahl RL. Over expression of Glut-1 glucose transporter in human breast cancer: an immunohistochemical study. Cancer 1993;72:2979.

79. Leskinen-Kallio S, Nagren K, Lehikoinen P, et al. Uptake of 11C-methionine in breast cancer studied by PET: an association with the size of S-phase fraction. Br J Cancer 1991;64:1121.

80. Wahl RL, Cody RL, Hutchins GD, et al. PET imaging of breast cancer with 18FDG. Radiology 1989;173:419.

81. Kubota K, Matsuzawa T, Amemiya A, et al. Imaging of breast cancer with [18F]fluorodeoxyglucose and positron emission tomography. J Comput Assist Tomogr 1989;13:1097.

82. Wahl RL, Cody R, Hutchins GD, et al. Primary and metastatic breast carcinoma: initial clinical evaluation with PET with the radiolabeled glucose analog 2-(F-18)fluoro-deoxy-2-D-glucose (FDG). Radiology 1991;179:765.

83. Hoh CK, Hawkins RA, Glaspy JA, et al. Cancer detection with whole-body PET using 2-(18F)fluoro-2-deoxy-D-glucose. J Comput Assist Tomogr 1993;17:582.

84. Wahl RL, Cody RL, August D. Initial evaluation of FDG PET for the staging of the axilla in newly-diagnosed breast carcinoma patients. J Nucl Med 1991;32:981.

85. Tse NY, Hoh CK, Hawkins RA, et al. The application of positron emission tomographic imaging with fluorodeoxyglucose to the evaluation of breast disease. Ann Surg 1992;216:27.

86. Adler LP, Crowe JP, al-Kaisi NK, et al. Evaluation of breast masses and axillary lymph nodes with (F-18) 2-deoxy-2-fluoro-D-glucose PET. Radiology 1993;187:743.

87. Zasadny KR, Wahl RL. Standardized uptake values of normal tissues in FDG/PET: variations with body weight and a method for correction: "SUV-lean". Radiology 1993;189:847.

88. Wahl RL, Zasadny KR, Hutchins GD, et al. Metabolic monitoring of breast cancer chemohormonotherapy using positron emission tomography (PET): initial evaluation. J Clin Oncol 1993;11:2101.

89. Ryan K, Dillman RO, DeNardo SJ, et al. Breast cancer imaging with In-111 human IgM monoclonal antibodies: preliminary studies. Radiology 1988;167:71.

90. Kramer EL, DeNardo SJ, Liebes L, et al. Radioimmunolocalization of metastatic breast carcinoma using indium-111-methyl benzyl DTPA BrE-3 monoclonal antibody: phase I study. J Nucl Med 1993;34:1067.

91. Waxman AD, Ramanna L, Memsic LD, et al. Thallium scintigraphy in the evaluation of mass abnormalities of the breast. J Nucl Med 1993;34:18.

92. Campeau RJ, Kronemer KA, Sutherland CM. Concordant uptake of ^{99m}Tc-sestamibi and Tl^{201} in unsuspected breast tumor. Clin Nucl Med 1992;17:936.

93. Khalkhani I, Mena I, Jouranne E, et al. Prone scintimammography in patients with suspicion of carcinoma of the breast. J Am Coll Surg 1994;178:491.

Diseases of the Breast, edited by Jay R. Harris,
Marc E. Lippman, Monica Morrow, and Samuel Hellman.
Lippincott-Raven Publishers, Philadelphia, © 1996.

5

Management of Common Breast Disorders

5.1

Etiology and Management of Breast Pain

V. SUZANNE KLIMBERG

Breast pain in women was first described in the early 19th century by Sir Astley Cooper, who suggested that women who sought advice for breast pain were "usually of a nervous and irritable temperament."[1] This sentiment has persisted despite reports like that of Preece and coworkers,[2] who said that women with breast pain were no more psychoneurotic than those having an operation for varicose veins. Mastalgia remains a poorly characterized, underreported syndrome, but it is among the most frequent reasons for breast consultation in general practice.[3] When questioned, nearly 66% of women report breast pain, 21% of which is severe.[4] Only half of those with severe pain consult their general practitioner. Because of increasing awareness of breast cancer and the possibility that mastalgia may indicate disease, more women now seek advice for breast pain. Most physicians are ill trained for treating mastalgia, which often consists of balancing the management of relatively minor complaints against the side effects of treatment. Overall, 92% of patients with cyclic mastalgia and 64% of patients with noncyclic mastalgia can obtain a clinically useful response using a combination of reassurance, evening primrose oil, danazol, and bromocriptine.[5]

Evaluation of Breast Pain

CLINICAL ASSESSMENT

Patient assessment begins with a thorough history that includes diet, new medications, and a report of recent stress. Clinical examination, mammography, ultrasonogra-

phy, and needle aspiration are performed if indicated. A diagnosis of cancer must be considered in patients presenting with well-localized recent onset of breast pain. Preece and coworkers[6] reported on the importance of pain as a presenting symptom of breast cancer in a series of 240 patients with operable breast cancer over a 4-year period; 15% had breast pain as a presenting symptom, and 7% presented with mastalgia alone.[6] Jenkins and associates[7] reported that nearly one third of patients with subclinical cancers present with pain. Breast pain secondary to cancer is usually unilateral, persistent, and constant in position. Once clinical investigations exclude an overt pathologic process, subsequent neoplasia is rare (0.5%).[7] After informed reassurance, 60% to 80% of patients with mastalgia need no further intervention. If therapy is required, the patient is asked to complete a breast pain chart for at least two menstrual cycles using a visual analogue scale. This provides a baseline measurement of pain severity and allows classification into cyclic and noncyclic mastalgia.[8] This distinction is important because the likelihood of response to drug treatment differs for the 2 conditions; noncyclic pain tends to be more resistant to treatment than cyclic mastalgia. Musculoskeletal pain may be improved by analgesics or local injection of steroid or anesthetic agents.

CLASSIFICATION

Initial evaluation excludes breast pain from localized benign lesions of the breast that require needle aspiration or surgical therapy including painful cysts, fibroadenomas, subareolar duct ectasia, lipomas, fibrocystic change, and cancer. Breast pain is then classified into cyclic, noncyclic, and other causes.[8] Cyclic mastalgia presents most commonly during the third decade of life. Although the character of cyclic breast pain is usually bilateral, dull, burning, or aching, it can be unilateral and sharp, with radiation to the axilla or arm. Cyclic mastalgia usually starts 7 to 10 days before, and accentuating until the onset of, menses, when the pain dissipates. With premenstrual exacerbation, however, pain can persist throughout the cycle. The condition tends to be chronic, with resolution of symptoms at menopause. Spontaneous resolution occurs in about 22% of patients. Noncyclic mastalgia tends to occur a decade later, and duration is usually shorter, with spontaneous resolution in 50% of patients.[9] True noncyclic breast pain is unilateral, occurs in upper outer quadrants of the breast, and is associated with nodularity. Chest wall pain is always felt on the lateral chest wall or the costochondral junction.[10] Pain bears no relation to the menstrual cycle, but it may be exacerbated or disappear for no apparent reason. Mastalgia from other causes includes costochondritis, lateral extramammary pain syndrome,[11] cervical radiculopathy[12] or other nonmammary causes. Of cases referred to a dedicated mastalgia clinic in England, 67% were cyclic, 26% were noncyclic, and 7% were due to costochondritis.[13]

Histologic Correlates

Watt-Boolsen and colleagues[14] found no histologic differences in women with cyclic and noncyclic mastalgia and in patients with no symptoms. Histologic changes included proliferation of intraductal and periductal connective tissue, adenosis, papillomatosis, duct ectasia, intraductal debris, and mast cells. Jorgensen and Watt-Boolsen[15] reported finding fibrocystic changes in 100% of 41 women with breast pain who underwent breast biopsy. Although a higher incidence of fibrocystic change was seen than in asymptomatic controls, a causative role of fibrocystic disease in mastalgia is far from proved. The total incidence of breast abnormalities did not differ between groups in the Jorgensen study. Moreover, fibrocystic changes have been identified in 50% to 100% of breast specimens from "normal" women at autopsy.[16–18]

Etiology of Mastalgia

ROLE OF DIET

A relation between diet and breast pain was originally described for methylxanthines. Minton and associates[19,20] hypothesized that methylxanthines caused cellular proliferation in the breast by increases in cyclic adenosine monophosphate (cAMP), either by inhibition of phosphodiesterase breakdown of cAMP or by increased catecholamine release. Tissue from patients with breast disease showed unchanged phosphodiesterase activity, but had increased levels of adenylate cyclase and increased responsiveness to biochemical stimulation by methylxan-

thines.[21] These studies spawned many trials of caffeine or total methylxanthine abstention.

As with breast cancer, mastalgia is less frequent in Asians and in Eskimos, whose diets are lower in fat. The theory that fat increases endogenous hormone levels, and thus breast pain, has led to fat-restriction studies.[22] In addition, women with breast pain may have low plasma levels of γ-linolenic acid (GLA), an essential fatty acid.[23,24] The δ-6 desaturation step between linoleic and GLA is severely rate-limiting and is inhibited by high levels of saturated fats.[25] A higher ratio of saturated to unsaturated fatty acids leads to a hypersensitive state because of increased receptor affinity. This phenomenon has been shown for estrogen and progesterone. This finding has led to the hypothesis that essential fatty acid deficiencies may affect the functioning of breast hormone receptors and may produce a supersensitive state.[23,24] Administration of essential fatty acids in the form of evening of primrose oil (9% GLA) bypasses the blocked metabolic step, leading to a gradual reduction in the proportions of the saturated fatty acids[24] and attenuating the abnormal sensitivity of the breast tissue. Ghent and colleagues[26] theorized that the absence of dietary iodine may render terminal intralobular duct epithelium more sensitive to estrogen stimulation. This is the basis for iodine replacement studies.

ROLE OF HORMONES

Hormonal factors clearly play a role in the origin of cyclic mastalgia, as evidenced by the manifestation of the condition primarily during the ovulatory years with menstrual cycle–related symptoms that intensify premenstrually and subside with menses.[27] Hormonal imbalances proposed include an excess of estrogen,[28] progesterone deficiency,[29] changes in progestin/estrogen ratio,[30] differences in receptor sensitivity,[23] disparate secretion of follicle-stimulating hormone (FSH) and luteinizing hormone (LH),[31] low androgen levels,[32] and high prolactin levels.[33] Definitive evidence of hormonal abnormality in women with breast pain has been difficult to obtain, however, because of daily and circadian variations in plasma hormone levels.[34,35] Patient selection and sampling regimens may also account for conflicting observations.

Sitruk-Ware and coworkers,[36] in 66 patients with mastalgia versus 50 controls, and Walsh and colleagues,[37] in 82 patients with mastalgia versus 206 controls, studied 3 luteal-phase samples that showed no estrogen elevation in patients with breast pain. In two large studies, however, Sitruk-Ware and associates[30,36] showed decreased progesterone levels in mastodynia patients. Several other studies, by Walsh and colleagues,[38] England and associates,[39] and Kumar and coworkers,[31] failed to show such a progesterone deficiency. Mauvais-Jarvis and colleagues[29] theorized that luteal-phase insufficiency or progesterone deficiency leads to unopposed estrogen activity and an imbalance between estrogen and progesterone in the second half of the menstrual cycle.[30] This theory has been the basis of antiestrogen and progesterone therapy. Results of other studies point toward a prolactin secretory hypersensitivity for estradiol in patients with cyclic mastalgia. Watt-Boolsen and colleagues[40] demonstrated that basal serum prolactin, although within the normal range, was significantly elevated in 20 patients with mastalgia versus 10 controls. Walsh and associates[37] demonstrated prolactin elevation in severe breast pain, but not in moderate to mild pain. Kumar and colleagues,[31,35] Sitruk-Ware and coworkers,[36] Ayers and associates,[41] and Golinger and colleagues all reported no prolactin elevation in patients with breast pain over controls. Conflicting results may come from the pulsatile nature of prolactin secretion, as well as changes in prolactin secretion during acute emotional stress.[35] Cole and colleagues[33] demonstrated that prolactin is involved in the regulation of water and electrolyte balance in nonlactating breast. Increased serum prolactin may cause an influx of water and electrolytes in the breast, thus increasing water tension and causing pain. Further support for this theory comes from the observation of Blitchert-Toft and coworkers that breasts become smaller, softer, and less tender during prolactin-suppressive therapy.[43]

Several studies have shown a marked increase in prolactin secretion in women with mastalgia versus controls when stimulated with thyrotropin-releasing hormone (TRH).[31,35,41] Relative estrogen dominance is suggested as a cause of increased prolactin responsiveness to TRH. Initial studies suggest that thyroid hormones may antagonize the effects of estrogen at the pituitary TRH–receptor levels of lactotrophs.[35] Kumar and associates[31] found a generalized hypothalamopituitary abnormality in patients with cyclic mastalgia, compared with controls, by using a combined TRH and gonadotropin-releasing hormone test. This evidence led to the treatment of mastalgia with bromocriptine, a prolactin inhibitor.

Treatment of Mastalgia

As might be anticipated, numerous remedies are suggested for this ubiquitous condition of unknown origin that has a poorly understood relationship with fibrocystic breast disease and cancer. Double-blind placebo-controlled trials are required to prove drug efficacy because breast pain may resolve spontaneously (22% to 50%).[9] Patients have reported marked placebo responses (19%).[44] Bromocriptine, danazol, GLA, iodine, and tamoxifen have all been shown by such trials to be useful in treating breast pain. The safety, efficacy, and availability of these therapies, and other less-proven therapies, are discussed.

NUTRITIONAL TREATMENT

Nutritional factors have been less well documented than other regimens for treating breast pain. Although the least expensive and least prone to cause side effects, dietary changes are often the most difficult to institute in the noncompliant patient.

Methylxanthines

Minton and associates reported "complete disappearance of all palpable nodules and other symptoms" following dietary exclusion of methylxanthines in 13 of 20 women (65%)[45] and later in 37 of 45 (82.5%) women.[20] These studies have been criticized for methodologic weaknesses, including lack of a control group, lack of blinding, and failure to control for extraneous variables. The data of Minton and associates are supported by nonrandomized studies including retrospective data from 90 pairs of twins,[46] case control studies by Boyle and colleagues,[47] and most recently studies by Bullough and coworkers.[48] Ernster and associates[49] randomly assigned 82 of 158 women to methylxanthine abstinence and 76 to no dietary restriction. Palpable breast differences were minimally, but significantly, less. Only anecdotal improvement in premenstrual breast tenderness with the caffeine-free diet was reported. To document the instability of such clinical findings, Heyden and Muhlbaier[50] prospectively observed 72 women for 6 months, keeping methylxanthine intake constant. In 87% of breasts, a change in breast nodule number or position was noted. In 15%, nodules disappeared completely by the study's termination. Of the 32 women in the study who initially reported pain, 31% reported complete remission, and 16% demonstrated the typical waxing and waning characteristic of this disease. Several case-controlled studies have failed to demonstrate a relation between dietary caffeine or methylxanthine intake and fibrocystic change.[51–54] In a 4-month, single-blind randomized trial of 56 women (control: no dietary restrictions; placebo: no cholesterol; and experimental: no caffeine), caffeine restriction was not shown to lessen breast pain and tenderness.[55] Many clinicians continue to suggest methylxanthine restriction to patients with mastalgia on the grounds that no large-scale, unflawed prospective study has measured methylxanthines from all sources and has used reliable, dependent variables to assess pain. Likewise, no definitive evidence indicates a therapeutic benefit from caffeine restriction in mastalgia.

Dietary Fat

Boyd and coworkers[22] have shown that reduction of dietary fat to less than 15% of total caloric intake significantly improves cyclic breast tenderness and swelling after 6 months. This dietary manipulation is difficult to achieve, is difficult to monitor, and requires extreme compliance, however.[56]

Evening Primrose Oil (γ-Linolenic Acid)

Clinical experience with evening primrose oil for persistent mastalgia at the Cardiff Mastalgia Clinic produced 58% and 38% response rates with cyclic and noncyclic mastalgia, respectively.[5] The overall efficacy is similar to that of bromocriptine, but it is less than that of danazol. Evening primrose oil produces few side effects (2%), making it attractive.[5,57] In a placebo-controlled trial, evening primrose oil, 3 g/day, significantly improved the symptoms of pain and nodularity over placebo after 4 months.[58] In a double-blind crossover trial, 36 women with severe cyclic mastalgia and 8 with severe noncyclic mastalgia were randomly assigned to active or placebo arms of the study.[59] Controls received placebo for 2 months with crossover to evening primrose oil for 2 months; 16 of 38 (42%) completing 2 months and 9 of 18 patients (50%) who completed 4 months of therapy had a clinically useful response. In view of the low incidence of side effects and retrospectively reported equal efficacy with bromocriptine, evening primrose oil should be considered as a possible first-line treatment for mastalgia.[5] It is readily available over the counter.

Iodine

Ghent and colleagues[26] tested molecular iodine in a prospective, controlled, crossover study (145 patients) and in a controlled, double-blind study (56 patients). Subjective and objective improvement was reported in 65% to 74% of patients who received molecular iodine, 0.07 to 0.09 mg/kg. In controls, 33% had subjective placebo effect and 3% had objective deterioration. Molecular iodine was found to be nonthyrotropic and beneficial for breast pain. Studies have halted at the Virginia Mason Clinic because of the temporary unavailability of molecular iodine.

Vitamins

In spite of an early positive report of vitamin E administration,[60] well-controlled trials have failed to show a therapeutic role for vitamin E in mastalgia. Double-blind placebo trials by Meyer and associates[61] (in 105 women receiving 600 IU/d for 3 months), London and colleagues[62] (in 128 patients receiving 150, 300, and 600 IU/d for 2 months), and Ernster and coworkers[63] (73 patients receiving 600 IU/d for 2 months) reported no benefit for vitamin E. Similarly, randomized, double-blind, controlled trials of supplementation with vitamins B_1 and B_6 showed no proven benefit for mastalgia.[64,65] Properly controlled trials have failed to demonstrate a role for vitamins in the treatment of breast pain.

HORMONAL TREATMENT

Danazol

Danazol, the 2,3-isoxazol derivative of 17-α-ethynyl testosterone (ethisterone), is an attenuated androgen and the only drug approved by the US Food and Drug Administration for the treatment of mastalgia. At doses of 100 mg/d, it inhibits the mid-cycle surge of LH.[66] LH and FSH remain normal during treatment. Gonadotropin-releasing hormone administration results in depressed gonadotropin response. Danazol competitively inhibits estrogen and progesterone receptors in breast, hypothalamus, and pituitary,[67] as well as ovarian steroidogenesis.[68]

The first double-blind crossover study in 21 women with mastalgia comparing danazol at 2 doses, 200 and 400 mg/d, with placebo demonstrated a significant decrease in pain and nodularity scores in women taking danazol. The higher dose of danazol produced a better and more rapid clinical response; 30% of the women reported amenorrhea and significant weight gain.[44] The Hjorring Project[69] looked at mammographic changes in women with moderate to severe breast pain during and after 6 months of treatment with 200 or 400 mg/d danazol and saw sig-

nificant reduction in mean pain scores and mammographic density. Relapse was sooner when danazol was discontinued (9.2 versus 12.2 months) and greater (67% versus 52%) in women taking 200 versus 400 mg danazol per day. Because of dose-related side effects, Harrison and colleagues[70] and Sutton and O'Malley[71] tested low-dose danazol regimens. Patients who responded to 200 mg/d were then given 100 mg/d after 2 months, then 100 mg every other day,[71] or only during the second half of the menstrual cycle.[70] Serial reduction of the dose was continued monthly while the response was maintained using Harrison's regimen. Symptoms were controlled without side effects at a total average monthly dose of 700 mg. A complete response was maintained in 55%. Of 20 women, 13 (65%) had previously reported side effects; none did so on the low-dose regimen.

Gateley and associates[72] reported on 126 patients with refractory mastalgia. The response rate of patients with cyclic mastalgia was studied prospectively. When compared with EPO and bromocriptine, danazol was confirmed to be the most effective therapy irrespective of treatment order. Recommendations for the use of danazol are to start and maintain therapy at 100 mg twice daily for 2 months while maintaining a record of breast pain. If an incomplete response or no response is obtained, the dose is increased to 200 mg twice daily. If still no response occurs, another drug should be tried. Therapy should not continue longer than 6 months and should be tapered.

Gestrinone

Gestrinone, a 19-nortestosterone derivative, has androgenic, antiestrogenic, and antiprogestagenic properties. Gestrinone has at least three sites of action in the treatment of cyclic mastalgia. At the hypothalamopituitary level, the mid-cycle gonadotropin surge is inhibited. Gestrinone acts directly on the pituitary gland, on the ovary, and at the estrogen receptor of the mammary gland.[73] The efficacy and safety in cyclic mastalgia of gestrinone have been investigated in a multicenter trial[74]: 105 patients were randomly assigned to receive gestrinone, 2.5 mg twice a week for 3 months, or placebo. In the gestrinone-treated group, 55% of patients had a clinical response and 22% had a complete response, versus 25% and 2% on placebo, respectively. As an androgen derivative, the action and side effects of gestrinone are similar to those of danazol; however, the gestrinone dose required is much lower than that of danazol, that is, 5 mg/wk, versus 1400 to 2800 mg/wk. Its major side effect is contraceptive. Further trials with gestrinone are indicated.

Tamoxifen

Tamoxifen is a nonsteroidal triphenylethylene derivative that is an estrogen agonist–antagonist that competitively inhibits the action of estradiol on the mammary gland. In 1985, Cupceancu[75] first reported a 98% improvement in breast pain in an uncontrolled prospective study of tamoxifen, at 20 mg/d for 10 to 20 days each menstrual cycle, for two to six cycles. In a double-blind, controlled, crossover trial of tamoxifen, 60 women were randomly assigned to receive 3 months of tamoxifen, 20 mg/d, or placebo; 71% of the tamoxifen group and 38% of the placebo group had relief of pain.[76] After crossover, 75% on tamoxifen and 22% on placebo had mastalgia relief. Side effects were reduced with equal efficacy when the tamoxifen dose was lowered to 10 mg/d for 3 to 6 months, 65% at 20 mg/d and 20% at 10 mg/d.[77] Some reports have associated tamoxifen with the development of endometrial carcinoma.[78] Short-course tamoxifen, if used at all, should be reserved for patients whose symptoms are severe and in whom all standard therapies have failed.

Luteinizing Hormone–Releasing Hormone Agonist

Luteinizing hormone–releasing hormone (LHRH) analogues are effective in most cases of severe mastopathy. Their mechanism of action is incompletely understood. The potent antigonadotropic action of LHRH agonists induces complete ovarian inhibition, resulting in low blood levels of estradiol, progesterone, ovarian androgens, and prolactin.[79] The first randomized studies of the octapeptide analogue of LHRH, nafarelin, as a nasal spray showed a 50% response rate in mastalgia.[80] Monosonego and colleagues[81] enrolled 66 patients in a nonrandomized trial. All patients received intramuscular injections of a sustained delivery system of LHRH agonist for 3 to 6 months. A complete response ($N = 29$) or a partial response ($N = 30$) was seen in all patients. Hamed and coworkers[82] demonstrated an 81% overall response rate with LHRH analogue in both refractory cyclic and noncyclic mastalgia. Side effects can include hot flashes, myasthenia, depression, vaginal atrophy, decreased libido, visual disorders, and hypertension, but they usually do not require therapy cessation. LHRH agonist induces significant loss of trabecular bone, however.[83] For this reason, LHRH analogues should be reserved for severe refractory cases of mastalgia and are not used routinely or for longer than 3 months.

Thyroid Hormone

Carlson and associates[84] showed a response to thyroid hormone replacement in 16 of 18 patients with mastodynia and elevated TRH-induced prolactin responses; 13 patients had endemic goiter. In 17 patients with mastalgia who were given 0.1-mg doses of levothyroxine for 2 months, Estes[85] demonstrated that 47% obtained complete and 26% partial relief without side effects. Further studies are required before levothyroid can be recommended for mastalgia.

Progesterones

Several placebo-controlled trials with progesterone have shown no significant benefit for the patients with mastalgia.[64,86,87] Maddox and colleagues,[88] with a randomized, controlled, double-blind crossover trial of 20 mg of medroxyprogesterone acetate, again showed no benefit for patients with mastalgia.

NONHORMONAL TREATMENT

Bromocriptine

Bromocriptine is an ergot alkaloid that acts as a dopaminergic agonist on the hypothalamic–pituitary axis; one result is suppression of prolactin secretion. Mansel and associates[89] originally reported a double-blind crossover study in a group of patients with mixed breast pain using bromocriptine. These investigators reported their patients with cyclic, but not noncyclic, breast pain had lowered prolactin levels and clinical response. In a double-blind, controlled trial of danazol and bromocriptine, Hinton and colleagues[44] reported a clinical response in two thirds of patients with cyclic pain, but in none of those with noncyclic pain; bromocriptine was not as effective as danazol. The European Multi-Center Trial[90] of bromocriptine in cyclic mastalgia confirms the efficacy of bromocriptine. Side effects occurred in 45% of patients and were sufficiently severe to stop therapy in 11%. Side effects noted, which were nausea, vomiting, dizziness, and headaches, were reduced by incremental dose increases over a 2-week period. Bromocriptine, however, which is not approved for use in mastalgia, was recently banned for use in lactation cessation. Reports of serious side effects included seizures in 63 patients, strokes in 31, and fatalities in 9.[91]

Analgesics

Prospective randomized trials using oral analgesics have not been published.

Diuretics

Preece and associates[92] demonstrated no rationale for diuretics in mastalgia; premenstrual fluid retention in women with breast pain is no different from that in normal women.

Abstention From Medications

Recent start of any medication, especially hormones or phenothiazines, coinciding with the onset of breast pain should be suspect. Withdrawal of estrogenic drive by means of estrogen medication often can produce dramatic relief.[93]

PSYCHIATRIC TREATMENT

It is improbable that psychiatric disorders manifest as breast pain. Preece and colleagues did identify a small subgroup of patients (4%) who failed to respond to reassurance and treatment.[2] They suggested that psychiatric questionnaires be used to identify patients who are poor responders to therapy. This approach has not been tested in a prospective study. As with any chronic pain disorder, however, severe or resistant mastalgia can produce psychiatric morbidity. Jenkins and coworkers[7] showed that, of 25 patients with severe, resistant mastalgia, 16 had major depressive disorders. Physicians should be aware of this propensity and should be ready to treat with counseling or antidepressants.

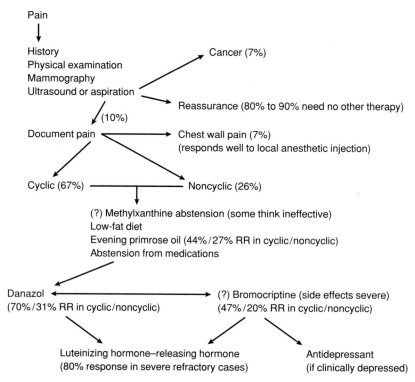

FIGURE 5.1-1 Algorithm for the management of mastalgia. RR, response rate.

SURGERY

Excision of discretely localized tender areas, known as trigger spots, shows a 20% failure rate.[94] Subcutaneous mastectomies, which were done more liberally in the past, should be reserved for the most refractory cases and should only follow considerable patient counseling. Surgery does not guarantee pain relief and carries the danger of replacing a painful area with a painful scar.

Treatment Algorithm

To establish the current treatment of cyclic mastalgia in the United Kingdom, Pain and Cahill[95] sent a postal questionnaire to 276 consultant general surgeons about their choices for persistent cyclic mastalgia after initial reassurance. Breast specialists tended to initiate treatments associated with fewer side effects (30% for evening primrose oil) and less cost, reserving danazol and bromocriptine for persistent pain. A suggested algorithm for breast pain management is shown in Figure 5.1-1.

MANAGEMENT SUMMARY

- The initial step in the evaluation of breast pain is a careful history to characterize the pain and a physical exam and mammogram (in women over age 35 years) to exclude the presence of a dominant breast mass.

- For women without a dominant mass, reassurance is sufficient therapy in about 80%.
- Patients seeking further therapy should keep a pain record for two menstrual cycles to quantitate the pattern and severity of pain and to allow a better estimate of the likelihood of a response to therapy.
- Evening primrose oil, danazol, and bromocriptine have all been shown to produce objective responses in women with mastalgia.

References

1. Cooper, A. Illustration of the diseases of the breast. London, Longman, 1829:1.
2. Preece PE, Mansel RE, Hughes LE. Mastalgia: psycho-neurosis or organic disease? Br Med J 1978;1:29.
3. Nichol S, Water WE, Wheeler MJ. Management of female breast disease by Southhampton general practitioner. Br Med J 1980; 281:1450.
4. Maddox PR, Mansel RE. Management of breast pain and nodularity. World J Surg 1989;13:699.
5. Gateley CA, Miers M, Mansel RE, et al. Drug treatments for mastalgia: 17 year experience in the Cardiff mastalgia clinic. J R Soc Med 1992;85:12.
6. Preece PE, Baum M, Mansel RE, et al. The importance of mastalgia in operable breast cancer. Br Med J 1982;248:1299.
7. Jenkins Pl, Jamil N, Gateley CA, et al. Psychiatric illness in patients with severe treatment-resistant mastalgia. Gen Hosp Psychiatry 1993;15:55.

8. Preece PE, Hughes LE, Mansel RE, et al. Clinical syndromes of mastalgia. Lancet 1976;2:670.

9. Gateley CA, Mansel RE. Management of painful nodular breast. Br Med J 1991;47:284.

10. Maddox PR, Harrison BJ, Mansel RE, et al. Non-cyclical mastalgia: improved classification and treatment. Br J Surg 1989;76:901.

11. Abramson DJ. Lateral extra mammary pain syndrome. Breast 1980;6:2.

12. LaBan MM, Meerschaert JR, Taylor RS. Breast pain: symptom of cervical radiculopathy. Arch Phys Med Rehabil 1979;60:315.

13. Wisbey JR, Kumar S, Mansel RE, et al. Natural history of breast pain. Lancet 1983;2:672.

14. Watt-Boolsen S, Emus H, Junge J. Fibrocystic disease and mastalgia. Dan Med Bull 1982;29:252.

15. Jorgensen J, Watt-Boolsen S. Cyclical mastalgia and breast pathology. Acta Chir Scand 1985;151:319.

16. Foote F, Stewart F. Comparative studies of cancerous versus noncancerous breasts. Ann Surg 1945;121:6.

17. Davis H, Simons M, Davis J. Cystic disease of the breast: relationship to cancer. Cancer 1964;17:957.

18. Rush BF, Kramer WM. Proliferative histologic changes and occult carcinoma in the breast of the aging female. Surg Gynecol Obstet 1962;117:425.

19. Minton JP, Foecking MK, Webster DJ, et al. Response of fibrocystic disease to caffeine withdrawal and correlation of cyclic nucleotides with breast disease. Am J Obstet Gynecol 1979;135:157.

20. Minton JP, Abou-Issa H, Reiches N, et al. Clinical and biochemical studies on methylxanthine-related fibrocystic disease. Surgery 1981;90:299.

21. Abou-Issa H, Bronn DG, Mousa S, et al. In vitro and in vivo effects of caffeine on cyclic nucleotide metabolism in mammary tissue. Fed Proc 1981;40:65.

22. Boyd NF, McGuire V, Shannon P, et al. Effect of a low-fat high-carbohydrate diet on symptoms of cyclical mastopathy. Lancet 1988;2:128.

23. Horrobin DF, Manku MS. Clinical biochemistry of essential fatty acids. In: Horrobin DF, ed. Omega-6 essential fatty acids: pathophysiology and roles in clinical medicine. New York, Wiley-Liss, 1990:21.

24. Horrobin DF. The effects of gamma-linolenic acid on breast pain and diabetic neuropathy: possible non-eicosanoid mechanisms. Prostaglandins Leuko Essent Fatty Acids 1993;48:101.

25. Sprecher H. Biochemistry of essential fatty acids. Prog Lipid Res 1982;20:13.

26. Ghent WR, Eskin BA, Low DA, et al. Iodine replacement in fibrocystic disease of the breast. Can J Surg 1993;36:453.

27. Andrews WC. Hormonal management of fibrocystic disease. J Reprod Med (Suppl) 1990;35:87.

28. Fechner RE. Benign breast disease in women on estrogen therapy. Cancer 1970;29:566.

29. Mauvais-Jarvis P, Sitruck-Ware AR, Kutten F, et al. Luteal insufficiency: a common pathophysiologic factor in the development of benign and malignant breast disease. In: Bulbrook RD, Taylor DJ, eds. Commentaries on research in breast disease. New York, Alan R Liss, 1979:25.

30. Sitruk-Ware AR, Sterkers N, Mowiszowicz I, et al. Inadequate corpus luteum function in women with benign breast diseases. J Clin Endocrinol Metabol 1977;44:771.

31. Kumar S, Mansel RE, Scanlon MF, et al. Altered responses of prolactin, luteinizing hormone and follicle stimulating hormone secretion to thyrotrophin releasing hormone/gonadotrophin releasing hormone stimulation in cyclical mastalgia. Br J Surg 1984;71:870.

32. Brennan MJ, Bulbrook RD, Dishponde N, et al. Urinary and plasma androgens in benign breast disease. Lancet 1973;1:1076.

33. Cole EM, Sellwood RA, England PC, et al. Serum prolactin concentrations in benign breast disease throughout the menstrual cycle. Eur J Cancer Clin Oncol 1977;13:597.

34. Mauvais-Jarvis P, Kuttenn F, Mowszowicz, et al. Mastopathies be-

nignes: etude hormale chez 125 malades. Nouv Presse Med 1977;6:4115.

35. Kumar S, Mansel RE, Hughes LE. Prolactin response to thyrotrophin-stimulating hormone stimulation in dopaminergic inhibition in benign breast disease. Cancer 1984;53:1311.

36. Sitruk-Ware R, Sterkers N, Mauvais-Jarvis P. Benign breast disease. I. Hormonal investigation. Obstet Gynecol 1979;53:457.

37. Walsh P, McDickens I, Bulbrook R, et al. Serum oestradoil-17β and prolactin concentrations during the luteal phase in women with benign breast disease. Eur J Cancer Clin Oncol 1984;20:1345.

38. Walsh P, Bulbrook R, Stell P, et al. Serum progesterone concentration during the luteal phase in women with benign breast disease. Eur J Cancer Clin Oncol 1984;20:1339.

39. England PC, Skinner LG, Cottrelle KM, et al. Sex hormones in breast cancer. Br J Surg 1977;62:809.

40. Watt-Boolsen S, Andersen AN, Blitchert-Toft M. Serum prolactin and oestradiol levels in women with cyclical mastalgia. J Horm Metab Res 1981;13:700.

41. Ayers J, Gidwani G. The "luteal breast" and hormonal and sonographic investigation of benign breast disease in patients with cyclic mastalgia. Fertil Steril 1983;408:779.

42. Zeppa R, Womack N. The role of histamine release in chronic cystic mastitis. Surgery 1962;52:195.

43. Blitchert-Toft M, Henriksen OB, Mygind T. Treatment of mastalgia with bromocriptine: a double-blind crossover study. Br Med J 1979;1:237.

44. Hinton CP, Bishop HN, Holliday HW, et al. Double blind controlled trial of danazol and bromocriptine in the management of severe cyclical breast pain. Br J Surg 1986;40:326.

45. Minton JP, Foecking MK, Webster DJT, et al. Caffeine, cyclic nucleotides and breast disease. Surgery 1979;86:105.

46. Odenheimer DJ, Zunzuneguie MV, King MC, et al. Risk factors for benign breast disease: a case controlled study of discordant twin. Am J Epidemiol 1984;120:585.

47. Boyle CA, Berkowitz GS, LiVolsi VA, et al. Caffeine consumption of fibrocystic disease: a case control epidemiologic study. J Natl Cancer Inst 1984;72:1015.

48. Bullough B, Hindei-Alexander M, Fetou HS. Methylxanthine and fibrocystic breast disease: a study of correlations. Nurse Pract 1990;15:36.

49. Ernster VL, Mason L, Goodson WH, et al. Effects of caffeine-free diet on benign breast disease: a randomized trial. Surgery 1982;91:263.

50. Heyden S, Muhlbaier LH. Prospective study of fibrocystic breast disease and caffeine consumption. Surgery 1984;96:479.

51. Lawson D, Jick H, Rothman K. Coffee and tea consumption and breast disease. Surgery 1981;90:801.

52. Marshall J, Graham S, Swanson M. Caffeine consumption and benign breast disease: a case control comparison. Am J Public Health 1982;72:610.

53. Lubin F, Wax Y, Black M, et al. A case-control study of caffeine and methylxanthines in benign breast disease. JAMA 1985;253:2388.

54. Schaierer C, Brinton LA, Hoover RN. Methylxanthines in benign breast disease. Am J Epidemiol 1986;124:603.

55. Allen SS, Froberg DG. The effect of decreased caffeine consumption of benign proliferative disease: a randomized clinical trial. Surgery 1987;101(6):720.

56. Vobecky J, Simard A, Vobecky JS, et al. Nutritional profile of women with fibrocystic disease. Natl J Epidemiol 1993;22:989.

57. Gateley CA, Pye JK, Harrison BJ, et al. Evening primrose oil (Efamol), a safe treatment option for breast disease. Breast Cancer Res Treat 1989;13:161.

58. Mansel RE, Pye JK, Hughes LE. Effects of essential fatty acids on cyclical mastalgia and non-cyclical breast disorders. In: Horrobin DF, ed. Omega-6 essential fatty acids: pathophysiology and roles in clinical medicine. New York, Wiley-Liss, 1990:557.

59. Gateley CA, Maddox PR, Pritchard GA, et al. Plasma fatty acid profiles in benign breast disease. Br J Surg 1992;79:407.

60. Abrams AA. Use of vitamin E in chronic cystic mastitis N Engl J Med 1965;272:1080.
61. Meyer EC, Sommers DK, Reitz CJ, Mentis H. Vitamin E in benign breast disease. Surgery 1990;107:549.
62. London RS, Sundaram GS, Murphy L, et al. Mammary dysplasia: a double-blind study. Obstet Gynecol 1985;65:104.
63. Ernster VL, Goodson WH, Hunt TKJ, et al. Vitamin E in benign breast disease: a double-blind randomized clinical trial. Surgery 1985;97:490.
64. Pye JK, Mansel RE, Hughes LE. Clinical experience of drug treatments for mastalgia. Lancet 1985;2:373.
65. Smallwood J, Ah-Kye D, Taylor I. Vitamin B6 in the treatment of pre-menstrual mastalgia. Br J Clin Pract 1986;40:532.
66. Greenblatt RB, Dmowski WP, Mahesh VB, et al. Clinical studies with the antigonadotrophin danazol. Fertil Steril 1971;22:102.
67. Chambers GC, Asch RH, Pauerstein CJ. Danazol binding and translocation of steroid receptors. Am J Obstet Gynecol 1980;136:426.
68. Barbieri RS, Canick JA, Makris A, et al. Danazol inhibits steroidogenesis. Fertil Steril 1971;22:102.
69. Tobiassen T, Rasmussen T, Doberl A, et al. Danazol treatment of severely symptomatic fibrocystic breast disease and long-term follow-up: the Hjorring Project. Acta Obstet Gynecol Scand 1984;123 (Suppl):159.
70. Harrison BJ, Maddox PR, Mansel RE. Maintenance therapy of cyclical mastalgia using low-dose danazol. J R Coll Surg Edinb 1989; 34:79.
71. Sutton GLJ, O'Malley UP. Treatment of cyclical mastalgia with low dose short-term danazol. Br J Clin Pract 1986;40:68.
72. Gateley CA, Maddox PR, Mansel RE. Mastalgia refractory to drug treatment. Br J Surg 1990;77:1110.
73. Snyder BW, Beecham GD, Winneker RC. Studies on the mechanism of action of danazol and gestrinone. Fertil Steril 1989;51:705.
74. Peters F. Multicentre study of gestrinone in cyclical breast pain. Lancet 1992;339:205.
75. Cupceancu B. Short tamoxifen treatment in benign breast diseases. Rev Roum Medendocrinol 1985;23:169.
76. Fentiman IS, Caleffi M, Brame K, et al. Double-blind, controlled trial of tamoxifen therapy for mastalgia. Lancet 1986;1:287.
77. Fentiman IS, Caleffi M, Hamed H, et al. Studies of tamoxifen in women with mastalgia. Br J Clin Pract 1989;43(Suppl 68):34.
78. Seoud MA-F, Johnson J, Weed JC. Gynecologic tumors in tamoxifen-treated women with breast cancer. Obstet Gynecol 1993;82:165.
79. Clayton RN. Gonadotrophin releasing hormone: from physiology to pharmacology. Clin Endocrinol 1987;26:361.
80. Roberts JV. Experience in the use of nafarelin for treatment of benign breast disease. Br J Clin Pract (Suppl) 1989;68:37.
81. Monosonego J, Destable MD, DeSaint FG, et al. Fibrocystic disease of the breast in premenopausal women: histohormonal correlation and response to luteinizing hormone releasing hormone analogue treatment. Am J Obstet Gynecol 1991;164:1181.
82. Hamed H, Caleffi M, Chaudary MA, et al. LHRH analogue for treatment of recurrent and refractory mastalgia. Ann R Coll Surg 1990;72:221.
83. Dawood MY, Lewis V, Ramos J. Cortical and trabecular bone mineral content in women with endometriosis: effective gonadotrophin-releasing hormone agonist and danazol. Fertil Steril 1989;52:21.
84. Carlson HE, Sawin CT, Krugman LG, et al. Effect of thyroid hormones on prolactin response to thyrotrophin releasing hormone in normal persons and euthyroid goiterous patients. J Clin Endocrinol Metab 1978;47:275.
85. Estes NC. Mastodynia due to fibrocystic disease of the breast controlled with thyroid hormone. Am J Surg 1981;142:764.
86. Dennerstein L, Spencer-Gardner C, Gotts G, et al. Progesterone and the premenstrual syndrome: a double-blind crossover trial. Br Med J 1985;290:1617.
87. Colin C, Gospard V, Lambotte. Relationship of mastodynia with its endocrine environment and treatment in a double blind trial with lynestrenol. Arch Gynecol 1978;225:7.
88. Maddox PR, Harrison BJ, Horrobin J, et al. A randomized controlled trial of medroxyprogesterone acetate in mastalgia. Ann R Coll Surg Eng 1990;72:71.
89. Mansel RE, Preece PE, Hughes LE. Double-blind trial of prolactin inhibitor bromocriptine in painful benign breast disease. Br J Surg 1978;65:724.
90. Mansel RE, Dogliotti L. A European multi-center trial of bromocriptine in cyclical mastalgia. Lancet 1985;335:192.
91. Arrowsmith-Lowe T. Bromocriptine indications withdrawn. FDA Med Bull 1994;24:2.
92. Preece PE, Richards AR, Owen CW, et al. Mastalgia and total body water. Br Med J 1975;4:498.
93. Maddox PR. Management of mastalgia in the UK. Horm Res 1989;32(Suppl 1):21.
94. Hinton CP. Breast pain. In: Blamey RW, ed. Complications and management of breast disease. London, Bailliere & Tindall, 1986:231.
95. Pain JA, Cahill CJ. Management of cyclical mastalgia. Br J Clin Pract 1990;44:454.

5.2
Nipple Discharge

DAVID P. WINCHESTER

Nipple discharge, although relatively common and usually benign in origin, can be frightening to women because of the widespread fear of breast cancer. It is difficult to estimate its true rate of occurrence because women seeking medical attention represent a subset of the population and are likely to be outnumbered by those not seeking attention. Spontaneous discharge from the nipple was reported in 10% of 2685 women undergoing routine health examination.[1] Because the most significant cause of nipple discharge is carcinoma of the breast, it is incumbent on physicians evaluating patients with nipple discharge to identify those requiring surgical evaluation.

Diagnostic Evaluation

Evaluation of the patient with nipple discharge should begin with a thorough history. It is important to differentiate spontaneous from induced discharge and unilateral from bilateral discharge. The character of the discharge should be categorized as potentially related to a neoplasm (serous, serosanguineous, bloody, or watery) or probably benign (various shades of green, gray, and brown). Persistent, nonpuerperal bilateral milky discharge may be caused by a pituitary adenoma, particularly when associated with amenorrhea, infertility, and visual field loss.[2] Further diagnostic evaluation should include determination of prolactin levels and, if persistently elevated, should be followed by computed tomography of the sella turcica region and visual field testing. Other endocrine causes of galactorrhea include hypothyroidism and various amenorrhea syndromes.[2,3] Other potential sources of galactorrhea are drugs (antihypertensives, oral contraceptives, phenothiazines, and tranquilizers) and transient hyperprolactinemia secondary to nipple stimulation and chest trauma, including thoracotomy.[4]

Physical examination of the breast for a mass associated with nipple discharge is important because the incidence of cancer increases with this finding.[5,6] Sequential quadrant compression and milking of the nipple–areola complex enables the examiner to determine whether the discharge is confined to one duct and to ascertain its location.

Guaiac testing of nipple discharge can identify occult blood and can aid in the categorization of the discharge as pathologic or physiologic.

The clinical features suggesting a benign or malignant neoplasm as the origin of nipple discharge and indicating the need for surgical evaluation include the following:

- Spontaneous discharge
- Unilateral localization
- Confinement to one duct
- Association with mass
- Bloody, serous, serosanguineous, or watery discharge
- Older age
- Male gender

Obviously, all these factors may not be present in the same patient, and a decision for surgical excision must depend on the judgment of the surgeon.

If the discharge is to be submitted for cytologic evaluation, an experienced cytopathologist must be available. The results of such testing, however, may be inconclusive

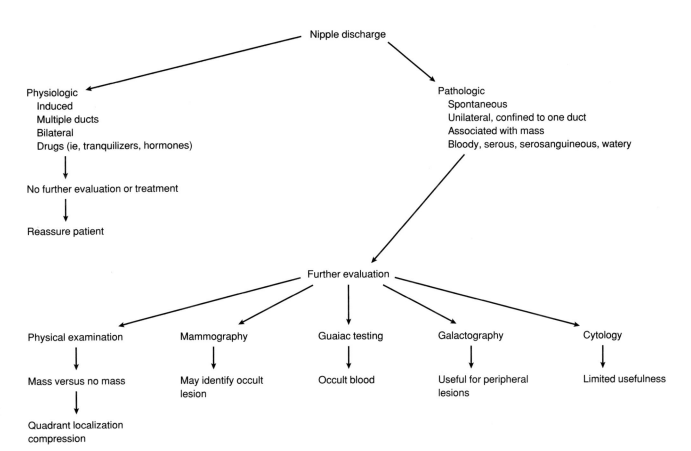

FIGURE 5.2-1   Evaluation of nipple discharge.

or misleading. In a collective review, Danforth and colleagues[7] reported a false-positive rate of 3% to 4% and a false-negative rate of 12% to 35% in patients with carcinoma. Based on 5305 cytologic examinations of nipple discharge, Ciatto and coworkers[8] advocated the selective use of cytology in patients with bloody nipple discharge. In this sample, 70% of the patients with carcinoma had bloody nipple discharge, most had positive cytologic results, and carcinoma was rarely detected in nonbloody nipple discharge. Cytology, however, will not accurately differentiate in situ from invasive breast cancers, and surgical excision should be done for persistent bloody nipple discharge, irrespective of cytologic findings. Thus, the clinical utility of this procedure is questionable.

Mammography should be part of the diagnostic evalua-

tion of nipple discharge of suspected neoplastic origin, but it is of little or no value in identifying lesions in patients with more frequent benign-type discharges.

Galactography, a specialized radiologic procedure involving contrast injection of the ductal system, is done in institutions where clinicians and radiologists have an interest in this technique. Advocates of this procedure[9–12] report accurate localization of lesions, allowing more conservative surgical excision. Accurate differentiation of benign from malignant lesions is not possible with galactography. The procedure is useful for distally or peripherally located lesions, which otherwise might be missed by standard major duct excision.

A negative galactographic, mammographic, or cytologic result should not deter surgical duct excision if a

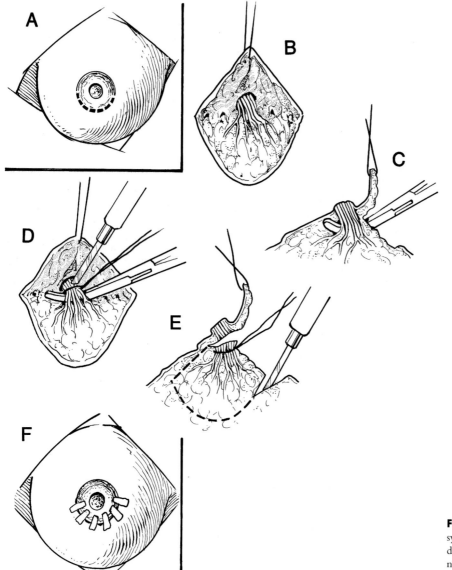

FIGURE 5.2-2 Excision of the major duct system. **A.** Circumareolar incision. **B.** Undermining areola. **C.** Isolating lactiferous sinuses. **D.** Transecting end of major duct system. **E.** Removing core of surrounding breast tissue. **F.** Closed incision.

FIGURE 5.2-3 Hematoxylin-eosin–stained histologic section of an intraductal papilloma of the breast (×16).

neoplasm is suspected. Figure 5.2-1 summarizes the evaluation of nipple discharge.

Surgical Treatment

Surgery for nipple discharge is indicated when a benign or malignant neoplasm is suspected. Surgical goals are to precisely define and treat the pathologic origin of the discharge and to eliminate a troublesome symptom.

The procedure can be done safely and comfortably in the outpatient setting and using only local anesthesia. Intravenous sedation is optional. The best cosmetic result can be expected from a circumareolar incision closed with a fine subcuticular suture. Re-approximation of breast tissue is neither necessary nor desirable. The placement of the incision may be influenced by preoperative clinical findings or galactography, but either complete terminal duct excision or single duct excision can be accomplished through a standard semicircular incision. The nipple flap is elevated and the ducts are divided close to the dermis to avoid missing the lesion. A selective duct excision is particularly appropriate for young women who desire

pregnancy and breastfeeding if the lesion can be completely excised. The technique for major duct excision is shown in Figure 5.2-2.

Pathology

The most common cause of nipple discharge identified from surgical specimens is solitary papilloma or papillomatosis, both of which are benign and seen in 35% to 48% of cases.[13–15] A papilloma is characterized by benign papillary epithelial cells (Fig. 5.2-3). Papillomas may be peripheral in location and may be missed by standard surgical duct excision. Ohuchi and colleagues[16] described 25 patients with peripheral papillomas, 6 of whom had concomitant ductal carcinoma in situ. Benign papillary lesions account for the infrequently observed patients with bloody nipple discharge during pregnancy.[17]

The next most common cause of pathologic nipple discharge is duct ectasia, a benign condition associated with loss of elastin within the duct walls and a chronic, usually plasma cell, inflammatory infiltrate. It has been reported in 17% to 36% of cases.[13–15,18]

The least observed cause of pathologic nipple discharge is carcinoma, which occurs with an incidence of 5% to 21%.[13–15,18] Generally speaking, when bloody nipple discharge is accompanied by a palpable mass, the tumor is invasive ductal carcinoma. Occult bleeding, however, is more often associated with ductal carcinoma in situ or papillary carcinoma.

References

1. Newman HF, Klein M, Northrup JD, et al. Nipple discharge: frequency and pathogenesis in an ambulatory population. NY State J Med 1983;83:928.
2. Kleinberg D, Noel G, Frantz A: Galactorrhea: a study of 235 cases, including 48 with pituitary tumors. N Engl J Med 1977;296.
3. Relkin R. Galactorrhea. NY State J Med 1965;65:2800.
4. Romrell L, Bland K. Anatomy and physiology of the normal and lactating breast. In: Bland K, Copeland E, eds. The breast: Comprehensive management of benign and malignant diseases. Philadelphia, WB Saunders, 1991;62.
5. Leis HP, Cammarata A, LaRaja RD, et al. Breast biopsy and guidance for occult lesions. Int Surg 1985;70:115.
6. Devitt JE. Management of nipple discharge by clinical findings. Am J Surg 1985;149:789.
7. Danforth D, Lichter A, Lippman M. The diagnosis of breast cancer. In: Lippman M, Lichter A, Danforth D, eds. Diagnosis and management of breast cancer. Philadelphia, WB Saunders, 1988;76.
8. Ciatto S, Bravetti P, Cariaggi P. Significance of nipple discharge: clinical patterns in the selection of cases for cytologic examination. Acta Cytol 1986;30:17.
9. Detraux P, Benmussa M, Tristant H, et al. Breast disease in the male: galactographic evaluation. Radiology 1985;154:605.
10. Osborne J. Galactography with contrast and dye: a two stage radiological/surgical approach to serous or bloody nipple discharge. Austral Radiol 1989;33:266.

11. Reid AW, McKellar NJ, Sutherland GR. Breast ductography: its role in the diagnosis of breast disease. Scot Med J 1989;34:497.
12. Baker KS, Davey DD, Stelling CB. Ductal abnormalities detected with galactography: frequency of adequate excisional biopsy. Am J Roentgen 1994;162:821.
13. Urban J, Egeli R. Non-lactational nipple discharge. CA Cancer J Clin 1978;28:3.
14. Leis H, Dursi J, Mersheimer W. Nipple discharge: significance and treatment. NY State J Med 1967;67:3105.
15. Murad T, Contesso G, Mouriesse H. Nipple discharge from the breast. Ann Surg 1982;195.
16. Ohuchi N, Abe R, Kasai M. Possible cancerous change of intraductal papillomas of the breast. Cancer 1984;54:605.
17. Kline TS, Lash SR. The bleeding nipple of pregnancy and postpartum period: a cytologic and histologic study. Acta Cytol 1964;8:336.
18. Chaudary M, Millis R, Daview G, et al. Nipple discharge: the diagnostic value of testing for occult blood. Ann Surg 1982;196:651.

5.3

Abnormalities on Physical Examination

JANET ROSE OSUCH

Although clinical breast examination (CBE) can detect a variety of abnormalities, by far the most common are those detected by palpation. This chapter provides a practical approach to the work-up and management of palpable breast abnormalities and describes ways to avoid the most common pitfalls in the timely diagnosis of breast cancer. Review Chapter 4.1, devoted to physical examination of the breast, to appreciate the careful, systematic approach CBE requires. However, nothing in the risk factor profile of an individual woman, nor in the clinical history of a self-discovered mass, rules out the possibility of breast cancer. In addition, the definition of a normal CBE is the absence of an abnormality, so interpretation of CBE can be challenging for even the most experienced clinicians.[1]

The clinical presentation of breast cancer can be subtle. Although it is correct that breast cancer presents as a three-dimensional hard mass, this understanding is incomplete. Any palpable finding not matched in a mirror-image location in the opposite breast is a reason for concern, including ill-defined asymmetric thickenings.[2-4] It is impossible to rule out breast cancer on clinical grounds alone. Failure to be impressed with physical examination findings was cited as the most common reason for a delay in the diagnosis of breast cancer in a 1990 study.[5]

Age Distribution of Palpable Abnormalities: General Guidelines

The four most common categories of breast masses are cysts, fibroadenomas, fibrocystic masses, and carcinoma.[2] The relative distribution frequency is age dependent, although all can occur at any age.[6] Fibroadenomas and fibrocystic masses are the most common causes of breast masses in women less than 25 years of age. It is uncommon for women in this age group to be diagnosed with either a breast cyst or breast cancer.[6,7] Fibroadenomas are perhaps the easiest breast mass to diagnose clinically, since the mass is smooth and mobile. In contrast, as women approach the fourth decade of life, breast cysts become common.

Although clinicians frequently reassure women that a self-reported breast mass is merely a cyst, it is impossible to distinguish a cyst from a solid mass by palpation alone.[4,7] One of the major responsibilities of the clinician is to establish that a palpable breast abnormality is a cyst and not a solid mass. This can be done with either needle aspiration or ultrasound, although needle aspiration is preferred because it provides simultaneous therapeutic drainage.[6,7] Palpable cysts should be drained for four reasons: (1) to establish the diagnosis of the cyst as benign, (2) to provide an expedient diagnosis, (3) to provide relief of pain in a woman who has a cyst under tension, and (4) to provide an optimal CBE interpretation free of interfering masses.

At the point in life when breast cysts become common, the incidence of breast cancer also rises steeply. During these perimenopausal years, the breast examination becomes difficult to interpret, and the cause of any palpable breast mass is impossible to predict with any certainty.[6] Postmenopausal women are much more straightforward. Any postmenopausal woman with a breast mass should be presumed to have carcinoma.[7] Before the widespread use of hormone replacement therapy (HRT), this clinical dictum was subject to little challenge. In some women, however, HRT influences postmenopausal breast tissue and converts it to perimenopausal breast tissue. This phenomenon has been shown clinically, mammographically, and histopathologically, but the explanation for its affecting only a subgroup of women remains elusive.[8]

Initial Diagnostic Work-Up of a Breast Mass

Initial management principles of a woman who presents with a breast mass are summarized in Figure 5.3-1 in algorithm format. The diagnostic approach to a breast mass varies only according to the age and menopausal status of the patient. Although suspicion that a breast mass may represent carcinoma may be low in premenopausal patients, this is a dangerous assumption. Although 78% of

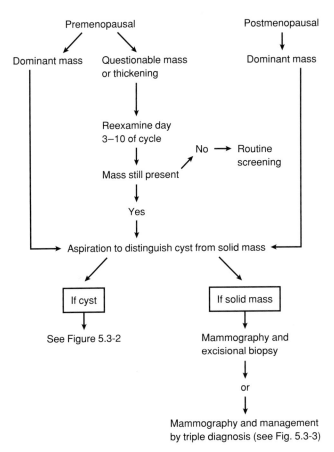

FIGURE 5.3-1 Initial evaluation of a breast mass.

women diagnosed with breast cancer are 50 years of age or older,[9] the sheer numbers of women diagnosed with the disease annually in the United States place a sobering perspective on its occurrence in premenopausal women. The American Cancer Society estimates that just over 40,000 women under 50 years of age were diagnosed with breast cancer in 1994. More women were diagnosed with breast cancer in this age group than with cervical and ovarian cancers across all age groups during that same year.[9] A recent review of the litigation literature found that 63% to 80% of women who sued physicians for a delay in the diagnosis of breast cancer were younger than 50 years.[4] This underscores the fact that any woman with a breast lump, no matter what her age, must have breast cancer included in the differential diagnosis.

Breast cancer can be an elusive diagnosis, especially in premenopausal women. It is more difficult to interpret CBE in premenopausal women, not only because the examination can differ markedly between women but also because the examination results can change depending on hormonal fluctuations in an individual woman's menstrual cycle. Because of this, the first step in evaluating a premenopausal woman with a potential abnormality is to examine her when ovarian hormones exert the least influence. Ideally, this is 3 to 10 days after the onset of menstruation.[2,3]

If a palpable asymmetric finding is present or persistent

in the above setting, full evaluation must ensue. This includes diagnostic mammography with the following caveat: in women less than 30 years of age, mammography is not recommended unless malignancy is strongly suspected.[10-12] Diagnostic mammography in a woman with a breast mass is ordered primarily to rule out occult lesions in noninvolved breast tissue and *not* to rule out cancer in the palpable abnormality.[6,7,10,13] Because mammography is less likely to demonstrate occult abnormalities in young women with dense breast tissue, and because the breast tissue of young women is much more susceptible to radiation exposure, the risks of mammography outweigh the benefits in this age group.[10-11] In women 30 years of age or over, diagnostic mammography is usually recommended. The work-up must proceed even if the mammogram is normal. False-negative results do occur, especially in premenopausal women, whose mammograms can be difficult to interpret secondary to dense glandular breast tissue.[4,5,7,10,11,13,14]

When work-up of a breast mass begins, the most important evaluation step is to distinguish whether the mass is cystic or solid. As discussed, this is most efficiently determined using fine needle aspiration.[3,7,11] This procedure requires no special skills other than stabilizing the mass so that needle aspiration can be done with precision. No special equipment is needed; a 22-gauge needle and a syringe suffice. There are no contraindications to this office procedure, which takes seconds and can usually be done without complications. Occasionally, hematoma formation can occur but can be avoided by applying firm pressure after the procedure. Pneumothorax can occur in inexperienced hands.[15]

If a clinician does not perform a definitive procedure to distinguish a cyst from a solid mass, the patient should be referred. It is unfortunate that the simple procedure of fine-needle aspiration is not routinely taught in medical school. It could save countless hours of anxiety for many women waiting to be seen by a specialist for a breast mass that proves to be a cyst.

The timing of needle aspiration of breast masses is important in relation to mammography. Documented false-positive mammograms have resulted in patients who had aspirations just before mammography due to small hematoma formation within the aspirated breast. If needle aspiration is done before mammography, the diagnostic mammogram should be delayed for 2 weeks after needle aspiration.[16] Although ultrasound is not recommended for evaluation of a palpable breast mass, similar false-positive results were found in a small series examining ultrasound findings after needle aspiration.[17]

Management of Breast Cysts

If the mass proves to be a cyst on aspiration, the fluid from it can be discarded unless it is grossly bloody, in which case it can be sent for cytopathologic examination. Excisional biopsy should be done, however, whenever gross blood is aspirated from a cyst to rule out intracystic carcinoma. It is important to document the exact location of the cyst before aspiration so that the excisional biopsy includes the involved area. The only other time that cytopathologic analysis of cyst fluid may be helpful is in postmenopausal patients who are not on HRT, since it is unusual for a woman to form a benign breast cyst in this setting.[6,7,10,11,18]

Other indications for excisional biopsy after cyst aspiration include a cyst that reaccumulates in the same location within 4 to 6 weeks of initial aspiration; this may be an indication of intracystic carcinoma as well. A routine part of the evaluation of every aspirated palpable breast cyst should be a 4- to 6-week follow-up examination that checks for cyst recurrence. Some clinicians reaspirate a rapidly recurring cyst once before open biopsy; if this is done, a second follow-up visit at a 4- to 6-week interval is necessary.

The objective of cyst aspiration is drainage of the entire cyst with subsequent collapse of the cyst wall. It is mandatory that palpation of the aspirated area occur after aspiration. If the mass has not totally disappeared, further work-up must commence; the residual mass needs to be treated the same as any solid mass.[6,7,10,11,18]

Principles of management of breast cysts are summarized as an algorithm in Figure 5.3-2.

Work-Up of a Solid Mass: Fine-Needle Aspiration Biopsy

When a mass is aspirated and found to be solid, excisional biopsy is usually the next step. Certainly, surgical referral is necessary at this point, unless the clinician is comfortable with and experienced in the application of fine-needle aspiration biopsy (FNAB) in the evaluation of a breast mass and uses it on a routine basis. The technique of FNAB differs significantly from simple fine-needle aspiration to determine whether a mass is cystic or solid. FNAB requires training in proper technique, experience to obtain optimal sampling of the cells composing a mass, and a skilled cytopathologist to accurately interpret the specimens and communicate the results. If these criteria can be met, FNAB results may be used to triage patients between biopsy and follow-up, especially if triple diagnosis is applied. If these circumstances cannot be met in a clinical setting, the procedure should not be used for triage purposes, and open biopsy should be performed instead.

The accuracy of FNAB in diagnosing malignancy has been established. The false-positive rate for the procedure is low, averaging approximately 0.17%.[19] The advantage of establishing the diagnosis of malignancy with FNAB is the rapidity of a definitive diagnosis, which offers the patient the simultaneous advantage of an expedient discussion of treatment options. Definitive surgery can be done using results of FNAB, although many surgeons perform an open biopsy and frozen section analysis to confirm the diagnosis at the beginning of the planned treatment procedure, especially if any clinical question exists as to its accuracy.[7,19]

On the other hand, the false-negative rate of FNAB (ie, benign results in the presence of malignancy) was quoted between 0.4% and 35% in an excellent review by Layfield and colleagues.[19] The most common reason for a false-negative result is inadequate sampling, usually as a result of inadequate experience on the part of the aspirator.[19,20] In a review of this topic, Bell and associates[21] reported an inadequate sampling rate between 6% and 32%, and a number of these cases ultimately proved malignant on follow-up. Any fine-needle aspiration of the breast reported by the cytopathologist to contain insufficient cells for interpretation must be repeated or excisional biopsy performed.

Other reasons for false-negative results include tumors 1 cm or less in size, for which the target tissue presumably has been missed by the aspirating needle.[20] Tumors containing a large degree of fibrosis also can result in false-negative aspiration results, as can large tumors with necrosis of the center or edema at the periphery.[20] However, even full awareness of these diagnostic pitfalls will not achieve 100% accuracy. Interpretive errors also occur, even by experienced cytopathologists. This is especially true in cases of well-differentiated tumors—tubular carcinoma, infiltrating lobular carcinoma, both in situ ductal and lobular carcinoma, colloid carcinoma, and papillary carcinoma are especially challenging in this regard.[19] To increase diagnostic accuracy and decrease the risk for false-negative results, any mass showing atypical changes cytologically should be excised.[22] In addition, the application of triple diagnosis of breast masses is especially important to achieve optimal diagnostic accuracy.

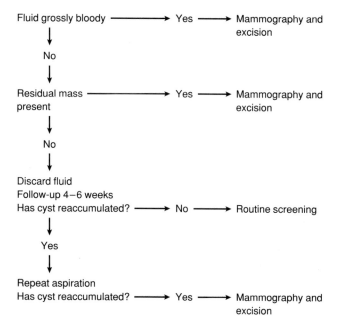

FIGURE 5.3-2 Management of breast cysts.

Use of Triple Diagnosis to Increase Diagnostic Accuracy

To increase the diagnostic accuracy of FNAB and eliminate as many false-negative results as possible, the use of triple diagnosis to triage patients between biopsy and follow-up has been used. *Triple diagnosis* refers to the application of three evaluation steps to a breast mass: clinical assessment by palpation, results of mammography, and results of FNAB. A summary of the principles of triple diagnosis can be found in Figure 5.3-3 in algorithm format. This approach to breast masses has been used for many years in the European community, but its acceptance among surgeons in the United States has been slow. No question exists that it requires less skill to simply remove any solid breast mass than to biopsy selected cases, and this approach may be the safest way for many surgeons to practice. For those who treat a large number of patients with breast disease, however, application of the triple diagnosis criteria to triage patients between biopsy and follow-up has become an accepted standard.

As has been stressed previously, accurate interpretation of CBE can be difficult, and documentation of false-negative interpretations can be readily found in summary form.[19] Clinicians who are able to gain immediate feedback in the operating room about the accuracy of their preoperative diagnosis enjoy a degree of expertise not available in other clinical settings. The most experienced surgeons, however, readily admit that preoperative assessment by palpation alone is too frequently inaccurate to be relied on with confidence. Diagnostic accuracy was only 73% in a study of concordance for the need for biopsy among four experienced surgeons in 15 patients who had malignant lesions.[23]

Mammography adds a second element to the diagnostic equation. To apply the concepts of triple diagnosis optimally, however, the examiner must personally review the mammograms during the clinical examination. Reading a report does not suffice, because the CBE and mammographic results must be synthesized so that any finding on CBE can be immediately correlated with mammographic findings in exactly the same location as the palpable abnormality.[7,19,24] Radiologists may not have results of the clinical examination when the mammogram is read, and it is the responsibility of the clinician applying the principles of triple diagnosis to correlate the mammographic findings with those of the CBE. A special note of caution is applicable in the case of a mammogram that does not show the palpable abnormality. Because no studies in the literature address the safety of the triple diagnosis technique to establish that a palpable breast mass is benign in the setting of a normal mammogram, and given the false-negative rate of fine-needle aspiration, it is safest for the patient to undergo excisional biopsy in this clinical setting.[19,24] This point is underscored by noting that 35% of all claimants had negative mammogram results in a review of medical malpractice closed claims cases alleging failure to diagnose breast cancer.[5]

The third component of triple diagnosis is FNAB, the accuracy of which has been discussed. Many studies have shown that, when the criteria of triple diagnosis is strictly applied, diagnostic accuracy is high. A strict principle of the triple diagnosis approach is that if discordance exists between any of the three diagnostic tests, open biopsy should be done. An extensive review has documented a greater than 99% predictive value for benign disease when all three diagnostic components are benign.[19] These data assume, of course, that all of the caveats listed earlier are heeded. Under these circumstances, a woman can be given an option of follow-up or biopsy. Those who choose follow-up are usually seen for at least one follow-up visit at 3 months, and visits can then be spaced out at 3- to 6-month intervals if CBE establishes that the mass is stable. Any breast mass monitored in this way should be evaluated by the same examiner at intervals for at least 1 year; many spontaneously resolve over time. If any change occurs on CBE or mammography, open biopsy is warranted.

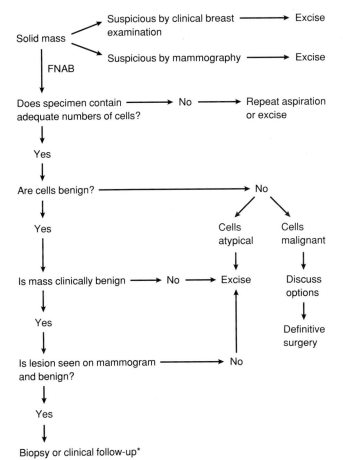

FIGURE 5.3-3. Management of solid breast masses by triple diagnosis. *Decisions about biopsy or follow-up should consider age and other breast cancer risk factors, and should recognize that follow-up has approximately a 1% risk of missing cancer. FNAB, fine-needle aspiration biopsy.

MANAGEMENT SUMMARY

- Any palpable breast mass must be evaluated to determine whether it is cystic or solid; neither CBE nor mammography can make this distinction.
- Women with successfully aspirated breast cysts require 4- to 6-week follow-up examinations to check for cyst recurrence.
- Any cytologic report indicating an inadequate sample should be repeated or open biopsy performed.
- Triple diagnosis reqirues confidence in interpretation of CBE, concomitant interpretation of CBE and mammography, and thorough knowledge of the pitfalls of FNAB results.
- When biopsy is deferred after triple diagnosis, careful follow-up is warranted.

References

1. Sienko DG, Osuch JR, Garlinghouse C, et al. The design and implementation of a community breast cancer screening project. CA Cancer J Clin 1992;42:258.
2. Haagensen C. Physicians' role in the detection and diagnosis of breast disease. In: diseases of the breast, ed 3. Philadelphia, WB Saunders, 1986:516.
3. Hughes LE, Mansel RE, Webster DJT. The approach to assessment and management of breast lumps. In: Benign disorders and diseases of the breast: concepts and clinical management. London, Bailliere Tindall, 1989:41.
4. Osuch JR, Bonham VL. The timely diagnosis of breast cancer. Cancer 1994;74:271.
5. Physician Insurers Association of America. Breast cancer study. Lawrenceville, NJ, Physicians Insurers Association of America, 1990.
6. Moore MP. Management of common breast disorders: mass: lump/cyst. In: Harris JR, Hellman S, Henderson IC, et al, eds. Breast diseases, ed. 2. Philadelphia, JB Lippincott, 1991:77.
7. Donegan WL. Evaluation of a palpable breast mass. N Engl J Med 1992;327:937.
8. Powell DE, Stelling CB. The normal breast: structure, function, and epidemiology. In: The diagnosis and detection of breast disease. St Louis, CV Mosby, 1994:3.
9. Boring CC, Squires TS, Tong T, et al. Cancer statistics, 1994. CA Cancer J Clin 1994;44:7.
10. Danforth DN, Lichter AS, Lippman ME. The diagnosis of breast cancer. In: Lippman ME, Lichter AS, et al. Diagnosis and management of breast cancer. Philadelphia, WB Saunders, 1988:50.
11. Donegan WL. Diagnosis. In: Donegan WL, Spratt JS, eds. Cancer of the breast, ed 3. Philadelphia, WB Saunders, 1988:125.
12. Zuckerman HC. Mammography in borderline cases. In: Ariel IM, Cahan AC, eds. Treatment of pre-cancerous lesions and early breast cancer. Baltimore, Williams & Wilkins, 1993:39.
13. Kinne DW, Kopans DB. Physical examination and mammography in the diagnosis of breast disease. In: Harris JR, Hellman S, Henderson IC, et al, eds. Breast diseases, ed 2. Philadelphia, JB Lippincott, 1991:81.
14. Ennis JT. Diagnostic radiological imaging for breast diseases. In: Bland KI, Copeland EM, eds. The breast: comprehensive management of benign and malignant disease. Philadelphia, WB Saunders, 1991:426.
15. Kline TS, Kline IK. Introduction: limitations and complications. In: Guides to clinical aspiration biopsy: breast. New York, Igaku-Shoin, 1989:3.
16. Sickles EA, Klein DL, Goodson WH, Hunt TK. Mammography after needle aspiration of palpable breast masses. Am J Surg 1983;145:395.
17. Svensson WE, Tohno E, Cosgrove DO, et al. Effects of fine needle aspiration on the US appearance of the breast. Radiology 1992;185:709.
18. Souba WW, Bland KI. Indications and techniques for biopsy. In: Bland KI, Copeland EM, eds. The breast: comprehensive management of benign and malignant disease. Philadelphia, WB Saunders, 1991:527.
19. Layfield LJ, Glasgow BJ, Cramer H. Fine-needle aspiration in the management of breast masses. Pathol Annu 1989;24:23.
20. Scopa CD, Koukouras D, Androulakis J, et al. Sources of diagnostic discrepancies in fine-needle aspiration of the breast. Diagn Cytopathol 1991;7:546.
21. Bell DA, Hajdu SI, Urban JA, et al. Role of aspiration cytology in the diagnosis and management of mammary lesions in office practice. Cancer 1983;51:1182.
22. Peterse JL, Koolman-Schellekens MA, van de Peppel, van de Ham T, van Heerde P. Atypia in fine-needle aspiration cytology of the breast: a histological follow-up study of 301 cases. Semin Diagn Pathol 1989;6:126.
23. Boyd NF, Sutherland HJ, Fish EB, et al. Prospective evaluation of physical examination of the breast. Am J Surg 1981;142:331.
24. Du Toit RS, Grobler SP, Brink C, et al. The role of mammography to evaluate palpable breast tumours. S Afr J Surg 1992;30:15.

5.4

The Abnormal Mammogram

MARK S. TALAMONTI · MONICA MORROW

Randomized studies have shown that the regular use of screening mammography reduces breast cancer mortality by 20% to 30% in women over 50 years of age.[1-5] This ability to affect breast cancer mortality has led to the development of mammographic guidelines for the routine screening of asymptomatic women.[6] Although debate continues on the optimal age at which to begin screening and the appropriate frequency of testing,[7,8] the number of women who have had at least one mammogram and who obtain subsequent follow-up studies continues to increase. The widespread use of screening has resulted in a concomitant increase in the number of breast biopsies recommended for clinically occult lesions. These trends have necessitated an examination of the mammographic findings most consistent with cancer and the indications for breast biopsy or follow-up radiographic studies in the management of nonpalpable breast lesions. In this chapter we review the mammographic signs of malignancy, the radiographic techniques used to evaluate nonpalpable breast abnormalities, and the indications for surgical biopsy.

Defining the Mammogram

Most women referred for evaluation of an abnormal mammogram have had screening mammography, two-view examinations of each breast consisting of craniocaudal and mediolateral oblique images.[9] The initial steps in the evaluation of the abnormal screening mammogram should include a careful physical examination to exclude the presence of any clinical breast abnormalities, comparison with prior mammograms to determine whether the abnormality in question is chronic, and diagnostic mammography. Although management recommendations for obvious abnormalities can frequently be made based on screening mammograms, more subtle findings require a diagnostic mammogram before determining the need for biopsy.

Diagnostic mammograms are done to further define the location of an abnormality detected during screening or to clarify the morphologic and radiographic characteristics of a vague, indeterminate lesion.[10,11] In addition to standard craniocaudal and mediolateral oblique images, exaggerated oblique projections and slightly rotated views of the breast facilitate localization of an abnormality. Small nodular densities can be defined more clearly by spot compression views, in which a focal area of the breast is compressed and the resultant pressure displaces some of the surrounding normal tissue. Spot or focal compression allows better visualization of the shape and margins of a mass lesion.[12,13] Microcalcifications are frequently evaluated using magnified spot views. The magnified images provide clearer views of size, morphology, density, and orientation, and thus help to determine the need for biopsy.[10,14]

Mammographic Abnormalities

The classic mammographic signs of malignancy are clustered microcalcifications and stellate masses. Other indirect signs of malignancy include areas of asymmetry and architectural distortion, dilated lactiferous ducts, and skin or nipple thickening or retraction.[10] The prevalence and predictive value of these findings vary considerably between series. Recent reviews illustrate the relative lack of specificity for many mammographic lesions. In Sickles'[14] review of 300 nonpalpable breast cancers, 36% presented with calcifications alone, 26% had dominant masses as the primary finding, and 20% presented with architectural distortion or asymmetric densities. Only half of these lesions were considered suggestive of carcinoma, however, and the others underwent biopsy because a diagnosis of cancer could not be completely excluded by mammography.[15]

The positive predictive value of mass lesions varies with their appearance. An irregular or spiculated margin is the most important indicator that a mass may be malignant.[16] Moskowitz[17] reviewed 40,431 screening mammograms and noted a predictive value of 74% for masses that were spiculated or stellate. Similarly high rates of malignancy were noted in studies by Tinnemans and colleagues[18] (67%), Meyer and associates[19] (55%) and Ciatto and coworkers[20] (75%). The presence of microcalcifications in a spiculated mass increases the liklihood of malignancy.[17] Spiculated lesions always require biopsy.

Mammographic masses with only slightly irregular margins or nodular, lobulated shapes may represent cancers such as papillary, medullary, or colloid tumors. Ultrasound and magnification views can clarify the need for biopsy in more than half of such indeterminate masses[16] (Fig. 5.4-1). In the review of screening mammograms by Moskowitz,[17] 593 noncalcified masses larger than 1 cm in diameter were identified, and more than half of these masses were shown by aspiration or ultrasonographic evaluation to be simple cysts requiring no further evaluation. An irregular mass that is determined to be solid after appropriate diagnostic studies may prove to be malignant in approximately 20% of cases, indicating the need for surgical biopsy or stereotactic biopsy to alleviate any remaining ambiguity.[21]

Well-circumscribed masses with smooth margins usually represent benign lesions including cysts, fibroadenomas, and intramammary lymph nodes. Only 4.5% of round densities reported by Bigelow and associates[22] were malignant, a rate similar to the 6% incidence of malignancy reported by Skinner and colleagues[23] and Meyer and coworkers.[19] Lesions considered to be benign and at a low risk for malignancy may be safely monitored using repeat imaging studies at 6-month intervals.[21] The decision to monitor selected patients with repeat mammographic studies and without breast biopsy has been shown to be safe when the status of any observed abnormalities is carefully interpreted.[24] Sickles[15] prospectively evaluated 3184 consecutive cases of nonpalpable abnormalities detected on screening mammograms. Initially, all abnormalities were believed to be benign. Follow-up included four mammograms during a 3- to 3.5-year period. During the follow-up period, 17 of these lesions (0.5%) were found to be cancerous. Fifteen of the 17 carcinomas were in situ or stage I tumors. Similarly, Erickson and coworkers[25] reviewed 214 patients over an 8-year period. Of the 214 patients, 114 were assigned to a follow-up arm. Only 2 of these patients were later diagnosed with breast cancer. These studies suggest that biopsy of all suspicious or possibly malignant abnormalities with careful mammographic follow-up of the remaining low-index cases is an appropriate management strategy. Mammographic changes that require biopsy after follow-up include masses that increase in size, circumscribed or dense masses with blurring or changes in the margins, microcalcifications that increase in number or density, masses that persist after ultrasonographic aspiration, and increased architectural distortions compared with the contralateral breast.

Classifying microcalcifications into specific risk categories has proved more difficult. Certain forms such as eggshell calcifications with lucent centers, calcified fibroade-

FIGURE 5.4-1   A. Mediolateral oblique mammograms suggesting a mass lesion in the left breast, also seen on the craniocaudal view. **B.** Mediolateral view demonstrating that the mass is actually asymmetric breast tissue not requiring surgical therapy.

nomas, calcifications of duct ectasia, and milk of calcium in small cysts are diagnostic of a benign process.[26] In contrast, punctate, pointed, irregular calcifications that are heterogeneous in size, located within a mass, or fine branching deposits that fill internal ducts indicate the presence of malignancy in 60% to 75% of cases.[16,17,26]

Small, clustered microcalcifications that are not obviously malignant pose a more complicated problem. If all such microcalcifications undergo biopsy, 20% to 30% prove to be malignant.[26] Several series have attempted to identify specific characteristics of microcalcifications that would allow them to be more accurately classified as benign or malignant.[27–29] In general, calcifications that are of similar size and shape and that are loosely grouped or scattered are frequently due to benign changes such as sclerosing adenosis or lobular hyperplasia.[30] Small calcifications that are associated with cancer more frequently appear irregular, jagged, linear, or branching, usually varying in size and shape.[31] Malignant microcalcifications tend to be distributed in tight clusters or in a segmental orientation. Despite these generalizations, most studies that have examined the incidence of malignancy in these small clusters of microcalcifications cite a preoperative specificity of 50% to 60% in distinguishing benign from malignant entities.[18–20,22,23,37–48]

Microspot magnification views can clarify the morphology and nature of indeterminate microcalcifications (Figs. 5.4-2 and 5.4-3). Sickles[14] reported the use of microfocal spot magnification views to further define indeterminate microcalcifications in 302 cases believed to be equivocal after two-view mammograms. One hundred eighty-four cases were thought to be benign after additional views, and only 49 underwent biopsy. No carcinomas were identified in this group. Diagnostic views showed signs of malignancy in 34 patients. Subsequent biopsy revealed malignancy in 33. Mammographic findings remained equivocal after magnification views in 84 patients. Biopsy was performed on 34 of these lesions, and malignancy was found in 9 patients. Of the original 302 abnormalities, 61% were shown to be benign by additional radiographic views, and 11% were shown to have malignant characteristics. Microcalcifications remained indeterminate after further imaging studies in 28%; however, in over 70%, the additional magnification views provided enough information to allow a definitive diagnosis—a diagnosis that was correct in all but 1 of the 83 cases for which pathologic proof later became available.[33] Similarly, Tabar and Gad[34] found that 62% of abnormalities identified on a single-view screening examination were found to be of no concern after additional views. Microcalcifications that remain indeterminate after magnification views should be considered for biopsy.

Other mammographic abnormalities that may be signs of malignancy are skin or nipple changes, asymmetry due

FIGURE 5.4-2 **A.** Indeterminate microcalcifications seen on craniocaudal mammogram (*arrow*). **B.** Magnified view demonstrating clearly benign nature of these skin calcifications.

to a density, and architectural distortions. Some 10% to 20% of breast cancers present with these abnormalities, which are often difficult to detect and diagnose.[16] Additional diagnostic views are usually necessary to assess the risk for malignancy in these patients. Calcifications associated with any of the above abnormalities strongly increase the risk for malignancy, and biopsy should be considered in these situations.[32]

Interpretation and Results

Most mammographic abnormalities do not have unequivocal signs of malignancy, and therefore variability in the interpretation of mammograms is a factor in determining the positive predictive value of any series.[35] The ability to consistently evaluate mammographic abnormalities and to report these findings in a clear and precise manner directly influences the number of biopsies being done and the rate at which these biopsies yield a diagnosis of cancer. Variability between radiologists is well documented. Ciatto and associates[20] compared the benign/malignant biopsy ratio for each of six radiologists over a 7-year period and found it to vary from 2.4:1 to 7.3:1. To avoid such wide variability in interpretations, Kopans[36] categorized radiographic recommendations according to the type of mammographic finding and the relative risk for malignancy, thereby establishing some justification for subsequent decisions to either monitor or perform biopsies on these lesions.[16] Findings considered as probably benign include multiple rounded densities, borderline calcifica-

FIGURE 5.4-3 A. Cluster of calcifications of indeterminate nature on craniocaudal mammogram. **B.** Magnified view showing irregularity of size and form of calcifications, confirming the need for surgical biopsy.

tions, and solitary round masses no larger than 8 to 10 mm in diameter. Appropriate radiographic recommendations for these low-risk lesions include additional imaging studies or follow-up in less than the usual time between screening films (usually 6 months). Malignant or suspicious radiographic findings warrant immediate biopsy and include spiculated masses or heterogeneous clustered microcalcifications as described earlier. Attempts to develop this type of internal consistency in mammographic reporting should result in a narrower range of positive biopsy rates between series while continuing to ensure that most cancers detected by mammography are either in situ or stage I lesions.

Critical analysis of recent experiences helps to define current trends in the management of nonpalpable mammographic abnormalities. Morrow[32] reviewed 5500 biop-

sies from 17 reports of 100 or more cases and found that 45% were done for microcalcifications alone, 43% for mass densities, 6% for masses containing microcalcifications, and 5% for asymmetric densities (Table 5.4-1). She noted considerable variability in the indications for biopsy between the series.[18–20,22,23,37–48] For example, mass lesions as the mammographic indication for biopsy ranged from 27% to 59%, suggesting considerable variation in the extent of evaluation before a recommendation for biopsy. As expected, differences were noted in the rates of positive biopsies when done for these various mammographic abnormalities (Table 5.4-2).

The incidence of positive biopsy results done for mammographic findings ranges between 9% and 65%,[34,48] with most authors reporting a positive biopsy rate of 15% to 30%.[32] The yield of positive biopsy results for a mammo-

TABLE 5.4-1
Mammographic Indications for Biopsy

Investigators	N	Cases With Cancer (%)	Biopsy Cases With Finding (%)			
			Microcalcification	Mass	Microcalcification and Mass	Asymmetric Density
Siemssen et al[47]	115	14	49	42	9	—
Chetty et al[37]	190	21	54	27	9	10
Bigelow et al[22]	150	16	33	55	12	—
Choucair et al[48]	103	9	42	49	4	6
Skinner et al[23]	179	23	34	48	18	—
Denning et al[38]	100	11	35	55	10	—
Graham & Bauer[39]	678	11.5	38	36	—	26
Lang et al[40]	122	8	36	42	22	—
Dershaw[41]	219	29	58	35	6	—
Gisvold & Martin[42]	343	27	36	54	10	—
Ciatto et al[20]	512	30	51	45	—	4
Schwartz et al[43]	1132	29	52	35	7	6
Tinnemanns et al[18]	359	33	52	34	14	—
Landercasper et al[44]	203	22	56	31	13	—
Rubin et al[45]	100	20	47	33	5	15
Symmonds & Roberts[46]	500	14	37	58	5	—
Meyer et al[19]	500	23	41	59	—	—

(Adapted from Morrow M. Management of nonpalpable breast lesions. Princ Pract Oncol Updates 1990;4:1)

TABLE 5.4-2
Incidence of Malignancy by Indication for Biopsy

Investigators	N	Cases With Malignancy (%)			
		Microcalcification	Mass	Microcalcification and Mass	Asymmetric Density
Chetty et al[37]	190	24	15	35	5
Bigelow et al[22]	150	24	—	33	—
Choucair[48]	103	5	12	0	0
Skinner et al[23]	179	13	22	42	—
Denning et al[38]	100	17	15	50	—
Graham & Bauer[39]	678	14	15	—	6
Lang et al[40]	122	14	2	7	—
Dershaw[41]	219	34	17	43	—
Gisvold & Martin[42]	343	30	25	67	—
Ciatto et al[20]	512	24	38	—	11
Schwartz et al[43]	1132	31	23	48	24
Tinnemanns et al[18]	359	32	35	29	—
Landercasper et al[44]	203	22	17	30	—
Rubin et al[45]	100	26	18	40	0
Symmonds & Roberts[46]	499	20	12	4	—
Meyer et al[19]	500	22	24	—	—

(Adapted from Morrow M. Management of nonpalpable breast lesions. Princ Pract Oncol Updates 1990;4:1) graphic abnormality depends not only on the radiographic criteria used to define cancer risk but also on other, often incalculable, factors. These confounding influences include patient age and risk factors in the population being screened, surgical expertise in obtaining the lesion in question, and accurate pathologic interpretation of frequently confusing lesions such as atypical hyperplasia and carcinoma in situ.[35] It is therefore impossible to define an appropriate rate of positive biopsy results in an absolute sense, when much of the management is based on subjective criteria. Attempts to improve the specificity of mammographic interpretation and thus the assessment of cancer risk will result in fewer biopsies being done for benign lesions yet will continue to ensure that most detected cancers are in situ or stage I lesions. Sickles[14] reported a positive biopsy rate of 32.5% when screening mammograms were interpreted as malignant or suggestive of malignancy. The mean size of the invasive lesions was only 16 mm, and 76% of the cancers detected were stage 0 or I.[35] Lesions that were initially monitored and that ultimately underwent biopsy because of interval changes showed similar findings in terms of size and stage.

Management Recommendations

Assuming that a high-quality screening mammogram has been done and interpretation of the mammographic abnormalities has been reasonable, certain treatment strategies can be suggested. Depending on the type of mammographic abnormality identified, additional mammographic films (including spot magnification views and compression images) may be appropriate. Ultrasound may be necessary to exclude cysts or to define other solid but well-circumscribed masses. Physical examination should be done to exclude palpable but nonvisualized breast abnormalities. After a careful diagnostic mammogram, certain lesions may be identified according to their risk for harboring malignancy. Treatment recommendations may then be made accordingly. Mammographic findings considered suspicious for malignancy and therefore at high risk include microcalcifications that are pleomorphic, that are greater than five in number, and that have either linear or clustered patterns; masses that are spiculated or stellate or that are associated with microcalcifications; asymmetric breast tissue, especially when associated with calcifications; and new architectural distortion compared with conditions observed on previous interval screening mammograms. These lesions warrant surgical biopsy. Indeterminate microcalcifications, nodular masses without calcifications, and asymmetric breast tissue not associated with calcifications all carry an intermediate risk for breast cancer, as previously described. Depending on other associated risk factors, stereotactic biopsy or surgical biopsy may be indicated in these lesions. Repeat diagnostic mammograms at 6-month intervals for benign-appearing calcifications or well-circumscribed masses may be indicated to ensure stability.

This type of critical approach to the evaluation of an abnormal screening mammogram can lead to cost-efficient yet clinically safe management of women with occult mammographic lesions. Morrow and colleagues[49] reviewed a recent experience using just such a systematic approach to abnormal mammograms. Two hundred sixty-seven consecutive patients were referred to a single surgeon for evaluation of nonpalpable mammographic abnormalities. The mammographic finding resulting in surgical consultation was a mass in 110 cases (42%), microcalcifications in 105 cases (39%), a mass containing microcalcifications in 14 cases (5%), and asymmetric density in 38 cases (14%). Mammograms were carefully reviewed and, according to the type of finding identified and other associated risk factors, assigned to defined categories of risk and management. One hundred eight women with suspicious mammographic findings and associated risk factors underwent immediate surgical biopsy, and 39 (36%) were found to have carcinoma. Other women with less obvious mammographic findings but who were assumed to harbor a 2% to 10% risk had stereotactic biopsy. The selective use of this new technology yielded 15 of 42 women with atypical or malignant cytologic results. Open biopsy was done, and 5 additional cancer cases were identified. Forty women were thought to have low-risk mammographic abnormalities, and 6-month follow-up studies were performed. Six of these patients demonstrated subsequent mammographic changes that were believed to require biopsy. In only 1 case was an invasive carcinoma seen on follow-up examinations. Thus, a total of 129 of 267 women evaluated (48%) underwent open breast biopsy at presentation or during the follow-up period. The positive biopsy rate was 36%. Of the 46 cancers identified, 23 were ductal carcinoma in situ, and 18 were stage I infiltrating carcinomas. The other 5 cancers were Stage II lesions with a mean tumor size of 1.5 cm. Of the 117 women assigned to annual or interval follow-up, 6 (5%) required biopsy, and 2 carcinomas (1.7%), 1 of which was ductal carcinoma in situ, were identified. The use of additional diagnostic studies, including stereotactic biopsy, and precise radiographic review were thought to be helpful in avoiding open biopsy in two thirds of women whose lesions were believed to be benign. In addition, a high rate of diagnostic accuracy was maintained in women with more suspicious findings.[49] Hamby and associates[50] reported similar results when low-probability lesions were managed with interval mammography rather than immediate biopsy. Sixty-seven patients were monitored for lesions considered at low risk for malignancy based on appropriate diagnostic studies. Classification criteria were similar to those used by Morrow and colleagues.[49] Biopsy was ultimately performed in 10%, and only two cases of cancer were found, both stage I. Sixty women had no evidence of progressive change on interval mammograms (median follow-up, 34 months) and were thus spared biopsy.

The algorithm in Figure 5.4-4 is proposed as a means to selectively manage patients referred with an abnormal mammogram. The objective is to enhance the true-positive rate for nonpalable mammographic lesions requiring biopsy while safely using nonsurgical approaches to manage low-risk findings. In situations in which stereotac-

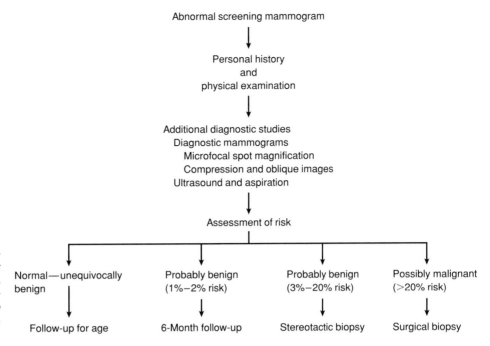

FIGURE 5.4-4 Approach to an abnormal screening mammogram. (After Morrow M., Schmidt RA, Cregger B, et al. Preoperative evaluation of abnormal mammographic findings to avoid unnecessary breast biopsies. Arch Surg 1994;129:1091)

tic biopsy is not available, lesions in the 3% to 20% category should be managed by interval follow-up mammography or surgical biopsy according to the individual level of risk.

References

1. Breen N, Kessler L. Increases in screening mammography: US women 40 and older. J Natl Cancer Instit 1992;84:1549.
2. Shapiro S, Venet W, Strax P, et al. Selection, follow-up and analysis in the Health Insurance Plan Study: a randomized trial with breast cancer screening. NCI Mongr 1985;67:65.
3. Tabar L, Fagerberg G, Duffy S, et al. Update of the Swedish two-country program of mammographic screening for breast cancer. Radiol Clin North Am 1992;30:187.
4. Verbeek KA, Hendriks J, Holland R, et al. Reduction of breast cancer mortality through mass screening with modern mammography: first results of the Nijmegan project 1975-1981. Lancet 1984;1:1222.
5. Anderson I, Aspergren K, Janzon L, et al. Mammographic screening and mortality from breast cancer: the Malmo mammographic screening trial. Br Med J 1988;297:944.
6. Shapiro S. Screening: assessment of current studies. Cancer [Suppl] 1994;74:231.
7. Smart CR. Highlights of the evidence of benefit for women aged 40–49 years from the 14-year follow-up of the Breast Cancer Detection Demonstration Project. Cancer [Suppl] 1994;74:296.
8. Kopans DB. Screening for breast cancer and mortality reduction among women 40–49 years of age. Cancer [Suppl] 1994;74:311.
9. American College of Radiology. Standards for the performance of screening mammography: mammography accreditation program. Reston, VA, American College of Radiology, 1990.
10. De Paredes ES. Evaluation of abnormal screening mammograms. Cancer [Suppl] 1994;74:342.
11. Sickles EA. Practical solutions to common mammographic problems: tailoring the examination. AJR 1988;151:31.
12. Berkowitz JE, Gatewood OMB, Gayler BW. Equivocal mammographic findings: evaluation with spot compression. Radiology 1989;1711:369.
13. De Paredes ES. Atlas of film–screen mammography. Baltimore, Williams & Wilkins, 1992.
14. Sickles EA. Microfocal spot magnification mammography using xeroradiographic and screen–film recording systems. Radiology 1979;131:599.
15. Sickles EA. Mammographic features of 300 consecutive nonpalpable breast cancers. AJR 1986;146:661.
16. McKenna RJ, Sr. The abnormal mammogram: radiographic findings, diagnostic options, pathology, and stage of cancer diagnosis. Cancer Suppl 1994;74:244.
17. Moskowitz M. The predictive value of certain mammographic signs in screening for breast cancer. Cancer 1983;51:1007.
18. Tinnemans J, Wobbes T, Holland R, et al. Mammographic and histopathologic correlation of nonpalpable lesions of the breast and the reliability of frozen section diagnosis. Surg Gynecol Obstet 1987;165:523.
19. Meyer J, Kopans D, Stomper P, et al. Occult breast abnormalities: percutaneous preoperative needle localization. Radiology 1984;150:335.
20. Ciatto S, Cataliotti L, Distante V. Nonpalpable lesions detected with mammography: review of 512 consecutive cases. Radiology 1987;165:99.
21. Schmidt RA. Stereotactic breast biopsy. CA Cancer J Clin 1994;44:172.
22. Bigelow R, Smith R, Goodman P, et al. Needle localization of nonpalpable breast masses. Arch Surg 1985;120:565.
23. Skinner M, Swain M, Simmons R. Nonpalpable breast lesions at biopsy. Ann Surg 1988;208:203.
24. Sickles E. Periodic mammographic follow-up of probably benign lesions: results in 3,184 consecutive cases. Radiology 1991;179.
25. Erickson EJ, McGreevy JM, Muskett A. Selective nonoperative man-

agement of patients with referred abnormal mammograms. Am J Surg 1990;6:659.

26. Sickles E. Breast calcifications: mammographic evaluation. Radiology 1986;160:289.

27. Murphy W, Deschryver-Kecskemeti K. Isolated clustered microcalcifications in the breast: radiologic–pathologic correlation. Radiology 1978;127:335.

28. Powell R, McSweeney M, Wilson C. X-ray calcifications as the only basis for breast biopsy. Ann Surg 1983;197:555.

29. Egan R, McSweeney M, Sewell C. Intramammary calcifications without an associated mass in benign and malignant diseases. Radiology 1980;137:1.

30. Pope TL Jr, Fechner RE, Wilhelm MC, et al. Lobular carcinoma in situ of the breast: mammographic features. Radiology 1988;168:63.

31. Tabar L, Dean PB. Teaching atlas of mammography. Stuttgart, Thieme Verlag, 1985.

32. Morrow M. Management of nonpalpable breast lesions. Princ Pract Oncol Updates 1990;4:1.

33. Sickles E: Further experience with microfocal spot magnification mammography in the assessment of clustered microcalcifications. Radiology 1980;137:9.

34. Tabar L, Gad A. Screening for breast cancer: the Swedish trial. Radiology 1981;138:219.

35. Sickles EA. Quality assurance: how to audit your own mammography practice. Radiol Clin North Am 1992;30:265.

36. Kopans DB. The positive predictive value of mammography. AJR 1992;158:521.

37. Chetty U, Kirkpatrick A, Anderson T, et al. Localization and excision of occult breast lesions. Br J Surg 1983;70:607.

38. Denning D, Farha G, McBoyle M. Role of needle localization of nonpalpable breast lesions. Am J Surg 1987;154.

39. Graham G, Bauer T. Early detection of occult breast cancer: the York experience with 678 needle localization biopsies. Ann Surg 1988;54:234.

40. Lang N, Talbert G, Shewmake K, et al. The current evaluation of nonpalpable breast lesions. Arch Surg 1987;122:1389.

41. Dershaw D. Nonpalpable, needle-localized mammographic abnormalities: pathologic correlation in 219 patients. Cancer Invest 1986;4:1.

42. Gisvold J, Martin J. Prebiopsy localization of nonpalpable breast lesions. AJR 1984;143:447.

43. Schwartz G, Feig S, Patchefsky A. Significance and staging of nonpalpable carcinomas of the breast. Surg Gynecol Obstet 1987;166:6.

44. Landercasper J, Gundersen S, Gundersen A, et al. Needle localization and biopsy of nonpalpable lesions of the breast. Surg Gynecol Obstet 1987;164:399.

45. Rubin E, Visscher D, Alexander R, et al. Proliferative disease and atypia in biopsies performed for nonpalpable lesions detected mammographically. Cancer 1988;61:2077.

46. Symmonds R, Roberts J. Management of nonpalpable breast abnormalities. Ann Surg 1987;205:520.

47. Siemssen O, Blichert-Toft M, Pedersen M, et al. Mammography directed wire marking of nonpalpable breast lesions. Acta Chir Scand 1981;147:525.

48. Choucair R, Holcomb M, Matthews R, et al. Biopsy of nonpalpable breast lesions. Am J Surg 1988;156:453.

49. Morrow M, Schmidt RA, Cregger B, et al. Preoperative evaluation of abnormal mammographic findings to avoid unnecessary breast biopsies. Arch Surg 1994;129:1091.

50. Hamby LS, McGrath PC, Stelling CB, et al. Management of mammographic indeterminate lesions. Am Surg 1993;59:4.

5.5

Abnormalities of the Breast in Pregnancy and Lactation

JEANNE A. PETREK

Distinguishing the normal but immense physiologic changes of gestation from those due to neoplasm is challenging.

Diagnosis of Breast Masses During Pregnancy and Lactation

PHYSICAL EXAMINATION

If the opportunity presents itself before pregnancy, a careful physical examination and baseline (or interval screening) mammography, as indicated by a patient's age and risk factors, are helpful and reassuring during the subsequent pregnancy.

The more common circumstance is the chance to perform a thorough breast examination at the first obstetric visit when the breasts have undergone the fewest physiologic changes. As pregnancy progresses, the breasts increase in volume, firmness, and nodularity. As the pregnancy continues, a mass may then feel similar to normal hypertrophic thickness, or a mass may be deeper in the breast because of the generalized greater volume, causing it to be nonpalpable.

The finding of a thickness or possible mass on physical examination during pregnancy brings different considerations than in the nonpregnant young woman. In a menstruating woman, one often reexamines the patient just after her next menstrual period. In a pregnant woman, no cycle exists, and the hormonal milieu intensifies steadily, causing greater breast volume and firmness. There is no recommended interval in which to reexamine, and one must be guided by the level of suspicion.

MAMMOGRAPHY AND ULTRASONOGRAPHY

Mammograms are not routinely performed because little information can be gained. The increased vascularity, cellularity, and water content of the pregnant breast and the additional presence of milk in the lactating breast all contribute to a generalized radiographic parenchymal density with loss of the contrasting fatty tissue. Ionizing radiation absorbed by the fetus is minimal, especially if the abdomen is shielded, so it is not a large consideration in cases where it might be helpful.

At Memorial Hospital in New York City, 78% of mammograms in 23 women with clinically evident pregnancy-associated breast cancer demonstrated radiologic signs of the cancer.[1] All of six ultrasonographic examinations performed in these patients with a palpable abnormality revealed a solid mass. In an older series, negative mammograms were found in 6 of 8 pregnant patients with breast mass and subsequent biopsy-proven cancer.[2] If mammography is deemed necessary in the lactating woman, it should be performed immediately after emptying the breast by nursing or pumping, and a serviceable radiographic image may be produced.

Breast ultrasonography is accurate and safe, as it is in nonpregnant women, in determining whether a palpable mass is fluid-filled or solid. It is not possible to distinguish a benign solid mass from a malignant one. Furthermore, no published literature on the normal gestational breast appearance aids in the ultrasonographic diagnosis of a questionable mass on physical examination.

NEEDLE ASPIRATION FOR CYTOLOGIC ANALYSIS

Aspiration, obtaining fluid, and noting the disappearance of the mass readily serve to differentiate a fluid-filled cyst or galactocele from a solid tumor. Cytologic interpretation of needle aspirates is notoriously difficult because of the hyperproliferative cellularity during pregnancy and lactation. Furthermore, as can occur in any patient, the needle tip can miss and aspirate cells adjacent to the mass, thereby causing false reassurance.

With the ever-increasing popularity of aspiration cytology in assessment of breast masses, several small reports concern pregnancy and lactation and address inherent problems.[3-5] False-positive aspiration cytodiagnosis has been documented during gestation for benign breast tissue and is probably due to frequent mitosis, increased cellularity, anisonucleosis, prominent nucleoli, and variable granular chromatin within a proteinaceous background. An experienced aspiration cytopathologist with knowledge of the clinical setting is required. With these warnings, aspiration cytology has a place in the workup of abnormal areas found in pregnant and lactating breasts.

DELAY IN DIAGNOSTIC BIOPSY

Many authors have attributed to delay of diagnosis the advanced disease and thereby the poor prognosis often characteristic of gestational breast cancer. Delays longer than in nonpregnant women seem to be common.[6-8] After a thickness or possible mass is found, the postponement of a surgical biopsy may be due to the greater complication rate expected in the pregnant or lactating woman.

A study of 63 patients in whom cancer was diagnosed while they were pregnant or within 1 year postpartum at Memorial Hospital suggests the reluctance to perform a biopsy during pregnancy.[8] In less than 20% of such patients

was the diagnosis made during pregnancy. In almost half, the diagnosis was made within 12 weeks of delivery. Even in patients with previously undocumented masses, the large size of the cancers at the time of postpartum diagnosis (median, 3.5 cm) makes it likely that a smaller mass was palpable during pregnancy.

SPECIAL CONSIDERATIONS OF BIOPSY IN THE PREGNANT OR LACTATING BREAST

In the pregnant woman, local anesthesia is theoretically always safer than other anesthetic techniques.[9] Monitored sedation or even general anesthesia, with an anesthesiologist experienced in obstetrics, is rarely required and is acceptable, especially in the later phases of pregnancy when teratogenesis is not of great concern. Further discussion of the effects of anesthesia are to be found in Chapter 24.5.

Although excisional biopsies performed under local anesthesia during pregnancy may occasionally be difficult, depending on the individual breast, an incisional biopsy is also an alternative. Excellent hemostasis is necessary because of the increased vascularity and likelihood of postoperative hematoma.

The patient should cease breastfeeding before biopsy is performed because of the significant risk of milk fistula or infection (milk is a good culture medium). Binding the breast and using ice packs may help. Lowering prolactin by bromocriptine has not been associated with breast cancer and has been advocated.[10]

If a woman will not stop nursing but accepts the risk of fistula or infection (best recorded in writing), the physician can proceed with biopsy, depending on the individual factors. Although no published data appear to be available, one can surmise that the risk of milk fistula increases from low in peripheral biopsies to high in central biopsies. Because the large ducts intercommunicate, an operative infection can involve the whole breast.

As concerns infection, if the woman stops nursing briefly, preoperative antibiotics can be given. The milk, containing the mother's antibiotics, can be expressed by breast pump and discarded. After a brief period of bottle feeding, the infant may then resume breastfeeding, assuming a benign diagnosis. The milk may be bloody, however, and the risk of milk fistula probably remains.

PATHOLOGIC DIAGNOSIS

In 105 benign biopsies during pregnancy, 71% of patients had conditions also found in nonpregnant women, and only a small proportion had changes peculiar to pregnancy, such as lobular hyperplasia, galactocele, lactational mastitis, and so on.[11] Benign lesions during pregnancy, in decreasing order of frequency, include fibroadenomas, lipomas, papillomas, fibrocystic disease, galactoceles, and inflammatory lesions. Moreover, localized breast infarcts can cause mass lesions during pregnancy, either from overgrowth of a preexisting fibroadenoma or spontaneously.[12-15] The likelihood of diagnosing cancer is similar to that in the nonpregnant population: Byrd and associates[11] reported that 22% of breast biopsies in pregnancy showed malignancy, compared with 19% in overall patients.

A more recent report also noted that the majority of breast lumps excised during the pregnancy were preexisting, although growth rate may be stimulated during pregnancy.[16] Morphologically, a preexisting underlying lesion was readily identified in 18 cases (7 fibroadenomas, 5 tubular adenomas, and 6 hamartomas). The other 12 cases were lobular hyperplasia and inflammation, with no evidence of a prepartum lesion.

Blood in Nipple Discharge

Nipple discharge with blood present either visibly or cytologically during pregnancy or lactation is common. In 20% of women with nipple discharge during pregnancy, and in 15% of asymptomatic lactating women, the presence of blood was confirmed by cytologic analysis of the nipple secretion.[17-18]

Two authors presented long-term followup of 12 women[6] and 5 women[19] with bloody nipple discharge while pregnant who developed neither cancer nor a benign lesion, such as intraductal papilloma, on postpartum follow-up. The possible cause, as related to rapid ductal proliferation and hypervascularity, is discussed in these reports.[6,17-19]

The clinical follow-up to bloody nipple discharge with a nonsuspicious physical examination includes cytologic study of nipple secretions. As noted previously, the cytologist must be aware of the clinical setting. If repeated cytologic analyses reveal no malignant cells, close follow-up is suggested. Women should be advised not to squeeze the nipple because they often "check to see what's there" and may be reinjuring the duct structure. If cytologic analyses demonstrate malignant cells, then mammography, ultrasonography, and possibly even a galactogram are indicated to localize the source.

Infection

Infection is uncommon during pregnancy, but common during breastfeeding. The symptoms of suppurative mastitis seldom appear before the first week after birth, and infection does not become common until the third or fourth week. With infection, the patient becomes febrile, and the whole breast becomes hard, reddened, and painful. In a small group of women, infection is subacute or almost chronic, and the first clinical indication is a fluctuant mass.

By far, the most common organism is *Staphylococcus aureus*, and streptococcal groups are second. Toxic shock has been reported.[20] The source is nearly always the nursing infant's nose and throat. The bacterial colonization of the infant may be totally asymptomatic or, in the neonate, may involve the umbilicus or the skin. The organism is thought to enter the nipple at a fissure or a minute abrasion. The possibility of entrance through the lactiferous ducts with intact integument has also been considered.[21] The organism can nearly always be cultured from breast milk.

Antibiotic therapy should be started as soon as possible after breast milk is obtained for culture. The initial choice of antibiotic is influenced by the current experiences with staphylococcal and streptococcal infections in the hospital and community.[9,21] Breastfeeding should be discontinued because it is painful, and the infant harbors the organism and can cause reinfection. Once established, resistant staphylococcal infections tend to recur in the family.

Repeated aspiration coupled with antibiotics may suffice for cellulitis, but formal incision and drainage are necessary for abscesses.[9] An incision, usually radial, should be placed over the most dependent area of the fluctuance overlying the infected ducts. Multiple abscesses require several incisions. The operation should ideally be performed under general anesthesia, allowing the manual breakdown of the loculations. The resulting cavity is loosely packed with gauze initially. The cavity should be irrigated and then packed with a smaller amount of gauze at least daily.

Inflammatory Cancer Versus Infection

Inflammatory cancer probably arises no more frequently in pregnant patients than in others,[22-23] despite earlier opinions to the contrary. Notwithstanding referral patterns that might attract more severe cases, only 3% of pregnant patients with breast cancer at Memorial Hospital had inflammatory breast cancer.[8] Nevertheless, the surgeon must not make the dire error of mistaking inflammatory cancer for common lactational mastitis or abscess, and it is useful to perform a biopsy of the skin and the indurated breast tissue at the time of incision and drainage.[24]

MANAGEMENT SUMMARY

Before pregnancy, careful physical examination and mammography, as indicated by the patient's risk factors, are useful. Most benign masses excised during pregnancy were present before pregnancy. Most often, however, the physician has the opportunity to perform an exacting physical examination only on the first obstetric visit.

During pregnancy, the work-up of a palpable abnormality can include the same techniques as in the nonpregnant woman, although the mammary changes of pregnancy bring special considerations:

Mammography: Radiographic images are poor overall and often useless because of gestational changes.

Ultrasonography: No published reports define the range of normal gestational appearance.

Fine-needle aspiration: The gestational cellular changes are hyperproliferative and may be misdiagnosed if the cytologist is unaware of the pregnancy.

Open surgical biopsy: The hypervascularity and increased volume of the breast in the setting of local anesthesia make these procedures difficult.

References

1. Liberman L, Giess CS, Dershaw DD, et al. Imaging of pregnancy-associated breast cancer. Radiology 1994;191:245.
2. Max MH, Klamer TW. Pregnancy and breast cancer. South Med J 1983;76:1008.
3. Bottles K, Taylor RN. Diagnosis of breast masses in pregnant and lactating women by aspiration cytology. Obstet Gynecol 1985;66:76S.
4. Gupta RK, McHutchinson AGR, Dowle CS, et al. Fine-needle aspiration cytodiagnosis of breast masses in pregnant and lactating women and its impact on management. Diagn Cytopathol 1993;9:156.
5. Novotny DB, Maygarden SJ, Shermer RW, et al. Fine needle aspiration of benign and malignant breast masses associated with pregnancy. Acta Cytol 1991;35:676.
6. Haagenson CD. Carcinoma of the breast in pregnancy. In: Haagensen CD, ed. Diseases of the breast, ed 2. Philadelphia, WB Saunders, 1971:74.
7. Zemlickis D, Lishner M, Degendorfer P, et al. Maternal and fetal outcome after breast cancer in pregnancy. Am J Obstet Gynecol 1992;166:781.
8. Petrek JA, Dukoff R, Rogatko A. Pregnancy-associated breast cancer. Cancer 1991;67:869.
9. Canter JW, Oliver GC, Zaloudek CJ. Surgical diseases of the breast during pregnancy. Clin Obstet Gynecol 1983;26:853.
10. Anderson JM. Mammary cancers and pregnancy. Br Med J 1979;1:1124.
11. Byrd BF, Bayer DS, Robertson JC, et al. Treatment of breast tumors associated with pregnancy and lactation. Ann Surg 1962;155:940.
12. Rickert RR, Rajan S. Localized breast infarcts associated with pregnancy. Arch Pathol 1974;97:159.
13. Jiminez JF, Rickey RO, Cohen C. Spontaneous breast infarction associated with pregnancy presenting as a palpable mass. J Surg Oncol 1986;32:174.
14. Majmudar B, Rosales-Quintana S. Infarction of breast fibroadenomas during pregnancy. JAMA 1975;231:963.
15. O'Hara MF, Page DL. Adenomas of the breast and ectopic breast under lactational influences. Hum Pathol 1985;16:707.
16. Slavin JL, Billson R, Ostor AG. Nodular breast lesions during pregnancy and lactation. Histopathology 1993;22:481.
17. Kline TS, Lash SR. The bleeding nipple of pregnancy and postpartum: a cytologic and histologic study. Am J Pathol 1964;8:336.
18. Kline TS, Lash S. Nipple secretion in pregnancy: a cytologic and histologic study. Am J Clin Pathol 1962;37:626.
19. Lafreniere R. Bloody nipple discharge during pregnancy: a rationale for conservative treatment. J Surg Oncol 1990;43:228.
20. Dixey JJ, Swanson DC, Williams TD, et al. Toxic-shock syndrome: four cases in a London hospital. Br Med J 1982;285:342.
21. Cunningham I, Gary F, Williams JW. Williams' obstetrics, ed 19. Norwalk, CT, Appleton & Lange, 1993.
22. Wallack MK, Wolf JA Jr, Bedwinek J, et al. Gestational carcinoma of the female breast. Curr Probl Cancer 1983;7:1.
23. Donegan WL. Pregnancy and breast cancer. Obstet Gynecol 1977;50:244.
24. White TT. Carcinoma of the breast in the pregnant and the nursing patient. Am J Obstet Gynecol 1955;69:1277.

5.6
Medicolegal Aspects of Breast Cancer Evaluation and Treatment

R. JAMES BRENNER

The clinical practice of medicine includes many forms of accountability, one of the more onerous being legal redress. When patients perceive that their medical care has been improper, they may pursue such claims by filing a lawsuit. Lawsuits may occur for many reasons, but the most common reason for a claim of malpractice is a form of civil law called negligence, in which a physician's conduct is questioned as departing from a standard of care involving the exercise of ordinary skill and care that would be reasonably applied by other physicians in similar circumstances.[1] The breach of this "duty" to the patient, if it bears a substantially causative relation ("cause in fact, proximate cause") to a patient's injury, may permit the patient to sue for damages, usually in the form of money, as a form of restitution.[2]

Delay in diagnosis of breast cancer, according to a national study in 1995 by a consortium of physician-owned insurance carriers, is the most common reason that physicians are sued and the second leading cause of indemnity payment.[3] Public awareness of the ability to intercept the natural history of this disease in many cases, high contingency fees afforded attorneys representing a large number of women suffering from this disease at a relatively early age, and preventable patterns of practice likely contribute to claims for "loss of chance of survival."

Reasonable conduct by physicians as evaluated from a legal perspective may be based on actual laws (statutes) or prior case decisions that have been appealed and reviewed by higher courts and are published nationally. The Mammography Quality Standards Act is an example of the former; the common notions of standards of care, as established by expert consultants to the court, are an example of the latter.[4] This chapter examines several areas of legal exposure in the evaluation of patients for and with breast cancer and indicates risk-management strategies that may be employed in each set of circumstances to avoid possible liability.

Patient Evaluation: Clinical Standards and Risk Management

History taking and physical examination are both art and science. Those involved in breast care may provide such services as primary care physicians, as consultants in conjunction with a primary care physician, or as temporary consultants. The ramifications of these different approaches are discussed later in this section.

The definition of a primary care provider is evolving and has traditionally included those involved in general medical practice (internal medicine and family practice) as well as obstetricians and gynecologists (whose designation as primary care providers versus specialists has at times been controversial). The role has been assumed by many surgeons and, recently, by radiologists who have afforded access to breast care by means of patient self-referral for women who do not have a regular clinical provider.[5] Regardless of the specialty, it is the duty of the clinician provider to perform a reasonable physical examination and evaluation of patient history (signs or symptoms of breast cancer). The parameters of a reasonable examination of the breast are beyond the scope of this discussion and are reviewed in Chapter 4.1.[6] In this context, however, the examination need be thorough, including not only the entire breast tissue but the axillary and clavicular nodal regions as well, regularly scheduled, and adequately documented.

From a medicolegal point of view, the last of these features not only deserves emphasis and ramification, but is probably the most important risk-management effort in the examination, assuming the examination is properly performed.

The institution of a medical malpractice lawsuit for delay in diagnosis of breast cancer occurs when a patient discovers or has reason to discover that there may have been an unreasonable delay at arriving at this diagnosis resulting from the conduct of those responsible for her care.[7] This event usually triggers a statute of limitations, a concept that is discussed later in this chapter. The discovery of breast cancer frequently follows a series of clinical interactions between the physician and patient, after which time the actual filing of the malpractice suit may be further delayed by 1 to 2 years. Consequently, the precise details of the clinical visits occurring long before the lawsuit will likely be unknown to the patient and the treating physician, or at least subject to different interpretations.

The medical record is the customary manner by which the clinical examination and history taking is documented. Although it is technically hearsay and is therefore subject to exclusion as evidence during court trial, the medical record is considered such a common exception to the hearsay rule as to be generally admissible in court. Justification for this exception is not relevant to the current discussion except to the extent that most courts presume a high degree of validity and reliability associated with the medical record, so long as it reflects a regular and customary entry immediately following the patient's examination.[8]

A well-documented medical record may thus substantiate and evidence reasonable care. As such, the record regarding breast evaluation should maintain certain standard parameters. It should be organized, complete, accurate, and legible. Vague descriptions of physical findings instead of objective parameters are ill advised. Although physicians may believe that they will escape accountability by vague notes, the converse is more likely the case. Ambiguity in the medical record affords an aggrieved plaintiff the opportunity to contend that the examination was not only suboptimally conducted, but that vaguely defined physical findings were in fact significant and not appropriately managed. Thus, in one appellate case in which the patient contended that a lump that was not removed was a cancer, the medical record was sufficiently clear to indicate that the eventual cancer arose in a location inconsistent with the lump earlier detected and documented, and the defendant physician prevailed.[9] Conversely, in the absence of such documentation, plaintiffs have prevailed.[10] More often than not, well-documented appropriate care and instruction to patients provide a basis for supporting reasonable care.[11]

Busy practices may find physicians struggling to document all instruction parameters thoroughly. Certain mechanisms may facilitate the accomplishment of goals without unnecessary hardship. Preprinted or stamped diagrams of the breast and nodal regions may provide a rapid basis for documenting clinical findings with near-anatomic reproducibility, for purposes of surveillance. Mnemonics, so long as they are used in a regular and appropriate manner, may be entered into the chart notes as evidence that certain elements of the history and patient instructions have been accomplished (Birney P, personal communication).

Medical records serve many risk-management purposes, in addition to the physician's personal notes. The record provides communication to others such as consulting physicians, insurance companies, and utilization review committees. Because photocopies of such records are frequently required, entries to the medical records should be made in black or blue pen and in regular sequential order with single-line entries receiving both date and personal identifying verification. Transcribed notes, when placed in the medical record, should be proofread. These elements of medical record keeping are applicable not only to breast care but to all medical care and are important in serving as a continuous record. As discussed later in this chapter, subsequent altering of these records should not occur.

The initial evaluation of a patient with lumpy breasts may be difficult, and the clinician is often prompted to assign an immediate benign or malignant impression to a given area prematurely. The situation invites both overuse of surgical intervention and delayed interception of breast cancer. In such context, repeat short-term interval clinical examinations may provide a more rational basis for continued surveillance or intervention.[12] This approach has been advocated for probably benign, clinically occult, mammographically detected lesions and has been used successfully in practice.[13,14] The medical record may thus provide not only a reference for documenting areas of concern, but also corroboration of the absence of worsening changes detected by physical examination. Such documentation is especially important if a malignant process emerges unrelated to the stable or transient physical findings documented by serial physical examinations.

When an area of concern is defined clinically, further evaluation is necessary. This does not necessarily translate into biopsy, although biopsy may be the favored alternative. Although the concept of further evaluation is beyond the scope of this discussion, certain recurring principles should be noted. Many courts have held that a diagnostic mammogram may be an important component of such further evaluation.[15,16] Appropriate referral, including surgical referral, may also be in order. Unless care for the patient is relinquished to a referral source, a process that must be well documented (discussed later), the primary care physician maintains responsibility for following the patient's course.

Indeed, the ordering of any referral, either for clinical examination or for imaging or pathologic consultation, requires that the treating physician be responsible for evaluating the results of that referral. Relinquishing the follow-up of such results to other individuals or systems, absent a convincing rationale, is ill-advised.

The Element of Duty: A Variable Concept

The discussion of negligence involved the establishment of a duty for reasonable conduct, the breach of which created a basis for legal liability. The element of duty should be seen as a variable or dynamic component rather than static one. This may seem obvious given the different presentations of patients to the clinical physician. The concept requires further discussion, however. Judge Learned Hand, one of the leading jurisprudential commentators regarding tort law, attempted to define standard of care mathematically as the product of two factors—namely, the likelihood of an untoward event and the severity of such an event.

The first component in Learned Hand's formula may be assessed in terms of age-related incidence of breast cancer.[17] Other risk factors such as family history or documented proliferative breast disease with atypia or lobular carcinoma in situ also become part of the equation.[18-21] Emerging concepts regarding a general tendency for more rapid growth of breast cancers in younger women also need be considered when arriving at decisions regarding surveillance and interventional management.[26]

The element of duty is not only variable for the range of risk factors described, but also for women who have a history of diagnosed breast cancer. Although the management of such patients is discussed elsewhere in this text, these women are clearly at higher risk not only for recurrent disease, but also for metastatic and contralateral disease. It follows then that the duty of evaluation and consequent methods of surveillance require a higher standard of care in such situations.

Inherent to the discussion of duty and causation is another legal concept called *forseeability*. In assessing negligence, the court focuses on the conduct of the defendant's actions, not the consequences of such conduct. The patient who presents clinically for the first time with metastatic disease and who is referred immediately for interventional therapy has little legal standing for malpractice even though her disease is diagnosed at a late stage and her prognosis may be poor. Rather, the issue of forseeability arises when the patient presents to the clinician with nonspecific complaints that may or may not be related to cancer. The operative standard for the clinical assessment may be stated thus: Is it reasonably foreseeable that a specific area of concern represents a breast cancer? Conversely, the question may be stated: Is it reasonably foreseeable that the breast abnormality of concern is likely to represent a benign condition that may lend itself to management that does not require immediate surgical removal? Certain conditions affect such decision making, the assessment of which depends on the particular circumstances.

A practical lesson derived from this legal consideration is that areas of concern to the patient or the physician should be discussed with the patient, and that discussion should be documented. Surveillance strategies require not only diligence on the part of the physician, but also reasonable compliance on the part of the patient. Most states have enacted business and professional codes in consonance with appellate court decisions that indicate a responsibility of the patient to comply with the physician's recommendations so long as they are properly communicated. The latter element is often the subject of litigation when patients contend that they were either not informed or inadequately informed in understandable lay terminology regarding the nature of their condition, and management plans were not developed consensually.[11] At times, it may be useful to include family members in such discussions, especially in discussions with surgical, medical, and radiation oncologists, when patients' fears and anxiety distract attention from the substance of the consultation.

Multiple additional duties attend oncologic consultation, for example, cytotoxic effects, consequences of radiation therapy, advisability of investigative protocols, which are beyond the scope of this discussion. In this context, however, appropriate communication is essential because estates of decedent patients may sue for damages for improper communication of prognosis, with alleged unnecessary hardships incurred in resolving subsequent affairs.[22]

Screening and Diagnostic Mammography

The duty to order screening mammography is controversial both by virtue of varying interpretations of clinical trials as well as because of conflict in specialty society recommendations. Although no appellate court has ruled on this matter as a standard of care, such duty may emerge as a liability issue, and it has certainly been raised by plaintiff counsel during trial in most of the United States. Because of an increased consensus regarding the advisability of screening mammography in women over the age of 50 years (the interval still subject to controversy), this standard of care may be more readily employed by an older plaintiff than a younger one. Such a decision needs to be tempered by the previously noted faster growth rates of tumors in younger women and the resultant need for even earlier intervention in this premenopausal population that accounts for a significant percentage of all cases of breast cancer. Future statutory or judicial direction may help resolve such issues.

The decision to obtain a screening or diagnostic mammogram, the latter of which often involves ancillary imaging procedures to define areas of clinical concern, is predicated on the initial clinical examination. Indeed, screening mammography is specifically defined for those women who have no signs or symptoms of breast cancer, a determination of which is best made by formal physical examination. A program that provides mammographic facilities to large populations of women in a low-cost, efficient public health–oriented manner may preclude on-site physical evaluation of the patient at the mammographic facility.[23,24] Unfortunately, many patients are evaluated by the clinician only after obtaining a screening mammogram. Two potential problems exist with this approach, which is used frequently, given the resource restrictions and time limitations often imposed in patient care.

The first problem is that a clinician may discover an abnormality that is unknown to the patient following a screening mammogram, a situation that renders the radiologic evaluation suboptimal. Specially tailored imaging examinations, based on suspicious clinical findings, may result in recommendations that vary from those rendered by a screening mammogram, a universally prescribed two-view study of all breast tissue. Theoretically, this situation may be remedied by the clinician's referring the patient back to the imaging facility for additional evaluation. A second potential problem of patients who obtain self-initiated screening mammograms before clinical evaluation is the possibility that the patient, on learning of a normal mammogram result, develops a sense of self-confidence and either delays or fails to seek a clinical examination. Screening for breast cancer is not synonymous with mammographic screening, and several studies, including notably the Breast Cancer Detection Demonstration Project, have documented the complementary roles of clinical examination and mammographic examination in detecting breast cancer.[25] This false sense of confidence has been observed in other screening trials, with a resultant delay in diagnosis in clinical breast cancer.[26] Clinicians are advised to employ recall mechanisms, similar to those suggested in the radiology literature, to ensure regular evaluations.[27]

The clinician who refers a patient to an imaging center for screening mammography, diagnostic imaging, or both should have some sense of the relative accuracy and expertise of the center. Perhaps needless to say—but too often taken (mistakenly) for granted—a mammographic examination is not tantamount to an automated blood test, but involves considerable subjective interpretation factors. Although this consideration is true for all imaging examinations involving the breast or other organ systems, the frequency of regular-interval mammography surveillance should underscore the need for familiarity with the center to which the patient is referred.

Lawsuit: Receiving a Summons and Complaint

Patient motivations for filing medical malpractice lawsuits against physicians are multifactorial and include need for money, anger, perceptions of poor patient–physician communication, encouragement by family and acquaintances, need for information, recognized cover-ups, desire to seek revenge or to protect others from harm, and inaccessibility of physicians who would listen to and consider problems.[28,29] The previous discussions have suggested the need for including the patient and even family members in management decisions. Indeed, the perception and even the reality of the hurried physician underlie many of the problems leading to legal repercussions.

Regardless of the reasons for the filing of a lawsuit, the receiving of a summons and complaint triggers a cascade of intellectual and emotional responses by the defendant physician. These responses need to be self-contained, and the physician is advised to "freeze the past action in place and time."[30] The matter should be referred immediately to the physician's insurance carrier and risk manager of the practice. The carrier ordinarily assigns administrative personnel and a defense attorney to the case.

Temptations to discuss the particular facts of the case with colleagues, and even patients, should be resisted. Once a malpractice claim is filed, all such discussions are "discoverable." The substance of seemingly innocuous conversations can be raised at trial unless the conversations occur in the presence of a defense attorney under specific circumstances. Too often, physicians believe that they will "quash" the complaint by trying to reason with the patient, a practice that has come back to haunt some individuals should the case go to trial. The period following the filing of a legal complaint is generally known as *discovery,* a time during which interrogatories or questionnaires and depositions or legal testimony are obtained. By such mechanisms, attorneys for both plaintiff and defendant assess initially the status of the case and devise respective strategies for seeking further facts relevant to the initial complaint. Discovery may be prolonged and, depending on the agreements of all parties, may extend for more than a year.

As mentioned earlier, statutory regulations by individual states define a finite period of time (usually 1 to 2 years) following the discovery of "actionable harm" or negligence by the defendant during which a plaintiff may file a legal complaint. So long as the lawsuit is filed within an appropriate time frame, any action regarding the case, regardless of when such actions occurred, may be subject to review. The rationale for statutes of limitations is beyond the scope of this discussion, but it includes the reliability of accessing information and testimony within a time frame reasonably proximal to the lawsuit. Most medical malpractice cases are settled before trial. The current requirements of reporting any money exchanged secondary to settlement to the National Practitioners Data Bank may affect this inclination for settlement in ways that cannot currently be predicted.

The trier of fact during trial may be either a judge or a jury. Determinations made at the trial of medical malpractice cases are not generally appealed. Appellate courts are more concerned with issues of law rather than fact and are reluctant to revisit the factual considerations arising at trial. Thus, physician defendants who are subjecting their conduct to a trial resolution should make every effort to prevail at this juncture. As a West Virginia court noted, "Ordinarily a juror's claim that he was confused over the law of evidence and therefore participated in the verdict on an incorrect premise is a matter that inheres in or is intrinsic to the deliberative process and cannot be used to impeach the verdict." Unless the jury or judge's verdict is believed to be plainly wrong—a decision uncommonly reached by an appellate court—the trial verdict is generally not overturned.[31]

Unlike many personal injury complaints, medical malpractice lawsuits usually involve the employment of physicians to serve as expert witnesses to help establish an appropriate standard of care for the lay jury or judge. Experts often disagree on such standards of care, and each case primarily depends on the factual circumstances. Defendant physicians may be afforded the opportunity to serve as their own experts if they maintain sufficient credentials to warrant such a designation. Regular appointments at academic centers of excellence or publications in peer-reviewed journals of material relevant to the case at bar may be useful considerations in attempting to establish the reasonableness of a given approach that is questioned in court.[30]

An unnecessary result of the legal adversarial approach to dispute resolution has been for experts to insist that only one approach is feasible when published reports support various approaches. This situation has caused one researcher to question whether expert witnesses act as partisans who think it is their job to win the case.[32] Perhaps the inclusion of previously overlooked legal aspects of medical practice in current medical school curricula will help to alleviate this problem.[33] The emergence of practice parameters by both medical specialty societies and governmental agencies such as the Agency for Health Care Policy and Research of the Department of Health and Human Services may affect the establishment of reasonable standards of care. Current considerations of such parameters, such as under investigation in the state of Maine, involve the use of such criteria as a basis for the defense and not as a mechanism by which the plaintiff attorney may impugn the actions of the defendant physician. Even the existence of such parameters is not necessarily binding on a physician if conduct at variance with such parameters can be established as reasonable. The eventual consequences of these approaches, especially in an era of managed care, will likely become an important component of risk-management strategies.

Other Legal Actions

FRAUD

Intentional misrepresentation is a problem for which both criminal and civil penalties apply. For example, the fraudulent filing of insurance claims may subject the physician to criminal penalties.

In the current discussion, however, fraud has a more relevant implication in terms of the previously described statute of limitations. The filing of a lawsuit must be completed within a time frame defined by when a patient discovers a wrongful act or negligence or should reasonably discover such act. If material or significant information is deliberately withheld or is misrepresented to a patient, such statute of limitations may be extended or "tolled" and consequently may subject the physician to unending legal exposure for a given course of conduct. Although efforts are often extended with best intentions to mitigate the anxiety of a patient who has discovered that she has breast cancer, the physician must be careful when relating the facts relevant to her care. Medical ethics dictate such standards, but the anxiety and fear imposed by the delayed discovery of breast cancer may prompt actions that, subject to interpretation, may expose the physician to unnecessary and severe legal consequences. Other technical legal doctrines, such as "continuous care," may also extend the period of legal exposure for the defendant physician, but may have only indirect relevance to risk-management strategies in the physician's office.

NEGLIGENT REFERRAL

The emphasis of the previous discussion has been establishing a reasonable standard of care for the conduct of a given physician. Attention has been drawn to the variable nature of the element of negligence called duty. We now consider the duty to refer a patient for care to another physician if the referring physician is unable to provide appropriate care. This duty to refer is itself subject to standard considerations of negligence. A "derivative" tort called *negligent referral* occurs when a physician refers a patient to another physician whom the first physician knows or has reason to know to be unable to care for the patient appropriately. Thus, if the consultant physician provides negligent care that should have been foreseeable to the referring physician, the referring physician may also be liable for any harm that may accrue because of the referral. The determination of how a referring physician should have known or have had reason to know is a factual determination for a judge or jury. Although suspension of medical staff privileges or extenuating economic relationships may be factors that enter into such an analysis, no prescriptive formula exists for making such a determination. Like any analysis in negligence, the issue is resolved by the particular facts of the case.

ABANDONMENT

The legal relationship of patient and physician is not one of parity. A patient may elect to discontinue care from a physician at any time and for any reason. In contrast, a physician who is responsible for the care of a patient must make some provision for the transfer of that care if he or she decides to terminate the relationship. The causes for a breakdown in a physician–patient relationship are variable, and it may not be in the best interest of either party to maintain a relationship under adversarial circumstances.

The extent to which a physician must go to provide such transference of care varies, depending on the circumstances of the patient. For example, the care of a well women with no medical problems may be transferred by relatively simple and documented means, provided both patient and physician understand the goals to be accomplished.

At the other extreme, the transference of care of a severely ill patient should be carefully documented, especially in terms of justifying the transference at that particular time and clearly defined acceptance of such care by another treating physician or facility. Specifically, fewer assumptions are likely to be held as reasonable for the transference of an acutely ill patient, as opposed to a well patient. The court looks critically at the circumstances surrounding such transfer and generally charges the physician with superior knowledge regarding the patient's condition. As always, the factual determinations surrounding such transfer of care are the basis for resolving the dispute.

Outcomes Review: Settlements and Cases

The cost of malpractice insurance for a physician varies from state to state and from specialty to specialty. One of the more significant elements in determining such rates is the presence of statutes limiting recovery for so-called *compensatory damages* of pain and suffering secondary to the delay in diagnosis of breast cancer. In addition, state courts may vary in assessing damages to be awarded secondary to the future loss of chance of survival.

The rationale for assigning medical malpractice rates based on medical practice experience is a subject of ongoing evaluation.[34,35] Nonetheless, it has been estimated that for every $100 paid to a physician, $11 are allocated for malpractice insurance.[36] Most of this money is allocated not to direct patient compensation, but rather to administrative costs and lawyer fees. Although health care reform may include systematic improvement in the resources available for restitution for harm to a patient caused by

physician negligence, the most direct intervention available to the practicing physician to diminish legal exposure is an evaluation of current practice patterns. This section attempts to establish the parameters by which such patterns are subject to legal accountability and to provide suggested strategies. The Physicians Insurers Association of America (PIAA) Breast Cancer Study of 1995, mentioned at the beginning of this chapter, reviewed a total of 487 claims directed against physicians for the delay in diagnosis of breast cancer in a report of the study performed in 1990.[3] On average, 1.88 physicians were included in lawsuits for negligence of cases reported. Primary care physicians were named most often, followed by radiologists in the 1990, but this order was reversed in the 1995 study. Average indemnity payments were variable, and both the frequency and indemnity rewards are reviewed in Table 5.6-1. From a liability standpoint, a disturbing observation in the PIAA study is the virtual inverse relation between frequency of lawsuits and amounts paid as a factor of patient age when compared with the frequency of cancer as a factor of age, a relation found in both the 1990 and 1995 studies (Tables 5.6-2 and 5.6-3). Although breast cancer in women under age 50 years accounts for less than one third of all cases, this group represented over two thirds of those seeking legal redress. The explanation is probably complex but likely reflects (1) a possible worsening of prognosis secondary to delay in diagnosis because of faster-growing tumors in this younger age group[20]; (2) a higher percentage of younger women having denser, firmer breasts for which earlier diagnosis may be more difficult; and (3) the potential amount of damages awarded to young women being likely higher (based on potential earnings lost, impact on family, and so forth), the measure by which attorneys are remunerated and thereby engage in case selection.

Pain was a presenting symptom in slightly over 27% of cases in the 1990 study and 9.2% of cases in the 1995 study. Clinicians should be alerted to this fact because a history of pain is often dismissed during clinical examinations, especially if breast pain is not carefully distinguished from referred chest wall pain. As might be expected, most

TABLE 5.6-1
Claims Counts and Indemnity by Specialty

Specialty	Claims	Total Indemnity ($)	Average Indemnity ($)
Radiology	165	30,079,579	182,300
Obstetrics and gynecology	154	42,736,849	277,512
Family practice	113	19,744,677	174,732
Surgical specialty	97	24,922,537	256,933
Internal medicine	61	10,760,277	176,397
Pathology	11	3,799,502	345,409
Other physician	31	5,084,276	164,009
Corporation	30	8,155,226	271,841
Hospital	13	1,528,167	117,551
TOTAL	675	146,811,040	217,498

TABLE 5.6-2
Percentage of Claimants by Menopausal Status

Status	Claimants (%)	
	1990	1995
Premenopausal	66.9	54.9
Perimenopausal	7.7	9.0
Postmenopausal	25.4	36.1

TABLE 5.6-4
Reasons for Delay in Diagnosis

Reason	Frequency
Physical findings failed to impress	169
Failure to follow up with patient	150
Negative mammographic report	125
Mammogram misread	110
Failure to do proper biopsy	110
Delay in or failure to consult	75
Failure to react to mammogram	60
Distracted by other health problems	55
Repeat examinations did not arouse suspicion	55
Failure to order mammogram	54
Inadequate communication	51
Poor examination by physician	50

patients in this study who sued for delay in diagnosis of breast cancer presented with a mass and no palpable lymph nodes (46.5%). Other symptoms included mass with palpable nodes, bleeding or nipple discharge, and mass with no palpable lymph nodes, as well as fixation of skin; 21.4% of the patients had no physical findings, but it is unknown how many of these patients had suggestive mammograms prompting a lawsuit. Thus, most patients who eventually sued for breast cancer malpractice demonstrated physical findings that, according to the initial discussion, may have prompted either short-term surveillance or immediate intervention. Although case-specific, a delay of 3 to 6 months may be reasonable, for example, for nonspecific complaints and unreasonable for an immovable dominant mass with skin retraction.

Table 5.6-4 indicates the frequency of reasons causing delay in diagnosis because of the physician. One lesson that may be derived is that physical findings that may not otherwise be impressive to the examining physician should allow for the possibility of a patient's procrastination and should perhaps prompt closer surveillance or even intervention. That a negative mammographic report has an impact on a delay in diagnosis reinforces the clinical dictum requiring physicians to evaluate palpable areas appropriately regardless of the mammographic findings.

Although clinical management of a palpable abnormality can be influenced by imaging studies (e.g., finding a cyst), the absence of imaging characteristics places the clinician as the sole arbiter in assessing future management.

TABLE 5.6-3
Comparitive Average Indemnity by Claimant Age

Age (y)	Indemnity ($)	
	1990	1995
20–29	286,000	375,000
30–39	330,000	358,000
40–49	194,000	334,000
50–59	135,000	262,000
60–69	73,000	197,000
70+	102,000	118,000

The findings of the PIAA are supported by a study of civil cases evaluated in a separate review of court cases, with a notable exception that the court case review indicates that radiologists were involved only 10% of the time.[37] This statistic may reflect the significant time lag in cases reaching the appellate court division.[30] The increasing use of mammography is likely to subject radiologists, already the most frequently named defendants, to increased legal exposure because lawsuits filed for delay in diagnosis of breast cancer generally name all physicians attending to the patient. Both studies indicated a mean average delay in diagnosis of approximately 14 months, the same period in the PIAA 1990 study.

My review of more than 60 cases in the appellate court literature demonstrates both recurrent errors in management as well as case-specific problems. The recurrent errors are discussed throughout this section, most prominently including the lack of appropriate documentation of physical findings, the lack of deliberate management plans, and the lack of communication regarding both of the foregoing to involve the patient. The review of appellate decisions shows a skewed population of cases reaching the courts for legal and not factual reasons. Other case-specific circumstances of lawsuits considered at the appellate level include situations such as the failure to obtain adequate consent for proposed surgical procedures and legal considerations regarding specific damage awards, areas that do not have universal importance to practicing physicians.

Summary

Expertise and experience in evaluating women for breast cancer are only as effective as their application in clinical practice. This latter parameter is the basis for legal accountability and the focus of practice patterns suggested in this chapter. Documentation is the essence of risk management, and the patient's history and physical examination need be committed to the medical record without ambiguity. When clinical circumstances are easily defined, appropriate referral and follow-up regarding resolution of the problem are indicated. When the examination or history is not clear, deliberate and reasonably close surveillance is required together, with appropriate ancillary testing such as imaging and even tissue sampling. Such medical plans, discussed with the patient, should be tailored to the individual clinical situation. When unanticipated circumstances emerge, management needs to be reassessed and again discussed directly with the patient. Routine screening may not only detect cancer at earlier stages, but it may also help to defeat speculative claims regarding delayed diagnosis.

Because the likelihood of being sued for delay in diagnosis of breast cancer is high, health care personnel should be sensitive to the careful response required to a lawsuit and the need to coordinate all activities with legal counsel. Although physicians may not always be able to prevent untoward outcomes, practice patterns that are validated from both a medical and a legal perspective offer the most successful approach for reducing the complications of breast cancer and defeating inappropriate legal redress.

References

1. Skettington v Bradley. 366 Mich 552, 115 NW 2d 303, 1962.
2. Brenner RJ. Medicolegal aspects of screening mammography. AJR 1989;153:53.
3. Physicians Insurers Association of America: The breast cancer study. Washington, DC, 1995.
4. Mammography Quality Standards Act, Publ L 102–539, 1992.
5. Monsees B, Destouet JM, Evens RG. The self-referred mammography patient: a new responsibility for radiologists. Radiology 1988;166:691.
6. Foster RS Jr, Limitations of physical examination in the early diagnosis of breast cancer. Surg Oncol Clin North Am 1994;3:55.
7. Steingart v White. 198 Cal App 33L 406, Cal Rprr 678, 1988.
8. Fed R. Evid 808(6).
9. Detimann v Flanary. 86 Wis 2D 728, 1979.
10. Deburkarte v Louvar. 393 NW 2d 131, Iowa, 1986.
11. Chudson v Ratra. 76 Md App 753, 1988.
12. Brenner RJ. Breast cancer evaluation: medical legal and risk management consideration for the clinician. Cancer [Supp] 1994;74:486.
13. Brenner RJ, Sickles EA. Acceptability of periodic follow-up as an alternative to biopsy for mammographically detected lesions interpreted as probably benign. Radiology 1989;171:645.
14. Sickles EA. Periodic follow-up of probably benign mammographic lesions: results for 3184 consecutive cases. Radiology 1991;179:463.
15. Beckcomb v United States. 584 F Supp 1471 (applying New York Law), ND, NY, 1984.
16. Barrenbrugge v Rich. 141 Ill App 3d 1046, 490 NE 2d 1368, 1st Dist, 1986.
17. Lipps v Downing. Ct of Appeals, Ohio, Slip op, 1988.
18. Kerilikowske K, Grady D, Barclay J. Positive predictive value of screening mammography by age: family history of breast cancer. JAMA 1993;270:2444.
19. Dupont WD, Page DL. Risk factors for breast cancer in women with proliferative breast disease. N Engl J Med 1985;312:146.
20. Colditz GA, Willet WC, Hunter DJ, et al: Family history, age and risk of breast cancer: prospective data from the Nurses' Health Study. JAMA 1993;270.
21. van Dijck JAAM, Petronella GMP, Hendricks JHCL. Age-dependent growth rate of primary breast cancer. Cancer 1993;71:3547.
22. Arato v Avedon. Calif Supr Ct, No so29049, 1993.
23. Bird RE, McLelland R. How to initiate and operate a low-cost screening mammography center. Radiology 1986;161:43.
24. Sickles EA, Weber WN, Galpin HD, et al. Mammographic screening: how to operate successfully at low cost. Radiology 1986.
25. The Breast Cancer Detection Demonstration Project and results. CA Cancer J Clin 1987;37:1.
26. Kopans DB, Feig SA. The Canadian National Breast Screening Study: a critical review. AJR 1993;161:755.
27. Brenner RJ. Evolving medical and legal concepts for clinicians and imagers in evaluation of breast cancer. Cancer [Supp] 1992;69:1950.
28. Waitzkin H. Doctor–patient communication: clinical implications of social science research. JAMA 1984;252:2441.
29. Hickson GB, Clayton GW, Githens PB, et al. Factors that prompted families to file medical malpractice claims following perinatal injuries. JAMA 1992;267:1359.
30. Brenner RJ. Mammography and malpractice litigation: current status, lessons and admonition. AJR 1993;161:931.
31. Livengood v Kerr. 391 SE 2d 371, 374, W Va, 1990.
32. Brent RL. The irresponsible expert witness: a failure of biomedical graduate education and professional accountability. Pediatrics 1982;70:754.
33. Beninger PR, Beninger ES, Fitzgerald FT. Survey on views and knowledge of house officers on medical legal issues. J Med Educ 1985;60:481.
34. Rolph JE, Kravitz RL, GoGuigan K. Malpractice claims data as a quality improvement tool: is targeting effective? JAMA 1991; 266:2093.
35. Sloan FA, Mergenhagen PM, Buatiek WB, et al. Medical malpractice experience of physicians: predictable or haphazard? JAMA 1989; 262:3291.
36. Domenici PV, Koop CE. Sue the doctor? There's a better way. New York Times 1991;June 6:A19,A25(611).
37. Kern KA. Causes of breast cancer malpractice litigation: a 20-year civil court review. Arch Surg 1992;127:542.

Diseases of the Breast, edited by Jay R. Harris,
Marc E. Lippman, Monica Morrow, and Samuel Hellman.
Lippincott-Raven Publishers, Philadelphia, © 1996.

Biopsy Techniques

6.1
Techniques for Diagnosis of Palpable Breast Masses

ROGER S. FOSTER, JR.

When physical examination of the breast shows a suspicious abnormality, either a definite mass or a thickening that is not unequivocally within the normal range, a biopsy for pathologic diagnosis should be done. Four different techniques are used to obtain pathologic material from a palpable lesion: fine-needle aspiration biopsy (FNAB), core-cutting needle biopsy, excisional biopsy, and incisional biopsy. Each of these procedures has advantages that may make it the most suitable for a particular patient. FNABs are usually done without an anesthetic, or with local anesthesia in the skin. Core-cutting needle biopsies and incisional biopsies require a local anesthetic. With appropriate technique, excisional biopsies may almost always be done comfortably while the patient is under local anesthesia. Some surgeons prefer to use a general anesthetic for most excisional breast biopsies.

Most patients are now treated using a two-step procedure. The first step is the biopsy, which can then be followed by a more extensive work-up and an informed discussion with the patient; the second step is the definitive surgical treatment. When the two-step procedure is accomplished using FNAB, costs are less than those incurred using an excisional biopsy, particularly if the excisional biopsy is done using general anesthesia.[1-3]

One of the past rationales for the one-step procedure was an emergency theory about the behavior of breast cancer; any delay in treatment was thought to decrease the patient's prognosis. Concern also existed that the biopsy procedure might disturb the cancer and lead to a lower survival rate if definitive surgery was not done. Both retrospective studies and data from the large prospective clinical trials show no difference in the survival rates between one- and two-step procedures.[4-7] Moreover, no evidence from these studies has shown delays of a month or even more between biopsy and definitive surgery have led to a poorer outcome.

Fine-Needle Aspiration and Fine-Needle Aspiration Biopsy

Fine-needle aspiration and FNAB of the breast are complementary procedures. Fine-needle aspiration of gross breast cysts is both diagnostic and therapeutic. If the suspected cyst proves to be a solid lesion, material for FNAB may obtained instead. Even if excision of a probably benign mass is planned and it is believed that FNAB would be redundant (eg, in a young woman with a dominant mass that is presumed to be a fibroadenoma), it is appropriate to perform an aspiration before the excision to exclude a tense cyst that may mimic a fibroadenoma on physical examination.

FNAB for the diagnosis of breast lesions has been used for more than six decades and has been an established procedure in Europe for many years.[8-11] Only in the past two or three decades, however, has it begun to become more widely accepted and used in the United States. When a skilled cytopathologist is available for interpretation of the specimen, FNAB has many advantages. For palpable breast masses, FNAB's advantages include simplicity, good accuracy, low morbidity, minimal patient discomfort, relatively low cost, and immediate availability as an office procedure that can be done at the time the patient is first seen in the surgeon's office.

If skilled cytopathologists are provided with adequate material, the diagnostic accuracy of FNAB should be high.[12] The apparent simplicity of FNAB can, however, lead to its application in unskilled hands.[13] A review of 31,340 FNABs in the medical literature indicates that the sensitivity and specificity of FNAB vary widely between reporting groups.[14] In that review, the reported sensitivity ranged from 65% to 98% and the specificity from 34% to 100%. No cytopathologist can make a reading unless adequate cellular material is aspirated from the lesion.

Before FNAB diagnosis of breast malignancy is used as the basis for definitive patient management, the track record of the cytopathologist should be known. A false-positive FNAB diagnosis by a skilled cytopathologist should be rare. Among experienced cytopathologists, the rate of false-positive results ranges from 0% to 0.4%, with an overall average of about 0.17%.[13,15,16] Rare false-positive readings also occur with open breast biopsies.

FNAB cannot always distinguish between an invasive carcinoma and noninvasive ductal carcinoma in situ. Pathologists should be encouraged to stratify their malignant diagnoses into "definite" and "probable" malignancy, with only a definitive diagnosis of malignancy supporting definitive therapy.[17] Histologic confirmation is required for the probable malignancy group. This approach not only avoids false-positive results but also tends to place in situ carcinomas and low-grade carcinomas requiring special clinical management into the probable group, ensuring that they are recognized before definitive treatment is begun.

False-negative rates in recent series have ranged from 0% to 4%.[12,18,19] A greater possibility of a false-negative interpretation exists for well-differentiated tumors such as tubular carcinomas and papillary carcinomas and for cases in which the tumor is paucicellular.[19] Most false-negative results are due to sampling errors, which tend to be associated with small tumor size, rather than misinterpretation by the cytopathologist.[12] The FNAB report needs to be interpreted in relation to the clinical examination and mammographic findings. If either the clinical examination or the mammogram is suggestive of possible malignancy, an incisional or excisional biopsy should be done.

TRIPLE-NEGATIVE DIAGNOSTIC TEST

The FNAB has been recommended as part of a triad of diagnostic procedures in women who present with asymmetric, thickened areas of the breast that are clinically believed to be probably benign yet raise a small element of suspicion.[20–22] If mammographic results are not suggestive, a negative FNAB that shows normal breast epithelial cells can provide additional reassurance. An FNAB that is acellular does not provide satisfactory reassurance that the sampling was adequate and should usually be repeated.

FINE-NEEDLE ASPIRATION BIOPSY OF SURGICAL SCAR LESIONS

Properly performed FNAB can be useful in evaluation of lesions detected in the scars after either breast-conserving surgery or total mastectomy. The sensitivity, specificity, and positive and negative predictive values are similar to those for the use of FNAB in patients with primary breast cancer.[23] Open biopsies for lesions in the breast treated by breast conservation surgery and irradiation are associated with a relatively high wound healing complication rate.[24]

TECHNIQUE OF FINE-NEEDLE ASPIRATION OF CYSTS

The skin of the breast is first treated with alcohol or an iodophor. A local anesthetic is not usually used because it requires a needle puncture, and the typical cyst can be aspirated with a single pass. Brief application of ethyl chloride spray, insufficient to freeze the skin but sufficient to distract the patient, can be used if available. I have found that a 1-inch no. 21 needle is satisfactory for most cysts. The size of the syringe chosen depends on the suspected volume of the cyst. Usual syringe sizes are 3 to 10 mL. Using universal precautions, the cyst is stabilized between two fingers of the nondominant hand so that the cyst may be punctured and aspirated with the dominant hand. The needle should be rotated, as it is slowly withdrawn, toward the completion of the aspiration to be certain that any cyst wall impinging on the bevel of the needle does not prevent complete aspiration. Palpation with the fingers of the nondominant hand can be used to determine whether the cyst has been completely emptied and whether an adjacent mass exists. Typical cyst fluid is thin and slightly opalescent, and varies from light tan to dark green. The fluid in a long-standing cyst may occasionally become thick and require a larger needle for complete evacuation. After aspiration, the patient is instructed to maintain pressure on the site for at least 5 minutes to prevent bleeding into the cyst cavity. Typical cyst fluid is discarded because large studies have shown that cytologic examination of typical cyst fluid is of little utility.[9,25,26] When malignant lesions are cystic, additional clinical factors usually indicate that the abnormality is not a typical gross cyst. In such cases, the fluid is bloody or a residual mass is present after aspiration of the fluid. On rare occasions, a unsuspected nonpalpable ductal or lobar carcinoma in situ has been detected on examination of apparently normal cyst fluid, just as such lesions are serendipitously identified adjacent to benign lesions that have been excised. If a bloody cyst is encountered, the fluid should be sent for cytologic examination to rule out cystic carcinoma.[27] The cystic mass should completely disappear. A persistent residual mass, multiple recurrences after aspiration of the same cyst, and a bloody aspirate are all indications to obtain adequate material for pathologic examination.

TECHNIQUE OF FINE-NEEDLE ASPIRATION BREAST BIOPSY

Adequate FNAB depends on skillful technique by both the operator and the cytopathologist. The operator must have the expertise to ascertain that the needle is within the lesion and that sufficient material for an adequate cytologic examination is obtained. Depending on the needs of the cytopathologist, the aspirated material must be immediately smeared on microscope slides or placed into a fixative for cell-block or cytospin preparations. The cytopathologist may request that the slides be immediately wet-fixed in 95% ethyl alcohol with no air-drying, that they be air-dried, or that both types of preparations be done.

FNAB is done after the skin has been cleaned with an antiseptic. The needles used for FNAB may vary in size from no. 21 to no. 27. If a cyst has been anticipated but the lesion proves to be solid, the no. 21 needle may be used to obtain the cytologic material. If the lesion is believed to be solid, a no. 25 needle may lead to less admixture of blood with the cells from the lesion. Some operators use a 20-mL syringe in a special holder designed to stabilize the syringe barrel, thus aiding one-handed withdrawal of the plunger to create the vacuum for aspirations. I and others have found it simpler to use a one-handed technique to withdraw the plunger of a standard 3-, 5-, or 10-mL hypodermic syringe. The needle is passed in and out of the lesion 3 to 10 times in various directions. A slight rotary motion allows the bevel of the needle to cut additional cells from the mass. The appearance of the aspirated material in the hub of the needle usually signals that an adequate amount of material has been aspirated. The suction on the plunger is released, and, after equilibration, the needle and syringe are withdrawn. The needle is disconnected from the syringe, and the syringe is filled with air. The needle is replaced, and a drop of the material is carefully expressed onto a glass microscope slide and immediately spread with another slide. Slides are immediately wet-fixed or air-dried as discussed previously.

Core-Cutting Needle Biopsy

Core-cutting needle biopsies provide histologic material that is usually suitable for interpretation by any pathologist[16,28] without requiring the special skills of a cytopathol-

ogist. Core-cutting needle biopsies may be processed for permanent sections or for frozen sections.

False-positive diagnoses obtained using core-cutting needle biopsies are rare but could occur with sclerosing ductal proliferations such as radial scars, where a pseudoinvasive mingling of proliferating epithelium and stroma is easier to diagnose using open biopsies that include the entire lesion. False-negative diagnoses with core-cutting needle biopsies are related to the same sampling problems encountered with FNAB. Sampling problems may even be slightly greater because of increased resistance to penetration of the larger needle into the tumor. In such cases, the needle may be deflected and thus sample tissue adjacent to, rather than within, the tumor.[29] Occasionally, the core biopsy sample may not provide sufficient material for diagnosis because of extreme desmoplasia or necrosis.

Although the likelihood of seeding the needle track with tumor cells during FNAB appears to be very low, some reports have described needle track seeding from core needle breast biopsies.[30] It is prudent to place the biopsy track so that the definitive treatment includes it. The depth of the biopsy should be adjusted to eliminate any chance of carrying malignant tissue into the chest wall or into other areas of the breast that would not be removed during the planned surgical procedure.

TECHNIQUE OF CORE-CUTTING NEEDLE BIOPSY

Core needle biopsies may be obtained with disposable needles such as the Tru-Cut (Fig. 6.1-1) or with the Bioptycut spring loaded device. The Tru-Cut needles have the advantage of being readily available and relatively inexpensive. Use of the Bioptycut device has the advantages of decreased pain, a slightly higher sampling success rate, a greater diagnostic sensitivity, and a somewhat better specimen quality than the Tru-Cut.[31] The Biopty device is relatively expensive, however, and therefore is less likely to be available in the outpatient office.

FIGURE 6.1-1 The Tru-Cut (Baxter) disposable core-cutting needle that can be used to obtain core biopsies of solid breast masses.

Excisional Biopsy

Excisional breast biopsy is the complete removal of a lesion, with or without a rim of surrounding normal parenchyma. The excisional biopsy is usually the definitive treatment of benign lesions. For malignant lesions, if a margin of normal tissue has been removed and if the pathologic examination confirms that the margins are not involved by cancer, no further breast surgery may be necessary.

TECHNIQUE OF EXCISIONAL BREAST BIOPSY

Local anesthesia, with or without supplemental sedation, can be used for excisional breast biopsies. General anesthesia entails greater cost, a slightly longer period of disability for the patient, and a small but finite risk associated with general anesthesia. Local anesthesia requires that the surgeon be skilled in infiltrating the anesthetic in a manner that causes minimal discomfort, that the surgeon be willing to communicate with the patient during the procedure, and that the surgery be done with minimal traction.

Adding 1 mL of 8.5% sodium bicarbonate to each 10 mL of 1% lidocaine without epinephrine creates a more neutral pH that causes less discomfort during infiltration. Discomfort can also be minimized by slowing the rate of infiltration, particularly during infiltration of the skin.

Although it is desirable to place the breast biopsy incision so as to obtain the best cosmetic result, consideration should also be given to further surgical management of

FIGURE 6.1-3 For larger excisions or when skin must be excised, radial incisions in the lower half of the breast and curvilinear incisions along the Langer lines in the upper half of the breast provide the best cosmesis.

FIGURE 6.1-2 Langer lines are the natural lines of skin tension and skin creasing. Incisions placed along the Langer lines usually produce the optimal cosmetic result. For larger lesions in the lower half of the breast, radial incisions may produce better cosmesis (see Fig. 6.1-3).

the patient if the lesion is suspected to be malignant. Liberal use of fine-needle aspirations before excisional biopsy minimizes the number of unexpected malignancies. Incisions along Langer lines usually produce the best cosmesis, particularly in the upper half of the breast (Fig. 6.1-2). In young women, in whom the lesion is most likely a benign fibroadenoma, it may be appropriate to use a periareolar incision, even where the lesion is a considerable distance from the areola. Incisions overlying the sternal area are particularly prone to the development of a hypertrophic scar. Most malignant lesions in the central and upper portions of the breast are best excised using transverse curvilinear incisions that are placed over the lesion. A radial incision is frequently preferred for malignant lesions in the lower half of the breast (Fig. 6.1-3). The potential problem with incisions along Langer lines in the lower half of the breast for larger lesions is that a greater cosmetic deformity is created if the removal of skin or tissue causes a shortening of the distance between the nipple–areolar complex and the inframammary crease than if the same volume of tissue were removed and the breast slightly narrowed.

The biopsy should be done using the cold knife rather than electrocautery. Thermal injury may confound histologic interpretation of the biopsy results, particularly assessment of the margins of excision. The heat from the electrocautery can also cause degradation of the estrogen receptor protein, leading to a falsely low or negative result. Specific bleeders encountered during the dissection may be electrocoagulated if necessary. After the lesion has been removed, hemostasis may be obtained using electrocoagulation.

Fibroadenomas may be excised with a small rim of normal breast tissue, or they may be enucleated, provided care is taken that the lesion is not morcellated.

Lesions that are shown or suspected to be malignant should be excised with a margin of apparently normal tissue. If malignancy is clearly established and if tumor-free margins exist, the patient will probably have had an adequate resection, should breast conservation be done. I prefer to remove a rectangular portion of apparently normal breast parenchyma around the lesion rather than a spheroid rim. The rectangular resection makes orientation of the margins easier and simplifies locating any area that requires reexcision because the margin is not tumor-free.

If the excisional biopsy includes a rim of apparently normal tissue around the lesion, orientation of the specimen margins relative to their location in the residual breast should be maintained. The specimen must be marked so that the cephalad (superior), caudad (inferior), dorsal, ventral, medial, and lateral margins can be identified by the pathologist. I usually use two sutures, one long lateral suture and one short superior suture.

The intact specimen should be examined by the surgeon to confirm that the biopsy contains the lesion. By moving the normal surrounding tissue over a suspected malignancy, the surgeon can usually determine whether an adequate margin has been removed. The surgeon should also manually examine the biopsy cavity to make sure no additional lesions are present.

After hemostasis is established, the incision is closed without a drain. It is almost always best to not try to approximate the breast parenchyma, as this creates distortion of the breast and poorer cosmesis. If the initial incision has been carried down through the subcutaneous fat and the superficial layer of the superficial fascia, closure of the superficial fascia provides good restoration of breast form. The skin is closed with a subcuticular suture.

Incisional Biopsy

Incisional biopsy is a diagnostic procedure that removes a portion of a mass for pathologic examination, where complete removal of the mass is unnecessary or might compromise future mastectomy. Unless larger amounts of tissue are required for pathologic examination, adequate material for diagnosis may be more simply obtained through FNAB or core needle biopsy.

Specimen Management After Incisional and Excisional Biopsy

The intact breast biopsy specimen should be transported promptly to the pathology laboratory. The specimen needs to be sent fresh, rather than in preservative, so that the pathologist can paint the outside of the specimen to aid in histologic examination of the margins if malignancy is confirmed (Fig. 6.1-4). If a delay of more than a few minutes is anticipated, any possibly malignant lesion should be placed on ice to prevent degradation of the estrogen receptor.

Skin Biopsy

Skin biopsy for histologic examination may be appropriate when lesions are either primary in the skin of the breast or originate within the breast but involve the skin. An incisional biopsy of the skin may sometimes be included when an incisional biopsy of an underlying breast mass is being done.

An excellent technique for obtaining a full-thickness skin specimen is to use a disposable punch biopsy tool. These biopsy specimens range in size from 2 to 6 mm, and the procedure is simple to perform with the patient under local anesthesia (Fig. 6.1-5). The circular biopsy hole assumes an elliptic shape in the direction of Langer

FIGURE 6.1-4 The specimen should remain intact and be marked so that the dorsal, ventral, cephalad, caudad, medial, and lateral surfaces can be identified by the pathologist. Rectangular margins are easier to orient than are ellipsoid margins. One convention for marking the specimen is to place a long suture on the lateral margin and a short suture on the superior (cephalad) margin. The fresh specimen is sent to the pathologist so that margins can be inked to aid in the histologic identification to determine whether the margin is tumor-free.

FIGURE 6.1-5 Disposable punch biopsies for full-thickness biopsy of skin lesions.

lines. The small biopsy incision can be closed with one or two fine sutures or with sterile tape.

Biopsy of Regional Adenopathy or Chest Wall Recurrence

All of the techniques described here can be used to obtain pathologic material for the evaluation of regional adenopathy that develops either in the absence of a breast mass or after previous treatment of the primary mass. The judgments relative to the selection of the optimum biopsy procedure are similar. Frequently, FNAB is used as the initial diagnostic procedure for regional adenopathy or subcutaneous recurrence. Punch biopsies are useful for obtaining histologic confirmation of a suspected cutaneous recurrence.

References

1. Walker GM, Foster RS Jr, McKegney CP, et al. Breast biopsy: a comparison of outpatient and inpatient experience. Arch Surg 1978;113:942.
2. Layfield LJ, Chrischilles EA, Cohen MB, et al. The palpable breast nodule: a cost-effectiveness analysis of alternate diagnostic approaches. Cancer 1993;72:1642.
3. Koss LG. The palpable breast nodule: a cost-effectiveness analysis of alternate diagnostic approaches: the role of the needle aspiration biopsy. Cancer 1993;72:1499.
4. Jackson PP, Pitts HH. Biopsy with delayed radical mastectomy for carcinoma of the breast. Am J Surg 1959;98:184.
5. Abramson DJ. Delayed mastectomy after outpatient biopsy. Am J Surg 1976;132:596.
6. Fisher ER, Sass R, Fisher B. Biologic considerations regarding the one- and two-step procedures in the management of patients with invasive carcinoma of the breast. Surg Gynecol Obstet 1985;161:245.
7. Bertario L, Reduzzi D, Piromalli D, et al. Outpatient biopsy of breast cancer: influence on survival. Ann Surg 1985;201:64.
8. Martin HE, Ellis EB. Biopsy by needle puncture and aspiration. Ann Surg 1930;92:169.
9. Franzen S, Zajicek J. Aspiration biopsy in diagnosis of palpable lesions of the breast: critical review of 3479 consecutive biopsies. Acta Radiol Ther Phys Biol 1968;7:241.
10. Zajdela A, Ghossein NA, Pilleron JP, et al. The value of aspiration cytology in the diagnosis of breast cancer: experience at the Foundation Curie. Cancer 1975;35:499.
11. Zajicek J, Caspersson T, Jakobsson, et al. Cytologic diagnosis of mammary tumors from aspiration biopsy smears: comparison of cytologic and histologic findings in 2111 lesions and diagnostic use of cytophotometry. Acta Cytol 1970;14:370.
12. Wollenberg NJ, Caya JB, Clowry LJ. Fine needle aspiration cytology of the breast: a review of 321 cases with statistical evaluation. Acta Cytol 1985;29:425.
13. Lee KR, Foster RS Jr, Papillo JL. Fine needle aspirate of the breast: importance of the aspirator. Acta Cytol 1987;31:281.
14. Hermans J. The value of aspiration cytologic examination of the breast: a statistical review of the medical literature. Cancer 1992;69:2104.
15. Feldman PS, Covell JL. Breast and lung. In: Fine needle aspiration cytology and its clinical application. Chicago, American Society of Clinical Pathologists, 1985:27.
16. Innes DJ Jr, Feldman PS. Comparison of diagnostic results obtained by fine needle aspiration cytology and Tru-Cut or open biopsies. Acta Cytol 1983;27:350.
17. Casey TT, Rodgers WH, Baxter JW, et al. Stratified diagnostic approach to fine needle aspiration of the breast. Am J Surg 1992;163:305.
18. Lannin DR, Silverman JF, Walker C, et al. Cost-effectiveness of fine needle biopsy of the breast. Ann Surg 1986;203:474.
19. OMalley F, Casey TT, Winfield AC, et al. Clinical correlates of false-negative fine needle aspirations of the breast in a consecutive series of 1005 patients. Surg Gynecol Obstet 1993;176:360.
20. Wanebo HJ, Feldman PS, Wilhelm MC, et al. Fine-needle aspiration cytology in lieu of open biopsy in management of breast cancer. Ann Surg 1984;199:569.
21. Ulanow RM, Galblum L, Canter JW. Fine-needle aspiration in the diagnosis and management of solid breast lesions. Am J Surg 1984;148:653.
22. Painter RW, Clark WE II, Deckers PJ. Negative findings on fine-needle aspiration biopsy of solid breast masses: patient management. Am J Surg 1988;155:387.
23. Malberger E, Edoute Y, Toledano O, et al. Fine-needle aspiration and cytologic findings of surgical scar lesions in women with breast cancer. Cancer 1992;69:148.
24. Pezner RD, Lorant JA, Terz J, et al. Wound-healing complications following biopsy of the irradiated breast. Arch Surg 1992;127:321.
25. Kline TS, Joshi JP, Neal MS. Fine-needle aspiration of the breast: diagnosis and pitfalls: a review of 3545 cases. Cancer 1979;1458.
26. Cowen PN, Benson GA. Cytologic study of fluid from benign breast cysts. Br J Surg 1979;66:209.
27. Devitt JE, Barr JR. The clinical recognition of cystic carcinoma of the breast. Surg Gynecol Obstet 1984;159:130.
28. Foster RS Jr. Core cutting needle biopsy for the diagnosis of breast cancer. Am J Surg 1982;143:622.
29. Shabot MM, Goldberg IM, Schick P, et al. Aspiration cytology is superior to "Tru-Cut" needle biopsy in establishing the diagnosis of clinically suspicious breast masses. Ann Surg 1982;196:122.
30. Harter LP, Curtis JS, Ponto G, et al. Malignant seeding of the needle track during stereotaxic core needle breast biopsy. Radiology 1992;185:713.
31. McMahon AJ, Lutfy AM, Matthew A, et al. Needle core biopsy of the breast with a spring-loaded device. Br J Surg 1992;79:1042.

6.2

Preoperative Imaging-Guided Needle Localization and Biopsy of Nonpalpable Breast Lesions

DANIEL B. KOPANS ▪ BARBARA L. SMITH

Randomized, controlled trials of breast cancer screening, as well as large-scale screening projects, have shown that screening can detect breast cancer earlier, reduce the size and stage at which cancers are diagnosed, and reduce the absolute mortality from breast cancer by 25% to 30%.[1,2] Mammography is the only screening modality shown in large, prospective trials to reliably detect clinically occult malignancy in women with no symptoms. Cancers detected by mammography alone are more likely to be at an earlier stage than clinically evident cancers and to have a correspondingly more favorable prognosis.[3] Excision of these nonpalpable cancers using needle-localized breast biopsy requires the coordinated efforts of the radiologist, surgeon, and pathologist.

Preoperative Needle Localization for Surgical Excision

Excisional biopsy after needle localization has been the "gold standard" for the diagnosis of clinically occult lesions detected by mammography. It is the most accurate method of separating benign from malignant lesions and is the only method that permits the pathologist to fully characterize malignant lesions. The combined procedure should be done with primary emphasis on the objectives of safety and accuracy. Whether the biopsy is done for primary diagnostic purposes or as primary therapy after diagnosis by needle biopsy, the positioning of guides for the surgeon, and the excision itself, should be carefully planned with the goal of minimizing the trauma for the patient while providing her with accurate and complete characterization of the mammographic lesion.

Guide placement for most clinically occult mammographically detected lesions can be easily accomplished using mammography. Ultrasound[4] and computed tomography[5] can also be used to place guides for the surgeon. Quadrant resection to remove nonpalpable lesions without imaging guidance is inappropriate. It is inaccurate and results in the removal of unnecessarily large amounts of tissue.

The radiologist and surgeon should recognize that it is difficult to deduce the actual position of a lesion when the patient is supine on the operating table, given mammograms obtained with the breast vigorously compressed and pulled away from the chest wall. Skin markers are therefore reliable only when the lesion is immediately beneath the skin.

To minimize the volume of tissue excised, accurate preoperative localization should position the guide through or alongside the lesion. Using the technique described below, a needle can be routinely placed within 5 mm of a lesion.[6] Any greater distance from a lesion should be unacceptable, and, if the guide is not within 5 mm of the abnormality, it should be repositioned or replaced.

THE CHOICE OF GUIDES

Numerous guides, each with particular advantages and disadvantages, have been developed to assist the surgeon in resecting a lesion that she or he can generally not palpate, even after the tissues have been entered. All rely on the positioning of a needle under imaging observation and guidance. The actual choice of the guide depends on the preferences of the radiologist and surgeon. Available systems range from standard hypodermic needles to specially designed localization devices.

Hypodermic Needles

The simplest guide for preoperative localization is a hypodermic needle inserted through or alongside the lesion (Fig. 6.2-1*A*) and taped in place. The needle must be of sufficient length to pass through and beyond the lesion and to maintain the target tissue during imaging with compression perpendicular to its course. A straight needle is the simplest guide to place in the breast. It can be palpated by the surgeon, and its course can be anticipated. It is also easily removed or repositioned if its relation to the lesion is suboptimal.

A disadvantage of a hypodermic needle is the protrusion of the needle hub above the skin, a factor which may result in inadvertently pulling the needle out of the breast. Although a straight needle may be sufficient, it only provides two-dimensional accuracy and requires that the surgeon estimate the distance of the lesion along its shaft. Movement of the breast may cause the lesion to slip off the needle.

Hookwire Systems

The guides most commonly used involve a wire with a hook on the end (see Fig. 6.2-1*B*). The hookwires are passed through a needle and the hook reforms when the needle is withdrawn over the wire, anchoring the wire in the tissue.[7] The needle is first positioned (or repositioned) to achieve a satisfactory relation to the lesion, and the wire is then engaged in the appropriate tissue volume. These devices can also be stiffened by sliding a cannula over them.[8]

The length of the wire guide is important. Wires that

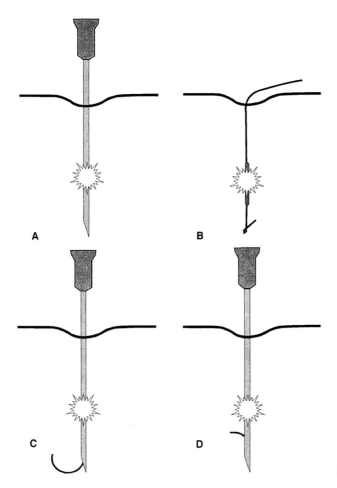

FIGURE 6.2-1 A. A simple hypodermic needle can be used transfixing or can be placed alongside a suspicious abnormality. **B.** Hooked wires are placed through needles that are first positioned in appropriate relation to the needle; the hook is then engaged, leaving a flexible wire for the surgeon to follow. **C.** Curved wires can be used to anchor needles, but their holding power is limited. **D.** Wires projecting from the side of a needle can be used to anchor a needle in position.

are too short should not be used because they may be enveloped by the breast when it changes position. Wires must be of sufficient length to ensure that, when the breast is in its natural position, the wire will not be drawn beneath the skin. The length of the wire should exceed by several centimeters the distance from the skin entry site to the lesion. If the length of wire is chosen properly and insertion is parallel to the chest wall, the protruding end of the wire need not be anchored. Firmly anchoring the wire is often not desirable because traction from breast movement may cause it to be pulled out of the lesion. These guides should be loosely taped to the skin.

Anchored Needles

Hookwires have been combined with needles to permit three-dimensionally accurate, surgically palpable guides. Instruments include curved-end wires that can be retracted

into the tip of the introducing needle, thus permitting the needle to be repositioned (see Fig. 6.2-1*C*). These lack holding power and may be fairly easily pulled from the targeted tissue. The most stable anchored needles are those in which the hook protrudes from the side of the needle (see Fig. 6.2-1*D*). A comparison of hook wires with stabilized needles has shown that a wire protruding from the side of a needle had 1.5 times the holding power of a flexible springhook wire anchor and 6 times the holding power of a curved wire protruding from the end of the needle.[9,10]

The major drawback to stabilized needle systems is the fact that they are not flexible. Three-dimensional positioning results in variable lengths of needle protruding from the breast, which must be protected to prevent them from being inadvertently hit and dislodged or from damaging the tissues.

Introduction of Dyes

The injection of vital dyes[11] and the deposition of inert carbon particles at a suspicious lesion[12] to stain the tissues and provide a track from the lesion to the skin have been useful for guiding biopsies. Dyes must be introduced fairly soon before surgery to prevent their absorption or diffusion into a large volume of tissue. The surgeon may have difficulty following a thin trail of dye to the lesion, and many who use this technique also leave a needle or wire guide in position.

Mammographically Guided Preoperative Needle Localization

LOCATING AN OCCULT LESION

Before the recommendation for a biopsy, the radiologist must have an accurate idea of the three-dimensional location of a lesion and be confident of the ability to place a needle tip at the lesion. If the location is uncertain, methods have been described to assist in confirmation and triangulation.[13,14] Lesions that are not clearly identified on two projections can often be localized using a parallax method.[15] If mammographic methods fail, ultrasound[16] or computed tomography can be used to direct the placement of guides.[17]

Given that the standard screening lateral projection is the mediolateral oblique, an additional straight lateral (orthogonal to the craniocaudal) image should be obtained before needle placement to provide true perpendicular coordinates to the craniocaudal view.

PATIENT PREPARATION

The procedure should be explained to the patient in detail so that she may be fully informed. It is important to provide compassionate support for the patient because these procedures can generate a great deal of anxiety. The patient should be attended at all times in the event that the rare vasovagal reaction occurs. Premedication is not recommended if it reduces the patient's ability to be fully cooperative for the localization procedure. Local anesthesia can be used, but it is not needed for most women and may be more painful than the localization itself.[18]

GENERAL CONSIDERATIONS

The radiologist, surgeon, and pathologist must work closely together. The radiologist should try to minimize the amount of dissection needed by choosing the shortest feasible distance to the lesion. Careful surgical dissection avoids dislodging needles or cutting wires.

All available methods require the placement of a needle either through or alongside the target lesion. Many surgeons prefer that needles be placed from the front of the breast. This is generally difficult to do with a high degree of accuracy, because it requires a free-hand needle localization that is extremely operator dependent. It is difficult to routinely position guides within 0.5 cm of a lesion using the free-hand method. Positioning guides from the front of the breast also risks causing a pneumothorax or entrance into the mediastinum.[19]

Regardless of the type of guide used, the development of dedicated mammography equipment has resulted in the ability to accurately position needles into or alongside the smallest mammographically detected abnormalities.[20] This is most accurately and safely accomplished by introducing the needle while the breast is held in the mammographic compression system and the needle introduced parallel to the chest wall.

GUIDES INTRODUCED PARALLEL TO THE CHEST WALL

Most complications associated with needle localization can be avoided if guides are placed parallel to the chest wall[31] using any standard mammographic system. This approach uses compression plates with a series of holes or a fenestration permitting access to the breast and a lesion while the breast is held in compression. The lesion is accessible through the fenestration. A single fenestration with calibrations along the sides is the most convenient and accurate.

To reduce the amount of tissue that must be traversed by the surgeon, the shortest distance to the lesion from the skin should be chosen for the introduction of the needle. Using the appropriate technique, the needle shaft should rarely (if ever) be more than 5 mm from the lesion.[21]

Wires with a 2-cm thickened segment just proximal to the hook are helpful for the surgeon. With these wires, the hook is ideally engaged 1.5 cm beyond the lesion so that the lesion is on the thickened segment just proximal to the hook. By placing the thickened segment of hookwire system through or alongside the lesion, the surgeon can use it as a marker to indicate that the level of the lesion has been reached and that the hook is 2 cm beyond. It is also helpful to place a radiopaque marker at the wire entry point on the skin for inclusion in the final picture of the wire and lesion to assist the surgeon in anticipating the depth of the lesion (allowing for distortion from the mammographic compression).

STEREOTACTIC NEEDLE PLACEMENT

The use of stereotactic devices to position needles for excisional biopsy is less accurate than the conventional method described here. Because the stereoscopic views obtained are not orthogonal, the inherent accuracy is less than that of conventional 90-degree projections. Although the technique is theoretically capable of 2- to 3-mm accuracy, if the identical point in a lesion is not targeted in the two views the depth calculation may be considerably off target. Even if the tip of a needle can be positioned accurately, proper engagement of a hookwire can be a problem because the breast is accordioned in the direction that the wire is passed, and the actual tissue plane that will be engaged by the hook cannot be accurately determined in the stereo device. These difficulties may explain why needle localizations using stereotactic devices have resulted in more failures in the excision of breast cancers than would be expected from accurate localizations.[22] Stereotactic devices are not necessary and are probably not desirable if the only need is the positioning of wire guides for surgical excision.

Surgical Approach to Nonpalpable Lesions

ANESTHETIC TECHNIQUES

Nearly all needle-localized breast biopsies can be done using local anesthesia alone or plus intravenous sedation. General anesthesia should be limited to patients who require biopsies of multiple sites or for those who have a deep central lesion in a very large breast, when the volume of tissue to be anesthetized raises concerns of toxicity due to the amount of local anesthesia required. Only rarely does a patient require general anesthesia because of extreme anxiety.

ACCURATE LOCALIZATION PERMITS ACCURATE EXCISION

The accurate placement of guides by the radiologist is critical. As described previously, the needle or wire should be either through the lesion or no more than 5 mm from it. This reduces the amount of tissue that must be removed and diminishes the probability that the lesion will be missed at surgery. Reports that suggest that as much as 40 mL of tissue must be removed during needle-localized biopsy come from series where free-hand localizations were done with the wire frequently 1 or more cm from the lesion. This approach required larger volumes of tissue to be removed and increased the likelihood that a cancer would be missed at surgical excision.[23] Not only does precise wire placement permit less tissue to be removed, but the failure to excise a breast cancer should be less than

1%. In our experience in excising 1000 cancers, the first localization resulted in a failure to excise only 5 cancers (.5%) necessitating repeat needle localization and surgical excision.

Communication between the radiologist and surgeon is critical for an accurate biopsy. It is important to recognize that the position of the breast in the operating room with the patient supine differs from the position of the breast during the localization procedure. In the supine position, the breast often falls laterally, altering the alignment of the wire and potentially drawing additional wire length into the breast. Therefore, although precise wire localization of the lesion by the radiologist is critical, it is equally important that the mammograms sent to the operating room allow the surgeon to determine the three-dimensional location of the lesion in the breast when the patient is supine, as well as the position of the lesion relative to the wire. Two images are used to orient the surgeon and should be available in the operating room—the image looking down the needle and the final, orthogonal image of the wire in place. A diagram, drawn by the radiologist, marking the positions of the wire and the lesion within the breast aids this orientation. This orientation process is also greatly facilitated by marking the skin entry site and the nipple clearly on the films. It is also helpful to provide the surgeon with an estimate of the distance in centimeters between the lesion and the skin entry site.

The position of the hook relative to the nipple remains fairly constant, despite movement of the breast into the supine position, and can be used to estimate the location of the lesion within the breast. The skin incision can then be placed as directly as possible over the lesion. The lesion itself should also be marked on the films, so that its distance from and position relative to the wire can be easily determined. This approach allows the surgeon to assess how much tissue to remove around the wire and on what side of the wire the greatest tissue volume should be excised. Wires with thickened segments are especially helpful in judging distances along the length of the wire and the distance to the hook within the breast tissue.[24]

SURGICAL PRINCIPLES

Although the excision of a nonpalpable, needle-localized breast lesion is technically more difficult than excision of a palpable lesion, the same general principles apply. Each lesion should be treated as if it were a malignancy and excised through an incision that could be contained within a mastectomy incision or converted into a cosmetically acceptable partial mastectomy (lumpectomy) incision. Given that most lesions requiring needle localization are small, an effort should be made to excise the lesion completely, with a rim of surrounding normal tissue. It is important to recognize, however, that most needle-localized breast biopsies ultimately prove to be benign. The volume of tissue excised should, therefore, be as small as possible, with wide excision reserved for lesions highly suspicious for malignancy or those already identified as malignant by needle biopsy techniques (see later).

Using these principles, the rules for the placement of the incision in needle-localized biopsy of a breast lesion are similar to those for a biopsy of a palpable lesion. The incision should be placed directly over the lesion, avoiding excessive tunneling through breast tissue, which increases the volume of tissue requiring a radiation boost. If the wire takes a long course through the breast tissue to reach the lesion, the incision should be moved along the expected course of the wire, away from the skin entry of the wire and over the expected location of the lesion (Fig. 6.2-2). The surgeon then dissects downward to identify the wire within breast tissue and then follows it to the thickened segment.

Circumareolar incisions should be used only when the lesion is close to the areolar border. Curvilinear incisions parallel to the areolar border are preferable for most locations, with radial incisions reserved for very medial or lateral lesions. The incision should be of sufficient length to provide adequate exposure, given that the vigorous retraction required with a very small incision may cause the wire to become dislodged. Skin should not be included in the biopsy specimen, even when the wire entry site is included in the incision.

The course of the wire is identified and followed to the thick segment. The tissue is then removed around the thick segment to encompass the lesion and a small amount of surrounding normal tissue (see Fig. 6.2-2*D*). For lesions shown to be malignant by fine-needle or core biopsy, an appropriately wide margin should be obtained. If the thick portion of the wire is encountered, the surgeon knows that he or she is very close to the lesion and can adjust the dissection accordingly.

After the appropriate portion of the wire has been identified, tissue on either side of the wire is grasped with clamps, and a core of tissue is taken around the wire. Caution must be used to avoid dividing the wire with scissors or cautery during the dissection. The amount of tissue taken around the wire depends on the actual distance of the lesion from the wire, as indicated on the localization films. In some cases, the lesion is palpable after its general position is identified by the wire. In such cases, complete excision of the lesion with a grossly clean margin is appropriate. If the preoperative placement of the guide has been accurate, only a small total volume of tissue must be excised.[24]

EXCISED SPECIMENS

Immediately after the surgical excision, the specimen should undergo radiography with some compression and magnification to confirm that the targeted abnormality has been removed.

If the radiologist does not see the lesion in the specimen and if the surgeon does not believe that the lesion was a cyst that ruptured during the excision, the surgeon may excise additional tissue around the track of the wire. If traction has occurred on the wire, it is possible that the lesion is further along the wire's previous course. If the lesion is not contained within the second specimen, it is generally best to close and obtain repeat

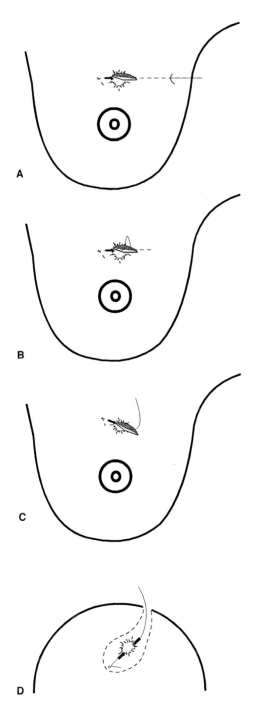

FIGURE 6.2-2   The relation of the wire entry point, the lesion, and the hook (**A**) should be understood by the surgeon so that the biopsy incision can be placed over the lesion, the wire located, and the lesion and tissue around the distal wire removed. After the wire is located, the distal end can be delivered into the incision so that the course of the wire is more accurately appreciated (**B** and **C**) and the tissue and wire can be excised en bloc (**D**).

mammographic views. In most cases, the patient can tolerate mammography 2 to 3 weeks after the biopsy attempt. It is neither necessary nor appropriate to wait several months before repeat imaging when the lesion may have been missed. On occasion, these repeat views show that the lesion has, in fact, been removed. If the lesion remains, another localization and biopsy should be done expeditiously.

After excision of the lesion has been documented, both the biopsy specimen and the specimen radiograph should be sent to the pathologist. As is the case for any breast biopsy, the margins of the specimen should be inked, and hormone receptor assays done. Receptor assays usually need to be done using immunohistochemical techniques because of the small size of the tumors identified.

The specimen radiograph helps the pathologist ensure that the area of the specimen containing the mammographic abnormality is appropriately sampled. If the biopsy was done for calcifications, it is important for the pathologists to be sure that the calcifications are seen in histologic tissue sections to ensure that the area containing the lesion has been examined. If the calcifications are not found on routine examination of tissue sections, roentgenographic images of the paraffin-embedded tissue blocks can be obtained to identify the sections containing the calcifications. Imaging the block on its side[25] can show that suspicious calcifications are deep in the block so that appropriate sections, at deeper levels, can be obtained.

If an area containing calcifications is found to contain a malignancy, many believe that it is important to ensure that all the calcifications are removed in the definitive wide excision. Magnified views of the breast that underwent biopsy are suggested if any concern about remaining calcifications exists. Any calcifications that remain may be wire localized for subsequent wide excision.

Summary

Accurate positioning of guides for the surgical removal of clinically occult lesions is required to ensure the safety of the patient and the accurate diagnosis of breast abnormalities with minimal cosmetic deformity. The radiologist, surgeon, and pathologist should have a close working relationship to ensure that the lesion is removed and appropriately analyzed. As with any interventional technique, a thoughtful approach to the particular lesion in question and an understanding of the procedures and their possible problems minimize the likelihood of complications.

References

1. Fletcher SW, Black W, Harris R, et al. Report of the International Workshop on Screening for Breast Cancer. J Natl Cancer Inst 1993;85:1644.
2. Smart CR. Highlights of the evidence of benefit for women aged 40–49 years from the 14-year follow-up of the Breast Cancer Detection Demonstration Project. Cancer 1994;74:296.
3. Bassett LW, Liu TH, Giuliano AE, et al. The prevalence of carcinoma in palpable vs impalpable mammographically detected lesions. AJR 1991;157:21.
4. Kopans DB, Meyer JE, Lindfors KK, et al. Breast sonography to guide aspiration of cysts and preoperative localization of occult breast lesions. AJR 1984;143:489.

5. Kopans DB, Meyer JE. Computed tomography guided localization of clinically occult breast carcinoma: the "N" skin guide. Radiology 1982;145:211.

6. Gallagher WJ, Cardenosa G, Rubens JR, et al. Minimal-volume excision of nonpalpable breast lesions. AJR 1989;153:957.

7. Kopans DB, Deluca S. A modified needle–hookwire technique to simplify the preoperative localization of occult breast lesions. Radiology 1980;134:781.

8. Kopans DB, Meyer JE. The versatile spring–hookwire breast lesion localizer. AJR 1982;138:586.

9. Urrutia EJ, Hawkins IF, Hawkins MC, et al. Clinical experience of a new retractable barb needle for breast lesion localization: the first 60 cases. Presented at the Radiologic Society of North America 73rd Scientific Assembly, Chicago, December 1987.

10. Czarnecki DJ, Berridge DL, Splittgerber GF, et al. Comparison of the anchoring strengths of the Kopans and Hawkins II needle–hookwire systems. Radiology 1992;183:573.

11. Horns JW, Arndt RD. Percutaneous spot localization of nonpalpable breast lesions. AJR 1976;127:253.

12. Svane G. A stereotaxic technique for preoperative marking of nonpalpable breast lesions. Acta Radiol 1983;24:145.

13. Berkowitz JE, Gatewood OMB, Gayler BW. Equivocal mammographic findings: evaluation with spot compression. Radiology 1989;171:369.

14. Swann CA, Kopans DB, McCarthy KA, et al. Practical solutions to problems of triangulation and preoperative localization of breast lesions. Radiology 1987;163:577.

15. Kopans DB, Waitzkin ED, Linetsky L, et al. Localization of breast lesions identified on only one mammographic view. AJR 1987;149:39.

16. Kopans DB, Meyer JE, Lindfors KK, et al. Breast sonography to guide aspiration of cysts and preoperative localization of occult breast lesions. AJR 1984;143:489.

17. Kopans DB, Meyer JE. Computed tomography guided localization of clinically occult breast carcinoma: the "N" skin guide. Radiology 1982;145:211.

18. Reynolds HE, Jackson VP, Musnick BS. Preoperative needle localization in the breast: utility of local anesthesia. Radiology 1993; 187:503.

19. Bristol JB, Jones PA. Transgression of localizing wire into the pleural cavity prior to mammography. Br J Radiol 1981;54:139.

20. Kopans DB, Meyer JE, Lindfors KK, et al. Spring–hookwire breast lesion localizer: use with rigid compression mammographic systems. Radiology 1985;157:505.

21. Gallagher WJ, Cardenosa G, Rubens JR, et al. Minimal-volume excision of nonpalpable breast lesions. AJR 1989;153:957.

22. Kopans DB. Review of stereotaxic large-core needle biopsy and surgical biopsy results in nonpalpable breast lesions. Radiology 1993;189:665.

23. Tinnemans JGM, Wobbes T, Hendricks JHCL, et al. Localization and excision of nonpalpable breast lesions: a surgical evaluation of three methods. Arch Surg 1987;122:802.

24. Kopans DB, Meyer JE. The versatile spring–hookwire breast lesion localizer. AJR 1982;138:586.

25. Cardenosa G, Eklund GW. Paraffin block radiography following breast biopsies: use of orthogonal views. Radiology 1991;180:873.

6.3
Stereotactic Core Breast Biopsy
W. PHIL EVANS III

The extensive use of mammography during the past decade has firmly established its efficacy in detecting small, nonpalpable invasive breast carcinomas.[1-3] Women with malignant lesions less than 1 cm in size have a long-term disease-free survival of more than 90% and a low incidence of axillary nodal metastases, the most important prognostic factor.[4] Randomized trials have shown a reduction in breast cancer mortality of up to 30% in groups screened using mammography.[5]

Screening mammography, however, identifies not only clinically occult malignancies but also many benign lesions. If widespread compliance with American Cancer Society screening guidelines could be achieved, almost half of all adult women would undergo annual screening mammography.[6] From 0.5% to 2.0% of these women could expect to receive a breast biopsy recommendation because of a mammographically detected lesion. Thus, compliance with screening guidelines could result in over 1 million breast biopsies per year in the United States.[7] Assuming a malignancy rate of 25%, some 750,000 biopsies would yield benign results.

In recent years, the usual pathway for diagnosis of a nonpalpable breast lesion has been discovery by screening mammography, characterization through diagnostic mammography or ultrasound, localization for surgical biopsy, excision with confirmation by specimen radiography, and final diagnosis by histologic assessment. Although surgical biopsy has been considered the gold standard by which all other diagnostic techniques are measured, it has several disadvantages. In this era of medical cost containment, expense is the most significant drawback, with surgical consultations and biopsies accounting for the largest category of induced costs in screening programs.[8] Other significant disadvantages include physical and psychological trauma, anesthetic risk, a failure rate of 0.2% to 22%,[9-12] removal of more tissue than necessary (in the case of benign lesions), and the creation of mammographic pseudolesions by postsurgical scarring.

To reduce the number of benign surgical breast biopsies, two approaches have been offered. First, based on careful review of previous mammograms, a meticulous imaging evaluation, or both, many lesions can be characterized as probably benign, having less than a 2% chance of malignancy. For these lesions, periodic mammographic follow-up (usually every 6 months for 2 to 3 years) as an alternative to surgical biopsy is reasonable and has been thoroughly reviewed by Sickles and Brenner.[13-15] Other lesions with a greater chance of malignancy require histologic diagnosis. The development of two devices has improved the accuracy and encouraged the use of needle biopsy in diagnosing nonpalpable breast lesions—stereotactic x-ray devices and automated biopsy guns with core biopsy needles.

Stereotactic Devices

All stereotactic mammographic devices use the principle of triangulation. By imaging an abnormality in two projections with a 30-degree tube shift, the precise location of the breast lesion can be determined in three dimensions. Two types of stereotactic equipment are available—devices that add on to standard upright mammography units and dedicated prone tables (Fig. 6.3-1). Although the add-on devices are relatively inexpensive and small, and allow multipurpose use, working space is limited, and the potential for vasovagal reaction exists. Moreover, it is difficult for patients to remain motionless while seated or standing upright. Dedicated prone stereotactic devices are expensive, require approximately twice the space of standard mammography rooms, and are single purpose; however, patient motion is minimal, the breast is in a dependent position, the patient cannot see the needle during the procedure, vasovagal reactions do not occur, and the units accommodate a core biopsy gun.[16] Most operators find the procedure easier and more accurate with the dedicated prone units.

The most significant cost with the prone unit, however, is not related to purchase price but to the single use. Few facilities perform enough biopsies for the unit to be used more than once or twice daily. Hence, an expensive piece of equipment in a large room will be idle most of the time. To expand its application, the stereotactic device can also be used for lesion localization and cyst aspiration, but these procedures are generally done more quickly and

accurately using a standard mammographic unit with alphanumeric grid or sonography.

Automated Biopsy Gun and Core Biopsy Needle

For core biopsy, a specially adapted 14-gauge cutting needle that fits into an automated spring loaded biopsy gun is used. The assembly consists of an inner tissue sampling needle and outer cutting needle. Four millimeters from the beveled tip of the inner needle is a 17-mm tissue slot. The outer needle covers the inner needle when the biopsy gun is in the prefire position. When the firing mechanism is activated, the springs in the gun cause the inner needle to advance. A sample of tissue becomes lodged in the slot. The outer needle then slides over the inner needle, cutting the tissue and securing it in the slot. This sequence of events occurs in a fraction of a second and is not visible except for the excursion of the entire needle. The "throw" of the biopsy gun refers to the distance the needle must travel to obtain a core of tissue. Some guns are equipped with variable throws, but the "long throw" (2.1 to 2.5 mm) is preferred because of greater tissue sampling.

PROCEDURE

The patient's mammogram is reviewed to determine the best approach to the lesion. In most cases, this is the skin surface closest to the lesion. The breast is compressed within the unit, and a scout image produced with the lesion visible in the 5×5-cm window of the compression paddle. The skin is pretreated with povidone-iodine. Stereo images are obtained with the tube shifted first 15-degrees to the left and then 15-degrees to the right (Fig. 6.3-2). Using a computed calculation,

FIGURE 6.3-1 Dedicated prone sterotactic core biopsy table.

the x, y, and z coordinates of a specific target within the lesion (usually the center) are calculated and relayed to the needle holder and assembly. The needle holder is positioned with respect to the x and y coordinates. The patient is given local anesthesia (1% lidocaine with epinephrine) and a small skin puncture is made using a no. 11 blade scalpel over the projected biopsy site. Using the z coordinate, the needle is advanced through the skin puncture to the center of the lesion. Stereo images are obtained to confirm placement of the needle within the target. Because of the biopsy gun's throw, the needle is retracted 5 to 10 mm, depending on lesion size, before the biopsy gun is fired to assure placement of the tissue slot within the center of the lesion. After the first firing, stereo views are obtained to document the needle traversing the lesion. The needle is removed, and the tissue core placed in formalin (Fig. 6.3-3). Additional cores (usually a total of 5 to 15) are obtained by simply retargeting various areas within the lesion. It

generally is not necessary to make a separate puncture for each pass because the skin nick can be moved without displacing the target within the breast. Core samples may be used to determine estrogen and progesterone receptor status and for flow cytometry studies, if indicated.

Each time the needle is removed from the breast, firm pressure is applied to the biopsy site. After the last biopsy, pressure is held for about 5 minutes or until bleeding has ceased. An ice pack may also help to minimize bruising.

Digital mammography is a major addition to the stereotactic biopsy procedure allowing the images to be viewed in a few seconds rather than several minutes (Fig. 6.3-4). The usual stereotactic biopsy is a 45- to 50-minute procedure, and the digital unit reduces average procedure time by 25%. Image quality is sufficient, and lesion visualization can be improved by varying the contrast, brightness, and magnification.

FIGURE 6.3-2 **A.** Mediolateral oblique view of left breast with a 1-cm mass. **B.** Stereo views with three lesion targets marked. **C.** Prefire views with core needle in place in the center of the target. **D.** Postfire views with needle passing through the target. The lesion has been sampled.

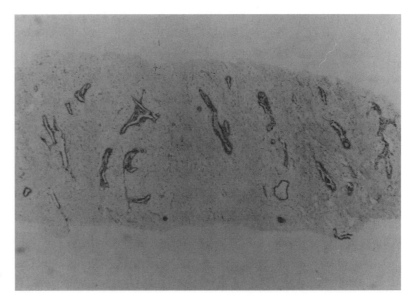

FIGURE 6.3-3 Microscopic histologic section showing fibroadenoma diagnosed by core biopsy.

Microcalcifications and Specimen Radiography

When performing stereotactic core biopsy to determine the etiology of microcalcifications, specific calcifications should be targeted within the segment or cluster. The cores are placed on a glass slide, moistened with a few drops of sterile saline, and labeled. A magnification radiograph of all cores is obtained to document removal of microcalcifications (Fig. 6.3-5). In some instances, the microcalcifications are noted histologically when not seen radiographically. The most sig-nificant pathologic diagnosis is usually found within the cores that contain the microcalcifications.[17] The cores without calcium are important as duct carcinoma in situ (DCIS) may be found adjacent to areas of benign calcification.

ACCURACY

The studies listed in Table 6.3-1 compare the agreement of stereotactic core biopsy with surgical biopsy. The concordance ranges from 71% to 99%, with the best results obtained using a 14-gauge core needle and removal of at least five cores per lesion.[18–24] In most series comparing

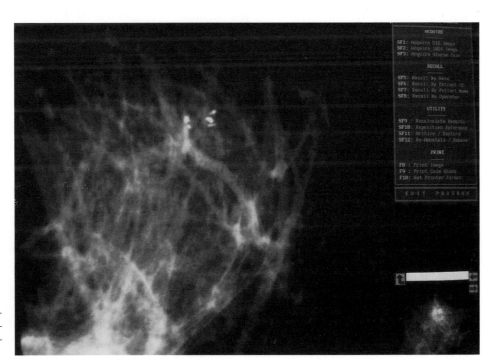

FIGURE 6.3-4 Digital mammography. Cluster of five microcalcifications imaged by digital mammography.

FIGURE 6.3-5 Specimen radiography. **A.** Magnified view of a cluster of microcalcifications. **B.** Specimen radiograph of cores from stereotactic needle biopsy. Calcium is seen in three of five cores.

TABLE 6.3-1
Stereotactic Core Biopsy:
Agreement With Surgical Biopsy

Investigators	Needle Gauge	Biopsies (N)	Agreement With Surgical Biopsy (%)
Parker et al, 1990[18]	14–18	102	87
Parker et al, 1991[19]	14	102	96
Dowlatshahi et al, 1991[20]	20	250	71
Dronkers, 1992[21]	18	53	91
Elvecrog et al, 1993[22]	14	100	94
Gisvold et al, 1994[23]★	14	104	90
Parker et al, 1994[24]†	14	1363	99

★ Cases with five cores.

† 23% of core biopsies performed using ultrasound guidance.

surgical with stereotactic biopsy, lesions diagnosed correctly by one technique will occasionally be missed by the other, suggesting that surgical biopsy is no longer a satisfactory gold standard for nonpalpable lesion diagnosis. Most experienced operators using stereotactic core biopsy can remove a satisfactory tissue sample almost 100% of the time with a sensitivity of 95% or better.[25]

COMPLICATIONS

The complications of stereotactic biopsy include hematoma, infection, and possible tumor seeding. In Parker and associates' multicenter experience,[24] 6 complications (0.2%) were reported in 3765 cases for which follow-up was available. Three hematomas required surgical drainage, and three infections required drainage, antibiotic treatment, or both. After more than 1000 core biopsies in our facility, no significant complications have occurred. Minor bruising around the biopsy site is common but can be minimized by maintaining pressure and using ice after the needle has been removed. Even if biopsy is done on a small artery, local pressure quickly stops any bleeding.

Patients receiving anticoagulant therapy can undergo biopsy if meticulous technique is used and the medication is reduced to the lowest acceptable level.

Seeding of the needle track was reported in a case of mucinous carcinoma that underwent core biopsy.[26] This possibility exists with any type of needle procedure, including fine-needle aspiration and needle localization, but the significance and incidence are not known. No cases were reported in the series of Parker and coworkers.[24]

MANAGEMENT

Proper management of a nonpalpable breast lesion begins with an appropriate imaging evaluation including spot compression, magnification, other special mammographic views, or ultrasound. To recommend biopsy, the radiologist should suspect a lesion to have a 2% or greater chance of malignancy and categorize it as either *high suspicion (HS)* or *low-intermediate suspicion (LS)*.[27] HS mammographic lesions, such as spiculated masses or irregular, pleomorphic, and casting calcifications, generally have an 80% or greater chance of malignancy. LS lesions, such as well-circumscribed or slightly lobulated masses more than 1 cm in diameter or granular microcalcifications, have a likelihood of malignancy averaging 10% (range, 2% to 80%).

Figure 6.3-6 shows the needle biopsy management algorithms used at our facility. LS and HS lesions are managed differently. With LS lesions, the radiologist should, after the imaging evaluation, have a brief list of possibilities with respect to lesion's histologic diagnosis. If the lesion's needle biopsy diagnosis correlates with the radiologic diagnosis, the lesion can be monitored mammographically. The recommended follow-up intervals are 6, 12, and 24 months. Surgical biopsy is recommended if the core histologic diagnosis and the mammographic diagnosis do not correlate, if a high-risk lesion (atypical ductal hyperplasia [ADH], atypical lobular hyperplasia [ALH], lobular carcinoma in situ [LCIS]) is found, or if the pathologist recommends excision. Patients with LS lesions proved malignant by core biopsy can proceed to appropriate therapy without surgical biopsy. Biopsies reported as insufficient or inadequate are uncommon and usually contain only fat and stroma. The cause for an insufficient sample (eg, superficial location of the lesion, inadequate targeting, gun failure) should be determined and the biopsy repeated using an appropriate surgical or stereotactic method.

HS mammographic lesions are usually malignant histologically. Therefore, the purpose of the stereotactic needle biopsy is to confirm the malignant mammographic impression and to give the surgeon enough information in most cases to perform definitive therapy with a single surgical procedure. Some of the HS lesions produce benign needle biopsy results, either because they are truly benign or (less probably) because of a needle biopsy miss. Because of the high probability of malignancy in this group, surgical biopsy is recommended despite benign needle biopsy find-

Nonpalpable, low- to intermediate-suspicion lesions (n = 469)

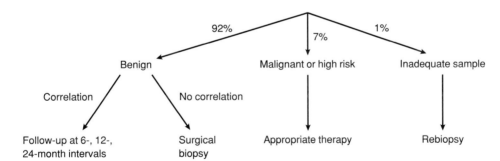

Nonpalpable, high-suspicion lesions (n = 117)

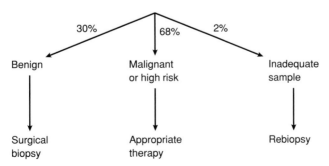

FIGURE 6.3-6 Management algorithm for stereotactic core needle biopsy used at the Susan G. Komen Breast Center, Dallas. Percentages refer to core needle biopsy results (June 1990 to May 1994).

ings. Some patients decline this recommendation and opt for mammographic follow-up. In these cases, the surgical biopsy recommendation and the patient's refusal should be clearly documented. As with LS lesions, needle biopsies with histologic results in the high-risk group should be recommended for surgical biopsy and those with results insufficient repeated with an appropriate biopsy method.

Follow-Up of Benign Lesions

Patients with LS lesions and benign histologic diagnoses by needle biopsy should receive recommendations for mammographic follow-up at 6-, 12-, and 24-month intervals. At 6 months, mammography of only the breast that underwent biopsy is done, followed at 12 and 24 months by a bilateral mammogram. Although changes can develop in benign lesions, surgical biopsy is recommended if any suspicious change such as mass enlargement or increasing microcalcifications occurs. Facilities should have predetermined follow-up reminder procedures to notify patients and physicians. Despite extensive follow-up efforts, some patients will not return at the appropriate time or at all. These follow-up attempts and refusals should be clearly documented in the patient's records.

Duct Carcinoma in Situ

For appropriate treatment of DCIS, it is important to determine accurately if a lesion is completely in situ without an invasive component. Jackman and colleagues[28] found that stereotactic core needle biopsy diagnosed DCIS but did not show invasive disease in 8 of 43 core biopsies (19%).[28] In the multicenter study reported by Parker and colleagues,[24] complete agreement between core and surgical histology occurred with 741 of 752 (98.5%) invasive lesions, 140 of 158 (89%) intermediate to high-grade DCIS lesions, and 116 of 173 (67%) lesions classified as low-grade DCIS, ADH, LCIS, or ALH. Accurate diagnosis of lesions in the last category from cores of tissue alone poses considerable difficulty for even experienced histopathologists. Therefore, surgical biopsy is usually recommended when the core biopsy diagnosis is DCIS, LCIS, ADH, or ALH.

Indications: Advantages, Disadvantages, and Problems

In today's medical and economic environment, surgical treatment of breast cancer is usually a two-step procedure. Surgical biopsy is followed by a definitive procedure—either lumpectomy with or without axillary dissection or mastectomy with or without reconstruction. However, because of core needle biopsy, this paradigm is changing.

The instances in which core breast biopsy offers clear advantages over surgery are as follows:

1. LS lesions. A definitive benign diagnosis by core biopsy essentially eliminates surgical biopsy.
2. HS lesions and a patient who wishes to have a mastectomy with or without reconstruction rather than lumpectomy. Such lesions can be definitively diagnosed by core biopsy, and surgical biopsy can be avoided.
3. Lesions characterized by multiple clusters of microcalcifications or multiple masses in different quadrants of the same breast. If two or more can be proven malignant by core biopsy, the patient is not a breast-conservation candidate and can proceed with mastectomy with or without reconstruction.

Because almost any breast lesion is suitable for stereotactic core needle biopsy, only a few instances exist in which generally it is *not* helpful: (1) the histologic diagnosis of the lesion by needle biopsy will not shorten the diagnostic process; (2) the removal of the entire lesion is necessary for diagnosis; and (3) the lesion cannot be successfully targeted.

Before biopsy, the radiologist and the referring physician should consider whether a specific tissue diagnosis by needle biopsy will improve patient care. If the procedure shortens the diagnostic process and potentially replaces surgical biopsy, it is valuable and should be done. LS lesions, particularly those with a level of suspicion of 20% or less, are ideal for needle biopsy.

The role of core biopsy, particularly with HS lesions, is controversial when breast conservation is the treatment of choice. Some surgeons prefer excisional biopsy as the first diagnostic and therapeutic maneuver. The patient can observe the lumpectomy's cosmetic result before axillary node dissection and radiation therapy. The presence or absence of an extensive intraductal component can be determined and the surgical margins assessed. If the surgical margins are not free of tumor, reexcision can be done before axillary dissection. As many as 76% of lumpectomies require reexcision because of involved margins.[29] In this two-step scenario, stereotactic core needle biopsy is an added expense. Other surgeons contend that a presurgical malignant diagnosis permits discussion of treatment options before surgery and performance of a "better" lumpectomy, increasing the likelihood of adequate margins with a single procedure. These differences seem to be related to surgical preference and the volume of breast tissue removed during lumpectomy. Based on data from our institution, it appears that, after core biopsy, surgical treatment of malignant lesions can be successfully done in most cases (88%) with one procedure (Table 6.3-2).

The histologic diagnosis of some lesions by core needle biopsy is particularly demanding. The radial scar (radial or complex sclerosing lesion), even when totally excised, may present a difficult histologic diagnosis. Its assessment, therefore, becomes an even greater (although not impossible) challenge from only core samples. Hence, if a lesion is suspected mammographically to be a radial scar, surgical biopsy rather than stereotactic biopsy is advised. Papillary

TABLE 6.3-2
Surgical Treatment of Malignant Lesions
Diagnosed by Stereotactic Core Biopsy★

Surgical Therapy	Total (N)	1 Surgical Procedure After Core Biopsy (N)	>1 Surgical Procedure After Core Biopsy (N)
Mastectomy	44	41	3
Lumpectomy and axillary dissection	31	26	5
Lumpectomy only	8	6	2
No surgery, chemotherapy only	2	2	0
Total	85	75 (88%)	10 (12%)

★ At the Susan G. Komen Breast Center, Dallas, June 1990 to May 1994. Eighty-eight percent had definitive surgical therapy with only one procedure after core biopsy.

lesions and some forms of sclerosing adenosis are also in this category.

Although small lesions can be accurately sampled, large areas of granular microcalcifications may be difficult to target stereotactically and require surgical biopsy for diagnosis. This lesion may also harbor low-grade DCIS unrelated to the microcalcifications.

Some patients or lesions may not be technically suited for stereotactic biopsy. Women who cannot lie prone or undergo extended breast compression are not candidates for the procedure. If the breast lesion is superficial or the breast compresses to 2 cm or less, the biopsy usually cannot be done. The long-throw biopsy guns have an excursion of 2.1 to 2.5 cm. With a superficial lesion or thinly compressed breast, the tip of the biopsy needle would have to begin its excursion outside the breast for the tissue slot to be at the proper position at the end of the excursion. Finally, some lesions situated far posteriorly in the breast cannot be imaged satisfactorily with the stereotactic device.

Stereotactic breast biopsy is no substitute for an excellent imaging evaluation. The same criteria used for determining the necessity of surgical biopsy should be used for core biopsy. Lesions classified as probably benign (having less than a 2% chance of malignancy) should usually undergo careful periodic mammographic follow-up rather than biopsy. In some circumstances, however, because of patient or physician anxiety, stereotactic core biopsy of such a lesion may be appropriate and necessary.[30]

COST OF STEREOTACTIC BIOPSY

In most institutions, the overall cost for stereotactic biopsy is one third to one fourth that of surgical biopsy. At the University of Chicago, Schmidt[25] reported that the "use

of stereotactic biopsy saved 86% of the patients a surgical biopsy or the anxiety of close follow-up, which translates into a cost savings of about 60%." The cost savings per biopsy in our institution and others has been estimated to be $1500 to $2000.[25] Given the 500,000 breast biopsies initiated by mammographic findings annually in the United States, the use of stereotactic breast biopsy could result in yearly savings of 750 million to 1 billion dollars.[31] Lindfors and Rosenquist[32] suggested through a theoretical model that use of stereotactic biopsy (instead of surgical biopsy) in a mammographic screening program could lower the marginal cost per year of life saved by a maximum of 23%, from $20,770 to $15,934.

Over 90% of women with suspicious, impalpable breast lesions are candidates for core biopsy. Appropriate use of this technique (rather than surgical biopsy) could result in tremendous cost savings. The extensive use of core biopsy for diagnosis of lesions classified mammographically as probably benign is inappropriate, however, and could potentially escalate costs.

Future Trends and Developments

About 55% of the core breast biopsies done at our facility use stereotactic guidance with microcalcifications as the predominant lesion. Ultrasound-guided core biopsy is used for nonpalpable masses. As imaging-guided breast biopsy gains greater acceptance, one predicts that fewer surgical biopsies will be needed to diagnose benign lesions and that the number of needle localizations will decrease. With further technologic improvements in minimally invasive procedures, physicians adept with these methods can expect to play a greater clinical role in the team approach to diagnosis and treatment of breast disease.

ACKNOWLEDGMENT

The author wishes to thank Mollie Standish for her invaluable assistance in the preparation of this chapter.

References

1. Shapiro S, Venet W, Strax P, et al. Ten-to fourteen-year effect of screening on breast cancer mortality. J Natl Cancer Inst 1982;69:349.
2. Tabar L, Fagerberg CJG, Gad A, et al. Reduction in mortality from breast cancer after mass screening with mammography. Lancet 1985;1:829.
3. Seidman N, Gelf SK, Silverberg E, et al. The Breast Cancer Detection Demonstration Project: end result. Cancer 1987;37:258.
4. Tabar L, Fagerberg G, Duffy SW, et al. Update of the Swedish two-county program of mammographic screening for breast cancer. Radiol Clin North Am 1992;30:187.
5. Shapiro S, Strax P, Venet L. Periodic breast cancer screening in reducing mortality from breast cancer. JAMA 1971;215:1777.
6. Hall FM. Screening mammography potential problems on the horizon. N Engl J Med 1986;314:53.
7. Hall FM, Storella JM, Silverstone DZ, et al. Nonpalpable breast

lesions: recommendations for biopsy based on suspicion of carcinoma at mammography. Radiology 1988;167:353.

8. Cyrlak D. Induced costs of low-cost screening mammography. Radiology 1988;168:661.

9. Yankaskas BC, Knelson MH, Abernethy ML, et al. Needle localization biopsy of occult lesions of the breast: experience in 199 cases. Invest Radiol 1988;23:729.

10. Homer MJ, Smith TJ, Safaii H. Prebiopsy needle localization: methods, problems, and expected results. Radiol Clin North Am 1992;30:139.

11. Kopans DB. Review of stereotaxic large-core needle biopsy and surgical biopsy results in nonpalpable breast lesions. Radiology 1993;189:665.

12. Norton LW, Zeligman BE, Pearlman NW. Accuracy and cost of needle localization biopsy. Arch Surg 1988;123:947.

13. Sickles EA. Periodic follow-up of probably benign mammographic lesions: results of 3184 consecutive cases. Radiology 1991;179:463.

14. Brenner RJ, Sickles EA. Acceptability of periodic follow-up as an alternative to biopsy for mammographically detected lesions interpreted as probably benign. Radiology 1989;171:645.

15. Brenner RJ. Follow-up as an alternative to biopsy for probably benign mammographically detected abnormalities. Curr Opin Radiol 1991;3:588.

16. Jackson VP. The status of mammographically guided fine needle aspiration biopsy of nonpalpable breast lesions. In: Radiol Clin North Amer, vol 30. Bassett LW, ed. Breast imaging: current status and future directions. Philadelphia, WB Saunders, 1992:155.

17. Liberman L, Evans WP, Dershaw DD, et al. Radiography of microcalcifications in stereotaxic mammary core biopsy specimens. Radiology 1994;190:223.

18. Parker SH, Lovin JD, Jobe WE, et al. Stereotactic breast biopsy with a biopsy gun. Radiology 1990;176:741.

19. Parker SH, Lovin JD, Jobe WE, et al. Non-palpable breast lesions: stereotactic automated large-core biopsies. Radiology 1991;180:403.

20. Dowlatshahi K, Yaremko ML, Kluskens LF, et al. Nonpalpable breast lesions: findings of stereotaxic needle-core biopsy and fine-needle aspiration cytology. Radiology 1991;181:745.

21. Dronkers DJ. Stereotaxic core biopsy of breast lesions. Radiology 1992;183:631.

22. Elvecrog EL, Lechner MC, Nelson MT. Non-palpable breast lesions: correlation of stereotaxic large-core needle biopsy and surgical biopsy results. Radiology 1993;188:453.

23. Gisvold JJ, Goellner JR, Grant CS, et al. Breast biopsy: a comparative study of stereotaxically guided core and excisional techniques. AJR 1994;162:815.

24. Parker S, Burbank F, Tabar L, et al. Percutaneous large core breast biopsy: a multi-institutional experience. Radiology 1994;193:359.

25. Schmidt RA. Stereotactic breast biopsy. CA Cancer J Clin 1994;44:172.

26. Harter LP, Curtis JS, Ponto G, et al. Malignant seeding of the needle track during stereotaxic core needle breast biopsy. Radiology 1992;185:713.

27. Sullivan DC. Perspective: needle core biopsy of mammographic lesions. AJR 1993;162:601.

28. Jackman RJ, Nowels KW, Shepard MJ, et al. Stereotaxic large-core needle biopsy of 450 nonpalpable breast lesions with surgical correlation in lesions with cancer or atypical hyperplasia. Radiology 1994;193:91.

29. Tafra L, Guenther JM, Guiliano AE. Planned segmentectomy: a necessity for breast carcinoma. Arch Surg 1993;128:1014.

30. Sickles EA, Parker SH. Appropriate role of core breast biopsy in the management of probably benign lesions. Radiology 1993;188:315.

31. Schmidt R, Morrow M., Bibbo M, et al. Benefits of stereotactic aspiration cytology. Admin Radiol 1990;9:35.

32. Lindfors KK, Rosenquist CJ. Needle core biopsy guided with mammography: a study of cost-effectiveness. Radiology 1994;199:217.

6.4

Ultrasound-Guided Percutaneous Needle Biopsy on Nonpalpable Breast Masses

BRUNO D. FORNAGE

The widespread use of screening mammography has resulted in the increased detection of nonpalpable breast lesions. The goal of guided percutaneous needle biopsy is to reduce the number of unnecessary open surgical biopsies for such lesions.[1] Needle biopsy also has the significant advantage of avoiding scarring that might affect follow-up imaging studies. The popularity of fine-needle aspiration biopsy (FNAB) has been challenged by the development of automatic biopsy devices for large-core needle biopsy (LCNB). Both FNAB and LCNB are effectively guided by real-time ultrasonography.[2-6] In experienced hands, any lesion that can be shown on sonograms can be successfully sampled under real-time ultrasonographic guidance. It must be remembered, however, that ultrasonography cannot visualize carcinomas that appear on mammograms as microcalcifications only or as solid masses 5 mm in diameter or smaller.

Ultrasound-guided needle biopsy is not without difficulty, and experience in every step is needed to yield optimal results. The success of ultrasound-guided biopsy of the breast depends on the following:

- The skills of the operator in hitting the target lesion
- Successful tissue extraction (which depends on the operator's technique and the nature of the tumor)
- Adequate preparation of the specimens
- Interpretation by an expert pathologist or cytopathologist.

Any factor compromising the success of any step will jeopardize the success of the procedure.

It is critical that ultrasound-guided needle biopsy be done after a meticulous review of recent mammograms. Doing such biopsies after mammography also avoids the risk of misinterpretation of a postbiopsy hematoma on subsequent mammograms.

Whatever the needle biopsy technique used, it is imperative to use state-of-the-art ultrasound equipment, that is, a high-frequency (7.5- or 10-MHz) linear-array transducer.

Ultrasound-Guided Fine-Needle Aspiration Biopsy

TECHNICAL CONSIDERATIONS

Instrumentation

Standard, 20- to 23-gauge (generally 22-gauge), 1.5-inch (3.8-cm) hypodermic needles are used. Rarely, a 2-inch needle is needed because of a deep lesion or large breast. If a needle guide is used, a longer needle such as a spinal needle must be used to compensate for the longer pathway.

The transducer is carefully cleansed and then soaked in a sterilizing solution for several minutes before the procedure. After the procedure, the probe is cleansed and decontaminated for 15 to 20 minutes in a glutaraldehyde solution (eg, Cidex).

Preparation of the Patient

The skin is prepared using rubbing alcohol, which also serves as an acoustic coupling medium. Depending on the location of the tumor, the patient is placed in a dorsal decubitus or oblique lateral position to spread the breast on the chest wall and thus shorten the needle's pathway. Local anesthesia is usually not necessary for FNAB.

Needle Insertion Technique

The most commonly used technique of needle insertion is the oblique insertion approach, in which the needle is inserted from the end of the transducer along the scan plane with an obliquity that depends on the depth of the target (Fig. 6.4-1). With this technique, not only the tip but most of the distal portion of the needle is visualized from the moment it enters the scan plane. In experienced hands, the oblique insertion technique is 100% accurate and safe.

Although needle guides that attach to the transducer and that maintain the oblique needle within the scan plane are available, the free-hand technique is often preferred for FNAB because it allows reorientation of the needle at different angles and therefore permits a larger volume to be sampled. The free-hand technique also allows an experienced operator to select virtually any site of needle entry and angle. The only technical limitation to ultrasound-guided fine-needle aspiration of the breast and regional lymph nodes is lack of visibility of the target lesion.

Sampling Technique

Sampling of solid masses is accomplished using to-and-fro and rotation (corkscrew) movements of the needle to dissociate the tumor tissue. With the no-aspiration sam-

FIGURE 6.4-1 Ultrasonography-guided fine-needle aspiration. **A.** Diagram showing the technique of oblique needle insertion. The needle is inserted obliquely from the end of the transducer (T) along the scan plane. The distal part of the needle is visualized, with its tip displayed in the center of the mass (M). **B.** Sonogram obtained during ultrasonography-guided fine-needle aspiration of a carcinoma smaller than 1 cm (*arrows*) shows the echogenic needle (*arrowheads*), the tip of which is clearly seen in the center of the mass.

pling technique,[4,7] capillarity spontaneously drives the dissociated cellular material into the lumen of the needle, which is not attached to a syringe and therefore remains in communication with the outer milieu. With the free-hand technique, every movement of the needle is monitored in real time on the video monitor. The sampling process takes about 20 to 30 seconds. It is recommended that the entire biopsy procedure be videotaped to document that samples were obtained from within the lesion. The appearance of material in the needle's hub confirms that the lumen of the needle probably contains adequate material. If necessary, brief suction with a syringe can be used to secure the specimen in the needle.

CYSTS AND FLUID COLLECTIONS

Cysts and other fluid collections can be readily aspirated with a fine needle. Occasionally, difficulties may arise in puncturing cysts. For example, a thickened wall may resist the passage of the needle. Cysts that are not under tension may show a significant deformation under the needle's pressure; penetration of the wall requires a brief and firm forward push of the needle. Also, small cysts in a fatty environment may move significantly under the needle. Increasing the pressure of the transducer on the skin may help keep lesions stationary. On occasion, an 18-gauge needle may be needed to drain an inspissated cyst, the contents of which typically appear as toothpaste-like material. In such cases, it may not be possible to drain the cyst completely; however, the typical appearance of the aspirate (which does not contain abnormal cells) and the fact that the cyst has been seen to partially deflate are diagnostic of this condition.

Cysts that require aspiration include those that do not have a typical sonographic pattern and those that appear as mammographically indeterminate densities. Symptomatic cysts are aspirated for therapeutic purposes. Asymptomatic typical cysts in a patient with fibrocystic disease do not require aspiration unless they show growth on repeat examination.

Typical (yellow-to-green) cystic fluid need not be analyzed; however, hemorrhagic fluid should be analyzed and a pneumocystogram done. Turbid fluid should be sent for both cytologic and bacteriologic analyses. When an intracystic tumor is suspected (based on sonograms) or when an unequivocal correlation with prebiopsy mammograms is needed, a pneumocystogram can be readily done by injecting into the cyst a volume of air about equal to the volume of the fluid aspirated and then obtaining standard mammographic views.[4] Pneumocystography has also been reported to have some therapeutic value, yet its mechanism is unclear.[8]

Postoperative hematomas or lymphoceles that have not resolved spontaneously can be drained under ultrasonographic guidance. The diagnosis of a breast abscess is readily confirmed by FNAB.

SOLID MASSES

Some solid masses may be difficult to sample by fine-needle aspiration. As a rule, an insufficient specimen must be regarded as a failure of the procedure, which must be repeated.[9]

Malignant Tumors

In infiltrating ductal carcinomas, the cytologic specimens are usually highly cellular, and, using ultrasonographic guidance, the diagnosis is established in most cases with a single needle pass. Other forms of breast malignancy, such as medullary or mucinous carcinomas, lymphomas, or metastases to the breast, can also be diagnosed cytologically. It must be emphasized that fine-needle aspiration cannot differentiate between invasive and noninvasive breast carcinoma. This differentiation requires histopathologic examination of a large core (see later).

In a series of 254 surgically verified, nonpalpable, noncystic lesions that were subjected to ultrasound-guided fine-needle aspiration, the sensitivity and specificity in the diagnosis of cancer were 91% (2% false-negative results) and 77% (1% false-positive results), respectively, with 11% of specimens deemed inadequate. When only lesions diagnosed as definitely benign or malignant were considered, the sensitivity and specificity of FNAB were 97% and 98%, respectively.[10] In another series of 36 carcinomas smaller than 1 cc, FNAB sensitivity was 94%, with 3% inadequate specimens.[3]

The hormonal receptor status of carcinomas is now routinely assayed in fine-needle aspirates.[11] Other new cytologic studies include the evaluation of proliferation markers (DNA ploidy, Ki-67) to determine the tumor's aggressiveness.[12]

Ultrasonographically guided fine-needle aspiration is also effective for diagnosing lymph node metastases in the axilla, the internal mammary chains, and the infraclavicular and supraclavicular regions.

Benign Lesions

With strict criteria, the cytologic diagnosis of fibroadenoma can be established with reliability. The major limitation of FNAB for diagnosing fibroadenomas is the relatively high incidence (up to 20%) of insufficient specimens; when fine-needle aspirates are insufficient, the operator should switch to LCNB. Cytologic examination can also readily establish a diagnosis of fat necrosis, acute inflammation, and intramammary lymph nodes.[4]

FAILURES AND LIMITATIONS OF ULTRASOUND-GUIDED FINE-NEEDLE ASPIRATION

A guidance failure may result in a missed target. Although such failures may occur while learning the technique, in experienced hands, ultrasonographic guidance is consistently successful in bringing the needle tip inside lesions larger than 6 to 7 mm visible on sonograms.

An insufficient smear represents a complete failure of the procedure and should prompt subsequent passes. Should this also fail, LCNB should be done. Otherwise, surgical excision must be considered after ultrasound-guided localization of the lesion.

False-negative cytologic diagnoses, although rare, may occur with paucicellular and markedly desmoplastic tumors such as infiltrating lobular carcinomas.[13] Tubular carcinomas also have the potential to mimic a fibroadenoma.[14] False-positive cytologic results are even rarer. They have been reported mostly in cases of hypercellular benign lesions such as papillomas, some tubular adenomas, and atypical ductal hyperplasia.[14] Radiation-induced changes can also mimic recurrent carcinoma.[15]

Ultrasound-Guided Large-Core Needle Biopsy

Recently, LCNB has been revived with the advent of automated spring-loaded devices that activate a 14- to 18-gauge cutting needle in a fraction of a second. These devices are much easier to use than the traditional Tru-Cut needle. Advantages of LCNB include a near 100% tissue recovery rate, even in fibrous masses, and the fact that tissue cores are readily interpreted by any pathologist.

INSTRUMENTATION

Numerous commercially available devices provide automatic propulsion of a cutting needle over a throw of about 2 to 4 cm. A clear understanding of the device and knowledge of the location from which the core will be taken are prerequisites to use of LCNB. Although the Biopty gun with 14-gauge Tru-Cut needle has been considered a standard for LCNB, new devices that cut full-cylinder cores (eg, Argovac) provide high-quality specimens with thinner (18-gauge) needles and less resultant trauma.[16]

PREPARATION OF THE PATIENT

Preparation of the patient for LCNB differs from that for FNAB. Because a small skin incision and generous local anesthesia are required when 14-gauge needles are used, the needle entry site must be carefully selected. Disinfection of the skin and transducer is achieved using povidone-iodine. Before the procedure is started, the firing mechanism of the biopsy device should be tested and the device cocked and locked in the safety position (when a lock is available). The procedure should be explained in detail to the patient.

NEEDLE INSERTION TECHNIQUE

Because of the throw of the needle (which may reach 4 cm with some devices), the cutting needle *must* be inserted as horizontally as possible, to prevent the needle from hitting the thoracic wall and possibly the lung (Fig. 6.4-2). This approach requires that the needle be inserted at a sufficient distance from the end of the transducer. Because the needle is nearly horizontal, its visualization is optimal. Under ultrasonographic guidance, and using the free-hand technique, the tip of the needle is brought into contact with the mass (see Fig. 6.4-2*A* and *C*); the perfect alignment of the needle with the scan plane is verified, and a hard copy of the prefiring position of the needle is taken. The mechanism is then fired, and a postfiring hard copy showing the needle traversing the target is also printed (see Fig. 6.4-2*B* and *D*). The needle is withdrawn and the core released from the cutting needle and placed in a solution of formalin (or saline if a frozen section is needed; eg, to obtain a diagnosis more rapidly). The procedure is repeated in different areas of the tumor until a sufficient number of satisfactory cores have been obtained.

Debate continues regarding the optimal number of cores to obtain. A large number of cores per lesion have been recommended for stereotactically guided LCNB with 14-gauge cutting needles, primarily to ensure correct sampling of the target. In our experience, however, when the transfixion of the target has been clearly documented with ultrasound and when cores appear to be of satisfactory size, no more than five cores are needed for diagnosis.

To avoid repeat passage through (and trauma to) the subcutaneous tissues when multiple cores are obtained, an introducer can be inserted first to the surface of the lesion, thus permitting rapid reinsertion of the needle for repeat passes and possibly reducing the risk for seeding of malignant cells along the needle track. Such an introducer has not been necessary in our experience with LCNB using 18-gauge needles.

Because currently no commercially available guide can guarantee the safe, nearly horizontal insertion of the needle along the ultrasound scan plane, LCNB has to be done with the free-hand technique. Because of the long needle path and the limited thickness of the breast when the patient is supine, the risk for injury to the thoracic wall and underlying lung should be constantly considered in selecting the entry site, monitoring the direction of the needle, and anticipating the postfiring position of the needle tip. As a result, LCNB requires more experience in ultrasonographic guidance of needles than does FNAB.

Ultrasound-Guided Fine-Needle Aspiration Biopsy Versus Ultrasound-Guided Large-Core Needle Biopsy

Major advantages of ultrasound-guided FNAB include its pinpoint accuracy, excellent tolerance by patients, and ability to aspirate or inject fluid or air. The outstanding accuracy is synonymous with total safety, and lesions that lie close to the chest wall or to breast implants can be safely aspirated.[17] Also, results can be obtained within minutes.

Disadvantages of FNAB include the risk for insufficient specimens, the inability to determine cancer invasiveness, and the need for an expert cytopathologist. On the other hand, LCNB has a very high tissue recovery rate in fibrous lesions, the large cores can be read by any pathologist, and the invasiveness of cancer can be determined. The procedure, however, takes longer than FNAB and is more invasive, with a higher rate of complications (including hematomas and, more infrequently, milk fistula and malignant seeding along the needle track).[18,19] Other disadvantages of LCNB are the need for multiple passes and the inability to aspirate fluid collections. Because of the sudden action of the device, problems also may occur in penetrating minute and mobile lesions. The slower, more controllable progression of the needle during ultrasound-guided FNAB is advantageous for penetrating such lesions. In institutions in which an expert cytopathologist is available, indications for ultrasound-guided LCNB remain limited to the failure of previous FNAB and assessment of invasiveness of the cancer.

FIGURE 6.4-2 Ultrasonography-guided large-core needle biopsy. **A.** Diagram showing the nearly horizontal prefiring position of the cutting needle, which has been placed into contact with the mass (M). The needle is aligned with the scan plane of the transducer (T). **B.** The postfiring location of the cutting needle, which has traversed the mass. **C.** Prefiring sonogram obtained during ultrasonography-guided lung core-needle biopsy of a 1-cm carcinoma (*arrows*) showing the echogenic 18-gauge cutting needle (*arrowheads*), the tip of which is near the mass. Note the nearly horizontal direction of the needle required because of the small size of the breast and the proximity of the thoracic wall. The adjustable throw of the needle has been set at 3 cm. L, lung; P, pectoralis major muscle; R, rib. **D.** Postfiring sonogram showing the echogenic cutting needle (*arrowheads*) traversing the tumor (*arrows*). **E.** Low-power photomicrograph showing three core biopsy specimens obtained from a carcinoma with an 18-gauge Argovac cutting needle (hematoxylin–eosin stain). The cores are of excellent quality, and there are no crushing artifacts.

Sonographic Versus Stereotaxic Guidance

Ultrasonography cannot be used to guide the biopsy of isolated microcalcifications (ie, without an associated mass); stereotaxic guidance is required for this purpose. For masses, most of which can be shown using high-resolution ultrasonography, advantages of ultrasonography over stereotaxic guidance include the ability to use the shortest route to the lesion, the unique real-time monitoring of both the placement of the needle *and* sampling of the lesion, the multidirectional sampling (with FNAB), the rapidity of the procedure, the comfort of the patient, the applicability to virtually any mass in the breast (even masses that lie at the periphery of the breast or next to a prosthesis)[17] and in node-bearing regions, and the wide availability of ultrasound equipment.[9] Ultrasonography is the only guidance technique for lesions visualized only by ultrasound, for example, lesions in dense breasts, in pregnant patients, and in women who refuse radiation exposure. Table 6.4-1 further compares the indications for and strengths of ultrasonographic and stereotaxic guidance of needle biopsy.

Radiologists in specialized breast centers should have both ultrasonography and stereotaxy available for guiding needle biopsy of nonpalpable masses and should be expert in using both. In dedicated centers so equipped, a reversal has occurred in the trend following the wave of popularity of stereotaxy, and most masses now undergo biopsy with ultrasonographic rather than stereotaxic guidance.[20]

Keys to Success

Ultrasound-guided needle biopsy of nonpalpable breast lesions requires teamwork. Progress can be made and experience accumulated only through ongoing communication between the radiologist, the pathologist, and the surgeon.

Because real-time ultrasonographic guidance is a meticulous procedure that requires excellent eye-hand coordination, proper training is essential. Simple phantoms have been described for this purpose.[21]

Cytologic diagnosis also requires solid experience. Therefore, these techniques work best in cancer centers, and implementation in the general medical community may be associated with some difficulties. Certainly, no one should undertake guided needle biopsy of nonpalpable breast lesions if the previously mentioned requirements cannot be met.

Summary

The impact on patient management of a definitely positive needle biopsy is to eliminate the need for open biopsy. At the other end of the spectrum, patients with cysts are

TABLE 6.4-1

Ultrasonographic Versus Stereotaxic Guidance for Needle Biopsy of Nonpalpable Breast Lesions

	Ultrasonographic Guidance	Stereotaxic Guidance
Indications		
Isolated calcifications	No	Yes
Mass (seen on both ultrasound and mammograms)	Yes	Yes
Mass seen only on ultrasound	Yes	No
Mass seen only on mammograms	No	Yes
Mass close to implant	Yes	Difficult
Mass at periphery of breast	Yes	No
Mass in pregnant patient	Yes	No
Regional lymph node	Yes	No
Real-time monitoring of needle penetration into lesion *and* of sampling	Yes	No
Accuracy	Very good	Very good
Safety	Optimal	Optimal
Duration of procedure	Several seconds	Several minutes
Number of passes required	Few	Several
Tolerance by the patient	Excellent	Good (occasional complaints related to prolonged breast compression)
Cost compared with open surgical biopsy	Moderate	Moderate

now treated expeditiously by FNAB and should no longer undergo surgery. The nonsurgical management of nonpalpable, solid breast masses diagnosed as benign by needle biopsy remains controversial and requires a shift in the attitude of surgeons, who will have to rely—at least in selected patients and with appropriate follow-up—on the negative result (ie, adequate specimen without evidence of suspicious or malignant tissue) of a perfectly guided needle biopsy. As a golden rule, however, a negative result of a needle biopsy in the face of a single suggestive finding—physical, mammographic, or sonographic—should not delay surgical excision.

References

1. Dixon JM, Clarke PJ, Crucioli V, et al. Reduction of the surgical excision rate in benign breast disease using fine-needle aspiration cytology with immediate reporting. Br J Surg 1987;74:1014.

2. Fornage BD, Faroux MJ, Simatos A. Breast masses: US-guided fine-needle aspiration biopsy. Radiology 1987;147:409.

3. Fornage BD, Sneige N, Faroux MJ, et al. Sonographic appearance and ultrasound-guided fine-needle aspiration biopsy of breast carcinomas smaller than 1 cm³. J Ultrasound Med 1990;9:559.

4. Fornage BD, Coan JD, David CL. Ultrasound-guided needle biopsy of the breast and other interventional procedures. Radiol Clin North Am 1992;30:167.

5. Gordon PB, Goldenberg SL, Chan NHL. Solid breast lesions: diagnosis with US-guided fine-needle aspiration biopsy. Radiology 1993;189:573.

6. Parker SH, Jobe WE, Dennis MA, et al. US-guided automated large-core breast biopsy. Radiology 1993;187:507.

7. Zajdela A, Zillhardt P, Voillemot N. Cytological diagnosis by fine-needle sampling without aspiration. Cancer 1987;59:1201.

8. Ikeda DM, Helvie MA, Adler DD, et al. The role of fine-needle aspiration and pneumocystography in the treatment of impalpable breast cysts. AJR 1992;158:1239.

9. Fornage BD. Percutaneous biopsies of the breast: state of the art. Cardiovasc Intervent Radiol 1991;14:29.

10. Sneige N, Fornage BD, Saleh G. Ultrasound-guided fine-needle aspiration of nonpalpable breast lesions: cytologic and histologic findings. Am J Clin Pathol 1994;102:98.

11. Lundy J, Lozowski M, Sadri D, et al. The use of fine-needle aspirates of breast cancers to evaluate hormone-receptor status. Arch Surg 1990;125:174.

12. Remvikos Y, Magdelenat H, Zajdela A. DNA flow cytometry applied to fine needle sampling of human breast cancer. Cancer 1988;61:1629.

13. Kline TS, Joshi LP, Neal HS. Fine-needle aspiration of the breast: diagnoses and pitfalls: a review of 3545 cases. Cancer 1979;44:1458.

14. Fischler DF, Sneige N, Ordonez NG, et al. Tubular carcinoma of the breast: cytologic features in fine-needle aspirations and application of monoclonal anti α-smooth muscle actin in diagnosis. Diagn Cytopathol 1994;10:120.

15. Peterse JL, Thunnissen FB, van Heerde P. Fine needle aspiration cytology of radiation-induced changes in nonneoplastic breast lesions: possible pitfalls in cytodiagnosis. Acta Cytol 1989;33:176.

16. Fornage BD. Ultrasound of the breast. Ultrasound Q 1993;11:1.

17. Fornage BF, Sneige N, Singletary SE. Masses in breasts with implants: diagnosis with US-guided fine-needle aspiration biopsy. Radiology 1994;191:339.

18. Schackmuth M, Harlow CL, Norton LW. Milk fistula: a complication after core breast biopsy. AJR 1993;161:961.

19. Harter LP, Swengros J, Ponto G, et al. Malignant seeding of the needle track during stereotaxic core needle breast biopsy. Radiology 1992;185:713.

20. Ciatto S, Catarzi S, Morrone D, et al. Fine-needle aspiration cytology of nonpalpable breast lesions: US versus stereotaxic guidance. Radiology 1993;188:195.

21. Fornage BD. A simple phantom for training in ultrasound-guided needle biopsy using the freehand technique. J Ultrasound Med 1989;8:701.

7

Diseases of the Breast, edited by Jay R. Harris,
Marc E. Lippman, Monica Morrow, and Samuel Hellman.
Lippincott-Raven Publishers, Philadelphia, © 1996.

Etiology and Pathogenesis of Breast Cancer

EPIDEMIOLOGIC FACTORS

7.1
Incidence, Demographics, and Environmental Factors

LOUISE A. BRINTON ▪ SUSAN S. DEVESA

Incidence, Mortality, and Survival

IMPACT IN THE UNITED STATES AND GENDER EFFECT

Breast cancer is the second most frequent cause of cancer death among American women, accounting for 18% of all cancer deaths among women and trailing only lung cancer.[1] Based on data from the National Cancer Institute's Surveillance, Epidemiology and End Results (SEER) program,[2] 32% of all incident cancers among women are breast cancer, the most frequently diagnosed cancer.[1] The American Cancer Society estimated that 182,000 cases and 46,000 deaths would occur among US women during 1994. Breast cancer is rare among men, with only 1000 cases and 300 deaths estimated for 1994 in the United States. Based on data from 1988 to 1990, the lifetime risk among US women of being diagnosed with breast cancer is 12.2%, or 1 in 8 women, and the lifetime risk of dying from breast cancer is 3.6%, or 1 in 28 women.[3]

INTERNATIONAL GEOGRAPHIC VARIATION

Internationally, mortality rates (per 100,000 woman-years, age-adjusted, world standard) varied five-fold during 1983 to 1987, from less than 6 in Japan to almost 30 in England and Wales.[4] Rates were also low (less than 15) in Mexico, Costa Rica, Chile, Hong Kong, and Singapore, around 20 in parts of Western Europe and the United States, and highest (more than 25) in the Netherlands, Denmark, Scotland, Ireland, and New Zealand. From the mid-1970s to the mid-1980s, mortality rates did not change greatly in many of the countries with high rates, whereas increases occurred in many of the countries with low rates, resulting in a narrowing of the international differences.

In contrast to mortality data that generally exist at the national level because death certificates are legal documents, incidence data from population-based cancer registries are not as widely available. Data from several dozen well-run registries around the world for 1983 to 1987 suggest that incidence rates (age-adjusted, world standard) varied four- to five-fold. Rates were lowest in parts of China, Japan, and India (less than 30), they were intermediate in South America, the Caribbean, and Eastern Europe, and they were highest in Western Europe, Canada, and North America (Fig. 7.1-1).[5] Geographic variation was apparent within many countries, but within-country differences were considerably smaller than those among countries. Rates in urban areas generally exceeded those in neighboring rural areas.[6]

MIGRANT STUDIES

Chinese women living in Shanghai had two thirds the risk of breast cancer compared with those in Hong Kong or Singapore, whereas the rates among Chinese women in California were more than twice as high (Table 7.1-1).[6] Similarly, Japanese women in Hawaii had rates double those in Japan. Within Israel, women born in Africa or Asia were at reduced risk compared with those born in Israel, Europe, or America. The risk of breast cancer among migrants approaches that of the native-born population and is affected by the time interval since migration; risk is further modified among subsequent generations.[7,8]

RACIAL AND ETHNIC GROUPS WITHIN THE UNITED STATES

Within the United States during 1978 to 1982, breast cancer incidence rates were highest among white women and Hawaiians (Table 7.1-2).[6] Rates among black women

TABLE 7.1-1
Variation in Breast Cancer Incidence Rates Among Women, 1978–1982

Group and Place	Rate* (%)
CHINESE	
Shanghai	19.1
Singapore	27.1
Hong Kong	28.7
Los Angeles	39.6
Bay Area	43.7
JAPANESE	
Osaka	19.7
Miyagi	22.0
Hawaii	50.1
ISRAELI	
Born Israel	70.2
Born Europe, America	69.8
Born Africa, Asia	62.8

* Per 100,000 woman-years, age-adjusted to the world standard.

(Muir C, Waterhouse J, Mack T, et al, eds. Cancer incidence in five continents, vol 5. IARC Scientific Publications no. 88. Lyon, IARC, 1987)

were lower. Rates among Asians and Hispanics were about half those of whites; American Indian women were at notably low risk.

GEOGRAPHIC VARIATION AMONG WHITES IN THE UNITED STATES

Considerable geographic variation in breast cancer mortality rates has been reported within the United States, with notably high rates in parts of the northeast and low rates across the south.[9] Figure 7.1-2 presents the ranked rates by state economic area for white women during 1970 to 1989. The age-adjusted (1970 US standard) rates varied more than two-fold, ranging from 15 to 34 per 100,000 woman-years; they were higher than 30 in urban areas of the northeast and midwest and 20 or lower across the south and mountain states. West of the Mississippi, only a few areas of Illinois, Wisconsin, and around San Francisco had rates in the top 10%. Reasons for these geographic variations are not well understood, but socioeconomic, reproductive, and perhaps dietary and environmental factors, to be discussed, may play a role. National data on survival rates among breast cancer patients are not available, but it is unlikely that geographic variations in survival greatly influence the mortality patterns.

AGE

The risk of breast cancer increases rapidly with age during childbearing years (Fig. 7.1-3). After menopause, rates continue to increase, but at a less rapid pace. Incidence

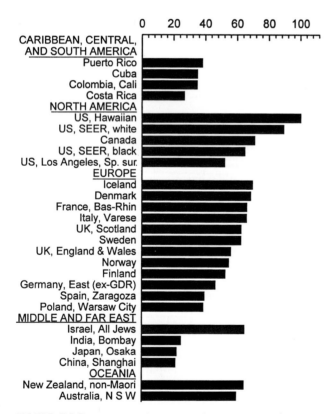

FIGURE 7.1-1 International variation in breast cancer incidence rates among women, 1983 to 1987, per 100,000 woman-years, age-adjusted to the world standard. (Parkin DM, Muir CS, Whelan SL, et al, eds. Cancer incidence in five continents, vol 6. IARC Scientific Publications no. 120. Lyon, IARC, 1992)

TABLE 7.1-2
Variation by Racial and Ethnic Group Within the United States in Breast Cancer Incidence Rates Among Women, 1978 to 1982*

	Bay Area	Detroit	Atlanta	Los Angeles	New Mexico	Hawaii
White	87.0	74.9	75.4	77.3	71.2	84.4
Black	66.4	63.4	56.6	59.1	NA	NA
Chinese	43.7	NA	NA	39.6	NA	57.5
Japanese	48.9	NA	NA	36.2	NA	50.1
Filipino	37.2	NA	NA	35.7	NA	32.0
Hispanic	NA	NA	NA	41.8	45.3	NA
American Indian	NA	NA	NA	NA	23.8	NA
Hawaiian	NA	NA	NA	NA	NA	93.9

NA, not available.

* Per 100,000 woman-years, age-adjusted to the world standard.

(Muir C, Waterhouse J, Mack T, et al, eds. Cancer incidence in five continents, vol 5. IARC Scientific Publications no. 88. Lyon, IARC, 1987)

rates were higher among blacks than whites during childbearing years, but substantial excesses among whites of up to 35% were apparent thereafter. Mortality rates also showed a crossover from an excess among blacks to whites, but at a later age—about 65 years for mortality compared with 45 years for incidence. Reasons for the crossover are not yet known.

TIME TRENDS

During the four decades from 1950 to 1989, age-adjusted breast cancer mortality rates among white women in the United States changed little, whereas rates increased among nonwhites, approaching those among whites in recent years.[10] During the past two decades, breast cancer mortality rates among blacks surpassed those among whites[11] (Fig. 7.1-4). In 1991, the rates were 32 and 27 per 100,000 woman-years among blacks and whites, respectively. Incidence rates during the past two decades generally have shown upward trends among both blacks and whites, with risk consistently about 20% higher among whites. The peaks during the early 1970s most likely were related to increased awareness and detection in response to the Breast Cancer Detection Demonstration Projects and to publicity surrounding the breast cancer diagnosis of several prominent women, whereas the steep increases during the 1980s may have been related to the increasing use of mammography.[12] Increases in mortality will lag behind those in incidence as the median survival time among women newly diagnosed with breast cancer is about 17 years.[11] Rising incidence has been more pronounced for estrogen receptor–positive tumors, particularly among older women.[13] Increases in breast cancer incidence and mortality have been noted internationally in many regions.[14]

The increases in invasive breast cancer incidence were

due largely to the diagnosis of localized cases, with rates increasing about 60% among both white and black women from 1975–1977 to 1988–1991 (Table 7.1-3). Rates for regional and distant disease did not change greatly. Although less frequently diagnosed than invasive disease, in situ carcinoma rates also rose rapidly. Increases in localized disease occurred among white women of all ages but were most pronounced among those aged 60 to 79 years. When the size of the tumor was considered, the diagnosis of cancers smaller than 2 cm rose much more rapidly than that of larger tumors.[12]

SURVIVAL

Five-year relative survival rates improved from 75% during the mid-1970s to 80% in the late 1980s among white women, but they changed little among black women, contributing to the observed incidence and mortality patterns.[11] Based on more than 50,000 cases diagnosed during 1983 to 1990,[11] 5-year relative survival rates for all breast cancer patients combined were 82% and 66% among white and black women, respectively (Table 7.1-4). More than half of breast cancers among white women were diagnosed at a localized stage, and slightly more than one third were diagnosed at a regional stage. The stage distribution among black women was not as favorable, with localized and regional stages each accounting for 40% to 45% of cases. Survival rates varied markedly by stage at diagnosis, being 86% or more for women with localized disease, in contrast to less than 20% among those with distant spread. The more favorable prognosis among whites compared to blacks persisted for patients within each stage category, perhaps because of differences in extent of disease within stage category or effectiveness of treatment.

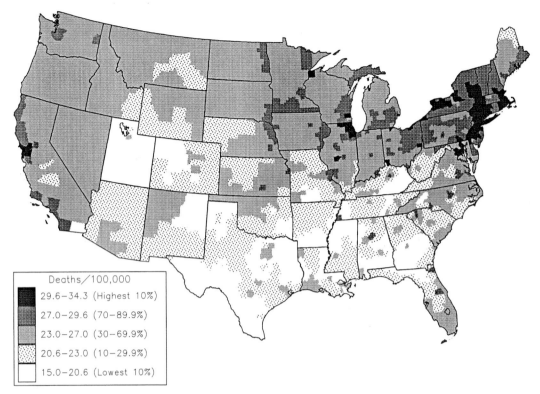

FIGURE 7.1-2 Breast cancer mortality rates among white women in the United States by state economic area, 1970 to 1989 (rates age adjusted using the 1970 US standard).

Risk Factors

DEMOGRAPHIC FACTORS

Breast cancer is generally recognized as a disease that occurs more often among women of the upper social classes, as measured by either educational status or family income.[15] Studies seem to indicate that these associations largely reflect the effect of correlated life-style factors, such as later ages at first birth.[16]

Never-married women over age 40 have been found to have a higher risk of breast cancer than women who have been married,[17] an association attributed to a reduced risk associated with childbearing. Similarly, nuns have been found to have a higher-than-average risk.[18]

There is common reference to the finding that Jewish women have high rates of breast cancer. The extent to which this association is due to the effects of correlated variables (eg, socioeconomic status) has not yet been adequately resolved.

FAMILIAL FACTORS

A family history of breast cancer in a first-degree relative is associated with approximately a doubling of risk.[19] If both the mother and a sister have had breast cancer, the risk is even higher. These familial effects are enhanced if the relative had either early-onset cancer or bilateral disease. In addition, familial effects predominate for early-onset cancers. The localization of a breast cancer gene to the q arm of chromosome 17 revolutionized research in this area.[20] The impact of identification of a breast cancer gene on prevention has yet to be determined, especially because only about 5% of all breast cancers are thought to result from a genetic predisposition.

REPRODUCTIVE RISK FACTORS

A late age at first birth is an important determinant of breast cancer risk. This was perhaps best demonstrated in MacMahon and colleagues' international study of breast cancer,[21] in which women with a first birth after age 30 years were shown to have approximately twice the risk of those with a first birth before age 18 years. Because nulliparous women have a risk similar to that of women with a first birth at around age 30 years, it is more hazardous to delay a first birth until after age 30 years than to remain childless. The protective effect of a pregnancy appears only after some delay, with a short-term increase in risk following delivery.[22] This transient adverse effect is greatest for women with later ages at first birth. Investigators have speculated that the short-term risk following delivery as well as the more adverse effect of a late pregnancy compared to nulliparity may result from a stimulation of cells that have already become initiated.

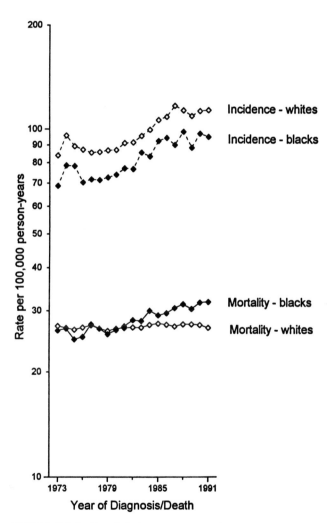

FIGURE 7.1-3 Age-specific breast cancer incidence (SEER program) and mortality (United States) curves by race, 1987 to 1991. (Ries LAG, Miller BA, Hankey BF, et al, eds. SEER Cancer Statistics Review, 1973–1991: tables and graphs. NIH publ no. 94-2789. Bethesda, USDHHS National Cancer Institute, 1994)

Although MacMahon and colleagues' study demonstrated that the relationship with number of births disappeared after adjustment for age at first birth, more recent studies suggest that there may indeed be an independent effect of parity for breast cancers detected after about ages 40 to 50 years. Before age 40 years, parity is associated with an increase rather than a decrease in risk,[17] presumably reflecting the influence of an adverse effect of a recent delivery. Limited evidence indicates that a late age at any birth and wide spacing of births are associated with some elevation in risk, but further clarification of these relationships is needed.

Several studies suggest that the protective effect of a pregnancy with later-onset breast cancers depends on the pregnancy's being full-term, with no protective effect exerted by shorter-term pregnancies.[23] In fact, several studies suggest that both induced abortions and miscarriages may have an adverse effect, although these relationships require further examination.[24] The effect on risk of a history of infertility also is in need of further evaluation. Of interest is not only how risk is influenced by the type of infertility (with a specific interest in certain types of hormonal deficiencies)[25] but also whether risk could be influenced by

ovulation-stimulating drugs.[26] Finally, of interest with respect to reproductive patterns is whether breastfeeding alters the subsequent risk of breast cancer. Several earlier studies dismissed this as an independent factor, but more recent investigations have shown that longer durations of breastfeeding may exert a protective effect.[27,28] Several of these studies suggest that the protective effect may be most profound for early-onset disease.

MENSTRUAL FACTORS

Numerous studies have shown that women with early onset of menarche are at an increased risk of breast cancer, and those who begin menstruating before age 12 years

FIGURE 7.1-4 Trends in breast cancer incidence (SEER program) and mortality rates among women in the United States by race, 1973 to 1991 (rates age adjusted using the 1970 US standard). (Ries LAG, Miller BA, Hankey BF, et al, eds. SEER Cancer Statistics Review, 1973–1991: tables and graphs. NIH publ no. 94-2789. Bethesda, USDHHS National Cancer Institute, 1994)

TABLE 7.1-3
Breast Cancer Incidence Trends by Race, Stage, and Age, SEER, 1975–1977 to 1989–1991

	Incidence		
	1975–1977	1989–1991	**Change**
WHITES BY STAGE			
In situ	4.5	16.4	11.9 (264.4%)
Invasive			
Total	87.4	111.9	24.5 (28.0%)
Localized	42.7	68.8	26.1 (61.1%)
Regional	34.0	33.5	−0.5 (−1.5%)
Distant	6.4	6.3	−0.1 (−1.6%)
Unstaged	4.3	3.4	−0.9 (−20.9%)
BLACKS BY STAGE			
In situ	2.9	12.5	9.6 (331.0%)
Invasive			
Total	73.5	93.7	20.2 (27.5%)
Localized	29.1	47.6	18.5 (63.6%)
Regional	32.3	32.4	0.1 (0.3%)
Distant	8.5	8.7	0.2 (2.4%)
Unstaged	3.6	4.9	1.3 (36.1%)
LOCALIZED STAGE AMONG WHITES BY AGE GROUP			
30–39 y	20.4	22.0	1.6 (7.8%)
40–49 y	73.3	95.3	22.0 (30.0%)
50–59 y	102.7	155.6	52.9 (51.5%)
60–69 y	130.3	246.9	116.6 (89.5%)
70–79 y	164.6	312.9	148.3 (90.1%)
≥80 y	171.5	286.8	115.3 (67.2%)

have approximately a 50% higher risk than those with menarche at age 15 years or later.[29] Some studies suggest that the effect may be greater for early-onset disease, but the extent to which this reflects better recall by younger women has yet to be resolved. Women who have an early age at menarche have an earlier onset of regular menstrual periods[30]; however, whether menstrual irregularities have an independent influence on breast cancer risk remains unresolved.

Women with late ages at menopause have been shown to be at an increased risk of breast cancer; the relative risk is approximately 2 for a natural menopause after age 55 years, compared with menopause before age 45 years.[29,31] Early menopause resulting from ovarian ablation is similarly associated with a reduction in risk. For instance, oophorectomy before age 40 years is associated with approximately a 50% reduction in risk, compared with natural menopause at age 50 years, the average age at menopause in the United States.[29] Some suggestion exists that bilateral oophorectomy at an early age exerts a stronger protective effect than natural menopause at the same age, possibly because of the more precipitous decline in hormones. Hysterectomy at an early age without ovarian ablation is not thought to alter risk further, but additional attention is warranted regarding the reasons for the hysterectomy, which could independently affect risk.

MEDICAL HISTORY

Although most studies indicate that women with a history of a biopsy resulting in a diagnosis of benign breast disease are at an increased risk of subsequent breast cancer, the interpretation of the association is complex. The association appears dependent not only on the indications for biopsy, but also on the histologic characteristics of the lesions. One study suggested that only proliferative forms of benign disease relate to subsequent breast cancer risk,[32] with atypical hyperplastic lesions being most predictive. The specific types of benign breast disease associated with the highest risk of subsequent breast cancer, however, have varied across studies,[33] possibly because of difficulties in standard classification of these lesions. Further examination of effects is needed, as well as evaluation of factors that might promote the progression of benign lesions to subsequent cancer.

The appearance of the breast mammographically has also been found to be a predictor of subsequent breast cancer risk. A parenchymal pattern classification system,

TABLE 7.1-4
Distribution of Breast Cancers and 5-Year Relative Survival Rates by Stage at Diagnosis Among White and Black Women, SEER, 1983 to 1990

	White	**Black**
Cases (*N*)	82,914	7,087
STAGE AT DIAGNOSIS (%)		
Total	100	100
Localized	56	45
Regional	34	40
Distant	6	10
Unstaged	4	5
5-YEAR RELATIVE SURVIVAL RATE (%)		
Total	81.6	65.8
Localized	95.0	86.0
Regional	74.8	59.5
Distant	19.0	13.2
Unstaged	53.9	41.5

(Ries LAG, Miller BA, Hankey BF, et al, eds. SEER cancer statistics review, 1973–1991: tables and graphs. National Institutes of Health publ no. 94–2789. Bethesda, MD, USDHHS National Cancer Institute, 1994)

which takes into account the amount of the breast composed of ductal prominence, was initially proposed,[34] but more recently, direct measurement of dense areas of the breast has been found to be a less subjective and stronger indicator of risk. In a recent study,[35] breasts with areas of density of 65% or more were associated with over a fourfold elevation in risk, a magnitude of risk as great if not greater than most other established risk factors.

Although other medical conditions have been suggested to relate to elevated breast cancer risks, inconsistencies prevail. Among those that have received the most attention are thyroid diseases, hypertension, and diabetes. Questions remain whether any observed elevations in risk associated with these conditions merely reflect the influence of correlated factors (eg, weight) or of prescribed medications (eg, rauwolfia derivatives). Of particular interest with respect to breast cancer risk has been the relationship with exogenous hormones (oral contraceptives and menopausal estrogens), a topic explored in Chapter 7.3.

Because silicone breast implants reportedly interfere with the detection of breast lesions, there has been interest in evaluating their relationship to subsequent breast cancer risk. Two investigations noted no elevations in risk,[36,37] but the absence of detailed information on patient characteristics limits interpretation of the findings.

MULTIPLE PRIMARY CANCERS

Cancer in one breast is associated with a relative risk of 2 to 4 for developing a second cancer in the contralateral breast, particularly in women with a family history of breast cancer.[38] Women with breast cancer also experience some increase in the risk of second cancers of the endometrium and ovary, and also possibly of melanoma and of colon, salivary gland, and thyroid cancers.[39] These associations may be due to shared risk factors.

PHYSICAL ACTIVITY

Despite the interest in the influence of both body size and dietary factors on breast cancer risk (topics explored in detail in Chapters 7.3 and 7.4), little attention has focused on the role of physical activity. One study found substantial reductions in risk of early-onset breast cancer associated with regular physical activity, an effect that appeared independent of body size.[40] Although the relationship is biologically plausible, given that physical activity can modify menstrual cycle patterns and alter the production of ovarian hormones, several studies have failed to support an effect on breast cancer risk of physical activity,[41,42] necessitating further confirmatory studies.

CIGARETTE SMOKING

Although cigarette smoking has been found to result in earlier ages at menopause, it has not generally been found to alter breast cancer risk.[43] However, investigators continue to be interested in the effects of smoking at young ages, hypothesized as a possible etiologic factor.

HAIR DYES

Reports of mutagenic effects of hair dyes have raised concern about their potential effect on breast cancer risk, but most studies that have examined the association have found no link.[41-46] Occupational exposures to hair dyes have also been examined in several small studies, with no consistent associations observed.[45]

PRENATAL EXPOSURES

Recent interest has focused on the role of a variety of prenatal exposures on subsequent breast cancer risk. Some evidence suggests an increased breast cancer risk to daughters born of mothers of advanced ages,[47,48] although data are not conclusive.[49] In addition, several studies have suggested that being a firstborn or of higher birthweight may confer an increased risk, although contradictions prevail.[50] Further, some evidence exists that dizygotic twins have elevated rates of breast cancer.[51] On the other hand, maternal preeclampsia during pregnancy has been associated with a decreased breast cancer risk in daughters.[52] These birth characteristics have been hypothesized to reflect effects of prenatal estrogenic exposures. One report showed a decreased breast cancer risk for daughters who were breastfed.[53] Whether this association reflects a protective effect of breastfeeding or of an adverse effect of supplements has yet to be determined.

IONIZING, ELECTROMAGNETIC, AND SOLAR RADIATION

From studies of women exposed to the atomic bombs in Japan and from observations of women exposed to medical treatments involving repeated exposure to radiation (eg, fluoroscopic chest radiography for tuberculosis and radiotherapy for acute postpartum mastitis, ankylosing spondylitis, scoliosis, or tinea capitis), it is well established that ionizing radiation to the chest in moderate to high doses (eg, between 1 and 3 Gy) before the age of 40 years increases breast cancer risk, and the higher the dose the greater the risk.[54] High rates of breast cancer have also been observed following radiotherapy for Hodgkin disease.[55] Further, second breast cancers have been linked to radiotherapy for primary breast cancer, but only among women under age 45 years at exposure.[56] Relatively few data are available regarding the effects of low radiation doses from medical or diagnostic exposures. An increase in breast cancer risk has been reported for radium dial painters,[57] exposed to a weekly dose of 0.001 to 0.004 Gy, and for medical diagnostic radiology workers.[58] Common diagnostic procedures, such as chest radiography and mammography, have a mean radiation dose to breast tissue of 0.0002 and 0.00015 Gy, respectively.[59] Less than 1% of breast cancer is estimated to result from general diagnostic radiographic procedures.[60] Because most women receive mammograms after age 40 years, when breast cancer risk associated with radiation appears small, the benefits of mammography are believed to far outweigh any potential risks.

The finding that male electrical line workers have an elevated breast cancer risk[61] has prompted interest in the etiologic role of electromagnetic fields for female breast cancer. One study of female electrical workers provided some support for the relationship,[62] but further confirmatory work is needed. Exposure to electric blankets has also been of interest, but a study of postmenopausal women showed no association.[63] Because both long-term exposure to 50- to 60-Hz electric fields and uninterrupted light reduce pineal production of melatonin, which can lead to increased production of estrogen and prolactin,[64] some interest has also been expressed in the role of light exposure to risk. One study found that women with profound bilateral blindness had half the risk of breast cancer of sighted women.[65]

The recognition of a distinct north–south gradient in breast cancer mortality rates and a correlation between these rates and solar radiation has led to the hypothesis that vitamin D or its metabolites might reduce breast cancer risk.[66] Analytic studies have yet to be reported.

OCCUPATIONAL EXPOSURES

The role of occupational exposures in women has only recently become of interest. Several studies have shown high rates of breast cancer in school teachers and nurses, probably owing to their higher socioeconomic status or unique reproductive histories. A recent conference on occupational risks among women suggested possible breast cancer links with employment in the printing and publishing, telephone, and electrical equipment manufacturing industries.[67]

ENVIRONMENTAL EXPOSURES

Recent attention has focused on the potential impact of environmental factors on breast cancer risk, with much of the interest stemming from the recognition of high breast cancer mortality rates in the industrialized northeastern United States. Of particular interest had been the relation of risk to organochlorine pesticides, notably DDT (2,2-bis(p-chlorophenyl)-1,1,1-trichloroethane) and polychlorinated biphenyls (PCBs), which have been demonstrated to induce cytochrome P-450 enzymes and to affect steroid metabolism, including the 2/16-hydroxylase pathway. Although one case control study noted significantly higher serum levels of dichlorodiphenyldichloroethylene (DDE) in breast cancer cases than in controls,[68] another study, which examined breast cancer risk using prediagnostic serum samples, found no consistent elevations in risk associated with either DDE or PCB levels.[69] Nonetheless, the relation of organochlorines with breast cancer risk remains of major interest, especially in view of the potential for these substances to interact with environmental phytoestrogens or other xenoestrogens. To understand reasons for the geographic variation in breast cancer rates, studies are also examining the relationship of risk with other environmental agents, including water contaminants, air pollution, toxic waste dumps, and other chemical exposures.

Summary

Table 7.1-5 summarizes the established and speculative risk factors for breast cancer and the magnitude of risks associated with these factors. Although breast cancer has

TABLE 7.1-5
Summary of Environmental Risk Factors for Breast Cancer*

Factors Influencing Risk	Estimated Relative Risk
ESTABLISHED RISK FACTORS	
Older ages (65–69 versus 30–34 y)	17
Residency in North America or Europe versus Asia	4–5
Residency in urban areas	1.5
Higher educational status or family income	1.5
Mother or sister with breast cancer	2–3
Nulliparity or late ages at first birth ($\geq$30 versus <20 y)	2–3
Absence of breastfeeding for long durations	1.5
Early ages at menarche (<12 versus $\geq$15 y)	1.5
Late ages at menopause ($\geq$55 versus natural menopause at <45 y or removal of ovaries at a comparable age)	2
Biopsy-confirmed proliferative breast disease	2–4
Mammographically dense breasts	2–4
Obesity (postmenopausal only) ($\geq$200 versus <125 lb)	2
Tallness ($\geq$68 versus <62 inches)	1.5–2
Radiation to chest in moderate to high doses	2–4
History of breast cancer in one breast	2–4
History of primary cancer in endometrium, ovary	1.5–2
SPECULATIVE RISK FACTORS	
Induced abortions or miscarriages	?
Infertility and associated treatment	?
Prenatal conditions involving high in utero estrogen levels	?
Postnatal exposures (breastfeeding)	?
Electromagnetic fields	?
Excessive light exposure	?
Restricted solar or vitamin D exposure	?
Organochlorines	?

* Exclusive of hormonal or dietary factors, which are discussed in Chapters 7.3 and 7.4.

been one of the most intensively studied cancers epidemiologically, much remains to be known about the disease. Despite the large number of identified risk factors, only about 55% of the cases of disease are explained by these factors.[70] This undoubtedly relates to our poor understanding of the biologic mechanisms underlying most of these factors. For instance, we have known for nearly three decades that a late age at first birth increases the risk of breast cancer, but whether this increase is due to changes in endogenous hormones, tissue changes, or some other factor has yet to be determined. Fortunately, more epidemiologic studies are integrating the evaluation of risk factors with biochemical markers, and they should assist in our understanding of biologic mechanisms. One hopes that this knowledge will eventually lead to a greater understanding of reasons for the occurrence of the disease of recent major epidemic proportions, and to more effective preventive interventions.

ACKNOWLEDGMENTS

The authors gratefully acknowledge Dan Grauman of the National Cancer Institute and Joan Hertel and Stella Semiti of IMS, Inc., for data development and figure generation.

References

1. Boring CC, Squires TS, Tong T, et al. Cancer statistics, 1994. CA Cancer J Clin 1994;44:7.
2. Miller BA, Ries LAG, Hankey BF, et al, eds. SEER Cancer Statistics Review 1973–1990: NIH publ no. 93–2789. Bethesda, USDHHS National Cancer Institute, 1993.
3. Hankey BF, Brinton LA, Kessler LF, et al. Breast. In: Miller BA, Ries LAG, Hankey BF, et al, eds. SEER Cancer Statistics Review 1973–1990. NIH publ no. 93–2789. Bethesda, USDHHS National Cancer Institute, 1993:1.
4. Aoki K, Kurihara M, Hayakawa N, et al, eds. Death rates for malignant neoplasms for selected sites by sex and five-year age group in 33 countries, 1953–57 to 1983–87. Nagoya, University of Nagoya, 1992.
5. Parkin DM, Muir CS, Whelan SL, et al, eds. Cancer incidence in five continents, vol 6. IARC scientific publ no. 120. Lyon, IARC, 1992.
6. Muir C, Waterhouse J, Mack T, et al, eds. Cancer incidence in five continents, vol 5. IARC scientific publ no. 88. Lyon, IARC, 1987.
7. Goodman MJ. Breast cancer in multi-ethnic populations: the Hawaii perspective. Breast Cancer Res Treat 1991;18:S5.
8. Ziegler RG, Hoover RN, Pike MC, et al. Migration patterns and breast cancer risk in Asian–American women. J Natl Cancer Inst 1993;85:1819.
9. Pickle LW, Mason TJ, Howard N, et al. Atlas of US cancer mortality among whites, 1950–1980: DHHS Publ No (NIH) 87-2900. Washington, US Govt Printing Office, 1987.
10. Devesa SS. Cancer patterns among women in the United States. Semin Oncol Nurs 1995;11:78.
11. Ries LAG, Miller BA, Hankey BF, et al, eds. SEER Cancer Statistics Review, 1973–1991: tables and graphs. NIH publ no. 94-2789. Bethesda, USDHHS National Cancer Institute, 1994.
12. Miller BA, Feuer EJ, Hankey BF: Recent incidence trends for breast cancer in women and the relevance of early detection: an update. CA Cancer J Clin 1993;43:27.
13. Glass AG, Hoover RN. Rising incidence of breast cancer: relationship to stage and receptor status. J Natl Cancer Inst 1990;82:693.
14. Coleman MP, Esteve J, Damiecki P, et al. Trends in cancer incidence and mortality. IARC scientific publ no. 121. Lyon, IARC, 1993.
15. Krieger N. Social class and the black/white cross-over in the age-specific incidence of breast cancer: a study linking census-derived data to population-based registry records. Am J Epidemiol 1990;131:804.
16. Jacobsen BK, Lund E. Level of education, use of oral contraceptives and reproductive factors: the Tromso Study. Int J Epidemiol 1990;19:967.
17. Janerich DT, Hoff MB. Evidence for a crossover in breast cancer risk factors. Am J Epidemiol 1982;116:737.
18. Fraumeni JF Jr, Lloyd JW, Smith EM, et al. Cancer mortality among nuns: role of marital status in etiology of neoplastic disease in women. J Natl Cancer Inst 1969;42:455.
19. Claus EB, Risch NJ, Thompson WD. Age at onset as an indicator of a familial risk of breast cancer. Am J Epidemiol 1990;131:961.
20. Friedman LS, Lynch ED, King MC. Two independent polymorphisms at the 17 beta-hydroxysteroid dehydrogenase (EDH17B) gene (17a21). Hum Mol Genet 1993;2:821.
21. MacMahon B, Cole P, Lin TM, et al. Age at first birth and breast cancer risk. Bull WHO 1970;43:209.
22. Lambe M, Hsieh C-C, Trichopoulos D, et al. Transient increase in the risk of breast cancer after giving birth. N Engl J Med 1994;331:5.
23. Brinton LA, Hoover R, Fraumeni JF Jr. Reproductive factors in the aetiology of breast cancer. Br J Cancer 1982;47:757.
24. Parazzini F, La Vecchia C, Negri E. Spontaneous and induced abortions and risk of breast cancer. Int J Cancer 1991;48:816.
25. Cowan LD, Gordis L, Tonascia JA, et al. Breast cancer incidence in women with a history of progesterone deficiency. Am J Epidemiol 1981;114:209.
26. Brzezinski A, Peretz T, Mor-Yosef S, et al. Ovarian stimulation and breast cancer: is there a link? Gynecol Oncol 1994;52:292.
27. Byers T, Graham S, Rzepka T, et al. Lactation and breast cancer: evidence for a negative association in premenopausal women. Am J Epidemiol 1985;121:664.
28. Newcomb PA, Storer BE, Longnecker MP, et al. Lactation and a reduced risk of premenopausal breast cancer. N Engl J Med 1994;330:81.
29. Brinton LA, Schairer CS, Hoover RN, et al. Menstrual factors and risk of breast cancer. Cancer Invest 1988;6:245.
30. Apter D, Vihko R. Early menarche, a risk factor for breast cancer, indicates early onset of ovulatory cycles. J Clin Endocrinol Metab 1983;57:82.
31. Trichopoulos D, MacMahon B, Cole P. Menopause and breast cancer risk. J Natl Cancer Inst 1972;48:605.
32. Dupont WD, Page DL. Risk factors for breast cancer in women with proliferative breast disease. N Engl J Med 1985;312:146.
33. Krieger N, Hiatt RA. Risk of breast cancer after benign breast diseases: variation by histologic type, degree of atypia, age at biopsy, and length of follow-up. Am J Epidemiol 1992;135:619.
34. Wolfe JN, Saftlas AF, Salane M. Mammographic parenchymal patterns and a quantitative evaluation of mammographic densities: a case-control study. AJR 1987;148:1087.
35. Saftlas AF, Hoover RN, Brinton LA, et al. Mammographic densities and risk of breast cancer. Cancer 1991;67:2833.
36. Berkel H, Birdsell DC, Jenkins H. Breast augmentation: a risk factor for breast cancer? N Engl J Med 1992;326:1649.
37. Deapen DM, Brody GS. Augmentation mammoplasty and breast cancer: a five year update of the Los Angeles study. Plast Reconstr Surg 1992;89:660.

38. Bernstein JL, Thompson WD, Risch N, et al. The genetic epidemiology of second primary breast cancer. Am J Epidemiol 1992;136:937.

39. Boice JD Jr, Storm HH, Curtis RE, et al, eds. Multiple primary cancers in Connecticut and Denmark. National Cancer Institute Monograph no 68: NIH publ no. 85-2714. Bethesda, National Cancer Institute, 1985.

40. Bernstein L, Henderson BE, Hanisch R, et al. Physical exercise and reduced risk of breast cancer in young women. J Natl Cancer Inst 1994;86:1402.

41. Dorgan JF, Brown C, Barrett M, et al. Physical activity and risk of breast cancer in the Framingham heart study. Am J Epidemiol 1994;139:662.

42. Paffenbarger RS Jr, Hyde RT, Wing AL. Physical activity and incidence of cancer in diverse populations: a preliminary report. Am J Clin Nutr 1987;45:312.

43. Palmer JR, Rosenberg L. Cigarette smoking and the risk of breast cancer. Epidemiol Rev 1993;15:145.

44. Green A, Willett WC, Colditz GA, et al. Use of permanent hair dyes and risk of breast cancer. J Natl Cancer Inst 1987;79:253.

45. Koenig KL, Pasternack BS, Shore RE, et al. Hair dye use and breast cancer: a case-control study among screening participants. Am J Epidemiol 1991;133:985.

46. Nasca PC, Baptiste MS, Field NA, et al. An epidemiologic case-control study of breast cancer and exposure to hair dyes. Ann Epidemiol 1992;2:577.

47. Janerich DT, Hayden CL, Thompson WD, et al. Epidemiologic evidence of perinatal influence in the etiology of adult cancers. J Clin Epidemiol 1989;42:151.

48. Thompson WD, Janerich DT. Maternal age at birth and risk of breast cancer in daughters. Epidemiology 1990;1:101.

49. Colditz GA, Willett WC, Stampfer MJ, et al. Parental age at birth and risk of breast cancer in daughters: a prospective study among US women. Cancer Causes Control 1991;2:31.

50. Gammon MD, John EM. Recent etiologic hypotheses concerning breast cancer. Epidemiol Rev 1993;15:163.

51. Hsieh C-C, Lan S-J, Ekbom A, et al. Twin membership and breast cancer risk. Am J Epidemiol 1992;136:1321.

52. Ekbom A, Trichopoulos D, Adami HO, et al. Evidence of prenatal influences on breast cancer risk. Lancet 1992;340:1015.

53. Freudenheim JL, Marshall JR, Graham S, et al. Exposure to breast milk in infancy and the risk of breast cancer. Epidemiology 1994;5:324.

54. John EM, Kelsey J. Radiation and other environmental exposures and breast cancer. Epidemiol Rev 1993;15:157.

55. Hancock SL, Tucker MA, Hoppe RT. Breast cancer after treatment of Hodgkin's disease. J Natl Cancer Inst 1993;85:25.

56. Boice JD Jr, Harvey E, Blettner M, et al. Cancer in the contralateral breast after radiotherapy for breast cancer. N Engl J Med 1992;326:781.

57. Stebbings JH, Lucas HF, Stehney AF. Mortality from cancer of major sites in female radium dial workers. Am J Ind Med 1984;5:435.

58. Wang J-X, Inskip PD, Boice JD Jr, et al. Cancer incidence among medical diagnostic x-ray workers in China, 1950 to 1985. Int J Cancer 1990;45:889.

59. Miller AB, Howe GR, Sherman GJ, et al. Mortality from breast cancer after irradiation during fluoroscopic examinations in patients being treated for tuberculosis. N Engl J Med 1989;321:1285.

60. Evans JS, Wennberg JE, McNeil BJ. The influence of diagnostic radiography on the incidence of breast cancer and leukemia. N Engl J Med 1986;315:810.

61. Demers PA, Thomas DB, Rosenblatt, et al. Occupational exposure to electromagnetic fields and breast cancer in men. Am J Epidemiol 1991;134:340.

62. Loomis DP, Savitz DA, Ananth CV. Breast cancer mortality among female electrical workers in the United States. J Natl Cancer Inst 1994;86:921.

63. Vena JE, Graham S, Hellmann R, et al. Use of electric blankets and risk of postmenopausal breast cancer. Am J Epidemiol 1991;134:180.

64. Stevens RG. Electric power use and breast cancer: a hypothesis. Am J Epidemiol 1987;125:556.

65. Hahn RA. Profound bilateral blindness and the incidence of breast cancer. Epidemiology 1991;2:208.

66. Garland FC, Garland CF, Gorham ED, et al. Geographic variation in breast cancer mortality in the United States: a hypothesis involving exposure to solar radiation. Prevent Med 1990;19:614.

67. Pottern LM, Zahm SH, Sieber SS, et al. Occupational cancer among women: a conference overview. J Occup Med 1994;36:809.

68. Wolff MS, Toniolo PG, Lee EW, et al. Blood levels of organochlorine residues and risk of breast cancer. J Natl Cancer Inst 1993;85:648.

69. Krieger N, Wolff MS, Hiatt RA, Breast cancer and serum organochlorines: a prospective study among white, black, and Asian women. J Natl Cancer Inst 1994;86:589.

70. Bruzzi P, Green SB, Byar DP, et al. Estimating the population attributable risk for multiple risk factors using case-control data. Am J Epidemiol 1985;122:904.

7.2
Familial Breast Cancer

BARBARA L. WEBER ▪ JUDY E. GARBER

Familial clustering of breast cancer was first described by physicians in ancient Rome.[1] The first documentation of familial clustering of breast cancer in modern times was published in 1866 by a French surgeon who reported 10 cases of breast cancer in 4 generations of his wife's family; 4 other women in this family died as a result of hepatic tumors.[2] Given the strong influence of molecular genetics in medicine in recent years, a tendency exists to assume that familial clustering of disease results from genetically inherited predisposition. Other explanations for familial clustering of breast cancer are possible, however, and include the following: (1) geographically limited environmental exposure to carcinogens that might affect an extended family living in close proximity; (2) culturally motivated behavior that alters risk-factor profile, such as age at first live birth; and (3) socioeconomic influences that, for example, might result in differing dietary exposures. In addition, multiple complex inherited genetic factors likely influence the extent to which a risk factor for breast cancer plays a role in any one individual; such modifying effects are likely to be shared among genetically similar members of an extended family. Although noninherited factors certainly play a role in familial clustering of breast cancer, recent advances have provided unequivocal evidence for the presence of breast cancer susceptibility genes responsible for 5% to 10% of all breast cancer. Yet much remains to be understood about the number of heritable factors, the function of such genes that, when functioning normally, appear to prevent the development of breast cancer, and the prevalence of such genetic mutations within various populations.

Inherited breast cancer has several distinctive clinical features—age of onset is considerably younger than in sporadic cases, the prevalence of bilateral breast cancer is higher, and the presence of associated tumors in affected individuals is noted in some families. Associated tumors may include ovarian, colon, prostate and endometrial cancers and sarcomas.[3,4] Inherited breast cancer does not appear to be distinguished by histologic type, morphologic grade, metastatic pattern, or survival characteristics, however. Although much has been learned about inherited breast cancer in the last 5 years, much more will be elucidated by ongoing and future work based on the foundation of epidemiologic and genetic data described in this chapter.

Epidemiologic Studies

The first attempts to determine the influence of family history on breast cancer risk were published in the first half of this century.[5-7] In general, these studies were performed by comparing breast cancer incidence in relatives of breast cancer patients with healthy controls. Familial clustering was noted in these early studies; however, these studies were often flawed by unverified diagnoses, lack of rigorously defined control groups, and the absence of adjustments for family size. In addition, these studies did not take into consideration the age of onset of breast cancer or the presence of other cancers in the family. These studies were followed by investigations in which control groups were more carefully defined or studies that used the general population from which families were derived as control subjects.[8-17] Although many of these studies also had methodologic flaws, they consistently demonstrated a two- to three-fold increase in breast cancer risk in mothers and sisters of breast cancer patients, figures compatible with current studies.[18-20] As noted previously, however, inherited susceptibility is only one of several possible explanations for familial clustering of disease. Breast cancer risk factors, other than family history, conferring a two- to three-fold increased risk include higher socioeconomic class, geographic country at birth, age at first term pregnancy, radiation exposure to chest, and alcohol intake.[18,21] Thus, an increase in risk of this magnitude does not exclude nongenetic causes for increased breast cancer risk in first-degree relatives of breast cancer patients.

Using modern epidemiologic methodology, several population-based studies have attempted to estimate breast cancer risk associated with a positive family history. The largest of these was a study conducted in Sweden[22] involv-ing 1330 women with a confirmed diagnosis of breast cancer in a defined geographic region and 1330 age-matched controls without a previous diagnosis of breast cancer. Data were obtained by mailed questionnaires. Within this study cohort, breast cancer in a first-degree relative was reported in 11.2% of breast cancer patients, as opposed to 6.7% of controls ($P < .01$), yielding a standardized relative risk (RR) of 1.7. When this observation was extended to include breast cancer in first- or second-degree relatives, the findings remained significant, with 19.8% of breast cancer patients and 12.9% of control women reporting an affected relative, yielding a standardized RR of 1.6. Although both previous and subsequent studies have reported an increased incidence of bilateral disease and a younger age of onset in patients with a family history of breast cancer,[23-28] these associations were not significant in this study. RRs of a similar magnitude were found in a Canadian population-based study[29] and the US Nurses' Health Study,[30] a large, retrospective case control study. Higher risks were reported in the Breast Cancer Detection Demonstration Project[31] and the American Cancer Society cohort.[32] These cohorts, although large, were composed of volunteers, so they may be biased.

Population-based studies have the advantage of avoiding selection bias in studying the contribution of risk factors to the occurrence of a specific disease; however, such an approach may dilute the effect of a strong association in a small subset of the study population. This was first demonstrated with regard to breast cancer by Anderson.[23] Anderson and others suggested that breast cancer was not a homogeneous disease, and as such, the occurrence of breast cancer was not influenced by genetic factors in a uniform manner. In such a setting, a small subset of families with a high risk of developing breast cancer as the result of genetic defects inherited in classic mendelian fashion might be obscured in large studies in which most breast cancer cases were multifactorial in origin. Anderson therefore assembled a data base enriched for kindreds with a family history of breast cancer, to emphasize the hereditary component if one were present.[33-37] Pedigrees were ascertained through breast cancer patients (primary probands) seen at the M.D. Anderson Cancer Center whose medical record indicated a diagnosis of breast cancer in at least one first- or second-degree relative. The original controls for studies based on these data were patients from the same institution with basal cell carcinoma, melanoma, or colon cancer who had a family history of malignant disease other than breast cancer. These studies were the first to demonstrate the heterogeneity of risk among breast cancer families. The primary factors that increased risk within families were premenopausal status at time of diagnosis and bilateral disease in the primary proband. Additionally, first-degree relatives of primary probands were found to be at higher risk than second-degree relatives. Data from these studies[33-39] are summarized in Table 7.2-1.

Calculation of risk in first-degree relative pairs (mother–daughter or sister–sister) derived from these observations yielded estimates of a 50% lifetime breast cancer risk in the presence of both premenopausal diagnosis and bilateral disease. This finding contrasts sharply with the

TABLE 7.2-1
Relative Risks for First–Degree Relatives of Women With Breast Cancer

Characteristics of Affected Mother or Sister	Relative Risk
Premenopausal diagnosis	3.0
Bilateral disease	5.0
Bilateral disease and premenopausal diagnosis	9.0
Postmenopausal diagnosis	1.5

(Data from Anderson DE. Genetic study of breast cancer: identification of a high risk group. Cancer 1974;34:1090; and Anderson DE, Badzioch MD. Risk of familial breast cancer. Cancer 1985;56:383)

7% calculated risk of breast cancer in first-degree relatives of women with postmenopausal diagnosis and unilateral disease,[24] a risk that does not differ significantly from the general population risk. These studies were confirmed by Ottman and colleagues, who reported an RR of 5 for sisters of patients with bilateral breast cancer diagnosed before age 50 years, an RR of 10.5 for sisters of patients with bilateral breast cancer diagnosed before age 40 years, and an RR of 2.5 for sisters of patients with unilateral breast cancer diagnosed before age 40 years.[40]

By 1980, a significant body of evidence supporting the presence of inherited factors responsible for familial clustering of breast cancer had accumulated, and efforts shifted to attempt to determine the inheritance pattern of breast cancer within these families. In 1984, Williams and Anderson[41] examined 200 Danish pedigrees obtained by contacting more than 300 breast cancer patients entered into the Danish Cancer Registry, a population-based registry based in Copenhagen. Ninety-five percent of cancer cases were confirmed. The Danish study provided evidence for an autosomal dominant breast cancer susceptibility gene with an age-related penetrance. This study was supported in 1988 by King and colleagues,[42] who studied 1579 nuclear families of breast cancer probands diagnosed before age 55 years. Again, all patterns of inheritance, with the exception of a highly penetrant susceptibility gene transmitted as an autosomal dominant trait, were excluded by this analysis. This hypothesis was proved correct in 1990 with the description of two such genes, BRCA1 and p53.[43–45]

NONWHITE POPULATIONS

Even though we are beginning to understand the influence of genetic factors on the incidence of breast cancer in largely white, Western populations of women, little is known about breast cancer risk attributable to inherited factors in other populations. The data in the medical literature consist of a small number of case control studies and case reports.

The few studies that have examined breast cancer risk

in African American women have concluded that a family history of breast cancer confers a magnitude of increased risk similar to that seen in white population-based studies.[46–48] Unfortunately, few African American families in which breast cancer fits an autosomal dominant pattern of inheritance have been described in the literature.[49,50] This could reflect a low prevalence of breast cancer–related inherited mutations in African Americans, but it is equally likely to be due to selection or referral biases.

Information on breast cancer incidence and family history collected on a large population of Hispanic women living in Laredo, Texas, from 1870 to 1981 suggest that familial clustering of breast cancer also appears in this population.[51] This study identified 13 families (of 11,740 genealogies) of which two or more members were reported to have died of breast cancer. This study used civil and church birth, marriage, and death records to reconstruct pedigrees and disease patterns within families, however. This approach allows for a significant margin of error, predominantly from underreporting of cases, particularly nonfatal cases or cases in which breast cancer is not recorded as the cause of death, and undocumented family relationships.

A single study of family history of Japanese women living in Japan has been reported in the English medical literature;[52] this study was a hospital-based case-control study incorporating 908 women with breast cancer. Controls were selected by identifying age-matched women seen at the same hospital within the preceding 3 years: 13.5% of patients reported at least one relative with breast cancer, as compared with 9% of controls; 1.5% of patients versus 0.9% of controls reported two or more relatives affected with breast cancer, less than is generally reported in Western studies.[18,19] The RR of developing breast cancer in women with two or more affected relatives was 2, comparable to studies involving primarily white women. Finally, a single study of breast cancer in Arab women included 73 breast cancer cases identified at a single hospital in Israel and found 15 patients (20%) who reported at least 1 affected family member.[53]

These studies provide only the most rudimentary look at genetic factors predisposing to breast cancer in nonwhite populations of women. These studies suggest that all populations of women may contain a subset of families with increased risk of developing breast cancer, but the amount of attributable risk, the spectrum of genetic mutations represented, and the ability of these genetic mutations to exert an effect remain unknown outside the largely white populations studied to date. The studies described here are subject to significant errors and, in addition, may suffer from cultural differences in the acceptability of discussing cancer and genetics. One hopes that the identification of breast cancer susceptibility genes and the ability to identify tumor-related gene mutations in archived specimens will provide a much more accurate look at the incidence of inherited breast cancer and the factors that modify the development of breast cancer in women of differing genetic heritage.

HOW MUCH BREAST CANCER IS INHERITED?

Given the overwhelming evidence that at least a small portion of breast cancer is inherited, recent studies have focused on determining the frequency of breast cancer–

related gene mutations in the general population and thus the percentage of breast cancer in the general population that is directly attributable to inherited genetic factors.[19,20,54] Unfortunately, available data addressing this question are limited. Among 225 consecutive breast cancer patients seen at the Creighton University Oncology Clinic, 5% had family histories considered consistent with hereditary forms of breast cancer.[55] This percentage increased to 11.4% with a strong family history among women diagnosed before age 50 years. Because of the recognized interest of these investigators in familial cancers, concern has been raised that this selected patient population is enriched for patients with a family history of breast cancer and may not have been representative of the population as a whole. Several subsequent studies have reported similar findings, however.

Two groups analyzed data from the Cancer and Steroid Hormone (CASH) Study,[18,54] a large, case-control study initiated in 1981 by the US Centers for Disease Control. This data set contains information on 4730 histologically confirmed breast cancer patients between the ages of 20 and 54 years from 8 geographic regions of the United States and 4688 age-matched controls from the same geographic regions. Family history information was obtained by personal interview. In this study group, 11% of breast cancer patients reported a first-degree relative with breast cancer, compared with 5% of controls.[18] Less than 1% of patients had both a mother and sister with breast cancer. Recognizing that some of these kindreds are likely to represent chance clustering of sporadic tumors, analysis of the CASH data set provides evidence for the existence of breast cancer–related gene mutations in approximately 0.33% of the population.[54] The effect of these mutations on breast cancer risk is a function of age; Claus and colleagues[54] estimated that 36% of breast cancer cases among women ages 20 to 29 years may be attributed to an autosomal dominant susceptibility gene (two of which have now been identified, with others sure to follow), with the attributable proportion of breast cancer decreasing to 1% by age 80 years. Caution must be exercised when considering the CASH data, which derive from predominantly early-onset breast cancer and are therefore enriched for families in which inherited factors are likely to play a role in the development of breast cancer.

In 1993, two additional studies attempting to calculate risk attributable to autosomal dominant breast cancer susceptibility genes were published. Colditz and associates[19] analyzed data from the Nurses' Health Study and suggested that 6% of all breast cancer occurred as a result of inherited genetic factors, and Slattery and Kerber[20] provided an estimate of 17% to 19% based on the Utah Population Data Base. Several explanations for the discrepancies have been noted;[56] these include the unique composition and large size of the families in the Utah data base and the small family size and absence of paternal data in the Nurses' Health Study cohort. It appears likely that the Nurses' Health Study data represent an underestimate, whereas the Utah Population Data Base provides an overestimate of risk of breast cancer attributable to inherited genetic factors, and the actual number lies somewhere between these

estimates. In addition, these studies are based on family history and do not take into account the occurrence of new mutations in predisposing genes, the rate of which is unknown but that could influence these estimates.

In summary, current estimates place the percentage of breast cancer cases directly attributable to inherited factors between 5% and 10%. The identification of the major breast cancer susceptibility genes based on ongoing investigations is expected eventually to allow a direct measurement of the percentage of breast cancers resulting from inherited mutations in breast cancer–related genes.

Genetics of Inherited Breast Cancer

AUTOSOMAL DOMINANT INHERITANCE

Mendelian diseases are defined as those diseases that are the result of a single mutated gene inherited in simple patterns described by Mendel in 1865 during his study of hybrid garden peas. Mendel described these principles in saying: "Those characteristics that are transmitted entire, or almost unchanged by hybridization . . . are termed dominant, and those that become latent in the process are termed recessive." All studies of familial breast cancer have suggested that the predominant breast cancer susceptibility genes are transmitted in an autosomal dominant manner. Many of the most common genetic disorders of adult life are autosomal dominant diseases; these include familial colon cancer syndromes, polycystic kidney disease, familial hypercholesterolemia, Huntington disease, and neurofibromatosis.

The pattern of autosomal dominant inheritance is illustrated in Figure 7.2-1. In general, an individual could have one of three possible genotypes: carrier of two nonmutant gene copies (alleles; homozygous normal) or carrier of one (heterozygous) or two (homozygote) mutant alleles and therefore affected or at risk of being affected based on the penetrance of the gene. Penetrance is the likelihood that the effect of a mutation will become clinically apparent. Individuals carrying two copies of an autosomal dominant disease–related gene are extremely rare, partially because of the mathematic probability of mating between heterozygotes and partially because of the potential for a lethal defect in a homozygote-affected fetus. As long as the gene examined is not on the X or Y sex-determining chromosomes, the sex of the carrier is irrelevant. In the case of autosomal dominant inheritance of breast cancer, however, significant differences are seen in the penetrance of mutations between male and female carriers. During meiosis, each gamete generated carries a single copy of the gene of interest, resulting in a 50% chance that any one offspring will inherit a mutant copy from the heterozygous parent. Thus, on average, 50% of the related individuals in a family carry the mutant gene. Therefore, the typical pedigree pattern for an autosomal dominant disease is striking, with vertical inheritance and half the children of an affected parent affected, whereas none of the offspring of a homozygous normal parent are affected. This phenomenon is illustrated in the pedigree

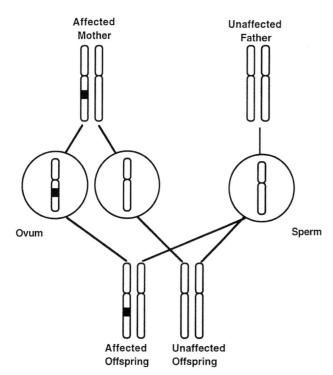

FIGURE 7.2-1 Autosomal dominant inheritance. A pair of chromosomes is shown from each parent. During gametogenesis, germ cells are formed that carry only one member of a chromosomal pair. In this example, all sperm are equivalent because the father is unaffected. In the genesis of ovum, half the germ cells carry a disease-related mutation and half do not. In the case of dominant inheritance, all offspring inheriting the disease-related mutation from the affected mother are also affected (assuming 100% penetrance). In the case of recessive inheritance, offspring must inherit two copies of a disease-related mutation, one from each carrier parent, to be affected.

shown in Figure 7.2-2, a typical pedigree of a family known to carry a mutation in the breast cancer susceptibility gene BRCA1. Because the defect in the BRCA1 gene that results in the development of breast cancer in women does not appear to cause breast cancer in male carriers, evidence for the presence of a gene mutation can be detected in 50% of family members (as would be expected for an autosomal dominant pattern of inheritance), but breast cancer appears in only the female gene mutation carriers. To date, no evidence has indicated an autosomal recessive or classic sex-linked (X or Y chromosome–linked) pattern of breast cancer inheritance, although a breast cancer susceptibility gene that was not associated with breast cancer in males (as BRCA1 and p53) that was present on the X chromosome would demonstrate an inheritance pattern identical to that which would occur if the same gene were not on a sex-determining chromosome.

GENETIC LINKAGE ANALYSIS

The traditional method of identifying the location of an unidentified disease-related gene is through genetic linkage analysis. This method has been used to identify im-

portant disease-related genes in recent years such as Huntington disease, cystic fibrosis, polycystic kidney disease, hereditary nonpolyposis colon cancer, and familial adenomatous polyposis, as well as the breast cancer susceptibility genes BRCA1 and, most recently, BRCA2. Efforts are currently underway to identify additional breast cancer–related genes by genetic linkage analysis, aided immensely by recent strides made as a result of the Human Genome Initiative. Linkage analysis relies on the finding that genes or genetic markers that lie near one another on a chromosome are inherited together with a likelihood that depends on the distance between the two loci. In other words, two segments of DNA that are immediately adjacent to one another have a low likelihood of being separated by a crossover event during meiosis, whereas DNA segments that are at opposite ends of a chromosome are separated during meiosis much more frequently.

The initial identification of genetic markers that lie near a disease locus is a time-consuming trial-and-error process that requires a collection of affected families scanned with large numbers of genetic markers of known chromosomal location. When a genetic marker is identified that travels with the disease in several pedigrees, the disease and the marker are said to be linked. The likelihood that the genetic marker tested is adjacent to a gene responsible for the occurrence of disease is reported as a lod score (abbreviated Z). The lod score, a "genetic *P* value," is the $\log_{10}$ of odds favoring linkage. Thus, if the lod score calculated for the linkage between a genetic marker and a disease locus is 2, the odds that this observation is occurring by chance alone are 1 in 100; if the lod score is 6, chance alone could have produced the observation only 1 in 1,000,000 times. A negative lod score is observed when the genetic marker and the disease loci are not close together, and as the lod score becomes increasingly more negative, the likelihood that the loci are close together becomes increasingly remote. A more complete mathematic description of the method of lod scoring can be found elsewhere.[57]

Linkage analysis has been the backbone of both the molecular genetic efforts to identify breast cancer–related genes and the pioneering work of providing genetic counseling to members of breast cancer families based on genetic analysis. When a clinically detectable disease, such as breast cancer, can be identified in a family pedigree, one can follow the responsible chromosomal segment through the family by following the inheritance of closely linked genetic markers (hence the term *linkage analysis*). This is illustrated in Figure 7.2-3, which shows a segment of the breast cancer family illustrated in Figure 7.2-2, which is known to carry a germline mutation in the breast cancer susceptibility gene BRCA1. This pedigree illustrates the following: (1) the ability to trace the chromosome carrying the mutant gene through several generations; (2) the ability to detect a meiotic recombination event within the family that allows narrowing the interval thought to contain the gene; and (3) the power of linkage analysis to predict which unaffected members of the family are at high risk of developing breast or ovarian cancer in the future and which members of the family are at no increased risk, as compared with the general popula-

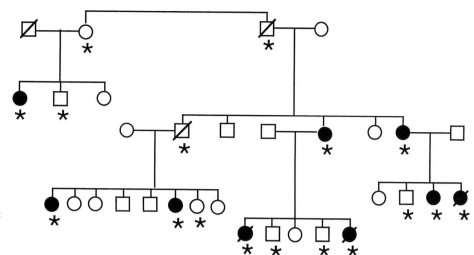

FIGURE 7.2-2 Kindred with a BRCA1 mutation. Open squares, unaffected males; open circles, unaffected females; filled circles, females with breast or ovarian cancer; *, known BRCA1 mutation carriers; diagonal line through symbol, deceased.

tion.[58,59] Linkage analysis is still the only means of identifying BRCA2 mutation carriers, whereas BRCA1 mutations can now be detected directly. Linkage analysis will also be critical in determining the location of BRCA3 and other breast cancer–related genes.

TUMOR-SUPPRESSOR GENES

Three fundamental types of genetic damage thought to be responsible for the development of the malignant phenotype are found in cancer cells: (1) activation of protooncogenes producing a gain of function in the affected cell, (2) inactivation of tumor-suppressor genes producing a loss of function in the cell, and (3) inactivation of genes that repair damaged DNA. Some tumor-suppressor genes

appear to be important in cell cycle regulation and normally function as checks on cell growth; others may be critical elements in DNA repair, by preventing the propagation of mutations in other critical genes. Mutated tumor-suppressor genes are thought to lose these regulatory functions and lead to malignant transformation. Many of the genes responsible for familial cancer syndromes appear to be tumor-suppressor genes. Evidence for the existence of this family of genes was first described by several groups following the observation that fusing chromosomes from a normal cell with a tumor cell line would result in suppression of the malignant characteristics of the tumor cell line. Thus, investigators hypothesized that genes existed whose normal function resulted in suppression of malignant cell growth; when the activity of these tumor-

FIGURE 7.2-3 Genetic linkage analysis. A portion of the family illustrated in Figure 7.2-2, showing genotyping with four genetic markers surrounding BRCA1. The chromosome carrying the disease-related mutation in this family can be traced in this family through three generations by following the markers associated with the occurrence of breast cancer, depicted in this figure as C-A-C-D and enclosed within a rectangle. This family also illustrates several of the clinical scenarios that arise during genetic testing for cancer susceptibility: (1) unaffected female carrier at high risk for developing breast or ovarian cancer; (2) unaffected female who would have previously been assigned a high risk of developing breast cancer based on family history but is now shown to be at no greater risk than the general population; (3) affected female carrier with a meiotic recombination event that narrowed the BRCA1 candidate interval during the effort to isolate BRCA1; and (4) male carrier, whose children each have a 50% risk of inheriting the disease-causing mutation. Another example of a male carrier is in generation I, the earliest identified carrier in this family.

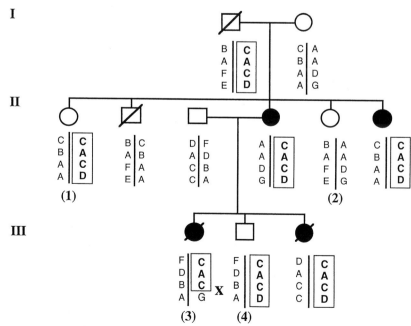

suppressor genes was lost, a clone of cells capable of malignant growth patterns emerged and resulted in the development of clinically detectable cancer.[60-62] Because all individuals are born with two copies of every gene, however, an explanation was needed for the development of cancer in large numbers of individuals who had only a single inherited mutation in a tumor-suppressor gene, with residual function remaining from the other copy. In 1971, Knudsen[63] put forth the two-hit hypothesis, suggesting that cancer occurred as a result of two genetic events occurring in the same cell, inactivating both copies of a given tumor-suppressor gene. In the case of sporadic, or noninherited, cancer, the likelihood that two events would occur in the same cell is low. Individuals from "cancer families" inherit an inactivating mutation in one allele of the implicated tumor-suppressor gene in all cells (ie, a germline mutation), however, so only one somatic (noninherited) event is required to inactivate the single remaining copy, making the development of cancer a much more common event than in individuals born without the "first hit."

The first evidence for the role for tumor-suppressor genes in the pathogenesis of human cancers was provided by the isolation of the retinoblastoma gene (Rb).[64,65] All patients with hereditary retinoblastoma carry a germline mutation in one allele of the Rb gene. Knudsen's two-hit hypothesis postulated the presence of a defect or mutation in the normal, or wild-type, allele arising in the tumor; this has proved to be the case with the Rb gene. Loss of the wild-type allele results in the inactivation of both Rb alleles: the first one by the inherited germline mutation, and the second by a somatic event. Thus, germline mutations in tumor-suppressor genes create highly susceptible groups of individuals for whom only one somatic event is required to produce complete inactivation of tumor-suppressor activity at a given locus. Of particular relevance to breast cancer are the tumor-suppressor genes p53, BRCA1, and presumably, BRCA2.

Identification of Tumor-Suppressor Genes Through Loss of Heterozygosity

Within familial cancer syndromes, the second hit can often be detected in tumor samples by the loss of genetic markers in the chromosomal region of interest; this phenomenon is termed *loss of heterozygosity* (LOH) and is illustrated in Figure 7.2-4. Consistent LOH for a genetic marker at a given locus in tumors from multiple patients has been considered strong evidence of the presence of a tumor-suppressor gene in that region. Nonrandom chromosome deletions and LOH at specific chromosomal regions have been identified in certain common human cancers, including carcinoma of the breast, a finding that supports this hypothesis. Analysis of individual breast tumors has provided additional clues to the role of tumor-suppressor genes in breast carcinoma.

A review of published studies of LOH in breast cancers suggests that potentially important breast cancer–related tumor-suppressor genes may be present on chromosomes 1p, 1q, 3p, 5p, 6q, 7q, 8p, 9q, 13q, 15q, 16q, 17p, 17q, and 18q.[66-68] More recent work examining LOH in familial breast cancers suggests that chromosomes 8p, 16q, 17p, 17q, and 19p exhibit LOH in at least 20% of tumors examined; 8p contained the area most frequently deleted in this series, with 33% LOH detected.[69] In addition, the availability of closely spaced genetic markers has allowed more detailed mapping in specific areas of interest. Chromosome 17 has been the focus of intensive investigation

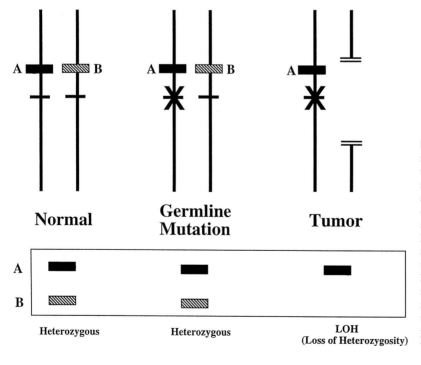

FIGURE 7.2-4 Loss of heterozygosity. Schematic representation of one mechanism of inactivation of a tumor-suppressor gene, leading to development of a malignant disease. The chromosome pair is represented as two vertical lines, the tumor-suppressor gene (one copy on each parental chromosome) by short horizontal lines, the genetic marker of variable size (A larger than B) adjacent to the tumor-suppressor gene as filled rectangles, the inactivation of one copy of the tumor-suppressor gene by an inherited mutation as an X through the gene, and the loss of the only remaining functional copy of the tumor-suppressor gene in a tumor by loss of a large chromosome segment containing the gene. The rectangle below the chromosomes depicts the DNA fragments of the genetic marker as would be seen on an electrophoresis gel.

because of the presence of three known tumor-suppressor genes: BRCA1 (17q), NF1(17q), and p53(17p), as well as the metastasis-suppressor gene nm23 (17q) and the breast cancer–associated oncogene HER-2/neu (17q). Detailed analysis of this chromosome suggests the presence of as many as five distinct regions of loss on chromosome 17[70–72]; two of these regions are known to encompass p53 and BRCA1, respectively. Finally, some indication exists that LOH in specific areas may be associated with distinct clinical characteristics. As an example of this phenomenon, LOH on chromosome 16q was significantly correlated with the occurrence of distant metastases in a subset of 82 breast carcinomas from patients with a family history of breast cancer.[73] Thus, LOH analysis may be a useful means of predicting clinical outcome as well as an important genetic tool in identifying breast cancer–related tumor-suppressor genes.

Hereditary Breast Cancer Syndromes

The work described previously has provided unequivocal evidence of the importance of genetic factors in the development of breast cancer. The further study of clinical syndromes that include an increased incidence of breast cancer extends these observations and provides insight into individual mechanisms by which genetic mutations result in the development of breast cancer. Examination of numerous pedigrees has resulted in the recognition of different syndromes in which dominantly inherited breast cancer may be featured. The most frequently identified pedigrees contain site-specific breast cancer and are thought to represent the effect of a single genetic abnormality; BRCA1 and BRCA2 are examples, and others are likely to be identified in the future. Breast cancer has also been noted to occur in association with other cancers; the occurrence of breast cancer in association with diverse childhood neoplasms in the Li-Fraumeni or (SBLA) syndrome (*s*oft tissue and *b*ony sarcomas, *b*rain tumors, *l*eukemias, and *a*drenocortical carcinomas) and the association between breast and ovarian cancer represent two of the most intensively studied examples. Finally, breast cancer may occur with increased frequency in patients with hereditary syndromes that include nonmalignant manifestations as well, such as Cowden and Muir syndromes. The genes whose primary phenotypic expression results in such disorders may also be involved in the development of breast cancer, or a separate gene important in breast cancer may be located on the chromosome near the genes for these syndromes. The preliminary observations of excess breast cancer among women presumed to be heterozygous for ataxia-telangiectasia (by virtue of having affected offspring) may be significant in this regard.[74]

BREAST–OVARIAN CANCER SYNDROME

The association between breast and ovarian carcinoma was first reported in 1971 by Lynch and Krush,[75] with additional families reported subsequently by these and other investigators.[76–78] The estimated cumulative risk of breast or ovarian cancer to daughters of affected mothers in 12 pedigrees reported by Lynch was 46%, consistent with transmission of a highly penetrant autosomal dominant trait. This finding was upheld by the identification of chromosome 17q21 as the location of a susceptibility gene for early-onset breast cancer, now termed *BRCA1*.[43,44] Within 6 months, Narod and colleagues[79] demonstrated unequivocal linkage between the genetic marker D17S74 on 17q21 (the same genetic marker linked to the appearance of breast cancer in families by King) and the appearance of ovarian cancer in several large kindreds. These data provided strong evidence that germline mutations in BRCA1 account for the clinical appearance of the breast–ovarian cancer syndrome. BRCA1 has now been isolated, confirming this hypothesis.[44] BRCA1 is a novel gene with homology to a zinc finger motif near the 5′ end of the gene, suggesting that BRCA1 may function as a transcription factor. The protein does not display homology to any other known motif or cloned gene. BRCA1 is extremely large, with a mRNA that is 7.8 kb in length, 24 exons that span almost 100 kb of genomic DNA, and a protein composed of 1863 amino acids (Fig. 7.2-5). Several reports

FIGURE 7.2-5 BRCA1 genomic structure and mutations. The 24 exons of BRCA1 are represented by vertical lines within the gene; the translation start and stop sites are as indicated. The 5′ region of homology to the RING finger motif found in a family of transcription factors is indicated by a shaded rectangle under the gene. The locations of five of the most common mutations are indicated above the gene. Exons 1 and 4 do not contain coding sequence; of particular note is the large exon 11, containing more than half the coding region.

were published shortly after the isolation of BRCA1 describing the spectrum of mutations in certain families predisposed to breast cancer and breast and ovarian cancer.[80-83] Unfortunately, the spectrum of mutations is large, spanning the entire length of the gene and clustering in only a few locations. This fact makes mutation screening as a diagnostic service difficult from a technical standpoint and sheds little light on regions of the BRCA1 protein that may be important.

Families in which breast and ovarian cancer are thought to result from BRCA1 mutations have now been identified by many groups. Inheritance in these families follows the classic mendelian pattern of autosomal dominant transmission, with 50% of children of carriers inheriting BRCA1 mutations. This inheritance pattern, as well as LOH studies in tumors from affected members of BRCA1-linked families, supports the hypothesis that BRCA1 fits the model of a classic tumor-suppressor gene, with loss of the normal, or wild-type, allele in the tumors of all informative cases.[50,84,85] Female mutation carriers are estimated to have an 85% lifetime risk of developing breast cancer[86] and 40% to 50% risk of ovarian cancer.[87] BRCA1 mutation carriers also have an increased incidence of bilateral breast cancer. It is estimated that 45% of families with apparent autosomal dominant transmission of breast cancer susceptibility, and approximately 90% of families with dominant inheritance of both breast and ovarian cancer, harbor BRCA1 germline mutations. The percentage of breast cancer–only families that are attributed to BRCA1 mutations rises to almost 70% if the median age of onset of breast cancer in the families is less than 45 years.[86]

A study of 33 families with evidence of germline mutations in BRCA1 was conducted by the Breast Cancer Linkage Consortium.[88] Families were contributed by 11 groups representing 6 different countries; families were eligible for inclusion if they contained at least 4 cases total of either breast or ovarian cancer diagnosed before age 60 years and demonstrated a lod score of at least 0.4 for families with breast and ovarian cancer or 1.0 for families with breast cancer only. This work presents evidence for risk heterogeneity among families though to carry BRCA1 germline mutations and suggests that various mutations may confer variable risks. Performing an analysis that allows for variable risk, the Breast Cancer Linkage Consortium data suggest that there may be at least 2 BRCA1 "subtypes," one conferring a breast cancer risk of 91% and an ovarian cancer risk of 32% by age 70 years and another conferring a breast cancer risk of 70% and an ovarian cancer risk of 84%. It is estimated that the first type represents 71% of all mutations. In addition, the Breast Cancer Linkage Consortium data suggest that the cumulative risk of developing a second breast cancer is 65% for mutation carriers that live to age 70 years.[87] Although estimates of the percentage of breast cancer cases that occur as a direct result of germline mutations in BRCA1 vary from 2% to 10%,[19,20] the estimate is a function of age. Thus, although less than 1% of all breast cancers in elderly women are likely to result from BRCA1 germline mutations, this fraction may approach 30% for women diagnosed with breast cancer under the age of 35 years.[27,54,86]

To determine whether tumors that arise as a result of BRCA1 mutations have clinical and pathologic characteristics that differ from those of sporadic tumors, Lynch and associates[89] analyzed 180 tumors from families with hereditary breast–ovarian or site-specific breast cancer. Ninety eight of the 180 tumors were analyzed as a subset more likely to result from BRCA1 mutations due to known linkage results or the presence of ovarian cancer in another family member. Both subgroups were significantly younger than the population average. The BRCA1 group was found to have more aneuploid and high S-phase tumors than the other group. Tubular and lobular cancers were more common in the group in which the presence of BRCA1 mutations was less certain; it now appears that these may be BRCA2-related tumors. Despite the findings of more ominous pathologic characteristics in the BRCA1 group, disease-free survival was longer in this group than in the group thought less likely to contain BRCA1 mutations. These investigators suggested that BRCA1 mutations may result in tumors with adverse pathologic indicators but a paradoxically better survival. This study was performed before it was possible to determine which tumors harbored BRCA1 mutations. The isolation of BRCA1 now makes this possible, and the collection of data on the clinical and pathologic characteristics of malignant tumors in BRCA1 mutation carriers will allow verification and refinement of this work.

Further analysis of the Breast Cancer Linkage Consortium data provides estimates for the risk of cancers other than breast and ovarian in the same 33 families discussed previously. Data published in 1993 from the study of a large Icelandic family with breast–ovarian cancer suggested that prostate cancer may be a component of this syndrome.[90] This finding was upheld by the Breast Cancer Linkage Consortium data in which significant excesses were observed for prostate cancer, with an estimated RR of 3.33 for males thought to carry BRCA1 germline mutations, and for colon cancer, with an estimated RR to mutation carriers of 4.11. The ages at diagnosis of prostate and colon cancer were not particularly early, however, as compared with the general population, in contrast to breast and ovarian cancer in these families. In addition, the excess colon cancer risk reflects the experience of only a few families, suggesting either low penetrance with regard to colon cancer or a limited number of specific mutations that increase colon cancer risk. No significant excesses were observed for cancers originating from other anatomic sites.[88] Specifically, male breast cancer does not appear to be a component tumor of this syndrome. An analysis of 22 pedigrees with a dominant inheritance pattern for female breast cancer and at least 1 case of male breast cancer provides strong evidence against linkage to BRCA1 in these families with a lod score of −16.63 (odds less than 1 in 10^{-16}).[91] These results indicated that a gene other than BRCA1 predisposes to early-onset breast cancer in women and confers an increased risk of male breast cancer, now confirmed with the finding of BRCA2 on chromosome 13.[92] Although estimates of the frequency of BRCA1 germline mutations in the general population will be difficult to determine with accuracy until population-based studies are completed, as many as 1 in 300 women in the United States may harbor germline mutations in breast cancer susceptibility genes and the associated increased risk of developing neoplastic disease, approximately half of which may be accounted for by BRCA1. Nonetheless, these preliminary studies, made possible by identification of the chromosomal location of BRCA1,[43] confirm the high penetrance of BRCA1 mutations suggested by earlier studies and provide the first estimates of overall cancer risk for mutation carriers, thus allowing counseling of families thought to be at risk.

Although breast cancer that can be attributed to a BRCA1 germline mutation probably accounts for only 3% to 5% of all breast cancers, identification of BRCA1 will likely have far-reaching consequences. First, the occurrence of breast cancer in 85% of women carrying BRCA1 mutations suggests that normal function of the BRCA1 gene product protects against the development of malignancy. The isolation of BRCA1 makes possible the studies needed to elucidate the function of BRCA1. Although early studies of LOH in the BRCA1 region, suggesting that 30% to 60% of noninherited breast cancers, would have BRCA1 mutations,[93–95] are not supported by the first report of BRCA1 mutation studies in tumors,[96] additional work will be needed to elucidate the role of BRCA1 in the development of sporadic cancers. Second, based on estimates of a susceptibility allele frequency of 0.033% in the general population[54] and the proportion of families linked to BRCA1,[86] as many as 1 in 600 women may carry BRCA1 germline mutations. A realistic option for women with 2 or more affected first-degree relatives is bilateral mastectomy in early adulthood. As many as 50% of these women may be at no greater risk than the general population, but genetic counseling based on linkage analysis or mutation detection is possible for few families.[58,59] The isolation of BRCA1 eventually will allow presymptomatic testing for any women desiring this information. Most important, isolation and cloning of BRCA1 should ultimately lead to a greater understanding of the causes of breast cancer and should lead to major advances in diagnostics and therapeutics benefiting all breast cancer patients.

LI-FRAUMENI SYNDROME

Li-Fraumeni syndrome was first identified as a syndrome in 1969 in a description of four kindreds in which cousins or siblings had childhood soft tissue sarcomas and other relatives had excessive cancer occurrence.[97] Subsequent epidemiologic efforts have resulted in enumeration of the major component neoplasms, including breast cancer, soft tissue and osteosarcomas, brain tumors, leukemias, and adrenocortical carcinomas, with several additional tumor types likely to merit inclusion.[98,99] Segregation analysis of families identified through a family member with sarcoma confirmed the autosomal dominant pattern of transmission of cancer susceptibility, with age-specific penetrance functions estimated to reach 90% by age 70 years.[100] Nearly 30% of tumors in reported families occur before age 15 years.[99]

The pattern of breast cancer in families with Li-Fraumeni syndrome is remarkable. Among 24 such families, 44 women had breast cancer, of whom 77% were between ages 22 and 45 years (Li FP, Garber JE, unpublished data). Bilateral disease was documented in 25% of these women; 11% had additional primary tumors. It has been suggested that males may have later-onset tumors in families with Li-Fraumeni syndrome because they do not get breast cancer, which is so dramatic among female family members.[101]

In 1990, germline mutations were identified in one copy of the p53 tumor-suppressor gene in affected members of families with Li-Fraumeni syndrome.[45,102] Mutations were clustered in the conserved sequences of the gene (exons 5 to 9), an observation that was thought to increase the significance of these findings. Additional families meeting the classic criteria for the clinical syndrome of Li-Fraumeni syndrome were subsequently evaluated for the presence of alterations in germline p53. Approximately 50% of such carefully defined families had alterations identified in the p53 gene. Although mutations are more frequently identified in hot spots within the conserved sequences, they have been seen throughout the gene;[103–107] p53 genes ostensibly normal by sequencing but with abnormal functional assays or expression have also been observed.[108–111] The degree of complexity in mutational analysis of this moderate-size gene has also become much more apparent.

The prevalence of germline p53 alterations among women with diagnosed breast cancer before age 40 years has been estimated at approximately 1%.[112,113] Therefore, this alteration is not a common explanation for breast cancer occurrence in the population; nonetheless, p53 alterations have permitted the first predisposition testing programs for breast cancer susceptibility to be developed. The technologic difficulties of p53 analysis and the low prevalence of the mutations in the general population have kept this genetic test from widespread application, however.

COWDEN SYNDROME

Multiple hamartoma syndrome or Cowden syndrome is a rare genodermatosis with multiple clinical features. The most consistent and characteristic findings are mucocutaneous lesions, including multiple facial trichilemmomas, papillomatosis of the lips and oral mucosa, and acral keratoses. Vitiligo and angiomas have also been reported. The syndrome is considered to be inherited in an autosomal dominant mode with variable expressivity.[114]

Benign proliferations in other organ systems are common in patients with Cowden syndrome, including thyroid goiter and adenomas, gastrointestinal polyps, uterine leiomyomas, and lipomas. Nonmalignant abnormalities of the breast are similarly noted in these patients and include fibroadenomas, fibrocystic lesions, areolar and nipple malformations, and ductal epithelial hyperplasia.[115,116]

A marked increase in breast cancer incidence as compared with the general population was observed in a series of published cases of Cowden syndrome.[115] Breast neoplasms occurred in 10 of the 21 female patients; lesions were bilateral in 4 women. Lesions were said to be exclusively intraductal in 2 of these 10 women; however, given the likelihood that these are true precursor lesions, these intraductal carcinomas are likely to represent a manifestation of the underlying genetic defect. Additional cases of Cowden syndrome have been published, bringing the total reported patients to 83, of whom 51 were female.[116] Thus, the number of women with breast cancer and Cowden syndrome totals 15 (29%), or 13 (25%) if the 2 known intraductal tumors are excluded, with bilateral invasive tumors in 4 women. Because many of the women in these families are still alive and are at risk of developing breast cancer, the number of these women with breast cancer is likely to increase, thereby increasing current estimates for the lifetime risk of developing breast cancer for women with this syndrome. On the other hand, increased recognition of Cowden syndrome could continue to increase the number of known patients with Cowden syndrome without breast cancer disproportionately and could ultimately reduce estimates of the breast cancer rate. Identification of a biologic marker of the syndrome will ultimately provide the most meaningful data on the association of breast cancer with this unusual condition.

MUIR SYNDROME

Muir syndrome, a variant of Lynch type II syndrome, is the eponym given to the association between multiple skin tumors and multiple benign and malignant tumors of the upper and lower gastrointestinal and genitourinary tracts.[117–119] Many of the manifestations are common lesions (basal cell carcinomas, keratoacanthomas, colonic diverticula) that occur at later ages in distributions similar to those in the general population. Inheritance of this syndrome is autosomal dominant, with high penetrance.[118] Females with the syndrome reportedly have an increased tendency to breast cancer, particularly after menopause, although lifetime risk has not been calculated.[119] Three genes responsible for inherited forms of colon cancer have been described,[120–125] including APC (responsible for familial adenomatous polyposis), MLH1, and MSH2 (responsible for hereditary nonpolyposis colon cancer). Muir syndrome results from germline mutations in the MSH2 and MLH1 loci, genes that affect the ability of cells to repair damaged DNA.

ATAXIA-TELANGIECTASIA

Ataxia-telangiectasia is an autosomal recessive disorder characterized by cerebellar ataxia, oculocutaneous telangiectasias, radiation hypersensitivity, and an increased incidence of malignant disease. Chromosomal fragility and resultant DNA rearrangements may be the result of the genetic defect that underlies the clinical AT syndrome. Characteristic of a disease with an autosomal recessive pattern of inheritance, individuals with ataxia-telangiectasia inherit a defective copy of the associated gene from both parents and are therefore homozygous. Ataxia-telangiectasia homozygotes, accounting for 3 to 11 live births

per million,[126] are estimated to have a risk of cancer 60 to 180 times greater than the general population;[127] cancers observed in association with ataxia-telangiectasia include non-Hodgkin lymphoma (nearly 100% lifetime risk) and significant but lower risks of breast cancer, ovarian cancer, lymphocytic leukemia, and malignant diseases of the oral cavity, stomach, pancreas, and bladder. In particular, breast cancer risk in ataxia-telangiectasia mutation carriers does not approach the risk observed in women with inherited mutations in p53 or BRCA1. Initially, reports of increased susceptibility to cancer were limited to homozygous ataxia-telangiectasia mutation carriers, representing approximately 0.2% to 0.7% of the general population in the United States.[127] A study published in 1987, however, suggested that ataxia-telangiectasia heterozygotes, who do not display the typical neurologic findings seen in homozygotes, have a five-fold increased incidence of breast cancer.[128] This finding was particularly significant given that ataxia-telangiectasia heterozygotes represent as much as 7% of the general population,[126] that screening mammography, a source of ionizing radiation, could possibly contribute to the increased breast cancer incidence seen in this population. This study has been criticized for methodologic flaws, including small sample size, appropriateness of the control group, and lack of quantitation of radiation exposure.[129] In addition, two groups analyzed a total of 80 families with evidence of an inherited form of breast cancer for linkage between breast cancer and genetic markers flanking the ataxia-telangiectasia locus on chromosome 11 with strong evidence against this association.[130,131] Both groups concluded that the contribution of ataxia-telangiectasia mutations to familial breast cancer is likely to be minimal. Nonetheless, if ataxia-telangiectasia results from an alteration in the ability to repair DNA damage, the hypothesis that ataxia-telangiectasia heterozygotes may have a decreased capacity to repair DNA as a result of one mutant ataxia-telangiectasia allele could explain an increased susceptibility to cancer in such individuals. The ataxia-telangiectasia gene has recently been identified on human chromosome 11q22. As noted previously, the ability to study the ataxia-telangiectasia gene and its gene product directly will likely answer some of the questions posed by these studies and will result in a further advance in our understanding of the factors that contribute to the development of breast cancer.

CONSTITUTIONAL 11q;22q CHROMOSOMAL TRANSLOCATIONS

A translocation between the long arm of chromosome 11 and the long arm of chromosome 22 is the most frequently reported heritable balanced translocation in humans, now described in more than 100 families.[132–134] Although descriptions of individuals carrying this translocation first appeared in the literature in 1980, no reports of associated neoplasia were published until 1994, when the appearance of breast cancer in a known carrier of the 11q;22q translocation prompted a review of 8 Swedish families with a total of 22 known carriers.[135] These 22 carriers consisted of 17 women and 5 men, consistent with the observation of a significant excess of phenotypically normal female carriers in the offspring of female carriers compared with the offspring of male carriers.[134] Family history of cancer was obtained by interview of a selected family member and was verified using medical records or a local cancer registry. Five of these 8 families had 1 case of breast cancer per family. In a sixth family, a malignant disease of unknown origin was diagnosed from biopsy of a chest wall nodule—the tumor was pathologically consistent with either breast or renal cell carcinoma, no primary source was identified, and the patient died 2 years later from metastatic disease. No additional cancers were reported. Even when excluding the index case that prompted this study and the carcinoma of unknown primary origin, the number of breast cancer cases observed was significantly greater than expected based on breast cancer incidence in the Swedish population as a whole, with a standardized RR of 9.8. If one includes these 2 cases, the RR rises even further to 14.6, similar to the risk observed in known carriers of BRCA1 germline mutations. Retinoblastomas, sarcomas seen with neurofibromatosis type 1, and renal cell carcinomas have been associated with gene disruption as a result of balanced translocation; this study suggests the presence of a breast cancer–associated gene on chromosome 11 or 22. No such gene has been described to date; however, efforts are underway in several laboratories to isolate the genes on both chromosomes affected by the translocation as well as to perform linkage studies of families with breast cancer.

Inheritance of Proliferative Breast Disease

Proliferative breast disease (PBD) is a term used to describe several benign breast lesions characterized on histologic examination by hyperplasia and cellular atypia but without evidence of cellular invasion through the basement membrane. Although the exact definitions of the various types of PBD remain controversial, and interobserver variation is significant, investigators have suggested that PBD represents a premalignant state for several reasons. This hypothesis stems from the findings that the involved cell type originates in the ductal–lobular unit and may morphologically resemble noninvasive cancer and that PBD is often found in mastectomy specimens obtained from breast cancer patients.[136] In addition, several studies have reported that women with PBD have a 2- to 5-fold increased risk of developing breast cancer.[137–139] One of these studies suggested that family history further increases the risk of breast cancer, as compared with PBD alone.[138] In 1990, results of a study examining the inheritance of proliferative breast disease suggested that genetic susceptibility was responsible for both PBD and breast cancer in the kindreds examined.[140] This study included 103 women from 20 breast cancer kindreds and 31 control women selected from the spouses of male family members. PBD was diagnosed by 4-quadrant fine-needle aspiration of both breasts of each of these women. These investigators reported that PBD, defined here as ductal hyperplasia with or without

atypia, was seen in 35% of clinically normal female first-degree relatives of breast cancer cases, as compared with 13% of the control women. Several genetic models that might explain this observation were tested; the only models not strongly rejected were those that allowed genetic susceptibility to PBD that was also expressed as increased breast cancer risk. This analysis could not distinguish between dominant and recessive modes of inheritance, given the low penetrance in women and the lack of penetrance in men. This study has been heavily criticized for the use of fine-needle aspiration to make a diagnosis of PBD, which can be difficult to classify even with a histologic specimen. Nonetheless, the study was carefully performed from a methodologic standpoint and adds weight to the hypothesis that PBD is a premalignant lesion that may be seen as a precursor lesion in individuals genetically predisposed to breast cancer.

Familial Male Breast Cancer

Although the study of the genetic aspects of female breast cancer is complicated by the high incidence of sporadic disease, the study of familial male breast cancer is even more difficult because of the rarity of any breast cancer in men and the even smaller number of cases that occur in first- or second-degree male relatives. The first published example of male breast cancer within a nuclear family appeared in 1889.[141] This case report described a father and son both diagnosed with breast cancer; no other family members with cancer were known, including female breast cancer. In the ensuing 100 years, only 16 additional families with 2 or more cases of male breast cancer were reported.[141–143] Analysis of these families suggests that familial male breast cancer is likely to be as heterogeneous as familial female breast cancer. In addition, more than half of these families with male breast cancer describe first-degree relatives with other types of cancers; these include oropharyngeal, ovarian, and female breast cancer.[142] Nine of the families on which data were available reported cases of female breast cancer.[143] Average age at diagnosis of breast cancer in female relatives (where data were available) was 46 years, considerably younger than the average age at diagnosis in the general population of 57 years,[144] and consistent with studies of familial breast cancer in females.

Epidemiologic case-control studies have also documented an increased risk of breast cancer in male relatives of affected males (RR, 6.1) and affected females (RR, 2.2), with risk to male relatives increasing with decreasing age at diagnosis of the affected relative.[145,146] Female relatives of affected males were similarly at increased risk, again suggesting an inherited component of male breast cancer. In 1992, a study provided evidence that inherited male breast cancer in one family was associated with germline mutations in the androgen receptor gene; this was subsequently confirmed in a second family.[147,148] This finding was of interest not only as the first direct evidence that susceptibility to male breast cancer could be inherited, but also because altered hormonal metabolism had been suggested by many investigators as a risk factor for male breast cancer. Indirect evidence for this hypothesis came from reports of an increased incidence of gynecomastia, exogenous estrogen usage, schistosomal liver fibrosis, orchitis, testicular atrophy, obesity, and Klinefelter syndrome among men diagnosed with breast cancer.[143] Evidence for the presence of inherited male breast cancer associated with a defective androgen receptor strengthens this hypothesis.

The most recent information on the genetics of familial male breast cancer comes from a linkage analysis of 22 families with female breast cancer with at least 1 case of male breast cancer; 12 of these families also had at least 1 individual diagnosed with ovarian cancer.[91] All 22 families were analyzed for linkage between breast cancer and genetic markers flanking the BRCA1 candidate region on chromosome 17. A maximum lod score of -16.63 was obtained, providing strong evidence against linkage to BRCA1 in these families; the estimate of the proportion of linked families was 0%. This study demonstrates that, at most, a small proportion of families with breast cancer characterized by at least 1 case of male breast cancer will be associated with germline mutations in BRCA1. These data argue strongly for the existence of at least one additional breast cancer susceptibility gene, now thought to be BRCA2.[92] Although one cannot determine the risk of male breast cancer to unaffected men in these families, inspection of the published pedigrees suggests that the penetrance of such a gene in men is low.

Interaction of Inherited Breast Cancer Risk With Other Factors

The effect of various risk factors on the incidence of breast cancer in the general population is controversial; the effect of these same risk factors in individuals with a family history of breast cancer is essentially unknown. Nothing is known about the interaction between genetic risk and diet. Several studies have attempted to look at the incidence of breast cancer in women with at least one affected first-degree relative as a function of oral contraceptive use or estrogen replacement therapy. Results of these studies are contradictory. The difficulty in such studies derives from two significant factors. The first problem is the relatively low number of women with inherited predisposition to breast cancer. Thus, even in a study in which all participants are defined by the diagnosis of breast cancer in at least one first-degree relative, the majority of the women studied will not be from families harboring significant breast cancer susceptibility. Additionally, even in such families, half the unaffected women would be expected to be at no greater risk of breast cancer than the general population, further diluting out the ability to determine the effect of exogenous hormones on breast cancer risk. Only now, when families can be studied in which genetic risk can be accurately assessed are such studies

likely to yield reliable results. At present, it may be wise to minimize exposure to exogenous estrogens in women likely to be at increased risk of breast cancer. Future studies will determine whether this precaution is unnecessary.

Estimating Risk of Breast Cancer in the Clinic

As a result of public awareness of the increasing incidence of breast cancer in Western women, combined with media coverage of recent advances in the genetics of breast cancer, women are increasingly concerned about their individual risk of developing breast cancer. Recognition of the contribution of heritable factors to the development of breast cancer has resulted in a role for genetic counseling in the care of women with a family history of the disease. Epidemiologic studies do not always provide accurate risk assessments for individual women, however. The complexities of genetic counseling for breast cancer risk have been well described.[58,59,149–151] The major categories of effort in providing risk assessment for women and families concerned about breast cancer include the collection of a detailed medical history of the extended family, interpretation of this history in light of available information to assess individual risk, and clear communication of this information to patient and family.

Family history information must include details of all cancers among blood relatives as well as the positions of these relatives within the family pedigree. Unaffected relatives should be included, because the distribution of normal and affected relatives within a pedigree is essential to the assessment of potential inheritance patterns. Ideally, family history data should be confirmed with medical or death records to ensure accuracy. Patients have been shown to identify the sites of primary cancer in first-degree relatives correctly 83% of the time, with significant declines in accuracy with increasing distance of relationship. Details such as age at diagnosis, tumor histologic features, laterality of breast tumors, and sites of primary tumors versus metastatic disease should be attained and verified whenever possible.

Recent dramatic advances in understanding of the molecular genetics of inherited breast cancer, specifically the isolation of BRCA1 and the localization of BRCA2, have allowed accurate determination of risk for a few individuals and have made risk counseling for most women more complex. Within families that can be directly studied for mutations in BRCA1, estimates of breast cancer risk can be made with a high level of accuracy. Previously, many women with a family history of breast cancer suggestive of dominant inheritance of susceptibility were told that they had a 50% lifetime risk of developing breast cancer, based on the 50/50 chance of inheriting the mutant allele of such a gene. In fact, individuals from these striking families either carry a mutant BRCA1 allele or they do not. Mutation carriers have an 85% lifetime risk of developing breast cancer; individuals with two normal copies of BRCA1 have a breast cancer risk equivalent to the general population and are essentially unaffected by their family history. Although the number of families in which mutations in BRCA1 can be identified with a high degree of certainty is small, these families have access to the most accurate breast cancer risk assessment available. Counseling families with apparent autosomal dominant inheritance of breast cancer in which BRCA1 mutations are not detected in affected family members, or in which linkage to BRCA2 cannot be determined, is more difficult. All the issues related to dominant inheritance of breast cancer susceptibility must be discussed, but little individual information can be given. Such individuals are left with the sense that their individual risk of developing breast cancer is either extremely low or extremely high, with no currently available means of making this significant determination. Finally, because all available data on families linked to BRCA1 are from a highly selected group of families, generally large families with at least four affected individuals, little is known about the contribution of this gene, or of other breast cancer susceptibility genes, to breast cancer in smaller families with fewer breast cancer cases.

For individuals without strong evidence for the transmission of a highly penetrant breast cancer susceptibility gene, two methods have been used to estimate risk of breast cancer based on family history. These studies provide results expressed as lifetime risk, rather than RR. The first approach is the assignment of empiric risk, based on the observed incidence of disease among relatives with a given family history, such as the frequency of breast cancer among a group of women who have a sister with breast cancer. This method of risk assessment requires no knowledge of, and makes no assumptions regarding, the mode of transmission of breast cancer among relatives. Such risk estimates have been calculated for several series of patients, each of which is subject to some limitations. These form the basis for the empiric risk column in Table 7.2-2, in which risk estimates are summarized for several categories of family history.

The alternative to empiric risk is analytic risk. Analytic risk is the calculated probability that an individual will be affected, given the observed distribution of disease among relatives. This approach requires the use of an underlying model that defines how the disease occurs among relatives. Estimation of analytic risk is standard practice for genetic counseling for most inherited disorders, but it has not become routine for breast cancer because of the absence of an accepted model of disease transmission, whether environmental, genetic, or multifactorial. The values for the analytic risk in Table 7.2-2 are based on calculations by Anderson and Williams;[151] another similar model, developed by Gail and colleagues,[152] has been widely used in the calculation of risk for the NSABP Breast Cancer Prevention Trial. These models are multifactorial, allowing the cumulative influences of genetic and environmental factors. The multifactorial model is appealing for breast cancer in light of the many risk factors likely to represent interactions between genetic and environmental influences (eg, parity, age at menarche, age at first pregnancy). The most heavily weighted parameters in these models are heritability, however. In general, analytic breast cancer risk estimates are more conservative than are the empiric risks.

The methods used to estimate analytic risk are imperfect because they are nonspecific and susceptible to sampling variation. The most important limitation is the absence of a model that characterizes the familial component of breast cancer accurately. As statistical and computer-assisted approaches to genetics continue to undergo refinement, development of such a model will permit more reliable risk estimates, using more data for individuals in unique pedigrees with complex risk factor profiles. Therefore, the numeric risks provided in Table 7.2-2 should be viewed only as estimates, and their limitations must be recognized

TABLE 7.2-2

Empiric and Analytic Risk of Developing Breast Cancer as a Result of Family History

Affected Relative	Clinical Features	Empiric Lifetime Risk* (%)	Analytic Lifetime Risk† (%)
Mother	Premenopausal or postmenopausal	18–27	13
Sister	Premenopausal	8–56	14
	Postmenopausal	18	12
Mother and sister	Premenopausal	33–85	23
	Postmenopausal	16–28	17
Two sisters	Premenopausal	18–50	20
	Postmenopausal	5	17
Mother and grandmother		27	10
Mother and aunt		14	16

* Empiric risk estimates represent the range of risk reported in the studies described in references 18 to 20 and 151.
† Data from reference 152.

by those who use them in the genetic counseling of women with family histories of breast cancer.

Even within each subgroup defined in Table 7.2-2, breast cancer risk as determined from population-based studies varies widely, and the need for caution in the application of these figures to the calculation of risk for individual women from the general population cannot be overemphasized. The study populations used to generate these estimates are selected, the ranges of risk estimates are broad, and application of the methods used by one group to data collected and analyzed by others often results in differing figures than obtained with the original data set. Further, such methods do not consider additional information present in a single pedigree, such as the distribution of breast cancers among more distant relatives (cousins or aunts) or the occurrence of such pertinent tumors as ovarian cancer or sarcoma.

Elucidation of the basic mechanisms in the genesis of breast cancer and numerous potential applications await further study of BRCA1, BRCA2, and other breast cancer susceptibility genes. Patients carrying germline mutations in such genes might be targeted for interventions designed to reduce or eliminate risk. Questions of genetic heterogeneity can be addressed: Do the various hereditary and nonhereditary forms of the disease involve the same or different loci? The mechanisms of the development of associated cancers in the various clinical syndromes associated with familial breast cancer also may be clarified. Finally, the influence of exogenous exposures may be addressed. The next several years should bring exciting developments in genetic epidemiology and molecular biology that may revolutionize present thinking about the role of hereditary factors in breast cancer and may provide new tools for the diagnosis and treatment of breast cancer in women affected with both inherited and sporadic forms of the disease.

References

1. Lynch HT. Introduction to breast cancer genetics. In: Lynch HT, ed. Genetics and breast cancer. New York, Van Nostrand Reinhold.
2. Broca P. Traite de tumeurs. Paris, Asselin, 1866.
3. Nelson CL, Sellers TA, Rich SS, et al. Familial clustering of colon, breast, uterine and ovarian cancers as assessed by family history. Genet Epidemiol 1993;10:235.
4. Anderson DE, Badzioch MD. Familial breast cancer risks: effects of prostate and other cancers. Cancer 1993;72:114.
5. Lane-Clayton JE. A further report on cancer of the breast, with special reference to its associated antecedent conditions. In: Reports of the Ministry of Health, no. 32. London, HM Stationery Office, 1926.
6. Wainwright JM. Comparison of conditions associated with breast cancer in Great Britain and America. Am J Cancer 1931;15:2610.
7. Wassink WF. Cancer et heredite. Genetika 1935;17:103.
8. Penrose LS, MacKenzie HJ, Karn MNA. Genetical study of human mammary cancer. Ann Eugenics 1948;14:234.
9. Smithers DW. Family histories of 459 patients with cancer of the breast. Br J Cancer 1948;2:163.
10. Bucalossi P, Veronesi U, Pandolfi A. Il problema dell'ereditarieta neoplastica nell'uomo: il cancro della mammela. Tumori 1954;40:365.
11. Martynova RP. Studies in the genetics of human neoplasms: cancer of the breast, based on 201 family histories. Am J Cancer 1937;29:530.
12. Jacobsen O. Heredity in breast cancer: a genetic and clinical study of two hundred probands. London, HK Lewis, 1946.
13. Tulinius H, Day NE, Bjarnason O, et al. Familial breast cancer in Iceland. Int J Cancer 1982;29:365.
14. Crabtree JA. Observations on the familial incidence of cancer. Am J Public Health 1941;31:49.
15. Anderson VE, Goodman HO, Reed SC. Variables related to human breast cancer. Minneapolis, University of Minnesota, 1950.
16. Macklin MT. Comparison of the number of breast-cancer deaths observed in relatives of breast-cancer patients, and the number expected on the basis of mortality rates. J Natl Cancer Inst 1959;22:927.
17. Papadrianos E, Haagensen CD, Cooley E. Cancer of the breast as a familial disease. Ann Surg 1967;165:10.
18. Sattin RW, Rubin GL, Webster LA, et al. Family history and the risk of breast cancer. JAMA 1985;253:1908.
19. Colditz GA, Willett WC, Hunter DJ, et al. Family history, age and risk of breast cancer. JAMA 1993;270:338.
20. Slattery ML, Kerber RA. A comprehensive evaluation of family history and breast cancer risk: the Utah population database. JAMA 1993;270:1563.
21. Kelsey JL, Berkowitz GS. Breast cancer epidemiology. Cancer Res 1988;48:5615.
22. Adami HO, Hansen J, Jung B, et al. Characteristics of familial breast cancer in Sweden: absence of relation to age and unilateral versus bilateral disease. Cancer 1981;48:1688.
23. Anderson DE. Some characteristics of familial breast cancer. Cancer 1971;28:1500.
24. Anderson DE, Badzioch MD. Bilaterality in familial breast cancer patients. Cancer 1985;56:2092.
25. Sakamoto G, Sugano H, Kasumi F. Bilateral breast cancer and familial aggregations. Prev Med 1978;7:225.
26. Mettlin C, Croghan I, Natarajan N, et al. The association of age and familial risk in a case-control study of breast cancer. Am J Epidemiol 1990;131:973.
27. Claus EB, Risch NJ, Thompson WD. Age at onset as an indicator of familial risk of breast cancer. Am J Epidemiol 1990;131:961.
28. Schneider NR, Chaganti SR, German J, et al. Familial predisposition to cancer and age at onset of disease in randomly selected cancer patients. Am J Hum Genet 1983;35:454.
29. Lubin JH, Burns PE, Blot WJ, et al. Risk factors for breast cancer in women in Northern Alberta, Canada, as related to age at diagnosis. J Natl Cancer Inst 1982;68:211.
30. Bain C, Speizer FE, Rosner B, et al. Family history of breast cancer as a risk indicator for the disease. Am J Epidemiol 1980;111:301.
31. Brinton LA, Williams RR, Hoover RN, et al. Breast cancer risk factors among screening program participants. J Natl Cancer Inst 1979;62:37.
32. Seidman H, Stellman SD, Mushinski MH. A different perspective on breast cancer risk factors: some implications of the nonattributable risk. CA Cancer J Clin 1982;32:301.
33. Anderson DE. Some characteristics of familial breast cancer. Cancer 1971;28:1500.
34. Anderson DE. A genetic study of human breast cancer. J Natl Cancer Inst 1972;48:1029.
35. Anderson DE. Genetic study of breast cancer: identification of a high risk group. Cancer 1974;34:1090.
36. Anderson DE. Genetic predisposition to breast cancer. Recent Results Cancer Res 1976;57:10.
37. Anderson DE. Breast cancer in families. Cancer 1977;40:1855.

38. Anderson DE, Badzioch MD. Risk of familial breast cancer. Cancer 1985;56:383.

39. Anderson DE, Badzioch MD. Combined effect of family history and reproductive factors on breast cancer risk. Cancer 1989;63:349.

40. Ottman R, Pike MC, King MC, et al. Familial breast cancer in a population-based series. Am J Epidemiol 1986;123:15.

41. Williams WR, Anderson DE. Genetic epidemiology of breast cancer: segregation analysis of 200 Danish pedigrees. Genet Epidemiol 1984;1:7.

42. Newman B, Austin MA, Lee M, et al. Inheritence of breast cancer: evidence for autosomal dominant transmission in high risk families. Proc Natl Acad Sci USA 1988;85:3044.

43. Hall JM, Lee MK, Newman B, et al. Linkage of early onset breast cancer to chromosome 17q21. Science 1990;250:1684.

44. Miki Y, Swensew J, Shattuck-Eidens D, et al. A strong candidate for the breast and ovarian cancer susceptibility gene BRCA1. Science 1994;266:66.

45. Malkin D, Li FP, Strong LC, et al. Germ line p53 mutations in a familial syndrome of breast cancer, sarcomas, and other neoplasms. Science 1990;250:1233.

46. Amos CI, Goldstein AM, Harris EL. Familiality of breast cancer and socioeconomic status in blacks. Cancer Res 1991;51:1793.

47. Schatzkin A, Palmer JR, Rosenberg L, et al. Risk factors for breast cancer in black women. J Natl Cancer Inst 1987;78:213.

48. Bondy ML, Fueger JJ, Vogel VG, et al. Ethnic differences in familial breast cancer. Proc Annu Meet Am Assoc Cancer Res 1991;32:A1316.

49. Siraganian PA, Levine PH, Madigan P, et al. Familial breast cancer in black Americans. Cancer 1987;60:1657.

50. Chamberlain JS, Boehnke M, Frank TS, et al. BRCA1 maps proximal to D17S579 on chromosome 17q21 by genetic analysis. Am J Hum Genet 1993;52:792.

51. Weiss KM, Chakraborty R, Smouse PE, et al. Familial aggregation of cancer in Laredo, Texas: a generally low-risk Mexican American population. Genet Epidemiol 1986;3:121.

52. Kato I, Miura S, Kasumi F, et al. A case-control study of breast cancer among Japanese women: with special reference to family history and reproductive and dietary factors. Breast Cancer Res Treat 1992;24:51.

53. Zidan J, Diab M, Robinson E. Familial breast cancer in Arabs. Harefuah 1992;15:767.

54. Claus EB, Risch N, Thompson WD. Genetic analysis of breast cancer in the cancer and steroid hormone study. Am J Hum Genet 1991;48:232.

55. Lynch HT, Guirgis HA, Brodkey F, et al. Genetic heterogeneity and familial carcinoma of the breast. Surg Gynecol Obstet 1976;142:693.

56. Weber BL, Garber JE. Family history and breast cancer: probabilities and possibilities. JAMA 1993;270:1602.

57. Gelehrter TD, Collins FC. Principles of medical genetics. Baltimore, Williams & Wilkins, 1990.

58. Biesecker BB, Boehnke M, Calzone K, et al. Genetic counseling for families with inherited susceptibility to breast and ovarian cancer. JAMA 1993;269:1970.

59. Lynch HT, Watson P, Conway TA, et al. DNA screening for breast/ovarian cancer susceptibility based on linked markers. Arch Intern Med 1993;153:1979.

60. Harris H. Suppression of malignancy by cell fusion. Nature 1969;223:363.

61. Stanbridge EJ, et al. Human cell hybrids: analysis of transformation and tumor genicity. Science 1982;215:252.

62. Klein, G. The approaching era of tumor suppressor genes. Science 1987;238:1539.

63. Knudsen AG. Mutation and cancer: statistical study of retinoblastoma. Proc Natl Acad Sci USA 1971;68:820.

64. Friend SH, Bernards R, Rogelj S, et al. A human DNA segment with properties of the gene that predisposes to retinoblastoma and osteosarcoma. Nature 1986;323:643.

65. Lee WH, Bookstein R, Hong F, et al. Human retinoblastoma susceptibility gene: cloning, identification, and sequence. Science 1987;235:1394.

66. Larsson C, Byström C, Skoog L, et al. Genomic alterations in human breast carcinomas. Genes Chromosom Cancer 1990;2:191.

67. Sato T, Tanigami A, Yamakawa K, et al. Allelotype of breast cancer: cumulative allele losses promote tumor progression in primary breast cancer. Cancer Res 1990;50:7184.

68. Devilee P, van Vliet M, van Sloun P, et al. Allelotype of human breast carcinoma: a second major site for loss of heterozygosity is on chromosome 6q. Oncogene 1991;6:1705.

69. Lindblom A, Skoog L, Rotstein S, et al. Loss of heterozygosity in familial breast carcinomas. Cancer Res 1993;53:4356.

70. Kirchweger R, Zeillinger R, Schneeberger C, et al. Patterns of allele loss suggest the existence of five distinct regions of loh on chromosome 17 in breast cancer. Int J Cancer 1994;56:193.

71. Saito H, Inazawa J, Saito S, et al. Detailed deletion mapping of chromosome 17q in ovarian and breast cancers: 2-cm region on 17q21.3 often and commonly deleted in tumors. Cancer Res 1993;53:3382.

72. Cornelis RS, Devilee P, van Vliet M, et al. Allele loss patterns on chromosome 17q in 109 breast carcinomas indicate at least two distinct target regions. Oncogene 1993;8:781.

73. Lindblom A, Rotstein S, Skoog L, et al. Deletions on chromosome 16 in primary familial breast carcinomas are associated with development of distant metastases. Cancer Res 1993;53:3707.

74. Swift M, Reitnauer PJ, Morrell D, et al. Breast and other cancers in families with ataxia-telangiectasia. N Engl J Med 1987;316:1289.

75. Lynch HT, Krush AJ. Carcinoma of the breast and ovary in three families. Surg Gynecol Obstet 1971;133:644.

76. Lynch HT, Harris RE, Guirgis HA, et al. Familial association of breast/ovarian carcinoma. Cancer 1978;41:1543.

77. Fraumeni JF Jr, Grundy GW, Creagan ET, et al. Six families prone to ovarian cancer. Cancer 1975;36:364.

78. Ferrell RE, Anderson DE, Chidambaram A, et al. A genetic linkage study of familial breast–ovarian cancer. Cancer Genet Cytogenet 1989;38:241.

79. Narod SA, Feuteun J, Lynch HT, et al. Familial breast–ovarian cancer locus on chromosome 17q12–23. Lancet 1991;338:82.

80. Castilla LH, Couch FJ, Erdos MR, et al. Mutations in the BRCA1 gene in families with early-onset breast and ovarian cancer. Nat Genet 1994;8:387.

81. Friedman LS, Ostermeyer EA, Szabo CI, et al. Confirmation of BRCA1 by analysis of germline mutations linked to breast and ovarian cancer families. Nat Genet 1994;8:392.

82. Simard J, Tonin P, Durocher F, et al. Common origins of BRCA1 mutations in Canadian breast and ovarian cancer families. Nat Genet 1994;8:399.

83. Shattuck-Eidens D, McClure M, Simard J, et al. A collaborative study of 82 mutations in the BRCA1 breast and ovarian cancer susceptibility gene: implications for presymptomatic screening and testing. JAMA 1995;273:535.

84. Smith SA, Easton DF, Evans DGR, et al. Allele losses in the region 17q12–21 in familial breast and ovarian cancer involve the wild-type chromosome. Nat Genet 1991;2:128.

85. Merajver SD, Frank TS, Xu J, et al. Loss of the wild type allele within the BRCA1 candidate region in tumors from early-onset breast/ovarian cancer families. Clin Cancer Res 1995;1:539.

86. Easton DF, Bishop DT, Ford D, et al. Genetic linkage analysis in familial breast and ovarian cancer: results from 214 families. Am J Hum Genet 1993;52:678.

87. Easton DF, Ford D, Bishop DT, et al. Breast and ovarian cancer incidence in BRCA1 mutation carriers. Lancet 1994;343:692.

88. Ford D, Easton DF, Bishop DT, et al. Risk of cancer in BRCA1 mutation carriers. Lancet 1994;343:962.

89. Lynch HT, Marcus J, Watson P, et al. Distinctive clinicopathologic features of BRCA1-linked hereditary breast cancer. Proc ASCO 13:56, 1994.

90. Arason A, Barkardottir RB, Egilsson V. Linkage analysis of chromosome 17 markers and breast–ovarian cancer in Icelandic families and possible relationship to prostatic cancer. Am J Hum Genet 1993;52:711.

91. Stratton MR, Ford D, Neuhausen S, et al. Familial male breast cancer is not linked to the BRCA1 locus on chromosome 17q. Nat Genet 1994;7:103.

92. Wooster R, Neuhausen S, Mangion J, et al. Localization of a breast cancer susceptibility gene, BRCA2, to chromosome 13q12–13. Science 1994;265:2088.

93. Leone A, McBride OW, Weston A, et al. Somatic allelic deletion of nm23 in human cancer. Cancer Res 1991;51:2490.

94. Sato T, Akiyama F, Sakamoto G, et al. Accumulation of genetic alterations and progression of primary breast cancer. Cancer Res 1991;51:5794.

95. Cropp CS, Nevanlinna HA, Pyrhonen S, et al. Evidence for involvement of BRCA1 in sporadic breast carcinomas. Cancer Res 1994;54:2548.

96. Futreal A, Liu Q, Shattuck-Eidens D, et al. BRCA1 mutations in primary breast and ovarian carcinomas. Science 1994;266:120.

97. Li FP, Fraumeni JF Jr. Soft-tissue sarcomas, breast cancer, and other neoplasms: a familial syndrome? Ann Intern Med 1969;71:747.

98. Li FP, Fraumeni JF, Mulvihill JJ, et al. A cancer family syndrome in 24 kindreds. Cancer Res 1988;48:5358.

99. Strong LC, Williams WR, Tainsky MA. The Li-Fraumeni syndrome: from clinical epidemiology to molecular genetics. Am J Epidemiol 1992;135:190.

100. Williams WR, Strong LC. Genetic epidemiology of soft tissue sarcomas in children. In: Muller HR, Weber W, eds. Familial cancer: First International Research Conference. Basel, S Karger, 1985:151.

101. Feunteun J. Personal communication.

102. Srivastava S, Zou Z, Pirollo K, et al. Germline transmission of a mutated p53 gene in a cancer-prone family with Li-Fraumeni syndrome. Nature 1991;348:747.

103. Law JC, Strong LC, Chidambaram A, et al. A germ line mutation in exon 5 of the p53 gene in an extended cancer family. Cancer Res 1991;51:6385.

104. Santibanez-Koref MF, Birch JM, Hartley AL, et al. p53 germline mutations in Li-Fraumeni syndrome. Lancet 1991;338:1490.

105. Srivastava S, Tong YA, Devadas K, et al. Detection of both mutant and wild-type p53 protein in normal skin fibroblasts and demonstration of a shared "second hit" on p53 in diverse tumors from a cancer-prone family with Li-Fraumeni syndrome. Oncogene 1992;7:987.

106. Brugieres L, Gardes M, Moutou C, et al. Screening for germ line p53 mutations in children with malignant tumors and a family history of cancer. Cancer Res 1993;53:452.

107. Sameshima Y, Tsynematsu Y, Watanabe S, et al. Detection of novel germ-line p53 mutations in diverse cancer-prone families identified by selecting patients with childhood adrenalcortical carcinoma. J Natl Cancer Inst 1992;84:703.

108. Frebourg T, Kassel J, Lam KT, et al. Germ-line mutations of the p53 tumor suppressor gene in patients with high risk for cancer inactivate the p53 protein. Proc Natl Acad Sci USA 1992;89:6413.

109. Frebourg T, Barbier N, Kassel J, et al. A functional screen for germ line p53 mutations based on transcriptional activation. Cancer Res 1992;52:6976.

110. Barnes DM, Hanby AM, Gillett CE, et al. Abnormal expression of wild type p53 protein in normal cells of a cancer family patient. Lancet 1992;340:259.

111. Toguchida J, Yamaguchi T, Dayton SH, et al. Prevalence and spectrum of germline mutations of the p53 gene among patients with sarcoma. N Engl J Med 1992;326:1301.

112. Sidransky D, Tolino T, Helzlsouer K, et al. Inherited p53 gene mutations in breast cancer. Cancer Res 1992;52:2984.

113. Borresen A-L, Andersen TI, Garber J, et al. Screening for germ type TP53 mutations in breast cancer patients. Cancer Res 1992;52:3234.

114. Wood DA, Darling HH. A cancer family manifesting multiple occurrences of bilateral carcinoma of the breast. Cancer Res 1943;3:509.

115. Brownstein MH, Wolf M, Bikowski JB. Cowden's disease: a cutaneous marker of breast cancer. Cancer 1978;41:2393.

116. Starink TM. Cowden's disease: analysis of fourteen new cases. J Am Acad Dermatol 1984;11:1127.

117. Muir EG, Yates-Bell AJ, Barlow KA. Multiple primary carcinomata of the colon, duodenum, and larynx associated with keratoacanthomata of the face. Br J Surg 1967;54:191.

118. Hall NR, Williams AT, Murday VA, et al. Muir-Torre syndrome: a variant of the cancer family syndrome. J Med Genet 1994;31:627.

119. Anderson DE. An inherited form of large bowel cancer. Cancer 1980;45:1103.

120. Kinzler KW, Nilber MC, Su LK, et al. Identification of FAP locus genes from chromosome 5q21. Science 1991;253:661.

121. Groden J, Thliveris A, Samowitz W, et al. Identification and characterization of the familial adenomatous polyposis coli gene. Cell 1991;66:589.

122. Papadopoulos N, Nicolaides N, Wei YF, et al. Mutation of mutL homolog in hereditary colon cancer. Science 1994;263:1625.

123. Bronner EC, Baker SM, Morrison PT, et al. Mutation in the DNA mismatch repair gene homologue hMLH1 is associated with hereditary non-polyposis colon cancer. Nature 1994;368:258.

124. Fishel R, Lescoe MK, Rao MRS, et al. The human mutator gene homolog MSH2 and its association with hereditary nonpolyposis colon cancer. Cell 1993;75:1027.

125. Leach FS, Nicolaides N, Papadopoulos N, et al. Mutations of a mutS homolog in hereditary nonpolyposis colon cancer. Cell 1993;75:1215.

126. Swift M, Morrell D, Cromartie E, et al. The incidence and gene frequency of ataxia–telangiectasia in the United States. Am J Hum Genet 1986;39:573.

127. Morrell D, Cromartie E, Swift M. Mortality and cancer incidence in 263 patients with ataxia–telangiectasia. J Natl Cancer Inst 1986;77:89.

128. Swift M, Morrell D, Massey RB, et al. Incidence of cancer in 161 families affected by ataxia–telangiectasia. N Engl J Med 1987; 325:1831.

129. Letters to the Editor. Risk of breast cancer in ataxia–telangectasia. N Engl J Med 1992;326:1357.

130. Cortessis V, Ingles S, Millikan R, et al. Linkage analysis of DRD2, a marker linked to the ataxia–telangiectasia gene, in 64 families with premenopausal bilateral breast cancer. Cancer Res 1993; 53:5083.

131. Wooster R, Ford D, Mangion J, et al. Absence of linkage to the ataxia-telangiectasia locus in familial breast cancer. Hum Genet 1993;92:91–94.

132. Fraccaro M, Lindsten J, Ford CE, et al. The 11q;22q translocation: A European collaborative analysis of 43 cases. Hum Genet 1980;156:21.

133. Zackai EH, Emmanuel BS. Site-specific reciprocal translocation t(11;22)(q23;q11) in several unrelated families with 3:1 meiotic disjunction. Am J Med Genet 1980;7:507.

134. Iselius L, Lindsten J, Aurias A, et al. The 11q;22q translocation: a collaborative study of 20 new cases and analyses of 110 families. Hum Genet 1983;64:343.

135. Lindblom A, Sandelin K, Iselius L, et al. Predisposition for breast

cancer in carriers of constitutional translocation 11q;22q. Am J Hum Genet 1994;54:871.

136. Wellings SR, Jensen HM. On the origin and progression of ductal carcinoma in the human breast. J Natl Cancer Inst 1973;50:111.

137. Black MM, Barclay THC, Cutler SJ, et al. Association of atypical characteristics of benign breast lesions with subsequent risk of cancer. Cancer 1972;29:338.

138. Dupont WD, Page DL. Risk factors for breast cancer in women with proliferative breast disease. N Engl J Med 1985;312:146.

139. Carter CL, Corle DK, Micozzi MS, et al. A prospective study of the development of breast cancer in 16,692 women with benign breast disease. Am J Epidemiol 1988;128:467.

140. Skolnick MH, Cannon-Albright LA, Goldgar DE, et al. Inheritance of proliferative breast disease in breast cancer kindreds. Science 1990;250:1715.

141. Williams WR. Cancer of the male breast: based on the records of 100 cases. Lancet 1889;2:261.

142. Kozak FK, Hall JG, Baird PA. Familial breast cancer in males: a case report and a review of the literature. Cancer 1986;12:2736.

143. Hauser AR, Lerner IJ, King RA. Familial male breast cancer. Am J Med Genet 1992;44:839.

144. Nemoto T, Vana J, Bedwani RN, et al. Management and survival of breast cancer: results of a national survey by the American College of Surgeons. Cancer 1980;45:2917.

145. Rosenblatt KA, Thomas DB, McTiernan A, et al. Breast cancer in men: aspects of familial aggregation. J Natl Cancer Inst 1991;83:849.

146. Cassagrande JT, Hanish RT, Pike MC, et al. A case-control study of male breast cancer. Cancer Res 1988;48:1326.

147. Wooster R, et al. A germline mutation in the androgen receptor in two brothers with breast cancer and Reifenstein syndrome. Nat Genet 1992;2:132.

148. Lobaccaro J-M, et al. Male breast cancer and the androgen receptor gene. Nat Genet 1993;5:109.

149. Anderson DE. Breast cancer in families. Cancer 1977;40:1855.

150. Hoskins KF, Stopfer JE, Calzone KA, et al. Assessment and counseling for familial cancer risk: a guide for clinicians. JAMA 1995;273:577.

151. Anderson DE, Williams WR. Familial cancer: implications for healthy relatives. In: Chaganti RSK, German J, eds. Genetics in clinical oncology. New York, Oxford University, 1985:241.

152. Gail MH, Brinton LA, Byar DP, et al. Projecting individualized probabilities of developing breast cancer for white females who are being examined annually. J Natl Cancer Inst 1989;81:1879.

7.3

Endogenous and Exogenous Hormonal Factors

BRIAN E. HENDERSON ▪ **LESLIE BERNSTEIN**

A substantial body of experimental, clinical, and epidemiologic evidence indicates that hormones play a major role in the etiology of breast cancer.[1,2] The known risk factors for breast cancer can be understood as measures of the cumulative exposure of the breast to estrogen and, perhaps, progesterone (Table 7.3-1). The actions of these ovarian hormones (and the hormones used in combination oral contraceptives [COCs] and hormone replacement therapy [HRT]) on the breast do not appear to be genotoxic, but they do affect the rate of cell division. Their effects on breast cancer rates are thus manifest in their effects on proliferation of the breast epithelial cell. Recent advances in the molecular genetics of cancer have provided a molecular basis for the concept that cell division is essential in the genesis of human cancer.

The activation of oncogenes and the inactivation of tumor-suppressor genes produce a sequence of genetic changes that leads to a malignant phenotype (Fig. 7.3-1). The activation of oncogenes, whether by mutation, translocation, or amplification, requires cell division. Genetic errors that precede the development of a fully malignant tumor also include the loss of inactivation during mitosis of several tumor-suppressor genes that function to control normal cellular behavior.[3–5] Germline mutations have been recently described with one such gene, the BRCA1 gene and have been associated with susceptibility to breast and ovarian cancer in certain kindreds.[6,7] Most of the models currently favored suggest that the first hit is the inactivation by a mutational event of one of the two alleles of a tumor-suppressor gene present in diploid cells, followed by a reduction to homozygosity of the faulty chromosome.[8] The initial mutagenic event and the loss of the wild-type allele of the tumor-suppressor gene (eg, TP53 or BRCA1) both require cell division. Thus, for expression of the full malignant phenotype, cells are absolutely required to divide.

The other genes critical to breast cancer risk are those that control the metabolism of estradiol (eg, 17-hydroxy-

TABLE 7.3-1
Risk Factors and Protective Factors for Breast Cancer

RISK FACTORS (INCREASED EXPOSURE TO ESTROGEN OR PROGESTERONE)

Early menarche

Late menopause

Obesity (postmenopausal women)

Hormone replacement therapy

PROTECTIVE FACTORS (DECREASED EXPOSURE TO ESTROGEN OR PROGESTERONE)

Early first-term pregnancy

Lactation

Physical activity

FIGURE 7.3-1 Estradiol and, to a lesser degree, other steroid hormones (eg, progesterone) drive cell proliferation, which facilitates fixation of genetic errors by loss of heterozygosity or leads to genetic changes that facilitate mutation by defects in DNA repair enzymes. Germline mutations in relevant tumor-suppressor genes accelerate the transformation to the malignant phenotype.

steroid dehydrogenase [17HSD]) and the activity of the estrogen receptor in the breast epithelial cell (Fig. 7.3-2). In breast tissue, at least two forms (types I and II) of 17HSD are present, one of which seems to favor the reductive conversion of estrone to estradiol.[9] The 17HSD type II gene is encoded by two autosomal codominant alleles, and there is some suggestion of an association between differences in exon 6 polymorphisms and the risk of breast cancer in a Finnish population.[10] Whether the 17HSD I gene is a separate or "pseudogene" is still not clear. The estrogen receptor gene is a large gene (more than 140 kb long),[11,12] and several polymorphisms and mutations have been described.[13,14] Substantial polymorphism has been reported for a TA repeat in the upstream promoter region of the gene as well.[15] The functional significance of these and presumably other polymorphisms yet to be described needs to be clarified.

Because endogenous hormones directly affect the risk of breast cancer, reason for concern exists about the effects on breast cancer risk if the same or closely related hor-

mones are administered for therapeutic purposes (eg, as COCs or HRT). It also follows that approaches to the prevention of breast cancer should focus on reducing the lifetime exposure of the breast to estrogen and progesterone, for example, reducing the number of ovulations through exercise or perhaps lowering steroid hormone levels by increasing the fiber content of the diet or by pharmacologic means.

Breast Cancer Risk Factors

AGE AT MENARCHE

Early age at menarche has been demonstrated as a risk factor for breast cancer in most case control studies. In general, about a 20% decrease in breast cancer risk results from each year that menarche is delayed. In a study of young women, we recorded not only age at onset of menstruation, but also age when regular (ie, predictable) menstruation was first established.[16] For a fixed age at menarche, women who established regular menstrual cycles within 1 year of the first menstrual period had more than double the risk of breast cancer of women who had a 5-year or longer delay in onset of regular cycles. Women with early menarche (age 12 or younger) and rapid establishment of regular cycles had an almost fourfold increased risk of breast cancer when compared with women with late menarche (age 13 or older) and long duration of irregular cycles.

These observations suggest that regular ovulatory cycles increase a woman's risk of breast cancer[17] and support results from an earlier study of circulating hormone levels in daughters of breast cancer patients and in age-matched daughters of controls. The daughters of the breast cancer patients, who as a group have at least twice the breast cancer risk of the general population, had higher levels of circulating estrogen and progesterone on day 22 of the

FIGURE 7.3-2 Metabolism and transport of estradiol (E$_2$) in breast epithelial cells. 17 HSD, 17-hydroxysteroid dehydrogenase; E$_1$, estrone.

menstrual cycle than did the controls.[18] This result was later confirmed.[19] Because cumulative estrogen levels are higher during the normal luteal phase than during a comparable period of a nonovulatory cycle, cumulative frequency of ovulatory cycles is an index of cumulative estrogen exposure (and of progesterone exposure as well).

Other supportive evidence for the concept that the cumulative number of ovulatory cycles (ie, cumulative estrogen exposure) is a major determinant of breast cancer risk comes from international studies of the frequency of ovulation in relation to age at menarche and the number of years since menarche in girls aged 15 to 19 years, selected from several populations at varying risk of breast cancer.[20] In all these populations, women with later menarche were more likely to have anovular cycles than women with early menarche, given the same number of elapsed years since menarche. Adjusting for years since menarche, the highest frequency of ovulatory cycles was observed in those populations with the highest breast cancer rates. Apter and Vihko,[21] in a longitudinal study of 200 schoolgirls, also found that those with early menarche established ovulatory cycles more quickly than did girls with later onset of menstruation.

During the past 100 years, age at menarche has progressively decreased both in the United States and in most other areas of the world. A series of extensive cross-sectional studies demonstrated that age at menarche is directly related to childhood growth patterns.[22] Attainment of a critical body weight–height ratio appears necessary for menarche to occur.[23] Chronic malnutrition during childhood delays the age at menarche, whereas the improved nutrition and control of infectious diseases of childhood of the past decades have combined to lower it.

PHYSICAL ACTIVITY

Strenuous physical activity may delay menarche. Girls who engage in regular ballet dancing, swimming, or running have a considerable delay in the onset of menses. In one study, ballet dancers had a mean age at menarche of 15.4

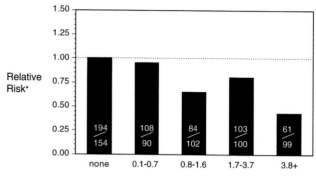

FIGURE 7.3-4 Average hours of physical exercise per week since menarche: breast cancer patients aged 40 years and under (*top number*) and controls (*bottom number*). Relative risk is adjusted for ages at menarche and first full-term pregnancy, number of full-term pregnancies, months of lactation and oral contraceptive use, first-degree family history of breast cancer, and Quetelet's index at reference date. Test for trend: 2-sided $P = .0001$. (Adapted from Bernstein L, Henderson BE, Hanisch R, et al. Physical exercise activity reduces the risk of breast cancer in young women. J Natl Cancer Inst 1994;86:1403)

years, compared with 12.5 years for controls.[24] Breast development was also delayed in the dancers, and they experienced intermittent amenorrhea throughout their teenage years, as long as they remained active dancers. Even moderate physical activity during adolescence can lead to anovular cycles. Girls who engaged in regular, moderate physical activity (averaging at least 600 kcal of energy expended per week) were 2.9 times more likely to be anovular than were girls who engaged in lesser amounts of physical activity[25] (Fig. 7.3-3). More recently, we reported that physical activity in adolescents and adults significantly reduces the risk of breast cancer in young women (up to 40 years of age).[26] The risk of breast cancer among women who averaged 4 or more hours per week of exercise activity during their reproductive years was nearly 60% lower than that of inactive women (Fig. 7.3-4).

AGE AT MENOPAUSE

The relationship between menopause and breast cancer risk has been known for some time. The rate of increase in the age-specific incidence rate of breast cancer slows at menopause, and the rate of increase in the postmenopausal period is only about one sixth the rate of increase in the premenopausal period.

Women who experience natural menopause (defined as cessation of menstrual periods) before age 45 are estimated to have only half the breast cancer risk of those whose menopause occurs after age 55[27] (Table 7.3-2). Another way of expressing this result is that women with 40 or more years of active menstruation have twice the breast cancer risk of those with fewer than 30 years of menstrual activity. Artificial menopause, by either bilateral

FIGURE 7.3-3 Relative risk (adjusted for gynecologic age and age at menarche) of ovulatory menstrual cycles in teenage girls by physical activity. Anovalatory/ovulatory menstrual cycles. Test for trend: 1-sided $P = .03$.

TABLE 7.3-2
Relative Risk of Breast Cancer by Age of Menopause

	Age at Menopause (y)			
	−44	45–49	50–54	55+
Artificial menopause★	0.77	1.00	1.34	—
Natural menopause	1.00	1.27	1.47	2.03

★ Bilateral oophorectomy.

(Trichopoulos D, MacMahon B, Cole P. The menopause and breast cancer risk. J Natl Cancer Inst 1972;48:605)

oophorectomy or pelvic irradiation, also reduces breast cancer risk. The effect appears to be just slightly greater than that of natural menopause, probably because surgical removal of the ovaries causes an abrupt cessation of hormone production, whereas some hormone production continues for a few months or years after the natural cessation of menses at menopause. Feinleib[28] showed that unilateral oophorectomy or simple hysterectomy produced little change in risk.

AGE AT FIRST FULL-TERM PREGNANCY

MacMahon and colleagues[29] made a major advance in our understanding of the role of pregnancy in altering breast cancer risk through their analysis of an international collaborative case-control study. Single and nulliparous married women were found to have the same increased risk of breast cancer, about 1.4 times the risk of parous married women. Among married women in each country, parous cases had fewer children than parous controls. These investigators clearly demonstrated, however, that this protective effect of parity was totally due to a protective effect of

early age at first birth. Those women with a first birth under age 20 years had about half the risk of nulliparous women. Controlling for age at first birth, subsequent births had no influence on the risk of developing breast cancer. More recent studies in other populations have observed a small residual protective effect of an increasing number of births, suggesting that, under certain circumstances, multiparity does offer some further protection. In a study in Shanghai, we observed a protective effect of multiple pregnancies that was most notable after the fifth pregnancy[30] (Table 7.3-3). The main protective effect is, however, undoubtedly associated with first full-term pregnancy.

Married women who have a late first full-term pregnancy are actually at an elevated risk of breast cancer, compared with nulliparous women.[29] This paradoxic effect of a late first full-term pregnancy has been confirmed repeatedly. A possible explanation for this effect is suggested by several related observations. In a hospital-based case-control study, the risk of breast cancer was substantially higher among women who had given birth during the 3 years before interview than among comparable women whose last birth occurred 10 years earlier (relative risk [RR], 2.66).[31] Further, we found that a first-trimester abortion, whether spontaneous or induced, before the first full-term pregnancy was associated with an increased risk of breast cancer.[32] This observation was confirmed in cohorts of Connecticut and New York women.[33,34]

We concluded that pregnancy has two contradictory effects on breast cancer risk that are particularly notable in the first pregnancy. This apparent paradox actually has a physiologic explanation based on estrogen secretion and metabolism during pregnancy. During the first trimester of pregnancy, the level of free estradiol rises rapidly, an effect that is more apparent in the first than in subsequent pregnancies.[35] The net effect of this early part of pregnancy, in terms of estrogen exposure to the breast, is equivalent to several ovulatory cycles over a relatively short time.

TABLE 7.3-3
Relative Risk of Breast Cancer by Number of Full-Term Pregnancies Among Parous Cases and Controls

Number of Full-Term Pregnancies	Cases	Controls	RR (95% Confidence Limits)	Adjusted RR★ (95% Confidence Limits)
1	116	77	1.00	1.00
2	113	100	0.61 (0.39, 0.96)	0.72 (0.45, 1.16)
3	78	74	0.47 (0.28, 0.79)	0.67 (0.38, 1.21)
4	55	61	0.33 (0.11, 0.34)	0.59 (0.30, 1.16)
5+	67	117	0.19 (0.11, 0.34)	0.39 (0.19, 0.80)

RR, relative risk.

★ Adjusted for age at menarche, age at first full-term pregnancy, parity, family history of breast cancer, and use of contraceptives.

(Yuan JM, Yu MC, Ross RK, et al. Risk factors for breast cancer in Chinese women in Shanghai. Cancer Res 1988;48,1949.)

In the long run, however, this negative effect of early pregnancy on breast cancer risk can be overridden by two beneficial consequences of a completed pregnancy. Several years ago, we reported that prolactin levels were substantially lower in parous compared with nulliparous women,[36] an observation that has been replicated.[37] In addition, we found that parous women had higher levels of sex hormone–binding globulin (SHBG) and lower levels of free (non–protein-bound) estradiol than their nulliparous counterparts[38] (Table 7.3-4).

LACTATION

Lactation has been increasingly reported to protect against breast cancer development. If the cumulative number of ovulatory cycles is directly related to breast cancer risk, a beneficial effect of long duration of nursing would be expected, because nursing results in a substantial delay in reestablishing ovulation following a completed pregnancy. With only a small proportion of mothers having a large cumulative number of nursing months, most previous epidemiologic studies have been unable to provide precise estimates of the effects of lactation on breast cancer risk.

TABLE 7.3-4
Geometric Mean Levels of Plasma and Urinary Hormones (Day 11) and Relevant Characteristics of Nulliparous and Parous Women With 24- to 32-Day Menstrual Cycles at Time of Sampling

Variable	Nulliparous Women (N = 59)	Parous Women (N = 47)	P Value*
PLASMA HORMONE			
Prolactin (ng/mL)	23.2	17.1	.001
E_1 (ng/dL)	8.7	8.0	.079
E_2 (ng/dL)	14.8	12.0	.001
SHBG (10^{-8} M)	3.8	4.2	.099
URINARY HORMONE *(pg/12 H)*			
E_1	4.9	4.0	.018
E_2	2.6	2.1	.008
E_3	5.7	4.6	.029
$E_1 + E_2 + E_3$	13.7	11.1	.010
CHARACTERISTIC			
Age (y)	33.3	33.3	.499
Weight (lb)	137.9	134.1	.200
Cycle length (d)	28.2	28.0	.307

E, estrone; E_2, estradiol; E_3, estrial; SHBG, sex hormone–binding globulin.

* One-sided significance levels after adjustment by analysis of covariance for cycle length (days) and age (years) and, in addition, for weight for SHBG.

(Bernstein L, Pike MC, Ross RK, et al. Estrogen and sex hormone–binding globulin levels in nulliparous and parous women. J Natl Cancer Inst 1985;74:741)

We recently completed a population-based case control study in China, a population in which long-duration nursing is the norm. In that study, a progressive reduction in breast cancer risk was observed with an increasing number of years of nursing experience[30,39] (Fig. 7.3-5).

WEIGHT

In addition to the menstrual and reproductive risk factors described in the foregoing sections, a strong relation exists between weight and breast cancer risk. The relation is critically dependent on age. Women under age 50 years have little or no increased risk associated with increased weight, but by age 60 years, a 10-kg increment in weight results in approximately an 80% increase in breast cancer risk[40] (Table 7.3-5).

Whether this weight effect is one of excess weight (body fat) or weight itself is unclear. Contradictory results have been reported, for example, on whether the Quetelet index (a measure of body mass) is correlated with breast cancer risk. Unadjusted weight appears to be as good an indicator of risk as any function of weight and height. In the postmenopausal period, the major source of estrogen is from extraglandular (largely adipose tissue) conversion of the adrenal androgen, androstenedione, to estrone.[41]

MODEL OF BREAST CANCER PATHOGENESIS

Pike and coworkers[42] developed a model of breast cancer incidence that incorporates all the reproductive and endocrine risk factors and provides an excellent fit to the actual age-specific incidence curves for breast cancer in different populations (Figs. 7.3-6 and 7.3-7). This model is based on the concept that breast cancer incidence does not increase proportionally with calendar age, but rather with breast tissue age raised to the power 4.5. The concept of breast tissue age is closely associated with the cell kinetics of breast tissue stem cells, which, in turn, are closely associated with exposure of breast tissue to ovarian hormones.

The model predicts relative risks that are remarkably consistent with the observed values for each of these risk factors, including the two contradictory effects of pregnancy. This model allows us to explore the degree to which variations in these risk factors among different populations may explain the large international variation in breast cancer rates, such as those between Japan and the United States.

As of 1970, age-adjusted incidence rates of breast cancer were five to six times higher in the United States than in Japan. Data on average age at menarche, first birth, and menopause among Japanese women are available from a 1970 survey.[43] The average age at natural menopause of Japanese women is similar to that of American women for these age groups, but fewer Japanese women had a surgical menopause. The data on menarche favor a lower breast cancer incidence rate in Japanese women: older Japanese women had a much later menarche than American women, but the data on age at first birth and nulliparity show that none of the decreased breast cancer rates in Japan can be attributed to these factors.

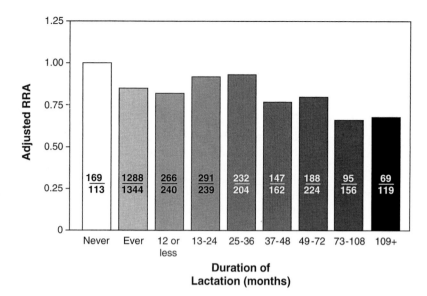

FIGURE 7.3-5 Duration of lactation among parous breast cancer patients (*top number*) and controls (*bottom number*) in China. RRA, relative risk adjusted for age at menarche, age at first full-term pregnancy, family history of breast cancer, and use of oral contraceptives. Test for trend: 2-sided $P < .01$. (Yuan JM, Yu MC, Ross RK, et al. Risk factors for breast cancer in Chinese women in Shanghai. Cancer Res 1988;48:1949)

Japanese breast cancer rates remain almost constant after age 50 years.[43] In model terms, this implies that no further breast tissue aging occurs in Japanese women in the postmenopausal period, probably as a reflection of body weight. In 1970, the average weight of postmenopausal women was less than 50 kg, and these women were unlikely to have been producing significant amounts of estrogen.

The model-predicted breast cancer incidence rates of Japanese women, which allow for their actual distribution of the established breast cancer risk factors, are still considerably lower than the observed rates for white women in the United States, whereas they are between 2.4- and 3.8-fold higher than observed Japanese rates. The late menarche in Japanese women would be expected to result in a substantial delay in the establishment of regular menstrual cycles compared with US women. Allowing for this delay, and incorporating the differences in average cycle length and the lower estrogen levels (see later) actually achieved during a typical ovulatory cycle in Asian women compared with US white women, the predicted Japanese rates are essentially identical to those observed in white women in the United States.

Endogenous Hormones

ESTROGEN

The association of breast cancer with cyclic ovarian activity implies that estrogen is important in the pathogenesis of this disease. We have discussed the rationale that hormones, and, in particular, estradiol, can directly increase the incidence of breast cancer.[2] A substantial amount of experimental work demonstrates the critical role of estrogens in breast cancer in experimental animals. Exogenous estrone, estradiol, and, under some conditions, estriol increase the incidence of mammary tumors in mice and rats. They also increase the tumor yield and decrease the time to induction following administration of dimethylbenzanthracine. Removing the ovaries or administering an antiestrogenic drug has the opposite effect.[44]

Attempts to understand and to quantify the role of estrogen in breast cancer development have been limited, to some extent, by our technical capability for measuring steroid hormones in human blood. A few studies of estrogen levels in premenopausal patients and controls had been reported. England and coworkers found a 15% average elevation of plasma total estrogens in patients with breast cancer,[45] and a similar increase was reported by others for total urinary estrogens.[20,45] Problems with such studies have been discussed. In particular, in some studies, urine collection was neither done on a fixed day of the cycle nor in a similar manner for cases and controls.[46] Moreover, close age matching is probably required in the premenopausal period.

The first substantial study of plasma estrogen levels in postmenopausal breast cancer patients and controls was

TABLE 7.3-5
Relative Risk of Breast Cancer by Body Weight

	Weight (kg)		
Age at Diagnosis (y)	<60	60–69	70+
35–49	1	0.94	1.16
50–59	1	1.22	1.43
60–69	1	1.61	1.81

(De Waard F, Cornelis J, Aoki K, et al. Breast cancer incidence according to weight and height in two cities of the Netherlands and in Aichi Prefecture, Japan. Cancer 1977;40:1269)

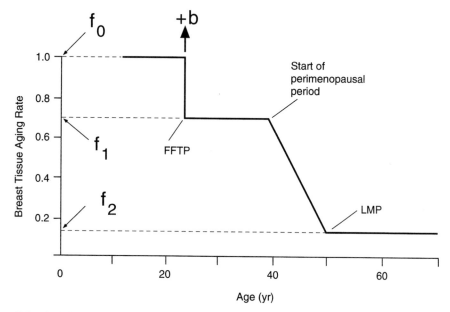

FIGURE 7.3-6 Model of rate of breast tissue aging. For most hormone-dependent cancers, the relation between incidence, I, and age, t, can be represented by the equation $I(t) = at^k$, which produces a straight line with slope k when the logarithm of incidence is plotted against the logarithm of age (t). Breast cancer incidence can be reconciled with a linear log-log plot of incidence against age if t in the formula is considered to be the cumulative effective mitotic rate of the breast epithelium. The fundamental idea is that aging of the breast relates directly to its cell kinetics. When the tissue is not undergoing cell division, the rate of aging is zero, whereas aging is maximum when the mitotic rate is maximal. To adapt the equation to breast cancer incidence, a simple model assumes that aging begins at menarche with rate $f_0 = 1$, is modified by first full-term pregnancy (FFTP) to $f_1 = .7$, is reduced further by the onset of the perimenopause at age 40, and eventually slows at the last menstrual period (LMP) to $f_2 = .1$. A small increase in risk of the initial part of pregnancy as mentioned in the text is represented by the value b. The value of k is set at 4.5. (Pike MC, Krailo MD, Henderson BE, et al. "Hormonal" risk factors, "breast tissue age" and the age incidence of breast cancer. Nature 1983;303:767)

reported by England and associates.[45] They studied the estradiol levels of 25 cases and 25 controls and found that, on average, the levels were 30% higher in cases. At least 12 additional studies have been conducted on plasma estrogens and 7 on urinary estrogens in postmenopausal breast cancer cases and controls.[46] Taken together, these studies support the finding of increased levels of estrogen and, in particular, estradiol reported by England and associates.[45]

Recent findings emphasize the possible importance of bioavailable estradiol fractions in the etiology of breast cancer. Siiteri and colleagues[41] studied a small group of breast cancer patients and controls matched on age, weight, height, and menopausal status; they found the known relations among obesity, SHBG, and increased free estradiol in both patients and controls. They also found that some normal-weight breast cancer patients with normal SHBG levels had an elevated percentage of free estradiol. These results suggest that in breast cancer patients, free estradiol in serum may be elevated by factors unrelated to SHBG concentration.

Moore and coauthors[47] compared total and non–protein-bound estradiol levels of 38 postmenopausal women with breast cancer with those of 38 controls of similar age and weight. Breast cancer patients had significantly higher levels of total estradiol and free estradiol than controls, and significantly less SHBG. In fact, the level of free estradiol in patients was nearly 4 times that of controls. Jones and coworkers[48] reported similar results comparing 32 women with breast cancer and 188 controls. The mean percentage of free estradiol and the percentage of albumin-bound estradiol were significantly higher in the patients.

The most careful international studies comparing estrogen levels in populations at differing risks of breast cancer also support a role of estrogens, particularly estradiol, in the pathogenesis of breast cancer. In the early 1970s, Mac-Mahon and associates[49] conducted a series of studies on teenagers and young women to investigate whether some aspect of estrogen metabolism was responsible for the large differences in breast cancer rates between Asia and North America. These investigators found that, in overnight urine samples collected on the morning of day 21 of the menstrual cycle, total urinary estrogen levels were 36% higher in the North American teenagers. In nulliparous women aged 20 to 24 years, total urinary estrogen levels were 49% higher on day 21 and 38% higher on day 10; similar differences were found among parous women aged 30 to 39 years. In two more recent studies, we characterized the relationship between serum estradiol levels and the international differences in breast cancer risk.[50,51] Geo-

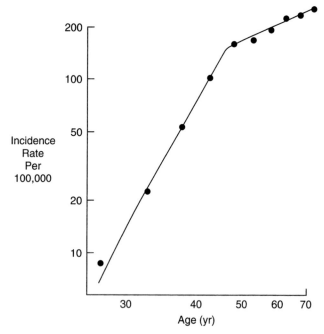

FIGURE 7.3-7 Age-specific incidence rates for breast cancer in US white women (Third National Cancer Survey, National Cancer Institute, 1969-1971). The dots are the actual incidence data, and the solid line marks the expected incidence rates calculated from the model in Figure 7.3-6.

metric mean estradiol levels were higher in breast cancer patients than in controls in Shanghai and Los Angeles, and estradiol levels were 20% higher in Los Angeles compared with Shanghai controls[50] (Table 7.3-6). In a comparison of postmenopausal women, the differences were even more striking, with estradiol levels 36% higher in Los Angeles

women than in their age-matched Japanese counterparts.[51] At least two possible explanations exist for these differences in estradiol levels: (1) physical activity, such as greater physical activity among Asians, that might alter the frequency of ovulatory cycles; and (2) higher dietary fiber intake in Asians, which might alter fecal excretion of enterohepatric steroids and thereby lower plasma estradiol levels.[52,53]

Much interest has focused on the issue of the relation of increased breast cancer risk and exposure to dietary phytoestrogens[54] and certain organochlorine compounds (particularly those commonly used in pesticides) and, possibly, other halogenated compounds.[55] The assumed mechanism by which these compounds influence breast cancer risk is their estrogenic effects. The observed estrogenicity of these compounds is relatively low, however. Hence, investigators have suggested that these compounds would provide only a small increase in exposure to estrogen among women. Investigators have proposed that differences in two alternative pathways of estradiol metabolism are associated with risk of breast cancer, with 16-α-hydroxylation (versus 2-hydroxylation) associated with elevated risk.[56,57] Metabolites resulting from these two metabolic pathways differ in biologic properties: 16-α-hydroxyestrone (16-OHE1) is a potent estrogen, whereas 2-hydroxyestrone (2-OHE1) is not. Several small studies have suggested that the extent of 16-α-hydroxyla-tion is greater among breast cancer patients than among controls.[56–58] Highly trained athletes who are amenorrheic also appear to metabolize more readily along the 2-hydroxylation pathway.[59] Although not all researchers agree that 16-α-hydroxylation is the critical pathway for breast cancer risk,[60,61] variations in estrogen metabolism could substantially influence the estrogenic effects of phytoestrogens and organochlorine compounds.

TABLE 7.3-6
Geometric Mean Values (With 95% Confidence Intervals) for Serum Estradiol and SHBG on Premenopausal Women With Breast Cancer and Individually Matched Control Women in Shanghai (39 Pairs) and Los Angeles (42 Pairs)

Variable	Study Group	Cases	Controls	P Value* Case Versus Control
Estradiol (pmol/L)	Shanghai Chinese	584 (509–671)	501 (444–565)	.089
	Los Angeles whites	669 (586–761)	604 (530–687)	.23
	P value* (control comparison)		0.036	
SHBG (nmol/L)	Shanghai Chinese	59.4 (50.3–70.2)	61.6 (55.4–68.6)	.71
	Los Angeles whites	54.1 (46.4–63.0)	59.1 (51.5–68.0)	.28
	P value* (control comparison)		0.63	

SHBG, sex hormone–binding globulin.

* Two-sided P value; paired *t*-test for matched case control comparisons and Student's *t*-test for comparison of controls.

(Bernstein L, Yuan JM, Ross RK, et al. Serum hormone levels in premenopausal Chinese women in Shanghai and white women in Los Angeles: results from two breast cancer case-control studies. Cancer Causes Control 1990;1:51)

PROGESTERONE

Evidence that elevated levels of the other major ovarian hormone, progesterone, may also be an important factor in increasing breast cancer risk has been summarized.[62] The mitotic activity of breast epithelium varies during the normal menstrual cycle, with peak activity occurring late in the luteal phase.[63,64] This finding suggests that progesterone, at least in the presence of estrogen, induces mitotic activity in breast epithelium. This effect of progesterone would be in sharp contrast to its effect on endometrial tissue, in which peak mitotic activity occurs in the estrogen-dominated follicular phase of the cycle. It strongly agrees, however, with the experimental findings that progesterone induces ductal growth in rodent breast tissue.[65] If progesterone does increase breast cancer risk, then regular ovulatory cycles should be more common in breast cancer patients than in controls. Breast cancer patients would be expected to have shorter cycles, on average, than controls, because differences in cycle length are almost completely due to differences in the length of the follicular phase. In ovulatory menstrual cycles, the shorter the cycle length, the greater the proportion of time a women spends in the luteal phase, with its associated high progesterone levels.[66] Although few studies have addressed these issues, they all provide support for this role for progesterone.[18,67]

Several studies have measured progesterone, or its major urinary metabolite pregnanediol, in premenopausal women. All four studies of pregnanediol, and five of six studies of progesterone, found lower levels in breast cancer patients than in controls.[62] Reason exists to suspect that early in the clinical course of breast cancer, the regularity of ovulation is disrupted, however, so such case-control comparisons may be misleading.[50] Furthermore, progesterone levels during the luteal phase are difficult to quantitate with spot samples, because the amount of progesterone detected in plasma or the amount of progesterone metabolites in urine depends specifically on the day of sampling in relation to the luteal phase peak. Yet, three prospective studies examined breast cancer incidence in women with clinical evidence of progesterone deficiency, and all reported elevated risks.[62] Thus, overall, little objective evidence supports the role of progesterone in the pathogenesis of breast cancer. More direct evidence to support or refute the role of progesterone should come from surveillance of women receiving medroxyprogesterone as a form of contraception or HRT.

Exogenous Hormones

ORAL CONTRACEPTIVES

Oral contraceptives have been widely used since the early 1960s. By 1978, the World Health Organization (WHO) estimated that more than 80 million women throughout the world had been exposed to these drugs. A substantial body of literature now exists on the relation between COC use and risk of breast cancer.[68] Although results have been published for 7 cohort studies and more than 20 case-control studies, the possible relationship between COC use and breast cancer continues to be controversial.[69-71] If one can draw any conclusion from these studies, it is that COCs do not protect against breast cancer.

Few studies have examined the association of COC use and breast cancer risk among perimenopausal women; only recently would this age group have had sufficient exposure to examine the effects of duration of COC use. Three of six studies that investigated the association of breast cancer risk and COC use in women over age 45 years at diagnosis show a positive association, but none is statistically significant (including the study by Kay,[72] in which COC users had 70% higher risk of breast cancer than nonusers, but which does not permit the calculation of a percentage of change in breast cancer risk per year of use)[73] (Table 7.3-7). The five studies that included information on duration of use are statistically consistent with each other, and overall, show no increase in breast cancer risk. What cannot be easily discerned from these studies is the effect on breast cancer risk from COC use during the perimenopausal years. One can argue that COC use during the perimenopausal period may increase breast cancer risk if COCs provide greater hormonal exposure to estrogens and progestogens than would occur naturally at this time, thereby masking the onset of menopause by producing a hormonal state approximating that of normal ovulation.

Numerous studies of younger women have been conducted to evaluate the risk of breast cancer associated with long-term use of COCs. To assess this relation adequately, women participating in case-control or cohort studies must have had access to COCs during the early years of their reproductive lives. Because oral contraceptives first became available during the 1960s, only studies completed during the 1980s or later, which evaluated risk for young women (under age 45 years) would have been adequate to assess risk associated with long-term use. The results of hospital-based case-control studies are not considered here because the magnitude of potential bias in such studies is large in relation to the size of the fairly modest COC–breast cancer association. Eight population-based studies conducted in the 1980s that evaluated total COC use and breast cancer risk among women younger than age 45 years at diagnosis are summarized in Table 7.3-8. All eight studies show an increased breast cancer risk among COC users. Although the results of the study by Kay[72] do not permit the calculation of percentage of change in risk per year of COC use, the risk comparing COC users with those who never took COCs was 1.1. The combined results of the remaining seven studies show a statistically significant 3.1% increase in breast cancer risk per year of COC use. Based on this analysis, young women who had taken COCs for 10 years had a 36% higher risk of breast cancer than women who had never used COCs (RR, 1.36).

The five case-control studies considered in Table 7.3-8 also provide data on breast cancer risk associated with COC use before first birth.[73] Of the four studies that found a positive association,[85-88] three were statistically significant[85,87,88] (Table 7.3-9). The duration effects of

TABLE 7.3-7
Population-Based Studies of Total Oral Contraceptive Use and Breast Cancer Risk in Women Over Age 45 Years

Investigators	Type of Study	Age Range (y)	Cases/Controls	Percentage of Controls Ever Exposed	Percentage of Change in Breast Cancer per Year of COC Use (95% Confidence Limits)	Relative Risk for 10 Years of COC Use
Brinton[74,a]	Case-control	—	962/858	22	+1.2 (−7.0, 10.2)	1.13
Stadel et al.[75,b]	Case-control	45–54	1021/883	52	−0.6 (−2.8, 1.7)	0.94
Paul et al.[76,c]	Case-control	45–54	242/327	63	−2.7 (−6.6, 1.2)	0.76
Kay[72,d]	Cohort	45–64	44/—	44	—	—
Vessey[77,e]	Cohort	45–64	63/—	32	−5.7 (−11.1, 0.0)	0.56
Romieu et al.[78,f]	Cohort	45–64	1301/—	30	+2.4 (−0.4, 5.2)	1.27
Weighted average[g]					−0.3 (−1.8, 1.2)	0.97

COC, combination oral contraceptives.

[a] Update of study by Brinton and coworkers.[79] All ages, 14.6% under age 45. Confidence limits calculated from crude analysis of published data because no "adjusted" trend statistic quoted in the paper.

[b] US Cancer and Steroid Hormone (CASH) study; other references are Centers for Disease Controls[80] and Wingo and coworkers.[81] The results shown in table are limited to parous women. Confidence limits calculated from crude analysis of published data because no adjusted trend statistic quoted in the paper.

[c] Update of certain aspects of this New Zealand study reported by Paul and coworkers.[82] Confidence limits calculated from crude analysis of published data because no adjusted trend statistic quoted in the paper.

[d] No data given on duration of use. The relative risk for ever use of COCs is 1.7 (0.3, 10.4).

[e] Update of study reported by Vessey and coworkers.[83]

[f] Update of study by Lipnick and coworkers.[84] Confidence limits calculated from crude analysis of published data because "adjusted" trend statistic not quoted in the paper.

[g] P value for heterogeneity is .12; if heterogeneity is considered significant, the best estimate of weighted average percentage of change is −0.8 (−3.3, 1.8). Relative risk for 10 years of COC use is 0.92.

(Pike M, Bernstein L, Spicer D: Exogenous hormones and breast cancer risk. In: Neiderhuber J, ed. Current therapy in oncology. St Louis, BC Decker, 1993)

these five studies are statistically consistent. Combined analysis of these studies shows that, on average, breast cancer risk increased 3.8% per year of COC use before first birth. This translates into an RR of 1.45 for women who took COCs for 10 years before their first birth, when compared with women with no such COC use. Based on the results in Tables 7.3-8 and 7.3-9, the effect of COC use before first birth in unlikely to differ from that after first birth. Two studies specifically investigated this issue and found little evidence of any difference.[85,87]

For COC use by women at high risk of breast cancer, no clear picture emerges. For example, within a breast cancer detection program, Brinton and coworkers reported that among women who had a sister with breast cancer, COC users were at higher risk of breast cancer than nonusers[79]; however, no increased risk was found among COC users whose mothers had a diagnosis of breast cancer. Results of studies that have examined the risk of breast cancer associated with COC use in women with benign breast disease are also inconsistent.

INJECTABLE CONTRACEPTIVES

Depot medroxyprogesterone acetate (DMPA), a progestogen, is a long-acting injectable contraceptive that has been used worldwide since the mid-1960s. It was not licensed for use in the United States until 1992 because of concerns

about a possible breast cancer risk. This concern stems, in part, from the results of animal studies that found increased numbers of malignant breast nodules in female beagle dogs,[93,94] as well as a high incidence of mammary tumors in female BALB/c mice treated with DMPA.[95]

Epidemiologic data related to breast cancer risk associated with DMPA use are limited. Early studies of the association are difficult to interpret because of design limitations; they were based on small samples, limited DMPA exposure, or inadequate comparison groups. Lee and associates[96] reported a statistically significant increased risk of breast cancer associated with DMPA use (RR, 2.6) in a study conducted in Costa Rica. Risk was elevated for all durations of use evaluated up to 6 years (less than 12 months, RR, 2.3; 12 to 23 months, 4.4; 24 to 71 months, 3.4). The results of this study have been questioned because the case response rate was only 66%, raising concern that selection bias may have produced spurious results.

Two studies, one conducted at five centers in three developing countries[97] and the other conducted in New Zealand,[98] showed no overall association between DMPA use and breast cancer, but both found some evidence of increased risk among women diagnosed before age 35 years, among recent users of DMPA, and among women who had used DMPA before 25 years of age. Both studies had similar prevalences of DMPA use among controls (just under 14%). The WHO Collaborative Study of Neoplasia

TABLE 7.3-8
Population–Based Studies of Total Oral Contraceptive Use and Breast Cancer Risk in Young Women

Investigators	Type of Study	Age Range (y)	Cases/Controls	Percentage of Controls Ever Exposed	Percentage of Change in Breast Cancer per Year of COC Use (95% Confidence Limits)	Relative Risk for 10 Years of COC Use
Bernstein et al.[85,a]	Case-control	≤36	439/439	85	+5.9 (1.5, 10.4)	1.77
Stadel et al.[86,b]	Case-control	≤44	1348/1307	82	+1.4 (−1.6, 4.5)	1.15
Paul et al.[82,c]	Case-control	≤44	191/570	88	+0.1 (−3.9, 4.3)	1.01
Meirik et al.[87,d]	Case-control	≤44	422/527	70	+3.6 (0.3, 6.9)	1.42
UK NCCSG[88,e]	Case-control	≤35	755/755	89	+8.6 (4.7, 12.7)	2.28
Kay[72,f]	Cohort	≤44	80/—	61	—	–
Vessey[77,g]	Cohort	≤44	126/—	62	+0.7 (−3.7, 5.3)	1.07
Romieu et al.[78,h]	Cohort	≤44	441/—	65	+1.4 (−2.6, 5.6)	1.15
Weighted average[i]					+3.1 (1.7, 4.6)	1.36

COC, combination oral contraceptives.

[a] Update of Los Angeles study reported by Pike and coworkers.[32,89]

[b] US Cancer and Steroid Hormone (CASH) study; other references are Centers for Disease Controls[80] and Wingo and coworkers.[81] The results shown in table are limited to parous women. Confidence limits calculated from crude analysis of published data because no adjusted trend statistic quoted in the paper.

[c] Update of New Zealand study reported by Paul and coworkers.[76]

[d] Update of this Swedish and Norwegian study may be found in Lund and coworkers.[90]

[e] See also Chilvers.[91]

[f] No data given on duration of use. The relative risk for ever use of COCs is 1.1 (0.8, 1.6).

[g] Update of study reported by Vessey and coworkers.[92]

[h] Confidence limits calculated from crude analysis of published data because adjusted trend statistic not quoted in the paper.

[i] P value for heterogeneity is .047; if heterogeneity is considered significant, the best estimate of weighted average percentage change is +3.1 (0.9, 5.4). Relative risk for 10 years of COC use is 1.36.

(Pike M, Bernstein L, Spicer D: Exogenous hormones and breast cancer risk. In: Neiderhuber J, ed. Current therapy in oncology. St Louis, BC Decker, 1993)

and Steroid Contraceptives, a hospital-based case control study, reported on 869 breast cancer patients and 11,890 controls.[97] The risk of breast cancer did not increase with increased duration of DMPA use, nor did it increase among women who had begun using DMPA more than 5 years previously. Among women under age 35 years, however, breast cancer risk was elevated (RR, 1.5), particularly among those who had begun DMPA use within the previous 4 years (RR, 2.2). Paul and colleagues[98] reported results of a population-based case-control study of breast cancer conducted among 891 patients and 1864 controls aged 25 to 54 years. A two-fold increased risk of breast cancer associated with DMPA use was observed in the youngest age group of women (25 to 34 years of age). Among women who had had 2 to 5 years of DMPA use before age 25 years, risk was significantly elevated (RR, 4.6). The 25- to 34-year age group also had a significantly elevated risk of breast cancer associated with COC use,[82] but adjustment for COC use did not affect the DMPA results.

If estrogens alone are a cause of breast cancer, then one would expect that DMPA would decrease breast cancer risk, because the regimen prevents ovulation and does not include any exposure to exogenous estrogen. After the administration of DMPA, estradiol levels vary between 20 and 50 pg/mL; these levels are slightly lower than normal early follicular phase levels.[99,100] The results of the foregoing epidemiologic studies suggest that DMPA offers no protection against breast cancer; one explanation for these observations is that progesterone (or progestins) plays some role in stimulating breast cell growth. These results are also consistent with the finding that progesterone and its synthetic analogues have no effect on the breast.

HORMONE REPLACEMENT THERAPY

More than 30 million postmenopausal women live in the United States. The advisability of long-term use of estrogen replacement therapy for such women remains controversial. Nonetheless, by the mid-1970s, over 28 million prescriptions of noncontraceptive estrogens were being filled annually in the United States. Concerns about the carcinogenic potential of estrogen replacement therapy on the endometrium, however, led to a 50% decline in the number of estrogen prescriptions by 1980.[101] Hence, a cyclic estrogen–progestogen regimen became widely recommended and prescribed. By 1983, prescriptions of estrogen had increased once again.

TABLE 7.3-9
*Population-Based Case Control Studies of Total Oral Contraceptive Use
Before First Full-Term Pregnancy and Breast Cancer Risk in Young Women*

Investigators	Type of Study	Age Range (y)	Cases/Controls	Percentage of Controls Ever Exposed	Percentage of Change in Breast Cancer per Year of COC Use (95% Confidence Limits)	Relative Risk for 10 Years of COC Use
Bernstein et al.[85,a]	Case-control	≤36	439/439	54	+2.4 (−3.5, 8.6)	1.27
Stadel et al.[86,b]	Case-control	≤44	1005/987	67	+2.5 (−2.1, 7.4)	1.28
Paul et al.[82,c]	Case-control	≤44	191/570	52	−7.7 (−18.8, 4.9)	0.45
Meirik et al.[87,d]	Case-control	≤44	422/527	36	+2.7 (−2.9, 8.6)	1.31
UK NCCSG[88,e]	Case-control	≤35	755/755	62	+10.8 (4.8, 17.2)	2.79
Weighted average[f]					+3.8 (1.1, 6.6)	1.45

COC, combination oral contraceptives; UK NCCSG, United Kingdom National Case-Control Study Group.

[a] Update of Los Angeles study reported by Pike and coworkers.[32,89]

[b] US Cancer and Steroid Hormone (CASH) study; other references are Centers for Disease Controls[80] and Wingo and coworkers.[81]

[c] Update of New Zealand study reported by Paul and coworkers.[76]

[d] Update of this Swedish and Norwegian study may be found in Lund and coworkers.[90]

[e] See also Chilvers[91] and UK NCCSG.[88]

[f] *P* value for heterogeneity is .11; if heterogeneity is considered significant, the best estimate of weighted average is +3.4 (−0.8, 7.8). Relative risk for 10 years of COC use is 1.40.

(Pike M, Bernstein L, Spicer D: Exogenous hormones and breast cancer risk. In: Neiderhuber J, ed. Current therapy in oncology. St Louis, BC Decker, 1993)

The most commonly prescribed HRT for menopausal women in the United States includes conjugated equine estrogens (CEE), with a preferred dose of 0.625 mg/d for 25 days in a 28-day treatment cycle. This dose is lower than those commonly prescribed during the 1970s. Progestogens, usually 10 mg/d of medroxyprogesterone acetate, are added during days 14 to 25.

Most early studies of the possible effects of estrogen replacement on risk of breast cancer were uncontrolled follow-up studies. The most credible cohort study was done by Hoover and coworkers.[102] Although these investigators reported only a 25% excess of breast cancer in their cohort of menopausal estrogen users, compared with the number expected based on general population rates (49 observed versus 39 expected), they did report a more substantial excess among women using high doses over a long time.

Early case-control studies that reported findings on menopausal estrogens and breast cancer were often limited by small numbers, insufficient data on dose and duration of use, and definite possibility of bias. A new round of carefully conducted case-control studies using healthy population controls and results of large cohort studies have been published. Overall, these studies found small to moderate increases in breast cancer risk after long-term use, although some variation exists across studies for ovarian status (intact versus removed) or antecedent surgical menopause.

Table 7.3-10 shows the results of 10 population-based epidemiologic studies of the use of HRT and breast cancer risk.[73] Nine of these studies show a positive association, and the results of 5 are statistically significant. Because the risk estimates from each of these studies are statistically significantly different from each other, the combined analysis allows for heterogeneity.[103] Based on these studies, the average annual increase in breast cancer risk is 3.1% per year of HRT. For women with 10 years of HRT, the risk of breast cancer is 1.36 times that of women who have never used these preparations. The studies conducted in the United States allow the estimation of breast cancer risk associated with use of a standard CEE dose of 0.625 mg/d[104–110]; based on these studies, the increase in breast cancer risk is estimated to be 2.2% per year of HRT. In fact, this figure may be an underestimation because some of these studies made inadequate adjustment for age at menopause. This would tend to produce estimates of breast cancer risk that are too low because the use of HRT is associated with early menopause, which is a protective factor for breast cancer.

On the basis of these population-based studies (see Table 7.3-10), we can conclude that long-term use of estrogen replacement therapy does carry with it an increase in breast cancer risk, although short-term use is not associated with such an increase. These results essentially agree with those of other published metaanalyses, which examined duration of use and breast cancer risk.[114–116] The estimated 2.2% increase in breast cancer risk associated with a CEE regimen of 0.625 mg/d translates into breast cancer RRs of 1.1 after 5 years of use, 1.2 after 10 years of use, and 1.4 after 15 years of use.

The estimated risk of breast cancer associated with HRT may be compared with the effect of endogenous

TABLE 7.3-10
Population-Based Studies of the Effect of Menopausal Hormone Replacement Therapy on Breast Cancer Risk

Investigators	Type of Study	Cases/Controls	Percentage of Controls Ever Exposed	Percentage of Change in Breast Cancer per Year of COC Use (95% Confidence Limits)	Relative Risk for 10 Years of HRT Use
Ross et al.[104,a]	Case-control	131/262	48	+10.3 (0.9, 20.4)	2.67
Hoover et al.[105,b]	Case-control	345/611	29	+6.7 (1.4, 12.3)	1.91
Hiatt et al.[106,b]	Case-control	119/119	90	+5.7 (−0.4, 12.3)	1.74
Brinton et al.[107,c]	Case-control	1960/2258	52	+1.9 (0.4, 3.4)	1.21
Nomura et al.[108,d]	Case-control	341/341	56	+0.7 (−3.9, 5.5)	1.07
Wingo et al.[78]	Case-control	1369/1645	32	+0.1 (−0.5, 0.7)	1.01
Ewertz[111,e]	Case-control	596/568	28	+9.3 (3.3, 15.7)	2.44
Rohan & McMichael[112]	Case-control	281/288	24	−2.3 (−20.6, 20.3)	0.79
Bergkvist et al.[113,f]	Case-control	219/653	100	+8.5 (0.4, 17.3)	2.26
Colditz et al.[110,g]	Cohort	722/—	47	+2.0 (−0.3, 4.3)	1.22
Weighted average[i]		All studies		+3.1 (1.2, 5.1)	1.36
		Studies permitting analysis for CEE at 0.625 mg/d		+2.2 (0.4, 3.9)	1.24

COC, combination oral contraceptives; HRT, hormone replacement therapy.

[a] Incomplete adjustment for age at menopause in oophorectomized patients.

[b] Medical chart study: one chart notation equated to 1 year of use. Oophorectomized women.

[c] Possibly inadequate adjustment for age at menopause.

[d] Weighted average of results for whites and Japanese in Hawaii. Possibly inadequate adjustment for age at menopause.

[e] Natural menopause data only.

[e] See also Chilvers.[91]

[f] No data given on duration of use. The relative risk for ever use of COCs is 1.1 (0.8, 1.6).

[g] Update of study reported by Vessey and coworkers.[92]

[h] Confidence limits calculated from crude analysis of published data because adjusted trend statistic not quoted in the paper.

[i] *P* value for heterogeneity is .047; if heterogeneity is considered significant, the best estimate of weighted average percentage of change is +3.1 (0.9, 5.4). Relative risk for 10 years of COC use is 1.36.

(Pike M, Bernstein L, Spicer D: Exogenous hormones and breast cancer risk. In: Neiderhuber J, ed. Current therapy in oncology. St Louis, BC Decker, 1993)

estrogens on breast cancer risk in postmenopausal women (about 2.1% increase in incidence per year of increasing age). In postmenopausal women in the United States, the mean serum level of bioavailable estradiol, the fraction of estradiol that is not bound to SHBG, is about 12 pg/mL.[62] The serum level of non–SHBG-bound estradiol in women receiving 0.625 mg/d of CEE is approximately 26 pg/mL,[62] about twice that of the normal postmenopausal level. Assuming that estradiol is the most important estrogen irrespective of its source, we predict that the incremental (additive) increase in breast cancer risk due to taking 0.625 mg/d of CEE should be about double that due to endogenous estrogens, similar to that predicted by the meta-analysis of population-based studies from the United States.

Certain subgroups of women are probably more susceptible to the carcinogenic effects of estrogens than others. In their metaanalysis, Steinberg and coworkers[115] showed that use of estrogen replacement therapy increased breast cancer risk irrespective of family history of breast cancer, parity, or history of benign breast disease. Although the effects of estrogen use were similar among nulliparous and parous women and among those with and without benign breast disease, the effects were enhanced among women with a family history of breast cancer.

Except for the study of Bergkvist and coworkers,[113] the breast cancer studies shown in Table 7.3-10 essentially evaluate the effect of estrogen replacement therapy alone, not combined estrogen and progestogen therapy. Persson and coworkers provided some data on the effect of combined therapy on breast cancer risk.[117] In their study, the RRs for long-term combination therapy users were higher than those for users of estrogen replacement therapy. For 6 years of follow-up or less, the RR for the combined regimen was 1.2, and for 7 to 11 years of follow-up, the statistically significant RR was 1.6.

In combination hormone therapy, progestogens may enhance the carcinogenic effect of estrogen therapy on the breast. Unlike the endometrium, for which maximal mitotic activity occurs during the follicular phase of the menstrual cycle, cell replication in breast epithelium peaks in the luteal phase.[63] This phenomenon suggests that progesterone, in conjunction with the luteal-phase estradiol peak, could stimulate breast cancer risk. A women's hormonal exposure to both estrogens and progestogens while receiving COCs is greater than that which occurs naturally during the perimenopausal period, precisely the situation that exists for estrogen–progestogen HRT given during the perimenopausal years. Finally, although not statistically significant, the Swedish results on combined therapy are consistent with the hypothesis that estrogen and progestogen are more carcinogenic to the breast than estrogen alone.[113]

The continuing controversy surrounding the advisability of long-term use of estrogen replacement therapy among postmenopausal women centers around three issues: (1) the potential benefits to be derived from such therapy compared with the potential risks, (2) the most favorable dose to maximize the benefit/risk ratio, and (3) the benefits and risks to be derived by adding a progestogen to the estrogen regimen.

Substantial epidemiologic and clinical evidence indicates that estrogens prevent osteoporosis and its most serious medical consequence, hip fracture. Women using estrogens for 5 years in the postmenopausal period approximately halve their risk of sustaining a nontraumatic osteoporotic fracture.[118] Case-control and cohort studies have provided compelling evidence that estrogens lower risk of coronary heart disease. This effect is most likely mediated through raised high-density and reduced low-density lipoprotein cholesterol levels in estrogen users. Because death rates from coronary heart disease among women in the United States are four times those from breast and endometrial cancer combined, this benefit alone could far outweigh any carcinogenic potential.[119]

References

1. Henderson BE, Ross RK, Pike MC, et al. Endogenous hormones as a major factor in human cancer. Cancer Res 1982;42:3232.
2. Henderson BE, Ross R, Bernstein L. Estrogens as a cause of human cancer: Richard and Hinda Rosenthal Foundation Award Lecture. Cancer Res 1988;48:246.
3. Stanbridge E. Identifying tumor-suppressor genes in human colorectal cancer. Science 1990;247:12.
4. Fearon E, Cho K, Nigro J, et al. Identification of a chromosome 18q gene that is altered on colorectal cancers. Science 1990;247:49.
5. Sager R. Tumor-suppressor genes: the puzzle and the promise. Science 1989;246:1406.
6. Miki Y, Swensen J, Shattuck-Eidens, et al. A strong candidate for the breast and ovarian cancer susceptibility gene BRCA1. Science 1994;266:66.
7. Futreal PA, Liu Q, Shattuck-Edens D, et al. BRCA1 mutations in primary breast and ovarian carcinomas. Science 1994;266:120.
8. Knudson A. Mutation and cancer: statistical study of retinoblastoma. Proc Natl Acad Sci USA 1971;68:820.
9. Poutanen M, Miettinen M, Vihko R. Differential estrogen substrate specificities for transiently expressed human placental 17β-hydroxysteroid dehydrogenase and an endogenous enzyme expressed in cultured COS-m6 cells. Endocrinology 1993;133:2639.
10. Mannermaa A, Peltoketo H, Winqvist R, et al. Human familial and sporadic breast cancer: analysis of the coding regions of the 17β-hydroxysteroid dyhydrogenase 2 gene (EDH17B2) using a single-strand conformation polymorphism assay. Hum Genet 1994;93:319.
11. Ponglikitmongkol M, Green S, Chambon P. Genomic organization of the human oestrogen receptor gene. EMBO J 1988;7:3385.
12. Piva R, Gambari R, Zoratao F, et al. Analysis of upstream sequences of the human estrogen receptor gene. Biochem Biophys Res Commun 1992;183:996.
13. Zuppan P, Hall J, Lee M, et al. Possible linkage of the estrogen receptor gene to breast cancer in a family with late-onset disease. Am J Hum Genet 1991;48:1065.
14. Yaich L, Dupont W, Cavener D, et al. Analysis of the PvuII restriction fragment-length polymorphism and exon structure of the estrogen receptor gene in breast cancer and peripheral blood. Cancer Res 1992;52:77.
15. del Senno L, Aguiari G, Piva R. Dinucleotide repeat polymorphism in the human estrogen receptor (ESR) gene. Hum Mol Genet 1992;1:354.
16. Henderson BE, Pike MC, Casagrande JT. Breast cancer and the oestrogen window hypothesis (letter). Lancet 1981;2:363.
17. Henderson BE, Ross RK, Judd HL, et al. Do regular ovulatory cycles increase breast cancer risk? Cancer 1985;56:1206.
18. Henderson BE, Gerkins VR, Rosario I, et al. Elevated serum levels of estrogen and prolactin in daughters of patients with breast cancer. N Engl J Med 1975;293:790.
19. Trichopoulos D, Brown J, Garas J. Elevated urine estrogen and pregnanediol levels in daughters of breast cancer patients. J Natl Cancer Inst 1981;67:603.
20. MacMahon B, Trichopoulos D, Brown J, et al. Age at menarche, probability of ovulation and breast cancer risk. Int J Cancer 1982;29:13.
21. Apter D, Vihko R. Early menarche, a risk factor for breast cancer, indicates early onset of ovulatory cycles. J Clin Endocrinol Metab 1983;57:82.
22. Tanner J. Growth at adolescence. Oxford, UK, Blackwell Scientific, 1962.
23. Frisch R, McArthur J. Menstrual cycles: fatness as a determinant of minimum weight for height necessary for their maintenance or onset. Science 1974;185:949.
24. Frisch R, Gotz-Welbergen A, McArthur J, et al. Delayed menarche and amenorrhea of college athletes in relation to age at onset of training. JAMA 1981;246:1559.
25. Bernstein L, Ross RK, Lobo RA, et al. Effects of moderate physical activity on menstrual cycle patterns in adolescence: implications for breast cancer prevention. Br J Cancer 1987;55:681.
26. Bernstein L, Henderson BE, Hanisch R, et al. Physical exercise activity reduces the risk of breast cancer in young women. J Natl Cancer Inst 1994;86:1403.
27. Trichopoulos D, MacMahon B, Cole P. The menopause and breast cancer risk. J Natl Cancer Inst 1972;48:605.
28. Feinleib M. Breast cancer and artificial menopause: a cohort study. J Natl Cancer Inst 1968;41:315.
29. MacMahon B, Cole P, Lin T, et al. Age at first birth and cancer of the breast: a summary of an international study. Bull WHO 1970;43:209.
30. Yuan JM, Yu MC, Ross RK, et al. Risk factors for breast cancer in Chinese women in Shanghai. Cancer Res 1988;48:1949.
31. Bruzzi P, Negri E, Vecchia CL, et al. Short-term increase in risk of breast cancer after full term pregnancy. Br Med J 1988;197:1096.
32. Pike MC, Henderson BE, Casagrande JT, et al. Oral contraceptive use and early abortion as risk factors for breast cancer in young women. Br J Cancer 1981;43:72.
33. Hadjimichael O, Boyle C, Meigs J. Abortion before first live birth and risk of breast cancer. Br J Cancer 1986;53:281.

34. Howe H, Senie R, Bzduch H, et al. Early abortion and breast cancer risk among women under age 40. Int J Epidemiol 1989;18:300.

35. Bernstein L, Depue RH, Ross RK, et al. Higher maternal levels of free estradiol in first compared to second pregnancy: a study of early gestational differences. J Natl Cancer Inst 1986;76:1035.

36. Yu MC, Gerkins VR, Henderson BE, et al. Elevated levels of prolactin in nulliparous women. Br J Cancer 1981;43:826.

37. Musey V, Collins D, Musey P, et al. Long-term effect of a first pregnancy on the secretion of prolactin. N Engl J Med 1987;316:229.

38. Bernstein L, Pike MC, Ross RK, et al. Estrogen and sex hormone-binding globulin levels in nulliparous and parous women. J Natl Cancer Inst 1985;74:741.

39. Ross R, Yu M. (Letter) N Engl J Med 1994;330:1683.

40. de Waard F, Cornelis J, Aoki K, et al. Breast cancer incidence according to weight and height in two cities of the Netherlands and in Aichi Prefecture, Japan. Cancer 1977;40:1269.

41. Siiteri P, Hammond G, Nishker J. Increased availability of serum estrogens in breast cancer: a new hypothesis. In: Pike M, Siiteri P, Welsh C, eds. Hormones and breast cancer. Cold Spring Harbor, NY, Cold Spring Harbor Laboratories, 1981.

42. Pike MC, Krailo MD, Henderson BE, et al. "Hormonal" risk factors, "breast tissue age" and the age incidence of breast cancer. Nature 1983;303:767.

43. Hoel D, Wakabayashi T, Pike M. Secular trends in the distributions of the breast cancer risk factors: menarche, first birth, menopause, and weight—in Hiroshima and Nagasaki, Japan. Am J Epidemiol 1983;118:79.

44. Dao T. The role of ovarian steroid hormones in mammary carcinogenesis. In: Pike M, Siiteri P, Welsh C, eds. Hormones and breast cancer. Cold Spring Harbor, NY, Cold Spring Harbor Laboratories, 1981.

45. England P, Skinner L, Cottrell K, et al. Serum oestradiol-17β in women with benign and malignant breast disease. Br J Cancer 1974;30:571.

46. Bernstein L, Ross R. Hormones and breast cancer. Epidemiol Rev 1993;15:48.

47. Moore J, Clark G, Bulbrook R, et al. Serum concentrations of total and non-protein bound oestradiol in patients with breast cancer and in normal controls. Int J Cancer 1982;29:17.

48. Jones L, Ota D, Jackson G, et al. Bioavailability of estradiol as a marker for breast cancer risk assessment. Cancer Res 1987;47:5224.

49. MacMahon B, Cole P, Brown J, et al. Urine oestrogen profiles of Asian and North American women. Int J Cancer 1974;14:161.

50. Bernstein L, Yuan JM, Ross RK, et al. Serum hormone levels in premenopausal Chinese women in Shanghai and white women in Los Angeles: results from two breast cancer case-control studies. Cancer Causes Control 1990;1:51.

51. Shimizu H, Ross RK, Bernstein L, et al. Serum oestrogen levels in postmenopausal women: comparison of American whites and Japanese in Japan. Br J Cancer 1990;62:451.

52. Aldercreutz H, Hockerstedt K, Bannwart C, et al. Effect of dietary components, including ligands and phytoestrogens, on enterohepatic circulation and liver metabolism of estrogens and on sex hormone binding globulin (SHBG). J Steroid Biochem 1987;27:1135.

53. Goldin B, Aldercreutz H, Gorbach S, et al. The relationship between estrogen levels and diets of Caucasian American and Oriental immigrant women. Am J Clin Nutr 1986;44:945.

54. Lee HP, Gourley L, Duffy SW, et al. Dietary effects on breast cancer risk in Singapore. Lancet 1991;337:1197.

55. Davis DL, Bradlow HL, Wolff M, et al. Medical hypothesis: xenoestrogens as preventable causes of breast cancer. Environ Health Perspect 1993;101:372.

56. Schneider J, Kinne D, Fracchia A, et al. Abnormal oxidative metab-

57. Fishman J, Schneider J, Hershkopf J, et al. Increased estrogen 16-alpha-hydroxylase activity in women with breast and endometrial cancer. J Steroid Biochem 1983;20:1077.

58. Osborne MP, Bradlow HL, Wong GYC, et al. Upregulation of estradiol C16α-hydroxylation in human breast tissue: a potential biomarker of breast cancer risk. J Natl Cancer Inst 1993;85:1917.

59. Snow RC, Barbieri RL, Frisch RE. Estrogen II: hydroxylase oxidation and menstrual function among elite oarswomen. J Clin Endocrinol Metab 1989;315:369.

60. Aldercreutz H, Fotsis T, Hockerstedt K, et al. Diet and urinary estrogen profile in premenopausal omnivorous and vegetarian women and in premenopausal women with breast cancer. J Steroid Biochem 1989;34:527.

61. Lemon HM, Heidel JW, Rodreguez-Sierra JF. Increased catechol estrogen metabolism as a risk factor for nonfamilial breast cancer. Cancer 1993;85:648.

62. Key T, Pike M. The role of oestrogens and progestogens in the epidemiology and prevention of breast disease. Eur J Cancer Clin Oncol 1988;24:29.

63. Ferguson D, Anderson T. Morphological evaluation of cell turnover in relation to the menstrual cycle in the "resting" human breast. Br J Cancer 1981;44:177.

64. Potten C, Watson R, Williams G, et al. The effect of age and menstrual cycle upon proliferative activity of the normal human breast. Br J Cancer 1988;58:163.

65. Dulbecco R, Hwenahan M, Armstrong B. Cell types of morphogenesis in the mammary gland. Proc Natl Acad Sci USA 1982;79:7346.

66. Aksel S. Hormonal characteristics on long cycles in fertile women. Fertil Steril 1981;36:521.

67. Olsson H, Landin-Olsson M, Gulberg B. Retrospective assessment of menstrual cycle length in patients with breast cancer, in patients with benign breast disease, and in women without breast disease. J Natl Cancer Inst 1983;70:17.

68. Malone K, Daling J, Weiss N. Oral contraceptives and breast cancer risk. Epidemiol Rev 1993;15:80.

69. Another look at the pill and breast cancer. (Editorial) Lancet 1985;2:985.

70. McPherson K, Neil A, Vessey M, et al. Oral contraceptives and breast cancer. (Letter) Lancet 1983;2:1414.

71. Stadel B, Rubin G, Wingo P, et al. Oral contraceptives and breast cancer in young women. (Letter) Lancet 1986;1:436.

72. Kay C. Results from the Royal College of General Practitioners' Oral Contraception Study. In: Mann R, ed. Oral contraceptives and breast cancer. Park Ridge, NJ, Parthenon, 1990.

73. Pike M, Bernstein L, Spicer D. Exogenous hormones and breast cancer risk. In: Neiderhuber J, ed. Current therapy in oncology. St Louis, BC Decker, 1993.

74. Brinton L. Update of the 1982 study among participants in the Breast Cancer Detection Demonstration Project and plans for a new study. In: Mann R, ed. Oral contraceptives and breast cancer. Park Ridge, NJ, Parthenon, 1990.

75. Stadel B, Webster L, Rubin G, et al. Oral contraceptives and breast cancer in young women. Lancet 1985;2:970.

76. Paul C, Skegg D, Spears G, et al. Oral contraceptives and breast cancer: a national study. Br Med J 1986;293:723.

77. Vessey M. Results from the Oxford Family Planning Association Study. In: Mann R, ed. Oral contraceptives and breast cancer. Park Ridge, NJ, Parthenon, 1990.

78. Romieu I, Willett W, Colditz G, et al. A prospective study of oral contraceptive use and the risk of breast cancer in women. In: Mann R, ed. Oral contraceptives and breast cancer. Park Ridge, NJ, Parthenon, 1990.

olism in women with breast cancer. Proc Natl Acad Sci USA 1982;79:3047.

79. Brinton L, Hoover R, Szklo M, et al. Oral contraceptives and breast cancer. Int J Epidemiol 1982;11:3136.

80. Centers for Disease Control. Oral contraceptive use and the risk of breast cancer. N Engl J Med 1986;315:405.

81. Wingo P, Lee N, Ory H, et al. Oral contraceptives and the risk of breast cancer. In: Mann R, ed. Oral contraceptives and breast cancer. Park Ridge, NJ, Parthenon, 1990.

82. Paul C, Skegg D, Spears G. Oral contraception and breast cancer in New Zealand. In: Mann R, ed. Oral contraceptives and breast cancer. Park Ridge, NJ, Parthenon, 1990.

83. Vessey M, Baron J, Doll R, et al. Oral contraceptives and breast cancer: final report of an epidemiological study. Br J Cancer 1983;47:455.

84. Lipnick T, Buring J, Hennedens C, et al. Oral contraceptives and breast cancer: a prospective cohort study. JAMA 1986;255:58.

85. Bernstein L, Pike MC, Krailo M, et al. Update of the Los Angeles Study of oral contraceptives and breast cancer: 1981–1983. In: Mann R, ed. Oral contraceptives and breast cancer. London, Parthenon Press in Association with The Royal Society of Medicine, 1990.

86. Stadel B, Schlesselman J, Murray P. Oral contraceptives and breast cancer. Lancet 1989;1:1257.

87. Meirik O, Lund E, Adami H, et al. Oral contraceptive use and breast cancer in young women. Lancet 1986;2:650.

88. UK National Case-Control Study Group. Oral contraceptive use and breast cancer risk in young women. Lancet 1989;1:973.

89. Pike MC, Henderson BE, Krailo MD, et al. Breast cancer in young women and use of oral contraceptives: possible modifying effect of formulation and age at use. Lancet 1983;2:926.

90. Lund E, Meirik O, Adami H, et al. Update of the Swedish–Norwegian case-control study on oral contraceptive use and breast cancer in young women: the possible role of bias. In: Mann R, ed. Oral contraceptives and breast cancer. Park Ridge, NJ, Parthenon, 1990.

91. Chilvers C. Oral contraceptives and breast cancer: the UK National Case-Control Study. In: Mann R, ed. Oral contraceptives and breast cancer. Park Ridge, NJ, Parthenon, 1990.

92. Vessey M, McPherson K, Villard-Mackintosh L, et al. Oral contraceptives and breast cancer: latest findings in a large cohort study. Br J Cancer 1989;59:613.

93. Finkel M, Berlinger V. The extrapolation of experimental findings (animal to man): the dilemma of systematically administered contraceptives. Bull Soc Pharmacol Environ Pathol 1973;4:13.

94. Geil R, Lamar K. FDA studies of oestrogen, progestogen and oestrogen–progestogen combinations. J Toxicol Environ Health 1977;3:179.

95. Lanari C, Molinolo A, Pasqualini C. Induction of mammary adenocarcinomas by medroxyprogesterone acetate in BALB/c female mice. Cancer Lett 1986;215:33.

96. Lee N, Rosero-Bixby L, Oberle M, et al. A case-control study of breast cancer and hormonal contraception in Costa Rica. J Natl Cancer Inst 1987;79:1247.

97. WHO collaborative study of neoplasia and steroid contraceptives: breast cancer and depot-medroxyprogesterone acetate: a multinational study. Lancet 1991;338:833.

98. Paul C, Skegg D, Spears G. Depot medroxyprogesterone (Depo-Provera) and risk of breast cancer. Br Med J 1989;229:759.

99. Jeppsson J, Johansson E, Ljungberg O, et al. Endometrial histology and circulating levels of medroxyprogesterone acetate (MPA): estradiol, FSH and LH in women with MPA-induced amenorrhoea compared with women with secondary amenorrhoea. Acta Obstet Gynecol Scand 1977;56:43.

100. Mishell D. Long-acting contraceptive steroids: postcoital contraceptives and antiprogestins. In: Mishell D, Davajan V, Lobo R, eds. Infertility, contraception and reproductive endocrinology. Boston, Blackwell Scientific, 1991.

101. Kennedy D, Baum C, Forbes M: Noncontraceptive estrogens and progestins: use patterns over time. Obstet Gynecol 1985;65:441.

102. Hoover R, Gray L, Cole P, et al. Menopausal estrogens and breast cancer. N Engl J Med 1976;295:401.

103. Der Simonian R, Laird N: Meta-analysis in clinical trials. Control Clin Trials 1986;7:177.

104. Ross RK, Hill AP, Gerkins VR, et al. A case-control study of menopausal estrogen therapy and breast cancer. JAMA 1980;243:1635.

105. Hoover R, Glass A, Finkle W, et al. Conjugated estrogens and breast cancer risk in women. J Natl Cancer Inst 1981;67:815.

106. Hiatt R, Bawol R, Friedman G, et al. Exogenous estrogens and breast cancer after oophorectomy. Cancer 1984;54:139.

107. Brinton L, Hoover R, Fraumeni J. Menopausal oestrogens and breast cancer risk: an expanded case-control study. Br J Cancer 1986;54:825.

108. Nomura A, Kolonel L, Hirohata T, et al. The association of replacement estrogens with breast cancer. Int J Cancer 1986;37:49.

109. Wingo P, Layde P, Lee N, et al. The risk of breast cancer in postmenopausal women who have used estrogen replacement therapy. JAMA 1987;257:209.

110. Colditz G, Stampfer M, Willett W, et al. Prospective study of estrogen and estrogen–progestin replacement therapy and risk of breast cancer in post-menopausal women. JAMA 1990;264:2648.

111. Ewertz M. Influence of non-contraceptive exogenous and endogenous sex hormones on breast cancer risk in Denmark. Int J Cancer 1988;42:832.

112. Rohan T, McMichael A. Non-contraceptive exogenous oestrogen therapy and breast cancer. Med J Aust 1988;148:217.

113. Bergkvist L, Adami H, Persson I, et al. The risk of breast cancer after estrogen and estrogen–progestin replacement. N Engl J Med 1989;321:293.

114. Grady D, Ernster V. Does postmenopausal hormone therapy cause breast cancer? Am J Epidemiol 1991;134:1396.

115. Steinberg K, Thacker S, Smith S, et al. A meta-analysis of the effect of estrogen replacement therapy on the risk of breast cancer. JAMA 1991;265:1985.

116. Sillero-Arenas M, Delgado-Rodriguez M, Rodigues-Canteras, et al. Menopausal hormone replacement therapy and the risk of breast cancer: a meta-analysis. Obstet Gynecol 1992;79:286.

117. Persson I, Yuen J, Bergkvist L, et al. Combined oestrogen–progestogen replacement and breast cancer risk (Letter). Lancet 1992;340:1044.

118. Paganini-Hill A, Ross RK, Gerkins VR, et al. Menopausal estrogen therapy and hip fractures. Ann Int Med 1981;95:28.

119. Henderson BE, Paganini-Hill A, Ross RK. Decreased mortality in users of estrogen replacement therapy. Arch Intern Med 1991;151:75.

7.4
Dietary Factors
DAVID J. HUNTER ▪ WALTER C. WILLETT

The incidence of breast cancer varies more than fivefold around the world,[1] and the offspring of migrants moving from countries with low breast cancer incidence to countries with high incidence acquire rates similar to those of the new country.[2,3] These observations suggest that environmental and life-style influences are important in the etiology of breast cancer. Diet has also been prominent among the putative environmental determinants of breast cancer. After several decades of study, however, few dietary constituents can be confidently associated with breast cancer. The dominant hypothesis linking diet to breast cancer has been that high fat intake increases risk. We review evidence of this relation, then turn our attention to data suggesting that body size and total energy balance during growth may be associated with breast cancer risk. We then review hypotheses relating micronutrients, anticarcinogenic phytochemicals, alcohol, and caffeine to breast cancer risk and briefly discuss the limited data relating diet to breast cancer recurrence. Relatively few studies have presented data on the associations between individual foods and breast cancer risk; thus, we concentrate on data for specific nutrients.

Dietary Fat and Breast Cancer

ANIMAL STUDIES

More than 50 years ago, Tannenbaum[4] showed that high-fat diets increased the occurrence of mammary tumors in rodents. The interpretation of these and other animal data, however, remain controversial. Fat is the most energy-dense macronutrient (9 kcal/g compared with 4 kcal/g for protein and carbohydrate); thus, high-fat diets tend to be higher in energy intake unless care is taken to keep energy intake constant. Many animal experiments have not done so, thereby confounding fat consumption by energy intake. In a metaanalysis of diet and mammary cancer experiments in mice, Albanes[5] observed a weak inverse association with fat composition (adjusted for energy), whereas total energy intake was positively associated with mammary tumor incidence. Freedman and colleagues[6] conducted a similar metaanalysis of experiments in both rats and mice and reported that both higher fat intake and higher caloric intake independently increased mammary tumor incidence. Further, the relevance of rodent models (in which animals are typically given potent-specific carcinogens to which humans are rarely exposed) to human experience is questionable. A large study of rats and mice fed substantially different amounts of fat as corn oil without administration of a carcinogen did not show any association between fat intake and spontaneous mam-

mary cancer incidence.[7] The clearest message from the animal data is the potential importance of total energy intake and the need to consider this factor in epidemiologic studies.

INTERNATIONAL CORRELATION (ECOLOGIC) STUDIES

The dietary fat hypothesis originated from the observation that national per capita fat consumption estimates are highly correlated with breast cancer mortality rates.[8] The quality of the existing data on average fat consumption is dubious, however, because such data are based on food disappearance estimates of the amount of fat in the food supply. For example, the fat intake of persons in the United States calculated from food disappearance data is at least 50% higher than the actual intake.[9] The most serious problem with ecologic comparisons of diet and breast cancer is the potential for confounding by known and suspected breast cancer risk factors. National fat consumption per capita correlates highly with level of economic development; the correlation between Gross National Product (GNP) per capita and breast cancer incidence is actually marginally stronger than that with fat consumption.[8] Prentice and colleagues[10] showed that the ecologic relation between fat disappearance and breast cancer incidence rates remains statistically significant after adjustment for GNP per capita and average age at menarche; however, other strong breast cancer risk factors, such as low parity and late age at first birth, are more prevalent in developed countries and would be expected to confound the apparent association with dietary fat intake.

SECULAR TRENDS

Both the estimates of per capita fat consumption based on food disappearance data and breast cancer incidence rates have increased substantially in the United States during this century. Surveys based on measures of individual intake, rather than food disappearance, however, indicate that consumption of energy from fat has actually declined in the past several decades,[11] a time during which breast cancer incidence has increased. Higher dietary fat consumption has been implicated in the increase in breast cancer incidence in Japan during this century;[12] however, this increase could also be due to the changing prevalence of reproductive risk factors, as well as higher energy intake during growth (consistent with a large secular increase in attained average adult height). Little increase in breast cancer mortality has occurred among Japanese women born before 1925,[13] a finding consistent with a birth cohort effect and suggestive of the hypothesis that adult fat intake does not substantially influence breast cancer risk. The dramatic increase in mortality at all ages due to colon cancer[13] suggests that older women have changed their diet and thus should be susceptible to an effect of increased fat intake on breast cancer risk.

SPECIAL POPULATIONS

Data from special populations with distinct dietary patterns are valuable, given that adherence to a particular diet over many years may represent a more stable long-term exposure than that applicable to most free-living adults whose diet may change substantially over time. These populations often have unusual distributions of nondietary potential risk factors such as alcohol consumption and reproductive behavior; thus, care must be taken in attributing differences in cancer rates to diet alone. Seventh-Day Adventists, who consume relatively small amounts of meat and other animal products, have substantially lower rates of colon cancer but only slightly lower breast cancer rates than US white women of similar socioeconomic status,[14] a finding compatible with observational data indicating that meat intake is strongly associated with colon cancer risk but not with breast cancer.[15] Breast cancer rates among British nuns who ate no (or very little) meat were similar to rates among single women from the general population,[16] also suggesting that no substantial association exists between animal fat and risk for breast cancer.

CASE-CONTROL STUDIES

In a typical case-control study of diet and breast cancer, the prediagnosis diet reported by women with breast cancer (cases) is compared with the diet of women from the population from which the cases were drawn but who have not been diagnosed with breast cancer. The largest such study is that of Graham and colleagues[17] who used a food frequency questionnaire to compare the fat intake of 2024 women with breast cancer to that reported by 1463 control women hospitalized with benign conditions. Animal fat and total fat intake were almost identical in the two groups. In a metaanalysis, Howe and colleagues[18] summarized the results from 12 smaller case-control studies comprising a total of 4312 cases and 5978 controls. The pooled relative risk (RR) for a 100-g increase in daily total fat intake was 1.35 ($P = .05$); the risk was somewhat stronger for postmenopausal women (RR, 1.48). Given that the average total fat consumption is estimated to be about 73 g/d for US women,[11] a reduction in fat intake as large as 100 g would be impossible for almost all women. The results of this pooled analysis suggest that, even if a positive association of this magnitude existed, the RR for readily achievable changes in total fat intake would be relatively small; the reduction in risk for a 20 g/d decrease among postmenopausal women (corresponding to a decrease from 40% to 29% of calories for a typical middle-aged woman), for example, would be about .9. Further,

TABLE 7.4-1

Prospective Studies (at Least 50 Incident Cases) of the Association Between Total Fat Intake and Risk of Breast Cancer

Investigator*	Population	Total Cohort (*N*)	Follow-Up (y)	Cases (*N*)	Total Fat Intake†	Relative Risk‡	95% Confidence Interval
Jones et al, 1987[110]	US	5,485	10	99	<30–≥42	0.62	0.33–1.19
Willet et al, 1987[111]	US	89,538	4	601	32–44	0.82	0.64–1.05
Mills et al, 1989[112]	California	20,341	6	193	NA	1.21§	0.81–1.81
Knekt et al, 1990[113]	Finland	3,988	20	54	NA	1.72	0.61–4.82
Howe et al, 1991[46]	Canada	56,837	5	519	31–47	1.30	0.90–1.88
Kushi et al, 1992[114]	US	32,080	4	408	27–41	1.13	0.84–1.51
Willet et al, 1992[19]	US	89,494	8	1,439	29–>49	0.86	0.67–1.08
Graham et al, 1992[27]	New York state	17,401	7	344	<26–>37	1.00	0.59–1.70
Byrne et al, 1992[115]	US	6,122	4	53	NA	1.10	0.50–2.40
Van den Brandt et al, 1993[116]	Netherlands	62,573	3	471	NA	1.08	0.73–1.59
Toniolo et al, 1994[117]	New York City	14,291	5	180	NA	1.49	0.89–2.48

NA, not available.

* For most studies, categories are quintiles of the intake distribution; in some, quartiles or tertiles are used.

† As a percentage of calories from fat.

‡ High versus low intake.

§ Estimate for animal fat intake only.

RRs of this magnitude in case-control studies may easily be due to selection bias (eg, women who participate as controls have a different distribution of fat intake than women who do not participate) or recall bias (the cases, knowing their diagnosis, misreport their prediagnosis diet).

COHORT STUDIES

In a cohort (prospective) study, the diet of a large group of women is assessed, and the diets of women who subsequently developed breast cancer are compared with the diets of women who did not. Selection bias should not be a problem because the population that gave rise to the cases is known (the original members of the cohort), and recall bias should not occur because dietary information is collected before knowledge of disease. The results from 10 prospective studies with at least 50 incident cases of breast cancer are shown in Table 7.4-1 and graphically in Figure 7.4-1. The number of breast cancer cases in these studies (3580) is similar to the number in the pooled analysis of case-control studies referred to previously, and the size of the comparison series (ie, noncases) is much larger. In no study has a significant association been observed (comparing the highest with the lowest category of total fat intake). The Mantel-Haenszel estimate (weighted by the inverse of the variance in each study) of the average RR for the 10 studies providing confidence intervals (CIs) is 1.06 (95% CI, 0.93 to 1.20). In the Nurses' Health Study (the largest prospective study to date), 89,494 women were monitored for 8 years, and 1439 cases of breast cancer were diagnosed.[19] The RR comparing the highest and lowest deciles of fat intake as a percentage of energy intake at baseline was 0.86 (95% CI, 0.67 to 1.08); the upper bound of this 95% CI excludes all but the smallest increases in risk.

The consistent absence of a significant positive associa-

tion between dietary fat intake and breast cancer in cohort studies has been attributed to nondifferential misclassification of the measures of dietary fat intake, leading to bias of RRs toward zero. The observed RR and its CI, however, can be corrected for this bias[20] if the relation between measured fat intake and true intake can be estimated from a validation study of the diet assessment instrument. Using this technique, Willett and colleagues[19] calculated the RR in the Nurses' Health Study for an increase of 24 g/d (30% to 44% of calories from fat). The original RR was 1.01 (95% CI, 0.92 to 1.1). After adjustment for measurement error, this estimate was 1 (95% CI, 0.79 to 1.27). Even the upper bound of this deattenuated confidence interval is still substantially less than the RRs of 1.4 to 1.5 predicted from the international correlation between fat intake and breast cancer risk.[21]

Thus, prospective studies provide strong evidence that no major relation exists between dietary fat intake of women in developed countries and breast cancer incidence for up to 10 years of follow-up. Two modifications of the original dietary fat and breast cancer hypothesis are not excluded by the available data. Almost all case-control and cohort studies address the influence of current diet in adults on fairly short-term (eg, 5 to 10 years) breast cancer risk. Dietary fat intake during childhood and adolescence may, however, affect breast cancer risk decades later (see later). The other possible modification of the hypothesis is that extremely low fat intake (by Western standards; eg, to less than 20% of calories from fat) may reduce this risk. The lowest cut-points for the lower categories of fat intake (usually quintiles) in the available studies are about 27% of calories from fat (see Table 7.4-1). Among women in the Nurses' Health Study who responded to a second food frequency questionnaire in 1984, however, the median intake for the lowest decile of intake was 23% of calories from fat.[19] Even at this low level, no evidence supported

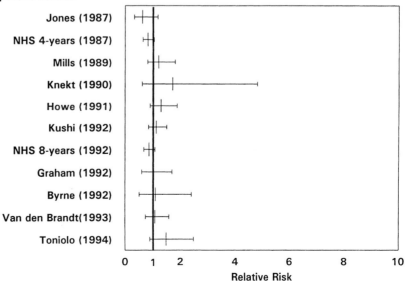

FIGURE 7.4-1 Prospective studies of the association between total fat intake and breast cancer risk. Vertical bars represent the relative risks for the highest category of intake (usually the highest quintile or quartile) versus the lowest; error bars represent the 95% confidence intervals.

a reduction in risk; indeed, the RR for the lowest decile (25% or fewer calories from fat) compared with the highest decile (over 40% calories from fat) was 1.2 (ie, a higher risk with lower fat intake). Cohort data are not available to test the possibility that a reduction in total fat intake to less than 20% of calories from fat may be associated with reduced breast cancer incidence. For this to be true, however, the association between fat intake and breast cancer would have to be highly nonlinear, with a threshold at about 20% of calories from fat. The ecologic comparisons of per capita fat consumption and breast cancer incidence suggest a linear association, however, and provide no evidence for the existence of such a threshold.

INTERVENTION STUDIES

It has been suggested that uncertainty about the association between dietary fat and breast cancer can be resolved only by randomized trials of fat reduction, and the Women's Health Initiative sponsored by the US National Institutes of Health has begun with the goal of enrolling and randomizing tens of thousands of women, half of whom will be instructed on how to reduce their total fat intake to 20% of calories from fat. This trial will not answer the most promising modification of the dietary fat hypothesis—that dietary fat reduction at an early age may reduce breast cancer risk decades later. Problems including the difficulty of maintaining compliance with a diet different from prevailing food consumption habits, as well as the gradual secular decline in total fat consumption already underway (which may reduce the size of the comparison in fat intake between intervention groups and controls), may severely compromise the ability of any trial to address the effect of reducing percent of fat from calories to 20%.[22]

Further, as pointed out by the Women's Health Initiative investigators, "women in the dietary intervention group will be counseled to adopt a dietary pattern that is high in fruits, vegetables, and grain products and low in total fat and saturated fat."[23] Thus, the trial will be unable to distinguish between a decrease in risk due to increased intake of fruit, vegetable, and grains, and a decrease due to lower fat intake.

Dietary Fiber and Breast Cancer

It has been suggested that diets high in fiber may protect against breast cancer, perhaps through inhibition of the intestinal reabsorption of estrogens excreted by the biliary system.[24] A high-fiber diet was associated with reduced incidence of mammary cancer in an animal study.[25] Dietary fiber includes crude fiber that is excreted unchanged as well as many soluble fiber fractions that may have different biologic effects. Epidemiologic assessment of fiber intake has been difficult because of the scarcity of data on the fiber content of individual foods and the controversy about the most appropriate methods of biochemical analysis to determine fiber content. In their metaanalysis of 10 case-control studies that included estimates of dietary fiber

intake, Howe and colleagues[18] observed a statistically significant RR of 0.85 for a 20-g/d increase in dietary fiber. In a case-control study of 519 cases nested in a prospective cohort, Rohan and coworkers[26] observed a marginally significant inverse association between dietary fiber and breast cancer risk; in another prospective cohort with 344 cases, Graham and colleagues[27] observed no suggestion of a protective association. In the largest prospective investigation (1439 cases), the Nurses' Health Study,[19] the association between total dietary fiber intake and subsequent breast cancer incidence was very close to zero, suggesting that any protective effect of dietary fiber is unlikely to be large. It remains possible, however, that certain subfractions of fiber intake may be relevant to breast cancer.

Height, Body Mass Index, and the Risk of Breast Cancer

Energy or protein restriction during childhood and adolescence stunts growth and results in reduced height. Height is positively correlated with international variations in breast cancer rates,[28] suggesting that childhood and adolescent energy intake may influence breast cancer risk decades later. As mentioned previously, energy restriction is a powerful intervention to reduce mammary tumor incidence in rodents.[5,6] This hypothesis is difficult to test directly in humans because estimates by adults of their dietary intake in the distant past are unlikely to be sufficiently valid and would also need to account accurately for physical activity. However, as children who experience energy deprivation during growth do not attain their full potential height, attained height may be used as a proxy for childhood energy intake.[29] In Japan, for example, a substantial increase in average height has occurred during the 20th century, presumably as a result of improved nutrition.[29]

Most of the case-control studies of this issue suggest a modest positive association between attained height and risk for breast cancer.[30] In addition, each of the available cohort studies supports a modest association between height and breast cancer risk (Fig. 7.4-2). De Waard and Baanders-van Halewijn,[31] in a follow-up of 7259 postmenopausal women in the Netherlands, observed a more than twofold increase in risk across a 15-cm difference in height. In a follow-up of the National Health and Nutrition Examination Surveys (NHANES) I, a population in which women at risk for malnutrition had been oversampled, Swanson and colleagues[32] observed a similar increase in risk. Among women in the Nurses' Health Study, a significant positive association was seen between height and breast cancer for postmenopausal women but not for premenopausal women.[33] Several large cohort studies have been conducted in Scandinavia and all have shown significant associations ranging from 1.1 (for a 5-cm increment) to 2 (for a greater than 8-cm increment).[34-37] In the studies of Vatten and Kvinnsland,[36,37] the positive trend between height and risk for breast cancer was most nearly linear in the birth cohort of women (1929

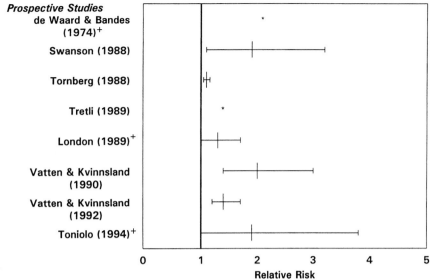

FIGURE 7.4-2 Prospective studies of the association between height and breast cancer risk. Vertical bars and asterisks represent the relative risks for the highest category of height versus the lowest; error bars represent the 95% confidence intervals. [+]Results for postmenopausal women only.

to 1932) who lived through their peripubertal period during World War II, a time in which food was scarce and the average attained height was reduced.

Thus, convincing evidence suggests that attained height is modestly associated with breast cancer risk. In the NHANES I study, height was positively associated with later age at menarche (protective against breast cancer) and late age at first birth, low parity, higher socioeconomic status, and alcohol use (risk factors for breast cancer), suggesting that height may be confounded by other breast cancer risk factors.[32] Controlling for these variables in multivariate analyses, however, had little influence on the association between height and breast cancer. It has also been suggested that height is a surrogate for mammary gland mass,[38] that higher energy intake during growth may result in increased gland mass, and that women with larger gland mass may be at higher risk. If growth restriction during childhood is shown to influence breast cancer risk, it is unlikely that energy restriction sufficient to stunt growth or to reduce mammary gland mass will be a practical public health intervention. However, this factor may contribute to understanding of the pathogenesis of this disease.

The association of body mass index (weight/height^2), a measure of obesity, appears to vary according to menopausal status. As reviewed elsewhere,[30,39,48] most studies support an inverse association among premenopausal women and a weak positive association among postmenopausal women.

Micronutrients

VITAMIN A

Vitamin A consists of preformed vitamin A (retinol, retinyl esters, and related compounds) from animal sources, and certain carotenoids that are partially converted to retinol in the intestinal epithelium (carotenoid vitamin A), found primarily in fruits and vegetables. Many carotenoids are potent antioxidants and thus may provide a cellular defense against reactive oxygen species that damage DNA.[40] Vitamin A is also a regulator of cell differentiation and may prevent the emergence of cells with a malignant phenotype.[41] Retinol inhibits the growth of human breast carcinoma cells in vitro,[42] and retinyl acetate reduces breast cancer incidence in some rodent models.[43-45]

Human studies of vitamin A intake and breast cancer have mostly been case-control investigations (Table 7.4-2); thus, their interpretation is limited by uncertainty about the extent to which selection and recall bias may have altered the observed effect estimates. All four of the studies that have reported data for total vitamin A intake (retinol plus carotenoid vitamin A) found a protective association. In the earliest and the largest case-control study, Graham and colleagues[17] observed a RR of 0.8 between the highest quartile of vitamin A consumption and the lowest, with a significant inverse trend in risk with increased vitamin A consumption. In their metaanalysis of nine other case-control studies with data on vitamin A intake, Howe and colleagues[18] reported a significant protective association between total vitamin A and breast cancer.

Of 9 case-control studies that have presented data for preformed vitamin A, 4 have reported RRs of 1 or above between the highest and lowest category of intake, and 5 0.9 or less. Of 14 studies with data for carotenoid vitamin A, RRs of 1 or above were observed in 4, whereas in 10 RRs of 0.8 or less were reported. Howe and colleagues[46] reported on a significant protective effect of β-carotene from the 8 studies with available data in their metaanalysis, whereas no significant association was present among 8 studies with data for preformed vitamin A. Thus, the data from case-control studies are more strongly supportive of a protective association for carotenoid vitamin A than for preformed vitamin A.

TABLE 7.4-2
Studies of Vitamin A Intake and Breast Cancer

Investigators	Population	Cases (N)	Comparison	Total Vitamin A		Preformed Vitamin A		Carotenoid Vitamin A		Factors Controlled For
				RR★	95% CI	RR★	95% CI	RR★	95% CI	
CASE-CONTROL										
Graham et al, 1982[17]	New York state	1803	Highest vs lowest quartile†	0.8	P trend <.05	—	—	—	—	—
La Vecchia et al, 1987[118]	Italy	1108	Highest vs lowest tertile†	—	—	0.9	0.7–1.1	0.8	0.6–1.1	Age, 1 or more breast cancer risk factors
Katsouyanni et al, 1988[119]	Greece	118	Highest vs lowest decile	0.5	0.3–0.8‡	0.6	0.4–1.0‡	0.6	0.3–1.0‡	Age, 1 or more breast cancer risk factors, calories, fat
Marubini et al, 1988[50]	Italy	214	Highest vs lowest quintile	—	—	0.7	0.4–1.5	1.2	0.6–2.5	Age, 1 or more breast cancer risk factors, calories, alcohol
Rohan et al, 1988[120]	Australia	451	Highest vs lowest quintile	—	—	1.2	0.8–1.8	0.8	0.5–1.2	Age
Toniolo et al, 1989[121]	Italy	250	Highest vs lowest quartile	—	—	1.2	P trend, .28	1.0	P trend, .89	Age, calories
Ewertz & Gill, 1990[122]	Denmark	1267	Highest vs lowest quartile	—	—	—	—	1.2	0.9–1.5	Age
Potischman et al, 1990[52]	New York state	83	Highest vs lowest quartile	0.7	0.3–2.0	—	—	0.8	0.3–2.3§	Age, 1 or more breast cancer risk factors
Van't Veer et al, 1990[78]	Holland	133	Highest vs lowest quartile	—	—	—	—	0.6	P trend, .23	Age, 1 or more breast cancer risk factors, calories, alcohol
Graham et al, 1991[68]	New York state	439	Highest vs lowest quartile	—	—	—	—	0.6	0.4–0.8	Age, 1 or more breast cancer risk factors
Ingram et al, 1991[123]	Australia	99	Above vs below median	—	—	1.0	0.6–1.7	0.8	0.5–1.4	Age
Lee et al, 1991[124]‖	Singapore	109	Highest vs lowest tertile	—	—	—	—	0.3	0.2–0.7	Age, 1 or more breast cancer risk factors, fat, red meat, protein
Richardson et al, 1991[125]	France	409	Highest vs lowest tertile	—	—	1.5	1.0–2.1	1.0	0.7–1.5	Age, 1 or more breast cancer risk factors
Zaridze et al, 1991[126]¶	Moscow	81	Highest vs lowest quartile	0.2	0.04–0.8	0.5	0.1–1.3	0.2	0.02–2.0	Age, 1 or more breast cancer risk factors, calories, vitamin C (carotenoid vitamin A)
London et al, 1992[51]	Boston	313	Highest vs lowest quintile	—	—	0.7	0.4–1.3	0.6	0.3–1.1	Age, 1 or more breast cancer risk factors, calories, alcohol
PROSPECTIVE										
Paganini-Hill et al, 1987[47]	California	123	Highest vs lowest tertile	0.8	NS trend	—	—	0.8	NS trend	Age
Graham et al, 1992[27]	New York state	344	Highest vs lowest quintile	1.0	0.7–1.3	0.9	0.7–1.3	0.9	0.6–1.3	Age, education
Rohan et al, 1993[26]	Canada	519	Highest vs lowest quintile	0.8	0.7–1.0	0.9	0.8–1.0	0.9	0.7–1.0	Age, 1 or more breast cancer risk factors, calories
Hunter et al, 1993[30,48]	US	1439	Highest vs lowest quintile	0.8	0.7–1.0	0.8	0.7–1.0	0.9	0.8–1.1	Age, 1 or more breast cancer risk factors, calories, alcohol

RR, relative risk; CI, confidence interval; NS, not significant.

★ High versus low intake.

† Evenly spaced categories rather than quintiles.

‡ 90% confidence interval.

§ Result is for vitamin A from vegetable sources.

‖ Results are for premenopausal women.

¶ Results are for postmenopausal women.

The limited prospective data available support a modest inverse association between vitamin A and breast cancer. In a follow-up of female residents of a California retirement community, 123 cases of breast cancer occurred, and the RR comparing the highest with the lowest tertile of vitamin A intake was 0.8[47] (for β-carotene this risk was also 0.8). In a prospective study in New York State (344 cases),[27] no significant association was observed. In a cohort of Canadian women (519 cases),[26] a marginally significant protective association between total vitamin A intake and breast cancer was observed with both preformed vitamin A and β-carotene, contributing to the inverse association. In the Nurses' Health Study, Hunter and colleagues[48] assessed these associations among the cohort of 89,494 women described in the discussion of dietary fat. A modest but significant (RR, 0.8), protective association for total vitamin A was apparent. This association was somewhat stronger for preformed vitamin A than for carotenoid vitamin A, and associations of a similar magnitude were seen based on 4 years of follow-up of a second food frequency questionnaire administered in 1984. Low intake of vegetables was itself associated with increased risk for breast cancer. Data from many of the prospective studies that have reported data for dietary fat (see Table 7.4-1) will soon be available.

An alternative to the dietary assessment of vitamin A intake is the measurement of vitamin A compounds in blood. Most studies have assessed blood retinol, however, and these are uninformative about vitamin A intake in well-nourished populations because the liver stores over 90% of body retinol and maintains relatively constant blood retinol concentrations.[49] Blood levels of β-carotene do, however, reflect β-carotene intake. Unfortunately, little consistency exists among these studies. Marubini and coworkers[50] and London and coworkers[51] observed no inverse association between higher levels of blood β-carotene and breast cancer risk in case-control studies in Italy and Boston. Potischman and colleagues,[52] in a case-control study in New York state, observed a significant inverse association. Of three prospective studies,[53–55] only one, which included 39 cases, reported an inverse association,[53] but the largest study had only 52 incident cases.[54,82]

Thus, available data are suggestive, but not conclusive, of a modest protective association between vitamin A intake and breast cancer. It is possible that other anticarcinogens in vitamin A–rich foods are responsible for the observed effect. The effect of vitamin A supplements, either in the form of preformed vitamin A or carotenoids, should be evaluated in randomized trials. A randomized trial of fenretinide, a powerful synthetic retinoid, in the prevention of contralateral breast cancer in women diagnosed with a first cancer in one breast is underway in Italy,[56] and a recently begun trial in the United States will test the effect of β-carotene among more than 44,000 postmenopausal women.

VITAMIN E

Vitamin E is also an antioxidant, and has inhibited mammary tumors in rodents in some[57,58] but not all[59] experiments. Relatively few available studies have assessed the association between dietary vitamin E intake and breast cancer, and none of the three published prospective studies has reported a significant inverse association. In the largest of these, the Nurses' Health Study,[30,48] an initially weak protective association with vitamin E disappeared entirely when control for vitamin A was undertaken, and no evidence suggested a protective association with consumption of vitamin E supplements even at high doses for long duration.

Blood levels of vitamin E reflect vitamin E intake, especially after controlling for blood lipid levels.[60] Two case-control studies comparing blood vitamin E in cases and controls have been done; in one, blood vitamin E was actually significantly higher in cases than in controls,[61] whereas, in the other, a weak protective association was reported.[51] An initial report from a cohort in Guernsey of lower serum vitamin E values among 39 women who subsequently developed breast cancer compared with controls[53] may have been due to differential degradation of vitamin E between cases and controls[62] and was not confirmed in further follow-up of this cohort. The two other prospective studies do not suggest that vitamin E is protective.[55,63] Although these data do not suggest that vitamin E supplement consumption is likely to alter breast cancer risk, emerging data suggest that vitamin E supplements may well lower risk for cardiovascular disease,[64] perhaps by increasing the resistance of low-density lipoprotein cholesterol to oxidation.[65]

VITAMIN C

Vitamin C (ascorbic acid) is also an antioxidant and can block the formation of carcinogenic nitrosoamines.[66] Few animal studies have assessed the effect of vitamin C on mammary cancer; a study in rats showed no effect of ascorbic acid on the growth of either transplanted or dimethylbenzanthracene-induced mammary tumors.[67]

In the largest case-control study reported, Graham and colleagues[17] observed no protective association for vitamin C; however, in a subsequent study by the same group,[68] a significant protective association was present (RR, 0.6 for highest versus lowest quartile). In their metaanalysis of nine other case-control studies with data on vitamin C, Howe and coworkers[18] observed a significantly inverse association (RR, 0.69 for each 300-mg/d increase in vitamin C).

Three prospective studies have reported on the relation of vitamin C and breast cancer[30,48] and only the study of Graham and coworkers[27] observed a (nonsignificant) inverse association. Thus, the existing data on intake of vitamin C and breast cancer risk are inconsistent. The available prospective data do not support an inverse association; however, more prospective data with longer periods of follow-up are needed.

SELENIUM

Selenium is an important component of the antioxidant enzyme glutathione peroxidase, inhibits cell proliferation,[69] and has been shown in animal studies (usually at high levels of intake) to consistently protect against various cancers.[70] Ecologic studies have shown strong inverse associations between county-specific (in the United States) and national measures of selenium exposure and breast cancer rates.[71–73] Selenium intake cannot be measured accurately by dietary assessment in geographically dispersed populations due to the high variability in the selenium content of individual foods depending on the geographic area in which the foods were grown.[74] Selenium levels in tissues such as blood and toenails, however, do reflect selenium intake.[75,76]

Several studies have used these biomarkers of selenium intake. Meyer and Verreault[77] observed a nonsignificant positive association between erythrocyte selenium and breast cancer. Van't Veer and colleagues[78] observed essentially no association comparing selenium levels in erythrocytes and toenails between cases and controls. In the largest prospective study, Hunter and colleagues[79] observed no association between toenail selenium and risk for breast cancer during 4 years of follow-up. Of four other prospective studies,[80–83] only the study of Knekt and colleagues[54,82] from Finland showed any evidence of an increased risk among women in the lowest category of selenium. Because Finland has the lowest dietary selenium levels of any of the countries in this table, this observation is consistent with the possibility that a threshold exists below which low selenium intake increases breast cancer risk. Although this possibility deserves further exploration, it seems unlikely that selenium is significantly associated with breast cancer for most women in countries with moderate or high levels of selenium intake.

Other Dietary Constituents

ALCOHOL

Although the association between alcohol and breast cancer has been controversial, substantial evidence has accumulated to support a positive association (Fig. 7.4-3). In a metaanalysis of 12 case-control studies, Longnecker and colleagues[84] estimated an RR of 1.4 (95% CI, 1 to 1.8) for each 24 g/d of alcohol (about two drinks). In their metaanalysis of 4 cohort studies, Longnecker and coworkers[84] calculated a pooled RR of 1.4 (95% CI, 1.1 to 1.7) for women drinking 12 g/d and of 1.7 (95% CI, 1.3 to 2.2) for those taking in 24 g/d. Data from 7 more prospective studies have been subsequently published. In the 2 smallest studies, the association was essentially zero; RRs for the highest category of alcohol consumption compared with zero consumption were 0.8 (95% CI, 0.5 to 1.2) based on 141 cases[85] and 1.1 (95% CI, 0.3 to 5) based on 87 cases.[86] In the 5 largest studies, which all controlled for major breast cancer risk factors, RRs for the highest category of alcohol consumption compared with zero consumption were 3.3 (95% CI, 1.2 to 9.3) based on 303 cases;[87] 1.6 (95% CI, 1 to 2.6) based on 2933 cases;[88] 1.5 (95% CI, 1 to 2) based on 493 cases;[89] 1.2 (95% CI, 0.8 to 1.9) based on 519 cases;[90] and 1.7 ($P = .05$) based on 422 cases.[91] Thus, an increased RR among women consuming alcohol is probably the best established dietary risk factor for breast cancer.

To translate this knowledge into advice for women seeking to avoid breast cancer, however, it is important to know whether reducing alcohol consumption in middle life is beneficial. Unfortunately, relatively few available data link age-specific drinking patterns with breast cancer risk. In a preliminary report from a large case-control study Longnecker and colleagues[92] reported that recent consumption of three or more drinks per day was associated with an RR of 2.2, whereas the RR was 0.9 for consumption of three or more drinks per day from age 16 to 29 years, suggesting that early adult drinking may be less important than drinking patterns later in life. In the study of Harvey and colleagues,[93] however, women who drank before age 30 years and who later stopped experienced a similar elevation in risk to those who con-

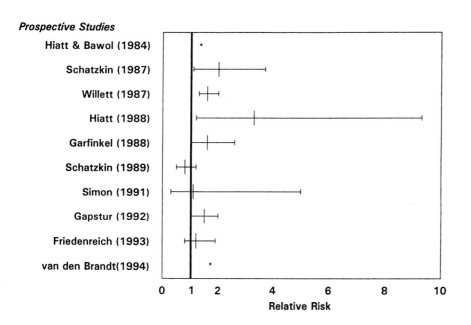

FIGURE 7.4-3 Prospective studies of the association between alcohol consumption and breast cancer risk. Vertical bars and asterisks represent the relative risks for the highest category of alcohol versus the lowest; error bars represent the 95% confidence intervals.

tinued to drink. Similarly, Hiatt and colleagues[94] observed an increase in risk among past drinkers compared with women who never drank (RR, 2.2; 95% CI, 1.3 to 3.9), although the age at quitting alcohol consumption was unspecified. In an intervention study, Reichman and colleagues[95] observed that consumption of about two alcoholic drinks per day increased total and bioavailable estrogen levels in premenopausal women, suggesting a mechanism by which alcohol may increase breast cancer risk.

The public health implications of this knowledge are complicated by the fact that consumption of one or two alcoholic beverages per day is almost certainly protective against cardiovascular disease.[96] Although specific data on the effect of quitting alcohol on cardiovascular risk are sparse, the mechanisms for the protective effect probably involve both a beneficial effect on high-density lipoprotein cholesterol levels[97] and short-term decreases in platelet aggregability,[98] suggesting that women who cease moderate alcohol consumption may experience a rapid increase in cardiovascular disease risk. Because cardiovascular disease is the leading cause of death among older women, the risk–benefit may favor moderate drinking, unless a women has other breast cancer risk factors or is at behavioral risk for excess drinking. This issue remains complex and controversial, however, and prospective studies of this risk–benefit are required to provide physicians with firmer grounds for giving practical advice.

CAFFEINE

Considerable speculation that caffeine may be a risk factor for breast cancer followed the report of Minton and colleagues,[99] which showed that women with benign breast disease experienced relief from symptoms after eliminating caffeine from their diet. Most case-control studies, however, have not observed evidence of a positive association with breast cancer. Among prospective studies, Snowden and Phillips[100] observed no increase in breast cancer risk among Seventh Day Adventist women who consumed coffee. Folsom and colleagues[101] observed no association among women living in Iowa, and Hunter and coworkers[102] actually observed a weak but significant inverse association between caffeine consumption and breast cancer risk. Thus, the epidemiologic evidence is not compatible with any substantial increase in breast cancer risk associated with coffee drinking.

ANTICARCINOGENIC PHYTOCHEMICALS

Various compounds in fruit and vegetables, other than those discussed here, have potential anticarcinogenic activity in vitro.[103] Some isoflavonoids, for example, appear to be antiestrogenic and thus may decrease breast cancer risk. In a case-control study in Singapore[104] intake of soy products, a major source of isoflavonoids, was associated with lower risk for breast cancer. High consumption of indole-3-carbinol, a compound found in cruciferous vegetables, appears to alter the balance of estrogen metabolism toward less potent forms.[105] Dietary supplementation with a large amount of soy product slightly lengthened menstrual cycle length, an effect which would be predicted to decrease breast cancer risk.[106] The possibility that phytochemicals that modulate estrogen metabolism may be a nontoxic means of altering breast cancer risk deserves further study, but the available evidence is limited.

Diet and Breast Cancer Survival

Whether or not diet is related to the occurrence of breast cancer, if postdiagnosis diet were related to risk of recurrence and breast cancer death, dietary modifications might assist in breast cancer treatment.

A number of studies (reviewed elsewhere[107]) have related dietary fat intake before breast cancer diagnosis to survival; results are inconsistent. All these studies have been conducted by monitoring the cases from breast cancer case-control studies. As the original interest in the case-control studies was the relation of diet to breast cancer incidence, the investigators were at pains to assess diet before diagnosis. This approach is unsatisfactory, however, if the question is whether diet after diagnosis has an influence on survival, because women may make major changes to their diet after receiving the diagnosis. In one study in which diet was evaluated after diagnosis (albeit in the 1 to 5 months immediately after the diagnosis) no association was seen between dietary fat intake and survival.[108] To investigate this issue, a randomized trial of a low-fat intervention among breast cancer patients is underway.[109]

Summary

Environmental and life-style factors appear to play important roles in the etiology of breast cancer; however, after several decades of study, the role of diet in breast cancer causation remains unclear. The enthusiasm for the hypothesis that increased dietary fat intake was responsible for increased breast cancer rates was based largely on the weakest form of epidemiologic evidence—international correlation studies. Results from prospective studies do not support the concept that fat intake in middle life has a major relation to breast cancer risk during up to 10 years of follow-up. The emerging hypothesis that energy intake and growth rate (rather than fat consumption) are most important, and that childhood and adolescence rather than middle life are the critical years of exposure, is also consistent with international correlations. Further, this hypothesis is supported by association of height with breast cancer risk in many studies. The possibility that vitamin A, or other compounds in vitamin A–rich foods, are protective deserves further consideration. Although the responsible substances are not yet defined, considerable evidence suggests that low intake of vegetables modestly increases the risk of breast cancer. Alcohol intake is the best established dietary risk factor for breast cancer in epidemiologic studies, and recent studies showing that even moderate alcohol intake alters estrogen metabolism provide a potential mechanism for this association, thus supporting a causal interpretation. The influence of adult diet on breast cancer should become clearer in the next few years as several major cohort studies present data. Hypotheses relating childhood and adolescent diet to breast cancer decades later is more difficult to test unless novel data sources or methods for measuring diet in the distant past are developed or unless radiographic, histologic, or other markers of breast cancer are found and validated for use as intermediate markers of breast cancer risk.

ACKNOWLEDGMENTS

Supported in part by NIH research grants CA 40456, CA 50598, and CA 55075, and a grant from the American Cancer Society (SIG-18). Dr. Hunter is partially supported by a Faculty Research Scholar Award from the American Cancer Society.

References

1. International Agency for Research on Cancer. Cancer incidence on five continents, vol 5. IARC scientific publ no. 88. Lyon, IARC, 1987:882.
2. Kelsey JL, Horn-Ross PL. Introduction: magnitude of the problem and descriptive epidemiology. Epidemiol Reviews 1993;15:7.
3. McMichael AJ, Giles GG. Cancer in migrants to Australia: extending descriptive epidemiological data. Cancer Res 1988;48:751.
4. Tannenbaum A. The genesis and growth of tumors: effects of a high fat diet. Cancer Res 1942;2:468.
5. Albanes D. Total calories, body weight, and tumor incidence in mice. Cancer Res 1987;47:1987.
6. Freedman LS, Clifford C, Messina M. Analysis of dietary fat, calories, body weight and the development of mammary tumor in rats and mice: a review. Cancer Res 1990;50:5710.
7. Appleton BS, Landers RE. Oil gavage effects on tumor incidence in the national toxicology program's 2-year carcinogenesis bioassay. Adv Exp Med Biol 1985;206:99.
8. Armstrong B, Doll R. Environmental factors and cancer incidence and mortality in different countries with special reference to dietary practices. Int J Cancer 1975;15:617.
9. Willett WC, Stampfer MJ. Dietary fat and cancer: another view. Cancer Caus Control 1990;1:103.
10. Prentice RL, Kakar F, Hursting S, et al. Aspects of the rationale for the Women's Health Trial. J Natl Cancer Inst 1988;80:802.
11. Stephen AM, Wald NJ. Trends in individual consumption of dietary fat in the United States, 1920–1984. Am J Clin Nutr 1990;52:457.
12. Hirayama T. Epidemiology of breast cancer with special reference to diet. Prevent Med 1978;7:173.
13. Aoki K, Kurihara M, Hayakawa N, et al. Death rates for malignant neoplasm for selected sites by age group in 33 countries. In: International union against cancer. Nagoya, University of Nagoya, 1992.
14. Phillips RL, Garfinkel L, Kuzma JL, et al. Mortality among California Seventh-Day Adventists. J Natl Cancer Inst 1980;65:1097.
15. Willett WC, Stampfer MJ, Colditz GA, et al. Relation of meat, fat, and fiber intake to the risk of colon cancer in a prospective study among women. N Engl J Med 1990;323:1664.
16. Kinlen LJ. Meat and fat consumption and cancer mortality: a study of strict religious orders in Britain. Lancet, 1982;1:946.
17. Graham S, Marshall J, Mettlin C, et al. Diet in the epidemiology of breast cancer. Am J Epidemiol 1982;116:68.
18. Howe GR, Hirohata T, Hislop TG, et al. Dietary factors and risk of breast cancer: combined analysis of 12 case-control studies. J Natl Cancer Inst, 1990;82:561.
19. Willett WC, Hunter DJ, Stampfer MJ, et al. Dietary fat and fiber in relation to risk of breast cancer. JAMA 1992;268:2037.
20. Rosner B, Spiegelman D, Willett WC. Correction of logistic regression relative risk estimates and confidence intervals for measurement error: the case of multiple covariates measured with error. Am J Epidemiol 1990;132:734.
21. Prentice RL, Sheppard L. Dietary fat and cancer: consistency of the epidemiologic data, and disease prevention that may follow from a practical reduction in fat consumption. Cancer Causes Cont 1990;1:81.
22. Michels KB, Willett WC. The women's health initiative: daughter of politics or science? In: DeVita VT, Hellman S, Rosenberg SA, eds. Cancer prevention. Philadelphia, JB Lippincott, 1992:1.
23. Freedman LS, Prentice RL, Clifford C, et al. Dietary fat and breast cancer: where we are. J Natl Cancer Inst 1993;85:764.
24. Goldin BR, Aldercreutz H, Gorbach SL, et al. Estrogen excretion patterns and plasma levels in vegetarian and omnivorous women. N Engl J Med 1982;307:1542.
25. Cohen LA, Kendall ME, Zang E, et al. Modulation of N-nitroso-methylurea-induced mammary tumor promotion by dietary fiber and fat. J Natl Cancer Inst 1991;83:496.
26. Rohan TE, Howe GR, Friedenreich CM, et al. Dietary fiber, vitamins A, C, and E, and risk of breast cancer: a cohort study. Cancer Causes Control 1993;4:29.
27. Graham S, Zielezny M, Marshall J, et al. Diet in the epidemiology of postmenopausal breast cancer in the New York State cohort. Am J Epidemiol 1992;136:1327.
28. Gray GE, Pike MC, Henderson BE. Breast cancer incidence and mortality rates in different countries in relation to known risk factors and dietary practices. Br J Cancer 1979;39:1.
29. Hirohata T, Shigematsu T, Nomura AM, et al. Occurrence of breast cancer in relation to diet and reproductive history: a case-control study in Fukuoka, Japan. Natl Cancer Inst Monogr 1985;69:187.
30. Hunter DJ, Willett WC. Diet, body size, and breast cancer. Epidemiol Rev 1993;15:110.
31. De Waard F, Baanders-van Halewijn EA. A prospective study in general practice on breast cancer risk in postmenopausal women. Int J Cancer 1974;14:153.
32. Swanson CA, Jones DY, Schatzkin A, et al. Breast cancer risk assessed by anthropometry in the NHANES I epidemiological follow-up study. Cancer Res 1988;48:5363.
33. London SJ, Colditz GA, Stampfer MJ, et al. Prospective study of relative weight, height, and risk of breast cancer. JAMA 1989;262:2853.
34. Tornberg SA, Holm L-E, Carstensen JM. Breast cancer risk in relation to serum cholesterol, serum beta-lipoprotein, height, weight, and blood pressure. Acta Oncol 1988;27:31.
35. Tretli S. Height and weight in relation to breast cancer morbidity and mortality: a prospective study of 570,000 women in Norway. Cancer 1989;44:23.
36. Vatten LJ, Kvinnsland S. Body height and risk of breast cancer: a prospective study of 23,831 Norwegian women. Br J Cancer 1990;61:881.
37. Vatten LJ, Kvinnsland S. Prospective study of height, body mass index and risk of breast cancer. Acta Oncol 1992;31:195.
38. Trichopoulos D, Lipman RD. Mammary gland mass and breast cancer risk. Epidemiol 1992;3:523.

39. Hunter DJ, Willett WC. Diet, body build, and breast cancer. Annu Rev Nutr 1994;14:393.

40. Peto R, Doll R, Buckley JD, et al. Can dietary beta-carotene materially reduce human cancer rates? Nature 1981;290:201.

41. Sporn MB, Roberts AB. Role of retinoids in differentiation and carcinogenesis. Cancer Res 1983;43:3034.

42. Fraker LD, Halter SA, Forbes JT. Growth inhibition by retinol of a human breast carcinoma cell line in vitro and in athymic mice. Cancer Res 1984;44:5757.

43. McCormick DL, Burns PJ, Albert RE. Inhibition of benzo-(a)pyrene-induced mammary carcinogenesis by retinyl acetate. J Natl Cancer Inst 1981;66:559.

44. Moon RC, Grubbs CJ, Sporn MB, et al. Retinyl acetate inhibits mammary carcinogenesis induced by N-methyl-N-nitrosourea. Nature 1977;267:620.

45. Moon RC, McCormick DL, Mehta RG. Inhibition of carcinogenesis by retinoids. Cancer Res 1983;43:2469.

46. Howe GR, Friedenreich CM, Jain M, et al. A cohort study of fat intake and risk of breast cancer. J Natl Cancer Inst 1991;83:336.

47. Paganini-Hill A, Chao A, Ross RK, et al. Vitamin A, beta-carotene and the risk of cancer: a prospective study. J Natl Cancer Inst 1987;79:443.

48. Hunter DJ, Manson JE, Colditz GA, et al. A prospective study of consumption of vitamins C, E and A and breast cancer risk. N Engl J Med 1993;329:234.

49. Willett WC, Stampfer MJ, Underwood BA, et al. Vitamin A supplementation and plasma retinol levels: a randomized trial among women. J Natl Cancer Inst 1984;73:1445.

50. Marubini E, Decarli A, Costa A, et al. The relationship of dietary intake and serum levels of retinol and β-carotene with breast cancer. Cancer 1988;61:173.

51. London SJ, Stein EA, Henderson IC, et al. Carotenoids, retinol, and vitamin E and risk of proliferative benign breast disease and breast cancer. Cancer Causes Control 1992;3:503.

52. Potischman N, McCullock CF, Byers T, et al. Breast cancer and plasma concentrations of carotenoids and vitamin A. Am J Clin Nutr 1990;52:909.

53. Wald NJ, Boreham J, Hayward JL, et al. Plasma retinol, beta-carotene and vitamin E levels in relation to the future risk of breast cancer. Br J Cancer 1984;49:321.

54. Knekt P, Aromaa A, Maatela J, et al. Serum vitamin A and the subsequent risk of cancer: cancer incidence follow-up of the Finnish Mobile Clinic Health Examination Survey. Am J Epidemiol 1990;132:857.

55. Comstock GW, Helzlsouer KJ, Bush TL. Prediagnostic serum levels of carotenoids and vitamin E as related to subsequent cancer in Washington County, Maryland. Am J Clin Nutr 1991;53:260S.

56. Formelli F, Clerici M, De Palo G, et al. Chronic oral administration of fenretinide, as a chemopreventive agent to breast cancer patients, does not affect plasma α-tocopherol concentration. Ann Oncol 1991;2:446.

57. Harman D. Dimethylbenzanthracene-induced cancer: inhibitory effect of dietary vitamin E. (Abstract) Clin Res 1969;17:125.

58. Lee C, Chen C. Enhancement of mammary tumorigenesis in rats by vitamin E deficiency. (Abstract) Proc Am Assoc Cancer Res 1979;20:132.

59. King MM, McCay PB. Modulation of tumor incidence and possible mechanism of mammary carcinogenesis by dietary antioxidants. Cancer Res 1983;43:2485S.

60. Willett WC, Stampfer MJ, Underwood BA, et al. Validation of a dietary questionnaire with plasma carotenoid and alpha-tocopherol levels. Am J Clin Nutr 1983;38:631.

61. Gerber M, Cavallo F, Marubini E, et al. Liposoluble vitamins and lipid parameters in breast cancer: a joint study in northern Italy and southern France. Int J Cancer 1988;42:489.

62. Wald NH, Nicolaides-Bouman A, Hudson GA. Plasma retinol, β-carotene and vitamin E levels in relation to future risk of breast cancer. Br J Cancer 1988;57:235.

63. Knekt P. Serum vitamin E level and risk of female cancers. Int J Epidemiol 1988;17:281.

64. Stampfer MJ, Hennekens CH, Manson JE, et al. Vitamin E consumption and the risk of coronary disease in women. N Engl J Med 1993;328:1444.

65. Esterbauer H, Dieber-Rotheneder M, Striegl G, et al. Role of vitamin E in preventing the oxidation of low-density lipoprotein. Am J Clin Nutr 1991;53:314S.

66. Dorgan JF, Schatzkin A. Antioxidant micronutrients in cancer prevention. Hematol Oncol Clin North Am 1991;5:43.

67. Abdul-Hajj YJ, Kelliher M. Failure of ascorbic acid to inhibit growth of transplantable and dimethylbenzanthracene induced rat mammary tumors. Cancer Lett 1982;17:67.

68. Graham S, Hellmann R, Marshall J, et al. Nutritional epidemiology of postmenopausal breast cancer in western New York. Am J Epidemiol 1991;134:552.

69. Medina D. Mechanisms of selenium inhibition of tumorigenesis. J Am Coll Toxicol 1986;5:21.

70. Ip C. The chemopreventive role of selenium in carcinogenesis. J Am Coll Toxicol 1986;5:7.

71. Shamberger RJ, Tytko SA, Willis CE. Antioxidants and cancer. VI. Selenium and age-adjusted human cancer mortality. Arch Environ Health 1976;31:231.

72. Clark LC. The epidemiology of selenium and cancer. Fed Proc 1985;44:2584.

73. Schrauzer GN, White DA, Schneider CJ. Cancer mortality correlation studies. III. Statistical associations with dietary selenium intakes. Bioinorg Chem 1977;7:23.

74. Levander OA. The need for a measure of selenium status. J Am Coll Toxicol 1986;5:37.

75. Hunter DJ. Biochemical indicators of dietary intake. In: Willett WC, ed. Nutritional epidemiology. New York, Oxford University, 1990;143.

76. Hunter DJ, Morris JS, Chute CG, et al. Predictors of selenium concentration in human toenails. Am J Epidemiol 1990;132:114.

77. Meyer F, Verreault R. Erythrocyte selenium and breast cancer risk. Am J Epidemiol 1987;125:917.

78. Van't Veer P, Kalb CM, Verhoef P, et al. Dietary fiber, β-carotene and breast cancer: results from a case-control study. Int J Cancer 1990;45:825.

79. Hunter DJ, Morris JS, Stampfer MJ, et al. A prospective study of selenium status and breast cancer risk. JAMA 1990;264:1128.

80. Van Noord PA, Collette HJ, Maas MJ, et al. Selenium levels in nails of premenopausal breast cancer patients assessed prediagnostically in a cohort-nested case-referent study among women screened in the DOM project. Int J Epidemiol 1987;16:318.

81. Coates RJ, Weiss NS, Daling JR, et al. Serum levels of selenium and retinol and the subsequent risk of cancer. Am J Epidemiol 1988;128:515.

82. Knekt P, Aromaa A, Maatela J, et al. Serum selenium and subsequent risk of cancer among Finnish men and women. J Natl Cancer Inst 1990;82:864.

83. Overvad K, Wang DY, Olsen J, et al. Selenium in human mammary carcinogenesis: a case-cohort study. Eur J Cancer 1991;27:900.

84. Longnecker M, Berlin JA, Orza MJ, et al. A meta-analysis of alcohol consumption in relation to breast cancer risk. JAMA 1988;260:642.

85. Schatzkin A, Carter CC, Green SB, et al. Is alcohol consumption related to breast cancer? results from the Framingham Heart Study. J Natl Cancer Inst 1989;81:31.

86. Simon MS, Carman LS, Wolfe R, et al. Alcohol consumption and the risk of breast cancer: a report from the Tecumseh Community Health Study. J Clin Epidemiol 1991;44:755.

87. Hiatt RA, Bawol RD. Alcoholic beverage consumption and breast cancer incidence. Am J Epidemiol 1984;120:676.

88. Garfinkel L, Bofetta P, Stellman SD. Alcohol and breast cancer: a cohort study. Prevent Med 1988;17:686.

89. Gapstur SM, Potter JD, Sellers TA, et al. Increased risk of breast cancer with alcohol consumption in postmenopausal women. Am J Epidemiol 1992;136:1221.

90. Freidenreich CM, Howe GR, Miller AB, et al. A cohort study of alcohol consumption and risk of breast cancer. Am J Epidemiol 1993;137:512.

91. van den Brandt PA, Goldbohm RA, Van't Veer P. A cohort study on alcohol consumption and breast cancer risk among postmenopausal women. (Abstract) Am J Epidemiol 1994;139:274.

92. Longnecker M, Newcomb PA, Mittendorf R, et al. Risk of breast cancer in relation to past and recent alcohol consumption. Am J Epidemiol 1992;136:1001.

93. Harvey EB, Schairer C, Brinton LA, et al. Alcohol consumption and breast cancer. J Natl Cancer Inst 1987;78:657.

94. Hiatt RA, Klatsky AL, Armstrong MA. Alcohol consumption and the risk of breast cancer in a prepaid health plan. Cancer Res 1988;48:2284.

95. Reichman ME, Judd JT, Lonscope C, et al. Effects of alcohol consumption on plasma and urinary hormone concentrations in premenopausal women. J Natl Cancer Inst 1993;85:722.

96. Stampfer MJ, Rimm EB, Chapman Walsh D. Commentary: alcohol, the heart, and public policy. Am J Publ Health 1993;83:801.

97. Stampfer MJ, Sacks FM, Salvini S, et al. A prospective study of cholesterol, apolipoproteins, and the risk of myocardial infarction. N Engl J Med 1991;325:373.

98. Kluft C, Hie AFH, Kooistra PK, et al. Alcohol and fibrinolysis. In: Veenstra J, van der Heij DG, eds. Alcohol and cardiovascular disease. Wageningen, The Netherlands, Pudoc, 1992:45.

99. Minton JP, Foecking MK, Webster DJ, et al. Response of fibrocystic disease to caffeine withdrawal and correlation of cyclic nucleotides with breast disease. Am J Obstet Gynecol 1979;135:157.

100. Snowden DA, Phillips RL. Coffee consumption and risk of fatal cancers. Am J Publ Health 1984;74:820.

101. Folsom AR, McKenzie DR, Bisgard KM, et al. No association between caffeine intake and postmenopausal breast cancer incidence in the Iowa Women's Health study. Am J Epidemiol 1993;138:380.

102. Hunter DJ, Manson JE, Stampfer MJ, et al. A prospective study of caffeine, coffee, tea, and breast cancer. Am J Epidemiol 1992;136:1000.

103. Steinmetz KA, Potter JD. Vegetables, fruits, and cancer. II. Mechanisms. Cancer Causes Cont 1991;2:325.

104. Lee HP, Gourley L, Duffy SW, et al. Dietary effects on breast cancer risk in Singapore. Lancet 1991;337:1197.

105. Michnovicz JJ, Bradlow HL. Induction of estradiol metabolism by dietary indole-3-carbinol in humans. J Natl Cancer Inst 1990;82:947.

106. Cassidy A, Bingham S, Carlson J, et al. Biological effects of plant estrogens in premenopausal women. (Abstract) FASEB J 1993; 7:A866.

107. Holmes M, Hunter DJ, Willett WC. Dietary guidelines. In: Stoll BA, ed. Reducing breast cancer risk in women. Boston, Kluwer Academic, 1995:135.

108. Newman SC, Miller AB, Howe GR. A study of the effect of weight and dietary fat on breast cancer survival time. Am J Epidemiol 1986;123:767.

109. Chlebowski RT, Nixon DW, Blackburn GL, et al. A breast cancer nutrition adjuvant study (NAS): protocol design and initial patient adherence. Breast Cancer Res Treat 1987;10:21.

110. Jones DY, Schatzkin A, Green SB, et al. Dietary fat and breast cancer in the National Health and Nutrition Examination Survey. I. Epidemiologic follow-up study. J Natl Cancer Inst 1987;79:465.

111. Willett WC, Stampfer MJ, Colditz GA, et al. Dietary fat and risk of breast cancer. N Engl J Med 1987;316:22.

112. Mills PK, Beeson WL, Phillips RL, et al. Dietary habits and breast cancer incidence among Seventh Day Adventists. Cancer 1989; 64:582.

113. Knekt P, Albanes D, Seppanen R, et al. Dietary fat and risk of breast cancer. Am J Clin Nutr 1990;52:903.

114. Kushi LH, Sellers TA, Potter JD, et al. Dietary fat and postmenopausal breast cancer. J Natl Cancer Inst 1992;84:1092.

115. Byrne C, Ursin G, Ziegler R. Dietary fat and breast cancer in NHANES I continued follow-up. Am J Epidemiol 1992;136:1024.

116. Van den Brandt PA, Van't Veer P, Goldbohm RA, et al. A prospective cohort study on dietary fat and breast cancer risk. Cancer Res 1993;53:75.

117. Toniolo P, Riboli E, Shore RE, et al. Consumption of meat, animal products, protein, and fat and risk of breast cancer: a prospective cohort study in New York. Epidemiology 1994;5:391.

118. LaVecchia C, Decarli A, Franceschi S, et al. Dietary factors and the risk of breast cancer. Nutr Cancer 1987;10:205.

119. Katsouyanni K, Willett W, Trichopoulos D, et al. Risk of breast cancer among Greek women in relation to nutrient intake. Cancer 1988;61:181.

120. Rohan TE, McMichael AJ, Baghurst PA. A population-based case-control study of diet and breast cancer in Australia. Am J Epidemiol 1988;61:173.

121. Toniolo P, Riboli E, Protta F, et al. Calorie-providing nutrients and risk of breast cancer. J Natl Cancer Inst 1989;81:278.

122. Ewertz M, Gill C. Dietary factors and breast cancer risk in Denmark. Int J Cancer 1990;46:779.

123. Ingram DM, Nottage E, Roberts T. The role of diet in the development of breast cancer: a case-control study of patients with breast cancer, benign epithelial hyperplasia and fibrocystic disease of the breast. Br J Cancer 1991;64:187.

124. Lee HP, Gourley L, Duffy SW, et al. Dietary effects on breast cancer risk in Singapore. Lancet 1991;337:1197.

125. Richardson S, Gerber M, Cenee S. The role of fat, animal protein and some vitamin consumption in breast cancer: a case-control study in Southern France. Int J Cancer 1991;48:1.

126. Zaridze D, Lifanova Y, Maximovitch D, et al. Diet, alcohol consumption and reproductive factors in a case-control study of breast cancer in Moscow. Int J Cancer 1991;48:493.

7.5
Molecular Epidemiology
BRUCE J. TROCK

Molecular epidemiology of cancer combines traditional epidemiologic methods for observational data with molecular biologic measurements of exposure and events in the etiologic pathway of cancer. Traditionally, epidemiology has focused on elucidating associations between risk factors and disease outcomes as a means of developing strategies for prevention and control. Because it was directed primarily against single exposures that produced large increases in disease risk, this approach has allowed important advances in disease control even when biologic mechanisms underlying disease pathogenesis were not well characterized.[1] Sporadic breast cancer is difficult to control, however, because it probably results from multiple, relatively weak causal factors (exogenous and endogenous) interacting against a background of variable susceptibility. Because of this difficulty, epidemiology has not had much success in defining the attributes that confer high risk for the majority of patients with sporadic breast cancer.[2] Molecular epidemiology represents an enhancement of the resolving power of epidemiologic studies. By studying how risk associated with specific molecules or biomarkers varies in the presence of other exposures and host factors in the natural setting, molecular epidemiology can clarify carcinogenic mechanisms and can provide improved assessment of individual risk. As such, it forms a bridge in the translation of basic scientific advances to clinical application.

It is useful to view molecular epidemiology from the context of a continuum between exposure and metastatic cancer (Fig. 7.5-1). Metabolic activation is important in determining both the internal dose and the biologically effective dose of exogenous carcinogens, and it also mediates oxidative DNA damage resulting from endogenous generation of active oxygen species. Variation in the fidelity of DNA replication and of repair processes determines the occurrence of mutation fixation, producing markers of early biologic effect. Individual differences in susceptibility to cancer probably reflect genetic and acquired factors that modulate metabolic activity and repair mechanisms. Mutation-driven clonal expansion of cell subpopulations, increased cellular proliferation, and genomic instability result in additional mutations, allelic loss and recombination, and gene amplification, with consequent alterations in molecular structures and functions.[3] These,

in turn, trigger alterations in growth control and acquisition of invasive and metastatic phenotypes.

Epidemiology usually operates at the extremes of the continuum. Characteristics associated with risk are usually fixed attributes identifiable before or near the time of exposure. Outcomes are incident cancer, metastatic behavior, and, less often, premalignant lesions. The magnitude of the association between exposure and outcome is attenuated by intervening factors (such as differences in carcinogen metabolism, DNA repair, endogenous mutation rates, and genetic instability) that modulate transition between events. This attenuation limits the ability of traditional studies to evaluate factors that do not produce large elevations in risk. By incorporating measurements of specific events along the continuum as both predictor variables and outcomes, molecular epidemiology enables one to refine exposure measures, more clearly to define risk groups based on host susceptibility factors and occurrence of intermediate endpoints in the neoplastic process, to evaluate factors that influence progression along the continuum, and to identify molecular markers to be used for early diagnosis. In addition, the ability to classify molecular subtypes of cancer (eg, p53 mutation spectra) allows for disease classification into more homogeneous subgroups, resulting in more specific etiologic inferences and increased statistical power.[3]

Despite great advances in the molecular biology of breast cancer, molecular epidemiologic research in breast cancer has only recently begun. Current research on the molecular epidemiology of breast cancer with regard to specific molecules and their occurrence along the continuum is discussed later in this chapter. The emphasis is on molecules that have been incorporated into epidemiologic studies and those likely to reflect specific exposures. Prognostic application of these molecules is considered in detail elsewhere in this book and is not emphasized here. Before discussing specific molecules, however, some methodologic issues important in all such studies are described.

Methodologic Issues

As research moves from the laboratory to the population, information on the occurrence of and variability in biomarker expression is required. Because a major goal in the

FIGURE 7.5-1   Events along continuum in the process of carcinogenesis.

use of biomarkers is to identify individuals without cancer who harbor premalignant changes or who are at high risk of malignant progression, normal background variation in expression of biomarkers must be characterized to enable molecular screening to be feasible. For example, overexpression of growth factors and their receptors (such as epidermal growth factor receptor [EGFR], transforming growth factors α and β [TGF-α, TGF-β], fibroblast growth factor [FGF] family[4–6]) occurs to varying degrees in normal tissue or body fluids, and oncogene amplification and mutant forms also occur (eg, erbB-2, ras oncoproteins, and rare alleles[7–9]). Markers of biologically effective dose or early biologic effect may be useful for planning preventive strategies directed against particular exposures. Because many such biomarkers can reflect exposure from more than one source (eg, DNA hydroxy adducts reflect free radical activation from both endogenous and exogenous sources[10]; dietary factors and environmental exposures may modulate estrogen 16-α-hydroxylase activity[11,12]; more than one exposure may produce similar p53 mutation spectra[13,14]), however, it will be necessary to determine the degree to which they are specific for particular exposures.

Use of biomarkers introduces additional sources of variability into epidemiologic studies. Intraindividual variation arises from random sampling variability and true biologic variability. The former is a component of all sampling processes and reflects differences between information provided by a sample and that associated with the entire organ or tissue compartment. The latter is composed of both time-dependent differences (eg, changes in levels of DNA hydroxy adducts with exposure and repair, growth factor variation associated with inflammatory processes or hormonal fluctuations) and heterogeneity of expression within tissues. Interindividual variation derives from many sources, including exposures, ethnicity, age, host-susceptibility factors, and laboratory factors (including measurement error, differences in techniques, reagents, and internal controls).[15] Studies of molecular factors, with the exception of prognostic factor studies, have often considered only the molecule of interest, and have not incorporated information about other, potentially confounding factors contributing to interindividual variability. Furthermore, laboratory artifacts, such as differences in antibody sensitivity and specificity in archival tissue, contamination by normal DNA, and false-positives and false-negatives associated with immunocytochemistry, contribute to inconsistent associations with particular molecules between studies.[16–18]

Small differences in assay sensitivity and specificity can have profound effects on observed associations with specific biomarkers. Molecular epidemiology relies heavily on case control studies, whether the outcome that defines a case is development of metastases, occurrence of cancer, or presence of a specific mutation. The odds ratio is the primary measure used in such studies to quantify associations between the outcome and an exposure or prognostic marker. Under some circumstances, however, minor decreases in assay sensitivity and specificity can introduce substantial bias in the observed odds ratio, resulting in

significant underestimation of the true association. Underestimation of the true odds ratio occurs (1) with small decreases in sensitivity when the prevalence of the marker is high (50% or higher), and (2) with small decreases in specificity when the prevalence of the marker is low (20% or lower).[19]

For example, if the true odds ratio is 10 and the prevalence of the biomarker in the population is 85% (eg, metabolic polymorphisms), an assay with extremely good sensitivity of 95%, and with perfect specificity, will result in an odds ratio of 3.3 for that study. For a similar true odds ratio with biomarker prevalence of 15% (eg, p53 serum antibodies, INT2 protooncogene), an assay with sensitivity and specificity both at 90% will produce an observed odds ratio of 5.6. In molecular epidemiologic studies, in contrast to traditional epidemiologic studies, true odds ratios of 10 or higher will not be uncommon, particularly when evaluating risk associated with susceptibility factors or markers of altered structure and function. This problem can be exacerbated in a multifactorial setting in which odds ratios are estimated for the simultaneous effects of multiple biomarkers, all with less than perfect assay methods. Thus, inconsistent risk associations observed across different studies may actually reflect minor differences in assay sensitivity. Furthermore, true genetic differences in biomarker prevalence across racial or ethnic groups can spuriously produce apparent racial differences in the magnitude of risk estimates associated with the marker.[19]

Finally, rigorous design of molecular epidemiologic studies is critical. Studies must have sufficient sample size to provide adequate statistical power to detect desired effects. This requires that the expected size of the effect (eg, differences in mutation prevalence between cases and controls) be specified ahead of time. If effects of the molecule of interest are expected to differ across subgroups of patients, then sample sizes in subgroups must be sufficient to detect *differences* in effect across subgroups. One must carefully define selection criteria for cases and controls entered into the study. Combining prevalent (existing disease) and incident (newly diagnosed) cases may cause one to identify effects associated with prognosis rather than cause. Patients should be representative of the cohort of patients (of the type of interest; eg, untreated premenopausal breast cancer) treated at the study center during a given period. Controls are often derived from women without cancer who are seen at breast clinics. Because they may share many of the risk factors of women with breast cancer, they may represent an overmatched control source, thereby reducing the statistical power of the study and potentially attenuating observed associations.

Markers of Oxidative Metabolism

An important use of biomarkers is to characterize biologically relevant exposures at the level of critical molecular targets. Measurement of exposure is a source of error in epidemiologic studies because it often depends on patient recollection of past events or habits or on exposure surrogates for environmental or workplace exposures. Such exposure estimates are subject to errors in absolute exposure levels and to misclassification, that is, classifying unexposed individuals as exposed and vice versa.[20] These problems can either attenuate or exaggerate the apparent association between the exposure and cancer. Associations with external exposure measurements are also complicated by the effects of unmeasured variability in metabolic and repair enzymes that modify susceptibility to the damaging effects of exposure. Markers of biologically effective dose or early biologic effect have the potential to reduce exposure measurement errors, although standardization of laboratory techniques and quality control are necessary to minimize the effect of technical errors. By integrating exposure from multiple sources with host variation in metabolic activity and DNA repair processes, these markers may provide clues to etiology and improved predictors of risk.

Oxidative DNA damage, caused by generation of active hydroxyl radicals, hydrogen peroxide, superoxide anions, and lipid peroxidation, is a putative source of carcinogenic mutations.[10,21–23] Reactive oxygen species may result from both endogenous factors (eg, redox reactions involving hormones) and exogenous exposures (eg, chlorinated organics, cigarette smoke).[10,22] Research has shown high concentrations of 8-hydroxyguanine and 8-hydroxyadenine base lesions in tumor and adjacent normal tissue from breast cancer patients, compared with control tissues from patients receiving reduction mammaplasty.[10,23] In particular, the ratio of 8-hydroxy base lesions to ring opening derivatives (2,6-diamino-4-hydroxy-5-formamidopyrimidine and 4,6-diamino-5-formamidopyrimidine) was particularly specific for tissue from cancer patients, but was not an artifact of inflammatory processes. This association was not influenced by differences in age between the two study groups.

The foregoing investigators suggested that hydroxyl radicals are generated as a consequence of hydrogen peroxide formed from redox cycling of hormones and chlorinated organics. Hydroxyl radical attack on purine bases can be followed by oxidative reactions to form mutagenic 8-hydroxy adducts or by reduction reactions to form non-mutagenic ring-opening derivatives.[10] Despite the small sample size of these studies, the results are provocative because of the propensity of chemical carcinogens for covalent binding to guanosines.[24] Furthermore, although serum studies of organochlorines and breast cancer have been inconclusive,[25,26] studies of adipose tissue from breast cancer patients have exhibited higher organochlorine concentrations than tissue from controls,[27–30] and organochlorines are commonly found in breast milk.[31,32] In addition, the lack of significant differences in base lesion concentrations between tumor tissue and adjacent normal tissue suggests a field effect, consistent with high risk of ipsilateral tumors. Because atypical hyperplasia and lobular carcinoma in situ have been postulated as markers of a possible field defect in breast epithelium, it would be informative to examine the occurrence of 8-hydroxy adducts in these lesions. If confirmed, these results would suggest a potential chemopreventive role for antioxidants and for the use of DNA base lesion profiles as an intermediate endpoint.

A shift in estradiol metabolism from the C2-hydroxylation pathway to the C16α-hydroxylation pathway has been associated with increased risk for breast cancer.[11,12,33] Although studies of this marker have been small and have not examined the influence of other breast cancer risk factors on the metabolic pathway, the results are suggestive because this shift is associated with increased formation of mutagenic 16α-hydroxyestrone, which may form DNA adducts in target tissues. Control of the C2 pathway appears to be mediated by the P-450 enzyme CYP1A2. The complexity of the risk relation is indicated by the finding that putative protective agents (dietary indoles) and putative genotoxic agents (polycyclic hydrocarbons, dioxins) and agents of uncertain breast cancer risk (cigarette smoke) all appear to enhance metabolism by the C2 pathway that is associated with decreased risk.[34,35] Specific enzymatic polymorphisms that mediate the 16α-hydroxylation pathway have not been identified, although treatment of mammary explants from breast cancer patients with benzo-(*a*)pyrene and ω-6 polyunsaturated fatty acids increased the activity of this pathway.[12]

The foregoing studies underscore the early stage of molecular epidemiologic research on markers of biologically effective dose and early biologic effect. Additional, larger studies must be performed to determine the specificity of these markers for particular exposures and the modulating influence of other risk factors and host factors. Studies incorporating other markers may also be useful. For example, 16α-hydroxyestrone is known to have alkylating properties. Alkylating agents preferentially cause GC−AT transitions at cytosine−guanine dinucleotides in p53, as discussed later. Thus, correlation of p53 mutations with C16α-hydroxylation could provide evidence for the mechanism underlying the increased risk associated with this pathway.

Although the potential of such markers is to reduce bias associated with error-prone exposure estimates in epidemiologic studies, first one must validate the associations among exposure, marker, and cancer occurrence. Two standard statistical methods can be applied to molecular epidemiologic data to derive inferences about the pathway from exposure to cancer: (1) calculation of the attributable proportion of cancer cases associated with the marker, and (2) estimation of exposure risk adjusted for the presence of the marker.

The attributable proportion (AP) associated with a particular marker estimates the proportion of cancer cases that acquire or exhibit the marker on the pathway from normal tissue to neoplasia. This is not simply the proportion of all cases that are positive for the marker, because the marker occurs in some cases even when the exposure of interest or the biologic events associated with the marker are not etiologic events for those cases (background levels). Thus, this measure indicates whether the marker is a contributing factor in a sufficient proportion of cases to be useful in evaluating etiologic associations with a particular exposure. The AP is defined in terms as follows:

$$AP = S \left(1 - 1/RR\right)$$

where S is the sensitivity of the marker (proportion of cases that are positive for the marker) and RR is the relative risk associated with the marker (ratio of cancer incidence among those with the marker to those without the marker).[20] Values of the marker approaching 1.0 suggest that most cases progress through the marker. Given the heterogeneity of breast cancer, values of AP are much lower than 1; however, use of AP can determine whether the marker is on the etiologic pathway in a sufficient proportion of cases to be a useful exposure or risk marker.

Once a marker has been demonstrated to be relevant to a significant proportion of tumors, one must examine the extent to which the marker truly represents a cellular event intervening between exposure and cancer. This is done using statistical adjustment methods such as stratification or regression. If the crude (ie, unadjusted) RR for the exposure of interest indicates a significant increase in risk, and the RR for exposure *adjusted* for the presence of the marker is reduced and nonsignificant, that suggests that the marker is linked to the pathway between exposure and cancer. If the effect of exposure occurs primarily through a pathway involving the marker, the marker-adjusted exposure effect is essentially eliminated; that is, the adjusted RR is close to 1.[20]

Figure 7.5-2A shows an example in which the RR associated with a particular exposure (E_1), adjusted for marker M_1, goes to 1. This is because all cases of cancer resulting from the exposure progress through M_1, even though a second carcinogenic pathway also exists. Note that because only a portion of cancers progress through M_1, the AP associated with M_1 is less than 1.

If the marker-adjusted exposure effect is smaller than the crude effect, but not close to 1, several possible mechanisms may be involved. First, the exposure may cause cancer through pathways involving more than one marker. This is indicated in Figure 7.5-2B, in which the effect of

exposure E_1 is mediated through markers M_1 and M_2. The smaller the adjusted effect, the greater the role played by M_1. A second reason for only partial reduction of the adjusted effect is depicted in Figure 7.5-2C, in which the marker (M) is not on the direct pathway to cancer, but occurs as a consequence of an unknown marker (U), which is the true intermediate between E and C. Some susceptibility markers may be examples of this situation. The marker-adjusted exposure effect decreases as the correlation between U and M increases. Finally, errors in measurement of the biologic marker can bias the estimate of the marker-adjusted effect away from a value of 1. Unfortunately, the statistical analyses alone do not allow these three alternatives to be readily distinguished. Incorporating auxiliary information about other markers and information about the error variance associated with the measurement may allow some discrimination among these pathways, but additional work on this methodologic approach needs to be done to allow full use of the method.[20]

Tumor-Suppressor Genes and Oncogenes

Oncogene activation and loss of suppressor function can result in selective growth pressures, loss of terminal differentiation, and programmed cell death. These lead, in a stochastic fashion, to clonal evolution and further genomic instability accompanied by gene amplification, chromosomal deletions, and allelic loss. This constellation of events is associated with altered structure and function and the development of intraepithelial neoplasia.[3] Because these mutations are associated with progression toward the malignant phenotype, they have great potential for use in molecular screening to define high-risk individuals and to detect preclinical neoplastic change.

Mutations in the p53 gene occur in 15% to 50% of sporadic breast cancers, with most estimates below 30%.[13,14,36] In its unmutated form, p53 acts as a tumor-suppressor gene, whose functions include cell-cycle regulation, transcriptional regulation, cell differentiation, and apoptosis,[37] although its role in breast cancer has not been determined. Mutation of p53 appears to be an early event in breast cancer, occurring in 13% to 25% of in situ carcinomas (primarily ductal carcinoma), and disproportionately occurring in biologically more aggressive large cell in situ lesions.[38,39] Alterations in p53 have shown significant associations with other markers of aggressive behavior, including estrogen receptor (*ER*) negativity, high nuclear grade, aneuploidy, and patient age under 50 years. However, p53 expression has not correlated with *erbB*-2 expression or with overall loss of heterozygosity, a marker of genomic instability.[36,38–40]

In several studies, serum antibodies to p53 oncoprotein were detected in 12% to 26% of breast cancer patients.[41–43] Antibody occurrence was significantly associated with positive p53 immunostaining in tumors, although 22% of seropositive patients lacked detectable p53 protein in tissue, whereas 36% of seronegative patients did have detectable protein levels in tissue. Serum antibodies

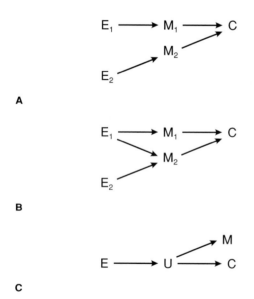

FIGURE 7.5-2 Pathways between external exposures (E), molecular biomarker (M), and cancer (C). **A.** Distinct exposure–biomarker–cancer pathways. **B.** Multiple overlapping pathways. **C.** Biomarker is a surrogate for an unobserved intermediate event (U).

occurred in all stages of disease progression, including in situ disease, and were correlated with histologic grade and lack of family breast cancer history. No associations were seen with tumor size, lymph node metastases, stage, age, parity, or menstrual status. In a small subset of patients in whom sequential samples were assayed before surgery and up to 6 months thereafter, serum antibody status did not change. Serum titers did not decrease even in patients with in situ disease who were subsequently assayed 6 months or more after surgery.[41] These results suggest the need for studies to validate the use of antibodies to p53 protein in serum and other accessible body fluids such as nipple aspirate fluid or urine as a marker for early detection.

The evaluation of p53 mutations in breast cancer exemplifies many of the difficulties of molecular epidemiology. Use of different antibodies, probes, and assay techniques leads to inconsistencies across studies. Immunohistochemical methods do not detect nonsense mutations or deletions, and protein stabilization may occur for reasons other than mutation.[18] Sequencing may detect mutations without functional significance. Heterogeneity of staining within tissues introduces additional variability,[40] and access to sufficient tissue may result in overrepresentation of large tumors (size bias). These problems require concerted efforts to standardize techniques and to define correspondences among different methods. Only then will studies to establish population variability and risk be feasible.

Because of the many types and locations of p53 mutations that have been identified, attempts have been made to determine whether particular carcinogens or classes of carcinogens are associated with specific patterns of mutation or mutational spectra. Most p53 mutations are missense mutations in which one base pair is substituted for another. Distinctive mutational spectra have been correlated with tobacco carcinogens in cancer of the lung and head and neck, with dietary aflatoxin B_1 in hepatocellular cancer, and with ultraviolet exposure in squamous cell skin cancer. The base-pair changes seen in these tumors are most consistent with direct adduct-driven mutagenesis rather than with indirect effects of increased cellular proliferation.[13,14,44,45]

Although fewer than half of sporadic breast cancers appear to harbor p53 mutations, analysis of mutation spectra strongly suggests that exogenous carcinogens may play an important role in a large fraction of breast cancer cases with p53 mutations. Evidence for this suggestion comes from examining the occurrence of p53 mutations on the nontranscribed (coding) strand of DNA. That repair of damaged DNA appears to occur preferentially on the transcribed (template) strand probably reflects an evolutionary response for maintaining the integrity of essential proteins.[14] Carcinogenesis studies in model systems have consistently shown that exogenous carcinogens induce mutations primarily on the nontranscribed strand (strand bias).[46,47]

Nearly half of p53 mutations in human breast cancer occur at sites associated with strand bias. Of these, the prevalence of strand bias is 89% for GC−TA transversions, 63% for GC−AT transitions at sites other than cytosine−guanine dinucleotides, and 75% for AT−GC transitions.[14] A role for exogenous carcinogens is also suggested by the frequency of mutations on guanosines on the nontran-

scribed strand, because chemical carcinogens in model systems selectively react with guanosines.[13,24] Differences in p53 mutational spectra have been observed between tumors from Japanese and those from Western women. In contrast to the foregoing rates, GC−TA transversions were rare, whereas AT−GC transitions occurred more frequently.[48,49] Rates of GC−TA transversions in US women also appear to be higher than those found among women from Scotland.[50] If borne out in larger samples, these contrasting mutational spectra could reflect different exposures, but they may also result from genetic polymorphisms in metabolic and repair processes or acquired susceptibility factors such as dietary micronutrients.[14]

Specific mutational spectra have also been associated with endogenous cellular events that produce mutations. The most characteristic of these is the GC−AT transition at cytosine−guanine dinucleotide sites; this lesion accounts for 23% of p53 mutations found in human breast cancer.[14]

The demonstration of specific mutational spectra may represent a molecular fingerprint of particular carcinogens or classes of carcinogens, providing a great opportunity for studies that can clarify the etiology of breast cancer. Correlation of individual carcinogen exposures with the prevalence of mutational spectra can indicate their relative contribution to cancer occurrence. Mutations associated with endogenous carcinogenesis should be correlated with known breast cancer risk factors related to ovarian function, for example, age at menarche, at first live birth, and at menopause. Such studies need to be large enough to include adequate numbers of patients with specific mutations. Cohort studies in populations of women with putative high-risk exposures (eg, women with high levels of environmental organochlorine exposure) may be able to use cells obtained from nipple aspirate fluid as a noninvasive means of serial monitoring for p53 mutations or antibodies.

The c-*erb*B-2 oncogene (also known as HER-2/*neu*) is a member of the EGFR family and is amplified or overexpressed in 20% to 30% of primary invasive breast cancers and in 50% to 60% of in situ lesions, particularly those with comedo-type histology.[51−53] The high prevalence of in situ lesion amplification and the concordance among expression levels in metastatic, invasive, and in situ tissues from the same individuals imply that this lesion is an early, genetically fixed marker that may characterize a specific subset of breast cancers.[52] The higher prevalence of *erb*B-2 overexpression may not be characteristic of in situ carcinoma in general, however, but rather may be an artifact of overrepresentation of specimens with comedo histology in any series of pure in situ specimens. Therefore, it is probably *not* the case that *erb*B-2 expression is down-regulated in the progression from in situ to invasive disease.[53a]

Amplification of *erb*B-2 has been significantly associated with advanced pathologic stage, number of positive axillary lymph nodes, histologic type, high S-phase fraction, and negativity of both ER and progesterone receptor (PR).[54,55] The mechanism by which *erb*B-2 oncoprotein affects cell growth has not been clearly determined, however.[51] The prognostic significance of *erb*B-2 amplification has been inconsistent and may be restricted to subsets of breast cancer.[56] Elevated levels of *erb*B-2 oncoproteins have been detected in serum from breast cancer patients, compared with controls, using antibodies to the shed extracellular domain.[57,58] Comparison of tumor and serum *erbB*-2 expression in the small subset of patients with both types of sample indicated that the tumor was the likely source of the oncoprotein.

Based on the similarity between clinicopathologic characteristics associated with the aforementioned *erbB*-2 amplification and those in tumors associated with oral contraceptive use at an early age,[59] a study was conducted examining the relation between reproductive factors and *erbB*-2 amplification. This study found that *erbB*-2 amplification in premenopausal breast cancer patients was significantly more likely among users of oral contraceptives up to age 20 years than among women who had never used oral contraceptives or those who first used oral contraceptives at age 20 years or older (odds ratio, 6.8 [95% CI, 1.3, 34.7]); adjusted for other breast cancer risk factors.[60] No significant association was found with duration of oral contraceptive use, early or late abortion, late age at first full-term pregnancy, parity, or progestin use.

Studies that have examined more than one oncogene in the same set of subjects have not observed concordance of marker expression. Studies of p53 have found little overlap with *erbB*-2 or overall loss of heterozygosity,[36,38–40] whereas *erbB*-2 amplification has not correlated with *myc* or INT2 amplification.[52,57,60] This implies the existence of multiple, unlinked pathways producing the same phenotype and is consistent with the heterogeneity of breast cancer and the concept of a stochastic process of clonal evolution or progression.[61] Given that both p53 mutation and *erbB*-2 amplification represent early, fixed events in breast cancer progression, and they correlate with similar clinicopathologic characteristics, it would be useful to identify factors that determine which of these biomarkers occurs in the progression pathway. Some possible explanations could involve differences in types of exposures, susceptibility factors, role of gene in normal cellular processes, control of transcription and replication, fidelity of repair mechanisms, genomic instability, or composition of tandem repeat sequences.

Certain other oncogenes have been found to be mutated or overexpressed in breast cancer, although few epidemiologic studies of these markers have been performed. Rare alleles of the HRAS protooncogene are the result of length polymorphisms in a sequence of tandem repeat bases (minisatellites) downstream from the HRAS coding region.[62] This region appears to provide an array of binding sites for transcriptional regulatory factors; binding to some rare alleles may enhance transcription to a greater degree than binding to common alleles.[63] Whether rare alleles also are a marker for genomic instability is not clear. Despite some inconsistency,[64,65] larger studies have shown rare HRAS alleles to be associated with increased breast cancer risk.[8,66,67] In the large molecular epidemiology study conducted by Garrett and colleagues,[66] rare alleles of HRAS were associated with a significant two- to three-fold increase in breast cancer risk, adjusted for other risk factors. Furthermore, the increase in risk was much higher in black women than in white women (odds ratio, 11 versus 1.7), and in women less than 50 years of age compared to those 50 years old or older (odds ratio, 3.7 versus 2.5). Rare alleles were also associated with ER and PR negativity but not with stage.[66] These findings are notable in that an increased predilection for ER- and PR-negative tumors has been observed in black women and in younger women.[68,69] This finding suggests that rare HRAS alleles may be a marker for an aggressive phenotype in black and younger patients. HRAS p21 oncoproteins have also been detected in serum from breast cancer patients with a significantly higher frequency than among controls (odds ratio, 11.1).[9]

Amplification of *c-myc* protooncogenes has been observed in 6% to 56% of breast tumors, whereas INT2 amplification occurs in 9% to 23% of breast tumors.[70] Overexpression of *c-myc* oncoprotein has also been observed in serum from breast cancer patients.[57] Associations between amplification of these oncogenes and prognosis have been inconsistent.[51,57] In the same study that showed a correlation between *erbB*-2 amplification and early use of oral contraceptives, INT2 amplification was significantly correlated with early abortion (odds ratio, 26.2) and progestin use (odds ratio, 17.4), but not with early contraceptive use or other reproductive risk factors.[60]

The use of oncogenes and their products as biomarkers of high risk or premalignant transition provides the potential for molecular screening. Additional characterization of the timing of these lesions remains to be done, as well as studies to determine the extent of variability associated with race and known risk factors. Because molecular screening would target healthy, asymptomatic women, noninvasive means of serial monitoring must be developed. The detection of ras, *erbB*-2, and *myc* oncoproteins and p53 antibodies in serum suggests the usefulness of monitoring body fluids. Nipple aspirate fluid, which can be obtained from nonlactating women with a simple pump apparatus, represents another potentially important medium. Studies of certain metabolites and growth factors show higher levels in nipple aspirate fluid than in serum, whereas exfoliated atypical epithelial cells can also be detected cytologically in nipple aspirate fluid.[71,72] Because nipple aspirate fluid represents a direct measure of the breast epithelial environment, and turnover in breast secretions is slow, this fluid may be a more sensitive medium for screening than serum or urine.

Growth Factors

Growth factors, discussed in detail elsewhere in this book, regulate normal breast epithelial proliferation and differentiation and appear to contribute to malignant transformation when their expression patterns are altered. In concert with growth regulatory oncogenes, growth factors mediate the effects of estrogens and progestins on neoplastic growth and promote tumor angiogenesis.[4,5,51,73–75] Most research in humans on these molecules has focused on their role as prognostic factors. These molecules are detectable in serum, urine, and nipple aspirate fluid, however, so they are potential markers for molecular screening. Because they are expressed variably in normal tissue, benign proliferative lesions, in situ disease, and invasive cancer, growth factors possess great potential for identification of early neoplastic changes and high-risk subsets of women. Additional work is necessary, however, to determine the timing of these changes and the extent of variability in normal women associated with other pathologic processes and breast cancer risk factors.

Summary

The tremendous advances in molecular biology offer the potential for identification of important carcinogens, for prediction of risk in individuals, and for molecular screening for early breast lesions that can be readily eradicated. Molecular epidemiology serves as the population laboratory that will be required to determine the behavior of variant molecules in the natural course of human breast carcinogenesis. Much research is still necessary for this objective to be reached. The accuracy, reliability, and interpretability of laboratory assay techniques must be improved, and standards must be developed for particular markers. Studies in normal women and in women at various stages of neoplastic progression must be undertaken to quantify intraindividual and interindividual variability. This will include examining the behavior of multiple markers in conjunction with other risk factors and the contribution of inherited and acquired susceptibility factors. Extension of existing tissue studies to more accessible body fluids such as serum, nipple aspirate fluid, and urine will facilitate serial monitoring of at-risk subgroups of women. These improvements will allow for resolution of etiologic questions and generation of new hypotheses for risk reduction and treatment.

References

1. Schulte PA. A conceptual and historical framework for molecular epidemiology. In: Schulte PA, Perera FP, eds. Molecular epidemiology: principles and practice. New York, Academic, 1993.
2. Baum M, Ziv Y, Colletta A. Prospects for the chemoprevention of breast cancer. Br Med Bull 1991;47:493.
3. Wogan GN. Molecular epidemiology in cancer risk assessment and prevention: recent progress and avenues for future research. Environ Health Perspect 1992;98:167.
4. Chrysogelos SA, Dickson RB. EGF receptor expression, regulation, and function in breast cancer. Breast Cancer Res Treat 1994;29:29.
5. Normanno N, Ciardiello F, Brand R, et al. Epidermal growth factor–related peptides in the pathogenesis of human breast cancer. Breast Cancer Res Treat 1994;29:11.
6. Wellstein A. Why monitor angiogenic factors in patients' urine? J Natl Cancer Inst 1994;86:328.
7. Wiener JR, Kerns BJM, Harvey EL, et al. Overexpression of the protein tyrosine phosphatase PTP1B in human breast cancer: association with p185$^{c-erb-2}$ protein expression. J Natl Cancer Inst 1994;86:372.
8. Krontiris TG, Devlin B, Karp DD, et al. An association between the risk of cancer and mutations in the HRAS1 minisatellite locus. N Engl J Med 1993;329:517.
9. Weissfeld JL, Larsen RD, Niman HL, et al. Evaluation of oncogene-related proteins in serum. Cancer Epidemiol Biomarkers Prev 1994;3:57.
10. Malins DC, Holmes EH, Polissar NL, et al. The etiology of breast cancer: characteristic alterations in hydroxyl radical–induced DNA base lesions during oncogenesis with potential for evaluating incidence risk. Cancer 1993;71:3036.
11. Osborne MP, Bradlow HL, Wong GYC, et al. Upregulation of estradiol 16α-hydroxylation in human breast tissue: a potential biomarker of breast cancer risk. J Natl Cancer Inst 1993;85:1917.
12. Telang NT, Bradlow HL, Osborne MP. Estradiol metabolism: an endocrine biomarker for chemoprevention of human mammary carcinogenesis. (Abstract) J Cell Biochem 1993;17G(Suppl):256.
13. Coles C, Condie A, Chetti U, et al. p53 mutations in breast cancer. Cancer Res 1992;52:5291.
14. Greenblatt MS, Bennett WP, Hollstein M, et al. Mutations in the p53 tumor suppressor gene: clues to cancer etiology and molecular pathogenesis. Cancer Res 1994;54:4855.
15. Hulka BS, Margolin BH. Methodological issues in epidemiologic studies using biologic markers. Am J Epidemiol 1992;135:200.
16. Press MF, Hung G, Godolphin W. Sensitivity of HER-2/*neu* antibodies in archival tissue samples: potential source of error in immunohistochemical studies of oncogene expression. Cancer Res 1994;54:2771.
17. Dhingra K, Sahin A, Supak J, et al. Chromosome *in situ* hybridization on formalin-fixed mammary tissue using non-isotopic, non-fluorescent probes: technical considerations and biological implications. Breast Cancer Res Treat 1992;23:201.
18. Wynford-Thomas D. p53 in tumour pathology: can we trust immunocytochemistry? J Pathol 1992;166:329.
19. Rothman N, Stewart WF, Caporaso NE, et al. Misclassification of genetic susceptibility biomarkers: implications for case-control studies and cross-population comparisons. Cancer Epidemiol Biomarkers Prev 1993;2:299.
20. Schatzkin A, Freedman LS, Schiffman MH, et al. Validation of intermediate end points in cancer research. J Natl Cancer Inst 1990;82:1746.
21. Floyd RA. The role of 8-hydroxyguanine in carcinogenesis. Carcinogenesis 1990;11:1447.
22. Shields PG, Harris CC. Molecular epidemiology and the genetics of environmental cancer. JAMA 1991;266:681.
23. Malins DC, Haimanont R. Major alterations in the nucleotide structure of DNA in cancer of the female breast. Cancer Res 1991;51:5430.
24. Kriek E, Engelse LD, Scherer E, et al. Formation of DNA modifications by chemical carcinogens: identification, localization and quantification. Biochim Biophys Acta 1984;738:181.
25. Wolff MS, Toniolo PG, Lee EW, et al. Blood levels of organochlorine residues and risk of breast cancer. J Natl Cancer Inst 1993;85:648.
26. Krieger N, Wolff MS, Hiatt RA, et al. Breast cancer and serum organochlorines: a prospective study among white, black, and Asian women. J Natl Cancer Inst 1994;86:589.
27. Dewailly E, Dodin S, Verreault R, et al. High organochlorine body burden in women with estrogen receptor-positive breast cancer. J Natl Cancer Inst 1994;86:232.
28. Mussalo-Rauhamaa H, Hasanen E, Pyysalo H, et al. Occurrence of beta-hexachlorocyclohexane in breast cancer patients. Cancer 1990;66:2124.
29. Falck F Jr, Ricci A Jr, Wolff MS, et al. Pesticides and polychlorinated biphenyl residues in human breast lipids and their relation to breast cancer. Arch Environ Health 1992;47:143.
30. Unger M, Kiaer H, Blichert-Toft M, et al. Organochlorine compounds in human breast fat from deceased with and without breast cancer and in biopsy material from newly diagnosed patients undergoing breast surgery. Environ Res 1984;34:24.
31. Bates MN, Hannah DJ, Buckland SJ, et al. Chlorinated organic con-

taminants in breast milk of New Zealand women. Environ Health Perspect 1994;102(Suppl 1):211.

32. Dewailly E, Ayotte P, Brisson J. Protective effect of breast feeding on breast cancer and body burden of carcinogenic organochlorines. (Letter) J Natl Cancer Inst 1994;86:80.

33. Bradlow HL, Hershcopf RJ, Martucci CP, et al. 16α-hydroxylation of estradiol: a possible risk marker for breast cancer. Ann NY Acad Sci 1989;464:138.

34. Nebert D. Elevated estrogen 16α-hydroxylase activity: is this a genotoxic or nongenotoxic biomarker in human breast cancer risk? J Natl Cancer Inst 1993;85:1888.

35. Michnovicz JJ, Bradlow HL. Induction of estradiol metabolism by dietary indole-3-carbinol in humans. J Natl Cancer Inst 1990;82:947.

36. Elledge RM, Fuqua SAW, Clark GM, et al. The role and prognostic significance of p53 gene alterations in breast cancer. Breast Cancer Res Treat 1993;27:95.

37. Deng G, Chen LC, Schott DR, et al. Loss of heterozygosity and p53 gene mutations in breast cancer. Cancer Res 1994;54:499.

38. Poller DN, Roberts EC, Bell JA, et al. p53 protein expression in mammary ductal carcinoma in situ: relationship to immunohistochemical expression of estrogen receptor and c-erbB-2 protein. Hum Pathol 1992;24:463.

39. Thor AD, Moore DH, Edgerton SM, et al. Accumulation of p53 tumor suppressor gene protein: an independent marker of prognosis in breast cancers. J Natl Cancer Inst 1992;84:845.

40. Thompson AM, Anderson TJ, Condie A, et al. p53 allele losses, mutations and expression in breast cancer and their relationship to clinico-pathologic parameters. Int J Cancer 1992;50:528.

41. Mudenda B, Green JA, Green B, et al. The relationship between serum p53 autoantibodies and characteristics of human breast cancer. Br J Cancer 1994;69:1115.

42. Davidoff AM, Iglehart JD, Marks JR. Immune response to p53 is dependent upon p53/HSP70 complexes in breast cancers. Proc Natl Acad Sci USA 1992;89:3439.

43. Schlichtholz B, Legros Y, Gillet D, et al. The immune response to p53 in breast cancer patients is directed against immunodominant epitopes unrelated to the mutational hot spot. Cancer Res 1992;52:6380.

44. Hollstein M, Sidransky D, Vogelstein B, et al. p53 mutations in human cancers. Science 1991;253:49.

45. Vogelstein B, Kinzler KW. Carcinogens leave fingerprints. Nature 1992;355:209.

46. Bohr VA, Phillips DH, Hanawalt PC. Heterogeneous DNA damage and repair in the mammalian genome. Cancer Res 1987;47:6426.

47. Ruggeri B, DiRado M, Zhang SY, et al. Benzo(a)pyrene-induced murine skin tumors exhibit frequent and characteristic G to T mutations in the p53 gene. Proc Natl Acad Sci USA 1993;90:1013.

48. Sasa M, Knodo K, Komaki K, et al. Frequency of spontaneous p53 mutations (CpG site) in breast cancer in Japan. Breast Cancer Res Treat 1993;27:247.

49. Tsuda H, Iwaya K, Fukutomi T, et al. p53 mutations and c-erbB-2 amplification in intraductal and invasive breast carcinomas of high histologic grade. Jpn J Cancer Res 1993;84:394.

50. Saitoh S, Cunningham J, De Vries EM, et al. p53 gene mutations in breast cancers in midwestern US women: null as well as missense-type mutations are associated with poor prognosis. Oncogene 1994;9:2869.

51. Dickson RB, Paik S. Regulation of proliferation and differentiation of normal and malignant breast: new factors and neu paradoxes. Breast 1993;2:83.

52. Liu ET. Oncogenes, breast cancer and chemoprevention. J Cell Biochem 1993;17G (Suppl):161.

53. Hubbard AL, Doris CP, Thompson AM, et al. Critical determination of the frequency of c-erbB-2 amplification in breast cancer. Br J Cancer 1994;70:434.

53a. Iglehart JD, Kerns BJ, Huper Gudrun, et al. Maintenance of DNA content and erbB-2 alterations in intraductal and invasive phases of mammary cancer. Breast Cancer Res Treat 1995;34:253.

54. Seshadri R, Firgaira FA, Horsfall DJ, et al. Clinical significance of HER-2/neu oncogene amplification in primary breast cancer. J Clin Oncol 1993;11:1936.

55. Tandon AK, Clark GM, Chamness GC, et al. HER-2/neu oncogene protein and prognosis in breast cancer. J Clin Oncol 1989;1120.

56. Osborne CK. Prognostic factors for breast cancer: have they met their promise? J Clin Oncol 1992;10:679.

57. Breuer B, DeVivo I, Luo JC, et al. erbB-2 and myc oncoproteins in sera and tumors of breast cancer patients. Cancer Epidemiol Biomarkers Prev 1994;3:63.

58. Kynast B, Binder L, Marx D, et al. Determination of a fragment of the c-erbB-2 translational product p185 in serum of breast cancer patients. Cancer Res Clin Oncol 1993;19:249.

59. Olsson H, Ranstam J, Baldetorp B, et al. Proliferation and DNA ploidy in malignant breast tumours in relation to early oral contraceptive use and early abortion. Cancer 1991;5:1285.

60. Ollson H, Borg A, Ferno M, et al. Her-2/neu and INT2 proto-oncogene amplification in malignant breast tumors in relation to reproductive factors and exposure to exogenous hormones. J Natl Cancer Inst 1991;83:1483.

61. Smith HS, Lu Y, Deng G, et al. Molecular aspects of early stages of breast cancer progression. J Cell Biochem 1993;17G (Suppl):144.

62. Capon DJ, Chen EY, Levinson AD, et al. Complete nucleotide sequences of the T24 human bladder carcinoma oncogene and its normal homologue. Nature 1983;302:33.

63. Trepicchio WL, Krontiris TG. Members of the rel/NF-κB family of transcriptional regulatory factors bind the hHRAS1 minisatellite DNA sequence. Nucleic Acids Res 1992;20:2427.

64. Sheng ZM, Guerin M, Gabillot ME, et al. C-Ha-ras-1 polymorphism in human breast carcinomas: evidence for a normal distribution of alleles. Oncogene Res 1988;2:245.

65. Barkardottir RB, Hohannsson OT, Arason A, et al. Polymorphism of the c-Ha-ras-1 proto-oncogene in sporadic and familial breast cancer. Int J Cancer 1989;44:251.

66. Garrett PA, Hulka BS, Kim YL, et al. HRS protooncogene polymorphism and breast cancer. Cancer Epidemiol Biomarkers Prev 1993;2:133.

67. Lidereau R, Escot C, Theillet C, et al. High frequency of rare alleles of the human c-ha-ras-1 proto-oncogene in breast cancer patients. J Natl Cancer Inst 1986;77:697.

68. Weston A, Vineis P, Caporaso NE, et al. Racial variation in the distribution of Ha-ras alleles. Mol Carcinog 1991;4:265.

69. Hulka BS, Chambless LE, Wilkinson WE, et al. Hormonal and personal effects on estrogen receptors in breast cancer. Am J Epidemiol 1984;119:692.

70. Callahan R. Genetic alterations in primary breast cancer. Breast Cancer Res Treat 1989;13:191.

71. Petrakis NL. Studies on the epidemiology and natural history of benign breast disease and breast cancer using nipple aspirate fluid. Cancer Epidemiol Biomarkers Prev 1993;2:3.

72. Connolly JM, Rose DP. Epidermal growth factor-like proteins in breast fluid and human milk. Life Sci 1988;42:1751.

73. Clarke R, Dickson RB, Lippman ME. Hormonal aspects of breast cancer: growth factors, drugs and stromal interactions. Crit Rev Oncol Hematol 1992;12:1.

74. Freiss G, Prebois C, Vignon F. Control of breast cancer cell growth by steroids and growth factors: interactions and mechanisms. Breast Cancer Res Treat 1993;27:57.

75. Nguyen M, Watanabe H, Budson AE, et al. Elevated levels of an angiogenic peptide, basic fibroblast growth factor, in the urine of patients with a wide spectrum of cancers. J Natl Cancer Inst 1994;86:356.

7.6

Oncogenes and Suppressor Genes

ROBERT B. DICKSON · MARC E. LIPPMAN

Genetic Alterations in Breast Cancer: General Principles

The study of genetic alterations in breast cancer is proceeding at a feverish pace. Inherited predispositions to the disease and the basis for progression of the disease from benign to malignant forms have their foundation in genetic alterations. Thus, multiple lines of investigation, including detection of chromosomal abnormalities in breast and nonbreast tissue of women at high risk of the disease, evaluations of breast tumors in their early stages, and characterization of highly malignant stages, are all contributing to the progress. The principal genetic lesions observed to date include gene amplifications, deletions, point mutations, loss of heterozygosity (LOH), and overall aneuploidy. Some of the earliest hints at a genetic basis for the disease were recorded by the ancient Romans, who noticed certain families at high risk for the disease. Two human genes have now been cloned (p53 and BRCA1) and another localized (BRCA2) whose function as tumor-suppressor genes are compromised when inherited as mutant alleles. This type of inherited lesion can allow early development to occur before loss of function of the second allele to elicit the disease. Thus, peripubertal LOH at the remaining allele of a breast tumor–suppressor locus can facilitate disease onset, usually in both breasts and at an early age. When genetic changes occur in breast tumors themselves, it now appears that a progressive cascade of genetic changes occurs. In the face of selective pressure, successive generations of tumor cells overgrow and dominate the tissue, eventually giving rise to clonal or nearly clonal metastatic disease.

Although breast cancer can exhibit a tremendous degree of genetic alteration, certain specific, common lesions have been described. The genes involved in a high proportion of these lesions are now recognized as the oncogenes and suppressor genes identified in many other cancers. Historically, few activated oncogenes have been identified in breast cancer by their ability to transform rodent fibroblasts in vitro. Instead, most oncogenes in breast cancer have been identified by detailed study of amplified and translocated chromosomal regions using cytogenetics. So far, point mutation does not appear to be a common mechanism for oncogenic activation in breast cancer. In contrast, tumor-suppressor genes are characterized primar-

ily by inactivating point mutations and LOH. In another evolving area of study, additional candidate oncogenes and suppressor genes have been proposed, based on their up- or down-regulation in the disease by nongenetic mechanisms. Although such nongenetic alterations of protooncogenes and suppressor genes have not classically been considered to have the same importance as genetic mechanisms, their roles in cancer progression deserve more study. Characterization of the major genetic changes in breast cancer will require many more years of study to complete (Table 7.6-1).

In this chapter, we organize our discussion of oncogenes and suppressor genes according to their functional hierarchy in the cascade of growth regulatory signals delivered to the nucleus from the cell surface. The reason is that the biochemical pathways of growth factor signal transduction and of the cell cycle contain most of the defined oncogenes and suppressor genes in cancer. An ever-increasing number of additional candidate oncogenes and suppressor genes include other important regulatory pathways, however, including steroid receptor genes and cell–cell and cell–substrate adhesion molecule genes.

EGF Receptor Family

Investigators have known for some 30 years that the receptor for epidermal growth factor (EGFR) is expressed in breast tissue, where it regulates mitogenesis and differentiation. In part because of the pioneering work of Cohen and colleagues,[5] this receptor has served as a prototype for understanding of tyrosine kinase signaling, receptor dimerization, and signal transduction cascades. Most important to the current discussion is that the mutation or amplification of this gene can convert its cognate protein to a form that confers increased cancer risk to experimental animals and humans. Our knowledge of the EGF family of growth factors and receptors has undergone rapid expansion in the past few years and continues to command the attention of many breast cancer researchers. The EGF family now includes transforming growth factor α (TGF-α), amphiregulin (AR), heparin-binding EGF (HbEGF), β-cellulin, the heregulins, crypto-1, and certain viral-encoded proteins. The EGFR family now has an additional three members, termed *erbB*-2, *erbB*-3, and *erbB*-4. Study

TABLE 7.6-1
Oncogenes and Suppressor Genes in Breast Cancer

ONSET OF FAMILIAL BREAST CANCER

Suppressor gene (mutated or lost)

    p53 (Li-Fraumeni syndrome)

Likely suppressor genes (mutated or lost)

    BRCA1 (breast and ovarian cancer families)

    BRCA2 (breast cancer families)

PROGRESSION OF BREAST CANCER

Oncogenes (amplified)

    erbB-2

    myc

    cyclin D₁

Suppressor genes (mutated or lost)

    cyclin E (?)

    Rb-1

    p53

Oncogene candidates

    ER

    PR

    EGFR

    c-Ras^H

Suppressor gene candidates

    MTS-1

    nm23

    α₆ integrin

    E-cadherin

    Brush 1

of this superfamily of factors and receptors has resulted in critical insights into regulation of the normal mammary gland, in identification of one of the most commonly activated oncogenes in the disease, in recognition of critical mechanisms of breast tumor promotion, in identification of mechanisms of resistance of the disease to therapy, in mechanisms of immune surveillance of breast cancer, and in new ideas for drug therapy of the disease. Although the *EGFR* gene is not generally considered to be an oncogene in breast cancer (eg, because its gene is seldom mutated nor amplified, as it is in many head and neck tumors), this receptor has many oncogene-like characteristics. Understanding its role is critical in evaluation both of mechanisms of tumor promotion and of the function of its close homologue, *erbB-2*, which is considered to be an extremely important oncogene in this disease.

EGF RECEPTOR–PROTOONCOGENE

Numerous studies comparing hormone-dependent and hormone-independent breast cancer cell lines and primary tumors have noted that the absence of the estrogen receptor (ER) is often coupled with expression of high lev-els of EGFR and with more aggressive states of the disease.[1-3] Although coexpression of the EGFR is seldom observed by immunohistochemistry for estrogen and progesterone, this is not the case in normal mammary luminal epithelial cells and fibroadenoma, in which coexpression of the three receptors is common.[4] EGFR is also commonly detected in normal myoepithelial cells and in fibroblastic stroma of the breast.[4] The EGFR is a 170-kd transmembrane glycoprotein that possesses intrinsic, ligand-regulatable tyrosine kinase activity.[5] Binding of EGF (or other family members) to the EGFR leads to kinase activation, autophosphorylation of EGFR, phosphorylation of other intracellular substrates,[6,7] internalization, and down-regulation of the receptor.[8] Molecular cloning of the *EGFR* gene has allowed exploration of its biologic role by gene transfer methods. Some of the earliest studies in this area explored the role of its overexpression for tumorigenic conversion of the cells. Overexpression of EGFR results in EGF-dependent phenotypic transformation of immortalized rodent fibroblasts,[9,10] implicating this growth factor–receptor system in the process of cellular transformation. Independent studies documenting extensive homology between mammalian *EGFR* and the avian erythroblastosis–derived v-*erbB* oncogene demonstrated that *EGFR* is the cellular homologue of this oncogene.[11] Although the exact molecular defects of the v-*erbB* oncogene (truncation and mutation) are seldom seen in the gene encoding the EGFR in human cancer, the gene encoding the EGFR is sometimes amplified (particularly in head and neck tumors) or overexpressed at the transcriptional and protein levels (breast cancer).

The EGFR serves to regulate the proliferation of multiple tissues during fetal development, in nonreproductive aspects of adult life, and in many aspects of spermatogenesis and pregnancy.[12] The ligand-receptor system appears to be ancient; all the ligands described to date are structurally related to *Drosophila notch, delta,* and *slit* genes and to nematode *lin-12* and *glp-1* genes.[13] The growth factors that make up the EGF family are thought to be synthesized from transmembrane precursors and to be cleaved by proteolytic enzymes to yield the fully processed, soluble forms. Although complete processing of the EGF family of growth factors to their soluble forms may predominate in many cell types, the uncleaved precursor can act on the receptor of an adjacent cell in a mode of action that has been termed *juxtacrine.* All members of this growth factor family, except the recently described cripto-1, possess a consensus array of three characteristic disulfide linkages that strongly define the three-dimensional structure of the protein and are required for growth factor action.[14]

The EGFR delivers its mitogenic signal to the cell coincident with growth factor binding and receptor dimerization within the plane of the membrane. Signal transduction itself is ultimately mediated through a cytoplasmic domain of the receptor that is homologous to the c-*src* oncogene kinase. Substrate specificity of the kinase involves protein–protein structural recognition by an additional cytoplasmic domain amino terminal to the kinase. Several primary kinase substrates and subsequent phosphorylated substrates that may participate in signal transduction by the EGFR have been identified: phospholipase C, phospholipase D, phosphoinositol-3-OH kinase (PI3K), GRB2–SOS, Ras–GAP, Raf-1 kinase, mitogen-activating protein (MAP) kinase, other kinases such as the ribosomal s-6 kinase,[15–17] and several growth factor receptors. These substrates are discussed in more detail later. Receptor function may be directly attenuated by cytoplasmic protein kinases, such as protein kinase C–mediated phosphorylation of a submembranous EGFR threonine residue[15] and later dampened in the signal transduction pathway by cyclic adenosine monophosphate (cAMP)-dependent protein kinase. Activated receptors are eventually internalized through a mechanism involving another short cytoplasmic region amino terminal to the kinase. Recognition of the receptors by adaptan proteins in coated pits results in their internalization into endosomes, their destruction in lysosomes, or their recycling back to the cell surface.[18]

The way in which genetic alterations during the process of breast tumorigenesis interact with EGFR signal transduction mechanisms is not fully clear. The function of the EGFR may change as a result of modulation of the kinetics of receptor turnover, heterodimeric coupling of the EGFR to another family member, aberrant modulation of phosphorylation of an EGFR kinase substrate, or more distal modulation of a signal transduction target. Specific examples of this consideration are presented later in connection with EGFR interaction with products of *c-myc* and other *c-erbB* family oncogenes.

In clinical studies of breast cancer, investigators have suggested that high levels of EGFR in breast tumors (in striking contrast to the type 1 insulin-like growth factor [IGF-1] receptor) correlate with a poor prognosis, even independently of ER status.[1–3] Most EGFR studies to date on clinical specimens have depended on a ligand-binding assay using tumor membrane. Future studies would benefit from further development of a standardized immunohistochemical approach to quantify EGFR in paraffin-fixed clinical specimens. As noted earlier, expression of high levels of EGFR are often accompanied by expression of low levels or complete lack of expression of ER. This finding may suggest that a mechanistic link exists between up-regulation of EGFR and hormone independence.[1–3] A similar inverse correlation is also well documented in many human breast cancer cell lines; EGFR expression levels have been shown to vary by more than two orders of magnitude comparing ER–positive with ER–negative cells.[19] The basis for the variations in EGFR expression appears to lie in a transcription-enhancing element located in the first intron of the EGFR gene. This element is selectively stimulated in ER–negative breast cancer cells.[18,20] Most hormones and drugs capable of regulation of expression of EGFR and ER (estrogen and phorbol esters such as TPA, for example) have opposing effects on these two receptors.[21–26] In vitro selection of ER– and PR–positive cell lines with chemotherapeutic drugs and radiation has also been shown to suppress ER and PR and lead to elevated levels of EGFR.[27,28] Elevated expression of TGF-α in human breast cancer is associated with endocrine resistance of the disease. The mechanism for this

effect remains unknown, however, because TGF-α expression in breast tumors is not closely related to expression of either ER or EGFR.[29] Expression of AR is also correlated neither with ER nor with EGFR. Expression of this factor was associated with a point-mutated *p53* tumor-suppressor gene (discussed later), however, with intralobular (but not intraductal) cancer.[30]

c-*erbB*-2 RECEPTOR–ONCOGENE, c-*erbB*-3 AND c-*erbB*-4

The protein encoded by the *c-erbB*-2 receptor–oncogene (also called p185, p185[erbB-2], p185[neu], p185[HER-2]) has substantial homology to EGFR. This protein was initially reported to be a receptor for a human TGF-α–related growth factor termed *heregulin-α*,[31] as well as its rat homologue NDF (neu differentiating factor).[32,33] More recent studies, however, have suggested that these ligands bind directly to different EGFR family members: erbB-4 and erbB-3.[34,35] Investigators have proposed that a different factor, termed *NAF* (neu activating factor), whose sequence is not yet known may bind directly to the erbB-2 protein.[36,37] It has been estimated that 10 to 30% of breast, gastric, and ovarian cancers overexpress the *c-erbB*-2 gene product at a sufficiently high level that the protein serves as an oncogene and can be easily detected using immunohistochemical staining with formalin-fixed and paraffin-embedded sections. Staining is usually uniform for the entire tumor. These characteristics have facilitated the rapid development of assays of the erbB-2 protein product as a tumor prognostic marker. The erbB-2 protein product has also been reported to be gene amplified and overexpressed in cancers from many other organ systems, including adenocarcinoma of the lung, ovaries, stomach,[38] and pancreas[39] and endometrial carcinoma.[40] The gene encoding erbB-2 is almost invariably amplified in connection with overexpression of the corresponding mRNA and protein product. The degree of its protein expression generally exceeds the degree of its gene amplification, however. This is not generally the case for the EGFR. It appears that both gene amplification and transcriptional mechanisms account for receptor overexpression. Whether the genes erbB-3 and erbB-4 are commonly amplified in human cancer is not yet known, but both possess transforming activity in fibroblast models in vitro. The function of the erbB-2 protein in normal tissues is not completely known. Studies have suggested its importance in neural and neuromuscular junction development. The function of the structurally related erbB-3 or erbB-4 receptors in normal development and physiology is even less certain.

As we noted previously, the literature is replete with confusing terminology used to identify the *c-erbB*-2 gene and its product. Both *c-erbB*-2[41] and *HER-2*[42] refer to the same human homologue of the rat *neu* oncogene.[41] We use the term erbB-2 protein in this review.

SIGNAL TRANSDUCTION FROM TYROSINE KINASES

A signal transduction cascade from the EGF receptor (Fig. 7.6-1) begins with receptor occupancy by one of its cognate ligands (eg, EGF, TGF-α, AR, HbEGF). Analogous

FIGURE 7.6-1 MAP kinase pathway.

cascades may be triggered from erbB-2 by NAF and from erbB-3 and erbB-4 by heregulin–NDF. Signal transduction results from an altered three-dimensional conformation of the receptor in the plasma membrane. A rapid result of this change is receptor dimerization, which activates receptor tyrosine kinase.[43,44] Kinase activation leads to autophosphorylation and a further conformational change to allow binding and phosphorylation of cellular substrates. A recent insight into function of the entire EGFR family is that heterodimerization among apparently all family members can occur; the nature of the dimer can determine the detailed nature of signal pathways activated.[45] Specifically, an EGFR–erbB-2 dimer can stimulate transformed growth of mammary epithelial cells,[46–48] and an EGFR–erbB-3 dimer can stimulate PI3K activity.[49] EGFRs with dominant negative mutations of their cytoplasmic (kinase) domains have been used to interfere with this dimerization and kinase activation process. These mutated receptors can have antiproliferative and antioncogenic activities.[50,51] As noted previously, kinase activation initially results in autophosphorylation of several C-terminal tyrosine residues of the EGFR. This appears to allow a conformational change to allow full exposure of the kinase active site for interaction with multiple exogenous substrates.

The next step in signal transduction involves interaction of receptor tyrosine phosphorylated residues with a domain termed *SH2* (*src*, homology 2) on a variety of cellular proteins. These proteins have been known for some time to be receptor-associated and have long been suspected of assisting the receptor in its functions. The SH2 domains of these proteins allow their direct receptor binding by receptor-associated phosphotyrosine residues or their indirect receptor binding by their interaction with a receptor-

docking protein such as insulin receptor substrate-1 (IRS-1, for the insulin or IGF-1 receptors), or the Shc protein for the EGFR or cytoplasmic tyrosine kinases.[52,53] The formation of receptor-signaling complexes appears to mediate the major effects of EGF receptor–ligand binding on ion fluxes, additional phosphorylation events, gene expression, DNA synthesis, and malignant growth. The principal components of this receptor-associated signaling complex are thought to be the Shc adaptor protein, the Src tyrosine kinase, phospholipase C-γ (PLC-γ), guanosine triphosphatase (GTPase)–activating protein (GAP),[54–61] and one or more protein phosphatases.[62,63] The growth factor receptor–binding protein 2 (GRB2) and an associated protein termed *SOS* have also been described as a dominant receptor–binding protein complex in mitogenic signaling.[64–67]

GRB2 is a cytoplasmic protein that exists in a heterodimeric complex with a protein termed *mammalian son of sevenless* (mSOS). The derivation of this name is the homologous protein in *Drosophila* that was discovered in the context of eye development. SOS is homologous to yeast protein kinase of central importance termed *CDC25*. When the EGFR is phosphorylated, the GRB2–SOS complex binds to the phosphotyrosine residues by its SH2 domains. The receptor–GRB2–SOS complex then binds to the Ras–guanosine diphosphate (GDP) complex. Ras–GDP is associated with the inner leaflet of the plasma membrane through a fatty acid residue incorporated in its structure. The formation of this high-order receptor complex serves to catalyze the Ras-activating exchange reaction of GTP for GDP.[68–70] Some G protein–coupled, non-EGF–related, non–tyrosine kinase receptors may also activate Ras in a similar manner.[71] Moreover, growth inhibitory actions of TGF-β may serve to activate Ras; however, subsequent steps in signal transduction appear to differ from those induced by tyrosine kinases.[72] A general mechanism of Ras deactivation involves the protein termed p120^GAP, which catalyzes the exchange of Ras–GDP for GTP to help end the signal transduction process.[73,74]

The next step of the EGFR pathway is binding of c-*raf*-1 protooncogene product Raf-1 or the PI3K protein into the receptor complex with Ras–GTP. Whereas p13K modulates lipid metabolism, Raf-1 may mediate a mitogenic signaling cascade. The way in which this complex formation serves to activate the Raf-1 kinase is still not fully defined.[75–79] Association of Raf-1 with Ras probably serves to localize Raf-1 in the plane of the plasma membrane, where it can respond to activational signals from the receptor.[80] Separate activational mechanisms for Raf-1 also appear to exist and involve protein kinase C (PKC) and a family of proteins termed the *14-3-3- family*.[81,82] The activated Raf-1 kinase triggers a subsequent phosphorylation cascade called the *mitogen-activated protein kinase* (MAP) cascade.[83] The best known kinase at the top of this cascade is a MAP kinase kinase termed *MEK*. MEK is phosphorylated by Raf-1 (and possibly other mechanisms); both Raf-1 and activated MEK phosphorylate the cytoplasmic–nuclear MAP kinases. A prominent member of the MAP kinase cascade was previously identified as the ribosomal S-6 kinase (p70^{S6K}). ERK-1, ERK-2, and JNK kinases are other MAP kinases. Phosphorylation of MAP kinases lead to their nuclear translocation where they modulate gene function by phosphorylation of transcription factors.[84-89]

The MAP kinase family is recognized as central to many mitogenic phosphorylation signals. A diverse series of phosphotyrosine, phosphoserine, and phosphothreonine kinase pathways, as well as some G protein–mediated pathways, mediate mitogenic signals in this manner.[90] MAP kinases phosphorylate the nuclear *c-myc, c-jun,* and *c-ets* protooncogene products. Phosphorylation of these nuclear proteins regulates their transcription activity.[91-93] The Myc and Fos proteins modulate transcription by heterodimer formation (exemplified by Myc–MAX, Fos–Jun); regulation of the other heterodimeric partner represents another site of possible modulation of the signal transduction cascade.[91,94] Mitogen-inducible phosphatases are thought to act in a regulatory fashion to attenuate MAP kinase activity.[95] Members of this cascade down to the level of the MAP kinase kinase have been demonstrated to have oncogenic potential in model systems or in various human cancers.[96] This is little evidence of this for breast cancer, however, except perhaps for the *c-ras*^{H} gene. A high level of protooncogene polymorphism (rare alleles) might suggest structural alterations in the Ras protein.[97]

Much current research is attempting to make the final links in signal transduction from transcription factors to mitosis. In yeast, the protein kinases at the end of the mitogenic pathways are cdc2 and CDC28; the mammalian homologue is termed *p34*^{cdc2}. Again, this represents a family of kinases forming complexes with activating members of the cyclin family and with inhibitory proteins. Cyclins are regulatory subunits of the kinases; different cyclin–kinase complexes catalyze different cell cycle–required phosphorylations, such as histones (for mitotic condensation), nuclear lamina (for mitotic dissolution of the nuclear membrane), and the retinoblastoma protein (Rb-1 for release of a mitotic blockade).[98-100] This system is discussed in greater detail in a later section of this chapter.

The details of the mitogenic regulatory cascades are now being defined specifically in breast cancer and other cancers. Both steroids and growth factors (including EGFR ligands) are known to induce nuclear protooncogenes and proteins termed *cyclins*. In addition, proliferation of breast cancer is associated with increased levels of EGFR, erbB-2, and Myc proteins.[101-104] As may be predicted, some of the most common mutations in breast cancer (amplification of the *erb*B-2, *myc,* and two of *cyclin* genes) are precisely in this pathway.[105-107] Additional complexity and understanding of this system will certainly emerge as studies in breast cancer proceed. An interesting example of such complexity is that of the EGF mitogenic pathway, which may be modulated by fatty acids.[108] This may be relevant to breast cancer onset because high-fat diets are under current scrutiny in this regard.

Drugs that target the mitogenic cascade could represent new classes of anticancer therapy.[109] Current approaches involve tyrosine kinase inhibitors such as tyrophostins[96,110]

and other classes and inhibitors of Ras farnesylation, which block its membrane localization.[111,112] Studies have also determined that a natural inhibitory pathway for the tyrosine kinase signal transduction cascade is regulated by cAMP. cAMP inhibits Ras activation of the Raf-1 kinase by inhibitory phosphorylations. Thus, protein kinase A–activating drugs may have potential as new anticancer therapeutics.[82,113-115] Much work remains to define the principal hormonal regulators of cAMP in normal and malignant breast tissue, however.

Recent work has also identified a separate signal transduction pathway shared by EGF, interferons, interleukins, other cytokines, and growth hormone. Receptor binding triggers autophosphorylation and activation of cytoplasmic Tyk and Jak tyrosine kinases. The molecular mechanisms receptor–Jak interaction are still under study. The activated Jak kinases phosphorylate STAT family proteins. Once phosphorylated, STAT proteins translocate to the nucleus and act as transcription factors to regulate genes containing GAS or ISRE sequences in their promoters.[116,117] Function of this pathway does not depend on the Ras protein.[118] The role of this pathway has not yet been defined in breast cancer; however, the pathway could conceivably be activated to mediate adverse responses of the tumor to cytokines of the immune system.

CLINICAL SIGNIFICANCE OF OVEREXPRESSION OF EGF RECEPTOR FAMILY AND LIGAND SYSTEMS

As described previously, the EGFR, a tyrosine kinase–associated protein, and some of its ligands (EGF, TGF-α, and AR) are closely associated, probably in a causal fashion, with mammary epithelial development and proliferation. TGF-α mRNA and protein have been detected in 70% or more of human breast cancer biopsies,[119] compared with 30% of benign breast lesions.[120] TGF-α has been detected by immunoassay both in fibroadenomas and in 25% to 50% of primary human mammary carcinomas.[121,122] An EGF-related protein of 43 kd has also been isolated from the urine of breast cancer patients.[123] It seems likely that detection of TGF-α and EGF in tumor biopsies, serum, or urine will eventually be found useful in determining prognosis or tumor burden, although this is not yet proved. Expression of AR and heregulin-α is also detected by immunohistochemistry in a significant proportion of primary breast tumors.[30,124,125] Other members of the EGF family of ligands (HbEGF, NAF, and cripto-1) are also produced in breast cancer, but their prevalence and functions are less clear.

The current data suggesting that EGFR is a clinical prognostic indicator and its inverse relationship with ER in both tumors and cell lines serve to point out our need to understand the mechanisms of regulation of EGFR in breast cancer.[3,19,126-128] Human breast tumor lines exhibit substantial variation in their level of EGFR, and the mechanisms responsible for elevated EGFR differ.[129-131] Cell lines have been identified that contain EGFR gene amplifications with or without gene rearrangements and with or without overexpression of EGFR in the absence of gene amplification. Human cell lines expressing a nonrearranged EGFR gene contain two major species of EGFR mRNA (10 and 5.6 kb); the levels of these transcripts and EGFR protein are usually closely correlated.[129] Differences in expression are controlled at least in part at the level of transcription; EGFR gene amplification appears to be a rare event (less than 5%) in breast cancer.[26,129–131] Overexpression of the EGFR also appears to signal poor tumor prognosis and poor response to tamoxifen therapy.[132,133]

Of the three other EGFR family members,[134] c-erbB-2, c-erbB-3, and c-erbB-4, all of which have also been detected in breast cancer, sufficient literature exists to implicate only the first in tumor growth, differentiation, and prognosis. Many studies have shown that 20% to 30% of primary, invasive breast cancers overexpress erbB-2 receptor protein. About 90% of tumors overexpressed the oncogene as a result of gene amplification. erbB-2 is overexpressed in a large proportion of cases of ductal carcinoma in situ[135,136] and in essentially 100% of comedo carcinomas at an early stage of malignancy. It is poorly expressed in lobular carcinomas in situ, however. Expression of erbB-2 is associated with a high cellular mitotic rate; it has been reported to correlate with poor clinical response to certain chemotherapeutic and antihormonal drugs (5-fluorouracil, methotrexate, cyclophosphamide, and tamoxifen-containing regimens) and insensitivity to tamoxifen in vitro.[137,138] Further study of tamoxifen sensitivity in a large population found no association of erbB-2 with response to tamoxifen, however.[139] Expression of erbB-2 is also associated with poor prognosis in patients not treated with chemotherapeutic or antihormonal drugs.[140–148]

Because c-erbB-2 amplification appears in breast tumors in situ and is associated with poor prognosis, it could hypothetically serve as a direct modulator of metastatic capacity. Based on data with tumor models, however, any effect of erbB-2 on metastasis would appear to be indirect and to require additional mutations.[149] Selected antibodies to the extracellular domain of the erbB-2 protein seem to sensitize cells to killing by cisplatin, carboplatinum, and doxorubicin in vivo. The mechanism of this effect is proposed to be interference with DNA repair mechanisms.[150–152] Other potentially interesting applications of erbB-2 are as a marker of tumor burden. Autoantibodies have been detected in the sera of tumor-bearing patients, and the shed extracellular domain of erbB-2 protein may represent an additional, useful blood-borne marker of the disease.[153,154] Finally, the erbB-2 protein, like the EGF receptor,[155] may be a new target of immunotherapy of cancer.[156–158] The real possibility of active targeting of erbB-2 protein for immunotherapy has been suggested by a study demonstrating that a lymphoplasmocytic infiltrate is indicative of good prognosis for an erbB-2–positive subset of patients. In this study, the authors observed that tumor growth–inhibitory antibodies were produced by peripheral lymphocytes from these patients.[159]

Although the prognostic significance of erbB-2 expression is well documented for node-positive patients, the biologic mechanism(s) for its apparent impact on the malignant process are less clear. Exogenous overexpression of erbB-2 in immortalized breast epithelial and breast cancer cell lines has suggested that it is only weakly trans-forming in vitro; c-erbB-2 gene transfection failed to induce or enhance a tumorigenic phenotype significantly in vivo in several studies.[160,161] Many established human breast cancer cell lines overexpressing erbB-2 are frequently poorly tumorigenic in the nude mouse. Possible explanations of this phenomenon could include a lack of coexpression of a heterodimeric partner or a ligand or coinduction of a suppressive phosphatase.[162] In the context of an actual mammary growth and development, however, a different result is obtained. In a transgenic mouse study, c-erbB-2 expression induced long-latency metastatic breast tumors.[163] Association with and activation of the c-src oncogene product by the erbB-2 product in this model has been proposed to be critical in the erbB-2–induced tumorigenic pathway.[17] Because the erbB-2 protein can heterodimerize with other receptor family members, cooverexpression of all their family members must be taken into account as future work in this area proceeds. So far, only erbB-2 and EGFR family members are clearly associated with poor prognosis. Recent preliminary studies have suggested erbB-4 and heregulin are indicators of good prognosis.[164] Much larger patient cohorts must be examined by multiple investigators to confirm these interesting observations fully, however.

Signal Transduction–Associated Nuclear Oncogenes

Regulation of nuclear protooncogenes occurs by both growth-promoting steroids and growth factors in many tissues. Nuclear protooncogenes may thus be regulated by convergent pathways of growth regulatory stimuli through direct steroid action, through growth factor induced MAP kinase, phospholipase C–PKC, or through cytokine-induced JAK–STAT pathways.[16,118,165–166] For example, protooncogene products of c-fos, c-myc, c-myb, and c-jun are commonly observed to be induced shortly following mitogenic treatment of cells. Many studies support a causal link between induction of this gene superfamily and proliferation processes. In breast cancer, the products of at least three nuclear protooncogenes (c-myc, c-fos, and c-jun) appear to be induced by both estrogen and progesterone.[165,166] Moreover, progestins induce c-junB, a c-jun–related protooncogene.[166] Antihormonal therapy may also modulate these genes; tamoxifen down-modulates c-Myc expression during treatment-induced tumor regression in patients.[167] In the context of proliferation of the normal gland, whether these nuclear protooncogenes are regulatory is not known. Induction of c-myc, c-fos, and c-jun has occurred in the rat uterus in response to estrogen treatment, however.[168,169] The protein products of the c-fos and c-jun genes contain specific domains that allow them to form a heterodimeric complex that can interact with a gene promoter consensus sequence termed AP-1. Similarly, the c-myc gene product dimerizes with another protein termed MAX (or MYN in the mouse) to modulate genes through a different consensus sequence. The Myc protein is also known to bind and inactivate the retinoblastoma tumor suppressor gene product (described later) as a part of its mechanism of action.[170] By using antisense oligonucleotides directed against the *c-myc* mRNA, the Myc protein has been demonstrated to be critical for estrogen induction of proliferation of breast cancer.[171]

Amplification of the gene for *c-myc,* although not widely appreciated, is one of the most common genetic alterations in breast cancer; approximately one third of breast cancers contain this genetic change.[172–175] A putative suppressor gene on 1p32-pter is proposed to control *c-myc* amplification in breast cancer.[176] Study of expression of the *c-myc* gene in breast cancer has been slow because of difficulties in measuring the protein in tumor biopsies. The protein has a short half-life. In addition is a lack of suitable monoclonal antibodies capable of staining paraffin sections. Several studies focusing on gene amplification have shown that c-*myc* is associated with poor prognosis,[171,175,177] high S-phase,[178] and postmenopausal disease.[179] Studies in various epithelial malignancies including those of the ovary and liver[180,181] have shown that c-*myc* amplification is associated with TGF-α overexpression. Dual stimulation of the EGFR pathway and Myc may serve a general cooperative function in epithelial transformation.

The Myc protein acts in multiple systems to regulate gene expression, to promote cell proliferation, to inhibit differentiation, to modulate cell adhesion, and to effect immune recognition.[182–184] Cellular proliferation appears modulated because Myc regulates initiation of DNA replication. The most clearly defined gene regulatory activities of the protein[185,186] are autosuppression and cell transformation; both involve the C-terminal portion of Myc. Although the *c-myc* protooncogene product can be used to immortalize fibroblasts[187] and modulate fibroblast responsiveness to growth factors,[188,189] only the latter effect is reported in mammary epithelium. Another interesting feature of c-*myc* amplification is that it may so disregulate the cell cycle (at least in fibroblasts) that programmed cell death results in a process that depends on the *p53* tumor-suppressor gene.[190] As studies have proceeded, a variety of biologic consequences of c-*myc* amplification have been described. Reports have suggested that expression of the c-*myc* gene may alter cellular resistance to cisplatin and other DNA strand scission–inducing drugs,[191] and it may act to suppress differentiation in association with the decrease of collagen gene transcription.[192] The Myc protein also inhibits transcription of the rat *neu* oncogene (c-*erbB*-2 homologue).[193] Although the importance of this interaction for human breast cancer is not yet known, the c-*myc* amplification is clearly not associated with c-*erbB*-2 amplification in primary breast cancer.[194] In addition, c-*myc* protooncogene may be related to breast cancer in older women. Increased amplification of the c-*myc* gene has been observed in human breast cancer tissue in postmenopausal patients. This may reflect cumulative proliferation-associated disregu-

lation and may contribute to aberrant mitogenic responses of the tissue in postmenopausal breast cancer.[172] Moreover, c-*myc* gene expression is enhanced in many other tissues as aging progresses.[195]

To study their role in transformation, the c-*myc* gene and other oncogenes were introduced into immortalized human or mouse mammary epithelial cells using an amphotrophic retroviral vector; *myc* or SV40T nuclear oncogene (but not v-*ras*^H or v-*mos*) allowed the cells to grow in soft agar in response to FGF-1, FGF-2, EGF, or TGF-α.[196,197] Because mammary fibroblasts produce EGF- and FGF-related growth factors,[198] and their conditioned media could support transforming growth of nuclear oncogene–transfected mammary epithelial cells,[197] these observations have supported a role in vivo for stromal–epithelial interactions. This synergy has been observed in vitro in TGF-α–*myc* bitransgenic mice. Expression of these two gene products allows rapid (10 weeks) onset of highly proliferative mammary tumors independent of sex hormones in either sex.[199] These data suggest that an amplified c-*myc* gene may function in early breast cancer lesions to allow growth factors or hormones to act to drive aberrant, transformed growth.

Tumor-Suppressor Genes

Broca[200] established in the 19th century that breast cancer may have a familial pattern of high incidence in 5% to 10% of cases. Families showing a high incidence of the disease sometimes have been noted to exhibit a high incidence of an additional cancer such as ovarian cancer. Such families have been thought to inherit a defective or lost allele encoding a tumor-suppressor gene. This supposition has been based largely on work by Knudson[201] who postulated the inactivation of two alleles of a gene in retinoblastoma, and by Harris and associates,[202] who demonstrated that certain chromosomes could suppress malignancy in cell–cell hybridization studies.

The first tumor-suppressor gene to be shown to have an association with inherited breast cancer was termed *p53* (on chromosome 17p13). Mutations in this locus were inherited in families with the rare breast cancer and sarcoma syndrome termed *Li-Fraumeni syndrome.*[203] The larger group of patients with an inherited pattern of breast or ovarian cancer has also been characterized by more recent studies. The specific gene responsible for the breast and ovarian syndrome has been reported. It is a zinc finger–containing DNA-binding protein whose gene is located on chromosome 17q21[204]; it is termed *BRCA1.*[205] A second genetic locus for a lower frequency, breast cancer–selective syndrome, termed *BRCA2,* is located on 13q12–13.[206]

During the malignant progression of breast cancer to its fully metastatic state, mutation, inactivation, loss, or down-regulated expression of tumor-suppressing genes may also occur. A gene termed the retinoblastoma gene (*Rb-1* on 13q14) and *p53* are mutated in 20% and 50% of cases, respectively.[207,208] A metastasis suppressor–candidate gene, with NDP-kinase activity, termed *nm23*, does not appear to be mutated, but its expression is down-modulated in metastatic breast cancer.[209] Three other such candidate, down-regulated suppressor genes are the genes encoding the cell–cell adhesion protein E–cadherin,[210] the integrin-α6 subunit,[211] and a gene termed *Brush 1*.[212] The function of each of these appears to be different.

Although *p53* is a tumor-suppressor gene, when mutated in one of several sensitive regions, the conformation of its encoded protein changes, its stability increases, and it functions as an inhibitor of unmutated p53. The *p53* gene is generally mutated in a distinct position in African-American women with high mortality from the disease compared with a corresponding white control population with breast cancer.[213] Although p53 is considered to be a nuclear protein, it has also been proposed that p53 may be excluded from the cell nucleus in some breast cancers by an unknown mechanism to prevent its function.[214] Moreover, p53 is known to be an oligomeric DNA-binding protein that regulates expression of DNA damage–response genes encoding MDM2 (a p53-binding antagonist), p21 (also called WAF-1, CIP1, SDI1, CAP-20, or PIC1, a cyclin-dependent kinase inhibitor), and bcl-2 (a suppressor of programmed cell death). The properties of *p53*, when transfected into cells, include cell cycle blockade at the G_1-S boundary, induction of apoptosis, and induction of differentiation. Thus, p53 appears to function in the context of DNA damage to slow cell growth and induce DNA repair. Loss of p53 function may contribute to the DNA instability of cancer.[215] Some programmed cell death pathways do not depend on p53, however. Furthermore, bcl-2 overexpression may suppress multiple types of apoptotic pathways in cancer.[216]

The *Rb-1* gene product is also a nuclear protein. When mutated in one of several specific regions, the function of its gene product is inactivated. The Rb-1 protein may also be functionally inactivated by phosphorylation (catalyzed by certain cyclin-dependent protein kinases, discussed later). Many cell cycle regulatory proteins such as members of the Myc and cyclin families, in addition to the transcription factor E2F-1, bind and inactivate the Rb-1 protein. Rb-1 function also appears to depend on binding to E2F-1 and to a protein termed BRG1 to form a transcription factor complex that regulates genes involved in G_1-S progression.[208,217,218]

Cyclins, Cyclin-Dependent Kinases, and Cyclin-Dependent Kinase Inhibitors

Stimulatory and inhibitory growth factors, sex steroids, and tumor suppressors primarily function in the G_1 phase of the cell cycle (Fig. 7.6-2). The cell cycle is tightly controlled by a series of cyclin-dependent kinases, their positive regulatory subunits (cyclins), and their inhibitors (cyclin–dependent kinase inhibitors). The early G_1 phase is driven by cyclin Ds bound to CDK2, CDK4, CDK5, and CDK6. Later, G_1-S is driven by cyclin E–CDK2.

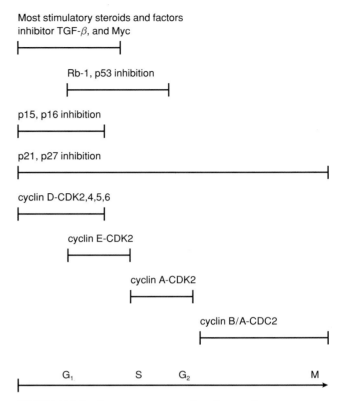

FIGURE 7.6-2 Tumor suppressor–cell cycle controls.

The S-phase is driven by cyclin A-CDK2, and G_2M is driven by cyclin B/A-CDC2. Tyrosine kinase–acting growth factors and sex steroids induce cyclin D1, whereas Myc suppresses D1 and induces cyclin E. The cyclin D1–CDK4/CDK6 complexes are inhibited by the protein p16 (or INK4, CDK4I, or MTS-1) and by p15 (or INK4B or MTS-2, which is induced by senescence, p53, and TGF-β and is overcome with SV40T antigen). Synthesis of CDK4 is inhibited by TGF-β; overexpression of CDK4 leads to TGF-β resistance. Cyclin D–CDK2 is inhibited by P16 and by another inhibitor p24 (CDI1–CIP2). Cyclin E–CDK2 is also inhibited by a phosphatase termed Cdi1–Cip2 and by p27 (or Kip1, which also inhibits CDK complexes with all other cyclins and somehow mediates TGF-β inhibition of cyclin E–CDK2). As noted earlier, Rb-1 is phosphorylated and inactivated by the cyclin D–CDK4/CDK6 kinases (and others). Thus, additional effects of TGF-β to activate Rb-1 may be mediated, at least in part, by down-regulation of the active cyclin D–CDK4/CDK6 complexes.

A major body of exciting work has begun to implicate cyclins as oncogenes and cyclin-dependent kinase inhibitors as tumor suppressors. Although studies in breast cancer are just beginning, the *cyclin D_1* and *cyclin E* genes appear to be commonly amplified in this disease. *Cyclin D_1* can function as a mammary cancer–inducing oncogene when driven by the MMTV promoter in the transgenic mouse. Recent studies have also implicated the cyclin inhibitor p16 as a major tumor suppressor, at least in cancer cell lines; the incidence of inactivation of this gene in primary tumors, such as breast cancer, is under investigation.[219-230]

Integration of Genetic Changes During Tumor Progression

Cancer is a process involving not only proliferative factors and activation of oncogenes but also loss of suppressor gene function. The role of germline deletion or mutation of suppressor genes in familial breast cancer and somatic mutation or deletion during breast tumor progression has been emphasized. Although numerous studies have focused on breast tumor oncogenes, identification of breast tumor—suppressor genes is likely in its infancy at present.

Malignant progression of breast cancer involves a transition from nearly normal mechanisms of proliferation in its early stages to highly abnormal regulation in metastatic disease.[231,232] Proliferative alterations early in the disease progression depend on systemic hormones (estrogen and progesterone) and local growth factors (such as TGF-α). Critical, additional damage or repair error event may then occur to compound the problem. Early genetic damage, in combination with proliferation, is thought to trigger gene amplification.[233] Amplification of c-erbB-2, c-myc, and *cyclin* genes in breast cancer may be critical in this respect. Mutations of *p53* and *Rb-1* suppressor genes and down-modulation of expression of other proposed suppressor genes also appear to be frequently associated with acquisition of poorer prognosis.[234-237] A major unknown is the determination of the stage in progression in which these genes become mutated or dysregulated, although it is becoming clearer that defects in c-erbB-2 and p53 occur relatively early. Proposed mechanisms for mutations and genetic instability in other cancers depend on overexpression of mutator genes such as *msh2*[238] and of the chromosomal stability—regulating enzyme telomerase.[239] These mechanisms for genetic instability have not been demonstrated to date, however. As multiple genetic alterations occur, cancer cells with the greatest capacity for growth, invasion, and survival will undergo positive selection.[240,241]

Studies using breast cancer cell lines in vitro are attempting to sort out the potential biologic roles and interactions of many potentially significant tumor prognostic factors. Certain common patterns of cytogenetic defects have also been described in breast tumors.[242] Examples were presented concerning the negative prognostic interaction of amplified *erbB*-2 or *myc* genes in the presence of an autocrine- or paracrine-activated EGFR system.[160,197] Moreover, c-erbB-2 amplification is particularly unfavorable in association with c-ras[H] overexpression[160,243] and mutation of the p53 gene.[244] Thus, the tyrosine kinase—ras—MAP kinase pathway is emerging as central in interaction with nuclear oncogenes in vitro, in transgenic mouse models of mammary cancer, and in prognosis of the disease in patients.[160,197,199,243,245] Another type of interaction is also reported to occur with c-myc amplification. As noted previously, the Myc protein is known to bind and inactivate the Rb-1 protein[170]; Myc may thus simultaneously stimulate proliferation and decrease tumor suppression.

Summary and Future Prospects

The study of interactions of growth regulatory pathways with mutations in genes involved in signal transduction and cell cycle pathways is in its infancy. Almost certainly, a major approach for the future understanding of these phenomenona will be the transgenic and gene knockout mouse models, with the eventual hope of establishing likely patterns of malignant progressions. At present, however, few studies have focused on combinations of oncogenes, growth factors, and loss of suppressor genes thought to be important in human disease. Future studies aimed at detailed characterization of the interaction of ERs, progesterone receptors, growth factors, and protooncogenes in these animal models are likely to shed much light on their interactive roles in onset and progression of breast cancer.

References

1. Fitzpatrick SL, Brightwell J, Wittliff J, et al. Epidermal growth factor binding by breast tumor biopsies and relationship to estrogen and progestin receptor levels. Cancer Res 1984;44:3448.
2. Sainsbury JRC, Farndon JR, Sherbert GV, et al. Epidermal growth factor receptors and oestrogen receptors in human breast cancers. Lancet 1985;1:364.
3. Klijn JGM, Berns PMJJ, Schmitz PIM, et al. The clinical significance of epidermal growth factor receptor (EGF-R) in human breast cancer: a review on 5232 patients. Endocr Rev 1992;13:3.
4. van Agthoven T, Timmermans M, Foekens JA, et al. Differential expression of estrogen, progesterone, and epidermal growth factor receptors in normal, benign and malignant human breast tissues using dual staining immunohistochemistry. Am J Pathol 1994; 144:1.
5. Cohen S, Ushiro H, Stoscheck C, et al. A native 170,000 epidermal growth factor receptor-kinase complex from shed plasma membrane vesicles. J Biol Chem 1982;257:1523.
6. Ushiro H, Cohen S. Identification of phosphotyrosine as a product of epidermal growth factor-associated protein kinase in A-431 cell membranes. J Biol Chem 1980;255:8363.
7. Hunter T, Cooper JA. Epidermal growth factor induces rapid tyrosine phosphorylation of proteins in A431 human tumor cells. Cell 1981;24:741.
8. Carpenter G, Cohen S. ^{125}I-labeled human epidermal growth factor (hEGF): binding, internalization, and degradation in human fibroblasts. J Cell Biol 1976;71:159.
9. Velu TJ, Beguinot L, Vass WC, et al. Epidermal growth factor dependent transformation by a human EGF receptor proto-oncogene. Science 1987;238:1408.
10. DiFiore PP, Pierce JH, Fleming TP, et al. Overexpression of the human EGF receptor confers an EGF-dependent transformed phenotype to NIH3T3 cells. Cell 1987;51:1063.
11. Downward J, Yarden Y, Mayes E, et al. Close similarity of epidermal growth factor receptor and v-erbB oncogene protein sequence. Nature 1984;307:521.
12. Fisher DA, Lakshmanan J. Metabolism and the effects of epidermal

growth factor and related growth factors in mammals. Endocr Rev 1990;11:418.

13. Luetteke NC, Lee DC. Transforming growth factor alpha expression, regulation and biological action of its integral membrane precursor. Semin Cancer Biol 1990;1:265.

14. Todaro GJ, Rose TM, Spooner CE, et al. Cellular and viral ligands that interact with the EGF receptor. Semin Cancer Biol 1990;1:257.

15. Nishibe S, Carpenter G. Tyrosine phosphorylation and the regulation of cell growth: growth factor-stimulated tyrosine phosphorylation of phospholipase C. Semin Cancer Biol 1990;1:285.

16. Roberts TM. A signal chain of events. Nature 1992;360:534.

17. Muthuswamy SK, Siegel PM, Dankort DL, et al. Mammary tumors expressing the neu proto-oncogene possess elevated c-Src tyrosine kinase activity. Mol Cell Biol 1994;14:735.

18. Segatto O, Leonardo F, Wexler D, et al. The Juxtamembrane regions of the EGF receptor and gp185erbB2 determine the specificity of signal transduction. Mol Cell Biol 1991;11:3191.

19. Davidson NE, Gelmann EP, Lippman ME, et al. Epidermal growth factor receptor gene expression in estrogen receptor-positive and negative human breast cancer cell lines. Mol Endocrinol 1987;1:216.

20. Murphey JM, Chrysogelos SA. Intron 1 elements are involved in EGFR gene regulation in breast cancer cells. (Abstract) Keystone Sympos Breast and Prostate Cancer II, Lake Tahoe, 1994.

21. Mukku VR, Stancel GM. Regulation of epidermal growth factor receptor by estrogen. J Biol Chem 1985;260:9820.

22. Lingham RB, Stancel GM, Loose-Mitchell DS. Estrogen regulation of epidermal growth factor receptor messenger ribonucleic acid. Mol Endocrinol 1988;2:230.

23. Saceda M, Lippman ME, Chambon P, et al. Regulation of the estrogen receptor in MCF-7 cells by estradiol. Mol Endocrinol 1988;2:1157.

24. Hudson LG, Santon JB, Gill GN. Regulation of epidermal growth factor receptor gene expression. Mol Endocrinol 1989;3:400.

25. Saceda M, Knabbe C, Dickson RB, et al. Post-transcriptional destabilization of estrogen receptor mRNA in MCF-7 cells by 12-O-tetradecanoylphorbol-13-acetate. J Biol Chem 1991;266:17809.

26. Chrysogelos SA, Dickson RB. EGF receptor expression, regulation, and function in breast cancer. Breast Cancer Res Treat 1994;29:29.

27. Schmidt-Ullrich RK, Valerie KC, Chan W, et al. Altered expression of epidermal growth factor receptor and estrogen receptor after single and repeated radiation exposure. Int J Rad 1994;29:813.

28. Vickers PJ, Dickson RB, Shoemaker R, et al. A multidrug-resistant MCF-7 human breast cancer cell line which exhibits cross-resistance to antiestrogens and hormone-independent tumor growth *in vivo*. Mol Endocrinol 1988;2:886.

29. Nicholson RI, McClelland RA, Gee JMW, et al. Transforming growth factor-α and endocrine sensitivity in breast cancer. Cancer Res 1994;54:1684.

30. Qi C, Liscia DS, Normanno N, et al. Expression of transforming growth factor alpha, amphiregulin, and cripto-1 in human breast carcinomas. Br J Cancer 1994;69:903.

31. Holmes WE, Sliwkowski MX, Akita RW, et al. Identification of heregulin, a specific activator of p185.[erbB2] Science 1992;256:1205.

32. Wen D, Peles E, Cupples R, et al. Neu differentiation factor: a transmembrane glycoprotein containing an EGF domain and an immunoglobulin homology unit. Cell 1992;69:559.

33. Peles E, Bacus SS, Koski RA, et al. Isolation of the neu/HER-2 stimulatory ligand: a 44 kd glycoprotein that induces differentiation of mammary tumor cells. Cell 1992;69:205.

34. Plowman GD, Culouscou J-M, Whitney GS, et al. Ligand-specific activation of HER4/p180,[erbB4] a fourth member of the epidermal growth factor receptor family. Proc Natl Acad Sci USA 1993;90:1746.

35. Plowman GD, Green JM, Culouscou JM, et al. Heregulin induces tyrosine phosphorylation of HER4/P180 (erbB$_4$). Nature 1993;366:473.

36. Samanta A, LeVea CM, Dougall WC, et al. Ligand and p185[c-neu] density govern receptor interactions and tyrosine kinase activation. Proc Natl Acad Sci USA 1994;91:1711.

37. Dobashi K, Davis IG, Mikami Y, et al. Characterization of a neu/c-erbB$_2$ protein-specific activating factor. Proc Natl Acad Sci USA 1991;88:8582.

38. Kern JA, Schwartz DA, Nordberg JE, et al. p185neu expression in human lung adenocarcinomas predicts shortened survival. Cancer Res 1990;50:5184.

39. Hall PA, Hughes CM, Staddon SL, et al. The c-erbB-2 proto-oncogene in human pancreatic cancer. J Pathol 1990;161:195.

40. Berchuck A, Rodriguez G, Kinney RB, et al. Overexpression of HER-2/neu in endometrial cancer is associated with advanced stage disease. Am J Obstet Gynecol 1991;164:15.

41. Semba K, Kamata N, Toyoshima K, et al. A v-erbB-related proto-oncogene, c-erbB-2, is distinct from the c-erbB-1/epidermal growth factor-receptor gene and is amplified in a human salivary gland adenocarcinoma. Proc Natl Acad Sci USA 1985;82:6497.

42. Coussens L, Yang-Feng TL, Liao YC, et al. Tyrosine kinase receptor with extensive homology to EGF receptor shares chromosomal location with neu oncogene. Science 1985;230:1132.

43. Ullrich A, Schlessinger J. Signal transduction by receptors with tyrosine kinase activity. Cell 1990;61:203.

44. Segatto O, Leonardo F, Wexler D, et al. The juxtamembrane regions of the EGF receptor and gp185erbB2 determine the specificity of signal transduction. Mol Cell Biol 1991;11:3191.

45. Carraway KL, Cantley LC. A new acquaintance for erbB$_3$ and erbB$_4$: a role for receptor heterodimerization in growth signalling. Cell 1994;78:5.

46. Goldman R, Levy RB, Peles E, et al. Heterodimerization of the erbB-1 and erbB-2 receptors in human breast carcinoma cells: a mechanism for receptor transregulation. J Biochem 1990;29:11024.

47. Quian XL, Decker SJ, Greene MI. p185-c-neu and epidermal growth factor receptor associate into a structure composed of activated kinases. Proc Natl Acad Sci USA 1992;89:1330.

48. Quian X, LeVea CM, Freeman JK, et al. Heterodimerization of epidermal growth factor receptor and wild-type or kinase-deficient Neu: a mechanism of interreceptor kinase activation and transphosphorylation. Proc Natl Acad Sci USA 1994;91:1500.

49. Soltoff SP, Carraway KL, Prigent SA, et al. ErbB$_3$ is involved in activating phosphatidylinositol 3-kinase by epidermal growth factor. Mol Cell Biol 1994;14:3550.

50. Quian X, Dougall WC, Hellma ME, et al. Kinase-deficient neu proteins suppress epidermal growth factor receptor function and abolish cell transformation. Oncogene 1994;9:1507.

51. Honegger AM, Schmidt A, Ullrich A, et al. Evidence for epidermal growth factor (EGF)-induced intermolecular antiphosphorylation of the TGF receptors in living cells. Mol Cell Biol 1990;10:4035.

52. Batzer AG, Rotin B, Urena JM, et al. Hierarchy of binding sites for Grb2 and Shc on the epidermal growth factor receptor. Mol Cell Biol 1994;14:5192.

53. Myers MG, Sun X-J, White MF. IRS-1 signalling system. Trends Biochem Sci 1994;19:289.

54. Panayotou G, Waterfield MD. The assembly of signalling complexes by receptor tyrosine kinases. Bioessays 1993;15:171.

55. Pazin MJ, Williams LT. Triggering signalling cascades by receptor tyrosine kinases. Trends Biochem Sci 1992;17:374.

56. Carpenter G. Receptor tyrosine kinase substrates: *src* homology domains and signal transduction. FASEB J 1992;6:3283.

57. Mangelsdorf-Soderquist A, Todderud G, Carpenter G. Elevated membrane association of phospholipase C-γ1 in MDA-468 mammary tumor cells. Cancer Res 1992;52:4526.

58. Feng G-S, Hui C-C, Pawson T. SH2-containing phosphotyrosine

phosphatase as a target of protein-tyrosine kinases. Science 1993;259:1607.

59. Davis RJ. The mitogen-activated protein kinase signal transduction pathway. J Biol Chem 1993;268:14553.

60. Margolis B. Proteins with SH2 domains: transducers in the tyrosine kinase signaling pathway. Cell Growth Different 1992;3:73.

61. Karin M, Smeal T. Control of transcription factors by signal transduction pathways: the beginning of the end. Trends Biochem Sci 1992;17:418.

62. Cohen P. Signal integration at the level of protein kinases, protein phosphatases and their substrates. Trends Biochem Sci 1992; 17:388.

63. Li N, Batzer A, Daly R, et al. Guanine-nucleotide–releasing factor hSos1 binds to Grb2 and links receptor tyrosine kinases to Ras signalling. Nature 1993;363:85.

64. Rozakis-Adcock M, Fernley R, Wade J, et al. The SH2 and SH3 domains of mammalian Grb2 couple the EGF receptor to the Ras activator mSos1. Nature 1993;363:83.

65. Egan SE, Giddings BW, Brooks MW, et al. Association of Sos Ras exchange protein with Grb2 is implicated in tyrosine kinase signal transduction and transformation. Nature 1993;363:45.

66. McCormick F. How receptors turn Ras on. Nature 1993;363:15.

67. Gale NW, Kaplan S, Lowenstein EJ, et al. Grb2 mediates the EGF-dependent activation of guanine nucleotide exchange on Ras. Nature 1993;363:88.

68. Medema RH, De Vries-Smits AMM, Van Der Zon GCM, et al. Ras activation by insulin and epidermal growth factor through enhanced exchange of guanine nucleotides on p21^{ras}. Mol Cell Biol 1993;13:155.

69. Bollag G, McCormick F. Regulators and effectors of *ras* proteins. Annu Rev Cell Biol 1991;7:601.

70. Chardin P, Camonis JH, Gale NW, et al. Human Sos 1: a guanine nucleotide exchange factor for Ras that binds to GRB2. Science 1993;260:1338.

71. Cresp P, Xu N, Simonds WF, et al. Ras-dependent activation of MAP kinase pathway mediated by G-protein $\beta\gamma$ subunits. Nature 1994;369:418.

72. Yan Z, Winnwer S, Friedman E. Two different signal transduction pathways can be activated by transforming growth factor β_1 in epithelial cells. J Biol Chem 1994;269:13231.

73. Liu X, Pawson T. The epidermal growth factor receptor phosphorylates GTPase-activating protein (GAP) at Tyr-460, adjacent to the GAP SH2 domains. Mol Cell Biol 1991;11:2511.

74. Ellis C, Moran M, McCormick F, et al. Phosphorylation of GAP and GAP-associated proteins by transforming and mitogenic tyrosine kinases. Nature 1990;343:377.

75. Rodriguez-Viciana R, Warne PH, Dhand R, et al. Phosphatidylinositol-3-OH kinase as a direct target of Ras. Nature 1994;370:527.

76. Dickson B, Sprenger F, Morrison D, et al. Raf functions downstream of Ras1 in the sevenless signal transduction pathway. Nature 1992;360:600.

77. Zhang X-F, Settleman J, Kyriakis JM, et al. Normal and oncogenic p21^{ras} proteins bind to the amino-terminal regulatory domain of c-Raf-1. Nature 1993;364:308.

78. App H, Hazan R, Zilberstein A, et al. Epidermal growth factor (EGF) stimulates association and kinase activity of Raf-1 with the EGF receptor. Mol Cell Biol 1991;11:913.

79. Warne PH, Viciana PR, Downward J. Direct interaction of Ras and the amino-terminal region of Raf-1 *in vitro*. Nature 1993;364:352.

80. Leevers SL, Paterson HF, Marshall CJ. Requirement for Ras in Raf activation is overcome by targeting Raf to the plasma membrane. Nature 1994;369:411.

81. Freed E, Symons M, Macdonald SG, et al. Binding of 14-3-3 proteins to the protein kinase Raf and effects on its activation. Science 1994;265:1713.

82. Hafner S, Adler HS, Mischak H, et al. Mechanism of inhibition of Raf-1 by protein kinase C. Mol Cell Biol 1994;14:6696.

83. Avruch J, Zhang X-F, Kyriakis JM. Raf meets Ras: completing the framework of a signal transduction pathway. Trends Biochem Sci 1994;19:279.

84. Hall A. A biochemical function for ras—at last. Science 1994;264:1413.

85. Kyriakis JM, App H, Zhang X-F, et al. Raf-1 activates MAP kinase–kinase. Nature 1992;358:417.

86. Lange-Carter CA, Pleiman CM, Gardner AM, et al. A divergence in the MAP kinase regulatory network defined by MEK kinase and RAF. Science 1993;260:315.

87. Dent P, Haser W, Haystead TAJ, et al. Activation of mitogen-activated protein kinase kinase by v-raf in NIH 3T3 cells and in vitro. Science 1992;257:1404.

88. Moodie SA, Willumsen BM, Weber MJ, et al. Complexes of Ras-GTP with Raf-1 and mitogen-activated protein kinase. Science 1993;260:1658.

89. Lane HA, Fernandez A, Lamb NJC, et al. p70^{s6k} function is essential for G1 progression. Nature 1993;363:170.

90. Nishida E, Gotoh Y. The MAP kinase cascade is essential for diverse signal transduction pathways. Trends Biochem Sci 1993;18:128.

91. Ransone LJ, Verma I. Nuclear proto-oncogenes FOS and JUN. Annu Rev Cell Biol 1990;6:539.

92. Kato GJ, Dang CV. Function of the c-Myc oncoprotein. FASEB J 1992;6:3065.

93. Franklin CC, Unlap T, Adler V, et al. Multiple signal transduction pathways mediate c-Jun protein phosphorylation. Cell Growth Different 1993;4:377.

94. Amati B, Dalton S, Brooks MW, et al. Transcriptional activation by the human c-Myc oncoprotein in yeast requires interaction with Max. Nature 1992;359:423.

95. Nebreda AR. Inactivation of MAP kinases. Trends Biochem Sci 1994;19:1.

96. Fry DW, Kraker AJ, McMichael A, et al. A specific inhibitor of the epidermal growth factor receptor tyrosine kinase. Science 1994;265:1093.

97. Garrett PA, Hulka BS, Kim YL, et al. HRAS protooncogenes polymorphism and breast cancer. Cancer Epidemiol Biomarkers Prev 1993;2:131.

98. Reed S. The role of p34 kinases in the G1 to S-phase transition. Annu Rev Cell Biol 1992;8:529.

99. Atherton-Fessler S, Parker LL, Geahlen R, et al. Mechanisms of p34^{cdc2} regulation. Mol Cell Biol 1993;13:1675.

100. Draetta G. Cell cycle control in eukaryotes: molecular mechanisms of cdc2 activation. Trends Biochem Sci 1990;15:379.

101. Musgrove EA, Hamilton JA, Lee CSL, et al. Growth factor, steroid, and steroid antagonist regulation of cyclin gene expression associated with changes in T-47D human breast cancer cell cycle progression. Mol Cell Biol 1993;13:3577.

102. Shrestha P. Proliferating cell nuclear antigen in breast lesions: correlation of c-erbB-2 oncoprotein and EGF receptor and its clinico-pathological significance in breast cancer. Virchows Arch 1992;421:193.

103. Kreipe H, Feist H, Fischer L, et al. Amplification of *c-myc* but not of c-*erb*B-2 is associated with high proliferative capacity in breast cancer. Cancer Res 1993;53:1956.

104. Monaghan P, Perusinghe NP, Nicholson RI, et al. Growth factor stimulation of proliferating cell nuclear antigen (PCNA) in human breast epithelium in organ culture. Cell Biol Int Reports 1991;15:561.

105. Hunter T, Pines J. Cyclins and cancer. Cell 1991;66:1071.

106. Lewin B. Oncogenic conversion by regulatory changes in transcription factors. Cell 1991;64:303.

107. Keyomarski K, Pardee AB. Redundant cyclin overexpression and gene amplification in breast cancer cells. Proc Natl Acad Sci USA 1993;90:1112.

108. Bandyopadhyay GK, Hwang S, Imagawa W, et al. Role of polyunsaturated fatty acids as signal transducers: amplification of signals from growth factor receptors by fatty acids in mammary epithelial cells. Prostagland Leukot Essent Fatty Acids 1993;48:71.

109. Sadowski HB, Shuai K, Darnell JE Jr, et al. A common nuclear signal transduction pathway activated by growth factor and cytokine receptors. Science 1993;261:1739.

110. Levitzki A. Tyrophostins: tyrosine kinase blockers as novel antiproliferative agents and dissectors of signal transduction. FASEB J 1992;6:3275.

111. James GL, Goldstein JL, Brown MS, et al. Benzodiazepine peptidomimetics: potent inhibitors of Ras farnesylation in animal cells. Science 1993;260:1937.

112. Kohl NE, Mosser SD, deSolms SJ, et al. Selective inhibition of ras-dependent transformation by a farnesyltransferase inhibitor. Science 1993;260:1934.

113. Wu J, Dent P, Jelinek T, et al. Inhibition of the EGF-activated MAP kinase signaling pathway by adenosine 3′,5′-monophosphate. Science 1993;262:1065.

114. Cho-Chung YS. Role of cyclic AMP receptor proteins in growth, differentiation, and suppression of malignancy: new approaches to therapy. Cancer Res 1990;50:7093.

115. Cook SJ, McCormick F. Inhibition by cAMP of Ras-dependent activation of raf. Science 1993;262:1069.

116. Darnell JE, Kerr IM, Starb GR. Jak-STAT pathways and transcriptional activation in response to IFNs and other extracellular signalling pathways. Science 1994;264:1415.

117. Sadowski HB, Shuai K, Darnell JE, et al. A common nuclear signal transduction pathway activated by growth factor and cytokine receptors. Science 1993;261:1739.

118. Silvennoinen O, Schindler C, Schlessinger J, et al. Ras-independent growth factor signalling by transcription factor tyrosine phosphorylation. Science 1993;261:1736.

119. Gregory H, Thomas CE, Willshire IR, et al. Epidermal and transforming growth factor α in patients with breast tumors. Br J Cancer 1989;59:605.

120. Travers MR, Barrett-Lee PJ, Berger U, et al. Growth factor expression in normal, benign, and malignant breast tissue. BMJ 1988;296:1621.

121. Perroteau I, Salomon D, DeBortoli M, et al. Immunological detection and quantitation of alpha transforming growth factors in human breast carcinoma cells. Breast Cancer Res Treat 1986;7:201.

122. Macias A, Perez R, Hägerström T, et al. Identification of transforming growth factor alpha in human primary breast carcinomas. Anticancer Res 1987;7:1271.

123. Eckert K, Granetzny A, Fischer J, et al. An Mr 43,000 epidermal growth factor−related protein purified from the urine of breast cancer patients. Cancer Res 1990;50:642.

124. Normanno N, Qi C-F, Gullick WJ, et al. Expression of amphiregulin, cripto-1 and heregulin α in human breast cancer cells. Int J Cancer 1993;2:903.

125. Le June S, Leak R, Horak E, et al. Amphiregulin, epidermal growth factor receptor, and estrogen receptor expression in human primary breast cancer. Cancer Res 1993;53:3597.

126. Fitzpatrick SL, Brightwell J, Wittliff J, et al. Epidermal growth factor binding by breast tumor biopsies and relationship to estrogen and progestin receptor levels. Cancer Res 1984;44:3448.

127. Sainsbury JRC, Farndon JR, Sherbert GV, et al. Epidermal growth factor receptors and oestrogen receptors in human breast cancers. Lancet 1985;1:364.

128. Fox SB, Smith K, Hollyer J, et al. The epidermal growth factor receptor as a prognostic marker: results of 370 patients and a review of 3009 patients. Breast Cancer Res Treat 1994;29:41.

129. Xu YH, Richert N, Ito S, et al. Characterization of epidermal growth factor receptor gene expression in malignant and normal human cell lines. Proc Natl Acad Sci USA 1984;81:7308.

130. King CR, Kraus MH, Williams LT, et al. Human tumor cell lines with EGF receptor gene amplification in the absence of aberrant sized mRNAs. Nucleic Acids Res 1985;13:8477.

131. Chrysogelos SA. Chromatin structure of the EGFR gene suggests a role for intron-1 sequences in its regulation in breast cancer cells. Nucleic Acids Res 1993;21:5736.

132. Klijn JGM, Cook MP, Portengen H, et al. The prognostic value of epidermal growth factor receptor (EGF-R) in primary breast cancer: results of a 10-year follow-up study. Breast Cancer Res Treat 1994;29:73.

133. Toi M, Tominaga T, Osaki A, et al. Role of epidermal growth factor receptor expression in primary breast cancer: results of a biochemical and immunochemical study. Breast Cancer Res Treat 1994;29:51.

134. Bargmann CI, Hung MC, Weinberg RA. The neu oncogene encodes an epidermal growth factor receptor-related protein. Nature 1986;319:226.

135. Gusterson BA, Machin LG, Gullick WJ, et al. Immunohistochemical distribution of c-*erb*B-2 in infiltrating and *in situ* breast cancer. Int J Cancer 1988;42:842.

136. Paik S, Hazan R, Fisher ER, et al. Pathologic findings from the National Surgical Adjuvant Breast and Bowel Project: prognostic significance of *erb*B-2 protein overexpression in primary breast cancer. J Clin Oncol 1990;8:103.

137. Benz CC, Scott GK, Sarup JC, et al. Estrogen-dependent, tamoxifen-resistant tumorigenic growth of MCF-7 cells transfected with Her2/neu. Breast Cancer Res Treat 1992;24:85.

138. Sunderland MC, McGuire WC. Oncogenes as clinical prognostic indicators. In: Lippman ME, Dickson RB, eds. Regulatory mechanisms in breast cancer. Boston, Kluwer, 1990:3.

139. Costantino J, Fisher B, Gunduz N, et al. Tumor size, ploidy, S-Phase, and erbB₂ markers in patients with node-negative, ER-positive tumors: findings from NSABP B-14. (Abstract) Annual Meeting of the American Association for Clinical Oncology, 1994.

140. Lippman ME, Weisenthal LM, Paik S, ErbB-2 positive specimens from previously untreated breast cancer patients have *in vitro* drug resistance profiles which resemble profiles of specimens obtained from patients who have previously failed combination chemotherapy. (Abstract) Annual Meeting of the American Association for Clinical Oncology, 1990.

141. Gusterson BA, Gelber RD, Goldhirsch A, et al. Prognostic importance of c-*erb*B-2 expression in breast cancer. J Clin Oncol 1992;10:1049.

142. Anbazhagen R, Gelber RD, Bettelheim R, et al. Association of c-*erb*B-2 expression and s-phase fraction in the prognosis of node positive breast cancer. Ann Oncol 1991;2:47.

143. Wright C, Cairns J, Cartwell BJ, et al. Response to mitoxantrone in advanced breast cancer: correlation with expression of c-*erb*B-2 protein and glutathione S-transferrase. Br J Cancer 1992;65:271.

144. Wright C, Nicholson S, Angus B, et al. Relationship between *erb*B-2 product expression and response to endocrine therapy in advanced breast cancer. Br J Cancer 1992;65:118.

145. Muss HB, Thor AD, Berry DA, et al. c-erbB₂ expression and response to adjuvant therapy in women with node positive breast cancer. N Engl J Med 1994;330:1260.

146. Allred DC, Clark GM, Tandon AK, et al. *Her-2/neu* in node negative breast cancer: prognostic significance of overexpression influenced by the presence of *in situ* carcinoma. J Clin Oncol 1992;10:599.

147. Toikkanen S, Helin H, Isola J, et al. Prognostic significance of

HER-2 oncoprotein expression in breast cancer: a 30-year follow up. J Clin Oncol 1992;10:1044.

148. Levine MN, Adrulis I. The *Her-2/neu* oncogene in breast cancers: so what is new? J Clin Oncol 1992;10:1034.

149. Yu D, Shi D, Scanlon M, et al. Reexpression of *neu*-encoded oncoprotein counteracts the tumor-suppressing but not the metastasis-suppressing function of E1A. Cancer Res 1993;53:5784.

150. Hancock MC, Langton BC, Chan T, et al. A monoclonal antibody against the c-erbB-2 protein enhances the cytotoxicity of cis-diamminedichloroplatinum against human breast and ovarian tumor cell lines. Cancer Res 1991;51:4575.

151. Pietras RJ, Scates S, Howell SB, et al. Monoclonal antibody to *HER-2/neu* receptor modulates DNA repair and platinum sensitivity in human breast and ovarian carcinoma cells. (Abstract) Proc Am Assoc Cancer Res 1992;33:547.

152. Pegram MD, Pietras RJ, Slamon DJ. Monoclonal antibody to *HER-2/neu* gene product potentiates cytotoxicity of carboplatin and doxorubicin in human breast tumor cells. (Abstract) Proc Am Assoc Cancer Res 1992;33:442.

153. Langton BC, Crenshaw MC, Chao LA, et al. An antigen immunologically related to the external domain of gp185 is shed from nude mouse tumors overexpressing the c-*erb*B-2 (*Her2/neu*) oncogene. Cancer Res 1991;51:2593.

154. Breuer B, DeVivo I, Luo J-C, et al. erbB-2 and myc oncoproteins in sera and tumors of breast cancer patients. Cancer Epidemiol Biomarkers Prev 1994;3:63.

155. Pastan I, Fitzgerald D. Recombinant toxins for cancer treatment. Science 1992;254:1173.

156. Wels W, Harweth IM, Mueller M, et al. Selective inhibition of tumor cell growth by a recombinant single-chain antibody-toxin specific for the *erb*B-2 receptor. Cancer Res 1992;52:6310.

157. King OR, Kraus M, DiFiore PP, et al. Implications of *erb*B-2 overexpression for basic science and clinical medicine. Semin Cancer Biol 1990;1:329.

158. Carter P, Presta L, Gorman CM, et al. Humanization of an anti-p185 HER2 antibody for human cancer therapy. Proc Natl Acad Sci USA 1992;89:4285.

159. Pupa SM, Menard S, Andreola S, et al. Prognostic significance of c-*erb*B-2 oncoprotein overexpression in breast carcinoma patients and its immunological role. (Abstract) Proc Am Assoc Cancer Res 1992;33:312.

160. Ciardiello F, Gottardis M, Basolo F, et al. Additive effects of c-*erb*B-2 c-Ha-*ras*, and transforming growth factor α genes in *in vitro* transformation of human mammary epithelial cells. Mol Carcinogen 1992;6:43.

161. Pierce JH, Arnstein P, DiMarco E, et al. Oncogenic potential of *erb*B-2 in human mammary epithelial cells. Oncogene 1991; 6:1189.

162. Zhai YF, Esselman W, Wang B, et al. Increased expression of LAR and PTPIB protein tyrosine phosphatases (PTPases) in human breast carcinoma cells neoplastically transformed by an activated *neu oncogene*. (Abstract) Proc Am Assoc Cancer Res 1992;33:380.

163. Guy C, Schuller M, Parsons T, et al. Induction of mammary tumors in transgenic mice expressing the unactivated c-*neu* oncogene. (Abstract) J Cell Biochem Suppl 1992;16D:100.

164. Baens SS, Plowman G, Yardin Y. Expression of erbB₂ receptor family and their ligands: implication to breast cancer biological behavior. Breast Cancer Res Treat 1994;32(Suppl):93.

165. Van Der Burg B, De Groot RB, et al. Oestrogen directly stimulates growth factor signal transduction pathways in human breast cancer cells. J Steroid Biochem Molec Biol 1991;40:215.

166. Alkahalf M, Murphy LC. Regulation of c-*jun* and *jun* B by progestins in T47D human breast cancer cells. Mol Endocrinol 1992;6:1625.

167. LeRoy X, Escot C, Browillet JP, et al. Decrease of c-erbB₂ and c-myc mRNA levels in tamoxifen-treated breast cancer. Oncogene 1992;6:431.

168. Chiappetta C, Kirkland JL, Loose-Mitchell DS, et al. Estrogen regulates expression of the *jun* family of protooncogenes in the uterus. J Steroid Biochem Mol Biol 1992;41:113.

169. Murphy LJ. Estrogen induction of insulin-like growth factors and myc proto-oncogene expression in the uterus. J Steroid Biochem Mol Biol 1991;40:223.

170. Rusty AK, Dyson N, Bernards R. Amino terminal domains of c-myc and N-myc proteins mediate binding to the retinoblastoma gene product. Nature 1991;352:541.

171. Watson PH, Pon RT, Shiu RPC. Inhibition of c-myc expression by phosphorothioate antisense oligonucleotide identifies a critical role for c-myc in the growth of human breast cancer. Cancer Res 1991;51:3996.

172. Escot C, Theillet C, Lidereau R, et al. Genetic alteration of the c-myc proto-oncogene in human primary breast carcinomas. Proc Natl Acad Sci USA 1986;83:4834.

173. Bonilla M, Ramirez M, Lopez-Cuento J, et al. *In vivo* amplification and rearrangements of c-myc oncogene in human breast tumors. J Natl Cancer Inst 1988;80:665.

174. Cline M, Battifora H, Yokota JJ. Protooncogene abnormalities in human breast cancer: correlations with anatomic features and clinical course of diagnosis. J Clin Oncol 1987;5:999.

175. Varlay JM, Swallow JE, Brammer VJ, et al. Alterations to either c-erb₂ (neu) short-term prognosis. Oncogene 1987;1:423.

176. Bieche I, Champeme M-H, Lidereau R. A tumor suppressor gene on chromosome 1p32-pter controls the amplification of MYC family genes in breast cancer. Cancer Res 1994;54:4274.

177. Berns EMJJ, Klijn JGM, Van Putten WLJ, et al. c-myc amplification is a better prognostic factor than HER2/neu amplification in primary breast cancer. Cancer Res 1992;52:1107.

178. Borg A, Baldetorp B, Ferno M, et al. c-myc amplification is an independent prognostic factor in postmenopausal breast cancer. Int J Cancer 1992;51:687.

179. Escot C, Theillet C, Lideream R, et al. Genetic alterations of the c-myc protooncogene in human breast carcinomas. Proc Natl Acad Sci USA 1986;83:4834.

180. Lee LW, Raymond VW, Tsao MS, et al. Clonal cosegregation of tumorigenicity with overexpression of c-myc and transforming growth factor α genes in chemically transformed rat liver epithelial cells. Cancer Res 1991;51:5238.

181. Hall JM, Lee MK, Newman B. Linkage of early onset familial breast cancer to chromosome 17q21. Science 1990;250:1684.

182. Jones N. Structure and function of transcription factors. Semin Cancer Biol 1990;1:5.

183. Prendergast GC, Lawe D, Ziff EB. Association of myn, the murine homologue of max with c-myc stimulating methylation-sensitive DNA binding and ras cotransformation. Cell 1991;65:395.

184. Meichle A, Philipp A, Eilers M. The functions of myc proteins. Biochem Biophys Acta 1992;1114:129.

185. Penn LJZ, Laufer EM, Land H. C-myc: evidence for multiple regulation functions. Semin Cancer Biol 1990;1:69.

186. Penn LJZ, Brooks MW, Laufer EM, et al. Negative autoregulation of c-myc transcription. EMBO J 1990;9:1113.

187. Kelekar A, Cole MD. Immortalization by c-myc, H-ras, and Ela oncogenes induces differential cellular gene expression and growth factor responses. Mol Cell Biol 1987;7:3899.

188. Leof EB, Proper JA, Moses HL. Modulation of transforming growth factor type B action by activated ras and c-myc. Mol Cell Biol 1987;7:2649.

189. Stern DF, Roberts AB, Roche NS, et al. Differential responsiveness of myc- and ras-transfected cells to growth factors: selective stimulation of myc-transfected cells by epidermal growth factor. Mol Cell Biol 1986;6:870.

190. Hermeking H, Eick D. Mediation of c-Myc–induced apoptosis by p53. 1994;265:2091.
191. Sklar MD, Prochownik EV. Modulation of cis-platinum resistance in friend erythroleukemia cells by c-myc. Cancer Res 1991; 51:2118.
192. Yang BS, Geddes TJ, Pogulis RJ, et al. Transcriptional suppression of cellular gene expression by c-myc. Mol Cell Biol 1991;11:2291.
193. Suen TC, Hung M-C. c-myc reverse new-induced transformed morphology by transcriptional repression. Mol Cell Biol 1991; 11:354.
194. Gullick WJ, Tuz NC, Kumar S, et al. c-erbB₂ and c-myc genes and their expression in normal tissues and in human breast cancer. Cancer Cells 1989;7:393.
195. Semsei I, Ma S, Culter RG. Tissue and age specific expression of the myc protooncogene family throughout the lifespan of the C57BL/6J mouse strain. Oncogene 1989;4:465.
196. Clarke R, Stampfer MR, Milley B, et al. Transformation of human mammary epithelial cells by oncogenic retroviruses. Cancer Res 1988;48:4689.
197. Valverius EM, Ciardiello F, Heldin NE, et al. Stromal influences on transformation of human mammary epithelial cells overexpressing c-myc and SV40T. J Cell Physiol 1990;145:207.
198. Cullen KJ, Lippman ME. Stromal-epithelial interactions in breast cancer. In: Lippman ME, Dickson RB, eds. Genes, oncogenes and hormones. Boston, Kluwer Academic, 1992:413.
199. Amundadottir LT, Johnson MD, Merlino GT, et al. Synergistic interaction between TGFα and c-myc in mouse mamman and salivary gland humorigenesis. Cell Growth Differ 1995;6:737.
200. Broca P. Traite des tumeurs. Paris, Asselin, 1866.
201. Knudson AG. Mutation and cancer: statistical study of retinoblastoma. Proc Natl Acad Sci USA 1971;68:820.
202. Harris H, Miller OJ, Klein G, et al. Suppression of malignancy by cell fusion. Nature 1969;223:368.
203. Malkin D, Li FP, Strong LC, et al. Germ line p53 mutations in a familial syndrome of breast cancer, sarcomas, and other neoplasms. Science 1990;250:1233.
204. Hall JM, Lee MK, Morrow J, et al. Linkage of early-onset familial breast cancer to chromosome 17q21. Science 1990;250:1684.
205. Miki Y, Swensen J, Shattuck-Eidens D, et al. A strong candidate for the breast and ovarian cancer susceptibility gene BRCA1. Science 1994;266:66.
206. Wooster R, Neuhausen SL, Mangion J, et al. Localization of a breast cancer susceptibility gene, BRCA2, to chromosome 13q12-13. Science 1994;265:2088.
207. Allred DC, Elledge R, Clark GM, et al. The p53 tumor-suppressor gene in human breast cancer. In: Dickson RB, Lippman ME, eds. Mammary tumorigenesis and malignant progression. Boston, Kluwer Academic, 1994:63.
208. Fung YK, T'Ang A. The role of the retinoblastoma gene in breast cancer development. In: Dickson RB, Lippman ME, eds. Genes, oncogenes and hormones. Boston, Kluwer Academic, 1992:59.
209. Steeg PS. Suppressor genes in breast cancer: an overview. In: Dickson RB, Lippman ME, eds. Genes, oncogenes and hormones. Boston, Kluwer, 1992:45.
210. Gamillo C, Palacios J, Suarez A, et al. Correlation of E-cadherin expression with differentiation grade and histological type in breast carcinoma. Am J Pathol 1993;142:987.
211. Sager R, Anisowicz A, Neveu M, et al. Identification by differential display of alpha 6 integrin as a candidate tumor suppressor gene. FASEB J 1993;7:964.
212. Schott DR, Chang JN, Deng G, et al. A candidate tumor suppressor gene in human breast cancers. Cancer Res 1994;54:1393.
213. Blaszyk H, Vaughn CB, Hartmann A, et al. Novel pattern of p53 gene mutations on an American black cohort with high mortality from breast cancer. Lancet 1994;343:1195.
214. Moll UM, Riou G, Levine AJ. Two distinct mechanisms alter p53 in breast cancer: mutation and nuclear exclusion. Proc Natl Acad Sci USA 1992;89:7262.
215. Cullotta E, Koshland DE. Molecules of the year: p53 sweeps through cancer research. Science 1993;262:1958.
216. Strasser A, Harris AW, Jacks T, et al. DNA damage can induce apoptosis in proliferating lymphoid cells via p53-independent mechanisms inhibitable by Bcl-2. Cell 1994;79:329.
217. Chellappan SP, Hiebert S, Madryj M, et al. The E₂F transcription factor is a cellular target for the Rb protein. Cell 1991;65:1053.
218. Dunaief JL, Strober BE, Guha S, et al. The retinoblastoma protein and BRG1 form a complex and cooperate to induce cell cycle arrest. Cell 1994;79:119.
219. Wang TC, Candiff RD, Zuckerbery L, et al. Mammary hyperplasia and carcinoma in MMTV-cyclin D₁ transgenic mice. Nature 1994;369:669.
220. Serrano M, Hannon GJ, Beach D. A new regulatory motif in cell-cycle control causing specific inhibition of cyclin D/CDK4. Nature 1993;366:704.
221. Kamb A, Gruis NA, Weaver-Feldhaus J, et al. A cell cycle regulator potentially involved in genesis of many tumor types. Science 1994;264:436.
222. Sutherland RL, Watts CKW, Musgrove EA. Cyclin gene expression and growth control in normal and neoplastic human breast epithelium. J Steroid Biochem Mol Biol 1993;47:99.
223. Hunter T. Braking the cycle. Cell 1993;75:839.
224. Peters G. Stifled by inhibitions. Nature 1994;371:204.
225. Koff A, Ohtsuki M, Polyak K, et al. Negative regulation of G1 in mammalian cells: inhibition of cyclin E-dependent kinase by TGF-β. Science 1993;260:536.
226. Keyomarsi K, Pardee AB. Redundant cyclin overexpression and gene amplification in breast cancer cells. Proc Natl Acad Sci USA 1993;90:1112.
227. Philipp A, Schneider A, Vasrik I, et al. Repression of cyclin D₁: a novel functioning of myc. Mol Cell Biol 1994;14:4032.
228. Pines J. Arresting developments in cell cycle control. Trends Biochem Sci 1994;19:143.
229. Polyak K, Lee M-H, Erdjument-Bromage H, et al. Cloning of p27ᴷⁱᵖ¹, a cyclin-dependent kinase inhibitor and a potential mediator of extracellular antimitogenic signals. Cell 1994;78:59.
230. Xu L, Sgroi D, Sterner CJ, et al. Mutational analysis of CDKN2 (MTS1/p16ⁱⁿᵏ⁴) in human breast carcinomas. Cancer Res 1994;54:5262.
231. Drake JW. Mutation rates. Bioessays 1992;2:137.
232. Cohen SM, Ellwein LB. Genetic errors, cell proliferation, and carcinogenesis. Cancer Res 1991;51:6493.
233. Tilsty TD, White AL, Sanchez J. Suppression of gene amplification in human cell hybrids. Science 1992;256:1425.
234. Thompson AM, Steel CM, Chetty U, et al. p53 gene mRNA expression and chromosome 17p allele loss in breast cancer. Br J Cancer 1990;61:74.
235. Davidoff AM, Kerns BJM, Pence JC, et al. p53 alterations in all stages of breast cancer. J Surg Oncol 1991;48:260.
236. Osborne RJ, Merlo GR, Mitsudomi T, et al. Mutations in the p53 gene in primary human breast cancers. Cancer Res 1991;51:6194.
237. Bevilacqua G, Sobel ME, Liotta LA, et al. Association of low nm23 RNA levels in human primary infiltrating ductal carcinomas with lymph node involvement and other histopathologic indicators of high metastatic potential. Cancer Res 1989;49:5185.
238. Fishel R, Lescoe MK, Rao MRS, et al. The human mutator gene homolog MSH2 and its association with hereditary nonpolyposis colon cancer. Cell 1993;75:1027.
239. Counter CM, Hirte HW, Bacchetti S, et al. Telomerase activity in human ovarian carcinoma. Proc Natl Acad Sci USA 1994;91:2900.
240. Moffett BF, Baban D, Bao L, et al. Fate of clonal lineages during neoplasia and metastasis studied with an incorporated genetic marker. Cancer Res 1992;52:1737.

241. Sato T, Akiyama F, Sakamoto G, et al. Accumulation of genetic alterations and progression of primary breast cancer. Cancer Res 1991;51:5794.
242. Callahan R, Cropp C, Merlo G, et al. Molecular lesions in sporadic human breast carcinomas. (Abstract) Proceedings of the Cold Spring Harbor Symposium on Genetics and Molecular Biology of Breast Cancer, Cold Spring Harbor, New York, 1992.
243. Dati C, Muraca R, Tazartes O, et al. c-erbB-2 and ras expression levels in breast cancer are correlated and show a cooperative association with unfavorable clinical outcome. Int J Cancer 1991;47:833.
244. Horack E, Smith K, Bromley L, et al. Mutant p53, EGF receptor, and c-erbB$_2$ expression in human breast cancer. Oncogene 1991;6:2277.
245. Sinn E, Muller W, Pattengale P, et al. Coexpression of MMTV/v-Ha-ras and MMTV/c-myc genes in transgenic mice: synergistic actions of oncogenes *in vivo*. Cell 1987;49:465.

7.7
Animal Models of Breast Cancer
ROBERT CLARKE

General Principles

Animal models of breast cancer have been widely used for many years and have contributed significantly both to our understanding of breast cancer biology and to the development of several new therapeutic strategies. Because the number of species that develop spontaneous breast tumors is limited, few good animal models of spontaneous breast cancer exist. For example, in addition to tumors in rats and mice, mammary tumors also arise spontaneously in dogs,[1,2] but the cost of these models is generally prohibitive. Most experimental animal models of breast cancer are limited to the rodents. Several different groups of rodent models are available for experimental breast cancer research, however. These include chemically induced rat mammary carcinomas (eg, 7, 12-dimethylbenz(a)anthracene [DMBA], *N*-nitrosomethylurea [NMU]), virally induced mammary tumors, human tumor xenografts, and transgenic mouse models.

Many aspects of experimental breast cancer research require the use of an appropriate animal model. For example, reproducing the complexity of the endocrinologic environment of the pituitary–adrenal–ovarian axis is beyond the scope of current in vitro technologies. Tumor–host interactions including immunologic effects, vascular and stromal effects, and host-related pharmacologic and pharmacokinetic effects also are relatively poorly modeled in vitro. Even a well-justified requirement for the use of living animals, however, imposes several ethical and scientific considerations. Investigators must give appropriate consideration to the health and welfare of experimental animals, for example, by providing adequate diet, space, health monitoring, and hygiene. Many of these concerns are of more importance than often realized. For example, almost all mammary animal tumor models are sensitive to (ie, inhibited by) caloric restriction.[3–5] Sufficient numbers of animals must be used to provide adequate statistical power and to ensure the validity of the study, but not such that animal usage is unnecessary.

Each rodent model has its own advantages and disadvantages, and a clear understanding of the limitations and utility of each model is critical for its appropriate application. In general, the major models for spontaneous breast cancer are the mouse strains susceptible to mouse mammary tumor virus (MMTV)–induced mammary neoplasia, and some transgenic mouse models. In these models, the mammary glands potentially express the transforming genes from early life onward (MMTV, neonatal; transgenics, fetal). For chemically induced tumors, initiation events are induced by the carcinogen. The spontaneous and chemically induced models are particularly useful for chemoprevention studies, because full transformation of the gland has either not occurred (young transgenic and MMTV-infected mice) or occurs within a reproducible time following carcinogenic insult (chemically induced tumors). In the human tumor xenografts, the malignant tissue is directly inoculated into host tissues. Thus, effects on early events (ie, initiation) are not amenable to study. These xenografts provide a good model for the study of malignant progression in the human disease and for screening drugs against established human tumors however. A major advantage of the xenografts is their human breast cancer origin, whereas a disadvantage of the rodent mammary models is their nonhuman origin. Choice of the appropriate model and a realistic assessment of its limitations are critical for adequate and appropriate experimental design. Siemann made a simple but important observation when he stated that a critical consideration is to ". . . choose the model to address the question rather than force the question on the tumor model."[6]

Chemically Induced Rodent Mammary Tumors

The mammary glands of several rat strains are susceptible to transformation by chemical carcinogens, most notably Sprague-Dawley,[7] Buf/N,[8] Fischer 344,[9] Lewis,[10] and to a lesser extent Wistar-Furth.[9] Other strains are relatively resistant, such as the Copenhagen rat.[11] Rats that have completed a full-term pregnancy or lactation, or have been treated with estrogen and progesterone before carcinogen administration, exhibit a reduced incidence of mammary tumors.[7] This may reflect an endocrine-induced differentiation that reduces the number of target undifferentiated stem cells.[12] For chemical carcinogens, the dose of carcinogen and the age of the rats are critical. The optimal age is 40 to 46 days old in virgin rats.

These mammary tumor models have been in constant use since their description by Huggins and associates in 1961,[13] and their use has provided critical insights into several aspects of breast cancer biology. For example, chemically induced tumors have been used to demonstrate the antitumor and chemopreventive effects of endocrine agents[14–16] and vitamins.[17] These models also are sensitive to dietary manipulations, particularly to apparently promotional events induced by diets high in n-6 polyunsaturated fats (eg, corn oil).[3,18–20] In contrast, diets high in fish oils (eg, menhaden oil) reduce tumor incidence.[21] Perhaps the most notable example of the use of chemically induced rodent models is their role in the preclinical development of the antiestrogen tamoxifen.

All chemically induced mammary tumors exhibit a low metastatic potential.[22] Although some local invasion is apparent, and occasional metastases have been reported, these are rarely sufficiently reproducible to provide a useful model of metastasis. The majority of tumors are initially prolactin dependent,[23] but a similar central role for prolactin in human breast cancer is not currently evident.[24] Chemically induced tumors also are initially estrogen responsive.[23] Progression to a hormone-unresponsive phenotype can occur rapidly in a significant proportion of tumors, however. These characteristics, and the high level of *ras* activation (eg, NMU-induced tumors), limit their applicability for some studies. In general, investigators should be cautious in designing experiments in which agents are coadministered with a chemical carcinogen, because effects on the carcinogen's pharmacokinetics can produce potentially artifactual observations specific for the carcinogen.

7,12-DIMETHYLBENZ(A)ANTHRACENE

DMBA is a potent inducer of mammary carcinomas. DMBA is generally administered by oral gavage, frequently as a solution in peanut oil; 20 mg/per animal produces a final incidence of 100% adenocarcinomas, generally within 10 to 15 weeks. The mammary tumors arise in the epithelium of the terminal end buds, which are comparable structures to the terminal ductal–lobular unit in the human breast.[7] The tumors are generally ductal carcinomas, papillary carcinomas, and intraductal papillomas.[7] The comparative biology of DMBA-induced mammary carcinomas has been extensively reviewed by Russo and coworkers.[7]

DMBA is highly lipophilic and requires metabolic activation for its carcinogenicity. Coadministration of agents that alter either its lipid biodisposition or its hepatic activation can influence subsequent tumor incidence. These apparent effects on tumorigenicity may be considered arti-factual, however, because they are pharmacologic effects specific to the carcinogen. The potential for such artifacts requires careful experimental study design when using DMBA, for example, in studies with agents that could alter hepatic function or in dietary studies utilizing high fat.

N-NITROSOMETHYLUREA

The ability of NMU to produce mammary tumors was reported by Gullino and colleagues 20 years ago.[25] NMU induces mammary carcinomas in rodents when the agent is administered subcutaneously or intravenously at 50 mg/kg. Tumor incidence and latency are comparable to that observed with DMBA administration, and tumors also exhibit steroid hormone and prolactin responsiveness.[26] Because NMU does not require metabolic activation, there are fewer concerns regarding coadministration artifacts than for DMBA. Approximately 75% of rodent mammary tumors induced by NMU exhibit altered *ras* expression and activation,[8] however, which occurs during initiation.[27] The incidence of altered *ras* expression in human breast cancer is approximately 20% and represents rare alleles or slight overexpression.[28] Furthermore, its role in human breast cancer initiation, promotion, and progression remains unclear.[28,29] This contrasts with the potent transforming *ras* mutations observed in NMU-induced rodent tumors.[8,27] The high incidence of *ras* activation potentially reduces the utility of NMU-induced tumors for signal transduction and mechanistic studies, because the probability that *ras*/G-protein–mediated pathways will predominate is high. The high incidence of activated *ras* increases the likelihood that data from such mechanistic studies could be heavily skewed. Although this also limits studies of the ability of agents (eg, tumor promoters) to increase the incidence of *ras* expression further, it may prove to be a good model for studying treatments that could either reduce *ras* expression or utilize *ras*-mediated signal transduction pathways.

Virally Induced Rodent Mammary Tumors

MMTV-INDUCED TUMORS

Several mouse strains are susceptible to mammary tumor virus (MMTV) infections that subsequently produce mammary tumors (eg, C3H, CD1, RIII, GR, SHN, BR6). Neonatal female mice are infected with MMTV through their mother's milk. Infected female mice of susceptible strains develop preneoplastic hyperplastic alveolar nodules that are generally apparent from at least 4 weeks of age. In C3H/OuJ[5] and C3H/HeJ mice,[30] mammary tumors begin to appear around 24 to 28 weeks of age. Approximately a 50% incidence in mammary tumors is achieved in virgin mice by about 35 weeks of age.[5] Many of the MMTV models exhibit a strong pregnancy- or progesterone-dependent increase in incidence.[31] In common with the chemically induced rat mammary tumor models described previously, these models also exhibit a strong prolactin dependence,[30] and they are responsive to retinoids.[31] Both ovariectomy and treatment with tamoxifen also induce regression in these spontaneous mammary tumors.[31]

The transforming potential of MMTV is almost certainly the result of virally induced mutational insertion.[32] MMTV proviral insertion occurs at four major chromosomal locations; *int-1/Wnt-1* (mouse chromosome 15), *int-2/FGF-3* (mouse chromosome 7), *int-3* (mouse chromosome 17), and *Wnt-3* (mouse chromosome 11). The most common insertions are observed at the *int-1* and *int-2/FGF-3* loci.[32] Different transcriptional and translational start sites and polyadenylation sites in different tissues can produce expression of various *int-2/FGF-3* mRNA species; however, each of these mRNAs can produce the same protein.[32] Although amplification of *int-2/FGF-3* and of *hst/FGF-4* is observed in both human and mouse mammary tumors (eg, approximately 30% of human breast tumors), their respective mRNAs and proteins are rarely expressed in the human disease.[33-35] MMTV-induced oncogene activation has been reviewed in detail.[32,36]

POLYOMA-INDUCED TUMORS

Mammary hyperplasia, dysplasia, and mammary tumors are observed in female mice infected with the polyoma WTA2 virus at 6 weeks of age.[37] Infected mammary glands exhibit an initial epithelial hyperplasia, followed by dysplasia 6 weeks after inoculum. Glands ultimately develop mammary adenocarcinomas of ductal origin (100% incidence) by 6 to 9 weeks after inoculum. Unlike MMTV- and chemically induced rodent models, polyoma-induced tumors are ovarian independent.[37] This model has been reviewed in detail.[38]

ADENOVIRUS-INDUCED TUMORS

One-day-old Wistar-Furth rats (less than 24 hours old) inoculated subcutaneously with human adenovirus type 9 develop benign mammary fibroadenomas, phylloides-like tumors, and solid sarcomas.[39,40] Palpable mammary lesions develop by 3 to 5 months of age, with the benign lesions apparently of primarily mammary fibroblastic origin, as determined by expression of type IV collagen and vimentin. Unlike the other rodent mammary tumor models, the areas of neoplasia are of myoepithelial and not of epithelial origin, as indicated by their continued expression of type IV collagen, vimentin, and muscle-specific actin. The tumors are estrogen-responsive, as indicated by an ovariectomy-induced inhibition of tumor development, induction by diethylstilbestrol, and the presence of estrogen receptor (ER) mRNA.[39]

Human Tumor Xenografts

The xenografting of human tumors into athymic nude mice has become almost routine during the past 10 years. The nude mouse is not the only immunocompromised rodent available, however. Mutations at approximately 30 loci have been shown to reduce immune function in mice.[41] The major mutations used to generate hosts for xenografts are the nude (*nu*), beige (*bg*), severe combined immune deficiency (*scid*), and X-linked immune deficiency (*xid*). Of these, the scid mouse is generally considered to exhibit the greatest degree of immunosuppression. The combined *bg/nu/xid* mutation strain (eg, NIH III) also produces severely immune compromised animals but has received less attention, perhaps as a result of a clotting disorder that reduces their utility in studies requiring survival surgery.

Human breast cancer cell lines inoculated into nude mice represent the majority of human breast tumor xenograft models. Relatively few xenografts have been in regular and widespread use other than MCF-7 (endocrine-responsive) and MDA–MB-231 (endocrine-unresponsive) cells, however. In part, this reflects the low success rate for establishing human breast tumors either directly as xenografts or as stable established cell lines in vitro.

Despite the ability to apply selective pressures resulting in variants with altered endocrine responsiveness,[42-44] the majority of endocrine-responsive xenografts are phenotypically stable, at least with respect to biologically important characteristics (eg, tumorigenicity, steroid hormone expression, hormone responsiveness). We have not observed any spontaneous loss of estrogen-dependence in MCF-7 cells (ER-positive; estrogen-dependent), gain of estrogen responsiveness in MDA–MB-435 cells (ER-negative, estrogen-unresponsive), or alteration in estrogen responsiveness of MCF-7/MIII cells (ER positive, estrogen-independent, and estrogen-responsive) maintained routinely in our laboratory in the absence of selective pressures. Indeed, the major phenotypic characteristics of hormone responsiveness, hormone receptor expression, antiestrogen responsiveness, tumorigenicity, and metastatic potential remain remarkably stable in the majority of human breast cancer cell lines. The stability of human tumor xenografts is widely reported.[45] Some minor phenotypic diversity is observed between laboratories and is not surprising because some of these cell lines have been in continuous culture for more than 15 years. Nevertheless, these models have the advantages of being human in origin and relatively reproducible with regard to their endocrine responsiveness and metastatic potential. A description of the characteristics of the major xenografts is provided in Table 7.7-1.

Many studies of endocrine agents, or studies using endocrine responsive xenografts, are performed in ovariectomized mice. The levels of circulating estrogens in these animals are low and closely approximate the levels found in postmenopausal women.[46-48] Because the major endocrine-responsive human breast cancer cells lines (eg, MCF-7, ZR-75-1, T47D) were derived from tumors in postmenopausal women,[49] the endocrine environment of the ovariectomized mouse is appropriate. Moreover, increasing evidence indicates that orthotopic implantation produces tumors with a more biologically relevant phenotype and greater tumor take rate.[50-53] Despite potential differences between the rodent mammary fat pad environment

TABLE 7.7-1
Characteristics of Representative Transplantable Mammary Tumor Cells

Cell Line	Origin/Derivation	Estrogen Responsiveness	Invasive/Metastatic	References
MCF-7	Human breast cancer cell line	Dependent	−/−	55, 138
ZR-75-1	Human breast cancer cell line	Dependent	−/−	139, 140
T47D	Human breast cancer cell line	Dependent	−/−	139, 140
MCF-7/MIII	MCF-7 variant	Independent/stimulated	+/±	42, 55
MCF-7/LCC1	MCF-7 variant	Independent/stimulated	+/±	55, 61
MCF-7/LCC2	MCF-7 variant	Independent/stimulated	ND	43
MCF-7/MKS-1	MCF-7 transfected with FGF-4	Independent/inhibited	+/+	137
ML-α	MDA-MB-231 transfected with estrogen receptor	Independent/inhibited	ND	69
T61	Human xenograft	Independent/inhibited	ND	141, 142
MCF-7[ADR]	MCF-7 variant selected for doxorubicin resistance	Independent/unresponsive	−/−	139, 143
MDA−MB-435	Human breast cancer cell line	Independent/unresponsive	+/+	68
MDA−MB-231	Human breast cancer cell line	Independent/unresponsive	+/+	68
Hs578T	Human breast cancer cell line	Independent/unresponsive	+/±	139

+, Phenotype observed reproducibly; −, phenotype rare; ±, phenotype observed occasionally; ND, no data available.

and the human breast,[7] the mammary fat pad provides an appropriate orthotopic site that is readily accessible. Although most human breast cancer cell lines grow adequately in almost any subcutaneous site (eg, the flank is widely used), inoculation into the mammary fat pad is the preferred site.

ENDOCRINE-RESPONSIVE XENOGRAFTS

Relatively few human breast cancer xenografts exhibit an endocrine-responsive phenotype, and all are ER–positive. Two categories of endocrine-responsive cells are recognized: (1) estrogen-dependent cells; and (2) estrogen-independent and estrogen-responsive cells.[54] The estrogen-dependent xenografts do not form proliferating tumors in the mammary fat pads of ovariectomized immunodeficient mice without estrogen supplementation, generally in the form of a 60-day release 0.72-mg 17β-estradiol pellet placed subcutaneously in the interclavicular region. Examples of estrogen-dependent xenografts include the MCF-7, ZR-75-1, T47D cell lines. Most of the estrogen-responsive xenografts produce well-differentiated adenocarcinomas,[55] are inhibited by tamoxifen,[56–60] and are poorly invasive and nonmetastatic.[55]

Several estrogen-independent and estrogen-responsive variants have been derived from estrogen-dependent cells in this[42,43,61] and other laboratories.[44] These variants form proliferating tumors in ovariectomized immunodeficient mice without estrogen supplementation. They grow more rapidly, however, in the presence of an estrogen pellet.[42,61] Examples of estrogen-independent and estrogen-respon-

sive xenografts derived from MCF-7 cells include MCF-7/MIII,[42] BSK-3,[42,44] MCF-7/LCC-1,[61] and MCF-7/LCC2 (tamoxifen resistant).[43]

Analysis of the growth and endocrine responsiveness of the various endocrine-responsive xenografts has provided useful information on the biology of malignant progression[62,63] and cross-resistance among antiestrogen therapies.[43,54] For example, the ability to isolate estrogen-independent cells from estrogen-dependent cells indicates a possible progression pathway to acquired estrogen independence in breast tumors arising in postmenopausal women.[54,62,64]

MCF-7/LCC2 cells are resistant to the inhibitory effects of 4-hydroxytamoxifen when growing both in vitro and in vivo.[43] MCF-7/LCC2 cells are not, however, cross-resistant to the steroidal antiestrogens ICI 182,780[43] and ICI 164,384.[65] These data would predict that patients in whom tamoxifen has induced a response but subsequently failed would respond to a steroidal antiestrogen. Preliminary data from a phase I trial of ICI 182,780 now demonstrate responses in patients in whom tamoxifen has failed.[66] Thus, the pattern of antiestrogen responsiveness exhibited by the MCF-7/LCC2 cells is an accurate prediction of a previously unknown pattern of clinical response.

MCF-7 human breast cancer cells transfected with an expression vector directing a high constitutive expression of FGF-4/kFGF produce highly vascular tumors that are inhibited by physiologic doses of estrogen and pharmacologic doses of tamoxifen[67]; the inverse response is exhibited by the parental MCF-7 cells.[59,60] These tumors produce a high incidence of lung and lymphatic metastases; however, ER-negative (estrogen-unresponsive) and metastatic MDA−MB-231 cells[68] transfected with the ER gene also exhibit an estrogen-inhibited phenotype.[69] These cells may provide potentially novel breast cancer metastasis models. MCF-7 tumors selected in vivo for resistance to tamoxifen also exhibit a tamoxifen-stimulated and estrogen-inhibited response pattern.[56,60]

Relevance of the inverted endocrine responsiveness of these models to the human disease is not immediately apparent, because tumors inhibited by physiologic estrogen concentrations could not arise in premenopausal women. Pharmacologic doses of estrogens produce remissions in hormone-responsive breast tumors,[70,71] and no clear evidence exists that either physiologic estrogen doses or hormone replacement therapy can produce remissions in postmenopausal breast cancer patients. These models do, however, suggest that withdrawal responses to tamoxifen may occur more frequently than previously reported. Despite the estimation that the total exposure to tamoxifen between 1971 and 1988 was greater than 1.5 million patient-years,[72] reports of tamoxifen withdrawal responses are relatively rare[70,73,74] and often represent individual case histories.[75-77] The underlying incidence of these withdrawal responses could be underestimated, because many patients would receive alternate treatments immediately on evidence of disease progression. This issue will remain controversial until sufficient clinical trials are conducted to specifically address the actual frequency of withdrawal responses to tamoxifen.

ENDOCRINE-UNRESPONSIVE XENOGRAFTS

The majority of human breast tumor xenografts are ER-negative and therefore are estrogen-unresponsive. These xenografts also tend to be more locally aggressive and exhibit a significantly increased metastatic potential. Two estrogen-unresponsive xenograft models (MDA−MB-231, MDA−MB-435) are capable of producing distant metastases in an apparently reproducible manner and with a sufficient incidence to be of use in the study of spontaneous metastasis.[68] The MDA−MB-435 model is sensitive to dietary manipulations.[78,79] My colleagues and I isolated an ascites variant of these cells (MDA435/LCC6) that is sensitive to a variety of cytotoxic drugs with proved efficacy in the human disease.[80] Most endocrine-unresponsive xenografts produce poorly differentiated tumors.

IMMUNODEFICIENT MOUSE MODELS

Mice homozygous for the nude (*nu*) mutation are athymic,[81] and they exhibit a defect in thymic-dependent B-cell maturation but possess apparently normal virgin B cells.[82] Primary responses to T-dependent antigens are low,[83] and they may be reversed by reconstitution of the mice with T cells.[84-86] Serum IgM levels are similar to those of their heterozygote littermates.[87] The number of cells making IgG and IgA is significantly decreased, however.[85] Despite their ability to maintain human tumor xenografts, nude mice retain considerable immunity. For example, these mice possess substantially *greater* numbers of NK cells than comparable heterozygotes, and this may contribute to the relatively low incidence of metastases from human tumor xenografts.[88,89] Nude mice possess a relatively normal primary response to T-cell−independent antigens,[87] and their splenocytes generate LAK cells at levels similar to those observed in normal mice.[90] The levels of macrophages are equivalent in *nu/nu* and *nu/+* mice and frequently exhibit tumoricidal properties.[91]

The severe combined immunodeficiency (*scid*) mutation is one of the few single mutations that produces viable severely immunodeficient mice. The *scid* mutation produces a deficiency in the rearrangement of genes coding for antigen-specific receptors on B and T cells.[92] Pre-B and B cells are absent, and remaining T cells are nonfunctional. Myeloid lineage cells appear normal, however.[93,94] Homozygotes generally have no detectable levels of IgGs 2a, 2b, and 3a[41] and IgA.[95] Some individual animals produce detectable levels of two or more IgG isotypes or IgM.[95] NK cells, macrophages,[96] and LAK activity are comparable to those in normal mice.[90]

Several immunodeficiency mutations have been combined to produce severely immunodeficient animals. The most widely used are mice bearing the combined *bg/nu/xid* mutations (eg, NIH III strain).[97] The *bg* mutation produces a significant block in NK function.[98,99] This is in marked contrast to the increased NK activity observed in mice homozygous for the *nu* mutation.[88,89] The *bg* mutation also produces functional defects in T cells, macrophages, and granulocytes.[41] The *xid* mutation in males (*xid*/Y) and homozygous females produces mice that cannot generate a humoral response to thymus-independent type II antigens.[41,100] In the *bg/nu/xid* combination, the *nu* mutation produces mice that are deficient in mature T cells, the *xid* mutation produces a deficiency in mature B cells,[101,102] and the *bg* mutation reduces the elevated NK activity conferred by the *nu* mutation.[98,99] Some NK activity remains detectable, however.[60,97] The *bg/nu/xid* strain is deficient in B-cell and T-cell activities and cannot produce detectable LAK activity.[97] Mice homozygous for *bg* also exhibit a clotting deficiency because of a platelet disorder. This latter characteristic can be problematic in *bg/nu/xid* mice if the experimental design requires survival surgery (eg, ovariectomy).

ENDOCRINE EFFECTS ON IMMUNE FUNCTION

Endocrine treatments are known to modulate immune function both in immunodeficient mice and in humans. ERs have been demonstrated on peripheral blood mononuclear cells and on splenic, thymus,[103] and CD8+ T cells.[104,105] Estrogens may alter B-cell function and increase IgM secretion.[106] Inhibition of T-suppressor function and T-helper maturation also have been reported.[107,108] Physiologic concentrations of estrogen stimulate pokeweed mitogen−induced Ig synthesis of B lymphocytes.[107,109] Pharmacologic administration of the progestin medroxyprogesterone acetate results in a reduced T4 + :T8 + ratio, perhaps as a result of its glucocorticoid activity.[110] The progestogen lynestrenol has been reported to stimulate active T-cell rosetting and phagocytosis by monocytes.[111]

The number of macrophages does not appear to be significantly modulated by E2 in nude mice;[112] several reports of altered NK cell activity exist. Thus, pharmacologic, but not physiologic, concentrations of E2 inhibit NK activity in athymic nude mice.[112–115] The effect of pharmacologic concentrations of E2 is biphasic: a stimulation of NK activity occurs within the first 30 days, inhibition being observed thereafter.[113] The delay in detecting an E2-induced suppression of NK activity is widely reported.[112–115] E2-induced effects on NK activity are unlikely to be responsible for E2's effects on breast tumor cell growth in vivo. The majority of breast tumor xenografts produce readily palpable tumors within 10 to 14 days, during which time the already high NK activity in nude mice is further elevated.[113] Furthermore, the concentrations of estrogens reported to suppress NK activity appear to exceed, by 10-fold or greater, the physiologic concentrations used to stimulate MCF-7 hormone–dependent breast tumor growth in nude mice.[42,46,116–118]

Tamoxifen stimulates NK activity both in vitro[119] and in vivo.[60] Other antiestrogens can increase pokeweed mitogen–induced Ig synthesis of B lymphocytes.[120] The aromatase inhibitor aminogluthemide reduces serum estrogens and increases NK activity in breast cancer patients.[121] Clearly, significant interactions exist between endocrine agents and effectors of cell-mediated immunity. The isolation of breast cancer cell variants with differing responsivities to both hormonal manipulations and immune response effectors will greatly improve our ability to determine the nature of these interactions and the way in which they may be manipulated to therapeutic advantage.

The ability of endocrine agents to perturb several effectors of cell-mediated immunity requires careful consideration for study design. For example, the ultimate reduction in NK activity by estrogens (at 30 or more days) depends on the dose of estrogen used and the length of the analysis. For example, long term in vivo experiments of more than 6 weeks' duration that use pharmacologic doses of estrogens could be influenced by perturbations in immunologic function. Although little direct evidence exists to the contrary, the relatively low estrogen levels (around 300 pg/mL estradiol)[122] released from the widely used 60-day release 0.72-mg estrogen pellets (Innovative Research of America, Toledo, OH) are probably insufficient to suppress NK activity to a level that would markedly influence tumorigenicity data.

Transgenic Mouse Models

Transgenic mice provide a powerful means to investigate the function of overexpression of a gene in vivo. Basically, the gene is inserted into a fertilized embryo that is then transplanted into an appropriate female. Reproductively viable homozygotes or heterozygotes can be mated to maintain the transgenic stock. This approach has several advantages and disadvantages. For models in which the transgene is expressed by a constitutive and nontissue-specific promoter, the gene is potentially expressed in every cell in the animal. For secreted factors (eg, some growth factors), it may become difficult to distinguish among endocrine, paracrine, and autocrine effects. The level of expression produced in transgenic mice can greatly exceed that observed in normal and malignant tissues.

Because all cells potentially express the gene, tumors can be multifocal or polyclonal. Polyclonality is rare in human breast tumors.[64] Expression can depend on the promoter construct used, with various tissues expressing different levels of the transgene. Mouse strain differences also may account for some of the apparently conflicting observations among groups generating transgenic mice with comparable transgene constructs. Several laboratories have attempted to use tissue-specific promoters, to restrict overexpression to the appropriate target tissue. For the mammary gland, this has generally involved use of the MMTV LTR (which is not totally specific for mammary gland),[123] or the whey acidic protein promoter that is expressed exclusively during lactation.[124]

The concept of these models relies to some extent on the ability of a single gene to produce a fully neoplastic phenotype that would include initiation, promotion, and progression events. It is not clear that cancer is a single gene–single hit phenomenon in humans. Thus, these models perhaps more accurately indicate what overexpression of a single specific gene *can* do, rather than what this gene *does* do in normal and malignant tissues. Despite the potential limitations inherent in transgenic mouse models, the ability to express an oncogene in the glandular or stromal tissues of otherwise normal breast tissues provides a unique and powerful technique to address the transforming potential of individual genes. In the next few years, it seems likely that more transgenic mouse models of breast cancer will be generated. How well these models will reflect the known biology of the human disease remains to be seen.

TGF-α TRANSGENIC MICE

The ability of a transgenic TGF-α to generate mammary tumors is less clear than for other genes. In one study, using the heavy metal–inducible metallothionine promoter, aberrant mammary gland development was observed, but no incidence of mammary adenocarcinomas was reported.[125] Another study, using a similar promoter construct, observed epithelial hyperplasia and breast carcinomas.[126] MMTV–TGF-α transgenic mice produce alveolar and terminal duct hyperplasia and have clear evidence of neoplasia.[127] The mammary adenocarcinomas generally occur with a long latency (longer than 6 months). TGF-α transgenic mice also exhibit increased serum E2 levels, reduced splenic NK cell activity,[128] and several behavioral modifications.[129,130]

c-erbB-2 TRANSGENIC MICE

The ability of MMTV–c-erbB-2 transgenic mice to generate a reproducible incidence of mammary tumors also is unclear. There have been two apparently conflicting studies. A high incidence of polyclonal mammary tumors arose with a short latency in one study.[131] In the other, monoclonal mammary adenocarcinomas arose with a longer latency (more than 5 months).[132] Despite these differences, it has been suggested that the ability of c-erbB-2 transgenic mice to develop mammary tumors is supportive of a major role for this oncogene in mammary tumorigenesis.[133]

v-Ha-ras TRANSGENIC MICE

Because v-Ha-ras expression is associated with chemically induced mammary tumors, it is not surprising that several groups have generated transgenic mice with this gene. Transgenic mice generated with a MMTV long terminal repeat construct generally develop a high incidence of mammary adenocarcinomas,[123,134] often arising as early as 1 month of age.[134] Use of the whey acidic protein promoter is less effective in inducing mammary carcinomas,[124] perhaps reflecting a lower capacity for inducing high levels of gene expression.[133]

c-myc TRANSGENIC MICE

MMTV-myc transgenic mice produce stochastic, well-differentiated mammary adenocarcinomas.[134] Whey acidic protein promoter−c-myc transgenic mice produce a higher incidence of histologically similar tumors, when compared with MMTV−c-myc mice.[134,135] Mating myc and ras transgenic mice can produce animals heterozygous for both transgenes.[135] Double transgenic animals do not, however, exhibit an altered incidence or latency of tumor appearance relative to the myc-alone transgenic mice.[135]

Future Directions

Many models for the study of breast cancer are available to the interested investigator. Each has its own advantages and disadvantages, and these should be clearly weighed and evaluated before their use. Because none of the models accurately reflects every aspect of the human disease, some studies may require the use of more than one model.

A need for more models exists in two areas. Currently, relatively few human xenograft models are ER-positive and E2-dependent. Because this represents an early phenotype, the ability to study malignant progression is restricted. Moreover, few reproducible metastatic models of breast cancer exist, particularly ER-positive and E2-dependent. The MDA−MB-231 and MDA−MB-435 xenografts are ER-negative,[136] and the MCF-7/FGF-4 transfectants are E2-inhibited and tamoxifen-stimulated.[137]

Although relatively new in terms of their use in breast cancer research, the polyoma and adenovirus models may provide us with new and important models for breast cancer research. Their further evaluation as models, and their similarities to and differences from the human disease should be clearly defined. If appropriate, they also could become an important component of our collection of animal models of breast cancer.

ACKNOWLEDGMENT

This work was funded in part by US Public Health Service grants R01-CA58022, 1P30-CA51008 and U01-CA51908.

References

1. Nerurkar VR, Chitale AR, Jalnapurkar BV, et al. Comparative pathology of canine mammary tumours. J Comp Pathol 1989;101:389.
2. Bartnitzke S, Motzko H, Caselitz J, et al. A recurrent marker chromosome involving chromosome 1 in two mammary tumors of the dog. Cytogenet Cell Genet 1992;60:135.
3. Kritchevesky D, Weber MM, Klurfeld DM. Dietary fat versus caloric intake in initiation and promotion of 7,12-dimethylbenz-(a)anthracene-induced mammary tumorigenesis in rats. Cancer Res 1984;44:3174.
4. Welsch CW. Enhancement of mammary tumorigenesis by dietary fat: review of potential mechanisms. Am J Clin Nutr 1987;45:192.
5. Engelman RW, Day NK, Chen R-F, et al. Calorie consumption level influences development of C3H/Ou breast adenocarcinoma with indifference to calorie source. Proc Soc Exp Biol Med 1990;193:23.
6. Siemann DW. Kallmann RF, ed. Rodent tumor models in experimental cancer therapy. New York, Pergamon, 1987:12.
7. Russo J, Gusterson BA, Rogers AE, et al. Biology of disease: comparative study of human and rat mammary tumorigenesis. Lab Invest 1990;62:244.
8. Sukumar S, Notario V, Martin-Zanca D, et al. Induction of mammary carcinomas in rats by nitroso-methylurea involves malignant activation of Ha-ras-1 locus by single point mutations. Nature 1983;306:658.
9. Gould MN. Inheritance and site of expression of genes controlling susceptibility to mammary cancer in an inbred rat model. Cancer Res 1986;46:1995.
10. Rivera EM, Vijayaraghavan S. Proliferation of ductal outgrowths by carcinogen-induced rat mammary tumors in gland-free mammary fat pads. J Natl Cancer Inst 1982;69:517.
11. Gould MN, Zhang R. Genetic regulation of mammary carcinogenesis in the rat by susceptibility and suppressor genes. Environ Health Perspect 1991;93:161.
12. Raynaud A. Observations sur les modifications provoquees pas les hormones oestrogenes, du mode de developpement des mamelons des foetus de souris. C R Acad Sci 1955;240:674.
13. Huggins C, Grand LC, Brillantes FP. Mammary cancer induced by a single feeding of polynuclear hyrocarbons, and its suppression. Nature 1961;189:204.
14. Chan PC, Cohen LA. Effect of dietary fat, antiestrogen and antiprolactin on the development of mammary tumors in rats. J Natl Cancer Inst 1974;52:25.
15. Ip C, Ip MM. Serum estrogens and estrogen responsiveness in 7,12-dimethylbenz(a) anthracene-induced mammary tumors as influenced by dietary fat. J Natl Cancer Inst 1981;66:291.
16. Zwiebel JA, Bano M, Nexo E, et al. Partial purification of transforming growth factors from human milk. Cancer Res 1986;46:933.
17. Lacroix A, Doskas C, Bhat PV. Inhibition of growth of established N-methyl-N-nitrosourea-induced mammary cancer in rats by retinoic acid and ovariectomy. Cancer Res 1990;50:5731.
18. Chan PC, Head JF, Cohen LA, et al. Influence of dietary fat on the induction of mammary tumors by nitrosomethylurea: associated

hormone changes and differences between Sprague-Dawley and F344 rats. J Natl Cancer Inst 1977;59:1279.

19. Dao TL, Chan PC. Effect of duration of high fat intake on enhancement of mammary carcinogenesis in rats. J Natl Cancer Inst 1983;71:201.

20. Ip C, Carter CA, Ip MM. Requirement of essential fatty acid for mammary tumorigenesis in the rat. Cancer Res 1985;45:1997.

21. Jurkowski JJ, Cave WT. Dietary effects of menhaden oil on the growth and membrane lipid composition of rat mammary tumors. J Natl Cancer Inst 1985;74:1145.

22. Briand P. Hormone-dependent mammary tumors in mice and rats as a model for human breast cancer. Anticancer Res 1983;3:273.

23. Manni A, Rainieri J, Arafah BM, et al. Role of estrogen and prolactin in the growth and receptor levels of N-nitrosomethyl-urea-induced rat mammary tumors. Cancer Res 1982;42:3492.

24. L'Hermite M, L'Hermite-Baleriaux M. Prolactin and breast cancer. Eur J Cancer Clin Oncol 1988;24:955.

25. Gullino PM, Pettigrew HM, Grantham FH. N-nitrosomethylurea as a mammary gland carcinogen in rats. J Natl Cancer Inst 1975;54:401.

26. Gottardis MM, Jordan CV. Antitumor actions of keoxifene and tamoxifen in the N-nitrosomethylurea-induced rat mammary carcinoma model. Cancer Res 1987;47:4020.

27. Zarbl H, Sukumar S, Arthur AV, et al. Direct mutagenesis of H-ras-1 oncogenes by N-nitroso-N-methylurea during initiation of mammary carcinogenesis in rats. Nature 1985;315:382.

28. Bos JL. ras oncogenes in human cancer: a review. Cancer Res 1989;49:4682.

29. Rochlitz CF, Scott GK, Dodson JM, et al. Incidence of activating ras oncogene mutations associated with primary and metastatic human breast cancer. Cancer Res 1989;49:357.

30. Welsch CW, Gribler C. Prophylaxis of spontaneously developing mammary carcinoma in C3H/HeJ female mice by prolactin. Cancer Res 1973;33:2939.

31. Osborne MP, Telang NT, Kaur S, et al. Influence of chemopreventive agents on estradiol metabolism and mammary preneoplasia in the C3H mouse. Steroids 1990;55:114.

32. Nusse R. Insertional mutagenesis in mouse mammary tumorigenesis. Curr Top Microbiol Immunobiol 1991;171:43.

33. Theillet C, Le Roy X, De Lapeyriere O, et al. Amplification of FGF-related genes in human tumors: possible involvement of HST in breast carcinomas. Oncogene 1989;4:915.

34. Lidereau R, Callaghan R, Dickson C, et al. Amplification of the int-2 proto-oncogene in DNA from primary breast carcinomas. Oncogene Res 1988;2:285.

35. Zhou DJ, Casey G, Cline MJ. Amplification of human int-2 in breast cancers and squamous carcinomas. Oncogene 1988;2:279.

36. Callahan R. Mammary tumor virus in rodent tumors. Breast Cancer Res Treat 1995 (in press).

37. Haslam SZ, Wirth JJ, Counterman LJ, et al. Characterization of the mammary hyperplasia, dysplasia and neoplasia induced in athymic female adult mice by polyomavirus. Oncogene 1992;7:1295.

38. Fluck MM, Haslam SZ. Mammary tumors induced by polyoma virus. Breast Cancer Res Treat 1995 (in press).

39. Javier R, Raska K, MacDonald GJ, et al. Human adenovirus type 9-induced rat mammary tumors. J Virol 1991;65:3192.

40. Javier R, Shenk T. Mammary tumors induced by adenovirus type-9. Breast Cancer Res Treat 1995 (in press).

41. Shultz LD. Single gene models of immunodeficiency diseases. In: Wu B, Zheng J (eds). Immune-deficient animals in experimental medicine. Basel, Karger, 1989:19.

42. Clarke R, Brünner N, Katzenellenbogen BS, et al. Progression from hormone dependent to hormone independent growth in MCF-7 human breast cancer cells. Proc Natl Acad Sci USA 1989;86:3649.

43. Brünner N, Frandsen TL, Holst-Hansen C, et al: MCF7/LCC2: A 4-hydroxytamoxifen resistant human breast cancer variant which retains sensitivity to the steroidal antiestrogen ICI 182,780. Cancer Res 1993;53:3229.

44. Katzenellenbogen BS, Kendra KL, Norman MJ, et al. Proliferation, hormonal responsiveness, and estrogen receptor content of MCF-7 human breast cancer cells grown in the short-term and long-term absence of estrogens. Cancer Res 1987;47:4355.

45. Fodstad Ø. Limitations for studies in human tumor biology. In: Boven E, Winograd B, eds. The nude mouse in oncology research. Boca Raton, CRC, 1991:277.

46. Seibert K, Shafie SM, Triche TJ, et al. Clonal variation of MCF-7 breast cancer cells in vitro and in athymic nude mice. Cancer Res 1983;43:2223.

47. van Steenbrugge GJ, Groen M, van Kreuningen A, et al: Transplantable human prostatic carcinoma (PC-82) in athymic nude mice. III. Effects of estrogens on the growth of the tumor. Prostate 1988;12:157.

48. Brünner N, Svenstrup B, Spang-Thompsen M, et al: Serum steroid levels in intact and endocrine ablated Balb/c nude mice and their intact litter mates. J Steroid Biochem 1986;25:429.

49. Clarke R, Leonessa F, Brünner N, et al. In vitro models of human breast cancer. In: Harris JR, Lippman ME, Morrow M, et al. Diseases of the breast. Philadelphia, Lippincott-Raven, 1995;245.

50. Meyvisch C: Influence of implantation site on formation of metastases. Cancer Metastasis Rev 1983;2:295.

51. Morikawa K, Walker SM, Nakajima M, et al. Influence of organ environment on the growth, selection, and metastasis of human colon carcinoma cells in nude mice. Cancer Res 1988;48:6863.

52. Volpe JPG, Milas L. Influence of tumor transplantation methods on tumor growth rate and metastatic potential of solitary tumors derived from metastases. Clin Exp Metastasis 1990;8:381.

53. Kozlowski JM, Fidler IJ, Campbell D, et al. Metastatic behavior of human tumor cell lines grown in the nude mouse. Cancer Res 1984;44:3522.

54. Clarke R, Thompson EW, Leonessa F, et al. Hormone resistance, invasiveness, and metastatic potential in human breast cancer. Breast Cancer Res Treat 1993;24:227.

55. Thompson EW, Brünner N, Torri J, et al. The invasive and metastatic properties of hormone-independent and hormone-responsive variants of MCF-7 human breast cancer cells. Clin Exp Metastasis 1993;11:15.

56. Osborne CK, Coronado EB, Robinson JP. Human breast cancer in athymic nude mice: cytostatic effects of long-term antiestrogen therapy. Eur J Cancer Clin Oncol 1987;23:1189.

57. Gottardis MM, Jordan VC. Development of tamoxifen-stimulated growth of MCF-7 tumors in athymic mice after long-term antiestrogen administration. Cancer Res 1988;48:5183.

58. Gottardis MM, Robinson SP, Satyaswaroop PG, et al. Contrasting actions of tamoxifen on endometrial and breast tumor growth in the athymic nude mouse. Cancer Res 1988;48:812.

59. Brunner N, Bronzert D, Vindelov LL, et al. Effect of growth and cell cycle kinetics of estradiol and tamoxifen on MCF-7 human breast cancer cells grown in vitro in nude mice. Cancer Res 1989;49:1515.

60. Gottardis MM, Wagner RJ, Borden EC, et al. Differential ability of antiestrogens to stimulate breast cancer cell (MCF-7) growth in vivo and in vitro. Cancer Res 1989;49:4765.

61. Brünner N, Boulay V, Fojo A, et al. Acquisition of hormone-independent growth in MCF-7 cells is accompanied by increased expression of estrogen-regulated genes but without detectable DNA amplifications. Cancer Res 1993;53:283.

62. Clarke R, Dickson RB, Brünner N. The process of malignant progression in human breast cancer. Ann Oncol 1990;1:401.

63. Leonessa F, Boulay V, Wright A, et al. The biology of breast tumor progression: acquisition of hormone-independence and resistance to cytotoxic drugs. Acta Oncol 1991;31:115.

64. Clarke R, Skaar T, Baumann K, et al. Hormonal carcinogenesis in breast cancer: cellular and molecular studies of malignant progression. Breast Cancer Res Treat 1994;31:237.

65. Coopman P, Garcia M, Brünner N, et al: Antiproliferative and antiestrogenic effects of ICI 164,384 in 4-OH-tamoxifen−resistant human breast cancer cells. Int J Cancer 1994;56:295.

66. Nicholson RI, Gee JMW, Anderson E, et al. Phase I study of a new pure antiestrogen ICI 182,780 in women with primary breast cancer: immunohistochemical analysis. Breast Cancer Res Treat 1993;27:135.

67. McLeskey SW, Honig S, Lippman ME, et al. MCF-7 cells transfected with an expression vector for fibroblast growth factor 4 exhibit opposite responses to tamoxifen in vivo and in vitro. Proc Am Assoc Cancer Res 1992;33:269.

68. Price JE, Polyzos A, Zhang RD, et al. Tumorigenicity and metastasis of human breast carcinoma cell lines in nude mice. Cancer Res 1990;50:717.

69. Jiang S-Y, Jordan VC. Growth regulation of estrogen receptor negative breast cancer cells transfected with estrogen receptor cDNAs. J Natl Cancer Inst 1992;84:580.

70. Gockerman JP, Spremulli EN, Raney M, et al. Randomized comparison of tamoxifen versus diethylstilbestrol in estrogen receptor-positive or -unknown metastatic breast cancer: a southeastern cancer study group trial. Cancer Treat Rep 1986;70:1199.

71. Kennedy BJ. Hormonal therapies in breast cancer. Semin Oncol 1974;1:119.

72. Litherland S, Jackson IM. Antioestrogens in the management of hormone-dependent cancer. Cancer Treat Rev 1988;15:183.

73. Vogel CL, East DR, Voigt W, et al. Response to tamoxifen in estrogen receptor-poor metastatic breast cancer. Cancer 1987;60:1184.

74. Howell A, Dodwell DJ, Anderson H, et al. Response after withdrawal of tamoxifen and progestogens in advanced breast cancer. Ann Oncol 1992;3:611.

75. Belani CP, Pearl P, Whitley NO, et al. Tamoxifen withdrawal response: report of a case. Arch Intern Med 1989;149:449.

76. Stein W, Hortobagyi GN, Blumenschein GR. Response of metastatic breast cancer to tamoxifen withdrawal: report of a case. J Surg Oncol 1983;22:45.

77. McIntosh IH, Thynne GS. Tumour stimulation by anti-oestrogens. Br J Surg 1977;64:900.

78. Meschter CL, Connolly JM, Rose DP. Influence of regional location of the inoculation site and dietary fat on the pathology of MDA-MB-435 human breast cancer cell-derived tumors growing in nude mice. Clin Exp Metastasis 1992;10:167.

79. Rose DP, Hatala MA, Connolly JM, et al. Effect of diets containing different levels of linoleic acid on human breast cancer growth and lung metastasis in nude mice. Cancer Res 1993;53:4686.

80. Wright A, Green D, Clarke R. An ascites model of human breast cancer (MDA435/LCC6): a potential new in vivo model for drug screening. Proc Am Assoc Cancer Res 1992;33:490.

81. Plantouris EM. Absence of thymus in a mutant mouse. Nature 1968;217:370.

82. Weisz P, Schrater AF, Lamm ME, et al. Immunoglobulin isotypes in plasma cells of normal and athymic mice. Cell Immunol 1979;44:343.

83. Kindred B. The inception of the response to SRBC by nude mice injected with various doses of congenic or allogeneic thymus cells. Cell Immunol 1975;17:277.

84. Jacobson EB, Caporale LH, Thorbecke GJ. Effect of thymus cell injections on germinal center formation in lymphoid tissues of nude (thymusless) mice. Cell Immunol 1974;13:416.

85. Guy-Grand D, Griscelli C, Vassalli P. Peyer's patches, gut IgA, plasma cells and thymic function: study in nude mice bearing thymic grafts. J Immunol 1975;115:361.

86. De Sousa M, Pritchard H. The cellular basis of immunological recovery in nude mice after thymus grafting. Immunology 1974;26:769.

87. Manning JK, Reed ND, Jutila JW. Antibody response to escherichia coli lipopolysaccharide by congenitally thymusless (nude) mice. J Immunol 1972;108:1470.

88. Herberman RB, Nunn ME, Holden HT, et al. Augmentation of natural cytotoxic reactivity of mouse lymphoid cells against syngeneic and allogenic tumors. Int J Cancer 1977;19:555.

89. Kiessling R, Klein E, Wagzell H. "Natural" killer cells in the mouse. I. Cytotoxic cells with specificity for mouse Moloney leukemia cells: specificity and distribution according to phenotype. Eur J Immunol 1975;72:2130.

90. Hasui M, Saikawa Y, Miura M, et al. Effector and precursor phenotypes of lymphokine-activated killer cells in mice with severe combined immunodeficiency (Scid) and athymic (Nude) mice. Cell Immunol 1989;120:230.

91. Johnson WJ, Balish E. Macrophage function in germ-free, athymic (nu/nu) mice and conventional flora (nu/+) mice. J Reticuloendo Soc 1980;28:55.

92. Schuler W, Weiler IJ, Schuler A, et al. Rearrangement of antigen receptor genes is defective in mice with severe combined immune deficiency. Cell 1986;46:963.

93. Dorshkind K, Keller GM, Phillips RA, et al. Functional status of cells from lymphoid and myeloid tissues in mice with severe combined immunodeficiency disease. J Immunol 1984;132:1804.

94. Custer RP, Bosma GC, Bosma MJ. Severe combined immunodeficiency (scid) in the mouse: pathology, reconstitution, neoplasms. Am J Pathol 1985;120:464.

95. Bosma GC, Custer RP, Bosma MJ. A severe combined immunodeficiency mutation in the mouse. Nature 1983;301:527.

96. Quimby FW: Immunodeficient rodents: a guide to their immunobiology, husbandry, and use. Washington, DC, National Academy, 1989.

97. Andriole GL, Mule JJ, Hansen CT, et al. Evidence that lymphokine-activated killer cells and natural killer cells are distinct based on an analysis of congenitally immunodeficient mice. J Immunol 1985;135:2911.

98. Roder JC. The beige mutation in the mouse. I. A stem cell predetermined impairment in natural killer cell function. J Immunol 1979;123:2168.

99. Roder JC, Duwe AK. The beige mutation in the mouse selectively impairs natural killer cell function. Nature 1979;278:451.

100. Ahmed A, Scher I, Sharrow SO, et al. B-lymphocyte heterogeneity: development and characterization of an alloantiserum which distinguishes B-lymphocyte differentiation alloantigens. J Exp Med 1977;145:101.

101. Azar HA, Hansen CT, Costa J. N:NIH(S)II-nu/nu mice with combined immunodeficiency: a new model for human tumor heterotransplantation. J Natl Cancer Inst 1980;65:421.

102. Karagogeos D, Rosenberg N, Wortis HH. Early arrest of B cell development in nude, X-linked immune-deficient mice. Eur J Immunol 1986;16:1125.

103. Danel L, Souweine G, Monier JC, et al. Specific estrogen binding sites in human lymphoid cells and thymic cells. J Steroid Biochem 1983;18:559.

104. Cohen JHM, Danel L, Gordier G, et al. Sex steroid receptors in peripheral T cells: absence of androgen receptors and restriction of estrogen receptors to OKT 8 positive cells. J Immunol 1983;131:2767.

105. Stimson WH. Oestrogen and human T cell lymphocytes: presence of specific receptors n the T-suppressor/cytotoxic subset. Scand J Immunol 1980;28:345.

106. Myers MJ, Peterson BH. Estradiol induced alterations in the immune system. I. Enhancement of IgM production. Int J Immunopharmacol 1985;7:207.

107. Paavonen T, Andersson LC, Adlercreutz H. Sex hormone regu-

lation of in vitro immune response: estradiol enhances human B cell maturation via inhibition of suppressor T cells in pokeweed mitogen stimulated cultures. J Exp Med 1981;154: 1935.

108. Ahmed AS, Dauphinee MJ, Talal N. Effects of short term administration of sex hormones on normal and autoimmune mice. J Immunol 1985;134:204.

109. Sthoeger ZM, Chiorazzi N, Lahita RG. Regulation of the immune response by sex steroids. I. In vitro effects of estradiol and testosterone on pokeweed mitogen-induced human B cell differentiation. J Immunol 1988;141:91.

110. Scambia G, Panci PB, Maccio A, et al. Effects of antiestrogen and progestin on immune functions in breast cancer patients. Cancer 1988;61:2214.

111. Wyban J, Govaerts A, van Dam D, et al. Stimulating properties of lynestrenol on normal human blood T-lymphocytes and other leucocytes. Int J Immunopharmacol 1979;1:151.

112. Seaman WE, Talal N. The effect of 17β-estradiol on natural killing in the mouse. In: Herberman RB, ed. Natural cell-mediated immunity against tumors. New York, Academic, 1980:765.

113. Screpanti I, Santoni A, Gulino A, et al. Estrogen and antiestrogen modulation of mouse natural killer activity and large granular lymphocytes. Cell Immunol 1987;106:191.

114. Seaman WE, Blackman MA, Gindhart TD, et al. β-estradiol reduces natural killer cells in mice. J Immunol 1978;121:2193.

115. Hanna N, Schneider M. Enhancement of tumor metastases and suppression of natural killer cell activity by β-estradiol treatment. J Immunol 1983;130:974.

116. Shafie SM, Grantham FH. Role of hormones in the growth and regression of human breast cancer cells (MCF-7) transplanted into athymic nude mice. J Natl Cancer Inst 1981;67:51.

117. Welsch CW, Swim EL, McManus MJ, et al. Estrogen-induced growth of human breast cancer cells (MCF-7) in athymic nude mice is enhanced by secretions from transplantable pituitary tumor. Cancer Lett 1981;14:309.

118. Clarke R, Brünner N, Thompson EW, et al. The inter-relationships between ovarian-independent growth, antiestrogen resistance and invasiveness in the malignant progression of human breast cancer. J Endocrinol 1989;122:331.

119. Mandeville R, Ghali SS, Chausseau JP. In vitro stimulation of NK activity by an estrogen antagonist (Tamoxifen). Eur J Cancer Clin Oncol 1984;20:983.

120. Paavonen T, Andersson LC. The oestrogen antagonists tamoxifen, FC-1157a display oestrogen like effects on human lymphocyte functions in vitro. Clin Exp Immunol 1985;61:467.

121. Berry J, Green BJ, Matheson DS. Modulation of natural killer cell activity in stage I postmenopausal breast cancer patients on low-dose aminogluthemide. Cancer Immunol Immunother 1987; 24:72.

122. Blumenthal RD, Jordan JJ, McLaughlin WH, et al. Animal modeling of human breast tumors: limitations in the use of estrogen pellet implants. Breast Cancer Res Treat 1988;11:77.

123. Trembley PJ, Pothier F, Hoang T, et al. Transgenic mice carrying the mouse mammary tumor virus fusion gene: distinct effects in various tissues. Mol Cell Biol 1989;9:854.

124. Andres AC, Schoenberger CA, Groner B, et al. Ha-ras oncogene expression directed by a milk protein gene promoter: tissue specificity, hormonal regulation, and tumor induction in transgenic mice. Proc Natl Acad Sci USA 1987;84:1299.

125. Jhappan C, Stahle C, Harkins RN, et al. TGFα overexpression in transgenic mice induces liver neoplasia and abnormal development of the mammary gland and pancreas. Cell 1990;61:1137.

126. Sandgren EP, Luetteke NC, Palmiter RD, et al. Overexpression of TGFα in transgenic mice: induction of epithelial hyperplasia, pancreatic metaplasia, and carcinoma of the breast. Cell 1990;61:1121.

127. Matsui Y, Halter SA, Holt JT, et al. Development of mammary hyperplasia and neoplasia in MMTV-TGFα transgenic mice. Cell 1990;61:1147.

128. Hilakivi-Clarke LA, Arora PK, Sabol MB, et al. Alterations in behavior, steroid hormones and natural killer cell activity in male transgenic TGF-α mice. Brain Res 1992;588:97.

129. Hilakivi-Clarke LA, Arora PK, Clarke R, et al. Opposite behavioral alterations in male and female transgenic TGFα mice: association with tumorigenesis. Br J Cancer 1993;67:1026.

130. Hilakivi-Clarke LA, Goldberg R. Tryptophan and 5-HT uptake inhibitors reverse alterations in depressive and aggressive behaviors in male transgenic TGFα mice. Eur J Pharm 1993;237:101.

131. Muller WJ, Sinn E, Pattengale PK, et al. Single-step induction of mammary adenocarcinoma in transgenic mice bearing the activated c-neu oncogene. Cell 1988;54:105.

132. Bouchard L, Lamarre L, Tremblay PJ, et al. Stochastic appearance of mammary tumors in transgenic mice carrying the MMTV/c-neu oncogene. Cell 1989;57:931.

133. Dickson RB, Gottardis MM, Merlino GT. Molecular insights into breast cancer from transgenic mouse models. Bio Essays 1991;13:591.

134. Sinn E, Muller W, Pattengale P, et al. Co-expression of MMTV/V-Ha-ras and MMTV/c-myc genes in transgenic mice: synergistic actions of oncogenes in vivo. Cell 1987;49:465.

135. Andres AC, van der Valk MA, Schoenberger CA, et al. Ha-ras and c-myc oncogene expression interferes with morphological and functional differentiation of mammary gland epithelial cells in single and double transgenic mice. Genes Dev 1988;2:1486.

136. Price JE, Zhang RD. Studies of human breast cancer metastasis using nude mice. Cancer Metastasis Rev 1990;8:285.

137. Kurebayashi J, McLeskey SW, Johnson MD, et al. Quantitative demonstration of spontaneous metastasis by MCF-7 human breast cancer cells cotransfected with fibroblast growth factor 4 and LacZ. Cancer Res 1993;53:2178.

138. Soule HD, Vasquez J, Long A, et al. Human cell line from a pleural effusion derived from a human breast carcinoma. J Natl Cancer Inst 1973;51:1409.

139. Thompson EW, Paik S, Brünner N, et al. Association of increased basement membrane-invasiveness with absence of estrogen receptor and expression of vimentin in human breast cancer cell lines. J Cell Physiol 1992;150:534.

140. Engel LW, Young NA. Human breast carcinoma cells in continuous culture: a review. Cancer Res 1978;38:4327.

141. Brunner N, Bastert GB, Poulsen HS, et al. Characterization of the T61 human breast carcinoma established in nude mice. Eur J Cancer Clin Oncol 1985;21:833.

142. Brunner N, Spang-Thomsen M, Vindelov L, et al. Effect of tamoxifen on the receptor-positive T61 and the receptor negative T60 human breast carcinomas grown in nude mice. Eur J Cancer Clin Oncol 1985;21:1349.

143. Vickers PJ, Dickson RB, Shoemaker R, et al. A multidrug-resistant MCF-7 human breast cancer cell line which exhibits cross-resistance to antiestrogens and hormone independent tumor growth. Mol Endocrinol 1988;2:886.

7.8

In Vitro Models of Breast Cancer

Robert Clarke ▪ Fabio Leonessa ▪ Nils Brünner ▪ Erik W. Thompson

Breast cancer cells that grow in vitro represent one of the most widely used experimental models of breast cancer. For many studies, these models provide the only means to address a specific hypothesis. Most breast cancer cell lines can easily be maintained and studied in vitro and are generally stable with respect to their endocrine responsiveness in vitro and in vivo. Our current understanding of the way in which breast cancer cells respond to estrogenic stimuli is, in no small part, the direct result of in vitro studies with human breast cancer cell lines.

Breast cancer cell lines are generally considered in terms of their estrogen receptor (ER) content, that is, ER-positive (ER+) or ER-negative (ER−). This largely reflects the clinical value of steroid hormone expression in predicting response to endocrine therapy. In addition, however, other characteristics of human breast tumors that tend to follow ER status are frequently exhibited in a similar pattern by cell lines growing in vitro and in vivo.[1]

A detailed and inclusive review of all breast cancer cell lines, their origin, their characteristics, and their uses is beyond the scope of this discussion. Consequently, we focus on the most widely used cell lines, some of their variants, and those models that express characteristics that closely reflect many of the properties of breast tumors in patients. We also include a brief description of cell lines with more unique properties or those cell lines best suited to specific studies, such as endocrine regulation, expression of growth factors, and oncogenes. The parental cell lines are readily available (eg, several are available through the American Type Culture Collection, Rockville, Maryland), and the variants can generally be obtained from their respective originators. For a more detailed description of the characteristics of several of these cell lines, the reader is referred to a review by Engel and Young.[2] Although this review is over 15 years old, it provides valuable information on the origin and characteristics of 22 breast cancer cell lines. The inclusion of the original citations for almost all these cell lines provides a valuable reference.

Steroid-Dependent (ER+/PR−) Breast Cancer Cell Lines

Approximately 30% of all breast cancer patients respond to endocrine manipulation. The overall response rate to antiestrogens increases to 70% or more in patients whose tumors express receptors for both estrogen and progesterone.[3–5] To define the mechanism of action of endocrine therapies and to develop and screen new agents and therapies require models that exhibit an endocrine response profile comparable to that found in breast cancer patients.

In this regard, the steroid-dependent breast cancer cell lines have been most useful in studying the growth regulatory effects of estrogens, antiestrogens, progestins, and antiprogestins. These cell lines are characterized by a dependence on estrogens for growth in vitro and in vivo and sensitivity to the growth inhibitory effects of antiestrogenic and progestational drugs. In general, steroid-dependent cell lines are poorly invasive and nonmetastatic in athymic nude mice.

MCF-7

The MCF-7 cell line is the most widely used and best characterized of all the human breast cancer cell lines. The mitogenic effects of E2 in human breast cancer cells in vitro were initially defined in these cells, as were the in vitro inhibitory effects of antiestrogens.[6,7] MCF-7 cells also are growth inhibited by luteinizing hormone–releasing hormone (LHRH) analogues[8] and retinoids.[9–11] The widely reported E2 dependence for exponential growth both in vitro and in vivo has provided this cell line with a central role in the study of endocrine responsiveness and malignant progression in vitro. Much of our current understanding of the mechanism of action of estrogens and antiestrogens and their role in regulating the proliferation of hormone-dependent breast cancer cells has been derived from work performed using this cellular model. Consequently, a full and detailed discussion of all the data generated using MCF-7 cells alone is beyond the scope of this chapter.

MCF-7 cells were established from a pleural effusion arising in a postmenopausal woman with breast cancer. The patient had received both radiotherapy and endocrine therapy before the appearance of the effusion.[12] In addition to the expression of ER,[12,13] MCF-7 cells express an E2-inducible PR,[13,14] as well as cellular receptors for androgens,[13] LHRH,[8,15] glucocorticoids,[13] insulin,[16] retinoic acid receptors (RAR-α and RAR-γ),[17] and prolactin.[18] The expression and secretion of several growth factors and their receptors also have been described in detail, including the insulin-like growth factors (IGFs),[19–22] the type I and type II IGF receptors[22–24] and several IGF-binding proteins,[25–27] transforming growth factor α (TGF-α) and epidermal growth factor receptor (EGFR),[28–30] several fibroblast growth factors (FGFs),[31] FGF receptors,[32] and platelet-derived growth factor (PDGF) but not PDGF receptors.[33] The expression of many of these growth factors, or their respective receptors, is strongly E2-regulated in MCF-7 cells.[34] The expression, secretion, and regulation of this wide variety of receptors and ligands have made MCF-7 cells a valuable model for the study of the role of growth factor and growth factor receptor expression in the proliferation of breast cancer cells.

E2 dependence for growth, antiestrogen sensitivity, and low metastatic potential of MCF-7 cells have led us to hypothesize that they represent an early breast cancer phenotype.[35,36] MCF-7 cells are an excellent model in which to study the process of malignant progression, because they can be subjected to appropriate endocrinologic and physiologic selective pressures for the derivation of variants with more progressed phenotypes. For example, we used the estrogenic requirement for tumorigenicity in immunocompromised mice to select for E2-independent MCF-7 variants, as discussed later. We also selected for antiestrogen resistant variants and determined the extent of induced cross-resistance among structurally diverse antiestrogens, as discussed later.

T47D

The T47D cells were established by Keydar and associates from a 54-year-old patient with an infiltrating ductal carcinoma.[37] The cells express ER, PR, androgen, glucocorticoid,[37] and insulin receptors.[38] Approximately 60% of the original cell line expressed casein.[37,39] The T47D cells are perhaps most notable for their high levels of PR and their remarkable genetic and phenotypic instability.[40–43] Furthermore, these cells exhibit significant growth regulatory responses to progestational agents.[44,45] It is not surprising that T47D cells and several T47D variants represent the major in vitro human breast cancer models for the study of the antiproliferative effects of progestins and antiprogestins and the regulation of PR expression.[42–46] T47D cells also express RAR-α and RAR-γ,[17] and they are sensitive to the growth inhibitory effects of retinoids and antiestrogens.[9,10]

The remarkable genetic instability of the T47D cells is in contrast to the other ER+−PR+ human breast cancer cell lines. Subtle differences in the phenotypic characteristics of all the ER+−PR+ cell lines are observed from laboratory to laboratory. These differences rarely extend to the pattern of expression of steroid hormone receptors, metastatic potential, antiestrogen responsiveness, the estrogen supplementation required for in vivo tumorigenicity, or metastatic potential, however. These are the major phenotypic characteristics of hormone-responsive breast cancer cells.[34–36] When significant divergent phenotypic responses in other ER+−PR+ cell lines are observed, this is almost always the result of an imposed selective pressure, such as in vivo or in vitro growth in the absence of E2 or selection for cytotoxic drug resistance. For example, no genuinely spontaneous ER or PR negative MCF-7 or ZR-75-1 cell lines have been described in detail, other than those generated by the imposition of selective pressures. In marked contrast, simple dilution cloning can produce T47D variants with fundamentally altered endocrine responsiveness including ER−−PR+, estrogen-unresponsive and, antiestrogen-resistant variants.[40–42] Many of these variants are unstable and readily revert to the wild-type phenotype.[40,43] Other T47D variants (eg, ER−/PR+ T47D$_{CO}$) have been stable for many years, as discussed later.

ZR-75-1

The ZR-75-1 cells were first described by Engel and colleagues in 1978.[47] These cell lines were established from ascites that developed in a 63-year-old woman with infiltrating ductal breast carcinoma. This patient had been receiving tamoxifen (TAM) for 3 months before the time when cells were removed to establish the ZR-75-1 cell line.[47] Although the ZR-75-1 cells are ER+ and PR+,[47,48] and their growth is stimulated by estrogens and is inhibited by antiestrogens in vitro,[47,49] the patient did not respond to TAM.[47] The expression of ER is up-regulated by interferons in these cells, and treatment with interferon-2α can increase sensitivity to TAM.[48] ZR-75-1 cells exhibit an eightfold overexpression of c-erbB-2 mRNA relative to normal fibroblasts.[50] This overexpression is E2-regulated in ZR-75-1 cells, a down-regulation being associated with E2-induced cell proliferation.[51] Both TAM-resistant and hormone-independent ZR-75-1 variants have been described.[49,52,53]

ZR-75-1 cells also express androgen and glucocorticoid receptors,[54] and they are growth inhibited in vitro by progestins[54,55] and somatostatin analogues.[56] They express the RAR-α and RAR-γ retinoic acid isoforms,[17] and they are growth inhibited by several retinoids.[9,10] ZR-75-1 cells also express low levels of EGFR, with altered EGFR expression associated with TAM resistance and hormone independence.[52,53] The ZR-75-1 cells appear to possess several steroid metabolism pathways.[57–59]

Steroid–Independent and Steroid–Responsive Breast Cancer Cell Lines

The estrogenic requirement of the MCF-7, T47D, and ZR-75-1 cells for growth in vitro or in vivo may not adequately reflect the endocrine environment of many breast tumors in postmenopausal women. Several breast cancer cell lines and variants of the MCF-7, ZR-75-1, and T47D cell lines have been generated that no longer require estrogenic supplementation for growth. These continue to express ER or PR, and many also retain responsiveness to endocrine agents. Several steroid-independent and steroid-responsive cell lines and variants exhibit properties that more closely resemble those of breast tumors in patients than those of the steroid-dependent cell lines.

MCF-7/MIII, MCF-7/LCC1: CELLS SELECTED FOR HORMONE INDEPENDENCE IN VIVO

Several aspects of the MCF-7 phenotype could be considered potentially inconsistent with the human disease. For example, these cells generally do not proliferate in cell culture media devoid of estrogens, and they do not form proliferating tumors when orthotopically transplanted into ovariectomized immunodeficient mice. If this dependence on estrogens for growth were to exist in a tumor cell in a postmenopausal woman, from which the MCF-7 cells were obtained,[12] the cells would not give rise to detectable disease. Despite their apparent metastatic site of origin, MCF-7 cells exhibit few characteristics associated with an invasive or metastatic phenotype. Thus, we suggested that the MCF-7 phenotype represents an early hypothetic breast cancer cell.[35,36]

We wished to determine whether by applying appropriate physiologic and endocrinologic selective pressures, we could obtain cells more representative of many of the ER+−PR+ cells apparent in the breast tumors of postmenopausal women. Thus, we selected MCF-7 cells by transplantation into the mammary fat pads of ovariectomized, athymic, nude mice. After approximately 6 months, we obtained cells (MCF-7/MIII) that were readily reestablished in vitro. MCF-7/MIII cells were determined to be of MCF-7 origin by karyotype and isozyme profile analyses.[14] A further selection of MCF-7/MIII cells produced a variant designated MCF-7/LCC1, which exhibits increased metastatic potential and a shorter lag time to tumor appearance when compared with MCF-7/MIII.[60,61]

We studied these cells for their respective responses to estrogens and antiestrogens both in vitro and in vivo. Both MCF-7/MIII and MCF-7/LCC1 cells proliferate in vivo and in vitro without estrogen supplementation,[14,60] and they are responsive to drugs representing each of the major classes of antiestrogens.[60,62] MCF-7/MIII cells also are inhibited by LHRH analogues.[63] Significantly, both variants exhibit an increased metastatic potential in vivo and in vitro,[14,61] although at a much lower level than ER− cell lines.[1,64] We interpret these observations as indicating that MCF-7/MIII and MCF-7/LCC1 cells exhibit a phenotype representative of many ER+−PR+ cells present in the tumors of postmenopausal breast cancer patients. The phenotype of these cells has been reviewed in detail.[35,36,65]

MCF-7 K3: CELLS SELECTED FOR HORMONE INDEPENDENCE IN VITRO

MCF-7 cells also can be selected in vitro for their ability to proliferate in the absence of estrogenic stimulation. For example, Katzenellenbogen and associates[66] selected MCF-7 cells in cell culture media devoid of estrogens. The resultant cells (MCF-7 K3) have a phenotype that is generally similar to the MCF-7/MIII cells.[14] In our studies, these cells also formed tumors in ovariectomized nude mice, but with a longer doubling time,[14] and without an apparently increased metastatic potential (unpublished data). Other, perhaps more subtle, differences appear to exist. For example, the estrogen-induced gene pS2 is constitutively expressed in MCF-7/LCC1 cells in vitro, but it retains some estrogen-inducible expression in vivo.[60] In MCF-7 K3 cells, pS2 mRNA expression appears to be inhibited by E2.[67] Some evidence indicates that MCF-7 K3 cells may be estrogen-supersensitive,[67] and estrogen-supersensitive MCF-7 cells have been previously reported by others.[68] We have no data for the in vivo selected cells (MCF-7/MIII; MCF-7/LCC1) that would clearly suggest that they have a supersensitive phenotype. The biologic significance of the apparent differences between in vivo

(eg, MCF-7/MIII) and in vitro selected cells (eg, MCF-7 K3) remains to be established.

MCF-7 MKS: CELLS TRANSFECTED WITH FGF-4

The FGFs are potent angiogenic growth factors, and several appear to be present in or secreted by human breast cancer cells. Transfection of cells with FGF-4 produces cells (MCF-7 MKS) that are able to generate proliferating tumors in the absence of estrogenic stimulation.[69,70] Although MCF-7 cells are generally nonmetastatic, MCF-7 MKS cells produce highly vascular tumors, from which both lymphatic and lung metastases arise with a high frequency. Unlike MCF-7 cells selected for an ability to grow in a low-estrogen environment, MCF-7 MKS cells are stimulated by TAM and are inhibited by physiologic concentrations of estrogen.[69] The extent to which this endocrine-inverted phenotype reflects a specific phenotype in human disease is unclear; however, these cells exhibit an endocrine response pattern similar to that of MCF-7 cells selected for in vivo resistance to TAM, as discussed later.

STEROID-INDEPENDENT (ER±/PR±) AND STEROID-UNRESPONSIVE BREAST CANCER CELL LINES

BT 20 (Mutant ER)

The BT 20 cell line is one of the older breast cancer cell lines, established in 1958 by Lasfargues and Ozzello.[71] The cell line was obtained from a breast cancer patient with infiltrating ductal carcinoma.[71] BT 20 cells were initially described as being ER− and PR−,[72] but subsequently ER mRNA was detected.[73] More recently, these cells were shown to express a novel ER mutant with an exon 5 deletion.[74] This produces a protein that does not bind E2 and would appear ER negative by ligand binding. Because some evidence indicates that exon 5 mutant ER proteins can be transcriptionally active,[75] BT 20 cells could be considered ER+, hormone-independent, and hormone-unresponsive. These cells also express GR,[72] and they have a 16-fold elevation in the mRNA levels of EGFR expression resulting from a 4- to 8-fold amplification.[50,76] BT 20 cells are tumorigenic but nonmetastatic when grown in athymic nude mice.[77]

BT474 (ER−/PR+)

BT474 cells were obtained from a solid primary infiltrating ductal carcinoma of the breast in a 60-year-old woman.[78] The cells express PR but not ER in vitro,[78] and they significantly overexpress c-erbB-2 because of an amplification in the c-erbB-2 gene.[50] The level of c-erbB-2 mRNA expression in BT474 cells is 128-fold that of normal fibroblasts, whereas EGFR is not overexpressed.[50]

T47D_CO (ER−/PR+)

These cells are a variant of the ER+/PR+ T47D cells,[37] and they were originally described by Horwitz and colleagues.[79] The most notable feature of these cells is their loss of ER but elevated and constitutive expression of PR.[38,45,79] The cells grow in vitro without E2 supplementation and are antiestrogen resistant.[79] Although the PR in T47D$_{CO}$ cells is E2-independent, insulin-receptor expression is up-regulated by progestins, despite their growth inhibitory effects.[45] The constitutive expression of PR in the absence of ER makes this an excellent in vitro model for screening progestins and antiprogestins, because no complicating requirement for E2 supplementation exists. For example, it was initially thought that the antiproliferative effects of the progestin R5020 in T47D cells reflected an antiestrogenic effect.[44] Subsequent data obtained in T47D$_{CO}$ cells demonstrated that progestins and antiprogestins exert direct growth inhibitory effects independent of ER-mediated events.[45]

Steroid-Unresponsive (ER−/PR−) Breast Cancer Cell Lines

The majority of human breast cancer cell lines are ER negative. Like ER+ cell lines, they exhibit characteristics that tend to reflect the nature of ER− tumors in breast cancer patients. For example, ER− tumors are generally faster growing,[80] more aggressive, and associated with a poorer prognosis,[81–83] and the ER− cell lines tend to produce rapidly growing tumors in nude mice; several of these tumors are highly invasive, and some can produce distant metastases.[1,64] None of these cell lines respond to the antiproliferative effects of estrogens and antiestrogens unless exposed to suprapharmacologic doses. The absence of response to steroids does not preclude responses to other noncytotoxic agents, however. Several ER− cell lines express retinoic acid receptors,[17] and they are growth inhibited by retinoids.[11,84]

MDA−MB-231 AND MDA−MB-435

The MDA−MB-231 cell line is among the most widely used ER− human breast cancer cell lines and is frequently used as a negative control in many laboratories studying the endocrine regulation of breast cancer cell growth. The MDA−MB-231 cells were established from a 51-year-old woman with breast cancer who developed a pleural effusion. The patient had received prior endocrine therapy (ovariectomy) and cytotoxic chemotherapy (initially 5-fluorouracil and then combined cyclophosphamide, methotrexate, and doxorubicin). She had received the combination regimen 3 weeks before the fluid was obtained from which the MDA−MB-231 cell line was isolated.[85] MDA−MB-231 cells are highly tumorigenic and can produce lung metastases from mammary fat pad tumors in nude mice.[64]

MDA−MB-435 cells were established from a pleural effusion in a 31-year-old white woman with metastatic breast cancer.[39,85] Unlike patients from whom other cell lines have been established, this patient had received no prior systemic therapy (Price J, personal communication).

Despite being initially described as nontumorigenic,[86] MDA−MB-435 is generally reported to be highly tumorigenic and is one of the few human breast cancer cell lines that produce lung metastases from solid tumors.[64,87] When growing as xenografts, the growth or metastasis of these cells also appears responsive to several dietary manipulations.[88–90] The study of metastasis from the MDA−MB-435 cell line has been greatly simplified by the introduction of a marker (β-galactosidase), which can facilitate visualization of micrometastases.[91]

We established an ascites variant of the MDA−MB-435 cells (MDA435/LCC6). We have routinely maintained these cells as ascites for several years and have assessed their sensitivity to a series of cytotoxic drugs. The ascites has a pattern of responsiveness to single agents that closely reflects the activity of these agents in breast cancer patients. The cells also are easily maintained in vitro and can be successfully reestablished as solid tumors or ascites in nude mice. The MDA435/LCC6 cells may provide an alternative to the L1210/P388 murine ascites (leukemia) for the screening of new agents for activity in breast cancer. The MDA435/LCC6 cells also respond to nanomolar concentrations of all-*trans*-retinoic acid, fenretinimide, and 9-*cis*-retinoic acid,[11] perhaps reflecting the expression of the RAR-α, RAR-β, and RAR-γ isoforms by the parental MDA−MB-435 cells.[17]

OTHER MDA−MB DESIGNATED CELL LINES

Up to 19 cell lines bear the MDA−MB designation, most derived by Cailleau and associates at the MD Anderson Hospital and Tumor Institute.[39] The basic characteristics and isozyme and karyotype patterns have been previously reported in some detail.[39,92] Most cell lines are ER−, with the notable exception of MDA−MB-134 and MDA−MB-175, which are ER+.[93] Several of these cell lines are of specific interest. The MDA−MB-468 cells overexpress EGFR,[50] and in contrast to other breast cancer cell lines, their growth is inhibited by exogenous EGF.[94] FGF receptors are overexpressed by MDA−MB-175 cells, which are growth inhibited by FGF.[95] The MDA−MB-175 cells also exhibit an 8-fold overexpression of c-erbB-2 relative to normal fibroblasts.[50] The MDA−MB-361 cells, which were obtained from a brain metastasis[39] and the MDA−MB-453 cells exhibit a 2- to 4-fold amplification of the c-erbB-2 gene, overexpressing the gene product by approximately 64-fold.[50] The external domain of c-erbB-2 is shed from MDA−MB-361 cells and can be detected in the serum of nude mice bearing these xenografts.[96] The MDA−MB-436 cell line was derived from a 43-year-old woman with metastatic breast cancer.[39] These cells are ER− and are sensitive to several cytotoxic drugs. We have used the MDA−MB-436 cells to investigate the effects of insulin and cell-seeding density on methotrexate metabolism[97,98] and on the non−ER-mediated effects of estrogens and antiestrogens on both the cytotoxicity of methotrexate[99,100] and cell membrane structure and function.[101]

SkBr3

SkBr3 cells were obtained from a pleural effusion that developed in a 43-year-old patient with breast adenocarcinoma.[102] These cells have been widely used in the study of c-erbB-2 expression because they overexpress c-erbB-2 128-fold relative to normal fibroblasts as a result of a 4- to 8-fold amplification of this gene.[50] SkBr3 cells also secrete a truncated c-erbB-2 into their cell culture medium.[103] The coexpression of EGFR and c-erbB-2 has enabled studies into the mechanisms of EGF-induced heterodimerization.[104]

Models of Acquired Antiestrogen Resistance (ER+ Cells)

Although acquired resistance to antiestrogens is one of the more pressing clinical problems in breast cancer, few in vitro models exist for the analysis of this aspect of malignant progression. The most common approaches to the isolation of antiestrogen resistant cells utilize an in vitro selection of hormone-dependent cells against either a high single dose of antiestrogen[105] or a stepwise selection against increasing concentrations of drug. These approaches have been widely used to generate resistant variants of cell lines to many antineoplastic agents. Unfortunately, several problems arise when this approach is applied to generating antiestrogen-resistant variants of estrogen-dependent breast cancer cells. For example, it has often been difficult to isolate resistant clones that retain stability for several years. Several laboratories have reported resistant variants that revert to a sensitive phenotype with a high frequency.[49,106–108] Some cell lines alter other critical aspects of their phenotype. The MCF-7 variant LY-2 has become nontumorigenic.[62] MCF-7 cells selected in vivo can become dependent or stimulated by tamoxifen.[109,110] Cells transfected with FGFs also flip-flop their endocrine responsiveness, becoming stimulated by tamoxifen and inhibited by physiologic concentrations of estrogens.[70]

LY-2: MCF-7 CELLS SELECTED AGAINST A BENZOTHIOPHENE (LY117018) IN VITRO

The MCF-7 variant LY-2 is perhaps the most stable antiestrogen-resistant variant, generated over 10 years ago.[105] These cells were selected in vitro in an anchorage-independent (soft agar) colony assay for resistance against LY117018.[105] We demonstrated that LY-2 cells are cross-resistant to drugs representative of the major structural classes of antiestrogens, including nafoxidine, 4-hydroxy-TAM, and ICI 164,384.[62] In addition to exhibiting a significant shift in their dose-response relationship for antiestrogens, LY-2 cells also exhibit a blunted mitogenic response to E2.[105] LY-2 cells have lost their ability to form proliferating tumors in ovariectomized or E2-supplemented nude mice,[62] however, limiting their utility to in vitro studies.

Although the precise resistance mechanism in LY-2 cells is unclear, these cells express ER levels approximately one third those of their parental MCF-7 cells, and they have become PR–.[105] A reduced level of ER expression would be expected to induce resistance to all antiestrogens, because interaction with ER is likely to be the most important early event in antiestrogen function. Thus, the altered ER levels or the reduced ability to mount an estrogenic response in the LY-2 cells may explain their antiestrogen-resistance pattern. LY-2 cells still express levels of ER that would be considered high in a breast tumor biopsy.[105] Furthermore, the remaining ER appears normal, not mutated or altered.[111] The LY-2 cells may mimic some aspects of the antiestrogen resistance profile in patients with ER+/PR– tumors.

MCF-7 CELLS SELECTED AGAINST TAMOXIFEN IN VIVO

Several groups have generated resistance models by selecting MCF-7 xenografts growing in nude mice against tamoxifen, an approach that would appear to mimic human disease more closely than an in vitro selection. MCF-7 cells do not form proliferating tumors in castrated female mice, however, an endocrine environment similar to that of postmenopausal women.[112–114] Because the xenografts would not be proliferating, their growth could not be further suppressed; tamoxifen is generally considered a cytostatic, not a cytotoxic, drug. Consequently, one may predict that the most efficient response to such a selective pressure would be a change in the cell's perception of tamoxifen from inhibition to the widely documented partial agonist (growth promotion at low concentrations) properties of tamoxifen.[115] Indeed, the resultant tumors exhibit a tamoxifen-stimulated–dependent phenotype,[109,110] suggesting that this "inverted" phenotype reflects a sensitization to the partial agonist (estrogenic) effects of the triphenylethylenes.[115] Tamoxifen dependence is evidenced by withdrawal responses to tamoxifen inducing regression of the xenografts.[109] More recently, an ER variant has been identified that may explain these changes in responses to antiestrogens.[116,117] Jiang and associates identified a glycine–valine mutation at amino acid position 400 in the ER protein. When transfected into breast cancer cells, this mutant confers a growth inhibitory response to estrogens and a growth stimulatory response to antiestrogens.[116,117]

A breast tumor in a patient with a tamoxifen-dependent phenotype could respond to removal of tamoxifen by exhibiting tamoxifen withdrawal. Withdrawal responses have been widely reported for other endocrine therapies, including high-dose estrogen and progestin treatment.[118] Whether this occurs for antiestrogens is unclear because the incidence of tamoxifen withdrawal responses has not been clearly defined and documented. Several anecdotal and single case reports of tamoxifen withdrawal responses have been published.[119–124] Several larger studies indicate a low incidence of tamoxifen withdrawal responses.[125,126] Thus, the data from these models may be either predicting a response yet to be clearly demonstrated in the clinic or an experimental artifact. Should these models be correct, the potential for a significant incidence of tamoxifen withdrawal responses could provide an important, and potentially underestimated, clinical response pattern.

SELECTION OF HORMONE-INDEPENDENT BUT RESPONSIVE CELLS AGAINST 4-HYDROXYTAMOXIFEN

Rather than use hormone-dependent cells and risk a loss of tumorigenicity (eg, the LY-2 phenotype), or select in vivo hormone-dependent cells and obtain a tamoxifen-stimulated phenotype, we hypothesized that cells already hormone-independent and responsive might provide a more appropriate starting point for the generation of resistant variants. These cells already proliferate in the absence of estrogenic stimulation both in vivo and in vitro and may more closely reflect the phenotype of endocrine-responsive tumors in postmenopausal women. To eliminate species-specific metabolic differences between rodents and humans, we chose to perform a stepwise selection of the MCF-7/LCC1 cells in vitro against the potent tamoxifen metabolite 4-hydroxytamoxifen. We obtained a stable resistant population designated MCF-7/LCC2. These cells are resistant to tamoxifen when growing either in vitro or as xenografts in nude mice,[127] and they have remained stably resistant in the absence of selective pressure for over 2 years.

We determined the likely cross-resistance profile of these cells by assessing their in vitro growth response to steroidal antiestrogens. Although resistant to tamoxifen, MCF-7/LCC2 cells are not cross-resistant to either ICI 182,780 or ICI 164,384.[127,128] This response pattern suggested that some patients who initially respond but ultimately have a relapse while receiving tamoxifen may retain the ability to respond to a steroidal antiestrogen. Subsequently, this resistance pattern has been observed in preliminary data from a phase I trial of ICI 182,780 in heavily tamoxifen-pretreated patients.[129] These data indicate that, as predicted by the MCF-7/LCC2 phenotype, patients who ultimately have a relapse while receiving tamoxifen can obtain responses to a subsequent steroidal antiestrogen treatment. Thus, an in vitro observation correctly predicted for a subsequent pattern of response in breast cancer patients. These data suggest that the clinical responses to ICI 182,780 probably represent a genuine direct antitumor effect, rather than a possible tamoxifen withdrawal response, and suggest that the MCF-7/LCC2 phenotype is not merely an in vitro artifact. The relevance of these cells and their phenotypes has been reviewed.[36,65]

CELLS SELECTED FOR RESISTANCE TO STEROIDAL ANTIESTROGENS

We have begun to characterize MCF-7/LCC1 cells selected against the steroidal antiestrogen ICI 182,780. We have used a similar in vitro stepwise selection to generate the MCF-7/LCC2 cells. The stable ICI 182,780-resistant population was designated MCF-7/LCC9. MCF-7/LCC9 cells are resistant to ICI 182,780 in vitro and in vivo.[130] Although preliminary, our data suggest that these cells exhibit cross-resistance to tamoxifen, even though these cells have not been exposed to a triphenylethylene antiestrogen. If correct, this pattern of in vitro resistance would suggest that patients may be better served if treated initially with tamoxifen, and subsequently with a steroidal antiestrogen, rather than vice versa. The validity of this prediction remains to be tested in patients.

Models for Studying Multidrug (MDR1/gp170) Resistance

Many breast tumors are often initially responsive to cytotoxic chemotherapy. Almost all develop a multidrug-resistant phenotype, however, and this is ultimately responsible for the failure of current cytotoxic regimens.[34] Acquired resistance is frequently associated with expression of the MDR1 gene and its gp170 glycoprotein product. The level or incidence of detectable MDR1/gp170 expression is significantly higher in the tumors of treated patients versus untreated breast cancer patients[131–133] and correlates with in vitro resistance to cytotoxic drugs.[133–135] Several in vitro models established to screen for new agents can reverse this form of multiple drug resistance.

CELLS SELECTED FOR RESISTANCE AGAINST DOXORUBICIN

Cell lines selected in vitro for resistance to doxorubicin (Adriamycin; ADR) frequently overexpress gp170, often as a result of amplification of the MDR1 gene. Among the most widely used cell lines are the MCF-7[ADR][136] and the HeLa (ovarian carcinoma) variant KbV series.[137] One problem with cells selected in vitro is that they frequently acquire multiple drug–resistance mechanisms. For example, we demonstrated that MCF-7[ADR], but not MDR1-transduced MCF-7 (CL 10.3), cells are cross-resistant to tumor necrosis factor.[138] Because both ADR and tumor necrosis factor can inhibit cells by the generation of free radicals,[139,140] this cross-resistance in MCF-7[ADR] cells strongly suggests the presence of ADR-resistance mechanisms in addition to gp170, including altered expression of manganous superoxide dismutase.[138] Indeed, MCF-7[ADR] cells also exhibit increased glutathione transferase and topoisomerase II activities,[141,142] and they have become estrogen-independent and antiestrogen resistant because of their loss of steroid hormone receptor expression.[136]

The complexity of the resistance phenotype in these cells may explain why the gp170-reversing potency of isomers of flupenthixol identified in MCF-7[ADR] cells could not be confirmed in MDR1-transfected NIH 3T3 cells,[143] suggesting a non–gp170-mediated mechanism. Although MCF-7[ADR] cells are clearly of considerable utility for screening new resistance-modifying agents and combinations, their utility for detailed mechanistic studies of resistance reversal may be limited. These cells are widely used and well characterized, however, and they provide an important benchmark for comparing data among different studies.

CELLS TRANSDUCED WITH THE MDR1 GENE

To obtain cells in which gp170 is the major multidrug resistance mechanism, we transduced a cloned, E2-dependent, MCF-7 human breast cancer subline with a retroviral vector directing the constitutive expression of the MDR1 gene.[144] Following selection in the presence of the gp170 substrate colchicine, cell populations (MCF-7^{MDR1}) were isolated, and their ability to produce gp170 was determined by radioimmunoprecipitation.[144] In this study we used one of the MCF-7^{MDR1} clones designated CL 10.3. Transduced cells expressed high levels of a 170-kd glycoprotein exhibiting immunoreactivity with specific anti-gp170 antibodies. Immunoreactivity was not detected in either the parental MCF-7 cells or in MCF-7 cells transduced with a control pSV2neo vector. We estimated the level of expression of MCF-7^{MDR1} cells to be within 2- to 3-fold of that expressed by the ADR-selected MCF-7^{ADR} cells.[144] The functionality of the expressed glycoprotein was confirmed by determining the sensitivity of parental and MCF-7^{MDR1} cells to both a gp170 substrate (ADR) and to a non-gp170 substrate (gossypol).[144,145] Transduced cells have a 10-fold greater IC$_{50}$ for ADR, whereas sensitivity to gossypol is equivalent in both parental and transduced cells.[145] In our unpublished observations, we (Clarke and Leonessa) have seen a similar relationship for colchicine and the non-gp170 substrate methotrexate.

The increase in resistance exhibited by the transduced MCF-7^{MDR1} cells would be expected to be sufficient to induce clinical resistance in tumors. We also have observed perturbations in energy metabolism in the MCF-7^{MDR1} cells that are not present in the parental cells.[145] MDR1 transduced cells retain ER and PR expression and sensitivity to the triphenylethylene antiestrogen 4-hydroxytamoxifen.[144] Expression of the estrogen-inducible pS2 and EGF-receptor genes is similar in parental and MCF-7^{MDR1} cells.[144] EGF receptor is up-regulated and pS2 expression is lost in MCF-7^{ADR} cells.[136,144] The data indicate that overexpression of the MDR1 gene alone confers a multiple drug–resistance phenotype, but it does not result in either cross-resistance to antiestrogens or loss of steroid hormone–receptor expression.[144]

More recently, we transduced the ascites variant MDA435/LCC6 of the ER− breast cancer cell line MDA−MB−435 (discussed earlier) with MDR1 cDNA. The MDA435/LCC6 ascites exhibits a pattern of responses to established cytotoxic drugs that closely reflects the activity of the agents when administered as single agents in previously untreated breast cancer patients. The MDR1-transduced cells (MDA435/LCC6^{MDR1}) provide an ER− model for comparing with the ER+ MCF-7^{MDR1} CL 10.3 cells. Our unpublished observations show that the ascites variants provide a viable alternative to the murine leukemia ascites models (eg, L1210, P388) for screening gp170-reversing agents.

Normal Breast Epithelial Cells and Their Derivatives

Several groups have attempted to isolate cell lines from normal human mammary epithelium.[146–148] The isolation of normal mammary epithelial cells has been a difficult and complex process, reflecting the difficulty in adapting these cells to in vitro growth. Several specialized cell culture media have greatly increased the success rate for establishing primary cultures. In general, these are semisynthetic media containing little or no serum, they have low levels of Ca^{2+}, and they are supplemented with various hormones, growth factors, and chemically undefined ingredients such as conditioned cell culture media and bovine pituitary extract.[146–149]

Although these cells represent primary cultures, that is, they have a finite life-span in vitro, they may be both immortalized by treatment with carcinogens and transformed by inducing an overexpression of several oncogenes. As with the neoplastic breast cell lines, several cautions should be borne in mind. For example, the primary and immortalized cells are adapted to in vitro growth, and some of their expressed (or repressed) characteristics may be more closely associated with this adaptation than their normal in vivo function. The immortalized cells are continually proliferating, a state different from the resting tissues from which their parental cells were derived. All the available cell lines established from normal mammary cells are ER−. Nevertheless, these potentially normal cells are important models that provide the opportunity to study aspects of the biology of normal mammary epithelial cells, to identify agents that may contribute to the malignant transformation of normal mammary cells, and to determine phenotypic and genotypic perturbations associated with this process.

BENZO(α)PYRENE-IMMORTALIZED 184 AND B5 LINEAGES FROM REDUCTION MAMMAPLASTIES

Stampfer and Bartley successfully established primary organoid cultures from normal reduction mammaplasty tissues.[149] The source tissues for these cultures were essentially resting, in that they were not obtained during a functional or active period, such as early pregnancy, lactation, or involution.[149] These cells can readily be immortalized by treatment with benzo(a)pyrene (eg, 184 cells). Immortalized normal mammary epithelial cells can exhibit evidence indicative of their breast epithelial origin. For example, the cells are clearly epithelial,[146] and they express several human milk fat globulin antigens and synthesize α-lactalbumin and β-casein.[149] Although they are immortalized, that is, they can be maintained continuously in vitro, these cells are not transformed by several criteria, including an inability to form tumors in nude mice or significant anchorage-independent growth.[149]

TRANSFORMATION OF IMMORTALIZED HUMAN MAMMARY EPITHELIAL CELLS WITH ONCOGENES

The introduction of viral or cellular oncogenes into benzo(a)pyrene-immortalized human mammary epithelial cell lines results in a stepwise progression from a normal to malignant phenotype.[149–152] Two distinct immortalized lineages (184A1N4 and 184B5) have been characterized after transformation by several viral oncogenes. Tumorigenicity in nude mice is observed after infection of the benzo(a)pyrene-immortalized 184A1N4 subline with v-Ha-ras (A1N4-H), but not v-mos (A1N4-M), c-myc (A1N4-myc), or SV40T (A1N4-T; after limited passaging of cells).[150] Although nontumorigenic, v-mos-, c-myc-, and SV40T-transformed cells do exhibit phenotypic transformation and autonomy from growth factors in vitro to varying degrees, combinations of v-Ha-Ras with v-mos (A1N4-MH) or SV40T (A1N4-TH) resulted in highly malignant tumors in the nude mouse.[150,151] Consistent with the effects of v-Ha-ras on the A1N4 cell line, infection of the 184B5 subline with v-Ki-ras (B5kTu cells) also confers tumorigenicity in nude mice.[149]

MCF-10A

Soule and associates[148] described a spontaneously immortalized "normal" human breast epithelial cell line (MCF-10). The cells were isolated from mastectomy tissue obtained from a 36-year-old premenopausal woman with fibrocystic disease. After 849 days in culture, a population designated MCF-10A was established. These cells exhibit a stable t(3:9)(3p13:9p22) translocation.[148] The MCF-10A cells resemble luminal epithelial cells, rather than myoepithelial cells, and express antigens for several keratins and epithelial sialomucins.[153] The cells are nontumorigenic in nude mice and do not exhibit anchorage-independent growth.[148] These cells have also been subjected to oncogenic transformation. Transformation with Ha-ras oncogene caused increased clonigenicity in vitro, but not tumorigenicity in nude mice.[154] MCF-10 cells cotransfected with the erbB-2 and Ha-ras oncogenes (MCF-10A HE) showed an even higher increase in soft agar clonigenicity, but still lacked tumorigenicity in nude mice.[155]

In Vitro Models for Studying Invasion and Metastasis

To metastasize effectively, cells must accomplish a complex compendium of activities, including escape from the primary lesion, avoidance of immune surveillance, and penetration of normal tissue at distant sites.[156] Invasion of extracellular matrices occurs repeatedly in this process, and basement membrane invasion in particular has received considerable attention.[157] The loss of basement membrane at the parenchymal–mesenchymal interface of locally invasive tumors has been closely associated with metastatic dissemination.[158–160] The uniformity of basement membrane composition and structure suggests that the molecular mechanisms in basement membrane recognition, attachment, degradation, and traversal may yield novel targets for cancer therapy. We have used several in vitro models to study the process of basement membrane invasion and its relationship with malignant progression.

IN VITRO ASSAYS FOR INVASIVE POTENTIAL

The development of Matrigel, a reconstituted basement membrane extract from the EHS sarcoma,[161] has been instrumental in facilitating compositional and functional analyses of basement membranes. Matrigel is liquid at 4°C, allowing various manipulations before it sets into a homogenous gel at 37°C. Matrigel contains the major basement membrane components, including laminin, collagen type IV and heparan sulfate proteoglycan. We have used Matrigel in two different assays to examine in vitro invasiveness of human breast cancer cells.[162]

The Boyden chamber chemoinvasion assay compares the ability of cells to traverse a Matrigel coated polycarbonate filter as they migrate toward different chemoattractants.[163] Invasive cells, stained on the lower filter surface, can be quantitated either by image analysis or by crystal violet staining.[164] Although originally developed in modified blind-well Boyden chambers, two-compartment chamber systems such as Transwell from Gibco and Bio-Coat wells from Collaborative Research have been successful. Other adaptations include prelabeling the cells with either a nontoxic fluorescent dye or radioactivity to facilitate quantitation of invaded cells.

The ability of cells to form invasive colonies when embedded in a three-dimensional gel of Matrigel is compared qualitatively in the Matrigel-outgrowth assay.[162,163] Cells dispersed in a three-dimensional layer of Matrigel are examined after culture for 2 to 10 days. Although dispersal of single cells throughout the upper layer of Matrigel provides the highest stringency for invasive outgrowth, characteristic morphologic features can be achieved more rapidly with cells sandwiched between two layers of Matrigel or simply plated on top of Matrigel.

The presence or lack of ER is an important determinant of both prognosis and choice of treatment of breast cancer. The hormone-responsive or hormone-dependent breast cancer cell lines represent a model system for the analysis of hormonal influences on the invasive process. Effects of estrogens, antiestrogens, and progestins on the in vitro invasiveness of steroid-dependent and steroid-responsive human breast cancer cells have been reviewed.[165,166,169,170] In addition, progression to hormone independence has implications for invasiveness and metastasis. For example, we demonstrated that MCF-7/MIII and MCF-7/LCC1 cells acquire an increased metastatic potential as they become estrogen-independent.[61] This increased metastatic potential is reflected in increased activity in the Boyden chamber,[62] but not in Matrigel outgrowth assays, increased local invasiveness in vivo, and an ability to produce occasional distant metastases in nude mice.[61]

To examine the hypothesis that ER— human breast cancer cell lines are constitutively more invasive than their ER+ counterparts, we examined many of the human breast cancer cell lines described previously for invasiveness in the Boyden chamber assay in vitro and for metastatic potential in the nude mouse. These studies clearly indicate that the majority of ER− cell lines are inherently more aggressive than ER+ cells both in vitro and in vivo.[1,162] Because the incidence of distant metastases is significantly lower and less reproducible than that observed in the MDA−MB-435 cells, the MCF-7/MIII and MCF-7/LCC1 cells appear to represent a phenotype intermediate between the poorly invasive MCF-7 and the metastatic MDA−MB-435.[61]

CELL LINES AND THE EPITHELIAL−MESENCHYMAL TRANSITION

An emerging development in progression studies for breast carcinoma is the immunocytochemical analysis of markers characteristic of epithelial or mesenchymal phenotypes. The mesenchymal intermediate filament glycoprotein vimentin (VIM) has been associated with lack of ER, high growth fraction, and poor nuclear grade in human breast cancer.[171−175] VIM expression in the tumor component is indicative of an epithelial−mesenchymal transition, which may occur during the process of malignant progression. Consistent with this notion, the epithelial marker E-cadherin, a homotypic cell adhesion molecule, is lost from more aggressive tumors.[176−178] Loss of E-cadherin and acquisition of VIM expression are events that characterize the epithelial−mesenchymal transition that occurs during embryogenesis.[179]

To begin to address this hypothesis, we compared the invasiveness of epithelial-like (VIM−) and mesenchymal-like (VIM+) human breast cancer cells in the Boyden chamber and Matrigel outgrowth assays. Irrespective of hormone responsiveness, VIM+ cells exhibited significantly higher levels of both in vitro invasiveness and metastatic potential when compared with the VIM− group.[1,162] VIM expression was not detected in cells containing ER and was present only in some of the cell lines lacking ER, whereas E-cadherin was expressed functionally in all cell lines expressing ER, as well as some that had lost ER expression and did not express VIM. These data suggest that the loss of E-cadherin expression is not linked to hormone independence, but that it occurs earlier than VIM expression in the progression cascade. VIM expression also appears to be downstream of hormone independence.

E-cadherin expression, indicative of an epithelial phenotype, associates with a compacted spherical morphology in VIM− cell lines.[180] E-cadherin is not present in any VIM+ cell lines. Absence of both E-cadherin and VIM is associated with a noninvasive cluster-type morphology. The MCF-7[ADR] cell line, derived from MCF-7 cells by stepwise selection for increasing resistance to the drug ADR, as previously discussed, is interesting in this regard. Derived from the E-cadherin+/ER+/VIM− MCF-7 phenotype, this subline has lost ER and E-cadherin, has gained VIM expression, and has become significantly more invasive. Examination of additional ADR- and vinblastine-resistant variants of the MCF-7 and ZR-75-1B cell lines shows that most drug-resistant sublines expressed VIM.[181] Understanding the relationships among drug resistance, VIM expression, and invasiveness may provide important clues for the optimization of chemotherapy for breast tumors.

The MCF-7/MIII and MCF-7/LCC1 variants retain ER and UVO expression and generally lack VIM expression, and they exhibit lower levels of invasiveness than VIM+ human breast cancer cells.[1,162] These observations support our hypothesis that these MCF-7 variants represent an intermediate point in the metastatic progression of breast cancer. The metastatic potential of MCF-7/MIII and MCF-7/LCC1 cells,[61] compared with ER−/VIM− cell lines (eg, MDA−MB-468) suggests, however, that metastatic potential may also develop independent of the epithelial−mesenchymal transition-like event, as previously reviewed.[182]

ONCOGENE EXPRESSION AND IN VITRO METASTATIC POTENTIAL

The effects of oncogenes on mammary cell invasiveness have been examined. The *ras* oncogene is perhaps best studied and can induce the invasive phenotype in a variety of both human and rodent epithelial systems. Transfection of human bronchial epithelial cells transfected with v-Ha-ras increased both invasiveness in vitro and metastatic potential in the nude mouse.[183,184] In NIH/3T3 cells, transfection with either *v*-Ha-*ras* or genomic DNA containing various forms of activated *ras* also resulted in increased invasiveness across the amniotic membrane in vitro and metastatic dissemination in vivo.[185,186]

MCF-7 cells transfected with *v*-Ha-*ras* show increased in vitro invasiveness of Matrigel, increased migration potential, and increased recognition of laminin,[187] but no apparent increases in metastatic potential in nude mice.[188,189] Although both 184 sublines (A1N4 and 184 B5) are transformed to a tumorigenic phenotype by expression of ras alone, only the initially more invasive A1N4 cells respond to ras transformation with increased invasiveness. The refractory nature of the 184B5 cells to ras-induced effects on invasiveness, despite the induction of tumorigenicity, suggests a possible lineage specificity for this response and begins to dissociate ras effects on tumorigenicity from invasiveness.

Differential induction of metastatic potential by v-Ha-ras was reported previously.[154,188−191] Detailed analysis of a highly stable rat mammary subclone after *ras* transduction implicated rapid phenotypic diversification rather than direct effects on a cascade of metastasis-effector genes.[192] No epithelial−mesenchymal transition-like changes were seen after ras transformation of A1N4 or B5 cells[166] or in ras-transfected MCF-7 cells.[165] In contrast, combined transformation of 184 A1N4 immortalized human mammary epithelial cells with v-Ha-ras and either SV40T or v-*mos* induces a VIM+, invasive phenotype indicative of the epithelial−mesenchymal transition event.[166]

We also further investigated the chemotactic activity and invasive property of the MCF-10A cells cotransfected with both Ha-ras and erbB-2 (MCF-10 HE cells) using

Matrigel-based assays. MCF-10A HE cells showed 10-fold higher invasiveness than nontransfected cells, formed branching colonies in Matrigel, and showed a high cloning efficiency in soft agar (Albini and Thompson, unpublished data). These attributes are indicative of VIM+ phenotype resulting from an epithelial–mesenchymal transition-like event.

Concluding Comments on in Vitro Models

Human breast cancer cell lines growing both in vitro and as human xenografts in vivo have a central role in most basic and preclinical breast cancer research. They have been widely used to investigate the cellular and molecular events associated with endocrine responsiveness, malignant progression, invasiveness, and metastatic potential. With the increasing restrictions imposed on the use of vertebrate animals, and the relatively limited number of species that develop spontaneous mammary carcinomas, it seems likely that the emphasis on the in vitro use of human breast cancer cell lines will increase in the coming decades. Consequently, it is critical both that additional representative human breast cancer cell lines be introduced, particularly hormone-responsive lines, and that the precautions associated with the use of in vitro models be realistically assessed and acknowledged.

SOME CAUTIONS REGARDING THE USE OF IN VITRO MODELS

Despite the widespread use of in vitro models and the useful and important data arising from this use, the use of these models has several potential limitations. There are relatively few well-characterized ER+ cell lines. Although these cell lines exhibit comparable estrogenic responses in the endpoints most widely applied, the extent to which these observations may be applied to all ER+ human breast tumors is unclear. Certainly, many of the most important attributes, such as growth inhibition by antiestrogens, are likely to reflect the human disease closely. Where responses differ markedly from predicted and observed responses in humans, such as growth inhibition by physiologic levels of E2, a greater degree of caution is clearly warranted. A clear deficit in the range of breast cancer cell lines currently available is the relatively small number of ER+ and E2-responsive cell lines.

The majority of steroid-responsive cell lines have been established, not from solid tumors, but from malignant effusions. Although such effusions occur with a 26% to 49% frequency in breast cancer patients,[193,194] they may not be fully representative of all solid tumors. Despite the likely metastatic origin of these cells, the ER+ cell lines from these sites are rarely metastatic in vivo, even in severely immunocompromised animals.

The most widely used cell lines have now been in use for 20 or more years. Subtle changes may have been acquired during this period, and these may not adequately reflect changes that occur in tumors in patients. Because the cells are clearly adapted to grow in vitro, the perturbations that have conferred this ability also may not occur in patients' tumors. Human breast tumors are highly heterogeneous and contain many subpopulations of cells with different phenotypic characteristics, including both ER+ and ER− cells.[195] In contrast, breast cancer cell lines are relatively homogeneous. This property can be viewed either as advantageous or disadvantageous. Whereas responses in a cell line may not fully reflect the response of a complex human tumor, they do provide the ability to study, in considerable detail and complexity, the responses of cells representative of tumor subpopulations.

In principle, cell lines are like any other experimental model. When their limitations are openly acknowledged and appropriately considered in experimental design and data analysis, they can provide useful and important tools. Otherwise, one risks overinterpretation of data or the pursuit of a potential in vitro artifact. As a generalization, observations from in vitro models that clearly reflect human disease are more likely to reflect real events and lead to new insights into mechanistic processes. When these models are used to generate hypotheses for future testing in humans, the validity of the observation awaits completion of the human trials. Thus, major strengths of in vitro models include the following:

- The ability to study a specific cell type and elucidate the mechanism of its response to agents at the cellular and molecular level
- The ability to identify mechanistic processes by comparing related cells with different phenotypic characteristics
- The ability to facilitate further hypothesis generation and testing in vivo when growing as xenografts
- The ability to generate hypotheses for testing in the ultimate model, the human being

ESTABLISHMENT AND CHARACTERIZATION OF NEW BREAST CANCER CELL LINES AND VARIANTS

Despite the presence of some breast cancer cell lines[2] and the emergence of new cell lines,[196] of those in common or widespread usage, only three (the parental MCF-7, T47D, and ZR-75-1) are clearly estrogen-dependent or estrogen-responsive. Few established cell lines are metastatic in nude mice, and those that metastasize with a high frequency are generally ER−. Thus, a need exists for new breast cell lines from malignant, solid metastatic (eg, bone, lung), and normal tissues, specifically steroid hormone–responsive cell lines. Unfortunately, breast cancer cells from patients' tumors are notoriously difficult to establish in vitro.[197,199] The take rate for xenografts of tumor tissue in immunocompromised rodents also is relatively poor, although it is generally higher than for direct in vitro growth.[200] In addition is a notable absence of a well-characterized panel of nonmalignant breast epithelial cell lines, which could be used for comparative studies. Of the normal cell lines available, none are steroid hormone–responsive.[146,149]

New breast cancer cell lines require careful description and characterization. When possible, the characteristics and history of the patient (eg, age, sex, race, treatment) and the known characteristics of the tumor (eg, histopathologic diagnosis, tumor grade, nodal status, ER, PR, S-phase–proliferative and any other pertinent information) should be provided. The human origin of the tissues should be confirmed, and a karyotype and isoenzyme profile should be reported. Typical polymorphic enzymes analyzed include lactate dehydrogenase, glucose-6-phosphate dehydrogenase (EC 1.1.1.49), phosphoglucomutase-1 (EC 2.7.5.1), phosphoglucomutase-3 (EC 2.7.5.1), esterase D (EC 3.1.1.1), mitochondrial malic enzyme (EC 1.1.1.40), adenylate kinase (EC 2.7.4.3), and glyoxalase (EC 4.4.1.5).[14] These data are particularly useful in confirming the origin of a variant as derived from its parental and in excluding contamination of a new cell line with cells of an established cell line. To this end, we have routinely used the services currently provided by Dr. Joseph Kaplan through the Cell Culture Laboratory of the Children's Hospital of Michigan in Detroit. This facility is currently maintained under National Cancer Institute contract to provide these services.

The general characteristics of the new cell line or variant should be clearly provided. This includes in vitro growth characteristics (eg, culture conditions, cell doubling time, split-ratio, and the passage number at which these data were obtained) and the hormone-receptor profile and endocrine responsiveness. A description of the morphologic features of the cells (eg, ultrastructural analyses), particularly where it addresses tissue origin or evidence of differentiated function (eg, secretory activity, production of milk proteins), is to be strongly encouraged.[2]

The tumorigenicity of a new cell line should be determined in at least one immunocompromised rodent model (preferably several) and reported. Different immunocompromised mice strains can exhibit different abilities to support xenografts, and the models in which tumorigenicity is assessed should be clearly indicated. The inability to form tumors in athymic nude mice may not indicate that the cells are nontumorigenic in other strains (eg, *scid:* see Chap. 7.7). The histologic features of any arising tumors should be compared with those of the original tumor when possible. The presence of any metastases and their histologic features also should be documented. When available, any other pertinent data also should be provided (eg, oncogene expression and amplification).

The designation of a cell line or variant should follow the guidelines of the Tissue Culture Association and should reflect both the tissue of origin and the laboratory where it was established.[201] For our variant cells, we have chosen to use a designation that appends our institution to that of the original (parental) cell line (eg MCF-7/LCC1).

CELL CULTURE CONDITIONS

The choice of culture conditions often can inadvertently influence the experimental outcome. For example, for many years insulin was routinely added to the cell culture media used to maintain breast cancer cells. Although insulin is a potent mitogen for many of these cells, it does not appear to be required for growth in vitro in serum-supplemented media for most human breast cancer cell lines. Insulin can down-regulate ER expression, however.[202] Both insulin and EGF have been added to serum-free media for breast cancer cells,[203] and both can influence the growth inhibitory effects of antiestrogens.[204,205] Phenol red is widely used as a pH indicator in cell culture media. A contaminant in phenol red is known to be estrogenic, and this activity can alter both growth and antiestrogen responsiveness.[206,207]

Serum contains various growth factors and steroid hormones. The steroids can be readily removed by treatment with dextran-coated charcoal.[208] MCF-7 cells also can use the steroid sulfates present in serum.[209] These steroid sulfates can be removed by prior treatment with sulfatase.[210] The growth factors and other proteins can be chemically inactivated to produce a growth factor–free serum.[210] The concentration of serum used also can be important. The dose-response relationship for antiestrogens is altered significantly by serum concentration.[211] We have found a final concentration of either 5% fetal calf serum or 5% dextran-coated charcoal serum to provide appropriate in vitro growth characteristics for most human breast cancer cell lines. Moreover, the concentrations of steroids, growth factors, and other constituents in serum may vary considerably from batch to batch.

Estrogens remain within cells for several days,[212] and when stripping cells of endogenous estrogens, it is often necessary to wash cell monolayers thoroughly and to maintain cells for several days in the absence of estrogens. We routinely wash cells at least three times with phenol red–free media supplemented with 5% dextran–charcoal-stripped serum and maintain the washed monolayers in this medium for a further 3 to 5 days to ensure adequate removal of endogenous steroids.[14,62]

The cell-seeding density also can have considerable effects on cellular growth and metabolism. We previously demonstrated that cells seeded at different densities exhibit both different cell population doubling times and differences in methotrexate poly-γ-glutamate formation.[98] In many instances, one must closely control for seeding density, proliferative capacity, confluence, and serum batch. The handling of cells also may be important, including duration of trypsinization and time at room temperature during passage or treatment. For some cell lines, one must pass a trypsinized cell suspension through a sterile needle to generate a single cell suspension.

These examples indicate the general importance of closely controlling cell culture conditions. The reader is referred to several excellent books on tissue culture techniques for a more detailed description of cell culture procedures.[213–215]

Summary

The development of stable cell lines derived from both malignant and normal human breast tissue has been of considerable use in breast cancer research, and it continues to occupy a central position in basic breast cancer research. These cell lines provide the ability to perform studies that could not easily be performed in experimental animals or in human beings. The ease of use, relatively low cost of maintenance, general reproducibility of phenotype, and ability to mimic properties seen in tumors in patients are considerable advantages. The use and applicability of cell lines are not without limitations, however. For example, these cell lines cannot be used to predict in vivo toxicity reliably or to assess the toxicologic properties of new agents. Cell lines also may be ineffective in establishing mechanisms of drug metabolism or in elucidating critical tumor—host interactions. Their metabolic adaptations to in vitro growth may not reflect adaptations that occur in vivo. Nevertheless, breast cancer cell lines have been used successfully for many years to generate new hypotheses, to screen new agents, and to study the biology of breast cancer. Many cell lines have the advantage of being tumorigenic and thereby can facilitate further studies in vivo in experimental animals. Provided their limitations are freely acknowledged, human breast cancer cell lines will continue to be one of the most powerful series of tools in breast cancer research.

ACKNOWLEDGMENTS

This work was funded in part by US Public Health Service grants R01-CA58022, R01-CA61344, and 1P30-CA51008.

References

1. Thompson EW, Paik S, Brünner N, et al. Association of increased basement membrane-invasiveness with absence of estrogen receptor and expression of vimentin in human breast cancer cell lines. J Cell Physiol 1992;150:534.

2. Engel LW, Young NA. Human breast carcinoma cells in continuous culture: a review. Cancer Res 1978;38:4327.

3. Magdelenat H, Pouillart P. Steroid hormone receptors in breast cancer. In: Sheridan PJ, Blum K, Trachtenberg MC, eds. Steroid receptors and disease: cancer autoimmune, bone and circulatory disorders. New York, Marcel Dekker, 1988;435.

4. McGuire WL, Clark GM. The prognostic role of progesterone receptor in human breast cancer. Semin Oncol 1983;10:2.

5. Ravdin PM, Green S, Dorr TM, et al. Prognostic significance of progesterone receptor levels in estrogen receptor-positive patients with metastatic breast cancer treated with tamoxifen: results of a prospective Southwest Oncology Group study. J Clin Oncol 1992;10:1284.

6. Lippman ME, Bolan G, Huff K. The effects of estrogens and antiestrogens on hormone responsive human breast cancer cells in long-term tissue culture. Cancer Res 1976;36:4595.

7. Lippman ME, Bolan G, Huff K. Interactions of antiestrogens with human breast cancer in long-term tissue culture. Cancer Treat Reports 1976;60:1421.

8. Yano T, Korkut E, Pinski J, et al. Inhibition of growth of MCF-7 MIII human breast carcinoma in nude mice by treatment with agonists or antagonists of LH-RH. Breast Cancer Res Treat 1992;21:35.

9. Fontana JA, Hobbs PD, Dawson MI. Inhibition of mammary carci-noma growth by retinoidal benzoic acid derivatives. Exp Cell Biol 1988;56:254.

10. Fontana JA. Interaction of retinoids and tamoxifen on the inhibition of human mammary carcinoma cell proliferation. Exp Cell Biol 1987;55:136.

11. Baumann K, Clarke R. Effects of all-*trans*-retinoic acid on proliferation and gene expression of human breast cancer cells *in vitro*. Proc Am Assoc Cancer Res 1994;35:275.

12. Soule HD, Vasquez J, Long A, et al. A human cell line from a pleural effusion derived from a human breast carcinoma. J Natl Cancer Inst 1973;51:1409.

13. Horwitz KB, Costlow ME, McGuire WL. MCF-7: a human breast cancer cell line with estrogen, androgen, progesterone and glucocorticoid receptors. Steroids 1975;26:785.

14. Clarke R, Brünner N, Katzenellenbogen BS, et al. Progression from hormone dependent to hormone independent growth in MCF-7 human breast cancer cells. Proc Natl Acad Sci USA 1989;86:3649.

15. Eidne KA, Flanagan CA, Harris NS, et al. Gonadotropin-releasing hormone (GnRH)-binding sites in human breast cancer cell lines and inhibitory effects of GnRH antagonists. J Clin Endocrinol Metab 1987;64:425.

16. Monaco ME, Lippman ME. Insulin stimulation of fatty acid synthesis in human breast cancer cells in long-term tissue culture. Endocrinology 1977;101:1238.

17. Swisshelm K, Ryan K, Lee X, et al. Down regulation of retinoic acid receptor β in mammary carcinoma cell lines and its upregulation in senescing normal mammary epithelial cells. Cell Growth Differ 1994;5:133.

18. Shafie SM, Brooks SC. Effect of prolactin on growth and estrogen receptor levels of human breast cancer cells (MCF-7). Cancer Res 1977;37:792.

19. Huff KK, Kaufman D, Gabbay KH, et al. Human breast cancer cells secrete an insulin-like growth factor-I-related polypeptide. Cancer Res 1986;46:4613.

20. Huff KK, Knabbe C, Lindsey R, et al: Multihormonal regulation of insulin-like growth factor-I-related protein in MCF-7 human breast cancer cells. Mol Endocrinol 1988;2:200.

21. van der Burg B, Isbrucker L, vasn Selm-Miltenburb AJP, et al. Role of estrogen-induced insulin-like growth factors in the proliferation of human breast cancer cells. Cancer Res 1990;50:7770.

22. Stewart A, Johnson MD, May FEB, et al. Role of insulin-like growth factors and the type I insulin-like growth factor receptor in the estrogen-stimulated proliferation of human breast cancer cells. J Biol Chem 1990;265:21172.

23. Furlanetto RW, DiCarlo JN. Somatomedin C receptors and growth effects in human breast cancer cells maintained in long-term tissue culture. Cancer Res 1984;44:2122.

24. Arteaga CL, Osborne CK. Growth inhibition of human breast cancer cells in vitro with an antibody against the type I somatomedin receptor. Cancer Res 1989;49:6237.

25. Yee D, Cullen KJ, Paik S, et al. Insulin-like growth factor–II mRNA expression in human breast cancer. Cancer Res 1988;48:6691.

26. Clemmons DR, Camacho-Hubner C, Coronado E, et al. Insulin-like growth factor binding protein secretion by breast carcinoma cell lines: correlation with estrogen receptor status. Endocrinology 1990;127:2679.

27. Yee D, Favoni R, Lupu R, et al. The insulin-like growth factor binding protein BP-25 is expressed by human breast cancer cells. Biochem Biophys Res Commun 1989;158:38.

28. Davidson NE, Gelmann EP, Lippman ME, et al. Epidermal growth factor receptor gene expression in estrogen receptor-positive and negative human breast cancer cell lines. Mol Endocrinol 1987;1:216.

29. Bates SE, Davidson NE, Valverius EM, et al. Expression of trans-

forming growth factor-α and its mRNA in human breast cancer: its regulation by estrogen and its possible functional significance. Mol Endocrinol 1988;2:543.

30. Clarke R, Brünner N, Katz D, et al. The effects of a constitutive production of TGF-α on the growth of MCF-7 human breast cancer cells in vitro and in vivo. Mol Endocrinol 1989;3:372.

31. Kern FG, Wellstein A, Flamm S, et al. Secretion of heparin binding growth factors by breast cancer cells and their role in promoting cancer cell growth. Cancer Chemother 1990;5:167.

32. Lehtola L, Partanen J, Sistonen L, et al. Analysis of tyrosine kinase mRNAs including four FGF receptors expressed in the MCF-7 breast cancer cells. Int J Cancer 1992;50:598.

33. Bronzert DA, Pantazis P, Antoniades HN, et al. Synthesis and secretion of platelet-derived growth factor by human breast cancer cell lines. Proc Natl Acad Sci USA 1987;84:5763.

34. Clarke R, Dickson RB, Lippman ME. Hormonal aspects of breast cancer: growth factors, drugs and stromal interactions. Crit Rev Oncol Hematol 1992;12:1.

35. Clarke R, Dickson RB, Brünner N. The process of malignant progression in human breast cancer. Ann Oncol 1990;1:401.

36. Clarke R, Skaar T, Baumann K, et al. Hormonal carcinogenesis in breast cancer: cellular and molecular studies of malignant progression. Breast Cancer Res Treat 1994;31:237.

37. Keydar I, Chen L, Karby S, et al. Establishment and characterization of a cell line of human carcinoma origin. Eur J Cancer 1979;15:659.

38. Horwitz KB, Friedenberg GR. Growth inhibition and increase of insulin receptors in antiestrogen-resistant T47Dco human breast cancer cells by progestins: implications for endocrine therapies. Cancer Res 1985;45:167.

39. Cailleau R, Olive M, Cruciger QVA. Long-term human breast carcinoma cell lines of metastatic origin: preliminary characterization. In Vitro 1978;14:911.

40. Reddel RR, Alexander IE, Koga M, et al. Genetic instability and the development of steroid hormone insensitivity in cultured T47D human breast cancer cells. Cancer Res 1988;48:4340.

41. Graham ML, Smith JA, Jewett PB, et al. Heterogeneity of progesterone receptor content and remodelling by tamoxifen characterize subpopulations of cultured human breast cancer cells: analysis by quantitative dual parameter flow cytometry. Cancer Res 1992;52:593.

42. Sartorius CA, Groshong SD, Miller LA, et al. New T47D breast cancer cell lines for the independent study of progesterone B- and A-receptors: only antiprogestin-occupied B-receptors are switched to transcriptional agonists by cAMP. Cancer Res 1994;54:3868.

43. Graham ML, Dalquist KE, Horwitz KB. Simultaneous measurement of progesterone receptors and DNA indices by flow cytometry: analysis of breast cancer cell mixtures and genetic instability of the T47D line. Cancer Res 1989;49:3943.

44. Vignon F, Bardon S, Chalbos D, et al. Antiestrogenic effect of R5020, a synthetic progestin in human breast cancer cells in culture. J Clin Endocrinol Metab 1983;56:1124.

45. Horwitz KB. The antiprogestin RU38 486: receptor-mediated progestin versus antiprogestin actions screened in estrogen-insensitive T47Dco human breast cancer cells. Endocrinology 1985;116:2236.

46. Mockus MB, Lessey BA, Bower MA, et al. Estrogen-insensitive progesterone receptors in a human breast cancer cell line: characterization of receptors and of a ligand exchange assay. Endocrinology 1982;110:1564.

47. Engel LW, Young NA, Tralka TS, et al. Establishment and characterization of three new continuous cell lines derived from human breast carcinomas. Cancer Res 1978;38:3352.

48. van den Berg HW, Leahey WJ, Lynch M, et al. Recombinant human interferon alpha increases oestrogen receptor expression in human breast cancer cells (ZR-75-1) and sensitises them to the anti-proliferative effects of tamoxifen. Br J Cancer 1987;55:255.

49. van den Berg HW, Lynch M, Martin J, et al. Characterization of a tamoxifen-resistant variant of the ZR-75-1 human breast cancer cell line (ZR-75-9a1) and stability of the resistant phenotype. Br J Cancer 1989;59:522.

50. Kraus MH, Popescu NC, Amsbaugh SC, et al. Overexpression of the EGF receptor-related proto-oncogene erbB-2 in human mammary tumor cell lines by different molecular mechanisms. EMBO J 1987;6:605.

51. Warri AM, Laine AM, Majasuo KE, et al. Estrogen suppression of erbB2 expression is associated with increased growth rate of ZR-75-1 human breast cancer cells in vitro and in nude mice. Int J Cancer 1991;49:616.

52. Long B, McKibben BM, Lynch M, et al. Changes in epidermal growth factor receptor expression and response to ligand associated with acquired tamoxifen resistance or oestrogen independence in the ZR-75-1 human breast cancer cell line. Br J Cancer 1992;65:865.

53. van Agthoven T, van Agthoven TL, Portengen H, et al. Ectopic expression of epidermal growth factor receptors induces hormone independence in ZR-75-1 human breast cancer cells. Cancer Res 1992;52:5082.

54. Poulin R, Baker D, Poirier D, et al. Androgen and glucocorticoid receptor-mediated inhibition of cell proliferation by medroxyprogesterone acetate in ZR-75-1 human breast cancer cells. Breast Cancer Res Treat 1989;13:161.

55. Poulin R, Baker D, Poirier D, et al. Multiple actions of synthetic "progestins" on the growth of ZR-75-1 human breast cancer cells: an in vitro model for the simultaneous assay of androgen, progestin, estrogen, and glucocorticoid agonistic and antagonistic activities of steroids. Breast Cancer Res Treat 1991;17:197.

56. Weckbecker G, Liu R, Tolcsvai L, et al. Antiproliferative effects of the somatostatin analogue octreotide (SMS 201-995) on ZR-75-1 human breast cancer cells in vivo and in vitro. Cancer Res 1992;52:4973.

57. Theriault C, Labrie F. Multiple steroid metabolic pathways in ZR-75-1 human breast cancer cells. J Steroid Biochem Mol Biol 1991;38:155.

58. Poulin R, Poirier D, Merand Y, et al. Extensive esterification of adrenal C19-delta-5 sex steroids to long-chain fatty acids in the ZR-75-1 human breast cancer cell line. J Biol Chem 1989;264:9335.

59. Roy R, Belanger A. ZR-75-1 breast cancer cells generate nonconjugated steroids from low density lipoprotein-incorporated lipoidal dehydroepiandrosterone. Endocrinology 1993;133:683.

60. Brünner N, Boulay V, Fojo A, et al. Acquisition of hormone-independent growth in MCF-7 cells is accompanied by increased expression of estrogen-regulated genes but without detectable DNA amplifications. Cancer Res 1993;53:283.

61. Thompson EW, Brünner N, Torri J, et al. The invasive and metastatic properties of hormone-independent and hormone-responsive variants of MCF-7 human breast cancer cells. Clin Exp Metastasis 1993;11:15.

62. Clarke R, Brünner N, Thompson EW, et al. The inter-relationships between ovarian-independent growth, antiestrogen resistance and invasiveness in the malignant progression of human breast cancer. J Endocrinol 1989;122:331.

63. Jones DY, Schatzkin A, Green SB, et al. Dietary fat and breast cancer in the National Health and Nutrition Examination Survey I epidemiologic follow-up study. J Natl Cancer Inst 1987;79:465.

64. Price JE, Polyzos A, Zhang RD, et al. Tumorigenicity and metastasis of human breast carcinoma cell lines in nude mice. Cancer Res 1990;50:717.

65. Clarke R, Thompson EW, Leonessa F, et al. Hormone resistance, invasiveness and metastatic potential in human breast cancer. Breast Cancer Res Treat 1993;24:227.

66. Katzenellenbogen BS, Kendra KL, Norman MJ, et al. Proliferation,

hormonal responsiveness, and estrogen receptor content of MCF-7 human breast cancer cells grown in the short-term and long-term absence of estrogens. Cancer Res 1987;47:4355.

67. Cho H, Ng PA, Katzenellenbogen BS. Differential regulation of gene expression by estrogen in estrogen growth-independent and -dependent MCF-7 human breast cancer cell sublines. Mol Endocrinol 1991;5:1323.

68. Natoli C, Sica G, Natoli V, et al. Two new estrogen-supersensitive variants of the MCF-7 human breast cancer cell line. Breast Cancer Res Treat 1983;3:23.

69. McLeskey SW, Kurebayashi J, Honig SF, et al. Fibroblast growth factor 4 transfection of MCF-7 cells produces cell lines that are tumorigenic and metastatic in ovariectomized or tamoxifen-treated athymic nude mice. Cancer Res 1993;53:2168.

70. Kurebayashi J, McLeskey SW, Johnson MD, et al. Quantitative demonstration of spontaneous metastasis by MCF-7 human breast cancer cells cotransfected with fibroblast growth factor 4 and LacZ. Cancer Res 1993;53:2178.

71. Lasfargues EY, Ozzello L. Cultivation of human breast carcinomas. J Natl Cancer Inst 1958;21:1131.

72. Horwitz KB, Zava DT, Thilagar AK, et al. Steroid receptor analyses of nine human breast cancer cell lines. Cancer Res 1978;38:2434.

73. Hall RE, Lee CSL, Alexander IE, et al. Steroid hormone receptor gene expression in human breast cancer cells: inverse relationship between oestrogen and glucocorticoid receptor messenger RNA levels. Int J Cancer 1990;46:1081.

74. Castles CG, Fuqua SA, Klotz DM, et al. Expression of a constitutively active estrogen receptor variant in the estrogen receptor-negative BT-20 human breast cancer cell line. Cancer Res 1993;53:5934.

75. Fuqua SAW, Fitzgerald SD, Chamness GC, et al. Variant human breast tumor estrogen receptor with constitutive transcriptional activity. Cancer Res 1991;51:105.

76. Kurokawa M, Michelangeli VP, Findlay DM. Induction of calcitonin receptor expression by glucocorticoids in T47D human breast cancer cells. J Endocrinol 1991;130:321.

77. Ozzello L, Sordat B, Merenda C, et al. Transplantation of a human mammary carcinoma cell line (BT 20) into nude mice. J Natl Cancer Inst 1974;52:1669.

78. Lasfargues EY, Coutinho WG, Redfield ES. Isolation of two human tumor epithelial cell lines from solid breast carcinomas. J Natl Cancer Inst 1978;61:967.

79. Horwitz KB, Mockus MB, Lessey BA. Variant T47D human breast cancer cells with high progesterone-receptor levels despite estrogen and antiestrogen resistance. Cell 1982;28:633.

80. Ballare C, Bravo AI, Laucella S, et al. DNA synthesis in estrogen receptor positive human breast cancer takes place preferentially in estrogen receptor-negative cells. Cancer 1989;64:842.

81. Shek LL, Godolphin W. Survival with breast cancer: the importance of estrogen receptor quantity. Eur J Cancer Clin Oncol 1989;25:243.

82. Clark GM, McGuire WL. Steroid receptors and other prognostic factors in primary breast cancer. Semin Oncol 1988;15:20.

83. Skoog L, Humla S, Axelsson M, et al. Estrogen receptor levels and survival of breast cancer patients. Acta Oncol 1987;26:95.

84. Halter SA, Fraker LD, Adcock D, et al. Effect of retinoids on xenotransplanted human mammary carcinoma cells in athymic mice. Cancer Res 1988;48:3733.

85. Cailleau R, Young R, Olive M, et al. Breast tumor cell lines from pleural effusions. J Natl Cancer Inst 1974;53:661.

86. Osborne CK, Coronado E, Allred DC, et al. Acquired tamoxifen resistance: correlation with reduced breast tumor levels of tamoxifen and isomerization of trans-4-hydroxytamoxifen. J Natl Cancer Inst 1991;83:1477.

87. Meschter CL, Connolly JM, Rose DP. Influence of regional location of the inoculation site and dietary fat on the pathology of MDA-MB-435 human breast cancer cell-derived tumors growing in nude mice. Clin Exp Metastasis 1992;10:167.

88. Rose DP, Connolly JM, Meschter CL. Effect of dietary fat on human breast cancer growth and lung metastasis in nude mice. J Natl Cancer Inst 1991;83:1491.

89. Rose DP, Hatala MA, Connolly JM, et al. Effect of diets containing different levels of linoleic acid on human breast cancer growth and lung metastasis in nude mice. Cancer Res 1993;53:4686.

90. Rose DP, Connolly JM. Influence of dietary fat intake on local recurrence and progression of metastases arising from MDA-MB-435 human breast cancer cells in nude mice after excision of the primary tumor. Nutr Cancer 1992;18:113.

91. Brünner N, Thompson EW, Spang-Thomsen M, et al. *lacZ* transduced human breast cancer xenografts as an in vivo model for the study of invasion and metastasis. Eur J Cancer 1992;28A:1989.

92. Siciliano MJ, Barker PE, Cailleau R. Mutually exclusive genetic signatures of human breast tumor cell lines with a common chromosomal marker. Cancer Res 1979;39:919.

93. Osborne CK, Lippman ME. Human breast cancer in tissue culture. In: McGuire WL, ed. Breast cancer advances in research and treatment. New York, Plenum, 1978:103.

94. Kaplan O, Jaroszewski JW, Faustino PJ, et al. Toxicity and effects of epidermal growth factor on the glucose metabolism of MDA-468 human breast cancer cells. J Biol Chem 1990;265:13641.

95. McLeskey SW, Ding IY, Lippman ME, et al. MDA-MB-134 breast carcinoma cells overexpress fibroblast growth factor (FGF) receptors and are growth-inhibited by FGF ligands. Cancer Res 1994;54:523.

96. Langton BC, Crenshaw MC, Chao LA, et al. An antigen immunologically related to the external domain of gp185 is shed from nude mouse tumors overexpressing the c-erbB2 (HER-2/neu) oncogene. Cancer Res 1991;51:2593.

97. Kennedy DG, Clarke R, van den Berg HW, et al. The kinetics of methotrexate polyglutamate formation and efflux in a human breast cancer cell line (MDA-MB-436): the effect of insulin. Biochem Pharmacol 1983;32:41.

98. Kennedy DG, van den Berg HW, Clarke R, et al. The effect of the rate of cell proliferation on the synthesis of methotrexate poly-τ-glutamates in two human breast cancer cell lines. Biochem Pharmacol 1985;34:3087.

99. Clarke R, van den Berg HW, Kennedy DG, et al. Reduction of the antimetabolic and antiproliferative effects of methotrexate by 17β-estradiol in a human breast carcinoma cell line (MDA-MB-436). Eur J Cancer Clin Oncol 1983;19:19.

100. Clarke R, van den Berg HW, Kennedy DG, et al. Oestrogen receptor status and the response of human breast cancer cells to a combination of methotrexate and 17β-estradiol. Br J Cancer 1985;51:365.

101. Clarke R, van den Berg HW, Murphy RF. Tamoxifen and 17β-estradiol reduce the membrane fluidity of human breast cancer cells. J Natl Cancer Inst 1990;82:1702.

102. Fogh J. Cell lines established from human tumors. In: Fogh J, ed. Human tumor cell lines in vitro. New York, Plenum, 1975:115.

103. Alpet O, Yamaguchi K, Hitomi J, et al. The presence of c-erbB-2 gene product-related protein in culture medium conditioned by breast cancer cell line SK-BR-3. Cell Growth Different 1990;1:591.

104. Goldman R, Levy MB, Peles E, et al. Heterodimerization of the erbB-1 and erbB-2 receptors in human breast carcinoma cells: a mechanism for receptor transregulation. Biochemistry 1990;29:11024.

105. Bronzert DA, Greene GL, Lippman ME. Selection and characterization of a breast cancer cell line resistant to the antiestrogen LY 117018. Endocrinology 1985;117:1409.

106. Nawata H, Chang MJ, Bronzert D, et al. Estradiol independent

growth of a subline of MCF-7 human breast cancer cells in culture. J Biol Chem 1981;256:6895.

107. Nawata H, Bronzert D, Lippman ME. Isolation and characterization of a tamoxifen resistant cell line derived from MCF-7 human breast cancer cells. J Biol Chem 1981;256:5016.

108. van den Berg HW, Clarke R. Preliminary characterization of a tamoxifen resistant variant of the oestrogen responsive human breast cancer cell line ZR-75-1. Br J Cancer 1985;52:421.

109. Gottardis MM, Jordan VC. Development of tamoxifen-stimulated growth of MCF-7 tumors in athymic mice after long-term antiestrogen administration. Cancer Res 1988;48:5183.

110. Osborne CK, Coronado EB, Robinson JP. Human breast cancer in athymic nude mice: cytostatic effects of long-term antiestrogen therapy. Eur J Cancer Clin Oncol 1987;23:1189.

111. Mullick A, Chambon P. Characterization of the estrogen receptor in two antiestrogen-resistant cell lines, LY2 and T47D. Cancer Res 1990;50:333.

112. Seibert K, Shafie SM, Triche TJ, et al. Clonal variation of MCF-7 breast cancer cells in vitro and in athymic nude mice. Cancer Res 1983;43:2223.

113. van Steenbrugge GJ, Groen M, van Kreuningen A, et al. Transplantable human prostatic carcinoma (PC-82) in athymic nude mice. III. Effects of estrogens on the growth of the tumor. Prostate 1988;12:157.

114. Brünner N, Svenstrup B, Spang-Thompsen M, et al. Serum steroid levels in intact and endocrine ablated Balb/c nude mice and their intact litter mates. J Steroid Biochem 1986;25:429.

115. Clarke R, Lippman ME. Antiestrogens resistance: mechanisms and reversal. In: Teicher BA, ed. Drug resistance in oncology. New York, Marcel Dekker, 1992:501.

116. Jiang SY, Parker CJ, Jordan VC. A model to describe how a point mutation of the estrogen receptor alters the structure–function relationship of antiestrogens. Breast Cancer Res Treat 1993;26:139.

117. Jiang SY, Langan-Fahey SM, Stella AL, et al. Point mutation of estrogen receptor (ER) in the ligand-binding domain changes the pharmacology of antiestrogens in ER-negative breast cancer cells stably expressing complementary DNAs for ER. Mol Endocrinol 1992;6:2167.

118. Engelsman E. Therapy of advanced breast cancer: a review. Eur J Cancer Clin Oncol 1983;19:1775.

119. Gockerman JP, Spremulli EN, Raney M, et al. Randomized comparison of tamoxifen versus diethylstilbestrol in estrogen receptor-positive or -unknown metastatic breast cancer: a southeastern cancer study group trial. Cancer Treat Rep 1986;70:1199.

120. Vogel CL, East DR, Voigt W, et al. Response to tamoxifen in estrogen receptor-poor metastatic breast cancer. Cancer 1987; 60:1184.

121. Howell A, Dodwell DJ, Anderson H, et al. Response after withdrawal of tamoxifen and progestogens in advanced breast cancer. Ann Oncol 1992;3:611.

122. Belani CP, Pearl P, Whitley NO, et al. Tamoxifen withdrawal response: report of a case. Arch Intern Med 1989;149:449.

123. Stein W, Hortobagyi GN, Blumenschein GR. Response of metastatic breast cancer to tamoxifen withdrawal: report of a case. J Surg Oncol 1983;22:45.

124. McIntosh IH, Thynne GS. Tumour stimulation by anti-oestrogens. Br J Surg 1977;64:900.

125. Canney PA, Griffiths T, Latief TN, et al. Clinical significance of tamoxifen withdrawal response. Lancet 1989;1:36.

126. Beex LVAM, Pieters GFFM, Smals AGH, et al. Diethylstilbestrol versus tamoxifen in advanced breast cancer. N Engl J Med 1981;304:1041.

127. Brünner N, Frandsen TL, Holst-Hansen C, et al. MCF7/LCC2: a 4-hydroxytamoxifen resistant human breast cancer variant which retains sensitivity to the steroidal antiestrogen ICI 182,780. Cancer Res 1993;53:3229.

128. Coopman P, Garcia M, Brünner N, et al. Antiproliferative and antiestrogenic effects of ICI 164,384 in 4-OH-tamoxifen-resistant human breast cancer cells. Int J Cancer 1994;56:295.

129. Nicholson RI, Gee JMW, Anderson E, et al. Phase I study of a new pure antiestrogen ICI 182,780 in women with primary breast cancer: immunohistochemical analysis. Breast Cancer Res Treat 1993;27:135.

130. Brünner N, Boysen B, Kiilgaard TL, et al. Resistance to 4OH-tamoxifen does not confer resistance to the steroidal antiestrogen ICI 182,780, while acquired resistance to ICI 182,780 results in cross resistance to 4OH-TAM. (Abstract) Breast Cancer Res Treat 1993;27:135.

131. Schneider J, Bak M, Efferth T, et al. P-glycoprotein expression in treated and untreated human breast cancer. Br J Cancer 1989;60:815.

132. Koh EH, Chung HC, Lee KB, et al. The value of immunohistochemical detection of P-glycoprotein in breast cancer before and after induction chemotherapy. Yonsei Med J 1992;33:137.

133. Sanfilippo O, Ronchi E, De Marco C, et al. Expression of P-glycoprotein in breast cancer tissue and in vitro resistance to doxorubicin and vincristine. Eur J Cancer 1991;27:155.

134. Salmon SE, Grogan TM, Miller T, et al. Prediction of doxorubicin resistance in vitro in myeloma, lymphoma and breast cancer by P-glycoprotein staining. J Natl Cancer Inst 1989;81:696.

135. Veneroni S, Zaffaroni N, Daidone MG, et al. Expression of P-glycoprotein and in vitro or in vivo resistance to doxorubicin and cisplatin in breast and ovarian cancers. Eur J Cancer 1994; 30A:1002.

136. Vickers PJ, Dickson RB, Shoemaker R, et al. A multidrug-resistant MCF-7 human breast cancer cell line which exhibits cross-resistance to antiestrogens and hormone independent tumor growth. Mol Endocrinol 1988;2:886.

137. Willingham MC, Cornwell MM, Cardarelli CO, et al. Single cell analysis of daunomycin uptake and efflux in multidrug resistant and sensitive KB cells: effects of verapamil and other drugs. Cancer Res 1986;46:5941.

138. Zyad A, Bernard J, Clarke R, et al. Human breast cancer cross-resistance to TNF and adriamycin: relationship to MDR1, MnSOD and TNF gene expression. Cancer Res 1994;54:825.

139. Doroshow JH, Akman S, Esworthy S, et al. Doxorubicin resistance is conferred by selective enhancement of intracellular glutathione peroxidase or superoxide dismutase content in human MCF-7 breast cancer cells. Free Radic Res 1991;12:779.

140. Iwamoto S, Takeda K. Possible cytotoxic mechanisms of TNF in vitro. Hum Cell 1990;3:107.

141. Batist G, Tuple A, Sinha BK, et al. Overexpression of a novel anionic glutathione transferase in multidrug-resistant human breast cancer cells. J Biol Chem 1986;261:15544.

142. Sinha BK, Mimnaugh EG, Rajagopalan S, et al. Adriamycin activation and oxygen free radical formation in human breast tumor cells: protective role of glutathione peroxidase in adriamycin resistance. Cancer Res 1989;49:3844.

143. Ford JM, Bruggemann EP, Pastan I, et al. Cellular and biochemical characterization of thioxanthenes for reversal of multidrug resistance in human and murine cell lines. Cancer Res 1990;50:1748.

144. Clarke R, Currier S, Kaplan O, et al. Effect of P-glycoprotein expression on sensitivity to hormones in MCF-7 human breast cancer cells. J Natl Cancer Inst 1992;84:1506.

145. Kaplan O, Jaroszewski JW, Clarke R, et al. The multidrug resistance phenotype: 31P NMR characterization and 2-deoxyglucose toxicity. Cancer Res 1991;51:1638.

146. Stampfer M, Hallowes RC, Hackett AJ. Growth of normal human mammary cells in culture. In Vitro 1980;16:415.

147. Smith HS. In vitro models in human breast cancer. In: Harris J, Hellman S, Henderson IC, et al. Breast diseases, ed 2. Philadelphia, JB Lippincott, 1994.

148. Soule HD, Maloney TM, Wolman SR, et al. Isolation and characterization of a spontaneously immortalized human breast epithelial cell line, MCF-10. Cancer Res 1990;50:6075.

149. Stampfer MR, Bartley JC. Human mammary epithelial cells in culture: differentiation and transformation. In: Lippman ME, Dickson RB, eds. Breast cancer: Cellular and molecular biology. Boston, Kluwer Academic, 1988:1.

150. Clark R, Stampfer MR, Milley R, et al. Transformation of human mammary epithelial cells with oncogenic viruses. Cancer Res 1988;48:4689.

151. Valverius EM, Ciardiello F, Heldin NE, et al. Stromal influences on transformation of human mammary epithelial cells overexpressing c-myc and SV40T. J Cell Physiol 1990;145:207.

152. Pierce JH, Arnstein P, DiMarco E, et al. Oncogenic potential of erbb-2 in human mammary epithelial cells. Oncogene 1991; 6:1189.

153. Tait L, Soule H, Russo J. Ultrastructural and immunocytochemical characterization of a immortalized human breast epithelial cell line, MCF-10. Cancer Res 1990;50:6087.

154. Ochieng J, Basolo F, Albini A, et al. Increased invasive, chemotactic and locomotive abilities of c-Ha-ras-transformed human breast epithelial cells. Invasion Metastasis 1991;11:38.

155. Ciardello F, Gottardis M, Basolo F, et al. Additive effects of c-erbB-2, c-Ha-ras, and transforming growth factor-α genes on in vitro transformation of human mammary epithelial cells. Mol Carcinog 1992;6:43.

156. Schirrmacher V. Cancer metastasis: experimental approaches, theoretical concepts and impacts for treatment strategies. Adv Cancer Res 1985;43:1.

157. Terranova VP, Hujanen ES, Martin GR. Basement membrane and the invasive activity of metastatic tumor cells. J Natl Cancer Inst 1986;77:311.

158. Barsky SH, Siegal GP, Jannotta F, et al. Loss of basement membrane components by invasive tumors but not by their benign counterparts. Lab Invest 1994;49:140.

159. Liotta LA, Rao CN, Barsky SH. Tumor invasion and the extracellular matrix. Lab Invest 1994;49:636.

160. Barsky SH, Togo S, Garbisa S, et al. Type IV collagenase immunoreactivity in invasive breast carcinoma. Lancet 1994;1:296.

161. Kleinman HK, McGarvey ML, Hassell JR, et al. Basement membrane complexes with biological activity. Biochemistry 1986; 25:312.

162. Bae S-N, Arand G, Azzam H, et al. Molecular and cellular analysis of basement membrane invasion by human breast cancer cells in matrigel-based in vitro assays. Breast Cancer Res Treat 1993; 24:241.

163. Albini A, Iwamoto Y, Kleinman HK, et al. A rapid in vitro assay for quantitating the invasive potential of tumor cells. Cancer Res 1987;47:3239.

164. Frandsen TL, Boysen BE, Jirus S, et al. Experimental models for the study of human cancer cell invasion and metastasis. Fibrinolysis 1992;6 (Suppl 4):71.

165. Thompson EW, Reich R, Shima TB, et al. Differential regulation of growth and invasiveness of MCF-7 breast cancer cells by antiestrogens. Cancer Res 1988;48:6764.

166. Thompson EW, Torri J, Sabol M, et al. Oncogene-induced basement membrane invasiveness in human mammary epithelial cells. Clin Exp Metastasis 1994;12:181.

167. Beatson GT. On the treatment of inoperable cases of carcinoma of the mamma: suggestions from a new method of treatment, with illustrative cases. Lancet 1896;2:104.

168. Campisi J, Pardee AB. Post-transcriptional control of the onset of DNA synthesis by an insulin-like growth factor. Mol Cell Biol 1984;4:1807.

169. Shi YE, Torri J, Yieh L, et al. Expression of 67 kDa laminin receptor in human breast cancer cells: regulation by progestins. Clin Exp Metastasis 1993;11:251.

170. Thompson EW, Katz D, Shima TB, et al. ICI 164,384: a pure antagonist of estrogen-stimulated MCF-7 cell proliferation and invasiveness. Cancer Res 1989;49:6929.

171. Cattoretti G, Andreola S, Clemente C, et al. Vimentin and P53 expression in epidermal growth factor receptor-positive oestrogen receptor-negative breast carcinomas. Br J Cancer 1988;57:353.

172. Raymond WA, Leong AS-Y. Co-expression of cytokeratin and vimentin intermediate filament proteins in benign and neoplastic breast epithelium. J Pathol 1989;157:299.

173. Raymond WA, Leong AS-Y. A new prognostic parameter in breast carcinoma? J Pathol 1989;158:107.

174. Domagala W, Lasota J, Bartowiak J, et al. Vimentin is preferentially expressed in human breast carcinomas with low estrogen receptor and high Ki67 growth fraction. Am J Pathol 1994;136:219.

175. Domagala W, Leszek W, Lasota J, et al. Vimentin is preferentially expressed in high grade ductal and medullary, but not in lobular breast carcinomas. Am J Pathol 1994;137:1059.

176. Gamallo C, Palacios J, Suarez A, et al. Correlation of E-cadherin expression with differentiation grade and histological type in breast carcinoma. Am J Pathol 1993;142:987.

177. Rasbridge SA, Gillett CE, Sampson SA, et al. Epithelial (E-) and placental (P-) cadherin cell adhesion molecule expression in breast carcinoma. J Pathol 1993;169:245.

178. Oka H, Shiozaki H, Kobayashi K, et al. Expression of E-cadherin cell adhesion molecule in human breast cancer tissues and its relationship to metastases. Cancer Res 1993;53:1696.

179. Thiery J-P, Boyer B, Tucker G, et al. Adhesion mechanisms in embryogenesis and in cancer invasion and metastasis. Ciba Found Symp 1988;141:48.

180. Sommers SL, Byers SW, Thompson EW, et al. Differentiation state and invasiveness of human breast cancer cell lines. Breast Cancer Res Treat 1994;31:325.

181. Sommers CL, Heckford SE, Skerker JM, et al. Loss of epithelial markers and acquisition of vimentin expression in adriamycin- and vinblastine-resistant human breast cancer cells. Cancer Res 1992;52:5190.

182. Brünner N, Johnson MD, Holst-Hansen C, et al. Acquisition of estrogen independence and antiestrogen resistance in breast cancer: association with the invasive and metastatic phenotype. Endocr Relat Cancer 1995;2:27.

183. Ura H, Bonfil RD, Reich R, et al. Expression of type IV collagenase and procollagen genes and its correlation with the tumorigenic, invasive and metastatic abilities of oncogene-transformed human bronchial epithelial cells. Cancer Res 1989;49:4615.

184. Bonfil DR, Reddel RR, Ura H, et al. Invasive and metastatic potential of a v-Ha-ras transformed human bronchial epithelial cell line. J Natl Cancer Inst 1989;81:587.

185. Simpson RJ, Smith JA, Moritz RL, et al. Rat epidermal growth factor: complete amino acid sequence. Eur J Biochem 1985; 153:629.

186. Thorgeirsson UP, Turpeenniemi-Hujanen T, Williams JE, et al. NIH/3T3 cells transfected with human tumor cDNA containing activated ras oncogenes express the metastatic phenotype in nude mice. Mol Cell Biol 1985;5:259.

187. Albini A, Graf J, Kitten GT, et al. 17β-estradiol regulates and V-Ha-ras transfection constitutively enhances MCF-7 breast cancer cell interactions with basement membrane. Proc Natl Acad Sci USA 1986;83:8182.

188. Sommers CL, Papageorge A, Wilding G, et al. Growth properties and tumorigenesis of MCF-7 cells transfected with isogenic mutants of rasH. Cancer Res 1990;50:67.

189. Van Roy F, Mareel M, Vleminckx K, et al. Hormone sensitivity *in vitro* and *in vivo* of v-ras-transfected MCF-7 cell derivatives. Int J Cancer 1990;46:522.

190. Muschel RJ, Williams JE, Lowy DR, et al. Harvey ras induction of metastatic potential depends upon oncogene activation and type of recipient cell. Am J Pathol 1985;121:1.

191. Taylor-Papadimitriou J, Stampfer MR, Bartek J, et al. Keratin expression in human mammary epithelial cells cultured from normal and malignant tissues: relation to *in vivo* phenotypes and influences of medium. J Cell Sci 1989;94:403.

192. Nicholson GL, Gallick GE, Sphon WH, et al. Transfection of activated c-Ha-rasEJ/pSV2neo genes into rat mammary cells: rapid stimulation of clonal diversification of spontaneous metastatic and cell surface properties. Oncogene 1992;7:1127.

193. De Vita VT. Principles of chemotherapy: In: De Vita VT, Hellman S, Rosenberg SA, eds. Cancer: principles and practice of oncology. Philadelphia, JB Lippincott, 1989:276.

194. Fracchia AA, Knapper WH, Carey JT, et al. Intrapleural chemotherapy for effusion from metastatic breast cancer. Cancer 1970;26:626.

195. Van Netten JP, Armstrong JB, Carlyle SS, et al. Estrogen receptor distribution in the peripheral, intermediate and central regions of breast cancers. Eur J Cancer Clin Oncol 1988;24:1885.

196. Meltzer P, Leibovitz A, Dalton W, et al. Establishment of two new cell lines derived from human breast carcinomas with HER2/neu amplification. Br J Cancer 1991;63:727.

197. Whitescarver J. Problems of in vitro culture of human mammary tumor cells. J Invest Dermatol 1974;63:58.

198. Foley JF, Aftonomos BT. Growth of human breast neoplasms in cell culture. J Natl Cancer Inst 1965;34:217.

199. Bastert G, Fortmeyer HP, Eichholz H, et al. Human breast cancer in thymus aplastic nude mice. In: Bastert GB, ed. Thymus-aplastic nude mice and rats in clinical oncology. New York, Springer-Verlag, 1981:157.

200. Berger DP, Winterhalter BR, Fiebig HH. Establishment and characterization of human tumor xenografts in thymus-aplastic nude mice. In: Fiebig HH, Berger DP, eds. Immunodeficient mice in oncology. Basel, Karger, 1992:23.

201. Federoff S, Evans VJ, Perry VP, et al, eds. Manual of the tissue culture association. 1975:53.

202. Gibson SL, Hilf R. Regulation of estrogen-binding capacity by insulin in 7,12-dimethylbenz(a)anthracene-induced mammary tumors in rats. Cancer Res 1980;40:2343.

203. Barnes D, Sato G. Growth of a human mammary tumor cell line in a serum free medium. Nature 1978;281:388.

204. Vignon F, Bouton MM, Rochefort H. Antiestrogens inhibit the mitogenic effect of growth factors on breast cancer cells in the total absence of estrogens. Biochem Biophys Res Commun 1987;146:1502.

205. Koga M, Sutherland RL. Epidermal growth factor partially reverses the inhibitory effects of antiestrogens on T47D human breast cancer cell growth. Biochem Biophys Res Commun 1987;146:738.

206. Berthois Y, Katzenellenbogen JA, Katzenellenbogen BS. Phenol red in tissue culture is a weak estrogen: implications concerning the study of estrogen-responsive cells in culture. Proc Natl Acad Sci USA 1986;83:2496.

207. Bindal RD, Carlson KE, Katzenellenbogen BS, et al. Lipophylic impurities, not phenolsulfonphthalein, account for the estrogenic properties in commercial preparations of phenol red. J Steroid Biochem 1988;31:287.

208. Darbre P, Yates J, Curtis S, et al. Effect of estradiol on human breast cancer cells in culture. Cancer Res 1983;43:349.

209. Vignon F, Terqui M, Westley B, et al. Effects of plasma estrogen sulfates in mammary cancer cells. Endocrinology 1980;106:1079.

210. van der Burg B, Ruterman GR, Blankenstein MA, et al. Mitogenic stimulation of human breast cancer cells in a growth factor-defined medium: synergistic action of insulin and estrogen. J Cell Physiol 1988;134:101.

211. Reddel RR, Murphy LC, Sutherland RI. Factors affecting the sensitivity of T-47D human breast cancer cells to tamoxifen. Cancer Res 1984;44:2398.

212. Strobl JS, Lippman ME. Prolonged retention of estradiol by human breast cancer cells in tissue culture. Cancer Res 1979;39:3319.

213. Freshney RI. Culture of animal cells: a manual of basic technique. New York, Wiley-Liss, 1991.

214. Hayflick L. Tissue culture. New York, Academic Press, 1973.

215. Methods in enzymology LVIII: cell culture methods. New York, Academic, 1979.

7.9

Estrogen and Progesterone Receptors and Breast Cancer

SUZANNE A.W. FUQUA

The purpose of this review is to highlight some of the recent advances in our understanding of the mechanism of action of steroid hormones in breast cancer. The discussion focuses on those alterations in the estrogen receptor (ER) that have been detected in human breast cancer biopsies, and data are presented that suggest that alterations in the ER might have important biologic and clinical consequences.

Background

Estrogens and progestins are considered the primary regulators of growth and differentiation of normal mammary tissue. Moreover, estrogens are thought to play an important role in the development and progression of breast cancer. This concept is based on several lines of evidence. First, epidemiologic evidence indicates a protective effect concomitant with ovariectomy and an increased risk of developing breast cancer among women treated with the estrogen diethylstilbestrol.[1,2] In addition, the mitogenic effects of estrogens on various breast cancer cell lines grown in culture, and in vivo in ovariectomized nude mice have been well documented in the literature.[3,4] Reports have also demonstrated that the use of oral contraceptives starting at a young age significantly increases the risk of breast cancer.[5] This cohort of women had a significant relationship between survival and exposure to oral contraceptives at a young age.[6] These results suggest that estrogens do indeed participate in tumor growth promotion and, later, in progression of the disease.

Estrogens and progestins exert their cellular effects through the binding and activation of specific nuclear receptors, the ER and the progesterone receptor (PR). When evaluating the role of these receptors in breast cancer, two issues are important. First, the absence of ER and PR predicts early recurrence and poor survival of breast cancer patients. Second, the presence of these receptors in tumors predicts the likelihood of benefit from endocrine therapy. Since the original publication suggesting the value of ER as a prognostic biomarker of delayed recurrence in primary breast cancer,[7] ER and PR assays have become standard practice in the management of breast cancer. As a single factor, PR has been shown to be a more powerful independent predictor of tumor recurrence than ER in certain subsets of patients, such as those with stage II breast cancer.[8] We now know that the correlation between ER and PR status and patient outcome is a general reflection of the intrinsic biologic behavior of receptor-positive tumors. ER- and PR-positive tumors are more likely to be highly differentiated, to be diploid, and to exhibit lower proliferative rates than are receptor-negative tumors.[9,10] The value of steroid receptors as single, independent prognostic biomarkers is limited, however, and they are most effectively used in combination with other prognostic biomarkers.[11,12]

Potentially of greater importance is the ability of ER and PR to predict response to endocrine therapy. The ER assay is most useful if the tumor is ER-negative; these patients seldom respond to endocrine therapy. The knowledge of ER and PR status together improves the ability to predict endocrine responsiveness. This finding is based on a hypothesis first published by Horwitz and associates,[13] suggesting that PR might be a better marker than ER for an intact endocrine response pathway because PR is a product of estrogen action. Indeed, this appears to be the case. Response rates higher than 70% are seen in metastatic ER-positive, PR-positive tumors.[14,15] In addition, a quantitative correlation appears to exist between receptor content and response, with some studies finding a quantitative correlation only with ER levels[16] and others finding correlations with both ER and PR levels.[17]

Predicting the probability of response in the discordant receptor phenotype, such as those tumors that are ER-negative and PR-positive, or those tumors that are ER-positive but PR-negative is more difficult. These tumors are intermediate in response, with response rates between 40% to 50% obtainable in advanced breast cancer.[14] The paradoxic behavior of the discordant receptor phenotype is further reflected in the data shown in Table 7.9-1. My colleagues and I have determined the proliferative rate in over 100,000 breast tumors contained within our SPORE Tumor Bank and National Resource using flow cytometric analysis of tumor powder remaining after steroid receptor assay.[18] We have shown that tumors containing both ER and PR exhibit low median S-phase fractions (SPF); conversely, tumors lacking these receptors exhibit high SPFs. Both discordant receptor phenotypes manifest significantly higher SPFs, as compared with tumors containing ER and PR. We hypothesized that the discordant receptor phenotype may be the result of a dysfunctional estrogen response pathway, or it may reflect the presence

TABLE 7.9-1
Estrogen Receptor and Proliferative Rate in Breast Tumors

Status	N	S-Phase Fraction
ER+, PR+	60,567	4.3
ER+, PR−	26,653	6.3
ER−, PR+	3,483	7.4
ER−, PR−	15,802	11.2

ER, estrogen receptor; PR, progesterone receptor.

of altered ERs.[19,20] These studies are fully discussed in the section of this chapter on ER variants. What is readily apparent from these data, however, is that an intact estrogen response pathway, as demonstrated by the majority of receptor-positive tumors, is an important determinant of tumor aggressiveness and endocrine response.

Estrogen and Progesterone Receptor Functional Domains

Since the original cloning of cDNAs for ER[21,22] and PR,[23] an explosion of information in the field of steroid hormone action has occurred. I do not attempt to review exhaustively those studies that have shaped our current understanding of steroid receptor structure and function,[23–25] but rather I focus on the pivotal studies that provide a background for evaluating the potential role of specific ER and PR alterations in breast cancer development and progression.

ER and PR belong to a superfamily of nuclear hormone receptors that function as transcription factors when they are bound to their respective ligand. On estrogen binding, the ER forms homodimers and binds to DNA with high affinity at specific sites, termed estrogen-responsive elements (or EREs).[26,27] EREs have classically been viewed as two inverted, palindromic half-sites separated by three variant nucleotides. Of interest is the recent discovery that novel sequences containing restricted homology to the canonical ERE half-site can function as EREs in mammalian cells.[28] This expansion of potential EREs could lead to the identification of new cellular targets of steroid hormone action, such as genes that are regulated by estrogen and could be possible candidates for future clinical intervention.

The ER influences the expression of estrogen-responsive genes, such as the PR, which are important in mitogenic signaling by incompletely understood mechanisms. Transcription is stimulated through at least two distinct transactivation domains located in the amino-terminal region and the carboxy-terminal hormone-binding region of the receptor.[29–31] These two ER regions appear to act in concert to produce full transcriptional activity on estrogen-responsive genes. The genomic organization of the human ER gene is complex, with eight exons spanning greater than 140-kb pairs of DNA.[32] The two ER transcriptional activation domains are not encoded within single exons, but rather encompass large regions of the receptor. A hormone-independent, amino-terminal ER activation domain is contained within exons 1 and 2 and is termed AF-1. A hormone-dependent, carboxy-terminal activation domain is contained within portions of exons 4 through 8 and is termed AF-2.[33] A region within AF-2 is highly conserved among nuclear hormone receptors and is composed of hydrophobic and charged residues critically important for hormone-dependent transcriptional activation.[34]

A third activation domain identified in the human ER within the N-terminal part of AF-2 has been designated AF-2a.[35] This region has either a constitutive transcriptional activating function or, alternatively, a stimulatory effect on AF-1. In addition, these authors identified a negatively acting domain just C-terminal to AF-2a.[35] This region is also involved in binding of heat shock protein 90, which helps to modulate receptor activation.[36-38] Similarly, a third potential activation domain has been identified within the amino terminus of the B form of the PR.[39] Thus, it appears that the steroid receptor–transactivation domains are more complex than previously appreciated, and further work will be required to delineate completely the various regions important for different transcriptional activating functions.

Individual residues distributed throughout the ER hormone-binding domain seem to be required for estrogen and antiestrogen binding. Site-directed mutagenesis and affinity-labeling studies have revealed that the hormone-binding pocket partially overlaps a region contained within the carboxy terminus required for dimerization of the receptor.[40] Cysteine 530 of the human ER is the major site labeled by both the estrogen ketononestrol aziridine, and the antiestrogen tamoxifen aziridine,[41] demonstrating that the regions for hormone and antiestrogen binding are coincident. This amino acid and other nearby cysteines, however, can be mutated without dramatically affecting estrogen binding,[40,42] illustrating that cysteine 530 is not absolutely required for binding, but rather that it must lie near those residues required. Danielian and colleagues have identified residues between amino acids 518 and 525 of the mouse ER (corresponding to residues 514 to 521 of the human ER) that, when mutated, reduce estrogen binding without affecting antiestrogen binding.[43] Similarly, mutation of lysines 529 and 531 of the human ER reduces estrogen binding, but not binding by the antiestrogen hydroxytamoxifen.[44] Thus, certain residues scattered through the C-terminal region of the hormone-binding domain confer differential sensitivity to estrogen and tamoxifen.

The important question, however, is whether specific alterations in ER or PR could account for some forms of clinical hormone resistance. Before detailing the alterations that have been found to date in these receptors, any alteration found must be analyzed in the context of other important cellular variables. An area of current research is focused on alternative pathways of steroid receptor activation. Cross-talk between the ER and the protein kinase A (PKA) pathway has been observed,[45-47] and stimulation of the PKA pathway has been found to activate the agonist activity of antiestrogens.[48] This finding has potential clinical importance in tamoxifen-resistant breast cancer if fluctuations in PKA activators, such as cyclic adenosine monophosphate (cAMP) are found to accompany the development of resistance. Similar results have been observed with antagonist-occupied PR[49]; one study suggests that this agonist–antagonist switch is specific only for the B form of the PR.[50] In addition, certain growth factors, such as insulin-like growth factor 1, can stimulate ER activity.[51]

Another factor to be considered in evaluating any specific ER or PR alteration in breast cancer is that both cellular and promoter context are important in dictating transcriptional activity.[52] On certain promoters, both AF-1 and 2 are required; on other promoters, these activation domains can function independently.[53] In the cervical carcinoma HeLa cell line, AF-1 exhibits only 5% of the transactivation activity of wild-type receptor; in chicken embryo fibroblast cells, it has about half.[31] Finally, it is now becoming evident that another level of complexity exists in interpreting steroid hormone action; specific accessory proteins directly interact with ER and PR. These receptor-associated proteins influence activity as negative regulators,[54] as enhancers of DNA binding,[55,56] and as necessary components of the activated receptor complex.[57,58] These data could help explain the paradoxic agonistic activity of antagonists in different cell systems.

Protein Studies

The loss of PR is a relatively frequent event associated with a poorer survival after endocrine therapy,[59] but a paucity of studies explores this clinical phenomenon. The simple loss of ER protein expression in tumors does not explain endocrine resistance, however; ER expression is maintained at recurrence in most cases.[60] Only a few studies have used protein-based, ER functional assays to address the question of whether specific ER defects are associated with particular tumor phenotypes or clinical outcome. Raam and associates[61] used an in vitro nuclear DNA-binding assay, coupled with immunohistochemical assessment, to demonstrate that ERs deficient in DNA or estrogen binding were present in a subset of endocrine-resistant breast tumors. Unfortunately, the technique used in this early study has not been validated in other studies to date, nor have these investigators reported the molecular basis for their observations.

Greene and colleagues were the first to report the preparation of a library of monoclonal antibodies to the human ER[62,63] and human PR,[64] antibodies that have been invaluable for a variety of techniques. Immunohistochemical evaluation with these antibodies has been found to correlate well with biochemical quantitations of ER and PR,[65,66] such that many clinical laboratories are now using these antibodies for routine immunohistochemical analysis or for enzyme immunoassay of receptor status in breast tumors.[67-69] When these ER-specific antibodies have been combined with gel-retardation analyses, sensitive detection of functional ER DNA binding from breast tumor samples has been reported.[70] This study is noteworthy because it demonstrates the presence of truncated forms of DNA-binding ER, and of non–DNA-binding ER, in human breast tumor samples that nevertheless express immunoreactive ER. These investigators have since determined that a significant percentage of ER-positive tumors, especially those with low ER protein levels, express the non–DNA-binding ER, and they have hypothesized that this defect results from posttranslational ER modifications.[70] Furthermore, these studies highlight that current immunohistochemical or biochemical ER assays used clinically are incapable of evaluating the functional capacity of the receptor and thus are limited for the evaluation of specific functional domains within the ER. Unfortunately, my own unpublished observations show that the first generation of receptor monoclonal antibodies has not proved useful in sensitive detection of putative receptor isoforms or truncated receptors from clinical samples in Western blot analysis. One hopes that the second-generation panel of monoclonal antibodies, recently available,[71] will prove more advantageous for Western blot analysis of breast tumor samples.

DNA Studies

As soon as cDNAs to the human ER became available for use, several groups quickly investigated whether genomic ER structure was altered in breast cancer, a likely possibility given the extensive cytogenetic changes documented in breast tumors. One of the central questions in all these studies was whether genomic deletion or rearrangement was the basis for the failure of some tumors to express ER. In a series of 188 primary breast tumor biopsies, my colleagues and I were unable to detect gross structural rearrangements of the ER gene using Southern hybridization analysis.[72] Subsequent studies have confirmed that large deletions, rearrangements, or gene amplifications in the ER are infrequent in breast cancer.[73,74] Our early genomic study also examined a PvuII restriction fragment length polymorphism (RFLP) and demonstrated that a particular allelotype was associated with ER-negative breast tumors.[72] The association of the PvuII RFLP with ER expression has not held up in two larger studies,[74,75] however, and because the RFLP is localized to an intronic region of the ER, our earlier results were probably spurious. Discrepancies such as this have led to the establishment of evaluation guidelines for potential prognostic biomarkers.[76] Unfortunately, few promising biomarkers, such as the ER PvuII RFLP, have been confirmed in independent, validation analyses.

Another plausible explanation for the absence of ER expression in ER-negative breast cancer cells is gene methylation. Studies examining this question again have

reached conflicting conclusions; some studies found no relationship between ER gene methylation patterns and ER expression in breast tumors,[73,77,78] but one study concluded that extensive methylation in the 5′ ER promoter region is associated with ER-negativity in breast cancer cell lines.[79] Because this last study actually examined a region known to be important for transcriptional control of gene expression, the cytosine-rich CpG islands, further work should be directed at determining whether abnormal methylation could indeed account for transcriptional inactivation of the ER, that is, ER-negativity.

In summary, it appears that the lack of ER expression in tumors is a transcriptional event, with evidence to date showing that ER-negative tumors are devoid of ER mRNA.[80] Thus, to delineate the elements within the 5′ ER region that are responsible for promoter activity in breast tumors will be important.[81,82] A negative element with strong silencing activity has been identified in the chicken ER promoter[83]; it is tempting to speculate that such negative elements may be involved in the transcriptional down-regulation of ER in human tumors. Two additional observations are of clinical interest. First, reported levels of measured ER in breast tumor biopsies have been rising, a rise that can not simply be explained by technical changes in assay conditions.[84] Shorter recurrence-free survival is associated with high ER levels in postmenopausal patients.[85] Thus, transcriptional control of the ER may prove important. Further work on the human promoter is definitely warranted and perhaps is overdue.

Estrogen Receptor Variants Isolated From Clinical Samples

Reports of altered ERs from breast cancer cells lines have been published[86-91]; however, this discussion focuses only on those altered ERs isolated from clinical samples. Several groups of investigators, using different recombinant DNA techniques, have reported variant forms of ER mRNA in human breast cancer biopsy samples; the locations of the ER variants isolated from clinical biopsy material are shown in Figure 7.9-1.

The first ER sequence alteration identified from human breast tumors was reported by Garcia and colleagues,[92] and it represents a silent polymorphism at codon 87 within the B region (exon 1) of the receptor.[93] This B-variant allele of ER has been shown to be associated with a history of spontaneous abortion in women with ER-positive, but not ER-negative, breast cancer.[94,95] A relationship does not appear to exist between the presence of the B-variant ER allele and breast cancer in women without a history of spontaneous abortion.[96] This group also reported a statistical association between the B variant and an increased height in women after adjusting for the effects of age and race.[97] Because the B variant represents a silent polymorphism, it has been hypothesized that a second mutation, either within the ER itself, or a neighboring gene, must be the important factor in the observed biologic associa-

FIGURE 7.9-1 The location of estrogen receptor (ER) alterations detected in human breast tumor biopsy specimens is diagrammed. Exons 1 through 8 are shown with the corresponding locations of the DNA and hormone binding domain of the ER. The locations of the B variant ER,[92] clones C.4, C.5, and C.26,[100] and the two ERs isolated from tamoxifen-resistant (TR) patients[103] are shown above the diagram. ER variants isolated by our group are shown below the diagram, and include a 6 bp insertion,[107] which is active in transactivation assays (+), an exon 3 deletion variant,[105] which is devoid of activity (≠), an exon 5 deletion variant,[19] which is a dominant-positive receptor (+), and an exon 7 deletion variant,[20] which is a dominant-negative receptor (−) in breast cancer cells.

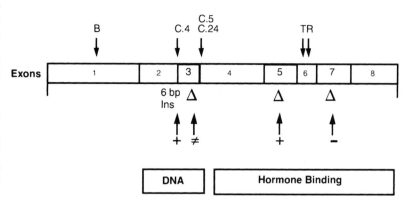

tions. In this regard, the first documented human estrogen resistance syndrome was due to a cytosine–thymine transition at codon 157, also within the B region of the ER, resulting in a premature stop codon.[98] In this report, the patient's mother had had three spontaneous abortions, and the authors hypothesized that heterozygous carriers of this mutation may have impaired fertility. Thus, certain alterations or distinct ER alleles may be subtly linked with clinical entities such as tall stature, spontaneous abortions, or infertility.

Murphy and associates analyzed 46 human breast tumor biopsies by Northern hybridization and detected smaller ER mRNAs, of 3.8 and 2.4 kb, that were coexpressed along with the wild-type 6.5-kb ER transcript.[99] The cDNAs for these variant ER mRNAs have now been cloned and represent either alternative or abnormal splicing of wild-type ER.[100,101] Some of the cDNAs, clones 5 and 24, were unique to a single breast tumor sample, whereas one cDNA, clone 4, was present in many of the tumors. Clones 5 and 24 are identical to wild-type ER up to the exon 3–intron boundary, at which their sequences diverge and are unrelated to ER (see Fig. 7.9-1). The origin of the unique sequences contained within ER variant clone 5 is unknown. The unique sequences of clone 24 have been localized to chromosome 12,[101] whereas human ER resides on chromosome 6.[102] This suggests that the clone 24 ER variant could have resulted from a *trans*-splicing mechanism because the majority of studies, as detailed earlier, have not shown major insertions, translocations, or rearrangements in the human ER gene.

The clone 4 ER variant contains wild-type ER sequences up to the exon 2–intron border, at which it diverges and contains sequences related to the long interspersed repetitive LINE-1 elements.[101] The origin of the introduced LINE-1 sequences in the clone 4 variant is unknown, but it appears likely that aberrant splicing may again play a role in the genesis of this variant transcript. These three variant ER mRNAs contain open reading frames that could encode proteins containing the entire (clones 5 and 24) or a portion (clone 4) of the DNA-binding domain of the receptor, but they would be missing the hormone-binding domain. In transient expression assays, both the clone 24 and the clone 4 ER variants were unable to activate an ERE-reporter construct in

COS cells.[100] Furthermore, these two variants were unable to modulate wild-type ER activity, indicating that they are nonfunctional, at least in this assay system.

To gain insight into a possible biologic role of the clone 4 ER variant in human breast cancer, its expression was measured in two groups of patients: those with a good prognosis and those with a bad prognosis, based on biologic factors such as ER–PR status, tumor size, ploidy, axillary lymph node status, and percentage of cells in S-phase (Murphy LC, Hilsenbeck SG, Dotzlaw H, and Fuqua SAW, unpublished observations). A total of 106 tumors were analyzed in this preliminary study. My colleagues and I determined that the clone 4 variant ER mRNA levels varied proportionally with wild-type ER mRNA levels, again suggesting that the variant results from alternative RNA splicing of wild-type ER. Regression analysis demonstrated that significantly higher levels of the variant were expressed relative to wild-type mRNA in tumors with poor prognostic biomarkers. Furthermore, the highest variant expression was found in the poor-prognosis, PR-negative tumors, suggesting a potential role for this variant in the development of hormone independence and progression in human breast cancer.

Reports of single base-pair changes within the ER have been few; however, Karnik and associates reported a 42 base-pair insertion and a single nucleotide deletion within exon 6 (see Fig. 7.9-1) of the ER from patients with tamoxifen-resistant breast cancer.[103] These alterations would both potentially result in carboxy-truncated receptors, but functional analyses of these two ER variants has not been reported. The authors examined a total of 20 tamoxifen-resistant tumors for ER alterations, and because alterations were found in only 2 of the tumors, they concluded that mutations in the ER occur at a low frequency and are not generally associated with tamoxifen resistance. Of issue in this study is the authors' definition of tamoxifen resistance. The time these patients received tamoxifen was not detailed; some of the relapses could have occurred before sufficient therapy had been given. The choice of primers used in this study may not have been optimal to identify alternatively spliced ER products, and furthermore, the method used, SSCP analysis, is known to be inadequate to identify all potential sequence alterations.[104] A similar study has been completed examining 30 patients who had received tamoxifen therapy for at least 6 months before disease recurrence (Zhang Q-X, Borg A, and Fuqua SAW, unpublished observations). In this study, direct sequencing of cDNA polymerase chain reaction (PCR) products was used, a sensitive method for detecting single base-pair alterations. Thus far, several ER alterations have been identified, and functional analyses are underway. Perhaps it may be premature to conclude that single base-pair ER alterations are really infrequent in breast cancer, especially among tamoxifen-treated patients.

Estrogen Receptor Variants Isolated From Breast Tumors With a Discordant Receptor Phenotype

To increase the likelihood of isolating ER variants, my colleagues and I began our investigation using specimens from patients who displayed a discordant receptor phenotype and that we already know display paradoxic clinical behaviors (Table 7.9-1). We originally proposed two different hypotheses in these patients (Fig. 7.9-2). First, we reasoned that alterations in the ER might occur whereby the receptor was capable of binding estrogen, but incapable of binding DNA and exerting control of estrogen-responsive genes, such as the PR. We predicted that this type of ER alteration would be found in ER-positive, PR-negative tumors, and these tumors would appear to be functionally ER-negative. Second, we hypothesized that we might detect alterations or truncations within the hor-

Functionally ER-negative?

Hormone independent?

FIGURE 7.9-2 A working model for estrogen receptor (ER) variants in either ER-positive, progesterone receptor (PgR)–negative (ER+/PgR−), or ER-negative, PgR-positive (ER−/PgR+) breast tumors. We hypothesize that ER variants are present in these lesions and are associated with dysfunctional estrogen responses or hormone-independent growth.

mone-binding domain of ER-negative, PR-positive tumors such that the ER would be unable to bind hormone and would thus appear ER-negative by hormone-binding assay, but would still be capable of independently stimulating estrogen-responsive genes such as PR. Furthermore, we hypothesized that these tumors might be hormone-independent.

ER-POSITIVE, PR-NEGATIVE TUMORS

Our first strategy was to focus on the DNA-binding domain of ER-positive, PR-negative tumors. We found, however, that most of these tumors contained ERs capable of DNA binding in gel-retardation analyses, and this conclusion was substantiated with direct sequence analysis of the DNA-binding region of selected tumors.[105] We concluded that the majority of these tumors do not contain mutations within the DNA-binding domain of the ER. Using gel-retardation analyses, however, we did identify tumors that contained an ER variant with an intact DNA-binding domain, but a truncation at the carboxy terminus.[20] The truncated variant is the result of a precise deletion of exon 7 in the hormone-binding domain of the ER (see Fig. 7.9-1).

We addressed the prevalence of exon 7 ER deletion variant RNA expression in ER-positive tumors and found that this variant was significantly more abundant in about half of the ER-positive, PR-negative breast tumors.[20] In addition, we showed that the variant was invariantly coexpressed along with wild-type receptor in these tumors. We next analyzed the transcriptional activity of this variant using a yeast transactivation assay system and found that it was devoid of transcriptional activity when expressed alone, but it exerted a potent dominant–negative effect on wild-type ER activity when coexpressed. Furthermore, we determined that this negative effect was due to its ability to inhibit the DNA-binding activity of wild-type receptor. We suggest that the overexpression of this variant plays a role in the genesis of certain breast tumors with the discordant ER-positive, PR-negative phenotype. We also propose that elevated levels of this naturally ocurring variant, as is frequently found in tumors (Zhang Q-X, Borg A, and Fuqua SAW, unpublished observation), may interfere with normal ER function and thus could render a tumor unresponsive to hormonal manipulations because the tumor is essentially ER-negative. A similar suggestion has been made with potent dominant–negative ERs constructed by site-directed mutagenesis.[106] This hypothesis awaits testing, but unfortunately it may prove difficult to pursue because overexpression of dominant–negative genes often results in growth inhibition.

ER-NEGATIVE, PR-POSITIVE TUMORS

Turning our attention to the ER-negative, PR-positive breast tumor subtype, we applied PCR amplification of cDNA to isolate an ER variant with a precise deletion of exon 5 of the hormone-binding domain[19] (see Fig. 7.9-1). Again, this variant appears to result from alternative splicing of wild-type ER and is coexpressed along with wild-type receptor. The exon 5 ER deletion variant displays about 10% to 15% activity of wild-type ER in one strain of yeast cells,[19] 40% to 50% in another strain of yeast[91] and almost 75% of wild-type ER activity in breast cancer cells.[107] Thus, its activity is highly dependent on the cellular environment in which it is expressed, not surprising given the available data on the transcriptional activity of AF-1 in different cell systems.[31,53] Constitutively active receptors, such as the exon 5 ER deletion variant, have been termed dominant–positive receptors.[108] Depending on the cell in which it is expressed, however, the levels of wild-type receptor coexpressed, and the overall transcriptional factor environment, it is conceivable that the exon 5 ER deletion variant may function either to *augment* (100% wild-type monomer ER activity plus 100% exon 5 variant monomer activity) or to *repress* (100% wild-type monomer ER activity plus 15% exon 5 variant monomer activity) the overall estrogen response, if functional heterodimers with wild-type ER are formed. Thus, it may be more appropriate to designate truncated ER variants as latent modulators of ER function in breast cancer cells that depend on the cellular milieu for signaling direction.

The exon 5 ER deletion variant was originally identified in the ER-negative, PR-positive breast cancer phenotype, which is a relatively rare subset of tumors.[109,110] My colleagues and I have observed, however, that it is almost always coexpressed at varying levels with wild-type ER in human breast cancers.[111] Its presence in ER-positive tumors suggests that it may play a crucial role in breast cancer progression. To address this question, we stably transfected ER-positive MCF-7 breast cancer cells with exon 5 ER deletion variant expression plasmids.[107] Another clinical problem we are trying to address is whether expression of the exon 5 ER deletion variant would modulate the growth of ER-positive breast cancer cells when they are exposed to antiestrogens, because the variant is missing the majority of the hormone domain of the receptor. We predict that cells coexpressing this variant might be resistant to the inhibitory effect of antiestrogens. We therefore tested the growth of our transfectants for anchorage-dependent growth in the presence of the nonsteroidal antiestrogens tamoxifen and 4-hydroxytamoxifen and the pure steroidal antiestrogen ICI 164,384. As expected, the growth of mock-transfected cells was inhibited by these agents; in contrast, the growth of the exon 5-transfected cells was unaffected by administration of either tamoxifen or 4-hydroxytamoxifen. These results suggest that cells expressing the exon 5 ER deletion variant, even when wild-type ER is coexpressed, are resistant to nonsteroidal antiestrogens.

My own unpublished observations show that the growth of the exon 5 ER transfectants was inhibited by the pure steroidal antiestrogen. This result was surprising, again because the exon 5 ER deletion variant is missing the majority of the hormone-binding domain of the receptor. A possible explanation for this observation is the data showing that the antiestrogen ICI 164,384 reduces cellular ER content by increasing its turnover and thus shortening its half-life in cells.[112] Furthermore, investigators have suggested that this antiestrogen impairs receptor dimeriza-

tion.[113] Therefore, the inhibitory action of the ICI 164,384 compound may be through the wild-type ER portion of an exon 5–wild-type ER heterodimer in transfected MCF-7 cells. This theory awaits confirmation in detailed DNA-binding studies with the exon 5 ER deletion variant.

These data tempt one to speculate that expression of the exon 5 ER deletion variant is involved in the hormone-independent breast cancer phenotype. Unfortunately, no reagents as yet are available to reliably measure its expression in a large number of clinical samples. Figure 7.9-3 represents an RNA-based technique that can be used to demonstrate variant expression in breast cancer samples; however, it is limited in its ability to measure the levels of the variant accurately, as compared with the levels of wild-type receptor in cells, because it involves PCR amplification. Regardless of the technique's limitations for absolute quantitation, it is apparent from this experiment that the exon 5 variant, although absent in the primary breast lesion, is abundantly expressed in the metastatic lesion from a patient undergoing tamoxifen therapy. The appearance during treatment of an ER variant with the ability to modulate ER activity and function in cells would be of obvious clinical concern. Future work should be directed at addressing this important question.

Breast Cancer Evolution

Unfortunately, little is known about the early events in breast carcinogenesis. A morphologic model of breast cancer evolution has been proposed,[114–116] based primarily on

FIGURE 7.9-3 The exon 5 estrogen receptor (ER) deletion variant is present in metastatic breast tumors. A primary and a metastatic (*met*) lesion were examined by polymerase chain reaction (PCR) amplification of ER cDNA. PCR primers were chosen such that both the wild-type (WT) ER product and the exon 5 ER deletion variant could be amplified. The metastatic lesion was a recurrence from a patient undergoing tamoxifen therapy. A nonspecific (NS) PCR fragment was also observed.

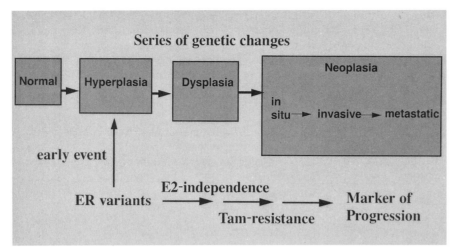

FIGURE 7.9-4 A model for breast cancer evolution that suggests that estrogen receptor (ER) variant expression may be an early event providing the environment for the series of genetic changes known to occur during tumor evolution. ER variant expression may also be a marker of estrogen independence, tamoxifen resistance (Tam-resistance), or tumor progression.

epidemiologic evidence.[113,117–120] In this model, diagrammed in Figure 7.9-4, human breast cancer is hypothesized as evolving through a series of genetic changes from normal epithelium to hyperplasia, to dysplasia, to carcinoma in situ, to invasive carcinoma, and finally, to metastatic carcinoma. Each lesion is predicted to be a nonobligatory precursor of the next, because some lesions may progress to the next stage and others may not. I would like to hypothesize further that either inappropriate expression of wild-type ER or expression of ER variants drives abnormal proliferation in premalignant hyperplasias, providing the environment for the genetic changes associated with the later evolutionary stages.

As detailed earlier, ample evidence indicates that estrogens play a role in the development and progression of breast cancer. Thus, ER expression may be a permissive event for breast cancer evolution. ER expression is low in normal breast epithelium.[121] Several studies indicate that ER expression is higher in adjacent premalignant or malignant lesions than in normal breast tissues.[122–124] One study even found that the incidence of ER expression paralleled the intensity of hyperplasia in some breast lesions.[125] One case-control study examining ER and PR expression in 51 patients with breast cancer and in 69 benign disease controls demonstrated that the presence of ER in benign breast epithelium was a significant risk factor for breast cancer development.[126]

With these historical data, my colleagues and I began a search for ER variants in breast hyperplasias. Using PCR amplification of cDNA, we isolated an ER variant from hyperplasias with an alteration (Lys 303 to Arg) in the beginning of the hormone-binding domain (Fuqua SAW, Wiltschke C, Allred DC, unpublished observations). When this ER variant is transiently transfected into the ER-negative MDA–MB-231 cell line, transcriptional activity of an ERE-reporter plasmid is elevated compared to wild-type ER. Furthermore, the variant is hypersensitive to superphysiologic levels of hormone. We are exploring whether this hypersensitivity and increased activity will similarly increase a breast cancer cell's proliferative response to hormone. We hypothesize that expression of

this ER variant may be one of the earliest events in breast cancer evolution.

Future Directions

Alternative splicing of the ER apparently is a frequent event in breast tumors. Alternative splicing is a mechanism whereby the primary transcript of the ER gene might be processed to yield mRNAs encoding proteins with specific functions in different cell types, and it might be an important mechanism of gene regulation in tumors. Unfortunately, nothing is known about the mechanisms underlying alternative splicing of the ER. The generation of truncated ERs, by alternative splicing or gene alteration, with the capability to enhance transcriptional activity even in the absence of hormone, may provide oncogenic potential in the early stages of tumor progression. Finally, single base-pair ER alterations, or polymorphisms, may play a role in estrogen independence or early breast disease. The molecular heterogeneity seen in the ER parallels the biologic diversity displayed by breast tumors, which has been clinically appreciated for many years. The ultimate significance of specific ER variant expression is only conjectural at present. Studies with sufficient power must be undertaken to determine the biologic significance of ER variants in breast cancer, because what we should have learned from the past is that conclusions drawn from small preliminary studies, especially if conducted with suboptimal reagents or techniques, are often reversed in larger clinical studies.

ACKNOWLEDGMENTS

The unpublished and in-press work referred to in this review was supported by NIH grants CA-52351, CA-30195, and CA-54171. The author would like to acknowledge the kind support and advice of her coworkers, Drs. D.C. Allred, R. Auchus, C.K. Osborne, D. Yee, D. Wolf, C. Castles, and C. Wiltschke.

References

1. Vessey MP. The involvement of oestrogen in the development and progression of breast disease: epidemiological evidence. Proc R Soc Edinb 1989;95B:35.
2. Henderson BE, Ross R, Bernstein L. Estrogens as a cause of human cancer. Cancer Res 1988;48:246.
3. Katzenellenbogen BS, Kendra KL, Norman MJ, et al. Proliferation, hormone responsiveness and estrogen receptor content of MCF-7 human breast cancer cells grown in the short-term and long-term absence of estrogens. Cancer Res 1987;47:4355.
4. Osborne CK, Hobbs K, Clark GM. Effect of estrogens and antiestrogens on growth of human breast cancer cells in athymic mice. Cancer Res 1985;45:584.
5. Olsson H, Moller TR, Ranstam J. Early oral contraceptive use and breast cancer among premenopausal women: final report from a study in southern Sweden. J Natl Cancer Inst 1989;81:1000.
6. Ranstam J, Olsson H, Garne J-P, et al. Survival in breast cancer and age at start of oral contraceptive usage. Anticancer Res 1991;11:2043.
7. Knight WA, Livingston RB, Gregory EJ, et al. Estrogen receptor as an independent prognostic factor for early recurrence in breast cancer. Cancer Res 1977;37:4669.
8. Clark GM, McGuire WL, Hubay CA, et al. Progesterone receptors as a prognostic factor in stage II breast cancer. N Engl J Med 1983;309:1343.
9. Clark GM, Osborne CK, McGuire WL. Correlations between estrogen receptor, progesterone receptor, and patient characteristics in human breast cancer. J. Clin Oncol 1984;2:1102.
10. Clark GM, McGuire WL. Steroid receptors and other prognostic factors in primary breast cancer. Semin Oncol 1988;15(Suppl 1):20.
11. McGuire WL. Estrogen receptor versus nuclear grade as prognostic factors in axillary node negative breast cancer. J Clin Oncol 1988;6(7):1071.
12. Osborne CK. Prognostic factors for breast cancer: have they met their promise? J Clin Oncol 1992;10:679.
13. Horwitz KB, McGuire WL, Pearson OH, et al. Predicting response to endocrine therapy in human breast cancer: a hypothesis. Science 1975;189:726.
14. Osborne CK, Yochmowitz MG, Knight WA, et al. The value of estrogen and progesterone receptors in the treatment of breast cancer. Cancer 1980;46:2884.
15. Bloom ND, Tobin EH, Schreibman B, et al. The role of progesterone receptors in the management of advanced breast cancer. Cancer 1980;45:2992.
16. Bezwoda WR, Esser JD, Dansey R, et al. The value of estrogen and progesterone receptor determinations in advanced breast cancer. Cancer 1991;68:867.
17. Ravdin PM, Green S, Dorr TM, et al. Prognostic significance of progesterone receptor levels in estrogen receptor-positive patients with metastatic breast cancer treated with tamoxifen: results of a prospective Southwest Oncology Group study. J Clin Oncol 1992;10:1284.
18. Wenger CR, Beardslee S, Owens MA, et al. DNA ploidy, S-phase, and steroid receptors in more than 127,000 breast cancer patients. Breast Cancer Res Treat 1993;28:9.
19. Fuqua SAW, Fitzgerald SD, Chamness GC, et al. Variant human breast tumor estrogen receptor with constitutive transcriptional activity. Cancer Res 1991;51:105.
20. Fuqua SAW, Fitzgerald SD, Allred DC, et al. Inhibition of estrogen receptor action by a naturally occurring variant in human breast tumors. Cancer Res 1992;52:483.
21. Greene GL, Gilna P, Walterfield M, et al. Sequence and expression of human estrogen receptor cDNA. Science 1986;231:1150.
22. Walter P, Green S, Greene G, et al. Cloning of the human estrogen receptor cDNA. Proc Natl Acad Sci USA 1985;82:7889.
23. Beato M. Gene regulation by steroid hormones. Cell 1989;56:335.
24. Gronemeyer H. Transcription activation by estrogen and progesterone receptors. Annu. Rev Genet 1991;25:89.
25. Parker MG. Steroid and related receptors. Curr Opin Cell Biol 1993;5:499.
26. Klein-Hitpass L, Ryffel GU, Heitlinger E, et al. A 13bp palindrome is a functional estrogen responsive element and interacts specifically with estrogen receptor. Nucleic Acids Res 1988;16:647.
27. Kumar V, Chambon P. The estrogen receptor binds tightly to its responsive element as a ligand-induced homodimer. Cell 1988;55:145.
28. Dana SL, Hoener PA, Wheeler DA, et al. Novel estrogen response elements identified by genetic selection in yeast are differentially responsive to estrogen and antiestrogen in mammalian cells. Mol Endocrinol 1994;8:1193.
29. Kumar V, Green S, Staub A, et al. Localisation of the oestradiol-binding and putative DNA-binding domains of the human oestrogen receptor. EMBO J 1986;5:2231.
30. Kumar V, Green S, Stack G, et al. Functional domains of the human estrogen receptor. Cell 1987;51:941.
31. Tora L, White J, Brou C, et al. The human estrogen receptor has two independent nonacidic transcriptional activation functions. Cell 1989;59:477.
32. Ponglikitmongkol M, Green S, Chambon P. Genomic organization for the human oestrogen receptor gene. EMBO J 1988;7:3385.
33. Webster NJG, Green S, Tasset D, et al. The transcriptional activation function located in the hormone-binding domain of the human oestrogen receptor is not encoded in a single exon. EMBO J. 1989;8:1441.
34. Danielian PS, White R, Lees JA, et al. Identification of a conserved region required for hormone dependent transcriptional activation by steroid hormone receptor. EMBO J. 1992;11:1025.
35. Pierrat B, Heery DM, Chambon P, et al. A highly conserved region in the hormone-binding domain of the human estrogen receptor functions as an efficient transactivation domain in yeast. Gene 1994;143:193.
36. Chambraud B, Berry M, Redeuilh G, et al. Several regions of human estrogen receptors are involved in the formation of receptor–heat shock protein 90 complexes. J. Biol Chem 1990;265:20686.
37. Picard D, Khursheed B, Garabedian MJ, et al. Reduced levels of hsp90 compromise steroid receptor action in vivo. Nature (Lond) 1990;348:166.
38. Inano K, Curtis SW, Korach KS, et al. Heat shock protein 90 strongly stimulates the binding of purified estrogen receptor to its responsive element. J Biochem 1994;116:759.
39. Sartorius CA, Melville MY, Hovland AR, et al. A third transactivation function (AF3) of human progesterone receptors located in the unique N-terminal segment of the B-isoform. Mol Endocrinol 1994;8:1347.
40. Fawell SE, Lees JA, White R, et al. Characterization and colocalization of steroid binding and dimerization activities in the mouse estrogen receptor. Cell 1990;60:953.
41. Harlow KW, Smith DN, Katzenellenbogen JA, et al. Identification of cysteine 530 as the covalent attachment site of an affinity-labeling estrogen (ketononestrol aziridine) and antiestrogen (tamoxifen aziridine) in the human estrogen receptor. J Biol Chem 1989;164:17476.
42. Reese JC, Wooge CH, Katzenellenbogen BS. Identification of two cysteines closely positioned in the ligand-binding pocket of the human estrogen receptor: roles in ligand binding and transcriptional activation. Mol Endocrinol 1992;6:2160.
43. Danielian PS, White R, Hoare SA, et al. Identification of residues

in the estrogen receptor that confer differential sensitivity to estrogen and hydroxytamoxifen. Mol Endocrinol 1993;7:232.

44. Pakdel F, Katzenellenbogen BS. Human estrogen receptor mutants with altered estrogen and antiestrogen ligand discrimination. J Biol Chem 1992;267:3429.

45. Cho H, Katzenellenbogen BS. Synergistic activation of estrogen receptor-mediated transcription by estradiol and protein kinase activators. Mol Endocrinol 1993;7:441.

46. Aronica SM, Kraus WL, Katzenellenbogen BS. Estrogen action via the cAMP signaling pathway: stimulation of adenylate cyclase and cAMP-regulated gene transcription. Proc Natl Acad Sci USA 1994;91:8517.

47. Ince BA, Montano MM, Katzenellenbogen BS. Activation of transcriptionally inactive human estrogen receptors by cyclic adenosine 3′,5′-monophosphate and ligands including antiestrogens. Mol Endocrinol 1994;8:1397.

48. Fujimoto N, Katzenellenbogen BS. Alteration in the agonist/antagonist balance of antiestrogens by activation of protein kinase A signaling pathways in breast cancer cells: antiestrogen selectivity and promoter dependence. Mol Endocrinol 1994;8:296.

49. Sartorius CA, Tung L, Takimoto GS, et al. Antagonist-occupied human progesterone receptors bound to DNA are functionally switched to transcriptional agonists by cAMP. J Biol Chem 1993;268:9262.

50. Sartorius CA, Groshong SD, Miller LA, et al. New T47D breast cancer cell lines for the independent study of progesterone B- and A-receptors: only antiprogestin-occupied B-receptors are switched to transcriptional agonists by cAMP. Cancer Res 1994;54:3868.

51. Aronica SM, Katzenellenbogen BS. Stimulation of estrogen receptor-mediated transcription and alteration in the phosphorylation state of the rat uterine estrogen receptor by estrogen, cyclic adenosine monophosphate, and insulin-like growth factor-I. Mol Endocrinol 1993;7:743.

52. Bocquel MT, Kumar V, Stricker C, et al. The contribution of the N- and C-terminal regions of steroid receptors in activation of transcription is both receptor and cell-specific. Nucleic Acids Res 1989;17:2581.

53. Tzukerman MT, Esty A, Santisomere D, et al. Human estrogen receptor transactivational capacity is determined by both cellular and promoter context and mediated by two functionally distinct intramolecular regions. Mol Endocrinol 1994;8:21.

54. McDonnell DP, Vegeto E, O'Malley BW. Identification of a negative regulatory function for steroid receptors. Proc Natl Acad Sci USA 1992;89:10563.

55. Prendergast P, Oñate SA, Christensen K, et al. Nuclear accessory factors enhance the binding of progesterone receptor to specific target DNA. J Steroid Biochem Mol Biol 1994;48:1.

56. Landel CC, Kushner PJ, Greene GL. The interaction of human estrogen receptor with DNA is modulated by receptor-associated proteins. Mol Endocrinol 1994;10:1407.

57. Halachmi S, Marden E, Martin G, et al. Estrogen receptor-associated proteins: possible mediators of hormone-induced transcription. Science 1994;264:1455.

58. Cavailles V, Dauvois S, Danielian PS, et al. Interaction of proteins with transcriptionally active estrogen receptors. Proc Natl Acad Sci USA 1994;91:10009.

59. Gross GE, Clark GM, Chamness GC, et al. Multiple progesterone receptor assays in human breast cancer. Cancer Res 1984;44:836.

60. Hull DF, Clark GM, Osborne CK, et al. Multiple estrogen receptor assays in human breast cancer. Cancer Res 1983;43:413.

61. Raam S, Robert N, Pappas CA. Defective estrogen receptors in human mammary cancers: their significance in defining hormone dependence. J Natl Cancer Inst 1988;80:756.

62. Greene GL, Nolan C, Engler JP, et al. Monoclonal antibodies to human estrogen receptor. Proc Natl Acad Sci USA 1980;77:5115.

63. Greene GL, Sobel N, King WJ, et al. Immunochemical studies of estrogen receptors. J Steroid Biochem Mol Biol 1984;20:51.

64. Greene GL, Sobel BN, WJK, et al. Purification of T47D human progesterone receptor and immunohistochemical characterization with monoclonal antibodies. Mol Endocrinol 1988;2:714.

65. Press MF, Greene GL. Immunocytochemical localization of estrogen and progesterone receptors. In: Advances in immunohistochemistry. DeLellis RA, ed. New York, Raven, 1988:341.

66. Allred DC, Bustamante MA, Daniel CO, et al. Immunocytochemical analysis of estrogen receptors in human breast carcinomas: evaluation of 130 cases and review of the literature regarding concordance with biochemical assay and clinical relevance. Arch Surg 1990;125:107.

67. Thorpe SM. Monoclonal antibody technique for detection of estrogen receptors in human breast cancer: greater sensitivity and more accurate classification of receptor status than the dextran-coated charcoal method. Cancer Res 1987;47:6572.

68. Pertschuk LP, Kim YD, Axiotis CA, et al. Estrogen receptor immunocytochemistry: the promise and the perils. J Cell Biochem Suppl. 1994;19:134.

69. Esteban JM, Ahn C, Mehta P, et al. Biologic significance of quantitative estrogen receptor immunohistochemical assay by image analysis in breast cancer. Anat Pathol 1994;102:158.

70. Scott GK, Kushner P, Vigne J-L, et al. Truncated forms of DNA-binding estrogen receptors in human breast cancer. J Clin Invest 1991;88:700.

71. Abbondanza C, Falco A, Nigro V, et al. Characterization and epitope mapping of a new panel of monoclonal antibodies to estradiol receptor. Steroids 1993;58:4.

72. Hill SM, Fuqua SAW, Chamness GC, et al. Estrogen receptor expression in human breast cancer associated with an estrogen receptor gene restriction fragment length polymorphism. Cancer Res 1989;49:145.

73. Watts CKW, Handel ML, King RJD, et al. Oestrogen receptor gene structure and function in breast cancer. J Steroid Biochem Molec Biol 1992;41:529.

74. Yaich L, Dupont WD, Cavener DR. Analysis of the PvuII restriction fragment-length polymorphism and exon structure of the estrogen receptor gene in breast cancer and peripheral blood. Cancer Res 1994;52:77.

75. Yaich LE, Dupont WD, Cavener DR, et al. The estrogen receptor PvuII restriction fragment length polymorphism is not correlated with estrogen receptor content or patient age in 260 breast cancers. Washington, DC, The Endocrine Society, 1991.

76. McGuire WL. Breast cancer prognostic factors: evaluation guidelines (Editorial). J Natl Cancer Inst USA 1990;83:154.

77. Piva R, Rimondi AP, Hanau S, et al. Different methylation of oestrogen receptor DNA in human breast carcinomas with and without oestrogen receptor. Br J Cancer 1990;61:270.

78. Fallette NS, Fuqua SAW, Chamness GC, et al. Estrogen receptor gene methylation in human breast tumors. Cancer Res 1990;50:3974.

79. Ottaviano YL, Issa J-P, Parl FF, et al. Methylation of the estrogen receptor gene CpG island marks loss of estrogen receptor expression in human breast cancer cells. Cancer Res 1994;54:2552.

80. Weigel RJ, deConinck EC. Transcriptional control of estrogen receptor in estrogen receptor-negative breast carcinoma. Cancer Res 1993;53:3472.

81. Grandien KFH, Berkenstam A, Nilsson S, et al. Localization of DNase I hypersensitive sites in the human oestrogen receptor gene correlates with the transcriptional activity of two differentially used promoters. J Mol Endocrinol 1993;10:269.

82. Keaveney M, Klug J, Dawson MT, et al. Evidence for a previously unidentified upstream exon in the human oestrogen receptor gene. J Mol Endocrinol 1991;6:111.

83. Nestor PV, Forde RC, Webb P, et al. The genomic organisation,

sequence and functional analysis of the 5′ flanking region of the chicken estrogen receptor gene. J Steroid Biochem Mol Biol 1994;50:121.

84. Pujol P, Hilsenbeck SG, Chamness GC, et al. Rising levels of estrogen receptor in breast cancer over 2 decades. Cancer 1994;74:1601.

85. Thorpe SM, Christensen IJ, Rasmussen BB, et al. Short recurrence-free survival associated with high oestrogen receptor levels in the natural history of postmenopausal, primary breast cancer. Eur J Cancer 1993;29A:971.

86. Graham ML, Krett NL, Miller LA, et al. T47D$_{co}$ cells, genetically unstable and containing estrogen receptor mutations, are a model for the progression of breast cancers to hormone resistance. Cancer Res 1990;50:6208.

87. Wang Y, Miksicek RJ. Identification of a dominant negative form of the human estrogen receptor. Mol Endocrinol 1991;5:1707.

88. Pfeffer U, Fecarotta E, Castagnetta L, et al. Estrogen receptor variant messenger RNA lacking exon 4 in estrogen-responsive human breast cancer cell lines. Cancer Res 1993;53:741.

89. Jiang S-Y, Langan-Fahey SM, Stella AL, et al. Point mutation of estrogen receptor (ER) in the ligand binding domain changes the pharmacology of antiestrogens in ER-negative breast cancer cells stably expressing cDNAs for ER. Mol Endocrinol 1992;6:2167.

90. Miksicek RJ, Lei Y, Wang Y. Exon skipping gives rise to alternatively sliced forms of the estrogen receptor in breast tumor cells. Breast Cancer Res Treat 1993;26:163.

91. Castles CG, Fuqua SAW, Klotz DM, et al. Expression of a constitutively active estrogen receptor variant in the estrogen receptor-negative BT-20 human breast cancer cell line. Cancer Res 1993;53:5934.

92. Garcia T, Lehrer S, Bloomer WD, et al. A variant estrogen receptor messenger ribonucleic acid is associated with reduced levels of estrogen binding in human mammary tumors. Mol Endocrinol 1988;2:785.

93. Taylor JA, Li Y, You M, et al. B region variant of the estrogen receptor gene. Nucleic Acids Res 1992;20:2895.

94. Lehrer S, Sanchez M, Song HK, et al. Oestrogen receptor B-region polymorphism and spontaneous abortion in women with breast cancer. Lancet 1990;335:622.

95. Lehrer S, Harlap S, Rabin J, et al. Estrogen receptor polymorphism, spontaneous abortion, and breast cancer risk. Intl J Oncol 1994;5:861.

96. Lehrer SP, Schmutzler RK, Rabin JM, et al. An estrogen receptor genetic polymorphism and a history of spontaneous abortion: correlation in women with estrogen receptor positive breast cancer but not in women with estrogen receptor negative breast cancer or in women without cancer. Breast Cancer Res Treat 1993;26:175.

97. Lehrer S, Rabin J, Stone J, et al. Association of an estrogen receptor variant with increased height in women. Horm Metab Res 1994;26:486.

98. Smith EP, Boyd J, Frank GR, et al. Estrogen resistance caused by a mutation in the estrogen-receptor gene in a man. N Engl J Med 1994;331:1056.

99. Murphy LC, Dotzlaw H. Variant estrogen receptor mRNA species detected in human breast cancer biopsy samples. Mol Endocrinol 1989;3:687.

100. Dotzlaw H, Alkhalaf M, Murphy LC. Characterization of estrogen receptor variant mRNAs from human breast cancers. Mol Endocrinol 1992;6:773.

101. Murphy LC, Dotzlaw H, Hamerton J, et al. Investigation of the origin of variant, truncated estrogen receptor-like mRNAs identified in some human breast cancer biopsy samples. Breast Cancer Res Treat 1993;26:149.

102. Gosden JR, Middleton PG, Rout D. Localization of the human oestrogen receptor gene to the chromosome 6q24->q27 by *in situ* hybridization. Cytogenet Cell Genet 1986;43:218.

103. Karnik PS, Kulkarni S, Liu X-P, et al. Estrogen receptor mutations in tamoxifen-resistant breast cancer. Cancer Res 1994;54:349.

104. Sarkar G, Yoon H-S, Sommer SS. Dideoxy fingerprinting (ddF): a rapid and efficient screen for the presence of mutations. Genomics 1992;13:441.

105. Fuqua SAW, Allred DC, Elledge RM, et al. The ER-positive/PgR-negative breast cancer phenotype is not associated with mutations within the DNA binding domain. Breast Cancer Res Treat 1993;26:191.

106. Ince BA, Zhuang Y, Wrenn CK, et al. Powerful dominant negative mutants of the human estrogen receptor. J Biol Chem 1993;268:14026.

107. Fuqua SAW, Wiltschke C, Castles C, et al. Endocrine-related cancer. 1995;2:19.

108. McGuire WL, Chamness GC, Fuqua SAW. Estrogen receptor variants in clinical breast cancer. Mol Endocrinol 1991;5:1571.

109. Pichon MF, Milgrom E. Oestrogen receptor–negative progesterone receptor–positive phenotype in 1,211 breast tumors. Br J Cancer 1992;65:895.

110. Keshgegian AA. Biochemically estrogen receptor-negative, progesterone receptor-positive breast carcinoma. Arch Pathol Lab Med 1994;118:240.

111. Zhang QX, Borg A, Fuqua SAW. An exon-5 deletion variant of the estrogen receptor frequently coexpressed with wild-type estrogen receptor in human breast cancer. Cancer Res 1993;53:5882.

112. Dauvois S, Danielian PS, White R, et al. Antiestrogen ICI 164,384 reduces cellular estrogen receptor content by increasing its turnover. Proc Natl Acad Sci USA 1992;89:4037.

113. Fawell SE, White R, Hoare S, et al. Inhibition of estrogen receptor-DNA binding by the "pure" antiestrogen ICI 164,384 appears to be mediated by impaired receptor dimerization. Proc Natl Acad Sci USA 1990;87:6883.

114. Dupont WE, Page DL. Risk factors for breast cancer in women with proliferative breast disease. N Engl J Med 1985;312:146.

115. Allred DC, O'Connell P, Fuqua SAW. Biomarkers in early breast neoplasia. J Cell Biochem 1993;(Suppl. 17G):125.

116. O'Connell P, Pekkel V, Fuqua S, et al. Molecular genetic studies of early breast cancer evolution. Breast Cancer Res Treat 1994;32:5.

117. London SJ, Connolly JL, Schnitt SJ, et al. A prospective study of benign breast disease and the risk of breast cancer. JAMA 1992;267:941.

118. Palli D, Roselli del Turco M, Simoncini R, et al. Benign breast disease and breast cancer: a case-control study in a cohort in Italy. Intl J Cancer 1991;47:703.

119. Dupont WD, Parl FF, Hartmenn WH, et al. Breast cancer risk associated with proliferative disease and atypical hyperplasia. Cancer 1993;71:1258.

120. Bodian CA, Perzin KH, Lattes R, et al. Prognostic significance of benign proliferative breast disease. Cancer 1993;71:3896.

121. Ricketts D, Turnbull L, Ryall G, et al. Estrogen and progesterone receptors in the normal female breast. Cancer Res 1991;51:1817.

122. Netto GJ, Cheek JH, Zachariah NY, et al. Steroid receptors in benign mastectomy tissue. Am J Clin Pathol 1990;94:14.

123. Allegra JC, Lippman ME, Green L, et al. Estrogen receptor values in patients with benign breast disease. Cancer 1979;44:228.

124. van Agthoven T, Timmermans M, Foekens JA, et al. Differential expression of estrogen, progesterone, and epidermal growth factor receptors in normal, benign, and malignant human breast tissues using dual staining immunohistochemistry. Am J Pathol 1994;144:1238.

125. Jacquemier JD, Rolland PH, Vague D, et al. Relationships between steroid receptor and epithelial cell proliferation in benign fibrocystic disease of the breast. Cancer 1982;49:2534.

126. Khan SA, Rogers MAM, Tamsen A. Estrogen receptor expression of benign breast epithelium and its association with breast cancer. Cancer Res 1994;54:993.

7.10

Autocrine and Paracrine Growth Factors in the Normal and the Neoplastic Breast

ROBERT B. DICKSON · MARC E. LIPPMAN

Studies during the past 10 years have begun to address mechanisms of action of estrogen and progesterone at the local tissue level in the early promotion and later progression of malignant disease of the breast. Tissue regulation by these hormones is modulated in a complex fashion by locally acting polypeptide hormones (growth factors), stage of cellular differentiation, cellular adhesion, and a poorly understood serum requirement.[1-4] Current research focuses on examination of the interaction of growth factors with defective or overexpressed growth regulatory genes (oncogenes or protooncogenes) in mediating or modulating endocrine steroid action in breast cancer. A second topic of concern is the possibility that an appropriate expression of positive-acting growth factors by fully or partially malignant cells may promote malignant progression in nearby tumor cells that would benefit from an additive proliferation advantage. A third important area of research is defective tumor–host interactions including stromal–epithelial communication to support estrogen-responsive growth, to induce aberrant stromal collagen synthesis (desmoplasia), and to induce vascular infiltration (angiogenesis) to promote metastasis. Finally, certain growth factors may suppress the host immune response to the tumor and may compromise the tumor's response to therapy (Table 7.10-1).

Early studies in the 1970s by Todaro, Sporn, Delarco, and others identified the transforming growth factors (TGFs) in conditioned media–transformed fibroblasts, in breast cancer, and in other cancers. In these pioneering studies, TGFs initially derived their name from their ability to reversibly induce the transformed phenotype (defined as the capacity for anchorage-independent or disordered focal growth of cellular monolayers) in certain rodent fibroblasts. This group of growth factors is now known to consist of several families of polypeptides that are synthesized and secreted by many normal and retrovirally, chemically, radiation-, or oncogene-transformed human and rodent cell lines.[5-10] Growth factors are proposed to have autocrine (self-regulatory), paracrine (regulatory of other local cells), and endocrine (regulatory of distant cells) actions.

Multiple Classes of Growth Factors

EGF FAMILY

Two major classes of structurally and functionally distinct TGF families are represented by prototypes TGF-α and TGF-β. Many factors of the TGF-α family compete with epidermal growth factor (EGF) for binding its cognate receptor (EGFR), to promote EGFR dimerization, to activate receptor tyrosine–kinase specific activity, and to stimulate proliferation or differentiation.[11-13] These EGF-related growth factors are all single-chain polypeptides, nearly all with a consensus pattern of three intrachain disulfide bonds. The family members that bind to the EGFR include TGF-α, EGF, amphiregulin (AR, a heparin-binding factor), heparin-binding EGF (HbEGF) and β-cellulin.[13-15] A factor termed *cripto-1* is related in structure,[16] but has an unknown receptor. A set of related, but virally encoded, factors, including vaccinia growth factor (VGF) and others have also been described as binding the EGFR.[13] Finally, a separate EGF-related, heparin-binding subfamily with members termed heregulin (from human) and *neu*-differentiating factor (NDF; from rat) has been identified and cloned.

Heregulin α, a prototype member of a major subclass of EGF-related molecules is 44 kd in size. The rat and human heregulin homologues have substantial regions of sequence identity and are representative of a large number of gene-splice variants, many of which are focused in neural and neuromuscular tissue.[17-21] This subfamily does not appear to bind to the EGFR, unlike most other EGF family members. Instead, NDF and heregulin were initially reported to bind to erbB-2 (HER-2/*neu*), an EGFR family member. Our knowledge of the EGFR family has rapidly expanded in the past few years; we now know that, in addition to EGFR and erbB-2, it also includes erbB-3 and erbB-4, two other closely related tyrosine kinase–linked receptors.[22-24] Contrary to initial interpretations of data on NDG–heregulin receptor specificity, more recent reports have suggested that heregulin–NDF binds directly to the erbB-4 and more weakly to erbB-3 receptors. Investigators have proposed that these factors may interact only indirectly with c-erbB-2 by receptor heterodimerization.[24-28] An additional factor of 15 to 17 kd, termed human *neu*-activating factor (NAF), has been proposed as an erbB-2–specific receptor ligand.[29,30] The sequence of this factor has not been reported, however, and whether it is part of the EGF family is not known. All four members of the EGFR family and all the EGF-related growth factors (except the viral family members and β-cellulin) have been detected in breast cancer. They are likely to play a central role in tumor growth, as well as in interactions of the tumor with the surrounding host tissue.

TGF-β FAMILY

The TGF-β family of growth factors consists of at least three related gene products, each forming 25-kd homodimeric or heterodimeric species. These species are found

Autocrine and Paracrine Factors in Progression of Breast Cancer

NORMAL

Tightly controlled epithelial growth and regression cycles by steroids and growth factors

Strongly compartmentalized tissue function controlled by cell–cell and cell–substrate interactions

EARLY PROGRESSION OF BREAST CANCER

Epithelial desensitization to inhibitory factors

Epithelial sensitization to stimulatory factors

Steroid regulation of growth factors

Stromal support of steroid effects

LATER PROGRESSION OF BREAST CANCER

Growth factor disruption of stromal architecture (desmoplasia)

Local invasion

Angiogenesis

Survival of distant metastases

Chemotherapeutic and antihormonal drug resistance

Immunosuppression

in the normal mammary epithelium and in breast cancer. A complex pattern of interaction of these TGF-β isoforms with at least two different soluble binding proteins and with three different molecular-weight classes of specific binding proteins is reported.[31–34] Members of each of the three classes of TGF-β binding proteins have been cloned and sequenced. Although one of these classes of binding proteins appears to represent a nonsignaling entity, the other two classes appear to be receptor subunits that deliver intracellular signals through their serine–threonine–specific kinase activities.[33,35–39] This entire multiple growth factor–receptor system is now known to be analogous to the receptor system for the related activin family of hormones that regulates reproductive function.[40] Indeed, type I and type II receptors may heterodimerize to form an active signaling complex. Four type I receptors have been cloned; each may associate with a type II receptor and with a protein termed immunophilin (FKBP-12).[41] The specific type II receptor used in a particular dimeric complex appears to recognize TGF-β directly and to determine relative affinity for each TGF-β species. The function of a given type II receptor is based on which type I receptor is recruited into dimer formation.[42] Separate pathways appear to exist for regulation of growth versus differentiation by TGF-β.[43] Growth-inhibitory effects of TGF-β on epithelial cells are now known to be mediated by effects on cell cycle–regulatory proteins CDK4 and p15 (ink4B).[42]

TGF-β (as well as TGF-α) family members have been found in many cancers, in the urine and pleural and peritoneal effusions of cancer patients,[44–47] and in many normal tissues.[48–51] Initial studies in vitro had suggested that TGF-β was inhibitory and differentiating in breast cancer cell lines in normal mammary epithelial cells and of most other normal and malignant epithelial cell types. TGF-β overexpression in breast tumor biopsies is associated with increased malignant progression of the clinical disease, however.[52,53] TGF-β is thus likely to have complex, additional effects on breast cancer in vivo, including immunosuppression and angiogenesis.[31,54] Other inhibitory factors may also be relevant to breast cancer, such as mammary-derived growth inhibitor (MDGI),[55] mammostatin,[56] α-lactalbumin,[57] and lactoferrin.[58] Neither receptors for these additional factors nor their role in cancer have been established at present. They are all unrelated to the TGF-β family and have not been thoroughly studied in clinical breast cancer.

OTHER FAMILIES OF GROWTH FACTORS

At least five other families of stimulatory growth factors are also found in breast cancer. These are insulin-like growth factors (IGF-1 and IGF-2, and at least six soluble binding proteins), platelet-derived growth factors (PDGF-A and PDGF-B, and fibroblast growth factors (FGF, a family of at least nine members and a soluble binding protein).[7–9] Each of these growth factor classes binds to one or more specific tyrosine kinase–encoding receptors. Vascular endothelial growth factor (VEGF), a member of a different family of tyrosine kinase receptor–binding factors,[59,60] pleiotrophin (a developmental, neurotropic factor), and scatter factor (also called hepatocyte growth factor [HGF]) and its tyrosine kinase–encoding receptor Met[61] are also produced by breast cancer. Finally, a factor termed *mammary-derived growth factor 1* (MDGF-1) has been found in human milk and in conditioned medium from human breast cancer cell lines.[48,49] This glycosylated, monomeric, non–disulfide-linked, 62-kd growth factor stimulates stromal collagen production and may also play a role in growth regulation of normal and malignant human mammary epithelium. The receptor for MDGF-1 is known to include a 130-kd protein that also stimulates tyrosine phosphorylation of a 180-kd cellular protein.[50,62] Thus, a widely diverse collection of growth factors is proposed to mediate a multitude of effects in breast cancer (Figs. 7.10-1 and 7.10-2).

Role of Growth Factors in Tumor Onset and Early Progression

An early hypothesis of cancer biology is that transformation of cells from normal to malignant may indirectly or directly result from increased production of growth-stimulatory factors or decreased production of growth-inhibitory factors. A revision of this hypothesis invokes altered responsiveness to either or both groups of negative- and positive-acting TGFs.[8,9] Testing of these hypotheses depends on our understanding of pathways of growth control both in neoplastic cells and in normal cells from which

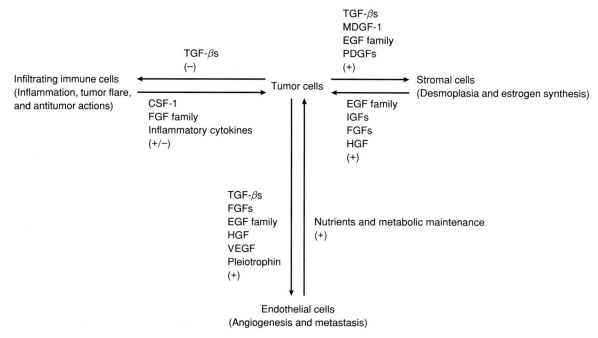

FIGURE 7.10-1 Proposed autocrine factors in breast cancer.

cancer derives. Development of serum-free culture conditions has facilitated the study of growth regulation in normal human mammary epithelial cells.[63,64] Although human mammary epithelial cells may be cultured in vitro, that the cultured subtype is of the lineage or differentiation type that gives rise to breast cancer in a woman is not yet clear. Receptors for estrogen and progesterone have not been demonstrated in these cells, and they appear to have a basal epithelial stem cell character.[63,64] More recently, relatively nonproliferative luminal cells and basal cells have been isolated, based on different antigenic markers and immortalized with SV40T antigen.[65–68] Other studies with primary mammary organoid–derived cultures and with milk-derived, shed epithelial cultures have used benzo-(a)pyrene, human papillomavirus, and prolonged culture in low-Ca^{2+} medium to achieve immortalization.[63,69,70] Further transformation of basal epithelial cells to full malignancy can occur in the presence of an overexpressed nuclear oncogene and an activated kinase–signal transduction oncogene.[63,71,72] Transformation of more differentiated luminal human mammary epithelial cells to full malig-

nancy by a series of defined oncogenic steps has not been described.

Steroid–growth factor interactions have been studied in human mammary tissue only in the context of malignant epithelium, although they are almost certainly crucial in the regulation of the normal gland as well. In hormone-responsive human breast cancer cells, estrogen-induced proliferation is accompanied by an increase in growth-stimulatory TGF-α, AR, and IGF-2, modulation of IGF-binding proteins, induction of EGF and IGF-1 receptors, and inhibition of TGF-β.[73–82] Antiestrogenic inhibition of proliferation of the same cell types in vitro and of primary breast tumors in vivo is paralleled by decreased levels of positive growth factors and augmented secretion of growth inhibitory TGF-β.[81] Analogous effects have been observed with progestins: TGF-α, EGF, IGF-1 receptor, and EGFRs were induced, whereas TGF-β was inhibited by natural or synthetic progestins. Antiprogestational drugs had effects opposite to those of progestins.[82–87] Growth-stimulatory steroids and growth factors also exert similar or additive effects on certain other genes such as those encoding c-Myc, pS2, and cathepsin D.[85] As one might expect, in hormone-independent breast cancer cell lines, the foregoing growth factors are constitutively produced, although their levels of secretion may not significantly exceed those of the normal tissue (with the exception of TGF-β).[87–89] As noted in Chapter 2, another level of steroid–growth factor interaction is in the function of steroid receptors themselves. Signal transduction pathways activated by growth factors and other hormones may directly modulate steroid receptor function at the level of the chromatin.

In cell lines in vitro and in experimental animal models

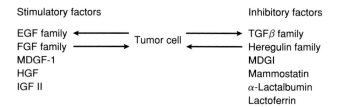

FIGURE 7.10-2 Proposed autocrine interactions in breast cancer.

in vivo, TGF-α has been directly implicated as a powerful modulator of cellular transformation. Transfection of a human TGF-α cDNA under a strong promoter into the immortal, but nontumorigenic, mouse mammary epithelial cell line NOG-8 induced anchorage-independent growth, but not full tumorigenicity.[90] A different study used MCF-10A, a spontaneously immortalized human breast ductal epithelial cell line, as recipient for an expression vector containing TGF-α gene; similar results were obtained.[91] In contrast, when fully malignant MCF-7 cells were used as a recipient for TGF-α transfection, no significant growth advantage to the cells was observed in tumors grown in vitro or in vivo in the nude mouse.[92] Divergent results have also been obtained when fibroblasts are transfected with the TGF-α gene. When immortalized rodent fibroblasts were used as recipients for the human or rat TGF-α cDNA, one study demonstrated that transformation to full tumorigenicity was achieved.[93] The closely related factor EGF was also observed to act as an oncogene-like molecule when transfected and overexpressed in immortalized rodent fibroblasts.[94] In contrast, TGF-α transfection into other fibroblasts induced increased proliferation but not full malignant progression to tumorigenicity.[95] The relative levels of secretion of TGF-α by breast cancer and by rodent fibroblasts are associated with the levels of expression of other oncogenes or protooncogenes. For example, a clear correlation among TGF-α production, c-ras[H] oncogene expression (after transfection of its cDNA), and malignant transformation has been demonstrated in MCF-10A mammary epithelial cells in vitro.[91] The function of TGF-α and other family members as oncogenic or tumor progression factors and the relations among growth factor and oncogene expression depend on the mammary epithelial cell type in question, its level of EGFRs, and its stage in malignant progression.[5] This type of complexity requires in vivo modeling to assess biologic relevance.

Several studies have addressed the effect of TGF-α overexpression (with mouse mammary tumor virus [MMTV] or metallothioneine promoters) in the mammary glands of transgenic mice. These studies clearly show that TGF-α–induced proliferation of the gland may be important in early stages of onset of mammary cancer. Using the metallothioneine promoter and an outbred mouse strain, one study found the mammary gland to be hyperproliferative and delayed in developmental penetration of the epithelial ducts into the stromal fat pad.[96] A similar block in glandular differentiation had previously been observed with local mammary implants of EGF.[97] Other TGF-α transgenic mouse studies using inbred strains demonstrated the TGF-α–transgenic glands to be hyperproliferative, resulting in mammary cancer after multiple pregnancies.[98,99] Another also suggested that expression of a TGF-α transgene accelerates the progression of carcinogen-induced mouse mammary tumors.[100]

Evidence in vitro of strong autocrine growth dependence on the TGF-α–EGFR system has only been seen using an EGFR-blocking antibody in the hormone-independent MDA MB-468 cell line. This cell line has a uniquely high expression of TGF-α because of an ampli-

fied gene encoding the EGFR. The level of expression of EGFR in this line is so high (in excess of 10^6 per cell) that exogenous EGF can have a growth inhibitory effect in vitro,[101] possibly by depletion of adenosine triphosphate (ATP). Using antibody strategies or antisense oligonucleotides complementary to TGF-α, estrogen-induced growth of hormone-dependent MCF-7 cells can also be attenuated.[102] Autocrine function of another EGF family, AR, has been demonstrated in nonimmortalized and carcinogen-immortalized human mammary epithelial cells in culture using antisense AR and heparin (which binds and blocks the factor).[103,104] These pilot studies suggest that the TGF-α–AR–EGFR system may play multiple roles both in hormone-dependent and in hormone-independent breast cancer. Recent work has demonstrated HbEGF in human mammary cancer cells.[105] HbEGF may be synthesized as a transmembrane which is released by proteolytic cleavage on protein kinase C (PKC) activation in the cell. Studies have also addressed the function of the erbB-3–erbB-4 ligand family, the heregulins, in breast cancer. This family of factors appears principally to act by growth inhibition of breast cancer, although weak stimulation has also been observed.[18,19] Heregulins also appear to induce casein synthesis in breast cancer cells.[19] As discussed later, overexpression of EGF family members in breast cancer may also contribute to aberrant tumor–host interactions. Current strategies using EGFR ligands or antibodies coupled to toxins or other therapeutic drugs and directed to the EGFR or erbB-2 also show promise for therapeutic utility, because a large portion of hormone-independent breast cancers express significant levels of these receptors.[89,101,106–108]

Another important family of growth-regulatory factors in the normal and malignant breast is the FGF family. When this family of growth factors binds to heparin, it requires a heparin cofactor for proper presentation to receptors, and it accumulates in the extracellular matrix following its secretion. Some FGF family members do not possess a signal sequence, but all forms appear to be released by cells. FGF-1, FGF-2, and FGF-7 have been detected in mouse mammary preneoplasias, tumors, and cell lines, but not in elevated levels. FGF-3 (int-2), however, a well-known oncogenic growth factor activated by MMTV insertional mutagenesis and FGF-4 (also called HST or K-FGF) has been associated with metastasis of the mouse mammary gland.[109] In the human gland, FGF-1 and FGF-2 have been detected, but not in high levels in human breast cancer. FGF-2 has been proposed as an autocrine growth factor in immortalized human mammary epithelial cells.[110] FGF-2 is also expressed in breast cancer, in which it is apparently correlated with good prognosis. In breast cancer, FGF-1 is localized primarily to macrophages.[111] The biologic role in breast cancer is not known; however, it could contribute to inflammation and angiogenesis, as discussed later. FGF receptors 1 to 4 are expressed in human breast cancer cells.[112,113]

The epithelial inhibitory TGF-β family is also found in normal and malignant mammary epithelium and in human milk.[31,46,114] It is clearly negative in its effect on growth ductal epithelial proliferation in the mouse mammary

TABLE 7.10-2
Sex Steroid–Regulated Growth Factors

Growth Factor or Binding Protein	Effect of Estrogen	Effect of Progesterone
TGF-α	+★	+
EGF	?	+
AR	+★	?
IGF-2	+	?
TGF-β1	−	−
TGF-β2	−★	?
TGF-β3	−	?
IGF BP-3	+	?
IGF-BP-4	−	?

TGF, transforming growth factor; EGF, epidermal growth factor; IGF, insulin-like growth factor; BP, binding protein; AR, amphiregulin.

★ Regulation at mRNA level or transcriptional level.

TABLE 7.10-3
Sex Steroid–Regulated Growth Factor Receptors

Growth Factor Receptor	Effect of Estrogen	Effect of Progesterone
EGF receptor	+	+
erbB-2 receptor	−	−
IGF-1 receptor	+	+

EGF, epidermal growth factor; IGF, insulin-like growth factor.

glands in vivo.[115] As noted previously, production of TGF-β seems to increase with breast cancer; its accumulation may be significant in the characteristic fibrous desmoplastic stroma of the disease,[116] in immunosuppression,[54] or in tumor angiogenesis.[9] Thus, while clearly serving a growth-inhibitory role in the normal gland, overproduction of TGF-β may contribute to aberrant tumor–host interactions in breast cancer.[114,117] In some breast cancer cell lines, TGF-β has been observed to stimulate cell invasion in vitro.[118] The significance of this observation in vivo awaits further study, however.

Steroid Hormone Regulation of Growth Factors and Their Binding Proteins in Breast Cancer

Studies in breast cancer have begun to evaluate the mechanisms and consequences of induction of TGF-α, its family members, its receptor, other growth factors and receptors, and growth factor binding proteins (Tables 7.10-2 and 7.10-3). TGF-α, AR, and TGF-β_2 mRNAs are under control by estrogen and antiestrogen. The transcriptional regulation of TGF-α by estrogen depends on a poorly defined region 5′ to the coding region of the gene.[119] A more recent study in breast cancer cells has also demonstrated transcriptional regulation of the TGF-α–related factor AR by estrogen.[120] Under standard monolayer growth conditions, estrogen stimulates, whereas progestins inhibit, proliferation of hormone-responsive breast cancer cell lines. Although growth factors are also regulated by progestins and antiprogestins, detailed mechanisms of their control have been less well characterized. Under anchorage-independent conditions, colony formation of breast cancer cells can be stimulated by both estrogen and

progesterone. Under such anchorage-independent conditions, investigators have shown, using anti–growth factor antibodies and antisense oligonucleotides, that estrogen- and progesterone-induced TGF-α and estrogen- and progesterone-inhibited TGF-β play at least a modulatory role in steroid control of growth.[13,15,31,102] The transcriptional regulation of TGF-α by estrogen depends on a poorly defined region 5′ to the coding region of the gene.[119] A more recent study in breast cancer cells has also demonstrated transcriptional regulation of the TGF-α–related factor AR by estrogen.[120] Under standard monolayer growth conditions, estrogen stimulates while progestins inhibit proliferation of hormone-responsive breast cancer cell lines.[121–123] AR can also have autocrine effects in human mammary epithelial cells partially transformed with oncogenes[124]; however, future studies will be needed to address its function in hormonally regulated growth. TGF-β is down-regulated by both transcriptional and posttranscriptional mechanisms by estrogens and progestins and induced by antiestrogens and antiprogestins.[73–79] A novel synthetic progestin, gestodine, inhibits anchorage-dependent growth of hormone-dependent breast cancer cells at least partially by TGF-β induction,[125] and retinoids acting through both RAR and RXR receptors can modulate TGF-β_1 transcription.[126]

A complex regulatory system is also emerging from studies of the IGFs. IGF-2 production, as well as cellular responsiveness to IGFs, is stimulated by estrogen and inhibited by antiestrogens in some hormone-dependent breast cancer cell lines. The cellular responsiveness to IGFs appears to be modulated by estrogens and antiestrogens as a result of regulation of the type I IGF receptor, IGF binding protein 3 (both of which are estrogen-induced), and IGF binding protein 4 (which is estrogen-inhibited).[80,127–131] The biologic functions of each of these binding proteins is fully understood, although BP-1 appears inhibitory of the actions of IGF-1.[132] A body of literature is developing on the roles of steroid regulation of growth factors in the uterus as well as the breast.[133]

A different strategy for study of the roles of growth factors has used growth factor and receptor gene transfection into hormone-responsive breast cancer cell lines such as MCF-7 and ZR-75-1 to assess possible effects on malignant progression. Although transfection of TGF-α or the EGF receptor has had little effect on MCF-7, slightly growth-enhancing effects have been reported for overexpression of the IGF-2 gene product and for the erbB-2 protooncogene product.[134-136] In dramatic contrast, strong enhancement of tumor growth and of metastasis was observed after transfection of FGF-1 and FGF-4 into MCF-7 cells (see next section). One mechanism of enhancement of tumorigenesis of these growth factors appears to be promotion of angiogenesis (described later).[137,138]

Studies in vivo in the nude mouse are also providing additional perspectives on the roles of growth factors in breast cancer proliferation. Continuous infusion of EGF or IGF-1 is capable of limited stimulation of MCF-7 tumor growth. Tumors briefly grew, but regressed after several weeks.[139] In testing the effects of TGF-β on breast tumors, the TGF-β–inhibited MDA MB-231 cell line was grown as tumors in the nude mouse, and the factor was continuously infused. Unexpectedly in these experiments, tumor growth was unaffected by TGF-β in vivo, but the animals exhibited cachexia, multiple-organ fibrosis, and splenic regression.[140] A later study further characterized the effects of release of endogenous TGF-β from hormone-independent breast tumors in vivo[141] and observed that neutralizing anti–TGF-β antibodies suppressed tumor growth and enhanced natural killer cell (NK) immune function. As noted before, TGF-β may have additional tumor progression–associated effects on angiogenesis and tumor invasion.[31,52,54,118]

A final consideration of growth factor action must include programmed cell death (apoptosis). Although estrogen and progesterone are known to promote growth and survival of the mammary epithelium, the role of growth factors in epithelial survival is not yet known. This may be particularly important in the context of c-*myc* amplification, in which cells appear to be sensitized to both growth- and death-inducing stimuli. In fibroblasts, for example, several growth factor families can promote survival of cells overexpressing the c-*myc* oncogene.[142] Similar results have been observed in transgenic mouse models.[143] Investigators have proposed that growth factors can prevent apoptosis by inducing the *bcl-2* gene.[144] These fascinating areas await study in human breast cancer.

In summary, local functions of growth factors in normal breast tissue may include stimulation of epithelial proliferation by TGF-α, IGF, and FGF family members and inhibition of epithelial proliferation by other factors, including TGF-β and heregulin. In cancer, aberrant growth factor overproduction, perturbation of signal transduction mechanisms, and loss of tissue compartmentalization may lead to tumor progression. Effects of tumor factor overpopulation may encompass angiogenesis (TGF-β, FGF), desmoplasia and collagen deposition (MDGF-1, TGF-α, TGF-β), and immunosuppression (TGF-β).

Growth Factors, Angiogenesis, and Metastasis

Regulation of local invasion and metastases by breast cancer is not fully understood.[145] Although some studies have suggested that metastatic identification of a specific, mutated gene is not yet certain,[146] c-*erbB*-2 is a protooncogene whose amplification is closely associated with poor prognosis of node-positive breast cancer, but as described earlier, its role at the cellular level may be complex and indirect. Cellular motility is almost certainly involved as well in the progression of breast cancer. Motility-promoting molecules proposed to act in disease progression are the FGF family members[147,148] and HGF, or scatter factor, which acts through the tyrosine kinase–encoding product of the c-*met* oncogene and TGF-β.[149] Metastasis probably also depends on formation of tumor cell emboli in the blood and their subsequent entrapment of cells in capillary networks of metastasis and organs. This process is thought to depend on platelet activation and adhesion of the embolus to endothelial cells by $\alpha_{IIb}\beta_3$ integrin. Because $\alpha_{IIb}\beta_3$ is under regulation by PKC and prostaglandin pathways, it may represent another target of growth factor enhancement of metastatic progression.[150,151] The greatest amount of interest in a suspected gene in breast cancer progression has involved the c-*erbB*-2 gene.

The reconstituted basement-membrane extract Matrigel has been extensively used in attempts to model the process of invasion in vitro. With this type of system, estrogen receptor (ER)-negative cells are generally more invasive than ER-positive ones, and estrogen increases invasiveness of ER-positive cell lines. Tamoxifen was sufficiently estrogenic to induce invasion of a breast cancer cell line in an in vitro model; the pure antiestrogen ICI 164,384 was suppressive.[152] The integrin $\alpha_2\beta_1$ appears to play a major role in adhesion and invasion of breast cancer cells. Although it is a receptor for laminin and collagen in ER-positive breast cancer, it appears to bind only collagen in ER-negative disease. PKC stimulation induces $\alpha_2\beta_1$-dependent invasion.[153,154] So far, that growth factors strongly regulate cellular invasion has not been clearly demonstrated, although TGF-β may be a candidate, as noted earlier. TGF-β may modulate invasion, like PKC, through the NfκB transcription factor.[155] TGF-β may regulate both growth and adhesion through the cyclin inhibitor p27.[156]

Invasive breast cancer is marked by abnormal stromal–epithelial interaction and deposition of tenascin, an embryonic matrix component.[157] Aspects of this dysfunction include increased motility of tumor fibroblasts[158] and altered growth factor secretion by fibroblasts in the area of the tumor. The growth factor IGF-2 is expressed by breast tumor–derived fibroblasts, whereas IGF-1 is expressed by normal breast fibroblasts.[159] Numerous other growth factors including FGF-1, FGF-2, and FGF-5, and possibly HGF are also secreted by breast fibroblasts, regardless of whether the source was tumor or normal.[159,160] Stromal fibroblastic production of the protease styromelysin III (MMP-11) is also an early marker of invasive breast cancer[158]; the regulation of this and other proteases in the area of the tumor probably involves growth factors. The role of the local growth factor environment is emerging as critical to the regulation of proteases in invasive breast cancer. For example, stromelysin III is strongly regulated by TGF-β.[161] The 72-kd gelatinase (MMP-2), as well as MMP-1 and MMP-3, is induced by a factor termed tumor cell–derived collagenase-stimulatory factor (TCSF).[162] The 92-kd gelatinase (MMP-9) is induced by a different growth factor.[163] Although these proteases may be important in tissue invasion itself, they may have critical roles in processing of growth factors (such as TNF-α).[164,165] A further role for growth factors is proposed in tumor cell invasion. Although, as noted previously, numerous growth factors my modulate motility, components of a more specific motility-inducing factor pathway (the autocrine motility factor receptor and autotaxin) have been characterized.[166,167]

Angiogenesis (blood vessel invasion into the tumor area) is an important event leading to full metastatic dissemination of breast cancer.[145,168] For many years, this process has been appreciated as necessary for tumor growth beyond a few millimeters in size because of tumor tissue requirements for a proper metabolic environment. FGFs, EGF-related factors, TGF-βs, HGF, pleiotrophin, and VEGF (perhaps acting through the *flk* oncogene) are all thought to have the capacity to mediate angiogenesis.[169-171] The most important angiogenesis-inducing factor in breast cancer has not been fully defined at present, however. Emerging antiangiogenic therapies use structural antagonists of growth factors,[172] whereas others, such as AGM 1470 (now called TNP 470), appear to block directly the endothelial cell cycle.[173-176] Chemotherapy is potentially synergistic with this type of therapy and will lead to future clinical trials.[177] The process of necrosis is the result of an improperly vascularized tissue, such as in the lumen of a large tumor.

Studies show that the degree of tumor metastases is also directly proportional to the number of capillaries infiltrating the tumor (neoangiogenesis). Probably, at least two mechanisms to explain this effect are possible. First, tumor size alone is known to be a poor prognostic indicator. Therefore, the ability of a tumor to recruit a high degree of local microvasculature clearly contributes to its large size. Large tumors facilitate a greater diversity of mutational events and an increased likelihood of highly aggressive, metastatic cells. A second angiogenic mechanism of tumor progression probably directly involves the vasculature (venous and lymphatic drainage) as a necessary escape route for tumor cells. Tumor cells preferentially accumulate early in metastasis in local lymph nodes and in organ capillary beds. Thus, biopsy of local lymph nodes is an accurate indicator of disease progression.[178] A close, perhaps causal, relationship between breast tumor neoangiogenesis and metastasis has been observed in breast cancer patients.[179-181] In some experimental models, existence of a primary tumor is closely associated with increased proliferation of distant metastases, implying the possibility of continued growth factor communication among tumor colonies following dissemination.[182] Potential growth factor mediators of such an effect have not yet been identified.

In vivo model systems of human breast cancer metastases have been developed. Hormone-independent breast cancer cells are generally more locally invasive than hormone-dependent cells in the nude mouse.[183] In particular, the MDA MB-435 cell line has been developed into a hematogenesis metastasis model in the nude mouse. This cell line is widely metastatic in 6 to 9 months.[184] The inoculation site and dietary fat content strongly modulate tumor growth and metastatic spread in experimental models of breast cancer.[185,186] The inoculation site effect may relate to local factor specificity in tumor progression; dietary fat may modulate levels of estrogenic hormones.

Angiogenesis and metastases may be strongly regulated by heparin-binding growth factors such as FGFs, VEGF, and pleiotrophin. In the multistep development of human fibrosarcoma and bladder carcinoma, FGF-2 alternate splicing and release are observed to be closely associated with angiogenesis.[187-189] In models of spontaneous metastasis of mouse mammary carcinoma, FGF-4 expression is closely associated with metastases in spontaneous mouse mammary carcinoma.[190] The genes for FGF-3 (Int-2) and FGF-4 are amplified with a 15% frequency in human breast cancer; both genes are located at 11q13. Expression of these two genes at the mRNA and protein levels is not common, however. Investigators now believe that a more important gene also exists on the amplicon. The most likely candidate (described earlier) is cyclin D1, a cell cycle–related gene.[191] Nevertheless, studies have shown that FGF-4 or FGF-1 transfection into human MCF-7 breast cancer cells strongly promotes tumor growth and lymphatic or hematogenous metastases.[137,138,192] These studies were facilitated by cotransfecting cells with a gene encoding a chromogenic enzyme (lacZ, which renders cells easily stainable). LacZ staining of an FGF-4–transfected MCF-7 cell line afforded clear indication of metastatic cells. Ipsilateral lymph nodes were 100% positive for metastases by 3 weeks; by 6 weeks other, more distant lymph nodes, lung, and kidney were positive, and by 12 weeks, multiple organs showed evidence of metastases.[137,138] Identification and mechanistic study of the principal metastasis-inducing growth factors for breast cancer will continue to be a priority for breast cancer research in the foreseeable future.

Summary and Future Prospects

Progression of the normal breast through early stages of malignancy to metastasis reflects a gross alteration in functionality of autocrine and paracrine growth factors. Although in mammary development, these factors are under tight regulation, both quantitatively and regionally, cancer represents a progressive perturbation in growth controls (see Table 7.10-1). One principal example is the altered regulation of cancer cell proliferation itself (see Fig. 7.10-1). The EGFR pathway is perturbed in the presence of an amplified c-*myc* or c-*erbB-2* gene to enhance malignant progression dramatically. In addition, the sex steroids regulate critical growth factor pathways (see Tables 7.10-2 and 7.10-3). Later progression appears to involve more changes in the epithelial cell that seem to abrogate the need for exogenous growth factors to drive the cell cycle and to block the ability of TGF-β to attenuate proliferation. One aspect of this further series of perturbations involves overproduction of growth factors. A good example is TGF-β, which may carry out multiple functions to enhance angiogenesis, to suppress malignant function, and to modulate the stromal environment (see Fig. 7.10-2). Better understanding of growth factor pathways will certainly enhance our chances for improved drug therapy in cancer. Indeed, secreted factors that compromise the host to the benefit of the tumor may represent a weakness in the defenses of breast cancer. Blockade of these activities such as with tyrosine kinase inhibitors should be a major goal for the future.[193,194]

References

1. Dickson RB, Lippman ME. Growth regulation of normal and malignant breast epithelium. In: Bland KI, Copeland EM, eds. The breast. Philadelphia, WB Saunders, 1991:363.
2. Maemura M, Dickson RB. Are cellular adhesion molecules involved in the metastasis of breast cancer? Breast Cancer Res Treat 1994;32:23.
3. Van Der Burg B, Kulkhoven E, Isbruecken L, et al. Effects of progestins on the proliferation of estrogen-dependent human breast cancer cells under growth factor-defined conditions. J Steroid Biochem Mol Biol 1992;42:457.
4. Zugmaier G, Knabbe C, Fritsch C, et al. Tissue culture conditions determine the effects of estrogen and growth factors on the anchorage independent growth of human breast cancer cell lines. J Steroid Biochem Mol Biol 1991;39:684.
5. Dickson RB, Lippman ME. Estrogenic regulation of growth and polypeptide growth factor secretion in humor breast carcinoma. Endocr Rev 8:29.
6. Paul D, Schmidt GH. Immortalization and malignant transformation of differentiated cells by oncogenes *in vitro* and in transgenic mice. Crit Rev Oncog 1989;1:307.
7. Heldin CH, Westermark B. Growth factors: mechanism of action and relations to oncogenes. Cell 1984;37:9.
8. Goustin AS, Leof EB, Shipley GD, et al. Growth factors and cancer. Cancer Res 1986;46:1015.
9. Sporn MB, Roberts AB. Peptide growth factors and inflammation, tissue repair, and cancer. J Clin Invest 1986;78:329.
10. Basilico C, Moscatelli D. The FGF family of growth factors and oncogenes. Adv Cancer Res 1992;59:115.
11. Massague J. Epidermal growth factor-like transforming factor. J Biol Chem 1983;258:13606.
12. Derynck R. Transforming growth factor α. Cell 1988;54:593.
13. Todaro GJ, Rose TM, Spooner CE, et al. Cellular and viral ligands that interact with the EGF receptor. Semin Cancer Biol 1990;1:257.
14. Higashigama S, Abraham JA, Miller J, et al. A heparin-binding growth factor secreted by macrophage-like cells that is related to EGF. Science 1991;251:936.
15. Bates SE, Davidson NE, Valverius EM, et al. Expression of transforming growth factor alpha and its mRNA in human breast cancer: its regulation by estrogen and its possible functional significance. Mol Endocrinol 1988;2:543.
16. Normanno N, Qi C-F, Gullick WJ, et al. Expression of amphiregulin, cripto-1, and heregulin α in human breast cancer cells. Int J Oncol 1993;2:903.
17. Holmes WE, Sliwkowski MX, Akita RW, et al. Identification of heregulin, a specific activator of p185[erbB2]. Science 1992;256:1205.
18. Wen D, Peles E, Cupples R, et al. Neu differentiation factor: a transmembrane glycoprotein containing an EGF domain and an immunoglobulin homology unit. Cell 1992;69:559.
19. Peles E, Bacus SS, Koski RA, et al. Isolation of the neu/HER-2 stimulatory ligand: a 44 kd glycoprotein that induces differentiation of mammary tumor cells. Cell 1992;69:205.
20. Falls DL, Rosen KM, Corfas G, et al. ARIA, a protein that stimulates acetylcholine receptor synthesis, is a member of the neu ligand family. Cell 1993;72:801.
21. Marchionni MA, Goodearl ADJ, Chen MS, et al. A new acquaintance for erbB₃ and erbB₄: a role for receptor heterodimerization in growth signalling. Cell 1994;78:5.
22. Cadena DL, Gill GN. Receptor tyrosine kinases. FASEB J 1992;6:2332.
23. Plowman GD, Culouscou J-M, Whitney GS, et al. Ligand-specific activation of HER4/p180[erbB4], a fourth member of the epidermal growth factor receptor family. Proc Natl Acad Sci USA 1993;90:1746.
24. Plowman GD, Green JM, Culouscou JM, et al. Heregulin induces tyrosine phosphorylation of HER4/P180 (erbB₄). Nature 1993;366:473.
25. Carraway KL, Cantley LC. A new acquaintance for erbB₃ and erbB₄: a role for receptor heterodimerization in growth signalling. Cell 1994;78:5.
26. Carraway KL, Slikowski MX, Akita R, et al. The erbB₃ gene product is a receptor for herregulin. J Biol Chem 1994;269:14303.
27. Slikowski MX, Schaefer G, Akita RW, et al. Coexpression of erbB₂ and erbB₃ proteins reconstitutes a high affinity receptor for herregulin. J Biol Chem 1994;26:14661.
28. Peles E, Ban-Lerg R, Tzahan E, et al. Cell-type specific interaction of Neu differentiation factor (NDF/HER regulation) with Neu/HER-2 suggests complex ligand-receptor relationships. EMBO J 1993;12:961.
29. Samanta A, LeVea CM, Dougall WC, et al. Ligand and p185[c-neu] density govern receptor interactions and tyrosine kinase activation. Proc Natl Acad Sci USA 1994;91:1711.
30. Dobashi K, Davis IG, Mikami Y, et al. Characterization of a neu/c-erbB₂ protein-specific activating factor. Proc Natl Acad Sci USA 1991;88:8582.
31. Wakefield LM, Colletta AA, Maccune BK, et al. Roles for transforming growth factors β in the genesis, prevention, and treatment of breast cancer. In: Dickson RB, Lippman ME, eds. Genes, oncogenes, and hormones. Boston, Kluwer Academic, 1992:97.
32. Murphy-Ullrich JE, Schultz-Cherry S, Hook M. Transforming growth factor-β complexes with thrombospondin. Mol Cell Biol 1992;3:181.
33. Bützow R, Fukushima D, Twardzik DR, et al. A 60-kD protein mediates the binding of transforming growth factor-β to cell surface and extracellular matrix proteoglycans. J Cell Biol 1993;122:721.
34. Cheifetz S, Bassols A, Stanley K, et al. Heterodimeric transforming growth factor β. J Biol Chem 1988;263:10783.
35. Ohtsuki M, Massague J. Evidence for the involvement of protein kinase activity in transforming growth factor-β signal transduction. Mol Cell Biol 1992;12:261.
36. Shibanuma M, Kuroki T, Nose K. Release of H_2O_2 and phosphorylation of 30 kilodalton proteins as early responses of cell cycle-dependent inhibition of DNA synthesis by transforming growth factor β_1. Cell Growth Differ 1991;2:583.
37. Massague J. Receptors for the TGFβ family. Cell 1992;69:1067.
38. Ebner R, Chen R-H, Shum L, et al. Cloning of a type 1 TGF-β receptor and its effect on TGF-beta binding to the type 2 receptor. Science 1993;260:1344.
39. Attisamo L, Caracomo J, Ventura F, et al. Identification of human activin and TGFβ type I receptors that form heteromeric kinase complexes with type II receptors. Cell 1993;75:671.
40. Mathews LS. Activin receptors and cellular signaling by the receptor serine kinase family. Endocr Rev 1994;15:310.

41. Wang T, Donahoe PK, Zervos AS. Specific interaction of type I receptors of the TGFβ family with the immunophilin FKBP-12. Science 1994;265:674.

42. Wrana JL, Attisano L, Wieser R, et al. Mechanism of activation of the TGFβ receptor. Nature 1994;370:341.

43. Chen R-H, Ebner R, Derynck R. Inactivation of the type II receptor reveals two receptor pathways for the diverse TGF-β activities. Science 1993;260:1335.

44. Stromberg K, Hudgins R, Orth DN. Urinary TGFs in neoplasia: immunoreactive TGF-α in the urine of patients with disseminated breast carcinoma. Biochem Biophys Res Commun 1987;144:1059.

45. Artega CL, Hanauske AR, Clark GM, et al. Immunoreactive alpha transforming growth factor (IrαTGF) activity in effusions from cancer patients: a marker of tumor burden and patient prognosis. Cancer Res 1988;48:5023.

46. Sairenji M, Suzuki K, Murakami K, et al. Transforming growth factor activity in pleural and peritoneal effusions from cancer and non-cancer patients. Jpn J Cancer Res 1987;78:814.

47. Ohmura E, Tsushima T, Kamiya Y, et al. Epidermal growth factor and transforming growth factor α induce ascitic fluid in mice. Cancer Res 1990;50:4915.

48. Bano M, Soloman DS, Kidwell WR. Purification of mammary-derived growth factor 1 (MDGF1) from human milk and mammary tumors. J Biol Chem 1985;260:5745.

49. Bano M, Lupu R, Kidwell WR, et al. Production and characterization of mammary-derived growth factor 1 in mammary epithelial cells. Biochemistry 1992;31:610.

50. Bano M, Worland P, Kidwell WR, et al. Receptor-induced phosphorylation by mammary-derived growth factor 1 in mammary epithelial cells. J Biol Chem 1992;267:10389.

51. Massaque J. The transforming growth factor β family. Annu Rev Cell Biol 1990;6:597.

52. Gorsch SM. Immunohistochemical staining for transforming growth factor beta associates with disease progression in human breast cancer. Cancer Res 1992;52:6949.

53. Samuel SK, Hurta RAR, Kondaiah P, et al. Autocrine induction of tumor protease production and invasion by a metallothionein-regulated TGF-β₁. EMBO J 1992;11:1599.

54. Enenstein J, Walek NS, Kramer RH. Basic FGF and TGFβ differentially modulate integrin expression of human microvascular endothelial cells. Exp Cell Res 1992;203:499.

55. Grosse R, Bohmer RD, Binas B, et al. Mammary-derived growth inhibitor. In: Dickson RB, Lippman ME, eds. Genes, oncogenes and hormones. Boston, Kluwer Academic, 1992:69.

56. Ervin PR, Kaminski M, Cody RL, et al. Production of mammostatin, a tissue-specific growth inhibitor, by normal human mammary cells. Science 1989;244:1585.

57. Thompson MP, Farrell HM, Mohanam S, et al. Identification of human milk α-lactalbumin as a cell growth inhibitor. Protoplasma 1992;167:134.

58. Hurley WL. *In vitro* inhibition of mammary cell growth by lactoferrin: a comparative study. Life Sci 1994;55:1955.

59. Ferrara N, Houck K, Jakeman L, et al. Molecular and biological properties of the vascular endothelial growth factor family of proteins. Endocr Rev 1992;13:18.

60. Ding IYF, Kern FG. Expression of vascular endothelial growth factor mRNA in human breast carcinoma and cell lines. (Abstract) Proceedings of the 84th Annual Meeting of the AACR. Orlando, 1993.

61. Rong S, Bodescot M, Blair D, et al. Tumorigenicity of the met proto-oncogene and the gene for hepatocyte growth factor. Mol Cell Biol 1992;12:5152.

62. Bano M, Kidwell WR, Lippman ME, et al. Characterization of MDGF-1 receptor in human mammary epithelial cell liver. J Biol Chem 1990;265:1874.

63. Stampfer MR, Bartley JC. Induction of transformation and contin-

64. Hammond SL, Ham RG, Stampfer MR. Serum-free growth of human mammary epithelial cells: rapid clonal growth in defined medium and extended serial passage with pituitary extract. Proc Natl Acad Sci USA 1984;81:5435.

65. Bartek J, Bartkova J, Kyprianou N, et al. Efficient immortalization of luminal epithelial cells from human mammary gland by introduction of simian virus 40 large tumor antigen with a recombinant retrovirus. Proc Natl Acad Sci USA 1991;88:3520.

66. Dundas SR, Ormerod MG, Gusterson BA, et al. Characterization of luminal and basal cells flow-sorted from the adult rat mammary parenchyma. J Cell Sci 1991;100:459.

67. Gusterson BA, Monaghan P, Mahendran R, et al. Identification of myoepithelial cells in human and rat breasts by anti-common acute lymphoblastic leukemia antigen antibody. J Natl Cancer Inst 1986;77:81.

68. Gusterson BA, Warburton MJ, Mitchell D, et al. Distribution of myoepithelial cells and basement membrane proteins in the normal breast and in benign and malignant breast disease. Cancer Res 1982;42:4763.

69. Band V, Zajchowski D, Kulesa V, et al. Human papilloma virus DNAs immortalize normal human mammary epithelial cells and reduce their growth factor requirements. Proc Natl Acad Sci USA 1990;87:463.

70. Soule HD, McGrath A. Simplified method for passage and long-term growth of human mammary epithelial cells *in vitro*. Cell Dev Biol 1986;22:6.

71. Clark R, Stampfer MR, Milley B, et al. Transformation of human mammary epithelial cells by oncogenic retroviruses. Cancer Res 1988;48:4689.

72. Valverius EM, Ciardiello F, Heldin NE, et al. Stromal influence on transformation of human mammary cells overexpressing c-myc and SV40 T. J Cell Physiol 1990;145:207.

73. Dickson RB, Huff KK, Spencer EM, et al. Induction of epidermal growth factor-related polypeptides by 17-beta estradiol in MCF-7 human breast cancer cells. Endocrinology 1986;118:138.

74. Liu SC, Sanfilippo B, Perroteau I, et al. Expression of transforming growth factor α (TGFα) in differentiated rat mammary tumors: estrogen induction of TGFα production. Mol Endocrinol 1987;1:683.

75. Knabbe C, Wakefield L, Flanders K, et al. Evidence that TGF beta is a hormonally regulated negative growth factor in human breast cancer. Cell 1987;48:417.

76. King RJB, Wang DY, Daley RJ, et al. Approaches to studying the role of growth factors in the progression of breast tumors from the steroid sensitive to insensitive state. J Steroid Biochem 1989;34:133.

77. Knabbe C, Zugmaier G, Schmal M, et al. Induction of transforming growth factor beta by the antiestrogens droloxifen, tamoxifen, and toremifen in MCF-7 cells. Am J Clin Oncol 1991;14 (Suppl 2):515.

78. Arrick BA, Korc M, Derinck R. Differential regulation of expression of three transforming growth factor-β species in human breast cancer cell lines by estradiol. Cancer Res 1990;50:299.

79. Murphy LC, Dotzlau H. Regulation of transforming growth factor β messenger ribonucleic acid abundance in T47D human breast cancer cells. Mol Endocrinol 1989;3:611.

80. Stewart AJ, Johnson MD, May FEB, et al. Role of insulin-like growth factors and the type I insulin-like growth factor receptor in the estrogen-stimulated proliferation of human breast cancer cells. J Biol Chem 1990;265:21172.

81. Butta A, MacLennan K, Flanders KC, et al. Induction of transforming growth factor β₁ in human breast cancer *in vivo* following tamoxifen treatment. Cancer Res 1992;52:4261.

82. Murphy JM, Chrysogelos S. Intron 1 elements are involved in

uous cell lines from normal human mammary epithelial cells after exposure to benzo-*a*-pyrene. Proc Natl Acad Sci USA 1985; 82:2394.

EGFR gene regulation in breast cancer cells. (Abstract) Keystone Symposium on Breast and Prostate Cancer II. Lake Tahoe, 1994.

83. Murphy LC, Murphy LJ, Dubik D, et al. Epidermal growth factor gene expression in human breast cancer cells: regulation of expression by progestins. Cancer Res 1988;48:4555.

84. Murphy LC, Dotzlau H. Regulation of transforming growth factor α messenger ribonucleic acid abundance in T47D, human breast cancer cells. Mol Endocrinol 1989;3:611.

85. Musgrove EA, Lee CSL, Sutherland RL. Progestins both stimulate and inhibit breast cancer cell cycle progression while increasing expression of transforming growth factor α, epidermal growth factor receptor, c-fos, and c-myc genes. Mol Cell Biol 1991;11:5032.

86. Goldfine ID, Papa V, Vigneri R, et al. Progestin regulation of insulin and insulin-like growth factor I receptors in cultured human breast cancer cells. Breast Cancer Res Treat 1992;22:69.

87. Bates SE, McManaway ME, Lippman ME, et al. Characterization of estrogen responsive transforming activity in human breast cancer cell lines. Cancer Res 1986;46:1707.

88. Artega CL, Tandon AK, Von Hoff DD, et al. Transforming growth factor β: potential autocrine growth inhibitor of estrogen receptor-negative human breast cancer cells. Cancer Res 1988;48:3898.

89. Dickson RB, Lippman ME. Control of human breast cancer by estrogen, growth factors, and oncogenes. In: Lippman ME, Dickson RB, eds. Breast cancer: cellular and molecular biology. Boston, Kluwer Academic, 1988:119.

90. Shankar V, Ciardiello F, Kim N, et al. Transformation of normal mouse mammary epithelial cells following transfection with a human transforming growth factor alpha cDNA. Mol Carcinog 1989;2:1.

91. Ciardiello F, McGready M, Kim N, et al. TGFα expression is enhanced in human mammary epithelial cells transformed by an activated c-Ha-ras but not by the c-neu protooncogene and overexpression of the TGFα cDNA leads to transformation. Cell Growth Differ 1990;1:407.

92. Clarke R, Brunner N, Katz D, et al. The effects of a constitutive production of TGFα on the growth of MCF-7 human breast cancer cells *in vitro* and *in vivo*. Mol Endocrinol 1989;3:372.

93. Rosenthal A, Lindquist PB, Bringman TS, et al. Expression in rat fibroblasts of a human transforming growth factor-α cDNA results in transformation. Cell 1986;46:301.

94. Stern DF, Hare DL, Cecchini MA, et al. Construction of a novel oncogene based on synthetic sequences encoding epidermal growth factor. Science 1987;235:321.

95. Finzi E, Fleming T, Segatto O, et al. The human transforming growth factor type α coding sequence is not a direct-acting oncogene when overexpressed in NIH3T3 cells. Proc Natl Acad Sci USA 1987;84:3733.

96. Jhappan C, Stahle C, Harkins RN, et al. TGFα overexpression in transgenic mice induces liver neoplasia and abnormal development of the mammary gland and pancreas. Cell 1990;61:1137.

97. Coleman S, Daniel CW. Inhibition of mouse mammary ductal morphogenesis and down regulation of the EGF receptor by epidermal growth factor. Dev Biol 1990;137:425.

98. Sandgren EP, Luetteke NC, Palmiter RD, et al. Overexpression of TGFα in transgenic mice: induction of epithelial hyperplasia, pancreatic metaplasia and carcinoma of the breast. Cell 1990; 61:1121.

99. Matsui Y, Halter SA, Holt JT, et al. Development of mammary hyperplasia and neoplasia in MMTV-TGFα transgenic mice. Cell 1990;61:1147.

100. Coffey RJ Jr, Meise KS, Matsui Y, et al. Acceleration of mammary neoplasia in transforming growth factor α transgenic mice by 7, 12-dimethylbenzanthracene. Cancer Res 1994;54:1678.

101. Ennis BW, Valverius EM, Lippman ME, et al. Anti EGF receptor antibodies inhibit the autocrine stimulated growth of MDA-MB-468 breast cancer cells. Mol Endocrinol 1989;3:1830.

102. Kenney N, Saeki T, Gottardis M, et al. Expression of transforming growth factor α (TGFα) antisense mRNA inhibits the estrogen-induced production of TGFα and estrogen-induced proliferation of estrogen-responsive human breast cancer cells. J Cell Physiol 1993;156:497.

103. Thorne BA, Plowman GD. The heparin-binding domain of amphiregulin necessitates the precursor pro-region for growth factor secretion. Mol Cell Biol 1994;14:1635.

104. Kenney N, Johnson G, Selvam MP, et al. Transforming growth factor α (TGFα) and amphiregulin (AR) as autocrine growth factors in nontransformed immortalized 184AIN4 human mammary epithelial cells. Mol Cell Differ 1993;1:163.

105. Raab G, Higashiyama S, Hetelekidis S, et al. Biosynthesis and processing by phorbol ester of the cell surface-associated precursor form of heparin-binding egf-life growth factor. Biochem Biophys Res Commun 1994;204:592.

106. Mendelsohn JD. The epidermal growth factor receptor as a target for therapy with monoclonal antibodies. Semin Cancer Biol 1990;1:339.

107. Pastan IH, Chaudhary V, Fitzgerald DJ. Recombinant toxins as novel therapeutic agents. Annu Rev Biochem 1992;61:331.

108. Fry DW, Kraker AJ, McMichael A, et al. A specific inhibitor of the epidermal growth factor receptor tyrosine kinase. Science 1994;265:1093.

109. Coleman-Krnacik S, Rosen JM. Differential temporal and spatial gene expression of fibroblast growth factor family members during mouse mammary gland development. Mol Endocrinol 1994;8:218.

110. Soutton B, Hamelin R, Crepin M. FGF-2 as an autocrine growth factor for immortal human breast epithelial cells. Cell Growth Differ 1994;5:615.

111. Coombes RC, Gomm JJ, Lugmani YA, et al. Acidic and basic FGF and their receptors in normal and malignant breast cells. (Abstract) Proc Am Assoc Can Res 1994;35.

112. McLeskey SW, Ding IYF, Lippman ME, et al. MDA-MB-134 breast carcinoma cells overexpress fibroblast growth factor (FGF) receptors and are growth-inhibited by FGF ligands. Cancer Res 1994;54:523.

113. Ding IYF, McLeskey SW, Chang K, et al. Expression of fibroblast growth factors (FGFs) and receptors (FGFRs) in human breast carcinomas. (Abstract) Proc Am Assoc Con Res 1992;31.

114. McCure BK, Mullin BR, Flanders KC, et al. Localization of transforming growth factor-β isotypes in lesions of the human breast. Hum Pathol 1991;23:13.

115. Daniel CW, Silberstein GB. Developmental biology of the mammary gland. In: Neville MC, Daniel CW, eds. The mammary gland. New York, Plenum, 1987:3.

116. Stampfer MR, Yaswen P, Alhadeff M, et al. TGFβ induction of extracellular matrix associated proteins in normal and transformed human mammary epithelial cells in culture is independent of growth effects. J Cell Physiol 1993;155:21.

117. Travers MT, Barrett-Lee PJ, Berger U, et al. Growth factor expression in normal, benign, and malignant breast tissue. Br Med J 1988;296:1621.

118. Welch DR, Fabra A, Nakajima M. Transforming growth factor β stimulates mammary adenocarcinoma cell invasion and metastatic potential. Proc Natl Acad Sci USA 1990;87:7676.

119. Saeki T, Cristiano A, Lynch MJ, et al. Regulation by estrogen through the 5'-flanking region of the transforming growth factor α gene. Mol Endocrinol 1991;5:1955.

120. Meith M, Boehmer FD, Ball R, et al. Transforming growth factor-β inhibits lactogenic hormone induction of casein expression in HC11 mouse mammary epithelial cells. Growth Factors 1990;4:9.

121. Manni A, Wright C, Buck H. Growth factor involvement in the multihormonal regulation of MCF-7 breast cancer cell growth in soft agar. Breast Cancer Res Treat 1991;20:43.

122. Ahmed SR, Badger B, Wright C, Role of transforming growth

factor-α (TGF-α) in basal and hormone-stimulated growth by estradiol, prolactin and progesterone in human and rat mammary tumor cells: studies using TGF-α and EGF receptor antibodies. J Steroid Biochem Mol Biol 1991;38:687.

123. Reddy KB, Yee D, Coffey RJ, et al. Inhibition of estrogen-induced breast cancer proliferation by reduction in autocrine transforming growth factor-α expression. Cell Growth Differ 1994;5:1275.

124. Normanno N, Selvam MP, Qi C, et al. Amphiregulin as an autocrine growth factor for c-Ha-ras and c-erbβ-2 transformed human mammary epithelial cells. Proc Natl Acad Sci USA, 1994;91:2790.

125. Colleta AA, Wakefield LM, Howell FV, et al. The growth inhibition of human breast cancer cells by a novel synthetic progestin involves the induction of transforming growth factor beta. J Clin Invest 1991;87:277.

126. Salbert G, Fanjul F, Piedrafita J, et al. Retinoic acid receptors and retinoid X receptor-α down-regulate the transforming growth factor-β_1 promoter by antagonizing AP-1 activity. Mol Endocrinol 1993;7:1347.

127. Freiss G, Rochefort H, Vignon F. Mechanisms of 4-hydroxytamoxifen antigrowth factor activity in breast cancer cells alterations of growth factor receptor binding sites and tyrosine kinase activity. Biochem Biophys Res Commun 1990;173:919.

128. Sheikk MS, Shao Z, Hussain A, et al. Regulation of insulin-like growth factor-binding protein 1,2,3,4,5, and 6: synthesis, secretion, and gene expression in estrogen receptor negative human breast carcinoma cells. J Cell Physiol 1993;155:556.

129. Pratt SE, Pollack MN. Estrogen and antiestrogen modulation of human breast cancer cell proliferation is associated with specific alterations in accumulation of insulin-like growth factor-binding proteins in conditioned media. Cancer Res 1993;53:5193.

130. Huynh HT, Tetenes E, Wallace L, et al. *In vivo* inhibition of insulin-like growth factor I gene expression by tamoxifen. Cancer Res 1993;53:1727.

131. Kim I, Manni A, Lynch J, et al. Identification and regulation of insulin-like growth factor binding proteins produced by hormone-dependent and -independent human breast cancer cell lines. Mol Cell Endocrinol 1991;78:71.

132. Yee D, Jackson JG, Kozelsky TW, et al. Insulin-like growth factor binding protein 1 expression inhibits insulin-like growth factor 1 action in MCF-7 breast cancer cells. Cell Growth Differ 1994;5:73.

133. Westley BR, May FEB. Role of insulin-like growth factors in steroid modulated proliferation. J Steroid Biochem Mol Biol 1994;51:1.

134. Daly RJ, Harris WH, Wang DY, et al. Autocrine production of insulin-like growth factor II using an inducible expression system results in reduced estrogen sensitivity of MCF-7 human breast cancer cells. Cell Growth Differ 1991;2:457.

135. Cullen KJ, Lippman ME, Chow D, et al. Insulin-like growth factor-II overexpression in MCF-7 cells induces phenotypic changes associated with malignant progression. Mol Endocrinol 1992;6:91.

136. Slamon DJ. Role of the Her-2/*neu* gene in human breast and ovarian cancer. (Abstract) Proceedings of the Cold Spring Harbor Meeting on Genetics and Molecular Biology of Breast Cancer, Cold Spring Harbor, NY, 1992.

137. McLeskey SW, Kurebayashi J, Honig SF, et al. Development of an estrogen-independent, antiestrogen resistant, metastatic breast carcinoma line by transfection of MCF-7 cells with fibroblast growth factor-4. Cancer Res 1993;53:2168.

138. Kurebayashi J, McLeskey SW, Johnson MD, et al. Spontaneous metastasis of MCF-7 human breast cancer cell line cotransfected with fibroblast growth factor-4 and bacterial lacZ genes. Cancer Res 1993;53:2178.

139. Dickson RB, McManaway M, Lippman ME. Estrogen induced factors of breast cancer cells partially replace estrogen to promote tumor growth. Science 1986;232:1540.

140. Zugmaier G, Paik S, Wilding G, et al. Transforming growth factor beta 1 induces cachexia and systemic fibrosis without an antitumor effect in nude mice. Cancer Res 1991;51:3590.

141. Arteaga CL, Carty-Dugger T, Moses HL, et al. Transforming growth factor β_1 can induce estrogen-independent tumorigenicity of human breast cancer cells in athymic mice. Cell Growth Differ 1993;4:193.

142. Harrington EA, Bennett MR, Fanidi A, et al. c-Myc–induced apoptosis in fibroblasts is inhibited by specific cytokines. Biochem Cell Nucleus Lab 1994;3286.

143. Christofori G, Nalk P, Hanahan D. A second signal supplied by insulin-like growth factor II in oncogene-induced tumorigenesis. Nature 1994;369:414.

144. Vaux DL, Cory S, Adams JM. Bcl-2 gene promotes hematopoietic cell survival and cooperation with c-myc to immortalize pre-B cells. Nature 1988;335:440.

145. McCormick BA, Zetter BR. Adhesive interactions in angiogenesis and metastasis. Pharmacol Ther 1992;53:239.

146. Davies BR, Barraclough R, Rudland PS. Induction of metastatic ability in a stably diploid benign rat mammary epithelial cell line by transfection with DNA from human malignant breast carcinoma cell lines. Cancer Res 1994;54:2785.

147. Valles AM, Tucker GC, Thiery JP, et al. Alternative patterns of mitogenesis and cell scattering induced by acidic FGF as a function of cell density in a rat bladder carcinoma cell line. Cell Regulat 1990;1:975.

148. Jouanneau J, Gavrilovic J, Caruelle D, et al. Secreted or nonsecreted forms of acidic fibroblast growth factor produced by transfected epithelial cells influence cell morphology, motility, and invasive potential. Proc Natl Acad Sci USA 1991;88:2893.

149. Rosen EM, Knesel J, Goldberg ID. Scatter factor and its relationship to hepatocyte growth factor and *met*. Cell Growth Differ 1991;2:603.

150. Schneider MR, Schirner M. Antimetastatic prostacylin analogs. Drugs Fut 1993;18:29.

151. Schirner M, Schneider MR. The prostacyclin analogue cicaprost inhibits metastasis of tumours of R 3327 MAT Lu prostate carcinoma and SMT 2A mammary carcinoma. J Cancer Res Clin Oncol 1992;118:497.

152. Thompson EW, Katz D, Shima TB, et al. ICI 164,384: a pure antiestrogen for basement membrane invasiveness and proliferation of MCF-7 cells. Cancer Res 1989;49:6929.

153. Maemura M, Johnson MD, Woods V, et al. Expression and function of $\alpha_2\beta_1$ integrin is regulated by protein kinase C. (Abstract) Proceedings of the American Society for Cell Biology, San Francisco, 1994.

154. Johnson MD, Torri JA, Lippman ME, et al. The invasiveness of MCF-7 human breast cancer cells is regulated by agents that act through protein kinase C. (Abstract) Proceedings of the 5th International Meeting of the Metastasis Research Society, Washington, DC, 1994.

155. Perez JR, Higgins-Sochaski KA, Maltese J-Y, et al. Regulation of adhesion and growth of fibrosarcoma cells by NfkB RelA involves transforming growth factorβ. Mol Cell Biol 1994;14:5326.

156. Polyak K, et al. p27^{Kip1}, a cyclin-Cdk inhibitor, links transforming growth factor-β and contact inhibition to cell cycle arrest. Genes Dev 1994;8:9.

157. Sakakura T, Ishihara A, Yatani R. Tenascin in mammary gland development: from embryogenesis to carcinogenesis. In: Lippman ME, Dickson RB, eds. Regulatory mechanisms in breast cancer. Boston, Kluwer Academic, 1991:365.

158. Lamacher JM, Podhajcer OL, Chenard MP, et al. A novel metalloproteinase gene specifically expressed in stromal cells of breast carcinomas. Nature 1990;348:699.

159. Cullen KJ, Smith HS, Hill S, et al. Growth factor mRNA expression by human breast fibroblasts from benign and malignant lesions. Cancer Res 1992;51:4978.

160. Sonnenberg E, Meyer D, Weidner KM, et al. Scatter factor/hepatocyte growth factor and its receptor, the c-met tyrosine kinase, can mediate a signal exchange between mesenchyme and epithelia during mouse development. J Cell Biol 1993;123:223.

161. Seslar SP, Nakamura T, Byers SW. Regulation of fibroblast hepatocyte growth factor/scatter factor expression by human breast carcinoma cell lines and peptide growth factors. Cancer Res 1993;53:1233.

162. Kataoka H, DeCastro R, Zucker S, et al. Tumor cell-derived collagenase-stimulatory factor increases expression of interstitial collagenase, stromelysin and 72-kDa gelatinase. Cancer Res 1993;53:3154.

163. Hyuga S, Nishikawa Y, Sakata K, et al. Autocrine factor enhancing the secretion of M_R 95,000 gelatinase (matrix metalloproteinase 9) in serum-free medium conditioned with murine metastatic colon carcinoma cells. Cancer Res 1994;54:3611.

164. Gearing AJH, Beckett P, Christodoulou M, et al. Processing of tumour necrosis factor-α precursor by metalloproteinases. Nature 1994;370:555.

165. McGeehan GM, Becherer JD, Bast RC Jr, et al. Regulation of tumour necrosis factor-α processing by a metalloproteinase inhibitor. Nature 1994;370:558.

166. Raz A. Autocrine motility factor receptor and invasion. (Abstract) Clin Exp Metastasis 1994;12:11.

167. Murata J, Clair T, Lee A, et al. cDNA cloning of the autotaxin. J Biol Chem 1994 (in press).

168. Liotta LA, Steeg PS, Stetler-Stevenson WG. Cancer metastasis and angiogenesis: an imbalance of positive and negative regulation. Cell 1991;64:327.

169. Millauer B, Wizigmann-Voos S, Schnürch H, et al. High affinity VEGF binding and developmental expression suggest Flk-1 as a major regulator of vasculogenesis and angiogenesis. Cell 1993;72:835.

170. Folkman J, Shing Y. Angiogenesis. J Biol Chem 1992;267:10931.

171. Wellstein A, Fang W, Khatri A, et al. A heparin-binding growth factor secreted from breast cancer cells is homologous to a developmentally regulated cytokine. J Biol Chem 1992;267:2582.

172. Kim I, Manni A, Lynch J, et al. Identification and regulation of insulin-like growth factor binding proteins produced by hormone-dependent and -independent human breast cancer cell lines. Mol Cell Endocrinol 1991;78:71.

173. Yamaoka M, Yamamoto T, Masaki T, et al. Inhibition of tumor growth and metastasis of rodent tumors by the angiogenesis inhibitor O-(chloroacetyl-carbamoyl) fumagillol (TNP-470; AGM-1470). Cancer Res 1993;53:4262.

174. Thorpe PE, Derbyshire EJ, Andrade SP, et al. Heparin-steroid conjugates: new angiogenesis inhibitors with antitumor activity in mice. Cancer Res 1993;53:3000.

175. Welch DR, Harper DE, Yohem KH. U-77,863: a novel cinnamamide isolated from *Streptomyces griseoluteus* that inhibits cancer invasion and metastasis. Clin Exp Metastasis 1993;11:201.

176. Vukanovic J, Passaniti A, Hirata T, et al. Antiangiogenic effects of the quinoline-3-carboxamide linomide. Cancer Res 1993;53:1833.

177. Teicher BA, Sotomayor EA, Huang ZD. Antiangiogenic agents potentiate cytotoxic cancer therapies against primary and metastatic disease. Cancer Res 1992;52:6702.

178. Blood CH, Zetter BR. Tumor interactions with the vasculature: angiogenesis and tumor metastases. Biochim Biophys Acta 1990;1032:89.

179. Widner N, Semple JP, Welsch WR, et al. Tumor angiogenesis and metastases-correlation in invasive breast carcinoma. N Engl J Med 1991;324:1.

180. Weidner N, Folkman J, Pozza F, et al. Tumor angiogenesis: a new significant and independent prognostic indicator in early-stage breast carcinoma. J Natl Cancer Inst 1992;84:1875.

181. Fox SB, Gatter KC, Bicknell R, et al. Relationship of endothelial cell proliferation to tumor vascularity in human breast cancer. Cancer Res 1993;53:4161.

182. Fisher B, Gunduz N, Coyle J, et al. Presence of a growth-stimulating factor in serum following primary tumor removal in mice. Cancer Res 1989;49:1996.

183. Thompson EW, Paik S, Brunner N, et al. Association of increased basement membrane-invasiveness with absence of estrogen receptor and expression of vimentin in human breast cancer cell lines. J Cell Physiol 1992;150:534.

184. Price JE, Polyzos A, Zhang RD, et al. Tumorigenicity and metastases of human breast carcinoma cell lines in nude mice. Cancer Res 1990;50:717.

185. Meschter CL, Connolly JM, Rose DP. Influence of regional location of the inoculation site and dietary fat on the pathology of MDA-MB-435 human breast cancer cell-derived tumors grown in nude mice. Clin Exp Metastasis 1992;10:167.

186. Naguchi M, Ohta N, Kifugawa H, et al. Effects of switching from a high-fat diet to a low-fat diet on tumor proliferation and cell kinetics of DMBA-induced mammary carcinoma in rats. Oncology 1992;49:246.

187. Kandel J, Bossy-Wetzel E, Radvanyi F, et al. Neovascularization is associated with a switch to the export of bFGF in the multistep development of fibrosarcoma. Cell 1991;66:1095.

188. Savagner P, Valles AM, Jouanneau J, et al. Alternative splicing in fibroblast growth factor receptor 2 is associated with induced epithelial-mesenchymal transition in rat bladder carcinoma cells. Mol Biol Cell 1994;5:851.

189. Gavrilovic J, Moens G, Thiery JP, et al. Expression of transfected transforming growth factor α induces a motile fibroblast-like phenotype with extracellular matrix-degrading potential in a rat bladder carcinoma cell line. Cell Reg 1990;1:1003.

190. Murakami A, Tanaka H, Matsuzawa A. Association of *hst* gene expression with metastatic phenotype in mouse mammary tumor cells. Cell Growth Differ 1990;1:225.

191. Schuuring E, Verhoven E, Mooi WJ, et al. Identification and cloning of two overexpressed genes U 21B31/PRAD 1 and ems-1 within the amplified chromosome 11q13 region in human carcinomas. Oncogene 1992;7:355.

192. Zhang L, Kharbanda S, Chen D, et al. MCF-7 breast carcinoma cells transfected with an expression vector for fibroblast growth factor 1 are tumorigenic and metastatic in ovariectomized or tamoxifen-treated nude mice. (Abstract) Proc Am Assoc Cancer Res 1994;35.

193. Reddy KB, Mangold GL, Tandon AK, et al. Inhibition of breast cancer cell growth *in vitro* by a tyrosine kinase inhibitor. Cancer Res 1992;52:3636.

194. Wakeling AE, Barker AJ, Davies DH, et al. Specific inhibition of epidermal growth factor receptor tyrosine kinase by 4-anilinoquinazolines. Breast Cancer Res Treat 1995 (in press).

7.11

Control of Invasion and Metastasis

PATRICIA S. STEEG

A hallmark of invasion and metastasis is complexity.[1-3] To invade locally, tumor cells must traverse the tumor border, host parenchyma, and basement membrane, using reversible adherence mechanisms, proteinases (produced by the tumor or stromal cells), and motility. Once locally invasive, tumor cells must intravasate, arrest, and extravasate the lymphatic or circulatory system, and they must avoid host immune responses. Angiogenesis must be initiated at the metastatic site and is itself an extraordinarily complex process. Because it necessitates endothelial cell migration, invasion, and proliferation, angiogenesis has been compared to the tumor invasion process, albeit with a more stable, differentiated endpoint.[2] Colonization of tumor cells at the metastatic site appears to encompass more than oncogene-induced tumor growth and may be regulated by complex tumor cell responses to paracrine signals.[4]

Breast cancer metastasizes primarily to the lymph nodes, lungs, bone, brain, and liver. Metastases cause direct organ failure, critical obstructions, and paraneoplastic syndromes such as hypercalcemia, and the treatment of metastatic disease often results in life-threatening infections. At diagnosis and surgery, about 38% of patients exhibit lymph node metastases, whereas 7% of patients have detectable distant metastases.[4] These data argue that the metastatic process has only been completed in a small percentage of patients at diagnosis, and in the majority of patients, antimetastatic therapy may have a preventive role. A more cautious view of these data, however, argues that only the last steps of the metastatic process may be relevant to therapeutic development. It is possible that, in early disease, occult micrometastases have already seeded to distant organs by the time of diagnosis and surgery. In this situation, only those portions of the metastatic process involved in the outgrowth of tumor cells at the metastatic site, such as angiogenesis and colonization, would prevent progression to detectable metastatic disease.

Regulation of Breast Cancer Metastasis

Study of the molecular mechanisms of invasion and metastasis has made use of human tumor cohorts, in which molecular events are quantitated and correlated with histopathologic or clinical course measures of metastatic potential. Additionally, rodent or human model systems are used, in which molecular events are contrasted in related tumors or tumor cell lines of low or high metastatic potential. Human or rodent breast carcinoma cell lines have also been used for transfection experiments, designed to test whether a particular molecular event is correlated with invasion and metastasis, or whether alternatively, it actually causes changes in tumor metastatic potential. cDNA is subcloned into an expression construct and is transfected into breast carcinoma cells; as controls, a side-by-side transfection is performed using the expression construct minus the metastasis-related gene. High-expression transfectants are identified, and the behavior of control- and metastasis-gene transfectants are compared in vitro and in vivo. Table 7.11-1 lists representative transfection studies documenting a cause-and-effect relationship between gene expression and breast cancer invasion and metastasis. As shown, few genes have been reported to stimulate or inhibit metastatic potential by transfection, owing to difficulty in producing stable, high-expression transfectants as well as the tedious nature of metastasis assays. Transfection studies can be complemented by other functional approaches, including gene knockouts, studies in transgenic mice, and antisense transfections.

Tumor cells often possess multiple redundant mechanisms to accomplish each of the phenotypic changes required in invasion and metastasis, as discussed later. Few individual molecular events are universally required for invasive and metastatic behavior, and their relative importance to breast cancer progression remains under study. This degree of redundancy also predicts that our attempts to counteract a particular phenotype (production of matrix metalloproteinases in invasion, for instance, by recombinant tissue inhibitor of metalloproteinases [TIMP] proteins) may be successful, but the tumor may evade TIMP inhibition by producing redundant proteinases such as plasminogen activators, cathepsins, and heparanases.

Adhesion

Tumor cells reversibly adhere to each other, to extracellular matrices, and to other cells at various points in invasion and metastasis. Four major families of cell surface adhesion receptor molecules have been described—integrins, members of the immunoglobulin superfamily, cadherins, and selectins—that may mediate these adhesive interactions.[3] The integrins, composed of a heterodimer of α and β subunits, mediate cell binding to extracellular matrix proteins. Integrins have been implicated in the regulation of normal cell differentiation and are often correlated with cell motility and aggressive behavior in metastasis. The immunoglobulin superfamily of cell adhesion molecules (CAMs), represented by NCAM, ICAM, carcinoembryonic antigen [CEA], and potential adhesion molecules such as DCC, are involved in homophilic as well as heterophilic cell–cell interactions, with effects on cellular morphology, differentiation, sorting and signaling. CD44, a glycopro-

TABLE 7.11-1
Genes Regulating Breast Cancer Invasion and Metastasis, Demonstrated by Transfection Studies

Gene	Cell Line*	Phenotypic Effect		References
		In Vivo	In Vitro	
E-cadherin	MDA–MB-435 (H)	—	D invasion	6
Estrogen receptor†	MDA–MB-231 (H)	D met	D invasion	93
Interferon-γ	TS/A (M)	D tum	I macrophage lysis	94
		I met		
ras^H	MCF-7 (H)	NE met	I invasiveness	76
FGF-4	MCF-7 (H)	I tum	I anchorage-independent growth	95
		I met		
p9Ka (mts1)	Rama 37 (R)	I met		96
nm23	MDA–MB-435 (H)	NE tum	D anchorage-independent growth	
		D met	D motility	
			I differentiation	56–58
maspin	MDA–MB-435 (H)	D met	D invasion	10
TSP-1	MDA–MB-435 (H)	D tum		
		D met		
		D ang		34

D, decreased; I, increased; NE, no effect; tum, tumorigenicity; met, metastasis; ang, capillary density; TSP-1, thrombospondin-1.

* Origin: human (H); rat (R); murine (M).

† In the presence of estrogen.

tein with properties of a CAM in cell–cell adhesion as well as binding to extracellular matrix, has been investigated in rat mammary cell lines. Variant mRNAs encoding CD44, generated by alternative splicing, were identified that were not expressed in nonmetastasizing mammary carcinoma cell lines. Transfection of the CD44 splice variant in a pancreatic cell line resulted in the acquisition of metastatic behavior.[5] Cadherins are Ca^{2+}-dependent CAMs that mediate homophilic interactions involved in normal cell sorting and the organization of epithelial cell polarity. Among a limited panel of human breast carcinoma cell lines, high expression of E-cadherin was correlated with a more epithelioid differentiation, and transfection of E-cadherin cDNA into human breast carcinoma cells resulted in decreased invasiveness in vitro.[6] Selectins bind carbohydrate ligands by lectin-like domains to mediate heterophilic interactions between or among blood and endothelial cells, such as lymphocyte and neutrophil trafficking. Although proposed to influence lymphocytic and hematogenous dissemination of tumor cells, this class of CAMs remains poorly studied.

Proteinases and Inhibitors

Proteolytic degradation of the basement membrane is a crucial part of the invasion process, and degradation of other extracellular matrices occurs at multiple points in metastatic dissemination. Many proteinases have been identified and characterized, such as metalloproteinases, plasminogen activators (PAs), stromelysins, cathepsins, heparanases, and trypsins, and they are a prime example of the redundancy of mechanistic alternatives in the metastatic process. A corresponding list of proteinase inhibitors has been identified, and the overall balance and localization of proteinase and inhibitor may be important to the metastatic phenotype.[3]

PAs, a set of serine-specific proteinases, convert inactive plasminogen to active plasmin, a trypsin-like enzyme with broad substrate specificity. High levels of urokinase PA (uPA) have been correlated with poor clinical course in several large breast carcinoma cohorts,[7,8] and the uPA receptor has been observed immunohistochemically on invasive breast carcinoma cells, as well as on tumor macrophages and endothelial cells.[9] High levels of PA inhibitor (PAI-I) have also been correlated with poor prognosis in breast cancer cytosolic preparations,[8] possibly by forming complexes with PA on the tumor cell surface and protecting it against proteolytic degradation or by an independent role in promoting angiogenesis. Maspin, a serpin serine proteinase inhibitor with homology to PA inhibitors, is expressed at reduced levels in human breast carcinoma cell lines, and its transfection into the MDA–MB-435 breast carcinoma cell line has inhibited primary tumor size and metastatic potential.[10]

Metalloproteinases are synthesized as latent proenzymes that require activation. The in vivo mechanisms of metalloproteinase activation are incompletely understood, and their activity is further regulated by inhibitory molecules, the TIMPs. Antibody inhibition and transfection studies have demonstrated a functional role for the matrix metalloproteinases and their inhibitors in invasion, mostly in rodent model systems unrelated to breast carcinoma.[11] Stromelysin-3 (ST3), a member of the metalloproteinase family, has exhibited a unique pattern of expression, detectable in fibroblastic cells surrounding the tumor.[12] A limited breast tumor cohort study correlated ST3 RNA levels, but not the metalloproteinase type IV collagenase, with malignancy and the presence of lymph node metastases.[13]

The cathepsins are aspartic proteases normally found inside cells in lysosomes. Secretion of cathepsin B from cells has been found in activated macrophages and I cell disease as a consequence of altered intracellular trafficking of lysosomal enzymes.[14] Also complicating the biologic elucidation of the cathepsins is the pH requirement for an acidic environment normally not observed extracellularly. Montcourrier and associates reported that breast carcinoma cell lines overexpress cathepsin D, and activated cathepsin D in acidic vesicles can degrade endocytosed extracellular matrix.[15] Cathepsin D overexpression in breast carcinoma cytosolic preparations was correlated with poor patient prognosis in cohort studies.[16] The biology of cathepsin D, however, must be interpreted in light of human breast tumor cohort and cell line immunohistochemical studies that found that tumor cell cathepsin D expression was associated with favorable prognosis and infiltrating macrophages were a significant contributor of cathepsin D protein in breast tumors.[17,18] These controversies highlight the need to evaluate proteinases by multiple mechanisms.

Motility

Having modified the extracellular matrix, tumor cells must migrate to complete the invasion process.[19,20] The molecular basis of tumor motility is incompletely understood, although in vitro cell biology studies indicate a tremendous redundancy in motility stimulators. In general, tumor cells can migrate directionally to a given stimulus or in a nondirectional, scattering fashion. Tumor cells can migrate in vitro to various extracellular matrix components, either in soluble or insoluble form. Multiple growth factors, including the insulin-like growth factor (IGF), platelet-derived growth factor (PDGF), fibroblast growth factor (FGF), transforming growth factor β (TGF-β), and hepatocyte growth factor (HGF) families, can induce motility. This observation forces the reinterpretation of our definition of a growth factor, and the mechanism of cell signaling by a cytokine whereby proliferation or motility is attained is a topic of intense research interest. Several cytokine motility factors have also been reported that have no growth factor activity, such as autocrine motility factor, autotaxin, and migration stimulating factor.[3,20]

Angiogenesis

The development of new capillaries from preexisting blood vessels is necessary for tumors to continue growth beyond a few millimeters in diameter. Angiogenesis is required at a metastatic site. The process of angiogenesis is complex, typically consisting of the following:

- Dissolution of the basement membrane, usually at a postcapillary venule
- Migration of endothelial cells toward the tumor
- Proliferation of endothelial cells at the trailing edge of migration
- Canalization, branching, and formation of vascular loops
- Formation of new basement membranes

Capillary cells respond to both soluble mediators and extracellular matrix signaling in this process. Other gross changes in vascular architecture associated with tumor progression include a progressive arteriolization, in which smooth muscle cells proliferate to encase the developing artery.[21,22]

The importance of angiogenesis to breast cancer metastasis has been documented in several tumor cohort studies. Most of these studies used endothelial cell–specific antibodies for immunohistochemistry. The number of microvessels was quantitated, typically in the primary tumor microscopic field exhibiting the densest concentration. "Hotspot" microvessel counts have been correlated with nodal metastases and poor patient survival, and their predictive value was independent of variables such as tumor size, estrogen receptor status, c-*erb*B-2 expression, ploidy, and age.[23–26]

Multiple factors are capable of inducing the angiogenic process, another example of the redundancy inherent in the metastatic process. These factors include FGFs, TGF-α, TGF-β, tumor necrosis factor α, vascular endothelial growth factor, platelet-derived endothelial cell growth factor, angiogenin, epidermal growth factor (EGF), and others.[21] Some of the known angiogenic factors act directly on endothelial cells, whereas others activate local inflammatory cells to induce angiogenesis.

Tumor angiogenesis may reflect changes in angiogenesis inhibitors as well as stimulators.[4] Endogenous inhibitors of angiogenesis, such as thrombospondin (TSP), cartilage-derived inhibitor, the TIMPs, platelet factor 4, interferon-α, and interferon-β, may act by multiple mechanisms. TSP is a multifunctional glycoprotein component of the extracellular matrix that modulates cell adhesion, motility, and proliferation.[27–29] TSP has been reported to inhibit endothelial cell migration and proliferation to FGF-β, in vitro cord formation, and angiogenesis in vivo.[30–33] Some of this effect may be due to binding of growth factors such as FGF-β by the heparin-binding domain of TSP. We have found that transfection of the human MDA–MB-435 breast carcinoma cell line with TSP-1 cDNA inhibited primary tumor size, metastatic potential, and capillary densities in vivo. Deletion of the

C-terminal portion of TSP-1 cDNA abrogated its suppressive effect, identifying a new portion of this protein as potentially relevant.[34]

The proteinase-inhibitory activities of cartilage-derived inhibitor and TIMP-1 have been postulated to prevent degradation of extracellular matrix necessary for capillaries to grow, sprout, and migrate.[35] Alternatively, TIMP-2 has been reported to exert anti-angiogenic effects through a proteinase-independent effect. Platelet factor 4 can inhibit the metalloproteinase type IV collagenase and is also capable of binding angiogenic factors through a heparin-binding domain, suggesting a multifunctional inhibition of angiogenesis. Interferon-α has been successfully used to treat hemangiomas in infants, but it has been less effective in older patients.[36,37] Interferon inhibition of angiogenesis has been thought to be independent of its antiproliferative effects and may be mediated through binding of angiogenic factors.

Colonization

Colonization of a metastatic site may encompass more than simple oncogene-induced growth of tumor cells.[4] Normal cells exist within an architecture of other cells and extracellular matrix and are exposed to both paracrine and locally produced growth factors. These same influences may exert significant growth-modulatory effects on transformed cells. In studies of rodent mammary adenocarcinoma cell clones, Kerbel and colleagues[38,39] reported that as cells attain metastatic potential, their production of, and responsiveness to, growth factors may be altered, leading to a more aggressive phenotype. The clonal-dominance hypothesis was first described by using genetically tagged clones of the rodent SP1 mammary adenocarcinoma cell line. Individual clones of SP1 were transfected with an antibiotic (neomycin)-resistance construct. Because each clone incorporated the construct in a different chromosomal location, hybridization of the neomycin-resistance probe to Southern blots of restricted genomic DNA from the transfectants showed fragments of unique sizes. Pools of 50 to 100 distinct clones were injected into mice, and at various times after injection, DNA was harvested and analyzed from primary tumors and metastases. Within the first few weeks of growth, primary tumors continued to exhibit multiple distinct clones on Southern blots. The primary tumors were eventually dominated by one or a few clones, however, and metastatic lesions were composed of these same dominant clones. Further studies indicated that the nonmetastatic clones in the initial mixture produced TGF-β, a cytokine with growth-inhibitory activity for many cell types. Surprisingly, the clonally dominant metastatic clones were growth-stimulated by TGF-β. It can be hypothesized that, in the final steps of metastasis, tumor cells must grow in a foreign organ devoid of the cell–cell and cell–extracellular matrix interactions and locally produced growth factors found in the primary tumor environment. Those tumor cells that can grow independently of exogenous stimuli, or alternatively that are growth-stimulated by widely available cytokines such as TGF-β, may possess an advantage in the final colonization step of metastasis. In agreement with this hypothesis, immunohistochemical analysis of TGF-β1 in breast carcinoma cohorts localized the protein to the advancing edges of primary tumors and lymph node metastases,[40] and high expression was directly correlated with poor disease-free survival.[41] Treatment of rat MTLn3 mammary adenocarcinoma cells with TGF-β increased their pulmonary metastatic potential in vivo.[42]

Variations of the clonal-dominance hypothesis, which could also generate more aggressive behavior, have been reported in breast and other model systems. The cytokine interleukin-6 (IL-6) inhibited the growth of less aggressive, estrogen-dependent breast carcinoma cell lines, but exerted no significant effect on more aggressive, estrogen receptor–negative cell lines.[43] Thus, a lack of inhibition rather than stimulation was observed. In melanoma, autocrine production of growth factors was correlated with metastatic competence.[44] Not all studies have confirmed the clonal-dominance hypothesis,[45] and its relevance to metastasis in vivo is not known. If confirmed in vivo, however, the hypothesis will indicate a complex series of changes in tumor cells, for growth factor production, abrogation of inhibitory responses to cytokines, and stimulatory responses to traditionally inhibitory cytokines, that favor the independent colonization of a distant organ.

Organ-Specific Metastasis

Although many tumors metastasize to the first capillary bed encountered, other cancer cell types exhibit organ specificity. The molecular mechanisms responsible for organ-specific metastasis remain poorly studied. The role of adhesion molecules mediating extravasation has been proposed to influence organ-specific metastasis.[1,46] For breast carcinoma, the $\alpha_6\beta_4$ integrin was reported to mediate tumor cell adhesion to hepatocytes.[47] Bellachene and coworkers[48] reported bone sialoprotein is overexpressed by breast carcinoma and postulated that it may mediate adhesion to the skeleton. In addition, tissue-specific growth or inhibitory factors may select for metastatic outgrowth in particular organs.[49] Doerr and associates[50] also reported evidence that glycosaminoglycans within the extracellular matrices of various organs may specifically influence the colonization of mammary cells, possibly by regulating tumor cell secretion of autocrine growth factors.

Coordinate Regulation of Invasion and Metastasis?

Experimental evidence in transfection studies has demonstrated that the multitude of individual mechanistic changes required for overt invasive and metastatic behavior can be regulated by the overexpression of a single gene. Using fibroblasts, transfection of the activated *ras* oncogene was shown to induce both tumorigenic and metastatic behavior in vivo and was associated with altered expression of several metastasis-associated genes. For instance, Su and colleagues[51] transfected fibroblasts with the activated *ras* oncogene to produce tumorigenic and metastatic variants, retransfected these cells with the *k-rev* suppressor gene to produce less metastatic cells, and isolated revertants of the double transfectants exhibiting high metastatic potential. Increases in overt metastatic behavior in this model system were coordinately accompanied by decreased expression of TIMP-1 and *nm23* and increased expression of the growth factor cripto, a 94-kd metalloproteinase, and stromelysin. These studies predicted that the complex phenotypic changes in invasion and metastasis may be coordinately regulated by gene cascades, in which one or a handful of genes results in the up- or down-regulation of multiple additional genes. Gene cascades have been investigated in normal embryonic development and differentiation, in which cells proliferate, migrate, and invade before differentiation,[52–54] and one can hypothesize that similar or identical gene cascades are aberrantly operative in invasion and metastasis. If true, these studies would suggest that identification of, and therapeutic intervention into, genes controlling cascades may provide an antimetastatic effect extending to multiple "downstream" phenotypic changes.

Of the genes demonstrated by transfection to modulate breast carcinoma invasion and metastasis, *nm23* has been shown to cause a series of "downstream" phenotypic effects and may occupy a position near or at the top of a gene cascade. *Nm23* was identified by its reduced expression in highly metastatic murine melanoma cell lines, as compared with related tumorigenic but poorly metastatic cell lines. Reduced expression of *nm23* has been correlated with lymph node metastases or poor patient survival in several breast tumor cohort studies.[55] Transfection of human *nm23-H1* cDNA into the metastatic MDA–MB-435 human breast carcinoma cell line had no effect on primary tumor size, but reduced metastatic potential in vivo by 50% to 90%, inhibited motility responses to serum, PDGF, and IGF, inhibited the clonally dominant colonization response to TGF-β, and stimulated morphologic and biosynthetic differentiation in response to basement membrane proteins.[56–58]

The mutated rat *neu* oncogene has been transfected into fibroblasts with resultant stimulatory effects on metastatic potential in vivo.[59] The *neu* gene is a mutated rat homologue of *c-erbB-2* or *Her-2,* which is overexpressed (in its wild-type form) in approximately 30% of infiltrating ductal carcinomas and in a higher proportion of comedo ductal carcinomas in situ. In infiltrating ductal carcinoma cohort studies, *c-erbB-2* overexpression has been correlated with poor patient survival.[60,61] We have observed that transfection of *c-erbB-2* into human MDA–MB-435 breast carcinoma cells increased their pulmonary metastatic potential by two- to five-fold (Steeg PS, Slamon DJ, personal communication.) Additionally, expression of the wild-type and mutated forms of *neu* in transgenic mice resulted in metastatic mammary carcinomas.[62,63] Altered

"downstream" phenotypes associated with increased metastatic potential in the fibroblast-transfection study included colonization, motility, and invasiveness, suggesting that this oncogene may also occupy a high position on a gene cascade.

Additional Genetic Events Associated With Invasion and Metastasis

To investigate the regulation of the metastatic process further, studies of differential gene expression and chromosomal alterations have been performed. Such studies may lead to the identification of new mechanistic or regulatory molecular events. Differential gene expression studies have typically used model systems to minimize variability and techniques such as subtraction hybridization, differential colony hybridization, and differential display. Several genes have been identified that are either up- or down-regulated between tumor cells of low and high metastatic potential, including *WDNM1, WDNM2,* fibronectin, *mts-1,* maspin, *mta-1,* and *nm23.*[10,64–69] Data pertaining to many of these genes have been reported in breast carcinoma model systems. Other genes identified by comparing normal with tumorigenic breast cells await further experimentation to determine their relevance to invasion and metastasis and include *Brush-1*[70] and breast differential display clones.[71]

A second avenue of investigation takes its lead from the observation that many suppressor genes require inactivation of both chromosomal copies. Allelic deletion (loss of heterozygosity) has been widely reported as one mechanism of suppressor-gene inactivation. Alternatively, oncogenes such as N-*myc* can be amplified at the genomic level. Studies have therefore surveyed multiple loci on each chromosome from the chromosomal DNA of breast tumors to identify regions with a high frequency of alterations, either allelic deletion or amplification. Several of these alterations have been correlated with lymph node metastases or poor patient survival in tumor cohort studies, suggesting that the target gene may have a metastasis-associated function. Allelic deletions on 13q include the *retinoblastoma*-suppressor gene and the *Brush-1* gene, and their relationship with breast cancer invasion and metastasis awaits further experimentation. Deletion of 16q has been associated with the development of distant metastases.[72] On chromosome 17p, two loci have been implicated by deletion and other studies. Alterations such as allelic deletion or mutation to *p53* at 17p13.1 have been correlated with poor prognosis in several cohort studies, whereas a more distal locus of allelic deletion at 17p13.3 has also been identified.[73] Chromosome 17q amplification at *c-erbB-2* has been correlated with poor prognosis,[60] and multiple loci on 17q 21-3, including *nm23,* the *BRCA1,* and other genes, may influence multiple aspects of cancer progression.[73]

Metastasis Research Techniques

Although invasion and metastasis represent an intriguing biologic problem with clinical applicability, the techniques and approaches needed to study the metastatic process are not in widespread use. Many human breast carcinoma cell lines have been established from metastatic lesions, but few actually metastasize on injection into immunocompromised mice. The reasons for this apparent discrepancy are unknown, but they could include an alteration in metastatic potential on establishment of a tissue culture cell line and nonspecific immunity in nude mice. Table 7.11–1 lists several human breast carcinoma cell lines that have been used successfully for metastasis assays. Other problems are relevant to the use of rodent model systems of mammary carcinoma for metastasis research. Although the cell lines and tumors metastasize more readily on injection or implantation, the molecular alterations driving these model systems are not always germane to those of human breast cancer. For instance, nonmetastatic and metastatic rat mammary tumors have been induced by injection of nitrosomethylurea and retain these phenotypes on reimplantation.[68] The principal molecular alteration in this system is a *ras* oncogene mutation, however, which is rarely observed in human breast carcinoma.

The only universally accepted indicator of tumor metastatic potential is in vivo data. Experimental metastasis experiments constitute a quick metastasis assay, in which tumor cells are injected intravenously and gross pulmonary metastases are counted several weeks after injection. This technique is rapid and easily quantitated, but it measures only the last steps of the metastatic process. Few human breast carcinoma cell lines produce pulmonary metastases by this method.

Spontaneous metastasis assays involve the injection of tumor cells into an organ, the formation of a primary tumor at the site of injection, and the formation of distant metastases. In addition to metastasis data, primary tumor size and incidence data are obtained. Disadvantages of this assay include its poor quantitation and relatively long time after injection required for metastasis formation. Orthotopic injection of cells (such as injection of breast carcinoma cells into the mammary fat pad) is preferable to subcutaneous injection, permitting tumor–stromal cell interactions and locally produced growth factors to exert regulatory influences. Among *nm23*- and control-transfected MDA–MB-435 breast carcinoma cell lines, we observed that spontaneous metastases were formed at higher frequencies by the control transfectants on subcutaneous or mammary fat pad injection, but the percentages of mice with metastases were lower by the subcutaneous route.[56] Mice at autopsy are examined for gross metastases, which must be confirmed by microscopic examination of sections stained with hematoxylin and eosin. For organs such as lungs, which are common sites of breast carcinoma metastasis, preparation and examination of multiple sections at random depths (step sections) to identify occult micrometastases can be performed. Data are typically shown as the percentage of mice with metastases, with the number of metastases per mouse as appropriate. Techniques designed to improve metastasis assays include the injection of tumor cells in Matrigel, a basement membrane extract,[74] and the use of *lac-z* transfection for identification of micrometastases.[75]

In vitro assays are available for several aspects of the metastatic process, including colonization, motility, and invasion. Many angiogenesis assays are in use, including in vitro assays of endothelial cell growth, migration, and cord formation, as well as in vivo assays in the rabbit cornea, chick chorioallantoic membrane, and so forth.[21] An example of the discordance sometimes observed between in vitro and in vivo data is the *ras*^{H} transfection of human MCF-7 breast carcinoma cells, which increased invasion in vitro without a significant effect on spontaneous metastatic potential in vivo[76] (see Table 7.11–1). These data underscore the need to supplement in vitro data with in vivo metastasis experiments.

Human tissues are increasingly used for analysis of metastatic potential, to eliminate all questions of relevance to human disease. These include prognostic studies of primary breast carcinomas, in which a phenotype is quantitated and is correlated to lymph node metastasis or clinical course data. One particularly interesting type of prognostic study uses immunohistochemistry to count microvessels, providing an indicator of primary tumor angiogenesis.[24] An emerging research strategy is the identification of rare tumor cells in bone marrow aspirates and axillary lymph nodes, as potential indicators of increased metastatic potential.[77–79] Both polymerase chain reaction (PCR) and antibody-based methods have been used for tumor cell detection, although significant questions about sensitivity and accuracy remain.

Development of Antimetastatic Therapy

Data have been presented arguing that distant metastases are observable in only 7% of breast cancer patients at the time of diagnosis and surgery; these data suggest that the metastatic process is open for therapeutic intervention in a large number of cases. These data cannot exclude the possibility that occult micrometastases have already left the breast, have completed intravasation and extravasation of the circulatory system, and are lacking only the angiogenesis and colonization steps needed for outgrowth and detection, however. Preclinical research may therefore be most rewarding when directed at those events mechanistically involved in, or regulating, angiogenesis and colonization. Other limitations of preclinical research include the redundancy of the metastatic process. Multiple factors have been reported to mediate adhesion and proteolysis and to induce migration, colonization, and angiogenesis. Unless one factor predominates in a given patient, the development of a therapeutic approach to a single factor may be offset by the tumor's response to another factor with redundant function. More optimism may be garnered for the identification of, and therapeutic intervention into, common intracellular signaling mechanisms mediating the tumor cell's motility or angiogenic or colonization responses to multiple signals. Additionally, the identification of, and pharmacologic potentiation of, gene expression at or near the top of suppressor cascades for the metastatic phenotype may represent another valuable target. Several targets for clinical development are described later in this chapter and reviewed elsewhere.[80]

For angiogenesis, several agents have been identified on the basis of their inhibition of growth factor stimulation of endothelial cell function. The drugs β-cyclodextrin tetradecasulfate or heparin in combination with steroids have been shown to inhibit neovascularization because of heparin-binding growth factors, but their development has been curtailed by side effects.[81] Suramin inhibited angiogenesis in animal models by blocking the binding of FGF-β and other growth factors to their receptors, but toxicity problems remain to be addressed in clinical trials.[82] Another heparin analogue, pentosan polysulfate (PPS), inhibited the growth of tumors in mice by inhibition of FGF and other angiogenic, heparin-binding growth factors.[83,84] A phase I trial of PPS in advanced refractory breast cancer noted no objective responses, with three patients exhibiting stable disease and dose-limiting toxicities of thrombocytopenia and elevated hepatic transaminases (Swain S, personal communication).

Other preclinical efforts have focused on antiangiogenic compounds unrelated to heparin-binding growth factors. The antibiotic fumagillin and its synthetic analogues have shown endothelial cell–specific, antiproliferative, and antimetastatic effects. Even though prolonged use of fumagillin is expected to be precluded by its toxicity and associated weight loss, analogues such as TNP-470 have been better tolerated in animal experiments.[85,86]

Perhaps the most rewarding antiangiogenic strategies will emanate from the development of natural angiogenesis inhibitors. An example of translational development of basic research data stems from the transfection of TSP-1 cDNA, which has inhibited primary tumor formation, metastatic potential, and angiogenesis in vivo.[34] TSP protein is found in the blood. Despite this fact, women are still developing progressive breast tumors. The reasons for this apparent discrepancy may include the following: (1) the large size of TSP, which may limit its diffusion out of the circulation to the area where endothelial cells are migrating toward tumor cells; (2) the presence of multiple functional domains on TSP, some of which may be stimulatory for tumor progression; and (3) the bioavailability of TSP, which may be significantly lower than its plasma concentration because of binding to other proteins. Preclinical research is addressing these potential problems by identifying those domains of TSP with antiangiogenic activity. If TSP peptides or protein fragments can be identified, they may lack the binding domains that limit bioavailability, as well as stimulatory domains. Furthermore, their smaller size could facilitate diffusion into the extracapillary space where angiogenesis occurs. Peptides directed to several regions of TSP have been tested in vitro,[87] and additional regions are under investigation. Invasion inhibitors such as the TIMPs may also exert an angiostatic effect.

Translational approaches to aberrant colonization are planned for *nm23,* as transfection of *nm23*-inhibited TGF-β stimulation of colonization in metastatic murine melanoma and human breast carcinoma cell lines.[56,88] The promoter for human *nm23-H1* has been cloned, and screening is planned to identify pharmaceutical compounds to activate *nm23-H1* transcription in breast tumor cells.

Other agents directed toward the signal transduction cascade are under development and may exert inhibitory effects on aberrant colonization. Compounds such as CAI have been reported to inhibit signal transduction.[89] Another important target in the signal transduction cascade is protein kinase C. Considerable evidence indicates protein kinase C involvement in the signal transduction pathways of multiple growth factor receptors and *ras,* and it may affect aberrant colonization. Bryostatin 1, a partial protein kinase C agonist, has entered phase I clinical trial.[90]

Monoclonal antibodies have been characterized to two important cell-surface receptors: (1) c-erbB-2, in which transfection of the cDNA has demonstrated increased metastatic potential; and (2) EGF receptor, whose ligands have been implicated in tumor cell motility and angiogenesis. Clinical trials of monoclonal antibodies, alone or in combination with conventional chemotherapy, are planned.[91,92] These and other strategies may provide new, less toxic clinical approaches, based on the tumor cell's biology, for the prevention of further metastatic dissemination.

References

1. Nicolson G. Molecular mechanisms of cancer metastasis: tumor and host properties and the role of oncogenes and suppressor genes. Curr Opin Oncol 1991;3:75.

2. Liotta LA, Steeg PS, Stetler-Stevenson WG. Cancer metastasis and angiogenesis: an imbalance of negative and positive regulation. Cell 1991;64:327.

3. MacDonald N, Steeg P. Molecular basis of tumor metastasis. Cancer Surv 1993;16:175.

4. Weinstat-Saslow D, Steeg P. Angiogenesis and colonization in the tumor metastatic process: basic and applied advances. FASEB J 1994;8:401.

5. Gunthert U, Hofmann M, Rudy W, et al. A new variant of glycoprotein CD44 confers metastatic potential to rat carcinoma cells. Cell 1991;65:13.

6. Frixen UH, Behrens J, Sachs M, et al. E-cadherin–mediated cell–cell adhesion prevents invasiveness of human carcinoma cells. J Cell Biol 1991;113:173.

7. Foekens J, Schmitt M, VanPutten W, et al. Prognostic value of urokinase-type plasminogen activator in 671 primary breast cancer patients. Cancer Res 1992;52:6101.

8. Grondahl-Hansen J, Christensen I, Rosenquist C, et al. High levels of urokinase-type plasminogen activator and its inhibitor PAI-1 in cytosolic extracts of breast carcinomas are associated with poor prognosis. Cancer Res 1993;53:2513.

9. Bianchi E, Cohen R, Thor A, et al. The urokinase receptor is expressed in invasive breast cancer but not in normal breast tissue. Cancer Res 1994;54:861.

10. Zou Z, Anisowicz A, Hendrix M, et al. Maspin, a serpin with tumor-

suppressing activity in human mammary epithelial cells. Science 1994;263:526.

11. Stetler-Stevenson W, Liotta L, Liotta DK Jr. Extracellular matrix 6: role of matrix metalloproteinase in tumor invasion and metastasis. FASEB J 1993;7:1434.

12. Wolf C, Rouyer N, Lutz Y, et al. Stromelysin 3 belongs to a subgroup of proteinases expressed in breast carcinoma fibroblastic cells and possibly inplicated in tumor progression. Proc Natl Acad Sci USA 1993;90:1843.

13. Kawami H, Yoshida K, Ohsake A, et al. Stromelysin-3 mRNA expression and malignancy: comparison with clinicopathological features and type IV collagenase mRNA expression in breast tumors. Anticancer Res 1993;13:2319.

14. Sloane BF, Moin K, Krepela E, et al. Cathepsin B and its endogenous inhibitors: the role in tumor malignancy. Cancer Metastasis Rev 1990;9:333.

15. Montcourrier P, Mangeat P, Salazar G, et al. Cathepsin D in breast cancer cells can digest extracellular matrix in large acidic vesicles. Cancer Res 1990;50:6045.

16. Tandon AK, Clark GM, Chambiss GC, et al. Cathepsin D and prognosis in breast cancer. N Engl J Med 1990;332:3904.

17. Johnson M, Torri J, Lippman M, et al. The role of cathepsin D in the invasiveness of human breast cancer cells. Cancer Res 1993;53:873.

18. Henry J, McCarthy A, Angus B, et al. Prognostic significance of the estrogen-regulated protein, cathepsin D, in breast cancer: an immunohistochemical study. Cancer 1990;65:265.

19. Stracke M, Aznavoorian S, Beckner M, et al. Cell motility, a principal requirement for metastasis. In: Goldberg ID, ed. Cell motility factors. Basel, Verlag, 1991:147.

20. Aznavoorian S, Stracke ML, Krutzsch H, et al. Signal transduction for chemotaxis and haptotaxis by matrix molecules in tumor cells. J Cell Biol 1990;110:1427.

21. Blood CH, Zetter BR. Tumor interactions with the vasculature: angiogenesis and tumor metastasis. Biochim Biophys Acta 1990; 1032:89.

22. Ingber DE, Folkman J. How does extracellular matrix control capillary morphogenesis? Cell 1989;58:803.

23. Weidner N, Folkman J, Pozza F, et al. Tumor angiogenesis: a new significant and independent prognostic indicator in early-stage breast carcinoma. J Natl Cancer Inst 1992;84:1875.

24. Weidner N, Semple JP, Welch WR, et al. Tumor angiogenesis and metastasis correlation in invasive breast carcinoma. N Engl J Med 1991;324:1.

25. Horak ER, Leek R, Klenk N, et al. Angiogenesis, assessed by platelet/endothelial cell adhesion molecule antibodies, as indicator of node metastases and survival in breast cancer. Lancet 1992;340:1120.

26. Bosari S, Lee AKC, DeLellis RA, et al. Microvessel quantitation and prognosis in invasive breast carcinoma. Hum Pathol 1992;23:755.

27. Lawler J. The structural and functional properties of thrombospondin. Blood 1986;67:1197.

28. Bornstein P. Thrombospondins: structure and regulation of expression. FASEB J 1992;6:3290.

29. Frazier WA, Prater CA, Jaye D, et al. In: Lahav J, ed. Thrombospondin. Boca Raton, CRC, 1993:92.

30. Good DJ, Polverini PJ, Rastinejad F, et al. A tumor suppressor-dependent inhibitor of angiogenesis is immunologically and functionally indistinguishable from a fragment of thrombospondin. Proc Natl Acad Sci USA 1990;87:6624.

31. Taraboletti G, Roberts D, Liotta LA, et al. Platelet thrombospondin modulates endothelial cell adhesion, motility, and growth: a potential angiogenesis regulatory factor. J Cell Biol 1990;111:765.

32. Iruela-Arispe ML, Bornstein P, Sage H. Thrombospondin exerts an antiangiogenic effect on cord formation by endothelial cells in vitro. Proc Natl Acad Sci USA 1991;88:5026.

33. Tolsma SS, Volpert OV, Good DJ, et al. Peptides derived from two separate domains of the matrix protein thrombospondin-1 have anti-angiogenic activity. J Cell Biol 1993;122:497.

34. Weinstat-Saslow D, Zabrenetzky V, VanHoutte K, et al. Transfection of thrombospondin-1 cDNA into a human breast carcinoma cell line reduces primary tumor growth, metastatic potential and angiogenesis. Cancer Res 1994;54:6504.

35. Moses MA, Langer R. A metalloproteinase inhibitor as an inhibitor of neovascularization. J Cell Biochem 1991;47:230.

36. Ezekowitz R, Mulliken J, Folkman J. Interferon-2α therapy for life-threatening hemangiomas of infancy. N Engl J Med 1992;326:1456.

37. Sidky YA, Borden EC. Inhibition of angiogenesis by interferons: effects on tumor- and lymphocyte-induced vascular responses. Cancer Res 1987;47:5155.

38. Kerbel RS. Growth dominance of the metastatic cancer cell: cellular and molecular aspects. Adv Cancer Res 1990;55:87.

39. Theodorescu D, Cornil I, Sheehan C, et al. Dominance of metastatically competent cells in primary murine breast neoplasms is necessary for distant metastatic spread. Int J Cancer 1991;47:118.

40. Dalal B, Keown P, Greenberg A. Immunohistochemical localization of secreted transforming growth factor-β1 to the advancing edges of primary tumors and to lymph node metastases of human mammary carcinoma. Am J Pathol 1993;143:381.

41. Gorsch S, Memoli V, Stukel T, et al. Immunohistochemical staining for transforming growth factor β1 associates with disease progression in human breast cancer. Cancer Res 1992;52:6949.

42. Welch D, Fabra A, Nakajima M. Transforming growth factor B stimulates mammary adenocarcinoma cell invasion and metastatic potential. Proc Natl Acad Sci USA 1990;87:7678.

43. Chiu JJS, Cowan K. Differential effect of interleukin-6 on estrogen receptor positive and negative breast carcinoma cell lines. (Abstract) Proc Am Assoc Cancer Res 1993;34:55.

44. Shih I-M, Herlyn M. Role of growth factors and their receptors in the development and progression of melanoma. J Invest Dermatol 1993;100:196.

45. Moffett B, Baban D, Bao L, et al. Fate of clonal lineages during neoplasia and metastasis studied with an incorporated genetic marker. Cancer Res 1992;52:1737.

46. Pauli B, Augustin-Voss H, Ei'Sabban M, et al. Organ-preference of metastasis: the role of endothelial cell adhesion molecules. Cancer Metastasis Rev 1990;9:175.

47. Kemperman H, Wijnands Y, DeRijk D, et al. The integrin α6β4 on TA3/Ha mammary carcinoma cells is involved in adhesion to hepatocytes. Cancer Res 1993;53:3611.

48. Bellachene A, Merville M-P, Castronovo V. Expression of bone sialoprotein, a bone matrix protein, in human breast cancer. Cancer Res 1994;54:2823.

49. Horak E, Darling D, Tarin D. Analysis of organ-specific effects on metastatic tumor formation by studies in vitro. J Natl Cancer Inst 1986;76:913.

50. Doerr R, Zvibel I, Chiuten D, et al. Clonal growth of tumors on tissue-specific biomatrices and correlation with organ site specificity of metastases. Cancer Res 1989;49:384.

51. Su Z, Austin VN, Zimmer SG, et al. Defining the critical gene expression changes associated with expression and suppression of the tumorigenic and metastatic phenotype in Ha-*ras*–transformed cloned rat embryo fibroblast cells. Oncogene 1993;8:1211.

52. Reid L. From gradients to axes, from morphogenesis to differentiation. Cell 1990;63:875.

53. Hynes RO, Lander AD. Contact and adhesive specificities in the associations, migrations, and targeting of cells and axons. Cell 1992;63:303.

54. Gumbiner B. Epithelial morphogenesis. Cell 1992;69:385.

55. Steeg PS, Rosa ADL, Flatow U, et al. Nm23 and breast cancer metastasis. Breast Cancer Res Treat 1993;25:175.

56. Leone A, Flatow U, VanHoutte K, et al. Transfection of human nm23-H1 into the human MDA-MB-435 breast carcinoma cell line:

effects on tumor metastatic potential, colonization, and enzymatic activity. Oncogene 1993;8:2325.

57. Kantor JD, McCormick B, Steeg PS, et al. Inhibition of cell motility after nm23 transfection of human and murine tumor cells. Cancer Res 1993;53:1971.

58. Howlett A, Petersen O, Steeg P, et al. A novel function for Nm23: overexpression in human breast carcinoma cells leads to the formation of basement membrane and growth arrest. J Natl Cancer Inst 1994;86:1838.

59. Yu D, Hung M-C. Expression of activated rat *neu* oncogene is sufficient to induce experimental metastasis in 3T3 cells. Oncogene 1991;6:1991.

60. Slamon D, Clark G, Wong S, et al. Human breast cancer: correlation of relapse and survival with amplification of the *HER-2/neu* oncogene. Science 1987;235:177.

61. Press M, Pike M, Chazin V, et al. Her-2/neu expression in node-negative breast cancer: direct tissue quantitation by computerized image analysis and association of overexpression with increased risk of recurrent disease. Cancer Res 1993;53:4960.

62. Muller W, Sinn E, Pattengale P, et al. Single step induction of mammary adenocarcinoma in transgenic mice bearing the activated c-*neu* oncogene. Cell 1988;54:105.

63. Guy C, Webster M, Schaller M, et al. Expression of the *neu* protooncogene in the mammary epithelium of transgenic mice induces metastatic disease. Proc Natl Acad Sci USA 1992;89:10578.

64. Schalken J, Eveling S, Issacs J, et al. Down modulation of fibronectin messenger RNA in metastasizing rat prostatic cancer cells revealed by differential hybridization analysis. Cancer Res 1988;48:2042.

65. Dear T, Ramshaw I, Kefford R. Differential expression of a novel gene in nonmetastatic rat mammary adenocarcinoma cells. Cancer Res 1988;48:5203.

66. Dear T, McDonald D, Kefford R. Transcriptional down-regulation of a rat gene, WDNM2, in metastatic DMBA-8 cells. Cancer Res 1990;50:1667.

67. Ebralidze A, Florenes V, Lukanidin E, et al. The murine mts1 gene is highly expressed in metastatic but not in non-metastatic human tumour lines. Clin Exp Metastasis 1990;8:35.

68. Steeg PS, Bevilacqua G, Kopper L, et al. Evidence for a novel gene associated with low tumor metastatic potential. J Natl Cancer Inst 1988;80:200.

69. Toh Y, Pencil S, Nicolson G. A novel candidate metastasis-associated gene, *mta-1*, differentially expressed in highly metastatic mammary adenocarcinoma cell lines. J Biol Chem 1994;269:22958.

70. Schott D, Chang J, Deng G, et al. A candidate tumor suppressor gene in human breast cancers. Cancer Res 1994;54:1393.

71. Liang P, Averboukh L, Keyomarsi K, et al. Differential display and cloning of messenger RNAs from human breast cancer versus mammary epithelial cells. Cancer Res 1992;52:6966.

72. Lindblom A, Rotstein S, Skoog L, et al. Deletions of chromosome 16 in primary familial breast carcinomas are associated with development of distant metastases. Cancer Res 1993;53:3707.

73. Steeg P. Suppressor genes in breast cancer: an overview. In: Dickson RB, Lippman ME, eds. Genes, oncogenes and hormones: advances in cellular and molecular biology of breast cancer. Boston, Kluwer Academic, 1991:45.

74. Schnaper HW, Kleinman HK. Regulation of cell function by extracellular matrix. Pediatr Nephrol 1993;7:96.

75. Brunner N, Thompson E, Spang-Thomsen M, et al. *lacz* transduced human breast cancer xenografts as an in vivo model for the study of invasion and metastasis. Eur J Cancer 1992;28A:1989.

76. Gelmann E, Thompson E, Sommers C. Invasive and metastatic properties of MCF-7 cells and ras^H^-transfected MCF-7 cell lines. Int J Cancer 1992;50:665.

77. Diel I, Kaufmann M, Costa S, et al. Monoclonal antibodies to detect breast cancer cells in bone marrow. In: De Vita VT, Hellman S, Rosenberg SA, eds. Important advances in oncology 1994. Philadelphia, JB Lippincott, 1994:143.

78. Ghalia A, Silva O, Vredenburgh J, et al. Advances in the detection of marrow micrometastases in breast cancer. Cancer Res Ther Control 1994;4:43.

79. Schoenfeld A, Luqmani Y, Smith D, et al. Detection of breast cancer micrometastases in axillary lymph nodes by using polymerase chain reaction. Cancer Res 1994;54:2986.

80. Goldfarb R, Brunson K. Therapeutic agents for treatment of established metastases and inhibitors of metastatic spread: preclinical and clinical progress. Curr Opin Oncol 1992;4:1130.

81. Yanase T, Tamura M, Fujita K, et al. Inhibitory effect of angiogenesis inhibitor TNP-470 on tumor growth and metastasis of human cell lines in vitro and in vivo. Cancer Res 1993;53:2566.

82. Myers C, Cooper M, Stein C, et al. Suramin: a novel growth factor antagonist with activity in hormone-refractory metastatic prostate cancer. J Clin Oncol 1992;10:881.

83. Wellstein A, Zugmaier G, Kern F, et al. Tumor growth dependent on Kaposi's sarcoma-derived fibroblast growth factor inhibited by pentosan polysulfate. J Natl Cancer Inst 1991;83:716.

84. Zugmaier G, Lippman ME, Wellstein A. Inhibition by pentosan polysulfate (PPS) of heparin-binding growth factors released from tumor cells and blockage by PPS of tumor growth in animals. J Natl Cancer Inst 1992;84:1716.

85. Ingber D, Fujita T, Kishimoto S, et al. Synthetic analogues of fumagillin that inhibit angiogenesis and suppress tumor growth. Nature 1990;348:555.

86. Yamaoka M, Yamamoto T, Ikeyama S, et al. Angiogenesis inhibitor TNP-470 (AGM-1470) potently inhibits the tumor growth of hormone-independent human breast and prostate carcinoma cell lines. Cancer Res 1993;53:5233.

87. Vogel T, Guo N, Krutzsch HC, et al. Modulation of endothelial cell proliferation, adhesion, and motility by recombinant heparin-binding domain and synthetic peptides from the type I repeats of thrombospondin. J Cell Biochem 1993;53:74.

88. Leone A, Flatow U, King CR, et al. Reduced tumor incidence, metastatic potential, and cytokine responsiveness of *nm23*-transfected melanoma cells. Cell 1991;65:25.

89. Kohn E, Sandeen M, Liotta L. In vivo efficacy of a novel inhibitor of selected signal transduction pathways including calcium, arachidonate, and inositol phosphates. Cancer Res 1992;52:3208.

90. Harris A, Horak E. Growth factors and angiogenesis in breast cancer. Recent Results Cancer Res 1993;127:35.

91. Shepard H, Lewis G, Sarup J, et al. Monoclonal antibody therapy of human cancer: taking the *HER2* protooncogene to the clinic. J Clin Immunol 1991;11:117.

92. Baselga J, Mendelsohn J. The epidermal growth factor receptor as a target for therapy in breast carcinoma. Breast Cancer Res Treat 1994;29:127.

93. Garcia M, Derocq D, Freiss G, et al. Activation of estrogen receptor transfected into a receptor-negative breast cancer cell line decreases the metastatic and invasive potential of the cells. Proc Natl Acad Sci USA 1992;89:11538.

94. Lollini P, Bosco M, Cavallo F, et al. Inhibition of tumor growth and enhancement of metastasis after transfection of the γ-interferon gene. Int J Cancer 1993;55:320.

95. McLeskey S, Kurebayashi J, Honig S, et al. Fibroblast growth factor 4 transfection of MCF-7 cells produces cell lines that are tumorigenic and metastatic in ovariectomized or tamoxifen treated athymic nude mice. Cancer Res 1993;53:2168.

96. Davies B, Barraclough R, Davies M, et al. Production of the metastatic phenotype by DNA transfection in a rat mammary tumor model. Cell Biol Int 1993;17:871.

Control of Angiogenesis

ANTON WELLSTEIN

Ample experimental evidence in the past two decades shows that tumor growth and metastasis depend on neovascularization. Unless neovascularization occurs, a solid tumor grows no larger than about 2 mm in diameter. Moreover, for tumor cells to metastasize, they must gain access to the vasculature, localize in the target organ, and induce angiogenesis in that organ to expand. Angiogenesis is therefore necessary both at the beginning and at the end of the metastatic cascade. This doctrine is based on countless experiments using various tumor models and animal species.[1-3]

In the past 5 years, clinical studies by different groups have demonstrated that this dogma can also be applied to human tumors, including breast cancer. After a pioneering study published early in 1991,[4] a series of subsequent independent studies in more than 1000 patients demonstrated that microvessel density in primary breast cancers is an indicator of disease outcome.[5-13] In these studies, microvessel density was quantitated using light microscopy and immunohistochemical staining of a factor VIII–related antigen or a platelet/endothelial cell adhesion molecule (PECAM, or CD31). In general, these observations support the notion that, in clinical breast cancer, metastasis and, therefore, fatal outcome of the disease are closely linked to the angiogenic capacity of the primary tumor. Corroborating evidence is provided by studies of other tumor types: non–small cell lung, prostate, and head and neck carcinoma all showed a similar association between microvessel counts in the primary tumors and patient prognosis.[14]

Tumor angiogenesis as reflected in microvessel density appears to be an independent prognostic indicator in breast cancer patients when tested against known parameters such as tumor size, estrogen receptor (ER), lymph node status and c-erbB-2 expression. Of particular significance are recent reports that, in patients with ER-positive tumors (and apparently good prognosis), high microvessel density of the tumors predicted a reduction in survival in a subgroup of the patients.[13]

Factors Regulating Tumor Angiogenesis

Neoangiogenesis requires the degradation of the basement membrane and extracellular matrix, as well as the migration, proliferation, and differentiation of endothelial cells to form tubes, which finally anastomose into capillary networks. This process is based on the interplay of growth factors and extracellular proteases that is appropriately balanced by the respective inhibitors (Fig. 7.12-1):

Positive Modulators of Angiogenesis
Angiogenic growth factors
Proteases

Negative Modulators of Angiogenesis
Thrombospondin-1
Interleukin-1
Protease inhibitors

Physiologic angiogenesis in adults is restricted to the female reproductive cycle (ovulation, menstruation, and placenta growth), and turnover time of endothelial cells in adult tissues is measured in years. However, angiogenic factors can induce endothelial cells to proliferate as fast as bone marrow cells, with resultant turnover times of only days. In animal models, 50- to 100-times higher uptake of thymidine (as a proliferation marker) was observed in placental or tumor endothelium than in other normal tissues.[15] A recent study demonstrated similar findings in breast cancer versus normal breast tissue samples. Intratumoral microvessels showed a 45-fold greater labeling index of a proliferation antigen (Ki-67) than adjacent benign breast tissues.[16] Polypeptide growth factors released from the tumor cells are believed to trigger these host responses.[3,17]

However, the acquisition by a tumor of an angiogenic phenotype involves not only the induction of positive factors but also the suppression of angiogenesis inhibitors. One example is the regulation of metalloprotease inhibitors by oncogenes and tumor suppressor genes.[18] Another example is thrombospondin-1, a potent inhibitor of angiogenesis.[19] Dameron and colleagues[19] reported that cultured fibroblasts from patients with Li-Fraumeni syndrome with a germ line p53 mutation switched to an angiogenic phenotype with the loss of their wild-type allele of the p53 tumor suppressor gene. This switch coincided with the reduced expression of thrombospondin-1. Additional studies suggest that wild-type p53 can directly up-regulate thrombospondin-1 gene transcription, thus providing a direct link between the loss of a suppressor gene and angiogenesis inhibiton.

GROWTH FACTORS

A conservative estimate indicates that more than a dozen distinct protein products are known to induce proliferation of endothelial cells in vitro or angiogenesis in vivo[1,20]:

Heparin–Binding Growth Factors
Fibroblast growth factors (FGFs; eg, aFGF, bFGF, K-FGF)
Hepatocyte growth factor, scatter factor
Pleiotrophin
Vascular endothelial cell growth factor (VEGF; vascular permeability factor)

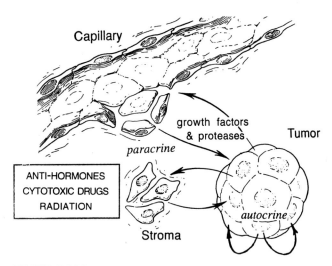

FIGURE 7.12-1 Interaction between tumor cells, stroma, and blood vessels. Growth factors and proteases (among other molecules) are released locally from the tumor cells and the surrounding host tissues. Systemic hormones and therapeutic interventions affect this local interaction.

Other Growth Factors
Interleukin-4
Interleukin-8
Transforming growth factor α

The most prominent and best-studied angiogenesis factors are members of the FGF family,[21] but a number of others also qualify as potential tumor angiogenesis factors. Furthermore, any combination of these proteins may be found expressed in tumor tissues or in tumor cell lines.[17] Thus, it is difficult to decipher which ones are only innocent bystanders and which are rate limiting during tumor angiogenesis.

One growth factor thought to play a role in breast cancer angiogenesis is VEGF, or vascular permeability factor.[22] VEGF is a heparin-binding growth factor with a selective activity toward vascular endothelial cells. VEGF expression was found to be widely distributed in different normal tissues. It appeared particularly high in areas of active vascular proliferation such as the corpus luteum and was localized to blood vessels in tumors.[22,23] A recent study demonstrated a good correlation between VEGF expression and microvessel density in breast cancer samples.[11] Furthermore, relapse-free survival for patients with VEGF-rich tumors was worse than that for patients with VEGF-poor tumors.

FGFs were the first endothelial cell growth factors characterized. Nine members of this heparin-binding growth factor family are known.[21] However, most work has been concentrated on aFGF and bFGF (also called FGF-1 and FGF-2). With respect to human tumors, bFGF levels have been found to be elevated in the urine of patients with breast cancer as well as other solid tumors.[24] This elevation was correlated with the activity state of the tumors, and it is possible that the growth factor becomes released into the circulation during invasion of the tumors into surrounding tissues.[25] We demonstrated that a novel heparin-binding growth factor, pleiotrophin, is expressed in a high portion of breast cancer samples, but a correlation with the disease state or prognosis has not yet been studied.[26]

In addition to the regulation of growth factors themselves, their receptors, which transduce the signal from the cell surface, are highly regulated. Furthermore, acceptor molecules for growth factors on the extracellular cell surface can modulate the bioavailability and activity of growth factors.[27] Finally secreted binding proteins (eg, for FGF[28]) or secreted receptor fragments (eg, the FGF receptor[29]) may also regulate the activity of these angiogenesis factors. Which of these molecules are the most significant with respect to tumor angiogenesis in breast cancer has not yet been established. It is conceivable that a few factors and their receptors will emerge as the major players in future clinical studies.

PROTEASES

Extracellular proteolysis is an essential component of the angiogenic process.[30] Appropriate balancing of proteolytic activities by endogenous protease inhibitors is required during this process to protect the extracellular matrix from excessive degradation. Endothelial cells are capable of activating the complete proteolytic and inhibitory machinery necessary to generate new blood vessels in response to angiogenic factors.[3] Endothelial cell–derived proteases include the urokinase-type plasminogen activator, metalloproteases, collagenases, gelatinases, and stromelysin.[31] In a cascade of events, plasmin degrades components of the extracellular matrix and at the same time activates the prometalloproteases. Secretion of plasmin activator inhibitor by migrating cells is generally stimulated by the same factors that induce production and secretion of the activator (eg, by bFGF or VEGF). Thus, fine tuning of the proteolysis of the matrix is maintained.[32] In general, the ratio between activator and inhibitor is tilted toward proteolysis in response to endothelial cell–activating factors such as FGFs and VEGF and toward antiproteolysis in response to endothelial cell–inhibitory growth factor such as transforming growth factor β. In line with this, plasminogen fragment (angiostatin) secreted from a primary tumor in rodents was recently shown to circulate in the bloodstream of tumor-bearing mice and to limit the growth of tumor metastases.[33] Finally, plasminogen activator and inhibitor were also extracted from breast cancer samples, and higher activites were associated with a poor prognosis of the patients.[34] The same correlation was shown for cathepsin D. These observations may reflect the different endothelial cell growth factor activities present in the tumor tissues that appear to regulate its proteolytic activities.

Conventional Therapies

Blood vessels in tumors are usually thin walled without smooth muscle cells and consist only of endothelial lining backed by a basement membrane.[1,2] As pointed out earlier, endothelial cells in breast cancer show high proliferation rates in areas of neoangiogenesis.[16] Areas of tumor cell and endothelial cell proliferation do not appear to coincide,[16,35] suggesting that different growth factors and inhibitors drive each process. Furthermore, the proliferating fractions of tumor cells and endothelial cells were similar and clearly distinct from those of normal control tissues. This observation warrants the speculation that much of the efficacy of conventional cytotoxic therapies may in fact have a major antiangiogenic component.[15,36] Evidence to support this notion is discussed later. Furthermore, the conventional understanding of drug resistance and appropriate models to search for effective anticancer drugs should be reevaluated, taking these findings into account.

CYTOTOXIC AGENTS

Cytotoxics agents are designed to kill cells by interfering with the normal process of DNA replication and cell division or by causing direct damage to the DNA. Proliferating endothelial cells in the tumor vasculature are also sensitive to damage by cytotoxic drugs. Furthermore, the poor organization of the tumor vessels should make endothelial cells more susceptible to damage and repair processes less efficient. Several drugs with proven clinical effects in diseases involving angiogenesis have been found to be inhibitors of angiogenesis, and this may be their primary mechanism of action. In particular, the antitumor activities of methotrexate[37] and of anthracyclines (eg, doxorubicin [Adriamycin])[38] can be explained in part by their antiangiogenic activities.

ANTIHORMONES AND HORMONES

Hormones that promote breast cancer growth can regulate polypeptide growth factor production, and these growth factors can in turn modulate the hormone action locally.[39,40] The application of this general rule to tumor angiogenesis was substantiated in studies with a hormone-sensitive breast cancer cell line in animal studies. Magnetic resonance spectroscopy revealed that tamoxifen treatment resulted in the inhibition of endothelial cell growth and enhanced necrosis and subsequent tumor regression.[41,42] These effects can be explained by the reduced production of endothelial cell growth factors by the hormone-sensitive tumor cells and subsequent death of growth factor–deprived tumor endothelium. To what extent the efficacy of other hormones and antihormones also relies on direct or indirect effects on the tumor–stroma interaction is not yet understood.

RADIATION THERAPY

Radiation-induced damage to cells becomes evident when the cells undergo mitosis. From the data on endothelial cell kinetics in tumors (discussed earlier), it can be expected that radiation-induced cell death will occur much earlier in tumor vessels and will be more abundant than in normal vessels. Effects of radiation therapy on tumor vasculature in combination with other treatments may be used to improve efficacy of the therapy.[15,36]

Novel Therapies

One unique property makes endothelial cell proliferation in tumors a promising target for the chemotherapy of malignant growth: in adults, the only physiologic conditions that require endothelial cell proliferation are wound healing and the female reproductive cycle. Endothelial cell proliferation in a growing primary tumor or a metastatic lesion, therefore, can hopefully be targeted with high selectivity. The selective endothelial cell proliferation in tumors should make selective inhibitors of endothelial cell proliferation effective anticancer drugs with only limited systemic effects on the host. It appears that the endothelial cell growth factors produced by tumor cells or released by tumor-derived enzymes from the surrounding stroma should be a convenient point of attack.

INHIBITORS OF SPECIFIC GROWTH FACTORS

Use of inhibitors of specific growth factors is still in the preclinical phase, but several hopeful candidate drugs have begun to emerge. Studies with blocking antibodies directed against VEGF demonstrated that this factor was rate limiting for the growth of selected model tumors in animals.[43] Similar studies with anti-bFGF antibodies showed only little efficacy.[44] Growth factor–toxin conjugates are still experimental[15] and are discussed elsewhere in text. The generation of peptide fragments or peptidomimetics that block receptor access has become more productive with the introduction of combinatorial peptide libraries.[46] However, this is still in preclinical drug development.

The inhibition of defined gene transcripts by antisense deoxyoligonucleotides has been used to dissect the role of growth factors and numerous other gene products.[47] The clinical application of these may become reality in the next few years, since problems of cheap and bulk synthesis of high-quality deoxyoligunucleotides have been solved. A new approach to the targeting of specific gene products is the use of ribozymes that cleave the targeted mRNA in a highly specific fashion. Using this approach, it has been shown that a tumor growth and angiogenesis factor (pleiotrophin) is a rate-limiting growth factor for some tumors.[49] This approach is still experimental, but with the emerging improvement of gene transfer methods, eventual clinical applications appear to be possible.

INHIBITORS OF HEPARIN-BINDING GROWTH FACTORS

Most endothelial cell growth factors have in common that they bind to heparin and can be summarized as heparin-binding growth factors (HBGFs). This laboratory observation is of high significance in vivo. The HBGFs bind to extracellular heparan sulfate proteoglycan molecules, and their biologic activities are modulated by this binding.[27]

Different molecules that mimic portions of heparan sulfate proteoglycans have been studied in detail with respect to their HBGF-inhibiting actions. Defined polysaccharides and heparin digests,[50–52] as well as different preparations of heparin-like substances in combination with steroids, were examined as inhibitors.[2] We searched for a compound that would bind HBGFs and block their activities instead of stabilizing the activity of HBGFs as observed with many preparations of heparin. The semisynthetic pentosanpolysulfate showed the most promising properties among various polysulfates with a selectivity ratio of more than 1000 comparing HBGF-specific inhibition versus nonspecific toxicity.[53] This compound is in clinical trial.[54] Recent studies demonstrate that binding of FGF molecules to monomeric heparin fragments can inhibit, and binding to polymeric heparin can promote, biologic activity of this growth factor.[55] This is a further lead to the systematic development of more effective HBGF inhibitors.

PROTEASE INHIBITORS

Inhibition of proteases to block invasion and metastasis, as well as in angiogenesis, is a field of intense drug development and is reviewed elsewhere.

INHIBITORS BASED ON ENDOTHELIAL CELL PROLIFERATION

The specific targeting of gene products expressed during endothelial cell proliferation seems to be an obvious choice for drug development,[56] but only a few promising leads have emerged. Expression of a specific vascular integrin, $\alpha(v)\beta(3)$, is required for angiogenesis in vivo.[57] This appears to be true for different angiogenic stimuli and points to a promising target for the generation of specific inhibitors of neoangiogenesis.[58] Furthermore, in a different experimental setting, the eradication of large solid tumors was possible using an immunotoxin directed against tumor vasculature.[59]

Finally, a derivative of the fungal product fumagillin, AGM-1470 (TNP-470),[60,61] was shown to inhibit proliferating endothelial cells with high specificity. This drug also inhibited tumor growth of hormone-independent human breast carcinoma cell lines in animal models.[62] Its mechanism of action seems to be suppression of specific functions of proteins that regulate the cell cycle in endothelial cells (cyclins and cdc2 kinases).[63,64] Clinical trials with this compound have begun at different sites.

THALIDOMIDE

Thalidomide is a hypnotic drug and a potent teratogen that causes dysmelia in offspring when administered during early pregnancy. Recent experiments revealed that the the teratogenicity of this drug can be explained by its antiangiogenic activity. No correlations of this effect with the sedative properties of thalidomide were found. The antiangiogenic activity of thalidomide was detected in animal studies using rabbit corneal neovascularization as a model. Ultrastructural changes due to thalidomide treatment observed in this classic angiogenesis model were similar to changes in the deformed limb bud vasculature of thalidomide-treated embryos. These findings suggest the potential use of thalidomide as an inhibitor of angiogenesis. In particular, the oral bioavailability of thalidomide and good safety profile in adults warrant further studies.[65]

Combination Therapies

Combinations of drugs that target tumor angiogenesis with conventional breast cancer treatments are an active area of preclinical studies. It is conceivable, for example, that antihormonal therapies (eg, tamoxifen) or cytotoxic treatment could remove the targeted proliferating tumor endothelium from a therapeutic attack by more specific antiangiogenic drugs and thereby require sequential treatment. Furthermore, anti–growth factor therapy could make radiation therapy or cytotoxic treatment less effective because of a reduction of the fraction of sensitive cells in the tumor.

Results with different tumor models suggest that a combination of cytotoxic agents with the endothelial cell inhibitor AGM-1470 may be beneficial in the treatment of solid tumors. Mostly additive effects were reported by different laboratories using AGM-1470 with doxorubicin, cisplatin, 5-fluorouracil, mitomycin, or taxol in rodent tumors.[62,66–69] These preclinical studies of combination therapies so far are encouraging and appear to suffice for the planning of clinical combination trials in the near future.

Outlook

Many current therapies have antiangiogenesis as an underlying mechanism of action. The combination of novel angiogenesis-targeted drugs with conventional therapies with different mechanisms of action is a promising approach to provide less toxic, more effective cancer treatments. In the current phase of ongoing preclinical development, more or less empiric combinations of antiangiogenic compounds and conventional cytotoxic drugs or radiation therapy need to be applied in defined tumor models. From this, the rational designs of future clinical studies should be derived.

References

1. Folkman J, Shing Y. Angiogenesis. J Biol Chem 1992;267:10931.
2. Folkman J. Antiangiogenesis. In: DeVita VT, Hellman S, Rosenberg SA, eds. Biologic therapy of cancer. Philadelphia, JB Lippincott, 1991:743.

3. Liotta LA, Steeg PS, Stetler-Stevenson WG. Cancer metastasis and angiogenesis: an imbalance of positive and negative regulation. Cell 1991;64:327.

4. Weidner N, Semple JP, Welch WR, et al. Tumor angiogenesis and metastasis: correlation in invasive breast carcinoma. N Engl J Med 1991;324:1.

5. Weidner N, Folkman J, Pozza F, et al. Tumor angiogenesis: a new significant and independent prognostic indicator in early-stage breast carcinoma. J Natl Cancer Inst 1992;84:1875.

6. Horak ER, Leek R, Klenk N, et al. Angiogenesis, assessed by platelet/endothelial cell adhesion molecule antibodies, as indicator of node metastases and survival in breast cancer. Lancet 1992;340:1120.

7. Bosari S, Lee AK, DeLellis RA, et al. Microvessel quantitation and prognosis in invasive breast carcinoma. Hum Pathol 1992;23:755.

8. Toi M, Kashitani J, Tominaga T. Tumor angiogenesis is an independent prognostic indicator in primary breast carcinoma. Int J Cancer 1993;55:371.

9. Obermair A, Czerwenka K, Kurz C, et al. Tumoral vascular density in breast tumors and their effect on recurrence-free survival. Chirurgie 1994;65:611.

10. Toi M, Hoshina S, Yamamoto Y, et al. Tumor angiogenesis in breast cancer: significance of vessel density as a prognostic indicator. Gan To Kagaku Ryoho 1994;21(Suppl 2):178.

11. Toi M, Hoshina S, Takayanagi T, et al. Association of vascular endothelial growth factor expression with tumor angiogenesis and with early relapse in primary breast cancer. Jpn J Cancer Res 1994;85:1045.

12. Weidner N, Gasparini G. Determination of epidermal growth factor receptor provides additional prognostic information to measuring tumor angiogenesis in breast carcinoma patients. Breast Cancer Res Treat 1994;29:97.

13. Fox SB, Leek RD, Smith K, et al. Tumor angiogenesis in node-negative breast carcinomas: relationship with epidermal growth factor receptor, estrogen receptor, and survival. Breast Cancer Res Treat 1994;29:109.

14. Weidner N. Tumor angiogenesis: review of current applications in tumor prognostication. Semin Diagn Pathol 1993;10:302.

15. Denekamp J. Angiogenesis, neovascular proliferation and vascular pathophysiology as targets for cancer therapy. Br J Radiol 1993;66:181.

16. Vartanian RK, Weidner N. Correlation of intratumoral endothelial cell proliferation with microvessel density (tumor angiogenesis) and tumor cell proliferation in breast carcinoma. Am J Pathol 1994;144:1188.

17. Cross M, Dexter TM. Growth factors in development, transformation, and tumorigenesis. Cell 1991;64:271.

18. Bouck N. Angiogenesis: a mechanism by which oncogenes and tumor suppressor genes regulate tumorigenesis. Cancer Treat Res 1992;63:359.

19. Dameron KM, Volpert OV, Tainsky MA, et al. Control of angiogenesis in fibroblasts by p53 regulation of thrombospondin-1. Science 1994;265:1582.

20. Fidler IJ, Ellis LM. The implications of angiogenesis for the biology and therapy of cancer metastasis. (Comment) Cell 1994;79:185.

21. Mason IJ. The ins and outs of fibroblast growth factors. Cell 1994;78:547.

22. Ferrara N, Houck KA, Jakeman LB, et al. The vascular endothelial growth factor family of polypeptides. J Cell Biochem 1991;47:211.

23. Berse B, Brown LF, Water LVD, et al. Vascular permeability factor (vascular endothelial growth factor) gene is expressed differentially in normal tissues, macrophages and tumors. Mol Biol Cell 1992;3:211.

24. Nguyen M, Watanabe H, Budson AE, et al. Elevated levels of an angiogenic peptide, basic fibroblast growth factor, in the urine of patients with a wide spectrum of cancers. J Natl Cancer Inst 1994;86:356.

25. Wellstein A. Why monitor angiogenesis factors in the urine of patients? (Editorial) J Natl Cancer Inst 1994;86:328.

26. Fang WJ, Hartmann N, Chow D, et al. Pleiotrophin stimulates fibroblasts, endothelial and epithelial cells, and is expressed in human cancer. J Biol Chem 1992;267:25889.

27. Aviezer D, Hecht D, Safran M, et al. Perlecan, basal lamina proteoglycan, promotes basic fibroblast growth factor–receptor binding, mitogenesis and angiogenesis. Cell 1994;79:1005.

28. Czubayko F, Smith RV, Chung HC, et al. A secreted binding protein can activate non-secreted FGF in tumors. J Biol Chem 1994;269:28243.

29. Hanneken A, Ying W, Ling N, et al. Identification of soluble forms of the fibroblast growth factor receptor in blood. Proc Natl Acad Sci USA 1994;91:9170.

30. Liotta LA. The role of cellular proteases and their inhibitors in invasion and metastasis. Introductory overview. Cancer Metastasis Rev 1990;9:285.

31. Menashi S, Lu H, Soria C, Legrand Y. Endothelial cell proteases: physiological role and regulation. Baillieres Clin Haematol 1993;6:559.

32. Pepper MS, Ferrara N, Orci L, et al. Vascular endothelial growth factor (VEGF) induces plasminogen activators and plasminogen activator inhibitor-1 in microvascular endothelial cells. Biochem Biophys Res Commun 1991;181:902.

33. O'Reilly MS, Holmgren L, Shing Y, et al. Angiostatin: a novel angiogenesis inhibitor that mediates the suppression of metastases by a Lewis lung carcinoma. Cell 1994;79:315.

34. Grondahl-Hansen J, Christensen IJ, Rosenquist C, et al. High levels of urokinase-type plasminogen activator and its inhibitor PAI-1 in cytosolic extracts of breast carcinomas are associated with poor prognosis. Cancer Res 1993;53:2513.

35. Fox SB, Gatter KC, Bicknell R, et al. Relationship of endothelial cell proliferation to tumor vascularity in human breast cancer. Cancer Res 1993;53:4161.

36. Denekamp J. Vascular attack as a therapeutic strategy for cancer. Cancer Metastasis Rev 1990;9:267.

37. Hirata S, Matsubara T, Saura R, et al. Inhibition of in vitro vascular endothelial cell proliferation and in vivo neovascularization by low-dose methotrexate. Arthritis Rheum 1989;32:1065.

38. Maragoudakis ME, Peristeris P, Missirlis E, et al. Inhibition of angiogenesis by anthracyclines and titanocene dichloride. Ann NY Acad Sci 1994;732:280.

39. Dickson R, Lippman ME. Estrogenic regulation of growth and polypeptide growth factor secretion in human breast carcinoma. Endocr Rev 1987;8:29.

40. Clarke R, Dickson RB, Lippman ME. Hormonal aspects of breast cancer: growth factors, drugs and stromal interactions. Crit Rev Oncol Hematol 1992;12:1.

41. Degani H, Furman E, Fields S. Magnetic resonance imaging and spectroscopy of MCF7 human breast cancer: pathophysiology and monitoring of treatment. Clin Chim Acta 1994;228:19.

42. Haran EF, Maretzek AF, Goldberg I, et al. Tamoxifen enhances cell death in implanted MCF7 breast cancer by inhibiting endothelium growth. Cancer Res 1994;54:5511.

43. Kim KJ, Li B, Winer J, et al. Inhibition of vascular endothelial growth factor–induced angiogenesis suppresses tumour growth in vivo. Nature 1993;362:841.

44. Matsuzaki K, Yoshitake Y, Matuo Y, et al. Monoclonal antibodies against heparin-binding growth factor II/basic fibroblast growth factor that block its biological activity: invalidity of the antibodies for tumor angiogenesis. Proc Natl Acad Sci USA 1989;86:9911.

45. Pai LH, Pastan I. Immunotoxins and recombinant toxins for cancer treatment. In: DeVita VT, Hellman S, Rosenberg SA, eds. Important advances in oncology 1994. Philadelphia, JB Lippincott, 1994:3.

46. Houghten RA. The broad utility of soluble peptide libraries for drug discovery. Gene 1993;7:432.

47. Wagner RW. Gene inhibition using antisense oligodeoxynucleotides. Nature 1994;372:333.

48. Cech TR, Bass BL. Biological catalysis by RNA. Annu Rev Biochem 1986;55:599.

49. Czubayko F, Riegel AT, Wellstein A. Ribozyme-targeting elucidates a direct role of pleiotrophin in tumor growth. J Biol Chem 1994;269:21358.

50. Ishihara M, Tyrrell DJ, Stauber GB, et al. Preparation of affinity-fractionated, heparin-derived oligosaccharides and their effects on selected biological activities mediated by basic fibroblast growth factor. J Biol Chem 1993;268:4675.

51. Aviezer D, Levy E, Safran M, et al. Differential structural requirements of heparin and heparan sulfate proteoglycans that promote binding of basic fibroblast growth factor to its receptor. J Biol Chem 1994;269:114.

52. Guimond S, Maccarana M, Olwin BB, et al. Activating and inhibitory heparin sequences for FGF-2 (basic FGF). J Biol Chem 1993;268:23906.

53. Zugmaier G, Lippman ME, Wellstein A. Inhibition by pentosan polysulfate (PPS) of heparin-binding growth factors released from tumor cells and blockade by PPS of tumor growth in animals. J Natl Cancer Inst 1992;84:1716.

54. Parker BW, Zugmaier G, Swain SS, et al. Detection of anti–growth factor activity in human serum after treatment of patients with pentosanpolysulfate. J Natl Cancer Inst 1993;85:1068.

55. Spivak-Kroizman T, Lemmon MA, Kikic I, et al. Heparin-induced oligomerization of FGF molecules is responsible for FGF receptor dimerization, activation and cell proliferation. Cell 1994;79:1015.

56. Denekamp J. The current status of targeting tumour vasculature as a means of cancer therapy: an overview. Int J Radiat Biol 1991;60:401.

57. Brooks PC, Clark RAF, Cheresh DA. Requirement of vascular integrin alpha(v)beta(3) for angiogenesis. Science 1994;264:569.

58. Brooks PC, Montgomery AMP, Rosenfeld M, et al. Integrin alpha(v)beta(3) antagonists promote tumor regression by inducing apoptosis of angiogenic blood vessels. Cell 1994;79:1157.

59. Burrows FJ, Thorpe PE. Eradication of large solid tumors in mice with an immunotoxin directed against tumor vasculature. Proc Natl Acad Sci USA 1993;90:8996.

60. Kusaka M, Sudo K, Fujita T, et al. Potent anti-angiogenic action of AGM-1470: comparison to the fumagillin parent. Biochem Biophys Res Commun 1991;174:1070.

61. Ingber D, Fujita T, Kishimoto S, et al. Synthetic analogues of fumagillin that inhibit angiogenesis and suppress tumour growth. Nature 1990;348:555.

62. Yamaoka M, Yamamoto T, Ikeyama S, et al. Angiogenesis inhibitor TNP-470 (AGM-1470) potently inhibits the tumor growth of hormone-independent human breast and prostate carcinoma cell lines. Cancer Res 1993;53:5233.

63. Abe J, Zhou W, Takuwa N, et al. A fumagillin derivative angiogenesis inhibitor, AGM-1470, inhibits activation of cyclin-dependent kinases and phosphorylation of retinoblastoma gene product but not protein tyrosyl phosphorylation or protooncogene expression in vascular endothelial cells. Cancer Res 1994;54:3407.

64. Hori A, Ikeyama S, Sudo K. Suppression of cyclin D1 mRNA expression by the angiogenesis inhibitor TNP-470 (AGM-1470) in vascular endothelial cells. Biochem Biophys Res Commun 1994;204:1067.

65. D'Amato RJ, Loughnan MS, Flynn E, et al. Thalidomide is an inhibitor of angiogenesis. Proc Natl Acad Sci USA 1994;91:4082.

66. Teicher BA, Sotomayor EA, Huang ZD. Antiangiogenic agents potentiate cytotoxic cancer therapies against primary and metastatic disease. Cancer Res 1992;52:6702.

67. Kato T, Sato K, Kakinuma H, et al. Enhanced suppression of tumor growth by combination of angiogenesis inhibitor O-(chloroacetyl-carbamoyl)fumagillol (TNP-470) and cytotoxic agents in mice. Cancer Res 1994;54:5143.

68. Oliver SJ, Banquerigo ML, Brahn E. Suppression of collagen-induced arthritis using an angiogenesis inhibitor, AGM-1470, and a microtubule stabilizer, taxol. Cell Immunol 1994;157:291.

69. Brem H, Gresser I, Grosfeld J, et al. The combination of antiangiogenic agents to inhibit primary tumor growth and metastasis. J Pediatr Surg 1993;28:1253.

7.13
Immunology and Immunotherapy of Breast Cancer

MALCOLM S. MITCHELL

Breast cancer is not often thought of as an immunologically responsive tumor, certainly not in the same context as melanoma or renal cell carcinoma. Moreover, because the chemotherapy of breast cancer predictably causes remissions, biologic therapy is not often entertained as an approach to the disease. Yet an increasing body of information suggests that perhaps breast cancer should be considered one of an increasing number of tumors for which different, immunologically based treatments may be useful by themselves or in combination with chemotherapy.

This discussion attempts to outline some of the information on the immunology of breast cancer that provides an insight into which types of immunologic treatment are likely to be of value. Factors that influence the host's immunologic response to breast cancer and the adverse consequences of the immune system on the course of breast cancer are also described. Finally, I discuss the recent application of immunologic methods to the early detection of micrometastases.

The fundamental aspects of tumor immunology and immunotherapy, which are extensively covered elsewhere,[1,2] are not considered here. Rather, the reader is presumed to understand about T lymphocytes, natural killer (NK) cells, and the like, and to be aware that tumor-associated, if perhaps not tumor-specific, antigens have been identified in several tumor systems.

Antigens of Breast Cancer

CARCINOEMBRYONIC ANTIGEN AND OTHER CARCINOFETAL ANTIGENS

One of the first antigens to be described for any human cancer was carcinoembryonic antigen (CEA). In a now-classic article, Gold and Freedman[3] described what they believed to be a tumor-specific antigen in adenocarcinomas of the gastrointestinal tract, but which later proved to be present in a variety of epithelial tumors. Although CEA did not prove to be absolutely tumor-specific, as no antigen is, its description provided a powerful impetus for investigations into tumor-associated antigens for this group as well as other tumors.

The value of CEA as a tumor marker is not discussed here. Rather, its role as a possible target for immunotherapy with antibodies or cells has been a more recent topic for study. Schlom and colleagues[4] have shown that recombinant vaccinia vaccines containing CEA as the immunogen are immunogenic in nonhuman primates as well as in rodents. This strategy has been proposed for the treatment of human adenocarcinomas that express CEA on their surface. Whereas the immunogenicity of CEA for mice is clear, a critical point to be proved is whether CEA is immunogenic in humans, and particularly whether it elicits cytolytic T lymphocytes. With those characteristics, CEA could then be considered a reasonable candidate antigen for active specific immunotherapy of breast cancer.

MUCINS AND BLOOD GROUP–RELATED ANTIGENS

Much excitement has been generated by the unique mucin shared by adenocarcinomas of the gastrointestinal tract and by breast, ovarian, and lung cancers. This polymorphic epithelial mucin (PEM)[5,6] is an approximately 400-kd glycoprotein composed of a central core protein with a series of 20 amino acid tandem repeats, on which are attached oligosaccharide side chains. Because glycosylation of the mucin by the breast cancer cells is aberrant, the saccharides are not the usual luxuriant, multibranched sugars characterizing normal epithelial mucin, but instead are truncated. Because of this truncation, not only are the saccharides unique to the tumor, but also the core of the PEM is unusually exposed to the immune system. Thus, two separate potential targets are available for immunologic attack. PEM is more highly expressed on carcinomas than on normal tissues, and the tandem repeats constitute repeated antigenic determinants (epitopes) per molecule.

Among the usually cryptic saccharides exposed in malignantly transformed cells are the Thomsen-Friedenreich (TF) antigen and the related saccharides Tn and sialyl-Tn. These antigens are related to the Lewis blood group antigens. The TF antigen is immunogenic, but it can act in vivo either as an immunogen or an immunosuppressive material, depending on the formulation used.[7] This is similar to findings with epiglycanin, a mucin-like glycoprotein from adenocarcinomas that contains TF and Tn epitopes, by the same investigative group.[8]

The MUC-1 peptide derived from the PEM has the structure PDTRPAPGSTAPPAHGVTSA.[5,6] The immunodominant B-cell–determinant region contains the structure PDTRPAP. This sequence is also either identical with, or overlaps, a T-cell epitope in humans. In fact, it is highly immunodominant for mice as well. Nearly all of the common mouse antibodies to serologic markers for breast cancer, such as CA 15-3 and B72.3, recognize the same region of the mucin. Linking this region to an influenza virus–hemagglutinin region recognized by T-helper

cells led to the induction of antibodies to MUC-1, with titers depending on the position of the T-cell determinant and matching of the class II haplotype recognizing that determinant.[9] This strategy was developed primarily to enable the production of potent monoclonal antibodies against MUC-1. Ding and associates[10] studied synthetic peptides from the PEM systematically, either conjugated to keyhole limpet hemocyanin (KLH) or clustered in a multiple antigenic peptide (MAP-4) configuration that included a malarial T-helper epitope. IgG antibodies were elicited in mice that bound MUC-1 and breast cancer cells that expressed MUC-1. The MAP-4 construct alone was less effective in inducing antibodies. Delayed-type hypersensitivity was induced well by all three constructs and could be detected either with synthetic peptides or MUC-1–transduced cells. Furthermore, irradiated MUC-1–transduced cells led to delayed-type hypersensitivity (DTH) that could be elicited by testing with synthetic peptides expressing the PDTRP sequence.

Another finding is also of great potential importance for the development of human vaccines. Finn and her colleagues have shown that cytotoxic T lymphocytes (CTL) react against MUC-1 and have the unusual property of being HLA-unrestricted.[11,12] The tandem repeats of the peptide may well account for that property, providing multiple epitopes on the same molecule and improving the strength of bonding between effector and target, as these investigators suggested. HLA-"nonfastidious" CTLs have also been identified in melanoma, however, in which tandem repeats have not been demonstrated,[13] and lesser degrees of HLA specificity are also a property of the CTLs found in elderly mice.

GENES AND ONCOGENES

p53

Overexpression of p53 occurs in about 25% of breast cancers and is associated with mutations in this suppressor gene. In one report, antibodies to wild-type and mutated p53 were detected in 23% of patients with breast cancer.[14] All the tumors of patients in whom antibodies were found had complexes between heat shock proteins (HSPs) and p53 protein, suggesting that the HSPs were involved in presenting this antigen to T-helper cells. When antibodies against p53 are detected in the serum, they portend a poor prognosis,[15] because they indicate the presence of the more immunogenic mutated gene.

HER-2/neu

The HER-2/neu oncogene encodes a protein tyrosine kinase that is homologous with human epidermal growth factor and is also termed *c-erbB-2*. Some controversy exists about the prognostic significance of the oncogene's presence, but the weight of evidence supports an important role. Patients whose tumors overexpress this oncogene have a poorer prognosis than counterparts with normal expression who have identical gross disease, including negative lymph nodes.[16] The response of these patients to endocrine treatment and chemotherapy may also be poorer than that of normal expressors of HER-2/neu. HER-2/neu is obviously of significance itself, but it may also serve as an important target for immunologic therapy.

The protein is 185 kd and has extracellular and transmembrane regions that are expressed on the surface of tumor cells bearing the oncogene. These include cells of adenocarcinomas of the breast and ovary, as well as melanoma to a lesser degree. The immunogenicity of p185HER2 has been demonstrated in nonhuman primates,[17] as well as in humans.[18,19] Both specific antibodies and T-cell proliferative responses have been identified in patients, although no one has yet identified CTLs spontaneously generated in vivo. CTLs have been produced in vitro by primary immunization with synthetic peptides, however.[20] HER-2/neu is an important antigen both as a target for monoclonal antibody (mAb)–based therapies and as a possible immunogen for active specific immunotherapy, as discussed later.

p21ras

p21ras is a common oncogene, present in approximately 20% of human malignant diseases, and was one of the earliest oncogenes identified in adenocarcinomas of the breast and gastrointestinal system. Early studies with mAbs found a significant concentration of oncogene-encoded protein in breast cancer cells. Notwithstanding that the ubiquity of the oncogene in normal tissues as well as tumors has made it unlikely to be a highly specific target for immunotherapy of breast cancer, Cheever and colleagues[22] attempted to use the mutated region as a target for immunotherapy. Mutations of p21ras usually occur at codons 12 or 61, leading to single amino acid substitutions. Peace and coworkers[21] reported that CTLs against p21ras mutated at position 61 were generated in rats immunized with synthetic peptides containing leucine substituted for glutamine ordinarily encoded by codon 61. These CTLs lysed syngeneic fibroblasts transformed by a mutated p21ras gene encoding the same substitution. Class II–restricted T-helper cells against the mutated segment of the p21ras were also generated by the same immunization.

MAGE-1

MAGE-1 is a melanoma-associated antigen (hence its name) described by Boon and his collaborators.[23] MAGE-1 represented the isolation of the first gene encoding a tumor-associated antigen and was duly heralded as a major step toward understanding the nature of such antigens. Epitopes of MAGE-1 are presented to CTLs by HLA-A1 molecules, which are found in approximately 20% of all whites; the gene itself is found in 40% of those patients. MAGE-1 is found not only on melanomas however, but also on breast cancers, in 20% of cases.[24] It is also present on some normal tissues as well, but to a lesser degree generally than on tumors. MAGE-1–based specific immunotherapy in melanoma and breast cancer is contemplated by several groups, who understand the limitations placed on its application by its limited distribution.

Immune Response to Breast Cancer

ROLE OF CD4 AND CD8 LYMPHOCYTES

CD4 Cytotoxic T Lymphocytes

Most CTLs are CD8+ cells with T-cell receptors composed of α and β chains. Whether these CTLs are important effectors in vivo is not completely resolved, but in vitro their activity has often correlated with clinical effectiveness of regimens designed to increase cell-mediated immunity to the tumor.

Other types of effector cells exist as well. Wang and colleagues showed that CD4 CTL with the unusual property of HLA class I restriction exist.[25] These CTLs recognize breast cancer antigens common to many cell lines and are inhibited only by antibodies to nonpolymorphous HLA determinants (β_2-microglobulin). Similar CTLs were described in melanoma patients by our group.[26,27] The assays required to demonstrate the CTLs are longer than those used for CD8 CTLs, and up-regulation by interferon-α or interferon-γ is important to ensure maximal expression of epitopes by the HLA class I molecule to permit these (presumably) weaker cytolytic cells to be demonstrable. Their role in vivo remains uncertain, but their scientific interest is considerable, because they show that at least some CD4 cells that usually recognize antigens in a class II context may recognize the same epitopes as their CD8 counterparts.

CD8 CTL Against HER-2/neu

CD8 CTLs against HER-2/neu were generated in vitro by two synthetic peptides that bound to HLA-A2.1, a common class I–restrictive element in antigen presentation, which is found in 40% to 50% of whites.[20] These peptides were made to contain HER-2/neu segments with amino acid motifs that were similar to published motifs for HLA-A2 binding. Beyond reaffirming that HER-2/neu is immunogenic for human T cells, this study may become a method for selective in vitro immunization with synthetic peptides of a large antigen that may prove useful in human T-cell–adoptive therapy.

γ-δ T cells

The α-β chains characterize most T-cell receptors, in which γ-δ chains are rare. Recognition of the 70-kd class of HSPs is a property often associated with γ-δ T cells. Studies showed that γ-δ T cells were cytotoxic to breast cancer cell lines and were found in the tumor-infiltrating lymphocytes of breast cancer metastases.[28,29] The T cells with γ-δ chains were invariably CD4−, but both CD8+ and CD8− cells had that type of T-cell receptor, usually CD8+. The proportion of γ-δ cells in lymph nodes, peripheral blood, and tumor infiltrate is invariably small, and whether such T cells play a major role in rejecting breast cancers in vivo is conjectural.

Possible Immunosuppressive Effects of CD4 T Cells

Tumor-infiltrating lymphocytes may be present in the process of rejecting breast cancers, but their presence should not be taken as evidence of rejection. CD4 T cells have been found in lesions where the tumor was not being rejected. Furthermore, suppressive effects of CD4 T cells have been demonstrated. At least two lymphokines produced by CD4 T cells have been shown to have immunosuppressive effects: TGF-β and interleukin-10 (IL-10). In addition, tumor cells themselves are capable of producing the same cytokines. Frey and Appleman,[30] in an important investigation in rats, showed that adenocarcinoma 13762 has tumor-rejection antigens eliciting cell-mediated immunity, but tumor-bearing rats could not mount an immune response to the tumor. CTLs were demonstrated by adoptive transfer techniques after immunization with irradiated tumor cells and were tumor-specific. Nevertheless, naive rats given viable tumor cells had progressive growth of the tumor. The tumor expressed high levels of major histocompatibility complex (MHC) class I antigens, eliminating poor target recognition as a mechanism. Moreover, the rats themselves could be immunized to many other antigens and were not systemically immunosuppressed. The authors concluded that the tumor itself exerted specific immunosuppression that blocked immunity against itself. In support of that contention, high levels of TGF-β were produced by the tumor in vitro.

In certain murine adenocarcinomas, epiglycanin, a mucin-like glycoprotein, is secreted by the tumor.[8] This material, when injected in adjuvant, elicits DTH against TF antigens. When injected by itself in nanogram doses, however, epiglycanin causes immunosuppression against DTH. This can be transferred with CD4 T cells and is abolished by anti-CD4. This type of immunosuppression leads to increased lethality of TA3-Ha cells that bear TF antigens, indicating that it is active in vivo. This elicitation of suppressor T cells is, then, another type of negative immunoregulation mediated by the tumor itself, and was noted in other systems in the 1970s, when suppressor T cells (then thought to be exclusively CD8) were first under investigation.

SUPERANTIGENS AND MOUSE MAMMARY TUMOR VIRUS TRANSMISSION

In mice, mouse mammary tumor virus (MMTV), a type B retrovirus, causes mammary cancer in C3H mice. Susceptibility to this virus depends on its recognition as a superantigen, which means that a permissive MHC class II molecule must be present on antigen-presenting cells in the mice. Superantigens attach to specific V β determinants, that is, the variable region of the T-cell receptor β chain, and cause specific deletion of T-helper cells bearing those T-cell receptors through nonspecific hyperproliferation. In transgenic mice expressing E α E β MHC class II molecules, MMTV has caused T-cell deletion and viral infection, but not in mice lacking that MHC molecule.[31,32] Although human breast cancer has not been proved to be of viral origin, these findings show an interesting new

pathway to viral infectivity and tumor causation through specific immunosuppression. That pathway and the principles that govern it may apply to those types of cancer that are eventually proved to be of viral origin in humans.

AN UNUSUAL ROLE OF MACROPHAGES

Suppressor Macrophages: GM-CSF

Lopez and her colleagues have shown that an immunosuppressive molecule produced by breast cancer cells is identical with granulocyte-macrophage–colony-stimulating factor (GM-CSF). The GM-CSF suppresses immunity by at least two mechanisms, directly and through the elicitation of suppressor macrophages. These investigators found that implants of breast adenocarcinoma cells grew more rapidly in mice treated with GM-CSF than in controls.[33] Suppressor macrophages elicited by GM-CSF made by the tumor down-regulated the proliferation of T cells, indirectly enhancing the growth of the tumor. These findings not only help to elucidate the way in which tumors may foster their own growth, but also provide a strong caution when hematopoietic growth factors are considered as adjuncts in the treatment of breast cancer. Because autologous bone marrow transplantation is increasingly performed to treat breast cancer, these observations take on special importance. Macrophages are generally important effector cells in rejecting tumors, however, and no detrimental effects of growth factors have been demonstrated in humans.

NATURAL KILLER CELLS: EFFECTS OF BEHAVIORAL INTERVENTIONS

NK cells may be involved in surveillance against the development of tumors, and in certain instances they may also be involved in the attack against established tumors, particularly when antigens on the tumor cross-react with the usual antigenic targets of those cells. The precise role of NK cells in the defense against breast cancer is still incompletely defined. Nevertheless, modifications of NK activity in breast cancer have been attempted in both directions: augmentation by behavioral modification and diminution by acute stress. NK cells do appear to be sensitive to the effects of behavioral modification and psychosocial support. For example, Levy and associates[34] found that NK activity predictably could be increased by emotional support, or its perception, from either the patient's family or the patient's physician. Actively seeking social support was also a predictor of higher NK activity. In another study, interventional modifications in behavior were attempted with biofeedback, relaxation, and guided imagery, to see whether nonspecific immunologic parameters were altered.[35] Improvement was seen not only in NK activity but also in T cell responses to mitogen (concanavalin A), mixed lymphocyte reactivity to alloantigens, and the number of peripheral blood lymphocytes. The major psychologic change was in a reduction of anxiety. Obversely, when Fischer rats were stressed acutely, NK cytotoxicity against a syngeneic mammary tumor was diminished in vitro,[36] and when challenged during this period, the rats had more lung metastases.

Physicians have often noted anecdotally that highly motivated patients who were attracted to phase I and phase II biologic therapy trials often did far better than unselected individuals in broader phase III trials. Whether increases in immunologic parameters were caused by better "attitude" and led to better response is an interesting question.

ROLE OF CYTOKINES AND CYTOKINE RECEPTORS ON THE CANCER

Cytokines appear to play an intimate role in the regulation of breast cancer. Receptors for a variety of cytokines are displayed on the surface of breast cancer cells. Included are receptors for estrogen, progesterone, epidermal growth factor (EGF), and several interleukins—both lymphokines and monokines.

Receptors for IL-4 are expressed on the surface of breast cancer cells.[37] IL-4 has had a cytostatic effect on the growth of breast cancer lines in vitro and has also up-regulated the expression of MHC class II antigens, particularly in-combination with interferon-γ. IL-6 also has effects on breast cancer, inhibiting proliferation in vitro in a manner similar to that of IL-4.[38] IL-6 also causes the breast cancer line to change phenotypically toward more normal (fibroblastoid) cells, with increased cell–cell separation, decreased adherent cell junctions, and increased motility. These changes have obvious clinical implications, but the two cytokines have not yet been tested in this context. Tumor cells genetically engineered to express IL-2 or IL-4 have been used, but their mode of action has involved more than simply direct down-regulation of cell growth.[39] Treatment with IL-2 has had limited clinical application, as mentioned later.

EGF receptors (EGFRs) are also present on breast cancer cells and have been the target for mAb-based therapies. Human cell lines overexpressing EGFRs have been inhibited in vitro by high-affinity rat mAbs specific for the extracellular domain of the human EGFR.[40,41]

Biologic Therapy

ANTIBODIES

Monoclonal Antibodies to HER-2/neu Protein, Alone and as Immunoconjugates

Among the defined targets of mAbs is p185HER2, against the extracellular domain protein of oncogene HER-2/neu. A humanized version of mouse antibody Ab4D5, constructed by investigators at Genentech, bound well to SKBR3 overexpressing the protein but did not inhibit its proliferation unlike the mouse mAb. A variant produced by molecular modeling, AB4D5-8, however, bound more tightly than either the humanized or mouse parental mAbs and did inhibit proliferation. In addition, the variant mAb-mediated ADCC did better than either.

Slamon and colleagues have been testing an immuno-

conjugate consisting of mAb 4D5 labeled with radioiodine (^{125}I) for the past several years. In vitro, the immunoconjugate was bound to NIH373 HER-2/neu cells, endocytosed, and rapidly catabolized intracellularly. Beige/nude mice bearing human tumors had a rapid falloff in uptake in the tumors within the first few days and rapid clearance of the material from the body, both of which limited efficacy. These problems have plagued much of immunoconjugate therapy and must be solved if this approach is to prove feasible.

Bispecific antibodies, with one chain engineered to recognize p185HER2 and the other to recognize CD3, were tested against breast cancers overexpressing the protein.[42] Those antibodies caused normal peripheral blood mononuclear cells to recognize and destroy breast cancers. Moreover, human T cells from breast cancer patients killed breast cancer cells four times as well in the presence of bispecific antibodies than in the absence of these antibodies. Despite its appeal as a strategy for improving CTL activity in vivo, proof of this approach in patients has not yet been reported.

Other Monoclonal Antibodies

The mAb L6 against a surface antigen on breast adenocarcinomas has been tested in a phase I trial in 18 patients. This mAb mediates antibody-dependent cell-mediated cytotoxicity (ADCC) and complement-dependent cytotoxicity in vitro and had bound well to tumors, as determined by biopsy. One complete remission of chest wall disease occurred in this trial, a finding that may lead to further testing of the mAb in this disease.[43]

The mAb DF3,[44] against a mucin-like epitope, coupled to ricin has been used in vitro to purge human bone marrow of breast adenocarcinoma cells, for use in bone marrow transplantation. A 30% reduction in bone marrow progenitor cells was also found, but at the same concentrations of the mAb effected from 1.6 to 2.8 logs of killing of various admixed breast cancer cell lines.

VACCINES

Mucin-Based Treatments

SIALYL-TN. Longenecker and colleagues[45] developed a synthetic epitope, NANA α (2-6) GalNAc alpha-O-crotyl (sialyl-Tn-crotyl), which mimics the natural O-linked epitope present on human adenocarcinoma cells, NANA alpha (2-6) Gal Nac, α-O-serine (sialyl-Tn-serine). This material was conjugated to KLH as a carrier and was injected with the adjuvant DETOX. In mice, this immunization elicited IgG antibodies in high titer that bound equally well to the native sialyl-Tn as to the synthetic saccharide.

When 100 μg was given to breast cancer patients, IgG antibodies were produced that reacted with sialyl-Tn from two sources. Small doses of the sialyl-Tn-crotyl generated DTH responses in the mice, inversely proportional to the antibody titers.

In phase I and limited phase II trials of this material in

patients with breast cancer, clinical responses suggested efficacy for the immunization scheme. Clinical trials in Canada with sialyl-Tn have shown long-term stability (over 6 months) of disease in 9 of 13 breast cancer patients and 2 true partial remissions lasting 6 months.[46] A confirmatory trial is in progress in the United States, with 1 partial remission and 1 instance of long-term (9+ months) stability among 16 patients. In these human clinical trials, increased titers of IgG and IgM antibodies to sialyl-Tn have been produced in nearly all patients, but they have not been correlated with clinical responses.

MUC-1. Because the MUC-1 tandem repeat peptide of PEM has been shown to act as a target for human CTL, vaccines based on it are under development. In fact, an early trial of MUC-1 immunotherapy for pancreatic carcinoma has just been initiated. Further trials in breast cancer and other adenocarcinomas are anticipated.

HER-2/neu Vaccines

A vaccine based on the p185 extracellular domain protein encoded by the HER-2/neu oncogene is immunogenic in rhesus monkeys.[17] A combination of p185 and the adjuvant DETOX in the nonhuman primates led to antibodies that neutralized the growth of human SKBR3 cells overexpresing p185, mediated ADCC, and restored sensitivity to macrophage-mediated cytotoxicity. Lymphocytes from immunized monkeys proliferated in the presence of p185 and were cytotoxic to human SKBR3, crossing species lines. These results suggest that HER-2/neu extracellular domain–protein or gene-based vaccines may be appropriate for humans, results that are reinforced by findings that the oncogene's products are immunogenic in patients.[19]

GENETICALLY ENGINEERED CELLS AS IMMUNOGENS

Insertion of Cytokine Genes

It has become possible and very common to insert cytokine genes into tumor cells in the hope of improving their ability to stimulate immunity in the host. Adjuvants act, in part, by stimulating the production of cytokines from antigen-presenting cells such as macrophages, and from lymphocytes, directly or through macrophages. Whether the insertion of a gene encoding the expression of a single cytokine gene will prove to be more effective than simply mixing the antigen with a potent adjuvant material has yet to be proved. The major value of the work with gene-engineered tumor cell vaccines is in its science, that is, the elucidation of which individual cytokines are important in generating an immune response to tumor antigens and therefore which should be included in a predetermined vaccine construct once the antigens are synthesized.

IL-2 has been inserted into a spontaneous BALB/c mouse mammary adenocarcinoma. These cells initially generated a potent nonspecific inflammatory response, but then led to systemic immunity and immunologic memory against the parental adenocarcinoma. The immune response was capable of preventing and, to a limited degree, treating viable adenocarcinomas. As the tumor size increased, this vaccination became less successful.[47,48] IL-4 was also inserted with similar results, but interferon-γ was less effective, although macrophages massively infiltrated the tumor and led to its rejection.[49] In fact, this group reported that interferon-γ enhanced metastases of this tumor, probably by inhibiting NK-mediated lysis.[50] Tsai and coworkers[51] were able to use mammary tumor virus–derived tumors transduced with the IL-2 gene as a vaccine to prevent outgrowth of the parental line in mice. This immunogen was more potent than the irradiated parental line, which, in fact, diminished the activity of the vaccine when admixed with IL-2–containing tumor cells. IL-2–transduced stromal fibroblasts did not produce a worthwhile vaccine in this system, but these results do not rule out further engineering of such fibroblasts (eg, with tumor antigens) as an alternative immunization strategy.

The new cytokine IP-10, whose secretion is induced by interferon-γ and lipopolysaccharide, has been engineered into breast cancer cells and has led in vivo to a marked inflammatory response of T cells, monocytes, and neutrophils.[52] The release of this material may account for some of the effects attributed to interferon-γ, which, as noted previously, causes a similar inflammatory infiltrate.

PEM DNA has been transfected into Epstein-Barr virus (EBV)–immortalized autologous and allogeneic B lymphocytes.[53] These cells have been used as a renewable source of antigen-presenting cells for in vitro immunization of CTLs. They have also served as convenient targets for testing the activity of CTLs. Although the authors did not propose this method as a strategy for vaccination, autologous or allogeneic transfected B cells (perhaps without EBV, however) could be used as vehicles for synthetic vaccines with difficult whole molecules such as the mucins.

CELLULAR AND CYTOKINE THERAPY

Interleukin-2 Therapy

Little has been done to study the effects of IL-2 on breast cancer. National Cancer Institute (NCI) trials of high-dose therapy with IL-2 together with adoptive cellular immunotherapy (LAK cells) showed little effect on breast cancer, and that tumor was omitted from most confirmatory trials. Rayner had at least one response to that therapy in his group's trials (Personal communication, 1988). Based on that result, and based on our success in melanoma with a low-dose regimen of IL-2, 21.6 million IU/m^2, preceded by low-dose cyclophosphamide, 300 mg/m^2,[54] my colleagues and I decided to investigate the same regimen in patients with breast cancer who had failed a doxorubin-containing regimen. In a trial that was aborted because of a temporary lack of IL-2 nationally, 13 patients were treated with the regimen. We observed three regressions of over 50%, one of which was a true partial remission lasting 7 months. The responses in the other 2 patients were short-lived, perhaps because of underaggressive treatment. Nevertheless, clear evidence exists for activity of

IL-2 alone in breast cancer.[55] Studies with IL-2–transduced tumor cells are not completely comparable, of course, but those results also support an effect of IL-2 on the rejection of breast cancers.

In Vitro and in Vivo Education Combined With Bone Marrow Transplantation

Bone marrow transplantation has been performed to replete hematopoietic cells after intensive chemotherapy for breast cancer, but it could subserve a different function: adoptive immunotherapy. Wingard has discussed this aspect of bone marrow transplantation, particularly with allogeneic cells.[56] Kennedy and Jones[57] reviewed autologous bone marrow transplantation as therapy for breast cancer and concluded that, although remission rates are high, the durations of remission remain short. Cyclosporin A can induce a syndrome resembling the graft-versus-host disease that occurs after allogeneic transplantation. This syndrome is augmented by interferon-γ. The authors suggest this as a strategy to use autologous bone marrow transplantation more thoroughly as treatment.

It is now technically possible to use in vitro stimulation of cytolytic and helper T cells (education) to produce or, preferably, to augment the immune response to tumors more specifically than with interferon-γ. Irradiated tumor cells or defined mucin antigens could be used for this purpose. Moreover, the combination of active immunization of patients at an appropriate interval before chemotherapy and autologous bone marrow transplantation can provide active T cells to be reinfused in the tumor-reduced host. This could create a setting akin to that seen after resection of early disease, which might be more conducive to a response to immunotherapy.

ROLE OF INTERFERONS AND TUMOR NECROSIS FACTOR

Up-Regulation of Antigens, Including HLA Antigens

I believe that the most important use of the interferons in immunotherapy will be as up-regulators of HLA molecules and the tumor-associated epitopes they present, to make the tumor more recognizable to the immune system in vivo. Metastases often lack discernible HLA molecules, either entirely or with specific allelic deletions, and hence tumor epitopes cannot be targeted by mAbs or T lymphocytes. Tumor necrosis factor (TNF)-α and IL-1 have the same property of up-regulation, but are more toxic than the interferons when given systemically. In the creation of whole-cell tumor vaccines, the same up-regulation in vitro may be important in ensuring optimal representation of antigens as immunogens. A precedent exists in melanoma for sequential use of active immunotherapy and interferon-α, with consequent improvement in response,[58] but this limited experience must be confirmed and extended in breast cancer.

Immunologic Detection of Tumor Markers

It is not the aim of this chapter to discuss tumor markers, but many of the antigens discussed are shed by breast cancer cells and are thus useful as markers. In this category are mucin-derived antigens, such as CA 15-3 and the identical antigen CA 27.29, TAG-72, and CA 125. The immunodominant epitope of all the mucin, described previously, led to mAbs directed against the same general region of the PEM protein in several laboratories. Diagnostic information gleaned from the use of several of these similar mAbs together is therefore not additive. This issue, as well as the entire field of tumor markers in breast cancer, is discussed elsewhere.[59] This discussion, however, deals briefly with an innovative use of immunodetection for bone marrow involvement that may be a useful measurement of visceral micrometastasis.

Cote and his collaborators have shown that mAbs against membrane and cytoskeletal antigens on epithelial cells in an immunohistochemical assay are capable of detecting one cancer cell among a million hematopoietic cells in bone marrow. These investigators found such cells in 35% (18 of 51) of patients with operable breast cancer, even in the absence of detectable cells by routine cytology; 27% of patients with negative lymph nodes had antigen-positive cells, whereas 41% with lymph node metastases had detectable cells.[60] When follow-up was performed on 49 of the 51 patients, the presence of bone marrow micrometastases was associated with early recurrence. At 2 years, a 3% recurrence rate was noted for those without bone marrow metastases, whereas 33% of those with detectable metastases had a relapse. Lymph node–negative patients who were also negative for bone marrow metastasis had 0% 2-year recurrence, but those who were lymph node–positive and bone marrow–positive had a 42% relapse rate (Cote RJ, personal communication, 1994). This finding strongly suggests that immunohistochemical detection of breast cancer cells in the bone marrow augurs for recurrence of disease and adds to the prognostic value of lymph node involvement.

Lymph node positivity was also detected by this procedure. When 251 patients with breast cancer with ostensibly negative lymph nodes were studied, additional staining of a paraffin section with antibodies to cytokeratins detected metastases in 60 patients who were otherwise lymph node–negative. At 5 years, the recurrence rate for the immunohistochemically detected group was 37% versus 27% for those with undetectable cells (Cote RJ, personal communication, 1994).

Whether immunologic detection can be used in vivo to attack occult metastases, perhaps through the use of immunoconjugates, is an intriguing question and would be a logical extension of the use of mAbs.

References

1. Mitchell MS. Principles of tumor immunology and their application to the biomodulation of cancer. In: Calabresi P, Schein, PS, eds. Medical oncology, ed 2. New York, McGraw-Hill, 1993:323.

2. Mitchell MS, ed. Biological approaches to cancer treatment: biomodulation. New York, McGraw-Hill, 1992.

3. Gold P, Freedman SO. Demonstration of tumor-specific antigens in human colonic carcinomata by immunological tolerance and absorption techniques. J Exp Med 1965;121:439.

4. Kantor J, Irvine K, Abrams S, et al. Immunogenicity and safety of a recombinant virus vaccine expressing the carcinoembryonic antigen gene in a nonhuman primate. Cancer Res 1992;52:6917.

5. Gendler S, Taylor-Papadimitriou J, Duhig T, et al. A highly immunogenic region of a human polymorphic epithelial mucin expressed by carcinomas is made up of tandem repeats. J Biol Chem 1988;263:12,820.

6. Price MR, Hudecz F, O'Sullivan C, et al. Immunological and structural features of the protein core of human polymorphic epithelial mucin. Mol Immunol 1990;27:795.

7. MacLean GD, Longenecker BM. Clinical significance of the Thomsen-Friedenreich antigen. Semin Cancer Biol 1991;2:433.

8. Fung PY, Longenecker BM. Specific immunosuppressive activity of epiglycanin, a mucin-like glycoprotein secreted by a murine mammary adenocarcinoma (TA3-HA). Cancer Res 1991;51:1170.

9. Denton G, Sekowski M, Price MR. Induction of antibody responses to breast carcinoma associated mucins using synthetic peptide constructs as immunogens. Cancer Lett 1993;70:143.

10. Ding L, Lalani EN, Reddish, M., et al. Immunogenicity of synthetic peptides related to the core peptide sequence encoded by the human MUC1 mucin gene: effect of immunization on the growth of murine mammary adenocarcinoma cells transfected with the human MUC1 gene. Cancer Immunol Immunother 1993;36:9.

11. Finn OJ, Barnd DL, Kerr LA, et al. Specific recognition of human tumor associated antigens by non-MHC-restricted CTL. In: Metzgar R, Mitchell MS, eds. Tumor antigens and specific tumor therapy. New York, Alan R Liss, 1989:157.

12. Jerome KR, Barnd DL, Bendt KM, et al. Cytotoxic T-lymphocytes derived from patients with breast adenocarcinoma recognize an epitope present on the protein core of a mucin molecule preferentially expressed by malignant cells. Cancer Res 1991;51:2908.

13. Kan-Mitchell J, Huang XQ, Steinman L, et al. Clonal analysis of in vitro-activated CD8+ cytotoxic T lymphocytes from a melanoma patient responsive to active specific immunotherapy. Cancer Immunol Immunother 1993;37:15.

14. Davidoff AM, Iglehart JD, Marks JR. Immune response to p53 is dependent upon p53/HSP70 complexes in breast cancers. Proc Natl Acad Sci USA 1992;89:3439.

15. Schlichtholz B, Legros Y, Gillet D, et al. The immune response to p53 in breast cancer patients is directed against immunodominant epitopes unrelated to the mutational hot spot. Cancer Res 1992;52:6380.

16. Dykins R, Corbett IP, Henry JA, et al. Long-term survival in breast cancer related to overexpression of the c-erbB-2 oncoprotein: an immunohistochemical study using monoclonal antibody NCL-CB11. J Pathol 1991;163:105.

17. Fendley B, Kotts C, Wong WLT, et al. Successful immunization of rhesus monkeys with the extracellular domain of p185^{HER2}: a potential approach to human breast cancer. Vaccine Res 1993;2:129.

18. Pupa SM, Menard S, Andreola S, et al. Antibody response against the c-erbB-2 oncoprotein in breast carcinoma patients. Cancer Res 1993;53:5864.

19. Disis ML, Calenoff E, McLaughlin G, et al. Existent T-cell and antibody immunity to HER-2/neu protein in patients with breast cancer. Cancer Res 1994;54:16.

20. Disis ML, Smith JW, Murphy AE, et al. In vitro generation of human cytolytic T-cells specific for peptides derived from the HER-2/neu protoonogene protein. Cancer Res 1994;54:1071.

21. Peace DJ, Smith JW, Chen W, et al. Lysis of ras oncogene-transformed cells by specific cytotoxic T lymphocytes elicited by primary in vitro immunization with mutated ras peptide. J Exp Med 1994;179:473.

22. Cheever MA, Chen W, Disis ML, et al. T-cell immunity to oncogenic proteins including mutated ras and chimeric bcr-abl. Ann NY Acad Sci 1993;690:101.

23. Van der Bruggen C, Traversari C, Chomez P, et al. A gene encoding an antigen recognized by cytolytic T lymphocytes on a human melanoma. Science 1991;254:1643.

24. Brasseur F. Human gene MAGE-1, which codes for a tumor-rejection antigen, is expressed by some breast tumors. (Letter) Intl J Cancer 1992;52:839.

25. Wang P, Vanky F, Klein E. MHC class-I–restricted auto-tumor–specific CD4+CD8-T-cell clones established from autologous mixed lymphocyte-tumor-cell culture (MLTC). Intl J Cancer 1992;51:962.

26. LeMay LG, Kan-Mitchell J, Goedegebuure P, et al. Detection of human melanoma-reactive CD4+ HLA class I-restricted cytotoxic T cell clones with long-term assay and pretreatment of targets with interferon-gamma. Cancer Immunol Immunother 1993;37:187.

27. Goedegebuure PS, Harel H, LeMay LG, et al. Cytotoxic CD4+ lymphocyte clones reactive with melanoma: the role of HLA and accessory molecules. Vaccine Res 1994;2:249.

28. Bank I, Book M, Huszar M, et al. V delta 2+ gamma delta T lymphocytes are cytotoxic to the MCF 7 breast carcinoma cell line and can be detected among the T cells that infiltrate breast tumors. Clin Immunol Immunopathol 1993;67:17.

29. Alam SM, Clark JS, Leech V, et al. T cell receptor gamma/delta expression on lymphocyte populations of breast cancer patients. Immunol Lett 1992;31:279.

30. Frey AB, Appleman LJ. Rat adenocarcinoma 13762 expresses tumor rejection antigens but tumor-bearing animals exhibit tumor-specific immunosuppression. Clin Immunol Immunopathol 1993;69:223.

31. Held W, Waanders GA, Shakhov AN, et al. Superantigen-induced immune stimulation amplifies mouse mammary tumor virus infection and allows virus transmission. Cell 1993;74:529.

32. Pucillo C, Cepeda R, Hodes RJ. Expression of a MHC class II transgene determines both superantigenicity and susceptibility to mammary tumor virus infection. J Exp Med 1993;178:1441.

33. Sotomayor EM, Fu YX, Lopez-Cepero M, et al. Role of tumor-derived cytokines on the immune system of mice bearing a mammary adenocarcinoma. II. Down-regulation of macrophage-mediated cytotoxicity by tumor-derived granulocyte-macrophage colony-stimulating factor. J Immunol 1991;147:2816.

34. Levy SM, Herberman RB, Whiteside T, et al. Perceived social and tumor estrogen/progesterone receptor status as predictors of natural killer cell activity in breast cancer patients. Psychosom Med 1990;52:73.

35. Gruber BL, Hersh SP, Hall NR, et al. Immunological responses of breast cancer patients to behavioral interventions. Biofeedback Self-Regul 1993;18:1.

36. Ben-Eliyahu S, Yirmiya R, Liebeskind JC, et al. Stress increases metastatic spread of a mammary tumor in rats: evidence for mediation by the immune system. Brain Behav Immun 1991;5:193.

37. Obiri NI, Siegel JP, Varricchio F, et al. Expression of high-affinity IL-4 receptors on human melanoma, ovarian and breast carcinoma cells. Clin Exp Immunol 1994;95:148.

38. Krueger J, Ray A, Tamm I, et al. Expression and function of interleukin-6 in epithelial cells. J Cell Biochem 1991;45:327.

39. Musiani P, Modesti A, Brunetti M, et al. Nature and potential of the reactive response to mouse mammary adenocarcinoma cells engineered with interleukin-2, interleukin-4, or interferon-gamma genes. Nat Immun 1994;13:93.

40. Modjtahedi H, Styles JM, Dean CJ. The human EGF receptor as a target for cancer therapy: six new rat mAbs against the receptor on the breast carcinoma MDA-MB 468. Br J Cancer 1993;67:247.

41. Fernandez A, Spitzer E, Perez R, et al. A new monoclonal antibody

for detection of EGF-receptors in western blots and paraffin-embedded tissue sections. J Cell Biochem 1992;49:157.

42. Shalaby MR, Shepard HM, Presta L, et al. Development of humanized bispecific antibodies reactive with cytotoxic lymphocytes and tumor cells overexpressing the HER2 protooncogene. J Exp Med 1992;175:217.

43. Goodman GE, Hellstrom I, Brodzinsky L, et al. Phase I trial of murine monoclonal antibody L6 in breast, colon, ovarian, and lung cancer. J Clin Oncol 1990;8:1083.

44. Tondini C, Pap SA, Hayes DF, et al. Evaluation of monoclonal antibody DF3 conjugated with ricin as a specific immunotoxin for in vitro purging of human bone marrow. Cancer Res 1990;50:1170.

45. Longenecker BM, Reddish M, Koganty R, et al. Immune responses of mice and human breast cancer patients following immunization with synthetic sialyl-Tn conjugated to KLH plus detox adjuvant. Ann NY Acad Sci 1993;690:276.

46. MacLean GD, Reddish M, Koganty RR, et al. Immunization of breast cancer patients using a synthetic sialyl-Tn glycoconjugate plus detox adjuvant. Cancer Immunol Immunother 1993;36:215.

47. Cavallo F, Di Pierro F, Giovarelli M, et al. Protective and curative potential of vaccination with interleukin-2-gene–transfected cells from a spontaneous mouse mammary adenocarcinoma. Cancer Res 1993;53:5067.

48. Cavallo F, Giovarelli M, Gulino A, et al. Role of neutrophils and CD4+ T lymphocytes in the primary and memory response to non-immunogenic murine mammary adenocarcinoma made immunogenic by IL-2 gene. J Immunol 1992;149:3627.

49. Musiani P, Modesti A, Brunetti M, et al. Nature and potential of the reactive response to mouse mammary adenocarcinoma cells engineered with interleukin-2, interleukin-4 or interferon-gammon genes. Nat Immun 1994;13:93.

50. Lollini PL, Bosco MC, Cavallo F, et al. Inhibition of tumor growth and enhancement of metastasis after transfection of the gamma-interferon gene. Int J Cancer 1993;55:320.

51. Tsai SC, Gansbacher B, Tait L, et al. Induction of antitumor immunity by interleukin-2 gene-transduced mouse mammary tumor cells versus transduced mammary stromal fibroblasts. J Natl Cancer Inst 1993;85:546.

52. Luster AD, Leder P. IP-10, a-C-X-C- chemokine, elicits a potent thymus-dependent antitumor response in vivo. J Exp Med 1993;178:1057.

53. Jerome KR, Domenech N, Finn OJ. Tumor-specific cytotoxic T cell clones from patients with breast and pancreatic adenocarcinoma recognize EBV-immortalized B cells transfected with polymorphic epithelial mucin complementary DNA. J Immunol 1993;151:1654.

54. Mitchell MS, Kempf RA, Harel W, et al. Effectiveness and tolerability of low-dose cyclophosphamide and low-dose intravenous interleukin-2 in disseminated melanoma. J Clin Oncol 1988;6:409.

55. Spicer DV, Kelley A, Herman R, et al. Low-dose recombinant IL-2 and low dose cyclophosphamide in metastatic breast cancer. Cancer Immunol Immunother 1992;34:424.

56. Wingard JR. Bone marrow transplantation: a form of adoptive immunotherapy. In: Mitchell MS, ed. Biological approaches to cancer therapy: biomodulation. New York, McGraw-Hill, 1993:554.

57. Kennedy MJ, Jones RJ. Autologous graft-versus-host disease: immunotherapy of breast cancer after bone marrow transplantation. Breast Cancer Res Treat 1993;26Suppl:S31.

58. Mitchell MS, Jakowatz J, Harel W, et al. Increased effectiveness of interferon alfa-2b following active specific immunotherapy for melanoma. J Clin Oncol 1994;12:402.

59. Fritsche HA, Mitchell MS, eds. The role of tumour markers in breast cancer. Etobicoke, Ontario, ADI Diagnostics, 1993.

60. Cote RJ, Rosen PP, Old LJ, et al. Detection of bone marrow micrometastases in patients with early-stage breast cancer. Diagn Oncol 1991;1:37.

8

Diseases of the Breast, edited by Jay R. Harris,
Marc E. Lippman, Monica Morrow, and Samuel Hellman.
Lippincott-Raven Publishers, Philadelphia, © 1996.

Breast Cancer Screening

BARBARA K. RIMER

The current generation of breast cancer screening interventions includes three modalities: mammography, clinical breast examination (CBE), and breast self-examination (BSE). CBE and mammography are reviewed in Chapters 4.1 and 4.2. The purpose of this chapter is to identify basic criteria that can be used to evaluate a screening intervention appropriate for widespread application, to discuss measures of effectiveness, and to review the evidence for the screening effectiveness of each of the three modalities alone and, in some cases, in combination. Of the three, mammography has been studied most widely and appears to offer the greatest potential for decreasing mortality from breast cancer among the largest group at risk for the disease—women aged 50 to 69 years. Regular mammograms can decrease breast cancer mortality rates for women aged 50 to 69 years by 30%. Issues related to adherence to breast cancer screening are reviewed briefly with an emphasis on the clinical implications.

Rationale for Screening

The purpose of breast cancer screening is to separate women who are clearly normal from those with abnormalities, not to diagnose disease. *Screening* refers to the application of a test to "people who are as yet asymptomatic for the purpose of classifying them as to their likelihood of having a particular disease."[1] The overall goal of breast cancer screening is to reduce morbidity and mortality due to breast cancer.[2] Although the potential of using outcome measures other than mortality has been suggested and is discussed later in this chapter, mortality reduction is considered the criterion in the evaluation of screening interventions.[3]

The goal of screening is to intervene in the disease process after biologic onset but before symptoms develop. The assumption is that earlier detection reduces cancer mortality. In breast cancer, this assumption has been proved clearly valid for women aged 50 to 69 years, but it is under debate for women 40 to 49 years old. To be a good candidate for screening, several other criteria must be met as well.[4] Prevalence of the detectable preclinical phase must be sufficiently high to make screening feasible. Under this criterion, breast cancer qualifies as appropriate for screening for women aged 50 years and older. The lifetime risk of breast cancer is 1 in 8. Some questions about the value of screening women under age 50 years relate to the lower likelihood of this group's being diagnosed with breast cancer, however. The annual risk of developing breast cancer is 1 in 3700 for a woman aged 30 to 34 years but 1 in 235 for a woman aged 70 to 74 years.[4] Because the incidence of breast cancer is higher for older than younger women, screening may be appropriate for women in their 50s but not for women in their 40s. It requires many screening examinations to save one life, even among older women. Tabar and colleagues[5] estimated that the deficit of 58 breast cancer deaths among women aged 50 to 69 years required 85,000 mammograms (1 death prevented per 1460 mammograms given) and 800 biopsies. Ultimately, the large number of examinations translates into few lives saved. Thus, Eddy and coworkers[6] estimated that if 25% of the women aged 40 to 49 years were screened every year, breast cancer mortality in the year 2000 would be reduced by only 373 deaths.

Evaluation of Screening Tests

Several criteria of a good screening test are accepted:

1. A good screening test should classify patients correctly. Women without preclinical disease should test negative and those with possible disease should test positive.[1]
2. The test should be acceptable to patients and physicians. Mammography is accepted widely, but its use still lags

far behind what is needed to exert a major impact on mortality.[7,8] The CBE and BSE are also acceptable to most patients and physicians but are similarly underused.[7] Nevertheless, in comparison with many other cancer screening tests, such as sigmoidoscopy and mammography, BSE and CBE have great acceptance.

3. The disease should be serious, or it is unlikely that the effort to screen for it would be worth the cost.[9] Obviously, breast cancer is a serious disease that would often be fatal if left untreated.

4. A good screening test should be precise, correctly classifying patients with the disease as test-positive and those without the disease as test-negative. Sensitivity and specificity are two indicators of precision. *Sensitivity* is defined as the probability of testing positive if the disease is truly present. Those cancers that are missed are called false-negatives. Overall, 10% to 15% of breast cancers are missed by mammography.[10] Sensitivity also refers to the percentage of patients found to have cancer within 1 year of screening who were diagnosed correctly on screening. *Specificity* is defined as the probability of screening negative if the disease is truly absent. One weakness of specificity is the problem of false-positives. In practice, this refers to the probability of an abnormal report when no cancer is present. No test is perfectly sensitive and specific. Rather, they are like two ends of a seesaw, operating in delicate balance. If one tries to avoid missing any case of breast cancer, one runs the risk of calling too many mammograms positive. Many of these results would be false-positives. This has important implications for the biopsy rate and all the attendant physical, economic, and psychosocial costs. As discussed later, mammography is highly sensitive and specific for women aged 50 to 69 years. It is less so for women in their 40s.[4]

5. The test should have a high positive predictive value. A high proportion of the women testing positive should, in fact, have the disease. Positive predictive value can range from 3% to 22%.[3] This is considered acceptable for a screening test. As discussed later, mammography is more sensitive and specific for women in their 50s and 60s than for those in their 40s. The reasons for this variability include the quality of mammography equipment, the competence of readers, and the limitations of radiographic technology in detecting abnormalities among younger women.

6. Finally, there would be little point in conducting population-based screening if effective treatment were not available.

Measures of Effectiveness

Four kinds of measures have been used to judge the effectiveness of breast cancer screening.

- Mortality rate from breast cancer in a screened versus an unscreened group
- Case fatality rate
- Survival (eg, number or proportion of women surviving 5 years)
- Case finding

The most definitive measure of the efficacy of a breast cancer screening program, and the least subject to bias, is breast cancer mortality rate, as determined by the comparison of screened and unscreened groups in a randomized clinical trial.[1] The ultimate question is, Are women who were screened less likely to die of breast cancer than those who were not screened? If the answer is no, some other compelling reason to screen must exist. It is not appropriate to use deaths from all causes as an outcome, because breast cancer screening is not thought to affect death from other diseases.[2] Excellent epidemiology texts[1,11] and reviews[2] discuss the measures in more detail than can be presented here.

Other outcome measures have been proposed, however, and these should be considered. Case finding and survival are two potential outcomes. Each has limitations. The problem with case finding is that it is subject to lead-time bias. *Lead-time bias* refers to an increase in survival as measured from disease detection until death, without lengthening of life.[11] Survival may appear to have been advanced, but this is only because cancer is found earlier in the screened group. *Length bias* refers to overrepresentation among screened groups of those with a long preclinical phase—slower-growing, less aggressive tumors than those detected without screening. Because of length bias, screening appears effective, but in fact, it has made no difference in mortality. This is because slow-growing cancers may contribute to the apparent success of the screened group. Thus, length bias undermines the value of survival data as a measure of outcome. Survival, in itself, does not establish that the natural history of the disease has been altered, or that mortality has been reduced.[11a]

Another potential consideration is *quality of life.*[12] Unfortunately, none of the international trials has good quality-of-life data, although this is an important area for further exploration. Cost per quality-adjusted life-year saved would be a good measure, but it has not been used.[13] QOL may also include a reduction in psychologic morbidity for a woman and her family.[14] Tabar and associates[5] argue that even if mammography does not reduce breast cancer mortality for women in their 40s, it may be beneficial because it avoids disfiguring and debilitating surgery. Harris[15] has expressed concern, however, that a woman's quality of life could be diminished by living longer with breast cancer.

The *randomized clinical trial* is the most powerful method for demonstrating the value of screening in comparison with an unscreened group.[16] Randomized clinical trials overcome the biases inherent in other designs. For example, women with symptoms should not be more likely to appear in one of the groups, and the age groups and risks of participants should be similar.[16] A randomized clinical trial with the endpoint of mortality avoids the two most important biases, lead-time and length.[17] Case control studies can also provide useful information, however, and may be used to supplement randomized clinical trial data.

Negative Consequences of Screening

A consideration of the negative consequences of screening is essential, because screening is offered to presumably healthy women.[2] The negative consequences should not override the potential benefits.

PSYCHOLOGIC CONSEQUENCES OF FALSE-POSITIVES. Eddy and colleagues[6] estimated that if a woman has a mammogram every year between the ages of 40 and 49 years, she has a 30% chance of receiving a false-positive result. Women who test positive but who do not prove to have cancer may experience some important negative sequelae.[3] Perhaps the most important is anxiety. Lerman and co-workers[18] found that even 3 months after women had abnormal mammograms that proved not to indicate cancer, they were experiencing adverse psychologic consequences. Symptoms included excessive worry, intrusive thoughts, and other symptoms similar to those seen in posttraumatic stress disorder.

OTHER CONSEQUENCE OF FALSE-POSITIVES. In addition to the psychologic consequences, many women undergo procedures that may, in fact, be unnecessary. These include ultrasound, magnification views, and biopsies. These procedures may inconvenience women and may result in financial costs and potential physical morbidity.[2]

FALSE-NEGATIVES. Women who are given a clean bill of health may derive a false sense of reassurance from a normal examination. If a lump or other physical symptom develops, they may be more likely to ignore it. This has been suggested as one of the reasons for excess mortality in the screened group in the Canadian trial.[4] Andersson and associates[19] also proposed false reassurance as a potential explanation for the higher death rates among women in their 40s in the Malmö trial.

LABELING. Once a woman has experienced a false-positive test result, she is subject to labeling phenomena. She may view herself as different, perhaps as a person who is not entirely well.[21] Her insurance company may view her negatively as well and may place her in a higher risk pool.

OVERDIAGNOSIS. Early detection also can be misleading when it results in the overtreatment of abnormalities.[13] Autopsy studies suggest that as many as 70% of breast cancers may never become clinically manifest.[2] Concern has been expressed that some early breast cancers diagnosed through mammography may represent the overtreatment of abnormalities.[20-21] Finding smaller and more node-negative cancers does not necessarily translate into a mortality reduction, as shown in the second Canadian National Breast Screening Study (NBSS2) trial.[22]

POTENTIAL CARCINOGENIC EFFECTS OF MAMMOGRAPHY. Feig[23] and others have estimated the potential for a radiation-induced breast cancer to result from regular mammograms. Feig[23] estimated that if one million women aged 30 years or older each received a mean breast dose of 1 rad, after 10 years, there would be an excess incidence of 3.5 cancers per year in the population. The subgroup of women who are heterozygous for the ataxia telangiectasia gene (about 1% of the population) appear to be at increased risk of breast cancer. These women appear to be especially sensitive to radiation.[16]

Principles for Evaluating Screening

Eddy[24] identified several principles that can be used in making decisions about mammography or other screening tests. To extend his principles, three criteria should be met before mammography is promoted:

1. Convincing evidence should show that, compared with no mammography, mammography is effective in improving health outcomes
2. Compared with no mammography, the beneficial effects of the test should outweigh harms.
3. The mammography should represent a good use of societal resources.

Eddy concluded, "I interpret the oath [Hippocratic] to mean that before we do things to patients, we should have reason to believe that they will be benefited."[24] These are useful principles with which to review the data about mammography and other breast screening interventions. Most important is the criterion of improved health outcomes compared with no treatment.

Overview of the Mammography Trials

Perhaps no topic has generated more controversy in the last several years than the question of *whom* to screen for mammography, at *what age,* and *how often.* Different investigators and organizations have examined the same data and have come to different conclusions about the scientific evidence. How is this possible? Part of the controversy rests on the criteria for evidence. Is an intervention effective until proved ineffective or considered ineffective until proved effective? What level of proof is adequate? Are other designs besides randomized clinical trials considered appropriate in terms of reaching conclusions about the value of an intervention? These are only some of the differing perspectives brought to bear on the evaluation of scientific evidence. This section of the chapter reviews the eight randomized trials that have been conducted during the past 31 years to assess the impact of mammography. Together, these trials include more than 500,000 women, with 180,000 women aged 40 to 49 years. Although randomized clinical trials are not the only source of data about the efficacy of mammography, most investigators would agree that they are the best source.

The eight international randomized clinical trials have varied greatly[4] (Table 8-1). Most have included women in their 40s, although two trials began accrual at patient age 45 years, and 1 of the Canadian trials (NBSS1) was designed to examine mammography with CBE versus usual care for women in their 40s with a separate study (NBSS2) to assess mammography with CBE versus CBE alone for women aged 50 to 59 years. As is evident from Table 8-1, the studies also varied in whether they used one-view or two-view mammography and in the screening interval, which varied from 12 to 24 months. Initial compliance ranged from 61% in the Edinburgh trial to 89% in the Swedish Two-County Study.[16] In all, the studies represent over 1.5 million patient-years of follow-up for women aged 40 to 49 years alone.

Summary of the International Breast Cancer Screening Trials

RANDOMIZED CLINICAL TRIALS

In this section, each of the major prospective, randomized international trials is summarized so the reader may understand the purpose, design, and major limitations of each. As noted previously, a wide variation in trial design exists. More detailed descriptions are available in the primary articles describing the trials (see Table 8-1).

Health Insurance Plan of New York

Although mammography was first reported in 1913, not until 1963 was the first randomized clinical trial commenced at the Health Insurance Plan of New York (the HIP Study). HIP included women aged 40 to 64 years at entry: nearly 62,000 women were randomly assigned to the study group (two-view mammography and CBE) or control group (usual care). Two-view mammography and physical examination were offered every 12 months during the 4-year study period, and follow-up was continued for 18 years.[25]

The HIP trial was ahead of its time in many ways. For example, an aggressive protocol existed, designed to enhance compliance by using letters and telephone calls. The trial enrolled 67% of eligible women in the first screen; the compliance rate for all four screens was 39.4%.[25] Although the separate contributions of mammography and CBE could not be assessed, CBE was believed to have made a major contribution.[26]

Swedish Trials

Four different trials have been conducted in Sweden.

SWEDISH TWO-COUNTY STUDY. This trial, in Kopparberg and Ostergotland, began in 1977 and 1978 with an enrollment of almost 135,000 women randomly assigned to undergo one-view mammography every 24 months (below age 50 years) or 33 months (over age 50 years). Within geographic areas, all women were invited to enroll by letters of invitation using the population registry list.

Screening continued for four rounds for younger women and three rounds for older women.[27] The Kopparberg arm of the trial used single-view mammography without grids; the other Swedish trials used a grid.[28] High compliance (89%) for the first screen and subsequent screens was achieved except for women in their 70s.

MALMÖ TRIAL. This trial was begun in 1976 in one city in Sweden.[19] It was one of only two trials that began screening at age 45 years, and it stopped entry at age 69 years. It used 2-view mammography every 18 to 24 months for five rounds; randomization was by cluster based on birth cohort. About 59,000 women were enrolled in this trial, with 74% of eligible women participating in the first screen. Some problems existed in the Malmö study. This response rate was lower than that of most of the other trials. Most notably, mammograms were free to the control group, and 24% had at least one.[29] Mean follow-up was 8.8 years.[16]

STOCKHOLM STUDY. This study began in 1981 and enrolled about 43,000 women aged 40 to 64 years who received single-view mammogram every 28 months. As in the Malmö trial, randomization was by birth cohort within clusters; 74% of eligible women participated. Written invitations and follow-up letters were used to obtain participants.[4]

The final Swedish study was conducted in Göteborg, starting in 1982. The trial began with nearly 50,000 women aged 40 to 59 years who received two-view mammography every 18 months; 84% of eligible women participated. Randomization of women aged 40 to 49 years was by individual, and clustered randomization was used for women aged 50 to 59 years. Results have not yet been published.[4]

EDINBURGH TRIAL. This trial was begun in 1978 as a randomized component of the larger, nonrandomized United Kingdom trial of The Early Detection of Breast Cancer (TEDBC). About 25,000 women aged 45 to 64 were randomly assigned to undergo two-view mammogram and CBE on either a 12-month or a 24-month schedule. The purpose was to assess the impact of mammography and CBE in reducing mortality due to breast cancer.[30] Randomization followed a cluster technique based on physicians' practices. This was necessary because there were no lists of eligible women who could be used for randomization. Medical practices were stratified by size; then all women within a given practice were assigned to the same group. The trial had three inherent problems. First, only 61% of eligible women participated. Second, the randomization resulted in some confounding by socioeconomic strata, not surprising given that medical practices in the British Health System are geographically defined. The investigators attempted, however, to control for this factor in analysis.[31,32] Finally, the quality of the mammography in the study has been criticized, but this allegation has not been substantiated.

TABLE 8-1
Selected Characteristics of the Design and Conduct of Eight Randomized Controlled Trials of Breast Cancer Screening

Study (Year Begun)	Age at Entry (y)	Screening Modality	Periodicity (mo)	Randomization	Sample Size Study	Sample Size Control	Percentage Screened at First Examination (%)
HIP (1963)	40–64	2-view MM + CBE	12	Individual	30,239	30,756	67
Sweden							
Two–County (1977)	40–74	1-view MM	24 (age < 50 y)	Cluster: geographic	78,085	56,782	89
			33 (age ≥ 50 y)				
Malmö (1976)	45–69	2-view MM	18–24	Cluster: birth cohort	21,088	21,195	74
Stockholm (1981)	40–64	1-view MM	28	Cluster: birth cohort	39,164	19,943	81
Göteborg (1982)	40–59	2-view MM	18	Individual (age 40–49 y)	20,724	28,809	84
				Cluster (age 50–59 y)			
Edinburgh (1976)	45–64	2-view MM + CBE initially (later, usually 1-view MM)	12 / 24	Cluster: physician	23,226	21,904	61
Canada NBSS1 (1980)	40–49	2-view MM + CBE	12	Individual: volunteers	25,214	25,216	~100*
Canada NBSS2 (1980)	50–59	2-view MM and CBE versus CBE only	12	Individual: volunteers	19,711	19,694	~100*

CBE, clinical breast examination; MM, mammography; HIP, Health Insurance Plan [of New York]; NBSS, National Breast Screening Study.

* Study design included randomization of volunteers after CBE; accordingly, virtually 100% had their first screening examination.

(Fletcher S, Black W, Harris R, et al. Special article: report of the International Workshop on Screening for Breast Cancer. J Natl Cancer Inst 1993;85:1644)

Canadian Trials

Two trials were conducted in Canada to answer different questions. NBSS1 was designed to examine the value of 2-view mammography and CBE compared with usual care in women aged 40 to 49 years. Nearly 53,000 women were enrolled starting in 1980 and received follow-up yearly for 5 years. Unlike the other trials, the women were recruited as volunteers and were then randomized. As Miller and coworkers[22] reported, these women differed from the general Canadian population in several ways; for example, they were less likely to smoke and had higher levels of education.

The second Canadian study, NBSS2, also begun in 1980, enrolled nearly 43,000 women aged 50 to 59 years and was designed to compare 2-view mammography and CBE against CBE only. In other words, the question was whether a benefit of mammography exists over and above CBE in this age group. This has been the only trial planned to assess the additive impact of mammography in addition to CBE. Again, volunteers were recruited. Compliance was high: 85% of the women in both groups continued after the first screening.[33] In both Canadian trials, women also were taught BSE.

Concerns have been raised about the quality of mammography in the NBSS trials from 1980 to 1984.[34,35] Critics also have suggested that problems existed with the mammogram units themselves as well as with interpretation in the early days of the trial. Finally, some women were included who had breast symptoms. It is unlikely, however, that these problems, if indeed they occurred, accounted for the lack of significance. Many of the criticisms have not held up under scrutiny.

NONRANDOMIZED CLINICAL TRIALS

In general, randomized clinical trials are preferred to non-randomized trials.[1] This is largely because of selection bias, lead-time bias, and length bias that can occur in nonrandomized clinical trials. One demonstration project and two case-control studies are reviewed here, however, because they provide additional information.

The largest study of mammography and CBE was the US Breast Cancer Detection Demonstration Project (BCDDP), for which 280,000 women aged 35 years and older were recruited and screened in 28 centers annually with mammograms and CBE during the 1970s.[17,29] Thermography was used initially but was dropped. The BCDDP was sponsored jointly by the National Cancer Institute (NCI) and the American Cancer Society (ACS). Because the BCDDP participants were not a random sample of the population, there were some important differences from women in the general population. Most notably, the BCDDP population was at higher risk, with a substantially higher incidence of breast cancer. Moreover, because it was not a randomized clinical trial, the patient fatality rate was used to assess the impact of screening.

A subset of women were monitored as part of a case control study conducted by Morrison and associates[36] to examine case-fatality rates within the BCDDP. Breast cancer mortality was about 20% less than expected from national data. A benefit was noted for younger women, but it was less than for older women.

Two case-control trials also have been conducted in the Netherlands; one in Utrecht and one in Nijmegen. The Nijmegen study began in 1975.[4] Women aged 35 to 65 years were invited, with 19,687 participating initially; an additional 30,502 women aged 40 years and older were subsequently included. The Nijmegen Study was originally a biennial single-view mammography screening program offered to women aged 35 to 65 years. Because participation declined over time, a case-control study approach was used for purposes of analysis.[2] The cases studied were women who had been invited to participate and who had died of breast cancer; they were compared with age-matched living controls.

The Utrecht (DOM) Study began in 1974 with 20,555 women aged 50 to 64 years participating. They received an initial mammogram and CBE with subsequent examinations at 12, 18, 24, and 48 months. A case-control strategy similar to that of the Nijmegen Study was used, except all breast cancer deaths after the introduction of screening were included.[2] Mortality was reduced by 30%.

A cohort study to compare mammography with or without CBE was conducted in the Miyagi Prefecture of Japan, from 1989 to 1991 among 9634 Japanese women aged 50 years and over. Higher detection rates were found among the women who had received mammography, especially those aged 60 years and over. The detection rate was 0.31% for mammograms and CBE, compared with 0.08% for CBE alone.[37]

Evidence for Mammography

There are now over 1.15 million person-years of observation for women aged 40 to 49 years at entry from the randomized clinical trials.[11a]

Figures 8-1 to 8-3 illustrate the mortality outcome for women of all ages, for those younger than 50 years old, and for those older than 50 years old at entry, with 10 years of follow-up for HIP, 10 years for the Edinburgh trial, and 5 years for the Canadian treatment and 7 to 13 years for the Swedish trials. The data show large variability in the relative risk (RR) of dying of breast cancer for women under age 50 years (see Fig. 8-1). Three trials (Ostergotland, NBSS1, and Stockholm) showed an increase in mortality for women in the screened group (RRs, 1.28, 1.04, and 1.36).[28,33,38] Five trials (Edinburgh, Malmö, Göteborg, Kopparberg, and HIP) had lower RRs associated with the screened group (RRs, 0.78, 0.51, 0.73, and 0.77).[19,25,28] Unfortunately, these RRs had wide confidence intervals. Thus, for example, the HIP Study had a 23% reduction in mortality rate for the screened group, but the confidence interval means that the true value could be anywhere between a 50% reduction and a 16% increase in mortality rate. Among women over age 50 years in the Edinburgh trial, Donovan and coworkers[20] concluded that mortality could be reduced by up to 50% but increased

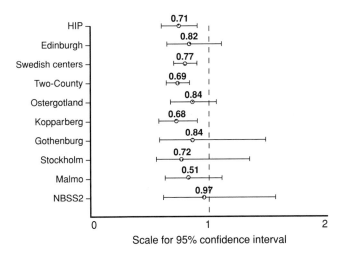

FIGURE 8-1 Mortality impact of the randomized clinical trials (all ages). HIP, Health Insurance Plan of New York; NBSS2, second National (Canada) Breast Cancer Screening Study.

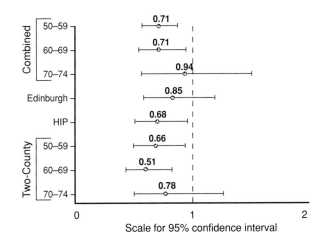

FIGURE 8-3 Mortality impact of the randomized clinical trials (women aged 50 years and over at entry). HIP, Health Insurance Plan of New York.

by up to 20%. In 1994, an analysis of 10-year data showed an 18% nonsignificant reduction in the breast cancer mortality for women in their 40s.[32] Thirteen-year data from the Swedish Two-County Study showed a reduction in mortality of 34% for women aged 50 to 74 years and 12% for women in their 40s.[28] The combined Swedish trials indicate a decrease in mortality of 30% for women aged 50 to 69 years but 12% for women aged 40 to 49 years.[38]

These nonsignificant results for women in their 40s are in great contrast to the effects for women aged 50 years and over, in whom all the RRs were less than 1 and ranged from 0.97 to 0.68. Significant reductions were found in the HIP and Swedish Two-County Study for women over age 50.[2] Only data for women aged 70 to

74 years in the combined Swedish trials and the Edinburgh trial included 1 in the confidence interval, in contrast with the data for women under age 50 years. What is striking is the differential benefit for women over and under age 50 years. None of the trials showed a statistically significant difference in mortality rates for women in their 40s, but nearly all the trials showed such a reduction for women their 50s, with the exception of the NBSS2.[33]

That mammography case finding does not necessarily lead to mortality reductions is illustrated in the NBSS2. Mammography did find more cancers than CBE alone, but this increase in case finding did not translate to a reduction in mortality.[22] In fact, more recent studies have had less dramatic effects on mortality than the HIP Study. The Swedish metaanalysis[38] found a reduction of 22% at 12 years of follow-up, and Alexander and associates[32] found about a 20% reduction in Edinburgh, a nonsignificant difference with wide confidence limits.

Figure 8-4 illustrates these age differences dramatically and shows the lack of mortality difference for women aged 40 to 49 years.[38] Only at about 8 years after randomization did the unscreened group begin to diverge from the screened group. This finding is in clear distinction to women in their 50s and 60s in whom an early and continued difference between the screened and unscreened groups is noted.[38] In this regard, the Canadian study is an exception because it did not find a reduced mortality rate among women who received mammography alone compared with mammography and CBE. In the latter group, however, the survival rate was highest among women whose cancers were diagnosed with mammography.[22] That the benefits of mammography take a long time to emerge for younger women means that such benefits are small and might be achieved by beginning screening around age 50 years.[32] On the basis of data from five studies, Day[39] estimated a 29% reduction in mortality for women aged 50 to 69 years, compared with a 4.7% reduction for women aged 40 to 49 years.[2] The latter is a small effect, indeed.

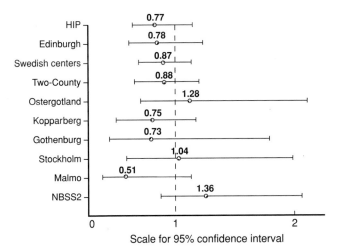

FIGURE 8-2 Mortality impact of the randomized clinical trials (women aged 40 to 49 years at entry). HIP, Health Insurance Plan of New York; NBSS1, first National (Canada) Breast Cancer Screening Study.

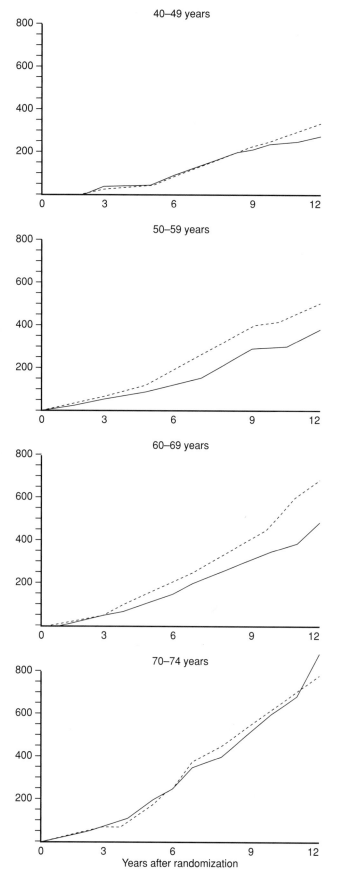

Four metaanalyses have examined the effect of the trials on women aged 40 to 49 years. When Elwood and associates,[16] in a metaanalysis that included all the data except for the controversial Canadian study, found an overall RR of 0.99, suggesting no difference between screened and control groups. With the Canadian data included, a slight increase was noted in the RR for the experimental group (RR, 1.16). The overall RRs found in the metaanalyses have ranged from 0.99 and 0.85 without the NBSS data to 0.93 and 1.08 with the NBSS data. None of the RRs were significant, and the upper and lower bounds suggest the potential for a reduction in mortality as great as 32% but an increase in mortality as large as 39% (Table 8-2).

Intermediate Measures of Screening Effectiveness

Although a significant reduction in morbidity and mortality from breast cancer is the most important outcome of breast cancer screening trials, certain intermediate markers can be used to gauge the quality of the trial. These include such measures as sensitivity, specificity, and positive predictive value (discussed earlier). These measures are described in greater detail elsewhere.[4]

As Table 8-3 shows, the trials themselves vary in their sensitivity, specificity, and positive predictive value. Moreover, age-related differences occur in the efficiency of screening. Mammography clearly is more sensitive and specific for women in their 50s and 60s than for women in their 40s. For example, 38% of the cancers in younger women (aged 40 to 49 years) may have been missed (ie, were false-negatives) in the Swedish Two-County Study, compared with 24% for women aged 50 to 59 years at entry.[4,28] The positive predictive value also varies, from 20% in the HIP trial and the NBSS1 to 70% in the Swedish Two-County Study.

Kerlikowske and coworkers[41] studied the results of nearly 32,000 mammograms using data from a large practice in California. They found lower positive predictive values for younger women compared with older women. In women aged 40 to 49 years, 2 cases of cancer were diagnosed per 1000 examinations and 48.3 diagnostic tests compared with 10 cancers per 1000 examinations and 14.8 diagnostic procedures in women aged 50 years and older. Only for higher-risk younger women was screening efficient. Elwood and associates[16] defined predictive value as the proportion of tumors diagnosed in the prevalence screen that would have come to clinical diagnosis later. These investigators concluded that the predictive value in the Swedish Two-County Study was 97% for women

FIGURE 8-4 Cumulative breast cancer mortality per 1000 in invited group (*solid line*) and control group (*dashed line*) by year since randomization and by age at randomization. (Nystrom L, Rutqvist LE, Wall S, et al. Breast cancer screening with mammography: overview of Swedish randomised trials. Lancet 1993;341:973)

TABLE 8-2
Metaanalyses of Trials for Women Aged 40 to 49 Years

Investigators	Description	Relative Risk	95% Confidence Interval	Reduction in Mortality Rate (%)
Miller et al, 1992[33]	Without NBSS data	0.85	0.68–1.08	15★
Eckhardt et al, 1994[40]	With NBSS data	0.93	0.76–1.15	7★
Elwood et al, 1993[16]	Without NBSS data	0.99	0.74–1.32	No difference
Elwood et al, 1993[16]	With NBSS data	1.08	0.85–1.39	No difference

NBSS, National (Canada) Breast Screening Study.

★ Nonsignificant.

aged 50 to 59 years, compared with 38% for women 40 to 49 years old at entry, suggesting a major overdiagnosis problem. One can detect many in situ cancers without changing mortality. The detection of small invasive cancers is most important.[16] Differences in standards for biopsy may help to explain these large international differences. In general, mammography appears to be specific if biopsy follows—96.6% to 99.9%.

Several studies have examined interval cancers, those that arise between screening examinations.[42] Some interval cancers represent human error; that is, they were visible on mammogram but were missed. Others truly represent cancers that developed between screenings; these tend to have a worse prognosis.[42] In the Edinburgh trial, screening resulted in a 70% reduction in interval cancers for women aged 45 to 54 years, compared with an 84% reduction for women older than 55 years.[43] This finding suggests a biologic difference in breast cancers in older and younger women.

Benefit of Mammography for Older Women

Most trials that have included women older than 70 years have found compliance to be lowest in the oldest group. In the Swedish trial, data were insufficient to permit analysis of older women.[4,28] Ironically, screening may be least acceptable to those who are most likely to benefit.[21] Thus, this creates a major problem in terms of making screening recommendations on the basis of data from randomized clinical trials. None are available, so extrapolation and clinical judgment must be used.

Wilson and coworkers[44] conducted a retrospective review of mammograms and records for women over age 75 years who were diagnosed at a large hospital. They concluded that screening mammography found significantly smaller (1.1 versus 2.1 cm; *P*=.0005) and earlier-stage disease.

Breast cancer screening is underused in women over age 70.[45–47] Morrow[45] concluded that screening is a cost-

effective but underused tool for older women. The Forum on Breast Cancer Screening[48] concluded that screening should be continued for these women unless contraindicated by significant comorbidity. This recommendation is based largely on the finding that breast cancer incidence continues to rise in women in their 70s.

The Mammography Controversy

Mammography has been more controversial than perhaps any other medical intervention. As noted, it may ultimately be a matter of philosophy—whether one believes a treatment is effective until proved ineffective or ineffective until proved effective. If one believes the first position, then studies that support the null hypothesis of no difference may not be convincing.

Another reason for disagreement relates to the type of evidence deemed acceptable. Reviews by Elwood,[16] the International Workshop on Breast Cancer Screening,[4] and the US Preventive Services Task Force[49] have given major weight to randomized clinical trial data. Mettlin and Smart[50,51] reviewed evidence that led the ACS to confirm its recommendation that women aged 40 to 49 years have mammograms every 1 to 2 years. These investigators emphasized the results of the BCDDP study and trend data showing reductions in tumor size observed through the Surveillance, Epidemiology, and End Results (SEER) program during the 1980s.[51] Finally, they argued that statistical significance should not be the only criterion by which results are judged.

Tables 8-4 and 8-5 summarize some of the arguments advanced to explain the lack of benefit of mammography for younger women and provide explanations for the lack of benefit. Arguments include the following:

- Insufficient sample size to detect small differences
- Quality concerns related to mammography
- Issues related to the different biology of the disease and response to treatment in younger women
- Limitations of mammography in younger women

TABLE 8-3
Estimates of Screening Test Performance and Other Intermediate Measures in Seven Randomized Controlled Trials

						Trial	Canada★ NBSS2 (Age 50–59 y) MM + CBE	Canada★ NBSS2 (Age 50–59 y) CBE Only
	HIP	Malmö	Swedish Two-County	Edinburgh★	Stockholm	Canada★ NBSS1 (Age 40–49 y)		
Sensitivity								
Detection method†	74	79	76	88	68	81	88	63
Incidence method‡	77	68	60–70	79	52–75	58	72	46
Prevalence§ per 1000 at first screen	2.72	7.5	6.0	6.2	4.0	3.89	7.20	3.45
Prevalence ratio‖	1.39	2.8	2.9	3.2	2.82	2.74	3.51	1.68
Specificity§	98.5	96–97	95–98	96–97	95–97	82–93	83–96	89–96
	99.8	NA	99.4–99.9	98.7–99.9	99.8–99.9	96.6–98.6	96.5–99.2	99.1–99.7
Positive predictive value (work-up) (%)	12	10–22	12	4–15	8–10	2	4–6	2–4
Positive predictive value (biopsy) (%)	20	33–61	50–75	36–64	62–78	12	20	28
Biopsy rate (per 1000 examinations)	10	NA	4–12	3–12.5	4–6	15–38	12–42	4–12
Benign/malignant ratio	3.9	NA	0.33–1	0.56–1.8	0.28–0.62	7.3	2.7–4.8	1.6–3.3
In situ (entire study group) (%)	12.8	15.8	8.4	10.1	10.5	18.9	16.7	5.8
Stage I (entire study group) (%)	56	50	53	32	65	NA	NA	NA
Node-negative (entire study group) (%)	57	NA	71	63	NA	65	69	67

CBE, clinical breast examination; MM, mammography; NBSS, National Breast Screening Study; NA, not applicable.

★ Estimates are based on the screening process as a whole. The individual contributions of MM and CBE are not included.

† Based on screen-detected and interval cancers from all rounds.

‡ Based on rate of interval cancers in study group and incidence rate in control group from all rounds.

§ Dependent on prevalence, spectrum of cancer in population, and sensitivity of screening.

‖ Based on each round.

(Fletcher S, Black W, Harris R, et al. Special article: report of the International Workshop on Screening for Breast Cancer. J Natl Cancer Inst 1993;85:1644)

TABLE 8-4

Potential Reasons for Lack of Effect of Mammography in Younger Women

1. The trials have not been designed to assess impact by age.[35,52]

2. Questions exist regarding quality of mammograms and patient selection in the NBSS1 trial.[52]

3. Mammography makes no difference in reducing breast cancer mortality for younger women.

4. Follow-up has not been long enough to observe a difference.

5. A biologic difference may exist in the response to therapy of disease detected in younger women.[16,17]

6. Detection of breast cancer earlier in younger women is more difficult because of the denser parenchyma.[38,53]

7. The small number of breast cancers in younger women makes screening inefficient.

8. Screening for women in their 40s is too infrequent; annual screening is needed because of the shorter sojourn time.[28]

9. The mammography units in the NBSS trial were not optimal.[35]

10. Participation rates and control group contamination could have affected the outcomes.[2]

11. Detection of in situ cancers that might not become invasive makes no contribution to a reduced mortality rate.[16]

12. One analysis showed that 40% of younger women with small lesions had positive lymph nodes.[11a]

13. Inconclusiveness should not be a reason to conclude that mammography is not beneficial (Osuch JR. Detection and Treatment Subcommittee on Breast Cancer. American Cancer Society, 1993).

- Study design issues
- The small number of cases of breast cancer in younger women

Plausible explanations exist for all these concerns, however.

To discount more than 30 years of research experience and more than 1.15 million woman-years of observation because the ideal trial has not been and may never be conducted would be a mistake. Even if the Canadian trial, which has been the most controversial, is omitted, the trial results are remarkably consistent—clear, significant reductions in the mortality rate for women over age 50 years and nonsignficiant results for women under age 50 years. If the Canadian trial were the exception, caution might be indicated; however, the Canadian trial was merely one in a series of disappointing results for women in their 40s.[4] As Nystrom and associates[38] concluded from a metaanalysis of the Swedish data, there is considerable age-related variation in screening. The largest benefit (29% reduction in mortality) was observed among women aged 50 to 59 years at entry. "Among women aged 40 to 49, the benefit was small (about a 13% reduction in mortality) and delayed."[11a] Miller and associates[33] and others[4,54] have advanced plausible explanations of the Canadian study that refute the charges of flawed randomization and poor quality. Moreover, how can it be that the same methodologic

flaws that hindered the finding of significant results for women aged 40 to 49 years did not affect outcomes for women aged 50 years and over? This is a troubling logical inconsistency.[11a]

It is remarkable that the reduction in mortality rate in women aged 50 to 69 years has remained so stable during more than 30 years of trials while the lack of impact on women aged 40 to 49 years also has been stable. The failure of modern mammography to produce greater decreases in mortality rate may simply be a limitation in radiographic technology.[4] The lack of an impact on women in their 40s may be a consequence of the greater density of breast tissue in younger women, differential biology, and differences in tumor type. For example, Tabar and others found a higher proportion of tumors in the groups with very good and very bad prognoses among younger women (unpublished observations). Mammography also had a lesser effect on tumor size for younger women.

Advocates of a costly screening procedure must have strong evidence of its effectiveness. Three expert panels (American College of Physicians, US Preventive Services Task Force, and the Canadian Task Force) reviewed the data on mammography and concluded that it does not reduce mortality rates for women aged 40 to 49 years.[49] Thus, they concluded, that no convincing evidence indicates that mammography benefits women aged 40 to 49 years who are at average risk.[49] This finding is consistent with the conclusion of the American Board of Family Practice and the report of the International Workshop on Breast Cancer Screening.[4] The latter summarized that, for women aged 40 to 49 years, randomized, controlled trials consistently demonstrated no benefit from screening in the first 5 to 7 years after study entry. Most medical organizations, however, including the American College of Radiology (ACR), ACS, and the American College of Obstetricians and Gynecologists, continue to recommend mammograms every 1 to 2 years for women in their 40s.[50]

TABLE 8-5

Responses to the Concerns Raised About the Canadian Trials

1. If the sample size must be hundreds of thousands to achieve adequate power, the effect sought must be small. The absolute benefit would be small.[26,54]

2. The Canadian study results are consistent with those of other trials.[4]

3. Although the Canadian trial had problems, more is known because the investigators were meticulous in auditing the trial and documenting problems. Undoubtedly, the other trials had problems as well, but the problems are not known.

4. Ederer[54] showed that women were similar across groups. Moreover, no evidence has been found of differential allocation of subjects based on abnormal findings.

5. Although image quality of mammography has improved, the mortality reductions remain consistent with the earliest trials—30% for women over age 50 years.[4] Improvements in technology have not necessarily translated into reductions in mortality.

Decisions about therapy for breast cancer should not be made on the basis of trends. Neither should decisions about cancer screening. Until a paradigmatic shift occurs in the scientific community, the randomized clinical trial is the best source of data about the efficacy of interventions. At this time, the evidence suggests a powerful and almost immediate impact of mammography for women aged 50 to 69 years. No trial has so far recorded convincing evidence of a reduction in mortality rate for women aged 40 to 49 years.[38] If there is an impact of mammography for women in their 40s, it is probably below a 15% reduction in mortality and does not occur for at least 7 years after trial entry. That translates into a great many mammograms to save a few lives.

Tabar and associates suggest that a 19% reduction in mortality might be possible if annual mammograms were used for women aged 40 to 49 years (unpublished observation). This suggestion is based on the hypothesis that the mean sojourn time for breast cancer is much shorter for women in their 40s. This argument is plausible, but it still remains hypothetic and cannot be proved within the context of any of the existing trials.

Clinical Breast Examination

More research has been devoted to mammography than to any other aspect of breast screening. Especially with the lack of evidence that mammography leads to mortality reductions in women aged 40 to 49 years, however, it is appropriate to ask whether a role exists for the clinical breast examination. Morrow and coworkers[55] reviewed the CBE as a modality, with the focus on CBE for screening. As discussed earlier, the results of the NBSS2 showed that mammography did not have an effect on mortality greater than that of CBE for women older than 50 years, although mammography did find smaller tumors. The HIP Study used both mammography and CBE, but the effects could not be separated. Evidence suggests that CBE did play an important role. For example, 44% of the cancers in women aged 50 to 59 years were found by mammogram alone, compared with only 19% among women aged 40 to 49 years.[22] Morrison and colleagues[36] concluded that a program of mammography alone could not be expected to have the same value as a program of mammography and CBE. It has been estimated from the HIP Study, the BCDDP, and the NBSS2 that breast palpation accounts for 50% to 67% of the value of CBE and mammography.[49]

CBE may add 5% to 20% of the number of cancers detected when combined with mammography; however, some of these cases represent women with symptoms. Ideally, CBE, BSE, and mammography should be viewed as complementary modalities.[56] Each provides a check and balance on the other methods. CBE can identify palpable masses that may be missed on mammography. This is especially true for younger women. Given the economic and human costs associated with mammography, CBE may be a reasonable alternative for younger women at average risk.

As with mammography, quality control of CBE is essential. One of the reasons the CBE arm of the study was so effective in the NBSS2 may have been the careful training of the nurse examiners. This resulted in a sensitivity, for the first round, of 80% and a specificity of 88% to 96%.[4,57] The positive predictive value of CBE alone was low, however, at 2.9% to 4.2%. These high rates are in contrast to the wide variation but generally lower rates in other trials; for example, CBE-only detection occurred in only 3.4% of screen-detected cancers in Edinburgh.[58]

Although mammography detects more cancers and earlier cancers than CBE, these advantages may not translate into a reduction in mortality rate.[58] The Canadian NBSS2 is the only trial that compares CBE and mammography, however. CBE has never been tested against an unexamined control group. CBE clearly has an important role, especially for younger women; however, much more attention should be paid to both training and quality control.

Breast Self-Examination

Adair[58] recommended in 1933 that women be taught to palpate their breasts occasionally. Over the years, most major medical organizations have advised women to practice BSE. Controversy has been considerable over whether BSE can reduce mortality from breast cancer. One of the earliest reviews concluded that BSE did find small cancers and could reduce mortality.[59] In Foster and Costanza's[59] often-cited study, however, BSE could not be separated from self-discovery. The combined group had lower cancer mortality than those who did not perform BSE. Moreover, as with CBE and mammography, important issues of quality control and proficiency exist.[60,61] All BSE is not alike. In addition are problems of compliance and questions regarding the validity of self-report. Most women practice BSE sporadically, and many women give up altogether.[13] Several reports of randomized trials have been conducted in countries other than the United States to assess the impact of BSE on mortality from breast cancer,[62–64] but most of these trials are ongoing.

Ellman and associates[62] reported on a substudy within the United Kingdom Trial of Early Detection to assess the impact of BSE centers with careful BSE training and subsequent practice on mortality. Mortality was not different in the BSE centers, compared with comparison centers. Some differences within the BSE centers may have confounded the results, however.

A randomized population-based BSE has been conducted in Leningrad (now St. Petersburg) since 1985, with final follow-up in 1999.[64] The study includes 120,310 women aged 40 to 64 years, half of whom were given personalized training and BSE calendars. Although more biopsies were conducted in the BSE group, so far this has not translated into a reduction in mortality. Moreover, no significant differences have been reported in the size of primary tumors or the presence of affected lymph nodes. The results, however, are still preliminary.

From 1973 to 1975, 28,785 women were taught BSE

in Finland as part of the MAMA program and were monitored to assess the impact of BSE on mortality using a historic cohort design.[63] The program included careful training, BSE calendars, and interaction with volunteers. The mortality rate for the BSE group was compared with that of the general Finnish population. Although stage differences did not appear to occur, the mortality rate was lower in the BSE group, with an observed death/expected death ratio of 0.75 for all ages. The effect was independent of age.

Some investigators have suggested that regular, competent BSE may increase survival rates. For example, a case-control study in the United Kingdom found that 73.1% of women in the BSE group, compared with 66.1% in the non–BSE group, survived.[65] As discussed earlier, increases in survival do not necessarily translate into reductions in the mortality rate.

Farwell and coworkers[66] conducted a case-control study to try to assess the contributions of BSE, CBE, and mammogram to mammography in Vermont. Only mammography was related to stage shifts. Kurioshi and associates[67] conducted a case-control study of about 1700 women in Japan, of 355 patients with BSE-detected breast cancer and 1327 patients with breast cancers detected by BSE incidentally; the BSE-detected cancers were significantly smaller.

Although some data are promising, the conclusion by O'Malley and Fletcher[68] reached in 1987 is still appropriate: evidence regarding BSE is lacking, and more data are needed. Morrison[69] found no data to support a recommendation that BSE be used in screening. The most positive conclusion would be that BSE has a small but measurable impact on earlier detection as measured by clinical stage and tumor size.[70] BSE is relatively low cost and low risk, although it is not sensitive.[56] If BSE is to be of any value, it should be taught carefully and consistently.[60,71] Moreover, the quality of practice should be checked on a return visit. Self-examination should never be considered a substitute for CBE or mammography. They are complementary modalities.[56]

Screening of High-Risk Women

Unfortunately, data from randomized trials do not provide direct evidence regarding the value of mammography in reducing the breast cancer mortality rate among high-risk women. With the exception of the NBSS1, most trials do not have good risk data about participants. As Elwood and coworkers[16] concluded, the higher risk does not suggest that the test will perform better for individuals or that earlier therapy will be more effective in higher-risk women. The study by Kerlikowske and associates[41] did show that mammography was more efficient in women at high risk, but no evidence indicates that this greater efficiency will translate into reductions in mortality rate.[62] It would be extremely helpful to have more information on this topic.

In the absence of data, it may be prudent to screen women at truly high risk more often.[72] To reach appropriate conclusions about risk status, a good family history is essential. It should include a personal history (eg, previous diagnosis of atypical hyperplasia), a family history, including a genealogy and relevant information about exposures.[73]

Adherence to Breast Cancer Screening

The barriers to mammography screening are reasonably consistent from study to study and are similar to those for Papanicolaou (Pap) tests.[74] The most important barrier is the lack of a recommendation by a woman's physician.[47,75–77] Older women, black women, and Hispanic women are less likely than middle-aged white women to report such a recommendation. Women report that their other most common reasons for not having mammograms, are that they believe there was no need because they had no breast problems and that mammograms are not needed in the absence of symptoms.

Other barriers exist, but they account for much less of the variance in explaining the behavior. These include concern about radiation and pain and anxiety about finding something. These barriers, however, may be important for individual women or for subgroups of women. For example, black and Hispanic women seem to be more concerned about pain. Some evidence suggests that older black women are more fatalistic about cancer in general, so this also should be addressed.[78] Calle and associates[79] also found that unmarried women were less likely to have had mammograms than married women.

Cigarette smokers are also less likely to have mammograms.[75,80] This may have more to do with their avoidance of health care in general, but it does make these women a special concern.

Other evidence suggests that access and environmental barriers may be important.[80] Women without health insurance are less likely to have mammograms or Papanicolaou tests.[7] Cost is not a major barrier reported by women, although it certainly is a barrier for some women, for example, women in their 50s and Hispanic women.[76] Studies show that even when the cost barrier is removed, however, other important psychologic barriers remain.[75] If these barriers are not removed, women still may not have regular mammograms.

Women who are advised by their physicians to have mammograms are indeed more likely to have them.[75,81] Women who know the recommended screening interval for their ages and who know the relationship between age and breast cancer screening also are more likely to have regular mammograms.[82,83] Evidence also indicates that women with strong social ties are more likely to have mammograms.[84]

Family history has been inconsistent as a predictor of screening. Some studies show that it increases the likelihood that women will have regular mammograms, but others do not.[85,86] In a review of the data, Lerman and Schwartz[87] showed that different studies found different kinds of relations between family risk and screening behavior, ranging from negative effect, to no effect, to positive effect. Many studies have used self-selected groups of women, however, who volunteered to participate in programs for women at high risk of breast cancer.

Summary

The data strongly support screening with women in their 50s and 60s, but not women in their 40s; however, certain important questions about breast cancer screening remain unanswered:

1. Is there an age during the 40s when screening should begin? None of the trials permit a conclusion about a specific age during the 40s at which screening should begin.
2. How should risk status modify advice about breast cancer screening?
3. Should early menopause dictate earlier screening? This is an important issue because age 50 often is used as a bellwether for menopause, but there is wide variability in the age when individual women experience menopause.
4. Do racial or ethnic differences influence the effectiveness of mammography?

Some of these questions could be answered by a proposed international breast screening trial designed to enroll women at ages 40 and 41 years. The answers will not be available for at least 10 years, however. In the meantime, an evidence-based approach, as proposed by Eddy[24] and others[49,88] would tend toward *not* recommending routine mammograms for women in their 40s. This is based on the use of mortality rate as an endpoint. Physicians who choose to use survival as an outcome, or who hold other values, may opt for guidelines such as those issued by the ACS and ACR instead.[14,50]

Women with a strong personal or family history of breast cancer should be screened in their 40s. Screening should include both mammography and a high-quality CBE for women aged 50 years and older, whereas the CBE is the minimum examination for women in their 40s who are at average risk. Although no evidence indicates that BSE reduces mortality from breast cancer, it seems prudent to teach BSE to women and to encourage its competent practice.

Controversy about breast screening makes it imperative that physicians engage in a partnership with women. The goal, however difficult, should be informed decision making.

References

1. Hennekens CH, Buring JE. Epidemiology in medicine. Boston, Little, Brown, 1987.
2. Hurley SF, Kaldor JM. The benefits and risks of mammographic screening for breast cancer. Epidemiol Rev 1992;14:101.
3. Kuni CC. Mammography in the 1990s: a plea for objective doctors and informed patients. Am J Prev Med 1993;9:185.
4. Fletcher S, Black W, Harris R, et al. Special article: report of the International Workshop on Screening for Breast Cancer. J Natl Cancer Inst 1993;85:1644.
5. Tabar L, Faberberg G, Duffy S, et al. The Swedish two-county trial of mammographic screening for breast cancer: recent results and calculation of benefit. J Epidemiol Community Health 1989;43:107.
6. Eddy D, Hasseiblad V, McGivney W, et al. The value of mammography screening in women under age 50 years. JAMA 1988;259:1512.
7. Breen N, Kessler L. Changes in the use of screening mammography: evidence from the 1987 and 1990 National Health Interview Surveys. Am J Public Health 1994;84:62.
8. Rakowski W, Rimer B, Bryant S. Integrating behavior and intention regarding mammography by respondents in the 1990 National Health Interview Survey of Health Promotion and Disease Prevention. Public Health Rep 1993;108:605.
9. Wong J, Feussner J. Screening for disease: screening mammography for breast cancer: a wise test when used in time. NC Med J 1993;54:257.
10. Miller AB. Incidence and demographics: radiation risk. In: Breast diseases, ed 2. Philadelphia, JB Lippincott, 1991.
11. Greenberg RS, Daniels SR, Flanders D, et al. In: Medical epidemiology. Norwalk, CT, Appleton & Lange. 1993.
11a. Baines CJ. A different view on what is known about breast screening and the Canadian National Breast Screening Study. (Submitted.)
12. Hakama M, Elovainio L, Kajantie R, et al. Breast cancer screening as public health policy in Finland. Br J Cancer 1991;64:962.
13. Ellman R. Clinical cost-benefit of screening programs. In: Stoll B, ed. Women at high risk to breast cancer. Boston, Wolters Kluwer, 1991.
14. Swanson GM. May we agree to disagree, or how do we develop guidelines for breast cancer screening in women? commentary. J Natl Cancer Inst 1994;86:903.
15. Harris R. Breast cancer among women in their forties: toward a reasonable research agenda. J Natl Cancer Inst. 1994;86:410.
16. Elwood JM, Cox B, Richardson AK. The effectiveness of breast cancer screening by mammography in younger women. Online J Curr Clin Trials 1993;32:93.
17. Miller A. Screening: clinical practice: mammography, reviewing the evidence, epidemiology aspect. Can Fam Physician 1993;39:85.
18. Lerman C, Trock B, Rimer BK, et al. Psychological and behavioral implications of abnormal mammograms. Ann Intern Med 1991;114:657.
19. Andersson I, Aspegren K, Janzon L, et al. Mammographic screening and mortality from breast cancer: the Malmo mammographic screening trial. BMJ 1988;297:943.
20. Donovan D, Middleton J, Ellis D. Letters to the editor: Edinburgh trial of screening for breast cancer. Lancet 1990;335:1298.
21. Peeters PH, Verbeek ALM, Straatman H, et al. Evaluation of overdiagnosis of breast cancer in screening with mammography: results of the Nijmegen Programme. Int J Epidemiol 1989;18:295.
22. Miller AB, Baines CJ, To T, et al. Canadian National Breast Screening Study. 2. Breast cancer detection and death rates among women aged 50 to 59 years. Can Med Assoc J 1992;147:1477.
23. Feig SA. Low-dose mammography: assessment of theoretical risk. In: Feig SA, McLelland R, ed. Breast carcinoma: current diagnosis and treatment. New York, Masson Publishing (alternate publisher American College of Radiology), 1983:69.
24. Eddy D. Clinical decision making: from theory to practice: principles for making difficult decisions in difficult times. JAMA 1994;271:1792.
25. Shapiro S, Venet W, Strax P, et al. Current results of the breast cancer screening randomized trial: the Health Insurance Plan (HIP)

of Great New York study. In: Screening for breast cancer. Toronto, Sam Huber Publishing, 1988.

26. Baines CJ. Perspectives: the Canadian National Breast Screening Study: a perspective on criticisms. Ann Intern Med 1994;120:326.

27. Tabar L, Fagerberg G, Duffy S, et al. Breast imaging: current status and future directions: update of the Swedish Two-County Program of Mammographic Screening for Breast Cancer. Radiol Clin North Am 1992;30:187.

28. Tabar L, Duffy S, Burhenne L. New Swedish breast cancer detection results for women aged 40–49. Cancer 1993;72:1437.

29. Smart C. The role of mammography in the prevention of mortality from breast cancer. Cancer Prev 1989;1.

30. Roberts MM, Alexander FE, Anderson TJ, et al. Medical science: Edinburgh trial of screening for breast cancer: mortality at seven years. Lancet 1990;335:241.

31. Alexander F, Roberts M, Lutz W, et al. Randomisation by cluster and the problem of social class bias. J Epidemiol Community Health 1989;43:29.

32. Alexander FE, Anderson TJ, Brown HK, et al. The Edinburgh randomised trial of breast cancer screening: results after 10 years of follow-up. Br J Cancer 1994;70:542.

33. Miller AB, Baines CJ, To T, et al. Canadian National Breast Screening Study. 1. Breast cancer detection and death rates among women aged 40 to 49 years. Can Med Assoc J 1992;147:1458.

34. Burhenne L, Burhenne H. The Canadian National Breast Screening Study: a Canadian critique. AJR 1993;161:761.

35. Kopans DB. The Canadian screening program: A different perspective: commentary. AJR 1990;155:748.

36. Morrison A, Brisson J, Khalid N. Breast cancer incidence and mortality in the Breast Cancer Detection Demonstration Project. J Natl Cancer Inst 1988;80:1540.

37. Ohuchi N, Yoshida K, Kimura M, et al. Improved detection rate of early breast cancer in mass screening combined with mammography. Jpn J Cancer Res 1993;84:807.

38. Nystrom L, Rutqvist LE, Wall S, et al. Breast cancer screening with mammography: overview of Swedish randomised trials. Lancet 1993;341:973.

39. Day NE. Screening for breast cancer. Br Med Bull 1991;47:400.

40. Eckhardt S, Badellino F, Murphy GP. UICC meeting on breast-cancer screening in pre-menopausal women in developed countries. Int J Cancer 1994;56:1.

41. Kerlikowske K, Grady D, Barclay J, et al. Positive predictive value of screening mammography by age and family history of breast cancer. JAMA 1993;270:1.

42. Frisell J, Eklund G, Hellstrom L, et al. The Stockholm breast cancer screening trial: 5 year results and stage at discovery. Breast Cancer Res Treat 1989;13:79.

43. Moss SM, Coleman DA, Ellman R, et al. Interval cancers and sensitivity in the screening centres of the UK trial of early detection of breast cancer. Eur J Cancer 1993;29A:255.

44. Wilson TE, Helvie MA, August DA. Breast imaging: breast cancer in elderly patient: early detection with mammography. Radiology 1994;190:203.

45. Morrow M. Surgery in the elderly patient. I. Breast disease in elderly women. Surg Clin North Am 1994;74:145.

46. Coleman EA, Feuer EJ, NCI Breast Cancer Screening Consortium Members. Breast cancer screening among women from 65 to 74 years of age in 1987–88 and 1991. Ann Intern Med 1992;117:961.

47. Rimer BK, Ross E, Cristinzio S. Older women's participation in breast screening. J Gerontol 1992;47:85.

48. Costanza ME, Zapka JG, Harris DH, et al. Impact of a physician intervention program to increase breast cancer screening. J Cancer Epidemiol Biomarkers Prevention 1992;1:581.

49. Sox HC Jr. Preventive health services in adults. N Engl J Med 1993;330:1589.

50. Mettlin C, Smart CR. Breast cancer detection guidelines for women aged 40–49 years: rationale for the American Cancer Society reaffirmation of recommendations. CA Cancer J Clin 1994;44:248.

51. Mettlin C, Smart C. The Canadian National Breast Screening Study: an appraisal and implications for early detection policy. Cancer 1993;72:1461.

52. Greenwald P, Kramer B, Weed D. Expanding horizons in breast and prostate cancer prevention and early detection (The 1992 Samuel C. Harvey Lecture). J Cancer Educ 1993;8:91.

53. Stacey-Clear A, McCarthy K, Hall D, et al. Breast cancer survival among women under age 50: is mammography detrimental? Lancet 1992;340:991.

54. Ederer F. Discussion of Canadian National Breast Screening Study. 2. Breast cancer detection and death rates among women aged 50–59 years. Bethesda, NCI National Workshop on Screening for Breast Cancer, February 24–25, 1993.

55. Morrow M. Locally advanced breast cancer. In: Harris JR, Hellman S, Henderson IC, et al, eds. Breast diseases, ed 2. Philadelphia, JB Lippincott, 1991:767.

56. Foster RS, Worden JK, Costanza MC, et al. Clinical breast examination and breast self-examination. Cancer 1992;69:1992.

57. Mittra I. Breast screening: the case for physical examination without mammography. Lancet 1994;343:342.

58. Baines CJ. Physical examination of the breasts: in screening for breast cancer. J Gerontol 1992;47.

59. Foster RS, Costanza MC. Breast self-examination practices and breast cancer survival. Cancer 1984;53:999.

60. Champion V. The role of breast self-examination in breast cancer screening. Cancer 1992;69:1985.

61. Stratton BF, Nicholson ME, Olsen LK, et al. Breast self-examination proficiency: attitudinal, demographic, and behavioral characteristics. J Women's Health 1994;3:185.

62. Ellman R, Moss SM, Coleman D. Breast self-examination programmes in the trial of early detection of breast cancer: ten-year findings. Br J Cancer 1991;68:208.

63. Gastrin G, Miller AB, To T, et al. Incidence and mortality from breast cancer in the MAMA Program for Breast Screening in Finland, 1973–1986. Cancer 1994;73:2168.

64. Semiglazov VF, Moiseyenko VM, Bavli JL, et al. The role of breast self-examination in early breast cancer detection (results of the 5-year USSR/WHO Randomized Study in Leningrad). Eur J Epidemiol 1992;8:498.

65. Le Geyte M, Mant D, Vessey MP, et al. Breast self-examination and survival from breast cancer. Cancer 1992;66:917.

66. Farwell MR, Foster RS, Costanza MC. Breast cancer and earlier detection efforts: realized and unrealized impact on stage. Arch Surg 1993;128:510.

67. Kurioshi T, Tominaga S, Ota J, et al. The effect of breast self-examination on early detection and survival. Jpn J Cancer Res 1992;83:344.

68. O'Malley MS, Fletcher SW. Screening for breast cancer with breast self-examination: a critical review. JAMA 1987;257:2197.

69. Morrison AS. Screening for cancer of the breast. Epidemiol Rev 1993;15:244.

70. Grady KE. The efficacy of breast self-examination. J Gerontol 1992;47:69.

71. McKenna Sr. RJ, Greene P, Winchester DP, et al. Breast self-examination and breast physical examination. 1992;69(Suppl):2003.

72. Garber JE. Familial aspects of breast cancer. In: Harris JR, Hellman S, Henderson IC, et al, eds. Breast diseases, ed 2. Philadelphia, JB Lippincott, 1991.

73. White LN, Spitz MR. Cancer risk and early detection assessment. Semin Oncol Nurs 1993;9:188.

74. Rimer BK. Adherence to breast cancer screening. In: Reintgen D, Clark R, eds. Cancer screening. St Louis, Mosby–Year Book (in press).

75. Rimer BK, Keintz MK, Keller HB, et al. Why women resist screen-

ing mammography: patient-related barriers. Radiology 1989; 172:243.

76. Fox SA, Murata PF, Stein JA. The impact of physician compliance on screening mammography for older women. Arch Intern Med 1991;51:50.

77. Burg M, Lane D, Polednak A. Age group differences in the use of breast cancer screening tests. J Aging Health 1990;2:514.

78. Rimer BK. Interventions to increase breast screening: lifespan and ethnicity issues. Cancer 1994;74:323.

79. Calle EE, Flanders WD, Thun MJ, et al. Demographic predictors of mammography and pap smear screening in US women. Am J Public Health 1993;33:51.

80. McBride CM, Curry SJ, Taplin S, et al. Exploring environmental barriers to participation in mammography screening in an HMO. J Cancer Epidemiol Biomarkers Prevention 1993;2:599.

81. Dawson DA, Thompson GB. Breast cancer risk factors and screening: United States, 1987, DHHS Publication No. (PHS) 900–1500. Hyattsville, MD, US Department of Health and Human Services, 1990:1.

82. Slenker SE, Grant MC. Attitudes, beliefs, and knowledge about mammography among women over forty years of age. J Cancer Educ 1989;4:61.

83. Champion VL. The relationship of selected variables to breast cancer detection behaviors in women 35 and older. Oncol Nurs Forum 1991;18:733.

84. King E, Resch N, Rimer BK, et al. Breast cancer screening practices among retirement community women. Prev Med 1991;22:1.

85. Costanza ME, Annas GJ, Brown ML, et al. Supporting statements and rationale. J Gerontol 1992;47:7.

86. Vogel VG, Peters GN, Evans WP: Design and conduct of a low-cost mammographic screening project: experience of the American Cancer Society, Texas division. Am J Roentgenol 1992;158:51.

87. Lerman C, Schwartz M. Adherence and psychological adjustment among women at high risk for breast cancer. Breast Cancer Res Treat 1993;28:145.

88. Kaluzny A, Rimer B, Harris R. Commentary: the National Cancer Institute and guideline development: lessons from the breast cancer screening controversy. J Natl Cancer Inst 1994;86:901.

9

Management of the High-Risk and the Concerned Patient

JUDY E. GARBER ▪ BARBARA L. SMITH

Diseases of the Breast, edited by Jay R. Harris, Marc E. Lippman, Monica Morrow, and Samuel Hellman. Lippincott-Raven Publishers, Philadelphia, © 1996.

Breast cancer is a common disease and a significant worry for many women and their physicians. A high level of awareness exists for various breast cancer risk factors; however, we know less about how these factors interact and still less about how their presence should influence recommendations regarding surveillance or prevention strategies. The designation of a woman as high risk causes anxiety for her and her physician, and may result in frequent physician visits and mammographic examinations, as well as multiple biopsies or even prophylactic surgery.[1] Given the range of risk-management options (from standard surveillance to prophylactic surgery), and the fact that few have proven efficacy, it seems reasonable that management options be appropriate to the level of risk. It is therefore imperative that physicians become familiar with breast cancer risk estimation so that reasonable recommendations about risk management can be made.

Although no consensus exists about what constitutes high risk or the effectiveness of various cancer surveillance or prevention options, the past few years have seen the beginning of substantial progress in both areas. The first incarnations of several sophisticated models have been developed to assist in more precise risk estimation.[2–4] Dramatic developments have also occurred in breast cancer genetics, as described in Chapter 3.2, which ultimately may permit the identification of groups of women with an exceptionally high risk for developing breast cancer.

In this chapter, we address issues in the identification of individuals at high risk for breast cancer, the quantification of risk estimation, and the controversies in risk management. We also review some of the current practical considerations in risk assessment programs and consider how the availability of testing for genetic predisposition to breast cancer may influence this area in the near future.

Understanding Risk

ABSOLUTE RISK

Risk is a probabilistic statement. *Absolute risk* is the chance of developing breast cancer during a specified time interval. It is often expressed as the cumulative risk, the sum of the annual risks to a specific point in time. Data on absolute risk can be compared with other statistical risks. For example, a woman's risk for developing breast cancer before 25 years of age is equivalent to the actuarial risk for drowning in 1 year.[5] For counseling purposes, one might consider providing breast cancer risk figures for various intervals, such as the next year, the next 10 years, and the lifetime. It is often difficult, however, to be certain that patients adequately distinguish among these statistics and do not experience risk as the lifetime risk estimate every year. As illustrated in Table 9-1, the risk of breast cancer development is always at least three-fold higher than is the risk of death from breast cancer, a potentially important fact for concerned women.[6]

RELATIVE RISK

Sometimes expressed as an odds ratio, *relative risk* (RR) is the number most often provided in epidemiologic studies of risk factors. The statistic expresses the comparison of the rate of disease in the population with the exposure under investigation against the rate in an unexposed, but otherwise similar, group. Interaction among various risk factors is poorly understood; complex statistical models addressing these issues may facilitate risk estimation.

RISK HISTORY

In preparation for risk counseling, a woman's status regarding number of risk factors should be determined, either because of the strength of the risk conferred by these

TABLE 9-1
Probability of Eventually Developing and Dying of Breast Cancer in White Women

Age Interval (y)	Risk of Developing Breast Cancer (%)	Risk of Developing Invasive Breast Cancer (%)	Risk of Dying of Breast Cancer (%)
Birth–110	10.2	9.8	3.6
20–30	0.04	0.04	0.00
20–40	0.49	0.42	0.09
20–110	10.34	9.94	3.05
35–45	0.88	0.83	0.14
35–55	2.53	2.37	0.56
35–110	10.27	9.82	3.56
50–60	1.95	1.86	0.33
50–70	4.67	4.48	1.04
50–110	8.96	8.66	2.75
65–75	3.17	3.08	0.43
65–85	5.48	5.29	1.01
65–110	6.53	6.29	1.53

(Seidman H, et al. Surveillance, Epidemiology, and End Results [SEER]: breast cancer—current trends in diagnosis and treatment. CA Cancer J Clin 1985;34:186)

factors or because consideration of their manipulation arises during risk management. Detailed discussions of these factors appear elsewhere in the text.

The risk factor history should not neglect basic risk factors such as a woman's age.[7] Data should be sought regarding age at menarche (increased if 12 years of age or less), age at menopause (age over 55 years has a risk more than three-fold greater than age under 45 years), age at first pregnancy (age under 20 years entails less than half the risk of age over 35 years), and histories of lactation, therapeutic abortion, and infertility and its treatment.[8–10] A hormonal history is incomplete without information on exogenous hormone use, both as oral contraceptives and as replacement after menopause, and should include duration of use, because prolonged use has been associated with greater increase in breast cancer risk.

A detailed discussion of histologic lesions and breast cancer risk is provided in Chapter 3.1. Women with lobular carcinoma in situ (LCIS) or atypical hyperplasia and a family history of breast cancer in at least one first-degree relative have a marked increase in breast cancer risk (RR, 7.3 to 11).[11,12] It is not yet known whether the presence of atypical hyperplasia or LCIS in a breast biopsy specimen from a woman with a strong family history should mark her as a carrier of the familial predisposition. The magnitude of risk associated with these two lesions, even in the absence of family history, suggests that knowledge of prior breast biopsy results is critical to risk estimation and may justify histologic review by an experienced breast pathologist.

Another exposure that may cause concern is radiation. Data on low-level exposure, such as that from usual diagnostic radiography, show little effect. Risk is largely extrapolated from models;[13] however, significant elevations in breast cancer risk have been found after moderate exposures, such as those associated with chest radiographs after pneumothorax treatment of tuberculosis.[14] High-dose radiation exposure, as might be accrued during the course of mantle radiation therapy for Hodgkin disease, has been shown to confer a significantly increased risk.[15] Age at radiation exposure should also be considered, given the particular sensitivity of the prepubertal and pubertal breast to the carcinogenic effects of radiation.[16]

The Gail Model of Risk Estimation

It has been recognized for some time that methods of quantitative estimation of an individual woman's risk for developing breast cancer are essential, particularly those capable of combining multiple risk factors into a comprehensible risk expression. Quantitative risk estimates may reduce the considerable variation in management recommendations among providers.

In response to these needs, the group at the National Cancer Institute, headed by Gail and Benichou,[17] have used data from the Breast Cancer Detection Demonstration Project (BCDDP)—a large observational study of white women willing to undergo annual mammographic examinations—to construct a model that permits computation of individualized absolute risk. The authors define this risk as the chance that a woman with specific risk factors at a given age will develop breast cancer in a specified future period.[17] The model has now been assessed in two other populations—the Texas Breast Screening

Project and the Nurses' Health Study—and has been found to be generally accurate, although some overestimation of risk occurs in specific subgroups.[18,19] A modified version is used to determine eligibility for the NSABP Breast Cancer Prevention Trial. The risk factors used in the model were determined and their relative risks estimated from a case-control study nested in the BCDDP. These include age, age at menarche, age at first birth, number of breast biopsies, and family history in first-degree relatives. A multiplier term is used for atypical hyperplasia. Controversy has surrounded the omission of some factors, such as alcohol use or age at menopause. Other factors, particularly the number of breast biopsies regardless of result, have been questioned for their inclusion. This factor may be particularly confounded, given that biopsies are recommended more often for women who are considered to be at higher risk.[20] The model calculates absolute risks over 20 or 30 years, for example, first by computing a relative risk based on the woman's age and individual risk factors, and then by combining this information with an estimate of baseline hazard rate for a woman with no risk factors.[17]

The computer program RISK, in which the Gail score is calculated, can be used to estimate a woman's risk over a defined period.[17] Figure 9-1 is an illustration of the data plotted for use in the Breast Cancer Prevention Trial for a hypothetical woman who might consider participation (model modified slightly for this application).

The Gail model provides a useful tool for risk estimation, but it is a model, and the numeric estimates it provides are intended as guides. All models are imperfect and have some limiting features that should be recalled as they are applied. In this case, the Gail model was developed for women who are undergoing examination annually, a feature that may itself select for women at increased risk. The risks among women in the BCDDP have been shown to be higher than those in analyses of population databases such as SEER.[20] The model may not apply absolutely to young women not undergoing regular mammography, to women known to be at reduced risk because of unrelated factors (such as immigration from low prevalence areas such as Asia), or to women with known strong risk factors such as a hereditary predisposition or therapeutic radiation exposure. The risk numbers generated on these clean curves are not yet expressed with confidence intervals (CIs), a modification soon to be forthcoming from the authors. The reliance on a single numeric estimate for risk counseling may not be wise in any case.

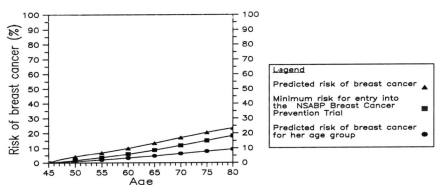

NATIONAL SURGICAL ADJUVANT BREAST PROJECT (NSABP) BREAST CANCER RISK PROFILE

Name   : JANE L. DOE   Social security number: 987654321
Address   : 1234 MAIN STREET
City   : PITTSBURGH   State/Province: PA   Zip/Postal Code: 12345
NSABP Center: NSABP Adjuvant Therapy Ctr., Pittsburgh

RISK FACTORS

Current age	: 45	Age at first live birth	: 28
Number of first degree relatives with breast cancer	: 1	Number of breast biopsies	: 2
Age at first menstruation	: 14	Atypical hyperplasia	: UNK

The following graph depicts the probability of developing breast cancer for Ms. DOE based on the risk factors listed above. Her estimated probability of developing breast cancer within the next 35 years is 23%.

Based on this risk profile, Ms. DOE is considered **eligible** for participation in the NSABP Breast Cancer Prevention Trial if all other entry criteria are met.

CONTROL # 999991

FIGURE 9-1 Data used to consider participation of a woman in the NSABP Breast Cancer Prevention Trial.

Family History

Women with family histories of breast cancer in close relatives have long been known to have an increased risk for developing the disease (see Chapter 7.2). Estimates from population-based series have consistently approached a two-fold risk increase for women with a mother or sister with the disease.[21,22] Epidemiologic studies have associated familial breast cancer with a family history of neoplasms of other sites, including cancers of the ovary, endometrium, colon, and prostate.[23] The identification of particular genes—including p53, BRCA1, and BRCA2, which are heritable in forms conferring marked breast cancer susceptibility—have permitted refined risk estimation for some families in which breast cancer occurrence is clearly excessive, presaging an era in which specific heritable risk for breast cancer can be identified for individuals.[24-26]

In risk estimation, one might consider evaluation of a family pedigree in light of the chance that it represents the action of a strong gene predisposing to cancer development. Segregation analysis is the formal application of statistical techniques to groups of pedigrees to assess the probability that a particular pattern of inheritance (eg, autosomal dominant or polygenic) might explain the pattern of disease. Several segregation analyses have concluded that rare autosomal dominant genes exist in evaluable kindreds, contributing to the development of perhaps 5% of breast cancers.[27,28] The models have suggested that these genes confer substantial risk—approximately 90% probability for developing breast cancer by age 80 years—and that they will be most likely to exert their effect in younger women.[29] The chance that a cancer susceptibility gene contributes to breast cancer development appears to be strongly influenced by age at diagnosis: 33% of those diagnosed at 20 to 29 years of age, 22% diagnosed at 30 to 39 years of age, and 13% diagnosed at 40 to 49 years of age, declining gradually to 1% by 80 years of age.[27] The implication is that a woman's risk for breast cancer is strongly related not only to the presence of a positive family history but also, and more specifically, to the number of family members affected, the genetic proximity of their relationships, and the ages at which they were diagnosed with the disease. It is useful to remember, however, that the model calculates the contribution of a gene based on age at diagnosis, not on family history: a very young woman without a family history of breast or related cancers may carry a germline mutation in a susceptibility gene that was not inherited from either parent but that occurred by chance during her own embryogenesis. Small family size with few female relatives makes patterns difficult to discern, and, less commonly, false paternity also contributes to the problems inherent in relying on family history to identify women at risk for heritable disease. Cancer history information for first-degree relatives has been shown to be accurate in over 80% of cases but is significantly less reliable for more distant relatives.[30] No data are available to assess reliability of information about age at diagnosis.

Claus Model of Risk Estimation in Families

The implications of a construct based on the described characteristics for considering a family history of breast cancer are significant. A recent publication by Claus and colleagues[3] used these considerations in the construction of a series of tables that can be used to estimate risk over a series of 10-year intervals by age for women with first-degree relatives (mothers, sisters, daughters) or second-degree relatives (grandmothers or aunts, maternal or paternal) with breast cancer. The calculations are based solely on genetic relationships: What is the chance that a woman with breast cancer has the disease because of an autosomal dominant susceptibility gene, given her age at diagnosis? What are the chances that she shares that gene with another close relative with breast cancer, based on biologic relationship and age of the second relative at diagnosis? Then, what are the chances that her at-risk relative shares this same gene, based on their biologic relationships? The calculations would predict that a woman whose mother was diagnosed with breast cancer at age 65 has perhaps half the risk of developing breast cancer at any age as does a woman whose mother was diagnosed at 35 years of age. Some examples of risk figures taken from this work appear in Table 9-2.

When applying the Claus model, it is also important to remember that *the relatives with breast cancer must be in the same lineage.* Risk for a woman whose mother and paternal grandmother had breast cancer should not be sought in the tables for first- plus second-degree affected relatives; instead, the table for one first-degree relative should be used.

Some additional caveats should be considered when applying these tables in practice. The model used to generate the risk estimates assumes that breast cancer risk is transmitted as an autosomal dominant trait. Evidence certainly shows that such genes exist (including BRCA1, BRCA2, and p53)[24-26] and that the risks they confer are strongly age specific, but they account for only perhaps 5% of breast cancers.[27,28] The model nonetheless underestimates risk if a predisposing gene originates in the paternal lineage or if a woman has no sisters. The model does not account for the possibility of modification of the effects of a strong susceptibility gene by other risk factors, such as parity or oral contraceptive use.[31] No role is considered for less powerful genetic influences on breast cancer risk, as may exist for the ataxia-telangiectasia gene or rare alleles of the *ras* oncogene.[32,33] Other markers of the effect of a strong breast cancer susceptibility gene, such as bilateral disease, are also absent from this construct.[34]

The Claus model may be best applied to families without strong features of a specific hereditary cancer syndrome. In families in which risk appears to be genetic but wherein no specific gene has been identified, risk may be calculated using the mendelian construct of a 50% risk for inheriting the same disease gene as the affected first-degree

TABLE 9-2
Absolute Risk, by Three Models, for Developing Invasive Breast Cancer by Age 60 Years for a Woman Aged 30 Years

Investigators	Risk Factor	Absolute Risk (%)
Feuer et al[7]	US woman, no risk factor information	4.3
Claus et al[3]	1 first-degree relative, diagnosed at age 65 y	3.4
	1 first-degree relative, diagnosed at age 35 y	7.5
	2 first-degree relatives, diagnosed at ages 38 and 48 y	19.4
Gail et al[4]	1 biopsy, menarche at age 12–13 y, first birth at age 25–29 y, 0 first-degree realtives	7.9
	1 biopsy, menarche before age 12 y, first birth before age 20 y, 2 first-degree relatives	32.7

relative, regardless of her age at cancer onset. Further refinement in the risk figure may be available if the age-specific risks for disease associated with gene carriers (penetrance) are known, as exist in limited form for p53 and BRCA1.[29,35] When results of direct genetic testing are available on a family member with a known hereditary predisposition, the model no longer applies to that individual, and risk figures should be taken from the gene- or mutation-specific estimates only.

Testing and Counseling for Genetic Risk

Testing for genetic susceptibility to breast cancer makes more accurate cancer risk assessment possible for a subgroup of women and their families. Because cancer-related genes do not cause cancer, but only confer susceptibility, testing of cancer-free women for these genes is called *predisposition* testing. Predisposition testing for breast cancer genes currently exists only on a limited scale but can be expected to become widely available as the genes are identified.

Information regarding an individual woman's genetic status has powerful implications for risk estimation. Women found to carry mutated versions of p53 or BRCA1 have a lifetime risk for cancer that approaches 90%, whereas their sisters who do not carry the gene presumably have the general population risk for breast cancer closer to 10%.[29,35] Given this new information on genetic status, women with strong family histories of breast cancer are able to assess their personal risk much more accurately, and they and their physicians are able to make management decisions accordingly.

Evaluation for genes that must be studied by linkage analysis, such as BRCA2, is possible only for large families with at least four affected members who are available to provide specimens and is generally done only in research laboratories. After a gene such as BRCA2 has been cloned, direct analysis of the gene in individuals is possible, albeit technically challenging. After the specific mutation has been identified in one person, analysis of blood from family members for the same alteration is much simpler. Interpretation of BRCA1 test results will be aided by data now being collected. BRCA1 is a large gene, and some alterations in its sequence have no functional significance. Some specific cancer risks may be associated with alterations in particular regions of the gene, and increased susceptibility to additional cancers may be recognized as more families are studied.

Quality-control standards for genetic testing, as exist for more routine laboratory tests, have not yet been established, so BRCA1 test results must be viewed with caution. Tests should be repeated several times, often on two independently collected specimens from a single patient. The characteristics of the tests themselves—false-positive and false-negative rates—can influence their use in clinical practice. Until better data about the accuracy of BRCA1 analysis are available it seems prudent to refer only the highest-risk individuals for testing, so that the prior probability that a BRCA1 alteration will be found is significant.

Wherever feasible, patients with breast or ovarian cancers should be tested first. At least two genes predisposing to breast cancer have already been identified, and more will probably follow. Women without cancer who have high-risk families have more informative tests if a specific alteration has been characterized in a family member who has had cancer. If the unaffected woman does not share the family BRCA1 alteration, for example, she does not have the increased family risk. If the BRCA1 status of at least one family member has not been determined, a positive test result (identification of a mutation in BRCA1) in a cancer-free woman is informative, but a negative test result becomes less informative. A negative result indicates either that the woman does not share the family risk if BRCA1 is the culprit, or that a different gene is the culprit, or that no hereditary predisposition exists; however, the correct interpretation cannot be determined. Individuals from large families with many relatives with breast or ovarian cancer should clearly be offered evaluation for BRCA1-related susceptibility. Women from small families with early-onset disease or bilateral breast cancer, or individual women diagnosed at exceptionally early ages (before 40 years of age) are also likely to carry predisposing genes and can be considered for evaluation. Families in which men have also had breast cancer may be evaluated for BRCA2 abnormalities; this is best accomplished by referral to a research center.[26,36] Ultimately, it will be possible to test all women diagnosed with breast cancer, as well as their at-risk family members, when the technology of molecular screening improves. Despite the power of genetic information, however, many women will continue to choose not to be tested.[37,38]

The impact of knowledge of an individual's genetic status can be powerful and requires that genetic testing be done with caution and counseling.[37,38] The largest experience with predisposition testing comes from Huntington disease. Unexpected adverse reactions (guilt, depression) have been seen in noncarriers and the partners of carriers of the Huntington disease gene.[39–41] The guilt felt by carriers who pass the disease genes to their children is significant; men must be educated to recognize that, despite their own low risk for breast cancer, they can pass the extraordinary susceptibility to their daughters and also through their sons to grandchildren. Prenatal testing is technically feasible but ethically complex. In addition, ethical dilemmas have arisen because hereditary information in an individual has obvious implications for family members, some of whom may not wish to know their status, even by inference. The lack of protection for genetic privacy has significant implications for testing and raises concerns about discrimination and stigmatization. Clinicians must recognize that current legislation does not prevent insurers from denying coverage for the surveillance or prevention strategies an individual would most need, or the breast cancer care an affected patient may require, based on the availability of genetic test results.[42] Recording of genetic test results in a patient's medical record may cost her continued insurance coverage.

Counseling of several families for BRCA1 linkage has been reported.[37,38,43] All programs have been characterized by prospective psychologic evaluation and extensive pretest education and counseling to help at-risk relatives make informed decisions about whether they wish to be tested; provision of test results and risk management recommendations are accompanied by additional counseling. The Human Genome Project and National Cancer Institute have allocated monies to study the best ways to offer predisposition testing and the impact of testing on various groups, factors which should provide additional guidance for the future. Predisposition testing is new, and much remains unknown. For the short term, women and their families should obtain genetic evaluation in a research program that provides adequate counseling.

Discussion of Risk

Accurate risk estimation, although challenging, is essential to providing appropriate recommendations for risk management. The discussion of risk is also not a straightforward process. A woman's recognition of her increased breast cancer risk often occurs because of a breast cancer diagnosis or death in a close family member or because of a premalignant tissue diagnosis in herself, and the emotional issues are likely to be significant. In a recent review, Lerman and Croyle[44] clearly summarized the psychologic issues that must be considered for women contemplating testing for genetic susceptibility. Many of these issues, however, also arise in less specific cancer risk counseling settings.[45] Reports have described significant adverse psychologic reactions among women in pertinent situations: after notification of abnormal mammographic results, after self-referral to a high-risk clinic, or after diagnosis of breast cancer in a first-degree relative.[45–47] These reactions include anxiety, depression, guilt, and reduced self-esteem. The overestimation of personal risk by women with a family history is well known. These reactions are not without consequences; women in such settings have been shown to have difficulty adhering to routine surveillance recommendations.[47]

Options for Management of High-Risk Patients

Three options are available to high-risk patients—close surveillance, prophylactic mastectomy, and participation in chemoprevention trials. Existing data on the efficacy of these options in reducing mortality in high-risk patients is limited. This uncertainty is of particular concern as our ability to identify high-risk patients improves, and concern about breast cancer risk is mounting among both patients and physicians.

CLOSE SURVEILLANCE

The option most often chosen by high-risk patients is close surveillance. Because screening has been found to be effective in reducing breast cancer mortality in women over 50 years of age, and perhaps in younger women as well, it is reasonable to extrapolate this concept to high-risk women.[48–50] As recent screening controversies have made clear, however, the efficacy of mammographic screening may be limited for younger women.[48] It is therefore unclear how effective mammographic screening will be in identifying early lesions in young, high-risk women.

The screening protocols in use for high-risk women are those proposed by Lynch and colleagues,[51] based on experience in caring for high-risk families. For families that appear to have a true cancer syndrome, it is recommended that screening consisting of annual mammography and twice-yearly physical examinations beginning at an age 10 years younger than that of the youngest affected relative. For women with weaker family histories, or increased risk due to nonfamilial causes, annual mammograms and twice-yearly physical examinations should begin when they are 5 years younger than the youngest affected relative, or no later than age 35.

For women found to be at increased risk for breast cancer by reasons other than family history, few data are available to guide screening regimens. For women with LCIS, mammograms can be done annually after diagnosis with twice-yearly physical examinations. For women with biopsy-proven atypical hyperplasia, annual mammography and at least annual physical examinations are recommended.

Table 9-3 summarizes the screening intervals and other management options used in patients with varying degrees of risk in our high-risk programs. It is hoped that, as greater numbers of patients are followed in high-risk programs, data collected will permit assessment of the efficacy of these follow-up regimens. It is important to recognize that part of the benefit of these regimens is the reassurance the patient feels as a result of regular visits to her physician.

No prospective trials have assessed the efficacy of these protocols in reducing breast cancer mortality in high-risk women, and it is not likely that such trials will ever be possible. As mentioned earlier, no evidence suggests that breast cancer risk is significantly increased by the additional radiation exposure resulting from earlier and more frequent mammograms in high-risk women, although this area remains of concern.

It is hoped that new imaging modalities, including magnetic resonance imaging (MRI), will help to overcome the limitations of standard mammography in high-risk women with dense breast tissue. Sensitive but more expensive breast imaging options, such as MRI, may actually prove cost-effective in women with sufficiently high breast cancer risk. MRI would also reduce any theoretical risk for increasing breast cancer risk with the radiation doses associated with frequent mammographic screening at an early age.

TABLE 9-3
Follow-Up Options for Women in Different Risk Categories

Risk Category	Lifetime Risk‡ (%)	Clinical Breast Examination Schedule§	Mammogram Schedule	Other Options
No risk factors	11–12	Annual after age 30 y	Every 1–2 y after age 40 y; annual after age 50 y	?Frequency of mammograms before age 50 y
Two or more reproductive or hormonal risk factors* and no family history	10–20	Annual after age 30 y	Annual after ager 40 y	
Weak family history†	15–20	Annual after age 30 y	Annual after age 40 y	
Strong family history†	>20	annual after age 25; twice yearly after age 30 y	Annual after age 35 y or 5 y younger than youngest affected relative	Chemoprevention trials, prophylactic mastectomy, ?genetic testing
Carrier of known breast cancer susceptibility gene *or* identifiable breast cancer syndrome *or* very strong family history†	20–85	Twice yearly after age 25 y	Annual after age 25 y	Chemoprevention trials, prophylactic mastectomy, ?genetic testing
Atypical hyperplasia with a negative family history	15–20	Annual after diagnosis	Annual after diagnosis	?Chemoprevention trials
Atypical hyperplasia with a positive family history	>20	Twice yearly	Annual after age 40 y; annual after diagnosis	Chemoprevention trials, ?prophylactic mastectomy
Lobular carcinoma in situ	20–30	Twice yearly	Annual after diagnosis	Chemoprevention trials, prophylactic mastectomy

* Reproductive and hormonal risk factors include menarche at age 11 y or earlier; menopause at age 55 y or later; nulliparity; first full-term pregnancy after age 30 y; current use of postmenopausal hormone replacement therapy.

† Weak family history is defined as two or fewer second-degree or more distant relatives with postmenopausal breast cancer. Strong family history is defined as any first-degree relative with breast cancer, three or more relatives with breast cancer, or any second-degree relative with breast cancer before 40 y. Very strong family history is defined as two or more first-degree relatives with breast or ovarian cancer, one or more first-degree relatives with breast cancer before age 40 y, or any first-degree relative with bilateral premenopausal breast cancer.

‡ Lifetime risk as calculated using the Gail, Claus, or other model of breast cancer risk. Risk figures for women with no risk factors and for those with lobular carcinoma in situ from historical data.

§ Monthly breast self-examination is recommended for women in all risk categories.

PROPHYLACTIC MASTECTOMY

The goal of prophylactic mastectomy is to reduce the chance for breast cancer development by removing the tissue at risk. It is hoped that, in addition to reducing risk, the procedure will also reduce anxiety for high-risk patients as compared with close surveillance alone. Prophylactic mastectomy has been done in response to various indications, not all of which are considered to be high-risk conditions by current standards. Patient selection has been based on individual physician's and patient's assessments of risk level, without any uniform system for risk quantitation. These facts make it difficult to determine the true efficacy of the procedure in reducing breast cancer risk. A number of reports in the literature have described breast cancer occurring on the chest wall or in the axilla after prophylactic mastectomy.[52–54] Standard prophylactic mastectomy techniques have been shown to leave a significant amount of breast tissue, which is presumed to be the source of subsequent malignancies. In a series of cadaver dissections, Goldman and Goldwyn[55] showed the presence of residual breast tissue in the subareolar and peripheral margins after subcutaneous mastectomy. Hicken[56] performed ductograms with methylene blue on a series of mastectomy specimens and showed that ducts had been divided at the margins of most mastectomy specimens, particularly in the axillary and subareolar regions, leaving breast tissue.

Results from a rat chemical carcinogenesis model raise the concern that risk reduction may not be directly proportional to the percentage of breast tissue removed.[57] In this model, female rats were exposed at puberty to the carcinogen dimethylbenzanthracene (DMBA) in doses at which all multifocal breast cancers or leukemias developed in all animals. Two weeks after exposure to DMBA, half to three quarters of breast tissue was surgically removed. Although a reduction was noted in the number of tumors appearing in the mastectomy sites, a concomitant increase was found to occur in the number of tumors arising in remaining breast tissue, so that the total number of tumors per animal was the same as that in the controls that did not undergo operation. Unfortunately, the study did not include a series of animals in which an attempt was made to remove all breast tissue, as is done in prophylactic mastectomies in humans. The applicability of this model to human breast cancer risk has also been questioned for other reasons.[58,59] Mammary carcinogenesis in rodents and humans differs in several significant ways, the doses of carcinogen required in this study were extremely high, and chemical carcinogens have not been shown to play a major role in the induction of human breast cancers.

The issue of whether prophylactic mastectomy is effective in reducing anxiety levels among high-risk patients has received less attention. Stefanek and colleagues[60] found a high level of satisfaction with the procedure among a small sample of 14 women who had undergone prophylactic mastectomy through a high-risk clinic.

It seems reasonable to reserve prophylactic mastectomy for highly motivated patients in the highest risk categories, including those patients with multiple risk factors, particularly those with very nodular and mammographically dense breasts, conditions which make early detection more difficult. It may also be useful to obtain a quantitative estimate of a woman's risk relative to the general population using mathematical models such as the Gail[4] or Claus[3] models to confirm the clinical impression that the woman has a significantly increased risk for breast cancer. Prophylactic contralateral mastectomy may also be considered for a high-risk woman who already has a breast cancer in one breast and for whom mastectomy is planned. This approach might be considered for women found to have BRCA1 alterations, whose risk of contralateral breast cancer approaches 87% by age 70 years.[61]

The optimal timing of prophylactic mastectomy in high risk women has not been studied. It is not known whether the age at which prophylactic mastectomy is done has an effect on the risk for malignancy in residual breast tissue, and the procedure's effects on quality of life have not been adequately assessed.

The patient considering prophylactic mastectomy must be made aware that some risk for developing breast cancer remains even after surgery. She must accept the change in body image that accompany bilateral mastectomy, even after reconstruction. It must also be recognized that some morbidity, and a low but measurable mortality risk are associated with a surgical procedure of this magnitude. The decision-making process must allow sufficient time for reflection and discussion, with psychologic evaluation and counseling as necessary. Patients whose central problem is actually an anxiety disorder with a focus on breast cancer risk are best treated with counseling or other therapy directed at the underlying anxiety disorder. Munchausen syndrome was diagnosed in a patient who presented with a fabricated family history of breast cancer and requested bilateral prophylactic mastectomy.[62]

The difficult and personal nature of these issues make the final decision as to the appropriateness of prophylactic mastectomy best made by the woman and her family, in conjunction with a sympathetic medical team. Women may also find it useful to discuss their feelings with other high-risk women, including both those who have chosen mastectomy and those who have chosen close surveillance. Patients are influenced in their decision making by their own personal experiences with breast cancer, by their observations of the disease course and outcome in family members, and by their degree of confidence that surveillance will achieve early detection. Stefanek and colleagues[60] reported that women choosing prophylactic mastectomy have higher anxiety levels and perform breast self-examination more frequently than do other high-risk women.

The subjective and emotional nature of these issues also makes it unlikely that a randomized trial will ever assess the efficacy of prophylactic mastectomy compared with that of close surveillance or chemoprevention. It would be reasonable, however, to establish a prospective registry to address the efficacy of prophylactic mastectomy in reducing the incidence of breast cancer in high-risk women.

With the availability of models for risk quantitation, it may be possible to compare the results of prophylactic mastectomy in reducing incidence and mortality with the efficacy of close surveillance in reducing breast cancer mortality in populations with similar risk levels.

If the patient and her physicians elect to proceed with prophylactic mastectomy, total mastectomy (which includes the nipple and areola) should be done. Flaps should be thin, and every effort should be made to remove all breast tissue, particularly in the periphery of the breast and in the axillary tail. Subcutaneous mastectomies are an inadequate procedure for prophylaxis and often leave an insensate nipple. Skin-sparing mastectomies, taking the nipple and areola, followed by immediate reconstruction are appropriate and can provide an excellent cosmetic result. Reconstruction may be achieved using bilateral subpectoral saline implants, bilateral TRAM flaps or bilateral latissimus dorsi flaps.

CHEMOPREVENTION

The possibility of preventing malignancy, rather than the hope of finding and treating a malignancy after it has developed, is one of the most exciting prospects in cancer management. Breast cancer chemoprevention trials using tamoxifen, retinoids, and other agents are already under way, and their results are eagerly awaited. Chemoprevention is discussed in detail in Chapter 10. It is important to recognize, however, that chemoprevention for high-risk women remains only a theoretic possibility, with risk/benefit ratios that remain unknown. It is therefore not appropriate to place high-risk patients on tamoxifen or other agents outside of a prospective, randomized clinical trial.

ORAL CONTRACEPTIVES IN HIGH-RISK WOMEN

Data from the general population suggest that no significantly increased risk for breast cancer exists among women who have used oral contraceptives.[63,64] Analysis of high-risk women as a separate cohort has not yet been done. In view of a potential increase in breast cancer risk seen with prolonged oral contraceptive use (particularly before the first full-term pregnancy),[63] however, it has been suggested that it would be prudent to avoid early and prolonged oral contraceptive use in young nulliparous women, including for noncontraceptive purposes as dysmenorrhea, menorrhagia, or breast pain.[65]

Oral contraceptives have been shown to reduce the risk for ovarian cancer even with only short durations of use.[66] The potential effect of this observation on women from families with clustering of both breast and ovarian cancer has not yet been determined.

In the absence of more specific data, it seems reasonable to use nonhormonal methods as the first-line contraceptive agents in high-risk women but to allow the use of oral contraceptives after a first term pregnancy or for short periods before the first full-term pregnancy if alternative methods are unsuitable.

POSTMENOPAUSAL HORMONE REPLACEMENT THERAPY IN HIGH-RISK WOMEN

Hormone replacement therapy provides many benefits to postmenopausal women. Estrogens relieve many of the troubling symptoms of menopause and appear to have a favorable effect on the cardiovascular system and on bone density. Hormone replacement therapy carries with it an increased risk for certain other problems, however, including thromboembolic disease, endometrial carcinoma, and, potentially, breast carcinoma. The balance between risks and benefits for women as a group, and for individual patients, has been the source of much recent discussion.[67]

A review of overall mortality among users and nonusers of postmenopausal hormone replacement showed a statistically significant decrease in mortality from all causes (RR, 0.8; $P < .0001$) among users compared with nonusers of hormone replacement therapy. This benefit seemed to be derived mainly from a reduction in mortality due to acute myocardial infarction (RR, 0.6, $P < .001$), but a trend toward decreased mortality from ischemic heart disease, stroke, and cancer of any type was also noted.[68]

When breast cancer risk is analyzed separately from other causes of morbidity and mortality, a trend toward increased risk for breast cancer is seen among women using hormone replacement therapy. Disagreement has been found among studies regarding the degree and magnitude of breast cancer risk associated with hormone replacement therapy and regarding the identification of individual subgroups of women at higher risk.

A recent metaanalysis of breast cancer risk and hormone replacement therapy found an approximate 10% overall increase in breast cancer risk among women using hormone replacement therapy compared with nonusers.[69] This value was of questionable statistical significance. Another metaanalysis done differently, using only studies that met certain criteria as to study design, found an RR of 1.3 for breast cancer among women using hormone replacement therapy for more than 15 years compared with nonusers.[70] A Swedish cohort study also found that risk increased with duration of use, finding an increased risk for breast cancer among users of hormone replacement therapy after 9 years of use.[71] The Nurses' Health Study also found an increase in breast cancer risk among current users of postmenopausal estrogen replacement therapy, particularly after prolonged use.[72] No increased risk for breast cancer was seen, however, among previous users of hormone replacement therapy. This finding suggested that the effect of estrogen on breast cancer risk may be reversible, since risks appeared to return to baseline nonuser levels within 2 to 3 years of cessation of hormone replacement therapy.

A metaanalysis of breast cancer risk with postmenopausal estrogen use, combined with other potential breast cancer risk factors, identified certain subsets of patients with significantly increased risk. In addition to a significantly increased risk among women with family histories of breast cancer (RR, 3.4), an increased risk was also identified among users of hormone replacement therapy who were nulliparous (RR, 1.5), among those with benign breast disease (RR, 1.7), and among those whose first pregnancy occurred after age 30 (RR, 1.7).[70]

In summary, a significant reduction in the mortality rate from all causes appears to be associated with the use of postmenopausal hormone replacement therapy, primarily through a reduction in deaths from cardiovascular disease. Reasonable evidence also seems to suggest a modest increase in the risk for breast cancer is associated with postmenopausal hormone replacement therapy, amounting to an approximately 10% increase in risk for the average woman. The increase in risk may be substantially higher for women with family histories of breast carcinoma or those with other breast cancer risk factors. In clinical practice, it seems prudent to weigh the individual woman's cardiovascular and perhaps osteoporotic risks against her preexisting risks for breast carcinoma before making a decision about the use of postmenopausal estrogens. For postmenopausal women with multiple risk factors for breast carcinoma, or for those who are reluctant to increase their breast cancer risk in any way, it may be most appropriate to address cardiovascular and osteoporotic risks through exercise, diet, and other nonhormonal means, rather than through hormone replacement therapy.

Development of a Program for Risk Assessment and Counseling

As the public has become more aware of and informed about breast cancer risk, increasing demand has focused on risk assessment and follow-up programs for high-risk patients. Several components should be included in any program for high-risk patients. The program should first include careful physical examination and mammography appropriate to the woman's age and risk level. Breast self-examination should be reviewed with the patient. An educational component should provide information about risk factors and should emphasize that most women who develop breast cancer do not, in fact, die of it. Patients should be reminded that familial breast cancer does not appear to have a poorer prognosis than does sporadic breast cancer. Many patients find it useful to receive a numerical estimate of their level of risk using the Gail[4] or Claus[3] models; however, optimal approaches to communication of risks to patients remain under study.

A follow-up component is also essential, with the options of careful surveillance, prophylactic mastectomy, and participation in chemoprevention trials discussed in detail. Because most patients will choose careful surveillance, recommendations for an appropriate screening schedule should be provided. Written recommendations should be provided to the patient and to her referring physicians. Patients should be provided access to formal counseling with a psychologist or therapist, as appropriate.

Summary

As our understanding of the etiology of breast cancer has improved, so has our ability to identify women at increased risk for developing breast cancer. Genetic syndromes associated with mutations in specific genes including BRCA1 and p53 have been identified, and testing for mutations or linkage to mutations is technically possible, although expensive and not yet widely available. Other genetic, histologic, reproductive, hormonal, and environmental factors associated with an increased risk for breast cancer have been identified. Determining the magnitude of risk for the individual woman remains complex, however, with uncertainty as to the ways various risk factors interact with or modify one another. Management options for women deemed to be at increased risk for breast cancer include careful surveillance, prophylactic mastectomy, and participation in chemoprevention trials. Selection among these options is largely based on the physician's best estimate of the woman's degree of risk, and the woman's own subjective interpretation of the threat posed by this risk. It is hoped that risk assessment in the future will be more precise both in identifying individuals at risk and in predicting the true magnitude of the individual's risk. It is hoped that new breast imaging modalities will facilitate early detection in high risk women and that genetic analysis will distinguish high-risk women from those with strong family histories but no additional risk factors. We are optimistic that chemoprevention strategies under investigation will prove effective in decreasing breast cancer risk.

References

1. Morrow M. Identification and management of the women at increased risk for breast cancer development. Breast Cancer Res Treat 1994;31:53.
2. Ottman R, Pike MC, King MC. Practical guide for estimating risk for familial breast cancer. Lancet 1983;2:556.
3. Claus EB, Risch N, Thompson WD. Autosomal dominant inheritance of early-onset breast cancer. Cancer 1994;73:643.
4. Gail MH, Brinton LA, Byar DP, et al. Projecting individualized probabilities of developing breast cancer for white females who are being examined annually. J Natl Cancer Inst 1989;81:1879.
5. Offit K, Brown K. Quantitating familial cancer risk: a resource for clinical oncologists. J Clin Oncol 1994;12:1724.
6. Seidman H, Mushinski M, Gelb S, et al. Probabilities of eventually developing or dying of cancer. United States, 1985. CA Cancer J Clin 1985;35:37.
7. Feuer EJ, Wun LM, Boring CC, et al. The lifetime risk of developing breast cancer. J Natl Cancer Inst 1993;85:892.
8. Henderson BE. Endogenous and exogenous endocrine factors. Hematol Oncol Clin North Am 1989;3:577.
9. Kelsey JL, Gammon MD, John EM. Reproductive and hormonal risk factors: reproductive factors and breast cancer. Epidemiol Rev 1993;15:36.

10. Bruzzi P, Negri E, LaVecchia C. Short-term increase in risk of breast cancer after full-term pregnancy. BMJ 1988;297:1096.

11. Dupont W, Page D. Risk factors for breast cancer in women with proliferative breast disease. N Engl J Med 1985;312:146.

12. London SJ, Connolly JL, Schnitt SJ, et al. A prospective study of benign disease and the risk of breast cancer. JAMA 1992;267:941.

13. Evans JS, Wenneberg JE, McNeil BJ. The influence of diagnostic radiography on the incidence of breast cancer and leukemia. N Engl J Med 1986;315:810.

14. Miller AB, Howe GR, Sherman GJ, et al. Mortality from breast cancer after irradiation during fluoroscopic examinations in patients being treated for tuberculosis. N Engl J Med 1989;321:1285.

15. Abrahamsen JF, Andersen A, Hannisdal E, et al. Second malignancies after treatment of Hodgkin's disease: the influence of treatment, follow-up time, and age. J Clin Oncol 1993;11:255.

16. Beir V. Committee on the biological effects of ionizing radiations: health effects of exposure to low levels of ionizing radiation. National Academy Press, 1990:253.

17. Gail MH, Benichou J. Epidemiology and biostatistics of the National Cancer Institute. J Natl Cancer Inst 1994;86:573.

18. Bondy M, Lustbader E, Halabi S, et al. Validation of a breast cancer risk assessment model in women with a positive family history. J Natl Cancer Inst 1994;86:620.

19. Speigelman D, Colditz GA, Hunter D, et al. Validation of the Gail et al model for predicting individual breast cancer risk. J Natl Cancer Inst 1994;86:600.

20. Pickle LW, Johnson KA. Estimating the long-term probability of developing breast cancer. J Natl Cancer Inst 1989;81:1854.

21. Colditz G, Willett WC, Hunter DJ, et al. Family history, age, and risk of breast cancer. JAMA 1993;270:338.

22. Bain C, Speizer FE, Rosner B, et al. Family history of breast cancer as a risk indicator for the disease. Am J Epidemiol 1980;111:301.

23. Andrieu N, Clavel F, Auquier A, et al. Association between breast cancer and family malignancies. Eur J Cancer 1991;27:244.

24. Malkin D, Li FP, Strong LC, et al. Germ line p53 mutations in a familial syndrome of breast cancer, sarcomas, and other neoplasms. Science 1990;250:1233.

25. Miki Y, Swensen J, Shattuck-Eidens D, et al. A strong candidate for the breast and ovarian cancer susceptibility gene BRCA1. Science 1994;266:66.

26. Wooster R, Neuhausen S, Mangion J, et al. Localization of a breast cancer susceptibility gene, BRCA2, to chromosome 13q12-13. Science 1994;265:2088.

27. Claus EB, Risch N, Thompson WD. Genetic analysis of breast cancer in the Cancer and Steroid Hormone Study. Am J Hum Genet 1991;48:232.

28. Newman B, Austin M, Lee M, et al. Inheritance of human breast cancer: evidence for autosomal dominant transmission in high-risk families. Proc Natl Acad Sci USA 1988;85:3044.

29. Easton D, Bishop D, Ford D, et al. Genetic linkage analysis in familial breast and ovarian cancer: results from 214 families. Am J Hum Genet 1993;52:678.

30. Love R, Evans A, Josten D. The accuracy of patient reports of a family history of cancer. J Chron Dis 1985;38:289.

31. Goldgar D, Fields P, Lewis C, et al. A large kindred with 17q-linked breast and ovarian cancer: genetic, phenotypic, geneological analysis. J Natl Can Inst 1994;86:200.

32. Swift M, Morrell D, Massey RB, et al. Incidence of cancer in 161 families affected by ataxia–telangiectasia. N Engl J Med 1991;325:1831.

33. Krontiris TG, Devlin B, Karp DD, et al. An association between the risk of cancer and mutations in the hras1 minisatellite locus. N Engl J Med 1993;329:517.

34. Anderson DE. Genetic study of breast cancer: identification of a high-risk group. Cancer 1974;34:1090.

35. Strong LC, Williams WR, Tainsky MA. The Li-Fraumeni syndrome: from clinical epidemiology to molecular genetics. Am J Epidemiol 1992;135:190.

36. Stratton M, Ford D, Neuhausen S, et al. Familial male breast cancer is not linked to the BRCA1 locus on chromosome 17q. Nat Genet 1994;7:103.

37. Biesecker B, Boehnke M, Calzone K, et al. Genetic counseling for families with inherited susceptibility to breast and ovarian cancer (published erratum appears in JAMA 1993;270:832.) JAMA 1993;269:1970.

38. Lynch HT, Watson P, Conway T, et al. DNA screening for breast/ovarian cancer susceptibility based on linked markers: a family study. Arch Intern Med 1993;153:1979.

39. Bloch M, Adam S, Wiggins S, et al. Predictive testing for Huntington disease in Canada: the experience of those receiving an increased risk. Am J Med Genet 1992;42:499.

40. Huggins M, Bloch M, Wiggins S, et al. Predictive testing for Huntington disease in Canada: adverse effects and unexpected results in those receiving a decreased risk. Am J Med Genet 1992;42:508.

41. Benjamin CM, Adam S, Wiggins S, et al. Proceed with care: direct predictive testing for Huntington disease. Am J Hum Genet 1994;55:606.

42. Ostrer H, Allen W, Crandall LA, et al. Insurance and genetic testing: where are we now? Am J Hum Genet 1993;52:565.

43. de Wit ACD, Meijers-Heijboer EJ, Tibben A, et al. Effect on a Dutch family of predictive DNA-testing for hereditary breast and ovarian cancer. Lancet 1994;344:197.

44. Lerman C, Croyle R. Psychological issues in genetic testing for breast cancer susceptibility. Arch Intern Med 1994;154:609.

45. Kash K, Holland J, Halper M, et al. Psychological distress and surveillance behaviors of women with a family history of breast cancer. J Natl Cancer Inst 1992;84:24.

46. Lerman C, Rimer B, Engstrom P. Cancer risk notification: psychosocial and ethical implications. J Clin Oncol 1991;9:1275.

47. Lerman C, Daly M, Sands C, et al. Mammography adherence and psychological distress among women at risk for breast cancer. J Natl Cancer Inst 1993;85:1074.

48. Fletcher SW, Black W, Harris R, et al. Report of the International Workshop on Screening for Breast Cancer. J Natl Cancer Inst 1993;85:1644.

49. Tabar L, Duffy SW, Warren BL. New Swedish breast cancer-detection results for women aged 40–49. Cancer 1993;72:(Suppl):1437.

50. Shapiro S. Periodic screening for breast cancer: the Health Insurance Plan Project and its sequelae, 1963–1986. Baltimore, Johns Hopkins University, 1988.

51. Lynch HT, Marcus JN, Watson P. Familial breast cancer, family cancer syndromes, and predisposition to breast neoplasia. In: Bland KI, Copeland EM III, eds. The breast: comprehensive management of benign and malignant diseases. Philadelphia, WB Saunders, 1991:262.

52. Holleb AI, Montgomery R, Farrow JH. The hazard of incomplete simple mastectomy. Surg Gynecol Obstet 1965;121:819.

53. Eldar S, Meguid MM, Beatty JD. Cancer of the breast after prophylactic subcutaneous mastectomy. Am J Surg 1984;148:692.

54. Zeigler LD, Kroll SS. Primary breast cancer after prophylactic mastectomy. Am J Clin Oncol 1991;14:451.

55. Goldman LD, Goldwyn RM. Some anatomical considerations of subcutaneous mastectomy. Plast Reconstr Surg 1973;51:501.

56. Hicken NF. Mastectomy: a clinical pathologic study demonstrating why most mastectomies result in incomplete removal of the mammary gland. Arch Surg 1940;40:6.

57. Jackson CF, Palmquist M, Swanson J, et al. The effectiveness of

prophylactic subcutaneous mastectomy in Sprague-Dawley rats induced with 7,12-dimethylbenzanthracene. Plast Reconstr Surg 1984;73:249.

58. Eggleston JC. The effectiveness of prophylactic subcutaneous mastectomy in Sprague-Dawley rats induced with 7,12-dimethylbenzanthracene. Plast Reconstr Surg 1984;73:256.

59. Giuliano AE. The effectiveness of prophylactic subcutaneous mastectomy in Sprague-Dawley rats induced with 7,12-dimethylbenzanthracene. Plast Reconstr Surg 1984;73:258.

60. Stefanek ME, Helzlsouer KJ, Wilcox PM, et al. Satisfaction with and predictors of bilateral prophylactic mastectomy. J Natl Cancer Inst (In press).

61. Ford D, Easton DF, Bishop DT, et al. Risks of cancer in BRCA1-mutation carriers. Lancet 1994;343:692.

62. Grenga TE, Dowden RV. Munchausen syndrome and prophylactic mastectomy. Plast Reconstr Surg 1987;119:119.

63. Romieu I, Berlin JA, Colditz GA. Oral contraceptives and breast cancer: review and meta-analysis. Cancer 1990;66:2253.

64. Wingo PA, Lee NC, Ory H, et al. Age specific differences in the relationship between oral contraceptive use and breast cancer. Obstet Gynecol 1991;78:161.

65. Henderson IC. Risk factors for breast cancer development. Cancer 1993;71(Suppl):2127.

66. Whittemore AS, Harris R, Intyre J, the Collaborative Ovarian Cancer Group. Characteristics relating to ovarian cancer risk. 2. Invasive epithelial cancers in white women. Am J Epidemiol 1992;136:1184.

67. Wood WC, Budman DR, Korzun AH, et al. Dose and dose intensity of adjuvant chemotherapy for stage II, node-positive breast carcinoma. N Engl J Med 1994;330:1253.

68. Henderson BE, Paganini-Hill A, Ross RK. Decreased mortality in users of estrogen replacement therapy. Arch Intern Med 1991;151:75.

69. Dupont WD, Page DL. Menopausal estrogen-replacement therapy. Arch Intern Med 1991;151:67.

70. Steinberg KK, Thacker SB, Smith SJ, et al. A meta-analysis of the effect of estrogen replacement therapy. JAMA 1991;265:1985.

71. Bergvist L, Adami HO, Persson I, et al. The risk of breast cancer after estrogen and estrogen−progestin replacement. N Engl J Med 1989;321:293.

72. Colditz GA, Stampfer MJ, Willett WC. Prospective study of estrogen replacement therapy and risk of breast cancer in post-menopausal women. JAMA 1990;264:2641.

Diseases of the Breast, edited by Jay R. Harris,
Marc E. Lippman, Monica Morrow, and Samuel Hellman.
Lippincott-Raven Publishers, Philadelphia, © 1996.

10

Prevention of Breast Cancer

10.1

Biologic Considerations in Breast Cancer Prevention

V. CRAIG JORDAN

Strategies to prevent breast cancer are focused either on dietary changes, based on epidemiologic studies, or on endocrine changes, again based on epidemiologic studies but with a strong biologic rationale from laboratory studies. The use of retinoids to prevent breast cancer draws on expertise from both the endocrinology of receptors and concepts in nutrition. The dietary approach advocates trials with reduced fat intake designed to mimic the diets of countries with low breast cancer incidence. Opponents of this approach argue that only a lifetime dietary change can decrease the risk of breast cancer. If this is true, major dietary changes now may not alter breast cancer incidence for another generation.

In contrast, endocrine dependency is a unique feature of breast cancer that can be manipulated to control growth[1] or prevent tumor development.[2,3] Unfortunately, our inability to predict precisely who will develop breast cancer has required broad, population-based strategies to prevent the disease. A successful strategy must be effective and acceptable to the majority of treated women who will not develop breast cancer. The goal has proved to be both difficult and controversial.

This chapter provides a synthesis of laboratory and clinical considerations to explain the biologic rationale for current hormonal approaches to prevent breast cancer. A fundamental issue in developing a strategy for breast cancer prevention is when carcinogenesis occurs. In laboratory models of mammary cancer, the timing of the carcinogenic insult is critical, and tumor development is influenced by the hormonal milieu. A series of experiments performed over 20 years in different strains of rat with different car-

cinogens[4-6] show that mammary cancer can only be induced by carcinogen administration during the first few months of puberty (Figure 10.1-1). Unfortunately, we are unaware of the nature and timing of the carcinogenic insult in women. Progress in the elucidation and cloning of the BRCA1 gene[7] may result in the identification of women who harbor germline breast cancer susceptibility. However these women, who have early-onset disease, are a minority (less than 10%) of all breast cancer cases. Most of our knowledge about carcinogenesis in the breast is based on small epidemiologic studies of known cancer-causing agents.

Data from irradiated women suggest a long period of promotion following initiation at a young age. In survivors of the atomic bombings, the greatest increase in breast cancer incidence was seen in women exposed during their early teens. However, breast cancer development in these women did not occur at an early age.[8] Additional support for a long period of hormonal promotion after an early carcinogenic insult is found in female infants undergoing thymic irradiation[9] and in adolescent girls irradiated during fluoroscopy for tuberculosis.[10] In both groups, a significant increase in breast cancer incidence is observed.

A Strategy to Prevent Mammary Cancer in the Laboratory

Animal models of mammary carcinogenesis have been studied extensively. High-incidence strains of mice that are infected with the mouse mammary tumor virus sponta-

FIGURE 10.1-1 The incidence of mammary cancer in groups of female rats given oral 3-methycholanthrene (66 mg/100 g; *squares*)[4]; intravenous 7,12-dimethylbenzanthracene (3 mg/100 g; *circles*)[5]; or intravenous nitroso-N-methylurea (5 mg/100 g; *triangles*)[6] at different days of age. Tumor incidence was evaluated at least 180 days after each administration of carcinogen.

neously develop tumors. The mice are particularly sensitive to tumorigenesis, through the activation of the integrated virus by progesterone. Thus, pregnancy enhances mammary carcinogenesis in this model. Early oophorectomy retards the development of mammary cancer.[11] This observation led Lacassagne in 1936 to suggest that because breast cancer appears to be due to a special heredity sensitivity to estrogen, perhaps a therapeutic inhibitor of estrogen accumulation can be found to prevent breast cancer.[12] Unfortunately, no therapeutic inhibitor was available at that time, and all of his suggestions were based on the use of oophorectomy. In modern times, tamoxifen has been studied in mouse models of carcinogenesis to provide a basis for clinical testing of the concept of prevention. Early, long-term tamoxifen therapy inhibits mouse mammary tumorigenesis,[13,14] and the therapy is superior to early oophorectomy. However, this is only one piece of laboratory evidence that can be used as a rationale to support the use of tamoxifen as a preventive measure in clinical trials.

The administration of chemical carcinogens to sensitive strains of young female rats causes mammary tumorigenesis. Unlike in mice, pregnancy or the administration of a suitable combination of progesterone and estrogen can prevent rat mammary carcinogenesis if this occurs at the time of the carcinogenic insult or soon after.[15-17] However, later pregnancy or progesterone administration can reduce the latency of rat mammary carcinogenesis and increase the growth rate of some tumors.[18,19] As in mice, oophorectomy can interfere with the process of chemical carcinogenesis in rats (Figure 10.1-2). The earlier it is

performed after the carcinogenic insult, the more effective is oophorectomy. Similarly, the administration of antiestrogens, for different times around the time of carcinogen administration, can alter carcinogenesis.[21,22] The coadministration of carcinogens and antiestrogens to female rats prevents mammary carcinogenesis.[21] Short-term (4-week) administration of tamoxifen a month after carcinogen administration only delays carcinogenesis, but it does reduce the number of mammary tumors produced.[23] In contrast, long-term treatment with low doses of tamoxifen after the carcinogenic insult can almost completely prevent the development of mammary tumors.[24] Paradoxically, progesterone can reverse the antitumor action of tamoxifen.[25]

Overall, the animal model systems demonstrate that intervention soon after initiation is the most effective form of breast cancer prevention. In addition, changes in the hormonal milieu can affect the process of carcinogenesis either by altering the receptivity of the epithelial tissue to carcinogens or by preventing the process of promotion to produce an invasive carcinoma.

Target Problems

Potential agents for breast cancer prevention must have a strong scientific basis and minimal toxicity. Ideally, a true preventive agent would block the carcinogenic insult in readily identifiable individuals and would have minimal side effects. However, this goal is not possible at present, and broad approaches are being suggested.

Figure 10.1-3 illustrates a sequence of events that can be exploited in a prevention strategy. In general, an intervention must be given over a prolonged period to protect the individual from repeated carcinogenic insults. The agent could either prevent metabolic activation of the carcinogen or change the hormonal balance necessary for the epithelium to be receptive to the carcinogen. Estrogen is key to consolidating the carcinogenic insult through promotion of the transformed cell. At this stage, the dividing cell population is directly or indirectly sensitive to estrogen stimulation through the estrogen receptor. However, as tumorigenesis progresses, the genetic instability of the transformed cells results in a mixed population of receptor-positive and receptor-negative breast cancer cells. To exploit this knowledge, a number of endocrine strategies have been proposed or are in clinical trial (Fig. 10.1-4). The use of a contraceptive that could protect young women from pregnancy and breast cancer would be the most effective strategy because, based on all our existing knowledge, it would be applied at the correct time during the process of tumorigenesis.

Pseudopregnancy

The observation that the repeated feeding of carcinogens to rats at the onset of pregnancy[15] or to other animals injected with large quantities of equine gonadotropins[26]

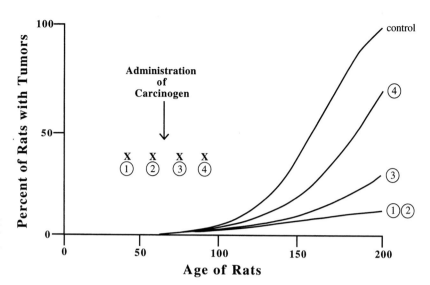

FIGURE 10.1-2 The effect of ovariectomy (X) at different times on the appearance of rat mammary cancer. 7,12-Dimethylbenzanthracene, 20 mg orally in 2 mL of peanut oil, was administered to groups of female Sprague Dawley rats at 55 days of age.

seldom results in mammary tumors provided the basis for the rigorous investigations of Russo and colleagues.[27] The administration of human chorionic gonadotropin can prevent both the initiation and progression of rat mammary carcinogenesis.[28] Russo and associates[27] hypothesize that human chorionic gonadotropin initiates ovarian estrogen and progesterone synthesis to induce differentiation of the mammary epithelium.[30] Unfortunately, the dosing schedules used reduced rat mammary tumorigenesis only by 50%,[30] and an optional treatment is needed. Although early pregnancy is known to reduce the risk of breast cancer, the development of a prevention strategy that administers gonadotropin to teenage girls has major societal implications.

Contraception

It is well established that women who use oral contraceptives, a combination of progestin and estrogen, have a reduced incidence of both endometrial and ovarian can-

cer.[31] In contrast, women who take oral contraceptives have either the same or a slightly higher relative risk for breast cancer compared with those who have never used birth control pills.[31] This may not be too surprising, since the breast responds to the administered estrogen. What is surprising is the fact that orally active progestins, which cause differentiation of the proliferating endometrium, do not protect the breast. The explanation for this observation is obscure, but the report that progestins have a proliferative effect on normal human breast tissue,[32] as well as the laboratory finding that many progestins used in oral contraceptives cause proliferation of breast cancer cells through an estrogen receptor–mediated mechanism,[33] suggests that these compounds have site-specific activity and may in fact promote breast cancer.

Recent studies suggest that gestodene, a new synthetic progestin, may have specific antiproliferative effects in breast cancer cells and stromal tissue while providing effective contraception.[34,35] The advantage of this strategy is that the early application of a hormonal agent might have

FIGURE 10.1-3 Diagram illustrating the potential process of carcinogenesis in the breast. The carcinogenic insult causes geronic alterations in the receptive epithelial cells, and then the insult is consolidated through promotion with estrogen. The estrogen receptor–positive cells then drift to become hormone independent and estrogen receptor–negative.

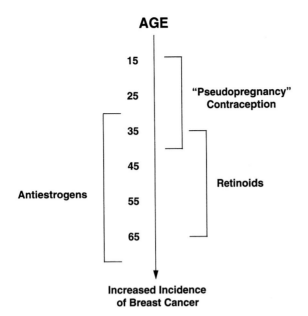

FIGURE 10.1-4 Potential windows of opportunity to apply prevention strategies.

an inhibitory effect on carcinogenesis. Unfortunately, the recent contradictory observation that gestodene causes an increase in breast cancer cell replication in the laboratory[36] must be carefully evaluated before gestodene or an analogue is proposed as an agent to prevent breast cancer. Nevertheless, a novel steroid could be devised to prevent breast cancer cell replication while also preventing ovulation.

An alternate contraceptive strategy has been proposed by Pike and coworkers.[37] Because early oophorectomy reduces breast cancer incidence, this strategy attempts to perform a "medical oophorectomy" by using a luteinizing hormone–releasing hormone superagonist (leuprolide, 7.5 mg every 28 days). To avoid the negative effects of premature menopause on cardiovascular risk and bone density, conjugated estrogens (0.625 mg orally) are administered for 6 days every week and medroxyprogesterone acetate (10 mg orally) is given for 13 days every fourth 28-day cycle.[38,39] This approach has the potential to reduce ovarian, endometrial, and breast cancer while maintaining bone density and a low cardiovascular risk.[40] It meets all the criteria for an effective preventive strategy. However, the precise dose of estrogen that will support physiologic functions without supporting the developing breast tumor is unknown.

Synthetic Retinoids

The rationale for using a retinoid to prevent cancer can be traced to early observations of increased epithelial cell replication in vitamin A–deficient animals.[41] Vitamin A and retinoids are known to cause suppression of DNA synthesis and to induce cellular differentiation. Although the precise mechanisms are not known, retinoids can increase the production of inhibitory growth factors of the transforming growth factor β family.[42] In the laboratory, retinyl acetate (vitamin A acetate) inhibits rat mammary carcinogenesis,[43] but its ability to cause severe liver damage[44,45] precludes its use as a preventive agent. The most promising analogue for prevention studies is N-(4-hydroxyphenyl retinimide (4HPR). Moon and coworkers[46] demonstrated that 4HPR is more potent and less toxic than retinyl acetate in preventing rat mammary carcinogenesis. As a first step in the evaluation of 4HPR as a preventive agent in humans, a clinical trial is being conducted in women with node-negative breast cancer (aged 35 to 65) to determine whether a decrease in second primary breast cancer is seen.[47]

Recent studies demonstrate that the retinoids can have direct effects on cell proliferation by interfering with estrogen responsiveness.[48,49] It can therefore be argued that preventive strategy will be valuable only in estrogen receptor–positive disease or during the early stages of promotion with estrogen. Again, early treatment might prove to be superior to later intervention. Nevertheless, retinoids may not be less toxic or as efficacious as antiestrogen therapy.

Antiestrogens

The successful use of adjuvant tamoxifen therapy for all stages of breast cancer[50] and the reported low incidence of side effects[51] prompted the evaluation of tamoxifen as a preventive agent in women. The biologic rationale to test tamoxifen is based on laboratory studies[21–23] and the clinical observation that tamoxifen prevents second primary breast cancers. In postmenopausal women, the drug maintains bone density and reduces fatal myocardial infarction, possibly by lowering circulating low-density lipoprotein cholesterol. The cases for and against testing tamoxifen as a preventive agent have already been presented.[52–56]

The carcinogenic potential of tamoxifen is a focus of a current debate for prevention trials. The increased risk (relative risk, 3) of endometrial carcinoma in tamoxifen-treated postmenopausal women is a major concern.[57] In athymic animals implanted with human breast and endometrial cancer, tamoxifen preferentially stimulates growth of the endometrial tumor,[58] and there is no reason to believe that tamoxifen prevents endometrial cancer growth in women. More than a hundred cases of endometrial cancer are recorded in the literature[59]; therefore, prevention trials become an evaluation of the net benefit to a cohort of women at risk for competing diseases. However, the detection and treatment of early-stage endometrial cancer, which has a lower incidence than breast cancer, is considered to be a less serious problem.

Tamoxifen induces liver tumors in rats,[60–62] and there is concern that tamoxifen has the potential to induce hepatocellular carcinoma in women. Current research is focused on the biologic differences between the metabolic route in rats and that in humans[63,64] to explain the formation of adducts to rat liver DNA[65,66] and mutations in p53.[67] The level of adduct formation in mouse systems is low,[66] and liver tumors are not produced in this species. That no increases in hepatocellular carcinoma have been noted in the clinical literature is encouraging and may support the hypothesis that rats are particularly sensitive to liver tumorigenesis because of inbred metabolic differences.

Three large clinical trials have been designed to test the worth of tamoxifen as a preventive agent in high-risk women.[50] Each is complementary and is designed to exploit various aspects of the biologic rationale. A vanguard study organized at the Royal Marsden Hospital to randomly assign 2000 healthy women at risk for breast cancer to placebo or tamoxifen treatment is now complete.[68] Most of the women are premenopausal (as young as 30 years old), because the plan is to apply the intervention early in the genesis of the disease. As a result, the concerns about the development of endometrial cancer are low, and incidence is estimated to be only three cases in the tamoxifen arm and two in the control arm by the year 2002.[69] A national trial has started in the United Kingdom to recruit up to 16,000 women.

In Italy, a prevention trial with tamoxifen is underway with women over the age of 45 years who have had hysterectomies. The recruitment goal is 20,000 women randomly assigned to receive a placebo or 5 years of tamoxifen, 20 mg/d. Concerns about the increase in endometrial cancer caused by tamoxifen were responsible for the prerequisite of hysterectomy.

In the United States, 16,000 high-risk premenopausal and postmenopausal women are being randomly assigned to receive tamoxifen, 20 mg/d, or placebo for 5 years. About one third of the women are high-risk, premenopausal women, so this trial will be able to evaluate the potential advantages for all age groups.

Future Considerations

The key to a successful prevention strategy appears to be early intervention to change the process of carcinogenesis for most women. The development of a new contraceptive would theoretically be the correct approach if it were used by the whole population. Based on present knowledge, a delay in applying an endocrine intervention will result in the protection of only a proportion of women at risk. The intervention will be too late for some women because occult disease will be hormone independent. The results from the three clinical trials of antiestrogens used at different times during carcinogenesis will serve to illustrate these concepts. The results will answer at least two important questions:

1. Can early tamoxifen treatment prevent premenopausal breast cancer and maintain the advantage for the rest of a woman's life?

2. Does postmenopausal tamoxifen treatment alter the course of the carcinogenic process in a proportion of women (estimated at 50%) or only delay the appearance of these tumors?

Clearly, if the answer to the first question is yes, the benefits of tamoxifen will be clearly demonstrated. However, if a proportion of postmenopausal women have an initial positive result that is ultimately found to be a delay rather than a cure, the period of gain and the associated effects on bones and lipids must be weighed against toxicologic considerations. If breast carcinogenesis is prevented, but tamoxifen is found to produce an unacceptable increase in primary liver and endometrial tumors, other potentially noncarcinogenic antiestrogens could be used.[70]

The major problem with all prevention strategies is the precise identification of target populations. It is not possible to state who will develop breast cancer with certainty, so prevention strategies have had to be applied to ill-defined groups of women. The knowledge about the positive effects of tamoxifen on bones and lipids[50] is being used to address breast cancer prevention from another direction. Results from the laboratory first demonstrated that the high-affinity antiestrogen raloxifene (originally named keoxifene) could maintain bone density in rats,[71] and the drug is to be tested in postmenopausal women as a treatment for osteoporosis. The compound inhibits rat mammary carcinogenesis[72] and lowers circulating cholesterol but has reduced estrogenic activity in the uterus compared with tamoxifen.[73] Based on present knowledge of structure–activity relations, raloxifene would be predicted to have little activity as a rat liver carcinogen. Therefore, the prolonged treatment of postmenopausal women for osteoporosis with new targeted antiestrogens could reduce the risk for breast cancer by up to 50% while also reducing the risks for coronary heart disease and endometrial carcinoma. This novel, indirect strategy could provide general improvements in womens' health, but the overall advantage would have to be assessed against hormone replacement therapy.

References

1. Boyd S. On oophorectomy in cancer of the breast. Br Med J 1900;2:1161.
2. Feinleib M. Breast cancer and artificial menopause: a cohort study. J Natl Cancer Inst 1968;41:315.
3. Trichopoulos DB, MacMahon B, Cole P. Menopause and breast cancer risk. J Natl Cancer Inst 1972;48:605.
4. Huggins SC, Grand LC, Brillantes FP. Mammary cancer induced by a single feeding of polynuclear hydrocarbons and their suppression. Nature 1961;189:204.
5. Dao TL. Mammary cancer induction by 7,12 dimethylbenzanthracene: relation to age. Science 1969;165:810.
6. Grubbs CJ, Peckham JC, Cato KD. Mammary carcinogenesis in rats in relation to age at time of nitroso-N-methyl urea administration. J Natl Cancer Inst 1983;70:209.
7. Bowcock AM. Molecular cloning of BRCA1: a gene for early onset familial breast and ovarian cancer. Breast Cancer Res Treat 1993;28:121.

8. Tokunaga M, Land CE, Yamamoto T, et al. Incidence of female breast cancer among atomic bomb survivors: Hiroshima and Nagasaki 1950–1980. Radiat Res 1987;112:243.

9. Hildreth N, Shore R, Dvukretski P, et al. The risk of breast cancer after irradiation of the thymus in infancy. N Engl J Med 1989;321:1281.

10. Miller AB, How G, Sherman G, et al. Mortality from breast cancer after irradiation during fluoroscopic examinations in patients being treated for tuberculosis. N Engl J Med 1989;321:1285.

11. Lathrop AEC, Loeb L. Further investigations on the origins of tumors in mice. III. Or the part played by internal secretions in the spontaneous development of tumors. J Cancer Res 1916;1:1.

12. Lacassagne A. Hormonal pathogenesis of adenocarcinoma of the breast. Am J Cancer 1936;27:217.

13. Jordan VC, Lababidi MK, Mirecki DM. The antiestrogenic and antitumor properties of prolonged tamoxifen therapy in C3H/OUJ mice. Eur J Cancer 1990;26:718.

14. Jordan VC, Lababidi MK, Langan-Fahey S. Suppression of mouse mammary tumorigenesis by long-term tamoxifen therapy. J Natl Cancer Inst 1991;83:492.

15. Dao TL, Sutherland H. Mammary carcinogenesis by 3-methylcholanthrene. 1. Hormonal aspects in tumor induction and growth. J Natl Cancer Inst 1959;23:567.

16. Dao TL, Bock FG, Greiner MJ. Mammary carcinogenesis by 3-methylcholanthrene. 2. Inhibitory effects of pregnancy and lactation on tumor induction. J Natl Cancer Inst 1960;25:991.

17. Huggins SC, Moon R, Morii S. Extinction of experimental mammary cancer. 1. Estradiol-17β and progesterone. Proc Natl Acad Sci USA 1962;48:379.

18. Jabara AC, Toyne PH, Harcourt AG. Effects of time and duration of progesterone administration on mammary tumours induced by 7,12-dimethylbenzanthracene in Sprague-Dawley rats. Br J Cancer 1973;27:63.

19. Grubbs CJ, Hill DL, McDonough KC, et al. N-nitroso-N-methylurea-induced mammary carcinogenesis: effect of pregnancy on preneoplastic cells. J Natl Cancer Inst 1983;71:625.

20. Dao TL. The role of ovarian hormones in initiating the induction of mammary cancer in rats by polynuclear hydrocarbons. Cancer Res 1962;22:973.

21. Jordan VC. Effect of tamoxifen (ICI 46,474) on initiation and growth of DMBA-induced rat mammary carcinomata. Eur J Cancer 1976;12:419.

22. Tsai TLS, Katzenellenbogen BS. Antagonism of development and growth of 7,12 dimethylbenzanthracene-induced rat mammary tumors by the antiestrogen U23,469 and effects on estrogen and progesterone receptors. Cancer Res 1977;37:1537.

23. Jordan VC, Allen KE. Evaluation of the antitumour activity of the non-steroidal antioestrogen monohydroxytamoxifen in the DMBA-induced rat mammary carcinoma model. Eur J Cancer 1980;16:239.

24. Jordan VC, Allen KE, Dix CJ. Pharmacology of tamoxifen in laboratory animals. Cancer Treat Rep 1980;64:745.

25. Robinson SP, Jordan VC. Reversal of the antitumor effects of tamoxifen by progesterone in the 7,12-dimethylbenzanthracene-induced rat mammary carcinoma model. Cancer Res 1987;47:5386.

26. Huggins C, Grand LC, Brillantes F. Critical significances of breast structure in the induction of mammary cancer in the rat. Proc Natl Acad Sci USA 1959;45:1294.

27. Russo J, Gusterson BA, Rogers AE, et al. Comparative study of human and rat mammary tumorigenesis. Lab Invest 1990;62:244.

28. Russo IH, Koszalka M, Russo J. Human chorionic gonadotropin and rat mammary cancer prevention. J Natl Cancer Inst 1990;82:1286.

29. Russo IH, Koszalka M, Gimotty PA, et al. Protective effect of chorionic gonadotropin on DMBA-induced mammary carcinogenesis. Br J Cancer 1990;62:243.

30. Russo IH, Koszalka M, Russo J. Effect of human chorionic gonadotropin on mammary gland differentiation and carcinogenesis. Carcinogenesis 1990;11:1849.

31. Prentis RL, Thomas DB. On the epidemiology of oral contraceptives and disease. Adv Cancer Res 1987;49:285.

32. Battersby S, Robertson BJ, Anderson TJ, et al. Influence of menstrual cycle parity and oral contraceptive use on steroid hormone receptors in normal breast. Br J Cancer 1992;65:601.

33. Jeng MH, Parker C, Jordan VC. Estrogenic potential of progestin in oral contraceptives to stimulate human breast cancer cell proliferation. Cancer Res 1992;52:6539.

34. Colletta AA, Harold FV, Baum M. A novel binding site for a synthetic progestin in breast cancer cells. J Steroid Biochem 1989;33:1055.

35. Colletta AA, Wakefield LM, Howell FV, et al. The growth inhibition of human breast cancer cells by a novel synthetic progestin is partly mediated by the induction of transforming growth factor beta. J Clin Invest 1991;87:277.

36. Catherino W, Jeng MH, Jordan VC. Norgestrel and gestodene stimulate breast cancer cell growth through an oestrogen receptor mediated mechanism. Br J Cancer 1993;67:945.

37. Pike MC, Ross RK, Lobo RA, et al. LHRH agonists and the prevention of breast and ovarian cancer. Br J Cancer 1989;60:142.

38. Spicer DV, Shoupe D, Pike M. GnRH agonists as contraceptive agents: predicted significantly reduced risk of breast cancer. Contraception 1991;44:289.

39. Spicer DV, Pike MC, Pike A, et al. Pilot trial of a gonadotropin hormone agonist with replacement hormones as a prototype contraceptive to prevent breast cancer. Contraception 1993;45:427.

40. Spicer DV, Pike MC. Breast cancer prevention through modulation of endogenous hormones. Breast Cancer Res Treat 1993;28:179.

41. Wolbach SB, Howe PR. Tissue changes following deprivation of fat soluble A vitamin. J Exp Med 1925;42:753.

42. Glick AB, McCure BK, Abdulkarem N, et al. Complex regulation of TGF-β expression by retinoic acid in the vitamin A-deficient rat. Development 1991;111:1081.

43. Moon RC, Grubbs CJ, Sporn MD, et al. Retinyl acetate inhibits mammary carcinogenesis induced by N-methyl-N-nitrosourea. Nature 1977;267:620.

44. Muenter MD, Perry HO, Ludwig J. Chronic vitamin A intoxication in adults: hepatic, neurologic and dermatologic complications. Am J Med 1971;50:129.

45. Smith FR, Goodman DS. Vitamin A transport and vitamin A toxicity. N Engl J Med 1976;294:805.

46. Moon RC, Thompson HJ, Becci PJ, et al. N-(4-hydroxy-phenyl) retinamide, a new retinoid for prevention of breast cancer in the rat. Cancer Res 1979;39:1339.

47. Veronesi U, Costa A. Chemoprevention of contralateral breast cancer with the synthetic retinoid fenretidine. Cancer Invest 1988;6:634.

48. Segars JH, Marks MS, Hirschfeld S, et al. Inhibition of estrogen-responsive gene activation by retinoid X receptor β: evidence for multiple inhibitory pathways. Mol Cell Biol 1993;13:2258.

49. Demirpence E, Balaguer P, Trousse F, et al. Antiestrogenic effects of all-trans retinoic acid and 1, 25-dihydroxy vitamin D3 in breast cancer cells occur at the estrogen response element level but through different molecular mechanisms. Cancer Res 1994;54:1458.

50. Jordan VC. Fourteenth Gaddum Memorial Lecture: a current view of tamoxifen for the treatment and prevention of breast cancer. Br J Pharmacol 1993;110:507.

51. Jordan VC, ed. Long-term tamoxifen therapy for breast cancer. Madison, University of Wisconsin, 1994.

52. Nayfield SG, Karp JE, Ford LG, et al. Potential role of tamoxifen in prevention of breast cancer. J Natl Cancer Inst 1991;83:1450.

53. Powles TJ. The case for clinical trials of tamoxifen for prevention of breast cancer. Lancet 1992;340:1145.

54. Jordan VC. Tamoxifen for breast cancer prevention. Proc Soc Exp Biol Med 1995;87:623.

55. Fugh-Berman A, Epstein S. Tamoxifen: disease prevention or disease substitution? Lancet 1992;340:1143.
56. Love RR. The National Surgical Adjuvant Breast Project (NSABP) breast cancer trial revisited. Cancer Epidemiol Biomarkers Prev 1993;2:403.
57. Fisher B, Costantino JP, Redmond CK, et al. Endometrial cancer in tamoxifen treated breast cancer patients: findings from the National Surgical Adjuvant Breast and Bowel Project (NSABP) B14. J Natl Cancer Inst 1994;86:527.
58. Gottardis MM, Robinson SP, Satyaswaroop PG, et al. Contrasting action of tamoxifen on endometrial and breast tumor growth in the athymic mouse. Cancer Res 1988;48:812.
59. Friedl A, Jordan VC. What do we know and what don't we know about tamoxifen in the human uterus. Breast Cancer Res Treat 1994;31:27.
60. Williams GM, Iatropoulos MJ, Djordjevic MV, et al. The triphenylethylene drug tamoxifen is a strong liver carcinogen in the rat. Carcinogenesis 1993;14:1993.
61. Greaves P, Goonetilleke R, Nunn G, et al. Two-year carcinogenicity study of tamoxifen in Alderley Park Wistar-derived rats. Cancer Res 1993;59:3919.
62. Dragan YP, Langen Fahey SM, Street K, et al. Studies of tamoxifen as a promoter of hepatocarcinogenesis in female Fisher F344 rats. Breast Cancer Res Treat 1994;31:11.
63. Styles JA, Davis A, Lim CK, et al. Genotoxicity of tamoxifen, tamoxifen epoxide and toremifene in human lymphoblastoid cells containing human cytochrome P450's. Carcinogenesis 1994;15:5.
64. Lim CK, Yuan Z-X, Lamb JH, et al. A comparative study of tamoxifen metabolism in female rat, mouse and human liver microsomes. Carcinogenesis 1994;15:589.
65. Han X, Liehr JG. Induction of covalent DNA adducts in rodents by tamoxifen. Cancer Res 1992;52:1360.
66. White INH, DeMatteis F, Davis A, et al. Genotoxic potential of tamoxifen and analogues in female Fischer 344/n rats, DBA/2 and C57BL/6 mice and in human MCL-5 cells. Carcinogenesis 1992;13:2197.
67. Vancutsem PM, Lazarus P, Williams GM. Frequent and specific mutations of the rat p53 gene in hepatocarcinomas induced by tamoxifen. Cancer Res 1994;54:3867.
68. Powles TJ, Jones AL, Ashley SE, et al. The Royal Marsden Hospital pilot tamoxifen chemoprevention trial. Breast Cancer Res Treat 1994;31:73.
69. Powles TJ, Ashley S. Endometrial cancer during tamoxifen treatment. Lancet 1994;343:978.
70. Jordan VC. Tamoxifen: toxicities and drug resistance during the treatment and prevention of breast cancer. Annu Rev Pharmacol Toxicol 1995;35:195.
71. Jordan VC, Phelps E, Lindgren JU. Effects of anti-estrogens on bone in castrated and intact female rats. Breast Cancer Res Treat 1987;10:31.
72. Gottardis MM, Jordan VC. Antitumor actions of keoxifene and tamoxifen in the N-nitrosomethylurea-induced rat mammary carcinoma model. Cancer Res 1987;47:4020.
73. Black LJ, Sata M, Rowley ER, et al. Raloxifene (LY139481 HCL) prevents bone loss and reduces serum cholesterol without causing uterine hypertrophy in ovariectomized rats. J Clin Invest 1994;93:63.

10.2
Clinical Considerations in Breast Cancer Prevention

VICTOR G. VOGEL

Clinical management of women at increased risk for breast cancer includes collecting risk information, quantifying cancer risk, communicating risk status, and providing a specific management plan. Published data indicate that women at increased risk for breast cancer are misinformed about their risks.[1] Unfortunately, communicating breast cancer risks potentially has adverse effects, including psychologic and emotional consequences, risks of breaches in confidentiality, and adverse economic and social consequences. On learning of their increased risk, some women experience an increased sense of denial, low self-esteem, anxiety, and guilt.[2] In this chapter, the elements of a clinical prevention strategy for managing breast cancer risk and for minimizing the psychologic consequences to a woman from knowing her risk are reviewed.[3] The features of this clinical approach are shown in Table 10.2-1.

Quantifying Risk

After age, the greatest risk factor for breast cancer is family history of the disease. Quantification of risk is possible using multivariate regression models,[4] but the available models may not accurately reflect the degree of risk experienced by women who are members of affected families. Simply counting affected first-degree relatives is not by itself an adequate assessment of the magnitude of familial risk because of the strong likelihood of vertical genetic transmission with more second- than first-degree relatives having breast cancer. Affected second-degree relatives (grandmothers, aunts, cousins) increase risk substantially without directly affecting quantitative risk assessments that merely count first-degree relatives.[5,6]

The availability of multivariate risk models allows the additional determination of a composite relative risk for breast cancer and the calculation of a cumulative lifetime risk of cancer adjusted for competing causes. There are, however, limitations to the generalization of risk estimates from multivariate models because of selection biases in the studied populations. Available models may not accurately estimate risk because they do not consider all risk factor information. Published data are largely from studies restricted to white women, and the generalizability of those data to other racial and ethnic groups is uncertain. The models were derived from case-control and screening studies, and inherent selection biases in the populations studied must be recognized. There may be a differential

TABLE 10.2-1
Considerations in the Clinical Prevention of Breast Cancer

Quantify risk in terms of the probability that a woman will develop breast cancer in her lifetime using either an empiric or an analytic estimate.

Review the benefits and limitations of mammographic screening in women under the ages of 40 and 50 years and recommend a specific screening schedule.

Discuss the possibility (if appropriate) of prophylactic mastectomy.

Discuss the impact of diet, exercise, and alcohol consumption on breast cancer risk.

Offer the possibility of participation in chemoprevention clinical trials to eligible women.

Review the risks and benefits of estrogen replacement therapy after menopause, and facilitate the process of deciding whether to accept or forgo replacement therapy.

Attend to the psychologic needs of the woman at risk and her family.

Adhere to ethical principles in the counseling process.

effect of family history by race or ethnicity, and multivariate risk models derived from minority populations have not been published.

The model developed by Gail and colleagues[4] is the most widely used method of quantifying risk to assist clinicians in counseling women about their probability of developing breast cancer. The model allows estimation of the likelihood that a woman of a given age with certain risk factors will develop breast cancer during a specified interval. Risk factors used in the model include age at menarche, age at first live birth, number of previous breast biopsies, and the number of first-degree relatives with breast cancer. The presence of a biopsy that shows atypical hyperplasia doubles the risk. Validation studies of multivariate risk models are important for ensuring accurate results, and recent validation studies of the model of Gail and associates indicate that the observed number of breast cancers agrees closely with the number predicted by the model.[7,8]

Regardless of how risk is quantified, it is also important to place an individual's risk in qualitative terms (eg, average, slightly elevated, moderately elevated) and to provide a specific plan to manage the risk.

Communicating Results From Risk Assessments

Women at increased risk for breast cancer tend to overestimate that risk.[9] Providing them with accurate information about their risk should heighten awareness while reducing anxiety. Although information about relative risk is useful to epidemiologists and perhaps to clinicians, formulating risk information in this way will be ambiguous for women at risk because the public does not routinely deal with comparative risk assessments.[10] A more useful strategy is

to use lifetime probability of disease, expressing risk as a proportion of women affected among a hypothetical group at similar risk over a fixed period (eg, 10 or 20 years). Proper communication of risk diminishes anxiety and improves compliance with screening recommendations.[11,12]

Risk assessment and counseling for women at increased risk for breast cancer include collection of family history data, calculation of cancer risks, communication of risk status, and education to reduce the risk of morbidity and mortality.[13,14] The patient's desire for information and the level at which the patient chooses to control decision making must be considered in clinical management of the risk.

It is inappropriate to assess a woman's risk for developing breast cancer without providing a plan to manage the risk. The sections that follow outline a strategy to provide mammographic screening; to discuss prophylactic mastectomy where appropriate; to review the impact of life-style changes in diet, alcohol consumption, and exercise habits; and to offer participation in chemoprevention clinical trials.

Mammographic Screening Prescriptions

An important component of risk management is a mammographic screening prescription. Although there is no conclusive proof that mammographic screening of women younger than 50 years reduces mortality from breast cancer,[15,16] there is no conclusive proof that it does not reduce mortality. Only one prospective randomized comparison of mammographic screening in women under 50 years of age has been published,[17] and technical limitations prevent acceptance of the trial's negative findings as definitive.[18] Because most younger women can have adequate mammographic visualization of their breast parenchyma, and because there is no sudden biologic change in the mammographic appearance of the breast at age 50, there is no reason to believe that mammographic screening of women younger than 50 years will be ineffective. In fact, the performance of any screening test is related not only to the performance characteristics of the test (eg, the sensitivity and specificity of the test) but also to the prevalence of the disease in the population being screened.[19] In a population of women under 50 years of age who are at increased risk of breast cancer, the prevalence of the disease is increased, so the performance outcomes of screening mammography should not differ from the outcomes of mammographic screening in older populations who have the same breast cancer prevalence based on age rather than a family history of the disease.[20]

These considerations underlie the screening strategy outlined in Figure 10.2-1. The initial consideration is whether a younger woman is attempting to become pregnant, is pregnant, or is lactating. Although the radiation dose to a fetus from a screening mammogram is minimal, the exposure must be avoided. Equally important, the benign nodular densities that appear in the breasts of lactating and pregnant women generate an increased number

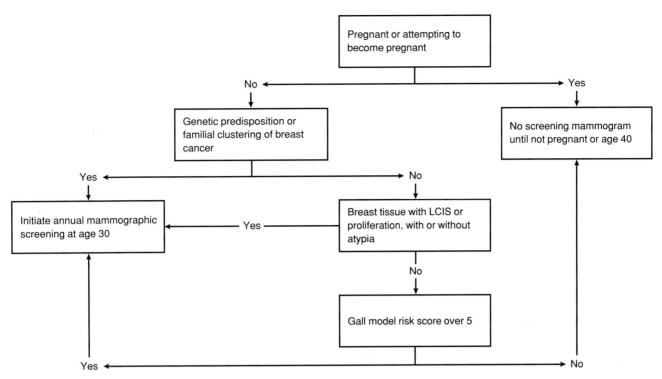

FIGURE 10.2-1 Mammographic screening algorithm for women younger than 40 years. The Gail model is described and referenced in the text. LCIS, lobular carcinoma in situ.

of false-positive mammographic readings that also must be avoided. Pregnant and lactating women who are at increased risk of breast cancer must delay initiation of screening mammography until they are no longer attempting to conceive children. Any symptomatic breast lesion in a pregnant woman who is at usual or increased risk of breast cancer must be evaluated aggressively to rule out the possibility of malignancy.

If a woman aged 30 years or older is not pregnant, and there is evidence of genetic predisposition or familial clustering of breast cancer, annual mammographic screening should begin. In a woman who has no genetic predisposition to breast cancer but who has had a breast biopsy showing either lobular carcinoma in situ or proliferative disease with or without atypia, initiation of annual mammographic screening is warranted after the positive biopsy. In women with none of these findings but who have Gail model risk scores of 5 or greater, initiation of annual mammographic screening at age 30 is advised based on the disease prevalence considerations explained earlier. Most of the women with elevated Gail model risk scores have multiple affected first-degree relatives or histories of breast biopsy, since these are the two factors with the greatest weight in the model.[4]

Two thirds of young women who are at increased risk for breast cancer have mammographic images of normal density that are amenable to usual radiologic interpretation (Vogel VG, Higginbotham E, unpublished data). Because adequate mammographic visualization can be difficult in young women with dense breasts,[21] ultrasonography

should accompany screening mammography to distinguish the frequent cystic lesions that occur in these young women from the solid lesions that require biopsy for diagnosis. This strategy minimizes the number of biopsies performed in young women who receive regular screening.

Mammographic screening offers several benefits as well as potential risks. The benefits include a demonstrated decrease in mortality for women older than 50 years, the ability to use conservative surgery for smaller, less advanced lesions, and the psychologic reassurance gained by a woman after a normal mammogram.[48] These benefits are accompanied by physical discomfort from compression techniques. Screening increases the likelihood of having to undergo additional investigations, including breast ultrasound, fine-needle aspiration, needle biopsy, or open biopsy. In addition, there is the possibility of overtreating lesions that are actually benign clinically and that would not have come to clinical attention in the absence of screening.[22] Unnecessary surgery and radiation therapy may be used to treat these lesions, which impose no threat to health.

Screening mammography has inherent limitations in its sensitivity, and up to 15% of negative mammograms may be false-negative.[23] The false reassurance that follows a negative mammogram may lead to decreased compliance with attendance at future scheduled screenings, and this issue has not been investigated in women who are at increased risk. There is also some psychologic morbidity associated with undergoing mammographic screening, with published studies showing that some women experience an increase in measured anxiety and psychologic distress immediately after mammographic screening.[2,24]

Clinicians should explain to anxious young women seeking mammographic screening that great controversy surrounds the assessment of benefit attributed to mammographic screening in women younger than 50 years. They should also explain that, of women whose breast cancer is not detected by screening, half die of complications of breast cancer. In women older than 50 years, screening mammography reduces breast cancer mortality by 30%,[15] and if screening in younger women were to reduce mortality from breast cancer by the same proportion, lives would be saved.[16] This remains a theoretical reduction in mortality, and this benefit has not been demonstrated conclusively. The cost of screening the entire population of younger women would be substantial, and patients must understand that they ultimately pay for mammographic screening whether they are insured, taxed, or pay costs themselves.[25]

Patients should understand that clinical limitations on the performance of screening mammography in younger women may impair its performance when compared with such screening in older women, and no published study has shown a benefit in mortality reduction from a selective screening strategy in women at increased risk. Clinicians should explain further that none of the completed mammographic screening studies has either sufficient methodologic rigor or significant statistical power to prove that screening is either beneficial or detrimental in women younger than 50 years. The uncertainties arising from this fact must be discussed openly.

Prophylactic Mastectomy

Prophylactic mastectomy for women at increased risk of breast cancer must be recommended cautiously and advisedly.[26] A prophylactic mastectomy is an operation that removes the total breast, tail of Spence, areola, and nipple.[27,28] It is typically followed by a reconstructive procedure for cosmetic reasons. There are several possible reasons that prophylactic mastectomy might appear to be a desirable clinical strategy for the control of breast cancer. These include elimination of the risk of developing breast cancer, removal of occult carcinomas, and improvement of psychologic distress related to unreasonable fears about the risk of developing breast cancer. Other chapters in this book review factors that increase the risk of breast cancer and that may lead patients to seek and physicians to recommend prophylactic mastectomy. These include genetic risk, proliferative benign breast disease with or without atypia, and lobular carcinoma in situ. Available data indicate, however, that prophylactic mastectomy does not offer complete protection from breast cancer without psychologic risk.

Experimental studies of prophylactic mastectomy in rats given chemical carcinogens show that tumors occur despite total mastectomy,[29] and similar observations have been made in mice that develop spontaneous breast malignancies without mammary carcinogens.[30] Pathologic examination of the chest wall and axilla in women undergoing mastectomy for breast cancer shows extension of breast tissue well into the axilla and pectoralis fascia,[31] indicating that total extirpation of the breast requires even more extensive surgery than a total mastectomy for cancer. Less extensive subcutaneous mastectomies are followed by invasive carcinomas in up to 1% of the cases.[32-34] Although as many as 5% of prophylactic mastectomy specimens contain occult carcinomas,[33] no data compare the outcomes of the patients treated with prophylactic mastectomy and those of a similar group of women at increased risk who were closely followed, including mammographic screening and timely biopsy when indicated clinically. Finally, rather than relieving anxiety, prophylactic mastectomy may increase it and cause other adverse psychologic consequences. After prophylactic mastectomy and reconstruction, 20% of women believed their breasts were either too small or in the wrong position, 100% lost erogenous sensitivity in the nipple–areola complex, and 60% reported markedly negative changes in their sex lives.[35] Based on these observations, it is difficult to argue in favor of prophylactic mastectomy as an effective preventive procedure with satisfactory clinical and psychologic outcomes.

The decision to undergo prophylactic mastectomy has profound physical and psychologic implications for women at increased risk. In a small subset of patients, it may be appropriate, and Figure 10.2-2 can assist clinicians in identifying patients for the procedure. The presence of lobular carcinoma in situ or atypical lobular or ductal hyperplasia in the setting of a history of breast cancer in first-degree relatives increases the risk of breast cancer significantly.[4,36] In these patients, the physician may initiate discussion of the possibility of prophylactic mastectomy with the understanding that half or more of the patients with these predisposing histologic lesions never develop breast cancer, making the procedure unnecessary for them.

Women who carry genes that increase the risk of breast cancer have a greater than 60% chance of developing breast cancer by age 50 years and may want to consider prophylactic mastectomy.[37,38] In women whose risk profiles show them to be at increased risk of breast cancer but who have negative genetic testing, a history of repeated breast biopsies in the presence of dense breast parenchyma, a history of proliferative benign breast disease on biopsy, or manifestations of extreme anxiety about developing breast cancer should lead the clinician to discuss prophylactic mastectomy. The physician should never force the decision on the patient and should explore carefully the relative advantages of the procedure, including the lack of certainty that the patient will develop breast cancer and the rare chance that a prophylactic procedure will not prevent breast cancer from occurring.[14] For some patients at increased risk, careful consideration of these risks and benefits leads to a decision to have prophylactic mastectomies

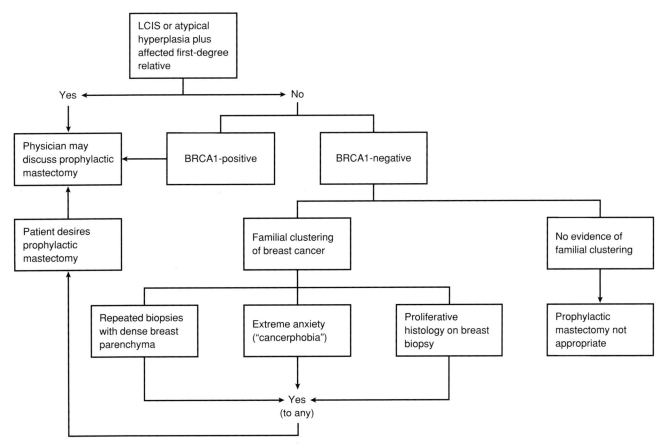

FIGURE 10.2-2 Algorithm to identify appropriate candidates for prophylactic bilateral mastectomy. LCIS, lobular carcinoma in situ; BRCA1, breast cancer 1 gene.

and reduces significantly the degree of anxiety they experience.

Life-Style Factors

DIET

The relation of major dietary components to the risk of breast cancer is reviewed elsewhere in this book. Here, the evidence that certain dietary components and micronutrients may have application in the prevention of breast cancer is reviewed.

The role of dietary fat in the etiology of breast cancer remains a point of debate, but there is both experimental and epidemiologic evidence that certain types of dietary fat may actually offer some protection against breast cancer. Some polyunsaturated fatty acids (such as linoleic acid) that are found in high levels in vegetable oil can be converted to arachidonic acid and serve as substrates for prostaglandin synthesis. Prostaglandins, in turn, are implicated in tumorigenesis.[39] Conversely, other polyunsaturated fatty acids with the double bond between the third and fourth carbon atoms (so-called ω-3 fatty acids) behave as competitive inhibitors of prostaglandin endoperoxidase

synthetase. It is possible, therefore, that ω-3 fatty acids such as eicosapentaenoic or docosahexaenoic acid may act as dietary inhibitors of carcinogenesis. This protective effect is suggested by the negative but nonsignificant association obtained when population-based disappearance of ω-3 fatty acids derived from consumption of fish oils is correlated with the age-standardized breast cancer incidence rates from countries around the world.[40,41] Such analyses are hampered by small amounts of fish oil consumed but are supported by experimental animal studies showing significant reductions in both tumor incidence and volume and prolongation of the tumor latent period in rats receiving both mammary carcinogens and diets rich in ω-3 fatty acids.[39,42] These data suggest a protective effect from fish oils, but additional studies in women are needed before dietary modification or supplementation can be recommended as a proven strategy for breast cancer prevention.

Similar suggestive, but unconfirmed, data exist for populations with increased dietary consumption of soybeans. Asians, for example, eat diets rich in soybean products and have breast cancer death rates one third to half those of women in the Western world.[43] Foods made from soybeans contain large quantities of the isoflavones genistein and daidzein, which are phytoestrogens with weak estrogen agonist activity that may interfere with the breast cancer–promoting effects of physiologic estrogen.[44] It has been reported that increased soy protein consumption is significantly correlated with a reduction in the risk of breast cancer.[45] Genistein inhibits the growth of both estrogen receptor–positive and estrogen receptor–negative breast cancer cells in culture, as well as cells showing overexpression of a multidrug resistance gene product.[44] These promising compounds merit additional clinical investigations.

Another group of substances thought to have potential preventive properties are the antioxidant vitamins (vitamins A, C, and E). Endogenous production of hydrogen peroxide has been associated with tumor cell proliferation, may confer a growth advantage to tumor cell populations, and may contribute to the malignant phenotype.[46] It has been hypothesized that antioxidant vitamins reduce the risk of cancer through their functions as free radical scavengers and blockers of nitrosation reactions.[47] Despite this plausible hypothesis, the epidemiologic evidence demonstrating a significant relation between either serum levels or dietary intake of vitamins C and E and reduced risk of breast cancer is limited and inconsistent.[47,48] The epidemiologic and prospective cohort data for vitamin A intake suggest a modest protective effect against breast cancer among women in the highest intake quartiles.[49,50] It is not yet known whether supplemental vitamin A reduces the risk of breast cancer for women with average dietary intakes of vitamin A, but prospective clinical studies are in progress to address that question.

ALCOHOL

Few risk factors for breast cancer have been studied as extensively as alcohol consumption. No fewer than 50 publications have reported studies of consumption patterns of alcohol and the subsequent development of breast cancer.[51,52] Although a specific mechanism whereby alcohol might enhance breast carcinogenesis has not been identified, several hypotheses have been proposed. These include induction of increased levels of circulating estrogen, stimulation of hepatic metabolism of carcinogens such as acetaldehyde, facilitation of transport of carcinogens into breast tissue, stimulation of pituitary production of prolactin, modulation of cell membrane integrity with an effect on carcinogenesis, production of cytotoxic protein products, impairment of immune surveillance, interference with DNA repair, production of toxic congeners, increased exposure to oxidants, and reduced intake and bioavailability of nutrients.[52–54]

Few of these mechanisms have been studied either in experimental animals or in humans with the exception of the effect of alcohol consumption on plasma and urinary hormone concentrations in premenopausal women.[55] When women volunteers aged 21 to 40 years were given a controlled diet that included 30 g of alcohol daily (equivalent to about two drinks) through three menstrual cycles, significant increases were seen in periovulatory plasma levels of dehydroepiandrosterone sulfate, estrone, and estradiol. Luteal phase increases in levels of urinary estrone,

estradiol, and estriol were also recorded. Although no changes were found in the percentage of bioavailable estradiol, the increased total estradiol levels in the periovulatory phase suggest elevated absolute amounts of bioavailable estradiol. These results imply that there are major effects of alcohol on both estrogen production and metabolism. Additionally, studies in breast cancer cases show increasing odds of having an estrogen receptor–positive breast cancer with increasing self-reported daily consumption of alcohol: the odds ratio of being estrogen receptor–positive with consumption of less than 1.5 g of alcohol daily were 1.18 but increased to 1.35 in women drinking over 15 g a day.[56] It is not clear whether increased levels of bioavailable estradiol increase either the risk of breast cancer or the chance that a breast cancer will contain measurable estrogen receptors, but it is clear that alcohol may play some role.

Metaanalysis of the published literature relating alcohol consumption and breast cancer shows strong evidence of a dose–response relationship with a very modest slope.[51] Relative risks of breast cancer associated with consumption of one, two, or three drinks per day are 1.11, 1.24, and 1.38, respectively, but the slope of the regression line relating the odds of breast cancer to alcohol consumption is only 0.0083 per gram of alcohol daily. Nearly all studies in the metaanalysis were adjusted for known breast cancer risk factors and socioeconomic factors. The metaanalyses have been criticized, however, for including hospital-based studies conducted in Europe and for being confounded by a number of biases.[54] Furthermore, the beneficial effects of light to moderate alcohol consumption on overall mortality[57,58] must be taken into consideration before abstinence can be recommended as a strategy to control breast cancer. Nevertheless, women who are at increased risk for breast cancer and at low risk of heart disease might benefit from a program of limited alcohol consumption.

EXERCISE

Studies in animals indicate that both the intensity and duration of exercise affect the development of experimentally induced breast cancer.[59] A decade ago, Frisch and colleagues[60] first proposed that moderate physical activity could have a protective effect against the development of breast cancer after observing a 50% lower prevalence of the disease among former college athletes compared with nonathletes. Subsequent studies did not always confirm the association,[61,62] showed nonsignificant protection afforded by physical activity, or showed unexpected increased levels of risk among the most physically active women with premenopausal[63] or postmenopausal[64] breast cancer. Studies of women with nonsedentary occupations suggest that physical activity at work lowers the risk of dying of breast cancer by approximately 15%,[65] but standardized incidence ratios for female breast cancer were found to be no different in Finnish physical education teachers than in language teachers.[66]

Some of these earlier studies may have been handicapped by an inability to control for other breast cancer risk factors, to accurately measure physical activity, or to account for changes in activity over time. More recent studies performed with greater methodologic rigor do show that the average number of hours spent in physical exercise activities per week from menarche to early middle age is a significant predictor of reduced breast cancer risk.[67] Women in Los Angeles who reported spending 3.8 or more hours per week in physical exercise activities experienced 58% less risk of breast cancer than inactive women. The effect was greatest for women who had at least one child, but the effect was not lost among obese women. The data indicate that women who spend 1 to 3 hours per week in physical activity could reduce their risk of breast cancer by 30% relative to inactive women, and that those who sustain at least 4 hours per week could reduce their risk by 50%.

That physical exercise may be biologically linked to breast cancer risk is plausible in that strenuous physical activity is associated with an increase in luteal phase defects and anovulation and depressed serum estradiol levels.[64] Exercise may also influence the prevalence of obesity, but large body mass has actually been associated with reductions in the risk of premenopausal breast cancer.[68] Both the timing of weight change in adulthood and body fat distribution may be important determinants of risk. Additional studies are needed to clarify the hormonal consequences of physical activity and obesity.

Preventive Medical Strategies

CHEMOPREVENTION

The use of drugs or other substances to prevent the development of cancer is known as chemoprevention.[69] Prevention of breast cancer in women who are at increased risk[70] is the focus of several active research studies involving the use of the antiestrogen tamoxifen.

Detailed information on the incidence of second primary breast cancers is available for some 10,000 women entered in eight randomized controlled clinical trials of adjuvant tamoxifen therapy for early-stage breast cancer.[71] An unexpected observation from these trials was the reduction in the incidence of contralateral breast cancers in patients receiving tamoxifen. Women taking tamoxifen adjuvant therapy experienced approximately one third fewer second primary breast tumors as the women taking placebo (2.4% versus 1.6%). A more comprehensive overview of the world's literature on the use of tamoxifen as adjuvant therapy for breast cancer included more than 18,000 women from 42 separate randomized, placebo-controlled trials for whom information about second primary breast cancers that occurred as long as 10 years after initial diagnosis is available. There were 184 cases (2%) of second primary breast cancers among 9135 women treated with placebo versus 122 second primary cancers (1.3%) among 9128 women who received 10 mg to 40 mg of tamoxifen for a median of 2 years.[72] A dose–response was observed for duration of tamoxifen therapy: for women

who received less than 2 years of therapy, the reduction in the actuarial odds of a second primary breast cancer was only 26% compared with a 37% reduction for women with exactly 2 years of therapy and 56% for women who received more than 2 years of adjuvant tamoxifen. Other studies demonstrate that short durations of tamoxifen adjuvant therapy (eg, 48 weeks) may not be sufficient to provide protection against the development of second primary breast cancers.[73]

Tamoxifen is an antiestrogen that binds to the estrogen receptor, resulting in altered RNA transcription, decreased cell proliferation, and partial estrogen agonist activity. It also causes mouse mammary cells in culture to become apoptotic rather than secretory and causes basement membrane alterations.[74] Additional mechanisms by which tamoxifen prevents the development of new primary breast cancers are complex and may include modulating production of transforming growth factors; decreasing circulating levels of insulin-like growth factor; increasing circulating levels of sex hormone–binding globulin, which may decrease the availability of free estrogen, removing a stimulus for tumor cell growth; and increasing levels of natural killer cells.

In addition to these observed reductions in the odds of developing second primary breast cancers, the overview data demonstrated a 12% reduction in non–breast cancer deaths ($P = .05$), a 25% reduction in vascular deaths, and a 9% reduction in other causes of death. A major proportion of the benefit in reduction of noncancer deaths was due to a reduction in cardiovascular disease mortality. In the Scottish Adjuvant Tamoxifen Trial,[75] for example, women receiving adjuvant tamoxifen experienced a 63% reduction in the hazard of dying of myocardial infarction compared with women receiving placebo. In another study,[76] women who took tamoxifen for 5 years experienced 32% fewer admissions for cardiac disease than women taking tamoxifen for only 2 years ($P = .03$), a 17% reduction in total cardiac mortality, and a 20% reduction in deaths due to myocardial infarction. These results are due, in part, to decreases in low-density lipoprotein (LDL) cholesterol observed as early as 2 months after the initiation of tamoxifen therapy that are followed at 6 months by increases in high-density lipoprotein (HDL) cholesterol.[77] In the Wisconsin Tamoxifen Study, a randomized comparison of tamoxifen, 20 mg daily, versus placebo in 140 postmenopausal women with early breast cancer, the average fall in cholesterol was 26% ± 3% after 3 months of tamoxifen therapy. These changes were associated with a 3% fall in HDL cholesterol, a 28% fall in LDL cholesterol, and a 23% increase in triglycerides.[78] Other small longitudinal studies of cholesterol changes associated with tamoxifen therapy show similar findings.[77,79–83] Additional data available from studies in women are limited but indicate that a 15% to 20% decrease in LDL cholesterol may result in a 6% to 20% decrease in coronary heart disease.[84,85] In addition to these effects are tamoxifen's known estrogenic effects on the liver, which may lead to increased synthesis of very low-density lipoprotein (VLDL) cholesterol and increased triglyceride levels, decreased levels of apolipoprotein B synthesis, decreased LDL cholesterol levels, and increased levels of apolipoprotein A-I synthesis, with resultant increased levels of HDL cholesterol.[86,87]

The effect of tamoxifen on the development of atherosclerotic cardiovascular disease may relate to its antithrombotic properties as well. Postmenopausal women taking tamoxifen show an average fall of only 10% in antithrombin III levels during therapy, whereas fibrinogen levels decline 16% or more.[88] Population studies demonstrate a relation between fibrinogen levels, myocardial infarction, and stroke, with lower levels associated with lower cardiovascular risk.[89,90] Concerns about the durability of these effects arise from studies of former users of tamoxifen that show reversal of the increases in HDL cholesterol at the cessation of tamoxifen therapy.[91] Additional prolonged observations of women taking tamoxifen are necessary to evaluate fully the duration of the observed benefits on cardiovascular morbidity and mortality.

The benefits of tamoxifen therapy are not restricted to the heart, blood vessels, and contralateral breast. Tamoxifen has also been shown to decrease the rate of resorption of trabecular bone, with a resulting net preservation of bone density.[92-95] Bone loss occurring in postmenopausal women is caused by increased bone resorption, leading to decreased bone density, osteoporosis, and fractures, which are a major cause of morbidity in women older than 55 years. In the Wisconsin Tamoxifen Study, bone mineral density in both the lumbar spine and radius increased 0.61% per year for 2 years in women taking tamoxifen, 20 mg daily, compared with a 1% per year decline in patients receiving placebo.[96] Serum osteocalcin and alkaline phosphatase levels (measures of active bone turnover and loss) decreased significantly ($P < .001$) in women treated with tamoxifen. These observations were confirmed in a Danish study that showed significant increases in lumbar spine bone mineral density after 1 year of tamoxifen therapy while decreases were observed in the control group.[97] Experimental data in vitro showing that tamoxifen blocks bone resorption induced by parathyroid hormone, prostaglandin E_2, and 1,25-dihydroxyvitamin D_3[98] support these clinical observations of benefit. In oophorectomized rats, tamoxifen also blocks both bone loss[92] and an increase in osteoclast number and activity.[94]

Tamoxifen therapy is associated with a variety of toxicities, including gynecologic symptoms (particularly hot flashes in perimenopausal women), ocular effects (including retinopathy), and hepatic neoplasms with doses of 40 mg daily.[71] Early reports of an increased risk of thrombotic events were not confirmed in subsequent prospective trials with prolonged periods of observation,[76] and no hepatic neoplasms have been reported in women taking the usually prescribed 20 mg daily. A well-established consequence of tamoxifen therapy is an increased incidence of endometrial carcinoma. In a randomized trial from Sweden that used 40 mg of tamoxifen daily, the incidence of uterine tumors (both endometrial carcinomas and uterine sarcomas) was 6.5 times higher in the women who received tamoxifen than in those who received placebo, and the cumulative frequency of uterine tumors was 0.4% in the control group, 0.9% in women who received tamoxifen for 2 years, and 5.5% in women treated with tamoxifen

for 5 years.[99,100] In another trial using tamoxifen, 30 mg daily for 48 weeks, the incidence ratio for endometrial carcinomas was 1.9, with a cumulative incidence after 10 years of 0.3% and 1% in the patients receiving placebo and tamoxifen, respectively.[73,101] Other smaller case series have suggested an increased incidence of endometrial carcinomas in women receiving tamoxifen.

Additional data are available from the National Surgical Adjuvant Breast and Bowel Project B-14 trial, which included 1419 women randomly assigned to receive tamoxifen, 1220 who entered the study on tamoxifen therapy after randomization closed, and 1424 placebo control patients. After an average study time of 5 to 8 years, two patients in the placebo group and 24 in the tamoxifen group had endometrial carcinoma.[102] The hazard rate in the placebo group was 0.2 per 1000 women compared with 1.6 per 1000 women in the tamoxifen group (relative risk, 7.5). There was a 46% reduction in breast cancer relapse in the patients who received tamoxifen, along with a 42% reduction of new primary cancers in the opposite breast. There was also a net benefit in 5-year event-free survival of 38% fewer relapses or new cancers among the women who received tamoxifen even when taking into account the occurrence of endometrial carcinomas. Because the observed benefits of tamoxifen substantially outweigh the demonstrated risks, the investigators recommended continued use of tamoxifen for treatment of breast cancer and its continued investigation in controlled trials for the prevention of breast cancer. The use of endometrial sampling and abdominal or vaginal ultrasound examination of the endometrium before and during tamoxifen therapy is under investigation.

The outcomes of interest in the clinical trials investigating tamoxifen as chemoprevention are the incidence of primary breast cancer, deaths due to stroke and myocardial infarction, and the incidence of fractures of the hip and wrist. Other outcomes of interest in the ongoing trials are the incidences of both symptoms and second primary malignancies related to tamoxifen toxicity.

Participation in these investigational studies offers women at increased risk[70] the potential of risk reduction while undergoing more intensive surveillance as part of the study protocol. For women who wish to take active steps to deal with their increased risk of developing breast cancer, participation in a chemoprevention trial affords them that opportunity. The informed consent process must include specific identification of the associated risks and the possibility that participants will receive the inactive placebo. Results from the studies in progress will be available in the next several years. It is inappropriate in the interim, however, to prescribe tamoxifen or any other agent with chemopreventive potential for the prevention of breast cancer until the studies in progress are completed and demonstrate a definite benefit from the active agent compared with placebo.

ESTROGEN REPLACEMENT THERAPY

The risk of breast cancer among women using replacement estrogen therapy after menopause is the subject of controversy and conflicting data in the medical literature.[103]

It is generally accepted that endogenous estrogens play some role in the causation of breast cancer,[104,105] but it has been difficult to prove that exogenous estrogens given at the time of menopause have a similar effect. Most studies that have evaluated estrogen replacement therapy and its possible role in the development of breast cancer found no overall increase in risk,[106–111] although several demonstrated a modest overall increase.[112,113]

Such studies may be confounded, however, by a bias in treatment selection that denies hormone replacement therapy to women with a family history of breast cancer.[114] If physicians are less likely to prescribe estrogen for women with family histories of breast cancer, a lack of association or a spurious inverse relation between estrogen use and breast cancer risk may appear. Nevertheless, the relative risk in published studies is related to the dose and duration of estrogen administration.[109]

The association of estrogen administration with the development of breast tumors is derived largely from in vitro or animal studies.[115] No prospective randomized trials have addressed the risks and benefits of estrogen replacement therapy in women at increased risk for breast cancer. Three metaanalyses to determine the effect of noncontraceptive estrogen replacement therapy on breast cancer risk have been published.[116–118] Two of the analyses did not find a positive association between estrogen replacement therapy and breast cancer in high-risk women, which included subjects with positive family histories.[117,118] One metaanalysis[117] included only American studies, whereas the other[118] included 27 American studies and 1 European study. Steinberg and associates[116] found that women with family histories of breast cancer who had ever used estrogen replacement had a significantly increased risk (relative risk, 3.4; 95% CI, 2–6). The increased risk among women with family histories in the latter analysis may be due to the difference in preparations of estrogen used in the United States and Europe.

Based on the results of these numerous and large epidemiologic studies, there is no definitive evidence that hormone replacement therapy with low-dose conjugated estrogens increases the risk of breast cancer, including therapy in high-risk women. The possibility remains, however, that the risk may be moderately increased with long durations of use (more than 15 years) and at higher doses, especially with unconjugated estrogens (eg, estradiol).

Most studies of oral contraceptive use show no associated increase in the risk of breast cancer,[119–121] and at least one study suggested a reduced risk in oral contraceptive users.[122]

The morbidity and mortality associated with estrogen deficiency in postmenopausal women is substantial. Estrogen deficiency causes hot flashes, genital atrophy with resultant dyspareunia, and mood swings, and the risk of death due to cardiovascular disease increases 18-fold after menopause.[123] Elevated levels of total cholesterol and LDL cholesterol have been causally related to an increased risk of coronary vascular disease. The use of estrogen replacement therapy after menopause has a favorable influence on HDL, LDL, and total cholesterol levels. Estrogen supplementation reduces the risk for coronary heart disease,[124] and estrogen replacement therapy has been reported to have a vascular protective effect.[125] Numerous studies have demonstrated that all-cause mortality and mortality from coronary heart disease and cerebrovascular disease is reduced in women who have ever used estrogen replacement therapy.[126]

Estrogen supplementation can reduce or prevent trabecular bone loss and the development of osteoporosis.[127,128] Other treatments for osteoporosis, including calcium supplementation, exercise, and fluoride administration, may not prevent osteoporosis when used alone.

Contrary to these arguments for the use of replacement estrogen therapy, substantial data show that breast cancer risk is lower among women who experience menarche at a later age, who have fewer ovulatory menstrual cycles during their lifetimes, or who are younger at menopause, whether the menopause is natural or surgical.[129,130] Anovulatory menstrual cycles and early menopause extract a price, however, through reduced bone mineral density and a higher risk of fracture.[131] Despite these observations, the lower risk of breast cancer among women who have lower endogenous estrogen levels does not necessarily imply an increased risk of breast cancer in women who receive replacement therapy at menopause.

In light of the published benefits of estrogen replacement therapy with regard to quality of life and reduction of cardiovascular morbidity and mortality, as well as reduction of morbidity and mortality attributable to osteoporosis, estrogen replacement therapy must be considered even in women known to be at increased risk for breast cancer.[132] It is unreasonable to reject such therapy as inappropriate for all women at increased risk.[133–135] In women who have undergone oophorectomy before natural menopause, low-dose estrogen replacement prevents the occurrences of stroke or myocardial infarction during an increased number of years at risk after premature menopause. To deny women who are at increased risk for breast cancer estrogen replacement therapy after menopause is to ignore the substantial competing risks of osteoporosis and heart disease, which both rise exponentially after menopause. Estrogen replacement therapy should be offered to these women after a careful discussion of the potential risks and known benefits.[126,136]

Psychologic Considerations

Patients are entitled to accurate and valid information about their risk, but women who seek that information harbor fears and anxieties as well as misinformation about risk factors. Studies show that mood disorders (including anxiety, depression, energy level, and sleep disturbances) are as common and severe in women at risk for breast cancer as they are in women with breast cancer.[137] Women who learn that their risk is low may express disbelief[138] or be subject to a troubling emotion called "survivor guilt," which is usually experienced by those who live through a disaster (eg, war, plane crash, earthquake) in which others, including loved ones, suffer or die. Because of these disorders, the clinician should provide ample opportunity for the patient to express her concerns and fears. Referral for psychologic counseling may be appropriate.[139]

Some women at risk seek information in an attempt to control and manage anxiety.[140] Information delivered in a supportive environment should lessen rather than heighten anxiety in those at risk. The greatest danger lies in clinicians' not delivering information to patients who need it because the clinicians either do not understand the factors that contribute to breast cancer risk or do not recognize the need to deliver the information.

It is also appropriate for physicians who treat women with breast cancer to offer risk assessment and counseling to patients' relatives. If a clinician is unable or unwilling to provide counseling for women at increased risk, the women should be referred to competent counselors. Counseling is difficult when family members live at a distance from the patient and cannot visit the clinic personally, but informational letters can be an effective mechanism for educating family members. The optimal strategy also involves notification of family members' primary care physicians with recommendations for appropriate screening interventions. When family members live in proximity to one another, family counseling visits are an effective means for transmitting information about risks and for outlining possible preventive interventions.

Research suggests that counseling about risk may have unwanted psychologic effects.[13] A substantial proportion of women who have abnormal mammograms but not cancer report significant impairments in mood and daily functioning.[2,24] More than one fourth of high-risk women may have clinically elevated levels of psychologic distress.[141] Psychologic distress can, in turn, interfere with adherence to recommended breast screening,[2] and heightened anxiety is associated with a reduced likelihood of adherence to mammography and clinical examinations in both high- and normal-risk populations.[137,141–143] Preliminary studies show a greater likelihood of having prior mammograms among women with higher self-perceived risks of breast cancer,[1] but more research is needed in this area. It is important to explore a woman's fears about breast cancer, and the clinician should ask each patient if her worries about breast cancer will impede her adherence to a recommendation to undergo screening. If simple reassurance and encouragement do not facilitate adherence, psychologic consultation is warranted.

Ever having had a mammogram is associated with higher perceived risk of developing breast cancer, whereas age is inversely related to perceived risk.[144] Daughters and sisters of breast cancer patients perceive their risk of developing breast cancer to be high,[1,9] and they are the women most likely to request risk assessment, predictive testing, and counseling.[145,146] They have more worries about cancer and more overall mood disturbances and are more likely to seek genetic testing, especially if they have an information-seeking coping style for dealing with stress.[140] The observation that measured mood disturbances are more likely in those seeking information indicates the need for the inclusion of someone with psychologic expertise in the counseling team, with referrals for psychiatric counseling when appropriate.

Cancer risk notification can have negative consequences on women at risk, including persistent worries, intrusive thoughts, depression, confusion, sleep disturbance, and avoidance of cancer-screening examinations.[13,137,146,147] The impact on the family of the woman at risk can be equally severe, leading to a collective sense of powerlessness, ambivalence, interdependence, role restructuring, and uncertainty.[148]

Ethical Implications of Risk Assessment and Management

Ethical issues arise in the management and counseling of women at increased risk for breast cancer.[139] The patient's comprehension of the risk information and the physician's disclosure to the patient of genetic testing data of uncertain significance create situations wherein harm is possible. Women at increased risk for breast cancer are understandably anxious, and they seek information that can assist them in modifying their risk and managing their clinical situations.

A program that seeks to provide clinical services to women at increased risk for breast cancer must embrace the Hippocratic mandate to "first, do no harm." Evaluating risk and labeling an individual as belonging to a high-risk group raise the possibility of causing emotional, financial, and social harm. Clinicians who counsel women can minimize the possibility for harm adhering to guidelines based on the ethical principles of autonomy, beneficence, justice, and confidentiality.

The physician must take special care to preserve the confidentiality of patients. This need is as great or greater in a healthy woman at risk as it is in a patient diagnosed as having cancer. This is difficult, by definition, when counseling individuals who are identified by family members who are themselves at risk or who have had breast cancer. The information obtained from an individual family member must be treated as privileged and confidential unless the woman specifically allows the release of information about her or her relatives. Disordered family dynamics and family psychosocial pathology may make disclosure a problem, especially if family members at risk are affected by substance abuse, psychiatric illness, or relational estrangement. The physician must preserve the autonomy of each family member even as he disseminates information to all family members at risk. This is achieved by asking each family member how much information can be shared with others and who in the family can be contacted.

The risk assessment process places an objective assessment of the patient's risk in the medical record. This should include a specific listing of each of the individual's risk factors, an overall qualitative and quantitative risk profile expressed in terms of relative risk of developing breast cancer and other site-specific malignancies, and a projection over 5 to 30 years of the probability that the patient will develop breast cancer or other cancers. The clinician must reassure each patient that, without written permission from the patient, no information about the risk assessment will be disclosed to employers, insurers, or others seeking information. The documentation in the medical record serves as a reference for other health care providers and as an educational tool for the patient. Clinicians must educate insurers and employers to recognize that this documentation does not by itself increase the risk experience of the patient. Each patient should be aware that the medical record is discoverable in the legal sense, and that the information cannot be suppressed if the patient gives written permission to a prospective employer or insurer to obtain medical records. When physicians receive such requests for information, a covering letter should explain that the process of risk assessment does not increase risk and that it is inappropriate to penalize women who seek counseling for their risks by denying them employment or insurance or by imposing other financial penalties. With these precautions in mind, physicians can provide clinical preventive services to women at risk for breast cancer without compromising the well-being or security of the patient.

References

1. Vogel VG, Graves DS, Vernon SW, et al. Mammographic screening of women with increased risk of breast cancer. Cancer 1990;66:1613.
2. Lerman C, Trock B, Rimer B, et al. Psychological side-effects of breast cancer screening. Health Psychol 1991;10:259.
3. Vogel VG, Yeomans A, Higginbotham E. Clinical management of women at increased risk for breast cancer. Breast Cancer Research Treat 1993;28:195.
4. Gail MH, Brinton LA, Byar DP, et al. Projecting individualized probabilities of developing breast cancer for white females who are being examined annually. J Natl Cancer Inst 1989;81:1879.
5. Claus EB, Risch NJ, Thompson WD. Age at onset as an indicator of familial risk of breast cancer. Am J Epidemiol 1990;131:961.
6. Claus EB, Risch N, Thompson WD. The calculation of breast cancer risk for women with a first degree family history of ovarian cancer. Breast Cancer Res Treat 1993;28:115.
7. Bondy ML, Lustbader ED, Halabi S, et al. Validation of a breast cancer risk assessment model in women with a positive family history. J Natl Cancer Inst 1994;86:620.
8. Spiegelman D, Colditz GA, Hunter D, et al. Validation of the Gail et al model predicting individual breast cancer risk. J Natl Cancer Ins 1994;86:600.
9. Bondy ML, Vogel VG, Halabi S, et al. Identification of women at increased risk for breast cancer in a population-based screening program. Cancer Epidemiol Biomarkers Prev 1992;1:143.
10. Newell GR, Vogel VG. Personal risk factors: what do they mean? Cancer 1988;62:1695.
11. Vogel VG, Graves DS, Coody DK, et al. Breast screening compliance following a statewide low-cost mammography project. Cancer Detect Prev 1990;14:573.
12. Vogel VG, Shepherd B, Craig K, et al. A randomized CCOP trial to improve mammographic screening compliance among women with family histories of breast cancer: trial design and preliminary results. (Abstract) Prev Med 1990;19:599.
13. Lerman C, Rimer BK, Engstrom PF. Cancer risk notification: psychosocial and ethical implications. J Clin Oncol 1991;9:1275.
14. King M-C, Rowell S, Love SM. Inherited breast and ovarian cancer: what are the risks? What are the choices? JAMA 1993;269:1975.
15. Hurley SF, Kaldor JM. The benefits and risk of mammographic screening for breast cancer. Epidemiol Rev 1992;14:101.
16. Vogel VG. Screening younger women at risk for breast cancer. J Natl Cancer Inst 1994;16:55.
17. Miller AB, Baines CJ, To T, et al. Canadian national breast screening study. 1. Breast cancer and death rates among women aged 40 to 49 years. Can Med Assoc J 1992;147:1459.
18. Sickles EA, Kopans DB. Deficiencies in the analysis of breast screening data. J Natl Cancer Inst 1993;85:1621.
19. Sackett DL, Haynes RB, Tugwell P. Clinical epidemiology: a basic science for clinical medicine. Boston, Little, Brown, 1985:59.
20. Mettlin C. Breast cancer risk factors: contributions to planning breast cancer control. Cancer 1992;69:1904.
21. Meyer JE, Kopans DB, Oot R. Breast cancer visualized by mammography in patients under 35. Radiology 1983;147:93.
22. Lantz PM, Remington PL, Newcomb PA. Mammography screening and increased incidence of breast cancer in Wisconsin. J Natl Cancer Inst 1991;83:1540.
23. Svane G, Potchen EJ, Siena A, et al. How to interpret a mammogram. In: Screening mammography: breast cancer diagnosis in asymptomatic women. St Louis, CV Mosby, 1993:148.
24. Lerman C, Rimer B, Trock B, et al. Psychological and behavioral implications of abnormal mammograms. Ann Intern Med 1991;114:657.
25. Mushlin AI, Fintor L. Is screening for breast cancer cost-effective? Cancer 1992;69:1957.
26. Love SM. Use of risk factors in counseling patients. Hematol Oncol Clin North Am 1989;3:599.
27. Bland KI, O'Neal B, Weiner LJ, et al. One-stage simple mastectomy with immediate reconstruction for high-risk patients. Arch Surg 1986;121:221.
28. Rubin LR. Prophylactic mastectomy with immediate reconstruction for the high-risk woman. Clin Plastic Surg 1984;11:369.
29. Wong JH, Jackson CF, Swanson JS, et al. Analysis of the risk reduction of prophylactic partial mastectomy in Sprague-Dawley rats with 7,12-dimethylbenzathracene-induced breast cancer. Surgery 1986;99:67.
30. Nelson H, Miller SH, Buck D, et al. Effectiveness of prophylactic mastectomy in the prevention of breast tumors in C3H mice. Plast Reconstr Surg 1989;83:662.
31. Temple WJ, Lindsay RL, Magi E. Technical considerations for prophylactic mastectomy in patients at high risk for breast cancer. Am J Surg 1991;161:413.
32. Goodnight JE, Quagliana JM, Mortoan DL. Failure of subcutaneous mastectomy to prevent the development of breast cancer. J Surg Oncol 1984;26:198.
33. Pennisi VR, Capozzi A. Subcutaneous mastectomy data: a final statistical analysis of 1500 patients. Aesthetic Plast Surg 1989;13:15.
34. Ziegler LD, Kroll SS. Primary breast cancer after prophylactic mastectomy. Am J Clin Oncol 1991;14:451.
35. Wapnir IL, Rabinowitz B, Greco RS. A reappraisal of prophylactic mastectomy. Surg Gynecol Obstet 1990;171:171.
36. Claus EB, Risch N, Thompson WD, et al. Relationship between breast histopathology and family history of breast cancer. Cancer 1993;71:147.
37. Biesecker BB, Boehnke M, Calzone K, et al. Genetic counseling for families with inherited susceptibility to breast and ovarian cancer. JAMA 1993;269:1970.
38. Miki Y, Swensen J, Shattuck-Eidens D, et al. A strong candidate for the breast and ovarian cancer susceptibility gene BRCA1. Science. 1994;266:66.

39. Jurkowski JJ, Cave WT Jr. Dietary effects of menhaden oil on the growth and membrane lipid composition of rat mammary tumors. J Natl Cancer Inst 1984;74:1145.

40. Kaizer L, Boyd NF, Kriukov V, et al. Fish consumption and breast cancer risk: an ecological study. Nutr Cancer 1989;12:68.

41. Hursting SD, Thornquist M, Henderson MM. Types of dietary fat and the incidence of cancer at five sites. Prev Med 1990;19:242.

42. Karmali RA, Marsh J, Fuchs C. Effect of omega-3 fatty acids on growth of a rat mammary tumor. J Natl Cancer Inst 1984;73:457.

43. Shimizu H, Ross RK, Bernstein L, et al. Cancer of the prostate and breast among Japanese and white imigrants in Los Angeles County. Br J Cancer 1991;63:963.

44. Barnes S, Peterson G, Grubbs C, et al. Potential role of dietary isoflavones in the prevention of cancer. In: Jacobs MM, ed. Diet and cancer: markers, prevention, and treatment. New York, Plenum, 1994:135.

45. Lee HP, Gourley L, Duffy SW, et al. Dietary effects on breast cancer risk in Singapore. Lancet 1991;337:1197.

46. Djuric Z, Everett CK, Luongo DA. Toxicity, single-strand breaks, and 5-hydroxymethyl-2′-deoxyuridine formation in human breast epithelial cells treated with hydrogen peroxide. Free Radical Biol Med 1993;14:541.

47. Knekt P. Vitamin E and cancer: epidemiology. Ann NY Acad Sci 1992;669:269.

48. Garland M, Willett WC, Manson JE, et al. Antioxidant micronutrients and breast cancer. J Am Coll Nutr 1993;12:400.

49. Hunter DJ, Manson JE, Colditz GA, et al. A prospective study of the intake of vitamins C, E, and A and the risk of breast cancer. N Engl J Med 1993;329:234.

50. Willett WC, Hunter DJ. Vitamin A and cancers of the breast, large bowel, and prostate: epidemiologic evidence. Nutr Rev 1994;52:S53.

51. Longnecker MP. Alcoholic beverage consumption in relation to risk of breast cancer: meta-analysis and review. Cancer Causes Control 1994;5:73.

52. Schatzkin A, Longnecker MP. Alcohol and breast cancer: where are we now and where do we go from here? Cancer 1994;74:1101.

53. Blot WJ. Alcohol and cancer. Cancer Res 1992;52:2119s.

54. Rosenberg L, Metzger LS, Palmer JR. Alcohol consumption and risk of breast cancer: a review of the epidemiologic evidence. Am J Epidemiol 1993;15:133.

55. Reichman ME, Judd JT, Longscope C, et al. Effects of alcohol consumption on plasma and urinary hormone concentrations in premenopausal women. J Natl Cancer Inst 1993;85:722.

56. Nasca PC, Liu S, Baptiste MS, et al. Alcohol consumption and breast cancer: estrogen receptor status and histology. Am J Epidemiol 1994;140:980.

57. Friedman LA, Kimball AW. Coronary heart disease mortality and alcohol consumption in Framingham. Am J Epidemiol 1986;124:481.

58. Klatsky AL, Friedman GD, Siegelaub AB. Alcohol and mortality: a ten-year Kaiser-Permanente experience. Ann Intern Med 1981;95:139.

59. Thompson HJ. Effect of exercise intensity and duration on the induction of mammary carcinogenesis. Cancer Res 1994;54:1960.

60. Frisch RE, Wyshak G, Albright NL, et al. Lower prevalence of breast cancer and cancers of the reproductive system among former college athletes compared to non-athletes. Br J Cancer 1985;52:885.

61. Paffenbarger RS Jr, Hyde RT, Wing AL. Physical activity and incidence of cancer in diverse populations: a preliminary report. Am J Clin Nutr 1987;45:312.

62. Paffenbarger RS Jr, Lee I-M, Wing AL. The influence of physical activity on the incidence of site-specific cancers in college alumni. In: Jacobs MM, ed. Exercise, calories, fat and cancer. New York, Plenum, 1992:7.

63. Albanes D, Blair A, Taylor PR. Physical activity and risk of cancer in the NHANES I population. Am J Public Health 1989;79:44.

64. Dorgan JF, Brown C, Barrett M, et al. Physical activity and risk of breast cancer in the Framingham Heart Study. Am J Epidemiol 1994;139:662.

65. Vena JE, Graham S, Zielezny M, et al. Occupational exercise and risk of cancer. Am J Clin Nutr 1987;45:318.

66. Pukkala E, Poskiparta M, Apter D, et al. Life-long physical activity and cancer among Finnish female teachers. Eur J Cancer Prevent 1993;2:369.

67. Bernstein L, Henderson BE, Hanisch R, et al. Physical exercise and reduced risk of breast cancer in young women. J Natl Cancer Inst 1994;86:1403.

68. Brinton LA. Ways that women may possibly reduce their risk of breast cancer. J Natl Cancer Inst 1994;86:1371.

69. Lippman SM, Benner SE, Hong WK. Cancer chemoprevention. J Clin Oncol 1994;12:851.

70. Vogel VG. High-risk populations as targets for breast cancer prevention trials. Prev Med 1991;20:86.

71. Nayfield SG, Karp JE, Ford LG, et al. Potential role of tamoxifen in prevention of breast cancer. J Natl Cancer Inst 1991;83:1450.

72. Early Breast Cancer Trialist' Collaborative Group: Systemic treatment of early breast cancer hormonal, cytotoxic, or immune therapy. Lancet 1992;339:1.

73. Andersson M, Storm HH, Mouridsen HT. Carcinogenic effects of adjuvant tamoxifen treatment and radiotherapy for early breast cancer. Acta Oncol 1992;31:259.

74. Vogel VG. Tamoxifen for the prevention of breast cancer. In: DeVita VT Jr, Hellman S, Rosenberg SA, eds. Important advances in oncology, 1995. Philadelphia, JB Lippincott (In press).

75. McDonald CC, Stevens HJ. Fatal myocardial infarction in the Scottish Adjuvant Tamoxifen Trial. BMJ 1991;159:312.

76. Rutqvist LE, Mattson A. Cardiac and thromboembolic morbidity among postmenopausal women with early-stage breast cancer in a randomized trial of adjuvant tamoxifen. J Natl Cancer Inst 1993;85:1398.

77. Bruning PF, Bonfrer JMG, Hart AAM, et al. Tamoxifen, serum lipoproteins and cardiovascular risk. Br J Cancer 1988;58:497.

78. Love RR, Newcomb PA, Wiebe DA, et al. Effects of tamoxifen therapy on lipid and lipoprotein levels in postmenopausal patients with node-negative breast cancer. J Natl Cancer Inst 1990;82:1327.

79. Powles TJ, Hardy JR, Ashley SE, et al. Chemoprevention of breast cancer. Breast Cancer Res Treat 1989;14:23.

80. Bertelli G, Pronzato P, Amoroso D, et al. Adjuvant tamoxifen in primary breast cancer: influence on plasma lipids and antithrombin III levels. Breast Cancer Res Treat 1988;12:307.

81. Sedlacek S. Estrogenic properties of tamoxifen on serum lipids in postmenopausal women with breast cancer. Breast Cancer Res Treat 1989;14:153.

82. Bogdade JD, Wolter J, Subbaiah PR, et al. Effects of tamoxifen treatment on plasma lipids and lipoprotein lipid composition. J Clin Endocrinol Metab 1990;70:1132.

83. Schapira D, Kumar M, Lyman GH. The effect of tamoxifen therapy on serum cholesterol. Proc Am Soc Clin Oncol 1990;9:49.

84. Bush T, Fried LP, Barrett-Connor E. Cholesterol, lipoprotein and coronary heart disease in women. Clin Chem 1988;34:60.

85. Yusuf SA, Wittes J, Friedman L. Overview of results of randomized clinical trials in heart disease. II. Unstable angina, heart failure, primary prevention with aspirin and risk factor modification. JAMA 1988;260:2259.

86. Windler E, Kovanen PT, Chao YS, et al. The estradiol stimulated lipoprotein receptor of rat liver: a binding site that mediates uptake of rat lipoproteins containing apoproteins B and E. J Biol Chem 1980;255:10464.

87. Stacls B, Anwer J, Chan L, et al. Influence of development, estro-

gens, and food intake on apolipoprotein A-I, A-III, and E in RNA in rat liver and intestine. J Lipid Res 1989;30:1137.

88. Love RR, Wiebe DA, Newcomb PA, et al. Effects of tamoxifen on cardiovascular risk factors in postmenopausal women. Ann Intern Med 1991;115:860.

89. Kannel WB, Wolf PA, Castelli WP, et al. Fibrinogen and risk of cardiovascular disease. JAMA 1987;258:1183.

90. Hoffman CJ, Miller RH, Lawson WE, et al. Elevation of factor VII activity and mass in young adults at risk of ischemic heart disease. J Am Coll Cardiol 1989;14:941.

91. Cuzick J, Allen D, Baum M, et al. Long-term effects of tamoxifen: biological effects of tamoxifen working party. Eur J Cancer 1993;29:15.

92. Jordan VC, Phelps E, Lingren JU. Effect of antiestrogens on bone in castrated and intact female rats. Breast Cancer Res Treat 1987;10:31.

93. Turner RT, Wakley GK, Hannon KS, et al. Tamoxifen prevents the skeletal effects of ovarian hormone deficiency in rats. J Bone Miner Res 1987;2:449.

94. Turner R-T, Wakley GK, Hannon KS, et al. Tamoxifen inhibits osteoclastimediated resorption of trabecular bone in ovarian hormone deficient rats. Endocrinology 1988;122:1146.

95. Wakley GK, Hannon KS, Bell NA, et al. The effects of tamoxifen on the osteopenia induced by sciatic neurotomy in the rat: histomorphometric study. Calcif Tissue Int 1988;43:383.

96. Love RR, Mazess RB, Borden HS, et al. Effects of tamoxifen on bone mineral density in postmenopausal women with breast cancer. N Engl J Med 1992;326:852.

97. Kristensen B, Ejlertsen B, Dalgaard P, et al. Tamoxifen and bone metabolism in post-menopausal low-risk breast cancer patients: a randomized study. J Clin Oncol 1994;12:992.

98. Stewart PJ, Stern PH. Effects of the antiestrogens tamoxifen and clomiphene on bone resorption in vitro. Endocrinology 1986;118:125.

99. Fornander T, Rutvqvist LE, Cedermark B, et al. Adjuvant tamoxifen in early breast cancer: occurrence of new primary cancers. Lancet 1989;1:117.

100. Fornander T, Hellstrom A-C, Moberger B: Descriptive clinicopathological study of 17 patients with endometrial cancer during or after adjuvant tamoxifen in early breast cancer. J Natl Cancer Inst 1993;85:1850.

101. Andersson M, Storm HH, Mouridsen HT. Incidence of new primary cancers after adjuvant tamoxifen therapy and radiotherapy for early breast cancer. J Natl Cancer Inst 1991;83:1013.

102. Fisher B, Costantino JP, Redmond CK, et al. Endometrial cancer in tamoxifen-treated breast cancer patients: findings from the National Surgical Adjuvant Breast and Bowel Project (NSABP) B-14. J Natl Cancer Inst 1994;86:527.

103. Hulka BS. Hormone-replacement therapy and the risk of breast cancer. CA Cancer J Clin 1990;40:289.

104. Kelsey JL, Berkowitz GS. Breast cancer epidemiology. Cancer Res 1988;48:5615.

105. Kelsey JL, Gammon MD. Epidemiology of breast cancer. Epidemiol Rev 1990;12:228.

106. Gambrell RD Jr, Maier RC, Sanders BI. Decreased incidence of breast cancer in postmenopausal estrogen–progestogen users. Obstet Gynecol 1983;62:435.

107. Brinton LA, Hoover R, Fraumeni JF Jr. Menopausal estrogens and breast cancer risk: an expanded case-control study. Br J Cancer 1986;54:825.

108. McDonald JA, Weiss NS, Daling JR, et al. Menopausal estrogen use and the risk of breast cancer. Breast Cancer Res Treat 1986;7:193.

109. Bergkvist L, Adami H-O, Person I, et al. The risk of breast cancer after estrogen and estrogen–progestin replacement. N Engl J Med 1989;321:293.

110. Kaufman DW, Palmer JR, de Mouzon J, et al. Estrogen replacement therapy and the risk of breast cancer: results from the case-control surveillance study. Am J Epidemiol 1991;134:1386.

111. Dupont WD, Page DL, Rogers LW, et al. Influence of exogenous estrogens, proliferative breast disease, and other variables on breast cancer risk. Cancer 1989;63:948.

112. Mills PK, Beeson WL, Phillips RL, et al. Prospective study of exogenous hormone use and breast cancer in Seventh-day Adventists. Cancer 1987;64:591.

113. Hunt K, Vessey M. Long-term effects of postmenopausal hormone therapy. Br J Hosp Med 1987;38:450.

114. Barrett–Connor E. Postmenopausal estrogen replacement and breast cancer. N Engl J Med 1989;321:319.

115. Lippman ME, Swain SM. Endocrine-responsive cancers of humans. In: Wilson JD, Foster DW, eds. Williams textbook of endocrinology, ed 8. Philadelphia, WB Saunders, 1992:1577.

116. Steinberg KK, Thacker SB, Smith SJ, et al. A meta-analysis of the effect of estrogen replacement therapy on the risk of breast cancer. JAMA 1991;265:1985.

117. Armstrong BK. Oestrogen therapy after the menopause: boon or bane? Med J Aust 1988;143:213.

118. Dupont WD, Page DL. Menopausal estrogen replacement therapy and breast cancer. Arch Intern Med 1991;151:67.

119. Schlesselman JJ, Stadel BV, Murray P. Breast cancer relation to early use of oral contraceptives: no evidence of a latent effect. JAMA 1988;259:1828.

120. Lipnick RJ, Buring JE, Hennekens CH, et al. Oral contraceptives and breast cancer: a prospective cohort study. JAMA 1986;255:58.

121. Sattin RW, Rubin GL, Wingo PA, et al. Oral-contraceptive use and the risk of breast cancer. N Engl J Med 1986;315:405.

122. Centers for Disease and Control Cancer and Steroid Hormone Study: long-term oral contraceptive use and the risk of breast cancer. JAMA 1983;249:1591.

123. Carr BR. Disorders of the ovary and female reproductive tract. In: Wilson JD, Foster DW, eds. Williams textbook of endocrinology, ed 8. Philadelphia, WB Saunders, 1992:733.

124. Barrett-Connor E, Bush TJ. Estrogen and coronary heart disease in women. JAMA 1991;265:1861.

125. Paganini-Hill A, Ross RK, Henderson BE. Postmenopausal oestrogen treatment and stroke: a prospective study. Br Med J 1988;297:519.

126. Grady D, Rubin SM, Petitti DB, et al. Hormone therapy to prevent disease and prolong life in postmenopausal women. Ann Intern Med 1992;117:1016.

127. Ettinger B, Genant HK, Conn CE. Postmenopausal bone loss is prevented by treatment with low-dose estrogen with calcium. Ann Intern Med 1987;106:40.

128. Kiel DP, Felson DT, Anderson JJ, et al. Hip fracture and the use of estrogens in postmenopausal women. N Engl J Med 1987;317:1169.

129. Henderson BE, Ross R, Bernstein L. Estrogens as a cause of human cancer: the Richard and Hinda Rosenthal Foundation Award Lecture. Cancer Res 1988;48:246.

130. Bernstein L, Ross RK, Henderson BE. Prospects for the primary prevention of breast cancer. Am J Epidemiol 1992;135:142.

131. Warren MP, Brooks-Gunn J, Hamilton LH, et al. Scoliosis and fractures in young ballet dancers: relation to delayed menarche and secondary amenorrhea. N Engl J Med 1986;314:1348.

132. Spicer D, Pike MC, Henderson BE. The question of estrogen replacement therapy in patients with a prior diagnosis of breast cancer. Oncology 1990;4:49.

133. Stoll BA. Hormone replacement therapy in women treated for breast cancer. Eur J Cancer Clin Oncol 1989;25:1909.

134. Theriault RL, Sellin RV. A clinical dilemma: estrogen replacement therapy in postmenopausal women with a background of primary breast cancer. Ann Oncol 1991;2:709.

135. Cobleigh MA, Berris RF, Bush T, et al. Estrogen replacement therapy in breast cancer survivors: a time for change. JAMA 1994;272:540.

136. American College of Physicians. Guidelines for counseling post-menopausal women about preventive hormone therapy. Ann Intern Med 1992;117:1038.

137. Lerman C, Schwartz M. Adherence and psychological adjustment among women at high risk for breast cancer. Breast Cancer Research Treat 1993;28:145.

138. Lynch HT, Watson P. Genetic counseling and hereditary breast/ovarian cancer. Lancet 1992;339:1181.

139. Vogel VG. Counseling the high risk woman. In: Stoll BA, ed. Reducing breast cancer risk in women. Boston, Kluwer Academic, 1995:69.

140. Miller SM. When is a little knowledge a dangerous thing? Coping with stressful events by monitoring versus blunting. In: Levine S, Ursin H, eds. Coping and health: proceedings of a NATO Conference. New York, Plenum, 1980:145.

141. Kash JM, Holland JC, Halper MS, et al. Psychological distress and surveillance behaviors of women with a family history of breast cancer. J Natl Cancer Inst 1992;84:24.

142. Alagna SW, Morokoff PJ, Bevett JM, et al. Performance of breast self-examination by women at high risk for breast cancer. Women Health 1987;12:29.

143. Lerman C, Rimer B, Trock B, et al. Factors associated with repeat adherence to breast cancer screening. Prev Med 1990;19:279.

144. Vernon SW, Vogel VG, Halabi S, et al. Factors associated with perceived risk of breast cancer among women attending a screening program. Breast Cancer Research Treat 1993;28:137.

145. Lynch HT, Watson P, Conway TA, et al. DNA screening for breast/ovarian susceptibility based on linked markers. Arch Intern Med 1993;153:1979.

146. Lerman C, Daly M, Masny A, et al. Attitudes about genetic testing for breast–ovarian cancer susceptibility. J Clin Oncol 1994;12:843.

147. Lerman C, Croyle R. Psychological issues in genetic testing for breast cancer susceptibility. Arch Intern Med 1994;154:609.

148. Lewis FM, Ellison ES, Woods NF. The impact of breast cancer on the family. Semin Oncol Nurs 1985;1:206.

11

Diseases of the Breast, edited by Jay R. Harris,
Marc E. Lippman, Monica Morrow, and Samuel Hellman.
Lippincott-Raven Publishers, Philadelphia, © 1996.

In Situ Carcinomas

11.1
Ductal Carcinoma in Situ

MONICA MORROW ▪ STUART J. SCHNITT ▪ JAY R. HARRIS

Ductal carcinoma in situ (DCIS), also known as intraductal carcinoma, is an entity distinct in both its clinical presentation and its biologic potential from lobular carcinoma in situ (LCIS), the other lesion classified as noninvasive carcinoma. Previously, DCIS was an uncommon lesion that was routinely cured by mastectomy, and little attention was given to defining its natural history or exploring alternative local treatments. The widespread use of screening mammography has resulted in a significant increase in the detection rate of DCIS, and the acceptance of breast-conserving therapy for the treatment of invasive carcinoma has raised questions about the routine need for mastectomy in a lesion that may only be precancerous. This combination of factors has made the management of DCIS one of the most widely debated issues in breast cancer therapy.

Presentation and Incidence

Ductal carcinoma in situ has various clinical presentations. In the past, most DCIS was gross or palpable. Gross DCIS accounts for only a small percentage of palpable breast cancers. An American College of Surgeons survey found only 2% of 10,000 ductal and lobular cancers reported in 1980 to be DCIS.[1] DCIS also presents as pathologic nipple discharge, with or without a mass, or can be identified as an incidental finding in a breast biopsy done to treat or identify another abnormality. Today, an abnormal mammographic result is the most common presentation of DCIS. DCIS usually appears as clustered microcalcifica-

tions, although nonpalpable masses may also represent DCIS. In many reports of mammographically directed biopsies, DCIS accounts for half or more of the malignancies identified.[2–5]

The use of screening mammography has resulted in a remarkable increase in the incidence of DCIS. Between 1979 and 1986, the incidence of DCIS in women aged 50 years and older increased 235%, compared with a 50% increase in the incidence of localized breast cancer.[6] For women under age 50 years, a 138% increase in the incidence of DCIS occurred during the same period.

Pathology

Ductal carcinoma in situ is characterized by a proliferation of presumably malignant epithelial cells within the mammary ductal-lobular system, without light microscopic evidence of invasion into the surrounding stroma.

CLASSIFICATION

The term *ductal carcinoma in situ* encompasses a pathologically heterogeneous group of lesions that differ in their growth pattern and cytologic features. In the traditional system for classifying DCIS, based primarily on the architectural pattern of the lesion, the most common types are designated comedo, cribriform, micropapillary, papillary, and solid.[7–9]

Comedo-type DCIS is characterized by prominent ne-

FIGURE 11.1-1 Comedo-type ductal carcinoma in situ. **A.** Prominent central necrosis and an area of coarse calcification (*arrow*) exist in this involved space. **B.** The cells constituting this lesion show considerable nuclear atypicality and nuclear pleomorphism, and mitotic figures are evident (*arrows*). Lesions of this type can also been classified as poorly differentiated ductal carcinoma in situ.[33]

crosis in the involved spaces (Fig. 11.1-1), which can often be appreciated on macroscopic examination as cords of pasty material exuding from the cut surface of the specimen or readily expressed from involved ducts by palpation. Microscopically, the cells of comedo DCIS are large and show nuclear pleomorphism. Mitotic figures, including abnormal mitoses, are usually evident and are often numerous. Many of the involved spaces contain necrotic cellular debris within their centers. This necrotic material frequently becomes calcified, and these calcifications may be detected mammographically, appearing characteristi-

cally as linear, branching (casting), and coarse granular calcifications.

Cribriform-type DCIS is characterized by a fenestrated, sieve-like growth pattern. The cells comprising this type of DCIS are typically small to medium in size and have relatively uniform hyperchromatic nuclei. Mitoses are relatively infrequent, and necrosis is limited to single cells or small cell clusters (Fig. 11.1-2). *Micropapillary-type* DCIS features small tufts of cells that are oriented perpendicular to the basement membrane of the involved spaces and that project into the lumina. The apical region of these small

FIGURE 11.1-2 Cribriform type ductal carcinoma in situ. **A.** The cells that make up this lesion grow in a fenestrated, sievelike pattern. Scattered, fine calcifications are present (*arrows*). **B.** The tumor cell nuclei are small and relatively uniform in shape and chromatin pattern. There is no mitotic activity. A single small calcification is present (*arrow*). Lesions of this type can also be classified as well differentiated ductal carcinoma in situ.[33]

FIGURE 11.1-3 Micropapillary ductal carcinoma in situ. **A.** The tumor cells form tufts that project into the lumens of the involved spaces. These tufts lack fibrovascular cores. **B.** The nuclei of the tumor cells are small and monomorphic. Lesions such as this can also be considered examples of well-differentiated ductal carcinoma in situ.[33]

papillations is frequently broader than the base, imparting a club-shaped appearance. The micropapillare lack fibrovascular cores. The cells constituting micropapillary DCIS are usually small to medium sized, and the nuclei show diffuse hyperchromasia. Mitotic figures are infrequent (Fig. 11.1-3). *Papillary* DCIS shows intraluminal projections of tumor cells that, unlike the micropapillary variant, show fibrovascular cores and thus constitute true papillations. In one variant of papillary DCIS, the tumor cells are primarily or exclusively present in a single cystically dilated space (intracystic papillary carcinoma).[10,11] In the *solid* type of DCIS, the tumor cells fill and distend the involved spaces and lack significant necrosis, fenestration, or papillations. Cytologically, the tumor cells may be large, medium, or small. The solid type is the least well defined of these subtypes. Less common variants of DCIS include "clinging" carcinoma,[7,12] intraductal signet-ring cell carcinoma,[13] and cystic hypersecretory duct carcinoma.[14,15] Similar to the comedo type, other DCIS variants may show calcifications that can be detected mammographi-

cally; however, the mammographic appearance of the microcalcifications associated with noncomedo DCIS is less distinctive than the pattern of calcifications seen in comedo lesions and overlaps with that of a number of benign processes.

Some authors believe it is useful to subdivide DCIS into two subgroups—the comedo type and the noncomedo type (which encompasses the other variants). This preference is based on the observation that comedo DCIS appears more malignant cytologically,[7–9] is more often associated with microinvasion,[16–18] and more often exhibits biologic markers indicative of high-grade malignant lesions than do the other types. For example, comedo lesions more frequently lack estrogen receptors,[19] have a high proliferative rate,[20] and exhibit aneuploidy,[21] overexpression of the HER2/*neu* (c-*erb*B-2) oncogene,[22–24] mutations of the p53 tumor suppressor gene with accumulation of its protein product,[25,26] and angiogenesis in the surrounding stroma.[27] Another difference reported for these two groups concerns the relation between the extent of mammographically evident microcalcifications and the histologic extent of the lesion. Using standard two-view mammography, the histologic extent of comedo DCIS correlates highly with the extent of the mammographically detected calcifications in most cases. In contrast, the mammographic extent of the calcifications associated with non-comedo DCIS frequently underestimates the pathologic extent of the lesion.[28] A recent study has indicated, however, that when standard mammographic images are supplemented with magnification views, a much better correlation exists between the extent of mammographic calcifications and the histologic extent of the lesion, even for noncomedo DCIS lesions.[29]

Unfortunately, both the traditional classification system and the dichotomous comedo–noncomedo classification system are oversimplifications because some DCIS lesions do not fit neatly into any of the described categories. For example, some DCIS lesions with small, uniform, low-grade nuclei display central comedo-type necrosis in the involved spaces, whereas others with cribriform, micro-

papillary, or papillary architectural patterns may be composed of cytologically malignant cells that exhibit large, high-grade nuclei. Further, some examples of DCIS have nuclear features intermediate between those of low- and high-grade lesions (Fig. 11.1-4). Classification of DCIS is further complicated by the fact that, in any one case, several patterns may coexist, particularly among larger lesions.[17] For example, in one study of 100 consecutive cases of DCIS reviewed in a consultation practice, 23 of 76 noncomedo lesions (30%) showed a mixture of histologic patterns, the most common being cribriform and micropapillary. Of 24 lesions with comedo DCIS, 10 (42%) also contained areas of noncomedo DCIS.[30]

A number of alternative classification schemes have been proposed in an attempt to overcome the limitations of the traditional classification system. Lagios and colleagues[31] proposed a system based primarily on nuclear grade. These investigators classify DCIS into one of four categories: comedo, cribriform with necrosis, cribriform with anaplasia, and micropapillary–cribriform. In this clas-

FIGURE 11.1-4 This example of ductal carcinoma in situ has a cribriform growth pattern (**A**), but, at higher power, (**B**), it shows more nuclear atypicality than the cribriform lesion in Figure 11.1-2. This type of lesion is an example of intermediately differentiated ductal carcinoma in situ.[33]

sification scheme, lesions categorized as comedo and cribriform with necrosis are both characterized by large cells with high-grade, pleomorphic nuclei and areas of comedo-type necrosis. These two types differ only in the architectural pattern of the viable tumor cells, which is solid in the former group and papillary or cribriform in the latter. The cribriform with anaplasia lesions are composed of large but more uniform cells with moderate nuclear atypia, a prominent cribriform pattern, and little or no necrosis.

Micropapillary–cribriform lesions are characterized by small cells with uniform nuclei, a micropapillary or cribriform growth pattern, and no necrosis. Investigators in Nottingham, England, developed a classification system for DCIS based primarily on the presence or absence of necrosis.[32] This group divides DCIS into three categories: pure comedo (lesions in which involved spaces show centrally necrotic debris surrounded by large, pleomorphic tumor cells in solid masses); DCIS with necrosis, also called nonpure comedo (lesions with necrotic neoplastic cells but with a cribriform or micropapillary pattern); and DCIS without necrosis (lesions with a cribriform papillary, micropapillary, or solid pattern and no necrosis). Finally, a group of European pathologists associated with the European Organization for Research and Treatment of Cancer (EORTC)[33] proposed classifying DCIS as well, intermediately, or poorly differentiated, based primarily on cytonuclear differentiation. Although these classification systems use different terminology, they have in common the recognition of three main categories of DCIS (ie, high, intermediate, and low grade) and they appear to be easily transposable (Table 11.1-1). The relative merits of these various classification systems with regard to their interobserver reproducibility and, more importantly, clinical utility, remain to be established. Ultimately, a classification system that includes both histologic features and molecular markers of biologic behavior may be necessary to provide the most clinically meaningful information about DCIS lesions.

Distribution of Tumor in the Breast and Axillary Lymph Node Involvement

The distribution of tumor in the breast, the incidence of unsuspected invasive carcinoma, and the incidence of axillary lymph node metastases are all important considera-tions in selecting appropriate therapy for patients with DCIS.

The reported incidence of multicentricity in mastectomy specimens from patients with DCIS varies considerably and has ranged from 9% to 47%.[34] Several factors have contributed to this variability, including differences in the definition of multicentricity and in the methods and extent of specimen sampling. Most authors define *multicentricity* as foci of DCIS in breast quadrants other than that harboring the index lesion (in contrast to *multifocality*, which denotes foci of DCIS in the same quadrant as the index lesion). Others define foci as multicentric if they are a specified distance from the index lesion (eg, 5 cm), regardless of the quadrant.[34] These studies of multicentricity were conducted before the widespread use of screening mammography, and it is unlikely that these data can be extrapolated to the small (often less than 1 cm), mammographically detected lesions commonly seen today. In these studies, the frequency of multicentricity appears to be related to the size of the index lesion. In one study, multicentricity was much more common in DCIS lesions larger than 2.5 cm (13 of 25 cases, 52%) than in smaller lesions (4 of 29 cases, 14%).[35] In another study, the frequency of multicentricity also correlated with the size of the lesion as determined by the number of involved ducts in the index lesion.[18] These investigators also noted a higher frequency of multicentricity in micropapillary lesions (8 of 10 cases, 80%) than in other types of DCIS (16 of 45 cases, 36%).[17] A similar association between micropapillary DCIS and frequent multiple quadrant involvement has also been recognized by others.[36] Because of the sampling methods used, however, it is not possible to determine whether the foci of DCIS characterized as multicentric in these studies are truly independent lesions or if they represent tumor that is, in fact, contiguous with the index lesion.

More recent studies suggest that, in most cases, true multicentricity in DCIS is rare. Holland and Hendriks[29] studied 119 mastectomy specimens containing DCIS by a subgross pathologic–mammographic technique. In all but one case, the tumor was confined to a single "segment" of the breast. Clear-cut multicentric distribution (defined in this study as foci of DCIS separated by 4 cm or more of uninvolved breast tissue) was found in only one patient. In another study using stereomicroscopic three-dimensional analysis to define the growth pattern of DCIS within the mammary duct system, Faverly and colleagues[37] studied 60 mastectomy specimens containing DCIS. They found that, within the segment of breast involved by DCIS, growth was continuous in some cases and discontinuous in others. Overall, half of cases showed a continuous growth pattern, and half showed a discontinuous pattern, characterized by uninvolved breast tissue between foci of DCIS (gaps). In most instances, these gaps were small (less than 5 mm in 82% of cases), and the likelihood of finding such gaps was related to the histologic type of the lesion. Although 90% of the cases of poorly differentiated DCIS grew in a continuous manner without gaps, only 30% of well-differentiated lesions and 45% of intermediately differentiated lesions were continuous. The

TABLE 11.1-1
Comparison of Recently Proposed Classification Systems for Ductal Carcinoma in Situ (DCIS)

Lagios et al[31]	Nottingham[32]	EORTC[33]
Micropapillary/ cribriform	DCIS without necrosis	Well differentiated
Cribriform with anaplasia	DCIS with necrosis (nonpure comedo)	Intermediately differentiated
Comedo/cribriform with necrosis	Comedo	Poorly differentiated

findings in these two studies indicate that, in most cases, DCIS involves the breast in a segmental distribution and that truly multicentric disease is uncommon. In some cases, however, the segment involved by DCIS may be large. For example, in the study of Holland and Hendriks,[29] although 86% of the DCIS lesions were nonpalpable and were detected mammographically, 46% were larger than 3 cm. A recent study of clonality in DCIS supports these conclusions, at least with regard to comedo lesions.[38] In that study, clonality was assessed in widely separated sites of comedo-type DCIS in the same breast. These widely separated sites were each found to be monoclonal, and each showed inactivation of the same X chromosome–linked phosphoglycerokinase allele, suggesting origin from the same clone.

The incidence of nipple involvement in patients with DCIS has been evaluated in few studies and appears to be related to the method of lesion detection. For example, among patients with DCIS presenting primarily with a palpable mass, nipple discharge, or Paget disease, Contesso and colleagues[39] found nipple involvement in 49% of 117 mastectomy specimens. In contrast, among 40 mastectomy specimens from patients with DCIS, most of whom presented with either mammographic calcifications or DCIS as an incidental finding, Lagios and colleagues[35] found involvement of the nipple in 8 cases (20%). This consisted of Paget disease in 5 cases and of lactiferous duct involvement in 3.

The incidence of occult invasion, either near the primary tumor or in other parts of the breast, has also been examined in mastectomy series. The reported incidence of occult invasion ranges from 0% to 26%[34]; however, these series are difficult to interpret for several reasons. The completeness of initial biopsy varies, and this variation affects the likelihood of finding residual cancer with invasion during mastectomy if the initial biopsy shows only noninvasive disease. Also, the extent of sampling of the initial biopsy specimen and of the remainder of the breast also differs substantially from series to series. The likelihood of finding occult invasion appears to be related to the size of the index lesion. In one series, patients with lesions larger than 2.5 cm were more likely to have occult invasion (16 of 55, or 29%) than were patients with smaller tumors (1 of 60, or 2%).[31] However, all four invasive tumors in the 90 patients with lesions 4.5 cm or smaller were found after inadequate initial excision. The frequency of occult invasion is also related to the method of DCIS detection. In one series, invasive cancer was identified in the mastectomy specimens of 6 of 54 patients (11%) with DCIS who presented with a palpable mass, nipple discharge, or Paget disease and in 1 of 16 patients who presented with mammographic microcalcifications or DCIS as an incidental finding.[40] In another series, 6 of 41 tumors (15%) that presented with a mass had occult invasion, compared with only 1 of 21 tumors (5%) detected only mammographically.[41] The incidence of occult invasion also appears to correlate with the histologic type of DCIS, being much more common in comedo-type lesions. For example, Patchefsky and colleagues[17] noted microinvasion in 12 of 19 (63%) comedo DCIS lesions and in only 4 of 36 (11%) noncomedo lesions.

About 1% of patients have axillary lymph node metastases when no evidence of stromal invasion is identified by light microscopic examination.[34] In such cases, invasion is undoubtedly present but either is not recognized by the pathologist or is undetected because of sampling error. Incidence rates reported for axillary nodal involvement in patients given the diagnosis of DCIS range from 0% to 7%,[7] with the higher rates noted in studies done during the premammographic era, when most patients with DCIS presented with palpable masses. In a recent series of 189 patients with DCIS, most of whose tumors were detected by mammography alone, none showed metastases on axillary dissection.[42]

Differential Diagnosis

In most instances, the pathologic diagnosis is straightforward, but occasional cases present diagnostic difficulties. At one end of the spectrum, low-grade (noncomedo) DCIS may sometimes be difficult to distinguish from atypical ductal hyperplasia. Although several authors have published criteria useful in making this distinction, some cases are subject to considerable interobserver variability in diagnosis, even with use of standardized criteria.[43,44] This issue is discussed in detail in Chapter 3.1.

At the other end of the spectrum, examples of pure DCIS may sometimes be difficult to distinguish from DCIS with focal stromal invasion (microinvasion) because of sampling error, distortion of the involved spaces by fibrosis or inflammation, or extension of DCIS into lobules (cancerization of lobules). Unfortunately, no universally accepted histologic criteria exist for the diagnosis of microinvasion. Fisher and colleagues[45] consider invasion to be present only when "unquestionable foci of well-recognized types of invasive carcinoma" are present.[45] Others restrict the diagnosis of invasion to cases in which tumor cells are present in stroma outside the immediate periductal or perilobular regions.[8] Although both electron microscopy and immunohistochemical staining for basement membrane proteins such as type IV collagen and laminin have been used to identify areas of invasion in DCIS, the practical value of these techniques for this purpose has not been clearly established.[46–48]

It may also be difficult to distinguish DCIS from frankly invasive breast cancer, because some breast cancers invade the stroma in rounded nests simulating DCIS (eg, invasive cribriform carcinoma).[49,50] Another less common diagnostic problem arises when one must distinguish nests of tumor cells in lymphatic or vascular spaces from DCIS.

Finally, although the distinction between DCIS and LCIS is usually not difficult to make, areas of overlap exist between these two lesions. As indicated, DCIS may extend into recognizable lobules,[51,52] LCIS may involve extralobular ducts,[53] and some lesions have cytologic features intermediate between the two disorders.[8,9] Further, DCIS and

LCIS may coexist in the same breast and even in the same ductal-lobular unit.[54]

Natural History

The major issue in the management of DCIS is the risk for progression to invasive carcinoma. Few clinically relevant data are available to address this question, primarily because DCIS has traditionally been treated with mastectomy. In addition, most DCIS treated in the past for which long-term follow-up is available was gross DCIS, a form that may not be equivalent to the mammographic DCIS more commonly seen today.

Long-term follow-up data are available for several small series of women found to have DCIS on review of biopsy specimens that were originally classified as benign. No attempt was made to assess margin status in these studies, and the completeness of excision remains uncertain. Page and associates[55] identified 25 such cases in a review of 11,760 breast biopsies. Invasive carcinoma developed in seven women (28%) at intervals of 3 to 10 years (mean 6.1 years) post biopsy. This incidence of carcinoma represents a relative risk of 11 compared with age-matched controls from the Third National Cancer Survey for white women in Atlanta. In a similar study, Rosen and colleagues[56] described 30 women with untreated DCIS, with complete follow-up available for only 15. Seven invasive cancers occurred at a mean of 9.7 years after the diagnosis of DCIS, an incidence of 27% if all cases are included, or 53% if only patients with complete follow-up are considered. In both the reports, all carcinomas were in the index breast, usually in the vicinity of the biopsy site. In a similar report, Eusebi and coworkers[12] described 28 cases of DCIS with a 11% incidence of invasive carcinoma at a median follow-up of 16.7 years. Eusebi and colleagues[57] subsequently reported on 80 cases of DCIS followed for a mean of 17.5 years, only 2 of which were high grade. Eleven patients developed invasive carcinoma, and 5 had recurrent DCIS, for a total recurrence rate of 20%. The risk for invasive carcinoma was twice that in the general population. Most cases included in all these studies were low-grade, noncomedo lesions, representing one extreme of the histologic spectrum of DCIS.

Further information on the natural history of DCIS can be obtained from autopsy studies. Alpers and Wellings[58] examined a series of 185 randomly selected breasts from 101 women examined by a subgross sampling technique. One or more foci of DCIS were found in 11 cases (6%). This finding was unrelated to age, with DCIS identified in 3 of 56 women (5%) 49 years of age or younger, in 7 of 70 women (10%) between the ages of 50 and 69 years, and in 1 of 59 women older than 70 years. In a study with similar methodology, Bartow and associates[59] examined the breasts of 519 women aged 14 years or older. Only one case of DCIS was identified, and five occult invasive carcinomas were found. An autopsy study from Denmark reported by Andersen and coworkers[60] found DCIS in 11 of 86 breasts examined (13%). As a group, these studies indicate that some, but not all, cases of DCIS progress to invasive carcinoma.

Treatment Options

The uncertainty about the natural history of DCIS has resulted in a wide range of treatments, ranging from excision alone to mastectomy. Making comparisons among reports is difficult because of differences in patient populations, lack of standardization of surgical and radiotherapeutic techniques, and changes in treatment practice over time.

Mastectomy is a curative treatment for about 98% of patients with DCIS, whether gross or mammographic.[61-64] Representative studies are summarized in Table 11.1-2. It is apparent that most of the series consist of relatively small numbers of patients followed for variable periods. In general, however, patients with initial biopsies that showed DCIS, but who later had invasive carcinoma identified in the mastectomy specimens, were excluded from these reports. This consideration is important when comparing survival after different methods of local therapy. The reported incidence of microinvasion after a biopsy showing DCIS varies. Silverstein and colleagues[16] reported on 208 intraductal carcinomas, 35% of which were detected mammographically. Microinvasion was found in 28% of cases. Microinvasion was seen in association with larger lesions, with only 4 of 82 tumors (5%) less than 1 cm in diameter having associated microinvasion compared with 24 of 126 tumors (19%) more than 1 cm in diameter. The mean tumor size for lesions with microinvasion was 3.8 cm, and 75% of the tumors that exhibited microinvasion were of the comedo subtype. In contrast, Rosen and coworkers[65] identified occult foci of invasive carcinoma in only 3 of 53 mastectomy specimens (6%) after a biopsy showing DCIS. These findings suggest that some women with DCIS treated with a breast-sparing approach will be understaged because of failure to identify occult foci of microinvasive carcinoma. Although more accurate staging may be responsible for some of the differences in recurrence and survival rates between women undergoing mastectomy and those treated with a breast-sparing approach, the ability to identify clinically occult foci of invasive carcinoma is one of the advantages of the treatment of DCIS by mastectomy.

Mastectomy is a highly effective treatment for DCIS, but it is a radical approach to a lesion that may not progress to invasive carcinoma during the patient's lifetime. It seems somewhat paradoxical that a woman with a palpable invasive carcinoma should be able to preserve her breast, whereas the "reward" for screening and early detection is a mastectomy. For this reason, breast-preserving approaches for DCIS (including excision alone and excision plus radiotherapy) have been studied.

Several investigators have examined the use of excision alone as a treatment for DCIS (Table 11.1-3). In general, patients treated with this approach are highly selected, usually on the basis of low histologic grade or small tumor

TABLE 11.1-2
Results of Treatment of Ductal Carcinoma in Situ With Simple Mastectomy

Investigators	Years	Patients	Follow-Up	Nonpalpable (%)	Recurrences
Von Rueden & Wilson[61]	1960–1981	45		7	0
Sunshine et al[62]	1960–1980	70	10 y	—	3
Schuh et al[64]	1965–1984	52	5.5 y	33	1
Silverstein et al[16]	1979–1989	97★	45 mo	35	2
Kinne et al[63]	1970–1976	82	11.5 y	—	1

★ Includes microinvasion.

size. The percentage of patients with DCIS in the study population meeting these selection criteria is usually not stated, making it unclear how many women with DCIS are candidates for this type of treatment. Lagios and colleagues[31] described 79 women with DCIS 25 mm or smaller (mean size, 6.8 mm) who were treated with wide excision alone. Thirteen local recurrences (16%) were noted at a mean of 124 months of follow-up. Six of the recurrences were invasive carcinoma, and 7 were DCIS.[66] Schwartz and coworkers[67] reported on 72 cases of DCIS treated by excision alone. Two thirds of the cases were detected as mammographic calcifications and one third as incidental findings. The patients were accrued between 1978 and 1990, indicating the highly selected nature of the population. All of the tumors measured less than 2.5 cm in greatest dimension, and reexcision was routinely used. At a mean follow-up of 49 months, 11 patients (15%) have had locally recurrent disease. In contrast, a 43% recurrence rate was noted at a mean follow-up of 85 months for 22 patients treated by local excision alone as part of NSABP Protocol BO6.[68] These women were initially diagnosed as having invasive carcinoma and were later reclassified as having DCIS. Only one of these cases was nonpalpable cancer, and tumor size averaged 2.2 ±

1.3 cm. These wide variations in local failure rates emphasize the importance of patient selection when attempting to treat women with DCIS by excision alone. In general, studies of the management of DCIS with excision alone show that, when local failure occurs, DCIS is present in about half the cases and invasive carcinoma in the other half.[31,66–73] The time course to local failure is prolonged, with studies with longer follow-up showing higher local failure rates. In the report of Gallagher and coworkers,[69] the median time to local failure was 47 months, and 4 of 8 patients monitored for more than 9 years had recurrent disease, emphasizing the importance of long-term follow-up.

Radiation therapy has been combined with excision in an attempt to improve local control in women with DCIS treated using a breast-conserving approach.[73–78] Solin and associates[74] reported the results of 259 women with 261 breasts treated with excision and irradiation at nine institutions in Europe and the United States. At a median follow-up of 78 months (range, 11 to 197 months), 28 failures were observed. The 10-year actuarial rate of local failure was 16%, and half of the failures represented invasive carcinoma. The median time to local failure was 50 months (range, 17 to 129 months), and the 10-year actuarial breast

TABLE 11.1-3
Results of Treatment of Ductal Carcinoma in Situ With Excision Alone

Investigators	Patients	Follow-Up (mo)	Recurrence	Invasive (%)
Arnesson et al[72]	38	60★	5 (13%)	40
Carpenter et al[71]	28	38†	5 (18%)	20
Lagios et al[31]	79	124†	13 (16%)	46
Schwartz et al[67]	72	49†	11 (15%)	27
Silverstein et al[70]	26	56★	2 (8%)	50
Fisher et al (B06)[68]	21	83†	9 (43%)	56
Fisher et al (B17)[73]	391	43†	64 (16%)	50

★ Median.
† Mean.

TABLE 11.1-4
Results of Treatment of Ductal Carcinoma in Situ with Excision and Radiation Therapy

Investigators	Patients	Follow-Up (mo)	Recurrences	Invasive (%)
Hiramatsu et al[75]	76	74★	7 (9%)	57
McCormick et al[76]	54	36★	10 (18%)	30
Ray et al[77]	56	67†	5 (9%)	20
Silverstein et al[70]	103	56★	10 (10%)	50
Solin et al[74]	261	78★	28 (9.3%)	50
Stotter et al[78]	42	92★	4 (9%)	100
Fisher et al (B06)[68]	27	83†	2 (7%)	50
Fisher et al (B17)[73]	399	43†	28 (7%)	40

★ Median.

† Mean.

cancer specific survival rate was 97%. Gross excision of the tumor was done in all cases, but only 15% underwent reexcision, and margin status was unknown in 120 cases (46%). The median whole breast dose delivered was 5000 cGy, and 164 of 261 cases (63%) received a boost to the primary tumor site. This study is noteworthy for the large number of patients and relatively long duration of follow-up. Despite variations in patient selection and technical details of surgery and radiation, the local failure rate was low. Other studies of excision and radiation are summarized in Table 11.1-4. The local recurrence rate after excision and radiation therapy is approximately 50% lower than the recurrence rate after excision alone. The pattern of recurrence is similar, with invasive carcinoma seen in half of recurrences, and most recurrent disease is at or adjacent to the site of the primary tumor (true recurrence or marginal miss). The time course to recurrence is protracted, with recurrences occurring at a steady rate throughout the follow-up period (Fig. 11.1-5).

Two studies from the NSABP have described treatment outcomes in women with DCIS who were randomized to receive excision alone or excision plus radiation therapy.[68,73] Protocol BO6[68] (discussed in the section on local treatment of invasive carcinoma) was designed to evaluate the local therapy of invasive carcinoma. On review of pathologic material, 78 patients with DCIS alone were identified. At a follow-up of 83 months, 12 of the 27 patients (7%) treated with irradiation and 9 of the 21 patients (43%) treated with lumpectomy alone had local failures. No local failures occurred in the 28 women treated with mastectomy. The NSABP has also reported the initial results of a prospective study designed to evaluate the role of radiation therapy in DCIS.[73] In this study, 818 women were randomized to excision alone or excision plus 5000 cGy of irradiation to the breast. Histologically negative surgical margins were required in both groups. Eighty percent of the women in the study had tumors detected by mammographic screening. At a median follow-up of 43 months, event-free survival was sig-

nificantly higher among women receiving irradiation (84% compared with 74%; $P = .001$). This difference was due to a 58.8% reduction in the annual incidence of ipsilateral breast cancer recurrence in the irradiated group. Sixty-four cancer recurrences (16%) were seen in the group receiving excision alone, and 28 recurrences (7%) occurred in the patients receiving radiation therapy. Although the incidence of both invasive and intraductal carcinoma was

FIGURE 11.1-5 Actuarial risk of local failure in 261 cases of ductal carcinoma in situ treated with excision and radiotherapy. The number at risk is the number of treated breasts at risk by 1-year intervals. (Solin LJ, Recht A, Fourquet A, et al. Ten-year results of breast-conserving surgery and definitive irradiation for intraductal carcinoma [ductal carcinoma in situ] of the breast. Cancer 1991;68:2340)

reduced by radiation (Fig. 11.1-6), the benefit of radiation was most evident for invasive recurrences. The 5-year cumulative incidence of recurrent invasive carcinoma was reduced from 10.5% to 2.9%, whereas the cumulative incidence of recurrent DCIS at 5 years was reduced from 10.4% to 7.5%. No difference in the incidence of contralateral breast carcinoma was noted between groups. Although the early results of this trial clearly indicate a reduction in the risk for breast cancer recurrence with radiation, longer follow-up is needed to determine whether this difference persists over time.

Because half of the local failures seen after breast-conserving therapy for intraductal carcinoma are invasive carcinoma, the outcome of salvage treatment of these recurrences is important. Solin and coworkers[79] described 42 cases of local failure in 274 cases of DCIS treated with excision plus irradiation. The median time to local failure was 5.1 years, and the median follow-up after salvage treatment was 3.7 years. Nineteen of the recurrences (45%) were intraductal carcinoma, and 14 of these were detected with mammographic findings alone. All of the women with intraductal recurrences remain free of disease after mastectomy with a median follow-up of 4.7 years. Five patients with invasive recurrence have developed distant metastases, either simultaneously with the recurrence (1 patient) or subsequently (4 patients). Chest wall recurrences were seen in three patients who had salvage mastectomy for an invasive recurrence, and all of these women developed distant metastases. Of the entire group of 42 women with recurrence, 36 patients (86%) were alive and free of disease, 4 patients (10%) died of disease, 1 patient is alive with disease and 1 patient died of other causes. Similarly high rates of salvage have been reported in other studies[68,73,80]; however, the ultimate breast cancer mortality resulting from breast preservation cannot yet be assessed. The 42 cases of recurrence reported by Solin and colleagues[78] occurred in a study population with a median follow-up of 78 months. Forty percent of the recurrences reported were seen between 5 and 10 years after treatment, and an additional 12% occurred after 10 years, indicating that a significant risk of further local recurrence exists among these women. In addition, the median follow-up after salvage therapy was only 3.7 years, too short an interval to determine the eventual risk of distant metastases.

PREDICTIVE FACTORS FOR TREATMENT SELECTION

It is apparent from the preceding discussion that identification of women with a high risk for developing invasive carcinoma after breast-conserving therapy for apparently localized DCIS would be extremely helpful. We are presently unable to differentiate tumors that will recur as invasive carcinoma from those that will recur as DCIS. Some studies have suggested, however, that infiltrating carcinoma that develops after high-grade DCIS is more likely to be poorly differentiated and associated with poor prognosis than infiltrating carcinoma that develops after low-grade DCIS.[57,81] Histologic subtype and grade of DCIS

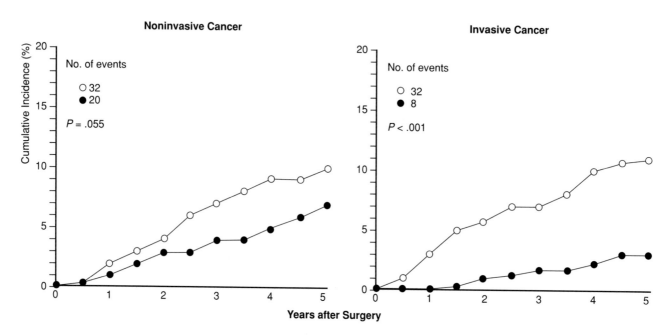

FIGURE 11.1-6 Cumulative incidence of noninvasive and invasive ipsilateral breast cancer in women treated by lumpectomy (*open circles*) or lumpectomy and radiotherapy (*filled circles*). (Fisher et al. N Engl J Med 1993;328:1585)

have generally been the most widely studied predictive factors for recurrence. The limitations of histologic subtyping are discussed in detail in the pathology section. Despite these limitations, evidence suggests that histologic subtype and nuclear grade, alone or in combination, may be predictive factors for local failure after treatment with excision alone or plus radiotherapy. In the study of Lagios and colleagues[31] of women treated with wide excision alone, a 33% recurrence rate (12 of 36) for patients with high-grade DCIS containing comedo type necrosis was noted, compared with 2% (1 of 43) in patients with intermediate or low-grade DCIS. Similar findings were reported by Schwartz.[67] After wide excision alone, 32% of patients with comedo histology experienced local recurrence, whereas only 3% of those with noncomedo histology had recurrent disease. Eusebi and associates[57] have observed that local failure occurs earlier with high-grade DCIS than with low-grade DCIS; long-term follow-up is needed to see whether these differences persist.

High nuclear grade and comedo-type histology have also been found to be predictors of local recurrence when radiation is added to excision. Silverstein and associates[16] reported an 11% rate of local recurrence in women with comedo DCIS compared with a 2% failure rate in non comedo DCIS in 96 women with a median follow-up of 45 months. However, an update of this study with longer follow-up (median, 62 months) showed no difference in the rate of local failure based on histologic subtype.[70] In 172 women from the multicenter study reported by Solin and associates,[74,79,82] pathology slides were available for review. Sixteen local recurrences occurred in the 172 patients studied.[82] A comparison of recurrence rates between the comedo and noncomedo subtypes showed no significant differences (14% compared with 6%). However, for patients with a tumor of the comedo subtype and a nuclear grade of 3, recurrence rates were significantly higher than for any other groups (20% compared with 5%; P = .009). Forty-four of the 172 patients studied had this combination of factors, and half of the observed local recurrences occurred in this group. A multivariate analysis including histologic subtype of the primary tumor, nuclear grade, amount of necrosis, final pathology margin, and the combination of histologic subtype of comedo carcinoma plus nuclear grade 3 found that only the combination of comedo carcinoma plus nuclear grade 3 correlated significantly with local control. These patients also had a shorter time to treatment failure (median, 38 months) than did patients without the combination of comedo subtype and nuclear grade 3 (median, 78 months). This finding, combined with the Silverstein data discussed earlier,[16,70] suggests that the importance of the comedo subtype in predicting local recurrence may be overemphasized in studies with short-term follow-up. The pathologic parameters studied had no impact on overall survival or freedom from distant metastases. The NSABP has reported the results of an analysis of the pathologic features of 573 of the 790 patients with DCIS enrolled in Protocol B17.[82a] Using a Cox analysis, the presence of moderate to marked comedo necrosis and unknown or involved margins was found to be associated with an increased risk of ipsilateral breast tumor recurrence. The risk

of a breast recurrence was reduced by the use of radiation therapy in all subgroups, regardless of the presence or absence of comedo necrosis or margin involvement. However, there appears to be a greater reduction in the number of recurrences with radiation therapy in patients with negative margins and moderate or marked comedo necrosis than in patients with negative margins and absent or slight necrosis (crude relative reduction, 0.22 versus 0.60).

TREATMENT SELECTION

The available information on DCIS suggests that, although all patients can be treated with mastectomy, many are candidates for treatment with excision and irradiation, and a smaller group may be appropriately treated with excision alone. In the absence of definitive information to guide treatment selection, it is useful to consider the risk for breast cancer recurrence, the risk for invasive breast cancer, and the risk for dying of breast cancer associated with breast-conserving treatment.

The available data on breast conserving treatment with irradiation show recurrence rates of 10% to 15% at 10 years. About half of these recurrences are invasive carcinoma, a risk of 5% to 7%. The risk of dying of breast cancer is about one third the risk of developing the disease, so the risk of breast cancer death is 2% to 3% at 10 years. The risk for death 10 years after a mastectomy for DCIS is 1% to 2%. It is likely, however, that the major force of breast cancer mortality after mastectomy will be evident in the first 10 years after treatment, given that death is presumably due to occult microinvasive disease present at the time of diagnosis. Local recurrences in DCIS continue to occur after 10 years, with additional breast cancer–associated mortality. Comparisons of breast cancer mortality rates 30 years after treatment may show greater differences in survival between women having mastectomy and those treated with excision and radiation than the 1% to 2% estimated here. Whether radiation is necessary for all patients with DCIS treated with a breast-sparing approach remains uncertain. Retrospective data indicate that highly selected patients usually with small, low-grade DCIS have a very low local failure rate after excision alone. The only results available from a prospective study are those from NSABP B17. Although this study indicates that radiation therapy reduces the risk of local recurrence in all subgroups of patients with DCIS, Page and Lagios[82b] have questioned whether a more detailed mammographic and pathologic evaluation would allow the identification of a subgroup of patients who will benefit from radiation.

It is becoming increasingly clear that DCIS, rather than being a singly entity, represents a spectrum of diseases of differing biologic potential. This clinical observation is supported by studies of biologic markers,[83,84] which indicate that characteristics of the malignant phenotype are more likely to be expressed in high-grade DCIS. While we await developments in molecular biology that will allow us to predict more precisely which tumors progress to invasive carcinoma, our efforts must be directed toward minimizing local recurrence in women treated with a breast-conserving approach. Because most patients with

DCIS have nonpalpable mammographic lesions, careful mammographic evaluation before treatment selection is critical. Holland and colleagues[28] have previously reported that the microscopic extent of poorly differentiated DCIS correlated well with the radiologic extent of the lesion, but the mammographic appearance of well-differentiated tumors substantially underestimated the microscopic extent. However, the routine use of magnification views as part of the mammographic evaluation allowed the detection of additional calcifications that reduced the discrepancy between the pathologic and the mammographic extent of well-differentiated DCIS.[36] Needle localization should be used to guide the biopsy, and, if the calcifications are extensive, bracketing wires are useful to aid in complete excision. Specimen mammography is essential to confirm the excision of calcifications. In cases where calcifications are extensive or approach the edge of the surgical specimen, postexcision mammograms are useful to confirm the removal of all suspicious calcifications. Gluck and coworkers[85] did postexcision mammograms, including spot compression views, on 43 women who required reexcision for positive or unknown margins after a diagnosis of breast carcinoma. Twenty-eight patients had DCIS, and the positive predictive value for residual calcifications as an indicator of residual tumor was 0.67, which increased to 0.9 when more than five calcifications were present.

A detailed pathologic evaluation is also needed and should include orientation and inking of the specimen before sectioning as well as measurement of both specimen and tumor size. Because accurate measurement of microscopic DCIS is often difficult, reporting the number of blocks in which DCIS is present, as well as its extent on a given slide, is often useful. The correlation of microcalcifications with DCIS (ie, DCIS present only in areas of calcification or in calcification and adjacent breast tissue) and the margin status should be noted. If margins are involved, the extent of involvement should be stated, and when negative, proximity of the lesion to the margin should be noted.

After a diagnosis of DCIS, treatment options and their risks and benefits should be discussed in detail. Although high nuclear grade and comedo subtype may be associated with an increased risk for local failure after breast preservation, most women with these factors do not have recurrent disease, and the presence of these factors should not be considered a contraindication to breast-conserving treatment. Residual microcalcifications on a postbiopsy mammogram and involved margins are indications for reexcision. However, failure to remove all calcifications or to achieve negative margins after a reexcision is an indication that such patients are poor candidates for breast-sparing approaches. A final consideration in treatment selection is the intensity of follow-up required for each approach. The optimal schedule for detecting recurrence at an early stage after breast preservation is unknown. We have used a baseline, posttreatment mammogram and films at 6-month intervals, usually with spot magnification views, for the first 2 postoperative years. Patients are examined three or four times a year for the first 5 postoperative years. In contrast, women undergoing mastectomy have annual mammography and physician visits every 6 months.

The final answers on the risk of breast-conserving therapy for DCIS will be obtained only after longer follow-up of available data and studies with greater numbers of patients with more precisely characterized tumors. The role of tamoxifen in reducing local failure is currently being studied, but no data are available. At this time, no indication exists for its use outside of a controlled clinical trial. The currently available data suggest that a woman's risk of dying of breast cancer with breast-conserving treatment of DCIS is only 2% to 3% at 10 years, but probably does not end at that point, whereas the risk for dying of breast cancer after mastectomy is 1% to 2% at 10 years. Regardless of whether mastectomy or breast preservation is chosen, patients should undergo lifetime surveillance for the development of an invasive cancer in the contralateral breast. Ultimately, the patient must make a careful assessment of the risks and benefits of each treatment option and select what she believes is the best form of therapy.

MANAGEMENT SUMMARY

- DCIS represents a heterogeneous group of lesions of varying malignant potential.
- Total (simple) mastectomy is associated with a cure rate of nearly 100% for all types of DCIS.
- Patients with localized DCIS are candidates for breast-sparing surgery and irradiation. Detailed mammography and careful pathologic evaluation are essential to confirm the localized nature of the lesion and judge the adequacy of resection.
- Excision alone may be an appropriate treatment for selected women with small (less than 1 to 2 cm) low-grade DCIS lesions.
- Axillary dissection is not indicated in DCIS. In women with large high-grade lesions undergoing mastectomy, a low axillary sampling obviates the need for reoperation if invasion is identified.
- A detailed discussion of the risks and benefits of the various options must be done to allow each woman with DCIS to make an informed treatment choice.

References

1. Rosner D, Bedwani RN, Vana J, et al. Noninvasive breast carcinoma: results of a national survey by the American College of Surgeons. Ann Surg 1980;192:139.
2. Morrow M, Schmidt R, Cregger B. Preoperative evaluation of abnormal mammographic findings to avoid unnecessary breast biopsy. Arch Surg 1994;129:1091.
3. Alexander HR, Candela F, Dershaw D. Needle localized mammographic lesions: results and evolving treatment strategy. Arch Surg 1990;125:1441.
4. Silverstein M, Gamagami P, Colburn W, et al. Non-palpable breast lesions: diagnosis with slightly over-penetrated screen-film mammography and hook wire-directed biopsy in 1014 cases. Radiology 1989;171:633.

5. Wilhelm MC, Edge S, Cole D, et al. Nonpalpable invasive breast cancer. Ann Surg 1991;213:600.

6. Kessler LG, Feur EJ, Brown ML. Projections of the breast cancer burden to US women: 1990-2000. Prev Med 1991;20:170.

7. Azzopardi JG. Problems in breast pathology. Philadelphia, WB Saunders, 1983.

8. Page DL, Anderson TJ. Diagnostic histopathology of the breast. Edinburgh, Churchill Livingstone, 1987.

9. Rosen PP, Oberman H. Tumors of the mammary gland. Washington, DC, Armed Forces Institute of Pathology, 1993.

10. Carter D, Orr SL, Merino MJ. Intracystic papillary carcinoma of the breast after mastectomy, radiotherapy, or excision alone. Cancer, 1983;52:14.

11. Lefkowitz M, Lefkowitz W, Wargotz ES. Intraductal (intracystic) papillary carcinoma of the breast and its variants: a clinico-pathological study of 77 cases. Hum Pathol 1994;25:802.

12. Eusebi V, Foschini M, Cook M, et al. Long term follow-up of in situ carcinoma of the breast with special emphasis on clinging carcinoma. Semin Diagn Pathol 1989;6:165.

13. Fisher ER, Brown R. Intraductal signet ring cell carcinoma: a hitherto undescribed form of intraductal carcinoma of the breast. Cancer 1984;55:2533.

14. Rosen PP, Scott M. Cystic hypersecretory duct carcinoma of the breast. Am J Surg Pathol 1984;8:31.

15. Guerry P, Erlandson RA, Rosen PP. Cystic hypersecretory hyperplasia and cystic hypersecretory duct carcinoma of the breast: pathology, therapy, and follow-up of 39 patients. Cancer 1988;61:1611.

16. Silverstein MJ, Waisman JR, Gamagami P, et al. Intraductal carcinoma of the breast (208 cases): clinical factors influencing treatment choice. Cancer 1990;66:102.

17. Patchefsky AS, Schwartz GF, Finkelstein SD, et al. Heterogeneity of intraductal carcinoma of the breast. Cancer 1989;63:731.

18. Schwartz GF, Patchefsky AS, Finklestein SD, et al. Nonpalpable in situ ductal carcinoma of the breast: predictors of multicentricity and microinvasion and implications for treatment. Arch Surg 1989;124:29.

19. Bur ME, Zimarowski MJ, Schnitt SJ, et al. Estrogen receptor immunohistochemistry in carcinoma in situ of the breast. Cancer 1992;69:1174.

20. Meyer JS. Cell kinetics of histologic variants of in situ breast carcinoma. Breast Cancer Res Treat 1986;7:171.

21. Killeen JL, Namiki H. DNA analysis of ductal carcinoma in situ of the breast: a comparison with histologic features. Cancer 1991;68:2602.

22. van de Vijver MJ, Peterse JL, Mooi WJ, et al. Neu-protein overexpression in breast cancer: association with comedo-type ductal carcinoma in situ and limited prognostic value in stage II breast cancer. N Engl J Med 1988;319:1239.

23. Bartkova J, Barnes DM, Millis RR, et al. Immunohistochemical demonstration of c-erbB-2 protein in mammary ductal carcinoma in situ. Hum Pathol 1990;21:1164.

24. Lodato RF, Maguire HC Jr, Greene MI, et al. Immunohistochemical evaluation of c-erbB-2 oncogene expression in ductal carcinoma in situ and atypical ductal hyperplasia of the breast. Mod Pathol 1990;3:449.

25. Poller DN, Roberts EC, Bell JA, et al. p53 protein expression in mammary ductal carcinoma in situ: relationship to immunohistochemical expression of estrogen receptor c-erbB-2 protein. Hum Pathol 1993;24:463.

26. O'Malley FP, Vnencak-Jones CL, Dupont WD. p53 mutations are confined to comedo type ductal carcinoma in situ of the breast: immunohistochemical and sequencing data. Lab Invest 1994;71:67.

27. Guidi AJ, Fischer L, Harris JR, et al. Microvessel density and distribution in ductal carcinoma in situ of the breast. J Natl Cancer Inst 1994;85:614.

28. Holland R, Hendricks J, Verbeek A, et al. Extent, distribution, and mammographic/histological correlations of breast ductal carcinoma in situ. Lancet 1990;335:519.

29. Holland R, Hendriks J. Microcalcifications associated with ductal carcinoma in situ: mammographic–pathologic correlation. Semin Diagn Pathol 1994;11:181.

30. Lennington WJ, Jensen RA, Dalton LW, et al. Ductal carcinoma in situ of the breast: heterogeneity of individual lesions. Cancer 1994;73:118.

31. Lagios MD, Margolin FR, Westdahl PR, et al. Mammographically detected duct carcinoma in situ: frequency of local recurrence following tylectomy and prognostic effect of nuclear grade on local recurrence. Cancer 1989;63:618.

32. Poller DN, Silverstein MJ, Galea M, et al. Ductal carcinoma in situ of the breast: a proposal for a new simplified histological classification association between cellular proliferation and c-erbB-2 protein expression. Mod Pathol 1994;7:257.

33. Holland R, Peterse JL, Millis RR, et al. Ductal carcinoma in situ: a proposal for a new classification. Semin Diagn Pathol 1994;11:167.

34. Fowble B. In situ breast cancer. In: Fowble B, Goodman RL, Glick JH, et al, eds. Breast cancer treatment: a comprehensive guide to management. St Louis, Mosby–Year Book, 1991.

35. Lagios MD, Westdahl PR, Margolin FR, et al. Duct carcinoma in situ: relationship of extent of noninvasive disease to the frequency of occult invasion, multicentricity, lymph node metastases, and short-term treatment failures. Cancer 1982;50:1309.

36. Bellamy CO, McDonald C, Salter DM, et al. Noninvasive ductal carcinoma of the breast: the relevance of histologic categorization. Hum Pathol 1993;24:16.

37. Faverly D, Holland R, Burgers L. An original stereomicroscopic analysis of the mammary glandular tree. Virchows Arch 1992;421:115.

38. Noguchi S, Motomura K, Inaji H, et al. Clonal analysis of predominantly intraductal carcinoma and precancerous lesions of the breast by means of polymerase chain reaction. Cancer Res 1994;54:1849.

39. Contesso G, Mouriesse H, Petit JY. Intraductal carcinoma studies on mastectomy specimens: preferential localization of DCIS: the nipple. Castle Marquette, The Netherlands, Proc EORTC In Situ Breast Cancer Workshop, 1988.

40. Gump FE, Jicha DL, Ozello L. Ductal carcinoma in situ (DCIS): a revised concept. Surgery 1987;102:790.

41. Fentiman IS, Fagg N, Millis RR, et al. In situ ductal carcinoma of the breast: implications of disease pattern and treatment. Eur J Surg Oncol 1986;12:261.

42. Silverstein MJ, Gierson ED, Waisman JR, et al. Axillary lymph node dissection for T1a breast carcinoma. is it indicated? Cancer 1994;73:664.

43. Rosai J. Borderline epithelial lesions of the breast. Am J Surg Pathol 1991;15:209.

44. Schnitt SJ, Connolly JL, Tavassoli FA, et al. Interobserver reproducibility in the diagnosis of ductal proliferative breast lesions using standardized criteria. Am J Surg Pathol 1992;16:1133.

45. Fisher ER, Sass R, Fisher B, et al. Pathologic findings from the National Surgical Adjuvant Breast Project (protocol 6). I. Intraductal carcinoma (DCIS). Cancer 1986;57:197.

46. Ozello L. Ultrastructure of intra-epithelial carcinomas of the breast. Cancer 1971;28:1508.

47. Barsky SH, Siegal GP, Jannotta F, et al. Loss of basement membrane components by invasive tumors but not by their benign counterparts. Lab Invest 1983;49:149.

48. Sakr WA, Zarbo RJ, Crissman JD. Immunohistochemical distribution of basement membrane in breast neoplasia. Surg Pathol 1988;1:3.

49. Page DL, Dixon JM, Anderson TJ, et al. Invasive cribriform carcinoma of the breast. Histopathology 1983;7:525.

50. Venable JG, Schwartz AM, Silverberg SG. Infiltrating cribriform carcinoma of the breast: a distinctive clinico-pathologic entity. Hum Pathol 1990;21:333.

51. Fechner RE. Ductal carcinoma involving the lobule of the breast: a source of confusion with lobular carcinoma in situ. Cancer 1971;28:274.

52. Kerner H, Lichtig C. Lobular cancerization: incidence and differential diagnosis with lobular carcinoma in situ of the breast. Histopathology 1986;10:621.

53. Fechner RE. Epithelial alterations in the extralobular ducts of breasts with lobular carcinoma. Arch Pathol 1972;93:164.

54. Rosen PP. Coexistent lobular carcinoma in situ and intraductal carcinoma in a single lobular-duct unit. Am J Surg Pathol 1980;4:241.

55. Page DL, Dupont WD, Rogers LW, et al. Intraductal carcinoma of the breast: follow-up after biopsy only. Cancer 1982;49:751.

56. Rosen PP, Braun D, Kinne D. The clinical significance of pre-invasive breast carcinoma. Cancer 1980;46:919.

57. Eusebi V, Feudale E, Foschini M, et al. Long term follow-up of in situ carcinoma of the breast. Semin Diagn Pathol 1994;11:223.

58. Alpers C, Wellings S. The prevalence of carcinoma in situ in normal and cancer associated breast. Hum Pathol 1985;16:796.

59. Bartow S, Pathak D, Black W, et al. Prevalence of benign, atypical, and malignant breast lesions in populations at different risk for breast cancer. Cancer 1987;60:2751.

60. Andersen J, Nielsen M, Christensen L. New aspects of the natural history of in situ and invasive carcinoma in the female breast: results from autopsy investigations. Verh Dtsch Ges Pathol 1985;69:88.

61. Von Rueden DG, Wilson RE. Intraductal carcinoma of the breast. Surg Gynecol Obstet 1984;158:105.

62. Sunshine JA, Moseley MS, Fletcher WS, et al. Breast carcinoma in situ: a retrospective review of 112 cases with a minimum 10 year follow-up. Am J Surg 1985;150:44.

63. Kinne DW, Petrek JA, Osborne MP, et al. Breast carcinoma in situ. Arch Surg 1989;124:33.

64. Schuh ME, Nemoto T, Penetrante RB, et al. Intraductal carcinoma: analysis of presentation, pathologic findings and outcome of disease. Arch Surg 1986;121:1303.

65. Rosen PP, Senie R, Schottenfeld D, et al. Noninvasive breast carcinoma: frequency of unsuspected invasion and implications for treatment. Ann Surg 1979;3:377.

66. Hetelekidis S, Schnitt SJ, Morrow M, et al. Management of ductal carcinoma in situ. CA Cancer J Clin 1995 (In press).

67. Schwartz GF, Finkel GC, Garcia JC, et al. Sub-clinical ductal carcinoma in situ of the breast: treatment by local excision and surveillance alone. Cancer 1992;70:2468.

68. Fisher E, Leeming R, Anderson S, et al. Conservative management of intraductal carcinoma (DCIS) of the breast. J Surg Oncol 1991;47:139.

69. Gallagher WJ, Koerner FC, Wood WC. Treatment of intraductal carcinoma with limited surgery: long-term follow-up. J Clin Oncol 1989;7:376.

70. Silverstein MJ, Cohlan BF, Gierson ED, et al. Duct carcinoma in situ: 227 cases without microinvasion. Eur J Cancer 1992;28:630.

71. Carpenter R, Boulter PS, Cooke T, et al. Management of screen detected ductal carcinoma in situ of the female breast. Br J Surg 1989;76:564.

72. Arnesson LG, Smeds S, Fagerberg G, et al. Follow-up of two treatment modalities for ductal cancer in situ of the breast. Br J Surg 1989;76:672.

73. Fisher B, Costantino J, Redmond C, et al. Lumpectomy compared with lumpectomy and radiation therapy for the treatment of intraductal breast cancer. N Engl J Med 1993;328:1581.

74. Solin LJ, Recht A, Fourquet A, et al. Ten-year results of breast-conserving surgery and definitive irradiation for intraductal carcinoma (ductal carcinoma in situ) of the breast. Cancer 1991;68:2337.

75. Hiramatsu H, Bornstein BA, Recht A, et al. Local recurrence after conservative surgery and radiation therapy for ductal carcinoma in situ: possible importance of family history. Cancer J Sci Am 1995;1:55.

76. McCormick B, Rosen PP, Kinne DW, et al. Ductal carcinoma in situ of the breast: an analysis of local control after conservation surgery and radiotherapy. Int J Radiat Oncol Biol Phys 1991;21:289.

77. Ray GR, Adelson J, Hayhurst E, et al. Ductal carcinoma in situ of the breast: results of treatment by conservative surgery and definitive irradiation. Int J Radiat Oncol Biol Phys 1993;28:105.

78. Stotter AT, McNeese M, Oswald MJ, et al. The role of limited surgery with irradiation in primary treatment of ductal in situ breast cancer. Int J Radiat Oncol Biol Phys 1990;18:283.

79. Solin LJ, Fourquet A, McCormick B, et al. Salvage treatment for local recurrence following breast conserving surgery and definitive irradiation for ductal carcinoma *in situ* (intraductal carcinoma) of the breast. Int J Radiat Oncol Biol Phys 1994;30:3.

80. Kuske RR, Bean JM, Garcia DM, et al. Breast conservation therapy for intraductal carcinoma of the breast. Int J Radiat Oncol Biol Phys 1993;26:391.

81. Lampejo OT, Barnes DM, Smith P, et al. Evaluation of infiltrating ductal carcinomas with a DCIS component: correlation of the histologic type of the in situ component with grade of the infiltrating component. Semin Diagn Pathol 1994;11:215.

82. Solin LJ, Yeh IT, Kurtz J, et al. Ductal carcinoma in situ (intraductal carcinoma) of the breast treated with breast-conserving surgery and definitive irradiation: correlation of pathologic parameters with outcome of treatment. Cancer 1993;71:2532.

82a. Fisher ER, Costantino J, Fisher B, et al. Pathologic findings from the National Surgical Adjuvant Breast Project (NSABP) Protocol B17: intraductal carcinoma (ductal carcinoma in situ). Cancer 1995;75:1310.

82b. Page DL, Lagios MD. Pathologic analysis of the National Surgical Adjuvant Breast Project (NSABP) B17 trial: unanswered questions remaining unanswered considering current concepts of ductal carcinoma in situ. Cancer 1995;75:1219.

83. Zafrani B, Leroyer A, Fourquet A, et al. Mammographically detected ductal in situ carcinoma of the breast analyzed with a new classification: a study of 127 cases: correlation with estrogen and progesterone receptors, p53 and C-erbB-2 proteins and proliferative activity. Semin Diagn Pathol 1994;11:208.

84. Bobrow LG, Happerfield LC, Gregory WM, et al. The classification of ductal carcinoma in situ and its association with biological markers. Semin Diagn Pathol 1994;11:199.

85. Gluck BS, Dershaw DD, Liberman L, et al. Microcalcifications on postoperative mammograms as an indicator of adequacy of tumor excision. Radiology 1993;188:469.

11.2

Lobular Carcinoma in Situ

MONICA MORROW · STUART J. SCHNITT

In 1941, Foote and Stewart[1] described a noninvasive lesion arising from the lobules and terminal ducts of the breast that they called *lobular carcinoma in situ* (LCIS). A review of 300 mastectomy specimens at Memorial Hospital in New York City resulted in only two examples of pure LCIS, and, in 12 additional cases, LCIS was identified in association with infiltrating carcinoma, leading Foote and Stewart[1] to conclude that LCIS was a rare entity. Despite the limited number of cases examined, their initial report identified three important features of LCIS. The lesion is an incidental microscopic finding that cannot be identified clinically or by gross pathologic examination, the lesion is multicentric in the breast, and the invasive carcinomas that develop after LCIS may be infiltrating-ductal or infiltrating-lobular tumors. Based on these observations Foote and Stewart[1] concluded that simple mastectomy was the appropriate treatment for LCIS. Additional information about LCIS gained since 1941 suggests that the lesion does not invariably progress to carcinoma and that the risk for subsequent cancer is roughly equal in both breasts. The uncertainties about the biologic significance of a diagnosis of LCIS have caused considerable confusion regarding its management.

Incidence

The true incidence of LCIS in the general population is unknown because of the lack of both clinical and mammographic signs. Page and colleagues[2] reviewed 10,542 benign breast biopsies done for clinical abnormalities and found only 48 cases (0.5%) that met strict diagnostic criteria for LCIS. In contrast, Haagensen and coworkers[3] reviewed 5000 patients who had breast biopsies between 1930 and 1972 and observed that 3.6% of the benign breast lesions were LCIS. Page and associates,[2] however, commented that some of the lesions in this series would not meet their diagnostic criteria for LCIS and would be classified as atypical lobular hyperplasia, illustrating a further problem in determining the incidence of LCIS. Wheeler and associates[4] noted LCIS in 0.8% of 3570 benign biopsies done for clinical problems, and Andersen[5] found a 1.5% incidence of LCIS in 3299 specimens. The variable incidence of LCIS reported in these series reflects differences in diagnostic criteria, the amount of normal breast tissue removed and examined, and differences in the patient populations undergoing biopsy. Although the exact incidence of LCIS varies, agreement exists that LCIS is an uncommon finding. Autopsy studies also suggest a low incidence of LCIS. Frantz and coworkers[6] found no cases of LCIS when studying the breasts of 225 women with a median age of 45 years. Alpers and Wellings[7] and Kramer and Rush[8] also found no evidence of LCIS in detailed autopsy studies. Nielsen and colleagues[9] examined 110 younger women and identified only four cases of lobular carcinoma in situ, confirming that LCIS is uncommon in the general population. In all reports, LCIS is noted to be more common in younger women with the mean age at diagnosis usually reported to be between 44 and 46 years,[2–5,10] with 80% to 90% of cases of LCIS occurring in premenopausal women.[2–5,10–12] This age distribution may be due to regression of LCIS in the absence of estrogen or may simply reflect the fact that benign breast abnormalities that require biopsy are more common in premenopausal women, resulting in more frequent identification of LCIS in this group. LCIS is reported to occur about 10 times more frequently in white women than black women in the United States.[13–15]

The frequency with which LCIS is diagnosed is increasing, with one series[16] reporting a 15% rise in the number of cases seen from 1973 to 1988. Although some of this increase is due to greater recognition of LCIS as a pathologic entity, the major factor responsible is the increasing use of screening mammography. A recent review[17] of 6287 mammographically generated biopsies showed that LCIS was present in 2.3% of total cases, accounting for 9.8% of mammographically detected lesions classified as malignancies. No specific mammographic findings are associated with LCIS.[18,19] Calcifications have frequently been the indication for surgery in cases where LCIS has been identified, but histologically the calcifications are located in normal epithelial cells adjacent to areas of lobular carcinoma in situ, rather than in the involved lobules.[18]

Several studies have examined the distribution of LCIS in an involved breast and the contralateral breast. Foote and Stewart[1] recognized the multicentric nature of LCIS in their original report, and subsequent reports[20–24] confirmed that multifocal LCIS is identified in 60% to 80% of mastectomy specimens. In addition, LCIS is frequently noted to be bilateral. Haagensen and associates[3] found bilateral LCIS in 19 of 73 women (26%) where bilateral breast tissue was available. Mirror-image biopsies done in patients with LCIS also provide an estimate of the incidence of bilateral disease. Newman[23] found contralateral LCIS in 6 of 26 women (23%) undergoing mirror image biopsy, and Urban[25] noted a 35% incidence of bilateral LCIS in 26 women. The incidence of bilaterality of LCIS has minimal clinical relevance, however, because the cancer risk associated with LCIS is bilateral, regardless of the presence of LCIS in the contralateral breast.

Pathology

Lobular carcinoma in situ is not detectable on macroscopic examination and is always an incidental microscopic finding in breast tissue removed for another reason. In contrast

FIGURE 11.2-1 Lobular carcinoma in situ. The acinar units are filled with and distended by a solid proliferation of relatively small monomorphic cells.

with ductal carcinoma in situ (DCIS), which is heterogeneous in its histologic appearance, the histologic features of LCIS show little variation and are usually easily recognized.[26–30]

LCIS is characterized by a solid proliferation of small cells, with small, uniform, round to oval nuclei, and variably distinct cell borders (Figure 11.2-1). The cytoplasm is clear to lightly eosinophilic; occasionally, the cells contain intracytoplasmic vacuoles that may be large enough to produce signet ring cell forms. Cell kinetic studies using thymidine labeling have shown that LCIS has a very low proliferative rate, similar to cribriform and micropapillary DCIS, and much lower than comedo-type DCIS or invasive cancers.[31] The cells of LCIS are also typically estrogen receptor–positive[32] and rarely, if ever, show overexpression of the c-*erb*B-2 (HER2/*neu*) oncogene.[33,34] LCIS is typically present in the terminal duct–lobular units and distends and distorts the involved spaces. In some instances, LCIS cells involve extralobular ducts. The growth within these ducts may be either solid or pagetoid (ie, the LCIS cells are insinuated between the duct basement membrane and the native ductal epithelial cells). Although some authors also recognize a cribriform pattern of involvement of extralobular ducts by LCIS,[35] in situ lesions with a cribriform pattern are probably best categorized as DCIS.

Differential Diagnosis

The cells composing atypical lobular hyperplasia (ALH) are similar to those that characterize LCIS, but, in ALH, the degree of involvement of the terminal ducts and lobules is less extensive. Unfortunately, no sharp dividing line exists between atypical lobular hyperplasia and LCIS.

Some authors require that at least half of the spaces in a given lobule be filled with and distended by the characteristic cells to warrant a diagnosis of LCIS.[27] In some patients, LCIS involves areas of breast tissue that have preexisting benign cellular alterations; for example, LCIS may involve foci of sclerosing adenosis and may produce a pattern that mimics invasive carcinoma.[36] However, low-power examination in such specimens usually shows the lobulocentric configuration characteristic of adenosis. Finally, as discussed in the section addressing the pathology of DCIS, distinguishing between LCIS and DCIS is sometimes a problem.[35,37–39]

Natural History and Treatment

The major issue in the management of LCIS is the risk for invasive carcinoma after a diagnosis of LCIS. Treatment strategies have varied, depending on whether LCIS was considered to be the anatomic precursor of invasive carcinoma, an obligate premalignant lesion, or simply a marker for an increased risk for breast cancer development. Five series[2–5,12] with long-term follow-up address the malignant potential of LCIS after biopsy alone (Table 11.2-1). Patients with LCIS and without associated invasive carcinoma were studied, although women with contralateral invasive carcinoma before a diagnosis of LCIS were included in some reports, making calculation of the incidence of invasive carcinoma difficult. The largest series, reported by Haagensen and associates,[3] included 287 women monitored for a mean of 16.3 years, with only 2 patients lost to follow-up. Breast cancer developed in 63 patients (21% of the series). If the 10 patients whose LCIS diagnosis followed treatment for contralateral invasive breast cancer are excluded, 18% of the women developed

TABLE 11.2-1
Follow-Up Studies of Lobular Carcinoma in Situ

Investigators	Cases	Invasive Cancer (%)	Follow-Up (y)	Relative Risk
Haagensen et al[3]	287	18.0	16.3	6.9
Rosen et al[12]	99	34.5*	24.0	9.0
Wheeler et al[4]	32	12.5	17.5	—
Andersen[5]	47	26.4†	15.0	12.0
Page et al[2]	44	23.0	18.0	9.0
Salvadori et al[40]	80	6.3	5.0	10.3
Ottesen et al[41]	69	11.6	5.0	11.0

* Percentage calculated for 85 patients with follow-up.

† Includes two patients with bilateral cancers counted separately.

carcinoma, an observed/expected ratio of 6.9:1. In a similar study from Memorial Hospital, Rosen and colleagues[12] identified 99 patients with LCIS monitored for a mean of 24 years, although complete follow-up was available for only 84 women. Twenty-nine women subsequently developed invasive carcinoma (34.5%), but, if all the patients lost to follow-up were considered free of disease, this figure falls to 29.2%. The relative risk for breast cancer development in this series was 9, the same level of risk observed by Page and coworkers[2] in a more recent report of 44 cases of LCIS followed for 18 years. Page's group, however, observed that the risk for developing infiltrating carcinoma was greatest during the first 15 years after biopsy (relative risk, 10.8) and decreased to 4.2 for those women remaining free of carcinoma for 15 years. In contrast, Rosen and associates[12] observed no decrease in the risk for development of invasive carcinoma during their 24-year follow-up period. Wheeler and coworkers[4] and Andersen[5] reported the development of invasive carcinoma in 12.5% and 26.4% of women monitored for 17.5 and 15 years, respectively. In two recently reported studies[40,41] similar levels of risk associated with LCIS were noted.

Salvadori and coworkers[40] reported 80 women with LCIS who were monitored for a median of 58 months. Five cases of invasive carcinoma (6.3%) were noted, an observed/expected ratio of 10.3. Sixty-nine cases of LCIS were identified in a prospective study by the Danish Breast Cancer Cooperative Group,[41] and, at a median follow-up of 61 months, 8 infiltrating carcinomas had occurred (11.6%). The relative risk for cancer development among women with LCIS in this study was 11.

The studies discussed agree that LCIS is associated with an increased risk for the development of breast carcinoma that is approximately 7 to 10 times that of the index population. In addition, the five studies with long-term follow-up periods agree that the risk for subsequent cancer development is equal in both breasts (Table 11.2-2). Most carcinomas that develop in women with LCIS are infiltrating ductal, not infiltrating lobular carcinoma. Infiltrating lobular carcinomas accounted for 25% to 37% of subsequent cancers in four of the six studies for which this information is available.[3,4,12,41] Page and colleagues[2] observed that 70% of the infiltrating carcinomas in their series that occurred after a diagnosis of LCIS were of lobular

TABLE 11.2-2
Laterality and Histology of Cancers After a Diagnosis of Lobular Carcinoma in Situ

Investigators	Cancer in Biopsied Breast	Cancer in Other Breast	Total Cancer Infiltrating Lobular (%)
Haagensen et al[3]	27/257 (10.5%)	26/258 (10.5%)	25.5
Rosen et al[12]	19/83 (22.9%)	19/83 (22.9%)	36.0
Wheeler et al[4]	1/25 (4.0%)	3/32 (9.7%)	25.0
Andersen[5]	9/44 (20.0%)	4/44 (9.1%)	—
Page et al[2]	5/44 (11.0%)	4/44 (9.1%)	70.0
Salvadori et al[40]	5/80 (6.3%)	0/80 (0.0%)	0.0
Ottesen et al[41]	8/69 (11.6%)	0/69 (0.0%)	37.0

histology, whereas none of the five cancers in the report of Salvadori and associates had infiltrating lobular histology (see Table 11.2-2). Although most cancers occurring after a diagnosis of LCIS are infiltrating ductal carcinomas, the incidence of infiltrating lobular carcinoma in this group of patients is significantly elevated compared with the 5% to 10% incidence observed among breast cancers in the general population. Wheeler and coworkers[4] estimated that invasive lobular carcinomas occur at 18 times the expected rate, whereas infiltrating ductal carcinomas occur at only 4 times their expected rate.

The observations that most women with LCIS do not develop breast cancer, that the risk for breast cancer is bilateral, and that most tumors are infiltrating ductal carcinomas gives credence to the hypothesis that LCIS is a risk factor for cancer development. One management option for the woman with LCIS is careful observation, as would be done for any woman known to be at increased risk for breast cancer development due to a positive family history or prior personal history of breast cancer. An alternative for women unwilling to accept the risk for breast cancer development of about 1% per year associated with a policy of careful observation is bilateral simple mastectomy, usually with immediate reconstruction. Treatment strategies addressing one breast, such as unilateral simple mastectomy with contralateral biopsy, would seem illogical because the risk of LCIS is bilateral regardless of the findings of the contralateral biopsy. The effectiveness of a program of careful follow-up in detecting potentially curable carcinoma in a population of high-risk women is uncertain. A metaanalysis of 389 reported cases of LCIS followed for a mean of 10.9 years reported a breast cancer mortality rate of 2.8%, although 16.4% of the group developed carcinoma.[42] In contrast, of 391 women treated initially with mastectomy, the breast cancer mortality rate was 0.9%. Frykberg and Bland,[17] analyzing data on 515 patients with LCIS treated with observation, reported a 7% breast cancer mortality rate. Many of these series antedate the use of modern mammography, however, and uniform clinical follow-up was not used. The large cohort of women with LCIS in the National Surgical Adjuvant Breast Project prevention trial will provide valuable information regarding the effectiveness of close clinical follow-up.

Wide surgical excision and histologically negative margins are not needed when follow-up is chosen, given that LCIS is known to be a multifocal lesion. Similarly, radiation therapy has no role in the management of LCIS. We examine women with LCIS at 4- to 6-month intervals and obtain annual diagnostic mammograms. When observation is elected, it must last for the patient's lifetime, because the increased risk of breast cancer persists indefinitely. Carson and colleagues[43] reported that 12 of 51 women (24%) monitored after a diagnosis of LCIS had a subsequent breast biopsy, although only 3 were found to have infiltrating carcinoma. Efforts to identify features of LCIS associated with a higher likelihood of the development of malignancy have been largely unsuccessful. Haagensen and coworkers[3] noted that the combination of LCIS and a family history of breast cancer increased the relative risk for breast cancer development to 8.5 (compared with 5.7 for women with LCIS alone). Page and colleagues,[2] however, did not find that a positive family history further increased risk in women with LCIS. Rosen and coworkers[12] extensively reviewed the histologic features of LCIS, including the amount of LCIS present, and were unable to identify any factors predictive of the subsequent development of invasive carcinoma, an observation similar to that made by Haagensen and coworkers.[3] Research using the tools of molecular biology to further define risk will provide critically important information for women with LCIS.

The choice between careful observation and bilateral prophylactic mastectomy can only be made by the patient who thoroughly understands the risk she assumes. Surgical treatment of LCIS is not an emergency, and detailed discussions of treatment options are important for patients to overcome the confusion often associated with this diagnosis. The use of mastectomy to treat LCIS appears to be decreasing.[11] In light of the increasing use of breast-preserving approaches for invasive carcinoma and ongoing clinical trials of breast cancer prevention, this trend is probably appropriate.

MANAGEMENT SUMMARY

- LCIS, which lacks clinical or mammographic signs, is a risk factor for bilateral breast cancer development.
- Careful clinical follow-up is appropriate for most women with LCIS and carries a risk of breast cancer development of about 1% per year. This risk persists indefinitely.
- Bilateral prophylactic mastectomy, usually with reconstruction, is an alternative approach for the woman unwilling to undergo follow-up.
- There is no role for excision to negative margins, radiation therapy, or systemic therapy for women with LCIS.

References

1. Foote FW Jr, Stewart FW. Lobular carcinoma in situ: a rare form of mammary carcinoma. Am J Pathol 1941;17:491.
2. Page DL, Kidd TE Jr, Dupont WD, et al. Lobular neoplasia of the breast: higher risk for subsequent invasive cancer predicted by more extensive disease. Hum Pathol 1991;22:1232.
3. Haagensen CD, Bodian C, Haagensen DE. Lobular neoplasia (lobular carcinoma in situ) breast carcinoma: risk and detection. Philadelphia, WB Saunders, 1981:238.
4. Wheeler JE, Enterline HT, Roseman JM, et al. Lobular carcinoma in situ of the breast: long-term follow-up. Cancer 1974;34:554.
5. Andersen JA. Lobular carcinoma in situ of the breast: an approach to rational treatment. Cancer 1977;39:2597.
6. Frantz VK, Pickren JW, Melcher GW, et al. Incidence of chronic cystic disease in so-called normal breasts: a study based on 225 post mortem examinations. Cancer 1951;4:762.
7. Alpers CE, Wellings SR. The prevalence of carcinoma in situ in normal and cancer associated breasts. Hum Pathol 1985;16:796.

8. Kramer WM, Rush BF Jr. Mammary duct proliferation in the elderly. Cancer 1973;31:130.

9. Nielsen M, Thomsen JL, Primdahl L, et al. Breast cancer and atypia among young and middle aged women: a study of 100 medicolegal autopsies. Br J Cancer 1987;56:814.

10. Singletary SE. Lobular carcinoma in situ of the breast: a 31 year experience at the University of Texas, M.D. Anderson Cancer Center. Breast Dis 1994;7:157.

11. Walt AJ, Simon M, Swanson GM. The continuing dilemma of lobular carcinoma in situ. Arch Surg 1992;127:904.

12. Rosen PP, Lieberman PH, Braun DW Jr, et al. Lobular carcinoma in situ of the breast. Am J Surg Pathol 1978;2:225.

13. Farrow JH. Current concepts in the detection and treatment of the earliest of early breast cancers. Cancer 1970;25:468.

14. Newman W. In situ lobular carcinoma of the breast: report of 26 women with 32 cancers. Ann Surg 1963;57:591.

15. Rosner D, Bedwani RN, Vana J, et al. Noninvasive breast carcinoma: results of a national survey by the American College of Surgeons. Ann Surg 1980;192:139.

16. Lemanne D, Simon M, Martino S, et al. Breast carcinoma in situ: greater rise in ductal carcinoma in situ vs lobular carcinoma in situ. Proc Am Soc Clin Oncol 1991;10:45.

17. Frykberg ER, Bland KI. In situ breast carcinoma. Adv Surg 1993;29.

18. Hutter RVP, Snyder RE, Lucas JC, et al. Clinical and pathologic correlation with mammographic findings in lobular carcinoma in situ. Cancer 1969;23:826.

19. Pope TL Jr, Fechner RE, Wilhelm MC, et al. Lobular carcinoma in situ of the breast: mammographic features. Radiology 1988;168:63.

20. Lewison EF, Finney GG Jr. Lobular carcinoma in situ of the breast. Surg Gynecol Obstet 1968;126:1280.

21. Donegan W, Perez-Mesa CM. Lobular carcinoma: an indicator for elective biopsy of the second breast. Am Surg 1972;176:178.

22. Carter D, Smith RL. Carcinoma in situ of the breast. Cancer 1977;40:1189.

23. Newman W. In situ lobular carcinoma of the breast: report of 26 women and 32 cancers. Ann Surg 1963;157:591.

24. Lambird PA, Shelley WM. The spatial distribution of lobular in situ mammary carcinoma. JAMA 1969;210:689.

25. Urban JA. Bilaterality of cancer of the breast: biopsy of the opposite breast. Cancer 1967;11:1867.

26. Azzopardi JG. Problems in breast pathology. Philadelphia, WB Saunders, 1983.

27. Page DL, Anderson TJ. Diagnostic histopathology of the breast. Edinburgh, Churchill Livingstone, 1987.

28. Rosen PP, Oberman H. Tumors of the mammary gland. Washington, DC, Armed Forces Institute of Pathology, 1993.

29. Wheeler JE, Enterline HT. Lobular carcinoma of the breast in situ and infiltrating. Pathol Annu 1976;11:161.

30. Frykberg ER, Santiago F, Betsill WL Jr, et al. Lobular carcinoma in situ of the breast. Surg Gynecol Obstet 1987;164:285.

31. Meyer JS. Cell kinetics of histologic variants of in situ breast carcinoma. Breast Cancer Res Treat 1986;7:171.

32. Bur ME, Zimarowski MJ, Schnitt SJ, et al. Estrogen receptor immunohistochemistry in carcinoma in situ of the breast. Cancer 1992;69:1174.

33. Ramachandra S, Machin L, Ashley S, et al. Immunohistochemical distribution of c-erbB-2 in in situ breast carcinoma: a detailed morphological analysis. J Pathol 1990;161:7.

34. Porter PL, Garcia R, Moe R, et al. c-erbB-2 oncogene protein in in situ and invasive lobular breast neoplasia. Cancer 1991;68:331.

35. Fechner RE. Epithelial alterations in the extralobular ducts of breasts with lobular carcinoma. Arch Pathol 1972;93:164.

36. Fechner RE. Lobular carcinoma in situ in sclerosing adenosis: a potential source of confusion with invasive carcinoma. Am J Surg Pathol 1981;5:233.

37. Fechner RE. Ductal carcinoma involving the lobule of the breast: a source of confusion with lobular carcinoma in situ. Cancer 1971;28:274.

38. Kerner H, Lichtig C. Lobular cancerization: incidence and differential diagnosis with lobular carcinoma in situ of the breast. Histopathology 1986;10:621.

39. Rosen PP. Coexistent lobular carcinoma in situ and intraductal carcinoma in a single lobular-duct unit. Am J Surg Pathol 1980;4:241.

40. Salvadori B, Bartolic, Zurrida S, et al. Risk of invasive cancer in women with lobular carcinoma in situ of the breast. Eur J Cancer 1991;27:35.

41. Ottesen GL, Graversen HP, Blichert-Toft M, et al. Lobular carcinoma in situ of the female breast: short-term results of a prospective nationwide study. Am J Surg Pathol 1993;17:14.

42. Bradley SJ, Weaver DW, Bowman DL. Alternatives in the surgical management of in situ breast cancer: a meta-analysis of outcome. Am Surg 1990;58:428.

43. Carson W, Sanchez-Forgach E, Stomper P, et al. Lobular carcinoma in situ: observation without surgery as an appropriate therapy. Ann Surg Oncol 1994;1:141.

12

Diseases of the Breast, edited by Jay R. Harris,
Marc E. Lippman, Monica Morrow, and Samuel Hellman.
Lippincott-Raven Publishers, Philadelphia, © 1996.

Natural History of Breast Cancer

JAY R. HARRIS • SAMUEL HELLMAN

The clinical behavior of breast cancer is characterized by a *long natural history* and by *heterogeneity* among patients in its clinical course. The prognosis of patients with breast cancer has been well documented in terms of the size of the tumor and the presence and extent of involvement of regional lymph nodes. However, patients diagnosed with breast cancer are at risk for metastases for extended time periods and the definition of *cure* in this disease is problematic. Models to describe the growth of breast cancer have been described, but they remain controversial. The treatment of breast cancer has been directed at the breast and regional lymph nodes locally and at sites of metastases systemically, but the importance of local treatment has been debated. This chapter reviews information related to these important aspects of the disease.

Plotting Survival in Untreated and Treated Breast Cancer

By documenting the natural history of untreated breast cancer, one can establish a baseline by which to judge the effects of treatment. Because breast cancer has been considered a treatable disease for at least the last several hundred years, series of untreated but well-documented patients are uncommon. One such series is from Middlesex Hospital in England, where one of the first cancer wards was established in 1792. Bloom and associates[1] reported on a group of 250 patients seen at Middlesex Hospital between 1805 and 1933. Patients generally were admitted to the hospital with locally advanced breast cancer. Seventy-four percent were in stage IV, 23% were in stage III, and only 2% were in stage II. Patients were not admitted to the hospital at the clinical onset of the disease but were for terminal care. No patient was treated with any form of surgery, radiation therapy (RT), or hormone therapy. Because of the meticulous medical records kept, it

was possible to estimate the onset of the disease with a fair degree of accuracy. Only 7% of the patients presented within 6 months of the initial symptom of the disease and only 39% within 1 year. Figure 12-1 shows the percentage of patients surviving, plotted from the time of the first onset of symptoms. The median survival time from the onset of symptoms was 2.7 years. Eighteen percent of untreated patients survived 5 years, and 4% survived 10 years. These figures indicate that survival of breast cancer patients can be lengthy, even if the disease is untreated.

The usefulness of plotting survival curves logarithmically is shown by Figure 12-1B. In this figure, the same survival data from the Middlesex Hospital given in Figure 12-1A are shown with survival plotted logarithmically. The approximately straight line in this figure indicates that the annual hazard or force of mortality (ie, the percentage of remaining patients who die each year) is constant. In this group of patients, about 25% of the patients at the start of any year died by the end of that year.

Compare the results in the Middlesex Hospital with results seen in modern times. Figure 12-2 shows the survival results collected by the End Results Section of the Biometry Branch of the National Cancer Institute (NCI) on a large group of patients with histologically confirmed breast cancer.[2] The results apply to patients who were treated for their cancer and are corrected for causes of death other than breast cancer. The biphasic shape of this survival curve has been interpreted as indicating that there are two subgroups of breast cancer patients. One subgroup is manifested by the curve past 10 years and represents patients who have a force of mortality rate of 2.5% per year. By backward extrapolation of this portion of the curve to time zero, one can estimate that this subgroup represents approximately 60% of the total group. The other subgroup has more aggressive disease, with a force of mortality rate of 25% per year, similar to that observed for untreated patients seen at Middlesex Hospital. There are, however, potential problems in making such a com-

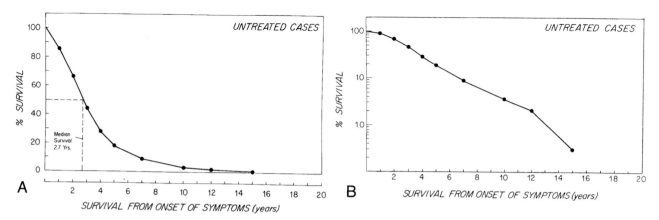

FIGURE 12-1   Survival of 250 untreated breast cancer patients from Middlesex Hospital plotted linearly (**A**) and semilogarithmically (**B**) (Bloom HJG, Richardson W, Harrier E. Natural history of untreated breast cancer [1805–1933]. BMJ 1962;2:213)

parison. The Middlesex Hospital experience represents a highly selected group of patients because only 250 patients were collected over 128 years, or approximately 2 per year. These patients were identified for inclusion in the series only if a postmortem examination had been performed, not at the onset of their disease. Given these caveats, the results seen in the NCI data indicate that breast cancer is a heterogeneous disease and that its natural history is even more protracted than was apparent in the Middlesex series. These data also suggest that there are clinically definable subsets of patients with a high annual hazard of death (more than 25%) and other subsets with low annual hazards of death (less than 2%). An alternative explanation is that breast cancer is a single, but heterogeneous, disease in which patients fall along a continuum of biologic aggressiveness.

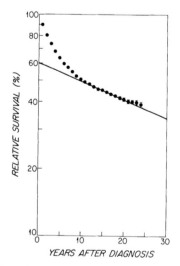

FIGURE 12-2   Relative survival rates of breast cancer patients (all stages) from the End Results Section, Biometry Branch, National Cancer Institute, 1977. (Fox MS. On the diagnosis and treatment of breast cancer. JAMA 1979;241:489)

An understanding of the survival curve for breast cancer patients is important in assessing prognosis in patient subgroups and assessing new therapies.[3] For most populations, the slope of the survival curve of treated patients becomes more shallow at 10 years (called the *inflection point*). The demonstration of a "cured" subgroup, therefore, requires follow-up of longer than 10 years. (Whether such patients are actually cured is discussed in the next section.) With long-term follow-up, it is possible to distinguish the disease's *virulence* and *metastagenicity*.[4] Virulence is the pace or rate of appearance of metastases or mortality, whereas metastagenicity is the ultimate likelihood of metastases. We[3] have also stressed elsewhere that improvements in the early portion of the survival curve by new therapies do not always result in an improvement in the survival curve past the inflection point. Conversely, in some cases, an early detrimental effect may obscure a benefit in long-term outcome. These considerations emphasize that effects seen on the early portion of survival curves may be premature and also misleading.

Curability of Breast Cancer

The protracted nature of the survival curve shown in Figure 12-2 raises the question of whether a patient with breast cancer is ever truly cured of her disease. Given that breast cancer has a relatively late age of onset and a long natural history, a large group of patients must be followed for a long time to address this question. Furthermore, the definition of *cure* is not straightforward, and a number of definitions have been proposed.[5] The most commonly used definition of cure is referred to as *statistical* cure. A group of treated patients can be considered statistically cured if their subsequent death rate from all causes is similar to that of a normal population group with the same age and sex distribution. *Clinical* cure for an individual refers to the apparent complete eradication of the disease. Clinical cure for a group occurs when long-term follow-up of the causes of death for the group shows that the risk of dying from breast cancer is the same as for women of the same age in the general population. An assessment of the likelihood of clinical cure involves determining the cause of death for treated patients. Inaccuracies in the information recorded on death certificates, however, limits the usefulness of this definition of cure. *Personal* cure for an individual refers to a patient living symptom-free from breast cancer and dying of other causes.

Attempts to assess statistical cure in breast cancer patients have all indicated a persistent excess risk of mortality. Brinkley and Haybittle[6] reported on a group of 704 breast cancer patients, from the Cambridge, England area, in whom the first diagnosis was made between 1947 and 1950. The minimum follow-up period for survivors was 31 years. Figure 12-3 shows the survival curves calculated by the life-table method and the expected curves for the normal population of the region with the same age distribution. The survival curves for breast cancer patients never become parallel with those for the normal population. There were eight deaths from breast cancer more than 25 years after treatment, which is 15 times the number that would be expected. Hibberd and associates[7] followed 2019 cases for 30 years and found a small excess of observed over expected deaths, even between 25 and 30 years. Rutqvist and Wallgren[8] presented follow-up on 458 patients 40 years of age or younger at diagnosis and found an excess mortality that persisted for at least 40 years. These studies all indicate a persistent excess risk of mortality after treatment for breast cancer.

Despite the lack of evidence for a statistical cure, a considerable percentage of patients experience a personal cure, as defined earlier. In the Brinkley and Haybittle report,[6] 176 (26%) of the 683 patients fell into this category. In the experience from Memorial Sloan-Kettering Cancer Center reported by Adair and coworkers,[9] 300 of the 1458 patients (21%) with operable breast cancer had

a personal cure of their disease. In a more recent report from Memorial Sloan-Kettering Cancer Center, Rosen and associates[10] reported on 382 patients with breast cancer 2 cm or smaller and axillary nodes negative for metastasis, who were treated with radical mastectomy and followed for a median of 18.2 years. Although recurrences were observed during the entire 20-year follow-up period, it was estimated that 80% of patients with tumors 1 cm or smaller had personal cures, and 70% of patients with tumors 1.1 to 2 cm had personal cures. This means that many patients treated for breast cancer will live out their normal life expectancy, free of further evidence of the disease. Similar findings were seen in the long-term follow-up of node-negative breast cancer patients from the University of Chicago; in addition, patients with small tumors and one to three involved axillary nodes similarly had an excellent prognosis.[4]

Growth Rate of Breast Cancer

The long natural history of breast cancer has been evaluated in terms of the clinical growth rate of the disease. The determination of clinical growth rate can provide information on the heterogeneity of the disease and has been used to estimate the time from oncogenesis to clinical presentation.

One of the ways in which the growth rate of breast cancer has been assessed is by the time required for a tumor to double its diameter, an amount equivalent to an eight-fold increase in volume. In 1956, Collins and colleagues[11] described the clinical growth rates of several human tumors, including carcinoma of the breast. They assumed an exponential model for tumor growth; that is, tumor cells divide at a constant rate over time. According to this model, a single cancer cell will grow to a nodule 1 mm in diameter in 20 doublings. Another 10 doublings

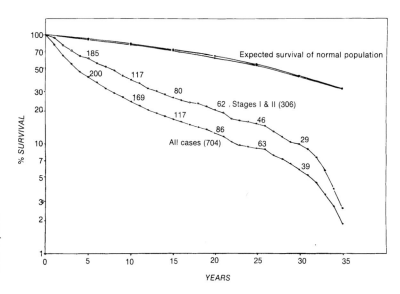

FIGURE 12-3 Survival rate curve for 704 breast cancer patients treated between 1947 and 1950 and observed for at least 31 years, compared with survival curve of the normal population. (Brinkley D, Haybittle JL. Long term survival of women with breast cancer. Lancet 1984;1:1118)

would produce approximately 1 kg of tumor tissue, an amount commonly observed at the time of death from the disease. Collins and associates plotted the clinical doubling time for a group of 24 patients with metastatic cancer involving the lungs, in whom measurements of tumor size could be performed on serial chest radiographs. The observed doubling times ranged from 28 to 164 days for patients with tumors of epithelial origin. The median volume doubling time for this group was 78 days. This study established the heterogeneity of clinical growth rates for human tumors and was used to estimate the duration of the preclinical phases of the disease. If one assumes this exponential model, a doubling time of 100 days, and that a primary and metastatic tumor have similar growth rates, then the time required for a single malignant cell to grow to a clinically detectable 1-cm mass would be slightly more than 8 years. This analysis suggests that there is ample time for spread, even before the earliest possible time of detection. Similar findings have been noticed by other investigators.[12-15] This model of exponential tumor growth provided the first theoretic basis for the use of cancer chemotherapy.[16,17]

It is also possible to estimate the interval between mammographic detectability and clinical detectability from data obtained from mammographic screening programs.[18] Using the data from the Health Insurance Plan of Greater New York study, the mean interval was estimated to be 1.7 years. Other estimates of the interval that used different mathematical models vary from 1.3 to 2.4 years.[19,20]

There are deficiencies, however, in the concept of exponential tumor growth. In fact, for breast cancer and other epithelial malignancies, tumor growth is better described by a Gompertzian rather than an exponential model.[21] In a Gompertzian model, the growth constant is exponentially slowing. Therefore, while the tumor mass increases in size, its doubling time becomes progressively longer. In vitro and in vivo studies have indicated that the human tumor cell cycle time is on the order of 2 days, not 100 days.[22] Gross tumor doubling times, in fact, represent a complex relationship between cell cycle time, the percentage of cells cycling (growth fraction), and the likelihood that a newly divided cell will not contribute to the tumor mass (cell loss factor). For breast cancer, the growth fraction is approximately 5%, and the cell loss factor is about 75%. Thus, most of a tumor is made of cells that are not cycling. Furthermore, each cell that is cycling does so at a very rapid rate, but most of its progeny do not survive. In this light, it is necessary to interpret volume doubling times as only a rough index of the aggressiveness of the tumor and as not valid for estimating the time from oncogenesis to clinical presentation. An improved knowledge of tumor growth can be exploited by devising new schemes using this knowledge for the treatment of breast cancer using chemotherapy (see Chap. 22.4).

The observed clinical growth rate of breast cancer ultimately needs to account for the evolving information on the molecular and genetic biology of the disease. As described in Chapter 3.6, breast cancer, similar to other malignancies for which more precise information is known, results from a series of mutations in growth-regulatory genes and other genes. It is unknown, however, whether these mutations need to occur in any particular order or how many separate pathways involving different genetic changes may eventually lead to the phenotype of breast cancer. The heterogeneity in the clinical behavior of breast cancer suggests that the genetic basis for the disease may be variable. These genetic changes result in growth under conditions that would be limiting for normal cells, and it is presumed that additional genetic changes favoring the survival of this clone, its uncontrolled growth, and its ability to change (genetic instability) are selected over time. Although this model of oncogenesis (clonal selection) was developed in the 1970s,[23] the details are just becoming available. By the time of clinical presentation, it is estimated that the extent of genetic change is large, as evidenced by the common finding of aneuploidy. A large variety of genetic changes have been described in the human breast cancers (see Chap. 3.6), although their pathogenetic significance has not been fully elucidated.

Even more complicated models of breast cancer growth have been proposed. In a model proposed by Speer[24] and Retsky[25] and their coworkers, tumor growth occurs in "spurts," during which Gompertzian growth pertains, separated by periods of little or no growth for varying lengths of time. It is possible to select specific values for the time between growth spurts and for their rates of growth that are consistent with well-described clinical data sets. Retsky and associates[25] have argued that their theory of tumor growth is consistent with tumor growth by clonal selection. They have hypothesized that additional genetic changes (such as for the ability to obtain new blood vessels for additional growth) can provide incremental spurts in tumor growth. These models are discussed in detail in Chapter 22.4.

Primary Cancer in the Breast

The spread of primary cancer through the breast occurs (1) by direct infiltration into the breast parenchyma, (2) along mammary ducts, and (3) by way of breast lymphatics. Direct infiltration of the cancer tends to occur by ramifying projections that give a characteristic stellate appearance on gross examination and on mammography. If untreated, direct involvement of overlying skin or deep pectoral fascia can occur. Involvement along ducts is observed frequently and may involve an entire segment of the breast. It is unclear, however, whether this intraductal involvement represents spread of a primary cancer along previously uninvolved ducts or the development of an invasive cancer or cancers from a diffuse area of ductal carcinoma in situ. Spread also can occur by the extensive network of breast lymphatics. Investigators have emphasized lymphatic spread vertically down to the lymphatic plexus in the deep pectoral fascia underlying the breast. In addition, spread to the central subareolar region has been described. These multiple mechanisms of spread through the breast emphasize the likelihood for cancer to be present in the breast wall beyond the palpable primary mass.

A detailed study of the distribution of cancer in a breast containing a localized tumor has been performed by Holland and colleagues.[26] They examined 264 specimens from patients with clinically unifocal breast cancer measuring 4 cm or smaller (see Fig. 17.1-1). In only 40% of cases was the cancer in the breast restricted to the palpable tumor. Nineteen percent of cases had additional foci of cancer but restricted to the immediate 2 cm around the tumor. Forty-one percent of the cases showed cancer foci further than 2 cm from the reference tumor, including 27% in which the additional foci were entirely intraductal and 14% in which they were invasive and intraductal. This study and its implications for breast-conserving treatment are further discussed in Chapter 17.1.

The primary site of breast cancer usually is described by its location by quadrant in the breast. In one series of 696 cases, 48% were located in the upper outer quadrant, 15% in the upper inner quadrant, 11% in the lower outer quadrant, 6% in the lower inner quadrant, and 17% in the central region (designated as within 1 cm of the areola).[27] An additional 3% were termed diffuse because of multicentric or massive involvement of the breast. The reason for the increased frequency of breast cancer in the upper outer quadrant is thought to be simply the greater amount of breast tissue in that quadrant. In this series of patients, no differences in survival based on quadrant location were observed. The relation between the location of the primary tumor in the breast and prognosis has also been examined in a large series of patients from the 1978 National Survey of the American College of Surgeons (ACS)[28] and by the National Surgical Adjuvant Breast Project (NSABP).[29] In the ACS study, outcome in 9401 patients was examined in relation to the size of the primary tumor, its location, and involvement of axillary nodes. Patients were treated with mastectomy without RT; the 5-year results are shown in Table 12-1. The distribution of tumor size for patients with medial and lateral tumors was nearly identical. Patients with medial tumors and node-negative breast cancer, however, did somewhat worse than patients with lateral tumors and node-negative disease (recurrence rates, 18% versus 14%, $P < .005$). The results for patients with node-positive breast cancer were not statistically different, based on tumor location. The results obtained in the NSABP study were similar. Patients with medial tumors and node-negative disease also did slightly worse than patients with lateral tumors who were node-negative (recurrence rates, 24% versus 19%). The number of patients in this study, however, was smaller, and the results did not reach statistical significance. Patients with node-positive disease had the same prognosis, regardless of location. The results from the ACS and NSABP studies suggest that patients with inner-half tumors and node-negative disease have a worse prognosis than patients with outer-half tumors and negative nodes. This observation is likely related to preferential involvement of internal mammary nodes (IMNs) with medial tumors, which is discussed further later.

The clinical size of the primary tumor is highly corre-lated with prognosis. The data from Koscielny and associates[30,31] of the Institut Gustave-Roussy illustrates this point. They examined the relationship between the size of the primary tumor and the likelihood of distant metastasis in 2648 patients with breast cancer treated at their institution between 1954 and 1972 (Fig. 12-4). Patients who presented with metastatic disease were included in the analysis; follow-up ranged from 10 years to over 25 years. The data, which were plotted using a logprobit coordinate system, indicate a direct relation between tumor size and the probability of metastasis. Similar findings have been reported in other studies.[9,32–35]

Regional Node Involvement

The most common sites of regional involvement of breast cancer are the axillary node, IMN, and supraclavicular lymph node regions. Knowledge of the likelihood of involvement of these sites and their significance is important for the staging and planning of treatment for patients with breast cancer.

AXILLARY NODE INVOLVEMENT

The axillary lymph node region is the major regional drainage site for the breast. Approximately 50% of patients with breast cancer that is evident on physical examination have histologic evidence of axillary node involvement. The likelihood of axillary nodal involvement is directly related to the size of the primary tumor. This was shown in studies by Nemoto and coworkers,[28] Haagensen,[35] and Fisher and associates[34] and documented in greater detail in the report from the Surveillance, Epidemiology and End Results (SEER) Program of the NCI[36] (Table 12-2). The SEER data examined the relationship between tumor size, axillary lymph node involvement, and 5-year relative survival in 24,740 patients with breast cancer. The data were taken from the nine SEER population-based tumor registries for patients diagnosed between 1977 and 1982 whose pathologic or operative tumor size was recorded and who had at least eight lymph nodes examined. Patients with distant metastases at diagnosis, carcinoma in situ, or prior cancer were excluded. The larger the primary tumor, the greater the risk of axillary node involvement. Even for the smallest tumors (less than 0.5 cm) the risk of axillary involvement was approximately 20%. As discussed in Chapter 17.1, patients with microinvasive breast cancer are the only subgroup in whom the risk of axillary nodal involvement is consistently reported to be less than 5%.

Evidence supports the theory that the location of the primary tumor in the breast influences the likelihood of axillary node involvement. Several studies have indicated that axillary nodes are more commonly involved when tumors are located in the lateral portion of the breast than when they are in the medial portion. In the 1978 National Survey of the ACS, 43% of patients with lateral-half tumors had node-positive node disease compared with 35% of patients with medial-half tumors.[28] Haagensen[35] de-

TABLE 12-1
Five-Year Recurrence Rates (RR) Related to Tumor Size, Tumor Location, and Involvement of Axillary Nodes

	Negative Nodes				Positive Nodes			
	Medial		Lateral		Medial		Lateral	
Tumor Size (cm)	N	RR (%)	N	RR (%)	N	RR (%)	N	RR (%)
0.1–1.0	141	12	408	10	19	32	83	21
1.1–2.0	471	16	1357	12	102	41	411	34
2.1–3.0	347	19	1034	13	114	43	424	36
3.1–5.0	227	20	721	17	102	47	406	45
≥5.1	54	34	191	21	46	33	166	57
All	1240	18	8711	14	383	42	1490	39

(Nemoto T, Natarajan N, Bedwani R, et al. Breast cancer in the medial half: results of the 1978 National Survey of the American College of Surgeons. Cancer 1983; 51:1333)

scribed similar results on the frequency of axillary node metastasis from his personal series of 917 patients treated with radical mastectomy. In this series, positive nodes were found in 47% of patients with upper outer quadrant tumors, 38% with lower outer quadrant tumors, 30% with upper inner quadrant tumors, and 23% with lower inner quadrant tumors. Similarly, Fisher and associates[29] found

that 52% of patients with lateral-half tumors had positive nodes compared with 39% of patients with medial-half tumors. In the previously noted ACS study, the results were examined in relation to tumor size and location (Table 12-3). In each category of tumor size, patients with medial tumors were less likely to have positive axillary nodes, compared with patients with lateral tumors. The increased likelihood of axillary involvement for lateral compared with medial tumors is most likely related to preferential drainage of some medial tumors to IMNs. As a result, regional lymph node involvement (either axillary nodes or IMNs) is similar for medial and lateral tumors.

The reported incidence of histologic involvement of axillary nodes is dependent, to some degree, on the extent of the axillary dissection performed and the thoroughness of the pathologic evaluation of the specimen. Radical mastectomy permits the most complete dissection of the axil-

FIGURE 12-4 Relation between clinical size of the tumor and the likelihood of distant metastasis for patients treated from 1954 to 1958 (O) and 1959 to 1972 (X). (Koscielny S, Tubiana M, Le M, et al. Breast cancer: relationship between the size of the primary tumor and the probability of metastatic dissemination. Br J Cancer 1984;49:709)

TABLE 12-2
Frequency of Axillary Node Involvement Related to Tumor Size

Tumor Size (cm)	Frequency of Axillary Node Involvement (%)
<0.5	20.6
0.5–0.9	20.6
1–1.9	33.2
2–2.9	44.9
3–3.9	52.1
4–4.9	60.0
>5.0	70.1

(Carter C, Allen C, Henson D. Relation of tumor size, lymph node status, and survival in 24,740 breast cancer cases. Cancer 1989;63:181)

TABLE 12-3
Incidence of Positive Axillary Nodes Relative to the Location and Size of the Primary Tumor

Tumor Size (cm)	Medial		Lateral	
	Patients	Positive (%)	Patients	Positive (%)
0.1–1.0	219	18	578	25
1.1–2.0	820	28	2212	35
2.1–3.0	691	35	1951	43
3.1–5.0	522	44	1651	53
>5.1	165	58	592	63
TOTAL	2417	35	6984	43

(Nemoto T, Natarajan N, Bedwani R, et al. Breast cancer in the medial half: results of the 1978 National Survey of the American College of Surgeons. Cancer 1983;51:1333)

lary contents and yields the greatest number of axillary nodes. Lesser surgical procedures, such as the modified radical mastectomy, typically give a less-complete axillary dissection and fewer axillary nodes. As a result of this variable extent of axillary dissection, the likelihood of histologic involvement must be viewed in terms of the surgical procedure performed. In one pathologic study of axillary specimens, it was observed that axillary node involvement after complete dissection would have been reduced by 29% if the axillary dissection had been extended only to the lateral border of the pectoralis minor muscle.[37]

Detection of axillary involvement by physical examination has both a high false-positive and false-negative rate[32,35,38,39] (Table 12-4). When axillary lymph nodes are palpable and suspect for cancer, histologic evidence of metastatic disease is found in about 70% of cases. Conversely, when axillary nodes are not palpable, histologic involvement is detected in approximately 30% of cases. These figures indicate the shortcomings of clinical evaluation in predicting histologic involvement.

Histologic involvement of axillary nodes has a high correlation with prognosis. Table 12-5 shows 10-year survival figures related to axillary involvement from seven separate series of patients treated with radical mastectomy.[32,40–45] Patients with histologically negative axillary nodes have markedly better survival rates than do patients with histologic involvement. Furthermore, patients with one to three nodes positive for metastasis do better than patients with four or more positive nodes. In fact, prognosis is directly related to the number of axillary nodes positive for disease. This is illustrated in the results obtained in the ACS survey[33] (Table 12-6). Prognosis showed a progressive decline with increasing numbers of positive nodes. Patients with one node positive for metastasis had a 63% 5-year likelihood of survival and a 33% risk of recurrence, compared with a 22% 5-year likelihood of survival and a 82% risk of recurrence for patients with 21 or more positive nodes. These data suggest that any comparison of prognosis that is based on dividing patients by a certain number of positive nodes is artificial because there are no clear dividing lines. However, such a division is practical. Many groups now divide patients into groups having 1 to 3 positive nodes, 4 to 9 positive nodes, or 10 or more positive nodes.

The axilla is commonly divided into three levels: level I or proximal, defined as tissue inferior and lateral to the lower border of the pectoralis minor muscle; level II or middle, tissue directly beneath the pectoralis minor; and level III or distal, tissue superior and medial to the pectoralis minor (see Fig. 17.1-6). Prognosis has been shown to be related to the level of axillary involvement.[32] Involvement of the distal level nodes carries a worse prognosis than involvement of the proximal level nodes. In a

TABLE 12-4
Accuracy of Physical Examination in Predicting Histologic Involvement of Axillary Nodes

Results	Bucalossi et al[39]	Butcher[38]	Haagensen[35]	Schottenfeld et al[32]
False-positive (%)	25	31	26	29
False-negative (%)	32	28	27	29

TABLE 12-5
Ten-Year Survival Rate by Axillary Node Status for Patients Treated With Radical Mastectomy

	Survival Rate (%)			
Study	Negative Nodes	Positive Nodes	1 to 3 Positive Nodes	4 or More Positive Nodes
Valagussa et al[40]	80	38	50	24
Haagensen[41]	76	48	63	27
Schottenfeld et al[32]	72	43	—	—
Fisher et al[42]	65	25	38	13
Spratt & Donegan[43]	68	27	—	—
Payne et al[44]	76	35	—	—
Ferguson et al[45]	72	39	52	27

study of 182 mastectomy specimens in which the axillary contents were completely examined (or cleared), involvement of nodes in the distal portion of the axilla was found in 15.[46] All 15 were associated with involvement of many nodes in the axilla (mean number of involved nodes was 16.2). In another study, axillary node involvement and survival were examined in 385 patients to determine whether the total number of involved nodes or the level of axillary node involvement was a better indicator of prognosis.[37] They found that for any given number of involved nodes, survival was independent of the level of involvement, and they concluded that prognosis was related more directly to the total number of nodes involved.

Involvement of the axilla is generally orderly relative to levels. This was examined in two large series of patients treated with radical mastectomy[47,48] and in other smaller series of patients treated with modified radical mastectomy[49-52] (see Table 17.1-11). In the two large series, isolated involvement at upper levels in the axilla in the absence of involvement at level I was uncommon. The results in the smaller series are more variable and are discussed in greater detail in Chapter 17.1.

The axillary nodes also can be subclassified into the following: (1) external mammary, (2) central, (3) scapular, (4) axillary vein, (5) apical or subclavicular, and (6) interpectoral (Rotter) lymph nodes (see Chap. 1). Haagensen[53] has documented sites of involvement by cancer in the axilla using this classification. He found that the most common site of involvement was the central group of nodes. When only one node was involved, in nearly all cases it was in the central group. The next most common site of involvement was the axillary vein group, followed by the scapular, interpectoral, and subclavicular groups.

The question of whether both the size of the primary tumor and the number of involved axillary nodes independently predict for prognosis has been addressed in several institutional studies and documented in greater detail in the SEER data (Table 12-7). The results indicate that these two factors are of independent prognostic value. Survival declines with increasing size when nodal status is held constant, and survival declines with increasing nodal involvement when tumor size is held constant. In fact, within each subgroup of axillary node involvement, the contribution of tumor size to mortality is roughly a linear function of the tumor size. The sole exception to this is the strikingly poor rate of survival for patients with tumors smaller than 2 cm who have four or more nodes positive for metastasis. Also, the effect of tumor size is greater for node-positive patients than for node-negative patients. These results on tumor size and nodal involvement are corroborated by results seen with longer follow-up. Adair and others[9] reported that for patients with node-negative disease, the 30-year relative survival rate was 61% when the primary tumor was 2 cm or smaller, 46% for tumors

TABLE 12-6
Five-Year Results Related to the Number of Axillary Nodes Pathologically Positive

Positive Axillary Nodes	Patients	Survival Rate (%)	Recurrence Rate (%)
0	12,299	72	19
1	2012	63	33
2	1338	62	40
3	842	59	43
4	615	52	44
5	478	47	54
6–10	1261	41	63
11–15	562	29	72
16–20	301	29	75
≥21	225	22	82

(Nemoto T, Vana J, Bedwani R, et al. Management and survival of female breast cancer: results of a national survey by the American College of Surgeons. Cancer 1980;45:2917)

TABLE 12-7

Five-Year Breast Cancer Survival Rates According to the Size of the Tumor and Axillary Node Involvement

Tumor Size (cm)	Patients Surviving 5 Years		
	Negative Nodes	1 to 3 Positive Nodes	4 or More Positive Nodes
<0.5	269 (99.2%)	53 (95.3%)	17 (59.0%)
0.5–0.9	791 (98.3%)	140 (94.0%)	65 (54.2%)
1.0–1.9	4668 (95.8%)	1574 (86.6%)	742 (67.2%)
2.0–2.9	4010 (92.3%)	1897 (83.4%)	1375 (63.4%)
3.0–3.9	2072 (86.2%)	1185 (79.0%)	1072 (56.9%)
4.0–4.9	845 (84.6%)	540 (69.8%)	727 (52.6%)
≥5.0	809 (82.2%)	630 (73.0%)	1259 (45.5%)

(Carter C, Allen C, Henson D. Relation of tumor size, lymph node status, and survival in 24,740 breast cancer cases. Cancer 1989;63:181)

between 2 and 5 cm, and 50% for tumors larger than 5 cm. For patients with involvement of level I axillary nodes, the 30-year relative survival rate was 40% when the tumor was 2 cm or smaller, 31% for tumors between 2 and 5 cm, and 14% for tumors larger than 5 cm. The results seen at the Institut Gustave-Roussy also are in general agreement.[30,31] This study population consisted of 2408 patients treated at the Institut Gustave-Roussy by initial radical or modified radical mastectomy between 1954 and 1979. For each patient, they systematically assessed the primary tumor size and the number of axillary nodes positive for metastasis. The authors used a probit analysis to estimate the distribution of tumor sizes at the times of axillary node involvement and distant metastases. As shown in other studies, they found that increasing tumor size was associated with an increasing likelihood and extent of axillary nodal involvement. Among all subsets of patients, a strong correlation was observed between the propensity for axillary nodal involvement and for distant metastasis (indicating that both reflect the biologic aggressiveness of a tumor). However, the capacity for nodal involvement was acquired at a smaller tumor size than the capacity for distant metastasis. For any group of patients, prognosis was better assessed using both tumor size and extent of axillary node involvement, rather than by one of these alone. These results stress that both tumor size and number of involved axillary nodes are useful in estimating prognosis and that a significant percentage of patients with involved axillary nodes have prolonged survival, without evidence of distant metastasis.

About 20% to 30% of patients with negative axillary nodes develop distant metastases within 10 years (see Table 12-5). This observation has important implications regarding the natural history of the disease. It suggests that metastases can travel directly from the primary tumor in the breast to distant sites by way of the bloodstream without

first involving the regional lymph nodes. A possible alternative explanation is that nodes that are called negative are in fact involved with metastases, but are undetected. There is known to be a sampling error in the detection of axillary metastases. It is possible to miss axillary nodes in the axillary dissection specimen unless a meticulous clearing method is employed, and it is possible to miss microscopic evidence of metastases in a given node unless it is thoroughly sectioned. In the United States, the routine method for detection of axillary nodal metastases does not involve clearing of the specimen and involves only a limited number of sections (typically only one per node). In 1984, Saphir and Amromin[54] reported that serial sectioning of the axillary nodes in 30 cases discovered metastases in 10 (33%) in which previous single-level sections had not shown metastases. However, this procedure does not necessarily identify those node-negative patients who have a recurrence. In one study by Pickren[55] of 51 patients reported to be node-negative cases by routine sectioning, 11 (22%) were positive on serial sectioning. The 5-year survival rate of these 11 patients was 91%. This was similar to that for patients without occult metastases on serial sectioning, and both were better than the 5-year survival rate of 53% for patients with metastases seen on routine sectioning. Similar results were found in studies by Fisher and coworkers[56] and by Wilkinson and associates.[57] In a more recent study, however, of 1680 breast cancers reported to be node-negative by routine sectioning, serial sectioning of axillary nodes revealed a single micrometastasis (defined as measuring 2 mm or less) in 120 cases (7%) and a single macrometastasis in 216 cases (13%).[58] With a median follow-up of 7 years, patients with either micrometastatic or macrometastatic involvement had a statistically significant worse disease-free and overall survival, although the magnitude of the differences was not large. In a multivariate analysis, the presence of macrometastatic involvement, but not micrometastatic involvement, remained in the final model for recurrence. Similar findings were seen in a study by the International (Ludwig) Breast Cancer Study Group.[59] These results indicate the following: (1) that histologic involvement of axillary nodes can be detected by serial sectioning in 10% to 20% of cases judged to be node-negative by routine sectioning; (2) that such involvement suggests a slightly worse prognosis compared with patients without involvement; and (3) that even in patients with negative nodes evaluated by serial sectioning, the 10-year recurrence rate is still 20% to 30%.

Attempts have been made to identify involvement in axillary nodes by the use of immunohistochemical techniques. A number of investigators have reported detection of metastases in 10% to 20% of allegedly negative nodes using a variety of monoclonal antibodies directed against epithelial cell antigens.[58,60–64] In the report by the Trojani group,[58] immunohistochemical staining (using a "cocktail" of five monoclonal antibodies directed against epithelial cell antigens) detected micrometastases in 37 cases of a group of 89 invasive lobular carcinomas (42%) and in 13 cases of a group of 129 invasive ductal carcinomas (10%). In the invasive lobular group, involvement had no prognostic value (median follow-up, 9.3 years). In the invasive ductal group, involvement was associated with a statistically significant decrease in relapse-free survival and overall survival (median follow-up, 15.6 years), although the difference in survival was modest. Similar to the findings with serial sectioning, the results using immunohistochemical staining indicate the following: (1) that histologic involvement in axillary nodes can be detected in 10% to 20% of cases of invasive ductal carcinoma judged to be node-negative by routine staining with hematoxylin and eosin; (2) that such involvement suggests a slightly worse prognosis compared with patients without involvement; and (3) that even in patients with negative nodes evaluated by immunohistochemical staining, the 10-year recurrence rate is still 20% to 30%. However, this technique is still limited by the sensitivity and specificity of currently available monoclonal antibodies, and its usefulness may change with the availability of better antibodies. It may also be possible to detect micrometastases by even more sensitive techniques of molecular biologic examination.[65,66]

A related issue is the prognostic significance of minimal axillary involvement, variously called *micrometastases* (involvement less than 2 mm) or *clandestine metastases* (involvement of small emboli of tumor cells in the sinuses of axillary nodes) detected by routine evaluation of axillary nodes. Information on this subject is available from two series with long follow-up. Investigators from Memorial Sloan-Kettering Cancer Center reported on 147 patients with T1 or T2 breast cancers and a single involved axillary lymph node followed for 10 years after treatment.[67] Overall, the 70 patients with micrometastases had fewer recurrences (24%) than did 77 patients with macrometastases (39%). A subset analysis yielding small numbers of patients suggested that micrometastasis and macrometastases had a similar prognosis in patients with T1 tumors (but worse than in patients without involvement). In patients with T2 tumors and a micrometastases, prognosis was similar to patients without involvement, but worse than in patients with a macrometastasis. The other study from Friedman and others[68] from the Institut Gustave-Roussy compared the rate of distant metastases among 41 patients with one node involved with a clandestine metastasis, 205 patients with one node involved with a parenchymal metastasis, and 637 patients without nodal metastases (median follow-up time, 118 months). The authors found that clandestine and parenchymal involvement of a single lymph node had similar prognostic value and conferred a worse prognosis than negative node results (relative risk, 1.7). The results of these two studies are limited by small numbers and are not consistent.

In summary, the axilla is the major lymph node region for carcinoma of the breast, and a histologic analysis of the axillary nodes provides a useful guide to a patient's prognosis.

INTERNAL MAMMARY NODE INVOLVEMENT

The second major nodal site of involvement in carcinoma of the breast is the IMN chain. This chain lies at the anterior end of the intercostal spaces by the side of the internal thoracic artery. Because of their intrathoracic loca-tion and their uncommon clinical presentation, the frequency of IMN involvement was not appreciated as early as axillary node involvement. One of the first to document this second route of spread was Handley,[69] who reported his results of IMN biopsy in 1000 patients in 1975 (Table 12-8). These results indicated the following: (1) overall, axillary lymph node involvement is more likely to occur than IMN involvement (54% versus 22%); (2) IMN involvement is more common when axillary nodes are involved than when uninvolved (35% versus 8%); and (3) IMN involvement is more common for inner quadrant or central primaries than for outer quadrant primaries. However, even in patients with inner or central tumors, axillary involvement was more common than IMN involvement (42% versus 28%). Furthermore, when axillary nodes were uninvolved, IMN involvement was uncommon, even with inner quadrant or central tumors.

Another large series of patients treated with IMN biopsy has been reported by Veronesi and colleagues.[70] In this series of 1119 patients, axillary involvement was seen in 50% of patients and IMN involvement was seen in 19%. They found that the likelihood of IMN involvement was related to axillary involvement (29% axillary node-positive, versus 9% node-negative, $P < .01$), and to patient age (40 years of age or younger, 28%; 41 to 50 years, 20%; and older than 50 years, 16%; $P = .01$). Unlike the findings of Handley,[69] however, IMN involvement was not related to the location of the primary tumor in the breast (19% inner versus 18% outer). Veronesi and associates[70] found that axillary involvement, tumor size, and patient age all influence the likelihood of IMN involvement. For a patient younger than 40 years of age with positive axillary node results and a primary tumor larger than 2 cm, the risk of IMN involvement was 44%. For a patient older than 50 years with negative axillary node results and a primary tumor smaller than 2 cm, the risk of IMN involvement was only 7%. In this study, the prognostic implication of IMN involvement was similar to that for axillary node involvement (Fig. 12-5). The 10-year disease-free survival rate was 73% when both axillary and IMNs tested negative, 47% when axillary nodes alone tested positive, 52% when IMNs alone tested positive, and only 25% when both areas tested positive.

Other investigators have examined the relation between tumor location and IMN involvement and, like Handley, have found that IMN involvement is more common for medial or central tumors. Haagensen[71] performed IMN biopsy in 1007 patients and found IMN involvement in 29% of patients with medial tumors, compared with 17% of patients with lateral tumors. Patients with central tumors and positive axillary nodes had a 43% risk of IMN involvement. Similarly, LaCour and colleagues[72] studied a group of 703 patients and reported IMN involvement in 24% of patients with medial or central tumors and 16% of patients with lateral tumors.

Overall, roughly 50% of patients have axillary node involvement and 20% of patients have IMN involvement. The most consistent finding in IMN involvement is its relation to axillary node involvement. When axillary nodes test negative, IMN involvement is uncommon (approxi-

TABLE 12-8
Internal Mammary Node Involvement Relative to Location of the Primary Tumor and Axillary Node Involvement

Axillary Node Status	Location of Primary Tumor					
	UIQ	LIQ	Central	UOQ	LOQ	All
Negative	10/143	2/36	5/76	7/170	2/40	8%
	14%	6%	7%	4%	5%	
Positive	47/105	18/25	65/140	47/212	10/53	35%
	45%	72%	46%	22%	19%	
All	27%	33%	32%	14%	13%	22%

UIQ, upper internal quadrant; LIQ, lower internal quadrant; UOQ, upper outer quadrant; LOQ, lower outer quadrant.

(Handley R. Carcinoma of the breast. Ann R Coll Surg Engl 1975;57:59)

mately 10%). When axillary nodes test positive, IMN involvement is approximately 30%. Furthermore, the greater the extent of axillary node involvement, the greater the likelihood of IMN involvement. However, the prognostic significance of IMN involvement is still apparent, even when adjusted for the extent of axillary node involvement.

SUPRACLAVICULAR LYMPH NODE INVOLVEMENT

Supraclavicular lymph node involvement is associated with extensive axillary node involvement. In one series of patients undergoing routine supraclavicular dissection, involvement of the supraclavicular region was found in 23 (18%) of 125 patients who had positive axillary nodes and in none of 149 patients whose axillary nodes did not test positive.[73] The significance of supraclavicular node involvement was first shown by Halsted,[74] who performed supraclavicular dissections in 119 patients: 44 patients were found to have involvement of these nodes, of whom only 2 were free of cancer at 5 years. Supraclavicular node involvement represents a late stage of axillary node involvement and carries a grave prognosis. Based on this,

more recent staging systems categorize supraclavicular node involvement as M1 or distant metastatic.

The Influence of Local Treatment on Survival

The treatment of breast cancer has been directed both at the breast and regional lymph nodes locally and at sites of metastases systemically, but the importance of local treatment has been debated. It is useful to examine this debate from a historical perspective.[75] Perhaps no other disease or its treatment has evoked such strong feelings as breast cancer. The reasons for this can be found both in our culture in general and in medicine in particular. The breast, in certain contexts, is the symbol of motherhood, nourishment, and security, whereas in others it represents beauty and femininity. There are equally compelling medical connotations that have made supporters of certain therapeutic alternatives act like religious zealots. Strongly held beliefs as well as the need for long-term follow-up

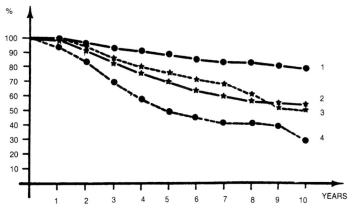

FIGURE 12-5 Ten-year overall survival rates in patients without node metastases (1), with axillary node metastases only (2), with internal mammary node metastases only (3), and with both groups involved (4) ($P = 10^{-9}$). (Veronesi U, Cascinelli N, Greco M, et al. Prognosis of breast cancer patients after mastectomy and dissection of internal mammary nodes. Ann Surg 1985;202:702)

have provided the ingredients for animated debate concerning the disease and its treatment.

In the middle of the 19th century, women with breast cancer typically were first seen by their physicians with locally advanced disease, not simply with an asymptomatic lump in the breast. There was no effective local therapy or any useful systemic anti-cancer treatment available at that time. Attempts at surgical extirpation generally resulted in a prompt return of the disease locally. The futility of therapy only reinforced the nihilistic attitude of the population toward the advisability of prompt treatment for suspicious breast masses.

The introduction of the radical mastectomy by Meyer[76] and Halsted[77] at the end of the 19th century was an important therapeutic advance and provided the first important therapeutic paradigm for the disease. The use of radical mastectomy was based on a model of cancer spread that was centrifugal. According to this view, a tumor started locally, infiltrated by way of the lymphatics in a direct and contiguous fashion to the regional lymph nodes, and only then spread to distant sites. In its most doctrinaire presentation, espoused by Halsted,[77] even distant metastases occurred by contiguous extension. This notion of the disease provided a rational basis for a radical operation designed to resect widely the tumor and contiguous tissues including the overlying skin, both of the underlying pectoral muscles, and all of the ipsilateral axillary lymph nodes. The rapid and widespread use of radical mastectomy was a result of the acceptance of this theory of disease spread and of improvements in surgical and anesthetic techniques that were required for the operation to be feasible.

The radical mastectomy was later expanded to extended radical and superradical operations, including dissections of the IMNs and supraclavicular lymph nodes. Radiation therapy was advocated as a further regional treatment to augment surgery in certain cases. Although these techniques may have improved the results for some patients, physicians became frustrated by the frequent appearance of distant metastasis despite proper application of this comprehensive regional treatment. In addition, laboratory studies performed on mastectomy specimens by Gray[78] demonstrated that lymphatics surrounding a primary tumor did not always show involvement, thereby weakening the concept of permeative spread of the disease. Such clinical and biologic observations suggested that, in many patients, metastases were present, but occult, at the time of a patient's initial presentation and were unaffected by local management.[79] This led to a new paradigm that hypothesized that there are two types of cancer: (1) one that remains local and rarely spreads, and (2) one in which occult micrometastases are already present when the patient is first seen.[80] In either of these circumstances, local therapy does not alter outcome. If the patient is in the former group, only minimal local therapy is needed. For the patient who already has micrometastases at original diagnosis, local therapy has no effect on the distant metastases already present.

This new paradigm, taken to its logical conclusion, denies the existence of a circumstance in which effective treatment to the local and regional area is important to survival. It suggests that metastatic spread never occurs during the clinical phase of disease evolution. The acceptance of this paradigm has led to less-aggressive local treatment and to efforts to discern the prognosis of individual patients. Such efforts were used to identify patients who already had occult metastases and those for whom breast cancer was a local condition. The pioneers of this new viewpoint were courageous surgeons who were anxious to move away from the mutilation of radical mastectomy and whose views were considered by many to be heresy.[80–82] Fisher[83] most clearly articulated the differences between these two views of breast cancer biology and provided strong support for the newer paradigm.

It is generally acknowledged that the halstedian view of breast cancer does not apply to *all* patients. The simple observation that 20% to 30% of node-negative patients develop metastases demonstrates that lymph node involvement is not a necessary precedent to more distant spread and that blood-borne dissemination occurs in at least some patients. Proponents of the importance of local therapy have replaced the halstedian model by a spectrum model of breast cancer spread, in which the disease is not viewed as systemic at its inception in all patients and, therefore, early diagnosis and effective local–regional treatment can affect survival in some patients.[4,75] The basis of this hypothesis is that metastases occur as a function of tumor growth and progression. This Spectrum view, however, stresses the importance of both local and systemic therapy. The contrasting elements of the Halsted and Systemic views are presented along with those for the Spectrum paradigm in Table 12-9.

The most important piece of evidence supporting the Spectrum view of breast cancer spread is the information derived from the randomized clinical trials testing the value of screening mammography. If metastases occur at the inception of a breast cancer, earlier detection will not be effective in preventing metastases or decreasing breast cancer mortality. Evaluation of this question requires the use of randomized clinical trials to avoid potential biases (avoid lead-time, length-time, selection, and over-diagnosis biases) in comparing cancers detected mammographically and those detected by physical examination. A number of screening trials have been performed and are reviewed in detail in Chapter 6. Overall, mammographic screening of asymptomatic women has been shown to result in about a 25% decrease in mortality from breast cancer.[84–86] This observation provides compelling evidence that breast cancer can metastasize during its clinical evolution.

A second, but less direct, support for the Spectrum view comes from clinical studies that demonstrate that as tumor size increases, the likelihood of metastases increases. As presented earlier in this chapter, the likelihood of metastasis increases with a sigmoid distribution when plotted against the logarithm of tumor volume.[30,87] This suggests that there is a critical volume for each tumor, which must be reached before distant metastasis occurs. This analysis enables the determination of a tumor diameter associated with a 50% probability of metastasis. In this series of patients, this tumor diameter was about 3.6 cm, well within

TABLE 12-9
Comparisons of the Various Models of Breast Cancer Spread

Halsted[77]	Systemic[83]	Spectrum[75]
Tumor spreads in an orderly manner based on mechanical considerations	There is no orderly pattern of tumor cell dissemination	In most patients, axillary nodal involvement precedes distant metastases
The positive lymph node is an indicator of tumor spread and is the instigator of distant metastases	The positive lymph node is an indicator of a host–tumor relationship that permits development of metastases, rather than the instigator of distant metastases	The positive lymph node is an indicator of a host–tumor relationship that is correlated with the subsequent appearance of distant disease
RLNs are barriers to passage of tumor cells	RLNs are ineffective as barriers to tumor cell spread	RLNs are ineffective as barriers to tumor spread, but involvement of RLNs is not always associated with distant metastases
The bloodstream is of little significance as a route of tumor dissemination	The bloodstream is of considerable importance in tumor dissemination	The bloodstream is of considerable importance in tumor dissemination
Operable breast cancer is a local–regional disease	Operable breast cancer is a systemic disease	Operable breast cancer is a systemic disease in many but not all cases
The extent and nuances of the operations are the dominant factors influencing a patient's outcome	Variations in local–regional therapy are unlikely to affect survival	Variations in local–regional therapy are unlikely to have a major influence on survival, but are of significance in some patients

RLNs, regional lymph nodes.

the range of clinical evolution. An alternative explanation, however, for the foregoing observation is that tumors have different growth rates, and it is generally the fast-growing (and, hence, more lethal) tumors that are large at diagnosis.

A third prima facie argument supporting the Spectrum paradigm is that many patients, including those with axillary node involvement, live for extended periods of time after effective local treatment. This is particularly true for small tumors measuring 2 cm or less, even when a limited number of axillary lymph nodes are involved.[4] Given the general level of awareness about breast cancer in the population and the widespread use of screening mammography, increasingly patients are being diagnosed with early-stage breast cancers. Another important point in evaluating these views of breast cancer spread is to determine whether variations in local–regional treatment affect outcome. If variations in local–regional treatment do not affect survival, then the case for breast cancer as a systemic disease is strengthened. The trials testing variations in local and regional treatment are discussed in Chapter 17-1. The ideal trial to evaluate these competing views is one that is properly conducted and accrues a large number of patients (about 1000 in each arm) with early-stage breast cancer randomly assigned to receive either effective local–regional treatment or to receive no or highly ineffective local–regional treatment without an opportunity for salvage treatment in the event of a local–regional failure. Such a trial would rightly be viewed as unethical. Virtually all available studies compare treatments with similar levels of effectiveness in obtaining local–regional control, allow for salvage, or have insufficient numbers of patients to eliminate small differences. As a result, these trials are inconclusive and have been used by advocates of both views as evidence in their favor.

The B-04[88] and B-06[89] trials by the NSABP are two of the major studies on the importance of local–regional treatment. The B-04 trial tested the value of axillary treatment. A total of 1159 breast cancer patients with clinically negative axillary nodes were randomly assigned to receive (1) radical mastectomy (RM), (2) total mastectomy and RT to the axilla and other draining lymph nodes (TMR), or (3) total mastectomy alone, without any axillary treatment (TM). The 10-year results of this trial do not show a statistically significant survival advantage for any of the treatment arms. This study does provide a clear comparison of effective axillary treatment to no axillary treatment (axillary recurrence rates were less than 5% for RM and TMR). The trial, however, allowed for salvage and by 10 years 18% of the TM group developed recurrence in the axilla and underwent delayed axillary dissection. There were also difficulties in the conduct of the trial, such that 35% of the patients assigned to total mastectomy, in fact, had a limited axillary dissection.[90] Also, it must be asked whether enough patients were included in the study to eliminate the possibility that axillary treatment has a small effect on survival.[91] It is possible to estimate the possible benefit of axillary treatment, given the data presented in this chapter. Some 360 patients were assigned to each treatment arm, and axillary metastases were found in 38.6% of patients undergoing RM. Because the value of axillary treatment is restricted to patients who have positive nodes, the critical population would be the 137 patients (38.6% of 360) who are presumed to have positive axillary nodes. Axillary treatment is also not of value in patients who have occult disease at the time of presentation. Overall, about one third of patients with positive axillary nodes are estimated to be free of occult distant disease. Therefore, the critical population is further restricted to the 48 patients (one third of 137) who have positive nodes and no occult distant spread, and could therefore possibly benefit from axillary treatment. In addition, one must consider the salvage potential of delayed axillary treatment. If one estimates that one third of patients initially treated by TM alone, who subsequently develop axillary adenopathy, are curable, then delayed axillary dissection is effective in an additional 16 patients. This leaves 32 patients who could possibly have benefited from initial axillary treatment, or 9% of the total group. To have a 90% chance of detecting a 9% difference between two treatment arms in a clinical trial at a statistically significant level of $P = .05$, about 1000 patients would be required. This analysis suggests that the results obtained in the NSABP trial B-04 do not prove that axillary treatment is of no value, but rather that the benefit, if present, must be small. The most recent report of this trial indicates a 10-year survival rate of 58% for the RM group and 59% for the TMR group, compared with 54% for the TM group, yielding a difference of 4% to 5%, which was not statistically significant.[88] This degree of benefit is roughly equivalent to a 10% reduction in mortality for axillary treatment. If this degree of benefit were shown to be valid and were applied to the general population of breast cancer patients, the absolute number of patients who benefit would be large. The case for effective axillary treatment is also supported by the results of the Guy's Hospital trial in which inadequate axillary treatment was associated with an increased rate of metastases and a decreased survival (see Chap. 17.1).

Similar considerations apply to effective control of the primary tumor, as analyzed in the NSABP B-06 trial.[89] In this trial, 1843 evaluable patients with early-stage breast cancer were randomly assigned to undergo TM, lumpectomy, or lumpectomy and RT. All patients underwent axillary dissection. The trial demonstrated a clear difference in control of the primary tumor (recurrence in the breast was 39% for the lumpectomy group and 10% for the lumpectomy and RT group [$P < .001$]), but no statistically significant difference in survival was observed. It is similarly possible to estimate the potential effect on survival by maximizing local tumor control. In approximately 60% of patients treated by lumpectomy, the use of RT is not of value because no residual disease is present in the breast. In addition, approximately one third of patients who have a recurrence in the breast are estimated to have had occult metastases at presentation and thus were incurable by local treatment from the onset. Also, one would anticipate that about 50% of the patients would be cured by mastectomy performed at the time of local recurrence. Given these estimates, the possible adverse effect on survival of the ineffective local tumor control would be only 5%. The 8-year results of the B-06 trial, in fact, show a 5.3% difference in survival among node-negative patients in favor of lumpectomy plus RT compared with lumpectomy alone, but this was not statistically significant.

This analysis of the NSABP B-04 and B-06 trials illustrates the shortcomings of such trials in attempting to distinguish between the paradigms of breast cancer spread. Variations in local–regional treatment are not likely to

TABLE 12-10
Sites of Metastases From Breast Cancer in Three Collected Series

Organ	160 Cases[93] (%)	43 Cases[94] (%)	100 Cases[71] (%)
Lung	59	65	69
Liver	58	56	65
Bone	44	—	71
Pleura	37	23	51
Adrenal glands	31	41	49
Kidneys	—	14	17
Spleen	14	23	17
Pancreas	—	11	17
Ovaries	9	16	20
Brain	—	9	22
Thyroid	—	—	24
Heart	—	—	11
Diaphragm	—	—	11
Pericardium	—	21	19
Intestine	—	—	18
Peritoneum	12	9	13
Uterus	—	—	15
Skin	39	7	30

produce a large difference in survival rates, because some local–regional recurrences can be effectively treated secondarily and others reflect a poor prognosis regardless of local–regional treatment. Large studies (about 1000 patients per arm) would be required to eliminate a small difference in survival. These issues were recognized by Fisher,[92] who stated in 1980 that "variations in effective local–regional treatment are unlikely to effect survival substantially."

Distant Metastases

Metastases from carcinoma of the breast can be seen in a variety of organs. The likelihood of organ involvement has been studied in a number of autopsy series[71,93,94] (Table 12-10). The most common sites of metastatic spread are bone, lung, and liver.

The time course to the appearance of clinically detected distant metastases can be extremely long. It is common for metastases to become manifest 10 years or more after initial diagnosis. Koscielny and colleagues[30] showed that the time course to distant metastases is influenced by the size of the primary tumor (Fig. 12-6). For patients with the smallest tumors (1 to 2.5 cm), the time course to the appearance of distant disease was the greatest. The cumulative proportion of patients with metastases reached half its ultimate value (median delay or median interval)

FIGURE 12-6 The cumulated proportions of patients with metastases as a function of the time after treatment in the different groups of patients defined by the clinical size of the tumor in centimeters. (Koscielny S, Tubiana M, Le M, et al. Breast cancer: relationship between the size of the tumor and the probability of metastatic dissemination. Br J Cancer 1984;49:709)

42 months after initial treatment. In contrast, the median interval was only 4 months for patients with tumors 8.5 cm or larger. The median interval between diagnosis and detection of first distant metastasis was 69 months for patients with axillary node–negative disease, 43 months when one to three axillary nodes were positive for metastasis, and 30 months when four or more axillary nodes were positive. Similarly, the median interval was 65 months for patients with histologic grade I tumors, 44 months for grade II tumors, and 21 months for grade III tumors. This inverse relation between initial stage and time to the appearance of distant metastases is also reflected in mortality statistics, as seen in the Edinburgh study[95] and in the study from the End Results Program of the NCI.[96]

Summary

The data presented in this chapter demonstrate that breast cancer is a heterogeneous disease that has a propensity for systemic involvement and commonly has a long natural history. Because of this long natural history and its onset typically at middle age, it is difficult to demonstrate, in a strict sense, that breast cancer is a curable disease. It is clear, however, that a considerable percentage of patients with treated breast cancer (particularly when detected at an early stage) live their lives without further evidence of the disease.

The axilla is the principal site of regional node involvement and the likelihood of axillary involvement is directly related to tumor size. Both tumor size and the presence and extent of axillary involvement are highly associated with survival. The proper view of breast cancer spread remains controversial. Some have argued that all breast cancer is a systemic disease at its inception, implying that local treatment does not influence survival. Others have argued that breast cancer metastasizes at some point in its clinical evolution. The major argument against breast cancer as a strictly systemic disease is the significant reduction in breast cancer mortality by the use of earlier detection using screening mammography.

References

1. Bloom H, Richardson W, Harrier E. Natural history of untreated breast cancer (1805–1933). BMJ 1962;2:213.
2. Fox M. On the diagnosis and treatment of breast cancer. JAMA 1979;241:489.
3. Harris J, Hellman S. Observations on survival curve analysis with particular reference to breast cancer treatment. Cancer 1986;57:925.
4. Hellman S. The natural history of small breast cancers. David A. Karnofsky Memorial Lecture. J Clin Oncol 1994;12:2229.
5. Haybittle J. The evidence for cure in female breast cancer. Comment Res Breast Dis 1983;3:181.
6. Brinkley D, Haybittle J. Long-term survival of women with breast cancer. Lancet 1984;1:1118.
7. Hibberd A, Harwood L, Well J. Long-term prognosis of women with breast cancer in New Zealand: study of survival to 30 years. BMJ 1983;286:1777.
8. Rutqvist L, Wallgren A. Long-term survival of 458 young breast cancer patients. Cancer 1985;55:658.
9. Adair F, Berg J, Joubert L. Long term follow-up of breast cancer patients: the thirty-year report. Cancer 1974;33:1145.
10. Rosen P, Groshen S, Siago P, et al. A long-term follow-up study of survival in stage I (T1N0M0) and stage II (T1N1M0) breast carcinoma. J Clin Oncol 1989;7:355.
11. Collins V, Loeffler R, Tivey H. Observations on growth rates of human tumors. Am J Roentgenol 1956;76:988.
12. Gershon Cohen J, Berger S, Klickstein H. Roentgenography of breast cancer moderating concept of "biological predeterminism." Cancer 1963;16:961.
13. Fournier D, Weber E, Hoeffken W, et al. Growth rate of 147 mammary carcinomas. Cancer 1980;45:2198.
14. Kusama S, Spratt J, Donegan W, et al. The gross rates of growth of human mammary carcinoma. Cancer 1972;30:594.
15. Pearlman A. Breast cancer: influence of growth rate on prognosis and treatment evaluation. Cancer 1976;38:1826.
16. Laird A. Dynamics of growth in tumors and in normal organisms. J Natl Cancer Inst Monogr 1969;30:15.
17. Skipper H, Schnabel F Jr, Lloyd H. Dose-response and tumor cell repopulation rate in chemotherapeutic trials. Adv Cancer Chemother 1979;1:205.
18. Walter S, Day N. Estimation of the duration of a preclinical disease state using screening data. Am J Epidemiol 1983;118:865.
19. Zelen M, Feinleib M. On the theory of screening for chronic diseases. Biometrika 1969;56:601.
20. Shapiro S, Goldbert J, Hutchinson G. Lead time in breast cancer detection and implications for periodicity of screening. Am J Epidemiol 1974;100:357.
21. Norton L. A Gompertzian model of human breast cancer growth. Cancer Res 1988;48:7067.
22. Tubiana M, Malaise E. Growth rate and cell kinetics in human tumors. In: Symington T, Carter RL, eds. On scientific functions of oncology. Chicago, Year Book, 1976:126.
23. Nowell P. The clonal evolution of tumor cell populations. Science 1976;194:23.
24. Speer J, Petrosky V, Retsky M, et al. A stochastic numerical model

of breast cancer growth that simulates clinical data. Cancer Res 1984;44:4124.

25. Retsky M, Swartzendruber D, Bame P, et al. A new paradigm for breast cancer. In: Senn H-J, Gelber R, Goldhirsch A, et al, eds. Adjuvant therapy of breast cancer, vol 4. Berlin, Springer-Verlag, 1993:13.

26. Holland R, Veling S, Mravunac M, et al. Histologic multifocality of Tis, T1-2 breast carcinomas. Cancer 1985;56:979.

27. Spratt J, Donegan W. Cancer of the breast. Philadelphia, WB Saunders, 1971:133.

28. Nemoto T, Natarajan N, Bedwani R, et al. Breast cancer in the medial half: results of the 1978 national survey of the American College of Surgeons. Cancer 1983;51:1333.

29. Fisher B, Slack N, Ausman R, et al. Location of breast carcinoma and prognosis. Surg Gynecol Obstet 1969;129:705.

30. Koscielny S, Tubiana M, Le M, et al. Breast cancer: relationship between the size of the primary tumor and the probability of metastatic dissemination. Br J Cancer 1984;49:709.

31. Koscielny S, Le M, Tubiana M. The natural history of human breast cancer: the relationship between involvement of axillary lymph nodes and the initiation of distant metastases. Br J Cancer 1989;59:775.

32. Schottenfeld D, Nash A, Robbins G, et al. Ten-year results of the treatment of primary operable breast carcinoma. Cancer 1976; 38:1001.

33. Nemoto T, Vana J, Bedwani R, et al. Management and survival of female breast cancer: results of a national survey by the American College of Surgeons. Cancer 1980;45:2917.

34. Fisher B, Slack N, Bross I, et al. Cancer of the breast: size of neoplasm and prognosis. Cancer 1969;24:1071.

35. Haagensen C. In: Diseases of the breast, ed 3. Philadelphia, WB Saunders, 1986:656.

36. Carter C, Allen C, Henson D. Relation of tumor size, lymph node status, and survival in 24,740 breast cancer cases. Cancer 1989;63:181.

37. Smith J, Gamez-Araujo J, Gallager H, et al. Carcinoma of the breast: analysis of total lymph node involvement versus level of metastasis. Cancer 1977;39:527.

38. Butcher H. Radical mastectomy for mammary carcinoma. Ann Surg 1969;170:833.

39. Bucalossi P, Veronesi U, Zingo L, et al. Enlarged mastectomy for breast cancer: review of 1213 cases. Am J Roentgenol Radium Ther Nucl Med 1971;111:119.

40. Valagussa P, Bonadonna G, Veronesi V. Patterns of relapse and survival following radical mastectomy. Cancer 1978;41:1170.

41. Haagensen C. Treatment of curable carcinoma of the breast. Int J Radiat Oncol Biol Phys 1977;2:975.

42. Fisher B, Slack N, Katrych D, et al. Ten-year followup results of patients with carcinoma of the breast in a cooperative clinical trial evaluating surgical adjuvant chemotherapy. Surg Gynecol Obstet 1975;140:528.

43. Spratt J, Donegan W. In: Carcinoma of the breast. Philadelphia, WB Saunders, 1971.

44. Payne W, Taylor W, Khonsari S, et al. Surgical treatment of breast cancer: trends and factors affecting survival. Arch Surg 1970;101:105.

45. Ferguson D, Meier P, Karrison T, et al. Staging of breast cancer and survival rates: an assessment based on 50 years of experience with radical mastectomy. JAMA 1982;248:1337.

46. Haagensen C. In: Diseases of the breast, ed 3. Philadelphia, WB Saunders, 1986:663.

47. Veronesi U, Rilke F, Luini A, et al. Distribution of axillary node metastases by level of invasion: an analysis of 539 cases. Cancer 1987;59:682.

48. Rosen P, Martin L, Kinne D, et al. Discontinuous or "skip" metastases in breast carcinoma: analysis of 1228 axillary dissections. Ann Surg 1983;197:276.

49. Pigott J, Nicols R, Maddox W, et al. Metastases to the upper levels of the axillary nodes in carcinoma of the breast and its implications for nodal sampling procedures. Surg Gynecol Obstet 1984;158:255.

50. Boova R, Bonanni R, Rosato F. Patterns of axillary nodal involvement in breast cancer: predictability of level one dissection. Ann Surg 1982;196:642.

51. Danforth DJ, Findlay P, McDonald H, et al. Complete axillary lymph node dissection for stage I–II carcinoma of the breast. J Clin Oncol 1986;4:655.

52. Schwartz G, D'Ugo D, Rosenberg A. Extent of axillary dissection preceding irradiation for carcinoma of the breast. Arch Surg 1986;121:1395.

53. Haagensen C. In: Diseases of the breast, ed 3. Philadelphia, WB Saunders, 1986:656.

54. Saphir O, Amromin G. Obscure axillary lymph metastasis in carcinoma of the breast. Cancer 1948;1:238.

55. Pickren J. Significance of occult metastases. Cancer 1961;14:1266.

56. Fisher E, Swamidoss S, Lee C, et al. Detection and significance of occult axillary node metastases in patients with invasive breast cancer. Cancer 1978;42:2025.

57. Wilkinson EJ, Hause LL, Kuzma JF, et al. Occult axillary lymph node metastasis in patients with invasive breast cancer. (Abstract) Lab Invest 1984;44,83A.

58. de Mascarel I, Bonichon F, Coindre J, et al. Prognostic significance of breast cancer axillary lymph node micrometastases assessed by two special techniques: reevaluation with longer follow-up. Br J Cancer 1992;66:523.

59. International (Ludwig) Breast Cancer Study Group. Prognostic importance of occult axillary lymph node micrometastases from breast cancers. Lancet 1990;335:1565.

60. Trojani M, de Mascarel I, Bonichon F, et al. Micrometastases to axillary lymph nodes from carcinoma of breast: detection by immunohistochemistry and prognostic significance. Br J Cancer 1983; 55:303.

61. Wells C, Heryet A, Brochier J, et al. The immunocytochemical detection of axillary micrometastases in breast cancer. Br J Cancer 1984;50:193.

62. Elson C, Kuf D, Scholm J, et al. Detection of occult foci of metastatic breast carcinoma in axillary lymph nodes using monoclonal antibodies B72.3 and DF3. (Abstract) Lab Invest 1988;58:27A.

63. Sedmak D, Meineke T, Knechtges D, et al. Prognostic significance of cytokeratin-positive breast cancer metastases. Mod Pathol 1989;3:516.

64. Nasser I, Lee A, Bosari S, et al. Occult axillary lymph node metastases in "node-negative" breast carcinoma. Hum Pathol 1993;24:950.

65. Noguchi S, Aihara T, Nakamori S, et al. The detection of breast cancer micrometastases in axillary lymph nodes by means of reverse transcriptase–polymerase chain reaction. Cancer 1994;74:1595.

66. Schoenfeld A, Luqmani Y, Smith D, et al. Detection of breast cancer micrometastases in axillary lymph nodes by using polymerase chain reaction. Cancer Res 1994;54:2986.

67. Rosen P, Saigo P, Braun D, et al. Axillary micro- and macro-metastases in breast cancer: prognostic significance of tumor size. Ann Surg 1981;194:585.

68. Friedman S, Bertin F, Mouriesse H, et al. Importance of tumor cells in axillary node sinus margins ("clandestine" metastases) discovered by serial sectioning in operable breast cancer. Acta Oncol 1988;27:483.

69. Handley R. Carcinoma of the breast. Ann R Coll Surg Engl 1975;57:59.

70. Veronesi U, Cascinelli N, Greco M, et al. Prognosis of breast cancer patients after mastectomy and dissection of internal mammary nodes. Ann Surg 1985;202:702.

71. Haagensen C. In: Diseases of the breast, ed 3. Philadelphia, WB Saunders, 1986:686.

72. LaCour J, Le M, Caceres E, et al. Radical mastectomy versus radical

mastectomy plus internal mammary dissection. Cancer 1983; 51:1941.

73. Dahl Iversen E. Recherches sur les metastases microscopiques des cancers du sein dans les ganglions lymphatiques parasternaux et sus-claviculaires. Mem Acad Clin 1952;78:651.

74. Halsted W. The results of radical operations for the cure of cancer of the breast. Ann Surg 1907;46:1.

75. Hellman S, Harris J. The appropriate breast carcinoma paradigm. Cancer Res 1987;2:339.

76. Meyer W. An improved method of the radical operation for carcinoma of the breast. Med Rec 1894;46:746.

77. Halsted W. The results of operations for the cure of cancer of the breast performed at the Johns Hopkins Hospital from June 1889 to January 1894. Johns Hopkins Hosp Bull 1895;4:297.

78. Gray J. The relation of lymphatic vessels to the spread of cancer. Br J Surg 1939;26:462.

79. Park W, Lee V. The absolute curability of cancer of the breast. Surg Gynecol Obstet 1951;93:129.

80. Fisher B. Breast cancer management: alternatives to radical mastectomy. N Engl J Med 1979;301:326.

81. Crile GJ. A biological consideration of the treatment of breast cancer. Springfield, IL, Charles C Thomas, 1967.

82. Keynes G. Carcinoma of the breast, the unorthodox view. Proc Cardiff Med Soc 1953–1954:40.

83. Fisher B. A commentary on the role of the surgeon in primary breast cancer. Breast Cancer Res Treat 1981;1:17.

84. Shapiro S. Determining the efficacy of breast cancer screening. Cancer 1989;63:1873.

85. Tabar L, Fagerberg C, Duffy S, et al. Update of the Swedish two-county program of mammographic screening for breast cancer. Radiol Clin North Am 1992;30:187.

86. Wald N, Frost C, Cuckle H. Breast cancer screening: the current position. BMJ 1991;302:845.

87. Tubiana M, Koscielny S. Natural history of human breast cancer: recent data and clinical implications. Breast Cancer Res Treat 1991;18:125.

88. Fisher B, Redmond C, Fisher E, et al. Ten-year results of a randomized clinical trial comparing radical mastectomy and total mastectomy with or without radiation. N Engl J Med 1985;312:674.

89. Fisher B, Redmond C, Poisson R, et al. Eight-year results of a randomized clinical trial comparing total mastectomy and lumpectomy with or without irradiation in the treatment of breast cancer. N Engl J Med 1989;320:822.

90. Fisher B, Wolmark N, Bauer M, et al. The accuracy of clinical nodal staging and of limited axillary dissection as a determinant of histologic nodal status in carcinoma of the breast. Surg Gynecol Obstet 1981;152:765.

91. Harris J, Osteen R. Patients with early breast cancer benefit from effective axillary treatment. Breast Cancer Res Treat 1985;5:17.

92. Fisher B. Laboratory and clinical research in breast cancer: a personal adventure: the David A. Karnofsky memorial lecture. Cancer Res 1980;40:3863.

93. Warren S, Witham E. Studies on tumor metastases: the distribution of metastases in cancer of the breast. Surg Gynecol Obstet 1933;57:81.

94. Saphir O, Parker M. Metastases of primary carcinoma of the breast with special reference to spleen, adrenal glands and ovaries. Arch Surg 1941;42:1003.

95. Langlands A, Pocock S, Kerr G, et al. Long-term survival of patients with breast cancer: a study of the curability of the disease. BMJ 1979;2:1247.

96. Hankey B, Steinhorn S. Long-term patient survival for some of the more frequently occurring cancers. Cancer 1982;50:1904.

Diseases of the Breast, edited by Jay R. Harris,
Marc E. Lippman, Monica Morrow, and Samuel Hellman.
Lippincott-Raven Publishers, Philadelphia, © 1996.

13

Invasive Mammary Carcinoma

PAUL PETER ROSEN

Invasive Duct Carcinoma

Invasive duct carcinoma is the single largest group of malignant mammary tumors, constituting 65% to 80% of mammary carcinomas.[1,2] The definition of this category offered in the World Health Organization (WHO) classification of tumors is one of exclusion: "Invasive ductal carcinoma is the most frequently encountered malignant tumour of the breast, not falling into any of the other categories of invasive mammary carcinoma."[3] Included under this heading are lesions characterized variously as duct carcinoma with productive fibrosis, scirrhous carcinoma, and carcinoma simplex. A generic term sometimes employed is *invasive duct carcinoma, not otherwise specified* (NOS). This is a useful designation because it considers the distinction between these tumors and the many other specific forms of duct carcinoma, such as tubular, medullary, metaplastic, colloid, and adenoid cystic carcinoma.

Invasive duct carcinoma includes many tumors that express, in part, one or more characteristics of the specific types of breast carcinoma but do not constitute pure examples of the individual tumors. Examples of this phenomenon are invasive duct carcinomas that have limited microscopic foci of tubular, medullary, papillary, or mucinous differentiation. The relatively favorable prognosis associated with specific histologic types has been found to apply only to those tumors composed entirely, or in large part, of the designated pattern. When these features are less extensively represented, the tumors are appropriately relegated to the broader group of invasive duct carcinoma, NOS. Tumors that consist of invasive duct carcinoma with associated Paget disease also are included in this category.

In one detailed review of 1000 carcinomas, about one third of the lesions characterized as invasive duct carcinoma expressed one or more combined features.[4] Slightly more than half of the combined tumors were invasive duct carcinoma with a tubular carcinoma component.

Combinations with invasive lobular carcinoma were detected in 6% of the tumors. A carcinoma with three distinct growth patterns is illustrated in Figure 13-1. Tumors that include invasive duct and invasive lobular carcinoma usually have been included in the duct carcinoma category. As a consequence, the clinical biology of these neoplasms has not been well defined. Thus far, prognostic differences have not been identified for most of the other combined histologic patterns and, as a consequence, they have been grouped together as invasive duct carcinoma. This section considers invasive duct carcinoma, NOS in the context of this broad definition.

The growth pattern, or cytologic features, of the intraductal component is sometimes reflected in the structure of an invasive duct carcinoma. Tubular carcinoma invariably arises from an orderly micropapillary or cribriform intraductal carcinoma that features cytologically low-grade nuclei. The intraductal component of medullary carcinoma is typically solid with poorly differentiated nuclei. Invasive poorly differentiated duct carcinoma (NOS) tends to develop from solid or comedo intraductal carcinoma. Comedo necrosis may occur in invasive areas of a tumor with solid or comedo intraductal carcinoma duplicating the intraductal pattern. It may be difficult in some areas of a tumor with solid or comedo intraductal carcinoma to distinguish between intraductal and invasive components. Moderately differentiated invasive duct carcinoma, NOS most often originates from cribriform or papillary intraductal components.

Invasive cribriform carcinoma is a subtype of invasive duct carcinoma with a prominent cribriform structure.[5] These tumors arise from cribriform intraductal carcinoma, and in these lesions, invasive components that mimic intraductal carcinoma can complicate the measurement of the invasive tumor area. Invasive lesions that are entirely cribriform and those with a mixture of cribriform and tubular components are relatively low grade and have a good prognosis. If less well-differentiated elements are present

FIGURE 13-1 Infiltrating duct carcinoma with heterogeneous histologic appearance in a 66-year-old woman treated by limited resection, axillary dissection, and radiotherapy. Different microscopic areas exhibited the following patterns: tubular (**A**), moderately differentiated infiltrating duct (**B**), and infiltrating lobular (**C**).

in the tumor, the prognosis is not as favorable. Invasive cribriform carcinoma is sometimes mistaken for adenoid cystic carcinoma.[6]

Breast carcinoma is an extremely heterogeneous disease clinically and pathologically. As observed by Sistrunk and MacCarty[7] more than 60 years ago, "It is impossible to foretell the duration of life of all patients with carcinoma of the breast, because the degree of malignancy varies widely, and persons react differently to the disease." Innumerable studies have assessed the prognosis of breast cancer patients on the basis of clinical and pathologic criteria. Because nearly three quarters of the patients have invasive duct carcinoma, the characteristics of these tumors have a considerable influence on laboratory, clinical, or pathologic studies.

The interval to recurrence and the length of survival are the basic measurements of prognosis. These are closely related; hence, factors associated with a high frequency of recurrence correlate with reduced survival. However, treatment that delays but does not reduce the overall frequency of recurrence may increase the duration of survival, without reducing mortality of the diseases in the long term. Evidence also indicates that the prognostic importance of a given pathologic variable does not apply uniformly throughout the course of follow-up. Some variables are more effective for predicting short-term outcome, whereas others exert an effect later. The time dependency of prognostic variables has not been thoroughly analyzed.[8,9]

The impact of primary treatment on the evaluation of prognostic factors must also be considered. Mastectomy was, until the 1960s, the most widely employed form of primary treatment. A large body of data was accumulated relative to the importance of stage at diagnosis, type of tumor, and other clinical and morphologic prognostic determinants in relation to this form of treatment. The past two decades have witnessed major changes in treatment with a shift from mastectomy to partial mastectomy, quadrantectomy, or limited resection combined with primary radiation therapy and axillary dissection. Evaluation of prognostic factors has been further complicated by the widespread use of adjuvant chemotherapy for women with stage II disease and for many with stage I disease. Reports documenting the follow-up of patients treated with various modalities suggest that pathologic prognostic variables determined to be significant for systemic recurrence and overall survival in populations treated by mastectomy also are applicable to patients treated by breast-conserving surgery combined with radiation therapy. The extent to which the assessment of the prognostic import of pathologic factors is influenced by adjuvant chemotherapy is less certain.

CLINICAL PRESENTATION

With rare exceptions, no clinical features are specifically associated with invasive duct carcinoma. The lesions occur throughout the age range of breast carcinoma, being most common in women in their middle to late 50s. An exception is palpable breast carcinoma associated with Paget disease of the nipple. The underlying invasive carcinoma in these cases is almost always of the duct type. However, in exceptional situations, Paget disease may derive from intraductal carcinoma limited to the lactiferous ducts. Coincidentally, there may be a palpable lesion formed by another separate carcinoma, possibly of a different histologic type, such as a tubular carcinoma.

GROSS PATHOLOGY

Invasive duct carcinoma invariably forms a solid tumor. The consistency and appearance of the cut surface vary considerably, depending on the composition of the lesion. Cystic change in this group of lesions is uncommon but it may be a manifestation of necrosis, usually accompanied by hemorrhage in the degenerated area. Noncystic areas of necrosis tend to be soft and chalky white. Tumors with a relatively abundant scirrhous or fibrotic stroma are firm to hard with a gray to white surface. When considerable elastosis of the stroma is present, a yellow tinge may be observed. Chalky white streaks in the tumor tissue usually indicate necrosis, calcification, or elastosis. Tumors with less-abundant stroma that are composed largely of neoplastic cells tend to be less firm and tan. The cut surfaces of such cellular neoplasms are likely to bulge slightly when bisected.

The measured gross size of a mammary carcinoma is one of the most critical prognostic variables. Numerous studies have shown that survival decreases with increasing tumor size, and that a coincidental rise in the rate of axillary nodal metastases occurs.[8,10–13] This phenomenon applies to the overall spectrum of primary tumor size and also within subsets, such as those defined by TNM staging. For example, among T1 breast carcinomas (2 cm or smaller in diameter), a significant relation exists between the size and frequency of nodal metastases when the tumors are stratified in 5-mm groups.[14–16]

Because most carcinomas have irregular shapes, measurement is reported in terms of the greatest diameter. The tumor must be submitted to the pathologist intact so that the configuration of the lesion can be assessed by palpation. This makes it possible to bisect the specimen in a plane that exposes the longest diameter. This measurement should be made before any samples are taken for frozen section, estrogen receptor analysis, or any other procedure. When a frozen section is prepared, the grossly measured diameter can be reported with the histologic diagnosis and entered as part of the frozen section record.

The gross measurement of a carcinoma is an approximation of the actual amount of invasive tumor present. Benign tissue with hyperplastic or reactive changes may contribute to the palpable lesion. In some tumors, a considerable part of the mass is composed of invasive carcinoma, whereas in other lesions of comparable gross size, most of the bulk may be intraductal tumor, with only microscopic invasion.

Most invasive ductal carcinomas can be assigned on the basis of gross tumor configuration to one of two groups: stellate (spiculated, infiltrative, radial, serrated), and circumscribed (rounded, pushing, encapsulate, smooth). About one third of the tumors have grossly circumscribed margins. A few tumors have indistinct borders and cannot be described in these terms. The gross appearance of the tumor generally duplicates the configuration visualized by mammography. However, tumors that appear to have circumscribed margins grossly or mammographically may exhibit an invasive growth pattern when studied microscopically. Fisher and associates[4] found microscopically invasive margins in slightly more than half of carcinomas that were described as grossly circumscribed.

Most investigators have observed a more favorable prognosis associated with circumscribed carcinomas, determined by mammography[17] or gross inspection of the tumor.[18] Infiltrative tumors tend to be larger when detected,[18,19] and they are more likely to have axillary lymph node metastases than those with circumscribed margins.[17,18] Tumors with a stellate configuration in which there is focal necrosis have an especially poor prognosis.[19]

MICROSCOPIC PATHOLOGY

Grading of carcinomas is an estimate of differentiation. Unless otherwise indicated, grading is limited to the invasive portion of the tumor. *Nuclear grading* is a cytologic evaluation in which the structural features of the tumor nuclei are compared with the nuclei of normal mammary epithelial cells. Because nuclear grading does not involve an assessment of the growth pattern of the tumor, this procedure is applicable to all types of mammary carcinoma. The most widely employed system for nuclear grading, introduced by Black and others,[20,21] reports three categories: well differentiated (grade 3), intermediate (grade 2), and poorly differentiated (grade 1) (Fig. 13-2). By convention, numerical designations used for nuclear grades have been recorded in a sequence that is the reverse of those used in histologic grading. It has been proposed that the numerical designations employed for nuclear grading be changed to conform with those used in histologic grading.[4]

Histologic grading takes into consideration the growth pattern of invasive ductal carcinomas and cytologic differentiation.[22,23] The parameters measured are the extent of tubule formation, nuclear hyperchromasia, and mitotic rate. Histologic grade is expressed in three categories: well

FIGURE 13-2 Nuclear grade. **A.** Low-grade cytologic appearance is characterized by small, round, uniform nuclei that lack nucleoli. **B.** High-grade nuclei are large, vesicular, and pleomorphic, and have prominent nucleoli.

differentiated (grade I), intermediate (grade II), and poorly differentiated (grade III) (Fig. 13-3).

The histologic and nuclear grades of a given tumor coincide in most invasive duct carcinomas. Studies have repeatedly demonstrated that patients with high-grade or poorly differentiated invasive duct carcinoma have a significantly greater frequency of axillary lymph node metastases, that they develop more recurrences, and that more of them die of metastatic disease than women with low-grade tumors.[8,15,20–30] Nuclear and histologic grade have been shown to be effective predictors of prognosis among patients stratified by stage of disease, especially among those without axillary lymph node metastases (stage I).[15,26,28,30–33] The absence of tubule formation is a particularly unfavorably histologic feature that, when combined with poorly differentiated nuclear cytologic features, was associated with 20 times the risk for recurrence as that for women who had neither variable.[26] Some investigators failed to find nuclear grade to be an effective predictor of prognosis in patients with early breast cancer,[34] whereas others found that grading based on nuclear cytologic examination and mitotic index was a more reliable indicator of prognosis than grading that included tubule formation.[33]

The impact of grade on prognosis in stage II patients is uncertain. Some authors have reported a significant correlation, noticing a more favorable outcome associated with low-grade lesions.[29,30] However, these analyses have not taken into consideration stratification on the basis of tumor size and the number of affected lymph nodes. In a carefully defined series of patients with stage T1, N1, M0 disease, neither histologic nor nuclear grade was significantly correlated with outcome.[16] On the other hand, a case–control analysis of patients who survived 25 years after radical mastectomy for invasive carcinoma revealed a significantly higher proportion of histologically grade 1 tumors (43%) among long-term survivors when compared with controls matched on the basis of tumor size, number

of lymph nodes with metastases, and age at diagnosis.[32] Histologic grade was reportedly a prognostically critical factor in the response of stage II patients to adjuvant chemotherapy.[35] Higher failure rates were observed in patients with higher grade tumors. This negative effect of grade was independent of nodal status, tumor size, hormone receptors, and several other prognostic factors. Histologic grade also was a strong indicator of response among patients who received endocrine treatment for systemic recurrence.[36,37] Histologic type of tumor (duct, lobular, or other) was not significantly related to response.

The prognostic import of *lymphoplasmacytic infiltration* in the stroma within and around invasive duct carcinomas has been the subject of interest and controversy. The reaction consists mainly of mature lymphocytes with a variable admixture of plasma cells. Rarely, plasma cells predominate, and these tumors usually are true medullary carcinomas. The moderate to marked lymphoplasmacytic reaction observed in medullary carcinoma also occurs in a small proportion of nonmedullary invasive duct carcinomas.[4,15] A subset of these tumors with some of the features of medullary carcinoma, referred to as atypical medullary carcinoma, may have a slightly more favorable prognosis than infiltrating duct carcinomas generally, but the difference is not statistically significant.[38] Most nonmedullary duct carcinomas with a prominent lymphocytic reaction tend to be poorly differentiated and have a circumscribed rather than infiltrative contour. This type of tumor is more common among blacks, and the mean age of these patients is relatively young.[39] Medullary carcinomas and invasive duct carcinomas with a marked lymphocytic reaction are almost always estrogen receptor− and progesterone receptor−negative.

Although the favorable prognosis of medullary carcinoma has been ascribed to the lymphoplasmacytic reaction that characterizes these tumors, it is less clear that the same conclusion can be drawn about the lymphoplasmacytic

FIGURE 13-3 Histologic grade. **A.** Low-grade invasive duct carcinoma, tubular type, featuring round, angular, or oval glands formed by a single layer of uniform cells. **B.** Moderately differentiated duct carcinoma with a complex invasive glandular pattern. **C.** Poorly differentiated duct carcinoma lacking glandular or papillary structures in the invasive tumor.

reaction in nonmedullary invasive duct carcinomas. Some investigators have found carcinomas with this host response to have a relatively favorable prognosis,[8,21,27,40,41] but others detected no significant difference or reported a less favorable outcome associated with the presence of a prominent lymphoplasmacytic infiltrate.[8,15,31,42]

Studies of the lymphocyte subgroups infiltrating mammary carcinomas indicate that they are largely T lymphocytes[43–45] consisting mainly of T4 and T8 cells.[43,44]

The intensity of mast cell infiltration in the substance or at the periphery of an invasive breast carcinoma is not significantly related to prognosis.[46]

The presence of *lymphatic tumor emboli* in the breast is an unfavorable prognostic finding. For this purpose, lymphatics are defined as vascular channels lined by endothelium without supporting smooth muscle or elastica (Fig. 13-4). Most do not contain red blood cells but, undoubtedly, some blood capillaries are included in this definition. Artifactual spaces are commonly formed around nests of tumor cells within an invasive carcinoma as a result of tissue shrinkage during processing. Because it

is difficult to distinguish these artifacts from true lymphatic spaces,[47] assessment for lymphatic invasion is more reliably accomplished in breast parenchyma adjacent to or well beyond the invasive tumor margin.[48] Efforts to identify intratumoral lymphatic spaces by using immunoperoxidase reagents associated with endothelial cells (factor VIII, blood groups antigens, CD34) have met with limited success.[49–51] Blood group isoantigens stain myoepithelial cells, which may be mistaken for endothelial cells when substantial tissue shrinkage occurs. Strong staining of tumor cells in artifactual spaces may be associated with diffusion of reactivity into the surrounding stroma that may be most intense at the margin of the space.[51,52] Factor VIII antigen has not been consistently and reliably demonstrable in all endothelial-lined capillary or lymphatic channels. False-negative immunohistochemical results usually can be recognized in extratumoral breast tissue, but the fact that they occur means these reagents are not reliable for detecting lymphatic tumor emboli within the tumor.

Extratumoral lymphatic tumor emboli in the breast are found to be associated with about 25% of invasive duct

FIGURE 13-4 Lymphatic invasion. **A.** A cluster of tumor cells in a lymphatic space adjacent to a small duct outside an invasive carcinoma. Nuclei of endothelial cells line the vascular channel, which has no discernible supporting muscular or stromal layer. **B.** Shrinkage artifact that simulates lymphatic invasion. A mass of invasive tumor cells has separated from supporting stroma but retains the identical shape. **C.** Endothelial cell nuclei are absent at high magnification.

carcinomas. This determination is made on the basis of routine sampling of biopsy and mastectomy specimens. Most of these patients also have axillary lymph node metastases, and it has not been determined whether the presence of lymphatic emboli alters their prognosis.

Lymphatic tumor emboli are found in the breast surrounding invasive duct carcinomas in 10% to 15% of patients who have pathologically negative lymph nodes. Several studies have shown that lymphatic invasion is prognostically unfavorable in node-negative patients treated by mastectomy.[15,42,48,53–56] The deleterious effect is most pronounced in women with T1, N0, M0 disease. In a 10-year follow-up study of 378 patients treated for T1, N0, M0 carcinoma, 33% of 30 women with lymphatic tumor emboli died of disease. Death from breast carcinoma was observed in 10% of the 348 women who did not have lymphatic invasion.[15] Another study comparing similar subsets of patients with stage T1, N0, M0 disease found recurrences in 32% of those with lymphatic invasion and in 10% of controls.[42] It has not been possible to demonstrate a statistically significant effect of lymphatic invasion on prognosis in node-negative patients with tumors larger than 2 cm (T2, N0, M0), although those with lymphatic invasion do experience a higher recurrence rate.[48] Recurrences that develop in node-negative patients who had peritumoral lymphatic emboli tend to occur more than 5 years after diagnosis, and they are almost always systemic. Lymphatic tumor emboli do not predispose to local recurrence in patients treated by mastectomy, but they are predictive of failure in the breast after breast conservation.

The unfavorable effect of lymphatic invasion in T1, N0, M0 patients probably is not because of occult metastases in their axillary lymph nodes. Metastases were detected in serial sections of lymph nodes in 9 of 28 patients whose disease originally was classified as T1, N0, M0 with lymphatic invasion in the breast. The recurrence rate was no higher among those with occult nodal metastases than in those in the subset with truly negative lymph nodes.[57]

The implication of lymphatic tumor emboli for prognosis in patients already proved to have lymph node metastases is uncertain. Among patients with stage T1, N0, M0 disease treated surgically before receiving adjuvant chemotherapy, lymphatic tumor emboli did not significantly influence disease-free survival at 10 years of follow-up.[58] One group of investigators[59] found that lymphatic invasion did not have an independent effect on disease-free survival at 10 years in patients who received adjuvant chemotherapy. Others have reported significantly lower overall and disease-free survival at 4 years in stage II patients with peritumoral vessel invasion in another adjuvant therapy trial.[60]

Blood vessel invasion is defined as penetration by tumor into the lumen of an artery or vein (Fig. 13-5). These vascular structures can be identified by the presence of a smooth muscle wall supported by elastic fibers. Usually, it is necessary to employ special histochemical procedures (eg, orcein or Verhoeff van Gieson stains) that selectively stain elastic tissue to detect this component of the vascular wall. Elastic fibers are often deposited around ducts that contain intraductal carcinoma within an invasive tumor, and the resulting appearance in an elastic tissue stain may be difficult to distinguish from vascular invasion. Because larger vascular components in the breast usually consist of a paired artery and vein, vascular invasion should be diagnosed with confidence only when the tumor is demonstrated within one or both of a pair of vessels demonstrated by elastic tissue stain.

The reported frequency of blood vessel invasion varies from 4.7% to 47.2%.[4,15,16,42,61–67] These divergent observations reflect major differences in these studies relative to the number of patients evaluated, clinical and pathologic characteristics of the study populations, and the methods by which blood vessel invasion was identified. These variations in study design and methodology are probably responsible for the different conclusions reached by the authors on the prognostic import of blood vessel invasion. Some have reported that blood vessel invasion denoted a poorer prognosis in node-positive patients[63] or only in those with two or more positive lymph nodes.[64] Others

concluded that this finding was prognostically indicative only in the absence of axillary lymph node metastasis.[66]

A thorough assessment of blood vessel invasion was provided by 10-year follow-up data for 524 women treated consecutively for invasive carcinomas 2 cm or less in diameter (T1) by modified or standard radical mastectomy.[15,16] It was possible to evaluate 502 tumors for blood vessel invasion by using one section per case stained to demonstrate elastic tissue. Blood vessel invasion was identified in 47 of 362 (13%) T1, N0, M0 cases. Recurrence of breast carcinoma was more frequent when blood vessel invasion was present (12 of 47; 26%) than in its absence (50 of 315; 16%), and death of disease also occurred more often among women with blood vessel invasion (present: 9 of 47, 19%; absent: 38 of 315, 12%). However, these differences in recurrence and death rates were not statistically significant. Visceral metastases occurred in 67% of patients with blood vessel invasion and in 35% when it was not present. Bone recurrences were more frequent in the absence of demonstrable blood vessel invasion. Others also have observed a similar trend toward a higher recurrence rate associated with blood vessel invasion in T1, N0, M0 disease.[42]

Blood vessel invasion was found in 23 of 117 (16%) stage II T1 tumors (T1, N0, M0).[16] Deaths of metastatic breast carcinoma occurred with significantly greater frequency among women with blood vessel invasion ($P < .03$), whether they had a single positive lymph node or two or more affected nodes.

The *angiogenic capacity* of breast carcinomas has attracted interest as a prognostic indicator. The capacity of neoplastic[68,69] and preneoplastic[70–72] tissues to induce angiogenesis is well documented. This property of proliferating tissues is attributed to the elaboration of angiogenic factors, such as vascular endothelial growth factor (VEGF) and basic

FIGURE 13-5 Blood vessel invasion. **A.** Routine section stained with hematoxylin–eosin in which vascular invasion can be suspected. A small, unaffected artery is seen on the right; on the left, a vein is filled with tumor cells. **B.** Comparable section for elastic tissue showing vascular structures. Invasive carcinoma can be seen in the surrounding stroma.

fibroblast growth factor (bFGF). Tumor growth is enhanced by increased perfusion associated with neovascularization and by the paracrine effects of growth factors produced by endothelial cells that promote tumor growth. Inhibition of tumor growth has been achieved experimentally with antibodies to VEGF[73] and to bFGF.[74] The angiogenic phenotype is expressed by a subset of cells in a carcinoma. Acquisition of this phenotype may be an important hallmark in the evolution of a carcinoma, and the presence or absence of this characteristic may be critical for promoting the viability of metastatic carcinoma cells. Expression of the angiogenic phenotype is probably mediated through complex molecular alterations. These seem to involve up-regulation of angiogenic peptides such as bFGF and concomitant down-regulation of inhibitors of endothelial cells and angiogenesis such as thrombospondin,[75,76] possibly through alterations in tumor-suppressor genes like p53.[76]

Pathologic studies of angiogenesis in breast carcinoma have examined the relevance of tumor vascularity to prognosis. To perform such studies, histologic sections or paraffin-embedded tissue are stained with immunohistochemical markers for endothelial cells such as factor VIII, CD34, and CD31. Vessel counts are recorded in foci of greatest vascular density, the so-called hotspot, by counting the number of immunostained structures in a predetermined number of fields at a fixed magnification.[77,78] Numeric microvessel counts have been analyzed by the comparison of cases above and below the mean number in a given study, or by comparing cases with fewer than or more than a mean of 100 microvessels per standardized field. In one study, analysis of microvessel count as a continuous numerical value revealed that more than 80 microvessels provided the optimal cutoff value for stratifying patients into relatively good and poor prognosis groups.

High microvessel density has been shown to be associated with a poor grade of histologic differentiation in invasive duct carcinomas[77,79,80] and with a greater probability of axillary nodal metastases.[79] Whereas some authors have found high microvessel counts to be associated with greater tumor size,[79] others have reported no significant relation with size.[77,80,81]

Angiogenesis has been reported to be an independent prognostic indicator by some investigators. High microvessel counts have been associated with a poor prognosis in node-negative[77,79,81] and in node-positive[79,81] breast carcinoma. However, others have failed to detect a significant relation to prognosis[80,82] or to recurrence in the breast after wide excision and breast conservation.[83]

Carcinomas arising in various organs exhibit a capacity, and in some instances, a proclivity to invade around and into nerves, *perineural invasion* (Fig. 13-6). This phenomenon is infrequently observed among invasive mammary carcinomas, perhaps in part because nerves of notable size are not numerous in mammary tissues. Perineural invasion can be found in about 10% of invasive duct carcinomas. It tends to occur in high-grade tumors, frequently associated with the presence of lymphatic tumor emboli, and has not been proven to have independent prognostic importance.

A variety of patterns have been described in the con-

FIGURE 13-6 Perineural invasion. Neoplastic glands surrounding and invading nerves are evident in the center and left parts of this photograph. A tumor gland lies just outside a nerve on the right.

nective tissue *stroma* formed in and around invasive duct carcinomas. Tumors vary considerably in the quantity and qualitative characteristics of their stroma. Extremes are represented by medullary carcinoma and cellular variants of invasive duct carcinoma, which contain virtually no fibrous stroma, and scirrhous carcinoma, characterized by marked collagenization. It is not clear if the character of stroma in an invasive duct carcinoma is an independent prognostic variable because there are clear associations between this and other prognostically important structural features of breast carcinomas. For example, tumors that contain minimal stromal reaction tend to have the following characteristics: circumscription, poorly differentiated nuclear and histologic grade, and marked lymphoplasmacytic reaction. They are usually estrogen receptor–negative. On the other hand, densely fibrotic or scirrhous carcinomas are more likely to be stellate, moderately differentiated, and to have little lymphoplasmacytic reaction. A greater proportion of these lesions are estrogen receptor–positive.

Attempts to assess the character or composition of stroma in invasive duct carcinomas have focused on the amount of elastic tissue present. Stromal elastic fibers can be detected with the same stains (orcein or Verhoeff van Gieson stains) used to demonstrate the elastic components in blood vessels. Although a minimal amount of elastic tissue is present in normal mammary stroma, increased amounts may be deposited around ducts in benign proliferative breast disease.[84,85] A similar phenomenon occurs commonly around intraductal carcinoma, particularly in the invasive portion of the tumor and, to a lesser extent, in the intervening stroma. The cellular source of elastin is uncertain. Because elastosis can develop in benign proliferative lesions, it is clearly not a specific product of carcinoma cells. It is likely that benign and malignant epithelial cells secrete a factor (or factors) that induces the production of elastin by stromal cells, thereby contributing to the development of elastosis.

In the absence of a widely accepted method for describing elastosis, various grading schemes have been adopted to convey quantitative estimates of the extent of this process. The frequency of the most extreme or marked degrees of elastosis described in certain reports varied from 17% to 23%,[4,86,88] whereas from 12% to 55% of tumors in the same studies were characterized by little or no elastosis.

Abundant elastosis is significantly associated with estrogen receptor positivity.[86-88] The import of elastosis as an independent prognostic variable remains controversial. Although marked elastosis has been described by some investigators as a favorable prognostic feature,[89,90] others found that abundant elastosis had a negative effect on outcome.[91,92]

Attention has been directed to the pattern and distribution of *intraductal carcinoma* as a prognostic variable in patients with invasive duct carcinoma. Tumors vary in the relative proportions of intraductal and invasive components from those with microscopic invasion that is not grossly measurable (Fig. 13-7) to lesions composed entirely of invasive carcinoma. The term *microinvasion* refers to invasion not easily measurable in microscopic dimensions, essentially a focus less than 1 mm in diameter. Silverberg and Chitale[93] observed a trend to decreased nodal metastases and a more favorable prognosis when the intraductal component in the tumor was relatively more abundant. In one report, little or no intraductal carcinoma was detected in sections from 72% of 974 tumors, and 11% were described as composed of at least 66% intraductal carcinoma.[4] These authors observed that lesions with a prominent intratumor intraductal component also tended to have invasive carcinoma in other quadrants of the breast. Although the distribution of invasive carcinoma in and around the primary tumor seems to correlate with the risk

for recurrence in the breast after lumpectomy and radiation therapy,[94] this feature has no bearing on the risk for systemic recurrence in women treated by mastectomy.[94] No independent association exists between the structural pattern of intraductal carcinoma (comedo, cribriform, papillary) in an invasive duct carcinoma and prognosis in patients treated by mastectomy. However, the pattern and amount of intraductal carcinoma influence the risk of recurrence in the breast after breast-conserving therapy. Recurrence occurs more frequently in the breast after lumpectomy and radiation therapy in women who have comedo intraductal carcinoma, or when there is extensive intraductal carcinoma defined as intraductal carcinoma within and around the tumor that comprises at least 25% of the neoplasm.

An array of *other histologic variables* has been assessed as potential prognostic indicators. Among these are the amount and type of mucin produced by the tumor cells, mucopolysaccharide content of tumor stroma, glycogen content of tumor cells, presence of calcifications in the tumor, and the influence of associated benign proliferative changes in the breast. None of these observations has been found to correlate strongly with prognosis or to be as useful in making therapeutic decisions as the other observations discussed in detail in this section.

IMMUNOHISTOCHEMICAL MARKERS

Interest has been growing in the application of immunohistochemical markers to tissue sections as potential indicators of prognosis (Table 13-1). Carcinoembryonic antigen (CEA) is the most extensively studied marker, perhaps because early studies suggested that elevated tissue and plasma CEA levels were indicative of a higher recurrence rate.[95] No consistent relation has been found between prognosis and the immunohistochemical demonstration of CEA activity in breast cancer.[51,96-102] Most of the other marker substances that can be detected in breast carcinoma cells by immunohistochemical methods have not been useful for routinely assessing prognosis.

FIGURE 13-7 Microinvasive duct carcinoma. The 1-cm tumor consisted of numerous clustered ducts with intraductal carcinoma seen on the right. A 1-mm focus of invasive carcinoma composed of small glands invading the stroma is present on the left.

Tubular (Well-Differentiated) Carcinoma

Tubular carcinoma, a morphologically distinctive form of mammary carcinoma, has been recognized for more than 100 years.[127] The term *tubular carcinoma*[128] describes the distinguishing microscopic feature of the lesion, which is composed of neoplastic elements resembling normal breast ductules. Alternative names, such as *orderly* and *well-differentiated*[129,130] carcinoma, are less specific and have not gained wide acceptance.

The precise pathologic definition of tubular carcinoma has been the subject of controversy, and this has influenced the reported frequency of the lesion. Elements of tubular carcinoma may be found in invasive duct carcinomas. As used in this section, tubular carcinoma refers to so-called pure tubular carcinoma. Most authors require that at

TABLE 13-1
Immunohistochemical Markers in Breast Carcinoma

Marker	% Tumors Immunoreactive	Comments	References
		ALA directly related to estrogen/	
ALA	56–75	progesterone receptors	103, 104
B-72.3 antibody	50–92		105–113
β-HCG	12–18	No correlation with tumor type	51, 98, 101, 114
CEA	34–90		51, 96–102, 115, 116
Cathepsin D		More often positive in medullary	538–540
GCDFP-15	72	More often positive in IDFC than IFLC	113
HER2/neu		Low frequency HER2 positive in medullary	541–543
p53		More often positive in medullary	544–546
Placental lactogen	30	No correlation with tumor type	51, 98
Pregnancy-specific β_1-glycoprotein (SP-1)	37–56	More often positive in IFDC than IFLC	51, 98, 101, 115, 117, 118
S-100 protein	50		119, 120
SC	25–50		103, 118, 121, 122
Vimentin	9	Vimentin-positive tumors have higher growth rate	123–126

ALA, α-lactalbumin; β-HCG, β-human chorionic gonadotropin; CEA, carcinoembryonic antigen; GCDFP-15, gross cystic disease fluid protein-15; IFDC, invasive duct carcinoma; IFLC, invasive lobular carcinoma; SC, secretory component.

least 75% of the tumor be tubular to qualify for this diagnosis.[131–136]

In its pure form, tubular carcinoma is uncommon, constituting not more than 2% of all breast carcinomas in most series.[131–133,137] Because tubular carcinomas are small, they are found with greater frequency in studies of early-stage breast cancer. In one series of 382 women with T1, N1, M0 breast carcinoma, treated between 1964 and 1969,[15] tubular carcinoma was present in 5%, occurring in 9% of patients with a tumor 1.0 cm or smaller in diameter and in 2% with a tumor measuring 1.1 to 2.0 cm. Only 1.5% of 142 patients with T1, N1, M0 disease had a tubular carcinoma.[16]

With the widespread use of mammography, emphasis on early breast cancer detection has contributed to increased interest in tubular carcinoma. These tumors constituted 8% of invasive carcinomas 1 cm or smaller in diameter, as found by a review of the Breast Cancer Detection Demonstration Projects.[138] Seven percent of 138 carcinomas detected in one US screening program were of the tubular variety,[139] all having been identified by mammographic and only 30% by clinical examination. In Malmö, Sweden, 21.5% of 116 breast carcinomas found in mammography screening were reportedly of the pure tubular variety.[140]

It has been suggested that tubular carcinomas are a stage in the evolution of a substantial number of breast cancers.[141,142] Authors who support this theory believe that tubular carcinomas arise from benign proliferative lesions, called radial scars, and that as they enlarge, tubular carcinomas are converted into ordinary invasive duct carcinomas. This subject remains controversial.[143,144]

CLINICAL PRESENTATION

Patients with tubular carcinoma have been mostly women.[135,136,145] Tubular carcinoma constitutes only about 1% of male breast carcinomas.[146,147] The clinical data presented here deals with women reported to have pure tubular carcinoma.

The age distribution at diagnosis ranges from 24 to 83 years,[133,136] with a median age in the middle to late 40s (range, 44 to 49 years). The presenting symptom for most patients is a palpable lesion and, in most cases, this proves to be the carcinoma. The reported duration of symptoms has been 1 week to 20 years (median, 2 months).[134–136] Skin retraction or fixation occurs in about 15% of cases; nipple discharge is rarely reported.[133] Several studies have compared patients treated for pure tubular carcinoma with women who had invasive carcinomas that contained tubular elements (mixed tubular carcinomas).[131–134] Other than a trend to younger age at diagnosis for pure tubular carcinoma, no consistent clinical differences have been observed. In one study, 40% of patients with tubular carcinoma reported a positive family history of breast carcinoma among first-degree relatives.[148]

GROSS PATHOLOGY

The reported size of tubular carcinomas ranges from 0.2 to 4 cm, except for one study in which the largest tumor measured 12 cm.[143] In two studies, 80%[135] and 87%[136] of tubular carcinomas were 1 cm or less in diameter, and in the latter series, the median size of 90 pure lesions was 0.8 cm. By contrast, these authors[136] described a size range of 0.4 to 2.1 cm for 55 mixed tubular carcinomas (median size, 1.1 cm) and noticed that 52% were 1 cm or less.

Grossly, tubular carcinoma produces a firm-to-hard tumor. The cut surface is gray to white. Rarely, a tan or pale yellow tinge may be found in lesions that have extensive elastosis. Tumor margins are ill defined or stellate. The cut surface tends to retract and become depressed in relation to surrounding breast parenchyma. Although tubular carcinoma may be suspected on gross inspection, the features are not specific enough to exclude some benign lesions or less well-differentiated invasive carcinomas of comparable size.

MICROSCOPIC PATHOLOGY

Tubular carcinoma is a variant of invasive duct carcinoma. As illustrated in Figure 13-8, the tumor is characterized microscopically by a proliferation of small glands to tubules that closely resemble nonneoplastic mammary ductules. These invasive tubular structures are haphazardly distributed and tend to form a stellate tumor with ill-defined boundaries. Stroma within the tumor is formed of dense collagenous tissue, with variable, sometimes abundant, amount of elastic tissue.[149,150] Calcifications are found in about 50% of cases, sometimes in the lumen of neoplastic tubules or in the stroma. More commonly, calcifications are detected in the intraductal component, which has been reportedly present in 60% to 84%[129,132,135,136,151] of the tumors. Most often, tubular carcinoma arises from papillary and cribriform intraductal carcinoma. Lobular carcinoma in situ has been found in association with tubular carcinoma in 0.7% to 40% of cases,[132,134,135,136,152] usually as part of the primary tumor.

FIGURE 13-8 Pure tubular carcinoma in a 57-year-old woman who had an asymptomatic lesion detected by mammography. Low-power view shows characteristic angular and oval invasive glands embedded in moderately cellular stroma. Micropapillary intraductal carcinoma fills a duct near the right margin.

Tubular carcinoma often is not accompanied by an appreciable lymphocytic reaction. Perineural invasion may be observed, but it is uncommon, and this form of carcinoma never has lymphatic tumor emboli detectable in histologic sections of the breast.[15]

Microscopically, tubular carcinoma must be distinguished from benign conditions such as sclerosing adenosis and microglandular adenosis. The proliferative pattern of sclerosing adenosis is lobulocentric. Consequently, at low magnification in sclerosing adenosis, multiple individual altered lobules can be identified, even when the process is sufficiently developed to clinically form a coalescent mass of adenosis tumor.[153] In contrast with the haphazardly dispersed, open, often angular glands of tubular carcinoma, the proliferation in sclerosing adenosis tends to be a compact whorled mixture of elongated and compressed glands interlaced with spindly myoepithelial cells. Histochemical studies have shown their presence in sclerosing adenosis and their absence in tubular carcinoma.[154,155] These differences have been confirmed by electron microscopic study.[156,157] The distinction between tubular carcinoma and microglandular adenosis, an uncommon tumor, is more difficult and depends on a careful assessment of fine cytologic details.[158]

Tubular carcinoma usually forms a single tumor clinically. However, in an undetermined number of patients, tubular carcinoma seems to grow as a more diffuse process, with multiple, separate foci in one or more quadrants of the breast. From 10% to 56% of patients with tubular carcinoma have been reported to have independent foci of carcinoma elsewhere in the breast,[132,134,136,148,151] including various types of in situ and invasive carcinoma. In one series of 120 patients treated by mastectomy, 20 (16.7%) had residual tubular carcinoma at the biopsy site, 6 (5%) had a second remote invasive carcinoma, 4 (3.3%) had multicentric intraductal carcinoma, and 3 (2.5%) had multicentric in situ lobular carcinoma.[136] Contralateral carcinoma has been reported in several series, with the percentage of cases varying from 0% to 38%.[132,148,159] The frequency of contralateral cancer in three studies was 9%, 10%, and 12%, respectively.[134,136] Most contralateral carcinomas were of the infiltrating duct type. Rare instances of bilateral tubular carcinoma have been observed.[133,134,151]

The tubular elements found in varying proportions in mixed tubular carcinomas, are indistinguishable from those in pure tubular carcinomas (Fig. 13-9). Trabecular, alveolar, and papillary growth, and nontubular gland formation constitute some of the components of infiltrating duct carcinoma found in mixed tubular lesions.

The diagnosis of tubular carcinoma may be suggested by the findings in a fine-needle aspiration specimen, but excisional biopsy is necessary to establish the diagnosis.[160]

Tubular carcinoma is frequently positive for estrogen and progesterone receptors when tested by immunohistochemical study.[161]

PROGNOSIS

The favorable prognosis attributed to tubular carcinoma is restricted to tumors composed of at least 75% tubular elements.[131–137] The reported frequency of axillary metastases

FIGURE 13-9 Mixed tubular carcinoma in a 70-year-old woman. Low-power view shows numerous invasive tubular glands and alveolar masses of invasive tumor with solid and laciform growth patterns.

ranges from none[133] to 25%,[130] with an average of 9%.[15,16,131,133,134,135,136,151] Involved lymph nodes rarely number more than three, they are usually located at level I, and the metastatic foci tend to have a tubular growth pattern. Axillary lymph node metastases have been reported in 21%[131] and 29%[134] of patients with mixed tubular carcinoma. In one study,[134] 21% of patients with stage II mixed tubular carcinoma had more than three lymph nodes involved.

Most patients with pure or mixed tubular carcinoma described in the literature have been treated by mastectomy, usually of the modified or radical type. Simple mastectomy or excisional treatment were employed in fewer than 10% of patients. Seven follow-up studies[130,132–136,151] describe 341 women with pure tubular carcinoma. Recurrences attributable to tubular carcinoma were reported in 12 patients (3.5%). Six of these were women who developed recurrences in the breast after simple excision. The interval to recurrence in the breast ranged from 2 to 22 years. Only one of these women had axillary nodal metastases at the time of recurrence, and none were reported to have systemic spread after mastectomy for the recurrence.

Recurrence after mastectomy was described in six cases. Three of these patients had had positive axillary lymph nodes at mastectomy. One developed a local recurrence, whereas the other two had fatal systemic metastases. Of two patients with negative axillary nodes, one developed systemic spread and another had persistent carcinoma. The sixth patient, whose nodal status was unreported, developed a local recurrence. Several patients had bilateral carcinoma whose death of metastatic disease seemed attributable to the contralateral lesion.[134,136] Among patients with mixed tubular carcinoma, 32% developed recurrence[133,134] and from 6% to 28% died of disease.[132–134]

Medullary Carcinoma

The term *medullary* has been used to describe mammary carcinomas for nearly a century. For much of this time, the name was employed to describe the clinical or gross pathologic appearance of large, solid, or papillary carcinomas that often produced axillary metastases. The name *medullary carcinoma* has been applied to a specific type of carcinoma since the 1940s.[162,163] Medullary carcinoma also has been referred to as solid circumscribed carcinoma.[164,165] These uncommon tumors constitute up to 7% of mammary carcinomas in most series.[1,166,167]

CLINICAL PRESENTATION

Patients with medullary carcinoma tend to be younger than those with other types of carcinoma. Moore and Foote[163] reported that 59% of the patients were younger than 50 years. Others found 40%,[168] 60%,[169] and 66%[165] of patients to be younger than 50 years. The mean age at diagnosis in several series was 46 to 54 years.[38,165,167,169] Medullary carcinoma constitutes 11% of carcinomas diagnosed in women 35 years of age or younger[39] and is relatively uncommon in elderly patients.[170]

Early clinical descriptions of patients with medullary carcinoma emphasized large tumor size, circumscription, and a tendency to cystic degeneration.[163,171] Fixation to the skin or chest wall and ulceration have been reported with larger tumors, mistaken clinically for fibroadenomas, especially in young women. Ultrasound has not yet provided diagnostic criteria specific for medullary carcinoma.[172]

Medullary carcinoma occurs in various parts of the breast, with a frequency similar to breast carcinoma in general. Because of its histologic and clinical characteristics, medullary carcinoma in the axillary tail of the breast may be mistaken for metastatic carcinoma in a lymph node.[173] Bilateral breast carcinoma has been reported in from 3% to 18% of patients who have medullary carcinoma in one breast.[159,165,167,170,174] Medullary carcinoma affecting both breasts, whether simultaneous or asynchronous, is uncommon.[159,170] Multicentric foci of carcinoma are found outside the primary quadrant in 8% to 10% of cases.[159,174]

Fewer than 10% of primary medullary carcinomas of the breast contain sufficient levels of estrogen or progesterone receptor to be regarded as testing positive.[175–178] The growth rate of medullary carcinoma, measured by thymidine incorporation, is among the fastest recorded among breast carcinomas,[179] an observation consistent with the rapid growth and short duration reported by many patients. Similar results are obtained by flow cytometric study.[179,180]

GROSS PATHOLOGY

In most series, the median size is between 2 and 3 cm. Medullary carcinoma has a well-defined contour that separates it from surrounding breast parenchyma. Close inspection of the cut surface of a bisected medullary carcinoma usually reveals a nodular architecture. The tumor is firm, but softer than the average breast carcinoma, and bulges above the surrounding tissue. Other notable features are a tendency to a pale brown or gray color and the presence of hemorrhage or necrosis in some tumors. The extent of necrosis tends to increase in proportion to tumor size, but may be prominent, even in small lesions. Necrotic tissue can have a granular, almost caseous appearance in medullary carcinomas. Lesions larger than 5 cm tend to undergo cystic degeneration.

MICROSCOPIC PATHOLOGY

Medullary carcinoma is defined by a complex constellation of histopathologic features.[163,170] The tumor must exhibit all of these elements to be diagnosed as a medullary carcinoma. Carcinomas that have most of the necessary microscopic components have been referred to as atypical medullary carcinomas. It is imperative that the histologic criteria for the diagnosis of medullary carcinoma be rigorously applied, because the prognosis of women with atypical medullary carcinoma is substantially less favorable than that of patients with medullary carcinoma.[38,174,181]

In addition to gross and microscopic circumscription, histopathologic features that define medullary carcinoma are intense lymphoplasmacytic reaction around and within the tumor; poorly differentiated nuclear grade (usually accompanied by a high mitotic rate among tumor cells); and a tendency for tumor cells to form broad sheets (syncytial pattern), rather than the trabecular, alveolar, or gland-forming patterns of ordinary invasive duct carcinoma (Fig. 13-10). Intraductal carcinoma is commonly present (46%) at the periphery of the tumor, often with involvement of the epithelium in adjacent lobules. An intense lymphoplasmacytic reaction occurs around the affected ducts and lobules. This reactive process also may extend to lobules and ducts, which are at a greater distance from the tumor, that do not contain recognizable tumor cells. It has been suggested that the expansile growth occurs at least partly because of coalescence of enlarging nodules of carcinoma in these peripheral ducts and lobules, a conclusion supported by the grossly nodular character of medullary carcinoma.[38]

Squamous metaplasia occurs in a substantial number (16%) of medullary carcinomas, and osteocartilaginous metaplasia and anaplastic giant cell formation also may be found. Medullary carcinoma is accompanied only rarely by intramammary lymphatic tumor emboli.

Electron microscopic study has revealed some distinctive ultrastructural features.[182–185] The tumor cells are rich in organelles and have a well-developed Golgi complex. Light and dark cells have been described, which differ in cytoplasmic density. Mucin secretory vacuoles are absent from the tumor cells.[185] Endothelial cells in the tumor stroma are prominent, and migration of lymphocytes has been observed through the endothelium of these channels.

Immunohistochemical study has shown that IgA plasma cells predominate in medullary carcinomas.[186–188] The tumor cells contain IgA and secretory component. By contrast, typical infiltrating duct carcinomas contain little or none of these substances and their associated plasma cells contain IgG. Cells with IgG also may be prominent in medullary carcinomas.[186–189] Lymphocytes and carcinoma cells in medullary carcinoma express HLA-DR more frequently than do other types of breast carcinoma.[190] Medullary carcinomas rarely show membrane immunoreactivity

for the HER2/neu oncogene, whereas they frequently exhibit nuclear immunoreactivity for p53.

PROGNOSIS

Moore and Foote[163] reported that 82.7% of the 52 patients with medullary carcinoma were alive and disease-free after radical mastectomy. Only 11.5% of their patients died of breast carcinoma within 5 years. They found axillary node metastases in 42% of cases and observed a 5-year survival rate of 50% in node-positive patients. Nine patients with a single lymph node metastasis survived disease-free for 5 years. Richardson's series[168] of 99 patients had a disease-free survival rate of 78% at 5 years. Death caused by disease was reported in 10%. Survival among 47 patients with 10 years of follow-up was 64%, with eight (17%) deaths of breast cancer and nine deaths (19%) of other causes. Richardson[168] confirmed Moore and Foote's[163] observation that axillary metastases were relatively infrequent (45%) and that prognosis was more favorable than among patients with ordinary stage II carcinoma.

Studies of medullary carcinoma also have reported a low frequency of axillary metastases[38,167,181] and, with few exceptions,[165,191] they have confirmed a favorable prognosis (Fig. 13-11A).[167,170] The size of the primary tumor and axillary nodal status are crucial determinants of survival (see Fig. 13-11B) for patients with medullary carcinoma.[167,170] Patients with tumors larger than 3 cm, accompanied by more than three involved lymph nodes, experience recurrence rates that are not appreciably different from patients with ordinary types of breast carcinoma. The outcome for women with node-negative medullary carcinoma seems to be especially favorable when the tumor is smaller than 3 cm,[15,38,167,192] and this probably applies to patients with small tumors when not more than three axillary lymph nodes are involved.[16,192] Recurrences may be local, as well as systemic, after modified or radical mastectomy. In one series, local recurrence was found in 25% of patients with recurrence.

Axillary lymph nodes in patients with medullary carcinoma tend to enlarge, even in the absence of nodal metastases, and this phenomenon may complicate clinical staging.[165] Microscopic examination reveals lymphoplasmacytic infiltration and follicular hyperplasia, with variable sinus histiocytosis. Because these hyperplastic lymph nodes are grossly conspicuous, the average number of lymph nodes obtained on pathologic dissection of the axillary contents exceeds that for other types of carcinoma.[193]

MUCINOUS CARCINOMA

In their pure or nearly pure form, these tumors constitute 1% to 2% of breast carcinomas.[138] About another 2% of carcinomas have areas of mucinous differentiation. The unusual microscopic appearance of this tumor, slow growth rate, and favorable prognosis have been recognized for more than a century.[194–196] Geschickter[197] emphasized the importance of distinguishing pure lesions from those containing mucinous and ordinary carcinoma elements. A tendency for metastases to become manifest late in the course of the disease has been reported in many studies.[197–201]

FIGURE 13-10 Medullary carcinoma in a 31-year-old woman who presented with a 1.5-cm tumor diagnosed clinically as a fibroadenoma. **A.** Histologic cross section of the tumor showing circumscribed margins and a multinodular structure. Cystic necrosis is visible in a nodule near the margin in the 10-o'clock position. **B.** Typical syncytial masses of tumor cells surrounded by an intense lymphoplasmacytic reaction that extends throughout the tumor, as well as around the periphery. **C.** Numerous mitotic figures are evident among the cytologically high-grade nuclei. Absence of distinct cell borders is typical in this syncytial growth pattern. **D.** Nodule at the periphery of the tumor in a different section. It appears to consist of several coalescent lobules and ducts surrounded by an intense lymphoplasmacytic infiltrate. Most of the round nests of tumor cells are composed of in situ tumor. **E.** A single lobule in which acinar units are expanded by tumor cells. Lymphoplasmacytic reaction is confined to the intralobular stroma, resulting in a sharply defined contour.

B

FIGURE 13-11 A. The overall prognosis of patients with medullary carcinoma is significantly more favorable than for patients with ordinary invasive duct carcinoma or for those who have invasive duct carcinoma with medullary features. The survival curves for nonmedullary and atypical medullary carcinoma patients are not significantly different. **B.** Survival curves of patients with typical medullary carcinoma and those with invasive duct carcinoma stratified by tumor size. The most favorable group includes those who have typical medullary carcinoma no larger than 3 cm.

CLINICAL PRESENTATION

Mucinous carcinoma occurs throughout the age range of breast carcinoma. Some authors have noticed an older mean age for patients with pure mucinous carci-

noma,[202–204] but this has not been reported in other studies.[199–201,203,205] Mucinous carcinoma constitutes about 7% of carcinomas in women older than 75 years of age and 1% in those younger than 35 years old at diagnosis.[170]

The initial symptom usually is a mass. Accompanying signs such as nipple discharge, fixation, and skin ulceration do not occur with exceptional frequency. The palpatory "swish" sign described by Halstead is rarely mentioned. A duration of symptoms exceeding 1 year has been observed in some elderly patients who have large pure mucinous carcinomas.[206] Mammography has enabled detection of small, clinically occult mucinous carcinomas. Calcifications that occur in some mucinous carcinomas may be detected in a mammogram. Mucinous carcinoma is not especially associated with bilaterality. About 60% of pure mucinous carcinomas are estrogen receptor–positive.[207,208] Nearly all pure mucinous carcinomas are diploid when studied by flow cytometric examination, whereas most mixed mucinous tumors were described as aneuploid.[209]

GROSS PATHOLOGY

Published studies of mucinous carcinoma have described tumors ranging in size from less than 1 cm to 20 cm or more. A widely held perception that pure mucinous carcinomas tend to be larger than other types of carcinomas[199,206,210] is based on observations made several decades ago. Experience suggests that mucinous carcinomas are not especially large.[211,212]

On gross inspection, pure mucinous carcinoma varies in consistency from soft and gelatinous to firm or hard, depending on the relative proportions of tumor and fibrous stroma present in the lesion. The mucinous character is readily appreciated on the cut surface, which appears moist and glistening. Margins of the tumor tend to be circumscribed, an impression often accentuated by a reddish zone of congested tissue at the periphery. Larger mucinous tumors may develop areas of cystic degeneration.

MICROSCOPIC PATHOLOGY

The distinguishing histopathologic feature is the accumulation of abundant extracellular mucinous secretion around clusters of tumor cells. In pure mucinous carcinoma, this pattern is seen in all histologic sections. However, the relative proportions of secretion and tumor cells varies from one patient to another, and even within a given tumor. One extreme variant is the tumor so disproportionately composed of mucin that numerous sections may be necessary to detect any carcinoma cells (Fig. 13-12).

Tumor cells usually are dispersed in the mucinous secretion in slender strands or in papillary clusters. Larger sheets of cells and zones of trabecular growth also are encountered. Gland formation is uncommon, and little intracellular mucin is evident on routine histologic examination. Signet-ring cells containing abundant cytoplasmic mucin, which are characteristic of infiltrating lobular carcinoma,[213] are rarely present in mucinous carcinoma. Mucin can be demonstrated within the cells by electron micro-

FIGURE 13-12 Mucinous carcinoma. **A.** Pure mucinous carcinoma composed almost entirely of extracellular mucin in a 73-year-old woman. After extensive study of numerous slides, a few clusters of tumor cells were found exemplified by glands in the upper right corner. **B.** A typical example of pure mucinous carcinoma from a 47-year-old woman who presented with a breast mass that features abundant tumor cells in a mucinous matrix. **C.** Mixed mucinous carcinoma composed in part of a solid invasive duct carcinoma as well as areas with a mucinous growth pattern.

scopic study.[213,214] The amount of secretion found in most cells of mucinous carcinoma is substantially less than in signet-ring cell carcinomas. However, a small number of cells that appear to accumulate abundant mucin are disrupted, discharging the secretion.[215] Acidic and neutral mucopolysaccharides have been detected in mucinous carcinomas. Generally, the type of mucin is homogeneous within a given tumor.[216,217]

Argyrophilic granules have been detected in the cytoplasm of tumor cells in 14% to 50% of mucinous carcinomas.[218–222] Mucinous carcinomas composed of cells arranged in sheets and trabeculae tend to contain argyrophilic granules and seem to occur more often in elderly women than do mucinous carcinomas with the papillary or festooned cell pattern. The content of the secretory granules has not been determined in most cases, but in some tumors they reportedly contained serotonin,[223,224] somatostatin, and gastrin.[224] In many instances, argyrophilic granules have proven to be intracytoplasmic mucin rather than endocrine secretory products. Argyrophilic granules in mucinous carcinoma do not seem to be prognostically significant.[222,225]

The classification of pure mucinous carcinoma as a vari-

ant of duct carcinoma is supported by finding an intraductal component in a substantial proportion of cases. The intraductal histologic pattern tends to be complementary to the growth pattern in the invasive tumor. Hence, mucinous carcinoma with a festooned or papillary structure usually derives from papillary, micropapillary, or cribriform intraductal carcinoma. Comedocarcinoma is more commonly associated with invasive mucinous carcinomas in which tumor cells form sheets and broad trabeculae in the mucinous secretion. Intracytoplasmic mucin secretion and signet-ring cells may be found in cells that form the intraductal component of mucinous carcinoma.

The differential diagnosis of mucinous carcinoma included certain forms of fibroadenoma and mucocele-like tumors. Histologic sections of fibroadenomas with edematous, myxoid stroma may be mistaken for mucinous carcinoma, especially at the time of frozen section. Most mucocele-like tumors are benign lesions composed of mucin-filled, cystically dilated ducts.[226] Disruption of these cysts may lead to extravasation of mucin to create a pattern that resembles mucinous carcinoma. The intracystic and extruded mucin in benign mucocele-like tumors is devoid of glandular cells, and the lining epithelium exhibits little or no hyperplasia. Few mucocele-like tumors feature atypical epithelial hyperplasia. In some cases, there are transitions to intraductal carcinoma and fully developed mucinous carcinoma.[227,228]

The diagnosis of mucinous carcinoma can be considered in material obtained by aspiration biopsy because the smears typically contain clusters of tumor cells and mucin.[229] However, some benign lesions, such as edematous fibroadenomas, some papillomas, and mucin-containing cysts also must be considered in this setting.

PROGNOSIS

Mucinous carcinoma is regarded as a prognostically favorable variant of duct carcinoma. With certain reservations, this conclusion seems warranted on the basis of reported data.[197–199,205,206,222,230] However, the disease occurs so infrequently that it has not been possible for one group of investigators to assemble enough cases to compare patients with mucinous and nonmucinous carcinoma when stratified by TNM stage. Because of differences in reporting among published series, combined data cannot be readily assembled.

Most studies of prognosis have compared patients treated for pure mucinous carcinoma with women who had mixed duct–mucinous carcinoma or ordinary invasive duct carcinoma. In these comparisons, pure mucinous carcinoma is associated with a lower frequency of metastases in axillary lymph nodes and fewer deaths resulting from breast carcinoma at 5 and 10 years, respectively, after treatment by mastectomy.[199–201,205,206,210,222,225,230] Tumor size and nodal status are the most important prognostic factors in patients with pure and with mixed mucinous carcinomas.

Systemic recurrences more than 10 years after mastectomy have been described by many investigators.[197–199,231] Geschickter[197] observed recurrences 6 to 18 years after diagnosis among 14 of 59 patients with pure colloid carcinoma, and he concluded that "a period of 5 to 10 years of freedom from symptoms following treatment does not necessarily indicate permanent cure." In a study of 41 patients with pure mucinous carcinoma followed for a mean of 16 years, 11 women (27%) developed recurrences and died of breast carcinoma, with 5 deaths occurring 12 years or more after diagnosis.[200] Most patients described in the literature were treated by radical or modified mastectomy. A few patients treated by simple or partial mastectomy also have done well, although follow-up was limited. Radiation treatment of a large unresected mucinous carcinoma that was diagnosed by incisional biopsy has been reported.[232] Ten patients with colloid carcinoma treated by primary radiation therapy have reportedly remained disease-free, with a median follow-up of 79 months.[233]

An unusual, fatal complication of mucinous carcinoma of the breast[234,235] and other organs is mucin embolism, which causes cerebral infarction.

Papillary Carcinoma

The problems in terminology associated with the diagnosis of papillary carcinoma have been reviewed by Fisher and coworkers[236] and Carter and associates.[237] Lesions classified as papillary carcinoma have included intraductal carcinoma with a papillary configuration involving multiple ducts, solitary papillary carcinomas that often have a cystic component, and invasive carcinomas with a papillary growth pattern. The WHO Histological Classification of Breast Tumors[238] defined papillary carcinoma as "a rare carcinoma whose invasive pattern is predominantly in the form of papillary structures. The same architecture is usually displayed in the metastases. Frequently foci of intraductal papillary growth are recognizable." Separately, the WHO classification states that "papillary carcinoma arising, and limited to a mammary cyst, is referred to as non-invasive intracystic carcinoma." Foote and Stewart,[162] who referred to intracystic carcinoma as "more distinctly a gross than a microscopic entity," noticed its papillary growth pattern and described the occurrence of invasive carcinoma in some cystic papillary carcinomas.

Thus, the term *papillary* usually is applied to carcinomas that form a mass in which there is predominantly a frond-forming growth pattern microscopically. Cyst formation is present in some papillary carcinomas, but this is not a requisite feature for diagnosis. Occasionally, such overgrowth of neoplastic epithelium occurs that frond formation is partially or entirely obliterated, leaving only the underlying branching structure of fibrovascular stroma. The compact epithelium in these areas is solid or cribriform. Such lesions are termed *solid papillary carcinomas*. Regardless of their structure, papillary carcinomas should be subclassified into noninvasive and invasive tumors. Overall, they constitute 1% to 2% of breast carcinomas in women.[236,237,239–241]

CLINICAL PRESENTATION

It has been reported that patients with papillary carcinoma tend to be older, on an average, than women with other forms of breast carcinoma.[236,237,239,240,242] In several series, the mean age at diagnosis for cystic papillary carcinoma ranges from 63 to 67 years. The mean age of patients with noncystic papillary carcinoma, reported in only one study, was 57 years. In a study of patients who were all 75 years of age or older, only 2 of 169 (1.2%) carcinomas were classified as papillary carcinomas, as defined in the foregoing discussion. Three other women had papillary intraductal carcinoma involving multiple ducts.[243] A disproportionate frequency of black or non-white patients[236] has been observed in some series of papillary carcinomas. However, this type of carcinoma occurs less frequently among Japanese women when compared with a predominantly white group of American patients.[244]

A duration of 1 year or more before diagnosis is commonly reported.[237,239,240,242] Nipple discharge occurs in 22% to 34% of patients,[237,239] and, although the frequency of central tumors is as high as 46%, Paget disease is rare. On clinical examination, a circumscribed, often lobulated tumor is palpated. The average clinical size is about 3 cm,[239] but cystic tumors that occupy the entire breast have been described.[240] Larger lesions may become fixed to and even invade the skin. Axillary lymph nodes tend to be enlarged and may be clinically suspicious, but even patients with invasive papillary carcinomas have a relatively low frequency of axillary nodal metastases.[236] Most papillary carcinomas are rich in estrogen receptors,[161] and they generally have a low growth rate.[245] Flow cytometric study has not been helpful for distinguishing between benign and malignant papillary tumors.[246] Mammography reveals a circumscribed, rounded tumor that may have a lobulated contour.[247,248] Invasion usually is manifested by loss of circumscription along part of the tumor margin.

GROSS PATHOLOGY

The tumors are frequently well circumscribed or may appear to be encapsulated, and are composed of soft to moderately firm fleshy tissue that is unusually tan, dark brown, or hemorrhagic. Friable, easily dislodged papillary fragments occur when the tumor has a cystic component. Large tumors that are entirely cystic are dramatic gross specimens, generally filled with partly clotted changed blood and fragments of papillary tumor. When the contents have been removed, much of the lining membrane has a smooth, glistening surface, but some papillary mural nodules remain attached to the surface. The cyst wall should be examined carefully for thickening, which may be indicative of invasive carcinoma.

MICROSCOPIC PATHOLOGY

The defining microscopic feature of these tumors is their frond-forming or papillary growth pattern (Fig. 13-13). This arrangement is found within the central portion of the tumor and also in ducts at the periphery and outside of the lesion, which are typically involved by intraductal extension of the lesion in many cases. When a papillary tumor is sufficiently low grade that it creates a diagnostic problem, the presence of these peripheral intraductal foci with papillary, cribriform, and comedocarcinoma patterns can be of considerable assistance. Intracystic papillary carcinomas are bounded microscopically by a zone of fibrosis, which constitutes part of the cyst wall.

Ultimately, the distinction between a papilloma and papillary carcinoma depends on the cytologic features of the cells and their growth pattern. It is not unusual to detect cribriform, micropapillary, solid, and comedocarcinoma foci within a papillary carcinoma. Supporting vascularized stroma may be found in benign and malignant papillary lesions. Invasive papillary carcinoma may retain the papillary pattern in part, but one or more other forms of growth, such as tubular, colloid, and ordinary infiltrating duct carcinoma, usually are also present. Coexistent foci of benign papilloma have been reportedly found in a few papillary carcinomas, and a review of the literature provides little evidence to indicate that benign papillomas

should be regarded as precancerous. Under some circumstances, papillary carcinomas probably develop from ordinary foci of intraductal carcinoma.

Papillary carcinoma cells may contain immunohistochemically demonstrable CEA.[249] This activity is absent in benign papillomas but may be found focally in papillomas that exhibit histologic evidence of transition to carcinoma.[250] Neurosecretory-type cytoplasmic granules are found in some papillary carcinomas, but not in papillomas.

Microscopic three-dimensional analysis of papillary tumors has revealed differences in the structural configuration of benign and malignant papillary duct tumors.[251,252] Ultrastructural differences exist between papillomas and papillary carcinomas,[253,254] but these reflect light microscopic findings. Myoepithelial cells are numerous in benign and hyperplastic papillary lesions and largely absent in carcinomas. Well-formed microvilli cover the luminal surfaces of epithelial cells in papillomas; these structures are usually short and poorly formed in papillary carcinomas. Electron microscopic study is not particularly useful in the differential diagnosis of borderline papillary lesions.

PROGNOSIS

Papillary carcinoma without invasion, whether cystic or not, may be regarded as a variant of intraductal carcinoma. In one study,[237] 11 of 29 patients with noninvasive tumors underwent mastectomy, including axillary dissection. None of the 11 had lymph node metastases. Sixteen were alive and disease-free after an average of 83 months and 13 died of other causes, with an average follow-up of 65 months. Another 11 patients were treated by excisional biopsy alone. Two developed ipsilateral invasive carcinomas, 3 and 6 years after diagnosis, respectively, and a third had recurrent noninvasive papillary carcinoma diagnosed after a 3-year interval. No disseminated carcinoma was found after treatment of the recurrences. Six patients treated only by excision were alive and disease-free after an average of 10 years (7 to 17 years). Two patients died of other causes without recurrence 6 and 11 years after treatment, respectively.

Fifteen patients with invasive papillary carcinoma also were studied.[237] All underwent mastectomy and axillary dissection. Two patients who had lymph node metastases died of breast carcinoma 5 and 7 years after diagnosis, respectively. Seven of the remaining 13 patients died of other causes without recurrence (mean follow-up, 42 months). Six were alive and disease-free for up to 232 months (mean, 94 months).

Fisher and others[236] reported on 35 women treated for invasive papillary carcinoma. Lymph node metastases were found in 32% of 22 patients whose treatment included axillary dissection. Two patients had four or more lymph nodes involved. At the time of the report, one patient had died of disease and two were alive with recurrence. Life-table analysis of the probability of disease-free survival showed an outcome similar to that of patients with tubular and mucinous carcinoma. Recurrences of invasive papil-

FIGURE 13-13 Papillary carcinoma in a 46-year-old woman who presented with a breast mass; aspiration yielded atypical epithelium. **A.** The lesion growing within a cystically dilated duct. The wall of the duct is at the lower margin of the picture. **B.** An enlarged view of papillary tumor fronds composed of orderly, cytologically low-grade cells without supporting stroma. Note the cribriform growth pattern within the tumor fronds.

lary carcinoma often become apparent more than 5 years after diagnosis of the primary tumor.

Other reports on papillary carcinoma do not distinguish between patients with noninvasive and invasive lesions. Haagensen[239] found that 20% of patients treated by radical mastectomy had axillary metastases, with four or more lymph nodes involved in 32% of positive node cases. Eight of 63 patients (13%) eligible for 10 years of follow-up were known to have died of disease. Included among the 63 were 9 patients initially treated by local excision. Two of the other seven who developed recurrences in the breast and underwent mastectomy died of metastases 13 and 16 years after initial treatment, respectively.

Studies of smaller groups of patients also fail to distinguish invasive from noninvasive papillary carcinomas. Czernobilsky[240] reported that 2 of 10 patients with intracystic carcinoma died of disease 9 and 10 years after simple mastectomy, respectively. Axillary metastases were found in specimens from two of eight patients treated with radical mastectomy. These eight patients remained disease-free with follow-up of 4 to 9 years. In a comparison group with noncystic papillary carcinomas, 25% of 23 patients had axillary metastases, the recurrence rate was 13.6%, and no deaths occurred from carcinoma.

Metaplastic Mammary Carcinoma

Carcinomas of the breast, arising as they do from glandular epithelium, are adenocarcinomas. In a small number of adenocarcinomas, the cancerous epithelium assumes a nonglandular appearance by a process termed *metaplasia*. The extent to which this phenomenon occurs varies from a few microscopic foci in an otherwise ordinary-appearing adenocarcinoma to complete replacement of the glandular elements. Metaplasia also may occur in the glandular epithelium of benign mammary tumors, such as fibroadenomas and papillomas, and in nonneoplastic breast epithelium (eg, ducts and cysts). The epithelium of many other glandular organs also is capable of metaplasia.

Two types of metaplastic mammary carcinoma are described: squamous and pseudosarcomatous. The former has been referred to as *homologous* because it retains an epithelial character, whereas the latter is termed *heterologous* because of its similarity to neoplasms of mesenchymal origin. The fact that squamous metaplasia may undergo further alteration to an undifferentiated spindle cell pseudosarcomatous pattern weakens the usefulness of this traditional distinction.[255]

The relative frequency of metaplastic carcinomas is difficult to ascertain because these neoplasms are not consistently described in routine pathologic reports. Small foci of squamous metaplasia may not be noticed in an otherwise typical mammary carcinoma. Some pathologists restrict the diagnosis for neoplasms that exhibit only pseudosarcomatous features, and others prefer alternative diagnostic terms, such as *carcinosarcoma* or *mixed tumor of the breast*. Squamous metaplasia occurs to some extent in about 2% of all mammary carcinomas, but it is a prominent feature in only a small fraction of these tumors. An exception to this is medullary carcinoma, 16% of which exhibit some squamous metaplasia.[38] Pseudosarcomatous metaplasia, which typically features the appearance of bone, cartilage, or undifferentiated spindle cell elements, generates greater interest and, therefore, this phenomenon is usually noted in the diagnosis. Metaplastic carcinomas constitute fewer than 1% of breast carcinomas. Metaplastic carcinomas tend to have low levels of estrogen receptors.[256,257]

The mechanism by which metaplasia occurs is not well understood. Early concepts that pseudosarcomatous metaplasia constitutes an alteration of the stroma induced by the adenocarcinoma have largely been abandoned, and it is not widely held that the process evolves from altered epithelial cells. The strongest support for the current interpretation comes from electron microscopic study.[255,258–261]

Uncertainty about the histogenesis of these carcinomas is reflected in confusing diagnostic terminology.[262] *Carcinosarcoma* is appropriate for malignant neoplasms that can be shown to contain distinct carcinomatous and sarcomatous components derived separately from epithelial and mesenchymal tissues, as, for example, carcinoma arising in a malignant cystosarcoma phyllodes with sarcomatous stroma. The term *mixed tumor* is not satisfactory because it creates confusion with neoplasms that more commonly develop in salivary glands than in the breast.

CLINICAL PRESENTATION

The initial symptom is almost always a mass. Secondary manifestations, such as fixation to the skin or underlying tissues, occur and skin ulcerations have been reported with large lesions. The duration of symptoms rarely exceeds a few months.[263] The age distribution and mean age at diagnosis correspond closely to breast carcinoma in general. Metaplastic carcinoma is not associated with bilaterality. Bone formation within the tumor may result in calcifications detectable by mammography, but not enough data are available to indicate a radiologic appearance specific for this type of carcinoma.

GROSS PATHOLOGY

Tumors ranging in size from less than 1 cm to more than 10 cm have been reported.[264–266,268] The size distribution approximates that of mammary carcinoma, with a mean size of 2 to 3 cm in the reported series. Gross appearance varies with the constituent parts, but most examples are described as hard, nodular, and well circumscribed. Cystic degeneration is common when there is extensive squamous metaplasia.[257,263]

MICROSCOPIC PATHOLOGY

Squamous metaplasia has been observed in many of the standard histologic variants of breast carcinoma (Fig. 13-14). In these cases, the microscopic description is determined by the basic configuration of the tumor (eg, medullary carcinoma with squamous metaplasia, or infiltrating duct carcinoma with squamous metaplasia). Metaplastic epithelium may form a mature, keratinizing tissue with keratohyaline granules. Various gradations of less-differentiated epithelium usually occur in the same specimen with transitions to a spindle cell pseudosarcomatous appearance commonly

FIGURE 13-14 Squamous metaplasia in invasive duct carcinoma that is manifested by three solid nodules of keratin pearl formation. Also evident are three glandular spaces containing mucinous secretion, which are indicative of the underlying adenocarcinoma. The patient is a 63-year-old woman who presented with a 2-cm tumor.

present.[255] Reports have drawn attention to a spindle cell variant of squamous metaplastic carcinoma, which is composed largely of less well-differentiated spindle cell elements and, therefore, may be mistaken for a sarcoma. The presence of squamous areas detectable through sampling, as well as epithelial features detected by electron microscopic and immunohistochemical study can be used to distinguish these lesions from sarcomas.[255,261]

Overt pseudosarcomatous differentiation is manifested by areas of cartilage or bone formation that may appear benign or malignant histologically (Fig. 13-15). Undifferentiated pseudosarcomatous areas with spindle or round cell features may coexist with osteocartilaginous metaplasia, or they may be the only metaplastic element. Matrix-producing carcinoma is a variant of heterologous metaplastic carcinoma in which osseous and cartilaginous elements seem to arise directly from adenocarcinoma, without associated spindle and giant cell components.[256] Angiosarcomatous and myosarcomatous metaplasia are rarely detectable. Infiltrating duct carcinomas that develop pseudosarcomatous metaplasia tend to be poorly differentiated, but metaplasia can occur in well-differentiated tumors. Metastases resulting from a metaplastic carcinoma may also have metaplastic foci, usually with the same patterns as the primary tumor, but more often they are entirely composed of adenocarcinoma.

Low-grade adenosquamous carcinoma,[267] an unusual variant of metaplastic carcinoma, tends to be a relatively small lesion, averaging 2.3 cm. These infiltrative lesions are composed of glandular elements with variable amounts of squamous differentiation. The growth pattern may have syringomatous features. Squamous cysts and foci of osteocartilaginous metaplasia are only rarely present.

PROGNOSIS

A proper assessment of prognosis requires sufficient cases to consider tumor size; histologic type; grade; nodal status; the type, amount, and differentiation of the metaplastic

FIGURE 13-15 Sarcomatous metaplasia in invasive duct carcinoma forming cartilage on the right and osteoid with osteoclasts on the left. A zone of undifferentiated spindle cell growth separates the two areas. At mastectomy, this 37-year-old patient had a 6-cm tumor and metastases in four axillary lymph nodes.

component; and the form of treatment. No published series has been large enough to evaluate these factors independently, and many reports do not provide the necessary data. Metaplasia does not confer a favorable prognosis, despite the relatively high frequency of stage I cases in most series. Pseudosarcomatous metaplasia probably has an unfavorable impact on outcome, especially in poorly differentiated carcinomas. Squamous metaplasia seems to have less effect prognostically, except for lesions with an extensive spindle cell component, which are especially aggressive.

Specific data on prognosis are based almost entirely on patients treated by mastectomy. In a study of 26 women with pseudosarcomatous metaplasia, overall survival was 44%, with an estimated 5-year survival for TNM stages I, II, and III of 56%, 26%, and 18%, respectively.[268] Axillary nodal metastases were detected in 25% of the patients. Responsiveness of metaplastic carcinoma to radiation and chemotherapy has not been determined. The 5-year disease-free survival in two other studies of patients with pseudosarcomatous metaplasia was 38%[264] and 40%.[263] Among women with carcinomas that exhibited squamous metaplasia, often with a spindle cell component, disease-free survival rates, generally for 5 years or longer have been 65%,[264] 63%,[257] and 50%.[263]

In one study,[267] four of eight women with low-grade adenosquamous carcinoma, who were initially treated by excisional biopsy, developed a recurrence in the breast requiring mastectomy 1 to 3.5 years later. None of these patients has had axillary lymph node or systemic metastases.

Apocrine Carcinoma

The apocrine glands are normal cutaneous appendages that are concentrated in the skin of the axilla, groin, anogenital region, and other sites. Histologically, the cells that form these glands have abundant pink, finely granular cytoplasm. At the luminal surface, the apical cytoplasm forms tufts or blebs characteristic of merocrine secretion. Nuclei, typically round with a small punctate nucleolus, are located near the base of the cell. Electron microscopic study has demonstrated the presence of cytoplasmic secretory granules and abundant mitochondria in apocrine cells.[269]

A variety of benign proliferative breast lesions may contain cells that are cytologically identical with those of the apocrine glands. The phenomenon by which duct or lobular epithelial cells undergo this structural alteration is referred to as apocrine metaplasia. Apocrine metaplasia occurs most often in the lining of cysts and in papillary duct hyperplasia, but it may be encountered in fibroadenomas, sclerosing adenosis, and in other benign lesions. Histochemical and ultrastructural studies have consistently shown that the cells of apocrine metaplasia in the breast have many characteristics in common with the cells of normal cutaneous apocrine glands.[269–272] Because of the pink, variably granular or vacuolated cytoplasm of cells in apocrine metaplasia, they also have been referred to as oncocytes or pale cells.

Apocrine metaplasia epithelium exhibits a spectrum of cytologic appearances that range from cells histologically identical with normal apocrine glands to cells exhibiting extreme cytologic atypia. Analysis of the DNA content of nuclei in apocrine metaplasia by Izuo and others[273] has shown that tetraploid cells become significantly more numerous with increasing atypia. The authors described one patient with aneuploid apocrine metaplasia who subsequently proved to have mammary carcinoma.

The precancerous significance of apocrine metaplasia has not been determined. Foote and Stewart[274] compared the distribution of benign proliferative changes in the breasts of women with and without carcinoma and, after finding no difference in the distribution of apocrine metaplasia, concluded that it was not a precancerous change. Page and associates[275,276] reported an association between papillary apocrine metaplasia in a benign breast biopsy specimen and an increased risk for subsequent carcinoma in one study,[275] but later concluded that apocrine metaplasia did not represent a reliable risk indicator.[276]

Apocrine differentiation is sufficiently conspicuous in 1% to 4% of carcinomas to qualify for the diagnosis of apocrine carcinoma. In some of these cases, the noncancerous breast contains areas of apocrine metaplasia that may exhibit varying degrees of atypia, but it is often difficult to demonstrate transitions from hyperplasia with apocrine metaplasia to carcinoma. However, intraductal apocrine carcinoma is a histologically distinct in situ variant of duct carcinoma that may exist alone or in conjunction with invasive apocrine carcinoma.[277] Electron microscopic study has demonstrated that the cells of apocrine carcinomas have many ultrastructural features in common with the cells found in apocrine metaplasia and the apocrine glands.[278,279]

The clinical features of apocrine carcinoma do not differ appreciably from conventional forms of duct carcinoma. The reported age at diagnosis ranges from 19 to 86 years with a slight predilection toward postmenopausal women.

Invasive tumors usually present as a mass, whereas intraductal apocrine carcinoma, which tends to develop calcifications, is increasingly detected by mammography.[280] The frequency of bilaterality is not exceptional, and both breasts rarely harbor apocrine carcinoma.

Apocrine carcinoma generally has a ductal growth pattern, but rarely can cells with this appearance be found in lobular carcinoma in situ.[281] Apocrine duct carcinoma tends to involve lobular epithelium by direct intraepithelial extension. Medullary[282] and tubular carcinomas[280] with apocrine features have been reported. Apocrine carcinoma has been described arising in the male breast.[283,284] Apocrine carcinoma was often classified under the heading of *sweat gland carcinoma of the breast*.[285,286] Although this term occasionally is still applied to breast carcinomas,[287] it is unsatisfactory because sweat gland carcinoma of the skin is a morphologically heterogeneous disease in which only a few tumors resemble mammary apocrine carcinoma.

Six examples of apocrine carcinoma studied by one group of investigators had low levels of estrogen and progesterone receptor protein,[278] but others have found that tumors are positive for estrogen or progesterone receptors.[281] In vitro studies have demonstrated enhanced metabolism of testosterone precursors by apocrine carcinomas when compared with other types of carcinoma.[288] This observation has not been correlated with levels of androgen receptors or clinical response to hormonal treatment, but is of considerable interest because the growth of cutaneous apocrine glands is stimulated by androgens[289] and some androgen metabolites are found concentrated in axillary secretions.[290] Apocrine carcinomas are strongly immunoreactive for gross cystic disease fluid protein-15.[291]

Prognostic data from many reports describing "sweat gland" carcinoma are difficult to interpret because of uncertainty about how many of the lesions were apocrine carcinomas. Frable and Kay[292] compared 18 apocrine carcinoma patients with 34 controls matched for clinicopathologic prognostic characteristics and observed no significant difference in outcome between the two groups. Similar results were obtained by d'Amore and colleagues[293] and Abati and coworkers,[280] who also compared matched series of patients with apocrine and nonapocrine carcinoma. Apocrine features were present in 2.2% of carcinoma studied by Fisher and associates[4]; this finding was not significantly correlated with prognosis. Data about pure apocrine carcinoma were not presented in their report.

Apocrine intraductal carcinoma seems to have the same clinical course as other forms of intraductal carcinoma. Abati and coworkers[280] studied 55 patients, including 33 (60%) treated by mastectomy and 22 (40%) whose surgery was limited to excisional biopsy. Breast recurrences were found in 3 of 20 (15%) who had only excisional surgery, but not in the 2 patients treated by excision and radiation. One patient treated by mastectomy had axillary metastases and later died of disease. All other patients with apocrine intraductal carcinoma remained disease-free at last follow-up, including those who required mastectomy for breast recurrence after lumpectomy.

Adenoid Cystic Carcinoma

Adenoid cystic carcinoma constitutes less than 0.1% of mammary carcinomas. Disproportionate interest in this type of carcinoma stems from its favorable prognosis and distinctive histopathologic appearance, identical with that of comparable tumors that originate in salivary glands. Adenoid cystic carcinoma arising in both sites is prone to microscopic invasion of perineural spaces.

Cylindroma, a term used synonymously with adenoid cystic carcinoma, was apparently introduced by Billroth to describe his concept that the tumor is composed of entwined cylinders of hyaline stroma and cylinders of tumor cells. Ewing[294] referred to adenoid cystic carcinoma of the salivary glands, and a similar term was first used with reference to mammary tumors by Geschickter[295] in 1945, when he described four breast lesions as adenocystic basal cell cancer. Foote and Stewart[162] referred to three examples of mammary adenoid cystic carcinoma in 1946. Reports of single cases were published in the succeeding two decades, until 1966 when Galloway and colleagues[296] summarized data on 9 new cases from the Mayo Clinic and 12 others previously reported.

CLINICAL PRESENTATION

The age distribution parallels that generally observed in breast cancer with cases diagnosed between 25 and 80 years.[296–306] The mean age at diagnosis in studies with five or more cases varied from 50 to 63 years. Most patients are women, but this type of carcinoma has been described in the male breast.[298,299] There does not seem to be a predilection for either breast, and the disease is not associated with bilaterality. However, carcinoma may develop in the opposite breast[300,301] or, rarely, elsewhere in the same breast.[302]

The presenting symptom is a tumor that is sometimes painful or tender. Large or superficial lesions can exhibit changes in the overlaying skin, such as ulceration, peau d'orange, or dimpling. Although any part of the breast may be affected, adenoid cystic carcinoma occurs with disproportionately high frequency in the central or subareolar region not associated with nipple discharge. Most patients report the tumor to have been present for days or weeks before seeking medical attention, but intervals of 18 months to 15 years have been described in a number of patients.[296,297] Most of the tumors analyzed have tested negative for estrogen and progesterone receptors.[303,306,307] One lesion was estrogen- and progesterone-positive, and another was positive for progesterone and negative for estrogen receptors.[306]

GROSS PATHOLOGY

Reported examples range in size from 2 mm to 12 cm, with most between 1 and 3 cm.[296,297,300,304] The gray to pale yellow cut surface reveals a neoplasm with well-defined margins that may appear circumscribed. Focal cystic areas can occur in tumors under 5 cm in diameter; larger lesions tend to undergo cystic degeneration.[296,305,306]

MICROSCOPIC PATHOLOGY

Figure 13-16 illustrates that characteristic microscopic appearance of adenoid cystic carcinoma, featuring a mixture of glandular (adenoid component) and stromal or basement membrane material (cystic, pseudoglandular, or cylindromatous component). Within a given tumor, substantial heterogeneity can be found in the organization of these elements. Some microscopic fields consist entirely of the adenoid elements, thereby bearing a close resemblance to cribriform carcinoma. Nearly half of the examples of adenoid cystic carcinoma reviewed in one study[308] proved to be misclassified, usually because of failure to distinguish accurately between cribriform and adenoid cystic carcinoma. Other portions of the lesion may be highly endowed with the stromal material and lacking in glandular elements. Such areas can be misinterpreted as scirrhous carcinoma. Because of this diversity, adenoid cystic carcinoma may not be recognizable in a small-needle biopsy sample unless the typical constellation of features is represented. Adenoid cystic carcinoma can be diagnosed in a needle aspiration smear when globules of cylindromatous material and adenoid gland clusters are present.[309–311]

Clusters of tumor cells at the invasive edges of adenoid cystic carcinoma tend to shrink and separate for the surrounding stroma. This creates an appearance that simulates the pattern of tumor invasion of lymphatics. True lymphatic invasion is extremely uncommon in adenoid cystic carcinoma.

Adenoid cystic carcinomas have been subdivided into three histologic grades determined by the proportion of solid growth within the lesion.[312] Tumors with no solid component were classified as low grade (I), those less than 30% solid as intermediate (II) and those with more than 30% solid areas as high grade (III). High-grade tumors were larger and more likely to recur locally than low-grade lesions. The only tumor to metastasize was high grade in the series reported by Rosen and coworkers.[306] In retrospect, the literature has insufficient documentation to grade most of the other adenoid cystic carcinomas that have metastasized.[306]

It has been claimed that electron microscopic study and mucin histochemical examination can be helpful in distinguishing between true glandular lumens and the cylindromatous element.[298,300,302,303,313] However, electron microscopic study may be misleading if the cylindromatous components is absent in the small sample studied from an otherwise typical adenoid cystic carcinoma. With an adequate number of histologic sections of an excised lesion, it is rarely necessary to employ histochemical studies to diagnose adenoid cystic carcinoma. The electron microscopic features of adenoid cystic carcinoma of the salivary glands and breast are identical.[314]

The cylindromatous element in adenoid cystic carcinoma contains noncollagenous glycoproteins associated with basal lamina, including laminin and fibronectin[315] and type IV collagen.[307] Xenographic transplants of adenoid cystic carcinoma in nude mice produce laminin and type IV collagen,[316] and similar results have been obtained with cultured tumor cells.[317]

Collagenous spherulosis is a microscopic benign proliferative duct lesion that has adenoid cystic features.[306,318] The hyperplastic duct epithelium forms glands, and it also contains round, acellular deposits of basement membrane–like material.[319,320] Thus far, no evidence supports that

FIGURE 13-16 Adenoid cystic carcinoma. **A.** The tumor consists of circumscribed masses of tumor cells. Because much of the lesion may have this growth pattern, it can be difficult to identify an intraductal component. In the upper central part of the picture, the adenoid structure of the lesion resembles cribriform, intraductal carcinoma. In the lower half, a cylindromatous component is more prominent. **B.** High-power view showing cylindromatous areas on the left, where tumor cells surround cords of basement membrane material, and adenoid pattern on the right, where tumor cells encircle round to oval glandular spaces containing mucin.

collagenous spherulosis is a precancerous process. It is found randomly in breast biopsy specimens with other benign proliferative lesions, or occasionally, coincidentally as a separate process in breast tissue from a patient with various types of carcinoma. It has not been associated with adenoid cystic carcinoma.

PROGNOSIS

With few exceptions, published data on prognosis relate to patients treated by modified or standard radical mastectomy. Axillary metastases have been described in three cases.[312,321,322] Recurrence has been reported in the breast more than 20 years[323] after treatment by local excision alone,[298,300,304,324] and chest wall recurrence has occurred after simple mastectomy.[325] Recurrences in the breast have been controlled by surgery. All patients with distant metastases have had pulmonary involvement with intervals of 6[326] to 12 years until the appearance of lung lesions.[327,328] Most patients with systemic metastases had negative lymph nodes.[300,311,313,324,326] Axillary nodal metastases were reportedly present at mastectomy in three cases,[312,321,322] and these patients developed pulmonary metastases. Metastases in bone,[312] the liver,[312] the brain,[314,327] and kidney[328] have been reported.

Squamous Carcinoma

To be regarded as an example of this extremely uncommon neoplasm, a mammary carcinoma must be composed entirely of squamous carcinoma. Because keratinizing epithelium is not a normal constituent of breast glandular tissue, the presence of squamous carcinoma in this organ must be regarded as a form of metaplasia. Pure squamous carcinoma of the breast is considered to be a pathologic entity separate from the group of metaplastic carcinomas in which adenocarcinoma is found giving rise to squamous or sarcomatous metaplasia. However, articles devoted to the subject of metaplastic carcinoma sometimes include lesions that are entirely squamous.[257]

The histogenesis of squamous carcinoma of the breast remains unexplained. It is likely that two pathways exist for these tumors to arise. Some lesions represent an extreme variant of metaplastic carcinoma. In these tumors, a residual component of the original adenocarcinoma from which the squamous carcinoma arose may be overlooked because of limited sampling, or it may have been destroyed by growth of the squamous component.

Metaplastic change to histologically benign squamous epithelium is probably a precursor to squamous carcinoma in some cases. Squamous metaplasia has been observed in the glandular epithelium of the breast associated with benign conditions such as fibroadenomas,[329] benign cystosarcoma phyllodes, papillomas,[330] and gynecomastia.[331] Benign squamous metaplasia occasionally is found in the epithelium of hyperplastic mammary ducts, in the lining of cysts in ordinary proliferative breast lesions (fibrocystic disease), and in extensive duct hyperplasia and papillo-

matosis.[332] It has been suggested that cyclic adenine nucleotide may be the primary mediator of benign squamous metaplasia in human breast epithelium. Tissues from patients who were in the early part of the menstrual cycle at the time of biopsy were less susceptible to the induction of squamous metaplasia than those obtained in the latter third of the cycle, an observation suggesting that progesterone or estrogen may promote the process.[333]

CLINICAL PRESENTATION

The clinical features of squamous carcinoma of the breast are not distinctive. The age distribution, 31 to 83 years, encompasses much of the range of breast carcinoma.[334,335] The average age in one review of 20 cases was 57 years, and half of the patients were 60 years or older.[334]

Two thirds of primary squamous carcinomas occur in the left breast.[335] Large tumors may be fixed to the skin or deep structures, and skin ulceration can occur. When this occurs, the distinction between a tumor originating from the overlying skin and squamous carcinoma arising in the breast may be difficult.[336] No consistent mammographic features have been described.[337,338] Calcification in the squamous tissue may be seen on radiographs. These tumors are estrogen receptor–negative.[334,339]

GROSS PATHOLOGY

Squamous carcinomas vary from 1 cm to more than 10 cm in diameter, but tend to be relatively larger than other forms of breast carcinoma. About half of reported cases were 5 cm or more in diameter. Cystic degeneration is common, especially in tumors larger than 2 cm. Hemorrhage and accumulated necrotic squamous debris fill the cavity. When keratinizing epithelium predominates, the tumor tissue will be relatively soft and granular. Extensive spindle cell metaplasia results in a firm to hard lesion.

MICROSCOPIC PATHOLOGY

The diagnosis of primary squamous carcinoma of the breast can be made only after excluding metastasis from an extramammary squamous carcinoma.[334] Metastatic squamous carcinoma in the breast is reported to have originated in the lung, uterine cervix, esophagus, urinary bladder, and other sites. Generally, the existence of an extramammary primary is known clinically. Unfortunately, this information may not be provided to the pathologist if the physician and surgeon do not consider a metastatic lesion when evaluating a patient with a breast tumor.

Squamous carcinoma of the breast is indistinguishable by light microscopic study from similar carcinomas that arise in numerous other sites. Many mammary squamous carcinomas are histologically well differentiated and produce substantial keratin. Ultrastructural studies have confirmed the squamous character of the tissue,[340] but intracellular canaliculi observed in some cells suggest that glandular features may persist in these tumors.[339] Immunohistochemical markers for intracellular keratin are strongly reactive with squamous mammary carcinoma. Degenerative changes with prominent cytoplasmic vacuolization characterize an unusual acantholytic variant of squamous carcinoma.[341]

Transformation from a squamous epithelial pattern to spindle cell pseudosarcomatous growth occurs, to some extent, in most squamous carcinomas of the breast. This phenomenon, which is also found in other sites,[342] may produce a tumor largely composed of the spindle cell component referred to as spindle cell carcinoma.[255,343] Extreme examples of this process are tumors virtually indistinguishable from a fibrosarcoma. Extensive sampling of the tumor, immunohistochemical studies, and electron microscopic examination may be necessary to determine that the tumor is a carcinoma. A needle or incisional biopsy of such a lesion is likely to be interpreted as sarcoma.

PROGNOSIS

Data describing the treatment and follow-up of these patients are variable or incomplete in reported cases. Most patients have been treated by mastectomy, usually with an axillary dissection. Postoperative radiation therapy and chemotherapy were given in some cases. Among 15 women without axillary lymph node metastases, 8 were alive and free of disease with follow-up ranging from 1 to 12 years, and 2 died of other causes 7 to 8 years after treatment. Five women who had negative axillary lymph nodes died of metastatic carcinoma 4 to 30 months after diagnosis. One patient with axillary lymph node metastases died 17 months after treatment, whereas two others were alive and well with 16 months and 6 years of follow-up, respectively. Local recurrence has been reported. Metastases usually involve bones and the lungs. The prognosis for patients with mammary squamous carcinoma is not markedly different from that of women with duct carcinoma of comparable stage.[344,345] It has been suggested that lesions exhibiting prominent spindle cell and acantholytic features may have a less favorable clinical course.[339,343,346]

Mammary Carcinoma With Osteoclast-Like Giant Cells

Carcinomas containing osteoclast-like multinucleated giant cells have been described in the pancreas, thyroid, lung, and breast. Fewer than 100 examples of such breast carcinomas have been reported. Although individual cases had been described previously,[347] it was not until 1979 that the first series was reported.[348] The giant cells are found within the stroma of the tumor, often associated with hemorrhage, lymphocytic reaction, and increased vascularity.[348] Electron microscopic and immunohistochemical studies have shown that the giant cells have histiocytic properties and are derived from stroma associated with the tumor.[347,349,350,351]

Patients with this type of carcinoma range in age from 32 to 84 years. The average age of patients included in

three reviews[348,350,351] was 53 years. Most of the tumors occur in the upper outer quadrant, but the lesion has been found in all quadrants. Mammographically, the well-circumscribed contour observed in many cases may suggest a benign lesion such as a cyst or fibroadenoma.[351]

The excised tumor usually has a striking, characteristic gross appearance when bisected. The dark brown or red-brown tumor tissue tends to bulge above the surrounding breast parenchyma, from which it is usually separated by a well-defined margin. On gross inspection, the lesion may suggest heavily pigmented metastatic melanoma, but it tends to be brown rather than black. The reported diameter in 22 cases ranged from 0.5 to 10 cm (average, 3.2 cm). Nine tumors were 2.0 cm or less in diameter.

Microscopically, most of these lesions are invasive duct carcinomas (Fig. 13-17). Uncommon examples of infiltrating lobular,[348] papillary,[348] mucinous,[350] tubular,[352] and metaplastic[352,353] carcinomas with osteoclast-like giant cells have been reported. The giant cells characteristically are closely approximated to the periphery of carcinomatous glands and may be found in the glandular lumens. Extravascular erythrocytes, hemosiderin, and lymphocytes are present in the surrounding highly vascular stroma. Erythrophagocytosis by the giant cells is uncommon. Inconspicuous metaplastic foci with spindle cells and squamous or osseous features have been described in a few cases.[352] The cytologic features of mammary carcinoma with osteoclast-like giant cells have been described.[354,355]

Osteoclast-like multinucleated giant cells have been observed within intralymphatic tumor emboli (Fig. 13-18) in regional lymph node metastases and in distant metastases, but not all metastatic foci contain these giant cells. Absence of factor VIII activity from giant cells suggests they are not of endothelial origin.[350] It has been postulated that one or more substances produced by the neoplastic

FIGURE 13-17 Infiltrating lobular carcinoma with osteoclast-like giant cells featuring multinucleated cells distributed among infiltrating small carcinoma cells. The patient was a 43-year-old woman with a 3.5-cm tumor present for 5 months. At mastectomy, a grossly circumscribed, reddish, firm lesion was found. There were no lymph node metastases. The patient died of metastatic disease years later.

FIGURE 13-18 Intralymphatic tumor embolus with osteoclast-like giant cells. This remarkable phenomenon indicates that histologically benign cells of stromal origin may be transported with metastasizing tumor cells.

cells in these tumors induces the formation of the giant cells and that same process is linked to the accompanying vascularity and hemorrhage.

Axillary lymph node metastases occur in about a third of cases. Follow-up is usually relatively short because this type of carcinoma has not been widely recognized. Local recurrence[351] and systemic metastases to the eye, liver, and other organs have been described.[348] Nearly two thirds of patients have been reported to be alive and well, but few patients have been followed for 5 years or longer.[352] Although most of these tumors have had low levels of estrogen receptor, many have remarkably high levels of progesterone receptors.[351,356]

Secretory Carcinoma

Breast carcinoma is an extraordinarily uncommon malignant tumor in children. Many of the various histologic types found in adults also have been described in children.[357] As one of the least common forms of mammary carcinoma, secretory or juvenile carcinoma is noteworthy for a tendency to occur relatively more frequently, but not exclusively, in children. Accordingly, the term *secretory* is preferable to *juvenile* in describing this tumor because its microscopic appearance is identical in children and adults. This is a morphologically distinctive tumor with a low-grade clinical behavior.

The first full description of secretory carcinoma was published in 1966 by McDivitt and Stewart[358] in a report based on seven patients who ranged in age from 3 to 15 years (average, 9 years). In 1972, Oberman and Stephens[359] referred to secretory carcinoma diagnosed in two women, 25 and 56 years of age, respectively, and Oberman[360] later described four additional instances in adult women 22 to

73 years old. A review of the experience at the Armed Forces Institute of Pathology yielded 19 patients described in a 1980 report.[361] Their median age was 25 years (range, 9 to 69 years) and 6 were 30 years of age or older. One patient was a 9-year-old boy. Additional adult cases have been described,[362–368] and there are reports of single cases in children.[368–371] A man[366] is reported to have developed regional and systemic recurrences 20 years after a simple mastectomy and to have died of disease shortly thereafter.

Secretory carcinoma does not occur with particular frequency in any part of the breast. A few lesions have been subareolar, and patients with such lesions may present with nipple discharge. Usually, the primary symptom is a painless mass that may be present for years before biopsy.[359] No clinical evidence of an associated hormonal abnormality has been reported. The development of these tumors has not been related to pregnancy or lactation in children, most of whom have been nulliparous. The excised tumor appears circumscribed or discrete in most cases, but infiltrative margins have been described. Color varies from white to gray or yellow to tan. Most tumors have been under 3 cm in diameter, but lesions up to 12 cm have been reported.

Microscopically, the tumor typically exhibits papillary and solid areas of growth. It is composed of cells with abundant pale to clear or amphophilic cytoplasm and small round, cytologically low-grade nuclei (Fig. 13-19). Abundant secretion that is positive with periodic acid–Schiff and mucin stains is found within tumor cells and glandular spaces formed by the tumor cells. Rarely, portions of the lesion may have granular eosinophilic cytoplasm and a nuclear cytologic appearance that suggests apocrine carcinoma. In most cases, the periphery exhibits a pushing or circumscribed margin microscopically, but invasive foci are not unusual. Intraductal carcinoma, generally with a secretory appearance, can be found within or at the pe-

FIGURE 13-19 Secretory carcinoma biopsy specimen, from the breast of an elderly woman, that exhibits a typical lobulated growth pattern composed of expanded ducts filled with small glands that contain secretion.

riphery of some tumors. Diagnosis of secretory carcinoma by aspiration cytologic study has been reported.[372]

Coexistence of secretory carcinoma with juvenile papillomatosis has been reported in two cases.[373] In one patient, secretory carcinoma appeared to arise from juvenile papillomatosis in the same breast. The other patients had juvenile papillomatosis in one breast and secretory carcinoma in the other breast.

The prognosis for these patients is favorable. Although most children and adults have been treated by mastectomy, a few have been free of disease 7 to 15 years after excisional biopsy.[358,359] Axillary metastases have been described,[361,362,366,368,369,370] but probably occur in no more than 20% of the cases and rarely involve more than three lymph nodes. About 50% the patients with positive lymph nodes have been older than 20 years of age. Recurrence in the breast after lumpectomy has been described by several authors,[358,359,361,365–367,369] and, in one case, axillary metastases were first manifest at the time of a local recurrence 7 years after local excision of the primary from a patient 19 years of age. Another patient developed a recurrence in the breast 21 years after initial excision, which was performed at 4 years of age.[356] Patients with axillary metastases have been reported to be well as long as 6 years after primary therapy. One patient, who had eight positive lymph nodes, developed distant metastases and died less than a year after diagnosis.[361]

Wide local excision is the preferred initial treatment in children found to have secretory carcinoma. Axillary dissection is indicated if clinical examination suggests nodal involvement. Long-term follow-up is imperative because of the indolent nature of the disease and the risk for late recurrence. In adult patients, local excision also may be appropriate, and this should be combined with dissection of the lower axillary lymph nodes. Adult patients treated by lumpectomy usually have not had postoperative radiation therapy,[366,367] and insufficient information exists to determine whether this would reduce the risk of local recurrence. For patients with large tumors or with unsatisfactory margins, mastectomy should be considered.

Lipid-Rich Carcinoma

Only a few examples of this rare variant of infiltrating duct carcinoma have been described.[374–377] It is composed of cells that contain abundant lipid, which, when processed for histologic study, is extracted, leaving clear, vacuolated cytoplasm. The tumor cells have been described as having small, round uniform nuclei, and, therefore, resemble the appearance of clear cell renal carcinoma. The presence of lipid can be demonstrated in frozen sections of fresh tissue, by electron microscopic study, or in tissue prepared by special processes that preserve cytoplasmic lipids. The disease was first described by Aboumrad and others[374] in a case report. Subsequently, these authors found one other example among 100 breast carcinomas and estimated the frequency of lipid-rich carcinoma to be 1%.

Ramos and Taylor[375] described 13 cases whom they

believed had the characteristic pattern of lipid-rich carcinoma, as demonstrated in routine histologic sections. However, they were able to demonstrate lipid in only four cases, which were available as unfixed specimens. The other nine were identified retrospectively among 900 cases on the basis of histologic pattern alone. Eleven of the 12 patients treated by radical mastectomy had axillary lymph node metastases. Follow-up revealed six patients dead of metastatic disease and two alive with recurrence. The remainder were alive and disease-free, with most having a follow-up shorter than 2 years.

Tsubura and colleagues[376] described an unusual variant of lipid-secreting carcinoma in patients who were treated with neuroleptic drugs for psychiatric disorders. Studies of more patients are required to determine if this is a clinically distinctive type of carcinoma.

Cystic Hypersecretory Carcinoma

First described in 1984,[378] cystic hypersecretory carcinoma is an uncommon multicystic variant of duct carcinoma of the breast. The patients, who have been 34 to 79 years old (mean, 56 years) have a mass at least 1 cm in diameter, with the largest tumor being 10 cm. There are no known specific clinical or epidemiologic features associated with this type of carcinoma.[378,379] Mammography in one case revealed a prominent ductal pattern and irregular density.[380] When examined grossly, the tumors were composed of numerous cysts containing viscid secretion that has been described variously as thyroid-like, colloid-like, and gelatinous.

Microscopic examination reveals dilated ducts and cysts containing homogeneous, eosinophilic material resembling thyroid colloid (Fig. 13-20). Histochemical study of the secretion yielded positive reactions for mucin, CEA,

FIGURE 13-20 Cystic hypersecretory carcinoma, characterized by cystically dilated ducts filled with homogeneous eosinophilic secretion and an intervening duct with micropapillary intraductal carcinoma.

and α-lactalbumin. It is uniformly negative for thyroglobulin. Many cysts are lined by flat, inconspicuous epithelial cells, but transitions to a micropapillary intraductal carcinoma growth pattern are found in the tumor. Generally, the best evidence of intraductal carcinoma occurs in nondilated ducts in the stroma between cysts, rather than in the cysts themselves. When biopsy, rather than excision, is performed on such a tumor, the sample obtained may consist largely of cysts, with few diagnostic foci of intraductal carcinoma. When these biopsy specimens have been diagnosed in the past as cystic disease, failure to excise the remainder of the tumor has been followed by continued growth of the lesion. The cytologic features of cystic hypersecretory carcinoma have been described.[380]

Invasive carcinoma that originated in cystic hypersecretory duct carcinoma has been observed in four cases. All have been poorly differentiated for histologic and nuclear grade. One woman, who presented with the clinical features of inflammatory carcinoma, died of systemic metastases. Two patients who had axillary lymph node metastases and a third with negative nodes remained disease-free.[379] All patients who had only intraductal carcinoma remained well after mastectomy when followed up for a mean of 8 years.[379] Too few patients have been treated by lumpectomy and radiation to evaluate the effectiveness of this treatment in this disease.

Infiltrating Lobular Carcinoma

In 1941, Foote and Stewart[381] published a description of lobular carcinoma in situ and observed that "when the tumor infiltrates, it is apt to do so in a peculiar fashion which permits one, after some experience, to recognize the high probability of such origin. . . ." The peculiar characteristics of infiltrating lobular carcinoma were an accompanying desmoplastic stromal reaction, the linear arrangement of tumor cells, and a tendency to grow circumferentially around ducts and lobules. The latter two patterns, commonly referred to, respectively, as Indianfile and targetoid growth, are important histologic features defining this type of invasive mammary carcinoma. In a subsequent description,[162] they noticed that growth featured "thread-like strands of tumor cells rather loosely dispersed throughout a fibrous matrix" with "no tendency for the cells to simulate atypical lobules," and they commented that "sheet like growth is distinctly uncharacteristic." The presence of central mucoid globules (signet-ring cells) and the small size of tumor cells, which could lead to an incorrect diagnosis of lymphoma, were additional features described by Foote and Stewart.[162,381]

Few studies of infiltrating lobular carcinoma appeared in the succeeding 25 years, and these consisted largely of case reports documenting progression from in situ lobular carcinoma.[382-386] In 1966, Newman[387] reported that infiltrating lobular carcinoma constituted 5% of 1436 carcinomas treated in a 17-year period at a single hospital. A review of more than 21,000 breast carcinomas diagnosed in the United States from 1969 to 1971 found that only 3% were classified as infiltrating lobular carcinoma.[388] At Memorial Hospital in New York City, 4.2% of carcinomas diagnosed from 1956 to 1970 were classified as a pure infiltrating lobular carcinoma.[389] With the less-restrictive microscopic criteria that have extended the diagnosis to so-called variant forms, the lesion has been reported to constitute 10% to 14% of invasive carcinomas.[213,390,391]

CLINICAL PRESENTATION

Infiltrating lobular carcinoma occurs throughout the age distribution of breast carcinoma (26 to 86 years). The median age at diagnosis in various series ranges from 45 to 56 years for pure forms.[387,389,390-396] In a study of carcinoma in patients of the extremes of age, classic infiltrating lobular carcinoma constituted only 2% of lesions diagnosed in women 35 years of age or younger and 11% of carcinomas found in women 75 years or older.[170] A review of 1024 patients treated at Memorial Hospital in the years 1976 to 1978 yielded 70 infiltrating lobular carcinomas (6.8%). The mean age of these patients was 57 years, identical with that of 676 women treated for infiltrating duct carcinoma.[169] One study,[393] which compared patients with pure and variant forms, found a younger median age of diagnosis for variant tumors (47 years) than for pure forms (53 years), but others[390] reported that patients with a solid variant were, on average, older (63 years) than women with classic infiltrating lobular carcinoma (56 years).

Virtually all patients present with a tumor, most frequently in the upper outer quadrant. The lesions tend to have ill-defined margins, and occasionally the only evidence is subtle thickening or induration. Skin retraction, fixation, and other signs of advanced local disease occur with large lesions. Nipple discharge and Paget disease are not symptoms of pure infiltrating lobular carcinoma, but may occur when there is a concurrent ductile carcinoma. Rarely, Paget disease results from direct extension of an underlying infiltrating lobular carcinoma to the nipple.

Calcifications are not ordinarily formed by infiltrating lobular carcinoma; therefore, this feature cannot be relied on for mammographic diagnosis.[397] However, calcifications may be present coincidentally in associated benign lesions such as sclerosing adenosis.[398] Lack of definite margins and a tendency to grow in multiple foci throughout the breast are other features that may obscure the lesion radiologically.[398]

Patients with infiltrating lobular carcinoma are especially prone to have bilateral carcinoma. Prior and concurrent carcinoma of the opposite breast has been reported in 6% to 28% of cases.[159,387,394-399] Subsequent contralateral carcinoma occurs in 9% to 14% of patients initially diagnosed as having infiltrating lobular carcinoma.[392,399]

Most synchronous and metachronous contralateral tumors have a lobular component or are pure lobular carcinomas, with 50% or more being invasive carcinomas.[159,394,399]

About half of the infiltrating lobular carcinomas studied biochemically are classified as estrogen receptor–positive, a proportion not significantly different from infiltrating duct carcinomas,[207] and the median estrogen receptor–

positive concentration in 55 tumors was 10 fmol/mg cytosol protein. The alveolar variant is reported to have especially high concentrations of estrogen receptor protein and many also had elevated levels of progesterone receptor.[400] When studied immunohistochemically, estrogen receptors can be detected at positive levels in classic and variant types of infiltrating lobular carcinoma.[401]

GROSS PATHOLOGY

Infiltrating lobular carcinomas range in size from microscopic lesions to tumors that diffusely infiltrate the entire breast. On average, the size of these lesions does not differ appreciably from infiltrating duct carcinomas. The excised carcinoma is usually firmer than the surrounding breast parenchyma, but the margins often tend to be indistinct, and the tumor tissue may not be visibly abnormal. Infiltrating lobular carcinoma is not prone to cyst formation, necrosis, hemorrhage, or calcification. Occasional lesions are distinctly tan, a feature associated with more cellular variants of the disease.

Uncommon and exceptional gross forms of infiltrating lobular carcinoma occur. One of these situations was described graphically by Foote and Stewart,[162] who noted that the "specimen may present no distinctly visible lesions and yet contain a palpable area of peculiar induration, the precise limits of which are vague. . . . After the diagnosis of cancer is made it is well to be prepared for querulousness from the operating surgeon who understandably would like to be operating for something more finite than indistinct induration."

The other gross manifestation of infiltrating lobular carcinoma may be minute, distinct, firm nodules that feel like grains of sand buried in the breast tissue. When such areas are the only evidence of carcinoma, the disease may be difficult to distinguish from sclerosing adenosis, both grossly and microscopically. Vague induration or minute sandlike nodules may be the only gross evidence of carcinoma in a specimen from a contralateral breast biopsy when the opposite breast showed normal results on clinical examination.

MICROSCOPIC PATHOLOGY

Newman,[387] who published the first series of patients with infiltrating lobular carcinoma, found that 142 tumors had features of infiltrating lobular carcinoma, but on further review, determined that only 73 fulfilled his criteria for a pure group (Fig. 13-21). In making this distinction, he sought to exclude cases in which there was a prominent duct-forming component or the growth pattern was not largely of the linear type originally described by Foote and Stewart.[162,381]

The difficulty Newman faced in assigning tumors to the category of infiltrating lobular carcinoma continues to persist. The histologic definition of this type of mammary carcinoma has been less precise than that of most major categories of breast carcinoma listed in classification schemes. Although some tumors are composed only of the histologic pattern described by Foote and Stewart, a subset of lesions exhibiting areas of classic infiltrating lobular carcinoma also have components with other variant features (Fig. 13-22). An additional group of tumors is composed largely, or occasionally entirely, of variant growth patterns. These structural variants of infiltrating lobular carcinoma, described as tubular, solid, trabecular, and alveolar forms of the lesion, have extended the diagnosis to a larger group of lesions in the last decade.[390,391,393,394,402] A series of 230 stage I and II patients with infiltrating lobular carcinoma included 54 (34%) women with variant lesions.[395]

Tubulolobular carcinoma contains glands of the type usually found in tubular carcinoma, within the growth pattern of infiltrating lobular carcinoma.[391,403] Fechner[393] described a variant group of tumors composed, in part, of trabeculae or broad sheets of tumor cells that had cytologic features identical with cells in other areas growing in the classic pattern. Other than the structural distinction, no outstanding clinical or pathologic differences were found between cases with pure and solid variant carcinomas. Others have commented on an alveolar arrangement of tumor cells in groups, which appear in histologic sections as rounded masses.[390,391,400] Finally, many tumors have combinations of mixtures of the classic and variant patterns. Dixon and associates[390] classified 103 cases of infiltrating lobular carcinoma as follows: classic 30%, mixed 29%, solid 22%, and alveolar 19%. Most authors require that at least 70% of a tumor exhibit a particular growth pattern to be classified under that category. More heterogeneous lesions constitute the subset with mixed patterns.

Cells with more abundant eosinophilic cytoplasm are found in some carcinomas with the pattern of invasive lobular carcinoma. This has been described as histiocytoid or pleomorphic lobular carcinomas.[404,405] The cytoplasmic features are a manifestation of apocrine differentiation in these carcinomas. Some authors have associated this histologic variant of lobular carcinoma with a poor prognosis,[404,405] but this conclusion is based on small series of cases studied retrospectively. The frequency of HER2/neu positivity in pleomorphic lobular carcinoma is reportedly much higher than in classic invasive lobular carcinoma.[404,406]

The cytologic nature of cells found within infiltrating lobular carcinoma has received less attention than the growth pattern of the tumor. In classic lesions, the invasive tumor cells are usually described as having small round nuclei, without prominent nucleoli, and with a limited amount of cytoplasm. Intracytoplasmic lamina, containing a mucinous secretion that reacts with mucicarmine and alcian blue stains, are found in a variable proportion of the cells.[407,408] When a cell contains a prominent, large cytoplasmic mucin vacuole that pushes the nucleus peripherally, the cell has a signet-ring cell configuration. The name signet-ring cell carcinoma has been applied to a group of tumors composed of such cells. Most are variants of infiltrating lobular carcinoma,[213,407-409] but this cytologic appearance also is found in duct carcinomas. Essentially the same cytologic features are found in classic and variant forms of infiltrating lobular carcinoma.

Dense-core neurosecretory granules have been found

FIGURE 13-21 In situ and infiltrating lobular carcinoma with the classic growth pattern. The patient, a 42-year-old woman, had a "lump" in the tail of the left breast and thickening of the right upper outer quadrant. Biopsy of the left breast revealed infiltrating duct carcinoma. These photographs are from the right breast lesion. **A.** Lobular carcinoma in situ fills a terminal duct and acinar units in the upper right; in the lower left corner, invasive tumor cells infiltrate the stroma. **B.** Magnified view showing cytologically identical cells in the in situ and invasive parts of the lesion. **C.** Classic linear growth of invasive lobular carcinoma.

FIGURE 13-22 Variants of infiltrating lobular carcinoma. **A.** Invasive carcinoma composed of small uniform cells with cytologic features of lobular carcinoma growing in a trabecular pattern on the right and in a more characteristic linear fashion on the left. **B.** An area from the same tumor featuring larger masses of cells that characterize the alveolar growth pattern.

by electron microscopic study in infiltrating lobular carcinoma.[401,410] It is possible that the recently described small cell neuroendocrine (oat cell) carcinoma of the breast is a variant of infiltrating lobular carcinoma.[411,412]

Immunoreactivity for CEA[400,401,413] tends to be directly related to the amount of mucin secretion, being most intense in tumors with prominent signet ring cell features. α-Lactalbumin reportedly has been detected in 19% to 100% of tumors studied.[401,413–415] A few casein-positive cells[401] can be found in most invasive lobular carcinomas. About 39% of these tumors also are immunoreactive for gross cystic disease fluid glycoprotein-15, with expression more pronounced in tumors with signet-ring cell features.[291]

Fibronectin, a noncollagenous glycoprotein, is associated with interstitial collagen and basement membranes. Although infiltrating duct carcinomas contain abundant stromal fibronectin, the concentration of this glycoprotein is substantially decreased in the stroma of infiltrating lobular carcinomas.[416] Because fibronectins contribute to cell adhesiveness,[417] decreased amounts of this substance may contribute to the dispersed growth pattern of infiltrating lobular carcinoma.

PROGNOSIS

When it metastasizes, infiltrating lobular carcinoma is predisposed to several unusual patterns of spread. Central nervous system metastases tend to be in the form of meningeal infiltration (carcinomatous meningitis), in contrast with duct carcinoma, which most often results in parenchymal deposits.[418,419] Intraabdominal metastases often diffusely involve the retroperitoneum and serosal surfaces.[409,420–422] Intestinal and ureteral obstruction have been reported to occur as a consequence. The operative findings may reveal only thickening of serosal, mesenteric, or retroperitoneal tissue, with no mass apparent.

Invasion of abdominal organs sometimes occurs coincidentally with diffuse serosal spread or as separate parenchymal metastases. Because the signet-ring cells of mammary and other types of carcinoma are morphologically indistinguishable, metastatic lobular carcinoma involving the gastrointestinal tract can cause considerable diagnostic difficulty.[421,423–425] Metastases in the stomach mimic primary gastric carcinoma and, when transmural, the clinical and pathologic findings are those of linitis plastica.[426,427] Under these circumstances, gastric and mammary carcinoma have an identical histologic appearance in a gastric biopsy specimen. A strongly positive immunohistochemical reaction for hormone receptor could be a helpful diagnostic procedure, especially if material from the original breast tumor is available for comparison. However, estrogen receptor has been detected in gastric adenocarcinoma with biochemical[428] and immunohistochemical[429] techniques.

Infiltrating lobular carcinoma also has a propensity to spread to the ovaries and uterus.[430] Because the carcinoma cells tend to blend with normal cells of the endometrial stroma, they may be overlooked in an endometrial biopsy performed for vaginal bleeding. A failure to inform the pathologist of a previously treated breast carcinoma in-

creases the likelihood that metastatic carcinoma will not be recognized in an endometrial or endocervical biopsy.

Metastatic lobular carcinoma has been mistaken for histiocytes.[431,432] Such a lesion in the eyelid can resemble a chalazion.[433,434] Similar problems have been encountered in other sites, such as the bone marrow. Histochemical studies for mucin secretion or the immunohistochemical demonstration of epithelial-associated antigen (epithelial membrane antigen or cytokeratins) usually resolve the issue.[435]

The prognosis of women with infiltrating lobular carcinoma has been described in several studies. In a series of women who underwent mastectomy for T1, N0, M0 carcinomas, death of disease at 10 years occurred in 6% with infiltrating lobular carcinoma and in 14% with infiltrating duct carcinoma.[15] Newman[387] reported that 14% of all node-negative patients with infiltrating lobular carcinoma died of disease, with follow-up averaging about 8 years. Death of disease occurred in nearly 50% of women who had lymph node metastases. Ashikari and associates[389] reported the overall 5- and 10-year survivals in node-negative patients, not stratified by tumor size, to be 86% and 74%, respectively. They found no significant differences in survival when patients having infiltrating lobular carcinoma were stratified by nodal status and compared with similar groups treated for infiltrating duct carcinoma.

Data on the prognostic significance of variant histologic patterns are inconclusive. Fechner[393] reported a lower frequency of axillary nodal metastases in women who had one of the variant forms of infiltrating lobular carcinoma, but he gave no follow-up data. Dixon and coworkers[390] reported that patients with classic infiltrating lobular carcinoma had a better prognosis than those with variant forms. In this series, most patients were treated by simple mastectomy, radiation, and occasionally, axillary lymph node biopsy or dissection. Because staging was based on the Manchester system in this series, there was a great deal of variation in the extent of disease among histologic types of infiltrating lobular carcinoma. In a study of 171 patients, du Toit and associates[436] reported a slightly more favorable prognosis for patients with classic as opposed to alveolar and solid variants of infiltrating lobular carcinoma. Patients with tubulolobular carcinoma had the best prognosis. The small groups of patients compared, limited staging data, and absence of uniform treatment weaken the reliability of these data.

A study at Memorial Hospital in New York evaluated 230 patients with pathologic stage I-II infiltrating lobular carcinoma treated by mastectomy and axillary dissection.[395] The series included 176 women with classic infiltrating lobular carcinoma and 54 women with variant growth patterns. The two groups did not differ significantly in the distribution of pathologic TNM stage. Median survival time and median time to recurrence were not significantly different in the two groups, although patients with classic lesions tended to have a better prognosis than those with variant tumors. In this[395] and other studies, patients with classic infiltrating lobular carcinoma did not exhibit a significant difference in prognosis from those with infiltrating duct carcinoma when stratified by stage at diagnosis and treated by excision and mastectomy.[437] The most important determinants of prognosis are primary tumor size and lymph node status. However, accurately distinguishing between invasive duct and infiltrating lobular carcinoma is important because of the higher frequency of bilaterality and multicentricity in the latter group.

Mammary Carcinomas With Endocrine Features

Some mammary carcinomas are able to synthesize hormones not considered to be normal products of the breast. This capacity to produce ectopic hormones may be considered endocrine or biochemical metaplasia. Such tumors have been found to contain peptide hormones, including human chorionic gonadotropic (HCG),[438] calcitonin,[439] and epinephrine.[440] These substances are detectable by biochemical analysis and also morphologically by immunohistochemical study of the tumor tissue.

In a few unusual instances, the microscopic growth pattern simulates the structure of nonmammary neoplasms that commonly contain the hormone in question, resulting in coincidental biochemical and structural metaplasia. A striking example of this combined metaplasia is mammary carcinoma with choriocarcinomatous differentiation.[438,441] In this type of mammary carcinoma, areas that microscopically look like syncytiotrophoblast and cytotrophoblast are strongly reactive for the β-unit of HCG. Carcinomas of the breast and other organs that exhibit structural choriocarcinomatous metaplasia have an aggressive clinical course, resulting in recurrence and death from disease.

Isolated carcinoma cells that are reactive immunohistologically for α- and β-HCG can be found in 15% to 21% of ordinary infiltrating duct carcinomas, respectively, that do not exhibit choriocarcinomatous metaplasia.[442] The reactive cells are otherwise morphologically indistinguishable microscopically from surrounding carcinoma cells that are not immunoreactive for HCG. The presence of these occasional HCG-positive cells does not seem to have prognostic significance,[442] and no functional effects have been described.

A more frequent form of biochemical and structural metaplasia occurs in mammary carcinomas that contain argyrophilic cytoplasmic granules that can be detected by light microscopic with histochemical techniques. The procedures most commonly used to demonstrate argyrophilic granules rely on reactions in which ammoniacal silver is reduced to particulate metallic silver that can be visualized with the light microscope.[443] Argentaffin granules, typically found in midgut carcinoid tumors, contain endogenous reducing substances. In the argyrophil reaction (eg, Grimelius stain), an exogenous reducing agent is added because some granules do not contain endogenous reducing substances. Because most cells with either argentaffin or argyrophilic granules are visualized with the argyrophil reaction, this is the preferable procedure. Breast neoplasms

that contain argyrophilic granules have been argentaffin-negative.[219,444,445]

The reported frequency of argyrophilia in female mammary carcinoma varies from 3% to 25%.[446] No systematic study of the frequency of argyrophilic granules in male breast carcinoma has been reported, but a few descriptions of argyrophil-positive tumors in men have been published.[440,447,448]

CLINICAL PRESENTATION

No specific clinical features are associated with mammary carcinomas that exhibit structural or histochemical evidence of endocrine differentiation. Because most of the lesions are invasive carcinomas, most of the patients present with a palpable tumor. The tumors may be detected in any part of the breast, but the most common location is the upper outer quadrant. Systemic evidence of ectopic hormonal secretion has been absent in all but a few cases. Individual case reports have described patients with symptoms attributable to ectopic ACTH,[449] parathormone,[450] calcitonin,[439] and epinephrine[440] secreted by mammary carcinomas.

Argyrophilia has been identified in breast carcinomas throughout the age distribution of the disease, extending from patients in their early 30s to women in their late 80s.[219,448,451,452] Men with argyrophilic carcinomas have been reported to range in age from 71 to 83 years old.

GROSS PATHOLOGY

Argyrophilic mammary carcinomas have not exhibited specific gross pathologic features. The invasive tumors measure 1 to 5 cm in diameter, with most between 1.5 and 3 cm. The tumors are likely to be grossly circumscribed, but in rare cases multiple foci of carcinoma were described in the breast.

MICROSCOPIC PATHOLOGY

Many of the tumors that contain argyrophilic granules have been described as infiltrating duct carcinomas, with varying degrees of differentiation. Argyrophilic cells can be found in the intraductal and the invasive portion of these tumors.[444,452] Argyrophilic intraductal carcinomas tend to have a distinctive solid papillary or organoid growth pattern,[444,453] whereas conventional cribriform and comedo intraductal carcinomas are typically nonargyrophilic.[453] In several studies,[219,220,448,454] the proportion of invasive mucinous carcinomas that were argyrophilic ranged from 8% to 80%.[454] The reported frequency of argyrophilic infiltrating duct carcinomas varied from 15%[219] to 71%[455] and, among infiltrating lobular carcinomas, 50%[219] to 100%[455] reportedly have been argyrophilic.

Some argyrophilic cancers have endocrine growth patterns resembling carcinoid tumors that arise in other organs. Recognition of this structural similarity led to a search for argyrophilic granules in mammary carcinomas. The term *primary carcinoid tumor of the breast* was introduced in 1977 by Cubilla and Woodruff[452] to characterize a group of neoplasms that they regarded as a new pathologic entity.[456] Although the investigators failed to detect argyrophilic granules in normal breast epithelium, they concluded that the primary mammary carcinoid was a neuroendocrine neoplasm of the breast derived from argyrophil cells of neural crest origin, presumed to have migrated to mammary ducts.

Not all carcinomas with an endocrine growth pattern contain argyrophilic cells, and it has not been possible to demonstrate polypeptide hormones or biogenic amines in most argyrophilic carcinomas.[219,454,457] Some argyrophilic mammary carcinomas are microscopically indistinguishable from argyrophil-negative mammary carcinomas. Despite the efforts of many investigators to find progenitor argyrophilic cells in normal mammary duct epithelium, such cells rarely have been detected, and then only in small numbers.[220,223,458]

Growing evidence supports that argyrophilic granules in benign cells and in carcinoma cells often are associated with nonhormonal products, and these granules are not necessarily indicative of endocrine differentiation. In 1982, Clayton and associates[457] reported that most of the argyrophilic carcinomas they studied also were reactive for lactalbumin. Intracytoplasmic localization of argyrophilia and lactalbumin showed a similar tendency to apical cytoplasmic staining in carcinomas and in tissue from a lactating breast. They concluded that argyrophilia might be evidence of lactational differentiation because "the secretory granules appear to contain milk secretory product rather than neuroendocrine polypeptides."[457] However, Bussolati and others[459] reported that the apparent immunoreactivity for α-lactalbumin found in argyrophilic carcinomas by Clayton and associates and other investigators was the result of a contaminant that had an affinity for endocrine cells.

These observations have led most investigators to conclude that neoplasms with argyrophilic granules do not constitute a specific histopathologic category of female mammary carcinoma. Although the idea of a primary mammary carcinoid tumor has been discredited, there is a group of mammary carcinomas capable of producing ectopic hormonal substances.

PROGNOSIS AND TREATMENT

When they are recognized, argyrophilic breast tumors are best diagnosed as mammary carcinomas with endocrine features. If ectopic hormones can be detected, they should be specified as, for example, *infiltrating duct carcinoma with endocrine features, argyrophil- and ACTH-positive*. The recognition of these tumors is necessary to more fully define their clinical characteristics. Nearly half of the patients have had axillary nodal metastases.[444,451,452,455,459] Although the stage at diagnosis is the major determinant of prognosis,[448] there have been no case-control studies comparing patients who have mammary carcinoma with endocrine differentiation with age- and state-matched control groups. Patients with argyrophilic mucinous carcinomas were more likely to have axillary nodal metastases (48%) than those with Grimelius-negative tumors (26%). They

also had a higher frequency of recurrence and death of breast carcinoma (65% versus 33%). In another study, the presence or absence of argyrophilic granules did not influence the prognosis of patients with mucinous carcinoma.[460]

The choice of primary treatment for mammary carcinomas with endocrine features should be determined by conventional clinical and pathologic criteria. Until further information becomes available, neither ectopic hormone production nor endocrine differentiation have been proved to be factors that critically influence prognosis or treatment.

Also recognize that metastases in the breast from a carcinoid that arose at another site may be mistaken for a primary mammary tumor.[461,462] The finding of an in situ component provides convincing evidence of breast origin.

Inflammatory Carcinoma

The clinical findings in primary inflammatory carcinoma are a superficial manifestation of an underlying invasive carcinoma. The primary carcinoma tends to be indistinct clinically and, on gross inspection of a mastectomy specimen, an exact size frequently is not recorded because the gross margins are not easily defined. The lesion may be described as diffusely involving the breast or simply as a large tumor.[463,464]

The WHO Report on the Histological Typing of Breast Tumors states that "inflammatory carcinoma does not constitute a histological type but rather a clinical entity."[465] Microscopically, there is usually a poorly differentiated infiltrating duct carcinoma. Rarely, the primary lesion is an invasive lobular or mucinous carcinoma. In virtually every case, there is some invasion of intramammary vascular spaces within and at the perimeter of the tumor. Usually, this is an extensive process throughout the breast, but in a few patients, parenchymal vascular invasion is inconspicuous. Because the vascular channels typically lack erythrocytes, they are usually regarded as lymphatics. However, tumor emboli can be found in vascular spaces containing red blood cells. Lymphoplasmacytic reaction to the tumor occurs with varying intensity but is generally inconspicuous.

Because of the striking clinical cutaneous findings, a great deal of attention has been directed to the pathologic characteristics of the skin. This is especially important because a biopsy of the skin is usually one of the first diagnostic procedures to be performed. In the typical case, microscopic examination of the skin reveals dilated dermal lymphatic channels, intralymphatic tumor emboli, and a lymphocytic reaction in the dermis that tends to localize around dilated vascular spaces (Fig. 13-23).

Considerable variation in clinical and pathologic features occurs from one patient to another. The intensity of erythema and edema does not correlate well with the amount of vascular dilatation, lymphoplasmacytic reaction, or the number of intravascular tumor emboli seen in microscopic sections of the skin. Biopsy specimens of skin

FIGURE 13-23 Inflammatory carcinoma. Skin biopsy from a patient who presented with a breast mass and inflammatory carcinoma clinically. Three dilated lymphatic channels contain tumor emboli. Lymphocytic infiltrate is present in the dermis, as is frequent in the skin of patients with inflammatory carcinoma.

within and outside the zone of erythema may have identical histopathologic features, including intralymphatic tumor emboli. It has not been possible to detect intralymphatic tumor emboli in the skin of all patients who have the typical clinical appearance of inflammatory carcinoma.[464,466–469] In one study, 8 of 16 patients had a negative result on skin biopsy.[467] A small group of long-term survivors among women treated for clinically diagnosed inflammatory carcinoma did not have dermal lymphatic tumor emboli in a skin biopsy specimen.[469] Consequently, no specific histologic picture can be consistently associated with the diagnosis of inflammatory carcinoma clinically or with the clinical findings in a particular case.

Another group of patients have cutaneous lymphatic tumor emboli in the absence of the clinical findings of inflammatory carcinoma, especially erythema.[464] In general, their presentation is otherwise similar to that of inflammatory carcinoma for tumor size, nodal involvement, and pathologic features of the underlying carcinoma. The prognosis in this condition, termed *occult* inflammatory carcinoma,[470] seems to be more favorable than that observed in women with the typical clinical features of inflammatory carcinoma.[464,465,469–471]

Invasion of the dermis and dermal lymphatics was encountered in 4% (38 of 946) of primary operable patients treated by mastectomy for invasive carcinoma not having inflammatory features clinically. Dermal lymphatic involvement alone was encountered in 1%. These tumors tended to be centrally located, generally were larger than 4 cm, and frequently they were multicentric.

When lymphatic tumor emboli are present in a skin biopsy specimen from a patient with inflammatory carcinoma, the tumor cells constitute a small percentage of the volume of the specimen. Most of these biopsy specimens have been reported to be estrogen receptor– and proges-terone receptor–negative,[208] as have biopsy specimens of the more cellular primary tumors.[472–474] When studied by immunohistochemical methods, most dermal lymphatic tumor emboli have been receptor-negative, and the same results have been obtained with corresponding samples of the primary tumor. Rarely, however, dermal tumor emboli may be immunohistochemically receptor-positive, despite negative results obtained when skin biopsy specimens were tested biochemically. Amplified expression of the HER2/neu oncogene has been found more often in inflammatory than in noninflammatory carcinomas.[475,476] In one study, HER2/neu expression was amplified most notably in node-positive estrogen receptor–negative tumors.[475] High levels of epidermal growth factor transcripts[475] and of cathepsin D[476] also have been detected in inflammatory carcinomas.

Recurrent mammary carcinoma involving the skin also can have inflammatory features clinically.[467,477] This type of recurrence generally occurs on the chest wall near the area of primary therapy or in the opposite breast. A review of the primary lesion in a series of patients with recurrent inflammatory carcinoma revealed that all were ductal in origin.[477] A relatively high proportion of the original tumors had the cytologic features of apocrine carcinoma. Intralymphatic tumor emboli were frequently present in the breast, nipple, or skin at the time of mastectomy, but usually the clinical presentation of the primary tumors did not have the typical appearance of inflammatory carcinoma.

Metastases to the Breast From Extramammary Malignant Tumors

Nearly one quarter of metastatic tumors in the breast are the presenting manifestation of an otherwise occult extramammary malignant tumor, usually a carcinoma. The most common primary site of an occult tumor presenting in this fashion is the lungs.[478–480] Clinically inapparent carcinoma of the kidneys, ovaries, stomach, and uterus, and intestinal carcinoid tumors may present as metastases in the breast. Among previously diagnosed lesions that most frequently give rise to metastases in the breast, detected clinically or at autopsy, are malignant melanoma and carcinomas of the lung, prostate, cervix, and urinary bladder. Metastatic ovarian carcinoma may simulate papillary or mucinous carcinoma of the breast.[481,482] The distinction between a metastasis from pulmonary oat cell carcinoma and primary lymphoma of the breast can be a difficult diagnostic problem. Adenocarcinoma of the colon and rectum is rarely the source of metastatic carcinoma in the breast, despite its relative frequency in the general population.[483] In children, metastases to the breast from medulloblastoma[484] and rhabdomyosarcoma[485] have been reported. Although sometimes included in reports of metastatic neoplasms in the breast, lymphoma involving the breast should be regarded as a primary breast neoplasm or as part of a systemic disease, depending on the clinical circumstances.

Metastatic prostatic carcinoma involved the breast in a substantial number of men with this neoplasm who were studied at autopsy.[486] Numerous clinical case reports describe palpable prostatic carcinoma metastases, often with bilateral involvement.[487,488] Although estrogen treatment has been implicated as a factor predisposing to the localization of prostate carcinoma in the breast, this is difficult to prove because of the widespread use of estrogens in this disease. Furthermore, a few patients not treated with estrogens have developed breast metastases. Patients with prostatic carcinoma rarely develop an independent primary mammary carcinoma.[489–491] These have all been unilateral lesions. Several reports that purport to illustrate cases of bilateral breast carcinoma after estrogen treatment for prostatic carcinoma appear, on review, to be examples of breast involvement by metastatic carcinoma.[492–494] In addition to histologic examination, immunohistochemical studies for prostatic-specific antigen and prostate-specific acid phosphatase identify prostatic carcinoma when results are positive. Estrogen receptor studies are not helpful, because estrogen receptor positivity may be present in both types of carcinoma.

For the pathologist, one of the most important aspects of metastatic tumor in the breast is to consider this possibility in the diagnosis when faced with a morphologically unusual breast lesion (Fig. 13-24). This requires sensitivity to morphologic patterns that are not typical for breast carcinomas. The pathologist should be provided with a complete history of previously treated neoplasms, but even when this information is given, primary tumor may be a new, occult tumor. The preoperative clinical work-up for a patient with a breast tumor who appears in good health is often perfunctory and cannot be relied on to exclude an extramammary primary. In this setting, it is especially difficult to recognize tumor metastatic from an occult nonmammary primary in an aspiration cytology specimen.

Other than an unusual histologic pattern and clinical information, few clues exist to identify a metastatic tumor in the breast. In situ carcinoma of ducts and lobules should be carefully sought, because this provides definitive evidence of mammary origin. Because an in situ component is not detectable in a substantial number of primary breast carcinomas, absence of this finding is not conclusive. Metastases may produce solitary or multiple tumor nodules in the breast. The latter circumstance should lead to suspicion of metastatic tumor, because primary breast carcinoma only rarely presents with two or more palpable tumors. Tumor emboli, when intramammary lymphatic spaces have been observed, are associated with metastases to the breast and with primary breast carcinomas. Metastatic tumor is suggested by the following combination of microscopic findings: a tumor composed of a homogeneous population of neoplastic cells without desmoplastic stromal reaction; no detectable in situ carcinoma of lobules or ducts; and a sharp transition at the periphery between tumor and entirely normal breast tissue, with no benign proliferative breast disease. In some difficult cases, electron microscopic study, lymphocyte marker analysis, immunohistochemical study, and estrogen receptor analysis may be helpful in assessing a tumor thought to be metastatic in the breast. The problems of distinguishing between mammary carcinoma with carcinoid features and metastatic carcinoid in the breast are discussed elsewhere in this chapter.

Distinguishing between a primary tumor of the breast and a metastasis to the breast is important for therapy and prognosis. When an occult extramammary neoplasm presents with a breast metastasis, work-up of the patients will be influenced by morphologic features of the tumor that may suggest particular primary sites. Only in exceptional circumstances would mastectomy be appropriate for metastatic tumor in the breast, and emphasis should be placed on systemic treatment appropriate to the primary lesion.

Pathologic Examination of Breast Specimens

This section highlights clinically important factors relating to the gross pathologic examination of breast specimens not discussed elsewhere in this or other chapters. Although some technical aspects of the laboratory processing of tissues are addressed, this is not a comprehensive presentation of differing points of view, nor should this material be regarded as sufficiently detailed to serve as a laboratory workbook. Additional information may be found in comprehensive reviews.[495,496,500]

BIOPSY

Small or Incisional Biopsy Specimens

Small-needle or incisional biopsy specimens usually are processed for histologic examination in their entirety. The operator who performs the biopsy should exercise care

FIGURE 13-24 Metastatic mucoepidermoid carcinoma of the parotid gland in the breast showing characteristic vacuolated mucin-containing cells. The primary salivary gland tumor was resected several years before the breast metastasis became apparent.

not to crush the specimens. A cautery-type scalpel should not be used in obtaining such a biopsy (see later discussion). Although these samples are suitable for frozen section, notice that limited information about the characteristics of a lesion is obtained from such small specimens, and the tissue should be saved for permanent sections.[498] The samples are usually too small to permit standard biochemical assays of hormone receptors but may be suitable for immunohistochemical receptor analysis. Unless frozen section or some other study that requires fresh tissue is intended, small biopsy specimens should be placed immediately in fixative for transport to the laboratory.

Excisional Biopsy Specimens

Many factors may influence the manner in which excisional biopsy specimens are handled in a given situation. Paramount among these are logistic considerations relating to when and where the biopsy is performed and the particular clinical circumstances. Hence, the material presented in this section should be regarded as a series of guidelines that may need to be modified in some situations.

GROSS EXAMINATION OF EXCISIONAL BIOPSY. The pathologist is responsible for describing the dimensions and character of the tissue removed from the patients. This can most accurately be accomplished if the excised specimen is delivered intact, promptly, and unfixed to the pathology laboratory.

The size of an excisional biopsy specimen should be recorded in centimeters in three dimensions, and the general shape (eg, ovoid, spherical) should be noted. Because the overall dimensions of an excisional biopsy cannot be determined after the tissue has been sliced open and dissected by the surgeon, the intact specimen should be delivered promptly to the laboratory. It is also useful to record specimen weight in grams.

It is preferable that the tissue remain unfixed to avoid precluding the possibility of performing a frozen section or obtaining material for receptor analysis, electron microscopic examination, or other studies. If a delay is anticipated, the tissue may be chilled, but freezing the entire specimen will compromise histologic examination. Even if a frozen section is not requested, the tissue should be dissected promptly by a pathologist to determine whether any grossly identifiable tumor is present. If such a lesion is found, the size should be recorded in centimeters. Because of the critical prognostic significance of tumor size, this measurement should be made before tissue is removed for frozen section or other studies, such as hormone receptor analysis. It is difficult to accurately measure the tumor if the specimen received has already been sliced by the surgeon. The gross character of the tumor (shape, consistency, appearance of cut surface) should be described. Whether or not a distinct lesion is found, the appearance of the breast parenchyma should be noted (consistency, relative proportions of fat and fibrous tissue, cysts, or other lesions).

The number of samples to be taken from an excisional biopsy for histologic examination varies with the clinical circumstances, gross appearance of the tissue, and results of frozen section, if performed. No fixed rule (eg, *x* number of specimens should be examined per 5 g of tissue) can be reasonably applied. If a frozen section is performed, the used tissue sample must be saved, processed into a paraffin section, and identified by a term such as the *frozen section control*. If a sample is removed for hormone receptor analysis, a corresponding specimen should be examined histologically as a *receptor control*. Distinct tumors that grossly appear to be carcinomas 2 cm or smaller in diameter can be entirely submitted for histologic assessment. Some sections should be taken to demonstrate the margin of the tumor and surrounding breast, which are examined microscopically for evidence of lymphatic tumor emboli and in situ carcinoma outside the lesion. When no distinct tumor is present, some laboratories advocate processing the entire specimen. This may be appropriate in some situations because of clinical or pathologic findings. However, the cost of applying this approach indiscriminately is prohibitive, and judgment must be exercised here and in the selection of other clinical or laboratory diagnostic procedures.

To establish criteria for sampling grossly negative specimens of breast biopsies, Schnitt and Connolly[499] carried out a retrospective study of 384 specimens entirely submitted for histologic examination from biopsies performed for clinically palpable lesions in which no distinct tumor was evident on gross pathologic examination. Carcinoma was found in 23 (6%) specimens and atypical hyperplasia in 3 others (0.8%). Eighty percent of the blocks with fibrous parenchyma contained all carcinomas, and two of the three contained atypical hyperplasias. By submitting up to 10 blocks per case, it would have been possible to detect 25 of the 26 significant lesions. Only a single microscopic focus of lobular carcinoma in situ was overlooked by this selection. The authors recommended submitting up to 10 samples of fibrous parenchyma or, if the specimen is composed entirely of fat, a similar number of samples. If carcinoma or atypical hyperplasia is found in the first set of slides, further sampling is recommended.

The description of the gross findings from a biopsy, mastectomy, or any other specimen becomes part of the pathologic report. Included in this report should be a listing of the tissue samples taken for microscopic examination, indicating the number of tissue blocks and providing a key to explain abbreviations used to designate individual samples. This information serves as an index, and it is particularly important to assist pathologists called on to review slides in other institutions when patients are referred for treatment. Most pathologic reports prepared in the United States do not provide this information or do so in a cursory, often confusing, manner.

ASSESSING MARGINS OF EXCISION. It is essential to accurately assess the margins of an excision that contains carcinoma.[500] Because the contours and orientation of tissue slices may be altered in the course of preparing histologic sections, the surfaces must be marked so that they can be identified microscopically. This is easily accomplished with finely particulate reagents, such as India ink or tatoo dyes, that remain adherent to the tissue throughout processing and are visible through the microscope (Fig. 13-25). These pigments adhere better to fresh tissue that has been blotted free of surface blood and moisture than to fixed tissue. If properly applied, the surface pigment should not contaminate the interior of the specimen where it could result in misleading conclusions about the margins. With experience, it is possible to ''ink'' the surface of an excisional biopsy in 1 to 2 minutes. Hence, this procedure is not a major impediment to performing a frozen section, nor does it appreciably delay obtaining tissue for receptor analysis.

An excisional biopsy specimen that has been sliced up by the surgeon cannot be reliably reassembled to ink the margins. This is a further reason why it is necessary that excisional biopsy specimens be submitted intact to the pathologist.

Once inked, the specimen should be split in a plane that will bisect a palpable tumor if present. It is possible to remove portions immediately for frozen section or receptor analysis. Frozen sections of margins are not appropriate unless the tumor appears close to a margin; intraoperative confirmation of this has an immediate impact on treatment.

It is not possible to orient an excisional biopsy specimen without guidance from the surgeon. This can be easily accomplished if the surgeon places a short suture at the superior margin and a long stitch laterally. At least two sections should be taken perpendicular to each of the six inked surfaces (superior, inferior, me-dial, lateral, superficial, and deep), with additional samples of margins determined by the gross findings.

No standardized system exists for reporting the microscopic appearance of margins. Tumor transected at an inked surface represents a clearly positive margin (Fig. 13-26). This criterion applies equally to in situ and to invasive carcinoma, but the type of tumor must be specified. Borderline situations occur in which the tumor closely approaches the margin, but is not truly transected. One useful convention in these situations is to regard foci within one high-power microscopic field (approximately 2 mm) as close to the margin.[500] The nature and amount of the tumor, and also the character of the tissue intervening to the margin, should be specified. It has not been determined whether the distinction between tumor transected at the margin or close to the margin, as defined here, is clinically important.

INTRAOPERATIVE THERMAL (ELECTROCAUTERY) DAMAGE TO BIOPSY SPECIMENS. Electrocautery instruments used to perform an excisional breast biopsy reduce the risk of hematoma formation in the biopsy cavity, and the operation can be completed in a shorter time. Unfortunately, the thermal effect may produce crucial changes in the tissues. Reduced estrogen receptor activity has been described,[501–503] with the decrease sufficient in some cases to result in a false-negative report.[504] Histochemical study of prostate and breast specimens after electrocautery treatment also reveals a decrease in fluorescent steroid binding,[501,502] and in immunohistochemical immunoreactivity, for estrogen and progesterone receptors.

FIGURE 13-25 Procedure for inking margins of an excisional biopsy. **A.** Intact excisional biopsy with short and long sutures, which indicate superior and lateral margins, respectively. India ink has been applied with wooden applicators. **B.** Specimen bisected after ink was completely applied. Applicator points to a carcinoma that does not extend to the margins.

FIGURE 13-26 Positive inked margin—invasive carcinoma. Clusters of poorly differentiated tumor cells infiltrating through fat extend to the ink-covered surface (*inset*) of this excisional biopsy from the breast of a 66-year-old woman.

The histologic effects of thermal damage caused by electrocautery on biopsy tissue are well known to pathologists. Thermal damage usually is limited to the surface of the specimen, generally penetrating not more than 1 mm. The manner in which the instrument is used, the character of the tissue, and the size of the specimen removed all influence the intensity and depth of the effect.[505] Two studies reported no significant differences in the proportion of hormone receptor–positive specimens among biopsies performed by cautery and noncautery methods.[505,506]

The histologic changes in the breast caused by thermal injury are similar to those seen at other sites (Fig. 13-27).

The most significant effect is severe alteration in cytologic detail. Microscopic architecture may be so distorted that the distinction between normal, hyperplastic, and neoplastic tissues can no longer be determined. Because the damage is maximal at the edges or marginal surfaces of the tissues, electrocautery artifacts severely limit the assessment of the margins of excision when mammary carcinoma is to be treated by limited resection and primary radiation therapy. If an excision is carried out with little or no breast parenchyma surrounding a carcinoma, thermal damage may occur in the tumor itself. This is a serious problem in the excision of recurrent or metastatic lesions. In addition to altering receptor activity, the histologic artifacts interfere with the assessment of microscopic prognostic features of the tumor, such as nuclear and histologic grade. As a result of damage of cells within ducts, it may be impossible to determine whether intraductal carcinoma is present in tissue outside of the tumor mass.

MASTECTOMY

The gross description of a mastectomy documents the extent of the operation and the tissue removed. A standard radical mastectomy can be oriented easily on the basis of landmarks in the specimen, especially the position of the muscle segments. This may not be so easily accomplished with various types of modified radical mastectomy, which have almost completely replaced the radical mastectomy. The surgeon must indicate if there is anything unusual about the specimen, and important landmarks such as levels of axillary lymph nodes, deep fascia, and segments of muscle must be identified. Tumor tissue can be taken for receptor analyses from the mastectomy if the specimen is submitted immediately to the laboratory and the pathologist has been alerted.

The external description of the specimen should in-

FIGURE 13-27 Thermal (electrocautery) damage in an excisional biopsy from a 40-year-old woman. **A.** View of a lobule showing considerable distortion, particularly smudging of nuclei. **B.** The lesion was a sclerosing tumor composed of small glands in proliferating stroma. This figure shows shedding of cells, which is another effect of thermal damage. Disruption of glandular elements made it impossible to distinguish between sclerosing adenosis and tubular carcinoma.

clude the following: overall size; dimensions and appearance of the skin, with measurement of scars or incisions; appearance of nipple and areola; presence of muscle and axillary tissue; and location of any distinct palpable lesion.

Dissection of the specimen is accomplished by placing it skin-side down and anatomically oriented to identify the quadrants. The deep surface should be inspected and palpated for evidence of tumor involvement and appropriately inked. The breast is dissected by a series of parallel incisions through the posterior surface up to the skin. A tumor should be described in the same fashion as for a biopsy specimen. The size and character of a prior biopsy site should be noted, including areas of induration. It is preferable that these areas not be identified as tumor, because the reaction in a healing biopsy cavity may be grossly indistinguishable from carcinoma. The appearance of the remaining breast parenchyma is also recorded, including relative proportions of fat and fibrous parenchyma; the size, location, and character of any discrete lesions; and the presence or absence of cysts. Samples for histologic examination are taken from the tumor or biopsy site, nipple, skin quadrants, and deep margin under the tumor.

One vertical section usually suffices to detect Paget disease or other forms of carcinoma[507] in the nipple. Generally, two sections are taken randomly per quadrant, but more extensive sectioning may be indicated by the gross findings, or if the mastectomy was performed for in situ lobular or intraductal carcinoma.

AXILLARY LYMPH NODES

It is impossible to determine by anatomic orientation alone the position or level of axillary lymph nodes in axillary contents received with a modified mastectomy specimen. If this information is desired clinically, the lymph node groups should be tagged or submitted as separately identified specimens. In properly oriented, complete axillary dissection specimens, the distribution of lymph node metastases almost always follows a consistent pattern. When lymph nodes are affected, metastases are found in a stepwise fashion in the low, middle, and upper or proximal axillary zones. Several authors reported that discontinuous or skip metastases that do not follow this distribution were found in fewer than 2% of all patients or in fewer than 5% of patients with axillary nodal metastases.[193,508,509] Others have described skip metastases in 6%[510] to 29%[511] of patients with axillary nodal involvement.

Careful manual dissection of the unfixed axillary fat is the most cost-effective method for isolating the lymph nodes for microscopic study. In this process, firm bits of fat and other tissue may be mistaken for lymph nodes. Although the gross description should include a count of tissue samples thought to be lymph nodes, which were submitted for histologic study, the final number of nodes is determined from those counted in tissue sections. The overall character and dimensions of lymph nodes should be described. Metastases should not be described as grossly present or absent, because uncertainty arises when the results of microscopic study differ from the gross impression. Lymph nodes distorted by inflammation or hyperpla-

sia, or those enlarged by fatty infiltration, are a common cause for a false-positive interpretation on gross pathologic and clinical examination.

A number of other elaborate procedures are available to identify lymph nodes in the fat. These methods include obtaining radiographs of the fat[512,513]; fixing the fat in Bouin solution, which stains fat intensely yellow but leaves the lymph nodes white; and clearing the fat by a process that renders it relatively transparent, so that solid structures such as lymph nodes stand out when the tissue is placed over a light source.[514]

These procedures increase the yield of lymph nodes obtained by locating small lymph nodes that may be missed on palpation. In a study of 42 axillary dissections, the mean number of lymph nodes found was increased by clearing from 20 to 26 in patients with stage I disease, and from 22 to 30 in patients with stage II disease.[515] Additional positive lymph nodes were found in the latter group, but not in cases originally assigned to stage I on the basis of manually dissected nodes. Hartveit and coworkers[516] cleared axillary tissue from 63 node-negative cases and found one node containing a micrometastasis that had not been found by routine processing. Although incorrect staging may occasionally occur in a patient because a positive node was missed in manual dissection, the likelihood of this is so small that it does not justify the considerable time and expense required for clearing.

In addition to detecting metastatic carcinoma in axillary lymph nodes and establishing the level of involvement, histologic examination provides other information about the metastatic foci. The number of lymph nodes that contain metastases should be documented. Prognosis is significantly decreased as the number of affected lymph nodes increases. Patients are stratified in the following three categories: 1 to 3, 4 to 9, and 10 or more affected lymph nodes.

Several investigators have assessed the prognostic significance of the size of metastatic foci in axillary lymph nodes. In these studies, micrometastases were 2 mm or less in diameter and larger metastases were macrometastases.[517–519] Studies that did not take the number of involved lymph nodes or the size of the primary tumor into consideration[517–519] led to the conclusion that patients with macrometastases had a less favorable prognosis than those with micrometastases. It was further suggested that the prognosis of women with micrometastases did not differ significantly from that of women with negative lymph nodes.[518]

Analyses that evaluate the size of metastases and number of affected lymph nodes are difficult to perform and practical only when limited to patients with single nodal metastases classified as either a macrometastasis or micrometastasis. When analysis was done for patients with T1, N1 disease with a single nodal metastasis, the disease-free survival of patients with a micrometastasis was nearly identical with that of patients with a macrometastasis, and both had a significantly worse prognosis than patients with negative lymph nodes.[520] The patients with T2 disease and negative lymph nodes or a single micrometastasis had survival rates that did not differ significantly throughout the 10-year follow-up. Each of these groups had an outcome significantly better than patients with macrometastases.

The prognostic significance of the spread of metastatic carcinoma from a lymph node to the surrounding axillary tissues, so-called extranodal extension, is uncertain. It has been difficult to analyze this feature independently of other factors, such as the number of involved lymph nodes or the size of the primary tumor. Two retrospective studies reported that extranodal extension was prognostically unfavorable.[521,522] In a prospective analysis, Fisher and associates[523] found that extranodal extension was significantly more frequent in patients who had four or more lymph nodes with metastases. Patients with extranodal extension had a significantly higher frequency of short-term relapse, but the analysis did not demonstrate that the tendency to treatment failure was independent of the extent of nodal involvement.

A series of 308 node-positive patients treated by mastectomy, without adjuvant radiation or chemotherapy, with 10 years of follow-up was evaluated at the Milan National Cancer Institute.[524] Extracapsular extension of nodal metastases had no impact on prognosis when only one lymph node was involved. When two or more lymph nodes were affected, extracapsular extension was associated with a significantly higher recurrence rate. In the group with two or more nodal metastases, the unfavorable effect of extranodal extension was independent of the number of lymph nodes involved by tumor.

Detection of Micrometastases

Immunohistochemical markers have been used to detect metastatic carcinoma cells that were inapparent in routine histologic sections of lymph nodes. Sloane and associates[525] employed a polyclonal anti–epithelial membrane antigen (EMA) antibody for this purpose and found that the yield of occult metastases was similar in new serial sections of negative lymph nodes from 26 cases and in duplicate slides stained with anti-EMA. Subsequently, Wells and others[526] reported finding occult metastases in lymph nodes from 4 of 12 (33%) node-negative patients with invasive lobular carcinoma with a monoclonal anti-EMA antibody. A lower yield (3 of 33 or 9%) was obtained in cases of infiltrating duct carcinoma. Another study of nearly 1000 patients in which serial sectioning was performed on lymph nodes that had been classified as negative by routine examination revealed micrometastases in 9% of cases.[527] Factors associated with the detection of micrometastases by serial sectioning or immunohistochemical study were larger tumor size, poor differentiation, and lymphatic tumor emboli in the breast.[527,528]

Trojani and colleagues[529] applied a mixture of five monoclonal antibodies to histologic sections of lymph nodes reported to be negative for metastasis, from 150 consecutive patients with an average follow-up of 10 years. Overall, 21 patients (14%) were found to have micrometastases. The yield of positive lymph nodes was greater in patients with invasive lobular (38%) than in those with invasive duct (11%) carcinoma. The finding of occult micrometastases was not related to tumor grade or lymphatic tumor emboli. Among patients with invasive duct carcinoma, death caused by disease was significantly more frequent in the group with micrometastases (23%) than in those with immunohistochemically negative lymph nodes (6.3%). The presence of micrometastases detected in lymph nodes by immunohistochemical study did not have a significant effect on survival in patients with invasive lobular carcinoma.[530]

Another clinically important application of the immunohistochemical detection of micrometastases is in the study of bone marrow. In 1980, Sloane and coworkers[525] described the use of EMA to identify micrometastases in tissue sections of bone marrow, increasing the positive yield by 21%. The authors found that conjugates of alkaline phosphatase were preferable to horseradish peroxidase and were able to effectively block endogenous alkaline phosphatase with 20% acetic acid. The procedure also was effective for examining smears of bone marrow aspirates.[440] The EMA-positive cells were detected in 15 aspirates, but malignant cells were recognized in only 8 Giemsa-stained samples from the same aspirates. The EMA-positive cells were found in marrow aspirates from 9 of 24 (38%) patients with known bone marrow metastases, 4 of 20 (20%) with nonosseous systemic metastases, and 2 of 30 (7%) not known to have metastatic disease.

In a subsequent study, Coombes and colleagues[497] reported finding EMA-positive cells in bone marrow aspirates from 60 to 269 patients (23%) with no clinical or radiologic evidence of systemic metastatic breast carcinoma. There was a significant relation between detection of micrometastases, stage of the primary tumor, estrogen receptor–negative tumors, and vascular invasion. After a median follow-up of 22 months, patients with micrometastases had relapsed at a significantly faster rate than those with negative bone marrow. The rate of relapse also was significantly related to the number of tumor cells detected.

Ginsbourg and associates[531] studied bone marrow aspirates from 200 patients to detect occult micrometastases and to determine the proliferative activity in the metastatic cells. The proportion of epithelial cells with nuclear labeling (S-phase cells) was nearly identical, regardless of whether the patients had known metastatic disease or were disease-free. These results suggest that the proliferative rate of micrometastatic breast carcinoma cells in the bone marrow is not dependent on the clinical status of the patient.

Although the antibody to EMA reacts with epithelial tissues and neoplasms, heterogeneous staining is observed in tissue sections, and some epithelial cells are not reactive. This observation has led to concern that this reagent might not detect all tumor cells in marrow aspirates, thereby resulting in false-negative diagnoses. The possibility of employing two or more antibodies to create a reagent "cocktail" has been investigated as a method for reducing false-negative marrow aspirates. Cote and colleagues[532] combined monoclonal antibodies C26 and T16 (which react with surface glycoproteins), and AE-1 (which reacts with acidic cytokeratin antigens), using an immunofluorescent labeling system. When tested with MCF-7 cells, the assay was sensitive enough to detect 10 tumor cells in 10^6 marrow cells with no false-positive results in control specimens.[533] Extrinsic cells were found in bone marrow aspirates from 18 of 51 (35%) patients examined by the monoclonal antibody method, but none were seen when portions of the same specimens were studied by routine cytologic examination.[532] A positive bone marrow result, detected by immunofluorescence, tended to occur more frequently in patients who had axillary nodal metastases and a more advanced stage at diagnosis. The presence of bone marrow micrometastases was significantly associated with earlier and more frequent relapse. The multiple monoclonal antibody cocktail has been adapted to the immunoalkaline phosphatase procedure[534] and proved capable of detecting one carcinoma cell among 1×10^5 bone marrow cells.[535] By using this method, one group of investigators reported finding tumor cells in the bone marrow of 18% of breast cancer patients.[536] The finding of tumor cells in the bone marrow was not significantly related to tumor size or axillary lymph node status. These authors also demonstrated that cells were labeled in vivo in the bone marrow by infusing an antibody, and subsequently, examining samples of bone marrow to detect antibody-labeled cells.

Immunohistochemical methods for detecting occult carcinoma cells may soon be replaced by molecular procedures. In one study, the reverse transcriptase polymerase chain reaction for cytokeratin 19 proved to be a sensitive method for detecting occult carcinoma cells in the peripheral blood and bone marrow.[537]

References

1. Rosen PP. The pathological classification of human mammary carcinoma: past, present and future. Ann Clin Lab Sci 1979;9:144.
2. Tulinius H, Bjarnason O, Sigvaldason H, et al. Tumours in Iceland. 10. Malignant tumours of the female breast: a histological classification, laterality, survival and epidemiological considerations. Acta Pathol Microbiol Immunol Scand 1988;96:229.
3. World Health Organization. Histological typing of breast tumours. In: International histological classification of tumours, ed 2. Geneva, World Health Organization, 1981:19.
4. Fisher ER, Gregorio RM, Fisher B, et al. The pathology of invasive breast cancer: a syllabus derived from findings of the National Surgical Adjuvant Breast Project (protocol no. 4). Cancer 1975;36:1.
5. Page DL, Dixon JM, Anderson TJ, et al. Invasive cribriform carcinoma of the breast. Histopathology 1983;7:525.
6. Wells CA, Ferguson DJP. Ultrastructural and immunocytochemical study of a case of invasive cribriform breast carcinoma. J Clin Pathol 1988;41:17.
7. Sistrunk WE, MacCarty WC. Life expectancy following radical amputation for carcinoma of the breast: a clinical and pathologic study of 218 cases. Ann Surg 1922;75:61.
8. Stenkvist B, Bengtsson E, Dahlqvist B, et al. Predicting breast cancer recurrence. Cancer 1982;50:2884.
9. Freedman LS, Edwards DN, McConnell EM, et al. Histological grade and other prognostic factors in relation to survival of patients with breast cancer. Br J Cancer 1979;40:44.
10. Smart CR, Myers MH, Gloecker LA. Implications for SEER data on breast cancer management. Cancer 1978;41:787.
11. Adair F, Berg J, Joubert L, et al. Long-term follow-up of breast cancer patients: the 30 year report. Cancer 1974;33:1145.
12. Fisher B, Slack NH, Bross ID. Cancer of the breast: size of neoplasm and prognosis. Cancer 1969;24:1071.
13. Say CC, Donegan WL. Invasive carcinoma of the breast: prognostic significance of tumor size and involved axillary lymph nodes. Cancer 1974;34:468.
14. Roger V, Beito G, Jolly PC. Factors affecting the incidence of lymph node metastases in small cancers of the breast. Am J Surg 1989;157:501.
15. Rosen PP, Saigo PE, Braun DW Jr, et al. Predictors of recurrence in stage I ($T_1N_0M_0$) breast carcinoma. Ann Surg 1981;193:15.
16. Rosen PP, Saigo PE, Braun DW Jr, et al. Prognosis in stage II ($T_1N_1M_0$) breast cancer. Ann Surg 1981;194:576.
17. Gold RH, Main G, Zippin C, et al. Infiltration of mammary carcinoma as an indicator of axillary metastases: a preliminary report. Cancer 1972;29:35.
18. Lane N, Giksel H, Salerno RA. Clinicopathologic analyses of the surgical curability of breast cancers: a minimum ten-year study. Ann Surg 1961;153:483.
19. Carter D, Pipkin RD, Shepard RH, et al. Relationship of necrosis and tumor border to lymph node metastases and 10 year survival in carcinoma of the breast. Am J Surg Pathol 1978;2:39.
20. Black MM, Speer FD. Nuclear structure in cancer tissues. Surg Gynecol Obstet 1957;105:97.
21. Cutler SJ, Black MM, Mork T, et al. Further observations on prognostic factors in cancer of the female breast. Cancer 1969;24:653.
22. Bloom HJG. Prognosis in carcinoma of the breast. Br J Cancer 1950;4:259.
23. Bloom HJG, Richardson WW. Histological grading and prognosis in breast cancer: a study of 1049 cases, of which 359 have been followed 15 years. Br J Cancer 1957;11:359.
24. Thoresen S. Histological grading and clinical stage at presentation in breast carcinoma. Br J Cancer 1982;46:457.
25. Andersen JA, Fischermann K, Hou-Jensen K, et al. Selection of high risk groups among prognostically favorable patients with breast cancer. An analysis of the value of prospective grading of tumor anaplasia in 1048 patients. Ann Surg 1981;194:1.
26. Parl FF, Dupont WD. A retrospective cohort study of histologic risk factors in breast cancer patients. Cancer 1982;50:2410.
27. Black MM, Barclay THC, Hankey BF. Prognosis in breast cancer utilizing histologic characteristics of the primary tumor. Cancer 1975;36:2048.
28. Fisher B, Redmond C, Fisher ER, et al. Relative worth of estrogen or progesterone receptor and pathologic characteristics of differentiation as indicators of prognosis in node negative breast cancer patients: findings from National Surgical Adjuvant Breast and Bowel Project Protocol B-06. J Clin Oncol 1988;6:1076.
29. Henson DE. The histological grading of neoplasms. Arch Pathol Lab Med 1988;112:1091.
30. Hopton DS, Thorogood J, Clayden AD, et al. Histological grading of breast cancer: significance of grade on recurrence and mortality. Eur J Surg Oncol 1989;15:25.
31. Bauer TW, O'Cealleigh D, Eggelston JC, et al. Prognostic factors in patients with stage I, estrogen receptor-negative carcinoma of the breast: a clinicopathologic study. Cancer 1983;52:1423.
32. Dawson PJ, Ferguson DJ, Karrison T. The pathologic findings of breast cancer in patients surviving 25 years after radical mastectomy. Cancer 1982;50:2131.
33. LeDoussal V, Tubiana-Hulin M, Friedman S, et al. Prognostic value of histologic grade/nuclear components of Scarff-Bloom-Richardson (SBR): an improved score modification based on a

multivariate analysis of 1262 invasive ductal carcinomas. Cancer 1989;64:1914.

34. Kister SJ, Sommers SC, Haagenson CD, et al. Nuclear grade and sinus histiocytosis in cancer of the breast. Cancer 1969;23:570.

35. Davis BW, Gelber RD, Goldhirsch A, et al. Prognostic significance of tumor grade in clinical trials of adjuvant therapy for breast cancer with axillary nodal metastases. Cancer 1986;58:2662.

36. Masters JRW, Millis RR, Rubens RD. Response to endocrine therapy and breast cancer differentiation. Breast Cancer Res Treat 1986;7:31.

37. Williams MR, Blamey RW, Todd JH, et al. Histological grade in predicting response to endocrine treatment. Breast Cancer Res Treat 1986;8:165.

38. Ridolfi R, Rosen PP, Port A, et al. Medullary carcinoma of the breast: a clinicopathologic study with 10 year follow-up. Cancer 1977;40:1365.

39. Rosen PP, Lesser ML, Kinne DW, et al. Breast carcinoma in women 35 years or younger. Ann Surg 1984;199:133.

40. Alderson MR, Hamlin I, Staunton MD. The relative significance of prognostic factors in breast carcinoma. Br J Cancer 1971;25:646.

41. Berg JW. Morphological evidence for immune response to cancer: an historical review. Cancer 1971;28:1453.

42. Roses DF, Bell DA, Flotte TJ, et al. Pathologic predictors of recurrence in stage 1 (T1N0M0) breast cancer. Am J Clin Pathol 1982;78:817.

43. Horny H-P, Horst H-A. Lymphoreticular infiltrates in invasive ductal breast cancer: a histological and immunohistological study. Virchows Arch 1986;409:275.

44. Whiteside TL, Miescher S, Hurlimann J, et al. Clonal analysis and *in situ* characterization of lymphocytes infiltrating human breast carcinomas. Cancer Immunol Immunother 1986;23:169.

45. Bilik R, Mor C, Haraz B, et al. Characterization of T-lymphocyte subpopulations infiltrating breast cancer. Cancer Immunol Immunother 1989;28:143.

46. Fisher ER, Sass R, Watkins G, et al. Tissue mast cells in breast cancer. Breast Cancer Res Treat 1985;5:285.

47. Gilchrist KW, Gould VE, Hirschl S. Interobserver variation in the identification of breast carcinoma in intramammary lymphatics. Hum Pathol 1982;13:170.

48. Rosen PP. Tumor emboli in intramammary lymphatics in breast carcinoma: pathologic criteria for diagnosis and clinical significance. Pathol Annu 1983;18:215.

49. Bettelheim R, Mitchell D, Gusterson BA. Immunocytochemistry in the identification of vascular invasion in breast cancer. J Clin Pathol 1984;37:364.

50. Saigo PE, Rosen PP. The application of immunohistochemical stains to identify endothelial-lined channels in mammary carcinoma. Cancer 1987;59:51.

51. Lee AKC, DeLellis RA, Wolfe HJ. Intramammary lymphatic invasion in breast carcinomas: evaluation using ABH isoantigens as endothelial markers. Am J Surg Pathol 1986;10:589.

52. Ordonez NG, Brooks T, Thompson S, et al. Use of *Ulex Europaeus* agglutinin I in the identification of lymphatic and blood vessel invasion in previously stained microscopic slides. Am J Surg Pathol 1987;11:543.

53. Nime F, Rosen PP, Thaler H, et al. Prognostic significance of tumor emboli in intramammary lymphatics in patients with mammary carcinoma. Am J Surg Pathol 1977;1:25.

54. Fracchia AA, Rosen PP, Ashikari R. Primary carcinoma of the breast without axillary lymph node metastases. Surg Gynecol Obstet 1980;151:375.

55. Merlin C, Gloor F, Hardmeier T, et al. Hat die intrammarare lymphangiosis Carcinomatosa bein nodel-negativen Mammakarziom eine prognostische Bedeutung? Schweiz Med Wochenschr 1980;110:605.

56. Bettelheim R, Penman HG, Thornton-Jones H, et al. Prognostic

significance of peritumoral vascular invasion in breast cancer. Br J Cancer 1984;50:771.

57. Rosen PP, Saigo PE, Braun DW Jr, et al. Occult axillary lymph node metastases from breast cancers with intramammary lymphatic tumor emboli. Am J Surg Pathol 1982;6:639.

58. Rosen PP, Groshen S, Saigo PE, et al. Pathologic prognostic factors in stage I ($T_1N_0M_0$) and stage II ($T_2N_1M_0$) breast carcinoma: a study of 644 patients with median follow-up of 18 years. J Clin Oncol 1989;7:1239.

59. Fisher ER, Sass R, Fisher B. Pathologic findings from the National Surgical Adjuvant Project for breast cancers (protocol no. 4). X. Discriminants of tenth year treatment failure. Cancer 1984;53:712.

60. Davis BW, Gelber R, Goldhirsch A, et al. Prognostic significance of peritumoral vessel invasion in clinical trials of adjuvant therapy for breast cancer with axillary lymph node metastases. Hum Pathol 1985;16:1212.

61. Sampat MB, Sirsat MV, Gangadharan P. Prognostic significance of blood vessel invasion in carcinoma of the breast in women. J Surg Oncol 1977;9:623.

62. Teel P, Sommers SC. Vascular invasion as a prognostic factor in breast carcinoma. Surg Gynecol Obstet 1964;118:1006.

63. Kister SJ, Sommers SC, Haagensen CD, et al. Reevaluation of blood vessel invasion and lymphocytic infiltrates in breast carcinoma. Cancer 1966;19:1213.

64. Weigand RA, Isenberg WM, Russo J, et al. Blood vessel invasion and axillary lymph node involvement as prognostic indicators for human breast cancer. Cancer 1982;50:962.

65. Friedell GH, Betts A, Sommers SC. Prognostic value of blood vessel invasion and lymphocytic infiltrates in breast carcinoma. Cancer 1965;18:164.

66. Bell JR, Friedell GH, Goldenberg IS. Prognostic significance of pathologic findings in human breast carcinoma. Surg Gynecol Obstet 1969;129:258.

67. Sato E, Kumagai N, Abe R. Significant prognostic factors in breast cancer of Japanese women: special reference to nuclear grade and sinus histiocytosis. Tohoku J Exp Med 1976;120:135.

68. Folkman J. Tumor angiogenesis: therapeutic implications. N Engl J Med 1971;285:1182.

69. Folkman J. What is the evidence that tumors are angiogenesis dependent? J Natl Cancer Inst 1990;82:4.

70. Brem SS, Jensen HM, Gullino PM. Angiogenesis as a marker of preneoplastic lesions of the human breast. Cancer 1978;41:239.

71. Jensen HM, Chen I, DeVault MR, et al. Angiogenesis induced by "normal" human breast tissue: a probable marker for precancer. Science 1982;218:293.

72. Folkman J, Watson K, Ingber D, et al. Induction of angiogenesis during the transition from hyperplasia to neoplasia. Nature 1989;339:58.

73. Kim KJ, Li B, Winer J, et al. Inhibition of vascular endothelial growth factor-induced angiogenesis suppresses tumour growth in vivo. Nature 1993;362:841.

74. Hori A, Sasada R, Matsutani E, et al. Suppression of solid tumor growth by immunoneutralizing monoclonal antibody against human basic fibroblast growth factor. Cancer Res 1991;51:6180.

75. Rastinejad F, Polverini P, Bouck NP. Regulation of the activity of a new inhibitor of angiogenesis by a cancer suppressor gene. Cell 1989;56:345.

76. Bouck NP. Tumor angiogenesis: the role of oncogenes and tumor suppressor genes. Cancer Cells 1990;2:179.

77. Gasparini G, Weidner N, Bevilaqua P, et al. Tumor microvessel density, p53 expression, tumor size, and peritumoral lymphatic vessel invasion are relevant prognostic markers in node-negative breast carcinoma. J Clin Oncol 1994;12:454.

78. Weidner N, Semple JP, Welch WR, et al. Tumor angiogenesis and metastasis-correlation in invasive breast cancer. N Engl J Med 1991;324:1.

79. Harris AL, Horak E. Growth factors and angiogenesis in breast cancer: recent results. Cancer Res 1993;127:35.

80. van Hoef MEHM, Knox WF, Dhesi SS, et al. Assessment of tumour vascularity as a prognostic factor in lymph node negative invasive breast cancer. Eur J Cancer 1993;29A:1141.

81. Toi M, Kashitani J, Tominaga T. Tumor angiogenesis is an independent prognostic indicator in primary breast carcinoma. Int J Cancer 1993;55:371.

82. Sightler HE, Borowsky AD, Dupont WD, et al. Evaluation of tumor angiogenesis as a prognostic marker in breast cancer. Lab Invest 1994;70:22A.

83. Cohen P, Guidi A, Harris J, et al. Microvessel density and local recurrence in patients with early stage breast cancer treated by wide excision above (WEA). Lab Invest 1994;70:14A.

84. Davies JD. Hyperelastosis, obliteration and fibrous plaques in major ducts of the human breast. J Pathol 1973;110:13.

85. Reyes MG, Bazile DB, Tosch T, et al. Periductal elastic tissue of breast cancer. Arch Pathol Lab Med 1982;106:610.

86. Humeniuk V, Forrest APM, Hawkins RA, et al. Elastosis and primary breast cancer. Cancer 1983;52:1448.

87. Masters JRW, Sangster K, Hawkins RA, et al. Elastosis and estrogen receptors in human breast cancer. Br J Cancer 1976;33:342.

88. Rasmussen BB, Pedersen BV, Thorpe SM, et al. Elastosis in relation to prognosis in primary breast carcinoma. Cancer Res 1985;45:1428.

89. Shivas AA, Douglas JG. The prognostic significance of elastosis in breast carcinoma. J R Coll Surg Edinb 1972;17:315.

90. Tamura S, Enjoji M. Elastosis in neoplastic and non-neoplastic tissues from patients with mammary carcinoma. Acta Pathol Jpn 1988;38:1537.

91. Anastassiades OT, Bouropoulou V, Kontogeorgos G, et al. Duct elastosis in infiltrating carcinoma of the breast. Pathol Res Pract 1979;165:411.

92. Glaubitz LC, Bowen JH, Cox ED, et al. Elastosis in human breast cancer. Correlation with sex steroid receptors and comparison with clinical outcome. Arch Pathol Lab Med 1984;108:27.

93. Silverberg SG, Chitale AR. Assessment of significance of proportions of intraductal and infiltrating tumor growth in ductal carcinoma of the breast. Cancer 1978;32:830.

94. Schnitt SJ, Connolly JL, Harris JR, et al. Pathologic predictors of early local recurrences in stage I and II breast cancer treated by primary radiation therapy. Cancer 1984;53:1049.

95. Mansour EG, Hastert M, Park CH, et al. Tissue and plasma antigen in early breast cancer: a prognostic factor. Cancer 1983;51:1243.

96. Gilchrist KW, Kalish L, Gould VE, et al. Immunostaining for carcinoembryonic antigen does not discriminate for early recurrence in breast cancer: the ECOG experience. Cancer 1985;56:351.

97. Halter SA, Fraker LD, Parmenter M, et al. Carcinoembryonic antigen expression and patient survival in carcinoma of the breast. Oncology 1984;41:297.

98. Horne CHW, Reid IN, Milne GD. Prognostic significance of inappropriate production of pregnancy proteins by breast cancers. Lancet 1976;2:279.

99. Robertson JFR, Ellis IO, Bell J, et al. Carcinoembryonic antigen immunohistochemistry in primary breast carcinoma. Cancer 1989;64:1638.

100. Smith SR, Howell A, Minawa A, et al. The clinical value of immunohistochemically demonstrable CEA in breast cancer: a possible method of selecting patients for adjuvant chemotherapy. Br J Cancer 1982;46:757.

101. Walker RA. Immunohistochemistry of biologic markers of breast carcinoma. In: DeLellis RA, ed. Advances in Immunohistochemistry. New York, Masson, 1984:223.

102. Walker RA. Demonstration of carcinoembryonic antigen in human breast carcinomas by the immunoperoxidase technique. J Clin Pathol 1980;33:356.

103. Bartek J, Tlaskalova-Hogenova H, Staskova Z, et al. Secretory component in differentiating normal epithelium, benign lesions and malignancy in the human breast as monitored by monoclonal antibodies. Histochemistry 1989;91:235.

104. Le Doussal V, Zangerle PF, Collette J, et al. Immunohistochemical detection of alpha-lactalbumin in breast lesions. Eur J Cancer Clin Oncol 1984;20:1069.

105. Bergeron C, Shatz P, Margolese R, et al. Immunohistochemical studies with monoclonal antibodies B72.3 and MH5 on histologic and cytologic specimens from benign and malignant breast lesions. Anal Quant Cytol Histol 1989;11:33.

106. Castagna M, Nuti M, Squartini F. Mammary cancer antigen recognized by monoclonal antibody B72.3 in apocrine metaplasia of the human breast. Cancer Res 1987;47:902.

107. Johnston WW, Szpak CA, Lottich SC, et al. Use of monoclonal antibody (B72.3) as a novel immunohistochemical adjunct for the diagnosis of carcinoma in fine needle aspirate biopsy specimens. Hum Pathol 1986;17:501.

108. Kline TS, Lundy J, Lozowski M. Monoclonal antibody B72.3: an adjunct for evaluation of suspicious aspiration biopsy cytology from the breast. Cancer 1989;63:2253.

109. Lundy J, Lozowski M, Mishriki Y. Immunocytochemistry with monoclonal antibody B72.3 applied to a spectrum of benign and malignant breast aspirates: strengths and pitfalls. Breast Cancer Res Treat 1988;12:259.

110. Nuti M, Teramoto YA, Mariani-Costantini R, et al. A monoclonal antibody (B72.3) defines patterns of distribution of a novel tumor-associated antigen in mammary carcinoma cell populations. Int J Cancer (Denmark) 1982;29:539.

111. Szpak CA, Johnston WW, Lottich C, et al. Patterns of reactivity of four novel monoclonal antibodies (B72.3, Df3, B1.1, B6.2) with cells in human malignant and benign effusions. Acta Cytol 1984;28:356.

112. Thor A, Ohuchi N, Szpak CA, et al. Distribution of oncofetal antigenic tumor-associated glycoprotein-72 defined by monoclonal antibody B72.3. Cancer Res 1986;46:3118.

113. Wick MR, Lillemoe TJ, Copland GT, et al. Gross cystic disease fluid protein-15 as a marker for breast cancer: immunohistochemical analysis of 690 human neoplasms and comparison with alpha-lactalbumin. Hum Pathol 1989;20:281.

114. Wachner R, Wittekind C, von Kleists S. Immunohistological localization of β-HCG in breast carcinomas. Eur J Cancer Clin Oncol 1984;20:679.

115. Kuhajda FP, Offutt LE, Mendelsohn G. The distribution of carcinoembryonic antigen in breast carcinoma. Cancer 1983;52:1257.

116. Shousa S, Lysiottis T, Godfrey VM, et al. Carcinoembryonic antigen in breast cancer tissue: a useful prognostic indicator. Br Med J 1979;1:777.

117. Grudzas Kas TG, Coombes RC, Ratcliffe JG, et al. Circulating levels of pregnancy specific β 1 glycoprotein in patients with testicular, bronchogenic and breast carcinomas. Cancer 1990;45:102.

118. Walker RA. Differentiation of human breast carcinomas: an immunohistological study of appropriate and inappropriate protein production. J Pathol 1981;135:87.

119. Dwarakanath S, Lee AKC, DeLellis RA, et al. S-100 protein sensitivity in breast carcinomas: a potential pitfall in diagnostic immunohistochemistry. Hum Pathol 1987;18:1144.

120. Nakajima T, Watanabe S, Sato Y, et al. An immunoperoxidase study of S-100 protein distribution in normal and neoplastic tissues. Am J Surg Pathol 1982;6:715.

121. Harris JP, South M. Immunohistochemical localization of secretory component in neoplastic disease. In: DeLellis RA, ed. Advances in Immunohistochemistry. New York, Masson Publishing, 1984:243.

122. Brooks JJ, Ernst CC. Immunoreactive secretory component of IgA in human tissues and tumors. Am J Clin Pathol 1984;82:660.

123. Azumi N, Battifora J. The distribution of vimentin and keratin in epithelial and nonepithelial neoplasms. Am J Clin Pathol 1987; 88:286.

124. Gould VE. Histogenesis and differentiation: a reevaluation of these concepts as criteria for the classification of tumors. Hum Pathol 1986;17:212.

125. Raymond WA, Leong AS-Y. Co-expression of cytokeratin and vimentin intermediate filament proteins in benign and neoplastic breast epithelium. J Pathol 1989;157:299.

126. Raymond WA, Leong AS-Y. Vimentin: a new prognostic parameter in breast carcinoma. J Pathol 1989;158:107.

127. Cornil V, Ranvier L. In: Manuel d'histologie pathologique. Paris, Germer Bailliere, 1869;1167.

128. Foote FW Jr. Surgical pathology of cancer of the breast. In: Parsons WH, ed. Cancer of the Breast. Springfield, Charles C Thomas, 1959;37.

129. Taylor HB, Norris HJ. Well-differentiated carcinoma of the breast. Cancer 1970;25:687.

130. Kouchoukos NT, Ackerman LV, Butcher HR. Prediction of axillary nodal metastases from the morphology of primary mammary carcinomas. Cancer 1967;20:948.

131. Carstens PHB. Tubular carcinoma of the breast: a study of frequency. Am J Clin Pathol 1978;70:204.

132. Cooper HS, Patchefsky AS, Krall RA. Tubular carcinoma of the breast. Cancer 1978;42:2334.

133. Peters GN, Wolff M, Haagensen CD. Tubular carcinoma of the breast: clinical pathologic correlations based on 100 cases. Ann Surg 1981;193:138.

134. Deos PH, Norris HJ. Well-differentiated (tubular) carcinoma of the breast. Am J Clin Pathol 1982;78:1.

135. Oberman HA, Fidler WJ Jr. Tubular carcinoma of the breast. Am J Surg Pathol 1979;13:387.

136. McDivitt RW, Boyce W, Gersell D. Tubular carcinoma of the breast: clinical and pathological observations concerning 135 cases. Am J Surg Pathol 1982;6:401.

137. Carstens PHB, Greenberg RA, Francis D, et al. Tubular carcinoma of the breast: a long-term follow-up. Histopathology 1985;9:271.

138. Beahrs O, Shapiro S, Smart C. Report of the working group to review the National Cancer Institute: American Cancer Society Breast Cancer Detection Demonstration Projects. J Natl Cancer Inst 1979;62:640.

139. Feig SA, Shaber GS, Patchefsky A, et al. Analysis of clinically occult and mammographically occult breast tumors. AJR 1977;128:403.

140. Andersson I. Radiographic screening for breast carcinoma. II. Prognostic considerations on the basis of short-term follow-up. Acta Radiol 1982;22:227.

141. Linell F, Ljungberg O. Breast carcinoma, progression of tubular carcinoma and a new classification. Acta Pathol Microbiol Immunol Scand 1980;88:59.

142. Linell F, Ljungberg O, Andersson I. Breast carcinoma. Aspects of early stages, progression and related problems. Acta Pathol Microbiol Immunol Scand 1980;272(Suppl):1.

143. Andersen JA, Carter D, Linell F. A symposium on sclerosing duct lesions of the breast. Pathol Annu 1986;21:145.

144. Wellings SR, Alpers CE. Subgross pathologic features and incidence of radial scars in the breast. Hum Pathol 1984;15:475.

145. Taxy JB. Tubular carcinoma of the male breast: report of a case. Cancer 1975;36:462.

146. Heller KS, Rosen PP, Schottenfeld D, et al. Male breast cancer: a clinicopathologic study of 97 cases. Ann Surg 1978;188:60.

147. Norris HJ, Taylor HB. Carcinoma of the male breast. Cancer 1969;23:1428.

148. Lagios MD, Rose MR, Margolin FR. Tubular carcinoma of the breast: association with multicentricity, bilaterality and family history of mammary carcinoma. Am J Clin Pathol 1980;73:25.

149. Eggor H, Dressler W. A contribution to the natural history of breast cancer. 1. Duct obliteration with periductal elastosis in the centre of breast cancers. Arch Gynecol 1982;231:191.

150. Tremblay G. Elastosis in tubular carcinoma of the breast. Arch Pathol Lab Med 1974;98:302.

151. Carstens PHB, Huvos AG, Foote FW Jr, et al. Tubular carcinoma of the breast: a clinicopathologic study of 35 cases. Am J Clin Pathol 1972;58:231.

152. Eusebi V, Betts CM, Bussolati G. Tubular carcinoma: a variant of secretory breast carcinoma. Histopathology 1979;3:407.

153. Haagensen CD. In: *Diseases of the breast,* ed 2. Philadelphia, WB Saunders, 1971:177.

154. Ekblom P, Miettinen M, Forsman L, et al. Basement membrane and apocrine epithelial antigens in differential diagnosis between tubular carcinoma and sclerosing adenosis of the breast. J Clin Pathol 1984;37:357.

155. Flotte TJ, Bell DA, Greco MA. Tubular carcinoma and sclerosing adenosis: the use of basal lamina as a differential feature. Am J Surg Pathol 1980;4:75.

156. Erlandson RA, Carstens PHB. Ultrastructure of tubular carcinoma of the breast. Cancer 1972;29:987.

157. Harris M, Ahmed A. The ultrastructure of tubular carcinoma of the breast. J Pathol 1977;123:79.

158. Rosen PP. Microglandular adenosis: a benign lesion simulating invasive mammary carcinoma. Am J Surg Pathol 1983;7:137.

159. Lesser ML, Rosen PP, Kinne DW. Multicentricity and bilaterality in invasive breast carcinoma. Surgery 1982;1:234.

160. Bondeson L, Lindholm K. Aspiration cytology of tubular breast carcinoma. Acta Cytol 1990;34:15.

161. Masood S, Barwick KW. Estrogen receptor expression of the less common breast carcinomas. Am J Clin Pathol 1990;93:437.

162. Foote FW Jr, Stewart FW. A histologic classification of carcinoma of the breast. Surgery 1946;19:74.

163. Moore OS Jr, Foote FW Jr. The relatively favorable prognosis of medullary carcinoma of the breast. Cancer 1949;2:635.

164. Haagensen CD. Circumscribed carcinoma. In: Diseases of the breast, ed 2. Philadelphia, WB Saunders, 1971:570.

165. Schwartz GF. Solid circumscribed carcinoma of the breast. Ann Surg 1969;169:165.

166. Bloom HJG, Richardson WW, Fields JR. Host resistance and survival in carcinoma of breast: a study of 104 cases of medullary carcinoma in a series of 1511 cases of breast cancer followed for 20 years. Br Med J 1970;3:181.

167. Maier WP, Rosemond GP, Goldman LI, et al. A ten-year study of medullary carcinoma of the breast. Surg Gynecol Obstet 1977;144:695.

168. Richardson WW. Medullary carcinoma of the breast: a distinctive tumor type with a relatively good prognosis following radical mastectomy. Br J Cancer 1956;10:415.

169. Rosen PP, Lesser ML, Senie RT, et al. Epidemiology of breast carcinoma. IV: Age and histologic tumor type. J Surg Oncol 1982;19:44.

170. Rosen PP, Lesser ML, Kinne DW. Breast carcinoma at the extremes of age: a comparison of patients younger than 35 years and older than 75 years. J Surg Oncol 1985;28:90.

171. Geschickter CF. In: Diseases of the breast: diagnosis, pathology, treatment, ed 2. Philadelphia, JB Lippincott, 1945:565.

172. Meyer JE, Amin E, Lindfors KK, et al. Medullary carcinoma of the breast: mammographic and US appearance. Radiology 1989; 170:79.

173. Haupt HM, Rosen PP, Kinne DW. Breast carcinoma presenting with axillary lymph node metastasis: an analysis of specific histopathologic features. Am J Surg Pathol 1985;9:165.

174. Rapin V, Contesso G, Mouriesse H, et al. Medullary carcinoma: a

reevaluation of 95 cases of breast cancer with inflammatory stroma. Cancer 1988;61:2503.

175. Rosen PP, Menendez-Botet CJ, Nisselbaum JS, et al. Pathological review of breast lesions analyzed for estrogen receptor protein. Cancer Res 1975;35:3187.

176. Ponsky JL, Gliga L, Reynolds S. Medullary carcinoma of the breast: an association with negative hormonal receptors. J Surg Oncol 1984;25:76.

177. Reiner A, Reiner G, Spona J, et al. Histopathologic characterization of human breast cancer in correlation with estrogen receptor status: a comparison of immunocytochemical and biochemical analysis. Cancer 1988;61:1149.

178. Stegner HE, Jonat W, Maass H. Immunohistochemicher Nachweis nuklearer Ostrogenrezeptoren mit monoclonalen Antikorpern in verschiednen Typen des Mammakarzinoms. Pathologe 1986; 7:156.

179. Patel JK, Nemoto T, Dao TL. Is medullary carcinoma of the breast hormone dependent? J Surg Oncol 1983;24:290.

180. Pedersen L, Holck S, Schiodt J. Medullary carcinoma of the breast. Cancer Treat Rev 1988;15:53.

181. Wargotz ES, Silverberg SG. Medullary carcinoma of the breast: a clinicopathologic study with appraisal of current diagnostic criteria. Hum Pathol 1988;19:1340.

182. Fisher ER. Ultrastructure of human breast and its disorders. Am J Clin Pathol 1976;66:291.

183. Ahmed A. The ultrastructure of medullary carcinoma of the breast. Virchows Arch 1980;388:175.

184. Gould VE, Miller J, Jao W. Ultrastructure of medullary intraductal, tubular and adenocystic breast carcinomas. Am J Clin Pathol 1975;78:401.

185. Harris M, Lessells MM. The ultrastructure of medullary, atypical medullary and non-medullary carcinomas of the breast. Histopathology 1986;10:405.

186. Ito T, Saga S, Nagayoshi W, et al. Class distribution of immunoglobulin-containing plasma cells in the stroma of medullary carcinoma of breast. Breast Cancer Res Treat 1986;7:97.

187. Sieinski W. Immunohistological patterns of immunoglobulins in dysplasia, benign neoplasms and carcinomas of the breast. Tumori 1980;66:699.

188. Hsu SM, Raine L, Nayak RN. Medullary carcinoma of breast: an immunohistochemical study of its lymphoid stroma. Cancer 1981;48:1368.

189. Jacquemier J, Robert-Vague D, Torrente M, et al. Mise en evidence des immunoglobulines lymphoplasmocytaires et epitheliales dans les carcinomes infiltrants a stroma lymphoid et les carcinomes medullaries du sein. Arch Anat Cytol Pathol 1983;31:296.

190. Yazawa T, Kamma H, Ogata T. Frequent expression of HLA-DR antigen in medullary carcinoma of the breast: a possible reason for its prominent lymphocytic infiltration and favorable prognosis. Appl Immunohistochem 1993;1:289.

191. Black CL, Morris DM, Goldman LI, et al. The significance of lymph node involvement in patients with medullary carcinoma of the breast. Surg Gynecol Obstet 1983;157:497.

192. Rosen PP, Groshen S, Saigo PE, et al. A long-term follow-up study of survival in stage I ($T_1N_0M_0$) and stage II ($T_1N_1M_0$) breast carcinoma. J Clin Oncol 1989;7:355.

193. Rosen PP, Lesser ML, Kinne DW, et al. Discontinuous or "skip" metastases in breast carcinoma. Ann Surg 1983;197:276.

194. Robinson RR. Gelatinous cancer of the breast. Trans Pathol Soc London 1852;4:275.

195. Lange F. Der Gallertkrebs der Brustdruse. Beitr Klin Chir 1896;16:1.

196. Larey M. Tumeur gelatiniforme ou colloide de la mamelle. Bull Soc Chir Paris 1853;3:545.

197. Geschickter CF. Gelatinous carcinoma of the breast. Arch Surg 1930;20:568.

198. Cheatle GL, Cutler M. Gelatinous carcinoma of the breast. Arch Surg 1930;20:568.

199. Lee BJ, Hauser H, Pack GT. Gelatinous carcinoma of the breast. Surg Gynecol Obstet 1934;59:841.

200. Rosen PP, Wang T-Y. Colloid carcinoma of the breast analysis of 64 patients with long-term follow-up. Am J Clin Pathol 1980; 73:30.

201. Veronesi U, Gennari L. Il carcinoma gelatinoso della mammella. Tumori 1960;46:119.

202. Haagensen CD. Secretory carcinomas of the breast. In: Diseases of the breast, ed 3. Philadelphia, WB Saunders, 1986:798.

203. Berg JW, Robbins GF. The histologic epidemiology of breast cancer. In: Breast cancer early and late. Chicago, Year Book, 1970:21.

204. Saphir O. Mucinous carcinoma of breast. Surg Gynecol Obstet 1941;72:908.

205. Melamed MR, Robbins GF, Foote FW Jr. Prognostic significance of gelatinous mammary carcinoma. Cancer 1961;14:699.

206. Silverberg SG, Kay S, Chitale AR. Colloid carcinoma of the breast. Am J Clin Pathol 1971;55:355.

207. Lesser ML, Rosen PP, Senie RT, et al. Estrogen and progesterone receptors in breast carcinoma: correlations with epidemiology and pathology. Cancer 1981;48:229.

208. Rosen PP, Menendez-Botet CJ, Senie RT, et al. Estrogen in receptor protein (ERP) and the histopathology of human mammary carcinoma. In: McGuire WL, ed. Hormones, receptors and breast cancer. New York, Raven Press, 1978:71.

209. Toikkanen S, Eerola E, Ekfors TO. Pure and mixed mucinous breast carcinomas: DNA stemline and prognosis. J Clin Pathol 1988;41:300.

210. Wulsin JH, Schreiber JT. Improved prognosis in certain patterns of carcinoma of the breast. Arch Surg 1962;85:791.

211. Rasmussen BB, Rose C, Christensen I. Prognostic factors in primary mucinous breast carcinoma. Am J Clin Pathol 1987;87:155.

212. Komaki K, Sakamoto G, Sugano H, et al. Mucinous carcinoma of the breast in Japan: a prognostic analysis based on morphologic features. Cancer 1988;61:989.

213. Steinbrecher JS, Silverberg SG. Signet ring cell carcinoma of the breast: the mucinous variant of infiltrating lobular carcinoma. Cancer 1976;37:828.

214. Jao W, Lau IO, Chowdhury LN, et al. Ultrastructural aspects of mucinous (colloid) breast carcinoma. Diagn Gynecol Obstet 1980; 2:83.

215. Harris M, Vasudev KS, Anfield C, et al. Mucin producing carcinomas of the breast: ultrastructural observations. Histopathology 1978;2:177.

216. Walker RA. Mucoid carcinomas of the breast: a study using mucin histochemistry and peanut lectin. Histopathology 1982;6:571.

217. Tellem M, Nedwick A, Amenta PS, et al. Mucin-producing carcinoma of the breast: tissue culture, histochemical and electron microscopic study. Cancer 1966;19:573.

218. Capella C, Eusebi V, Mann B, et al. Endocrine differentiation in mucoid carcinoma of the breast. Histopathology 1980;4:613.

219. Fetissof F, Dubois MP, Arbeille-Brassart B. Argyrophilic cells in mammary carcinoma. Hum Pathol 1983;14:127.

220. Fisher ER, Palekar AS. Solid and mucinous varieties of so-called mammary carcinoid tumors. Am J Clin Pathol 1979;72:909.

221. Rasmussen BB, Rose C, Thorpe SM, et al. Argyrophilic cells in 202 human mucinous breast carcinomas: relation to histopathologic and clinical features. Am J Clin Pathol 1985;84:737.

222. Toikkanen S, Kujari H. Pure and mixed mucinous carcinomas of the breast: a clinicopathologic analysis of 61 cases with long-term follow-up. Hum Pathol 1989;20:758.

223. Feyrter F, Hartmann G. Uber die carcinoide Wuchsform des Carcinoma mammae, insbesondere das Carcinoma solidum (gelatinosum) mamma. Frandf Z Pathol 1963;73:24.

224. Hull MT, Warfel KA. Mucinous breast carcinomas with abundant

intracytoplasmic mucin and neuroendocrine features: light microscopic, immunohistochemical and ultrastructural study. Ultrastruct Pathol 1987;11:29.

225. Rasmussen BB. Human mucinous carcinomas and their lymph node metastases: a histological review of 247 cases. Pathol Res Pract 1985;180:377.

226. Rosen PP. Mucocele-like tumors of the breast. Am J Surg Pathol 1986;10:464.

227. Ro JY, Sneige N, Saluni AA, et al. Mucocele-like tumor of the breast associated with atypical ductal hyperplasia or mucinous carcinoma. Arch Pathol Lab Med 1991;115:137.

228. Fisher CJ, Millis RR. A mucocele-like tumour of the breast associated with atypical ductal hyperplasia and mucoid carcinoma. Histopathology 1992;21:69.

229. Duane GB, Kanter MH, Branigan T, et al. A morphologic and morphometric study of cells from colloid carcinoma of the breast obtained by fine needle aspiration. Acta Cytol 1987;31:742.

230. Snyder M, Tobon H. Primary mucinous carcinoma of the breast. Breast 1977;3:17.

231. Scharnhorst D, Huntrakoon M. Mucinous carcinoma of the breast: recurrence 30 years after mastectomy. South Med J 1981;81:656.

232. Wasserman TH, Sickles EA, Phillips TL. Primary radiation treatment of colloid carcinoma: a case report. Cancer 1981;48:1972.

233. Kurtz JM, Jacquemier J, Torhorst J, et al. Conservation therapy for breast cancers other than infiltrating ductal carcinoma. Cancer 1989;63:1630.

234. Towfighi J, Simmonds MA, Davidson EA. Mucin and fat emboli in mucinous carcinoma: cause of hemorrhagic cerebral infarcts. Arch Pathol Lab Med 1983;107:646.

235. Deck JHN, Lee MA. Mucin embolism to cerebral arteries: a fatal complication of carcinoma of breast. Can J Neurol Sci 1978;5:327.

236. Fisher ER, Palekar AS, Redmond C, et al. Pathologic findings from the National Surgical Adjuvant Breast Project (Protocol No. 4). VI. Invasive papillary cancer. Am J Clin Pathol 1980;73:313.

237. Carter D, Orr SL, Merino MJ. Intracystic papillary carcinoma of the breast after mastectomy, radiotherapy or excisional biopsy alone. Cancer 1983;52:14.

238. World Health Organization. Histological typing of breast tumors. Tumori 1982;68:181.

239. Haagensen CD. The papillary type of mammary carcinoma. In: Diseases of the breast, ed 2. Philadelphia, WB Saunders, 1971:528.

240. Czernobilsky B. Intracystic carcinoma of the female breast. Surg Gynecol Obstet 1967;124:93.

241. Devitt JE, Barr JR. The clinical recognition of cystic carcinoma of the breast. Surg Gynecol Obstet 1984;159:130.

242. Hunter CE Jr, Sawyers JL. Intracystic papillary carcinoma of the breast. South Med J 1980;73:1484.

243. Schaefer G, Rosen PP, Lesser ML, et al. Breast carcinoma in elderly women: pathology prognosis and survival. Pathol Annu 1984; 19:195.

244. Rosen PP, Ashikari R, Thaler H, et al. A comparative study of some pathologic features of mammary carcinoma in Tokyo, Japan and New York, USA. Cancer 1977;39:429.

245. Meyer JS, Bauer WC, Rao BR. Subpopulations of breast carcinoma defined by S-phase fraction, morphology and estrogen receptor content. Lab Invest 1978;39:225.

246. Tiltman AJ. DNA ploidy in papillary tumours of the breast. South Afr Med J 1989;75:379.

247. Estabrook A, Asch T, Gump F, et al. Mammographic features of intracystic papillary lesions. Surg Gyncol Obstet 1990;170:113.

248. Silva R, Ferrozi F, Patics C. Invasive papillary carcinoma in elderly women: sonographic and mammographic features. AJR 1992; 159:898.

249. Papotti M, Gugliotta P, Eusebi V, et al. Immunohistochemical analysis of benign and malignant papillary lesions of the breast. Am J Surg Pathol 1983;7:451.

250. Papotti M, Gugliotta P, Ghiringhello B, et al. Association of breast carcinoma and multiple intraductal papillomas: an histological and immunohistochemical investigation. Histopathology 1984;8:963.

251. Ohuchi N, Abe R, Kasai M. Possible cancerous change in intraductal papillomas of the breast: a 3-D reconstruction study of 25 cases. Cancer 1984;54:605.

252. Ohuchi N, Abe R, Takahashi T, et al. Three-dimensional atypical structure in intraductal carcinoma differentiating from papilloma and papillomatosis of the breast. Breast Cancer Res Treat 1985; 5:57.

253. Tsuchiya S, Takayama S, Higashi Y. Electron microscopy of intraductal papilloma of the breast: ultrastructural comparison of papillary carcinoma with normal large duct. Acta Pathol Jpn 1983;33:97.

254. Ahmed A. Ultrastructural aspects of human breast lesions. Pathol Annu 1980;15:411.

255. Fisher ER, Gregorio RM, Palekar AS, et al. Mucoepidermoid and squamous cell carcinomas of breast with reference to squamous metaplasia and giant cell tumors. Am J Surg Pathol 1984;7:15.

256. Wargotz ES, Norris HJ. Metaplastic carcinomas of the breast. I. Matrix-producing carcinoma. Hum Pathol 1989;20:628.

257. Wargotz ES, Norris HJ. Metaplastic carcinoma of the breast. IV. Squamous cell carcinoma of ductal origin. Cancer 1990;65:272.

258. Llombart-Bosch A, Peydro A. Malignant mixed osteogenic tumours of the breast: a ultrastructural study of two cases. Virchows Arch 1975;366:1.

259. An T, Grathwohl M, Frable WJ. Breast carcinoma with osseous metaplasia: an electron microscopic study. Am J Clin Pathol 1983;80:127.

260. Kahn LB, Vys CJ, Dale J, et al. Carcinoma of the breast with metaplasia to chondrosarcoma: a light and electron microscopic study. Histopathology 1978;2:93.

261. Battifora H. Spindle cell carcinoma: ultrastructural evidence of squamous origin and collagen production by the tumor cells. Cancer 1976;37:2275.

262. Rottino A, Wilson K. Osseous, cartilaginous and mixed tumors of the human breast: a review of the literature. Arch Surg 1945; 50:184.

263. Oberman HA. Metaplastic carcinoma of the breast: a clinicopathologic study of 29 patients. Am J Surg Pathol 1987;11:918.

264. Huvos AG, Lucas JC Jr, Foote FW Jr. Metaplastic breast carcinoma. NY State J Med 1973;73:1078.

265. Smith BH, Taylor HB. The occurrence of bone and cartilage in mammary tumors. Am J Clin Pathol 1969;51:610.

266. Haagensen CD. Special pathological forms of breast carcinoma: carcinoma with squamous metaplasia. In: Diseases of the breast, ed 2. Philadelphia, WB Saunders, 1971:600.

267. Rosen PP, Ernsberger D. Low-grade adenosquamous carcinoma: a variant of metaplastic mammary carcinoma. Am J Surg Pathol 1987;11:351.

268. Kaufman MW, Marti JR, Gallager HS, et al. Carcinoma of the breast with pseudosarcomatous metaplasia. Cancer 1984;53:1908.

269. Charles A. An electron microscopic study of the human axillary apocrine gland. J Anat 1959;93:226.

270. Archer F, Omar M. Pink cell (oncocytic) metaplasia in a fibroadenoma of the human breast: electron microscopic observations. J Pathol 1969;99:119.

271. Pier WJ Jr, Garancis JC, Kuzma JF. The ultrastructure of apocrine cells in intracystic papilloma and fibrocystic disease of the breast. Arch Pathol 1970;89:446.

272. Ahmed A. Apocrine metaplasia in cystic hyperplastic mastopathy: histochemical and ultrastructural observations. J Pathol 1975; 115:211.

273. Izuo M, Okagaki T, Richart RM, et al. DNA content in "apocrine metaplasia" of fibrocyte disease of the breast. Cancer 1971;27:643.

274. Foote FW Jr, Stewart FW. Comparative studies of cancerous versus noncancerous breasts. Ann Surg 1945;121:6,197.

275. Page DL, Van der Zwaag R, Rogers LW, et al. Relation between component parts of fibrocystic disease complex and breast cancer. J Natl Cancer Inst 1978;61:1055.

276. Page DL, Jensen RA, Dupont WD. Papillary apocrine change of the breast: cancer risk indicator. Lab Invest 1994;70:26A.

277. Yates AJ, Ahmed A. Apocrine carcinoma and apocrine metaplasia. Histopathology 1988;13:228.

278. Mossler J, Barton TK, Brinkhous AD, et al. Apocrine differentiation in human mammary carcinoma. Cancer 1980;46:2463.

279. Roddy HJ, Silverberg SG. Ultrastructural analysis of apocrine carcinoma of the human breast. Ultrastruct Pathol 1980;1:385.

280. Abati AD, Kimmel M, Rosen PP. Apocrine mammary carcinoma: a clinicopathologic study of 72 patients. Am J Clin Pathol 1990;94:371.

281. Eusebi V, Betts C, Haagensen DE, et al. Apocrine differentiation in lobular carcinoma of the breast: a morphologic, immunologic and ultrastructural study. Hum Pathol 1984;15:134.

282. Burt AD, Seywright MM, George WD. Mixed apocrine-medullary carcinoma of the breast. Acta Cytol 1987;31:322.

283. Bryant J. Male breast cancer: a case of apocrine carcinoma with psammoma bodies. Hum Pathol 1981;12:751.

284. Haagensen CD. Carcinoma of the male breast. In: Diseases of the breast, ed 2. Philadelphia, WB Saunders, 1974:779.

285. Lee BJ, Pack GT, Scharnagel I. Sweat gland cancer of the breast. Surg Gynecol Obstet 1933;54:975.

286. Wald M, Kakulas BA. Apocrine gland carcinoma (sweat gland carcinoma) of the breast. Aust NZ J Surg 1964;33:200.

287. Betrand G, Bidabe M-C, Betrand AF. Le carcinome mammaire a stroma reaction giganto-cellulare. Arch Anat Cytol Pathol 1982;30:5.

288. Miller WR, Telford J, Dixon JM, et al. Androgen metabolism and apocrine differentiation in human breast cancer. Breast Cancer Res Treat 1985;5:57.

289. Wales NAM, Ebling FJ. The control of apocrine glands of the rabbit by steroid hormones. J Endocrinol 1971;51:763.

290. Labows JN, Preti G, Hoelzle E, et al. Steroid analysis of human apocrine secretion. Steroids 1979;34:249.

291. Mazoujian G, Bodian C, Haagensen DE Jr, et al. Expression of GCDFP-15 in breast carcinomas: relationship to pathologic and clinical factors. Cancer 1989;63:2156.

292. Frable WJ, Kay S. Carcinoma of the breast: histologic and clinical features of apocrine tumors. Cancer 1968;21:756.

293. d'Amore ESG, Terrier-Lacombe MJ, Travagli JP, et al. Invasive apocrine carcinoma of the breast: a long term follow-up study of 34 cases. Breast Cancer Res Treat 1988;12:37.

294. Ewing J. Neoplastic diseases, ed 3. Philadelphia, WB Saunders, 1919:780.

295. Geschickter CF. Diseases of the breast: diagnosis, pathology, treatment, ed 2. Philadelphia, JB Lippincott, 1945:824.

296. Galloway JR, Woolner LB, Clagett OT. Adenoid cystic carcinoma of the breast. Surg Gynecol Obstet 1966;122:1289.

297. Anthony PP, James PD. Adenoid cystic carcinoma of the breast: prevalence, diagnostic criteria and histogenesis. J Clin Pathol 1975;28:647.

298. Quizilbash AH, Patterson MC, Oliveira KF. Adenoid cystic carcinoma of the breast. Arch Pathol Lab Med 1977;101:302.

299. Hjorth S, Magnusson PH, Blomquite P. Adenoid cystic carcinoma of the breast. Acta Chir Scand 1977;143:155.

300. Peters GN, Wolff M. Adenoid cystic carcinoma of the breast: report of 11 new cases. Cancer 1982;52:680.

301. Friedman BA, Oberman HA. Adenoid cystic carcinoma of the breast. Am J Clin Pathol 1970;54:1.

302. Koss LG, Brannan CD, Ashikari R. Histologic and ultrastructural features of adenoid cystic carcinoma of the breast. Cancer 1970;26:1271.

303. Zaloudek C, Oertel YC, Orenstein JM. Adenoid cystic carcinoma of the breast. Am J Clin Pathol 1984;81:297.

304. Cavanzo FJ, Taylor HB. Adenoid cystic carcinoma of the breast: an analysis of 21 cases. Cancer 1969;24:740.

305. Lerner AG, Molnar JJ, Adam YG. Adenoid cystic carcinoma of the breast. Am J Surg 1974;127:585.

306. Rosen PP. Adenoid cystic carcinoma of the breast: a morphologically heterogeneous neoplasm. Pathol Annu 1989;24:237.

307. Düe W, Herbst H, Loy V, et al. Characterization of adenoid cystic carcinoma of the breast by immunohistology. J Clin Pathol 1989;42:470.

308. Sumpio BE, Jennings TA, Merino MJ, et al. Adenoid cystic carcinoma of the breast: data from the Connecticut Tumor Registry and a review of the literature. Ann Surg 1987;205:295.

309. Lamovec J, Us-krasovec M, Zidar A, et al. Adenoid cystic carcinomas of the breast: a histologic, cytologic and immunohistochemical study. Semin Diag Pathol 1989;6:153.

310. Oertel YC, Goldblum LI. Fine needle aspiration of the breast: diagnostic criteria. Pathol Annu 1983;18:375.

311. Nayer HR. Cylindroma of the breast with pulmonary metastases. Dis Chest 1957;31:324.

312. Ro JY, Silva EG, Gallager HS. Adenoid cystic carcinoma of the breast. Hum Pathol 1987;18:1276.

313. Harris M. Pseudoadenoid cystic carcinoma of the breast. Arch Pathol Lab Med 1977;101:307.

314. Orenstein JM, Dardick I, van Nostrand AWP. Ultrastructural similarities of adenoid cystic carcinoma and pleomorphic adenoma. Histopathology 1985;9:623.

315. d'Ardenne AJ, Kirkpatrick P, Wells CA, et al. Laminin and fibronectin in adenoid cystic carcinoma. J Clin Pathol 1986;39:138.

316. Barsky SH, Layfield L, Varki N, et al. Two human tumors with high basement membrane-producing potential. Cancer 1988;61:1798.

317. Sobue M, Takeuchi J, Niwa M. Establishment of a cell line producing basement membrane components from an adenoid cystic carcinoma of the human salivary gland. Virchows Arch 1989;57:203.

318. Clement PB, Young RH, Azzopardi JG. Collagenous spherulosis of the breast. Am J Surg Pathol 1987;11:411.

319. Clement PB. Collagenous spherulosis. (Letter) Am J Surg Pathol 1987;11:907.

320. Grignon DJ, Ro JY, MacKay BN, et al. Collagenous spherulosis of the breast: immunohistochemical and ultrastructural studies. Am J Clin Pathol 1989;91:386.

321. Wells CA, Nicoll S, Ferguson DJP. Adenoid cystic carcinoma of the breast: a case with axillary lymph node metastasis. Histopathology 1986;10:415.

322. Verani RR, Vander Bel-Kahn J. Mammary adenoid cystic carcinoma with unusual features. Am J Clin Pathol 1976;59:653.

323. Lusted D. Structural and growth patterns of adenoid cystic carcinoma of breast. Am J Clin Pathol 1970;54:419.

324. Lim SK, Kovi J, Warner OG. Adenoid cystic carcinoma of breast with metastasis: a case report and review of the literature. J Natl Med Assoc 1979;71:329.

325. Wilson WB, Spell JP. Adenoid cystic carcinoma of breast: a case of recurrence and regional metastasis. Ann Surg 1967;166:861.

326. Eisner B. Adenoid cystic carcinoma of the breast. Pathol Europ 1970;3:357.

327. Koller M, Ram Z, Findler G, et al. Brain metastasis: a rare manifestation of adenoid cystic carcinoma of the breast. Surg Neurol 1986;70:470.

328. Herzberg AJ, Bossen EH, Walter PJ. Adenoid cystic carcinoma of the breast metastatic to the kidney: a clinically symptomatic lesion requiring surgical management. Cancer 1991;68:1015.

329. Salm R. Epidermoid metaplasia in mammary fibro-adenoma with formation of keratin cysts. J Pathol Bacteriol 1957;74:221.

330. Flint A, Oberman HA. Infarction and squamous metaplasia of intra-

ductal papilloma: a benign breast lesion that may simulate carcinoma. Hum Pathol 1984;15:764.

331. Hassan MO, Olaizola MY. Ultrastructural observations on gynecomastia. Arch Pathol Lab Med 1979;103:624.

332. Soderstrom K-O, Toikkanen S. Extensive squamous metaplasia simulating squamous cell carcinoma in benign breast papillomatosis. Hum Pathol 1983;14:1081.

333. Schaefer FV, Custer RP, Sorof S. Squamous metaplasia in human breast culture: induction by cyclic adenine nucleotide and prostaglandins and influence of menstrual cycle. Cancer Res 1983; 43:279.

334. Rostock RA, Bauer TW, Eggleston JC. Primary squamous carcinoma of the breast: a review. Breast 1984;10:27.

335. Shousha S, James AH, Ferandez MD, et al. Squamous cell carcinoma of the breast. Arch Pathol Lab Med 1984;108:893.

336. Carnog JL, Mobini J, Steiger E, et al. Squamous carcinoma of the breast. Am J Clin Path 1971;55:410.

337. Hasleton PS, Misch KA, Vasudev KS, et al. Squamous carcinoma of the breast. J Clin Pathol 1973;31:116.

338. Bogomoletz WV. Pure squamous cell carcinoma of the breast. Arch Pathol Lab Med 1982;106:57.

339. Woodard BH, Brinkhaus AD, McCarty KS, et al. Adenosquamous differentiation in mammary carcinoma. Arch Pathol Lab Med 1980;104:130.

340. Toikkanen S. Primary squamous cell carcinoma of the breast. Cancer 1981;48:1629.

341. Eusebi V, Lamovec J, Cattani MG, et al. Acantholytic variant of squamous cell carcinoma of the breast. Am J Surg Pathol 1986; 10:855.

342. Lane N. Pseudosarcoma (polypoid sarcoma-like masses) associated with squamous cell carcinoma of the mouth, fauces and larynx: report of 10 cases. Cancer 1957;10:19.

343. Bauer TW, Rostock RA, Eggleston JC, et al. Spindle cell carcinoma of the breast: four cases and review of the literature. Hum Pathol 1984;15:147.

344. Lafreniere R, Moskowitz LB, Ketchain AS. Pure squamous cell carcinoma of the breast. J Surg Oncol 1986;31:113.

345. Eggers JW, Chesney TMcC. Squamous cell carcinoma of the breast: a clinicopathologic analysis of eight cases and review of literature. Hum Pathol 1984;15:526.

346. Gersell DJ, Katzenstein AA. Spindle cell carcinoma of the breast: a clinicopathologic and ultrastructural study. Hum Pathol 1981; 12:550.

347. Factor FM, Biempica L, Ratner I, et al. Carcinoma of the breast with multinucleated reactive stromal giant cells: a light and electron microscopic study of two cases. Virchows Arch 1977;374:1.

348. Agnantis NT, Rosen PP. Mammary carcinoma with osteoclast-like giant cells. Am J Clin Pathol 1979;72:383.

349. Sugano I, Nagao K, Kondo Y, et al. Cytologic and ultrastructural studies of a rare breast carcinoma with osteoclast-like giant cells. Cancer 1983;52:74.

350. Nielsen BB, Kiaer HW. Carcinoma of the breast with stromal multinucleated giant cells. Histopathology 1985;9:183.

351. Holland R, Van Haelst VJGM. Mammary carcinoma with osteoclast-like giant cells: additional observations on six cases. Cancer 1984;53:1963.

352. Tavassoli FA, Norris HJ. Breast carcinoma with osteoclast-like giant cells. Arch Pathol Lab Med 1986;110:636.

353. Boccato P, Briani G, d'Atri C, et al. Spindle cell and cartilaginous metaplasia in breast carcinoma with osteoclast-like stromal cells: a difficult fine needle aspiration diagnosis. Acta Cytol 1988;32:75.

354. Gupta RK, Wakefield StJ, Holloway LJ, et al. Immunocytochemical and ultrastructural study of the rare osteoclast-type carcinoma of the breast in a fine needle aspirate. Acta Cytol 1988;32:79.

355. Douglas-Jones AG, Barr WT. Breast carcinoma with tumor giant cells: report of a case with fine needle aspiration cytology. Acta Cytol 1989;33:109.

356. Bertrand G, Bidabe M-C, Bertrand AF. Le carcinome mammaire a stroma reaction giganto-cellulare. Arch Anat Cytol Pathol 1982;30:5.

357. Ashikari H, Jun MY, Farrow JH, et al. Breast carcinoma in children and adolescents. Clin Bull 1977;7:55.

358. McDivitt RW, Stewart FW. Breast carcinoma in children. JAMA 1966;195:388.

359. Oberman HA, Stephens PJ. Carcinoma of the breast in childhood. Cancer 1972;30:420.

360. Oberman HA. Secretory carcinoma of the breast in adults. Am J Surg Pathol 1980;4:465.

361. Tavassoli FA, Norris HJ. Secretory carcinoma of the breast. Cancer 1980;45:2404.

362. Akhtar M, Robinson C, Ali MA, et al. Secretory carcinoma of the breast in adults: light and electron microscopic study of three cases with review of the literature. Cancer 1983;51:2245.

363. Roth JA, Discafani C, O'Malley M. Secretory breast carcinoma in a man. Am J Surg Pathol 1988;12:150.

364. d'Amore ESG, Maisto L, Gatteschi MB, et al. Secretory carcinoma of the breast: report of a case with fine needle aspiration biopsy. Acta Cytol 1986;30:309.

365. Sullivan JJ, Magee JJ, Donald KJ. Secretory (juvenile) carcinoma of the breast. Pathology 1977;9:341.

366. Krausz T, Jenkins D, Grontoft O, et al. Secretory carcinoma of the breast in adults: emphasis on late recurrence and metastasis. Histopathology 1989;14:25.

367. Tournemaine N, Audouin AF, Anguill C, et al. Le carcinome secretoire juvenile: cinq nouveaux cas chez des femmes d'age adulte. Arch Anat Cytol Pathol 1986;34:146.

368. Rosen PP, Cranor ML. Secretory carcinoma of the breast. Arch Pathol Lab Med 1991;115:141.

369. Botta G, Fessia L, Ghiringhello B. Juvenile milk protein secreting carcinoma. Virchows Arch 1982;395:145.

370. Byrne MP, Fahey MM, Gooselaw JG. Breast cancer with axillary metastasis in an 8-½ year old girl. Cancer 1972;31:726.

371. Romdhane KB, Ayed B, Labbane N, et al. Carcinome secretant juvenile du sein: a propos d'une observation chez une fille de 4 ans. Ann Pathol 1987;3:227.

372. Gupta RK, Lallu SD, Fauck R, et al. Needle aspiration cytology, immunocytochemistry, and electron microscopy in a rare case of secretory carcinoma of the breast in an elderly woman. Diagn Cytopathol 1992;8:388.

373. Rosen PP, Holmes G, Lesser ML, et al. Juvenile papillomatosis and breast carcinoma. Cancer 1985;55:1345.

374. Aboumrad MH, Horn RC, Fine G. Lipid-secreting mammary carcinoma: report of a case associated with Paget's disease of the nipple. Cancer 1963;16:521.

375. Ramos CV, Taylor HB. Lipid-rich carcinoma of the breast: a clinicopathologic analysis of 13 examples. Cancer 1974;33:812.

376. Tsubura A, Hatano T, Murata A, et al. Breast carcinoma in patients receiving neuroleptic therapy: morphologic and clinicopathologic features of thirteen cases. Acta Pathol Jpn 1991;7:494.

377. Lin-Co RY, Gisser SD. Unusual variant of lipid-rich mammary carcinoma. Arch Pathol Lab Med 1978;102:193.

378. Rosen PP, Scott M. Cystic hypersecretory duct carcinoma of the breast. Am J Surg Pathol 1984;8:31.

379. Guerry P, Erlandson RA, Rosen PP. Cystic hypersecretory hyperplasia and cystic hypersecretory duct carcinoma of the breast: pathology, therapy and follow-up of 39 patients. Cancer 1988; 61:1611.

380. Colandrea JM, Shmookler BM, O'Dowd GJ, et al. Cystic hypersecretory duct carcinoma of the breast: report of a case with fine needle aspiration. Arch Pathol Lab Med 1988;112:560.

381. Foote FW Jr, Stewart FW. Lobular carcinoma *in situ*: a rare form of mammary cancer. Am J Pathol 1941;17:491.

382. Barnes JP. Bilateral lobular carcinoma in situ: report of two cases. Texas State J Med 1959;55:581.

383. Benfield JR, Jacobson M, Warner NE. In situ lobular carcinoma of the breast. Arch Surg 1965;91:130.

384. Godwin JT. Chronology of lobular carcinoma of the breast: report of a case. Cancer 1952;5:259.

385. Miller HW Jr, Kay S. Infiltrating lobular carcinoma of the female mammary gland. Surg Gynecol Obstet 1956;102:661.

386. Haagensen CD. Lobular carcinoma of the breast: a precancerous lesion? Clin Obstet Gynecol 1962;5:1093.

387. Newman W. Lobular carcinoma of the female breast: report of 73 cases. Ann Surg 1966;164:305.

388. Henson D, Tarone R. A study of lobular carcinoma of the breast based on the Third National Cancer Survey in the United States of America. Tumori 1979;65:133.

389. Ashikari R, Huvos AG, Urban JA, et al. Infiltrating lobular carcinoma of the breast. Cancer 1973;31:110.

390. Dixon JM, Anderson TJ, Page DL, et al. Infiltrating lobular carcinoma of the breast. Histopathology 1982;6:149.

391. Martinez V, Azzopardi JG. Invasive lobular carcinoma of the breast: incidence and variants. Histopathology 1979;3:467.

392. Haagensen CD. Small cell carcinoma. In: Diseases of the breast, ed 3. Philadelphia, WB Saunders, 1986:816.

393. Fechner RE. Histologic variants of infiltrating lobular carcinoma of the breast. Hum Pathol 1975;6:373.

394. Fechner RE. Infiltrating lobular carcinoma without lobular carcinoma *in situ*. Cancer 1972;29:1539.

395. DiCostanzo D, Rosen PP, Gareen I, et al. Prognosis in infiltrating lobular carcinoma: an analysis of "classical" and variant tumors. Am J Surg Pathol 1990;14:12.

396. Richter GO, Dockerty MB, Clagett OT. Diffuse infiltrating scirrhous carcinoma of the breast: special consideration of the single filing phenomenon. Cancer 1967;20:363.

397. Newstead GM, Bante PB, Toth HK. Invasive lobular and ductal carcinoma: mammographic findings and stage at diagnosis. Radiology 1992;184:632.

398. Mendelson EB, Harris KM, Doshi N, et al. Infiltrating lobular carcinoma: mammographic patterns with pathologic correlation. AJR 1989;153:265.

399. Shousha S, Backhous CM, Alaghband-Zadeh J, et al. Alveolar variant of invasive lobular carcinoma of the breast. Am J Clin Pathol 1986;85:1.

400. Dixon JM, Anderson TJ, Page DL, et al. Infiltrating lobular carcinoma of the breast: an evaluation of the incidence and consequence of bilateral disease. Br J Surg 1983;70:513.

401. Nesland JM, Holm R, Johannessen JV. Ultrastructural and immunohistochemical features of lobular carcinoma of the breast. J Pathol 1985;145:39.

402. Van Bogaert L-J, Maldaque P. Infiltrating lobular carcinoma of the female breast: deviations from the usual histopathologic appearance. Cancer 1980;45:979.

403. Fisher ER, Gregorio RM, Redmond C, et al. Tubulolobular invasive breast carcinoma: a variant of lobular invasive cancer. Hum Pathol 1977;8:679.

404. Eusebi V, Magalhaes F, Azzopardi JG. Pleomorphic lobular carcinoma of the breast: an aggressive tumor showing apocrine differentiation. Hum Pathol 1992;23:655.

405. Weidner N, Semple JP. Pleomorphic variant of invasive lobular carcinoma of the breast. Hum Pathol 1992;23:1167.

406. Porter PL, Garcia R, Moe R, et al. C-erbB-2 oncogene protein in *in situ* and invasive lobular breast neoplasia. Cancer 1991;68:331.

407. Gad A, Azzopardi JG. Lobular carcinoma of the breast: a special variant of mucin secreting carcinoma. J Clin Pathol 1975;28:711.

408. Breslow A, Brancaccio ME. Intracellular mucin production by lobular breast carcinoma cells. Arch Pathol Lab Med 1976;100:620.

409. Merino MJ, LiVolsi VA. Signet ring carcinoma of the female breast: a clinicopathologic analysis of 24 cases. Cancer 1981;48:1830.

410. Gould VE, Chejfec G. Lobular carcinoma of the breast with secretory features. Ultrastruct Pathol 1980;1:151.

411. Jundt G, Schulz A, Heitz PU, et al. Small cell neuroendocrine (oat cell) carcinoma of the male breast. Virchows Arch 1984;213.

412. Wade PM, Mills SE, Read M, et al. Small cell neuroendocrine (oat cell) carcinoma of the breast. Cancer 1983;52:121.

413. Lee AK, DeLellis RA, Rosen PP, et al. Alphalactalbumin as an immunohistochemical marker for metastatic breast carcinomas. Am J Surg Pathol 1984;8:93.

414. Clayton F, Ordonez NG, Hanssen GM, et al. Immunoperoxidase localization of lactalbumin in malignant breast neoplasms. Arch Pathol Lab Med 1982;106:268.

415. Toyoshima S, Inoshita S, Enjoji M. Invasive lobular carcinoma of the breast: an analysis of 29 cases. Acta Pathol Jpn 1986;36:161.

416. d'Ardenne AJ, Barnard NJ. Paucity of fibronectin in invasive lobular carcinoma of breast. J Pathol 1989;157:219.

417. Yamada KM, Olden K. Fibronectins: adhesive glycoproteins of cell surface and blood. Nature 1978;275:179.

418. Smith DB, Howell A, Harris M, et al. Carcinomatous meningitis associated with infiltrating lobular carcinoma of the breast. Eur J Surg Oncol 1985;11:33.

419. Olsen ME, Chernik NL, Posner JB. Infiltration of the leptomeninges by systemic cancer: a clinical and pathologic study. Arch Neurol 1974;30:122.

420. Harris M, Howell A, Chrissohou M, et al. A comparison of the metastatic pattern of infiltrating lobular carcinoma and infiltrating duct carcinoma of the breast. Br J Cancer 1984;50:23.

421. Klein MS, Sherlock P. Gastric and colonic metastases from breast cancer. Am J Dig Dis 1972;17:881.

422. Feun L, Drelichman A, Singhakowinta A, et al. Ureteral obstruction secondary to metastatic breast carcinoma. Cancer 1979;44:1164.

423. Hartman S, Schliftman R, Bennett B. Correlation conferences in radiology and pathology: gastric rigidity and breast masses. NY State J Med 1977;77:1120.

424. Hartmann WH, Sherlock P. Gastroduodenal metastases from carcinoma of the breast: an adrenal steroid induced phenomenon. Cancer 1961;14:426.

425. Kondo Y, Akita T, Sugano I, et al. Signet ring cell carcinoma of the breast. Acta Pathol Jpn 1984;34:875.

426. Cormier WJ, Gaffey TA, Welch JM, et al. Linitis plastica caused by metastatic carcinoma of the breast. Mayo Clin Proc 1980;55:747.

427. Yoshida Y. Metastases and primary neoplasms of the stomach in patients with breast cancer. Surgery 1973;125:738.

428. Matsui M, Kokima O, Uehara Y, et al. Characterization of estrogen receptor in human gastric cancer. Cancer 1991;68:305.

429. Harrison JD, Morris DL, Ellis IO, et al. The effect of tamoxifen and estrogen receptor status on survival in gastric carcinoma. Cancer 1989;64:1007.

430. Kumar NB, Hart WR. Metastases to the uterine corpus from extragenital cancers: a clinicopathologic study of 63 cases. Cancer 1982;50:2163.

431. Allenby PL, Chowdhury LN. Histiocytic appearance of metastatic lobular breast carcinoma. Arch Pathol Lab Med 1986;110:759.

432. Warren RB. Infiltrating lobular carcinoma metastatic to bone marrow: an unusual morphologic pattern. Breast 1985;11:16.

433. Weinstein GW, Goldman JN. Metastatic adenocarcinoma of the breast masquerading as chalazion. Am J Ophthamol 1970;69:259.

434. Hood CI, Font RI, Zimmerman LE. Metastatic mammary carcinoma in the eyelid with histiocytoid appearance. Cancer 1973;31:793.

435. Dearnaley DP, Sloane JP, Ormerod MG, et al. Increased detection

of mammary carcinoma cells in marrow smears using antisera to epithelial membrane antigen. Br J Cancer 1981;44:85.

436. du Toit RS, Locker AP, Ellis IO, et al. Invasive lobular carcinomas of the breast: the prognosis of histopathological subtypes. Br J Cancer 1989;60:605.

437. Schnitt SJ, Connolly JL, Recht A, et al. Influence of lobular histology on local tumor control in breast cancer patients treated with conservative surgery and radiotherapy. Cancer 1989;64:448.

438. Saigo PE, Rosen PP. Mammary carcinoma with "choriocarcinomatous" features. Am J Surg Pathol 1981;5:773.

439. Coombes RC, Easty GC, Detre SI, et al. Secretion of immunoreactive calcitonin by human breast carcinomas. Br Med J 1975;4:197.

440. Kaneko H, Hojo H, Ishikawa S, et al. Norepinephrine-producing tumors of bilateral breasts: a case report. Cancer 1978;41:2002.

441. Green DM. Mucoid carcinoma of the breast with choriocarcinoma in its metastases. Histopathology 1990;16:504.

442. Lee AK, Rosen PP, DeLellis RA, et al. Tumor marker expression in breast carcinomas and relationship to prognosis: an immunohistochemical study. Am J Clin Pathol 1985;84:687.

443. Smith DM Jr, Haggitt RC. A comparative study of generic stains for carcinoid secretory granules. Am J Surg Pathol 1983;7:61.

444. Partanen S, Syrjanen J. Argyrophilic cells in carcinoma of the female breast. Virchows Arch 1981;391:45.

445. Chabon AB, Costales F. Estrogen receptor activity in primary argyrophil carcinoma of the breast. Diagn Gynecol Obstet 1980;2:93.

446. Nesland JM, Holm R, Johannessen JV. A study of different markers for neuroendocrine differentiation in breast carcinomas. Pathol Res Pract 1986;181:524.

447. Gill IS. Carcinoid tumour of the male breast. J R Soc Med 1990;83:401.

448. Toyoshima S. Mammary carcinoma with argyrophil cells. Cancer 1983;52:2129.

449. Woodard BH, Eisenbarth G, Wallace NR, et al. Adrenocorticotropin production by a mammary carcinoma. Cancer 1981;47:1823.

450. Mavligit GM, Cohen JL, Sherwood LM. Ectopic production of parathyroid hormone by carcinoma of the breast. N Engl J Med 1971;285:154.

451. Azzopardi JG, Muretto P, Goddeeris P, et al. Carcinoid tumors of the breast: the morphological spectrum of argyrophil carcinomas. Histopathology 1982;6:549.

452. Cubilla AL, Woodruff JM. Primary carcinoid tumor of the breast: a report of eight patients. Am J Surg Pathol 1977;1:283.

453. Cross AS, Azzopardi JG, Krausz T, et al. A morphological and immunocytochemical study of a distinctive variant of ductal carcinoma in situ of the breast. Histopathology 1985;9:21.

454. Min K-W. Argyrophilia in breast carcinomas: histochemical, ultrastructural and immunocytochemical study. Lab Invest 1983;48:58A.

455. Nesland JM, Memoli VA, Holm R, et al. Breast carcinomas with neuroendocrine differentiation. Ultrastruct Pathol 1985;8:225.

456. Cubilla AL, Woodruff JM. Primary carcinoid tumor of the breast: a new pathologic entity. Lab Invest 1978;38:340.

457. Clayton F, Sibley RK, Ordonez NG, et al. Argyrophilic breast carcinomas: evidence of lactational differentiation. Am J Surg Pathol 1982;6:323.

458. Bussolati G, Gugliotta P, Sapino A, et al. Chromogranin-reactive endocrine cells in argyrophilic carcinomas ("carcinoids") and normal tissue of the breast. Am J Pathol 1985;120:186.

459. Bussolati G, Papotti M, Sapino A, et al. Endocrine markers in argyrophilic carcinomas of the breast. Am J Surg Pathol 1987;11:248.

460. Rasmussen BB, Rose C, Thorpe SM, et al. Argyrophilic cells in 202 human mucinous breast carcinomas: relation to histopathologic and clinical features. Am J Clin Pathol 1985;84:737.

461. Kashlan RB, Powell RW, Nolting SF. Carcinoid and other tumors metastatic to the breast. J Surg Oncol 1982;20:25.

462. Ordonez NG, Manning JT Jr, Raymond K. Argentaffin endocrine carcinoma (carcinoid) of the pancreas with concomitant breast metastasis: an immunohistochemical and electron microscopic study. Hum Pathol 1985;16:746.

463. Meyer AC, Dockerty MB, Harrington SW. Inflammatory carcinoma of the breast. Surg Gynecol Obstet 1948;87:417.

464. Lucas FV, Perez-Mesa C. Inflammatory carcinoma of the breast. Cancer 1978;41:1595.

465. World Health Organization. International histological classification of tumours. 2. Histological typing of breast tumours, ed 2. Geneva, World Health Organization, 1981:21.

466. Barker JL, Nelson AJ III, Montague ED. Inflammatory carcinoma of the breast. Radiology 1976;121:173.

467. Droulias CA, Sewell CW, McSweeney MB, et al. Inflammatory carcinoma of the breast: a correlation of clinical radiologic and pathologic findings. Ann Surg 1976;184:217.

468. Nussbaum H, Kagan AR, Gilbert H, et al. Management of inflammatory breast carcinoma. Breast 1977;3:25.

469. Ellis DL, Teitelbaum SL. Inflammatory carcinoma of the breast: a pathologic definition. Cancer 1974;33:1045.

470. Saltzstein SL. Clinically occult inflammatory carcinoma of the breast. Cancer 1974;34:382.

471. Levine PH, Steinhorn SC, Ries LG, et al. Inflammatory breast cancer: the experience of the surveillance, epidemiology, and end results (SEER) program. J Natl Cancer Inst 1985;74:291.

472. Schäfer P, Alberto P, Forni M, et al. Surgery as part of a combined modality approach for inflammatory breast carcinoma. Cancer 1987;59:1063.

473. Kokal WA, Hill RL, Porudominsky D, et al. Inflammatory breast carcinoma: a distinct entity? J Surg Oncol 1985;30:152.

474. Noguchi S, Miyauchi K, Nishizawa Y, et al. Management of inflammatory carcinoma of the breast with combined modality therapy including intraarterial infusion chemotherapy as an induction therapy: long-term follow-up results of 28 patients. Cancer 1988;61:1483.

475. Guerin M, Gabillot M, Mathieu M-C, et al. Structure and expression of c-erbB-2 and EGF receptor genes in inflammatory and non-inflammatory breast cancer: prognostic significance. Int J Cancer 1989;43:201.

476. Charpin C, Bounier P, Khouzami A, et al. Inflammatory breast carcinoma: an immunohistochemical study using monoclonal anti-pHER-2/neu, pS2, cathepsin, ER and PR. Anticancer Res 1992;12:591.

477. Robbins GF, Shah J, Rosen P, et al. Inflammatory carcinoma of the breast. Surg Clin North Am 1974;54:801.

478. Nielsen M, Andersen JA, Hendricksen FW, et al. Metastases to the breast from extramammary carcinomas. Acta Pathol Microbiol Immunol Scand 1981;89:251.

479. Hadju SI, Urban JA. Cancers metastatic to the breast. Cancer 1972;29:1691.

480. McCrea ES, Johnston C, Haney PJ. Metastases to the breast. AJR 1983;141:685.

481. Frauenhoffer EE, Ro JY, Silva EG, et al. Well differentiated serous ovarian carcinoma presenting as a breast mass: a case report and flow cytometric DNA study. Int J Gynecol Pathol 1991;10:79.

482. Yamasaki H, Saw D, Zdanowitz J, et al. Ovarian carcinoma metastasis to the breast: case report and review of the literature. Am J Surg Pathol 1993;17:193.

483. Alexander HR, Turnbull AD, Rosen PP. Isolated breast metastases from gastrointestinal carcinomas. J Surg Oncol 1989;42:264.

484. Brutschin P, Culver GJ. Extracranial metastases from medulloblastoma. Radiology 1973;107:359.

485. Howarth GB, Caces JN, Pratt CB. Breast metastases in children with rhabdomyosarcoma. Cancer 1980;46:2520.

486. Salyer WR, Salyer DC. Metastases of prostatic carcinoma to the breast. J Urol 1973;109:671.

487. Scott J, Robb-Smith AHT, Burns I. Bilateral breast metastases from carcinoma of the prostate. Br J Urol 1974;46:209.

488. Hartley LCJ, Little JH. Bilateral mammary metastases from carcinoma of the prostate during oestrogen therapy. Med J Aust 1971;1:434.

489. Moldwin RM, Orihuela E. Breast masses associated with adenocarcinoma of the prostate. Cancer 1989;63:2229.

490. Abramson W, Warshawsky H. Cancer of the breast in the male secondary to estrogenic administration: report of a case. J Urol 1948;59:76.

491. Wilson SE, Hutchinson WB. Breast masses in males with carcinoma of the prostate. J Surg Oncol 1976;8:105.

492. Campbell JH, Cummins SD. Metastases simulating mammary cancer in prostatic cancer under estrogenic therapy. Cancer 1951;4:303.

493. Jakobsen AHI. Bilateral mammary carcinoma in the male following stilboestrol therapy. Acta Pathol Microbiol Immunol Scand 1952;31:61.

494. Graves GY, Harris HS. Carcinoma of the male breast with axillary metastasis following stilbestrol therapy: report of a case treated by radical mastectomy. Ann Surg 1952;152:411.

495. National Cancer Institute. Standardized management of breast specimens: recommended by Pathology Working Group, Breast Cancer Task Force. Am J Clin Pathol 1973;60:789.

496. Schmidt WA. The breast. In: Principles and techniques of surgical pathology. Stoneham, MA, Butterworths, 1983:362.

497. Coombes RC, Berger U, Mansi J, et al. Prognostic significance of micrometastases in bone marrow in patients with primary breast cancer. In: Adjuvant chemotherapy and endocrine therapy for breast cancer. Natl Cancer Inst Monogr 1986;1:51.

498. Assoc of Directors of Anatomic and Surgical Pathology. Immediate management of mammographically detected breast lesions. Am J Surg Pathol 1993;12:850.

499. Schnitt SJ, Connolly JL. Processing and evaluation of breast excision specimens: a clinically oriented approach. Am J Clin Pathol 1992;98:125.

500. Connolly JL, Schnitt SJ. Evaluation of breast biopsy specimens in patients considered for treatment by conservative surgery and radiation therapy for early breast cancer. Pathol Annu 1988;23:1.

501. Bloom ND, Johnson F, Pertshuck L, et al. Electrocautery: effects on steroid receptors in human breast cancer. J Surg Oncol 1984;25:21.

502. Pertshuck LP, Tobin EH, Tanapat P, et al. Histochemical analyses of steroid hormone receptors in breast and prostate carcinoma. J Histochem Cytochem 1980;28:799.

503. Rosenthal LJ. Discrepant estrogen receptor protein levels according to surgical technique. Am J Surg 1979;138:680.

504. Rosen PP. Electrocautery induced artifacts in breast biopsy specimens: an iatrogenic source of diagnostic difficulty. (Letter) Ann Surg 1986;204:612.

505. Glen PM, Margulies D. Electrocautery and hormone receptor status in breast biopsy. Am J Surg 1989;158:6.

506. Pilnik S, Steichen F. The use of the hemostatic scalpel in operations upon the breast. Surg Gynecol Obstet 1986;162:589.

507. Menon RS, van Geel AN. Cancer of the breast with nipple involvement. Br J Cancer 1989;59:81.

508. Lloyd LR, Waits RK, Schroder D, et al. Axillary dissection for breast carcinoma: the myth of skip metastases. Ann Surg 1989;55:381.

509. Veronesi V, Rilke F, Luini A, et al. Distribution of axillary node metastases by level of invasion: an analysis of 539 cases. Cancer 1987;59:682.

510. Schwartz GF, Rosenberg AL, Danoff BF, et al. Lumpectomy and level I axillary dissection prior to irradiation for "operable" breast cancer. Ann Surg 1984;200:554.

511. Danforth DN, Findlay PA, McDonald HD, et al. Complete axillary lymph node dissection for stage I–II carcinoma of the breast. J Clin Oncol 1986;4:655.

512. Anderson J, Jensen J. Lymph node identification: specimen radiography of tissue predominated by fat. Am J Clin Pathol 1977;68:511.

513. Groote AD, Oosterhuis JW, Molenaar WM, et al. Radiographic imaging of lymph nodes in lymph node dissection specimens. Lab Invest 1985;52:326.

514. Durkin K, Haagensen CD. An improved technique for the study of lymph nodes in surgical specimens. Ann Surg 1980;191:419.

515. Morrow M, Evans J, Rosen PP, et al. Does clearing of axillary lymph nodes contribute to accurate staging of breast carcinoma? Cancer 1984;53:1329.

516. Hartveit F, Samonsen G, Tanqen M, et al. Routine histological investigation of the axillary lymph nodes in breast cancer. Clin Oncol 1982;8:121.

517. Huvos AG, Hutter RVP, Berg JW. Significance of axillary macrometastases and micrometastases in mammary cancer. Ann Surg 1971;173:44.

518. Attiyeh FF, Jensen M, Huvos AG, et al. Axillary micrometastases and macrometastases in carcinoma of the breast. Surg Gynecol Obstet 1977;144:839.

519. Fisher ER, Palekar A, Rockette H, et al. Pathologic findings from the National Surgical Adjuvant Breast Project (protocol no. 4). V. Significance of axillary nodal micro- and macrometastases. Cancer 1978;42:2032.

520. Rosen PP, Saigo PE, Braun DW, et al. Axillary micro- and macrometastases in breast cancer: prognostic significance of tumor size. Ann Surg 1981;194:585.

521. Mambo NC, Gallager HS. Carcinoma of the breast: the prognostic significance of extranodal extension of axillary disease. Cancer 1977;39:2280.

522. Hultborn KA, Tornberg B. Mammary cancer: the biologic character of mammary carcinoma studied in 517 cases by a new form of malignancy grading. Acta Radiol 1960;(Suppl)196:1.

523. Fisher ER, Gregorio RM, Redmond C, et al. Pathologic findings from the National Surgical Adjuvant Breast Project (Protocol No. 4). III. The significance of extranodal extension of axillary metastases. Am J Clin Pathol 1976;65:439.

524. Cascinelli N, Greco M, Bufalino R, et al. Prognosis of breast cancer with axillary node metastases after surgical treatment only. Eur J Cancer Clin Oncol 1987;23:795.

525. Sloane JP, Ormerod MG, Imrie S, et al. The use of antisera to epithelial membrane antigen in detecting micrometastases in histological sections. Br J Cancer 1980;42:392.

526. Wells CA, Heryet A, Brochier J, et al. The immunocytochemical detection axillary micrometastases in breast cancer. Br J Cancer 1984;50:193.

527. International (Ludwig) Breast Cancer Study Group. Prognostic importance of occult axillary lymph node micrometastases from breast cancers. Lancet 1990;1:1565.

528. Nasser IA, Lee AKC, Bosari S. Occult axillary lymph node metastases in "node-negative" breast carcinoma. Hum Pathol 1993;24:950.

529. Trojani M, de Mascarel I, Bonichon F, et al. Micrometastases to axillary lymph nodes from carcinoma of breast: detection by immunohistochemistry and prognostic significance. Br J Cancer 1987;55:303.

530. de Mascarel I, Bonichon F, Coindre JM, et al. Prognostic significance of breast cancer axillary lymph node micrometastases assessed by two special techniques: reevaluation with longer follow-up. Br J Cancer 1992;66:523.

531. Ginsbourg M, Musset M, Misset JL, et al. Simultaneous detection in the bone marrow of mammary cancer metastatic cells and of

their labelling index as respective markers of the residual minimum submacroscopic disease and its proliferative condition (preliminary results). Biomed Pharmacother 1986;40:386.

532. Cote RJ, Rosen PP, Hakes TB, et al. Monoclonal antibodies detect occult breast carcinoma metastases in the bone marrow of patients with early stage disease. Am J Surg Pathol 1988;12:333.

533. Osborne MP, Asina S, Wong GY, et al. Immunofluorescent monoclonal antibody detection of breast cancer in bone marrow: sensitivity in a model system. Cancer Res 1989;49:2510.

534. Cordell JL, Falini B, Erber WN, et al. Immunoenzymatic labeling of monoclonal antibodies using immune complexes of alkaline phosphatase and monoclonal anti-alkaline phosphatase (APAA complexes). J Histochem Cytochem 1984;32:219.

535. Taha M, Ordonez NG, Kulkarni S, et al. A monoclonal antibody cocktail for detection of micrometastatic tumor cells in the bone marrow of breast cancer patients. Bone Marrow Transplant 1989;4:297.

536. Schlimok G, Funke I, Holzmann B, et al. Micrometastatic cancer cells in bone marrow: *in vivo* detection with anti-cytokeratin and *in vivo* labelling with anti-17-1A monoclonal antibodies. Proc Natl Acad Sci USA 1987;84:8672.

537. Datta YH, Adams PT, Drobyski WR, et al. Sensitive detection of occult breast cancer by the reverse transcriptase polymerase chain reaction. J Clin Oncol 1994;12:475.

538. Armas OA, Gerald WL, Lesser ML, et al. Immunohistochemical detection of cathepsin D in $T_2N_0M_0$ breast carcinoma. Am J Surg Pathol 1994;18:158.

539. Domagala W, Striker G, Szadowska A, et al. Cathepsin D in invasive ductal NOS breast carcinoma as defined by immunohistochemistry: no correlation with survival at 5 years. Am J Pathol 1992;141:1003.

540. Pujol P, Maudelonde T, Daures JP, et al. A prospective study of the prognostic value of cathepsin D levels in breast cancer cytosols. Cancer 1993;71:2006.

541. Rosen PP, Lesser ML, Arroyo CD, et al. Immunohistochemical detection of HER2/neu in node-negative breast carcinoma: a study of epidemiologic risk factors, histologic features and prognosis. Cancer 1995;75:1320.

542. Marx D, Schauer A, Reiche C, et al. c-erbB2 Expression in correlation to other biological parameters of breast cancer. J Cancer Res Clin Oncol 1990;116:15.

543. Gusterson BA, Machin LG, Gullick WJ, et al. Immunohistochemical distribution of c-erbB-2 in infiltrating and in situ breast cancer. Int J Cancer 1988;42:842.

544. Rosen PP, Lesser ML, Arroyo CD, et al. P53 on node-negative breast carcinoma: an immunohistochemical study of epidemiologic risk factors, histologic features and prognosis. J Clin Oncol 1995;13:821.

545. Poller DN, Hutchings CE, Galea M, et al. p53 Protein expression in human breast carcinoma: relationship to expression of epidermal growth factor receptor, c-erbB-2 protein overexpression, and oestrogen receptor. Br J Cancer 1992;66:583.

546. Walker RA, Dearing SJ, Lane DP, et al. Expression of p53 protein in infiltrating and in-situ breast carcinomas. J Pathol 1991;165:203.

Diseases of the Breast, edited by Jay R. Harris,
Marc E. Lippman, Monica Morrow, and Samuel Hellman.
Lippincott-Raven Publishers, Philadelphia, © 1996.

14

Molecular Pathology of Breast Carcinoma

ANN D. THOR · DAVID W. YANDELL

Anatomic pathology of the breast is generally classified by characteristic gross and microscopic abnormalities. A multitude of other subcellular (nuclear, cytoplasmic, and membranous) alterations may also occur that are not detectable by routine histopathologic analysis. Recent developments in cytogenetics and molecular genetics, including the polymerase chain reaction (PCR) and microassays that can be performed on minute tissue samples, have facilitated identification of many defects, including a variety of nonrandom genetic lesions in breast cancer. Identification of these genetic alterations may become an important step in the diagnosis of breast carcinoma and may eventually allow tumor subtyping beyond standard histologic and clinical groups. Ultimately, the hope for these technologies is that they will improve our ability to determine prognosis and optimal therapeutic interventions for individual patients and will lead to a better understanding of human breast carcinogenesis.

The process of cellular transformation (conversion to a state of unrestrained growth resembling a tumorigenic condition) involves multiple single events. This sequence of changes, which is often tissue-specific, leads to a progressive increase in cell growth and a decrease in cellular responsiveness to the normal growth controls. Phenotypic (morphologic) alterations recognized by routine techniques (such as gross or microscopic atypia) may not be present during these phases or may not correlate with sequential genetic changes that occur with neoplastic transformation and clonal evolution.

Investigators have hypothesized that the biology and clinical progression of any single tumor are due to these progressive genetic alterations, and it is generally accepted that alteration of a single gene is not sufficient to induce neoplastic transformation of breast epithelium. Several nonexclusive models have been proposed to explain the heterogeneity of genetic lesions identified in breast cancers, including a stochastic model of genetic instability[1] and a morphologic model of breast cancer evolution.[2]

Each of these models depicts a multistep process of carcinogenesis that includes multiple genetic or morphologic alterations, nonobligatory precursor lesions, and generally increasing dysplasia during the transition from benign to malignant. Each model also includes early lesions believed to occur many years before the development of frank carcinoma. Because of the tremendous clinical, biologic, and genetic heterogeneity observed among breast cancers, many different pathways probably can lead to the disease, and with better tools to measure these differences, additional clinically relevant disease subgroups will likely be recognized. This premise has fostered the development of prognostic markers as an active area of research.

Gene abnormalities have been identified in both benign and malignant breast lesions, although these abnormalities are far more common in carcinomas. Therefore, the presence of genetic alterations should not be used to diagnose malignancy. Abnormalities of several genes are usually identified in malignant cells, in contrast to single-gene alterations associated with many inherited human genetic disorders.[3] The spectrum of genetic abnormalities unique to a single neoplasm may be used to fingerprint tumors for subclassification, identification of occult lesions, or investigation of clonality. Furthermore, genetic instability is commonplace in neoplasia, and carcinoma of the breast appears to be no exception. Secondary (ie, subsequent to carcinogenesis), and perhaps random, gene abnormalities may be difficult to distinguish from those critical to the development of cancer. This is particularly true when molecular genetic studies are performed on tissues representing the final phase of carcinogenesis (ie, large invasive breast cancers), rather than a hyperplastic or atypical hyperplastic lesion or carcinoma in situ.

Subtle differences in DNA transcription and RNA translation may also occur within breast epithelial hyperplasia and carcinoma cells. Our understanding of the regulatory factors underlying these changes in gene expression, however, is in its infancy. Many host and exogenous fac-

445

tors influence breast epithelial cell growth as well, and these factors may play a key role in carcinogenesis. As a result, studies that focus only on a specific genetic alteration, without analysis of the encoded RNA transcript and protein, can be difficult to interpret and are often misleading. Furthermore, studies that lack detail regarding ascertainment of specimens and at least a modicum of clinical, histologic, and outcome information are difficult to interpret with respect to potential clinical relevance.

Given the complexity of genetic and epigenetic factors to study in a single tumor and the severe limitation of tissue availability for research, the development of new investigational methods such as comparative genomic hybridization (CGH) is particularly exciting. CGH allows identification of multiple genetic abnormalities using a single assay system and a small tissue sample. Advanced technologies have facilitated a greater understanding of the diverse and complex nature of the molecular pathology of breast cancer and may be particularly useful in differentiating random alterations from those specific to the neoplastic process. In addition, because of the microscopic size of most preinvasive lesions, most forms of genetic analysis were prohibitively difficult until recently. Molecular genetic techniques using the PCR are sufficiently robust to detect genetic alterations reliably in specimens of fewer than 100 cells; use of these methods to describe genetic alterations in specimens of 10 or fewer cells is increasingly common. Until recently, however, much of what has been reported in the molecular pathology of breast cancer represents later stages of carcinogenesis, either invasive primary carcinoma (particularly large lesions) or metastatic tumors.

This chapter focuses on newer molecular genetic techniques and slide-based or tissue-based assay systems to investigate the molecular pathology of breast cancer and precursor lesions. Following a brief discussion of each method, highlights of the pathologic features identified using these techniques are summarized. (For more extensive discussions of oncogenes or prognostic markers, see Chapters 7.6 and 16.) A discussion of breast tissue heterogeneity, tumor acquisition issues, and laboratory quality assurance as they apply to molecular diagnostics has been added where applicable.

The field of molecular genetics has grown enormously in the past decade and can be complex and confusing to the uninitiated. The techniques in use today did not exist when the majority of clinicians now practicing were trained. An understanding of the basic principles of gene structure, function, and regulation is necessary to appreciate the explosive growth of the field (see Chap. 27.1).[4,5]

Cytogenetics

Cytogenetics (the study of cellular genetics) can be broadly divided into traditional and molecular branches. Traditional cytogenetic methods require growth of cells in media, interruption and arrest of cells undergoing mitosis, and examination of individual chromosomes from these mitotic cells for deletions, translocations, or alterations of ploidy. Cytogenetic studies of breast cancers have been limited because it is difficult to obtain primary cultures of breast carcinomas (not overgrown by stromal fibroblasts) with adequate cellular proliferation to provide sufficient mitotic cells for examination. Tumor-associated chromosomal (karyotypic) abnormalities identified with this technique are most commonly ploidy alterations in breast neoplasia, none of which are specific for breast cancer.[6] (Ploidy alterations identified by flow cytometry are discussed in Chapter 16.)

Molecular cytogenetics includes three relatively new methods: (1) fluorescence in situ hybridization (FISH); (2) primed in situ labeling (PRINS); and (3) CGH.

Fluorescence in Situ Hybridization

Fluorescence in situ hybridization[7-10] is a powerful tool to evaluate specific regions of the genome using either metaphase or interphase cells.[11] Although the technique is most commonly used to study DNA, RNA analysis can be performed as well.[12] It has proved useful for detection of many abnormalities, from chromosomal abnormalities (eg, translocations, numeric abnormalities, and deletions) to gene alterations (deletions, rearrangements, amplification, and other large-scale genetic changes).[13] Briefly, FISH requires chromosomal denaturation to produce single-stranded DNA, recognition and hybridization of a labeled DNA probe to the denatured DNA, and microscopic visualization of the signal. Probes may be tagged with a variety of different photoreactive dyes, or fluors, allowing color-coded labeling of the chromosomal sequences (Fig. 14–1). Probes for specific chromosomal regions are often used parallel to centromeric probes labeled with a different color. The use of several probes that hybridize with geographically clustered regions and even whole-chromosome painting using hundreds of probes is now common.[9]

Advantages of FISH include the possibility of routine microscopic analysis for cellular phenotype and molecular genetic analysis on the same cells, simultaneous use of multiple probes for detection of concordant genetic changes, and detection of genetic changes in single cells such that the frequency of genetic changes per cell can be measured and alterations of low frequency can be identified. Although sequences smaller than a kilobase can sometimes be detected,[10] targets of 25 kb or larger are optimal. The disadvantages of FISH include tissue requirements (eg, single cell preparations—touch preparations, cell suspensions, and so forth), a lack of robustness when using paraffin-embedded fixed tissues, limited probe availability, low hybridization efficiency of small target regions, and imperfect correspondence between "the number of hybridization signals and the number of target chromosomes."[10]

Significant observations have been made using FISH technology in the molecular pathology of breast carcinomas. Chromosomal aberrations have been reported to be

Denaturation of DNA to Single Strand

Hybridization to Labeled Oligonucleotide

Molecular Marker Binding to Label

FIGURE 14-1 DNA Fluorescence in situ hybridization requires denaturation to single-stranded DNA and hybridization of the labeled oligonucleotide probe to the test DNA. Several classes of probes may be used, such as repetitive probes, whole-chromosome probes, and locus-specific probes, as described in detail.[8,13] Detection methods include fluorescent as well as hapten or enzyme labeling of the oligonucleotide. The last two methods allow binding of secondary reagents and the formation of precipitates that may enhance the signal when illuminated by transmitted or reflected light microscopy.

common, with aneusomy involving at least one chromosome in nearly all malignant tumors.[14] Amplification of the oncogene *erb*B-2 (HER2/neu) detected by FISH correlates with *erb*B-2 data derived using other methods (Southern blot, immunohistochemistry) and occurs in approximately one third of cancers.[14] Marked cell–cell heterogeneity of *erb*B-2 amplification can be detected within tumor–subcellular populations, some of which contain highly amplified levels (more than 25 copies) of the gene.[14] Tumors without gene amplification also showed heterogeneous but low levels of *erb*B-2 (1 to 5 copies per cell).[14] This cell–cell heterogeneity for *erb*B-2 gene copy number is an unexpected finding and may explain, at least in part, the heterogeneous expression of *erb*B-2 p185 protein noted in many immunohistochemical studies.[15] Finally, physical deletion has been shown to be a common mechanism leading to loss of heterozygosity (LOH) at 17p, a region harboring many genes of interest in breast cancers.[16]

The oncogene *erb*B-2 is amplified and overexpressed in at least one third of breast cancers. This alteration is of probable independent prognostic significance, particularly in patients with nodal metastases. The prognostic significance of *erb*B-2 alterations in patients with lymph node–negative disease is more controversial. Reports suggest that *erb*B-2 amplification and overexpression may be associated with improved survival in patients treated with dose-intensive cyclophosphamide, doxorubicin, and 5-fluorouracil[15] and relative chemoresistance in patients treated with cyclophosphamide, methotrexate, and 5-fluorouracil (CMF).[17,18]

Of biologic significance, Micale and coworkers[19] used FISH technology and pericentromeric probes for chromosomes 1, 16, 17, 18, and X to investigate aneusomy in proliferative breast disease (believed by many to represent precursor lesions to carcinoma). Fixed paraffin-embedded tissue sections were used to preserve tissue architecture and to facilitate pathologic classification of cell populations. Surgically resected breast tissues containing normal breast, adenosis, moderate or florid hyperplasia, ductal or lobular hyperplasia with atypia, ductal or lobular carcinomas in situ, and invasive carcinomas were studied. Chromosomal aberrations were not identified in normal tissues or adenosis. Losses (deletions) of chromosomes 17 and 18 were identified in over half of ductal or lobular hyperplasias as well as in situ or invasive lesions. Chromosome 17 is of particular interest in molecular genetic studies of breast cancers because the genes *erb*B-2, nm23, BRCA1, p53, and estradiol dehydrogenases colocalize there. Losses of 17 and 18 in early lesions suggest that one or more genes from these regions may contribute to carcinogenesis. Gains of chromosome 1 were found in in situ and invasive neoplasia, whereas losses were not identified. Hence, alteration of chromosome 1 appears to be a relatively late event.

Primed in Situ Labeling

Primed in situ labeling is an extension of FISH technology with increased "speed and specificity."[8] It is particularly useful to identify genomic regions where mutations or microdeletions are common (eg, the p53 gene in human breast cancers).[20] Briefly, PRINS involves hybridization of a short, synthetic oligonucleotide to single-stranded DNA. A short oligonucleotide priming sequence is extended using DNA polymerase and labeled nucleoside triphosphates (Fig. 14–2). Visualization of labeled sequences is then similar to FISH. This technique may be particularly useful in breast cancers as the method is further developed.

Comparative Genomic Hybridization

Comparative genomic hybridization differs from FISH and PRINS in that probes to specific gene sequences are not required and the entire genome can be screened for gene

Denaturation of DNA

**Binding of Short Oligonucleotide Primer
to Target DNA**

Incorporation of Labeled Nucleotides During Extension by DNA Polymerase

FIGURE 14-2 Primed in situ labeling uses denatured single-stranded DNA and a short oligonucleotide primer that binds to the target sequence. The primer is then extended using DNA polymerase and labeled nucleotides. Primed in situ labeling is more sensitive, because subtle sequence changes (deletions or mutations) do not prevent probe binding. Detection methods are similar to fluorescence in situ hybridization.

copy number alterations.[8,21,22] Briefly, CGH uses dual-color fluorescence in situ hybridization methods and DNA from three sources. DNA from the test cell population (labeled with one fluorochrome) and a comparison–normal cell population (labeled with a second fluorochrome) are hybridized to normal human cell DNA in a metaphase spread (Fig. 14-3). Relative amounts of test and comparison DNA are determined by the color and intensity of the fluorochrome labels bound to the metaphase spread. For example, if the test DNA is labeled yellow and the comparison DNA is labeled red, a strongly yellow region on the metaphase spread indicates an increased gene copy number in the test DNA. A red region on the metaphase spread would indicate decreased copy number in the test DNA. By comparison of the color ratios (determined by fluorescence photomicroscopy and computer processing), regions of increased or decreased copy number are identified on the entire genome simultaneously.[23]

The sensitivity of CGH for detecting gene amplifications depends on the size of the amplicon as well as on the level of amplification.[8] Hence, CGH has two major advantages: (1) probes are not required, so previously unmapped regions or alterations may be detected; and (2) the entire genome can be analyzed in a single experiment. Disadvantages include the semiquantitative nature of the

assay, failure of the assay to identify specifically altered genes (eg, mutated), and a loss of sensitivity when contaminating normal cells or genetic heterogeneity is present in the test cell population.

In a landmark article, Kallioniemi and associates[24] described CGH results on 5 breast cancer cell lines and 33 primary breast cancers. Two thirds of primary tumors and most cell lines showed increased DNA sequence copy number affecting 26 chromosomal subregions. Sequences from 17q22–q24 and 20q13 showed the highest frequency of amplification, and many new areas of gene amplification were identified.[24] These studies identified many new chromosomal areas for the quantitative investigation of breast cancers using more specific methods such as FISH or PRINS. These investigators further suggested that in many chromosomal regions, contiguous genes might be important because larger-than-expected sequences were often amplified.[24]

Southern Blot

The Southern blot, named for its inventor (Southern), is a technique used to quantitate and evaluate specific DNA sequences.[25] A full discussion of this method and the scien-

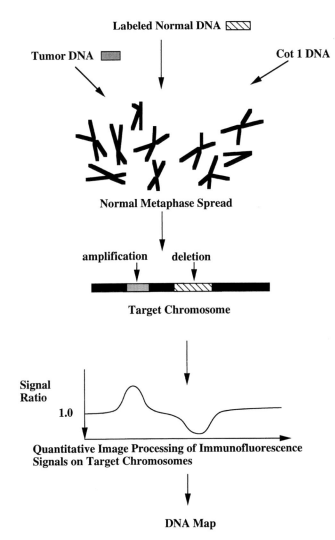

Labeled Normal DNA

Tumor DNA

Cot 1 DNA

Normal Metaphase Spread

amplification   deletion

Target Chromosome

Signal Ratio

1.0

Quantitative Image Processing of Immunofluorescence Signals on Target Chromosomes

DNA Map

FIGURE 14-3 Comparative genomic hybridization allows detection of DNA amplification anywhere on the tumor genome. The technique uses differentially labeled tumor and normal DNA that bind to competitively bind a normal metaphase spread. Cot-1/DNA is used to block binding of repetitive sequences. Counterstaining with diamino-2-phenylindole produces a banding pattern that facilitates chromosomal identification. Label binding is quantitatively determined by photography and digital image analysis.

tific principles that underly its application are found in Chapter 27.1. For breast cancers, commonly amplified gene sequences such as *erb*B-2 (see Chaps. 7.6 and 16) can be evaluated using Southern blots.[14,26] This method has also sometimes been used to identify areas of LOH (loss of one of two distinct or heterozygous alleles), a frequent mechanism of genetic alteration. LOH occurs commonly in several distinct loci in breast cancers, including 1p, 1q, 3, 3p, 6, 8, 11p, 13q, 16q, and 17p.[27] Areas of LOH frequently contain tumor-suppressor genes, several of which have been implicated in breast carcinogenesis. For example, the p53 gene (located at 17p13) encodes a 53-kd nuclear phosphoprotein believed to confer tumor-suppressor activity. The p53 gene is altered either through

LOH or by point mutation in 30% to 45% of primary breast carcinomas.[28,29] Most studies have shown no direct association between LOH at 17p and p53 gene mutation in breast carcinomas, unlike in some other tumor types that have been studied. Both mechanisms may result in altered p53 and therefore independently affect the tumor-suppressive activity of the 53 gene, either through simple dosage or by direct alteration of the gene.

Southern blot analysis has also been used to identify mutations of dominant oncogenes in breast carcinomas. Mutations of the *myc* oncogene have been found using this method, including such changes as amplification of one *myc* gene and rearrangement of the other in an invasive ductal carcinoma; normal tissues from this same patient did not show these changes.[30] In other studies, amplifications and rearrangements of *myc* were found in a high fraction of breast tumors,[31] and amplification of *myc* has been found to be associated with progesterone receptor–negative status in high-grade tumors in at least one study.[32] Southern blot analysis has also been used to characterize amplification of the *hst/int* 2 sequences; amplification was found to be present in 10% to 20% of breast cancers.[33] Further studies have not demonstrated a clear correlation of these changes with clinical parameters related to diagnosis or prognosis, however.[34]

In spite of the many contributions this method has made in the study of breast cancer, the limitations of this approach have led to a search for alternative methods. Southern blots require a relatively large amount of tissue; lower limits are in the range of several cubic millimeters. When compared with the more modern PCR-related techniques, Southern blotting requires (and irretrievably expends) three to four orders of magnitude more of the clinical specimen. Usage of larger tissue samples invariably increases the likelihood of heterogeneity within the sample. This heterogeneity may be anatomic (eg, inclusion of other epithelial lesions, such as hyperplasia and stromal or inflammatory cells), genetic (eg, subclones of breast cancer cells with *erb*B-2 amplification as discussed previously), or physiologic (eg, tissue growth factors, vascularity, and other factors). Breast cancer analysis is particularly prone to contamination by stromal, inflammatory, and benign epithelial cells because of the admixture of all cell types in tissue samples. In principle, contamination of malignant cells by unwanted (or unrelated) specimens or cell types should be detected in a quantitative manner with this technology. For example, if LOH is studied in a specimen containing more than 50% stromal or other nonmalignant cells, loss of signal intensity resulting from LOH in the malignant cells (50% of the signal in the tumor specimen) will be reduced by at least 25% on the Southern blot, increasing the possibility that LOH will be undetected. Although this can be accounted for in part by careful microscopic examination and identification of nonmalignant cell types in a representative portion of the specimen, the tissue used cannot be examined in its entirety. This represents a major problem with the Southern blot analysis of human tumor specimens. It is particularly a problem when microscopic confirmation of malignancy in the tissue sample or quantitation of the fraction of contaminating nonmalignant stromal, epithelial, or inflammatory cells has not been microscopically performed, regrettably a common practice in many laboratories. Interpretation of Southern blot data in which the normal cell content is over 25% should be considered unreliable. Tumors from which extracts are made may also vary in cellularity, histologic subtype, grade, and so forth, and this variability should be considered when the data are analyzed.

A second major disadvantage of Southern blotting for clinical applications in breast cancer has to do with the routine use of isotopic labels. Although nonisotopic methods have been developed, the sensitivity of these techniques has only recently begun to approach the sensitivity of isotopic methods.

Southern blotting is also notoriously susceptible to contamination of the sample DNA with parts of the cloned probe, which is isolated from a bacterial host. This common methodologic problem can produce an overwhelming artifact known as plasmid contamination. Plasmid contamination occurs when the cloned probe sequences contaminate, through laboratory reagents, DNA from clinical specimens. This type of contamination can only be controlled by scrupulous segregation of reagents in the molecular pathology laboratory, including an isolated location for culture and purification of DNA plasmid probes. Southern blotting from embedded tissues is rarely possible because of degradation of the DNA in the embedded specimen. Finally, assay-related issues (cell preparation, fixation, storage, cell viability) must always be considered. Each of the foregoing factors may significantly affect the data and may induce bias (particularly false-negatives) that may alter the conclusions.

Northern Blot

Use of the Northern blot for analysis of molecular alterations in breast cancers is also commonplace. Northern blotting is similar in every respect to Southern blotting, except the substrate analyzed is RNA rather than DNA. The RNA can be a crude extract from a breast tumor or a "normal" specimen (sensitive to contamination of stroma or other cell types similar to Southern blotting), and may be further fractionated according to its function (eg, messenger RNAs, which encode gene sequences, can be separated from total cellular RNA). Studies based on this technique detect alterations in a gene transcript and more particularly can be used to quantify the level of RNA transcript present in a breast tumor specimen accurately. Quantitative analysis of transcription in breast tumors has been carried out on a variety of genes including *myc,*[32] HER2/neu,[35] p53,[36] and the Rb gene.[37] Although application of Northern blotting to the study of breast carcinomas has considerable value, its limitations are similar to those of Southern blotting. An additional limitation of this technique is that RNA is intrinsically unstable and can be degraded quickly both in vivo and in vitro. Tissue specimens must be prepared by snap freezing or other rapid preparation techniques that are not required for recovery

of DNA. Furthermore, natural contaminants in the laboratory that degrade RNA require a much higher level of care in handling clinical specimens that will be used for Southern blotting; because of this, Northern blotting of embedded tissue is possible only in rare circumstances.[12] The problem of sample size that plagues Southern blotting for analysis of small specimens is accentuated with Northern blotting; the amount of tumor tissue required to do a good Northern blot is two- to threefold greater than that for the Southern blot (a total of 1 mL or more is required for Northern blotting). This technique is equally susceptible to plasmid contamination and must be scrupulously controlled in diagnostic molecular pathology laboratories when clinical specimens are studied.

Polymerase Chain Reaction

The techniques discussed in this section and following sections have been widely applied to study molecular pathology of the breast and rely on the PCR. This technology uses small amounts of DNA and has been particularly useful for recovering DNA or RNA from extremely small specimens, microdissecting small cell subpopulations from a significantly larger background, and extracting usable DNA from degraded tissues such as those that have been fixed or embedded. Many permutations on this technique have evolved since it was first developed in 1987.[38] Although many possible applications of this technology to the study of breast cancer exist, only those with potential clinical application are covered here.

The principle underlying the PCR is successive denaturation of double-stranded DNA, annealing of a specific oligonucleotide primer to the denatured sequence, and replication of the target sequence using a heat-stable DNA polymerase.[39] In principle, this reaction doubles the quantity of the target sequence in each round and can be cycled

TABLE 14-1
Polymerase Chain Reaction DNA Amplification

Polymerase Chain Reaction Round	Theoretic Amplification		Actual Amplification	
1		2		1.7
2		4		2.9
3		8		4.9
10		1,024	×(1.7)—	202
15	×(2.0)—	32,768		2,862
20		1.05×10^6		40,642
25		3.36×10^7		5.77×10^5
30		1.07×10^9		3.10×10^6
35		3.43×10^{10}	×(1.4)—	1.67×10^7
40		1.10×10^{12}		9.00×10^7

for as many as 40 rounds before its usefulness is limited as reagents are exhausted and competition of the product with the substrate occurs. Table 14-1 illustrates the potential of this technique for amplification of small quantities of material. In practice, the efficiency of the reaction varies from the early rounds to the later rounds, with an overall average efficiency of 1.7 (a 70% increase in the amount of product over template in each round) typical in early rounds, and a reduction to 1.4 (40% increase per round) in later rounds. Even under these constraints, the potential for this technique is enormous when studying small breast lesions or microscopic specimens.

Because PCR methods are particularly useful for small specimens, it is tempting to apply these to archival materials and thin sections in which a close correlation with tissue morphology can be preserved. A limitation of this application arises from degradation of DNA in many tissue specimens that have been formalin-fixed and paraffin-embedded.[40–42] This degradation may occur before the time of fixation, as with autopsy specimens or specimens that are refrigerated for long periods before acquisition, or it may occur due to fixation. Fixatives including heavy metals preclude the later use of PCR. In spite of these problems, PCR is a useful method for analysis of breast cancers and has been widely applied. Because of the inherent tissue heterogeneity (mixture of benign and malignant epithelium as well as stromal cells discussed already) in breast cancers, PCR can be combined with light microscopic–guided microdissection. This approach facilitates analysis of the earliest stages of the disease, such as focal epithelial hyperplasias and in situ lesions.[40,41]

PCR can also be performed in situ (ie, on the slide).[43,44] For example, methods have been developed in which DNA from cells that are not of interest on the slide can be selectively destroyed by ultraviolet irradiation,[45] preserving only a microfocus of epithelium (eg, in situ carcinoma within a terminal duct–lobular unit) for PCR. Further expanded PCR methods, such as multiplex PCR (which is similar to traditional PCR except that primers are synthesized that simultaneously amplify several fragments of DNA) and PCR for mRNA[46] continue to be developed and give PCR-based techniques even greater utility.

Quality control is of paramount importance using the PCR. Frequent methodologic problems arise even with careful handling. Because of the extreme sensitivity of this technique to detect and amplify sequences at low concentration in a sample, PCR methods are also good at amplifying rare contaminants in the laboratory or specimens that are unrelated to the tissue analyzed. As seen from Table 14–1, the enhancement in concentration of 10^6- to 10^7-fold of the target sequence results in a final product with a high concentration of the target (the volume stays constant). The product of this PCR reaction, having concentrated the target up to seven orders of magnitude, now has the potential for totally obscuring any target sequences in the next sample that is to be studied if only a minor volume of product–contaminant is accidentally introduced into the sample. Aerosols produced during pipetting can become an overwhelming contaminant in such studies. This phenomenon is called *carryover contamination*. Rigid quality assurance practices in the molecular pathology laboratory are essential in dealing with these problems. These include positive displacement pipettors, the use of nested primer pairs (in which the product of one reaction is no longer a substrate for the second reaction), and the introduction of ultraviolet-sensitive nucleotide analogues in the reaction, so decontamination can be carried out using ultraviolet illumination.[47] Although all these measures are helpful, no substitute exists for physical separation of the areas where PCR is conducted and where the initial tissue preparation is performed. It is not only prudent, but essential, that a PCR-free "clean room" is set up for the initial handling of specimens. No PCR reagents or equipment should be allowed to enter this room. A detailed discussion of measures to protect against carryover contamination can be found elsewhere.[48]

Gene Level Analysis Using Polymerase Chain Reaction

PCR-based methods have been particularly useful for the detection of mutations in oncogenes and tumor-suppressor genes and therefore have become "invaluable in the elucidation of mechanisms of carcinogenesis."[49] These methods are increasingly used for studying breast carcinogenesis, using invasive and noninvasive carcinomas as well as precursor lesions. For example, the tumor-suppressor gene p53 has been extensively amplified (at least exons 5 to 9) and analyzed using PCR-based techniques. In brief, these investigations have shown that exons 5 to 9 contain the major mutational hotspots in this disease, germline p53 mutations are rare in comparison with tumor-associated mutations,[49–53] more than one mutation can occur in a single p53 allele,[52] and mutations in exons 5 and 6 are associated with an increased proliferative rate.[54] Most of the mutations that have been characterized in one large series of breast cancers were single nucleotide substitutions and missense mutations with G:C to A:T transitions most prevalent and G:C to T:A transversions next common.[55] Statistically significant associations between missense mutations of p53 and nuclear accumulation of the encoded protein (as detected by immunohistochemical assay) have been reported by several groups.[28,29,56–58] PCR-based methods are discussed elsewhere.[59,60]

Abnormalities of p53 were initially reported in breast carcinomas as early as 1982 by Crawford and coworkers,[61] who reported that approximately 9% of breast cancer patients had circulating anti-p53 antibodies. Missense p53 mutations, in which an amino acid is changed, generally result in an aberrant protein with a prolonged half-life, resulting in protein accumulation and detectability by immunohistochemical assays.[28,29] More recently, inherited p53 mutations have been found to underlie the Li-Fraumeni syndrome,[50,51] an inherited disorder with increased incidence of many cancers including carcinoma of the breast often occurring in the patients' 20s and 30s.

Abnormalities of p53 have also been shown to be an independent marker of poor clinical outcome in breast cancer patients, particularly those with lymph node–negative disease.[16,28,29,62–65] The prognostic significance of p53 alterations has not been confirmed by all investigators,[66–68] however, so clinical applications may be premature.[29] A complicating factor in these studies is that intragenic mutations that result in a total loss of function of p53 through introduction of a new stop codon (termed *nonsense mutations*) are not easily detected by immunohistochemistry. Because many studies have focused on immunohistochemical methods to analyze p53, and many of these may have underestimated the frequency of nonsense mutations in breast carcinomas, it is possible that a more standardized approach to molecular analysis of these lesions will lead to a consensus on the prognostic significance of these defects.

The normal cellular role of p53 is discussed in detail elsewhere.[69,70] One of its more important functions is to regulate cell cycle progression including apoptosis (programmed cell death).[71] Regulation of apoptosis occurs principally through down-regulation of the bcl-2 gene.[72] As noted previously, LOH at 17p (site of the p53 gene) does not correlate with p53 mutations in primary breast carcinomas.[73] An association between LOH at two other specific loci, 3p24-26 and 17q31 with p53 mutation, has been reported in breast cancers, although this observation is of uncertain biologic or clinical significance.

DNA Sequencing of Polymerase Chain Reaction Products

DNA sequence analysis of PCR products has been possible since 1987. In principle, sequence can be derived from any specimen that can be amplified using the PCR. A more thorough discussion of this method appears in Chapter 27.1. The limitations of this technique, in analysis of breast carcinoma, include the following: (1) the size of the region that can be studied is restricted to 500 to 700 base pairs or less; and (2) it can only be carried out on genes of known sequence. A major advantage of this technique is that it represents a 10-fold reduction in effort and cost over previous DNA sequencing methods that relied on cloning. PCR-based sequencing also has the inherent advantage that both copies of an autosomal gene are studied at the same time, with no need for separate isolation and characterization. Direct sequence analysis of genes related to the development of breast cancer has been an important step forward in the past few years, as our understanding of the critical genes has increased.

Mutation Screening Methods

Although DNA sequence analysis of the PCR products, or of cloned fragments of genes, is adequate to detect mutations in genes relative to breast cancer development, these methods are relatively labor-intensive. To avoid the labor-intensive aspects of DNA sequencing, several approaches have been devised for screening large numbers of specimens that will allow the detection of variants among these. Once again, a detailed discussion of the methodologic aspects of these screening techniques, and their scientific basis, appears in Chapter 27.1. These screening methods use the PCR and are therefore subject to the previously described constraints and potential artifacts typical of PCR. Because many of the screening techniques have been developed for research, in which a lower level of sensitivity is acceptable as a trade-off for higher throughput, their application in a clinical diagnostic laboratory should be approached with caution. For the analysis of breast tumors in particular, with a clinical endpoint such as diagnosis or prognosis, these techniques may have limited value.

The most widely used mutation screening method is called single-strand conformation polymorphism analysis (SSCP). This method is used to screen for mutations in DNA or in a reverse-transcribed mRNA sequence (mRNA that has been converted to its cDNA using an enzyme called reverse transcriptase).[73,74] Single base-pair differences between two fragments produce altered mobility that can be detected as distinguishably different patterns after electrophoresis (Fig 14-4). Unfortunately, this approach is highly empiric in that it is extremely sensitive to ambient temperature, gel conditions, and buffer concentrations; because of this, the appearance of the SSCP pattern from a single PCR fragment may vary from day to day. It is thus only useful when used with appropriate positive and negative control specimens. The sensitivity of this approach is adequate for most screening methods, and under carefully controlled conditions may be in the middle to upper 90% range for PCR fragments less than 350 base pairs in size.[75–77] So far, SSCP analysis has been used primarily as an investigative tool and has had little application in the clinical molecular pathology laboratory. Likewise, denaturant gradient gel electrophoresis (DGGE), and variations on this method, have been used for investigational mutation screening in many tumor types, including breast carcinoma. This method is technically difficult and is prone to errors in inexperienced hands. As with SSCP, the sensitivity and specificity of this technique are not well characterized, limiting the usefulness of this method in the diagnostic molecular pathology laboratory. Similarly, RNAse mismatch analysis has been applied to mutation screening, but the sensitivity of this technique may ultimately limit its application to clinical problems.[78,79] On the average, the sensitivity of this assay system to detect unknown point mutations is approximately 50%.[78–80]

Summary

Recent advances in molecular genetics have facilitated a revolution in our understanding of breast cancer pathology. Methods with increased sensitivity that can be used to

FIGURE 14-4 Single-strand conformation polymorphism analysis is used to detect genetic sequence variations. The mobility of fragments run on acrylamide is determined by the DNA sequence; any variation in sequence results in altered mobility. Here, three members of a large family (lanes 5, 7, 10) carry a variant form of a gene causing cancer. The altered mobility is a clue that a sequence variation is present in this polymerase chain reaction fragment. Confirmation is carried out by DNA sequencing. Lane 1, control specimen; lane 2, blank; lanes 3 to 11, family member's blood; lanes 12 to 14, blank controls; lane 15, nondenatured control.

identify genetic alterations and our burgeoning knowledge base on the relative clinical significance of various different genetic alterations that occur in breast carcinoma raise the expectation that this new molecular genetic information will soon be clinically applicable. The path from investigational application of these technologies to their responsible integration in a clinical setting is tortuous, however.[81]

Two major obstacles must be overcome before these recent advances in molecular genetics will translate into clinically meaningful tests in the molecular pathology laboratory. First, methods must be both cost effective and reproducible in clinical laboratories, where the standards for utility are different from those in the research laboratories where the methods were developed. Second, the clinical significance of specific alterations must be repeatedly demonstrated through validation studies to warrant testing of clinical samples. Translation requires extensive multiinstitutional testing and studies with clinical correlation. Hence, clinical integration is both time consuming and expensive.

PCR-based techniques, for example, may hold great promise for distinguishing microscopically similar yet genetically and biologically distinct subsets of breast lesions (eg, invasive breast carcinoma adjacent to ductal carcinoma in situ). Presumably, identifiable genetic alterations distinguish these two cell populations. PCR-based approaches

might enable rapid and definitive testing for these genetic alterations. These might be particularly useful on cell preparations where architectural detail is unavailable and hence routine histologic criteria cannot be used, such as fine-needle aspiration biopsy. In these cytologic preparations, a definitive diagnosis of invasive as opposed to in situ carcinoma can be difficult. Potential utility such as this will require extensive testing and raises many additional issues. What would the sensitivity, specificity, and cost of a PCR-based screening method be, as compared with the immunohistochemical methods for the same marker? What are the trade-offs in moving from a relatively insensitive but established tissue-based technology to one that increases sensitivity three to four orders of magnitude but is unproved in the clinical laboratory? Is it fair to base our estimates of these factors on the investigational applications from which most of our current data are derived? Clearly, further validation of these newer research methods will be required before they can be integrated into the molecular pathology laboratory for routine application.

In looking to the future with respect to clinical application of modern molecular pathologic methods to breast cancer, it is useful to examine the status of integration of these methods into other areas of molecular pathology, or molecular diagnostics. New molecular methods are in various stages of clinical integration in four areas of pathology: microbiology, hematopathology, inherited disease testing, and solid tumor analysis. Of these, the best established and most widely accepted has been in hematopathology, in which analysis of clonality for diagnosis of hematopoietic neoplasia and analysis of specific translocations characteristic of various leukemias are common. Methods for quality control, including clinical survey materials and laboratory procedure guidelines, have been developed and are widely available, but whereas PCR-based methods allow an unprecedented level of sensitivity for identifying minimal residual disease in a treated leukemic patient, for example, the clinical implications of this finding—and appropriate clinical action—are not always clear. For genetic (inherited) disease testing, molecular diagnostic techniques are also well accepted, although they have a shorter history of application for most disorders. Questions regarding interpretation, accuracy, and the relative value of presymptomatic genetic testing versus clinical diagnosis at the onset of disease are abundant at this point. Ethical issues related to data reporting are also problematic. Application of these methods in the microbiology laboratory has been slowed primarily by questions of cost-effectiveness. Nonetheless, one might predict that, of the four areas listed previously, molecular diagnostic technologies may have the greatest impact on the clinical microbiology laboratory in the next 5 years as newer, cheaper assays are developed.

Of the four areas listed previously, solid tumor analysis is probably the farthest behind in terms of clinical application. The complexity of the genetic events that occur during carcinogenesis and the extreme variability of the genetic targets in different tumor types have prevented all but the earliest investigations of clinical validity and applicability. The molecular diagnostic technologies discussed here are likely to have little role in the routine clinical care of breast cancer patients during the next 2 to 5 years unless some unforeseen studies demonstrate significant clinical applicability. Some of the most promising prognostic or diagnostic markers, such as p53 alteration as a prognostic marker in women with node–negative disease or *erb*B-2 alterations as predictors of poor outcome in node-positive cancer patients or chemotherapeutic responsiveness, are still in the process of validation and clinical testing. This will involve rigorous standardization of the methods, assessment of cost-effectiveness, technical and interpretive difficulties, and clinical significance. Nonetheless, we predict that, over the next few years, these and other methods yet to be developed will lead to research that will take our knowledge and clinical investigation of breast carcinoma far beyond the routine microscopic categorization of lesions.

References

1. Smith HS, Lu Y, Deng G, et al. Molecular aspects of early stages of breast cancer progression. J Cell Biochem 1993;17G:144.
2. Allred DC, O'Connell P, Fuqua SAW. Biomarkers in early breast neoplasia. J Cell Biochem 1993;17G:125.
3. Johnston J. Human genetic disorders. J NIH Res 1992;4:153.
4. Benz EJ. The molecular genetics of cancer: introduction to principles of recombinant DNA technology. Cancer 1990;65:731.
5. Dracopoli NC, Haines JL, Korf BR, et al, eds. Current protocols in human genetics. New York, John Wiley & Sons, 1994.
6. Trent JM, Yang JM, Thompson FH, et al. Chromosome alterations in human breast cancer. In: Sluyser M, eds. Oncogenes and hormones in human breast cancer. Chichester, England, Ellis Horwood, 1987:142.
7. Trask B, Pinkel D. Fluorescence *in situ* hybridization with DNA probes. Methods Cell Biol 1990;33:383.
8. Gray JW, Kallioniemi A, Kallioniemi O, et al. Molecular cytogenetics: diagnosis and prognostic assessment. Curr Opin Biotechnol 1992;3:623.
9. Wolman SR. Fluorescence *in situ* hybridization: a new tool for the pathologist. Hum Pathol 1994;25:586.
10. Gray JW, Pinkel D. Molecular cytogenetics in human cancer diagnosis. Cancer 1992;69:1536.
11. Anastasi J. Interphase cytogenetic analysis in the diagnosis and study of neoplastic disorder. Am J Clin Pathol 1991;95(Suppl 1):S22.
12. DeLellis RA. *In situ* hybridization techniques for the analysis of gene expression: applications in tumor pathology. Hum Pathol 1994;25:580.
13. Pinkel D, Sakamoto M, Matsumura K, et al. Application of fluorescence *in situ* hybridization to detection of chromosomal aberrations. Cytom Res 1992;2:1.
14. Kallioniemi O-P, Kallioniemi A, Kurisu W, et al. *erb*B-2 amplification in breast cancer analyzed by fluorescence *in situ* hybridization. Proc Natl Acad Sci USA 1992;89:5321.
15. Muss HB, Thor AD, Berry DA, et al. c-*erb*B-2 expression and response to adjuvant therapy in women with node-positive early breast cancer. N Engl J Med 1994;330:1260.
16. Matsumura K, Kallioniemi A, Kallioniemi O, et al. Deletion of chromosome 17p loci in breast cancer cells detected by fluorescence *in situ* hybridization. Cancer Res 1992;52:3474.
17. Allred DC, Clark GM, Tandon AK, et al. HER-2/*neu* in node-negative breast cancer: prognostic significance of overexpression influenced by the presence of *in situ* carcinoma. J Clin Oncol 1992;10:599.
18. Gusterson BA, Gelber RD, Goldhirsch A, et al. Prognostic importance of c-*erb*B-2 expression in breast cancer. J Clin Oncol 1992;10:1049.
19. Micale MA, Visscher DW, Gulino SE, et al. Chromosomal aneuploidy in proliferative breast disease. Hum Pathol 1994;25:29.
20. Koch J, Mogensen J, Pedersen S, et al. Fast one-step procedure for the detection of nucleic acids *in situ* by primer-induced sequence specific labeling with fluorescein-12-d UTP. Cytogenet Cell Genet 1992;60:1.
21. Kallionemi A, Kallionemi O, Sudar D, et al. Comparative genomic hybridization for molecular cytogenetic analysis of solid tumors. Science 1992;258:818.
22. Thompson CT, Gray JW. Cytogenetic profiling using fluorescence *in situ* hybridization (FISH) and comparative genomic hybridization (CGH). J Cell Biochem 1993;17G:139.
23. Kallioniemi O, Kallioniemi A, Sudar D, et al. Comparative genomic hybridization: a rapid new method for detecting and mapping DNA amplification in tumors. Cancer Biol 1993;4:41.
24. Kallioniemi A, Kallioniemi O, Piper J, et al. Detection and mapping of amplified DNA sequences in breast cancer by comparative genomic hybridization. Proc Natl Acad Sci USA 1994;91:2156.
25. Southern EM. Detection of specific sequences among DNA fragments separated by gel electrophoresis. J Mol Biol 1975;98:503.
26. Slamon DJ, Clark GM, Wong SG, et al. Human breast cancer: correlation of relapse and survival with amplification of the HER-2/*neu* oncogene. Science 1987;235:177.

27. Bernstam VA. Handbook of gene level diagnostics in clinical practice. Ann Arbor, MI, CRC, 1992:271.

28. Thor AD, Moore II DH, Edgerton SM, et al. Accumulation of p53 tumor suppressor gene protein: an independent marker of prognosis in breast cancers. J Natl Cancer Inst 1992;84:845.

29. Thor AD, Yandell DW. Prognostic significance of p53 overexpression in node-negative breast carcinoma: preliminary studies support cautious optimism. (Editorial) J Natl Cancer Inst 1993;85:176.

30. Morse B, South VJ, Rothberg PG, et al. Somatic mutation and transcriptional deregulation of *myc* in endemic Burkitt's lymphoma disease: heptamer-nonamer recognition mistakes? Mol Cell Biol 1989;9:74.

31. Bonilla M, Ramirez M, Lopez-Cueto J, et al. *In vivo* amplification and rearrangements of *c-myc* oncogene in human breast tumors. J Natl Cancer Inst 1988;15:665.

32. Adnane J, Gaudray P, Simon MP, et al. Protooncogene amplification and human breast tumor phenotype. Oncogene 1989;4:1389.

33. Varley JM, Walker RA, Casey G, et al. A common alteration in the *int-2* protooncogene in DNA from primary breast carcinomas. Oncogene 1988;3:87.

34. Borg A, Sigurdsson H, Clark GM, et al. Association of INT2/HST1 coamplification in primary breast cancer with hormone-dependent phenotype and poor prognosis. Br J Cancer 1991;63.

35. Read LD, Keith D Jr, Slamon DJ, et al. Hormonal modulation of HER2/*neu* protooncogene messenger ribonucleic acid and p185 protein expression in human breast cancer cell lines. Cancer Res 1990;50:3947.

36. Thompson AM, Steel CM, Chetty U, et al. p53 gene mRNA expression and chromosome 17p allele loss in breast cancer. Br J Cancer 1990;61:74.

37. Lee EY-HP, To H, Shew J-Y, et al. Inactivation of the retinoblastoma susceptibility gene in human breast cancers. Science 1988;241:218.

38. Mullis KB, Faloona F. Specific synthesis of DNA *in vitro* via a polymerase-catalyzed chain reaction. Methods Enzymol 1987;155:335.

39. Innis MA, Gelfand DH, Srinsky JJ, eds. PCR protocols: a guide to methods and applications. San Diego, Academic Press, 1990.

40. Bianchi AB, Navone NM, Conti CJ. Detection of loss of heterozygosity in formalin-fixed paraffin-embedded tumor specimens by the polymerase chain reaction. Am J Pathol 1991;138:279.

41. Mies C. Molecular biological analysis of paraffin-embedded tissues. Hum Pathol 1994;25:555.

42. Greer CE, Peterson SL, Kiviat NB, et al. PCR amplification from paraffin-embedded tissues: effects of fixative and fixation time. Am J Clin Pathol 1991;95:117.

43. Nuovo GJ, Gallery F, Hom R, et al. Importance of different variables for optimizing *in situ* detection of PCR-amplified DNA. PCR Methods Appl 1993;2:305.

44. Chen RH, Fuggle SV. *In situ* DNA polymerase chain reaction: a novel technique for detecting MRNA expression. Am J Pathol 1993;143:1529.

45. Shibata D. Extraction of DNA from paraffin-embedded tissue for analysis by polymerase chain reaction: new tricks from an old friend. Hum Pathol 1994;25:561.

46. Eliyahu D, Goldfinger N, Pinhasi-Kimhi O, et al. Meth A fibrosarcoma cells express two transforming mutant p53 species. Oncogene 1988;3:313.

47. Sarkar G, Sommer SS. Shedding light on PCR contamination. Nature 1990;343:27.

48. Kwok S, Higuchi R. Avoiding false positives with PCR. Nature 1989;339:237.

49. Kovach JS, McGovern RM, Cassady JD, et al. Direct sequencing from touch preparations of human carcinomas: analysis of p53 mutations in breast carcinomas. J Natl Cancer Inst 1991;83:1004.

50. Malkin D, Li FP, Strong LC, et al. Germline p53 mutations in a familial syndrome of breast cancer, sarcomas, and other neoplasms. Science 1990;250:1233.

51. Srivastava S, Zou ZQ, Pirollo K, et al. Germline transmission of a mutated p53 gene in a cancer-prone family with Li-Fraumeni syndrome. Nature 1990;348:747.

52. Osbourne RJ, Merlo GR, Mitsudomi T, et al. Mutations in the p53 gene in primary human breast cancers. Cancer Res 1991;51:6194.

53. Merlo GR, Bernardi A, Diella F, et al. In primary human breast carcinomas mutations in exons 5 and 6 of the p53 gene are associated with a high s-phase index. Int J Cancer 1993;54:531.

54. Prosser J, Thompson AM, Cranston G, et al. Evidence that p53 behaves as a tumour suppressor gene in sporadic breast tumours. Oncogene 1990;5:1573.

55. Mazars R, Spinardi L, Ben Cheikh M, et al. p53 mutations occur in aggressive breast cancer. Cancer Res 1992;52:3918.

56. Hurlimann J, Chaubert P, Benhattar J. p53 gene alterations and p53 protein accumulation in infiltrating ductal breast carcinomas: correlation between immunohistochemical and molecular biology techniques. Mod Pathol 1991;7:423.

57. Jacquemier J, Molès JP, Penault-Llorca F, et al. p53 immunohistochemical analysis in breast cancer with four monoclonal antibodies: comparison of staining and PCR-SSCP results. Br J Cancer 1994;69:846.

58. Tsuda H, Hirohashi S. Association among p53 gene mutation, nuclear accumulation of the p53 protein and aggressive phenotypes in breast cancer. Int J Cancer 1994;57:498.

59. Loda M. Polymerase chain reaction-based methods for the detection of mutationsin oncogenes and tumor suppressor genes. Hum Pathol 1994;25:564.

60. Farkas DH, ed. Molecular biology and pathology: a guidebook for quality control. New York, Academic, 1993.

61. Crawford LV, Pim DC, Bulbrook RD. Detection of antibodies against the cellular protein p53 in sera from patients with breast cancer. Int J Cancer 1982;30:403.

62. Stenmark-Askmalm M, Stål O, Sullivan S, et al. Cellular accumulation of p53 protein: an independent prognostic factor in stage II breast cancer. Eur J Cancer 1994;30A:175.

63. Friedrichs K, Gluba S, Eidtmann H, et al. Overexpression of p53 and prognosis in breast cancer. Cancer 1993;72:3641.

64. Riou G, Lê MG, Travagli JP, et al. Poor prognosis of p53 gene mutation and nuclear overexpression of p53 protein in inflammatory breast carcinoma. J Natl Cancer Inst 1993;85:1765.

65. Isola J, Visakorpi T, Holli K, et al. Association of overexpression of tumor suppressor protein p53 with rapid cell proliferation and poor prognosis in node-negative breast cancer patients. J Natl Cancer Inst 1992;84:1109.

66. Hurlimann J. Prognostic value of p53 protein expression in breast carcinomas. Pathol Res Pract 1993;189:996.

67. Gasparini G, Bevilacqua P, Boracchi P, et al. Prognostic value of p53 expression in early-stage breast carcinoma compared with tumour antiogenesis, epidermal growth factor receptor, c-*erb*B-2, cathepsin D, DNA ploidy, parameters of cell kinetics and conventional features. Int J Oncol 1994;4:155.

68. Hanzal E, Gitsch G, Kohlberger P, et al. Immunohistochemical detection of mutant p53-suppressor gene product in patients with breast cancer: influence on metastasis-free survival. Anticancer Res 1992;12:2325.

69. Stürzbecher H-W, Deppert W. The tumor suppressor protein p53: relationship of structure to function. (Review) Oncol Reports 1994;1:301.

70. Levine AJ, Perry ME, Chang A, et al. The 1993 Walter Hubert Lecture: the role of the p53 tumour-suppressor gene in tumorigenesis. Br J Cancer 1994;69:409.

71. Hoffman B, Liebermann DA. Molecular controls of apoptosis: differentiation/growth arrest primary response genes, proto-oncogenes,

and tumor suppressor genes as positive and negative modulators. Oncogene 1994;9:1807.

72. Haldar S, Negrini M, Monne M, et al. Down-regulation of bcl-2 by p53 in breast cancer cells. Cancer Res 1994;54:2095.

73. Deng G, Chen L-C, Schott DR, et al. Loss of heterozygosity and p53 gene mutations in breast cancer. Cancer Res 1994;54:499.

74. Orita MY, Iwahana H, Kanazawa H, et al. Detection of polymorphisms of human DNA by gel electrophoresis as single-strand conformation polymorphisms. Proc Natl Acad Sci USA 1990;86:2766.

75. Orita MY, Sekiya T, Hayashi K. Rapid and sensitive detection of point mutations and DNA polymorphisms using the polymerase chain reaction. Genomics 1989;5:874.

76. Hayashi K, Yandell DW. How sensitive is PCR-SSCP? Hum Mutat 1993;2:338.

77. Sarkar G, Yoon H-S, Sommer SS. Screening for mutations by RNA single-strand conformation polymorphism (rSSCP): comparison with DNA-SSCP. Nucl Ac Res 1992;20:871.

78. Myer RN, Fishcer SG, Lerman LS, Maniatis T. Nearly all single base substitutions in DNA fragments joined to a CG-clamp can be detected by denaturing gradient gel electrophoresis. Nucleic Acids Res 1985;13:3131.

79. Myer RM, Lumelsky N, Lerman LS, et al. Detection of single base substitutions in total genomic DNA. Nature 1985;313:495.

80. Gibbs RA, Caskey CT. Identification and localization of mutations at the Lesch-Nyhan locus by ribonuclease A cleavage. Science 1987;236:303.

81. Curiel DT, Buchhagen DL, Chiba I, et al. A chemical mismatch cleavage method useful for the detection of point mutations in the p53 gene in lung cancer. Am J Respir Cell Mol Biol 1990; 3:405.

82. Fenoglio-Preiser CM. Selection of appropriate cellular and molecular biologic diagnostic tests in the evaluation of cancer. (Supplement) Cancer 1992;69:1607.

15

Diseases of the Breast, edited by Jay R. Harris,
Marc E. Lippman, Monica Morrow, and Samuel Hellman.
Lippincott-Raven Publishers, Philadelphia, © 1996.

Staging of Breast Carcinoma

JAY R. HARRIS

Staging refers to the grouping of patients according to the extent of their disease. It is useful in (1) determining the choice of treatment for individual patients, (2) estimating their prognosis, and (3) comparing the results of different treatment programs. Staging can be based on either clinical or pathologic findings.

The first clinical staging system widely used in the United States was the Columbia Clinical Classification. This system was developed by Dr. Cushman Haagensen and coworkers and was based primarily on patients treated by radical mastectomy between 1915 and 1942 at Columbia-Presbyterian Hospital[1,1a] (Table 15-1).

Currently, staging of cancer is determined by the American Joint Committee on Cancer (AJCC), which is jointly sponsored by the American Cancer Society, the National Cancer Institute, the College of American Pathologists, and the American Colleges of Physicians, Radiology and Surgeons. The AJCC system is a clinical and pathologic staging system and is based on the TNM system, in which *T* refers to tumor, *N* to nodes and *M* to metastasis. The current edition, the fourth, published in 1992,[2] differs substantially from previous versions and its implications are discussed below.

Clinical staging (designated cTNM or TNM) according to the 1992 AJCC system is based on all information available prior to the first definitive treatment and includes the findings on physical examination, imaging studies, operative findings, and pathologic examination of the breast or other tissues. The extent of tissues examined pathologically for clinical staging is less than that required for pathologic staging. Operative findings that are appropriate for clinical staging include the size of the primary tumor, the presence of chest wall invasion, and the presence of regional or distant metastases. The clinical stage is useful in selecting and evaluating therapy.

Pathologic staging (designated pTNM) includes all data used for clinical staging and surgical resection as well as pathologic examination of the primary carcinoma and axillary lymph nodes. A tumor is inevaluable for pathologic staging (pTX) if the excision of the primary carcinoma reveals tumor in any margin of resection by *gross* pathologic examination. Regional nodes are inevaluable for pathologic staging (pNX) if less than the low axillary lymph nodes (level I) have been resected. Metastatic nodules in the fat adjacent to the mammary carcinoma, without evidence of residual lymph node tissue, are considered regional lymph node metastases. The pathologic stage provides the most precise data to estimate prognosis and to calculate end results.

There are several important rules and definitions for the use of the current staging system:

cT size: The clinical measurement used for classifying the primary tumor should be the one judged most accurate (eg, physical examination or mammography).

pT size: The pathologic tumor size is a measurement of the invasive component. Specifically, if there is a large in situ component and a small invasive component, the tumor is classified by the size of the invasive component.

Multiple, simultaneous, ipsilateral (infiltrating, grossly measurable) cancers: One should use the largest lesion to classify T stage and should specify that this is a case of multiple lesions. Such cases should be analyzed separately.

Simultaneous bilateral breast cancers: These should each be staged separately.

Paget disease of the nipple: Without an associated tumor mass (clinical) or invasive carcinoma (pathologic), this is classified as Tis. Paget disease with a demonstrable mass (clinical) or invasive component (pathologic) is classified according to the size of the mass or invasive component.

Dimpling of the skin or nipple retraction: This or any other skin change except those described under T4b and T4d can occur in T1, T2, or T3 without changing the classification.

TABLE 15-1
Columbia Clinical Classification

Stage	Description
A	No skin edema, ulceration, or solid fixation of the tumor to the chest wall. Axillary nodes are not involved clinically.
B	No skin edema, ulceration, or solid fixation of the tumor to the chest wall. Axillary nodes are involved clinically.
C	Any one of the five grave signs of advanced breast carcinoma: Edema of the skin of limited extent (involving less than one third of the skin over the breast) Skin ulceration Solid fixation of the tumor to the chest wall Massive involvement of axillary lymph nodes (measuring 2.5 cm or more in transverse diameter) Fixation of the axillary nodes to overlying skin or deeper structures of the axilla.
D	All other patients with more advanced breast carcinoma, including: A combination of any two or more of the five grave signs listed for stage C Extensive edema of the skin (involving more than one third of the skin over the breast) Satellite skin nodules The inflammatory type of carcinoma Clinically involved supraclavicular lymph nodes Internal mammary metastases as evidenced by a parasternal tumor Edema of the arm Distant metastases

Chest wall: This includes the ribs, intercostal muscles, and serratus anterior muscle, but not the pectoral muscles.

Inflammatory carcinoma: This is a clinicopathologic entity characterized by diffuse brawny induration of the skin of the breast with an erysipeloid edge, usually without an underlying palpable mass. This clinical presentation is due to tumor embolization of dermal lymphatics.

If there is doubt concerning the correct T, N, or M category to which a particular case should be allotted, then the lower (less advanced) category should be chosen.

Definitions for classifying the primary tumor (T) are the same for clinical and for pathologic classification. If the measurement is made by physical examination, the examiner should use the major headings (T1, T2, or T3). If other measurements, such as mammographic or pathologic, are used, the examiner can use the subsets of T1. The primary tumor (T) is classified as follows:

Tx—Primary tumor cannot be assessed
T0—No evidence of primary tumor
Tis—Carcinoma in situ: intraductal carcinoma, lobular carcinoma in situ or Paget disease of the nipple with no tumor
T1—Tumor 2 cm or less in greatest dimension
  T1a—0.5 cm or smaller

T1b—More than 0.5 cm but not more than 1 cm in greatest dimension
T1c—More than 1 cm but not more than 2 cm in greatest dimension
T2—Tumor more than 2 cm but not more than 5 cm in greatest dimension
T3—Tumor more than 5 cm in greatest dimension
T4—Tumor of any size with direct extension to chest wall or skin
  T4a—Extension to chest wall
  T4b—Edema (including peau d'orange), ulceration of the skin of the breast, or satellite skin nodules confined to the same breast
  T4c—Both (T4a and T4b)
  T4d—Inflammatory carcinoma (see previous definition)

The regional lymph nodes (N) are classified clinically as follows:

Nx—Regional lymph nodes cannot be assessed (eg, previously removed)
N0—No regional lymph node metastasis
N1—Metastasis to one or more movable ipsilateral axillary node
N2—Metastasis to one or more ipsilateral axillary lymph node fixed to one another or to other structures
N3—Metastases to ipsilateral internal mammary lymph node(s)

The regional lymph nodes are classified pathologically as follows:

pNx—Regional lymph node metastasis cannot be assessed
pN0—No regional lymph node metastasis
pN1—Metastasis to one or more movable ipsilateral axillary node
  pN1a—Only micrometastasis (none larger than 0.2 cm)
  pN1b—Metastasis to one or more lymph node, any of which is larger than 0.2 cm
    pN1bi—Metastases in one to three lymph nodes, any of which is larger than 0.2 cm in greatest dimension
    pN1bii—Metastases to four or more lymph nodes, any of which is larger than 0.2 cm and all of which are less than 2 cm in greatest dimension
    pN1biii—Extension of tumor beyond the capsule of a lymph node metastasis less than 2 cm in greatest dimension
    pN1biv—Metastasis to a lymph node 2 cm or more in greatest dimension
pN2—Metastasis to ipsilateral axillary lymph nodes that are fixed to one another or to other structures
pN3—Metastasis to one or more ipsilateral internal mammary lymph node

Distant metastasis (M) is classified as follows:
Mx—Presence of distant metastases cannot be assessed
M0—No distant metastasis
M1—Distant metastasis (including metastases to one or more ipsilateral supraclavicular node)

TABLE 15-2
Stage Grouping

Stage	TNM Grouping
0	Tis, N0, M0
I	T1, N0, M0
IIA	T0, N1, M0
	T1, N1,* M0
	T2, N0, M0
IIB	T2, N1, M0
	T3, N0, M0
IIIA	T0, N2, M0
	T1, N2, M0
	T2, N2, M0
	T3, N1, M0
	T3, N2, M0
IIIB	T4, any N, M0
	Any T, N3, M0
IV	Any T, any N, M1

* The prognosis of patients with stage N1a disease is similar to that of patients with stage pN0 disease.

Stage grouping is as shown in Table 15-2.

The current AJCC system differs significantly from previous versions[3–7] in allowing all information available prior to when the first definitive treatment is used, including the operative findings and pathologic examination of the resected breast specimen with the primary tumor. In earlier systems, clinical staging was restricted to findings available before surgery—namely, physical examination and imaging studies. The many changes in the AJCC system over time and its complexity have greatly limited its use and usefulness. In addition, the current system does not address present-day issues in clinical decision making, such as a patient's suitability for breast-conserving treatment or the risk of distant relapse with and without systemic therapy. In practice, most clinicians simply use the tumor size and histologic findings of axillary dissection, often grouped for convenience into negative nodes, 1 to 3 positive nodes, 4 to 9 positive nodes, and 10 or more positive nodes. Attempts are underway to develop more useful staging systems.[8]

References

1. Haagensen C. Diseases of the breast, ed 3. Philadelphia, WB Saunders, 1986:852.
1a. Haagensen CD, Stout AP. Carcinoma of the breast: results of treatment. Ann Surg 1942;116:801.
2. American Joint Committee on Cancer. Breast. In: Beahrs OH, Henson DE, Hutter RVP, et al, eds. Manual for staging of cancer, ed 4. Philadelphia, JB Lippincott, 1992:149.
3. American Joint Committee on Cancer Staging and End Results Reporting. Clinical staging system for cancer of the breast. Chicago, 1962.
4. American Joint Committee on Cancer Staging and End Results Reporting. Clinical staging system for carcinoma of the breast, rev ed. Chicago, 1973.
5. American Joint Committee on Cancer Staging and End Results Reporting. Breast. In: Beahrs OH, Henson DE, Hutter RVP, et al, eds. Manual for staging of cancer. Philadelphia, JB Lippincott, 1977.
6. American Joint Committee on Cancer Staging and End Results Reporting. Breast. In: Beahrs OH, Henson DE, Hutter RVP, et al, eds. Manual for staging of cancer, ed 2. Philadelphia, JB Lippincott, 1983.
7. American Joint Committee on Cancer. Breast. In: Beahrs OH, Henson DE, Hutter RVP, et al, eds. Manual for staging of cancer, ed 3. Philadelphia, JB Lippincott, 1988.
8. Yarnold J, Dixon J, Greco M. Consensus document on staging for breast cancer. Breast 1994;3:238.

Diseases of the Breast, edited by Jay R. Harris,
Marc E. Lippman, Monica Morrow, and Samuel Hellman.
Lippincott-Raven Publishers, Philadelphia, © 1996.

16

Prognostic and Predictive Factors

GARY M. CLARK

The diagnosis of breast cancer presents several dilemmas for the patient and her physician. What type of surgery should be performed? Is radiation therapy necessary? Should additional systemic adjuvant therapy be used? If so, which therapy is best for this particular patient? To address these questions, one must first determine the likelihood that this patient will have a recurrence of her disease in the future if no additional therapy is administered. Then, the efficacy of the available therapies must be estimated and weighed against the potential side effects to determine the probable benefit for this patient. Unfortunately, the clinical course of primary breast cancer varies from patient to patient. Some patients have long disease-free survival, whereas others experience a rapid deterioration with early recurrence of breast cancer, followed shortly by death. Some of this variability is undoubtedly explained by differences in tumor growth rates, invasiveness, metastatic potential, and other mechanisms that we do not yet fully understand. To have biomarkers that could measure these functions, either directly or indirectly, would obviously be useful so individual patients could be classified into subsets with varying risks of disease recurrence.

Throughout this chapter, I use the terms *prognostic factor* and *predictive factor*. A *prognostic factor* is defined as any measurement available at the time of diagnosis or surgery and is associated with disease-free or overall survival in the absence of systemic adjuvant therapy. Potential prognostic factors include demographic characteristics (eg, age, menopausal status, ethnicity), tumor characteristics (eg, axillary lymph node status, tumor size, pathologic subtype), biomarkers that measure or are associated with biologic processes purportedly involved in tumor progression (eg, altered oncogenes, tumor suppressor genes, growth factors, measures of proliferation), and other factors. Prognostic factors can be used to predict the natural history of the tumor. A *predictive factor* is defined as any measurement associated with response or lack of response to a particular

therapy. An example of a predictive factor is the estrogen receptor (ER) status of a tumor, which predicts response to hormonal therapy in the adjuvant setting and in metastatic disease.

This chapter describes the current standard prognostic and predictive factors for primary breast cancer and details several newer markers that are being evaluated but have the potential for becoming standard factors in the future. I also describe pitfalls to be considered when evaluating these new markers.

Historical Perspective

The role of prognostic factors in optimizing treatment for breast cancer patients has clearly changed with the trend toward general use of systemic adjuvant therapy. Several years ago, patients with axillary node–negative breast cancer were considered to have a relatively good prognosis, and few received adjuvant therapy after local surgery. In 1985, a National Cancer Institute (NCI) Consensus Development Conference concluded that no standard therapy existed for patients with node-negative breast cancer.[1] Some of these patients were destined to have early recurrences of their disease, but despite attempts by several groups to identify subsets of patients at an increased risk of disease recurrence and death using prognostic factors, a consensus could not be reached concerning the identity of such high-risk patients. With the publication of early results from several randomized clinical trials showing a benefit from adjuvant therapy for patients with node-negative breast cancer,[2-5] and the publication of the overview analysis by the Early Breast Cancer Trialists' Collaborative Group,[6] however, many clinicians began to adopt the treatment strategy of administering systemic adjuvant therapy to all breast cancer patients regardless of their prognostic factors. A subsequent NCI Consensus Development

461

Conference in 1991[7] recognized that clinical outcomes varied among patients with primary breast cancer, but the investigators generally concluded that, aside from the standard factors of nodal status, tumor size, and histopathologic subtype, none of the newer prognostic factors had been proved to have clinical utility. Thus, one might question whether we really need any new prognostic factors for breast cancer.

Today, prognostic factors would be useful in at least three clinical situations.[8] The first is to identify patients whose prognosis is so good following local surgery that the addition of systemic adjuvant therapy would not be cost-beneficial. The second is to identify patients whose prognosis is so poor with conventional treatment that other forms of more aggressive therapy might be warranted. The third, perhaps the most useful, is to indicate which patients are or are not likely to benefit from specific therapies.

The standard prognostic factors currently in use for primary breast cancer include the following:

- Axillary lymph node status
- Histologic subtype
- Tumor size
- Nuclear or histologic grade
- Estrogen and progesterone receptor status
- Measure of proliferation

Unfortunately, at the present time, none of these factors alone, or in combination, completely separates patients who are cured by local therapy from those whose cancer is destined to recur and who will die without intervention. Therefore, to accomplish this objective, we need to consider newer markers that have not yet been fully evaluated. Caution must be taken when interpreting results of published studies that have evaluated potential prognostic and predictive factors. McGuire[9] proposed guidelines for the design and conduct of prognostic factor studies, and Gasparini and associates[10] gave more details on evaluation of these factors.

Statistical *P* values, especially those from univariate analyses, can be misleading because they depend on the number of patients included in the study. In this chapter, whenever possible, other statistics including relative risks (RRs) or absolute survival or recurrence rates are presented to give the reader some estimates of the magnitude of the effects that have been observed with the various factors. In addition, emphasis is placed on multivariate analyses that at least partially take into account the prognostic significance of the established factors and often of newer putative prognostic factors.

Histopathologic Features

HISTOLOGIC TYPE

Infiltrating ductal and infiltrating lobular carcinomas, either in their pure form or in combination with other tumor types, are the most common types of breast cancer.

When cells of two or more histologic types are present, the tumor is usually evaluated according to its most malignant-appearing elements, although Fisher and colleagues[11] have questioned the appropriateness of this practice. Patients with infiltrating ductal tumors generally have a higher incidence of positive axillary lymph nodes and poorer clinical outcomes than patients with the less common types of infiltrating tumors. With increased usage of mammography and other screening programs, more and more noninvasive breast tumors are diagnosed. Although these tumors generally portend a favorable clinical outcome, some do recur as invasive carcinomas. Considerable interest exists in identifying prognostic factors for these noninvasive tumors. Because of the low relapse rates and relatively long disease-free survival, however, large studies must be conducted to address this question, and definitive results are not available at this time. The remainder of this chapter focuses on invasive, infiltrating ductal carcinomas.

AXILLARY LYMPH NODES

The presence or absence of metastatic involvement in the axillary lymph nodes is the most powerful prognostic factor available for patients with primary breast cancer. Although most clinical trials stratify patients into three nodal groups (those with negative nodes, those with one to three positive nodes, and those with four or more positive nodes), several groups have demonstrated a direct relationship between the number of involved nodes and clinical outcome.[12–14] Figure 16-1 displays disease-free survival as a function of number of positive lymph nodes for patients in the San Antonio Data Base. Although lymph node involvement is associated with larger tumors, it is relatively independent of other biomarkers, including steroid receptors and measures of proliferation, leading to the conjecture that axillary node status may merely reflect the relative chronologic age of the tumor, and the various biologic prognostic factors might influence prognosis through other mechanisms.[15]

Although axillary lymph node dissection provides important prognostic information, debate exists about its therapeutic utility for local–regional control. Some studies have found a modest benefit, whereas others have not. Consensus has been reached, however, that not all patients need undergo this procedure. Patients with small, pure, noninvasive, ductal carcinoma in situ derive little benefit from an axillary dissection because their incidence of axillary involvement is low and their clinical prognosis is good. The value of axillary dissection in patients who present with systemic, metastatic disease is also questionable.

Several investigators have conducted studies to determine whether available prognostic factors could be used to replace axillary dissection in subsets of patients with primary breast cancer.[16–18] Ravdin and coworkers[18] showed that, in addition to tumor size, other factors such as the patient's age, S-phase fraction by flow cytometry, and ER concentration refined the prediction of nodal status by tumor size alone, but they could not identify any patient subsets with at least a 95% chance of being node-

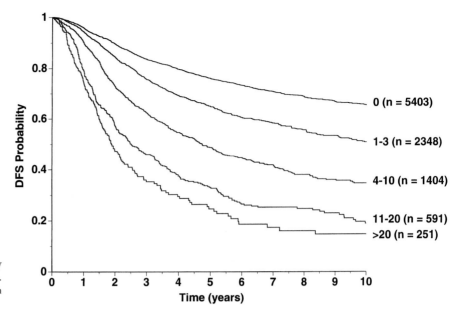

FIGURE 16-1 Disease-free survival by number of positive axillary lymph nodes. Data from San Antonio Data Base; median follow-up, 51 months.

negative or node-positive. Possibly, some of the newer factors discussed in this chapter might permit the creation of more powerful multivariate prediction models. If ongoing clinical trials of neoadjuvant therapies suggest advantages of systemic therapy before surgery, then the number of involved lymph nodes and tumor size will no longer be available, and other factors may have to be reexamined to replace the loss of prognostic information provided by these two powerful factors.

Standard practice is to administer systemic adjuvant therapy to all patients with node-positive breast cancer unless otherwise contraindicated. Thus, little need exists for new prognostic factors for this subset of patients. Indeed, evaluation of new markers prospectively in untreated node-positive patients will be nearly impossible. Therefore, this chapter concentrates on prognostic factors for patients with node-negative breast cancer. A great need remains for new predictive markers for all patients with primary breast cancer, however, and this discussion includes predictive factors for both node-negative and node-positive patients.

TUMOR SIZE

Within the subset of patients with node-negative breast cancer, tumor size is the most powerful and consistent predictor of breast cancer recurrence. Several large studies have examined the relationship between tumor size and clinical outcome.[19-27] Disease recurrence generally increases as the tumor size increases, but some studies have found that extremely large tumors tend to have better outcomes than tumors of intermediate size.[21] One might hypothesize that tumors that have grown to a large size without killing the patient or resulting in nodal involvement might have a lower potential for metastatic spread. Data from the San Antonio Data Base, however, suggest

a plateau in the risk of recurrence for tumors between 3 and 6 cm in diameter, and a significant decrease in disease-free survival for node-negative patients with tumors larger than 6 cm (Table 16-1).

McGuire and Clark[28] have suggested that tumor size and histopathologic subtype might be used to make treatment decisions for up to 50% of all node-negative patients. Table 16-2 outlines criteria for adjuvant therapy in node-negative breast cancer, including tumor size. Data from Memorial Sloan-Kettering Cancer Center indicate that patients with tumors less than 1 cm in diameter have a 20-year relapse rate of only 12%.[26,27] A study from the National Surgical Adjuvant Breast Project (NSABP), however, reported a 25% recurrence rate among untreated, node-negative, ER-negative patients.[29] These results confirm the necessity to examine several factors before estimating disease recurrence probabilities for individual patients.

TABLE 16-1
Actuarial 5-Year Disease-Free Survival by Tumor Size for Node-Negative Patients*

Tumor Size (cm)	N	5-y Disease-Free Survival
1–2	2014	79±1
2–3	1162	77±1
3–4	536	72±2
4–5	276	74±3
5–6	134	72±5
>6	144	57±5

* San Antonio Data Base; median follow-up, 3.8 y.

TABLE 16-2
Frequency of Adjuvant Therapy in Node-Negative Breast Cancer, According to Various Criteria

Variable	Adjuvant Therapy		
	Unlikely★	Possible	Probable
Percentage of patients	25	50	25
Patients per year	30,500	61,000	30,500
Tumor size (cm)	<1	1–3	>3
Eventual recurrence rate (%)	1–10	~30	>50
Patients receiving adjuvant therapy	Few	Unknown	Most or all

★ Therapy is also unlikely if the tumor is ductal carcinoma in situ, pure tubular, papillary, or typical medullary.

(McGuire WL, Clark GM. Prognostic factors and treatment decisions in axillary node–negative breast cancer. N Engl J Med 1992;326:1756)

Although retrospective studies consistently confirm the excellent prognosis of patients with tumors less than 1 cm in diameter, the increased use of mammography and other early detection systems has already changed the distribution of tumor sizes at diagnosis. Whether a 1-cm tumor detected mammographically will have the same natural history as a 1-cm tumor detected on physical examination is unclear. Perhaps some of the small tumors detected by early screening intrinsically have high proliferative capacity and metastatic potential, and other factors will have to be measured before the prognostic significance of a small tumor can be determined.

TUMOR GRADE

Tumor grade is a standard component of the pathology report, and several investigators have proposed that it is a powerful predictor of the course of a breast cancer. Indeed, when tumor grading is performed at single institutions by trained pathologists, most grading systems do correlate well with clinical outcomes. The primary difficulties with tumor grading are poor reproducibility and lack of agreement among different observers.[30–34] Some grading systems use only nuclear features and produce a nuclear grade. Others combine nuclear features with assessments of the architecture of the tumor and report a histologic grade. The most widely used grading systems for breast cancer are the Scarff-Bloom-Richardson (SBR) classification[35,36] and Fisher's nuclear grade,[37] although both systems are frequently used in modified versions.

The SBR grading system consists of three components (degree of differentiation, extent of pleomorphism, mitotic index), each scored on a scale from 1 to 3. The degree of differentiation is evaluated according to the ability of the tumor to form tubular, glandular, or papillary formations. Pleomorphism describes the shape of the nuclei, with par-

ticular attention to irregular cells distorted in size. The mitotic index evaluates the number of mitoses found in the tumor specimen. The scores for the three components are summed and categorized as grade 1 (well differentiated), grade 2 (moderately differentiated), or grade 3 (poorly differentiated). A modified SBR (MSBR) uses only the extent of pleomorphism and the mitotic index and rearranges the scoring system to yield five classifications of nuclear grade.[38]

Fisher's grading system includes a combined assessment of nuclear grade and the presence of tubule or gland formation. Nuclear grade considers nuclear size, shape, nucleolar content, chromatin pattern, and mitotic rate. Although histologic grading is only applicable to the invasive component of ductal carcinomas, the nuclear grade can be determined on all components of all histologic types of breast cancer.

Many published studies demonstrate the prognostic significance of individual grading systems.[38–48] Despite these observations, the Surveillance, Epidemiology and End Results (SEER) Program of the NCI reported that only 25.1% of breast tumors in the SEER registry were graded.[49] Even though several different types of grading systems were used, survival analyses of the 29,642 patients in the SEER registry with graded tumors revealed that, within each stage of disease, grade provided additional prognostic information.

A standardized grading system likely could be one of the most powerful prognostic factors for breast cancer, and reproducibility of grading breast cancers probably can be achieved using grading schemes with specific guidelines.[34]

OTHER HISTOLOGIC FACTORS

Several other histologic factors, including an extensive intraductal component, lymphatic vessel invasion, tumor necrosis, and mononuclear inflammatory cell reaction, have been associated with clinical outcome in one or more studies. A biologic hypothesis supports the use of each of these factors, but no factor has yet been fully validated as prognostic or predictive.

Patient Characteristics

AGE AT DIAGNOSIS

The influence of age and menopausal status at diagnosis on the prognosis of patients with primary breast cancer remains controversial. Some studies have found that younger patients have worse clinical outcomes than older patients,[50–59] others have reported that younger patients have a more favorable outcome,[60–63] and others have found no relation with age.[64–66] Explanations for these conflicting results have included small numbers of patients in the studies, differences in patient selection, and differences in the age groupings used in the analyses.

Two large studies carefully analyzed the clinical outcomes of young patients with breast cancer.[58,59] Both concluded that breast cancer patients younger than 35 years of age have a worse prognosis than older patients. Nixon and associates[58] found highly significant trends for the prevalence of poor prognostic features (grade 3 histology, extensive intraductal component, lymphatic vessel invasion, necrosis, mononuclear inflammatory cell reaction) to decrease with increasing age. Albain and colleagues[59] also observed increases in lymph node involvement, tumor size, steroid receptor negativity, S-phase fractions, and p53 abnormalities in patients younger than 30 to 35 years of age. Multivariate analyses were performed in each study, and both concluded that young age remained a significant predictor of recurrence and death after adjustment for other prognostic factors. This might suggest that breast cancer in some young women is biologically different from breast cancer in older women. The identification of the BRCA1 and BRCA2 genes implicated in some forms of familial breast cancer may help to establish the biologic basis of the disease in relation to age at diagnosis.[67–69]

At the other end of the age spectrum, controversy also exists about the appropriate therapy for older women with breast cancer. The metaanalysis by the Early Breast Cancer Trialists' Collaborative Group did provide some guidance on the efficacy of hormonal and chemotherapy within menopausal groups.[6] In older, postmenopausal women, tamoxifen significantly decreases mortality, and the magnitude of the effect generally increases with increasing concentrations of ER in the tumor. Chemotherapy is much less effective than tamoxifen in this age group. Because of the effectiveness of tamoxifen and its relatively few side effects, some physicians have questioned whether it could be used as primary treatment with only minimal local–regional therapy in elderly breast cancer patients. Rubens[70] summarized a series of studies that address this issue and described several disadvantages of this approach, including increased rates of local recurrence, the need for frequent monitoring, and the possibility that patients may not be fit for surgery or the tumor may have become inoperable. He concluded that, irrespective of age, the treatment of breast cancer should be designed to give the best chance of both local and distant control of the disease in the long term.

ETHNICITY

Survival after the diagnosis of breast cancer is poorer among black and Hispanic women than among white women.[71–76] Minorities tend to present with higher-stage or more advanced disease. An analysis of more than 100,000 women from the SEER program found significant increases in the incidence of early-stage breast cancers between 1983 and 1989.[77] Although increases were observed for both white and black women, black women had substantially lower rates of the least extensive breast cancers, leading the investigators to conclude that a major explanation for the increase might be the increased prevalence of breast cancer screening among women in the United States. Other researchers found, however, that even after adjusting for stage of disease, survival rates were lower for blacks,[78,79] but not for Hispanics.[75] Differences

in treatment might account for a portion of the poorer survival, but evidence indicates that black patients who receive the same or similar therapy still have a worse outcome.[78] Other factors such as the lower socioeconomic status of minority women are also associated with a worse prognosis; however, the precise cause of this association is unknown.[80,81] A delay in diagnosis related to lack of access to medical care or to cultural beliefs about cancer might contribute to a worse survival, but at least one study found no clinically significant interval between symptom recognition and medical consultation between whites and blacks.[82]

Elledge and coworkers[76] compared several prognostic factors among 4885 white, 1016 black, and 777 Hispanic women. White women were older, presented with smaller tumors, had less lymph node involvement, had higher incidences of steroid receptor positivity, and had lower S-phase fractions than Hispanic or black women. No clinically important differences in DNA ploidy, histologic type, HER2/*neu*, and p53 expression were found among the three groups. After adjustment for these poor prognostic factors, no significant differences were seen in disease-free survival or overall survival for node-negative patients, although blacks tended to have a worse prognosis. For node-positive or locally advanced disease and for metastatic disease, however, blacks had significantly worse disease-free and overall survival than did white or Hispanic women.

Measures of Proliferation

Growth fraction, or proliferative capacity, is important in the evolution of breast cancer. This has led many investigators to develop new techniques for evaluating potential markers of tumor cell proliferation that are expressed in various phases of the cell cycle (Table 16-3). Mitotic index (MI) has been an important component of all histologic

TABLE 16-3
Measures of Proliferation

Marker	G_0	G_1	S	G_2	M
Mitotic index	–	–	–	–	+
Thymidine labeling-BRdU	–	–	+	+	+
S-phase fraction	–	–	+	–	–
Ki67/MIB1	–	±	+	+	+
Mitosin	–	–	–	±	+
Histones (H2, H3)	–	–	+	±	–
Topoisomerase II	–	–	±	+	+
DNA polymerases (α, δ)	–	±	+	+	±
Cyclins (PCNA, A, D, E)	–	±	+	±	±

BRdU, bromodeoxyuridine; PCNA, proliferating cell nuclear antigen.

TABLE 16-4
Technical Considerations for Measuring Proliferation

Method	Markers	Advantages	Disadvantages
Flow cytometry	S-phase	Specific for S-phase Quickly analyzes large numbers of cells	Expensive Admixture of stromal elements Variable reproducibility
Autoradiography	TLI BRdU	Specific for S+G_2M	Requires viable tissue Exposure to radioactivity Slow
IHC frozen	Ki67	Requires only 1 slide Sensitive Specific for S+G_2M in tumor cells	Logistics (difficult shipping, handling, storage) Scoring tedious How to score?
IHC permanent	MiB1	Requires only 1 slide Specific for S+G_2M in tumor cells Logistics (easy shipping, handling, storage)	Variable immunostaining sensitivity Scoring tedious How to score?

IHC, immunohistochemistry; TLI, thymidine labeling index; BRdU, bromodeoxyuridine.

grading systems. Newer methods such as the thymidine labeling index (TLI) and bromodeoxyuridine (BRdU) have been applied to fresh breast cancer tissue, and flow cytometry has been used to determine the fraction of cells in various phases of the cell cycle in fresh, frozen, and paraffin-embedded tumors. Several antibodies now available recognize specific cell cycle–associated antigens.

Rather than measure cell proliferation directly, many investigators have evaluated factors that may regulate cell proliferation. One such factor is the tumor-suppressor gene, p53, described in more detail later in this chapter. Studies designed to evaluate its prognostic significance have also demonstrated a strong relationship between expression of aberrant p53 protein and tumor proliferation rates. In vitro experiments have now demonstrated that other markers such as p21 and p16 are positively regulated by p53. Cell proliferation during various phases of the cell cycle appears to be controlled by a series of multiprotein complexes that involve several cyclin-dependent kinases, p21, p16, D-type cyclins, and other factors including the retinoblastoma protein. Classic prognostic factor studies can be used to help elucidate some of these complex pathways.

One of the criticisms of measures of proliferation is the lack of standardization of the various methods. For some markers, multiple antibodies are available, each with its own sensitivity and specificity. In addition, different techniques such as immunohistochemistry (IHC), immunoblotting, and measurement of enzymatic activity have been used. Table 16-4 presents some technical considerations for some of these techniques. Immunohistochemistry can reliably be performed on small amounts of archival material. This will become increasingly important as smaller and smaller tumors are diagnosed by mammography or other early detection methods. IHC has several disadvantages, however, including the variability in the fixation of the tissue, which can lead to differences in

staining, and the subjectivity of the interpretation of the staining. Table 16-5 gives some of the advantages and disadvantages of various scoring systems that have been used to measure tumor proliferation by IHC.

MITOTIC INDEX

The MI is determined by counting mitotic figures using light microscopy on paraffin-embedded tumor specimens stained with hematoxylin–eosin. It has been described as the oldest, easiest, fastest, and cheapest way of assessing proliferation.[83] Mitotic activity is usually expressed as the number of mitoses per high-power field (HPF), although other scoring systems have been suggested, such as relating number of mitoses to tumor cellularity, tumor volume index, and area in square millimeters. Each of these systems has been correlated with clinical outcome, at least in uni-

TABLE 16-5
Immunohistochemical Scoring Systems

Method	Advantages	Disadvantages
Absolute counting (light microscopy)	Sensitivity Specificity Reproducibility	Extreme slowness
Point counting (light microscopy)	Sensitivity Specificity	Slowness Variable reproducibility
Semiquantitative (light microscopy)	Sensitivity Specificity Speed	Variable reproducibility
Image analysis (computer)	Sensitivity	Slowness Variable specificity Variable reproducibility

variate analyses. Expression of mitotic activity by dividing the number of mitoses by the number of cancer cells eliminates variability in the size of HPFs from one microscope to another, variation in tumor cellularity, and variation in tumor size. Reproducibility of the MI was demonstrated in the Multicenter Morphometric Mammary Carcinoma Project,[84] which included 14 pathology laboratories throughout the Netherlands. Correlation coefficients between 0.81 and 0.96 were obtained on tissues from 2469 patients with invasive breast cancer.

Only a few studies have included the MI in multivariate analyses of clinical outcome and have reported multivariate RRs. Russo and associates[85] reported RRs of 1.59 and 2.12, respectively, for disease recurrence and death, for patients with higher mitotic grades. Clayton[86] found that patients with more than 4.5 mitotic figures per 10 HPFs had a 2.8-fold increased risk of death in multivariate analyses. Aaltomaa and colleagues[87] found that volume-corrected MI is a more powerful predictor of clinical outcome than uncorrected MI. The MI is a component, in combination with other histopathologic features, of several prognostic indices. For example, both the Nottingham Prognostic Index[88] and the Multivariate Prognostic Index of Baak and colleagues[89] combine the MI with lymph node status and tumor size. Both indices have been shown to be more powerful prognostic factors than any of the individual components.

THYMIDINE LABELING INDEX

The TLI is determined autoradiographically by counting the number of labeled nuclei on autoradiographed microsections following incubation of the tumor specimen with tritiated thymidine. The TLI is independent of extent of disease at the time of diagnosis, axillary involvement, and tumor size, but is inversely correlated with steroid receptor levels.[90–97] Silvestrini[90] reviewed the clinical utility of cell kinetics, with particular emphasis on TLI in node-negative

patients. Most of the studies cited found an advantage in relapse-free survival for patients with slowly proliferating tumors. Table 16-6 presents an updated list of correlative studies in node-negative breast cancer. The RR of relapse based on multivariate analyses reported in these studies is approximately 2.

As with any new assay, methodologic standardization and reproducibility of results have been criticisms of TLI. Initially, the requirement for fresh tumor material was a limitation of the technique. The availability of a kit for in vitro incubation with [³H]dT and histologic fixation of solid tumor specimens has contributed to the methodologic simplification and standardization of the technical procedure, however.[98] In addition, Silvestrini and colleagues have conducted quality-control studies throughout Italy. Despite the relatively labor-intensive counting of labeled nuclei on autoradiographed microsections, correlation coefficients ranging from 0.78 to 0.99 within and among laboratories have been reported.[90]

The role of TLI as a predictive factor is being evaluated. Bonadonna and coworkers[99] used TLI as a stratification factor in a randomized clinical trial of high-risk, node-negative patients. One might hypothesize that adjuvant chemotherapy would be more effective against tumors with high TLI; however, a benefit from adjuvant cyclophosphamide, methotrexate, and 5-fluorouracil (CMF) therapy was observed in all subgroups. In another study of cytoreductive chemotherapy before surgery in patients with locally advanced breast cancer, no correlation was noted between pretreatment TLI and objective clinical response, which was inversely related to posttreatment cell kinetics.[100] Thus, the role of TLI as a predictive factor remains to be determined.

S-PHASE FRACTION BY FLOW CYTOMETRY

DNA flow cytometry can be performed on fresh tissue specimens, frozen biopsy samples, needle aspirates taken directly from the tumor, or paraffin-embedded tissues.

TABLE 16-6
Prognostic Significance of Thymidine Labeling Index (TLI) in Node-Negative Patients

Investigators	N	Follow-Up (mo)	Cutpoint	High TLI (%)	Univariate P Value		Multivariate P Value	
					DFS	OS	DFS	OS
Héry et al[91]	76	74	1.14	50	.02	<.001	—	—
Meyer & Province[92]★	148	49	3.0/8.0	67/33	.001	.001	—	—
Silvestrini et al[93]	354	62	2.8	48	<.0001	.0005	.0009	.0098
Tubiana et al[94]★	125	>180	0.25/3.84	67/17	<.01	<.01	.01	<.05
Courdi et al[95]	167	—	2.14	50	.01	—	.37	—
Cooke et al[96]	185	>93	7.25	50	.11	—	NS	—
Silvestrini et al[97]	340	48	2.8	?	.00	—	.009	—

DFS, disease-free survival; OS, overall survival; NS, not significant.

★ Used two cutpoints that produced three subsets of patients.

TABLE 16-7
Correlation of S-Phase Fraction With Other Prognostic Factors

	Diploid and Near-Diploid Tumors		Aneuploid Tumors	
	N	Median S-Phase	N	Median S-Phase
STEROID RECEPTORS				
ER+/PR+	37,173	3.1	23,289	6.5
ER+/PR−	14,107	3.7	12,492	11.4
ER−/PR+	1,712	3.9	1,756	13.0
ER−/PR−	6,175	5.1	9,560	15.3
POSITIVE NODES				
0	6,611	3.2	4,686	10.0
1–3	2,043	3.8	1,898	10.7
4–10	927	4.0	1,076	10.8
>10	475	4.4	583	11.6
TUMOR SIZE (CM)				
≤1	1,734	3.1	827	8.1
1–2	4,448	3.2	3,159	9.7
2–5	3,640	3.8	3,990	11.2
>5	531	3.9	614	12.2
AGE (Y)				
<35	280	4.9	305	14.4
35–65	5,864	3.6	5,260	11.4
>65	5,248	3.2	3,631	8.8

ER, estrogen receptor; PR, progesterone receptor.

(Adapted from Wenger CR, Beardslee S, Owens MA, et al. DNA ploidy, S-phase and steroid receptors in more than 127,000 breast cancer patients. Breast Cancer Res Treat 1993;28:9)

This technique produces a DNA histogram from which a measure of DNA content (DNA ploidy) and cell cycle components can be estimated. Traditionally, the cell populations are classified into three cell cycle compartments. Theoretically, the G_0-G_1 compartment consists of normal nondividing (G_0) or quiescent cells (G_1); the S-phase fraction is composed of cells undergoing replication or cell synthesis; and the G_2-M compartment includes cells in the postsynthetic phase (G_2) and cells in mitosis (M).

A strong correlation exists between high S-phase fraction and other prognostic factors, including poor histologic or cytologic grade. Wenger and associates[101] reported correlations among S-phase fractions, DNA ploidy, and steroid receptor status in more than 127,000 patients with breast cancer. They also found correlations with the number of positive lymph nodes, tumor size, and age of the patient (Table 16-7).

The clinical utility of DNA cytometry in carcinoma of the breast was the topic of a consensus conference that reviewed 43 published papers.[102] Despite the lack of stan- dardized methods and suboptimal measurement of S-phase fraction, that literature clearly supported an association between high S-phase fraction and increased risk of recurrence and mortality for patients with both node-negative and node-positive invasive breast cancer. The investigators noted that S-phase fraction is a continuous biologic variable, rather than a dichotomous function, and each laboratory must validate the prognostic significance of its own S-phase values. At a minimum, each laboratory should establish its own distribution of S-phase values and interpret individual results in the context of these distributions rather than by comparison with published cutoff points established by other laboratories. The optimal separation of patients into different risk groups by S-phase fraction has not been established, but the use of three rather than two risk groups may lessen the chance of misclassifying tumors with near-borderline values.

Herman and colleagues[103] reviewed some of the limitations of single-parameter DNA flow cytometry. A major limitation is the variable admixture of stromal elements in clinical samples. This produces DNA histograms that are composites of normal and malignant cells. This problem is greatest with DNA diploid tumors when, because of complete overlap between the two populations, the measured S-phase fraction is highly dependent on the percentage of normal host cells in the sample, in addition to the proliferation kinetics of the tumor cells. Combined staining with fluorescein-labeled anticytokeratin antibodies allows the DNA content of epithelial cells to be separated from that of other elements, and although definitive studies have not yet been published, this will probably further improve the prognostic significance of the S-phase fraction in breast cancer.

One is tempted to conclude that cell cycle–specific cytotoxic agents might work best against tumors with high S-phase fractions. Indeed, Remvikos and coworkers[104] noted that tumor responsiveness to neoadjuvant chemotherapy was directly related to S-phase fractions in 50 premenopausal women. S-phase fractions in studies of adjuvant therapies have not been predictive of response to chemotherapy, however. Dressler and associates[105] performed flow cytometry on tumor specimens from node-negative patients enrolled in a large randomized Intergroup study comparing CMF therapy and observation. The chemotherapy was equally effective for patients with low and high S-phase fractions. Muss and colleagues[106] evaluated S-phase fractions on tumors from node-positive patients enrolled in a Cancer and Leukemia group B study designed to study dose intensification of cyclophosphamide, doxorubicin, and 5-fluorouracil (CAF). Although the dose-intensity hypothesis was confirmed in this study, S-phase fraction did not predict response to therapy either alone or in combination with other predictive factors. A recently completed Intergroup study of patients with node-negative breast cancer used S-phase fraction as a stratification factor. Patients with high S-phase fractions were randomized to receive CMF or CAF. This study will help to establish whether S-phase fraction is indeed a predictive factor for these patients. Additional retrospective and prospective clinical trials with well-defined treatment regimens that also measure S-phase fraction will be required to address this issue.

Ki67

Ki67 is a monoclonal antibody developed by Gerdes and associates[107] that is specific for a nuclear antigen that is expressed only in proliferating cells (late G_1, S, M, and G_2 phases of the cell cycle). This antibody can be used with fresh or frozen sections of breast tissue and can be detected by a rapid IHC assay. Newer antibodies, polyclonal Ki67 and MIB1, have been raised against peptides from recombinant fragments of the gene for the Ki67 antigen and are effective in fixed, archival sections following microwave irradiation.[108,109] Ki67 staining correlates directly with tumor size, histologic grade, vascular invasion, and axillary lymph node status and inversely with steroid receptors.[110–113] Ki67 correlates well with TLI,[114,115] but poorly with S-phase fraction and proliferating cell nuclear antigen (PCNA).[116]

Several studies investigated the prognostic significance of Ki67, and most found a correlation with clinical outcome in univariate analyses.[90,113,116–125] Most studies had relatively few patients, were composed of heterogeneous groups of node-negative and node-positive patients who received a variety of treatments, and had short follow-up intervals. Table 16-8 presents the results of studies that either focused on node-negative patients or reported a subset analysis within this group of patients. Although few studies reported RRs of disease recurrence or death, inspection of the survival curves presented suggests that the increased risk of disease recurrence in patients with high Ki67 may be in the same range as for patients with high TLI or increased S-phase fraction. Additional studies with multivariate analyses are needed to define the role of Ki67 as a prognostic factor.

PROLIFERATING CELL NUCLEAR ANTIGEN

PCNA is a nuclear protein associated with DNA polymerase ∂, which is present throughout the cell cycle in proliferating cells. The monoclonal antibody PC10 recognizes an epitope of human PCNA in fixed breast cancer tissue. Most studies have found only weak correlations with other prognostic factors,[90,126–129] and associations with clinical outcomes have been disappointingly poor, especially in node-negative patients.

COMPARISON OF MEASURES OF PROLIFERATION

Relatively few studies have compared different measures of proliferation in head-to-head prognostic studies. Rose and associates[130] compared five antibodies for IHC assessment of growth fraction in formalin-fixed, paraffin-embedded tissues (MIB1, polyclonal Ki67, monoclonal Ki67, PC10, JC1). Based on evaluations of the staining performance of the different antibodies, these researchers concluded that MIB1 and polyclonal Ki67 are the best proliferation markers in conventional histologic preparations, and the other markers could not be recommended for routine use. Gasparini and colleagues[116] directly compared the prognostic significance of S-phase fraction, Ki67, and PCNA in a series of 168 breast cancer patients and concluded that S-phase fraction was the strongest prognostic factor. Neither Ki67 nor PCNA was an independent prognosticator in their study. Brown and coworkers[113] reported that both S-phase fraction and Ki67 are significant predictors of disease recurrence, and they can be combined, in a complex manner depending on tumor size, to provide additional prognostic information.

Steroid Receptors and Estrogen-Regulated Factors

ESTROGEN AND PROGESTERONE RECEPTORS

Steroid receptor status determined by ligand-binding assays has been used to make treatment decisions for patients with advanced breast cancer for many years. Nearly 20 years ago, the first report of the prognostic significance

TABLE 16-8
Prognostic Significance of Ki67 in Node-Negative Patients

Investigators	N	Follow-Up (mo)	Cutpoint	High Ki67 (%)	Univariate P Value		Multivariate P Value	
					DFS	OS	DFS	OS
Brown et al[113]	673	52	7	21	.005	NS	<.05	NS
Bouzubar et al[117]	77	88	4/13	71/33	<.01	—	—	—
Weikel et al[118]	76	24	10/20	76/45	<.01	—	—	—
Sahin et al[120]	42	20	20	25	.01	—	—	—
Veronese et al[123]	71	42	20	25	.01	—	—	—
Gaglia et al[125]	197	31	9	50	.01	—	—	—

DFS, disease-free survival; OS, overall survival; NS, not significant.

of the ER was published.[131] Although conflicting results have appeared in the literature, the larger studies with longer follow-up consistently demonstrate that patients with ER-positive tumors have longer disease-free intervals than patients with ER-negative tumors. Data from San Antonio and the NSABP indicate that the disease-free survival advantage is about 10% at 5 years.[132] The additional knowledge gained by measuring progesterone receptors (PRs) in patients with node-negative disease is not clear. Theoretically, PR is an indicator of an intact estrogen-response pathway because it is produced by estrogen stimulation.[133] In multivariate analyses of node-negative patients, however, either ER or PR, but seldom both, is a significant predictor of clinical outcome. Often, ER is a stronger predictor of disease-free survival, whereas PR is more closely associated with overall survival, perhaps because it is a better indicator of response to endocrine therapy following disease recurrence.

Some studies have reported that disease-free survival curves tend to merge with longer follow-up,[134,135] suggesting that ER status is a reflection of proliferative capacity rather than metastatic potential. Figure 16-2 demonstrates a similar phenomenon for both ER and PR in untreated, node-negative patients from the San Antonio Data Base. Both ER and PR levels are strongly inversely correlated with measures of proliferation,[90,101] and they are directly related to histologic grade. ER concentrations increase almost linearly with increasing age, whereas PR levels depend more on menopausal status.[136]

A large Danish study of 952 untreated postmenopausal women with breast cancer found an unusual relationship between ER levels and clinical outcome.[137] Patients with extremely high ER levels had as poor a prognosis as ER-negative patients, whereas patients with intermediate ER levels had the longest disease-free intervals. The investigators hypothesized that overexpression of ER might signify the progression of the tumor from a fully hormone-dependent to a hormone-independent state by a hormone-responsive state. In contrast to the poor disease-free survival

in patients with extremely high ER levels, this group derives the greatest benefit from adjuvant treatment with hormonal therapies.

Because of the decreasing size of newly diagnosed breast cancers and the inability of biochemical assays to assess intratumoral heterogeneity, histochemical techniques have been proposed for determining steroid receptor levels. Despite the growing popularity of histochemical assays, few comparative studies have been performed. Kinsel and coworkers[138] reported a correlation of 0.63 between biochemical and histochemical ER levels in a series of 257 breast cancer patients. ER by both techniques correlated with disease-free and overall survival, but only the immunochemical values remained significant after 5 years of follow-up. Berger and associates[139] reported a correlation of 0.78 between PR levels determined by biochemical and immunocytochemical techniques, but they did not assess the prognostic significance of PR levels determined by either assay. Foekens and colleagues[140] compared ER and PR determined by biochemical and by enzyme immunoassay in 205 patients and reported correlations of 0.94 and 0.88, respectively, for ER and PR when the assays were performed on the same cytosols. Survival analyses showed that both methods were equally useful for predicting disease-free and overall survival. A limitation of this study is that the cutoffs used to define assay positivity were derived from the same data used to compare the assays. Andersen and coworkers[141] compared biochemical ER values with IHC assays in frozen and paraffin-embedded tissue from 130 postmenopausal high-risk breast cancer patients with a median follow-up of 75 months. The biochemical assay was slightly more sensitive (80% positive) than the IHC assay in frozen tissue (73% positive), which was more sensitive than the assay in paraffin-embedded tissue (60% positive). Correlations among the three assays ranged from 0.61 to 0.85. The RRs of relapse for patients with ER-negative tumors determined by biochemical assay, IHC assay in frozen section, and IHC assay

FIGURE 16-2 Disease-free survival by estrogen (**A**) and progesterone (**B**) receptor status. Data from San Antonio Data Base; median follow-up, 62 months. Relative risks of recurrence (95% confidence intervals): 1.31 (1.12 to 1.53), *P*=.0008; 1.17 (1.00 to 1.37), *P*=.04, respectively, for estrogen and progesterone receptors.

in paraffin-embedded tissue were 3.12, 2.90, and 1.94, respectively.

The cutoffs used to define ER positivity depend on the objective of the assay. If the intent is to identify patients who are likely to benefit from hormonal therapy, then high cutoffs that result in lower percentages of ER-positive patients would be preferred. On the other hand, if the intent is to identify patients who will not benefit from hormonal therapy, then lower cutoffs might be optimal. The general tendency for IHC assays to be less sensitive than biochemical assays suggests that they might be more useful as predictive factors for response to endocrine therapies rather than as markers of resistance. Additional studies with standardized methods and definitions of receptor positivity are needed to adequately address this question.

pS2

The pS2 gene was first identified in a human breast cancer cell line in response to estrogen stimulation.[142] The pS2 protein is a small (6450-kd), secreted protein of unknown function. The gene has been cloned and isolated to 21q, and sequencing has revealed homologies with a porcine pancreatic protein known to inhibit gastrointestinal mobility and secretion,[143] and with human insulin-like growth factors I and II.[144] Investigators have suggested that pS2 expression could reflect the functional status of ER, and it might be both a prognostic factor and predictive factor in primary breast cancer.[145]

Several studies have demonstrated strong associations between pS2 concentrations in human breast tumors and ER and PR status. Most studies have found no significant relation with nodal status or tumor size, however.

An initial study by Foekens and associates[145] found that patients whose tumors expressed high levels of pS2 determined by a radioimmunoassay had significantly better disease-free and overall survival in both univariate and multivariate analyses. Using a data-derived cutpoint, 27% of patients were classified as pS2-positive. Subsequent studies by the same group, however, found that this prognostic significance disappeared when newer cytosolic factors, including cathepsin D, urokinase-type plasminogen activator (uPA), and plasminogen activator inhibitor-1 (PAI-1) were measured simultaneously. Other studies using radioimmunoassays have produced conflicting results. Predine and colleagues[146] reported increased risks of relapse (RR, 1.80) and death (RR, 2.56) for patients whose tumors had absent or low pS2 concentrations (15% of all patients). Attempts to validate the higher cutpoint used by Foekens and coworkers[145] failed to achieve statistical significance. A study by Gion and associates[147] did find strong prognostic significance for both disease-free and overall survival, however, and a study by Spyratos and coauthors[148] reported that pS2 positivity was associated with longer overall survival, particularly in patients who received hormone therapy, but was not related to disease-free survival.

Four studies determined pS2 status by IHC techniques.[149–152] Even though similar rates of pS2 positivity were observed compared with studies using radioimmunoassays, none of these studies found associations between pS2 status and clinical outcome. In some studies, trends were found for better overall survival for pS2-positive patients, findings suggesting that these patients might be responding to hormonal therapy after disease recurrence. Investigators have hypothesized that expression of pS2 is not related to the ability of breast tumors to recur or to form metastases, but rather to the aggressiveness of recurrences and metastases, perhaps through their stage of differentiation.[148]

pS2 will probably be most useful as a predictor of response to hormone therapy for both primary and advanced breast cancer, especially when used in concert with ER and PR.

HEAT SHOCK PROTEINS

Heat shock proteins (hsps) are produced in response to environmental stresses (eg, exposure to heat, heavy metals, or oxidants) and physiologic stresses (eg, viral and microbial infections, inflammation, ischemia, exposure to certain antineoplastic agents).[153] Several different hsps are normally expressed in cells and are differentially expressed or regulated during the cell cycle by hormones at different stages of development and differentiation. Members of the hsp family are usually identified by their molecular weights (eg, hsp27, hsp60, hsp70, hsp90, hsp100).

Initial studies by Chamness and associates[154] and Tandon and colleagues[155] suggested that hsp27, hsp70, and hsp90 might be prognostic factors, especially for time to recurrence of node-negative breast cancer patients. A follow-up study by Ciocca and coworkers,[156] however, which attempted to confirm the original findings in 345 node-negative patients was unable to do so for hsp27 and hsp90. Nonetheless, hsp70 continued to be an independent predictor of disease recurrence in multivariate analyses.

Thor and associates[157] found striking associations between hsp27 overexpression and ER content, nodal metastases, large tumor size, and lymphatic or vascular invasion. In univariate analyses, hsp27 correlated with shorter disease-free survival, but in multivariate analyses, it was not a statistically significant independent prognostic factor for clinical outcome. Love and King[158] measured hsp27 in 361 patients with primary breast cancer and found a strong correlation with ER but not PR. It was also unrelated to age, menstrual status, and tumor size. In univariate analyses, hsp27 predicted a short disease-free interval, but longer survival from first relapse. In multivariate analyses, however, hsp27 was not an independent predictor of clinical outcome.

Data reported by Ciocca and colleagues[159] suggest that hsp27 may be involved in cellular resistance to cytotoxic drugs, particularly doxorubicin. When cancer cell lines were exposed to heat shock treatment, significant elevations of hsp27 were observed. Subsequent treatment with doxorubicin showed increased resistance, compared with control cells. This resistance, however, was not seen with other drugs such as colchicine and methotrexate. Oesterreich and associates[160] conducted a series of experiments to determine whether hsp27 expression is *directly* involved in heat-induced doxorubicin resistance. They introduced hsp27 expression vectors into cells that express low levels of hsp27 and cells that express high levels of hsp27 as a result of gene amplification. When the low hsp27–expressing cells were then transfected with a full-length cDNA, the cells displayed a threefold elevated resistance to doxorubicin. When the high hsp27–expressing cells were transfected with an antisense hsp27 construct, they became threefold more sensitive to doxorubicin. These results suggest that hsp27 specifically confers doxorubicin resistance in human breast cancer cells, and manipulation of hsp27 levels, either genetically or pharmacologically, may be useful in reversing this drug resistance in breast cancer patients.

Thus, although the hsps may not be powerful prognostic factors, they may eventually have clinical utility for predicting response to therapy. In addition, they may provide targets of opportunity for new therapeutic strategies.

Growth Factors and Receptors

The epithelial cells of the breast are under the influence of a variety of hormones and growth factors. The tyrosine kinase growth factor receptors are among the best studied, and they have been subclassified into nine different families based on the structure of their extracellular ligand-binding and intracellular kinase domains and the nature of their activating ligands.[161] The type I growth factor receptors include the epidermal growth factor receptor (EGFR) family, which contains several polypeptides that are expressed in the breast and are involved in the development of breast cancer. Members of this family are EGFR (also known as c-erbB-1), HER-2/neu (also known as c-erbB-2), HER-3 (also known as c-erbB-3), and HER-4 (also known as c-erbB-4). The specific ligands have yet to be identified for some of these receptors, but Table 16-9 displays what is known today.

TABLE 16-9
Type I Growth Factor Receptor Family and Their Known Ligands

Growth Factor Receptor	Ligands
EGFR	EGF, TGF-α, amphiregulin, heparin-binding EGF, viral growth factors, β cellulin
HER-2/neu	Unknown
c-erbB-3	Heregulin (?)
c-erbB-4	Heparin-binding c-erbB-4 stimulatory factor, heregulin
Unknown	Cripto (?)

EGF, epidermal growth factor; EGFR, EGF receptor; TGF-α, transforming growth factor α.

(Adapted from Rajkumar T, Gullick WJ. The type I growth factor receptors in human breast cancer. Breast Cancer Res Treat 1994;29:3)

HER-3 and HER-4 have only recently been discovered, and definitive information is not yet available concerning the prognostic or predictive significance of either of these receptors. Several studies have been conducted to evaluate EGFR and HER-2/neu, however, and these factors are discussed in more detail.

EPIDERMAL GROWTH FACTOR RECEPTOR

The EGFR is a 170-kd transmembrane glycoprotein translated from mRNAs of 6 and 10 kb encoded by a gene on chromosome 7q21. EGFR has been identified by several methods including radioligand-binding assays, autoradiography, immunocytohistochemistry, immunoenzymatic assays, and measurement of EGFR transcripts. An entire issue of the journal *Breast Cancer Research and Treatment* (volume 29, no. 1, 1994) was devoted to the biologic, prognostic, and therapeutic roles of EGFR in breast cancer. EGFR is present at low levels on normal breast epithelial cells and in other tissues, including the liver. Approximately 35% to 60% of primary breast cancers overexpress EGFR. No clear differences in EGFR positivity are seen among the various assay techniques, although EGFR positivity tends to be lowest when measured by immunologic methods. Nearly all studies have reported a negative relation between EGFR and steroid receptor status, with EGFR positivity twice as high in ER-negative or PR-negative tumors. Most published reports have found statistically significant associations or trends for direct relation to worse tumor grade and increased proliferation indices. Only a few published studies have reported associations with age, menopausal status, histologic type, tumor size, or axillary nodal status. Studies suggest that EGFR may be correlated with overexpression of abnormal p53 and angiogenesis factors.

The relation between EGFR and clinical outcome remains controversial. Several reviews have summarized the results of many studies with more than 3000 patients.[162–164] Care must be taken when summarizing these studies because several publications are updated analyses of previously published studies. Most of the studies show a significant relation between EGFR status and disease-free or overall survival using univariate analyses. In some studies, however, the results apply only to node-negative or node-positive patients. In studies with longer follow-up, the initial significant separation of disease-free or overall survival curves tends to diminish with time. Multivariate analyses have been performed in few of the published studies. Another confounding factor is the variable systemic adjuvant therapies that the patients have received.

In summary, EGFR is probably an important prognostic factor for primary breast cancer, but the lack of standardization of the assay methods, the small numbers of patients and short follow-up intervals in most of the studies, and the general lack of multivariate analyses make it impossible to draw firm conclusions about the optimal role of EGFR in determining prognosis for the individual breast cancer patient.

On the other hand, the role of EGFR as a predictive factor for hormone resistance or responsiveness is better defined. Several groups have clearly shown that tumors expressing EGFR are more likely to be resistant to endocrine therapy. Conversely, EGFR-negative tumors, especially if they are also ER-positive, tend to have high response rates. Nicholson and colleagues[165] reported an 80% response rate for EGFR-negative–ER-positive patients, with 45% achieving complete or partial remission.

Perhaps the most exciting use of EGFR is as a target for new therapies. Mendelsohn and associates[166] have been the leaders in this area and have developed several monoclonal antibodies directed against EGFR. Some of these antibodies have been evaluated in clinical trials, and novel combinations of chemotherapeutic agents and anti–EGFR monoclonal antibodies are being evaluated.

HER-2/neu

The HER-2/neu gene is located on chromosome 17q21 and is transcribed into a 4.5-kb mRNA, which is translated into a 185-kd glycoprotein. The HER-2/neu protein is expressed at low levels in the epithelial and myoepithelial cells of normal breast tissue. It is overexpressed in comedo, large cell, ductal carcinoma in situ, but relatively low levels are found in papillary and cribriform in situ tumors.

Seven years after the initial studies of the prognostic value of HER-2/neu in breast cancer, its role is still being defined. Ravdin and Chamness[167] reviewed the published literature concerning HER-2/neu, and they concluded that the interpretation of studies on the use of this gene and its protein product in prognostic and predictive tests for breast cancer is complicated by multiple methods and inherent difficulties in many of the studies. The work has moved beyond the stage at which small studies with short follow-up (useful for hypothesis generation) are of value, to the stage in which large studies with sufficient statistical power to find significant correlations are central. These larger studies do not lend support for the use of HER-2/neu in the evaluation of patients with negative axillary lymph nodes, the group of breast cancer patients for whom refinement of prognostic estimates is now most important. Hints exist, however, that HER-2/neu may have value in predicting response to certain treatments, although the studies so far are too few, often too small, and too conflicting to confirm this reliably.

The first studies addressing the possible prognostic significance of HER-2/neu measured gene amplification. HER-2/neu amplification was generally found to be predictive of poorer disease-free and overall survival in node-positive patients, but seldom in the node-negative subgroups.[168–177] Later studies measured expression of the HER-2/neu protein product rather than gene amplification. Protein expression correlates well with gene amplification,[170,172,178,179] but one might hypothesize that gene expression would more directly relate to tumor cell behavior. Both immunoblotting and IHC have been used to measure HER-2/neu protein levels, although most of the work has been done with the IHC, because if appropriate antibodies are used, this technique can be performed on paraffin-embedded archived material. Immunoblotting is more technically involved, requires fresh or frozen mate-

rial, and is far less feasible for most centers. The two methods have been compared in a large series of patients with 95% concordance.[180]

Most of the published studies have used IHC, and this test is commercially available from several reference laboratories. Ravdin and Chamness[167] summarized the results from 18 studies with at least 3 years of follow-up and more than 100 patients. Some studies found that overexpression of HER-2/neu had prognostic utility, although others did not. Not surprisingly, the univariate analyses were more positive than the multivariate analyses. Two of the studies that appeared to be positive in univariate analyses were negative in multivariate analyses, perhaps because of the inclusion of other uncommon prognostic variables. The reviewers concluded that overexpression of HER-2/neu by IHC adds little to the prediction of disease-free survival, but may add something to the prediction of overall survival.

Examination of 11 studies in node-negative patients (Table 16-10) suggests little clinical utility in this group.[178,181–190] Only 1 of these 11 studies notes a positive finding in multivariate analysis. Even in the univariate analyses, the correlations appear weak. Thus, little support seems to exist for the use of HER-2/neu in node-negative patients, the group for which prognostic factors are most important for making adjuvant treatment decisions.

Assay method is a major problem in this field. Different studies have used different antibody preparations for HER-2/neu detection, and different definitions were used for scoring HER-2/neu positivity, ranging from continuous scoring of the percentage of positively stained cells to simply scoring a case as positive if any staining was detectable. Different antibodies or tissue preparations (fresh or frozen versus fixed) may explain some of the differences among studies.[177,189] The number of different antibody preparations used complicates assessment of whether a particular antibody can be used with more valid prognostic results. Certainly, particularly in node-negative disease, no consistent pattern emerges in the studies to support use of a given antibody or tissue preparation protocol. The inconsistencies among studies suggest that method may be important, and the prognostic significance of HER-2/neu has not yet been adequately validated.

Recent studies suggest that HER-2/neu may have some association with resistance to certain therapeutic agents. Têtu and Brisson[191] found that HER-2/neu was not a significant predictor of clinical outcome for untreated node-positive patients, but it was a powerful predictor of disease-free and overall survival for patients treated either with adjuvant chemotherapy or with hormone therapy. Allred and associates[186] measured HER-2/neu in node-negative patients randomized to receive adjuvant CMF chemotherapy versus observation. CMF therapy was effective for prolonging time to recurrence if the tumor contained no or low levels of the oncogene. The therapy was not effective, however, if the tumor overexpressed HER-2/neu. A similar result was reported by Gusterson and colleagues[188] from randomized trials of both node-negative and node-positive patients.

Not all studies agree that HER-2/neu is more pre-

TABLE 16-10

Prognostic Significance of HER-2/neu by Immunohistochemistry in Node-Negative Patients: Studies With More Than 3 Years of Follow-Up and More Than 100 Patients

Investigators	N	Follow-Up (mo)	Univariate P Value		Multivariate P Value	
			DFS	OS	DFS	OS
Thor et al[178]	141	102	NS	NS	—	—
Lovekin et al[181]	250	~60	—	NS	—	—
McCann et al[182]	113	48	—	NS	—	—
Kallioniemi et al[183]	174	118	—	.01	—	.03
Tanner et al[184]	105	36	NS	NS	—	—
Yuan et al[185]	101	>120	.002	.003	NS	NS
Allred et al[186]	453	61	NS	NS	—	—
Noguchi et al[187]	151	~60	NS	NS	NS	NS
Gusterson et al[188]	760	42	.22	0.0	NS	.08
Press et al[189]	210	108	.0004	—	—	—
Bianchi et al[190]	230	>84	.03	.0007	NS	NS

DFS, disease-free survival; OS, overall survival; NS, not significant.

(Adapted from Ravdin PM, Chamness GC. The c-*erbB*-2 proto-oncogene as a prognostic and predictive marker in breast cancer: a paradigm for the development of other macromolecule markers. Gene [in press])

dictive in the more heavily treated patients, however. A report by Muss and coworkers[106] of a trial randomizing node-positive patients to different intensities of adjuvant CAF chemotherapy found a significant dose-response effect among patients whose tumors overexpressed HER-2/neu, but not among patients with normal HER-2/neu. Whether this apparent discrepancy between different trials is due to differences in the types of chemotherapy used, the relative doses, statistical aberrations, or other factors is unclear at this time.

Direct preclinical and clinical evidence indicates that HER-2/neu may be a predictor of treatment resistance. Benz and associates[192] showed that, in animal models, transfection of breast tumor cells with HER-2/neu results in treatment resistance to tamoxifen. Wright and colleagues[193] studied the effect of HER-2/neu overexpression on resistance to tamoxifen in 65 patients with recurrent metastatic breast cancer. Response rates were 7% in the HER-2/neu–positive patients and 37% in the HER-2/neu–negative patients ($P < .05$). Although the subsets were small, HER-2/neu expression appeared predictive of treatment failure in ER-positive patients, with response rates of 20% (1 of 5) in the ER-positive–HER-2/neu–positive patients and 48% (12 of 25) in the ER-positive–HER-2/neu–negative patients. The work of Klijn and coworkers[194] is consistent with these tamoxifen results. Paradoxically, these investigators also found that HER-2/neu overexpression was a predictor of good response to CMF chemotherapy in patients with metastatic disease. A study by Wright and associates[195] in 68 patients with metastatic breast cancer treated with mitoxantrone showed a marginally poorer response rate in patients who were HER-2/neu overexpressors (50% versus 58%), however,

and survival was significantly but only marginally shorter. The ability of HER-2/neu to predict treatment responsiveness will have to be evaluated more carefully in studies of specific treatment regimens.

Tumor-Suppressor Genes

p53

The p53 tumor-suppressor gene is located on chromosome 17p13 and encodes a 53-kd nuclear phosphoprotein. Alterations in this gene are the most frequent genetic changes found in many malignant diseases, including breast cancer.[196] Mutations are most prevalent in five conserved exons, resulting in a conformationally altered and nonfunctional, but apparently more stable, nuclear protein. Mutant protein accumulates to high concentrations that can be detected by IHC staining. Alternatively, mutations can be detected by DNA-based methods such as single-strand conformation polymorphism (SSCP) analysis.[197]

Overexpression of p53 is relatively independent of axillary lymph node status and menopausal status, is weakly related to tumor size, but is strongly associated with DNA ploidy and measures of proliferation, steroid receptors, and nuclear grade.[197–204] The incidence of p53 mutations detected by SSCP is significantly less than the overexpression rates by immunochemistry,[205,206] and only one of the two studies using this technique reported significant correlations with clinical outcome (Table 16-11). At least seven studies have examined the prognostic significance of p53 measured by IHC in node-negative patients. De-

TABLE 16-11
Prognostic Significance of p53 in Node-Negative Patients

Investigators	Antibodies	N	Follow-Up (mo)	High p53 (%)	DFS RR	DFS P Value	OS RR	OS P Value
IMMUNOHISTOCHEMISTRY								
Thor et al.[198]	1081	127	84	24	2.7	.018	2.8	.057
Isola et al[199]	CM1/Tab250	127	102	14	—		2.7	<.0001
Allred et al[200]	1081/240	70	54	52	2.5	.002	1.7	.03
Barnes et al[201]	CM1	103	120	19	—	.009	—	<.001
Silvestrini et al[202]	1081	256	72	44	3.95	<.0001	3.10	.0001
Marks et al[203]	1081	147	61	27	—	.03	—	.01
Gasparini et al[204]	1081	254	62	28	3.08	.004	NS	.024
SSCP								
Elledge et al[205]		200	71	14	2.2	.01	—	
Caleffi et al[206]		78	48	15	—		—	NS

DFS, disease-free survival; OS, overall survival; RR, relative risk; NS, not significant; SSCP, single-strand conformation polymorphism.

spite using a variety of antibodies with differing sensitivities, all these studies demonstrated the prognostic significance of p53. In one study, p53 lost statistical significance when S-phase fraction was included in the analysis,[199] but in two other studies, p53 and a marker of proliferation were both significant factors in multivariate analyses.[200,202] This finding suggests that despite the strong direct association between accumulation of mutant p53 and proliferation, p53 has other biologic functions in addition to cell cycle regulation. Not all tumors that exhibit positive staining with the various p53 antibodies have mutations of the p53 gene,[207] nor is it likely that all mutations are equal in their contribution to the aggressiveness of breast tumors.[208]

At least 13 different monoclonal antibodies induced by the product of the human p53 gene are available.[209] Two studies compared panels of antibodies. Elledge and associates[210] evaluated 5 different antibodies (240, 1801, 421, BP53-12, CM1) and mutations determined by SSCP in 169 node-negative patients. The staining rates for the different antibodies ranged from 18% to 36%. A cocktail of both 1801 and 240 produced a p53-positive rate of 45% and was the only technique that was associated with worse clinical outcome. Jacquemier and colleagues[211] compared 4 antibodies (240, 1801, DO7, DO1) and SSCP in 106 tumors from a heterogeneous group of primary breast tumors. Staining was observed in 17% to 30% of the tumors, depending on the antibody. Unfortunately, the median follow-up was only 10.7 months, so correlations with clinical outcomes were not observed for any of the antibodies. The investigators did not draw any conclusions regarding which antibody or combination of antibodies might be most useful in a clinical setting.

The associations observed between IHC staining and clinical outcomes are exciting, and one might be tempted to add p53 to the list of biomarkers that should be routinely obtained for treatment decisions. Much remains to be learned about the function of p53 and its interactions with other genes and their products, however. Standardized assays and guidelines for interpretation of the results need to be developed, and interlaboratory studies need to be conducted before we can be confident of the clinical utility of measuring p53 in breast cancers.

nm23

The nm23 gene was originally identified by Steeg and coworkers[212] by screening cDNA libraries from murine melanoma cell lines of varying metastatic potential. Investigators proposed that nm23 may function as a suppressor gene for tumor metastasis. The product of the nm23-H1 gene has been identified as the nucleoside diphosphate (NDP) kinase A.[213] Contradictory findings have been reported regarding correlations with other prognostic factors, especially lymph node status and tumor grade. Several small studies have reported a significant relation between expression of nm23 mRNA and longer disease-free or overall survival in patients with primary breast cancer.[214–217] None of these studies performed multivariate analyses among node-negative patients, however. A more recent study of 197 breast cancer patients found no relation between NDP kinase activity and clinical outcome.[218]

Perhaps NDP kinase activity of nm23 protein does not correlate well with nm23 protein levels, and the biochemical mechanism of nm23-suppressive activity is not due to its NDP kinase activity, association with GTPase-activating proteins, or secretion from cells.[219] Additional studies must be conducted to understand the biologic significance and prognostic utility of nm23.

Measures of Invasiveness

Cancer invasion and metastasis are multifactorial processes involving complex interactions of a variety of proteolytic enzymes, growth factors, and cell–cell and cell–substrate adhesion molecules. A special issue of the journal *Breast Cancer Research and Treatment* (volume 23, no. 3, 1993) reviewed several invasion and metastasis factors in breast cancer. Several factors have been studied using in vitro and in vivo model systems to gain a better understanding of some of these interactions. Few have been evaluated as potential prognostic factors for primary breast cancer, however.

CATHEPSIN D

Cathepsin D is a glycoprotein that is originally translated and glycosylated to produce a 52-kd form, which is then processed to a 48-kd form, which, on further processing, produces a 34-kd and a 14-kd protein. The 52-kd proenzyme and the processed 48- and 34-kd forms are all enzymatically active at acidic pHs, with an optimal pH of 3.5, but have little or no enzymatic activity at physiologic pH. Cathepsin D has been proposed as a marker of estrogenic activity, to act as a growth factor through the insulin II receptor, and to play a role in tumor invasion as a protease by degrading the basement membrane and enhancing the processing or release of peptide growth factors. Thus, it is an attractive candidate for a prognostic marker for invasion and metastasis.

Ravdin[220] reviewed many of the studies conducted to evaluate its prognostic utility in breast cancer. Interpretation of these studies is hampered by the use of different antibodies and different assay techniques and by the use of optimized cutpoints that were obtained from the same data sets without validation in subsequent studies. Four different types of assays have been used in published studies: enzyme-linked immunoassay, Western blotting, enzymatic assay, and IHC. Although most studies were declared to be positive by their authors, nearly all found statistical significance only in specific subsets of patients after optimizing their cutpoint for their particular group of patients. The reviewer concluded that cathepsin D is a potentially important prognostic marker whose clinical application awaits further definition.

Subsequent to this review, results from at least eight studies were published.[147,221–227] None of the studies that used IHC techniques found any relation between tumor staining and clinical outcomes.[222–224,226,227] Têtu and associates[223] reported that although cancer-cell immunostaining was not associated with prognosis, positive staining of stromal elements was related to shorter metastasis-free survival. These researchers suggested that stromal cells may play a key role in local invasion and metastatic dissemination of the tumor. The discrepancy between immunostaining and other techniques has been noted by others and is consistent with findings from Johnson and colleagues,[228] whose work with cell lines also suggested that the poor prognosis of

some tumors with high levels of cathepsin D is probably due to high levels of cathepsin D in the stromal components of the tumor such as infiltrating inflammatory cells. If this is the case, then additional work must be done before the prognostic role of cathepsin D will be clear.

PLASMINOGEN ACTIVATORS AND INHIBITORS

Several teams of investigators have studied the uPA pathway of plasminogen activation in breast cancer and its involvement in the process of tumor cell invasion.[221,225,229–233] uPA is a serine protease that catalyzes the conversion of plasminogen into the active enzyme plasmin. Plasmin can activate type IV collagenase, which then degrades collagen and proteins of the basement membranes. uPA binds to its receptor, uPAR, which is a glycolipid-anchored cell surface protein. uPA is controlled by two specific, naturally occurring inhibitors, PAI-1 and PAI-2. Inhibition of uPA activity leads to inhibition of invasion in several experimental systems, and PAI-1 inhibits receptor-bound uPA nearly as well as uPA in solution.

Both uPA and PAI-1 have been evaluated as potential prognostic factors in primary breast cancer. As with other new prognostic markers, slightly different assays with different antibodies have been used in these studies. Consequently, the median levels of uPA and PAI-1 activity have varied, different cutpoints have been used to define assay positivity, and the percentage of positive assays differs among studies (Table 16-12).

Duffy and coworkers[232] reported a significant relation between uPA and both disease-free and overall survival in univariate analyses of 166 patients with more than 5 years of median follow-up. Similar results were found for the 75 patients with node-negative disease ($P < .05$ for disease-free survival, $P = 0.055$ for overall survival).

Janicke and colleagues[231] performed multivariate analyses of uPA and PAI-1 in 229 patients with a median follow-up of 30 months. Using optimized cutpoints of 2.97 and 2.18 ng/mg protein for uPA and PAI-1, respectively, 39% of all tumors were positive for uPA and 17% were positive for PAI-1. Strong statistical significance of uPA and a weaker relation to PAI-1 were reported. Subset analyses of 101 node-negative patients, however, revealed that the multivariate RRs of relapse were 5.5 and 4.9, respectively, for uPA and PAI-1. Using these factors in combination permitted the identification of a subset of node-negative patients with less than a 10% probability of relapse at 3 years.

Grondahl-Hansen and colleagues[230] measured uPA and PAI-1 in international and interim units, respectively, by calibration with standard preparations and defined assay positivity as values above the median. Using 191 high-risk breast cancer patients with a median observation time of 8.5 years, both factors were found to correlate with relapse-free and overall survival. Because all patients were participants in clinical trials and randomization was based on menopausal status, separate multivariate analyses were reported by menopausal status. uPA was an independent predictor of overall survival in premenopausal patients

Percentage of Patients With High Urokinase-Type Plasminogen Activator or High Plasminogen Activator Inhibitor 1

Investigators	All Patients		Node-Negative Patients		Node-Positive Patients	
	N	High uPA/PAI-1 (%)	N	High uPA/PAI-1 (%)	N	High uPA/PAI-1 (%)
Foekens et al[225,229]	657	32/44	273	32/43	379	31/45
Grondahl-Hansen et al[230]	191	50/50	23	—/—	168	—/—
Janicke et al[231]	229	39/17	101	40/16	128	38/19
Duffy et al[232]	166	50/—	75	40/—	74	58/—
Bouchet et al[233]	314	32/26	146	34/30	168	31/23

uPA, urokinase-type plasminogen activator; PAI-1, plasminogen activator inhibitor-1.

(RR, 2.0), and PAI-1 was an independent predictor in postmenopausal women (RR, 2.9).

Foekens and coworkers[225,229] measured uPA and PAI-1 in nearly 700 breast cancer patients with 48 month median follow-up. Using optimally determined cutoffs of 1.15 ng/mg protein and 17 ng/mg protein, respectively, for uPA and PAI-1, 32% of their patients were positive for uPA, and 44% were positive for PAI-1. Both factors were significant predictors of relapse-free and overall survival for both node-negative and node-positive patients. In multivariate analyses, the estimated RRs of relapse for uPA-positive and PAI-1–positive patients were 1.47 and 3.10, respectively, for node-negative patients, and 1.50 and 1.80 for node-positive patients. No differences were observed by menopausal status.

Bouchet and associates[233] measured uPA, PAI-1, and PAI-2 in tumor specimens from 314 patients with primary breast cancer. Using a clustering technique that is independent of clinical outcome, their cutpoints were 0.52, 3.0, 14.5 ng/mg protein, respectively, for uPA, PAI-1, and PAI-2, which yielded rates of positivity of 32%, 26%, and 14%. None of these factors was related to clinical outcome for node-positive patients. In multivariate analyses of 146 node-negative patients, both PAI-1 and PAI-2, but not uPA, were predictive of disease-free and metastasis-free survival. High PAI-1 was associated with worse outcomes (RRs, 2.0 and 4.8 for disease-free and metastasis-free survival), but high PAI-2 was associated with prolonged survival (RR, 0.1 for both clinical outcomes). The authors concluded that PAI-1 provided prognostic information similar to that of uPA, and it does not appear to play a role as an inhibitor. In contrast, PAI-2 enhanced the prognostic value of PAI-1 in node-negative women.

These results are promising, but additional validation studies must be performed that use the same assay methods and the same cutpoints before we will know the role of these biomarkers as prognostic factors for breast cancer.

Possibly, the uPA pathway of plasminogen activation might provide new therapeutic approaches. For example, the proteolytic activity of the tumor cell might be modified by blockade of uPA or uPA receptor or inhibition of uPA–uPA receptor synthesis.[234] Thus, these factors might

become useful predictive factors regardless of their eventual role as prognostic factors.

LAMININ RECEPTORS

The laminin receptor is a 67-kd cell-surface protein that has been hypothesized to be involved in invasion and penetration of cancer cells through the basement membranes of endothelial vessels.[235] Expression of laminin receptors is associated with involved lymph nodes and young patient age, and a weak relation to tumor size may exist. Steroid receptor status and proliferative rate appear to be unrelated to laminin receptor levels, but in vitro experiments suggest that expression of the laminin receptor may be modulated by estrogen and progestins.[236]

Three studies have examined the prognostic significance of laminin receptors, with mixed results. Marques and associates[237] measured laminin receptor expression in 235 consecutive patients with primary breast cancer and found that patients whose tumors expressed laminin receptors had a 40% less risk of recurrence than those with no expression of these receptors. Daidone and colleagues[238] reported no associations between laminin receptor expression and disease-free or overall survival in a series of 187 node-negative patients, but they did find that high levels were strong indicators of local–regional diffusion of the disease. Martignone and coworkers[239] measured laminin receptor expression in 1160 tumor specimens from patients with node-negative disease who received no systemic adjuvant therapy. They found a small, but statistically significant increased RR of death (1.33) among patients whose tumors expressed laminin receptors. Thus, whereas laminin receptors probably have a role in the metastatic process, they will have little clinical utility unless new treatment strategies are developed that would decrease expression of these receptors.

Angiogenesis

Considerable experimental evidence indicates that tumor growth depends on the induction of new capillary blood vessels, or angiogenesis.[240] After a new tumor has grown to a few millimeters in diameter, further expansion of the tumor cell population requires neovascularization. Although endothelial cells are actively proliferating within the tumor, intratumoral microvessel density and intratumoral endothelial cell proliferation are independent of each other and of tumor cell proliferation.[241] Investigators have proposed that counting microvessel formation in tumors might provide prognostic information for predicting distant disease recurrence. Investigators have detected tumor-associated neovascularization by different methods, including staining with a polyclonal antiserum against factor VIII–related antigen and immunoperoxidase staining with a monoclonal antibody that recognizes the cell adhesion molecule CD31.

Several studies have reported correlations with clinical outcomes in primary breast cancer, and several of these have been reviewed by Craft and Harris.[242] Weidner and colleagues[243] originally demonstrated a correlation between the number of microvessel counts per 200× field and distant metastasis in 49 patients. In a follow-up study of 165 patients, these investigators found that microvessel count was an independent predictor of disease-free and overall survival when compared with lymph node status, tumor size, ER status, S-phase fraction, c-erbB-2 expression, Ki67, EGFR expression, and cathepsin D. Bosari and associates[244] studied 120 patients and found associations among microvessel count, axillary metastasis, and disease-free and overall survival.

Horak and colleagues[245] reported a strong correlation between tumor-associated vascular counts and axillary lymph node metastasis in 103 patients; however, they found no association between vascular counts and ER status, EGFRs, c-erbB-2, or p53. Despite the small number of patients and relatively short follow-up, these investigators found a significant relationship with overall survival. Toi and colleagues[246] evaluated 220 tumors from Japanese women by immunostaining to factor VIII antigen. A multivariate analysis demonstrated that vessel density was an independent prognostic factor that was as potent as nodal status.

Two studies have focused on node-negative breast cancer. Gasparini and coworkers[204] reported that microvessel density was the strongest independent predictor of disease-free survival in 254 node-negative patients with a 5.78 RR of relapse after a median follow-up of 62 months. Other significant factors in their multivariate analysis included peritumoral lymphatic vessel invasion, p53 mutation, and tumor size. By changing the cutoff from 80 vessels to 70 vessels, it was also a strong predictor of overall survival with a RR of death of 3.27. Fox and associates[247] studied 109 node-negative patients with a short median follow-up of only 25 months. Despite the short follow-up, the multivariate RRs of relapse and survival were 3.5 and 6.6, respectively.

The results of these studies are impressive, but the number of patients is small, and the follow-up interval is relatively short to determine the precise clinical utility of angiogenesis as a prognostic factor. Tumor-associated angiogenesis is a particularly appealing putative prognostic factor because it appears to be a marker of invasion, rather than of differentiation or proliferation, as are most of the currently available biomarkers.[248]

An attractive feature of angiogenesis is that it offers a target for novel therapeutic interventions. Over the past 10 years, several antiangiogenic agents have been developed and evaluated in a variety of systems. Classes of antiangiogenic agents include the following[248]:

- Polysulfated glycosamines, peptidoglycans, polyglycosylated lipids
- Enzymes that control the vascularization process
- Steroids and steroid-related substances
- Antibiotics and synthetic antibiotic derivatives
- Specific immunotherapeutics
- Nonspecific biologic response modifiers

Clinical trials are being designed to test these therapies as single agents and in combination. Successful regimens may have their greatest efficacy early in the course of the disease, most likely in the adjuvant setting.

Prognostic Factor Models

Given the number and diversity of the potential prognostic factors, physicians and patients have difficulty synthesizing and integrating the information that they provide. A special issue of the journal *Breast Cancer Research and Treatment* (volume 22, no. 3, 1992) was devoted to prognostic factor integration. Factor integration techniques include simply adding points for each adverse factor (eg, histologic grading systems), multiple regression equations usually from Cox survival models (eg, the Nottingham Prognostic Index), decision trees,[249] and neural networks.[250] No matter how sophisticated the model might be, however, it is only as good as the data used to construct and validate it.

Most of the information in this chapter is derived from retrospective studies that have included relatively few factors. Some of these studies involved large numbers of patients, but most had small to modest sample sizes with relatively short follow-up. Small studies that include patients who have received heterogeneous treatments are unlikely to answer any of the questions about new prognostic factors. Definitive studies in node-negative breast cancer, in which only about 30% of patients have a recurrence, require large numbers of patients followed for long periods to evaluate new prognostic factors adequately. Each study has its own particular selection biases, and all the usual precautions concerning the interpretation of retrospective analyses pertain to most of these studies. A particular concern is the lack of multivariate analyses in the evaluation of potential prognostic factors. Many of these factors are related to each other and may in fact be alternative representations of the same biologic phenomena. Without adjustments for these statistical correlations, the results of univariate correlative analyses may be misleading. One should always ask whether the new factor adds any information to what can be learned from the standard prognostic factors.

Another problem is lack of standardization of assay

methods, scoring systems, and antibodies used to measure new biomarkers. Even though many of the new, potential prognostic factors have been evaluated in several studies, few have been conducted under standardized conditions that would permit a true validation of previous results. Particularly worrisome is the use of different cutpoints to define assay positivity, especially when these cutpoints are derived from the same patients used to evaluate the new factor. Hilsenbeck and associates[251] demonstrated that performing multiple analyses on the same data set to find the optimal cutpoint for a new prognostic factor results in substantial type I errors. Validation of results on a truly independent, external population of patients using standardized methods is a necessity before any new factor can be considered ready for clinical use.

On one hand, the prognostic factor field might appear discouraging. Despite the plethora of potential prognostic factors, the list of established factors is short and has been unchanged for more than a decade. On the other hand, many of these studies have shed new light on the complex system of pathways that regulate human breast cancer. We are just now beginning to see new therapeutic approaches evolve that have become possible as a by-product of our search for new biomarkers. The goal of the future is to not only determine which patients should receive adjuvant therapy, but more important, what specific therapy is optimal for an individual patient.

References

1. Adjuvant chemotherapy for breast cancer. JAMA 1985;254:3461.
2. Fisher B, Redmond C, Dimitrov NV, et al. A randomized clinical trial evaluating sequential methotrexate and fluorouracil in the treatment of patients with node-negative breast cancer who have estrogen-receptor–negative tumors. N Engl J Med 1989;320:473.
3. Fisher B, Constantino J, Redmond C, et al. A randomized clinical trial evaluating tamoxifen in the treatment of patients with node-negative breast cancer who have estrogen-receptor-positive tumors. N Engl J Med 1989;320:479.
4. Mansour EG, Gray R, Shatila AH, et al. Efficacy of adjuvant chemotherapy in high-risk node-negative breast cancer: an Intergroup study. N Engl J Med 1989;320:485.
5. The Ludwig Breast Cancer Study Group. Prolonged disease-free survival after one course of perioperative adjuvant chemotherapy for node-negative breast cancer. N Engl J Med 1989;320:491.
6. Early Breast Cancer Trialists' Collaborative Group. Systemic treatment of early breast cancer by hormonal, cytotoxic, or immune therapy. Lancet 1992;339:1, 71.
7. Consensus Development Panel. Consensus statement: treatment of early-stage breast cancer. J Natl Cancer Inst Monogr 1992;11:1.
8. Clark GM. Do we really need prognostic factors for breast cancer? Breast Cancer Res Treat 1994;30:117.
9. McGuire WL. Breast cancer prognostic factors: evaluation guidelines. J Natl Cancer Inst 1991;83:154.
10. Gasparini G, Pozza F, Harris AL, et al. Evaluating the potential usefulness of new prognostic and predictive indicators in node-negative breast cancer patients. J Natl Cancer Inst 1993;85:1206.
11. Fisher ER, Gregorio RM, Fisher B, et al. The pathology of invasive breast cancer. Cancer 1975;36:1.
12. Berg JW, Robbins GF. Factors influencing short and long-term survival of breast cancer patients. Surg Gynecol Obstet 1966;122:1311.
13. Fisher B, Bauer M, Wickerham DL, et al. Relation of number of positive axillary nodes to the prognosis of patients with primary breast cancer: an NSABP update. Cancer 1983;52:1551.
14. Saez RA, Clark GM, McGuire WL. Prognostic factors in breast cancer. Semin Surg Oncol 1989;5:102.
15. Mittra I, MacRae KD. A meta-analysis of reported correlations between prognostic factors in breast cancer: does axillary lymph node metastasis represent biology or chronology? Eur J Cancer 1991;27:1574.
16. Chadha M, Chabon AB, Friedmann P, et al. Predictors of axillary lymph node metastases in patients with T1 breast cancer: a multivariate analysis. Cancer 1994;73:350.
17. Silverstein MJ, Gierson ED, Waisman JR, et al. Axillary lymph node dissection for T1a breast carcinoma: is it indicated? Cancer 1994;73:664.
18. Ravdin PM, De Laurentiis M, Vendely T, et al. Prediction of axillary nodal status in breast cancer patients by use of prognostic indicators. J Natl Cancer Inst 1994;86:1771.
19. Carter CL, Allen C, Henson D. Five year survival of breast cancer by histology, tumor size, and extent of axillary lymph node involvement. Proceedings of the 14th International Cancer Congress 1987;3:53.
20. Fisher B, Slack NH, Bross DM, et al. Cancer of the breast: size of neoplasm and prognosis. Cancer 1969;24:1071.
21. Adair F, Berg J, Joubert L, et al. Long-term follow-up of breast cancer patients: the 30-year report. Cancer 1974;33:1145.
22. Nemoto T, Vana J, Bedwani RN, et al. Management and survival of female breast cancer: results of a national survey by the American College of Surgeons. Cancer 1980;45:2917.
23. Koscielny S, Tubiana M, Le MG, et al. Breast cancer: relationship between the size of the primary tumour and the probability of metastatic dissemination. Br J Cancer 1984;49:709.
24. Moon TE, Jones SE, Bonadonna G, et al. Development and use of a natural history data base of breast cancer studies. Am J Clin Oncol 1987;10:396.
25. Carter CL, Allen C, Henson DE. Relation of tumor size, lymph node status, and survival in 24,740 breast cancer cases. Cancer 1989;63:181.
26. Rosen PP, Groshen S, Saigo PE, et al. Pathological prognostic factors in stage I (T1N0M0) and stage II (T1N1M0) breast carcinoma: a study of 644 patients with median follow-up of 18 years. J Clin Oncol 1989;7:1239.
27. Rosen PP, Groshen S, Saigo PE, et al. A long-term follow-up study of survival in stage I (T1N0M0) and stage II (T1N1M0) breast carcinoma. J Clin Oncol 1989;7:355.
28. McGuire WL, Clark GM. Prognostic factors and treatment decisions in axillary node–negative breast cancer. N Engl J Med 1992;326:1756.
29. Fisher B, Redmond C, Wickerham DL, et al. Systemic therapy in patients with node-negative breast cancer. Ann Intern Med 1989;111:703.
30. Delides GS, Garas G, Georgouli G, et al. Intralaboratory variations in the grading of breast carcinoma. Arch Pathol Lab Med 1982;106:126.
31. Gilchrist KW, Kalish L, Gould VE, et al. Interobserver reproducibility of histopathological features in stage II breast cancer: an ECOG study. Breast Cancer Res Treat 1985;5:3.
32. Theissig F, Kunze KD, Haroske G, et al. Histological grading of breast cancer: interobserver, reproducibility and prognostic significance. Pathol Res Pract 1990;186:732.
33. Harvey JM, de Klerk NH, Sterrett GF. Histological grading in breast cancer: interobserver agreement, and relation to other prognostic factors including ploidy. Pathology 1992;24:63.

34. Dalton LW, Page DL, Dupont WD. Histologic grading of breast carcinoma: a reproducibility study. Cancer 1994;73:2765.

35. Bloom HJ, Richardson WW. Histological grading and prognosis in breast cancer. Br J Cancer 1957;11:359.

36. Scarff RW, Torioni H. Histological typing of breast tumors. Geneva, WHO, 1968:13.

37. Fisher ER, Redmond C, Fisher B. Histologic grading of breast cancer. Pathol Ann 1980;15:239.

38. le Doussal V, Tubiana-Hulin M, Friedman S, et al. Prognostic value of histologic grade nuclear components of Scarff-Bloom-Richardson (SBR): an improved score modification based on a multivariate analysis of 1262 invasive ductal breast carcinoma. Cancer 1989;64:1914.

39. Davies BW, Gelber D, Goldhirsh A, et al. Prognostic significance of tumor grade in clinical trials of adjuvant therapy for breast cancer with axillary lymph node metastasis. Cancer 1986;58:2662.

40. Contesso G, Mouriesse H, Friedman S, et al. The importance of histologic grade in long-term prognosis of breast cancer: a study of 1,010 patients, uniformly treated at the Institut Gustave Roussy. J Clin Oncol 1987;5:1378.

41. Rank F, Dombernowsky P, Jespersen NC, et al. Histologic malignancy grading of invasive ductal breast carcinoma: a regression analysis of prognostic factors in low-risk carcinomas from a multicenter trial. Cancer 1987;60:1299.

42. le Doussal V, Tubiana-Hulin M, Hacène K, et al. Nuclear characteristics as indicators of prognosis in node negative breast cancer patients. Breast Cancer Res Treat 1989;14:207.

43. Fisher B, Redmond C, Fisher ER, et al. Relative worth of estrogen or progesterone receptor and pathologic characteristics of differentiation as indicators of prognosis in node negative breast cancer patients: findings from National Surgical Adjuvant Breast and Bowel Project Protocol B-06. J Clin Oncol 1988;6:1076.

44. Chevallier B, Mosseri V, Dauce JP, et al. A prognostic score in histological node negative breast cancer. Br J Cancer 1989;61:436.

45. Elston CW, Ellis IO. Pathological prognostic factors in breast cancer. I. The value of histological grade in breast cancer: experience from a large study with long-term follow-up. Histopathology 1991;19:403.

46. Dawson AE, Austin RE, Weinberg DS. Nuclear grading of breast carcinoma by image analysis: classification by multivariate and neural network analysis. Am J Clin Pathol 1991;95(Suppl 1):S29.

47. Henson DE, Ries L, Freedman LS, et al. Relationship among outcome, stage of disease, and histologic grade for 22,616 cases of breast cancer: the basis for a prognostic index. Cancer 1991;68:2142.

48. Schumacher M, Schmoor C, Sauerbrei W, et al. The prognostic effect of histological tumor grade in node-negative breast cancer patients. Breast Cancer Res Treat 1993;25:235.

49. Henson DE. The histological grading of neoplasms. Arch Pathol Lab Med 1988;112:1091.

50. Crosby CH, Barclay THC. Carcinoma of the breast: surgical management of patients with special conditions. Cancer 1971;28:1628.

51. Stoll BA. Does the malignancy of breast cancer vary with age? Clin Oncol 1976;2:73.

52. Ribeiro GG, Swidell R. The prognosis of breast carcinoma in women aged less than 40 years. Clin Radiol 1981;32:231.

53. Noyes RD, Spanos WJ, Montague ED. Breast cancer in women aged 30 and under. Cancer 1982;49:1302.

54. Adami HO, Malker B, Meirik O, et al. Age as a prognostic factor in breast cancer. Cancer 1985;56:898.

55. Host H, Lund E. Age as a prognostic factor in breast cancer. Cancer 1986;57:2217.

56. de la Rochefordiere A, Asselain B, Campana F, et al. Age as prognostic factor in premenopausal breast carcinoma. Lancet 1993;341:1039.

57. Fowble BL, Schultz DJ, Overmoyer B, et al. The influence of young age on outcome in early stage breast cancer. Int J Radiat Oncol Biol Phys 1994;30:23.

58. Nixon AJ, Neuberg D, Hayes DF, et al. Relationship of patient age to pathologic features of the tumor and prognosis for patients with stage I or II breast cancer. J Clin Oncol 1994;12:888.

59. Albain KS, Allred DC, Clark GM. Breast cancer outcome and predictors of outcome: are there age differentials? J Natl Cancer Inst Monogr 1994;16:35.

60. Hakama M, Rihimaki H. End results of breast cancer patients in Finland 1953–1968. Ann Clin Res 1974;6:115.

61. Langlands AO, Pocock JP, Keww GR, et al. Long-term survival of patients with breast cancer: a study of the curability of the disease. Br Med J 1979;2:1247.

62. Rutqvist LE, Wallgren A. The influence of age on outcome in breast cancer. Acta Radiol Oncol 1983;22:289.

63. Mueller CB, Ames F, Anderson GD. Breast cancer in 3558 women: age as a significant determinant in the rate of dying and causes of death. Surgery 1978;83:123.

64. Cutler SJ, Axtell LM. Adjustment of long-term survival rates for deaths due to intercurrent disease. J Chron Dis 1969;22:485.

65. Wallgren A, Silfersward C, Hulthorn A. Carcinoma of the breast in women under 30 years of age: a clinical and histopathological study of all cases reported as carcinoma to the Swedish Cancer Registry 1958–1968. Cancer 1977;40:916.

66. Hibberd AD, Horwood LJ, Wells JE. Long term prognosis of women with breast cancer in New Zealand: study of survival to 30 years. Br Med J 1983;286:1777.

67. Miki Y, Swenson J, Shattuck-Eidens D, et al. A strong candidate for the 17q-linked breast and ovarian cancer susceptibility gene, BRCA-1. Science 1994;266:66.

68. Futreal PA, Pingham L, Shattuck-Eidens D, et al. BCRA1 mutations in primary breast and ovarian carcinomas. Science 1994;266:120.

69. Wooster R, Neuhausen SL, Mangion J, et al. Localization of a breast cancer susceptibility gene, BRCA2, to chromosome 13q12-13. Science 1994;265:2088.

70. Rubens RD. Age and the treatment of breast cancer. J Clin Oncol 1993;11:3.

71. Freeman HP, Wasfie TJ. Cancer of the breast in poor black women. Cancer 1989;63:2562.

72. Bain RP, Greenberg RS, Whitaker JP. Racial differences in survival of women with breast cancer. J Chron Dis 1986;39:631.

73. Westbrook KC, Brown BW, McBride CM. Breast cancer: a critical review of a patient sample with a ten-year follow-up. South Med J 1975;68:543.

74. National Cancer Institute. Five-year relative survival rates by primary site and racial/ethnic group, SEER Program, 1973–81. In: Cancer among blacks and other minorities statistical profiles. DHEW Publ No. (NCI)86-278S. Bethesda, National Cancer Institute, 1986.

75. Daly MB, Clark GM, McGuire WL. Breast cancer prognosis in a mixed Caucasian–Hispanic population. J Natl Cancer Inst 1985;74:753.

76. Elledge RM, Clark GM, Chamness GC, et al. Tumor biologic factors and breast cancer prognosis among white, Hispanic and black women in the United States. J Natl Cancer Inst 1994;86:705.

77. Swanson GM, Ragheb NE, Lin C-S, et al. Breast cancer among black and white women in the 1980s. Cancer 1993;72:788.

78. Pierce L, Fowble B, Solin LJ, et al. Conservative surgery and radiation therapy in black women with early stage breast cancer: patterns of failure and analysis of outcome. Cancer 1992;69:2831.

79. National Cancer Institute. Annual Cancer Statistics Review, Including Cancer Trends: 1950–1985. Washington, DC, US Government Printing Office, 1988.

80. Vernon SW, Tilley BC, Neale AV, et al. Ethnicity, survival, and

delay in seeking treatment for symptoms of breast cancer. Cancer 1985;55:1563.

81. Gordon NH, Crowe JP, Brumberg DJ, et al. Socioeconomic factors and race in breast cancer recurrence and survival. Am J Epidemiol 1992;135:609.

82. Coates RJ, Bransfield DD, Wesley M, et al. Differences between black and white women with breast cancer in time from symptom recognition to medical consultation. Black/White Cancer Survival Study Group. J Natl Cancer Inst 1992;84:938.

83. Baak JPA. Mitosis counting in tumors. Hum Pathol 1990;21:683.

84. van Diest PJ, Baak JPA, Matze-Cok P, et al. Reproducibility of mitosis counting in 2,469 breast cancer specimens: results from the Multicenter Morphometric Mammary Carcinoma Project. Hum Pathol 1992;23:603.

85. Russo J, Frederick J, Ownby HE, et al. Predictors of recurrence and survival of patients with breast cancer. Am J Clin Pathol 1987;88:123.

86. Clayton F. Pathologic correlates of survival in 378 lymph node-negative infiltrating ductal breast carcinomas: mitotic count is the best single predictor. Cancer 1991;68:1309.

87. Aaltomaa S, Lipponen P, Eskelinen M, et al. Predictive value of a morphometric prognostic index in female breast cancer. Oncology 1993;50:57.

88. Galea MH, Blamey RW, Elston CW, et al. The Nottingham Prognostic Index in primary breast cancer. Breast Cancer Res Treat 1992;22:207.

89. van der Linden JC, Lindeman J, Baak JPA, et al. The Multivariate Prognostic Index and nuclear DNA content are independent prognostic factors in primary breast cancer patients. Cytometry 1989;10:56.

90. Silvestrini R. Cell kinetics: prognostic and therapeutic implications in human tumours. Cell Prolif 1994;27:579.

91. Héry M, Gianni J, LaLanne CM, et al. The DNA labeling index: a prognostic factor in node-negative breast cancer. Breast Cancer Res Treat 1987;9:207.

92. Meyer JS, Province M. Proliferative index of breast carcinoma by thymidine labeling: prognostic power independent of stage, estrogen and progesterone receptors. Breast Cancer Res Treat 1988;12:191.

93. Silvestrini R, Daidone MG, Valagussa P, et al. Cell kinetics as a prognostic indicator in node-negative breast cancer. Eur J Cancer Clin Oncol 1989;25:1165.

94. Tubiana M, Pejovic MH, Koscielny S, et al. Growth rate, kinetics of tumor cell proliferation and long-term outcome in human breast cancer. Int J Cancer 1989;44:17.

95. Courdi A, Héry M, Dahan E, et al. Factors affecting relapse in node-negative breast cancer: a multivariate analysis including the labeling index. Eur J Clin Oncol 1989;25:351.

96. Cooke TG, Stanton PD, Winstanley J, et al. Long-term prognostic significance of thymidine labelling index in primary breast cancer. Eur J Cancer 1992;28:424.

97. Silvestrini R, Daidone MG, Del Bino G, et al. Prognostic significance of proliferative activity and ploidy in node-negative breast cancers. Ann Oncol 1993;4:213.

98. Silvestrini R. Feasibility and reproducibility of the [³H]-thymidine labelling index in breast cancer. Cell Prolif 1991;24:437.

99. Zambetti M, Bonadonna G, Valagussa P, et al. Adjuvant CMF for node-negative and estrogen receptor-negative breast cancer patients. J Natl Cancer Inst Monogr 1992;11:77.

100. Daidone MG, Silvestrini R, Valentinis B, et al. Changes in cell kinetics induced by primary chemotherapy in breast cancer. Int J Cancer 1991;47:380.

101. Wenger CR, Beardslee S, Owens MA, et al. DNA ploidy, S-phase and steroid receptors in more than 127,000 breast cancer patients. Breast Cancer Res Treat 1993;28:9.

102. Hedley DW, Clark GM, Cornelisse CJ, et al. Consensus review of the clinical utility of DNA cytometry in carcinoma of the breast. Cytometry 1993;14:482.

103. Herman CJ, Duque RE, Hedley D, et al. DNA cytometry in cancer prognosis. Princ Pract Oncol Updates 1993;7:3.

104. Remvikos Y, Beuzeboc P, Zajdela A, et al. Correlation of pretreatment proliferative activity of breast cancer with the response to cytotoxic chemotherapy. J Natl Cancer Inst 1989:81:1383.

105. Dressler LG, Eudey L, Gray R, et al. Prognostic potential of DNA flow cytometry measurement in node-negative breast cancer patients: preliminary analysis of an Intergroup study (INT0076). J Natl Cancer Inst Monogr 1992;11:167.

106. Muss HB, Thor AD, Berry DA, et al. c-erbB-2 expression and response to adjuvant therapy in women with node-positive breast cancer. N Engl J Med 1994;330:1260.

107. Gerdes J, Schwab U, Lemke H, et al. Production of mouse-monoclonal antibody reactive with a human nuclear antigen associated with cell proliferation. Int J Cancer 1983;31:13.

108. Key G, Petersen JL, Becker MHG, et al. New antiserum against Ki-67 antigen suitable for double immunostaining of paraffin wax sections. J Clin Pathol 1993;46:1080.

109. Cattoretti G, Becker MHG, Key G, et al. Monoclonal antibodies against recombinant parts of the Ki-67 antigen (MIB1 and MIB3) detect proliferating cells in microwave-processed formalin-fixed paraffin sections. J Pathol 1992;168:357.

110. Charpin C, Andrac L, Vacheret H, et al. Multiparametric evaluation (SAMBA) of growth fraction (monoclonal Ki67) in breast carcinoma tissue sections. Cancer Res 1988;48:4368.

111. Walker RA, Camplejohn RS. Comparison of monoclonal antibody Ki-67 reactivity with grade and DNA flow cytometry of breast carcinomas. Br J Cancer 1988;57:281.

112. Gasparini G, Dal Fior S, Pozza F, et al. Correlation of growth fraction by Ki-67 immunohistochemistry with histologic factors and hormone receptors in operable breast carcinoma. Breast Cancer Res Treat 1989;14:329.

113. Brown RW, Allred DC, Clark GM, et al. Prognostic significance and clinical–pathological correlations of cell-cycle kinetics measured by Ki-67 immunocytochemistry in axillary node-negative carcinoma of the breast. Breast Cancer Res Treat 1990;16:191.

114. Gerdes J, Lemke H, Baisch H, et al. Cell cycle analysis of a cell proliferation-associated human nuclear antigen defined by the monoclonal antibody Ki-67. J Immunol 1984;133:1710.

115. Kamel OW, Franklin WA, Ringus JC, et al. Thymidine labeling index and Ki-67 growth fraction in lesions of the breast. Am J Pathol 1989;134:107.

116. Gasparini G, Boracchi P, Verderio P, et al. Cell kinetics in human breast cancer: comparison between the prognostic value of the cytofluorimetric S-phase fraction and that of the antibodies to Ki-67 and PCNA antigens detected by immunocytochemistry. Int J Cancer 1994;57:822.

117. Bouzubar N, Walker RJ, Griffiths K, et al. Ki-67 immunostaining in primary breast cancer: pathological and clinical associations. Br J Cancer 1989;59:943.

118. Weikel W, Beck T, Mitze M, et al. Immunohistochemical evaluation of growth fractions in human breast cancers using monoclonal antibody Ki-67. Breast Cancer Res Treat 1991;18:149.

119. Wintzer H-O, Ziffel I, Schulte-Monting J, et al. Ki-67 immunostaining in human breast tumors and its relationship to prognosis. Cancer 1991;67:421.

120. Sahin AA, Ro J, Ro JY, et al. Ki-67 immunostaining in node-negative stage-I/II breast carcinoma. Cancer 1991;68:549.

121. Gasparini B, Pozza F, Bevilacqua P, et al. Growth fraction (Ki-67 antibody) determination in early stage breast carcinoma: histologic, clinical and prognostic correlations. Breast 1992;1:92.

122. Gottardi O, Scanzi F, Zubidda S, et al. Clinical and prognostic usefulness of immunohistochemical determination of Ki-67 in breast cancer. Breast 1993;2:33.

123. Veronese SM, Gambacorta M, Gottardi O, et al. Proliferation index as a prognostic marker in breast cancer. Cancer 1993;71:3926.

124. Railo M, Nordling S, von Boguslawsky K, et al. Prognostic value of Ki-67 immunolabelling in primary operable breast cancer. Br J Cancer 1993;68:579.

125. Gaglia P, Bernardi A, Venesio T, et al. Cell proliferation of breast cancer evaluated by anti-BrdU and anti-Ki-67 antibodies: its prognostic value on short term recurrences. Eur J Cancer 1993;29A:1509.

126. Bianchi S, Paglierani M, Zampi G. Prognostic value of proliferating cell nuclear antigen in lymph node-negative breast cancer patients. Cancer 1993;72:120.

127. Thomas M, Noguchi M, Kitagawa H, et al. Poor prognostic value of proliferating cell nuclear antigen labelling index in breast carcinoma. J Clin Pathol 1993;46:525.

128. Cummings MC, Furnival CM, Parsons PG, et al. PCNA immunostaining in breast cancer. Aust NZ J Surg 1993;63:630.

129. Aaltomaa S, Lipponen P, Syrjanen K. Proliferating cell nuclear antigen (PCNA) immunolabeling as a prognostic factor in axillary lymph node negative breast cancer. Anticancer Res 1993;13:533.

130. Rose DSC, Maddox PH, Brown DC. Which proliferation markers for routine immunohistology? a comparison of five antibodies. J Clin Pathol 1994;47:1010.

131. Knight WA III, Livingston RB, Gregory EJ, et al. Estrogen receptor as an independent prognostic factor for early recurrence in breast cancer. Cancer Res 1977;37:4669.

132. Clark GM, McGuire WL. Steroid receptors and other prognostic factors in primary breast cancer. Semin Oncol 1988;15:20.

133. Horowitz KB, McGuire WL, Pearson OH, et al. Predicting response to endocrine therapy in human breast cancer: a hypothesis. Science 1975;189:726.

134. Adami H-O, Graffman S, Lindgren A, et al. Prognostic implication of estrogen receptor content in breast cancer. Breast Cancer Res Treat 1985;5:293.

135. Mason BH, Holdaway IM, Mullins PR, et al. Progesterone and estrogen receptors as prognostic variables in breast cancer. Cancer Res 1983;43:2985.

136. Clark GM, Osborne CK, McGuire WL. Correlations between estrogen receptor, progesterone receptor, and patient characteristics in human breast cancer. J Clin Oncol 1984;2:1102.

137. Thorpe SM, Christensen IJ, Rasmussen BB, et al. Short recurrence-free survival associated with high oestrogen receptor levels in the natural history of postmenopausal, primary breast cancer. Eur J Cancer 1993;29A:971.

138. Kinsel LB, Szabo E, Greene GL, et al. Immunocytochemical analysis of estrogen receptors as a predictor of prognosis in breast cancer patients: comparison with quantitative biochemical methods. Cancer Res 1989;49:1052.

139. Berger U, Wilson P, Thethi S, et al. Comparison of an immunocytochemical assay for progesterone receptor with a biochemical method of measurement and immunocytochemical examination of the relationship between progesterone and estrogen receptors. Cancer Res 1989;49:5176.

140. Foekens JA, Portengen H, van Putten WLJ, et al. Prognostic value of estrogen and progesterone receptors measured by enzyme immunoassays in human breast tumor cytosols. Cancer Res 1989;49:5823.

141. Andersen J, Thorpe SM, King WJ, et al. The prognostic value of immunohistochemical estrogen receptor analysis in paraffin-embedded and frozen sections versus that of steroid-binding assays. Eur J Cancer 1990;26:442.

142. Masiakowski P, Breathnah R, Bloch J, et al. Cloning of cDNA sequences of hormone-regulated genes from the MCF-7 human breast cancer cell line. Nucleic Acids Res 1982;10:7895.

143. Rio MC, Bellocq JP, Daniel JY, et al. Breast cancer–associated pS2 protein: synthesis and secretion by normal stomach mucosa. Science 1988;241:705.

144. Jakowlew SB, Breathnach R, Jeltsch JM, et al. Sequence of the pS2 mRNA induced by estrogen in the human breast cancer cell line MCF-7. Nucleic Acids Res 1984;12:2861.

145. Foekens JA, Rio MC, Sequin P, et al. Prediction of relapse and survival in breast cancer patients by pS2 protein status. Cancer Res 1990;50:3832.

146. Predine J, Spyratos F, Prud'homme JF, et al. Enzyme-linked immunosorbent assay of pS2 in breast cancers, benign tumors, and normal breast tissues. Cancer 1992;69:2116.

147. Gion M, Mione R, Pappagallo GL, et al. PS2 in breast cancer: alternative or complementary tool to steroid receptor status? Evaluation of 446 cases. Br J Cancer 1993;68:374.

148. Spyratos F, Andrieu C, Hacéne K, et al. pS2 and response to adjuvant hormone therapy in primary breast cancer. Br J Cancer 1994;68:394.

149. Henry JA, Piggott NH, Mallick UK, et al. pNR-2/pS2 immunohistochemical staining in breast cancer: correlation with prognostic factors and endocrine response. Br J Cancer 1991;63:615.

150. Thor AD, Koerner FC, Edgerton SM, et al. pS2 expression in primary breast carcinomas: relationship to clinical and histological features and survival. Breast Cancer Res Treat 1992;21:111.

151. Cappelletti V, Coradini D, Scanziani E, et al. Prognostic relevance of pS2 status and proliferative activity in node-negative breast cancer. Eur J Cancer 1992;28A:1315.

152. Soubeyran I, Coindre J-M, Wafflart J, et al. Immunohistochemical determination of pS2 in invasive breast carcinomas: a study on 942 cases. Breast Cancer Res Treat (In press).

153. Ciocca DR, Oesterreich S, Chamness GC, et al. Biological and clinical implications of heat shock protein 27000 (Hsp27): a review. J Natl Cancer Inst 1993;85:1558.

154. Chamness GC, Ruiz A, Fulcher L, et al. Estrogen-inducible heat shock protein hsp27 predicts recurrence in node negative breast cancer. Proc Am Assoc Cancer Res 1989;30:252.

155. Tandon AK, Clark GM, Chamness GC, et al. Clinical significance of heat-shock/stress-response proteins in breast cancer. Breast Cancer Res Treat 1990;16:146.

156. Ciocca DR, Tandon AK, Fuqua SAW, et al. Heat shock protein hsp70 with axillary lymph node-negative breast cancer: prognostic implications. J Natl Cancer Inst 1993;85:570.

157. Thor A, Benz C, Moore D II, et al. Stress response protein (srp-27) determination in primary human breast carcinomas: clinical, histologic, and prognostic correlations. J Natl Cancer Inst 1991;83:170.

158. Love S, King RJ. A 27 kDa heat shock protein that has anomalous prognostic powers in early and advanced breast cancer. Br J Cancer 1994;69:743.

159. Ciocca DR, Fuqua SAW, Lock-Lim S, et al. Response of human breast cancer cells to heat shock and chemotherapeutic drugs. Cancer Res 1992;52:3648.

160. Oesterreich S, Weng C-N, Qiu M, et al. The small heat shock protein hsp27 is correlated with growth and drug resistance in human breast cancer cell lines. Cancer Res 1993;53:4443.

161. Rajkumar T, Gullick WJ. The type I growth factor receptors in human breast cancer. Breast Cancer Res Treat 1994;29:3.

162. Klijn JGM, Berns PMJJ, Schmitz PIM, et al. The clinical significance of epidermal growth factor receptor (EGF-R) in human breast cancer: a review on 5232 patients. Endocr Rev 1992;13:3.

163. Klijn JGM, Berns PMJJ, Schmitz PIM, et al. Epidermal growth factor receptor (EGF-R) in clinical breast cancer: update 1993. Endocr Rev 1993;1:171.

164. Fox SB, Smith K, Hollyer J, et al. The epidermal growth factor receptor as a prognostic marker: results of 370 patients and review of 3009 patients. Breast Cancer Res Treat 1994;29:41.

165. Nicholson RI, McClelland RA, Gee JMW, et al. Epidermal

growth factor receptor expression in breast cancer: association with response to endocrine therapy. Breast Cancer Res Treat 1994;29:117.

166. Baselga J, Mendelsohn J. The epidermal growth factor receptor as a target for therapy in breast carcinoma. Breast Cancer Res Treat 1994;29:127.

167. Ravdin PM, Chamness GC. The c-*ERBB*-2 proto-oncogene as a prognostic and predictive marker in breast cancer: a paradigm for the development of other macromolecule markers. Gene (in press).

168. Slamon DJ, Clark GM, Wong SG, et al. Human breast cancer: correlation of relapse and survival with amplification of the HER-2/*neu* oncogene. Science 1987;235:177.

169. Ali IU, Campbell G, Lidereau R, et al. Lack of evidence for the prognostic significance of c-*erb*B-2 amplification. Oncogene Res 1988;3:139.

170. Slamon DJ, Godolphin W, Jones LA, et al. Studies of the HER-2/*neu* proto-oncogene in human breast and ovarian cancer. Science 1989;244:707.

171. Tsuda H, Hirohashi S, Shimosato Y, et al. Immunohistochemical study on overexpression of c-*erb*B-2 protein in human breast cancer: its correlation with gene amplification and long-term survival of patients. Jpn J Cancer Res 1990;81:327.

172. Borg Å, Tandon AK, Sigurdsson H, et al. HER-2/*neu* amplification predicts poor survival in node-positive breast cancer. Cancer Res 1990;50:4332.

173. Winstanley J, Cooke T, Murray GD, et al. The long term prognostic significance of c-*erb*B-2 in primary breast cancer. Br J Cancer 1991;63:447.

174. Paterson MC, Dietrich KD, Danyluk J, et al. Correlation between c-*erb*B-2 amplification and risk of recurrent disease in node-negative breast cancer. Cancer Res 1991;51:556.

175. Clark GM, McGuire WL. Follow-up study of HER-2/*neu* amplification in primary breast cancer. Cancer Res 1991;51:944.

176. Berns EM, Klijn JG, van Putten WL, et al. c-*myc* amplification is a better prognostic factor than HER2/*neu* amplification in primary breast cancer. Cancer Res 1992;52:1107.

177. Press MF, Pike MC, Chazin VR, et al. Her-2/*neu* expression in node-negative breast cancer: direct tissue quantitation by computerized image analysis and association of overexpression with increased risk of recurrent disease. Cancer Res 1993;53:4960.

178. Thor AD, Schwartz LH, Koerner FC, et al. Analysis of c-*erb*B-2 expression in breast carcinomas with clinical follow-up. Cancer Res 1989;49:7147.

179. Ciocca DR, Fujimura FK, Tandon AK, et al. Correlation of HER-2/*neu* amplification with expression and with other prognostic factors in 1103 breast cancers. J Natl Cancer Inst 1992;84:1279.

180. Molina R, Ciocca DR, Tandon AK, et al. Expression of HER-2/*neu* oncoprotein in human breast cancer: a comparison of immunohistochemical and western blot techniques. Anticancer Res 1992;12:1965.

181. Lovekin C, Ellis IO, Locker A, et al. c-erbB-2 oncoprotein expression in primary and advanced breast cancer. Br J Cancer 1991;63:439.

182. McCann AH, Dervan PA, O'Regan M, et al. Prognostic significance of c-*erb*B-2 and estrogen receptor status in human breast cancer. Cancer Res 1991;51:3296.

183. Kallioniemi O-P, Holli K, Visakorpi T, et al. Association of c-*erb*B-2 protein over-expression with high rate of cell proliferation, increased risk of visceral metastasis and poor long-term survival in breast cancer. Int J Cancer 1991;49:650.

184. Tanner B, Friedberg T, Mitze M, et al. C-erbB-2-oncogene expression in breast carcinoma: analysis by S1 nuclease protection assay and immunohistochemistry in relation to clinical parameters. Gynecol Oncol 1992;47:228.

185. Yuan J, Hennessy C, Givan AL, et al. Predicting outcome for patients with node negative breast cancer: a comparative study of the value of flow cytometry and cell image analysis for determination of DNA ploidy. Br J Cancer 1992;65:461.

186. Allred DC, Clark GM, Tandon AK, et al. HER-2/*neu* in node-negative breast cancer: prognostic significance of overexpression influenced by the presence of in situ carcinoma. J Clin Oncol 1992;10:599.

187. Noguchi M, Koyasaki N, Ohta N, et al. C-*erb*B-2 oncoprotein expression versus internal mammary lymph node metastases as additional prognostic factors in patients with axillary lymph node-positive breast cancer. Cancer 1992;69:2953.

188. Gusterson BA, Gelber RD, Goldhirsch A, et al. Prognostic importance of c-*erb*B-2 expression in breast cancer: International [Ludwig] Breast Cancer Study Group. J Clin Oncol 1992;10:1049.

189. Press MF, Hung G, Godolphin W, et al. Sensitivity of HER-2/*neu* antibodies in archival tissue samples: potential source of error in immunohistochemical studies of oncogene expression. Cancer Res 1994;54:2771.

190. Bianchi S, Paglierani M, Zampi G, et al. Prognostic significance of c-erbB-2 expression in node negative breast cancer. Br J Cancer 1993;67:625.

191. Têtu B, Brisson J. Prognostic significance of HER-2/neu oncoprotein expression in node-positive breast cancer: the influence of the pattern of immunostaining and adjuvant therapy. Cancer 1994;73:2359.

192. Benz CC, Scott GK, Sarup JC, et al. Estrogen-dependent, tamoxifen-resistant tumorigenic growth of MCF-7 cells transfected with HER2/*neu*. Breast Cancer Res Treat 1992;24:85.

193. Wright C, Nicholson S, Angus B, et al. Relationship between c-erbB-2 protein product expression and response to endocrine therapy in advanced breast cancer. Br J Cancer 1992;65:118.

194. Klijn JG, Berns EM, Bontenbal M, et al. Cell biological factors associated with the response of breast cancer to systemic treatment. Cancer Treat Rev 1993;19(Suppl B):45.

195. Wright C, Cairns J, Cantwell BJ, et al. Response to mitoxantrone in advanced breast cancer: correlation with expression of c-*erb*B-2 protein and glutathione S-transferases. Br J Cancer 1992;65:271.

196. Hollstein M, Sidransky D, Vogelstein B, et al. p53 mutations in human cancers. Science 1991;253:49.

197. Elledge RM, Fuqua SAW, Clark GM, et al. The role and prognostic significance of p53 gene alterations in breast cancer. Breast Cancer Res Treat 1993;27:95.

198. Thor AD, Moore DH II, Edgerton SM, et al. Accumulation of p53 tumor suppressor gene protein: an independent marker of prognosis in breast cancers. J Natl Cancer Inst 1992;84:845.

199. Isola J, Visakori T, Holli K, et al. Association of overexpression of tumor suppressor protein p53 with rapid cell proliferation and poor prognosis in node-negative breast cancer patients. J Natl Cancer Inst 1992;84:1109.

200. Allred DC, Clark GM, Elledge R, et al. Association of p53 protein expression with tumor cell proliferation rate and clinical outcome in node-negative breast cancer. J Natl Cancer Inst 1993;85:200.

201. Barnes DM, Dublin EA, Fisher CJ, et al. Immunohistochemical detection of p53 protein in mammary carcinoma: an important new independent indicator of prognosis? Hum Pathol 1993;24:469.

202. Silvestrini R, Benini E, Daidone MG, et al. p53 as an independent prognostic marker in lymph node-negative breast cancer patients. J Natl Cancer Inst 1993;85:965.

203. Marks JR, Humphrey PA, Wu K, et al. Overexpression of p53 and HER-2*neu* proteins as prognostic markers in early stage breast cancer. Ann Surg 1994;219:332.

204. Gasparini G, Weidner N, Bevilacqua P, et al. Tumor microvessel density, p53 expression, tumor size, and peritumoral lymphatic vessel invasion are relevant prognostic markers in node-negative breast carcinoma. J Clin Oncol 1994;12:454.

205. Elledge RM, Fuqua SAW, Clark GM, et al. Prognostic significance

of p53 gene alterations in node-negative breast cancer. Breast Cancer Res Treat 1993;26:225.

206. Caleffi M, Teague MW, Jensen RA, et al. p53 gene mutations and steroid receptor status in breast cancer: clinicopathologic correlations and prognostic assessment. Cancer 1994;73:2147.

207. Battifora H. p53 immunohistochemistry: a word of caution. Hum Pathol 1994;28:435.

208. Callahan R. p53 mutations, another breast cancer prognostic factor. J Natl Cancer Inst 1992;84:826.

209. Legros Y, Lacabanne V, d'Agay MF, et al. Production of human p53 specific monoclonal antibodies and their use in immunohistochemical studies of tumor cells. Bull Cancer 1993;80:102.

210. Elledge RM, Clark GM, Fuqua SAW, et al. p53 protein accumulation detected by five different antibodies: relationship to prognosis and heat shock protein 70 in breast cancer. Cancer Res 1994;54:3752.

211. Jacquemier J, Molès JP, Penault-Llorca F, et al. p53 immunohistochemical analysis in breast cancer with four monoclonal antibodies: comparison of staining and PCR-SSCP results. Br J Cancer 1994;69:846.

212. Steeg P, Bevilacqua G, Kopper L, et al. Evidence for a novel gene associated with low tumor metastatic potential. J Natl Cancer Inst 1988;80:200.

213. Gilles AM, Presecan E, Vonica A, et al. Nucleoside diphosphate kinase from human erythrocytes. J Biol Chem 1991;266:8784.

214. Hennessy C, Henry JA, May FE, et al. Expression of the antimetastatic gene nm23 in human breast cancer: an association with good prognosis. J Natl Cancer Inst 1991;83:281.

215. Barnes R, Masood S, Barker E, et al. Low nm23 protein expression in infiltrating ductal breast carcinomas correlates with reduced patient survival. Am J Pathol 1991;139:245.

216. Tokunaga Y, Urano T, Furukawa K, et al. Reduced expression of nm23-H1, but not of nm23-H2, is concordant with the frequency of lymph-node metastasis of human breast cancer. Int J Cancer 1993;55:66.

217. Cropp CS, Lidereau R, Leone A, et al. NME1 protein expression and loss of heterozygosity mutations in primary breast tumors. J Natl Cancer Inst 1994;86:1167.

218. Sawan A, Lascu I, Veron M, et al. NDP-K/nm23 expression in human breast cancer in relation to relapse, survival, and other prognostic factors: an immunohistochemical study. J Pathol 1994;172:27.

219. Steeg PS, De La Rosa A, Flatow U, et al. Nm23 and breast cancer metastasis. Breast Cancer Res Treat 1993;25:175.

220. Ravdin PM. Evaluation of cathepsin D as a prognostic factor in breast cancer. Breast Cancer Res Treat 1993;24:219.

221. Spyratos F, Martin P-M, Hacène K, et al. Multiparametric prognostic evaluation of biological factors in primary breast cancer. J Natl Cancer Inst 1992;84:1266.

222. Remmele W, Sauer-Manthey J. Comparative biochemical and immunohistochemical studies on the cathepsin D content of human breast cancer. Virchows Arch A Pathol Anat Histopathol 1993;422:467.

223. Têtu B, Brisson J, Cote C, et al. Prognostic significance of cathepsin-D expression in node-positive breast carcinoma: an immunohistochemical study. Int J Cancer 1993;55:429.

224. Armas OA, Gerald WL, Lesser ML, et al. Immunohistochemical detection of cathepsin D in T2N0M0 breast carcinoma. Am J Surg Pathol 1994;18:158.

225. Foekens JA, Schmitt M, van Putten WLJ, et al. Plasminogen activator inhibitor-1 and prognosis in primary breast cancer. J Clin Oncol 1994;12:1648.

226. Gasparini G, Boracchi P, Bevilacqua P, et al. A multiparametric study on the prognostic value of epidermal growth factor receptor in operable breast carcinoma. Breast Cancer Res Treat 1994;29:59.

227. Ravdin PM, Tandon AK, Allred DC, et al. Cathepsin D by western blotting and immunohistochemistry: failure to confirm correlations with prognosis in node-negative breast cancer. J Clin Oncol 1994;12:467.

228. Johnson MD, Torri JA, Lippman ME, et al. The role of cathepsin D in the invasiveness of human breast cancer cells. Cancer Res 1993;53:873.

229. Foekens JA, Schmitt M, van Putten WLJ, et al. Prognostic value of urokinase-type plasminogen activator in 671 primary breast cancer patients. Cancer Res 1992;52:6101.

230. Grondahl-Hansen J, Christensen IJ, Rosenquist C, et al. High levels of urokinase-type plasminogen activator and its inhibitor PAI-1 in cytosolic extracts of breast carcinomas are associated with prognosis. Cancer Res 1993;53:2513.

231. Janicke F, Schmitt M, Pache L, et al. Urokinase (uPA) and its inhibitor PAI-1 are strong and independent prognostic factors in node-negative breast cancer. Breast Cancer Res Treat 1993; 24:195.

232. Duffy MJ, Reilly D, McDermott E, et al. Urokinase plasminogen activator as a prognostic marker in different subgroups of patients with breast cancer. Cancer 1994;74:2276.

233. Bouchet C, Spyratos F, Martin PM, et al. Prognostic value of urokinase-type plasminogen activator (uPA) and plasminogen activator inhibitors PAI-1 and PAI-2 in breast cancers. Br J Cancer 1994;69:398.

234. Graeff H, Harbeck N, Pache L, et al. Prognostic impact and clinical relevance of tumor-associated proteases in breast cancer. Fibrinolysis 1992;6:45.

235. Hand PH, Thor A, Schlom J, et al. Expression of laminin receptor in normal and carcinomatous human tissues as defined by a monoclonal antibody. Cancer Res 1985;45:2713.

236. Castronovo V, Taraboletti G, Liotta LA, et al. Modulation of laminin receptor expression by estrogen and progestins in human breast cancer cell lines. J Natl Cancer Inst 1989;81:781.

237. Marques LA, Franco ELF, Torloni H, et al. Independent prognostic value of laminin receptor expression in breast cancer survival. Cancer Res 1990;50:1479.

238. Daidone MG, Silvestrini R, D'Errico A, et al. Laminin receptors, collagenase IV and prognosis in node-negative breast cancers. Int J Cancer 1991;48:529.

239. Martignone S, Ménard S, Bufalino R, et al. Prognostic significance of the 67-kilodalton laminin receptor expression in human breast carcinomas. J Natl Cancer Inst 1993;85:398.

240. Folkman J. What is the evidence that tumors are angiogenesis dependent? J Natl Cancer Inst 1990;82:4.

241. Vartanian RK, Weidner N. Correlation of intratumoral endothelial cell proliferation with microvessel density (tumor angiogenesis) and tumor cell proliferation in breast carcinoma. Am J Pathol 1994;144:1188.

242. Craft PS, Harris AL. Clinical prognostic significance of tumour angiogenesis. Ann Oncol 1994;5:305.

243. Weidner N, Semple J, Welch WR, et al. Tumor angiogenesis and metastasis: correlation in invasive breast carcinoma. N Engl J Med 1991;324:1.

244. Bosari S, Lee AKC, DeLellis RA, et al. Microvessel quantitation and prognosis in invasive breast carcinoma. Hum Pathol 1992;23:755.

245. Horak ER, Leek R, Klenk N, et al. Angiogenesis, assessed by platelet/endothelial cell adhesion molecule antibodies, as indicator of node metastases and survival in breast cancer. Lancet 1992;340:1120.

246. Toi M, Hoshina S, Yamamoto Y, et al. Tumor angiogenesis in breast cancer: significance of vessel density as a prognostic indicator. Gan To Kagaku Ryoho 1994;21:178.

247. Fox SB, Leek RD, Smith K, et al. Tumor angiogenesis in node-negative breast carcinomas: relationship with epidermal growth

factor receptor, estrogen receptor, and survival. Breast Cancer Res Treat 1994;29:109.

248. Hayes DF. Angiogenesis and breast cancer. Breast Cancer 1994;8:51.

249. Albain KS, Green S, LeBlanc M, et al. Proportional hazards and recursive partitioning and amalgamation analyses of the Southwest Oncology Group node-positive adjuvant CMFVP breast cancer data base: a pilot study. Breast Cancer Res Treat 1992;22:273.

250. Ravdin PM, Clark GM. A practical application of neural network analysis for predicting outcome of individual breast cancer patients. Breast Cancer Res Treat 1992;22:285.

251. Hilsenbeck SG, Clark GM, McGuire WL. Why do so many prognostic factors fail to pan out? Breast Cancer Res Treat 1992;22:197.

17

Treatment of Early-Stage Breast Cancer

Diseases of the Breast, edited by Jay R. Harris,
Marc E. Lippman, Monica Morrow, and Samuel Hellman.
Lippincott-Raven Publishers, Philadelphia, © 1996.

17.1

Local Management of Invasive Breast Cancer

JAY R. HARRIS ▪ MONICA MORROW

The local treatment of breast cancer has long been a source of controversy. For many years, local treatment was considered the domain of the surgeon. However, changes in our understanding of the biology of the disease, the detection of smaller tumors over time, an increasing emphasis on systemic therapy, and greater patient participation in the decision-making process have radically changed our approach to the local treatment of breast cancer during the past 20 years. Local treatment of breast cancer involves a collaborative effort between surgeons, radiation oncologists, reconstructive surgeons, radiologists, pathologists, and medical oncologists. This chapter reflects this multimodality approach by addressing the use of surgery and radiation therapy (RT) in a coordinated fashion as well as considering the integration of local and systemic treatment. The history of local treatment of breast cancer, the rationale for the current approach to local treatment, and the studies that support this approach are discussed. In addition to providing the theoretical basis for local treatment, this chapter addresses practical issues in the local treatment of breast cancer, including the following:

▪ Guidelines for patient selection
▪ Timing of surgery
▪ Indications for, techniques, and complications of axillary surgery
▪ Indications for postoperative RT
▪ Sequencing of RT and systemic therapy
▪ Management of microinvasive breast cancer
▪ Breast-conserving surgery without RT
▪ Tamoxifen as primary treatment in elderly patients

▪ Technique and complications of breast-conserving surgery
▪ Technique and complications of modified radical mastectomy, including oncologic considerations in the use of immediate breast reconstruction
▪ Technique of RT
▪ Complications of RT

History of Surgical Treatment

The modern era of breast cancer surgery began with the popularization of the radical mastectomy by William Halsted in 1894.[1,2] The development of the radical mastectomy was based on a theory of breast cancer spread that emphasized the local spread of the disease, particularly through the lymphatics. Radical mastectomy, an en bloc resection of the breast, the overlying skin, the pectoral muscles, and the entirety of the axillary contents, had two major advantages. It was technically possible in most women with breast cancer, even in the advanced cancers seen in the first half of the century, and it was an effective means of obtaining local control of the primary tumor. Of 1640 women seen at Memorial Hospital[3] from 1940 to 1943, 89% were considered candidates for radical mastectomy. However, of the 1458 patients who underwent radical mastectomy, only 13% survived 30 years free of cancer, with 57% patients dying of breast cancer, 24% dying of other causes, and 6% lost to follow-up.

The failure of radical mastectomy to cure many patients

with breast cancer was initially thought by some surgeons to be because of its failure to extirpate all of the draining lymphatics of the breast. It was recognized in the 1950s that one quarter of the lymphatic drainage of the breast is through the ipsilateral internal mammary nodes, and that this drainage occurs from all quadrants of the breast.[4] To address this, the extended radical mastectomy was developed. The extended radical mastectomy is a radical mastectomy combined with en bloc removal of the internal mammary nodes. Nonrandomized studies suggested that survival might be improved in selected patients by this more radical procedure.[5,6] However, a prospective randomized trial comparing radical and extended radical mastectomy failed to show any difference in disease-free or overall survival between the two treatment groups.[7] This is not surprising, since metastases to the internal mammary nodes in the absence of axillary node involvement are uncommon, occurring in only 5% of 7070 patients in whom both axillary and internal mammary nodes were sampled.[8] Based on these results, the extended radical mastectomy is an operation of historic interest. The failure of this more extensive procedure to improve survival cast doubt on the validity of Halstedian principles and the need for radical mastectomy itself.

Modified radical mastectomy is the most common operative treatment for patients with invasive breast cancer in the United States.[9–11] The term *modified radical mastectomy* is used to describe a variety of surgical procedures, but all involve complete removal of the breast, the underlying pectoral fascia, and some of the axillary nodes. Whereas the modified radical mastectomy may not seem to differ significantly from the radical mastectomy, it represented a major departure from Halstedian principles of en bloc cancer surgery. The switch to modified radical mastectomy occurred when it became recognized that treatment failure after breast cancer surgery usually is because of the systemic dissemination of cancer cells before surgery, rather than an inadequate operative procedure. In addition, by the 1970s, fewer patients with large tumors with fixation to the pectoral muscle were being seen, making modified radical mastectomy feasible for most women. Several retrospective studies[12,13] demonstrated no difference in survival between patients treated with modified radical and radical mastectomy. These findings were confirmed in two prospective randomized trials. In the Manchester study,[14] 534 patients with clinical stage I or II breast carcinoma were randomized to treatment with radical mastectomy or modified radical mastectomy. At 5 years, no differences were observed in overall survival, disease-free survival or local recurrence rates. In a similar study involving 311 patients treated at a single institution, Maddox and coauthors[15] failed to demonstrate any significant benefit in survival or local control for patients undergoing radical mastectomy. Although only two randomized studies directly compared radical and modified radical mastectomy, further evidence that radical en bloc surgery did not prolong survival came from several randomized trials comparing radical mastectomy with simple mastectomy and RT. An overview analysis[16,17] of patients treated in four randomized trials demonstrated equivalent

survival for patients treated with radical mastectomy and those treated with simple mastectomy combined with RT.

Today there are few indications for radical mastectomy. If the pectoral fascia has been violated at the time of biopsy or if the tumor abuts the pectoral fascia or even invades a small portion of the pectoral muscle, it is preferable to resect a small portion of the muscle directly beneath the tumor to obtain a negative deep margin of resection. Large tumors that involve greater amounts of the pectoral muscle are best treated with chemotherapy or RT, not radical surgery, as the initial approach. After a response to the initial therapy, a standard modified radical mastectomy with primary skin closure frequently can be done in these cases.

Some of the same principles that led to the use of the modified radical mastectomy contributed to the development of breast-conserving treatment. These included recognition that adherence to the Halstedian principle of en bloc extirpation of the breast and its draining lymphatics failed to cure many patients with breast cancer, the increasingly frequent identification of small breast cancers by mammography, and the success of moderate-dose RT in eliminating subclinical foci of breast cancer after mastectomy. An initial objection to the use of breast-conserving treatment was the known multicentricity of breast carcinoma. The reported incidence of multicentricity ranged from 9% to 75%, depending on the definition employed, extent of tissue sampling, and the techniques of pathologic examination used.[18–20] These studies were used to argue against anything less than complete mastectomy as optimal local treatment for breast cancer.

The strategy behind breast-conserving treatment is to remove the bulk of the tumor surgically and to use moderate doses of radiation to eradicate any residual cancer. A key element in the successful application of this approach is the preservation of a good cosmetic appearance of the treated breast. The application of this strategy requires an understanding of the extent and distribution of cancer in a breast with an apparently localized tumor. Considerable clarification of this issue has occurred as a result of the work of Holland and coauthors.[21,22] In their initial study,[21] mastectomy specimens with primary tumors 4 cm or less in size were studied. In all cases, the tumors were considered unicentric based on clinical and radiographic assessment. Detailed evaluation of the breast was carried out using 5-mm sections, radiography of these thin slices, and an average of 20 blocks per specimen for histologic evaluation. This technique allowed precise mapping of the extent and distribution of residual carcinoma in relation to the primary (or reference) tumor. Only 39% of specimens showed no evidence of cancer beyond the reference tumor. In 20%, there was additional cancer but confined to within 2 cm of the reference tumor. Forty-one percent of cases had residual cancer more than 2 cm from the reference tumor; of these, two thirds had pure intraductal carcinoma and one third had mixed intraductal and invasive carcinoma (Fig. 17.1-1). The percentage of cases with residual cancer more than 2 cm from the reference tumor corresponds well to the rate of local failure reported in patients treated with excision of the primary tumor

FIGURE 17.1-1 Frequency of additional cancer foci at increasing distance from a clinically unifocal reference tumor.[21] Two hundred sixty-four mastectomy specimens were studied from patients with breast cancers measuring 4 cm or less and judged to be unifocal based on clinical findings. Thirty-nine percent of cases (group A) showed no additional cancer foci beyond the reference tumor. In 20% of cases (group B), additional foci were found but restricted to within 2 cm of the reference tumor. Forty-one percent of the cases showed cancer foci further than 2 cm from the reference tumor, including 27% in which the additional foci were entirely intraductal (group C) and 14% in which they were invasive and intraductal (group D).

alone.[23–27] In these series, local recurrence in the breast occurs at or near the site of the primary tumor in most cases, also emphasizing that multifocal breast cancer commonly remains after an excision of the tumor and that this multifocal involvement is biologically important. This is true even if the margins of surgical resection are assessed to be negative.

In a subsequent study, Holland and others[22] quantitated the amount of residual intraductal carcinoma at various distances from the primary tumor. Prominent intraductal carcinoma was defined as a total of six or more low-power fields of intraductal carcinoma measured using a 6-mm field and a 2.5× objective. Approximately 10% of patients had prominent intraductal carcinoma extending more than 2 cm from the reference tumor, and approximately 5% of patients had prominent intraductal carcinoma extending more than 3 cm. These studies of Holland and associates indicate that the extent and amount of multifocal cancer in the vicinity of a primary tumor is variable. In some patients, there seems to be minimal multifocal involvement, whereas in others there is extensive intraductal disease. These results imply that the extent of surgical resection required in breast-conserving treatment varies from patient to patient. These issues are considered in more detail later in this chapter.

History of Radiation Therapy for Breast Cancer

The use of RT for breast cancer began at nearly the same time as surgical treatment. In 1895, Wilhelm Roentgen, using a primitive cathode-ray tube, discovered a new form of radiation that was able to penetrate various materials and darken photographic plates. To distinguish this new form of radiation from others, he chose to call it *x-rays*.

In the next year, Henri Becquerel demonstrated that some naturally occurring material in uranium crystals emitted a form of radiation similar to x-rays. Three years later, Marie and Pierre Curie reported their discovery of a new radioactive substance found in pitchblende, which they named *radium*. These physicists provided the basic tools to be used in the treatment of cancer by RT: x-rays, created by the bombardment of accelerated electrons on a target, and gamma rays, emitted by radium and other radioactive materials. X-rays and gamma rays are, in reality, both photons, differing primarily in origin.

Within 1 year after Roentgen reported his discovery, patients with cancer were treated with x-rays. Early practitioners of this modality demonstrated the ability of x-rays to shrink and, in some cases, to eliminate cancerous growths completely. These practitioners were limited, however, by the rudimentary equipment available at that time and by the absence of a technique and treatment schedule able to deliver RT to the tumor while sparing normal tissues. The energy of x-ray machines available before 1920 was in the range of 120 to 135 kvp, compared with greater than 4000 kvp (4 MV) typically used today. These older x-ray machines delivered their maximal dose at the skin surface with a rapid falloff into deeper tissues. Because of the poor penetration of these low-energy x-rays, doses were limited to what the skin could tolerate, whereas tumors situated at deeper levels were spared. X-ray machines with energies over 1 MV (commonly referred to as *supervoltage*) were not commercially available in large numbers until the 1960s. The major form of supervoltage machine has become the linear accelerator, which typically provides the option of delivering an electron beam. This form of radiation permits penetration to a depth determined by the energy of the electrons. This property makes it an ideal method for treating limited superficial regions, such as "boosting" the tumor bed in the breast or on the chest wall.

It was soon realized that the optimal use of RT depends on extending the course of treatment over time. Large single exposures to radiation result in significant and progressive adverse effects on normal tissues. Careful observation of treated patients determined that best results were achieved by delivering relatively small doses of radiation daily over an extended period. This fractionation and protraction of treatment allows greater recovery of normal tissues and still permits killing of tumor cells. Worldwide experience since has generally established that a dose in the range of 1.8 to 2 Gy given once a day provides optimal results. (The current official unit of radiation dose absorbed in tissue is the gray [Gy]; 1 Gy = 100 cGy [centigray] = 100 rad [the previous unit of absorbed dose]. The roentgen (R) is a unit of "exposure," or ionization induced in air, and generally corresponds to less than 1 cGy.)

Among the first to document the dose of radiation required to achieve local tumor control of breast cancer was Gilbert Fletcher.[28] He examined the incidence of supraclavicular node relapse in patients with positive axillary nodes treated with radical mastectomy. Prior retrospective reports had indicated a relapse rate of 20% to 25% when no postoperative RT was given. Fletcher found that the rate of supraclavicular relapse was 3% when 30 to 35 Gy was delivered in 4 weeks and was only 1.3% when 50 to 55 Gy in 4 weeks was used. These inferential data provide support for the use of 45 to 50 Gy in 4.5 to 5 weeks to eradicate "subclinical" deposits of breast cancer in a high percentage of cases. In a test of this concept, a trial of historical importance was conducted in Copenhagen from 1951 to 1957. In this trial, 559 patients were randomly assigned to undergo either an extended radical mastectomy or a total mastectomy and postoperative RT. The technique of RT used in the trial was orthovoltage treatment as developed by Robert McWhirter from Edinburgh. Despite the limitations of the RT techniques available at that time, long-term results reported by Kaae and Johansen[29] revealed equivalent local tumor control and survival for the two treatments. This trial was the first to demonstrate the effectiveness of RT in treating areas of subclinical involvement.

The concept of combining conservative surgery (CS) with RT as a substitute for mastectomy is not new. Geoffrey Keynes[30] in London and M. Vera Peters[31] in Toronto were early proponents of this approach before supervoltage irradiation was available. Keynes,[30] a surgeon at St. Bartholomew's Hospital, began to treat patients with operable carcinoma of the breast in this manner as early as 1924. M. Vera Peters, a radiation oncologist at the Princess Margaret Hospital in Toronto, began her large series in 1939.[31] With the development of supervoltage irradiation, it became feasible to pursue this breast-conserving therapy with the goal of preserving highly satisfactory cosmetic results. Developers of this approach were Robert Calle of the Institut Curie, Bernard Pierquin of the Henri Mondor Hospital, J.M. Spitalier of the Marseilles Cancer Institute in Europe, Eleanor Montague of M.D. Anderson Cancer Center, and Samuel Hellman at the Harvard Joint Center for Radiation Therapy in the United States. Formalized clinical trials to evaluate its effectiveness in comparison with mastectomy

were initiated by Umberto Veronesi at the National Cancer Institute of Italy in Milan and Bernard Fisher of the National Surgical Adjuvant Breast and Bowel Project (NSABP).

Results of Clinical Trials of Conservative Surgery and Radiation Therapy

Because of the almost universal acceptance of the Halstedian dogma regarding breast cancer, a relatively large number of randomized clinical trials were conducted to determine if survival after breast-conserving treatment equalled survival after mastectomy. Two of the initial trials comparing mastectomy and conservative surgery combined with RT were conducted at Guy's Hospital, London[32-34] and illustrate that inadequate local–regional treatment can result in a lower rate of survival. In the initial trial,[32] 376 patients with clinical stage I or II breast cancer were randomly assigned to undergo (1) wide excision of the tumor (without axillary dissection) followed by low-dose RT to the breast (38 Gy) and axilla (27 Gy) or (2) radical mastectomy and RT to the supraclavicular and internal mammary nodes (IMNs). In the second trial, carried out from 1971 to 1975, 250 patients with clinical stage I disease were randomly assigned to undergo either wide excision or radical mastectomy, both combined with RT.[33] A high rate of axillary recurrence was observed in the wide excision arms of both of these studies. In the first study, node-positive patients were found to have a higher rate of survival after radical mastectomy and RT compared with node-positive patients treated with wide excision and RT.[32] In the second trial, radical mastectomy and RT resulted in a survival benefit for the node-negative patients (Fig. 17.1-2). A reanalysis of the second trial[34] indicated that the improvement in survival after radical mastectomy and RT was confined to patients with T1 cancer. These results emphasize that local control in the axilla may affect survival in patients with favorable cancers in whom the risk of distant metastases at presentation is low. However, they provide little practical information for modern clinical practice because of the inadequacies of the treatments employed.

Since 1970, there have been six prospective randomized trials[35-41] using modern radiation techniques in which CS and RT have been compared with mastectomy (Table 17.1-1). At the National Cancer Institute of Italy in Milan, 701 women with clinical stage I breast carcinoma (tumor less than 2 cm, clinically negative axillary nodes) were randomized to treatment with CS or radical mastectomy.[35,36] CS consisted of a quadrantectomy, including removal of the skin overlying the tumor, a full quadrant of breast tissue oriented in a radial fashion, and the fascia of the pectoralis major muscle. A complete axillary dissection also was performed. After CS, RT was administered to the breast alone through two opposing tangential fields giving a dose of 50 Gy in 5 weeks. Another 10 Gy was given to the tumor bed by orthovoltage radiation. After

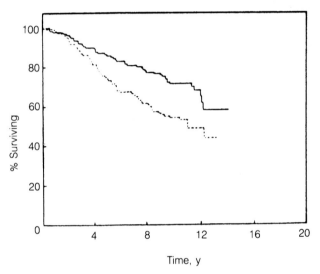

FIGURE 17.1-2 Results from the second Guy's Hospital trial comparing conservative surgery (without axillary dissection) combined with radiation therapy (RT) (*dashed lines*) and radical mastectomy (*solid lines*) in clinically node-negative patients.[34] The dose of RT used to treat the axilla was low, and a substantial rate of axillary recurrences was seen. This increased rate of axillary recurrence was associated with an increased rate of distant failure (*top*) and a decreased rate of survival (*bottom*) in the patients treated with conservative surgery and RT.

1975, all patients with histologically positive axillary lymph nodes received 12 cycles of cyclophosphamide, methotrexate, and 5-fluorouracil (CMF). The latest report of this trial was published in 1990.[36] No differences in relapse-free or overall survival rates were noticed, and this was true for node-positive and node-negative patients (Fig. 17.1-3). With a minimum follow-up of 10 years, ipsilateral breast recurrence occurred in 3% of the patients treated with quadrantectomy. There were 19 cases of contralateral breast carcinoma in the quadrantectomy group and 20 in the mastectomy group.

The National Surgical Adjuvant Breast and Bowel Project (NSABP) began a randomized three-arm trial (protocol B-06) in 1976 comparing mastectomy to lumpectomy with or without RT.[27,37] A total of 1843 evaluable patients with clinical stage I or II carcinoma whose tumors were 4 cm or less in greatest diameter were entered. Of these, 174 patients refused their assigned treatment and were excluded from analysis. All patients underwent axillary dissection, and those with histologically involved lymph nodes received adjuvant systemic therapy. The surgery differed from that performed in the Milan study in both concept and extent. In the NSABP trial, the breast resection was not designed to remove an anatomic segment of breast tissue and there was no effort to perform an en bloc resection of skin and fascia. Lumpectomy involved removal of the tumor with enough grossly normal breast tissue around it to ensure that the microscopic margins of the specimen were tumor-free. Margins were defined as tumor-free if cancer cells were not present on the inked edges of the resected breast specimen. In 10% of the patients randomized to lumpectomy, tumor-free margins were not obtained, and in these patients, total mastectomy was carried out. RT was delivered to the breast alone with supervoltage equipment using opposed tangential fields, often without wedge filters to compensate for the slope of the breast, to a dose of 50 to 53 Gy in 5 to 6 weeks. No boost was given to the tumor site. Patients have now been followed for a mean of 102 months,[37] and no differences in distant disease-free survival or overall survival rates were observed between patients undergoing mastectomy and those undergoing lumpectomy with or without RT. (Fig. 17.1-4 shows the 9-year results comparing mastectomy to lumpectomy and RT.) Although the use of RT was not associated with an improvement in survival, it significantly reduced the incidence of local recurrence in the breast. The 9-year probability of a recurrence in the breast was 12% for patients who received RT and 42% for those who did not. The benefit of RT in terms of local control was seen both in patients with positive and negative nodes and was independent of both tumor size and patient age.

Another trial testing the value of breast-conserving treatment was performed by the European Organization for Research and Treatment of Cancer (EORTC). Between 1980 and 1986, 148 patients with stage I and 755 with stage II breast cancer were entered into a trial comparing mastectomy with conservative surgery, axillary dissection, and RT.[38] The breast surgery removed 1 to 2 cm of grossly normal breast tissue around the tumor. RT to the breast consisted of 50 Gy to the breast over 5 weeks, and a boost dose of 25 Gy was given using iridium interstitial implantation. Indications for adjuvant chemotherapy varied among institutions participating in the study. No differences in the rates of local recurrence, distant recurrence, or overall survival have been observed between the two treatment groups. Results from the Danish Breast Cancer Cooperative Group Trial[42] and the National Cancer Institute (US) Early Breast Cancer Trial[40] also demonstrate no survival differences at 5 years between patients treated with mastectomy and those given breast-conserving treatment.

Emphasis has been placed on the problem of recurrence in the breast after breast-conserving treatment. In the ran-

TABLE 17.1-1

Survival Results in the Modern Randomized Trials Comparing Conservative Surgery (CS) and Radiation Therapy (RT) With Mastectomy *

Trial	Years	Patients	Time (y)	Mastectomy (%)	CS and RT (%)
Institut Gustave-Roussy[41]	1972–1979	179	10	79	78
NCI—Milan[36]	1973–1980	701	13	69	71
NSABP trial B-06[27]	1976–1984	1843	8	71	76
NCI—US[40]	1979–1987	237	5	85	89
EORTC[38]	1980–1986	903	7	75	75
Danish Breast Cancer Group[42]	1983–1987	905	6	82	79

EORTC, European Organization for Research and Treatment of Cancer; NCI, National Cancer Institute; NSABP, National Surgical Adjuvant Breast and Bowel Project.

* None of the differences in survival were statistically significant.

domized studies presented, with widely varying surgical and RT techniques, the rates of recurrence in the breast at 8 to 10 years ranged from 4% to 20%.[36–38,40–42] In the corresponding patients treated with mastectomy, 2% to 9% of patients developed local recurrence, emphasizing that mastectomy does not guarantee freedom from local recurrence, even in women with clinical stage I and II breast carcinoma (Table 17.1-2).

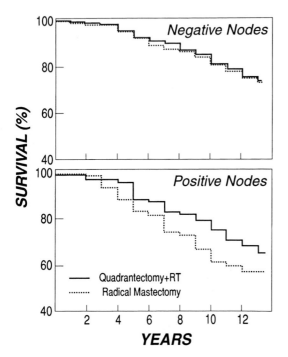

FIGURE 17.1-3 Thirteen-year survival results for the 520 pathologic node-negative and the 181 node-positive patients in the Milan I trial comparing radical mastectomy with quadrantectomy, axillary dissection, and radiation therapy. No statistically significant differences occurred in survival between the two treatment arms for all patients in the trial or in the two subsets of patients according to axillary node status.[63]

Retrospective Studies of Conservative Surgery and Radiation Therapy

The goal of breast-conserving treatment using CS and RT is to provide survival equivalent to mastectomy with preservation of the cosmetic outcome and a low rate of recurrence in the treated breast. Since the 1970s, numerous reports from centers in Europe and North America on the use of CS and RT have demonstrated high rates of local tumor control with satisfactory cosmetic results.[43–52] The long follow-up available for many of these retrospective studies has helped to document the time course and pattern of recurrence in the breast, factors which may be associated with an increased risk of recurrence in the breast, and information regarding cosmetic and psychologic outcomes after breast-conserving therapy. This information is useful in determining the optimal approach to CS and RT, in providing guidelines for patient selection, and in providing patients treated with CS and RT with important information on their expected outcome.

LOCAL RECURRENCE

Retrospective studies have helped to establish the incidence of local recurrence and its time course. Ten-year local recurrence rates ranging from 8% to 20% have been reported.[43–46,48–53] These rates are similar to the local recurrence rates seen in the randomized trials of CS and RT. However, the nonrandomized studies with the longest follow-up emphasize the prolonged time course to local recurrence in some patients undergoing breast-conserving treatment.[49,50,54] Kurtz and coworkers[50] noticed that the actuarial incidence of recurrence in the treated breast increased from 7% at 5 years to 14% at 10 years and 20% at 20 years after treatment. These findings were similar to other reports describing a persistent risk of recurrence in the breast through 20 years of follow-up.[49,54] These results

FIGURE 17.1-4 Nine-year results of the NSABP trial B-06 comparing total mastectomy (TM) with lumpectomy (L) plus breast irradiation (XRT), both combined with axillary dissection. Disease-free survival, distant disease-free survival, and overall survival were similar for the two arms.[37]

have been contrasted to those seen after mastectomy, in which most local failures occur in the first 3 years after surgery.

Other studies have examined both the time course of local recurrence and the pattern of treatment failure.[55–58] Most investigators have classified recurrences in the breast by their location in relation to the original tumor. Recurrences at or near the primary site (presumably representing a recurrence of the original tumor) are classified as either a true recurrence (TR; within the boosted region) or a marginal miss (MM; adjacent to the boosted region). Other categories of recurrence include those elsewhere in the breast (occurring at a distance from the original tumor and presumably representing a new primary), those primarily involving the skin, and those which are unclassifiable or diffuse in the breast. Gage and others[58] reported on 1628 patients with clinical stage I or II invasive carcinoma treated with gross tumor excision and RT including a

dose of at least 60 Gy to the primary site. The median follow-up time in survivors was 116 months. Table 17.1-3 shows the annual incidence rates for all sites of recurrence, both local and distant. The annual incidence rate for a TR/MM recurrence was between 1.3% and 1.8% for years 2 through 7 after treatment, and then decreased to 0.4% by 10 years after treatment. In contrast, the annual incidence rate for recurrence elsewhere in the breast increased slowly to a rate of approximately 0.7% per year at 8 years and remained stable. Kurtz and coauthors[57] similarly noticed that 32% of breast recurrences seen after 5 years occurred at a distance from the primary tumor compared with only 14% of recurrences seen during the first 5 years. The risk of recurrence elsewhere in the breast after the first 5 years after treatment is remarkably similar to the risk of developing a contralateral breast carcinoma.[59] This suggests that although whole-breast irradiation is effective at eradicating multicentric breast carcinoma, it does

TABLE 17.1-2

Local Recurrence Rates in Modern Randomized Trials Comparing Conservative Surgery (CS) and Radiation Therapy (RT) With Mastectomy

Trial	Follow-Up	Local Recurrence (%)		Type CS	Boost	Boost Dose
		Mastectomy	CS and RT			
Gustave-Roussy[41]	10	9	7	2-cm gross margin	Yes	15 Gy
NCI—Milan[36]	10	2	4	Quadrantectomy	Yes	10 Gy
NSABP B-06[27]	8	8	10	Lumpectomy	No	
NCI—US[40]	8	6	20	Gross tumor excision	Yes	15–20 Gy
EORTC[38]	8	9	13	1-cm gross margin	Yes	25 Gy
Danish Breast Cancer Group[42]	6	4	3	Wide excision	Yes	10–25 Gy

EORTC, European Organization for Research and Treatment of Cancer; NCI, National Cancer Institute; NSABP, National Surgical Adjuvant Breast and Bowel Project.

TABLE 17.1-3
Annual Incidence of Recurrence by Site in Years After Treatment, JCRT Series, 1968–1986

Site of Recurrence	Years After CS and RT									
	1	2	3	4	5	6	7	8	9	10
Ipsilateral breast										
TR/MM	0.4	1.3	1.9	1.4	1.8	1.6	1.5	0.7	0.4	0.4
Elsewhere	0.1	0.3	0.3	0.1	0.2	0.4	0.4	0.7	0.7	0.5
Skin/unclassifiable	0.1	0.4	0.2	0.2	0.1	0.1	0.1	0.2	0.0	0.0
Distant or regional	3.2	5.0	4.6	3.2	2.4	2.1	2.5	1.6	1.0	2.4
Dead of other causes	0.2	0.7	0.6	0.7	1.4	0.5	1.0	1.0	0.9	1.6
Patients at risk	1628	1567	1438	1324	1245	1158	1056	879	698	550

CS, conservative surgery; JCRT, Joint Center for Radiation Therapy; Pts, patients; RT, radiation therapy; TR/MM, true recurrence–marginal miss (recurrence at or near the primary site).

* Incidence figures are percentages.

(Gage I, Nixon A, Gelman R, et al. Long-term outcome following breast-conserving surgery and radiation therapy. Int J Radiat Oncol Biol Phys [in press])

not prevent the subsequent development of new cancers. Patients who elect breast-conserving therapy require life-long follow-up to screen for the development of new cancers in both the treated and the contralateral breast.

COSMETIC OUTCOME

A major goal of breast-conserving treatment is the preservation of a cosmetically acceptable breast. To standardize grading of the cosmetic outcome, observer-based scales comparing the degree of deformity of the treated breast with the untreated breast have been developed. In the scoring system employed at the Joint Center for Radiation Therapy (JCRT), an *excellent* score is assigned when the treated and untreated breast are essentially identical, *good* signifies that treatment effects are minimal but easily identifiable, *fair* indicates obvious treatment effects, and *poor* is used when there are severe changes in the normal breast tissue.[60] Pezner and coauthors[61] found that there was significant interobserver and intraobserver variability in the application of observer-based cosmetic scores, even with experienced observers. These differences were most marked for early stage cases. Pezner and coworkers concluded that although good and poor results could be distinguished grossly, specific cosmetic changes should be analyzed. Several studies[62–65] have attempted to quantitate the cosmetic outcome more objectively by measuring the degree of breast retraction, extent of telangiectasia, or alteration in breast contour in a reproducible fashion. However, what remains most important in the evaluation of cosmetic outcome is the patient's and, to a lesser extent, the physician's perception of the appearance of the breast.

The long-term cosmetic outcome after CS and RT has been evaluated in a number of studies from the JCRT.[60,66–72] Elements of the cosmetic outcome were assessed by the physician, including breast edema, retraction, fibrosis, telangiectasia, and arm edema, as well as the overall cosmetic appearance. In a study of patients treated between 1968 and 1981, the overall cosmetic result 5 years after treatment was excellent in 65% of patients, good in 25%, fair in 7%, and poor in 3%.[69] During the first 3 years after treatment, overall cosmetic results declined, paralleling the development of breast retraction. After 3 years, and through 7 years of follow-up, the results stabilized. Breast edema was most pronounced in the first year after treatment, with 33% of patients having mild edema and 6% demonstrating moderate to severe edema. By 3 years, the incidence rate of mild edema was 20%, with only 1% having moderate to severe edema. The incidence of breast edema was related to the use of axillary node dissection. Three years after treatment, 24% of patients who underwent axillary dissection had some degree of breast edema compared with 11% of those who did not have a dissection ($P > .007$). In contrast to the early development of breast edema, breast retraction and telangiectasia occurred more slowly. At 1 year, 40% of evaluated patients had some degree of breast retraction, but this increased to 57% at 7 years. Retraction seemed to be the most important determinant of overall cosmetic outcome. Of the 36 patients with fair or poor results at 3 years, 78% had moderate or severe retraction compared with only 6% of 266 patients with good or excellent cosmetic scores. Telangiectasia developed even more slowly than breast retraction, first being observed 12 to 18 months after treatment in most patients. Moderate or severe telangiectasia was uncommon, occurring in only 8% of patients at 5 years. Although treatment-related changes in the treated breast stabilize at 3 years, other factors that primarily affect the *untreated* breast, such as change in size because of weight gain and the normal ptosis seen with aging, continue to affect the symmetry between a patient's breasts.

Although a variety of patient, tumor, and treatment factors have been reported to influence the cosmetic result, the amount of breast tissue resected seems to be the major factor. This is most convincingly demonstrated in the randomized trial performed at the National Cancer Institute of Milan[63,73] comparing quadrantectomy combined with RT to gross tumor excision (lumpectomy) combined with RT. One hundred forty-eight consecutive patients participated in a cosmetic evaluation 18 to 24 months after treatment. Twenty-one percent of patients in the quadrantectomy group had a greater than 3 cm difference in height between the nipples compared with 7% of patients in the lumpectomy group. Similar discrepancies in the inferior profile of the breast and the distance from the midline to the nipple were observed, and these differences are summarized in Table 17.1-4. Similar findings in retrospective studies have been observed by others (Table 17.1-5).[62,72,74] In a small series of patients evaluated both before and after RT, Matory and associates[75] found that surgery was the main contributor to breast distortion. In that series, the cosmetic outcome was graded by a general surgeon, a radiation oncologist, and a plastic surgeon. The general surgeon and radiation oncologist rated 80% of the results as good or excellent, whereas the plastic surgeon considered only 50% to be good or excellent. However, the patients' assessments of cosmetic outcome correlated well with those of the general surgeon and radiation oncologist, suggesting that minor discrepancies in breast appearance are of limited significance.

Breast size also has been shown to influence the cosmetic outcome. Clarke and others[76] observed a decrease in the likelihood of an excellent cosmetic result with increasing breast size as measured by cup size. Excellent results were observed in 100% of patients with an A cup, 84% of patients with a B cup, 78% of patients with a C cup, and 50% of patients with a D cup ($P = .02$). Dose inhomogeneity and increased fat content of large breasts were postulated as the cause of the worse cosmetic results. Inhomogeneity of radiation dose is known to be a greater problem in patients with large breast size, but this is improved with the use of higher photon energy.[77] Gray and associates[78] also examined cosmetic outcome in relation to breast size. Women were classified as having large breasts on the basis of a weight of 80 kg or more, bra size 40 inches or larger, cup size D or larger, or tangent separa-

tion 23 cm or more. Other patients were considered to have average breast size. At 1 year after treatment, the average breast size group had a significantly better overall cosmetic outcome, and scored higher on five of seven indices (symmetry, edema, skin thickening, fibrosis, retraction). At 3 and 5 years after treatment, only symmetry and retraction remained significantly different. At 3 years, patients with large breast size had a mean cosmetic score of 7.69 on a scale of 10, compared with 8.45 for patients with average breast size. Thus, although the cosmetic outcome was slightly worse in patients with large breasts than those with smaller breasts, it was still satisfactory. To avoid the problems associated with irradiation of patients with extremely large breasts, bilateral reduction mammoplasty has been described in conjunction with lumpectomy.[79]

Cosmetic outcome has been related to a number of other tumor factors. Studies of the influence of tumor location on the cosmetic outcome are inconclusive. Van Limbergen and associates[64] reported poor cosmetic results for patients with lesions in the medial breast, whether superior or inferior. Pezner and coworkers[62] found that primary tumors in the upper breast were associated with a worse cosmetic outcome. Other studies have not shown a relation between tumor location and cosmetic outcome.[74,78] Cosmetic outcome has been shown to be dependent on tumor size because of its relationship to the amount of breast tissue that must be resected.[72,74] In practice, a variety of factors must be considered together (the size of the patient's breast, the size of the tumor, the depth of the tumor within the breast, and the quadrant of the breast in which the tumor is located) to judge the feasibility of a cosmetically acceptable resection. For example, although the removal of a large tumor in the lower portion of the breast often results in distortion of the breast contour, this is only apparent with the arms raised, and is acceptable to most women. A similar distortion in the upper inner quadrant of the breast, which is visible in most types of clothing, might not be as acceptable.

The technique of RT also is important in preserving the cosmetic appearance. Early studies from the JCRT[60] demon-

TABLE 17.1-4

Outcome in Milan II Trial Comparing Quadrantectomy With Lumpectomy, Both Combined With Radiation Therapy

	Quadrantectomy (%)	Lumpectomy (%)
Local recurrence[73]	5.3	13.3
Cosmetic results[63]		
>3 cm difference in height between nipples	21	7
>3 cm difference in height, inferior profile of breasts	11	3
>1.5 cm difference in length, nipple to midline	17	5

(Veronesi U, Volterrani F, Luini A, et al. Quadrantectomy versus lumpectomy for small size breast cancer. Eur J Cancer 1990;26:671; Veronesi U, Luini A, Galimberti V, et al. Conservation approaches for the management of stage I/II carcinoma of the breast: Milan Cancer Institute trials. World J Surg 1994;18:70)

TABLE 17.1-5

Major Factors Influencing Cosmetic Outcome at 3 Years Among Patients Treated at JCRT, 1982–1985: Use of Chemotherapy (CT) and Volume of Breast Tissue Resected

		Cosmetic Score at 3 Years			
Factors	Patients	Excellent (%)	P Value	Good (%)	P Value
RT alone	279	77		97	
Sequential RT–CT	57	65	.09	95	NS
V<35	85	86		96	
V=36–85	78	78	<.01	97	NS
V>86	70	51		94	

JCRT, Joint Center for Radiation Therapy; V, volume of breast tissue resected (cm³); RT, radiation therapy; CT, chemotherapy.

(de la Rochefordiere A, Abner A, Silver B, et al. Are cosmetic results following conservative surgery and radiation therapy for breast cancer dependent on technique? Int J Radiat Oncol Biol Phys 1992;23:925)

strated that total dose and daily fractionation influence the cosmetic outcome. Increasing total breast dose correlates with a greater degree of retraction and fibrosis, with a significant increase in retraction and fibrosis seen at doses above 50 Gy.[60] Fraction sizes of 1.8 to 2 Gy/d seem to be associated with the best cosmetic outcome.[60,76,80] Another factor found to adversely affect cosmetic outcome is the use of a third treatment field to treat the axillary and supraclavicular nodes. Small variations in patient set-up and movement in patients treated with a three-field approach can result in areas of matchline fibrosis where the three fields meet. In the early JCRT experience, 69% of patients treated with a three-field technique had an excellent outcome compared with 89% of patients treated with tangents alone.[70] Clarke and associates[76] also showed significantly worse cosmetic results because of matchline fibrosis and telangiectasia when patients are treated with a supraclavicular and axillary field. A high boost dose[81] also has been shown to worsen cosmetic outcome. However, the technique of the boost does not seem to be a significant factor. The cosmetic outcome has been shown to be similar with electron beam and with interstitial implantation.[72,82]

To assess the effect of improved technique on the cosmetic outcome, two cohorts of patients treated at the JCRT were compared.[72] The first cohort was treated between 1970 and 1981, and the second was treated between 1982 and 1985. In the later cohort, treatment modifications based on the findings described above were carried out. The whole breast dose was limited to 45 to 46 Gy with a daily dose not greater than 2 Gy, boost doses of 18 Gy or less were used, and a more accurate matching technique was employed.[83] In addition, sequential, rather than concurrent, chemotherapy was administered. An excellent cosmetic result at 3 years was seen in 58% of the patients in the earlier cohort compared with 73% of patients in the later cohort ($P < .0001$). Excellent or good results were seen in 86% and 96% of the groups, respectively. No differences in the 5-year actuarial rates of recurrence in the breast were observed between groups.

These findings suggest that when modern treatment techniques are used, an acceptable cosmetic outcome can be achieved in almost all patients without compromise of local tumor control. Table 17.1-5 shows the major factors influencing the cosmetic outcome among the patients treated from 1982 to 1985.

A final factor that has been suggested to influence cosmetic outcome is the use of adjuvant chemotherapy. In studies from the JCRT,[68,71] the effects of chemotherapy given either sequentially or concurrently with RT were assessed. Patients treated with sequential chemotherapy (typically CMF) and RT had a small decrease in their cosmetic outcome compared with patients not treated with chemotherapy, whereas patients treated with concurrent chemotherapy and RT had a large decrease in their cosmetic outcome. Increased breast retraction seemed to be the factor responsible for this difference. A similar decrease in the cosmetic result after treatment with concurrent CMF and RT was described by Ray and others.[84] Similarly, other studies have not found that the use of sequential chemotherapy and RT significantly affected the cosmetic outcome.[74,81] Investigators at the University of Pennsylvania found no significant decrease in the cosmetic outcome related to the use of concurrent CMF chemotherapy and RT when methotrexate was dropped during the period of irradiation. This issue is discussed in greater detail in the section on sequencing of RT and adjuvant chemotherapy.

RISK FACTORS FOR LOCAL RECURRENCE

The identification of risk, or prognostic, factors associated with local recurrence has at least three possible purposes:

- To identify patients who might benefit from an altered form of breast-conserving treatment (such as more extensive breast resection or more aggressive irradiation) or from mastectomy

- To obtain a better understanding of the pathophysiology and significance of local recurrence; in particular, it would be useful to determine which factors reflect the inherent biological aggressiveness of the cancer and which reflect extensive local involvement of the cancer that might be remediable by more extensive local treatment
- To inform patients who choose breast-conserving treatment about their expected prognosis with regard to control in the breast

A large number of studies have been published attempting to identify such prognostic or risk factors. In examining this literature, a number of methodologic considerations are worth mentioning that contribute to some confusion in the area. First, many of the reports examining this issue differ with regard to patient selection, the techniques of surgery and RT, and the use of adjuvant systemic therapy. The risk factors observed to be important in each study may differ accordingly. In addition, the risk factors themselves may be defined differently in different series. For example, studies may vary in the definition of pathologic factors, such as lymphatic vessel invasion, histologic grade, or an extensive intraductal component. Furthermore, many reports are limited in numbers of patients or length of follow-up, resulting in a small number of patients with local recurrence. A limited number of local recurrences in a study limits the ability of the study (ie, its statistical power) to identify risk factors.

A second problem is that estimating the risk of local recurrence is complicated by the competing risk of distant recurrence. Consider, for example, a group of patients with a virulent form of breast cancer such that all patients manifest distant recurrence and die within 1 year without evidence of local recurrence. Is the true rate of local recurrence in this group 0%, or are some local recurrences masked by the rapid onset of distant recurrence and death? This problem cannot be solved by using actuarial methods (such as Kaplan-Meier plots) to estimate curves of time to local recurrence. This statistical method was developed for analysis of survival data and is not well suited for analysis of local recurrence. With such methods, patients who recur first in distant sites or die before local recurrence can occur are eliminated from the analysis or, more technically, are considered "censored" for local recurrence. To be useful, actuarial methods require the assumption that the time to local recurrence and the time to distant recurrence are statistically independent. For most human malignancies (including breast cancer) this is not a reasonable assumption, because there are some patient subgroups at high risk for both local and distant failure and some patient subgroups at low risk for either type of failure. Without independence of local and distant failure, the curve for time to local recurrence distribution is not well defined. This problem is referred to as *competing risks,* because the various types of failure (local and distant) are competing in the same patient. Consequently, the effect of a particular factor on local recurrence *cannot* be assessed separately from its effect on distant recurrence. Because of this, it has been recommended that authors of reports on risk factors for local recurrence provide crude rates of both local and distant recur-

rence to allow the reader to assess this.[85] A second, but more trivial, problem with the use of Kaplan-Meier estimates is their misuse in projecting estimates too far in time. This is especially true when analyzing time to local recurrence in breast cancer patients treated with CS and RT, because the time course to local recurrence is protracted. In the experience at the JCRT, early Kaplan-Meier plots seriously underestimated the true incidence of local recurrence observed when longer follow-up of patients was obtained. As a general rule, estimates beyond the median follow-up time are unreliable. In this section, we provide results in terms of crude incidence (when available) and indicate the length of follow-up. In some cases, only actuarial curves are available or they are provided for comparison.

A third consideration is that different types of local recurrence may have different risk factors. As previously described, most investigators have classified recurrences by their location in the breast in relation to the primary tumor. It seems likely, for example, that recurrences at sites distant from the original tumor will have risk factors similar to those associated with opposite breast cancer (such as young patient age and lobular histologic findings), whereas those primarily involving the skin will have risk factors similar to those associated with local recurrence after mastectomy (such as nodal involvement). It is also likely that these types of local recurrence may have different consequences. As a result, combining all types of local recurrence may obscure important relationships.

Fourth, it is important to distinguish between risk factors that are *prognostic* and those that are *predictive*. As discussed in Chapter 16 with regard to distant recurrence, a prognostic factor is used to estimate outcome, whereas a predictive factor is used to estimate the differential effect of a particular treatment. Therefore, if a factor has been reported as a risk factor for local recurrence after breast-conserving treatment but is also known to be a risk factor for local recurrence after mastectomy, then this factor is prognostic, not predictive; that is, it is of no assistance in selecting the best form of local treatment for a patient with that factor.

Finally, few of the risk factors identified so far reliably divide patients into groups having different risks of local recurrence. In considering the general literature on risk factors for local recurrence, it is rare to find any factor associated with both a sensitivity and a specificity of over 50%.

Risk factors for recurrence after breast-conserving treatment can be subdivided as follows: patient factors, such as age; tumor factors, such as tumor size or location, nodal status, multiple primaries, and various histopathologic features; and treatment factors, such as the extent of breast resection, the use of a boost to the primary site, and the use of adjuvant systemic therapy.

PATIENT RISK FACTORS

Young patient age has consistently been observed to be associated with an increased risk of local recurrence after breast-conserving surgery and RT.[37,49,86-90] As shown in Table 17.1-6, in the experience of the JCRT, younger

TABLE 17.1-6
Incidence of Pathologic Features of Breast Cancer and 5-Year Crude Rates of Failure Stratified by Age Group, JCRT Series, 1969–1985★

	Age Group				
	<35 y	35–50 y	51–65 y	>65 y	P Value†
Patients with histologic review	103	474	356	202	
FEATURES					
EIC+	23	24	19	13	.0014
LVI+	36	33	23	23	.0004
Necrosis	30	25	21	14	.0006
MCR+	31	23	15	8	<.0001
Grade 3	47	50	38	24	<.0001
SITE OF FAILURE					
None	64	74	78	75	
Ipsilateral Breast	15	11	5	4	
TR/MM	13	8	4	3	
Elsewhere	2	2	0	1	
Other	0	1	1	0	
Regional	1	1	1	0	
Distant	20	15	15	21	
Total patients	106	562	440	234	

EIC, extensive intraductal component; LVI, lymphatic vessel invasion; MCR, mononuclear cell reaction; TR/MM, true recurrence–marginal miss; +, positive; JCRT, Joint Center for Radiation Therapy.

★ Incidence figures are percentages.

† Chi-square test for trend; chi-square = 25.77 with 6 df; P = .0002.

age was associated with an increased frequency of various adverse pathologic features, such as lymphatic vessel invasion, grade 3 histology, absence of estrogen receptors (ERs), and the presence of an extensive intraductal component (EIC). However, even when correction was done for the differing incidence of the pathologic features of the primary tumor between the age groups, younger age still was associated with an decreased survival rate and an increased likelihood of recurrence in the breast.[87,91] In the series from Marseille, which also examined both age and the histologic features of the primary tumor, younger patients were also more likely than older patients to have grade 3 tumors, a mononuclear cell reaction in the stroma, and an extensive intraductal component. In that study, the final model in a multivariate analysis contained the pathologic features, but not age.[92] On the other hand, the effect of patient age eliminated pathologic features as a prognostic factor in a multivariate analysis in the Institut Curie series.[49] Hence, whereas young patient age clearly is correlated with various adverse pathologic features, this does not entirely explain the worse outcome in these patients.

Young patient age has similarly been described as an important factor associated with a worse outcome after mastectomy. A marked increase in local failure in younger patients was seen in a study of patients treated with radical mastectomy.[93] In a retrospective analysis from the M.D. Anderson Hospital,[89] patients 35 years of age or younger did worse than older patients, but there was no difference in local recurrence, disease-free survival, or overall survival rates between young patients treated with tumorectomy and irradiation and young patients treated with mastectomy. In a review of 1703 premenopausal patients with stage I to III breast cancer treated at the Institut Curie between 1981 and 1985, very young age (younger than 34 years) was associated with a worse outcome independent of type of local treatment.[94] The data from the two randomized trials with longest follow-up do not specifically address the issue of patients younger than 35 years, but do not show an advantage for one form of local treatment for younger patients. In the Milan trial, survival was similar after treatment with quadrantectomy and RT or mastectomy among patients younger than 45 years, and in the NSABP trial B-06, survival was similar after treatment with lumpectomy and RT or mastectomy among premenopausal patients. Thus, the available information suggests that young patient age is a prognostic factor, but does not seem helpful in selecting the best form of local treatment.

TUMOR RISK FACTORS

Tumor size has not been shown to be a major factor associated with recurrence in the breast after CS and RT.[27,46,47,95] It is possible that the small mammographically detected lesions, which are being detected with greater frequency, may have a more favorable recurrence rate. When comparing T1 and T2 lesions, however, tumor size has little effect on the recurrence rate. For example, among 783 patients with stage I or II breast cancer (all histologic types) treated with excisional biopsy and RT including a boost to the primary site, the rate of recurrence in the breast was 13% for T1 lesions and 12% for T2 lesions (median follow-up, 91 months).[96] This observation is consistent with data from Holland and coworkers,[21] which indicated that the likelihood and extent of additional tumor foci in the breast after simulated excision of the tumor is similar for T1 and T2 lesions. Thus, the tumor burden remaining in the breast after CS to be eradicated by irradiation is similar for T1 and T2 lesions. In addition, in the two randomized trials with longest follow-up, patients with T1 or T2 tumors[27] or with T1 tumors either less than or greater than 1 cm[36] had similar outcomes whether treated with CS and RT or treated with mastectomy. The location of the tumor within the breast also has not been shown to be a major factor associated with recurrence in the breast after CS and RT.[87,97]

Involvement of axillary nodes does not seem to be a major factor associated with recurrence in the breast after CS and RT.[46,47,87] However, this issue is difficult to evaluate because of the greater competing risk of distant recurrence in patients with involved nodes than in patients with uninvolved nodes (thus possibly obscuring local recurrence in node-positive patients) and the formerly common practice of routinely giving adjuvant systemic therapy to patients with involved nodes, but not to patients with uninvolved nodes. (The effect of adjuvant systemic therapy on local recurrence is addressed later in this chapter.) Notice that although involvement of axillary nodes is a recognized risk factor for local recurrence after mastectomy, in the two randomized trials with longest follow-up, node-positive patients treated with CS and RT did at least as well with regard to survival as did node-positive patients treated with mastectomy.[27,43]

A number of studies have examined the relationship between the presence of various histologic features of the cancer and the rate of local recurrence after CS and RT. The results from the JCRT have suggested that the presence of an extensive intraductal component, in particular, is an important risk factor for local recurrence. These studies, however, were performed during a time when the microscopic margins of resection were not routinely evaluated. An EIC applies to infiltrating duct carcinomas in which (1) intraductal carcinoma is prominently present within the tumor, *and* (2) intraductal carcinoma is present in sections of grossly normal adjacent breast tissue. In addition, tumors that are predominantly intraductal but have

foci of invasion are considered to have an EIC. The JCRT has previously reported on the outcome of 732 patients treated between 1968 and 1982, during which time high-quality mammography was not routinely performed and patients typically underwent a limited excision of the tumor without attention paid to the microscopic margins of resection.[52] Among the 584 patients with histologic slides evaluable for EIC, EIC-positive cancers constituted 28% of the infiltrating ductal carcinomas and were associated with a 21% 5-year crude incidence of local recurrence. In contrast, EIC-negative cancers were found in 72% of evaluable cases and were associated with a 5-year crude incidence of local recurrence of only 6% ($P < .0001$). The corresponding 5-year crude incidence of distant or regional failure was 13% for EIC-positive cancers and 20% for EIC-negative cancers. In examining the pattern of local recurrence, EIC-positive cancers were associated with a higher rate of true recurrences or marginal misses than EIC-negative tumors. EIC-positive cancers were not associated with an increased rate of recurrence elsewhere in the ipsilateral breast or in the opposite breast, compared with EIC-negative cancers. This observation suggests that the problem in treating EIC-positive cancers with gross excision and RT is one that is localized to the vicinity of the tumor, rather than one that is diffusely present through the breast or throughout breast tissue. Also notice that EIC-positive cancers have, if anything, a lower rate of distant recurrence than EIC-negative cancers; thus, the higher rate of local recurrence seen in EIC-positive cancers is not because of a biologically more aggressive form of breast cancer compared with EIC-negative cancers.

The association between EIC-positive cancers and recurrence in the breast has been evaluated in a number of other studies. The presence of an EIC also was found to be associated with an increased rate of local failure in a series of patients treated at the Marseille Cancer Institute.[98] As in the JCRT series, patients in this series underwent a gross resection of the tumor and the margins of resection were not routinely inked. The RT treatment protocol also was similar to that used in the JCRT series. Overall, 21% of patients had an EIC-positive cancer. With a median follow-up time of 71 months, the crude local recurrence rate was 21% for patients with an EIC-positive cancer and 10% for patients with an EIC-negative cancer ($P < .001$) In both series, the increased risk was seen only in patients with both prominent intraductal cancer within the tumor *and* intraductal cancer present in the adjacent breast tissue; the presence of only one of these features was not associated with an increased risk. In a subset analysis of the Marseille series, the association between an EIC and local recurrence was only observed among premenopausal patients. In a series from the University of Pennsylvania, only 23 of 275 patients were classified as having an EIC-positive cancer; however, those patients had a 5-year actuarial rate of local recurrence of 22% compared with 4% in EIC-negative patients. Among patients treated in the Milan II trial with tumorectomy and RT, the 5-year cumulative incidence rate of local recurrence was about 30% for patients with an EIC-positive cancer and about 10% for patients with an EIC-negative cancer. In contrast, among patients treated in the Milan II trial with quadrantectomy and RT, the 5-year cumulative incidence rate of local recurrence was about 10% for patients with an EIC-positive cancer and about 5% for patients with an EIC-negative cancer.[73] In a series of patients treated at the Netherlands Cancer Institute, the overall 5-year actuarial local recurrence rate was 4%.[99] Patients in this series underwent more extensive breast resections and received higher doses of RT (75 Gy) than are typically used in the United States, and this may account for their low rate of local recurrence. Of the 45 local recurrences seen in this series, only 13 (29%) occurred in the same quadrant as the primary tumor. Young patient age (younger than 40 years), the presence of an EIC, lymphatic vessel invasion, and involvement of microscopic margins of resection were all associated with local recurrence on univariate analysis. On multivariate analysis, the major risk factors were young patient age and the presence of vascular invasion. These results are similar to those of the Curie Institute series.[49] These studies again indicate that patient age and the presence of an EIC are interrelated. Both factors are generally associated with local recurrence on univariate analysis. Whether one factor or another or both persist on multivariate analysis may be related to the details of the surgery and RT and the role of margin assessment in patient selection for CS and RT. These treatment factors are discussed in greater detail later. The presence of an EIC is not a risk factor for local recurrence after mastectomy[100] and therefore may potentially be useful in selecting local treatment for an individual patient.

Previous studies have addressed possible reasons for a higher rate of recurrence in the breast for EIC-positive cancers than EIC-negative cancers after treatment with a simple gross excision and RT. In a study of patients who underwent reexcision of the primary tumor site after an initial gross excision because of positive or close margins of resection, it was found that patients with EIC-positive cancers had a greater incidence of residual tumor in the reexcision specimen than did patients with EIC-negative cancers (88% versus 48%, P = .002).[101] For patients with an EIC-positive cancer, the residual tumor often was widespread and was composed predominantly of intraductal carcinoma, whereas residual tumor in patients with an EIC-negative cancer usually consisted of only scattered microscopic foci of infiltrating or intraductal carcinoma. Similar findings were noticed in a study of mastectomy specimens by Holland and others.[22] The frequency of residual cancer in the breast after simulated gross excision was significantly greater for EIC-positive cancers than for EIC-negative cancers (74% versus 42%, P < .00001). This residual cancer was either infiltrating, intraductal, or intralymphatic, with intraductal carcinoma being the predominant type. Of particular interest, approximately 30% of patients with EIC-positive cancers had prominent residual intraductal carcinoma (six or more low-power fields) at least 2 cm beyond the edge of the primary tumor, compared with only 2% of patients with EIC-negative cancers (Fig. 17.1-5; P < .0001). This incidence of prominent residual intraductal carcinoma is similar to the incidence of a TR or MM for patients with EIC-positive and EIC-

FIGURE 17.1-5 Frequency of prominent intraductal carcinoma (defined as six or more low-power fields) as a function of the distance from the reference tumor in relation to the presence or absence of an extensive intraductal component (EIC) in the reference tumor.[22] About 30% of EIC-positive tumors have prominent residual intraductal carcinoma 2 cm beyond the reference tumor.

negative cancers, respectively. Furthermore, in the Holland study, residual microscopic cancer was most often located in the vicinity of the primary tumor, rather than randomly located throughout the remainder of the breast. These observations provide support for the hypothesis that in many patients with an EIC-positive cancer treated with a simple gross excision, there is a large residual tumor burden in the remainder of the breast and that doses of RT consistent with a satisfactory cosmetic result are not able to eradicate it. This information also suggests that a larger breast resection in patients with an EIC-positive cancer might result in a smaller residual tumor burden and, therefore, might lower the risk of recurrence in the breast.

The problem of recognizing cancers with such extensive intraductal involvement has been greatly facilitated by the use of mammography.[102] The intraductal component in these lesions frequently shows calcium deposits, and their presence and extent can be detected on high-quality mammograms, particularly with the use of magnification views. The problem of recognizing EIC-positive cancers also has been facilitated by the routine evaluation of the microscopic margins of resection; this is discussed in detail later.

The pathophysiology of EIC-positive cancers has not been fully clarified. These cancers are more common in premenopausal patients than in older patients (see Table 17.1-6), suggesting a hormonal influence. It is not certain if there is extensive intraductal involvement first with subsequent invasion or if some invasive cancers show intraductal extension. A study for clonality (using restriction fragment length polymorphism of the X chromosome–linked phosphoglycerokinase gene) in three cases of EIC-positive breast cancers with multiple areas of involvement showed that all three cases were monoclonal.[103]

Some, but not all studies have identified LVI as an important pathologic risk factor for local recurrence after CS and RT.[49,99] LVI also is known to be an adverse prognostic factor with regard to survival and has been shown to be a risk factor for local recurrence after mastectomy as well.[104,105] Thus, lymphatic vessel invasion, like node involvement, may be more useful in assessing overall prognosis than in selecting local treatment for patients with this factor.

Some information is available regarding histologic tumor types other than infiltrating ductal and the uncommon finding of multiple tumors as possible risk factors for local recurrence after CS and RT. Infiltrating lobular carcinomas account for 5% to 10% of invasive breast cancers and, in most studies, are associated with a local recurrence rate similar to that seen for infiltrating ductal carcinomas.[106-110] In the JCRT experience, the presence and extent of associated lobular carcinoma-in-situ was *not* related to the rate of local recurrence.[106] Updated results from the JCRT on 1121 patients with infiltrating ductal carcinoma and 80 patients with infiltrating lobular carcinoma treated between 1968 and 1985 show a 10-year actuarial rate of local recurrence of 16% for patients with ductal histologic type and 14% for patients with lobular histologic type (median follow-up about 9 years; unpublished data). Given the diffuse infiltration seen with infiltrating lobular carcinomas, however, a wide resection with clearly negative microscopic margins of resection is generally advised. Limited experience[107,108] (including unpublished data from the JCRT) with less common histologic types such as colloid, medullary, and tubular, which are known to be more favorable with regard to survival, suggests that the rate of local recurrence is lower than that for the common form of infiltrating ductal carcinoma. However, some tubular and colloid carcinomas are associated with an extensive intraductal component. There is some evidence that the presence of multiple macroscopic tumors is associated with a higher local recurrence rate compared with a single macroscopic tumor.[111-113] Multiple tumors are more common in EIC-positive cancers and in the presence of lymphatic vessel invasion. Breast-conserving therapy is generally reserved only for those patients with multiple tumors in the same quadrant in whom negative microscopic margins of resection can be achieved.

MARGIN INVOLVEMENT

Surprisingly little long-term information exists relating tumor involvement at the microscopic margins of resection (or margins) and recurrence in the breast after CS and RT. There are significant technical considerations and limitations in the use of margins.[114] The pathologist needs to put ink on the margins of resection before cutting the specimen so that the margins can be clearly identified on microscopic examination. If the tumor is resected in two or more specimens, it is often not possible to orient the specimens to determine the true margins. Even if ink is used to mark the margins of the specimen, there is a tendency for the ink to track down into the interstices of the specimen through defects in the surface.

This may create difficulties in defining the true margins on histologic examination. In addition, the surfaces of breast excision specimens are often fatty and irregular and the surface area may be large. Therefore, any method used to examine the margins is highly subject to sampling error. There are also considerable differences among institutions regarding the method and extent of margin evaluation. At the JCRT, for example, there has been an evolution in the evaluation of margins among its member hospitals. Margin assessment was first routinely begun in the early 1980s, at which time a number of radial sections of the margin were taken. Such an approach, however, is highly subject to sampling error. More recently, margins have been assessed by the shaved-margin technique, which increases the chances of detecting any margin involvement.[114] Another major difficulty in the evaluation of margins is the lack of a uniformly accepted definition of a positive margin. Investigators from the NSABP consider a margin to be positive only if cancer cells are present directly at an inked surface. Others consider a margin positive if cancer cells are present within some arbitrary distance from an inked surface (such as a millimeter or two). Finally, the importance of tumor involvement at or close to the margins may be dependent on the technical details of the surgery and RT.

Despite these limitations, the available data suggest that an assessment of margin involvement is of use in predicting the risk of local recurrence (Table 17.1-7). The NSABP has demonstrated that use of its definition results in an acceptably low rate of local recurrence and a survival rate comparable with that achieved with the use of mastectomy.[27] Furthermore, the NSABP investigators, as well as those from Duke, have not found the presence of an EIC to be of prognostic value for local recurrence among patients with uninvolved margins.[37,115] Other investigators also have found that local recurrence is uncommon when the margins of resection are uninvolved.[49,73,116] The results of a study from the JCRT are consistent with these findings.[117] The study population was limited to 181 patients with an infiltrating ductal carcinoma who received a radiation dose to the surgical site of 60 Gy or greater, whose final microscopic margins of resection were evaluable and who had at least 5 years of follow-up. Margins were assessed by the radial technique. A positive margin was defined as tumor present at the inked margin of resection, a close margin as tumor within 1 mm of the inked margin, and a negative margin as no tumor within 1 mm of the inked margin. A focally-positive margin was defined as tumor at the margin in three or fewer low-power fields. In 157 patients (87%), the tumor was evaluable for the presence or absence of an EIC. The median follow-up time was 86 months. The results are shown in Table 17.1-8. Taken together with the results from the NSABP and from Duke, these results indicate that the presence of an EIC per se should not be a contraindication to breast-conserving therapy. Patients with an EIC-positive cancer and uninvolved margins of resection are adequately treated with breast-conserving therapy, and patients with a EIC-positive cancer and positive margins on an initial resection can be

TABLE 17.1-7
Local Recurrence Rates in Relation to the Microscopic Margins of Resection*

		Status of Microscopic Margins (%)			
Investigator	Interval (y)	Positive	Negative	Close	Unknown
Van Dongen et al[363]	8	20	9		
Veronesi et al[73]	5	17.4	8.6		8.9
Anscher et al[115]	5	10	2		10
Schnitt et al[117]	5	15	3		
Schmidt-Ullrich et al[360]	10	1.3	1.3		1.3
Solin et al[116]†	5	2	7	11	7

* Recurrence rates are percentages.

† In these series, the dose of radiation was adjusted in relation to margin status.

considered for a reexcision of the primary tumor site to obtain negative margins.

The use of breast-conserving therapy in patients with positive margins is controversial. The results in the JCRT series suggest that when patients with an EIC-negative cancer are treated with breast irradiation, including a boost to the primary tumor site, focal involvement of the margins is associated with a low rate of a local recurrence. This is consistent with the prior observation that EIC-negative cancers are rarely associated with prominent residual cancer in the breast following a limited breast resection.[22,101] These results suggest that it is reasonable to offer patients with an EIC-negative cancer and only focal margin involvement the option of breast-conserving therapy if a reexcision is not considered feasible. Whereas the value of a boost has not been clearly demonstrated in patients with negative margins, it seems prudent to use a boost in these patients as part of breast-

conserving therapy. Given the limited number of patients with an EIC-negative cancer and more than focally involved margins treated with CS and RT, additional breast surgery (either reexcision or mastectomy) seems most appropriate in this setting. More experience relating margin involvement in the absence of an EIC to the rate of local recurrence is required.

TREATMENT FACTORS

The rate of local recurrence after CS and RT potentially can be influenced by a number of treatment factors, including the extent of breast resection, the technical details of the RT, and the use of adjuvant systemic therapy. The extent of breast resection has a clear association with local recurrence. The rate of local recurrence is much greater after an incisional biopsy than after an excisional biopsy.[55,118,119] Based on this, gross excision, at a minimum, is

TABLE 17.1-8
Five-Year Crude Rate of Recurrence in Relation to Microscopic Margin Status, JCRT Series

				Site of First Recurrence			
Margin Status	Patients	NED	Dead < 5 y	Breast, TR/MM	Breast, Other	Regional Nodes	Distant Metastases
Negative	70	52 (74%)	5 (7%)	0 (0%)	2 (3%)	1 (1%)	10 (14%)
Close	25	19 (76%)	3 (12%)	1 (4%)	0 (0%)	0 (0%)	2 (8%)
Positive	86	45 (52%)	3 (3%)	11 (13%)	2 (2%)	1 (1%)	24 (28%)
Focally positive	48	29 (60%)	2 (4%)	3 (6%)	2 (4%)	0 (0%)	12 (25%)
More than focally positive	38	16 (42%)	1 (3%)	8 (21%)	0 (0%)	1 (3%)	12 (32%)

NED, no evidence of disease; Dead < 5 y, dead without recurrence with less than 5 years of follow-up; TR/MM: true recurrence–marginal miss; breast, other, recurrence elsewhere in breast, in skin of breast, or unclassifiable breast recurrence; JCRT, Joint Center for Radiation Therapy.

(Schnitt S, Abner A, Gelman R, et al. The relationship between microscopic margins of resection and the risk of local recurrence in breast cancer patients treated with conservative surgery and radiation therapy. Cancer 1994;74:1746)

considered mandatory before RT. Beyond gross excision, however, considerable controversy exists regarding the optimal extent of breast resection. In North America, a more limited resection (lumpectomy) is typically performed, whereas in Europe, a wider resection (quadrantectomy) is more common. Quadrantectomy was designed to address the segmental nature of involvement of the cancer in the breast; however, the precise limits of these segments are not apparent at the time of surgery. Increasing the volume of breast resection is associated with a decrease in the rate of local recurrence but, as previously discussed, also has an adverse effect on the cosmetic result.[63]

The results from the JCRT have been analyzed to examine the associations between the extent of breast resection and both local recurrence and the cosmetic result. The extent of breast resection was the major factor in determining the cosmetic outcome among more recently treated patients (see Table 17.1-5).[72] In a separate study, the association between the volume of resected breast tissue and the rate of local recurrence was examined in relation to the presence or absence of an extensive intraductal component.[120] These results indicated that the risk of local recurrence was related to both the presence of an EIC and the extent of breast resection. For EIC-negative cancers, a limited breast resection (the tumor plus 1 to 2 cm of grossly tumor-free adjacent breast tissue) was associated with a low risk of local recurrence (and a high likelihood of a satisfactory cosmetic result), whereas for EIC-positive cancers, a more extensive breast resection was commonly required to assure a low rate of local recurrence. Similar results were seen in the Milan II trial.[73] Taken together with the information on margin assessment and local recurrence, these results suggest that a knowledge of margin involvement and the presence or absence of an extensive intraductal component can be used to individualize the volume of resected breast tissue needed to reduce a patient's risk of local recurrence to an acceptable level.

Surprisingly little is established concerning the association between radiation treatment factors and recurrence in the breast. As a result, information on the possible importance of radiation factors comes from comparisons within a retrospective review or comparisons between different retrospective reviews, both of which are subject to the potential confounding of treatment factors with other important variables. In a report by Kurtz and associates,[92] local recurrence was more common among patients treated with inadequate RT (defined as weekly RT doses less than 8 Gy) than among patients treated with conventionally delivered RT. At the Royal Marsden Hospital, a high rate of local recurrence also was seen with a weekly dose of 8 Gy or less.[121]

Uncertainty exists about how great an interval between last breast surgery and the start of irradiation (in the absence of intervening chemotherapy) is acceptable. It seems logical that excessive delays will allow sufficient regrowth of cancer cells to increase the rate of local recurrence. Clarke and others[46] showed in a retrospective review that the rate of local recurrence was 5% for patients who started irradiation within 7 weeks of breast surgery compared with 14% for patients who started 7 or more weeks later.

In a multivariate analysis, however, this factor was not statistically significant. In another retrospective review, Slotman and coworkers[122] similarly found that local recurrence rate was 1.7% for patients who started irradiation within 50 days compared with 5.6% for patients who started 50 or more days after surgery. This factor was statistically significant in multivariate analysis. In a recent retrospective review from the JCRT, the rate of local recurrence was examined among a homogeneous group of node-negative patients with clinical stage I or II breast cancer who had not received adjuvant systemic therapy.[123] The interval from last breast surgery to the start of irradiation was not predetermined systematically, but rather was set by logistic considerations or by delays in wound healing. Two hundred eighty-three patients started irradiation within 4 weeks and 308 started 5 to 8 weeks after last breast surgery. These two groups were well balanced with regard to various clinical and pathologic characteristics. Within this range (0 to 8 weeks), there was no statistically significant association between the interval between surgery and RT and the risk of overall recurrence (or the sites of failure), on either univariate or multivariate analysis. These results suggest that such delays of up to 8 weeks are not associated with an increased risk of recurrence. The influence of delays beyond 8 weeks is less certain.

The need for supplemental irradiation to the primary tumor site (or boost) has been controversial. Many have argued that because the rate of local recurrence in the NSABP B-06 trial (in which a boost was not employed) is comparable with that of other series in which a boost is routinely employed, a boost is not required in patients with negative margins of resection. On the other side are the arguments that only a very large study could demonstrate the small improvement in local recurrence that might be expected from a policy of routinely using a boost and that the use of a boost does not greatly increase the rate of complications or decrease the cosmetic outcome. Such a large trial testing the value of a boost is being performed by the EORTC and is expected to close by January 1996. In this trial, patients with negative microscopic margins of resection receive 50 Gy to the whole breast and then are randomized to receive either no boost or a boost of 15 Gy by interstitial irradiation or 16 Gy by external beam techniques; patients with positive microscopic margins of resection receive 50 Gy to the whole breast and then are randomized either to a low-dose boost of 10 Gy or to a high-dose boost, either 25 Gy by interstitial irradiation or 26 Gy by external beam techniques. Results from this trial will be helpful in settling this controversy.

Evidence suggests that the use of adjuvant chemotherapy is an important factor associated with recurrence in the breast when used in conjunction with CS and RT. The rate of recurrence in the breast in the NSABP B-06 trial was lower for patients treated with CS and RT who received chemotherapy than for those who did not.[27] Similar results have been seen in other retrospective series.[90,124] In these series, however, the effect of chemotherapy was assessed by indirect comparisons, because the patients who received chemotherapy generally were node-positive, and patients who did not generally were node-negative.

The NSABP B-13 trial, comparing outcome for node-negative patients who received chemotherapy with that of a no-treatment control group, permits a more scientifically valid assessment of the effect of chemotherapy on local recurrence. In this trial, 32% of the 579 patients were treated with CS and RT. With a median follow-up of about 3 years, the rate of recurrence in the breast was 7.4% in the CS and RT group compared with 1.7% in the CS, RT, and chemotherapy group.[125] Although additional information on this issue is required, the available results suggest that chemotherapy reduces the risk of recurrence in the breast when used in conjunction with CS and RT.

The issue of the effect of adjuvant systemic therapy on local recurrence is complicated by whether the particular sequencing of RT and chemotherapy also influences the rate of local recurrence. Limited retrospective data suggest that delayed initiation of RT after CS and chemotherapy is associated with an increase in the rate of local recurrence compared with early initiation of RT after CS.[126] This issue is addressed later in this chapter.

There is similar evidence that adjuvant tamoxifen also may reduce the risk of recurrence in the breast when used in conjunction with CS and RT. This was examined in the NSABP B-14 trial, which compared outcome after adjuvant tamoxifen with that of controls among 2644 node-negative patients, 38% of whom received CS and RT. With a median follow-up time of about 3 years, the rate of recurrence in the breast was 3.5% in the CS and RT group compared with 1.9% in the CS, RT, and tamoxifen group. Here too, however, additional follow-up is required before firm conclusions can be reached.

SUMMARY OF RISK FACTORS FOLLOWING CONSERVATIVE THERAPY AND RADIATION THERAPY AND THE SIGNIFICANCE OF LOCAL RECURRENCE

The significance of local recurrence of the primary tumor after CS and RT still is an unresolved issue. (Recurrences elsewhere in the treated breast likely have a different set of risk factors and prognosis.) In most reported series, local recurrence after CS and RT seems to have a better prognosis than local recurrence after mastectomy (see Chap. 21). Local recurrence after CS and RT is associated with a worse prognosis than that for apparently similar patients who do not develop a local recurrence. A multivariate analysis from the NSABP trial B-06, in which local recurrence after CS was entered as a time-covariate, indicated that local recurrence is associated with an increased relative risk of distant metastases of about 3, even when other known prognostic factors also were considered.[127] Other studies have shown similar results.[128] One explanation for these findings is that there are two types of local recurrence after CS and RT: one that reflects the inherent biologic aggressiveness of the cancer (and is not altered by the type of local treatment) and one that reflects a particular local manifestation of the cancer, either extensive involvement in the breast or an intrinsic radioresistance, such that the cancer was not eradicated by the local treatment employed.

The information on risk factors after CS and RT bears on this issue. Some risk factors, such as lymphatic vessel invasion and young patient age, reflect an inherently more aggressive biologic character and are also known to be risk factors for local recurrence after mastectomy and for distant metastases after local treatment of any kind. Advances in basic science likely will help to identify molecular or genetic risk factors in addition to these clinical and pathologic risk factors. Such risk factors are not useful in selecting local therapy for an individual patient with that factor. Other risk factors, such as the presence of an extensive intraductal component with involvement of the margins of resection, reflect a type of breast cancer that is locally extensive and not well controlled with conventional RT. An extensive intraductal component with involvement of the margins of resection is not a risk factor for local recurrence after mastectomy and is not associated with a greater likelihood of subsequent metastases. In addition, local recurrences in patients with an extensive intraductal component with involvement of the margins of resection who are treated with CS and RT are commonly entirely or predominantly composed of intraductal carcinoma, and the prognosis after mastectomy in these patients is excellent.[51] Therefore, the presence of an extensive intraductal component in a patient in whom it is not feasible to obtain negative margins of resection may be a useful factor in selecting local treatment. Such patients clearly have a better rate of local tumor control when treated with mastectomy than when treated with CS and RT; whether or not they have a better survival rate with mastectomy is uncertain.

The last decade has seen a number of improvements in pretreatment evaluation and management, including more detailed mammographic evaluation, more precise pathologic assessment with regard to margin involvement and the presence of an extensive intraductal component, and an increased use of reexcision. These changes will result in a lower percentage of treated patients having an EIC-positive cancer (because those with extensive local disease are preferentially being treated with mastectomy) and a lower rate of local recurrence for patients with an EIC-positive cancer treated with CS and RT compared with historical series. It is also likely, however, that as a result of these improvements a higher proportion of local recurrences of the primary tumor in patients thus treated will reflect an inherently more aggressive biologic character and be associated with a poor prognosis. In a 1994 report from Memorial Sloan-Kettering Cancer Center,[129] outcome after treatment for local recurrence was compared for 72 patients initially treated with CS and RT and 50 patients initially treated with mastectomy; at 5 years, there was no difference in disease-free or overall survival between the two groups.

PSYCHOLOGIC OUTCOME OF BREAST SURGERY

A large number of studies have compared the psychologic morbidity of mastectomy to that of breast-conserving surgery. The impact of breast cancer therapy on the patient can be measured by assessing psychologic discomfort (usually depression, anxiety, and anger), changes in life patterns, or fears and concerns.[130] Most studies comparing psychologic distress between patients undergoing mastectomy and patients undergoing breast-conserving therapy[131–139] have found no significant differences. This is particularly striking in view of the different methodologies used, varying times of evaluation, and the fact that some studies evaluate patients who had no role in treatment selection whereas others involve patients who selected their local therapy. The studies that do demonstrate differences in psychologic distress do not agree on which operative procedure is associated with a greater degree of distress. Levy and others[140] prospectively evaluated 98 women who chose their own form of local treatment. Seventy-two percent of the patients chose breast-conserving surgery. At a 3-month follow-up visit, patients who chose breast-conserving surgery were found to be more distressed and more depressed than patients who underwent mastectomy. In contrast, Lasry and coauthors[141] reported significantly less depression in women treated with breast-conserving therapy than in those treated with mastectomy as part of a randomized trial. These studies demonstrate that patients treated for breast cancer have psychologic distress primarily related to the diagnosis and its implications, and that this is little affected by the choice of local treatment.

Although the operative procedure chosen does not seem to influence overall psychologic outcome, most studies evaluating body image find fewer problems in patients undergoing breast-conserving treatment than in patients undergoing mastectomy.[134–136,139,141,142] Several studies have also reported better sexual adjustment in patients treated with breast-conserving treatment,[142–144] although Schain and others[144] observed that these differences disappeared as the time from surgery increased. The impact of the operative procedure on fear of recurrence also has been evaluated. Six of eight reported studies[134–136,141,145,146] showed no difference in the fear of recurrence measured from 3 months to 9 years after treatment between patients undergoing mastectomy and those having breast-conserving treatment. Two studies reported an increased fear of recurrence in patients undergoing mastectomy,[142,147] whereas Fallowfield and others[137] noticed that 10% of patients treated with breast-conserving treatment developed obsessive checking of their breasts for recurrence.

In general, it seems that most patients undergoing breast cancer surgery do not have major psychologic sequelae, regardless of the operative procedure, emphasizing that no single local treatment is right for all patients. Characteristics of patients who are likely to have psychologic morbidity include a prior history of psychiatric treatment,[148] emotional lability,[149] a perception of a low level of social support,[150] and a history of unemployment.[151] Efforts should be directed toward identifying such patients preoperatively and providing psychologic counseling to aid them in the choice of local therapy and in their adjustment after surgery.

Guidelines for Patient Selection

Based on the information available from prospective and retrospective studies, a general consensus on the criteria for patient selection for the use of breast-conserving treatment has been developed. As described earlier, multiple studies have established that in most cases breast-conserving treatment results in a cosmetically satisfactory breast and that it provides survival rates equivalent to those seen after mastectomy. The National Cancer Institute Consensus Conference[152] on the treatment of early-stage breast cancer held in 1990 concluded that "breast-conservation treatment is an appropriate method of primary therapy for the majority of women with Stage I and II breast cancer and is preferable because it provides survival equivalent to total mastectomy and axillary dissection while preserving the breast."

Patient selection for breast-conserving treatment involves an assessment of whether the primary tumor can be successfully removed with an acceptable cosmetic result, an estimate of the risk of local recurrence after breast-conserving treatment and mastectomy, and an evaluation of the patient's desires and expectations. Evaluation of these factors requires a medical history and physical examination, a detailed mammographic evaluation (ideally with magnification views and prior to surgical biopsy) to exclude the presence of other lesions in the breast and to help define the extent of the primary tumor, and careful pathologic evaluation of the resected breast specimen. Adequate evaluation of the specimen is dependent on the surgeon and the pathologist; the elements of a complete pathologic evaluation include the following:

- Measurement of the dimensions of the intact gross specimen
- Inking of the surface (margins) of the specimen
- On gross examination, measurement of the size of the tumor and the closest distance between the tumor and the margin of resection
- Obtaining tissue for hormone receptors; if the tumor is small, this is best done using an immunohistochemical technique
- Microscopic description, including the proximity, presence, and extent of cancer cells at inked margins, as well as identification of the margins involved

Careful mammographic evaluation, in particular, helps to ensure that patients who elect breast-conserving treatment are not found to require mastectomy after breast-conserving surgery. Wolberg and others[153] reported that 20% of patients selected for breast-conserving treatment required mastectomy based on the histologic findings in the resected breast specimen. In contrast, among a group of patients carefully evaluated with mammography, the conversion rate was only 2.8% (Morrow M, unpublished data).

In 1991, representatives from the American College of Surgeons, the American College of Radiology, the College of American Pathologists, and the Society of Surgical Oncology met to develop standards of care for breast-conserving treatment.[154] Absolute and relative contraindications to breast-conserving treatment as determined by the panel are listed in Table 17.1-9. Whereas little debate exists regarding the absolute contraindications to breast-conserving treatment, a number of the relative contraindications deserve comment. Although a large tumor-to-breast ratio may produce an unacceptable cosmetic result, the suitability of large tumors for breast-conserving treatment is dependent on several factors, including the quadrant of the breast in which the tumor is located and the depth of the tumor within the breast. Large lesions in the inferior breast and those that can be excised with preservation of the subcutaneous fat often can be removed with a good cosmetic result. In addition, the value to a patient of preserving her own breast with sensation intact, even if the cosmetic appearance is not perfect, should not be underestimated. Several studies have indicated that patients tend to score their cosmetic results more favorably than their physicians do.[60,76,155] Similarly, a tumor located beneath the nipple should not be a contraindication to breast-conserving treatment if the patient understands the anticipated deficit and desires the procedure. Although excision of the nipple–areolar complex may be necessary to achieve negative margins, the patient is still left with a sensate breast, and nipple reconstruction can be performed after the completion of RT. Mastectomy, with or without reconstruction, also removes the nipple–areolar complex and leaves the patient with an insensate chest wall or breast mound. Extremely large breast size is not a contraindication to breast preservation, provided that RT technical resources are adequate to immobilize the breast and to obtain dose homogeneity. Connective tissue disease is considered a contraindication because of a number of anecdotal reports of severe fibrotic reactions to irradiation in patients with lupus and scleroderma.[156–159] The number of patients with these conditions who did not develop unusual radiation reactions is not stated, so it is difficult to estimate the prevalence of this problem. In one series of patients with connective tissue disease treated with RT, no increased incidence of complications occurred.[160]

Another factor to consider when selecting the type of local therapy is the risk of local recurrence. The risk of local recurrence that is acceptable to a patient to preserve her breast varies from individual to individual. Factors that affect local recurrence have been reviewed earlier; however, if all of the gross tumor has been excised, the predictive value of these other factors is low. Because even a high rate of recurrence in the breast has not been shown to alter breast cancer mortality,[27] caution must be exercised in excluding women from breast-conserving therapy on the basis of a small increase in the risk of local recurrence. On the other hand, the psychologic morbidity associated with fear of local recurrence or further surgery may be unacceptable to some women.[137] When considering the potential impact of a recurrence in the treated breast, it is also useful to consider the patient's risk of systemic failure and the risk of local recurrence after mastectomy. In patients with axillary node involvement (particularly if more than four nodes are positive), the risk of distant metastases frequently outweighs the risk of a recurrence in the breast. Patients with multiple positive axillary nodes also are at high risk for chest wall recurrence after mastectomy.

A final, and critical, factor in the selection of local therapy is patient desire. Several studies indicate that more than 50% of patients in the United States with stage I or II breast cancer are treated with mastectomy.[9,11,161] Potential explanations for this include the presence of medical contraindications to breast-conserving treatment, lack of access to such therapy on the basis of income or geography, patient preference for mastectomy, and physician bias. In one study, a multidisciplinary team of physicians prospectively evaluated 456 patients with ductal carcinoma in situ and clinical stage I or II breast cancer seen at the University of Chicago between 1988 and 1991.[162] Medical contraindications to breast preservation were present in only 26% of patients. The most common medical contraindication, comprising half of the patients deemed to have a medical contraindication, was multifocality. This included patients with multiple primary tumors or diffuse microcalcifications, or patients whose tumors could not be excised with histologically negative margins. The next most common contraindication was having a tumor too large to be excised with a cosmetically acceptable outcome (40% of ineligible patients, 10% of entire group). Of the 337 medically eligible patients who were offered a choice between breast-conserving treatment, mastectomy, or mastectomy with immediate reconstruction, 81% chose breast-conserving treatment. Patient preference for breast-conserving treatment was corroborated in a study of patients with stage I or II breast cancer evaluated at the University of Vermont between 1989 and 1990 in which 80% elected breast-conserving treatment.[163] These data suggest that medical contraindications and patient bias

TABLE 17.1-9
Absolute and Relative Contraindications to Breast-Conserving Treatment*

ABSOLUTE CONTRAINDICATIONS

First or second trimester of pregnancy

Two or more gross tumors in separate quadrants of the breast

Diffuse indeterminate or malignant-appearing microcalcifications

History of therapeutic irradiation of the breast region

RELATIVE CONTRAINDICATIONS

Large tumor/breast ratio

History of collagen vascular (connective-tissue) disease

Large breast size

Tumor location beneath the nipple

* Joint Committee of the American College of Surgeons, American College of Radiology, College of American Pathologists, and Society of Surgical Oncology.

(Winchester D, Cox J. Standards for breast conservation treatment. CA Cancer J Clin 1992;42:134) are not the primary reasons for the low national rates of breast-conserving treatment. Rates of breast-conserving treatment did not vary by ethnicity in the National Cancer Data Base,[164] a finding similarly noticed in the study from the University of Chicago.[162] Some studies suggest that physician bias or their misunderstanding of the contraindications to breast-conserving treatment may be a major factor accounting for high rates of mastectomy. Tarbox and others[165] surveyed 134 general surgeons in Colorado as to whether they believed that the survival rate after breast-conserving treatment was equal to the rate after mastectomy for patients with T1 breast cancer. Twenty-two percent of surgeons surveyed believed that mastectomy was superior to breast-conserving treatment and 34% believed that although the treatments were probably equal, they biased their presentations to patients toward mastectomy. Surgeons who ascribed to either belief performed mastectomy significantly more often than breast-conserving treatment. Tate and researchers[166] investigated the reasons why only 10% to 20% of patients in their Kentucky community underwent breast-conserving treatment. Reasons cited as medical contraindications to breast-conserving treatment included large breast size, centrally located tumors, axillary adenopathy, and dense fibrocystic disease. Eighty-two percent of medically eligible patients elected mastectomy, with fear of RT being the most commonly cited reason. This suggests a problem with patient education as well as confusion on the part of some surgeons regarding contraindications to breast-conserving treatment.

With the availability of medically equivalent options in the local management of breast cancer, the role of the physician has shifted from that of informing the patient with a newly diagnosed breast cancer of her treatment to helping to educate her regarding her treatment options. Each patient should be informed of the options of mastectomy alone, mastectomy with immediate reconstruction, and breast-conserving treatment, including what each treatment entails, the risks and complications, and the follow-up procedures. If there are medical contraindications to one of these procedures, these should be discussed. For the patient who is undecided after this initial discussion with the surgeon, multidisciplinary consultation often is valuable, as is contact with support groups staffed by women who have faced this difficult choice. Time for reflection is particularly important for many patients. Patients should be advised that the surgical treatment of breast cancer is not an emergency and that a delay of several weeks to consider carefully the risks and benefits of the various options is reasonable. There is no single "right" treatment for all patients with breast cancer and each patient should be given the opportunity to participate in the decision-making process.

Timing of Breast Surgery

In 1989, Hrushesky and others[167] reported the results of a retrospective study of 41 premenopausal patients with breast cancer, suggesting that the timing of surgery in relation to the menstrual cycle was an important, independent predictor of survival. In that study, patients who underwent resection during the perimenstrual period (days 0 to 6, 21 to 36) had a 95% survival rate at 10 years compared with 78% for women who had surgery at other times of the menstrual cycle. Since this report, six additional studies have been published[168-174] suggesting a relationship between the timing of surgery and survival (Table 17.1-10). However, nine other studies[175-183] failed to demonstrate a correlation between phase of the menstrual cycle, timing of surgery, and patient outcome.

Davidson and Abeloff[184] have reviewed in detail the problems with the available data. All of these reports, with the exception of the Ville study,[174] assigned time of the menstrual cycle according to the date of the last menstrual period in the medical record. In many of the reports, multiple surgical procedures were undertaken over varying periods of time, and it is not clear whether the biopsy, the mastectomy, or the axillary dissection is the critical surgical procedure. When one considers these methodologic problems, it is not surprising that a wide variety of results has been obtained. However, even within the positive studies, surgery on different days of the menstrual cycle has been shown to correlate with poor outcome. Senie and others[170] found no relation between menstrual cycle timing and outcome when analyzing the intervals defined by Hrushesky and coworkers.[167] Instead, their results suggest that surgery during the follicular phase (days 7 to 14) is associated with worse outcome, but this effect was limited to patients with positive lymph nodes. Badwe and associates[168] reported a similar effect on node-positive patients treated during the same period, whereas Sainsbury and associates[171] identified a third interval (within 10 days of the last period) as being the most favorable time for surgery.

McGuire and others[183] hypothesized that the range of positive associations noticed in these reports might simply be due to chance. The impact of testing multiple windows on a single data set was studied by randomly assigning menstrual dates to 675 patients in the San Antonio data base and by dividing the menstrual cycle into two 14-day windows. The experiment was repeated 100 times with different random assignments of menstrual dates, and a significant prognostic period was identified in 28% of the experiments.

In summary, the available data are insufficient to draw any firm conclusions regarding a prognostic effect of timing of surgery. This question can only be answered by a prospective, randomized trial with sufficient numbers of patients to control for other known prognostic variables including the use of adjuvant systemic therapy. Menstrual cycle timing must be more precisely defined with biochemical determination of hormone levels, and the surgical procedure under study (biopsy, mastectomy, axillary dissection) must be clarified.

Indications for, Techniques, and Complications of Axillary Surgery

A variety of surgical procedures have been described for the removal of the axillary nodes, ranging from an anatomic dissection of all nodal tissue (complete dissection) to

TABLE 17.1-10
Studies of the Effect of Timing of Surgery During the Menstrual Cycle

| | | Poor Outcome | | |
	Patients	Interval (d)	Endpoint	10-y Advantage (%)
POSITIVE STUDIES				
Hrushesky et al[167]	41	0–6, 21–36	OS	95 vs 78
Badwe et al[168]	249	3–12	OS	84 vs 54
Badwe et al[169]	150	3–13	DFS	70 vs 38
Senie et al[170]	283	7–14	DFS	69 vs 58
Sainsbury et al[171]	139	0–2, 13–32	OS	72 vs 54
Spratt et al[172]	40	0–6	OS	71 vs 20
Sadd[173]	86	1–12	OS	74 vs 39
NEGATIVE STUDIES				
Powles et al[175]	313			
Powles et al[176]	81			
Gelber & Goldhirsch[177]	245			
Low et al[178]	125			
Goldhirsch et al[179]	225			
Sigurdsson et al[180]	382			
Rageth et al[181]	224			
Ville et al[174]	165			
Nathan et al[183]	132			
Total	1892			

OS, overall survival; DSF, disease-free survival.

attempts to identify and remove individual axillary lymph nodes. The appropriateness of each of these operations depends on the purpose for which the procedure is being done. As concepts of breast cancer spread and management have changed, so have concepts regarding what constitutes appropriate axillary surgery.

The extent of axillary surgery is commonly described in relation to the levels of the axilla. The axillary triangle is bordered by the axillary vein superiorly, the latissimus dorsi laterally, and the serratus anterior medially. Within this space, the axillary contents are divided into three levels: level I (proximal), which is the tissue inferior and lateral to the pectoralis minor muscle; level II (middle), the nodes posterior to the pectoralis minor and below the axillary vein; and level III (apical), the nodes medial to the pectoralis minor against the chest wall (Fig. 17.1-6).

As dictated by the Halstedian concept of breast cancer spread, axillary dissection was considered a critical component of the surgical cure of breast cancer, and the en bloc resection of the entirety of the draining lymphatics in the axilla was standard surgical practice. The axillary nodes were considered the "filter" before spread of cancer cells to distant sites could occur. The importance placed on the complete removal of all lymph nodes is emphasized by studies using the pathologic technique of clearing of lymph nodes to increase the number of nodes identified. Durkin and Haagensen[185] demonstrated that clearing of the axillary

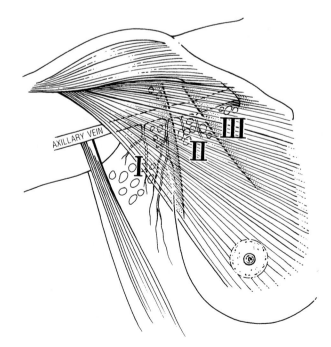

FIGURE 17.1-6 Axillary lymph nodes by level. Levels I (low axilla), II (mid-axilla), and III (apex of the axilla) are defined in relation to the pectoralis minor muscle (fan-shaped muscle superficial to level II nodes).

fat in cedar oil increased the axillary lymph node yield to a mean of 32.9 nodes per case compared with 19.4 nodes when manual dissection was done. A major impetus for clearing was to explain the appearance of distant metastases in some patients with histologically negative axillary nodes, a finding contrary to the Halstedian view of the spread of the disease. However, the percentage of patients who had axillary metastases identified with the clearing technique was similar to that using the manual dissection, and this was confirmed in other studies.[186–188] For this reason, this time-consuming and expensive technique was not widely adopted. Moreover, the failure of clearing to explain distant metastases in node-negative patients provided a serious contradiction to the Halsted hypothesis.

By the 1970s, there was increasing evidence that axillary lymph node metastases were more an indicator than an instigator of decreased survival (see Chap. 16), and axillary dissection came to be regarded as a staging, rather than a therapeutic, procedure. The limited impact of axillary dissection on survival was most convincingly demonstrated in the NSABP trial B-04. In that trial, patients with clinically negative axillary nodes were randomized to radical mastectomy, total mastectomy with observation of the axillary nodes and a delayed dissection if positive nodes appeared, or total mastectomy with RT to the regional lymphatics.[189] No statistically significant difference in the 10-year survival rate was found among the groups, despite the fact that about 40% of the patients undergoing axillary dissection had positive nodes, and a similar percentage were presumed to have positive nodes in the observation-only arm. Although this study emphasizes that axillary dissection is not of survival benefit for the majority of patients, the number of patients in this trial was insufficient to rule out a small, but clinically important survival benefit.[190] Also notice that 25% to 30% of the 20-year survivors reported in a number of series of patients treated with radical mastectomy alone had positive axillary nodes.[3,191–193] suggesting that for a small number of patients, axillary dissection may be therapeutic.

With the general recognition that axillary node involvement is principally a marker of risk for the development of systemic disease, rather than the cause of systemic disease, studies were undertaken to determine the extent of axillary surgery needed to determine whether nodes were positive or negative. Many of these studies examined the likelihood of skip metastases, that is, involvement of nodes in the upper axilla in the absence of involvement in the lower (level I) nodes. Rosen and others[194] reviewed 1228 specimens of complete axillary dissection, 429 of which contained positive nodes. Isolated metastases to the level III nodes were found in only 0.2% of cases. In another large series, Veronesi and coworkers[195] evaluated 539 specimens of complete axillary dissection in patients with positive axillary nodes, and similarly found a 0.4% incidence of skip metastases to level III. The low incidence of skip metastases to level III is not surprising considering that Veronesi identified a mean of only 2.2 lymph nodes per patient in level III. Additional studies of the frequency of skip metastases are summarized in Table 17.1-11.[194–200] These data demonstrate that in contrast to the uniformly low incidence of skip metastases to level III, there is considerable variability in the risk of skip metastases to level II. Much of this variability may be because of variations in the definition of which nodal tissue constitutes levels I and II. These disparate observations have led some authors to conclude that a level I dissection provides accurate staging information,[195,200] whereas others have concluded that removal of both levels I and II is required.[197,199]

The procedures described above are based on the removal of an anatomically defined volume of tissue in the axilla. A number of lesser and less precisely defined procedures also have been studied. *Axillary sampling* refers to the removal of some of the lower axillary contents, often without reference to anatomic structures. Kissin and associates[201] performed axillary sampling to the level of the intercostobrachial nerve followed by a level I and II dissection in 50 consecutive patients. The mean number of nodes removed with the sampling was 4 compared with 14 for the anatomic dissection. Overall, a 24% error rate in staging was observed with the sampling procedure. In five of the sampling cases (10%), no nodes were recovered. In contrast, Steele and others[202] randomized 401 patients to axillary dissection or to axillary sampling and found no significant difference in the incidence of positive nodes

TABLE 17.1-11
Frequency of Skip Metastases to Upper Levels in the Axilla When Lower Levels Are Negative

Investigators	Patients With Axillary Metastases	Negative Level I/ Positive Level II (%)	Negative Levels I and II/ Positive Level III (%)
Rosen et al[194]	429	2	0.2
Veronesi et al[195]	539	1.5	0.4
Smith et al[196]	309	16	10
Danforth et al[197]	65	29	3.1
Chevinsky et al[198]	93	7	2
Pigott et al[199]	72	23.6	1.4
Boova et al[200]	80	7.5	1.3

between the two groups. Only one patient in the node-sampling group had no nodes identified. A subset of 67 patients underwent node sampling followed by dissection. Although the number of nodes recovered increased from 4.1 to 19.7 by the larger procedure, no patient's stage was changed. These findings support the earlier report of Forrest and coworkers,[203] who compared node sampling to complete dissection in a randomized study of 298 patients and found that the percentage of patients with positive nodes was the same in both groups, although more patients with four or more positive nodes were identified by complete dissection. The most likely explanation for the conflicting results in these studies is the difference in the amount of axillary tissue removed. Large sampling procedures are similar to a level I axillary dissection and will accurately stage the majority of patients.

Another role of axillary dissection is to maintain local control in the axilla. Complete axillary dissection provides excellent local control for both the clinically positive and negative axilla. In NSABP trial B-04, isolated axillary recurrences after complete axillary dissection were seen in only 1.4% of clinically node-negative patients and 1% of clinically node-positive patients.[189] Haagensen[204] noticed only two axillary recurrences among 794 Columbia stage A and B patients (0.25%) treated with complete axillary dissection. Among patients treated with a level I-II dissection as part of breast-conserving treatment, axillary recurrence rates of less than 3% have been reported.[205-208] When patients undergo axillary sampling procedures, however, the likelihood of local recurrence is related to the number of lymph nodes removed (Table 17.1-12). The Danish Breast Cancer Group analyzed the relation between number of lymph nodes removed with axillary sampling and the risk of axillary recurrence in 3128 clinically node-negative patients.[209,210] The 5-year probability of an axillary recurrence was 19% in patients with no lymph nodes examined, 10% when one to two negative nodes were removed, 5% when three to four negative nodes were removed and 3% when more than five negative nodes were seen. Similar findings were observed by Fowble and others[208] and among the patients in the simple mastectomy–alone arm of the NSABP trial B-04, many of

whom, in fact, had some degree of nodal sampling.[189] The latest results from the Danish Breast Cancer Group[211] among 7145 patients with early-stage breast cancer treated without adjuvant therapy suggest that at least 10 nodes should be removed to avoid misclassification and optimize local control in the axilla. Thus, nodal sampling runs the risk of failing to accurately stage the patient and failing to maintain local control in the axilla unless at least 5 to 10 nodes are removed. As larger numbers of nodes are excised, the distinction between sampling and dissection becomes blurred. However, formal identification of the axillary vein and the thoracodorsal and long thoracic nerves allows these structures to be protected during the surgical procedure. A level I and II dissection accurately stages the patient and provides excellent local control. When grossly positive axillary nodes are identified intraoperatively, a level III dissection usually is carried out to maximize local control.

Major complications of axillary dissection are infrequent and include injury or thrombosis of the axillary vein and injury to the motor nerves of the axilla. Minor complications are much more common and include seroma formation, shoulder dysfunction, loss of sensation in the distribution of the intercostobrachial nerve, and edema of the arm and breast. Seroma formation is the most frequent complication, and closed suction drainage is employed by most surgeons in an effort to prevent this problem. Siegel and associates[207] described 259 women who underwent level I and II axillary dissection without drains as part of breast-conserving therapy. They reported a 4.2% incidence of seroma formation. However, patients were considered to have seromas only if the fluid accumulation was bothersome, and the average amount of fluid aspirated was 100 mL. Somers and coworkers[212] performed a randomized study of 227 axillary dissections in which patients were randomized to receive an axillary drain for 24 hours or to be followed expectantly. Any palpable fluid collections were aspirated. The use of a drain was found to decrease the time to seroma resolution, the mean number of aspirations required, and the mean volume of fluid aspirated. The incidence of many of the other complications of axillary dissection is probably underestimated, since they are not life-threatening and do not require hospitalization. Ivens and others[213] evaluated 106 patients at least 6 months after axillary dissection without RT. The most common complaints were numbness (70%), pain (30%), and weakness (25%), although less than 15% of respondents believed that their symptoms were sufficiently severe to interfere with daily living. Lin and associates[214] evaluated 122 patients at least one year after surgery and found that 78% had numbness in the intercostobrachial nerve distribution, 22% had numbness and pain, and 17% had greater than or equal to 15 degrees of restriction of shoulder motion. Hladiuk and coworkers[215] prospectively assessed subjective feelings of pain and stiffness as well as objective measures of strength and mobility in 63 patients undergoing axillary dissection using preoperative arm function as a control. Overall, 42% of patients had subjective or objective impairment of arm function 1 year after surgery. Pain and reduced grip strength were the most

TABLE 17.1-12

Risk of Axillary Recurrence After Nodal Sampling in Relation to the Number of Axillary Nodes Removed*

Study	Nodes Removed				
	0	<3	<5	>5	>10
Danish Breast Cancer Group[209]	19	10	5	3	—
NSABP[246]	21	—	12	0	—
Fowble et al[208]	—	21	—	5	2

NSABP, National Surgical Adjuvant Breast and Bowel Project.

* Risk figures and percentages.

common problems and were each seen in 16% of patients. Gutman and others[216] compared range of motion in patients undergoing quadrantectomy, axillary dissection, and RT and those undergoing modified radical mastectomy. In the early postoperative period, range of motion in the quadrantectomy group was 70% of baseline in 81% of women in the quadrectomy group, compared with 33% of patients in the modified radical mastectomy group. However, range of motion in all patients returned to baseline by 3 months. Lotze and others[217] compared the effects of early (postoperative day 1) versus late (postoperative day 7) physical therapy on range of motion in 36 patients (21 with breast cancer) undergoing axillary dissection. No significant differences in the percentage of patients achieving functional range of motion were identified at 1, 3, or 6 months after operation. An increase in the number of days in which a drain was required and in wound complications was observed in the early-motion group. Petrek and associates[218] failed to confirm this adverse effect of early arm motion on lymphatic drainage.

In addition to problems with arm function, axillary dissection seems to contribute to the breast edema seen after breast-conserving surgery, but this effect is largely transient.[69,219] Lymphedema of the arm, the most widely recognized complication of axillary dissection, is discussed in detail in Chapter 24.7.

ROLE OF AXILLARY DISSECTION

With the demonstration that survival could be prolonged for patients with node-positive breast cancer with the use of adjuvant systemic therapy, surgical staging of the axilla became a routine method of determining postoperative therapy. However, changing trends in the management of patients with node-negative breast cancer, the increasing use of breast-conserving treatment, and the increasing numbers of patients with small, mammographically detected cancers have caused a reexamination of the need for axillary dissection in all patients with invasive breast cancer.[214,220–222] Two general approaches have been taken: (1) to identify patients with tumors having such a low risk of nodal metastases that axillary dissection is not warranted, (2) to identify patients whose therapy would not be altered by axillary dissection. The incidence of axillary nodal involvement is known to be related to tumor size. However, axillary node metastases have been seen in 12% to 37% of tumors measuring 1 cm or less in size,[211,220,221,223–227] and, in a number of studies, the incidence of metastases did not decrease appreciably even with tumors 0.5 cm or smaller.[211,224,226] Silverstein and coworkers,[221] on the other hand, reported nodal metastases in only 3% of 96 patients with tumors 0.5 cm or smaller, but 50% of these patients had ductal carcinoma in situ (DCIS) with areas of microinvasive carcinoma. Preliminary data from these authors also suggest that for tumors between 0.5 and 1 cm in size, the risk of axillary nodal involvement is related to the method of tumor detection, with mammographically detected tumors having a 7% incidence rate of nodal metastases and palpable tumors, a 24% incidence rate of metastases.[228] A review of 456 patients treated at the University of Chicago

found no difference in the incidence rate of nodal metastases by method of tumor detection, with 19% of clinically detected T1 lesions and 18% of mammographically detected T1 lesions having positive nodes (Morrow M, unpublished data). Wilhelm and others[229] similarly noticed no decrease in the incidence of nodal metastases in mammographically detected breast cancers.

Some investigators have evaluated whether a combination of tumor size and other pathologic characteristics of the primary tumor could be used as a predictor of axillary nodal metastases. Chadha and coworkers[225] found that the combination of tumor size and lymphatic or vascular invasion correlated with the presence of axillary nodal metastases. Of 79 patients with tumors smaller than 1 cm and without LVI, only 9% had nodal metastases. In comparison, 68% of patients had metastases when the tumor showed LVI and measured between 1 and 2 cm. Ravdin and associates[230] analyzed data from 11,964 patients to determine whether tumor size, age, S-phase fraction, receptor status, and ploidy could accurately predict axillary nodal involvement. No subsets of patients with a less than 10% or greater than 75% risk of involvement were identified. The addition of epidermal growth factor receptor, HER2 neu expression, and cathepsin D to the model in 324 patients did not improve its predictive value. The only group of patients with invasive carcinoma regularly identified as having nodal metastases in fewer than 5% of cases are those with microinvasive tumors[231–234] and those with pure tubular carcinomas less than 1 cm in size.[235,236]

An alternative approach is to identify patients whose therapy would not be altered by the findings on axillary dissection (ie, patients who would receive adjuvant chemotherapy regardless of their axillary status). Based on recent information from the overview analysis on the use of adjuvant systemic therapy, this therapy is routinely recommended for patients with tumors measuring 1 cm or larger.[237,238] Lin and others[214] retrospectively reviewed the records of 240 clinically node-negative patients to determine the impact of axillary dissection on the use of adjuvant therapy. Sixty-three percent of patients were considered to require adjuvant therapy on the basis of primary tumor size, receptor status, ploidy, or S-phase. Of the remaining 88 patients, 11 (13%) were found to have nodal metastases. Overall, the findings at axillary dissection were the deciding factor in the recommendation for systemic therapy for only 5% of the clinically node-negative patients.

Although axillary dissection may not be needed to direct the use of adjuvant therapy, it is still of value in obtaining local control in the axilla and in providing patients with important prognostic information. As discussed in Chapter 16, the number of involved axillary nodes remains the single most reliable indicator of prognosis. It may, however, be possible to identify node-positive patients by the removal of a "sentinel node," as is done in patients with melanoma.[239] Giuliano and coworkers[240] have reported that this technique accurately staged 95% of patients. A learning curve for the technique was clearly present because the sentinal node was identified in only 96 of 152 cases (63%), but in all of the last 68 cases in the series. This technique has the potential to allow axillary dissection to be limited to patients with nodal involvement who require axillary dissection for local control and for quantification of the number of involved nodes.

An alternate method of maintaining local control in the axilla is the use of axillary irradiation. Axillary recurrence rates of 3% or less have been reported in clinically node-negative patients undergoing CS and RT without axillary dissection.[206,241–243] The incidence of lymphedema of the arm and breast after axillary radiation alone seems to be lower than after surgical dissection,[69,243] but as discussed later in this chapter, there are other uncommon complications from axillary irradiation that must be considered, particularly when RT is given in conjunction with adjuvant chemotherapy.

A randomized trial examining the value of axillary dissection in 658 clinically node-negative patients treated with CS and RT has been reported.[244] Patients were randomized to lumpectomy with RT to the breast and draining lymph node regions or to lumpectomy, axillary dissection, and breast irradiation. Patients randomly assigned to undergo axillary dissection had their treatment modified based on the histologic findings of the dissection. In particular, patients with histologically positive axillary nodes also received adjuvant chemotherapy. Axillary recurrences were uncommon in both the axillary RT and the axillary dissection groups. The 5-year survival rate was better in the axillary dissection group (97% versus 93%, $P = 0.01$). The authors concluded that these findings justify routine axillary dissection. However, the selective use of adjuvant chemotherapy in the axillary-dissection group makes it difficult to draw any firm conclusions from this study.

In summary, the role of axillary dissection is in evolution. Axillary dissection can be eliminated for patients with DCIS or with DCIS and small areas of microinvasion, and for those with pure tubular carcinoma less than 1 cm in size, because the risk of nodal involvement is extremely low. Most clinically node-negative patients with tumors larger than 2 cm who undergo breast-conserving treatment receive adjuvant therapy regardless of histologic nodal status; for these patients, irradiation of levels I and II of the axilla is a reasonable alternative to dissection for obtaining local control. Many patients continue to benefit from axillary dissection, including those who have the following:

- Mastectomy as operative procedure
- Patient desire for prognostic information
- Therapy changed by identification of the number of positive nodes
- Tumor smaller than 1 cm
- Tumor 1 to 2 cm in size with favorable prognostic features
- Different adjuvant therapy for node-positive and node-negative tumors
- Participation in clinical trials requiring axillary node dissection

Aggressive adjuvant treatment strategies, such as high-dose chemotherapy, are being investigated for patients with high numbers of positive nodes. If these strategies are successful for certain groups of patients identified on the basis of nodal involvement, then axillary dissection may again be necessary for all patients to select the most appropriate systemic treatment.

Indications for Postoperative Radiation Therapy

The term *postoperative RT* refers to RT to the chest wall and draining lymph node regions used as an adjuvant treatment after definitive surgery (mastectomy). There are two possible reasons for the use of prophylactic postoperative RT. The first is to reduce the rate of local or regional tumor recurrence (ie, recurrence on the chest wall or in the axillary, internal mammary, or supraclavicular lymph nodes) by treating residual microscopic disease that has spread beyond the margin of surgical resection. It has been well documented that in the absence of postoperative RT, there is a substantial risk of local recurrence after modified radical or radical mastectomy. This risk is principally related to the presence and extent of axillary nodal involvement; if axillary nodes are involved, local recurrence is seen in about 25% of patients, whereas if axillary nodes are uninvolved, local recurrence is seen in only about 5% of patients.[245,246] Once a local recurrence is clinically manifest, it can be effectively controlled in only about half of patients.[247–249] In addition, it is often distressing for afflicted patients. Thus, postoperative RT can benefit high-risk patients by preventing local recurrence. The second potential rationale for postoperative RT is to improve survival. It is possible that residual local disease after mastectomy may be the only site of persistent cancer and a source of subsequent distant metastases. Obviously, patients without residual local disease or patients who already have distant metastases fail to show any improvement in survival with this form of adjuvant therapy.

The addition of postoperative RT to radical mastectomy has been shown to decrease the risk of local recurrence in a number of retrospective series,[250,251] and this has been confirmed in a number of randomized clinical trials discussed later. Despite this clear-cut improvement in local control, the effect of adjuvant RT on survival remains uncertain. Assessing the survival value of postoperative RT requires evaluation within prospective randomized clinical trials. However, there are significant methodologic considerations in performing such a study properly. A major consideration is that the technical aspects of the RT must be carefully monitored. Postoperative RT can be effective only if the correct volume is treated with the correct dose. Many of the earlier series used techniques that either did not ensure adequate coverage of the entire tumor volume, including the draining lymph nodes and chest wall, or did not use a sufficient dose. Some of those trials also used techniques, since considered outmoded, that irradiated large portions of the heart resulting in excess late cardiac mortality. Another major consideration is the large number of patients required for such a study. As will be discussed later, the survival benefit from postoperative RT, if it exists, is likely to be small, on the order of 5% to 10%. Two thousand patients would be required for a study to have a 90% chance of detecting a 7% difference between two treatment arms at a significance level of $P = .05$. Finally, randomization in these trials must be strict. In some earlier, less controlled studies, it was possible for clinicians to avoid RT for patients perceived to have a good prognosis and to select RT for patients with a poor prognosis. Because the expected survival benefit, if it exists, is likely to be small, such deviations from true randomization could obscure a benefit from postoperative RT.

The trials testing the value of RT after radical or modified radical mastectomy can be subdivided into those in which adjuvant systemic therapy was not used and those in which postoperative RT was used in conjunction with systemic therapy.

TRIALS OF POSTOPERATIVE RADIATION THERAPY WITHOUT SYSTEMIC THERAPY

There are five published trials in which patients were randomized after radical or modified radical mastectomy to postoperative RT or no further treatment in the absence of systemic therapy. Table 17.1-13 provides the details of treatment and patient accrual for these trials. Some of these are among the earliest clinical trials performed in medicine. In many of these trials, RT was given using orthovoltage equipment and in most, techniques were used that delivered considerable dose to the heart and are considered outmoded. The use of prophylactic postoperative RT clearly reduced the incidence of local recurrence, but none of these trials demonstrated a clear-cut improvement in the survival rate. As discussed below, many of these trials showed a late increase in cardiac mortality in patients treated with RT compared with unirradiated patients.

The most modern of these trials was conducted at the Radiumhemmet in Stockholm between 1971 and 1976.[252-254] Three hundred twenty-one patients with operable breast cancer were randomized to modified radical mastectomy alone and 323 patients to modified radical mastectomy and postoperative RT. The latest results of the Stockholm trial were published in 1993 with a median follow-up time of 16 years.[254] Table 17.1-14 shows outcome and an analysis of sites of failure for the two groups, analyzed by the pathologic status of the axillary lymph nodes. For node-negative patients, the use of postoperative

TABLE 17.1-13
Patient Accrual and Treatment Details of Randomized Trials of Postoperative Radiation Therapy (RT) Without Systemic Therapy in Overview Report

Trial	Period of Entry	Date of Last Follow-Up	Type of RT	Dose (Gy)	No. Fractions	Duration (d)	Patient-Years 10+
RADICAL MASTECTOMY ± RT							
Manchester-Q[462]	1949–52	12/82	250 kV	35–40	15	21	1590
Manchester-P[462]	1952–55	12/82	250 kV	32.5–42.5	15	21	1884
Oslo I[463]	1964–68	12/87	200 kV	18–36	20	28	1783
Oslo II[463]	1968–72	12/87	^{60}Co	50	20	28	1201
Heidelberg[464]	1969–72	10/89	^{60}Co	54	30	42	171
Stockholm[256]	1971–76	12/89	Nodal, ^{60}Co	45	25	35	1217
SUBTOTAL							7846
TOTAL MASTECTOMY ± RT							
Manchester Regional I[257]	1970–75	4/91	300 kV or nodal	37	15	21	1335
			(4 MeV)	40	15	21	
				30	15	21	
CRC[258]	1970–75	12/91	Ortho or MeV	32.5–46	—	21–42	5567
				35.7–50.6	—	21–42	
NSABP B-04[189]	1971–74	12/86	MeV	40–50	25	35	725
Edinburgh[259]	1974–79	8/92	4 MeV	42.5	10	28	497
SUBTOTAL							8124
TOTAL							15,970

Ortho, orthovoltage radiation therapy; MeV, megavoltage radiation therapy; kV, kilovoltage radiation therapy; NSABP, National Surgical Adjuvant Breast and Bowel Project; CRC, Cancer Research Campaign.

(Cuzick J, Stewart H, Rutqvist L, et al. Cause-specific mortality in long-term survivors of breast cancer who participated in trials of radiotherapy. J Clin Oncol 1994;12:447)

TABLE 17.1-14
Stockholm Trial of Postoperative Radiation Therapy

	Postoperative Radiation Therapy		Surgery Alone		Rate Ratio (95% Confidence Interval)	P Value (Log-Rank)
	Patients	Events (%)	Patients	Events (%)		
PATHOLOGICALLY NEGATIVE NODES	204		197			
Treatment failure*		74 (36%)		99 (50%)	0.65 (0.48–0.88)	<.01
Local–regional recurrence		10 (5%)		45 (23%)	0.25 (0.15–0.42)	<.001
Distant metastases		52 (26%)		49 (25%)	1.02 (0.69–1.50)	.94
Death		66 (33%)		74 (38%)	0.87 (0.63–1.21)	.40
Breast cancer death		47 (23%)		43 (22%)	1.05 (0.70–1.59)	.80
PATHOLOGICALLY POSITIVE NODES	118		120			
Treatment failure*		76 (64%)		94 (78%)	0.64 (0.47–0.87)	<.01
Local–regional recurrence		18 (15%)		58 (48%)	0.29 (0.18–0.45)	<.001
Distant metastases		61 (52%)		83 (69%)	0.66 (0.48–0.92)	.02
Death		72 (61%)		84 (70%)	0.82 (0.60–1.12)	.21
Breast cancer death		59 (50%)		81 (68%)	0.70 (0.50–0.98)	.04

* Treatment failure defined as local–regional recurrence, distant metastases, or death without recurrence.

(Rutqvist L, Pettersson D, Johansson M. Adjuvant radiation therapy versus surgery alone in operable breast cancer: long-term follow-up in a randomized clinical trial. Radiat Oncol 1993;26:104)

RT was associated with a decrease in local recurrence, but had no effect on distant metastases or survival. For node-positive patients, the use of postoperative RT was associated with a decrease in local recurrence, but also with a decrease in distant metastasis ($P = .02$). The 15-year survival rate was 31% for node-positive patients treated with mastectomy alone compared with 40% for node-positive patients treated with mastectomy and postoperative RT ($P = .21$). In contrast to the results seen in the Manchester trials, the proportion of patients with persistent local–regional disease at death or last follow-up was greater in the unirradiated group than the irradiated group (16% versus 6%, $P < .01$). A similar reduction in persistent local recurrence was noticed in a separate trial performed in southern Sweden.[255]

Rutqvist and others[256] provided additional information on the Stockholm trial with regard to the technique of irradiation and its association with cause-specific mortality. The overall results indicated that breast cancer mortality was lower in irradiated than unirradiated patients (relative risk [RR], 0.8; $P = .07$), but that mortality from ischemic heart disease was higher in irradiated patients (RR, 1.39; $P = .38$). Postoperative and preoperative RT was given either by cobalt-60 or by electron beam. The dose and volume of heart irradiated was estimated for each of the techniques and patients were grouped as having either low dose-volume (right-sided tangential cobalt-60 fields), intermediate (electron beam fields to either side), or high (left-sided tangential cobalt-60 fields). When cause-specific mortality was examined in relation to radiation dose-volume to the heart, increased mortality from isch-

emic heart disease was higher than for unirradiated patients only in the high group (RR, 3.2; $P < .05$ by trend). The reduction in breast cancer mortality was similar in all three groups. This study suggests that the increased cardiovascular mortality associated with adjuvant irradiation can be avoided by the use of appropriate techniques without compromising the effectiveness of RT in treating breast cancer.

In addition to the trials examining the value of giving RT after radical mastectomy, there are a number of trials testing the value of RT after total or "simple" mastectomy. These are not discussed in detail here as they are no longer relevant to clinical practice. They are, however, relevant to an understanding of the natural history of breast cancer and are discussed in greater detail in Chapter 12. The oldest of these studies are the Manchester Regional I trial,[257] the Cancer Research Campaign trial from the United Kingdom,[258] NSABP trial B-04,[189] and the Southeast Scottish (or Edinburgh) trial[259] (see Table 17.1-15).

An overview of randomized trials of postoperative RT after either simple or radical mastectomy was first published in 1986.[16] Included in this study were the results from the Manchester trials, the Oslo trials, the Stockholm trial, and an unpublished small trial from Heidelberg, all of which used radical mastectomy, and the four trials noted above, which used simple mastectomy. The results of these various trials were combined by the use of a summary log-rank statistic (Mantel-Haenzel) obtained by adding together across trials the difference between observed and "expected" deaths. No difference was seen in the summary observed-minus-expected deaths when patients treated with RT were compared with those treated without RT over the first 10 years after surgery. After 10 years, there was a lower rate of survival associated with the use of RT. The results obtained after 10 years, however, were heavily weighted by the results from the oldest trials, particularly the Manchester trials. In addition, this overview did not provide an analysis of cause of death.

An update of this overview was published in 1994[17] in which many more patients from the later trials had more than 10 years of follow-up (see Table 17.1-13). To explain the excess mortality seen previously, cause-specific mortality data were collected for all of the trials, except the NSABP B-04, for which this information was not available. The previously reported lower overall survival rate for patients treated with RT was no longer significant, because the more recent trials had found a trend to improved survival associated with RT (Fig. 17.1-7). An excess of cardiac deaths among patients treated with RT was apparent in both the early and more recent trials (*P* < .001), but this was offset by a reduced number of deaths from breast cancer, especially in the more recent trials (Fig. 17.1-8). A more detailed discussion of the relation between RT technique and late cardiac effects is provided in the section on complications of RT later in this chapter.

It remains undetermined whether there is a subset of patients who would derive a long-term survival benefit from postoperative RT. The authors of the overview comment that their study "suggests that radiation therapy may have a value beyond the clearly established improvements obtainable for local control."[17] This issue is moot for the most part, given the demonstrated value of adjuvant systemic therapy. The critical issue is whether it is of value to add RT to adjuvant systemic therapy, and this is discussed in the next section.

USE OF POSTOPERATIVE RADIATION THERAPY WITH SYSTEMIC THERAPY

The results presented thus far on the use of postoperative RT emphasize the limitations of local treatment (beyond mastectomy) and the importance of systemic involvement in determining curability for most patients. An appreciation of these results has led to the development of adjuvant systemic therapy, including chemotherapy and hormone therapy. The status of the use of adjuvant systemic therapy is presented later in this chapter.

The effect of adjuvant chemotherapy on local tumor control has been assessed in several clinical trials testing the value of adjuvant chemotherapy. In general, they have demonstrated only a modest effect. In the Milan trial, comparing patients treated with CMF with an untreated control group, the 10-year probability of relapse-free survival was 43% for CMF patients and 31% for controls (*P* < .01).[260] The 10-year local recurrence rate in the CMF group was 11.6% compared with 14.5% for untreated control patients (*P* = NS). In NSABP trial B-05, comparing patients treated with melphalan (L-phenylalanine mustard; L-PAM) with a control group, the cumulative incidence of local recurrence as the site of first failure at 10 years was 14% in the patients who received L-PAM and 24% in the patients who received a placebo.[261] Five-year results of two separate trials from the United Kingdom have been reported.[262,263] In the first, node-positive patients received either melphalan or no treatment. First failure occurred in a local site by 5 years in 18% of patients who received chemotherapy compared with 27% of controls (*P* = NS). In the second trial, node-positive patients were randomly assigned to receive CMF or to no treatment. The crude local failure rate was 9% in the CMF group and 21% in the control group (*P* = .007). Other trials with long-term follow-up, notably those from Japan[264] and the British West Midlands,[265] do not show a reduction in local recurrence after mastectomy for patients treated with chemotherapy. Overall, the results from these studies suggest that adjuvant chemotherapy, by itself, given after mastectomy has only a modest effect on the frequency of local recurrence as a first site of failure. In contrast, the use of adjuvant tamoxifen seems to be associated with a more significant decrease in local recurrence.[266-268]

Other studies have examined the rate of local recurrence in patients treated with mastectomy and adjuvant chemotherapy, but without RT. In a study of patients treated with CMF by Stefanik and others,[269] the local recurrence rate was 9% in patients with one to three positive nodes and 36% for patients with four or more positive

FIGURE 17.1-7 Percentage difference in the death rates from all causes after 10 years in the overview analysis of trials testing the value of postoperative breast irradiation (XRT) after radical mastectomy (*upper*) and total or simple mastectomy (*lower*).[17] The size of the square is related to the number of events after 10 years shown with its 95% confidence intervals. Diamond-shaped symbol represents combined results.

FIGURE 17.1-8 Standardized mortality ratios, a measure of cause-specific death rates (breast cancer mortality, *left*; cardiac mortality, *right*) after 10 years in the overview analysis of trials testing the value of postoperative breast irradiation (XRT) after radical mastectomy (*upper*) and total or simple mastectomy (*lower*).[17] The size of the square is related to the number of events after 10 years shown with its 95% confidence intervals. Diamond-shaped symbol represents combined results.

nodes. Fowble and others[270] examined the rate of local recurrence in 627 node-positive patients entered into Eastern Cooperative Oncology Group adjuvant systemic therapy trials between 1978 and 1982. Premenopausal patients were randomly assigned to receive CMF, CMF and prednisone (CMFP), or CMFP and tamoxifen (CMFPT). Postmenopausal patients were randomly assigned to observation, CMFP, or CMFPT. At 3 years, 225 patients had experienced relapse, and in 70 (31% of relapses, 11% of all patients), the initial relapse was in an isolated local site, that is, without evidence of distant metastases. Local recurrence was not significantly influenced by the use or type of adjuvant systemic therapy, but was influenced by the number of positive nodes. The 3-year rate of local recurrence was 7% for patients with one to three positive nodes, 15% with four to seven positive nodes, and 15% with eight or more positive nodes. Because of the increasing rate of distant metastases in patients with increasing numbers of positive nodes, the percentage of initial relapses that were in isolated local sites was 29% for patients with one to three positive nodes, 42% with four to seven positive nodes, but only 24% with eight or more positive nodes. This study again demonstrates the high risk of local recurrence in patients treated with adjuvant systemic therapy, particularly when four or more nodes are involved,

and suggests that patients with four to seven positive nodes might derive the greatest benefit from adjuvant RT.

There are reasons to suspect that adjuvant chemotherapy might be less effective in decreasing local recurrence after mastectomy than in eradicating systemic micrometastases. One reason is that the local tumor burden (in the remaining regional nodes and chest wall) is likely to be considerable when many axillary nodes are involved. It is also possible that the surgery itself may alter the blood supply to the region, thereby preventing adequate levels of drugs from being delivered to the region. If these speculations on the magnitude of the local tumor burden are correct, they provide a rationale for the use of postoperative RT in conjunction with adjuvant systemic therapy. This rationale is based on a concern over drug resistance: when the tumor burden exceeds a certain level, drug resistance of tumor cells is commonly observed.[271] Adjuvant RT may be critical in reducing the residual local tumor burden sufficiently to avoid the emergence of drug-resistant tumor cells, thereby allowing adjuvant chemotherapy to eradicate systemic micrometastases more effectively.

A number of studies have examined the issue of adding postoperative RT to adjuvant chemotherapy (Table 17.1-15). In a trial from British Columbia, 318 node-

TABLE 17.1-15
Randomized Trials Testing the Value of Postoperative RT Used in Conjunction With Adjuvant Systemic Therapy

Trial	Treament Arms	Patients	Years	Type RT	Follow-Up (y)	Survival Rate (%)	P Value
DFCI/JCRT[285]	CT	100	1974–1984	Supervoltage	5	72	.20
	CT + RT	106				66	
SEG[465]	CMF × 6	133	1976–1981	Supervoltage	10	36	.55
	CMF × 12★	61				22†	
	RT + CMF × 6	137				44	
Danish Breast Cancer Group[274]	CMF	856	1982–1989	Supervoltage	7	55	.003
	CMF + RT	852				62	
Danish Breast Cancer Group[275]	Tam	689	1982–1989	Supervoltage	7	53	.59
	Tam + RT	686				53	
Mayo Clinic[315]	L-Pam	81	1974–?	Supervoltage	5	NS	
	CFP	104					
	RT + CFP	108					
Piedmont Oncology[466]	CT	86	1977–?	Supervoltage	10	53	.91
	RT + CT	72				53	
Glasgow[467]	RT	103	1976–1982	Orthovoltage	5	59‡	
	RT + CMF	111				68‡	
	CMF	108				63‡	
British Columbia[272]	CMF	156	1979–1985	Supervoltage	10	57	.3
	CMF + RT	162				60	
Helsinki[468]	CAFt	52	1981–1984	?	8	56	NS
	RT	50				55	
	CAFt-RT	47				65	
	CAFt-RT-Tam	50				67	

RT, radiation therapy; CT, chemotherapy with L-PAM or CMF; CMF, cyclophosphamide, methotrexate, and 5-fluorouracil; Tam, tamoxifen; CFP, cyclophosphamide, 5-fluorouracil, prednisone; CAFt, cyclophosphamide, doxorubicin, ftorafur; SEG, Southeastern Cancer Study Group; JCRT, Joint Center for Radiation Therapy; DFCI, Dana Farber Cancer Institute.

★ ≥4 positive nodes.

† Percentage estimated from curves.

‡ Disease-related mortality.

positive premenopausal patients treated with modified radical mastectomy were randomly assigned to undergo adjuvant CMF chemotherapy and postoperative RT or chemotherapy alone.[272] The 10-year disease-free survival rate was improved for the CMF and RT group (68% versus 53%, $P = .02$), but the difference in the 10-year survival rates (60% versus 57%; $P = .3$) was not statistically significant. In a subset analysis, the largest improvements in disease-free and overall survival were noted in patients with the most extensive disease. Patients with four or more positive nodes had greater benefit than patients with one to three positive nodes, and patients with eight or more positive nodes appeared to benefit more than patients with four to seven positive nodes. Among the 70 patients with extensive extracapsular spread, the 10-year disease-free survival rate was 55% for patients who received CMF and RT compared with only 13% for patients who received CMF alone ($P = .0003$). The corresponding

10-year survival rates were 52% and 33%, respectively ($P = .03$).

The results of the two Danish trials may be the most relevant to this issue because of their study design and large number of patients. A report published in 1990 described a total of 1473 premenopausal high-risk patients treated with mastectomy who were randomly assigned to receive CMF or CMF and RT, and a total of 1202 postmenopausal high-risk patients who were randomly assigned to receive tamoxifen or tamoxifen and RT.[273] (High-risk was defined as either involvement of the axillary nodes or a T3 or T4 primary tumor.) The RT was given after the first cycle of chemotherapy. For premenopausal patients, the 5-year local recurrence rate was 9% for the CMF and RT group compared with 28% for the CMF group ($P < .0001$). The 5-year survival rate was 68% for the CMF and RT group compared with 63% for the CMF group ($P = .0028$). For postmenopausal patients, the 5-year local recurrence rate was 36% for the tamoxifen group and 6% for the tamoxifen and RT group ($P < .0001$). At 5 years, an advantage was noted in disease-free survival for the tamoxifen and RT group, but no difference in survival was found. Updated results with a greater number of patients and longer follow-up have been reported.[274,275] The large reduction in local recurrence seen with the addition of RT was still observed in both trials. The trial for premenopausal and perimenopausal patients included a total of 2028 patients and had a median follow-up time of 88 months. The 7-year survival rate was 62% for the CMF and RT group compared with 55% for the CMF group ($P = .003$). The trial for postmenopausal patients included a total of 2030 patients and had a median follow-up time of 90 months. The 7-year survival rate was similar (53%) for the tamoxifen and RT group and the tamoxifen alone group ($P = .59$). The results of this study indicate that adjuvant systemic therapy alone is considerably less effective at preventing local recurrence after mastectomy than is the combination of adjuvant systemic therapy and RT. In addition, the results of the study suggest that in premenopausal patients the addition of RT to adjuvant chemotherapy increases the survival rate.

There is also a trial from the Stockholm Breast Cancer Group directly comparing chemotherapy (CMF) and RT (with or without tamoxifen). The trial was initiated in 1976 and a preliminary report on the first 706 patients was published in 1989.[276] At a mean follow-up of 6.5 years, there was no significant difference in relapse-free survival between the two groups. However, postmenopausal patients fared better with RT ($P < .01$), and premenopausal patients fared slightly better with chemotherapy ($P = .33$). In a recent abstract, high S-phase fraction and absence of c–erbB-2 overexpression in premenopausal patients in this trial predicted for greater benefit from chemotherapy than from RT.[277]

There are practical considerations in treating patients with both adjuvant chemotherapy and RT, including the integration of the two modalities. Prompt initiation of postoperative RT may be favored to minimize the absolute number of tumor cells exposed to chemotherapy, thus reducing the likelihood of subsequent drug resistance. On the other hand, adjuvant chemotherapy may need to be given promptly for maximal benefit to be obtained. There is also concern that initial RT may inhibit the ability to administer full doses of chemotherapy. This issue is controversial; many institutions have found it feasible to deliver full-dose chemotherapy after RT[278–281] but others have not.[282,283] Notice that in the studies that have shown interference with drug delivery a direct anterior field was used to treat the IMNs, whereas in studies that have not shown interference tangential fields were used.[284] Also, when chemotherapy is used after RT, modification of the drug dose levels should be based on the neutrophil count and not the total white-cell count. RT is known to reduce the lymphocyte count significantly, and this can persist for many months after completion of treatment.

One reasonable method of integrating chemotherapy and RT is to use postoperative RT after adjuvant chemotherapy. As part of the Dana-Farber Cancer Institute–JCRT adjuvant chemotherapy trial,[285] patients completing chemotherapy were randomly assigned to receive postoperative RT or no further therapy. As in other studies, patients with four or more positive nodes had a high rate of local recurrence after chemotherapy alone, but RT given after chemotherapy reduced the rate of local recurrence to a level comparable with that seen with immediate postoperative RT. This study provides support for the use of RT after completion of adjuvant chemotherapy in patients treated with mastectomy.

Patients with 10 or more positive nodes entered onto trials testing the value of high-dose chemotherapy employing bone marrow transplantation routinely receive postoperative RT after completion of chemotherapy. This is based on a high early local failure rate when patients were not irradiated and, with short follow-up, the apparent safe and effective use of RT in this setting.[286]

Technique of Irradiation

The technique of postoperative irradiation is similar to that for RT after conservative surgery. The target volume to be irradiated includes the chest wall and the ipsilateral internal mammary nodes, axillary apex, and supraclavicular fossa. The typical dose is 45 to 50 Gy given in 25 to 28 fractions over 5 weeks. Several points concerning this treatment are worth stressing. Bolus is typically used periodically (such as every other day) when treating the chest wall with tangential fields. Also, it is simpler to treat the IMNs after mastectomy than after breast-conserving surgery. With breast-conserving surgery, the presence of the intact breast frequently makes it difficult to treat the breast and the IMNs without serious overdosage or underdosage in the medial portion of the breast. In contrast, after mastectomy this is rarely a problem unless an immediate reconstruction has been performed. Also, notice that treatment of the IMNs is one of the major theoretic goals of postoperative treatment and, therefore, the IMNs should be included in the target volume. Computed tomography scanning or lymphoscintigraphy can identify the location of the IMNs. In many patients, it may be preferable to use a direct anterior field to treat the IMNs. The importance of *not* using a photon beam for the entire course of such treatment (particularly for left-sided lesions) because of the risk of late cardiac effects has been stressed.[287] It is preferable to use a mixture of photon beam and electron beam in this situation. An alternative technique to photon irradiation for chest wall treatment is the use of multiple electron beams; however, care must be given to avoid overlap between abutting radiation fields. For patients treated with a full axillary dissection, axillary irradiation should be avoided.

In conclusion, the use of postoperative RT remains controversial. Evidence suggests that such treatment may reduce breast cancer mortality, but it is also possible that the late detrimental effects of treatment on the heart may mitigate or outweigh this benefit. However, evidence also suggests that currently used techniques are not associated with an increase in late cardiovascular mortality. There is no consensus of informed opinion. Additional studies are required to resolve this issue. Postoperative RT is not indicated in patients with uninvolved axillary nodes unless there is clear evidence of disease extending locally beyond the deep margins of resection. In patients with involved axillary nodes, particularly when four or more are positive, RT will greatly reduce the likelihood of local recurrence (even in patients treated with adjuvant systemic therapy).

Sequencing of Chemotherapy and Radiation Therapy in Patients Treated With Breast-Conserving Treatment

Clinical trials have demonstrated both the effectiveness of adjuvant systemic therapies in prolonging survival and the equivalence of breast-conserving treatment and mastectomy in terms of survival; consequently, clinicians are commonly faced with the necessity of combining RT and systemic therapy in patients after CS. In this section, the available information regarding the integration of RT and chemotherapy (CT) after CS are reviewed first. After this, issues related to the combination of RT and tamoxifen are discussed.

It is useful at the start to state the goals, options, and issues in combining RT and CT. The chief goal is to obtain the highest rate of survival; additional important goals are to maintain a low rate of local recurrence, a low rate of complications, and a high rate of satisfactory cosmetic results. The options for combining RT and CT are the following sequences: RT first followed by CT; CT first followed by RT; RT and CT simultaneously; or some number of cycles of CT, then RT, and then more CT (commonly referred to as "sandwich" therapy).

In considering this issue of combining RT and CT, it would be useful to know the answers to a number of questions, such as whether a delay in either CT or RT decreases its effect, whether RT and CT can be given simultaneously without an increase in complications or a decrease in the cosmetic outcome, and whether prior RT affect the ability to give maximal doses of CT. In addressing these questions, one must remember that there are differences in the implementation of breast-conserving surgery, RT, and CT from center to center; therefore, the optimal combination of RT and CT may differ from center to center.

It seems intuitively logical that delays in the initiation of CT may decrease its effectiveness; however, firm data demonstrating this are not available. Efforts to address this have focused on the possible benefit of perioperative CT and on the results obtained in patients treated with mastectomy. In the International Breast Cancer Study Group trial testing the value of perioperative CMF treatment,[288] node-positive patients were randomly assigned to undergo one cycle of perioperative CMF (within 36 hours of surgery), this treatment followed by six cycles of conventionally timed CT, or six cycles of conventionally timed CT alone. With a median follow-up of 42 months, disease-free survival rates were equivalent for patients treated with

conventionally timed CT with or without one cycle of perioperative CT, and both of these groups had better disease-free survival rates than patients treated with one cycle of perioperative CT alone. These results suggest that very prompt initiation of CT is not required. Similar results have been reported in a study from Austria[289] and in a study from Italy using perioperative epidoxorubicin.[290]

Sequencing was evaluated in a randomized clinical trial in which patients treated with *mastectomy* were randomly assigned to undergo RT followed by CT (six cycles of CMF), CT followed by RT, or a sandwich approach using three cycles of CT initially, RT, then completion of the CT. With a relatively small number of patients in each arm (about 80), the best results were observed in patients treated with the sandwich approach.[291] Retrospective reviews of patients treated either with mastectomy or breast-conserving treatment examining the influence of the delay of CT on outcome have demonstrated conflicting results.[126,292–295]

It is also possible that a delay in the initiation of RT to give CT first may decrease its effectiveness. The information available on this issue is also not definitive. As discussed before, among a group of patients treated at the JCRT without adjuvant chemotherapy, the rate of local recurrence was similar for patients treated with RT that was started 4 to 8 weeks after CS and patients treated within 4 weeks.[123] In addition, the JCRT previously reported on a retrospective analysis of 295 node-positive patients treated with RT and CT using a variety of sequences that were not randomly assigned.[126] In that series of patients treated between 1976 and 1985, careful mammographic and pathologic evaluation was not routinely performed, and the extent of breast resection was typically limited to a gross excision of the tumor with a small rim of adjacent breast tissue. Many of these patients likely had involvement of the margins of resection. These results have been updated and there is a median follow-up time of 99 months among surviving patients.[296] Patients who received RT more than 16 weeks after surgery had a 5-year actuarial local recurrence rate of 28% compared with 5% for patients who received RT within 16 weeks of surgery ($P < .05$). This apparent difference in local recurrence rates was not seen until after the first 3 years after treatment. The distribution of clinical and pathologic features was compared for the groups treated within 16 weeks and treated after 16 weeks. The two groups were balanced with regard to patient age, the percentage of tumors with infiltrating duct histologic type, tumor size, the percentage of tumors with an extensive intraductal component, and the frequency of reexcision of the primary site before RT. These groups were not balanced with regard to the number of positive nodes; patients with four or more positive nodes were more likely to have received delayed RT. These results suggest that a delay in the initiation of RT beyond 16 weeks to give CT first may result in an increased rate of local recurrence.

There are a number of important caveats regarding this finding. First, the study is based on a retrospective analysis involving small numbers of patients, especially those with long delays. Second, the study does not evaluate the most important endpoint (namely, survival) in relation to sequencing. Finally, even if these results were to be confirmed in randomized clinical trials, they may not apply to patients undergoing wider resections as opposed to the limited ones performed here.

A number of other institutions have examined this issue. Some have found that delays in the initiation of RT were associated with an increased rate of local recurrence,[297,298] whereas others have not.[299–301] It seems that in the three studies with negative results, more extensive breast resections were performed, with greater attention paid to obtaining negative margins of resections than in the studies with positive results. This suggests that the importance of delay may be related to the tumor burden remaining after breast-conserving surgery. In patients treated with more extensive breast resections and attention to obtaining negative margins of resections, only a small tumor burden may be present and a delay of 4 to 6 months may not be detrimental to local control. All of these studies, however, are limited by the retrospective nature of the data and by relatively small numbers of patients.

Prospective randomized clinical trials are required to test formally the effect of sequencing of RT and CT on outcome. In 1984, a trial was initiated at the JCRT in which 244 patients at moderate or high risk for relapse (typically node-positive) were randomly assigned to receive either RT followed by four cycles of CAMFP or this CT followed by RT. With a median follow-up of 58 months, the 5-year actuarial overall rate of distant failure was higher in the RT-first arm (37% versus 25%, $P = .05$). The 5-year crude rate of local failure was higher in the CT-first arm (13% versus 5%, $P = .07$ for pattern of failure).[301a]

Another important question regarding sequencing is whether RT and CT can be given simultaneously without an increase in complications or a decrease in the cosmetic outcome. The use of simultaneous RT and CT has the advantage of eliminating the necessity for delaying one of the modalities and also might provide an additive or synergistic interaction between the RT and CT. The available information on the effects of simultaneous treatment is conflicting; this is likely because of differences in the details of the RT and CT protocols used (eg, the number, types, and doses of drugs, the daily and total doses of RT, the machine energy, the use of two versus three RT fields, and the specific details by which RT and CT are given simultaneously). In some studies, patients treated with simultaneous treatment have had greater skin reactions compared with patients treated sequentially,[302–306] but this has not been seen in other studies.[307–311] In the experience at the JCRT, acute skin reactions were more pronounced with simultaneous treatment compared with sequential treatment, particularly in patients who received full doses of RT and four injections of methotrexate during RT.[302] It was also found that patients given simultaneous treatment had an increased rate of radiation pneumonitis (particularly when a third field was used to treat the axillary or supraclavicular nodal areas or both)[312] and a decrease in the long-term cosmetic result.[71] In contrast, Glick and colleagues[278] reported that neither an increase

in radiation pneumonitis nor a decrease in the cosmetic outcome was seen when patients were treated with simultaneous RT and CMF in which methotrexate was omitted during the RT. An increase in cardiac complications was reported by the Milan group for patients treated with simultaneous RT and doxorubicin (Adriamycin)-containing CT,[308] but this has not been reported by others. Thus, the use of simultaneous RT and CT has potential advantages, but the precise details of the administration of these two modalities are important to ensure its safety. The JCRT is investigating the use of simultaneous full-dose CMF and a modified program of RT in patients with zero to three positive nodes. The RT is restricted to the breast alone and is given at 180 cGy/d to a total dose of 3960 cGy to the whole breast followed by a boost of 1600 cGy.

A final question about sequencing is whether prior RT affects the ability to give full doses of CT. The available information on this question is also conflicting and, here too, this is likely because of differences in the specifics of the RT and CT used. Two randomized trials comparing breast-conserving treatment with mastectomy are useful to assess the impact of prior irradiation on CT doses. In the study from the US National Cancer Institute,[313] no significant difference was found in CT doses between the patients treated with breast-conserving treatment and those treated with mastectomy, whereas in the Guy's Hospital trial,[314] patients treated with mastectomy were able to receive greater amounts of CT. In the Guy's Hospital trial, however, at least some patients received irradiation of the internal mammary nodes through a separate direct anterior field and drug dose reductions were made based on the total white cell count and were not reescalated if counts improved. Experience has shown that dose reductions should be made based on the granulocyte count because irradiation can result in a large reduction in the lymphocyte count and that reescalation of CT doses is possible. The results from other randomized studies have found that CT doses are only slightly lower when RT is added.[315–317]

In conclusion, the available information regarding the optimal sequencing of CT and RT is limited, based entirely on retrospective reviews, and often conflicting. Differences in the details of the treatment (surgery, RT, and CT) may explain some of the conflicting results. There are concerns about delaying the initiation of CT in patients at high risk for metastases and the possibility that a delay in the initiation of RT may be associated with an increase in the rate of local recurrence. It may be possible to deliver RT and CT simultaneously in a safe and effective manner, but the precise details for this have not been established. Additional data from randomized clinical trials addressing this important issue are required and will be available during the next few years. In the meantime, clinicians faced with this issue might modify the sequence in an individual patient based on both the patient's risk of metastases and the closeness of cancer cells to the margin of resection. In patients with small tumors, negative nodes, and close margins of resection, it may be prudent not to delay greatly the initiation of RT, whereas in patients with many positive nodes and clearly negative margins of resection, the major focus should be on prompt initiation of CT.

Concern has also been raised about the sequencing of tamoxifen and RT. There is a hypothetical concern that the concurrent use of tamoxifen and RT might result in a decreased sensitivity to irradiation if cancer cells are made noncycling by tamoxifen. The results from laboratory studies that have examined this possible effect have been conflicting and do not convincingly demonstrate a decrease in radiation sensitivity in the presence of tamoxifen.[318-320] In addition, there is no clinical evidence that giving RT and tamoxifen concurrently has an adverse effect on local control. In the NSABP trial B-14, node-negative ER-positive patients were randomized to receive tamoxifen or a placebo. Among patients given breast-conserving treatment, tamoxifen was started after surgery and continued during RT. Patients who received tamoxifen had a lower rate of local recurrence than did patients who received a placebo.[125] Some evidence shows that tamoxifen worsens the cosmetic result after breast-conserving treatment,[74] but this is not known for certain, nor is the role of sequencing known in this possible interaction. There is also little information about the timing of the initiation of tamoxifen and its effects on survival. The available data on this issue are so limited that it is reasonable for clinicians to give tamoxifen with RT or to wait until RT is completed.

Microinvasive Carcinoma

Microinvasive carcinoma is a poorly defined pathologic entity that is characterized by the presence of DCIS with microscopic or limited invasion. (Microinvasive breast cancer corresponds to one of the definitions of an invasive breast cancer with an EIC described in detail earlier in this chapter.) Similar to DCIS, it is being diagnosed more frequently because of the increased use of screening mammography. To properly treat patients with microinvasive carcinoma, it is necessary to know whether this lesion behaves like DCIS, invasive carcinoma, or something in between. The behavior of microinvasive carcinoma is difficult to determine because it was considered part of the diagnostic group called *minimal breast cancer*. Minimal breast cancer, as originally described by Gallagher and Martin,[321] consisted of lobular carcinoma in situ, DCIS, and invasive carcinomas with a volume less than that of a sphere 0.5 cm in diameter. This definition was later expanded by McDivitt[322] to include infiltrating tumors less than 1 cm in diameter. The heterogeneous nature of the lesions grouped as minimal breast cancer makes it difficult to draw any firm conclusions regarding the behavior of the group as a whole, and this has lead to the abandonment of the use of this diagnostic group.

There are varying definitions of microinvasive carcinoma used, including DCIS with only a few cells penetrating the basement membrane,[231] DCIS with one or two foci of invasion measuring not more than 1 mm in diameter,[323] and DCIS with invasion present in less than 10%

of the histologic sections.[324] Disagreements also exist about the diagnostic criteria for distinguishing DCIS with microinvasion from pure DCIS, as described in Chapter 11. Microinvasion has been reported to occur more frequently in DCIS that is high grade[323-325] or extensive.[324,325] Lagios and colleagues[325] found no instances of microinvasion in 29 cases of DCIS less than 25 mm in size (median, 8 mm), compared with 11 cases of microinvasion in 24 cases of DCIS larger than 25 mm (median, 56 mm). Silverstein and coworkers[323] reported microinvasion in 26% of comedo-type DCIS cases, and Schwartz and associates[324] found microinvasion in 53% of such cases.

Axillary lymph node metastases are infrequent in microinvasive carcinoma. Wong and others[231] found no axillary node metastases in 33 patients undergoing axillary dissection. Solin and others[232] found positive nodes in 2 of 37 patients (5%), and Kinne and associates[326] reported positive nodes in 4 of 41 patients (10%) with microinvasive carcinoma. In contrast, Schuh and colleagues[327] reported that 6 of 30 patients (20%) with microinvasive carcinoma had axillary metastases. These differences likely reflect variations in the definition of microinvasive carcinoma.

The limited available long-term follow-up data on patients with microinvasive carcinoma suggest that the prognosis after surgical treatment is excellent. Rosner and coworkers[328] reported 36 cases of DCIS with microinvasion treated between 1976 and 1987. Thirty-three patients underwent mastectomy, and at a mean follow-up time of 57 months, all patients remained free of disease. Wong and coworkers[231] also observed no treatment failures at a median follow-up of 47 months, and Kinne and colleagues[326] reported a 94% disease-free survival rate with a median follow-up of 11.5 years. Most patients in these reports were treated with mastectomy. Solin and coauthors[232] reported on the outcome of 39 patients treated with breast-conserving surgery and RT. With a median follow-up time of 55 months, the overall survival rate was 97%. However, nine patients (23%) developed a recurrence in the breast. Outcome was compared for patients with microinvasive carcinoma, patients with DCIS, and patients with node-negative invasive carcinoma treated during the same period. Patients with microinvasive carcinoma were found to have a higher local recurrence rate than those with pure DCIS or those with invasive carcinoma, and a survival rate intermediate between the two groups.

From the limited information available on microinvasive carcinoma, several tentative conclusions may be drawn. First, because of variability in the definition of microinvasion, results from the literature are applicable to an individual patient only if microinvasion is defined in the same way. The incidence of axillary node metastases is low, and axillary dissection is not routinely indicated. Survival in patients with microinvasive carcinoma seems to be intermediate between that for DCIS and that for small invasive carcinomas. The use of breast-conserving treatment in these patients should follow the same guidelines for careful mammographic and pathologic evaluation with the requirement for negative margins of resection as for patients with an EIC-positive invasive carcinoma.

TABLE 17.1-16

Patient Characteristics in the Trials Comparing Conservative Surgery With and Without Radiation Therapy

Trial	Years	Patients	Tumor Size	Nodal Status	Type of Surgery	Final Margins	Adjuvant Therapy
NSABP B-06[37]	1976–1984	1140	≤4 cm	+/−	Lumpectomy	−	Chemotherapy for node-positive patients
Swedish[336]	1981–1988	381	≤2 cm	−	Sector resection	−	None
Ontario[331]	1984–1989	837	≤4 cm	−	Lumpectomy	−	None
Milan III[332]	1987–1989	567	<2.5 cm	+/−	Quadrantectomy	−/+	Chemotherapy for some node-positive patients

NSABP, National Surgical Adjuvant Breast and Bowel Project.

Conservative Surgery Without Radiation Therapy

An unresolved question is whether RT is necessary in all patients with invasive breast cancer after CS. Four randomized clinical trials with published results compare CS alone to CS and RT in patients with early-stage breast cancer.[27,37,128,329–332] These trials, summarized in Table 17.1-16, vary with regard to patient selection, the details of the surgery and RT, the use of adjuvant systemic therapy, and the length of follow-up. The results of these various trials are shown in Table 17.1-17. These trials all show a large reduction in the rate of local recurrence after RT, with an average crude rate of reduction of about 85% (range, 75% to 97%). None of the four trials shows a significant survival benefit for RT; however, in the three trials with published data, the survival rate is slightly better for irradiated patients than for nonirradiated patients. In a multivariate analysis of survival in the Ontario trial, for example, the use of RT was associated with a 15% reduction in the relative risk of dying (RR, 0.85), but this was not statistically significant (95% CI, .59 to 1.23). As previously noted, a very large trial (or perhaps a metaanal-

ysis of multiple smaller trials) is necessary to detect a small, but clinically significant difference in survival, if it in fact exists. None of these four trials has the statistical power to eliminate a 5% to 10% difference with confidence.

It may be possible to identify a subgroup of patients (based on various clinical and histologic features) who have a low risk of local recurrence after CS alone. It was not possible to identify such a subgroup within the Canadian and NSABP randomized trials,[37,331] although the local recurrence rate was lower in trials using more extensive surgery than in those using lumpectomy and in older patients than younger patients. In the Milan trial, with a follow-up time of 39 months, the 3-year rate of local recurrence after quadrantectomy was 17.5% in patients aged 55 years or younger, but only 3.8% in patients older than 55 years.[332] Other institutions have also attempted to identify such a subgroup. The JCRT completed a prospective single-arm trial in which very favorable patients were offered the option of CS alone.[333] The criteria for entry into this protocol were tumor size of 2 cm or less, histologically negative axillary nodes, absence of both lymphatic vessel invasion and an extensive intraductal component in the cancer, and no cancer cells visualized within 1 cm of inked margins. Almost all patients had a negative reexci-

TABLE 17.1-17

Outcome in the Trials Comparing Conservative Surgery (CS) With and Without Radiation Therapy (RT)

Trial	Median Follow-Up (mo)	Local Recurrences		Survival		Analysis
		CS (%)	CS + RT (%)	CS (%)	CS + RT (%)	
NSABP B-06[37]	102	40	10	68	69	9-y actuarial
Swedish[330]	64	18	2	90	91	5-y actuarial
Ontario[331]	66	29	7	85	87	5-y* actuarial
Milan III[332]	39	8.8	0.3	No difference		Crude

NSABP, National Surgical Adjuvant Breast and Bowel Project.

* Estimated from curves.

sion. The median age of patients in this trial was 67 years. This trial was stopped shortly before reaching its accrual goal of 90 patients because of stopping rules ensuring against an excessively high local recurrence rate. The average annual rate of local recurrence was 3.6% and the 3-year crude rate of local failure was 8%. In a reference group of 45 patients treated with breast irradiation between 1983 and 1986 with similar pathologic criteria, the 3-year crude rate of local recurrence was 0%. Based on these results, it was concluded that even in a highly selected group of breast cancer patients, there is a substantial risk of early local recurrence after treatment with wide excision alone. Efforts are underway at the JCRT to see if molecular markers can be used, in addition to clinical and histologic features, to identify patients who are at low risk of local recurrence after CS alone. Similar results using CS alone were also seen in a prospective one-arm trial from Erlangen[334] and in some retrospective studies in the United States.[220,335,336] In the Erlangen study, 241 patients with cancers that were negative for both lymphatic vessel invasion and EIC and had clear margins of 1 to 2 cm were treated with quadrantectomy. With a median follow-up of 5 years, local recurrence was seen in 23 patients (9.5%). This local recurrence rate is lower than that seen in the JCRT series and likely reflects the more extensive breast resection used in this series of patients.

The use of adjuvant CT does not seem to reduce greatly the rate of local recurrence after CS alone. In the NSABP trial B-06, node-positive patients treated with lumpectomy, without RT, but with adjuvant chemotherapy had a 9-year rate of recurrence in the breast of 46% compared with only 10% for patients treated with lumpectomy, RT, and chemotherapy ($P < .001$).[37] In a preliminary report of the Scottish trials examining the use of adjuvant systemic therapy in patients treated with CS with or without RT, patients with ER-negative cancers were treated with adjuvant CMF chemotherapy. With a median follow-up time of about 2.5 years, the crude rate of local–regional recurrence was 25% among patients treated without RT compared with only 4% among patients treated with RT.[337] In a trial conducted in Ontario comparing two different adjuvant chemotherapy regimens, the subgroup of patients treated with lumpectomy and a 12-week course of adjuvant chemohormonal therapy without RT had a 32% rate of recurrence in the breast; the rate was 20% among patients who received the same local treatment and a 36-week course of adjuvant multiagent chemotherapy.[338]

Additional evidence suggests that the use of wide excision in patients aged 70 years or older with small tumors is associated with a low risk of local recurrence, particularly when combined with tamoxifen. In a retrospective review of 122 patients treated with wide excision and adjuvant systemic therapy, 23 patients (19%) had a recurrence in the breast at a median follow-up time of 4 years.[339] Most patients older than 50 years of age received tamoxifen. Patients with an extensive intraductal component were excluded, and all patients had negative margins of resection. The rate of recurrence in the breast was related to the size of the tumor and to patient age. There were no local recurrences among the 15 patients with tumors

smaller than 1 cm compared with 17% among the 58 patients with tumors between 1 and 2 cm, and 32% among the 41 patients with tumors between 2 and 5 cm. Only 1 of the 31 patients aged 70 years or older had a recurrence in the breast compared with 40% of patients aged 30 to 39 years, 26% of patients aged 40 to 59, and 11% of patients aged 60 to 69. Similar results were observed in a retrospective study from Canada.[340] Of 97 postmenopausal, node-positive, ER-positive patients treated with wide excision, 53 did not receive RT and 44 did. With a median follow-up time of about 3 years, the 39-month rate of recurrence in the breast was 21% for patients who did not receive RT and 5% for patients who received RT. However, none of the 22 patients aged 70 years or older who did not receive RT developed a recurrence in the breast. In a retrospective study from Oxford, 49 patients aged 70 years or older (or medically frail) were treated with wide excision and tamoxifen; RT was added only if a patient was deemed to be high risk, which included having positive margins or multifocal involvement.[341] The 8-year crude rate of local–regional (breast or axilla) recurrence was 4% for patients with T1 tumors and 32% for patients with T2 or T3 tumors. The corresponding rates for high-risk patients who were treated with RT were 5% and 10%, respectively. In the preliminary report of the Scottish trials examining the use of adjuvant systemic therapy in patients treated with CS alone or with RT, ER-positive patients younger than 70 years were treated with adjuvant tamoxifen. With a median follow-up time of about 2.5 years, the crude rate of local–regional recurrence was 7% among patients who did not get RT compared with 0% among patients treated with RT.[337] Further follow-up is needed on this study. The NSABP trial B-21 opened in 1989 and randomized patients with tumors smaller than 1 cm and with negative margins to either RT, tamoxifen, or both. Accrual to this trial, however, was not adequate and the trial was closed prematurely in 1993.

In conclusion, the use of breast irradiation after CS is associated with a large reduction in the rate of local recurrence. It is not yet fully established whether RT after CS is associated with a small improvement in survival. The available data from the randomized trials do not show a survival benefit; however, none of the available trials has the statistical power to eliminate a small survival difference with confidence. If one assumes that RT is associated only with an improvement in local control, it is unclear how to balance this improvement against the risk of complications and the cost and inconvenience of such treatment. Although the cost, inconvenience, and complications are not trivial, a number of arguments are in favor of RT. RT is useful to minimize the risk of mastectomy and to increase the recurrence-free interval. Any recurrence after primary breast cancer treatment is psychologically devastating, and this is equally so for a recurrence in the treated breast. The rate of complications after breast irradiation is low (but not zero). Finally, there may be subgroups of patients at low risk of local recurrence after CS for whom RT can be safely omitted. The most consistently identified subgroup is patients aged 70 years or older with a T1,

ER-positive tumor treated with wide resection (such as quadrantectomy including negative margins of resection) and adjuvant tamoxifen.

Tamoxifen as Primary Therapy for Elderly Patients

Concerns regarding the morbidity and mortality of conventional surgical therapy for breast cancer in elderly patients with comorbid conditions have resulted in a number of studies examining the efficacy of tamoxifen as a primary treatment. In 1982, two pilot studies were reported of tamoxifen as the sole primary treatment for localized breast cancer. In the study by Preece and others,[342] 67 consecutive patients older than 75 years received tamoxifen, 20 to 40 mg/d. Seventy-three percent of patients had a complete or partial response, although 18% did not achieve maximum response until treated for more than 12 months. In the study by Helleberg and colleagues,[343] responses were observed in 21 of 27 patients (81%) taking tamoxifen (40 mg daily). The mean time to complete response was 14 months. In 15 cases, a complete response by both radiologic and clinical criteria was seen. In a larger study of 100 patients, Allan and coauthors[344] observed complete responses in 39% of patients with a median duration of response of 19 months. Of 14 deaths occurring in this study, only 5 were because of breast carcinoma. Auclerc and colleagues[345] reported a median duration of response of 35 months in their group of patients treated with tamoxifen and found that more than half of the deaths in the series were due to causes other than breast cancer. Overall, the reported rates of complete response range from 10% to 55% with a failure of response or progression of disease occurring in 19% to 58% of cases.

Studies of the value of hormone receptor levels in predicting response to primary tamoxifen therapy are surprisingly limited and yield conflicting results. Fondraine and associates[346] did not find a relation between ER or progesterone receptor status and tumor response in the 19 patients for whom these data were available. In contrast, Gaskell and coworkers[347] observed a 26% response rate and no instances of tumor progression in 31 patients whose tumors showed greater than 25% of cells staining for the ER by immunocytochemical study, compared with no responses and a 100% progression rate in 9 patients in whom no staining was observed. Further studies on larger numbers of patients are needed to clarify this point.

Three randomized trials have been reported comparing treatment with tamoxifen alone to some form of surgical therapy in elderly patients with operable breast cancer. Gazet and others[348] randomly assigned 200 patients aged 70 years or older to undergo treatment with tamoxifen, 10 mg/d, or surgical resection without systemic therapy. Of the 100 patients in the surgery arm, 64 were treated with local excision of the tumor (lumpectomy) alone. At a median follow-up of 6 years, no difference in survival was observed between the two groups. However, isolated local progression of disease occurred in 56 of the patients in the tamoxifen arm compared with 36 of the patients in the surgery arm. Twenty-one of the patients in the tamoxifen arm underwent surgical salvage and have remained free of disease. The surgical arm of this study does not represent the best available conventional therapy because RT was not used in the lumpectomy group and no systemic therapy was given. Despite this, local control was superior in surgically treated patients than in those treated with tamoxifen alone.

In a larger study, Bates and coauthors[349] randomly assigned 381 patients aged 70 and older to receive tamoxifen, 40 mg/d, or to undergo optimal surgery combined with tamoxifen. Optimal surgery was either wide excision alone or mastectomy at the discretion of the surgeon. At a median follow-up of 34 months, 64 local recurrences (35%) were seen in the tamoxifen group compared with 21 (13%) in the surgery group. Of the 21 local recurrences in the surgical patients, only 1 occurred after mastectomy. Again, however, no difference in breast cancer mortality was observed between the two treatment groups. Quality of life was compared for the two groups at a mean of 1 year after diagnosis. The groups were well matched for demographic characteristics and approximately 50% of patients in each group lived alone. No differences were observed between treatment groups in the incidence of physical malaise, anxiety, social dysfunction, or depression.

The third randomized trial assigned 135 patients aged 70 years or older to receive tamoxifen, 40 mg/d, or to undergo wedge mastectomy, defined as the removal of the pendulous portion of the breast at its base without creating skin flaps or performing an axillary dissection. Sixty-seven percent of the patients in the tamoxifen group achieved a response, but at 5 years, 40 patients (59%) had local or regional progression of disease, primarily in the breast. Only 20 local or regional recurrences were seen in the surgery group and half of these occurred in untreated axillary nodes. Although local control in the surgery patients was significantly better ($P < .001$) compared with the tamoxifen patients, no difference in survival was noted between the two groups at a mean follow-up of 65 months. However, the high rate of local or regional recurrence in the patients treated with tamoxifen led the authors to conclude that in elderly patients able to tolerate surgery, mastectomy should be done to maintain local control.

The three randomized trials of patients with operable breast cancer comparing treatment with tamoxifen alone to surgery with or without tamoxifen fail to demonstrate a survival advantage in favor of surgery. Although the operative procedures used do not represent the best available therapy, significant improvements in local control were seen in the patients treated with surgery in all three studies. There are additional reasons to use more standard treatment in elderly patients if possible. The use of primary tamoxifen requires close follow-up for a number of years to monitor its response. Although the response rates to primary tamoxifen are high, there is a high likelihood of local progression of disease with long-term follow-up requiring surgical salvage. Mastectomy is well tolerated in elderly patients, with 30-day operative mortality rates of less than 2% reported in most studies.[350] Alternatively, no increase has been reported in the incidence of radiation side effects in elderly patients compared with younger patients treated with RT after tumor excision.[351,352] The need to use RT after CS has already been discussed. Because mastectomy or lumpectomy and RT are well tolerated by most elderly patients and provide a high level of local tumor control, there is no reason to substitute tamoxifen as a routine treatment. However, for the elderly patient with a limited life-span and a high risk of operative mortality because of comorbid conditions, tamoxifen is a reasonable alternative as a primary therapy.

Technique and Complications of Breast-Conserving Surgery

The goal of breast-conserving surgery is to minimize the risk of local recurrence while leaving the patient with a cosmetically acceptable breast. The most common form of breast-conserving surgery used in the United States is referred to as *lumpectomy*. The surgical technique of lumpectomy differs from that used for mastectomy in that lumpectomy is not a en bloc cancer operation. Quadrantectomy is another type of breast-conserving surgery that is designed to remove an anatomic segment of breast tissue and frequently includes removal of the overlying skin and underlying pectoral fascia. The rationale and results of this procedure are discussed in detail elsewhere in this chapter. Because excision of a large amount of breast tissue is the major factor responsible for a poor cosmetic outcome after breast-conserving treatment,[62,63,72] lumpectomy is considered the appropriate initial surgical approach in the United States. Other surgical factors that influence the cosmetic appearance are the size and placement of the incision, the management of the lumpectomy cavity, and the extent of axillary dissection.

A number of technical aspects of lumpectomy are worth emphasizing. In general, the incision should be placed directly over the area of the tumor. This is true even when a biopsy is performed for a mammographically detected lesion. Whereas tunneling for short distances is acceptable to avoid incisions in areas of the breast that may be exposed, extensive tunneling can make it difficult to assess the extent of tumor and to obtain meticulous hemostasis. In the upper part of the breast, incisions should be curvilinear or transverse and follow the natural skin creases (Langer lines) of the breast. In the lower part of the breast, the choice of a curvilinear or radial incision depends on the contour of the patient's breast, the distance from the skin to the tumor, and the amount of breast tissue to be resected. It is not necessary to remove skin (except for very superficial tumors) or to remove needle tracks from core needle biopsies or fine-needle aspirations.[353] In particular, skin removed with a curvilinear incision in the inferior breast distorts the breast contour and should be avoided.[354] Preservation of the subcutaneous fat and the avoidance of thin skin flaps is also important in maintaining normal

breast contour.[154] Raising flaps is necessary only to allow access to the tumor; tumors located deep within the breast parenchyma should be approached by incising the breast tissue superficial to the tumor without raising flaps. Meticulous hemostasis is important, because a large hematoma distorts the appearance of the breast and makes reexcision and follow-up evaluation more difficult. The presence of a postbiopsy hematoma, however, is not a contraindication to breast-conserving treatment. It is best to avoid reapproximation of the breast tissue, especially in the upper part of the breast. Reapproximation of the breast tissue can result in distortion of the breast contour, which may not be apparent with the patient supine on the operating table. The best cosmetic results usually are obtained by allowing the lumpectomy cavity to fill in with serum and fibrin. For this reason as well, drainage of the lumpectomy cavity should be avoided. Finally, the incision should be closed with a subcuticular suture to avoid cross hatching of the skin.

A critical step in lumpectomy is the evaluation of the completeness of excision of the tumor. Gross assessment of tumor removal is important, but histologic verification of margin status must also be obtained. To allow adequate histologic evaluation, the specimen should be removed as a single piece of tissue and should not be transected unless the pathologist is present. The use of marking sutures to orient the specimen for the pathologist allows reporting of the status of individual margins. This helps to avoid reexcision of large amounts of normal breast tissue if a single margin is found to be positive. Gross inspection of the specimen in the operating room allows identification of positive or close margins, facilitating immediate reexcision. Frozen-section histologic study is sometimes useful to evaluate grossly suspicious areas, but the routine use of frozen sections to evaluate grossly normal margins is of doubtful value, because it represents a minimal sampling that does not preclude the presence of tumor on permanent section. Intraoperative touch-preparation cytologic study may be useful for margin assessment if a cytologist experienced in this technique is available.[355,356] The ideal amount of grossly normal breast tissue around the tumor that should be resected as part of a lumpectomy is uncertain. The resection of 0.5 to 1 cm of grossly normal breast tissue resulted in histologically negative margins in 95% of 239 patients in the experience at the University of Chicago.[357] Larger resections may be necessary for invasive ductal carcinomas with an extensive intraductal component[73,101,120] and for infiltrating lobular carcinomas.[358]

When axillary dissection is performed as part of breast-conserving surgery, a separate incision should be used, except in patients with tumors high in the tail of the breast. A curvilinear incision at the edge of the hair-bearing axillary skin provides the best cosmetic result. The incision should not extend anterior to the fold of the pectoralis major or posterior to the latissimus dorsi. Incision across these muscles does not improve access to the apex of the axilla and worsens the cosmetic result. In patients with a narrow axilla, a U-shaped incision rather than a transverse one should be employed.

INDICATIONS FOR REEXCISION

The primary indications for a reexcision are positive or unknown histologic margins of resection on the initial excision. Several studies have demonstrated residual carcinoma in about half of cases when reexcision is performed for positive or unknown margins,[101,357,359] with little difference in the incidence between those patients with positive and those with unknown margins (Table 17.1-18). Schmidt-Ullrich and coauthors[360] observed that the likelihood of residual carcinoma in a reexcision specimen done for positive or unknown margins was related to the histologic type of the primary tumor. Sixty-seven percent of invasive tumors with associated DCIS had residual disease compared with 50% of infiltrating lobular carcinomas and only 35% of cases with infiltrating ductal carcinoma without associated DCIS. Schnitt and others[101] also found that invasive ductal carcinomas with an EIC predicted a greater likelihood of residual tumor in reexcisions (88% for EIC-positive versus 48% for EIC-negative, $P = .002$).

The question of what is an acceptable margin status for a lumpectomy has not been resolved. Remember when evaluating this issue that even when margins are determined to be negative, residual cancer is present in a significant number of mastectomy specimens.[21,361,362] As shown in Table 17.1-4, a randomized trial by Veronesi and associates[63,73] comparing quadrantectomy with lumpectomy, both combined with RT (Milan II), demonstrated that removal of a larger margin of grossly normal breast tissue reduces the rate of local recurrence, but also decreases the cosmetic outcome. Table 17.1-6 shows reported studies on the incidence of local recurrence in relation to the histologic status of the margins. Within the lumpectomy group in the Milan II trial, there was a 17.4% incidence rate of local recurrence in patients with histologically positive margins compared with a 8.6% incidence rate with negative margins.[73] Similar findings were described by others.[115,117,363] In contrast, Solin and colleagues[116] and Schmidt-Ullrich and coauthors[360] observed no differences in local recurrence among patients with microscopically positive, negative, close, or unknown margins. However, in both of these studies, radiation doses were adjusted based on margin status. In the Solin report,[116] patients with positive margins received a median of 65 Gy compared with 60 Gy in patients with negative margins, and in the Schmidt-Ullrich report,[360] patients with positive margins received a boost of 20 Gy compared with a 10-Gy boost for patients with negative margins. These studies suggest, but do not establish, that increased radiation doses (above 60 Gy) are important in patients with positive margins. A study to test this formally is under way by the EORTC. Several studies have suggested that local recurrence rates are higher in patients with an invasive ductal carcinoma that contains an extensive intraductal component.[52,92] However, these studies were done at a time when the margins of resection were not routinely evaluated. Patients with an invasive ductal carcinoma that contains an extensive intraductal component are more likely to have positive margins after lumpectomy.[117] However, when patients with EIC-positive cancers undergo sufficient breast resection to obtain negative margins of resection, local recurrence rates are low.[115,117,331,364] Thus, the presence of an extensive intraductal component per se should not be a contraindication to breast-conserving treatment.

Reexcision should be undertaken in patients with unknown margins and in patients with gross tumor or extensive amounts of microscopic cancer at the margins of resection. The need for reexcision in patients with focal microscopic involvement at the margin of resection is less clear. Whether reexcision or an increased dose of radiation is the optimal method of maintaining local control in this circumstance requires further evaluation. Cases should be assessed on an individual basis to determine whether reexcision or an increased radiation dose will have a less adverse impact on the cosmetic outcome. In addition to margin status, histologic features of the primary tumor should be considered in the decision for reexcision. In patients with an EIC-positive cancer or an infiltrating lobular carcinoma,[358,365,366] reexcision should be strongly considered in patients with focally positive or even close margins of resection.

No consensus exists on the best technique for reexcision. When reexcision is done within 1 to 2 weeks of the biopsy, it is not usually possible to reexcise an entire biopsy cavity as a single specimen without sacrificing large amounts of breast tissue, and this technique should be attempted only for small biopsy cavities in patients with moderate- to large-sized breasts. My technique of reexcision (M.M.) in most cases is to reexcise each of the walls of the biopsy cavity separately. If the initial specimen was

TABLE 17.1-18

Finding of Residual Cancer on Reexcision in Relation to the Microscopic Margins of Resection on the Initial Specimen

Investigators	Cases With Positive Margins on 1st Excision	Incidence of Residual Cancer on Reexcision (%)	Cases with Unknown Margins on 1st Excision	Incidence of Residual Cancer on Reexcision (%)
Schnitt et al[101]	29	69	33	64
Gwin et al[359]	54	65	100	45
Kearney & Morrow[357]	42	45	48	42

marked with orienting sutures, reexcision can be limited to the involved margins. Otherwise, thin pieces of tissue are shaved off each wall of the biopsy cavity and sent as separate specimens, with the new margin surface marked for the pathologist. When longer intervals have elapsed between the biopsy and the time of reexcision, contraction of the biopsy cavity may allow excision of the entire cavity as a single specimen without sacrificing excessive amounts of breast tissue. The presence of residual tumor in the reexcision is not a contraindication to breast-conserving treatment. The status of the final margin should be used to determine the patient's suitability for breast-conserving treatment. Kearney and Morrow[357] found that 86 of 90 patients undergoing reexcision for positive or unknown margins were satisfactory candidates for breast-conserving treatment.

There are relatively few complications of breast-conserving surgery. Lumpectomy by itself can be performed as an outpatient procedure under local anesthesia with supplemental sedation as needed. Wound infection is infrequent, although rates of infection may be increased when reexcision is performed. The late occurrence of breast abscess after breast-conserving treatment has been reported, and I (M.M.) have observed four such cases in 420 patients. Keidan and coworkers[367] noticed a 6% incidence of delayed breast abscess in 112 patients undergoing lumpectomy and RT. The median time to abscess development was 5 months (range, 1.5 to 8 months). The use of prophylactic antibiotics, postoperative chemotherapy, the surgeon involved, and whether the excision was primary or secondary did not correlate with abscess formation. The only factor found to correlate with abscess formation was larger size of the lumpectomy specimen. Necrosis of marginally viable fat in the lumpectomy site may be the cause of this problem. Cellulitis of the breast occurring at a median of 4 months after breast-conserving therapy also has been reported in about 3% of cases.[368] Altered lymphatic drainage in the breast after axillary dissection and breast irradiation may be an etiologic factor.

Technique and Complications of Mastectomy

The term *modified radical mastectomy* encompasses several different operative procedures, depending on the management of the pectoral nerves, the extent of the axillary dissection, and whether the pectoralis minor muscle is preserved, removed, or divided. All of the operations share the complete removal of the breast tissue, the underlying fascia of the pectoralis major muscle, and the removal of some of the axillary lymph nodes. The modified radical mastectomy initially described by Patey and Dysin[369] is identical to the radical mastectomy except that the pectoralis major muscle and the lateral pectoral nerve are preserved. In this operation, the pectoralis minor muscle is removed and the medial pectoral nerve is sacrificed. In contrast, the modified radical mastectomy popularized by

Auchincloss[370] preserves the pectoralis minor and the pectoral nerves. Other modifications involving splitting the pectoralis major[371,372] or dividing the tendon of the pectoralis major[373] to improve access to the apex of the axilla have also been described.

Modified radical mastectomy is performed through an elliptical transverse incision, which encompasses the nipple–areolar complex and the biopsy scar if an open biopsy has been performed. The abandonment of the Halstedian concepts of en bloc surgery also has led to abandonment of the idea that large (4 cm) areas of skin adjacent to the tumor must be excised. The nipple–areolar complex and the biopsy incision must be removed, but the remainder of the skin of the breast can be preserved in early-stage breast cancer if needed for breast reconstruction. With a skin-sparing procedure, additional exposure to allow complete excision of the breast tissue is achieved by incision rather than excision of the skin. Skin flaps are created in the plane between the subcutaneous fat and the underlying breast tissue. Because of the variability in the amount of subcutaneous fat, no single thickness is appropriate for all skin flaps. To encompass all breast tissue, the dissection should extend superiorly to the inferior border of the clavicle, medially to the lateral border of the sternum, inferiorly to the superior extent of the rectus sheath, and laterally to the latissimus dorsi muscle. After skin flaps have been raised, the breast is taken off the chest wall in a superior-to-inferior direction, with the fascia of the pectoralis major muscle as the posterior margin of the specimen. The fascia of the pectoralis major muscle was initially thought to represent an anatomic barrier to the spread of breast cancer. However, the demonstration that lymphatics from the breast penetrate this fascia renders this concept invalid,[4] and the fascia can safely be preserved when needed for breast reconstruction. In general, however, excision posterior to the fascia provides a convenient plane for ensuring removal of most of the breast tissue. At this point, with the breast attached inferiorly and laterally, axillary dissection is carried out. At the conclusion of the procedure, closed suction drains are placed in the apex of the axilla and beneath the inferior skin flap. Skin closure is accomplished with a subcuticular suture. Pressure dressings are not needed with suction drains, and may compromise the blood supply to marginally viable skin flaps.

The term *total mastectomy* refers to the removal of the entire breast, with the same limits of dissection as described for the modified radical mastectomy. Care must be taken to remove the axillary tail of Spence, so identification of the latissimus dorsi muscle is important. Both pectoral muscles and the axillary nodes are preserved. Because of the importance of axillary dissection as a staging procedure, total mastectomy has not been considered a standard approach to the management of infiltrating carcinomas. The indications for total mastectomy include patients with DCIS who elect mastectomy, patients undergoing prophylactic surgery to prevent the development of breast cancer, patients who develop a recurrence in the breast after breast-conserving treatment that had included an axillary dissection, and, on occasion, patients with metastatic disease undergoing toilet mastectomy for local control of the primary tumor.

Mastectomy is an extremely safe operative procedure. A review of the Surveillance, Epidemiology, and End Results (SEER) data for 10,056 patients treated between 1967 and 1973 noted a 30-day operative mortality rate of 0.35%, and even for patients older than 75 years, the 30-day operative mortality rate was 0.87%.[374] For patients with serious comorbid conditions who are at an unacceptably high risk for general anesthesia, mastectomy can be done using a combination of local anesthesia, intercostal blocks, and intravenous sedation.

The reported incidence rate of wound infection with mastectomy ranges from 6% to 14%.[375,376] Infections in the early postoperative period tend to present as cellulitis, whereas those seen later tend to present as abscess formation. The most common organisms are streptococcus or *Staphylococcus aureus*.[376] Factors that predispose to infection include the use of a two-step procedure (ie, open biopsy preceding mastectomy) and prolonged suction catheter drainage.[376] Beatty and others[377] observed an 8% incidence rate of wound infection in patients undergoing mastectomy, with a 5% incidence rate for patients undergoing biopsy and mastectomy as a single procedure compared with a 12% rate of infection for patients undergoing a two-step procedure. Platt and associates[378,379] analyzed the effect of a single dose of antibiotics (86% cephalosporin) on wound infection rates after breast surgery. Their study included 2587 breast operations, including 606 that were part of a randomized trial of antibiotic prophylaxis. Forty-six percent of the operations were mastectomies, 41% lumpectomies, 10% reduction mammoplasties, and 4% axillary node dissections. Wound infection was defined as a wound with purulent drainage, a wound that was opened, or a wound with erythema and drainage. Because erythema alone was not considered to be infection, the incidence of infections in the mastectomy group might have been underestimated. The overall incidence rate of infection was 3.7%. After adjustment for type and duration of procedure, the relative risk of infection in the group receiving prophylaxis was .62, a 38% reduction in the risk of infection (*P* = .03). However, because the overall incidence of infection in these patients was so low, the cost effectiveness of routine antibiotic prophylaxis for all patients undergoing mastectomy has not been established. A selective policy of antibiotic administration to high-risk patients (eg, prior biopsy, anticipation of long operating time) seems to be most appropriate.

Necrosis of the skin flaps is a relatively uncommon problem today, but was reported in 8% to 60% of cases, particularly in earlier series of patients undergoing radical mastectomy.[380,381] Chilson and coworkers[382] reported an 18% incidence rate in 351 patients treated between 1983 and 1990. Factors associated with skin-flap necrosis include denuding the subcutaneous fat from the flaps, closure under tension, infection, and occlusive pressure dressings.[375,376] Vertical incisions, rarely employed today, significantly increase the risk of flap necrosis.[383] Most of these factors are avoidable. Skin incisions should be planned to allow tension-free closure, and if tension is noticed, full-

thickness flaps may be raised onto the abdominal wall and above the clavicle. Pressure dressings are not necessary when suction drains are used, and suspected cellulitis should be promptly treated with antibiotics. If skin necrosis develops at the suture line it can usually be managed with conservative debridement after demarcation and closure by secondary intention.

Seroma formation occurs in 100% of patients after mastectomy and should be considered a side effect, rather than a complication, of the procedure. In a prospective randomized trial, Petrek and coworkers[218] demonstrated that extensive axillary node involvement was the greatest predictor of prolonged lymphatic drainage after mastectomy, followed by obesity and the performance of a two-step procedure. Prolonged seroma formation, in addition to requiring multiple physician visits, may be associated with delayed wound healing and an increased risk of infection.[375,376,380] Seroma formation can be minimized by leaving drains in place until their combined output is less than 40 mL/24 h, rather than arbitrarily removing them on a predetermined day. Fluid collections should be managed by aspiration every other day to seal the skin flaps against the chest wall. Chilson and associates[382] have reported on the use of tacking sutures to obliterate the axillary dead space and attach the skin flaps to the pectoral muscle. In a retrospective review of 351 cases, a decrease (39% versus 25%) in seroma formation was noticed in patients having the tacking procedure. However, a number of other variables that could influence these results were not evaluated in this study, making it difficult to conclude that flap-tacking is of value.

Phantom breast syndrome was first recognized by Ambrose Parè.[384] As many as 50% of patients who undergo mastectomy experience some sensation of a residual breast after mastectomy. The most common complaint is pain, but itching, nipple sensation, erotic sensations, and premenstrual-type breast soreness also are described. Kroner and colleagues[385] prospectively evaluated a group of patients 3 weeks, 1 year, and 6 years after mastectomy. Phantom pain was reported in 13% of patients at 3 weeks, and nonpainful phantom sensations were present in 15%. At 1 year, these incidences were 13% and 12%, respectively; at 6 years, they were 17% and 12%, respectively. This suggests that symptoms are relatively constant over time. The cause of this syndrome is unknown. However, patient education before mastectomy outlining the possible changes in chest wall sensation and the possibility of phantom breast syndrome may help to relieve patient anxiety if symptoms develop.

ONCOLOGIC CONSIDERATIONS IN IMMEDIATE RECONSTRUCTION

The switch from radical mastectomy to modified radical mastectomy and advances in plastic surgical technique have made immediate breast reconstruction an option for most patients who undergo mastectomy. The technical aspects of immediate reconstruction are discussed in detail in Chapter 19. This discussion considers the impact of immediate reconstruction on breast cancer therapy and its outcome. Concerns about immediate reconstruction have included the potential for the following: (1) an increased incidence of local failure, (2) a delay in the diagnosis of local failure, and (3) a delay in the administration of adjuvant chemotherapy because of wound healing problems.

There have been no prospective randomized trials comparing patients undergoing immediate reconstruction with patients undergoing mastectomy alone. A number of retrospective studies have assessed the incidence of local failure in patients undergoing breast reconstruction in comparison with patients treated by mastectomy alone. Webster and coworkers[386] compared 85 patients undergoing immediate reconstruction using a variety of techniques with 85 controls treated with mastectomy alone who were matched for age, stage, number of involved nodes, and ER status. No differences in the incidence of local or distant recurrence were seen at 30 months. Johnson and others[387] reported a 6% incidence of local failure in 118 patients treated with mastectomy and immediate reconstruction, and 5-year survival rates for reconstructed patients also did not differ from those of historical controls treated by mastectomy alone at the same institution. Petit and colleagues[388] compared 146 patients treated with both immediate and delayed silicone-gel implant reconstruction with a control group of patients treated with mastectomy alone. The groups were matched for age, year of diagnosis, stage, histologic tumor type and grade, and nodal status. The 10-year rate of local recurrence was 8% for the reconstructed patients and 15% for the patients having mastectomy alone. Kroll and others[389] analyzed 87 patients having 100 reconstructions who were followed a mean of 23 months to determine the impact of skin preservation on the rate of local failure. The nipple–areolar complex and the biopsy scar, if present, were removed, but the remaining skin of the breast was preserved. Two patients developed local recurrences, one of which was associated with widespread metastases. This low rate of local recurrence is consistent with the observation that the extent of skin excision is not a major determinant of the risk of chest wall recurrence after mastectomy alone.[390] Thus, the available data do not indicate a higher risk of local failure in patients undergoing immediate reconstruction, although it is possibly subject to selection bias. Concerns that a breast reconstruction may prevent the detection of local recurrence also are not confirmed by the available data. Noone and coworkers[391] reported on 306 patients who had immediate reconstruction and were followed a mean of 6.4 years. Local recurrence as the first site of treatment failure occurred in 5.2% of the group. Fourteen of the 16 isolated local recurrences were in the skin or subcutaneous fat, and 4 involved the pectoral muscle superficial to the implant. Eberlein and others[392] also saw no delay in the detection of local recurrence in a study of 216 patients undergoing mastectomy and immediate reconstruction. Thirty-four percent of the patients in this study received chemotherapy, and no delay in the administration of chemotherapy because of complications of reconstruction was observed, a finding also reported by Noone and others.[393]

In summary, immediate breast reconstruction has not been shown to increase the incidence of local failure or impede the detection of local recurrence. In the hands of an experienced reconstructive surgeon, the incidence of complications associated with the procedure is low (see Chap. 19), and the need for postoperative systemic therapy should not be considered a contraindication to immediate reconstruction. In patients with locally advanced breast cancer or clinically positive nodes, where there is a high likelihood that postoperative chest wall RT will be administered, it may be prudent to delay reconstruction because RT has been observed to increase the risk of implant loss and capsular contracture[394] and may result in fat necrosis after reconstruction with autologous tissue.

Technique of Radiation Therapy

Radiation therapy after breast-conserving surgery typically consists of tangential irradiation of the whole breast designed to minimize lung and heart exposure using supervoltage equipment and an isocentric technique in which the deep edges of fields are co-planar. The dose to the whole breast should be in the range of 45 to 50 Gy (delivered in 4.5 to 5 weeks), because higher doses cause significant breast retraction and fibrosis.[60]

There has been interest in identifying a shorter (and hence less expensive) fractionation schedule than 45 to 50 Gy given in 1.8- to 2-Gy fractions that provides a comparable rate of local tumor control, cosmetic outcome, and risk of complications. Preliminary data from the British Columbia Cancer Agency suggest that 44 Gy given in 16 fractions might achieve this goal (Olivotto I, unpublished data, 1994). A clinical trial was performed in the United Kingdom between 1986 and 1992 in which 719 patients with T1-2, N0-1, M0 carcinoma of the breast were randomized after local excision to one of three fractionation schedules delivered over 5 weeks: 50 Gy in 25 fractions, 42.9 Gy in 13 fractions, and 39 Gy in 13 fractions. Preliminary results suggested that the probability of having a late tissue response was similar for 50 Gy in 25 fractions and 42.9 Gy in 13 fractions, and both were greater than for 39 Gy in 13 fractions.[396] Further evaluation of these investigations is required before firm conclusions are possible.

The patient set-up should be accurately reproduced on a daily basis. A system for reproducible immobilization of the patient can be achieved by the use of a commercially available arm board or by use of a plaster or styrofoam cast that uniformly positions the patient's head and arm. At the JCRT, patients are treated in the supine position with both arms up. Occasionally, an angle board is needed for patients with a steep sternal angle. For patients with large or pendulous breasts, netting is used for immobilization. Others have described other methods for immobilization in this situation, including the use of a polyvinyl-chloride tube formed into a ring around the breast.[397] If the two-field tangential technique is used, the arms can be brought up as high as comfortably possible to allow full coverage of the superior portion of the breast. If a three-field technique is used, the arm position should be lower (slightly higher than perpendicular to the patient's body) to minimize skin folds in the supraclavicular area.

In setting up the tangential fields, some distance should be allowed for penumbra and daily variation in patient set-up. About a 2-cm margin should be given anteriorly above the highest point of the breast and 1 to 1.5 cm allowed for the inferior, superior, medial, and lateral borders. Typically, the lateral border is at the mid-axillary line, the medial border is at midline and the superior border is at the lower portion of the head of the clavicle. To help ensure consistency of set-up on a daily basis, small permanent skin marks (tattoos) are placed at field edges at the time of simulation. At the JCRT, tattoos are placed at the superior, central-axis, and inferior entrance points of the medial field and the central-axis and inferior entrance points of the lateral field. Photographs of the patient in the treatment position also are taken for documentation and to aid in set-up. Even more precise and reproducible set-ups may be achieved using on-line electronic portal imaging devices.[398]

One important consideration in breast irradiation is minimizing the risk of radiation pneumonitis. It is important to make the deep edges of the tangential fields co-planar. At the time of simulation, it is possible to estimate the amount of lung irradiated by the tangential fields using the demagnified perpendicular distance from the posterior field edge to the posterior part of the anterior chest wall at the center of the field (referred to as the central lung distance [CLD]).[399] A CLD of 1.5 cm predicts that about 6% of the ipsilateral lung is treated, a CLD of 2.5 cm about 16%, and a CLD of 3.5 cm about 26%. Firm guidelines for tolerable lung volumes to be irradiated have not been established. At the JCRT, the CLD is generally less than 3.0 cm.

Another important technical aspect of breast irradiation is achieving dose homogeneity within the target volume. At a minimum, the dose distribution should be calculated through the plane of the central axis and inhomogeneity should not be greater than 10%. For nearly all patients, this requires the use of wedges as tissue compensators. In patients younger than 45 years, it is generally preferable to use a single lateral wedge and to avoid the use of a beam splitter to minimize the dose to the opposite breast.[400] Homogeneity of radiation dose, particularly when viewed in three dimensions, is also influenced by photon energy.[77,400,401] The greater the energy, the better the homogeneity, but at the expense of decreased dose to the skin of the breast. For most patients, 6-MV irradiation is the best compromise in terms of homogeneity and skin dose. Cobalt-60 and 4 MV are acceptable for patients with small chests. In patients with large separations, there is experience using 8-MV irradiation (without bolus) without an increase in skin recurrences (JCRT, unpublished data).

A number of different systems have been described for simulating a patient's treatment.[83,402-405] Most of these systems have used a breast bridge to measure the separation and the angle from horizontal of the line that connects the medial and lateral entrance points. However, a system has been described that uses the more accurate capabilities available on the simulator to achieve this.[406] Using any of these systems, the simulation should include a careful visual inspection of the tangential fields to ensure coverage of all breast tissue, particularly when the primary tumor is located peripherally in the breast.

Computed tomographic scanning used in conjunction with simulation has demonstrated that dose distributions in planes off the central axis may be different from the distribution in the plane through the central axis. In one study using computed tomography–based simulation for 5.8-MV photon irradiation, dose inhomogeneity off the central axis was typically ±20%, even though the dose inhomogeneity through the central axis was less than 10%.[407] This is because of significant alteration in the anatomy of the breast and irradiation geometry as one examines planes superior and inferior to the plane of the central axis. The highest dose inhomogeneity is typically seen at the inferior margin of the breast where the entrance–exit distance of the two beams is significantly shorter than for the central axis.[77,401] The use of computed tomographic scanning also allows for more accurate dose distribution by correcting for the actual lung density. Correcting for lung density increases the dose in the lung and the "hot spots" on either side of the lung. This increase varies between 3% and 25% depending on the photon energy, lung density, and length of lung traversed.[77,400] Routine three-dimensional treatment planning, however, would necessitate a three-dimensional dose-calculation algorithm with the use of lung density corrections and a system to fabricate three-dimensional compensators. Such systems are not widely used because of their expense and their lack of demonstrated clinical advantage.

The location at which the dose is prescribed (normalization point) varies from institution to institution. For example, the NSABP guidelines for RT call for prescribing the dose at a point two thirds of the distance between the skin and the base of the tangential fields at the midseparation. At other institutions, the dose is normalized to an isodose line identified by the physician that encompasses the target volume. At the JCRT, the normalization point is 1.5 cm from the deep edges of the tangential fields along the line that is perpendicular to this plane and extends through the isocenter. This point was picked based on a phantom study that showed that the points 1 cm away from this reference point generally varied by less than 1%.[77] This normalization point agrees with that selected by Fraass and others[400] through a different analysis.

Controversy exists about the need for a supplemental dose of irradiation (boost) to the primary site. The usefulness of a boost should be considered in relation to the extent of surgical resection, the proximity of cancer cells to the inked margins of resection, and the histologic characteristics of the cancer. It is likely that a boost is more important after lumpectomy than after wide excision or quadrantectomy. There are several rationales for the use of a boost in patients treated with limited breast surgery. Most local recurrences are at or near the primary site and would be encompassed in a boost field. A histologic study of mastectomy specimens has shown that cancer cells are commonly found in the breast after a simulated lumpectomy, and these cancer cells are primarily located in the breast tissue surrounding the primary tumor.[21] Furthermore, the morbidity of a boost of moderate size and dose is small whether delivered by electron beam or interstitial implantation.[72] As discussed earlier in this chapter, an EORTC randomized clinical trial is being performed to address this issue. Given that breast resections are typically limited at the JCRT, an electron beam is used in most patients to deliver an additional 16 Gy (specified at the 80% isodose) in eight fractions. The reproducibility of the electron beam fields is aided by photographs of the set-up and by a clear film template on which the field borders are drawn and landmarks and tattoos are noted. The field typically measures 8 × 8 cm and encompasses the region of resection with a margin of several centimeters as determined by a review of the surgeon's and patient's description of the location of the primary, the presenting mammogram, and the location of the healing ridge in the breast. (In many patients, the location of the scar is *not* a good indication of the location of the tumor bed.) Because the involvement of the cancer in the breast tends to be segmental, the boost is typically directed at the involved quadrant and commonly includes the nipple. The electron energy is selected based on the thickness of the breast tissue from the skin surface to the anterior chest wall as determined by ultrasonography. The energies chosen are typically in the range of 7 to 12 MeV. Other institutions use different techniques for localizing the tumor bed. At many institutions, the surgeon places opaque clips at the margins of the tumor bed,[408,409] whereas at others ultrasonography[410,411] or computed tomographic scans[412] are used.

It is likely that a boost is not required in all patients. This is suggested by the acceptably low rate of local recurrence seen in the NSABP B-06 trial among patients with negative margins treated to a whole breast dose of 50 Gy without a boost to the primary site.[37] Based on this, some institutions routinely do not use a boost in patients with negative margins of resection. At other institutions, the boost is omitted or the boost dose is reduced in patients who undergo a reexcision that shows no residual cancer. The most favorable subgroup consists of patients with an EIC-negative and LVI-negative cancer whose reexcision is negative and who start RT within 8 weeks of the reexcision. In such patients, it is reasonable either to treat the whole breast with 44 to 46 Gy and use a reduced boost dose or to treat the whole breast to 50 Gy.

Another area of controversy concerns the irradiation of the axillary, supraclavicular, and IMN areas. As previously discussed, a survival benefit for such treatment has not been established. When additional information becomes available regarding the possible survival benefit of postmastectomy RT, this issue may need to be reconsidered. This issue must be considered in relation to the use and extent of axillary dissection and the use of adjuvant systemic therapy to assess the risks and benefits of such treatment for an individual patient (see Complications of Radiation Therapy). Also, as previously discussed, the use of axillary dissection is being reevaluated in light of the more general use of systemic therapy, even in node-negative patients. Axillary dissection is still indicated in patients with clinically suspicious nodes because the dose of RT required to control such nodes is considerably higher than that required to control subclinical involvement and is associated with a much greater risk of complications.

Among patients undergoing axillary dissection, the most common procedure is a level I/II dissection, as described in the section on surgery in this chapter. There is still some variation, however, in the extent of the dissection, even when this term is applied. Therefore, when considering nodal irradiation, the radiation oncologist must communicate with the surgeon directly to clarify this. If axillary nodes are histologically negative after a level I/II dissection, the risk of nodal recurrence is low and nodal irradiation is not indicated.[27,205,206,208] Even in patients with one to three positive nodes, the risk of nodal recurrence is still low and nodal irradiation is not usually advised.[205,206] Less settled is the need for axillary-supraclavicular irradiation in patients with four or more positive nodes. The use of a third field reduces the risk of nodal recurrence but is also associated with a small but significant risk of complications. The results of the randomized trials from Milan and the NSABP comparing mastectomy with CS and RT were achieved without nodal irradiation, thus establishing this approach as a reasonable option. Whether some subgroups (eg, patients with greater than 50% of nodes involved or with extensive extracapsular spread) derive more benefit from such treatment is not established, but nodal irradiation is more commonly used in these patients to reduce the risk of local recurrence. Given the limited extent of axillary dissection at the JCRT, a third field is used in patients with four or more positive nodes. If the dissection did not include removal of tissue around the axillary vein (level I dissection), both the axillary and supraclavicular regions are treated. This field is treated to a dose of 45 to 46 Gy specified at a depth of 5 cm. If the dissection did include this tissue, only the supraclavicular region is irradiated. This field is treated to a dose of 45 to 50 Gy specified at a depth of 3 cm. When a third field is added, a treatment plan that assures a good geometric match with the tangential fields is required.[83,402] In patients who do not undergo axillary dissection or who undergo a more limited sampling procedure, a third field is added. In selected patients, it may be possible to include most of the axilla using tangents that are extended superiorly (high tangents).

There are other technical considerations in the use of a third field. The daily set-up is greatly aided by the use of a protractor with pegs placed along the matchline to help visualize that the match is correct on a daily basis. The third field should be angled approximately 10 degrees from the vertical to avoid treating the cervical spinal cord. At the JCRT, the superior border of this field is typically at the superior aspect of the first rib, and an effort is made not to clear skin (flash) in the supraclavicular region. The lateral border is placed at a point two thirds of the mediolateral distance through the humeral head when the intention is to treat the full axilla. The lateral border is placed at the lateral edge of the coracoid process (the insertion of the pectoralis minor) when the intention is to treat only the axillary apex and supraclavicular region. Occasionally, it is necessary to give a dose above 45 to 46 Gy to the axilla. At the JCRT, this additional dose is typically given by an en face axillary boost. The patient is positioned supine and flat on the table with the arm positioned 10 to 20 degrees above perpendicular to the body. The couch, gantry, and collimator are angled to direct the beam from the axilla toward the supraclavicular fossa. The anterior edge of the field should be at the midportion of the pectoralis major muscle. The typical field size is 6×8 cm. The dose is usually prescribed at a depth of 3.5 cm, although this may vary from case to case. Either photons or high-energy electron beam may be used, although the skin dose is higher with electron beam. An alternative method is the posterior axillary boost.[413] This has the disadvantage of traversing more normal tissue than the en face boost, and also of giving additional dose to the pectoralis major. However, the set-up may be easier than for the en face boost. The superior border is just above the clavicle, the inferior border is blocked to match the tangents, the medial border includes 1 to 2 cm of the lung, and the lateral border includes one third of the humeral head. In some situations, the use of opposed anterior and posterior fields may be warranted.

The treatment of IMNs in the context of CS and RT is technically difficult. In addition to the concern of avoiding excessive irradiation of the lung and heart, there is also the difficulty of attempting to match radiation fields along the medial aspect of the breast. It is possible to treat IMNs with an obliquely incident electron beam field and the breast with abutting photon tangential fields.[414,415] However, great technical care is required to avoid an overlap or an underdosage using this technique and it is not commonly performed in the United States. It is also possible to try to include the IMNs using wide tangential fields. Some institutions have used the guideline of putting the medial entrace point for the tangents 3.0 cm across the midline; however, this guideline is limited in its usefulness because of the variability in the position of the IMNs from patient to patient.[416] It is also possible to use computed tomographic data to simulate wide tangents to include the IMNs and to use customized blocks that allow treatment of the superior IMNs (which are most likely to be involved), but shield a large portion of the heart inferiorly.[417] At the JCRT, patients at high risk for IMN involvement undergo a computed tomographic scan before simulation to determine the position of IMNs and the anatomy of the normal tissues. This allows the clinician to judge the additional amount of lung and heart that would be irradiated by the inclusion of the IMNs in the tangential fields. Given the uncertainty of the value of IMN irradiation, the emphasis at the JCRT is placed on avoiding complications. As a result, IMNs are included only if this can be done without excessive irradiation of normal tissues.

Complications of Radiation Therapy

Possible complications of RT include arm edema, brachial plexopathy, decreased arm mobility, soft tissue necrosis, rib fractures, radiation pneumonitis, carcinogenesis (eg, contralateral breast cancer and sarcoma), and radiation-related heart disease. The data on complications after both postoperative RT and RT as part of breast-conserving treatment are presented here. However, the risks of the various complications may be different after these two uses of RT.

The methodology for assessing the risk of a complication varies by the particular complication being assessed. Some complications, such as arm edema, are not otherwise commonly observed and their incidence can be evaluated simply in a cohort of treated patients. Other complications, such as induced cancers, may be difficult to separate from those that occur in the absence of RT. The risk of these complications requires evaluation either within a randomized clinical trial comparing mastectomy and CS and RT or by using epidemiologic techniques within a large population-based registry. If such a complication is uncommon, an increased risk may not be detectable in the available clinical trials, given their relatively small numbers of patients and length of follow-up. The use of epidemiologic techniques typically provides relative risk as the measure of the increased risk for irradiated patients compared to unirradiated patients. However, in clinical medicine, the increased absolute risk is usually more useful in assessing the magnitude of the risk. If the condition is rare, increases in relative risk of even 5 to 10 are still associated with a small absolute number of additional cases. Whenever possible, both relative and absolute risk are provided.

The most frequent complication of RT for breast cancer encountered in the past was arm edema. The issue of arm edema is discussed in greater detail in Chapter 24.7. The etiology of the disorder is poorly understood, but is probably related to obliteration of lymphatics in the axilla by surgery or RT and enhanced by scarring secondary to thrombophlebitis and infection. Bretton and Nelson[418] reported the incidence of arm edema after radical mastectomy from 14 separate series. The incidence rate of arm edema averaged 20% to 25% and was clearly increased with the use of postoperative RT. Precise volumetric measurements of the arm were made for patients in the Stockholm trial for each of three treatment groups (modified radical mastectomy alone, modified radical mastectomy and postoperative RT, and preoperative RT and modified radical mastectomy).[419] RT was delivered to the entire axilla for a total dose of 45 Gy in 5 weeks. In all three treatment groups, some arm edema was observed. Modified radical mastectomy alone resulted in a 2.2% volume increase compared with a volume increase of 4.5% after preoperative RT and 4.8% after postoperative RT. Severe arm edema was uncommon in all treatment groups: 1% of the patients treated with mastectomy alone, 2% of the postoperative RT patients, and 3% of the preoperative RT patients. The risk of arm edema was reviewed in a group of patients treated with CS and RT at the JCRT.[420] The entire axilla was irradiated in most patients during this period. The risk of arm edema was found to be related to the use and extent of axillary surgery. The actuarial risk of arm edema at 6 years was 4% for patients treated without axillary surgery and 13% for patients treated with axillary surgery ($P = .006$). Patients treated with a combination of a full axillary dissection (defined as including a stripping of the axillary vein) and axillary irradiation had a 37% risk of arm edema at 6 years, whereas patients who underwent a lesser axillary dissection and axillary irradiation had only a 7% risk of arm edema ($P < .001$). Arm edema in this series was either mild or moderate with no patient having severe edema. Similar results were reported by Dewar and others[421] from the Institut Gustav-Roussy. The available results indicate that both the extent of axillary surgery and the use of axillary irradiation influence the risk of arm edema. In particular, the use of a full axillary dissection *and* postoperative RT that includes treatment of the axilla significantly increases the risk of arm edema.

One of the possible complications of treatment to the axillary and supraclavicular regions is injury to the brachial plexus. Classic radiation-induced brachial plexopathy is characterized by discomfort in the shoulder and by paresthesias and weakness in the arm and hand and is usually progressive. Typically, there is evidence of soft tissue fibrosis in the supraclavicular and infraclavicular regions. It is sometimes difficult to distinguish radiation-induced plexopathy from plexopathy caused by involvement by cancer, and this is discussed in greater detail in Chapter 23.4. The classic radiation-induced injury is dose related and rarely occurs with doses less than 50 Gy given in 5 weeks.[422,423] In a randomized trial conducted at the Royal Marsden Hospital, the incidence of brachial plexus neuropathy was related to fraction size.[424] Patients who received 56 Gy in 15 fractions to the axilla had a 5.9% probability of brachial plexus injury at 6 years compared with only 1% for patients who received 54 Gy in 30 fractions ($P < .01$). Another form of radiation-related brachial plexus injury called *reversible brachial plexopathy* occurs at doses less than 50 Gy, has a short latency period (median, 4.5 months), and is characterized by transient paresthesias and weakness.[425] Neither of these radiation-induced injuries to the brachial plexus has any recognized therapy.

The updated results from the JCRT regarding the incidence and risk factors for brachial plexopathy are shown in Table 17.1-19.[426] Twenty of the 1624 patients (1.2%) treated between 1968 and 1985 developed brachial plexopathy. The median time to its appearance was 10.5 months (range, 1.5 to 77 months). The median age of patients with plexopathy was 44 years old, which was younger than that of the entire group. In 16 of the patients (80%), the plexopathy was mild and resolved within 1 year. Plexopathy was restricted to patients who were treated with a third radiation field, and was more common with doses above 50 Gy and with the use of adjuvant chemotherapy. Similar findings were observed in a study from Denmark.[427]

The use of postoperative RT can be associated with alterations of soft tissues and bones in the treatment volume. This complication, however, is rare when modern techniques and dose fractionation (2 Gy/d) are used. Studies from both Sweden[419] and Denmark[428] have shown decreased range of movement about the shoulder joint in patients treated with mastectomy, axillary dissection, and postoperative RT compared with patients treated without RT. These changes are more common in patients treated twice a week than in patients treated five times a week and in patients older than 60 years compared with younger patients.[429] In the study by Bentzed and others,[429] this complication was correlated with the development of subcutaneous fibrosis, and the routine use of posttreatment physical therapy was effective at reducing its frequency.

The updated results from the JCRT regarding the incidence and risk factors for rib fractures are shown in Table 17.1-20.[426] Twenty-nine of the 1624 patients (1.8%) treated between 1968 and 1985 developed a rib fracture. The median time to its occurrence was 12 months (range,

TABLE 17.1-19

Incidence of Brachial Plexopathy in Relation to Radiation Technique, Dose, and Chemotherapy (CT)

	Incidence		
	No CT	CT	Total
TECHNIQUE			
Two-field	0% (0/458)	0% (0/49)	0%
	↑ *P*=NS ↓	↑ *P*=NS ↓	
Three-field	0.6% (5/787) ←*P*<.0001→	4.5% (15/330)	1.8%
THREE-FIELD TECHNIQUE ONLY (AXILLARY DOSE)			
≤50 Gy	0.4% (3/724) ←*P*=.0002→	3.7% (10/267)	1.3%
	↑ *P*=.05 ↓	↑ *P*=NS ↓	↑ *P*=.004 ↓
>50 Gy	3.2% (2/63) ←*P*=NS→	7.9% (5/63)	5.6%

(Pierce S, Recht A, Lingos T, et al. Long-term radiation complications following conservative surgery [CS] and radiation therapy [RT] in patients with early stage breast cancer. Int J Radiat Oncol Biol Phys 1992;23:915)

TABLE 17.1-20
Incidence of Rib Fracture in Relation to Dose to the Whole Breast and Machine Energy and Use of Chemotherapy (CT)

	Machine Energy			
Whole-Breast Dose	4 MV	*P* Value	6 or 8 MV	**Total**
≤45 Gy	0.4% (1/279)		0% (0/131)	0.2%
>45–<50 Gy	1.4% (10/725) *P*=.003		0.8% (1/120)	1.3%
≥50 Gy	5.7% (17/296)	NS	0% (0/25)	5.3%
Total	2.2% (28/1300)	.05	0.4% (1/276)	1.8%

	Use of CT		
	No CT		CT
<50 Gy	0.5% (5/990)	.01	2.3% (7/331)
≥50 Gy	4.7% (12/225)	NS	7.4% (5/68)

(Pierce S, Recht A, Lingos T, et al. Long-term radiation complications following conservative surgery [CS] and radiation therapy [RT] in patients with early stage breast cancer. Int J Radiat Oncol Biol Phys 1992;23:915)

1 to 57 months). Rib fracture was rare in patients treated on a 6- or 8-MV machine, but more commonly observed in patients treated on a 4-MV machine. (This is presumably because of the greater dose inhomogeneity seen with 4-MV irradiation compared with higher energy irradiation, resulting in increased dose to the lateral rib cage in particular.) Among patients treated on a 4-MV machine, the likelihood of rib fracture was related to radiation dose given to the entire breast and the use of adjuvant chemotherapy.

Soft tissue necrosis is a rare complication after moderate-dose RT, but its incidence can be increased by increasing the radiation dose or by altering the fractionation schedule. Montague[430] documented the likelihood of soft tissue complications for patients treated with postoperative RT. Patients were treated with either 2 Gy/d given five times a week of 3.3 Gy/d given three times weekly. Patients treated only three times a week received the same weekly dose and the same total dose and yet had a marked increase in soft tissue complications. Similar results were described by Kim and others.[431] In the experience at the JCRT, among 1624 patients treated with CS and RT between 1968 and 1985, 3 (0.4%) developed soft tissue necrosis that required surgical correction.[426] In two of these patients, the necrosis was located in the region of an interstitial implant boost. Among patients treated at the University of Pennsylvania, where interstitial implantation was less commonly performed, there were no cases of necrosis seen among 697 patients.[47] Investigators at the M.D. Anderson Hospital have reported that long-term soft tissue reactions are more common and more severe in patients with connective tissue disease.[157] As discussed previously in this chapter, however, the precise level of increased risk associated with RT in patients with connective tissue disease has not been established.

Radiation pneumonitis is a recognized complication of thoracic RT. Patients with radiation pneumonitis typically present 6 to 18 months after treatment with a dry cough, shortness of breath, and low-grade fever. The likelihood and severity of this complication is directly related to the volume of lung irradiated and the dose used. Small segments of lung can be irradiated to 60 Gy without symptomatic pneumonitis, whereas 20 Gy to an entire lung is likely to result in pneumonitis. Symptomatic radiation pneumonitis is an uncommon complication of RT for breast cancer. The results from the JCRT regarding the incidence and risk factors for radiation pneumonitis are shown in Table 17.1-21.[312] Seventeen of the 1624 patients (1%) treated between 1968 and 1985 developed radiation pneumonitis. In all cases, the symptoms were transient, and no patient developed permanent respiratory problems. The likelihood of pneumonitis was related to the use of a third radiation field and to the use of adjuvant chemotherapy, particularly when given concurrently with RT. A case–control analysis was performed to see if the volume of lung irradiated in the tangents (as measured by the CLD[399]) was predictive of pneumonitis. Among these patients in whom the CLD was limited to 3 cm or less, there was no apparent correlation between CLD and the appearance of pneumonitis.

A number of studies have examined pulmonary function testing in patients undergoing RT. In one study, the percentage of lung volume irradiated was estimated from computed tomographic scans.[432] The irradiated lung vol-

TABLE 17.1-21
Incidence of Radiation Pneumonitis in Relation to the Use and Sequencing of Chemotherapy (CT) and Use of a Third Field

	CT			Sequencing of CT and RT		
	No CT	*P* Value	CT	Sequential CT	*P* Value	Concurrent CT
Two-field	1/457 (0.2%)		0/51 (0%)	0/46 (0%)		0/3
Three-field	5/788 (0.6%)	.001	11/328 (3.3%)	3/236 (1.3%)	.002	8/92 (8.8%)

RT, radiation therapy.

(Lingos T, Recht A, Vincini F, et al. Radiation pneumonitis in breast cancer patients treated with conservative surgery and radiation therapy. Int J Radiat Oncol Biol Phys 1991;21:355)

ume was kept to 10% or less of the total lung volume (corresponding to a CLD of about 2 cm). Twenty-two patients were treated with two-field tangential breast irradiation and 7 patients were also treated with a third field to the regional nodal areas. There was generally an acute drop in the diffusing capacity of carbon monoxide (DLCO), but this returned to normal levels by 24 months. At 5 years, there was no discernible decrement in pulmonary function as measured by spirometrics, lung volume, or DLCO. Two patients developed radiation pneumonitis and both had baseline deficits in DLCO and had more than 10% of the lung irradiated. In another study, patients were irradiated with a technique that treated a greater percentage of lung, although CT scans were not done to quantify this.[433] Sixteen patients were treated with two-field tangential breast or chest wall irradiation, and 85 patients also were treated with a third field to the regional nodal areas. Twenty-two patients (26%) treated with local–regional RT developed symptoms of radiation pneumonitis compared with two patients (13%) treated with local RT. These patients, particularly those treated with three fields, also showed persistent small changes in pulmonary function tests at one year.

The use of RT to treat the supraclavicular and axillary region is typically associated with subsequent radiographic changes in the irradiated lung.[434] These changes are characterized by fibrosis and pleural thickening corresponding to the treated area, but are not necessarily associated with symptomatic pneumonitis. These radiographic changes can be confused with evidence of metastatic disease or with lung cancer by physicians unfamiliar with them. Such changes also can be seen on CT scans in the area treated by tangential irradiation.[435]

One possible complication of RT is the induction of a breast cancer. Breast tissue is known to be sensitive to radiation carcinogenesis (see Chap. 3.1). The latency period between exposure and the detection of induced cancers is about 10 years, and this risk is apparent for many decades after that.[436] Two important factors, radiation dose and age at exposure, influence the likelihood of radiation carcinogenesis in breast tissue. The influence of dose on the risk of carcinogenesis is illustrated in a study from Sweden of young women who received irradiation for

benign breast conditions.[437,438] The risk of carcinogenesis increases linearly with doses up to 10 Gy. With doses above 10 Gy, there seems to be a bending of the curve and a decrease, or at least a levelling off, in the risk of carcinogenesis. When doses in the therapeutic range are used (greater than 45 Gy), the risk of carcinogenesis seems to be small. To explain this phenomenon, it has been hypothesized that radiation results in two competing processes: carcinogenesis and cell inactivation.[439] Carcinogenesis has a linear relationship with radiation dose, whereas cell inactivation occurs as an exponential process with an initial shoulder region. Based on these relations, there is a relatively greater risk of carcinogenesis at lower doses. At higher dose levels, cell inactivation becomes dominant, and the relative risk of carcinogenesis decreases. Because the dose to the opposite breast from a course of RT is in the range of 1 to 3 Gy,[440] tumor induction in the contralateral breast is of greater potential concern than in the ipsilateral breast. Age at exposure to radiation is the other important risk factor for carcinogenesis in human breast tissue.[436,441] The highest risk occurs in females exposed at the youngest age. With increasing age, the risk of carcinogenesis declines. The risk for women older than 40 years of age seems to be negligible, but not zero.[438,441]

A number of studies have addressed the risk of contralateral breast cancer after postoperative RT. Boice and colleagues[442] conducted a case–control study in a cohort of 41,109 patients diagnosed with breast cancer between 1935 and 1982 in Connecticut. During this time period, RT was principally used after mastectomy rather than as part of breast-conserving treatment. Medical records were reviewed for the 655 patients in whom a contralateral breast cancer developed 5 or more years after the initial tumor, and their radiation exposure was compared with that of 1189 matched controls from the cohort that did not develop a contralateral cancer. Overall, 23% of the women who had a contralateral breast cancer and 20% of the controls had received RT. The average dose of radiation to the contralateral breast, estimated from the original RT records, was 2.82 Gy. Among women who survived for at least 10 years, RT was associated with a small, but marginally significant, elevation in the risk of a contralateral breast cancer (RR, 1.33). Over the range of radiation doses to the contralateral breast, the risk increased significantly with dose. The increased risk associated with RT was evident among women who were younger than 45 years of age when they were treated (RR, 1.59), but not among older women (RR, 1.01). In another case–control study from Denmark,[443] the incidence of a second primary breast cancer in the contralateral breast was examined among 56,540 women with a first primary breast cancer diagnosed between 1943 and 1978 and entered into the national registry. In that study, RT was not associated with an increased risk of contralateral breast cancer (RR, 1.04). These data provide additional evidence that the risk of radiation-induced breast cancer associated with RT is small.

It is possible to estimate the increased absolute risk of contralateral breast cancer given the elevated risk for patients aged 45 or younger seen in the study by Boice and others. (The risk may actually be lower as suggested by the Danish study.) For patients aged 45 years or younger, the risk of contralateral breast cancer within 15 years is about 11% without RT and increased to about 12% to 13% with the addition of RT. The risk of contralateral breast cancer within 30 years is about 22% without RT and increased to about 25% to 26% with RT. Thus, the risk of contralateral breast cancer in young patients, which is already higher than that for older patients, is likely to be further increased to a small extent by the use of RT. Given this, it seems prudent to reduce the dose to the contralateral breast in young patients to as low as possible.

Sarcomas of soft tissue or bone are a rare but well-documented complication of RT. In a report from Memorial Sloan-Kettering Cancer Center, a total of 48 patients with a prior history of breast cancer and a subsequent treatment-related sarcoma were seen at the institution between 1948 and 1991.[444] Lymphangiosarcoma of the extremity accounted for 22, or 46% of the series. Most of these patients had been treated with radical mastectomy and postoperative RT. The other 26 sarcomas occurred within an RT treatment field and were considered radiation related. Twenty-one of these 26 patients were diagnosed with a soft tissue sarcoma and 5 with a bone sarcoma. The median latency interval between the diagnosis of breast cancer and the development of sarcoma was 11 years (range, 4 to 44) and was similar for the two types of sarcomas. The survival of these patients was poor. Because the institution is a major referral source for patients with sarcoma, it was not possible to calculate an actuarial risk for this event. In a series from France, 9 of 7620 patients treated for breast cancer developed a sarcoma within the irradiated fields.[445] The mean latency period was 9.5 years. The cumulative incidence after initial treatment was 0.2% at 10 years, 0.43% at 20 years, and 0.78% at 30 years. Kurtz and others[446] reported on 2850 patients with clinical stage I or II breast cancer treated with CS and RT who had survived 5 years without recurrence. Two of these patients (0.1%) developed a chest wall sarcoma and this represented 9 cases per 100,000 patient-years of observation. Similar findings were observed in series from the JCRT[426] and from the Milan Cancer Institute.[447] Of particular interest is that a high percentage of

sarcomas after treatment with CS and RT are angiosarcomas.[448] The typical initial clinical appearance of this sarcoma is reddish, purplish, or bluish nodules or discolorations of the skin that are often multiple. These initial findings can be subtle and diagnosis is commonly not made until more advanced signs are present.

Acute nonlymphocytic leukemia is also a well-described, but rare, complication of RT. The median latency period for its appearance is shorter than that for solid tumors, generally 4 to 7 years after exposure.[449] The amount of bone marrow irradiated seems to be a factor influencing risk.[450] The risk of acute nonlymphocytic leukemia is greater after local–regional irradiation than after more localized breast irradiation. Radiation dose is also a factor in the risk of leukemia. An excess of leukemia cases has been seen after low doses of RT (1 to 10 Gy) to the pelvis given for benign conditions,[451–453] but is less common after therapeutic levels of RT (40 Gy or greater). Although a small increase in acute nonlymphocytic leukemia has been seen in some cohorts of breast cancer patients treated with postoperative RT, in a case–control study reported by Curtis and coworkers[454] using the Connecticut Tumor Registry, an increased risk of leukemia associated with RT could not be detected (RR, 1.16; 90% CI, 0.6 to 2.1). Adjuvant chemotherapy (especially with alkylating agents) is also known to be associated with a small increased risk of acute nonlymphocytic leukemia, and the use of local–regional RT in conjunction with chemotherapy seems to increase this risk further.[450]

Lung cancer also appears to be increased in patients irradiated for breast cancer. The latency period from RT to diagnosis is about 10 years. In a case–referent study reported by Inskip and others[455] using the Connecticut Tumor Registry, there was a small increased risk of lung cancer among 10-year survivors of breast cancer associated with the use of postoperative RT (RR, 1.8; 95% CL, 0.8 to 3.8). The RR for the period 15 years or more after RT was 2.8 (95% CI, 1.0 to 8.2); however, it can be difficult to distinguish a late metastasis of breast cancer to lung from a new primary lung cancer even with a tissue specimen. This increased relative risk suggests that there would be approximately nine cases of RT-induced lung cancer per year among 10,000 breast cancer patients who survived at least 10 years. Similar findings were noted in a study using the SEER data base.[456] Another study from this same group suggested that the effects of smoking and RT are multiplicative,[457] although this relation has not been established with certainty.[458] These studies all examined the risk of lung cancer after local–regional irradiation, and this risk may be greater than that seen after more localized breast irradiation.

Injury to the heart is a possible complication after RT, but its likelihood seems related to the technique of RT used. As discussed earlier in this chapter, the long-term results from the trials of postoperative RT show an increased risk of cardiac mortality. In the updated overview of these trials,[17] an excess of cardiac deaths was apparent in both early and more recent trials, but this was offset by a reduced number of deaths because of breast cancer, especially in the more recent trials. (see Fig. 17.1-8) Data from the Stockholm trial relating to the technique of irradiation and its association with cause-specific mortality suggests that increased mortality from ischemic heart disease was evident only in patients treated with an old technique in which a large percentage of heart was irradiated, but that the reduction in breast cancer mortality was similar in all groups.[256] This study suggests that the increased cardiovascular mortality associated with RT can be avoided by the use of appropriate techniques without compromising its effectiveness in treating breast cancer. However, the dose to the left anterior descending artery (but not the other coronary arteries) remains high in patients treated for left-sided cancers, even with the modern technique.[459,460] Further follow-up on patients treated with limited RT fields is still required.

It is also possible that RT may increase the risk of cardiomyopathy in patients treated with doxorubicin. In a study from Milan, 4 of 114 patients who were treated with concurrent doxorubicin and left-sided RT developed subacute symptomatic congestive heart failure.[461] Similar findings have not been reported in patients treated with tangential breast irradiation and sequential doxorubicin, but further follow-up is needed, especially because there is the potential for late cardiac problems after doxorubicin in the absence of RT.

References

1. Halsted W. The results of operations for cure of cancer of the breast performed at Johns Hopkins Hospital. Johns Hopkins Hosp Bull 1894;4:497.
2. Halsted W. The results of radical operations for the cure of carcinoma of the breast. Ann Surg 1907;46:1019.
3. Adair F, Berg J, Joubert L, et al. Long term follow-up of breast cancer patients: the 30-year report. Cancer 1974;33:1145.
4. Turner-Warwick R. The lymphatics of the breast. Br J Surg 1959;46:574.
5. Urban J. Management of operable breast cancer: the surgeon's view. Cancer 1978;42:2066.
6. Meir P, Ferguson D, Harrison T. A controlled trial of extended radical mastectomy. Cancer 1985;55:880.
7. Veronesi U, Valagussa P. Inefficacy of internal mammary nodes dissection in breast cancer surgery. Cancer 1981;47:170.
8. Morrow M, Foster R. Staging of breast cancer: a new rationale for internal mammary node biopsy. Arch Surg 1981;116:748.
9. Lazovich D, White E, Thomas D, et al. Underutilization of breast-conserving surgery and radiation therapy among women with stage I or II breast cancer. JAMA 1991;266:3433.
10. Samet J, Hunt W, Farrow D. Determinants of receiving breast conserving surgery: the surveillance, epidemiology and end results program, 1983–1986. Cancer 1994;73:2344.
11. Nattinger A, Gottlieb M, Veum J, et al. Geographic variation in the use of breast-conserving treatment for breast cancer. N Engl J Med 1992;326:1102.
12. Robinson D, Van Heerden J, Payne W, et al. The primary surgical treatment of carcinoma of the breast: a changing trend toward modified radical mastectomy. Mayo Clin Proc 1976;51:433.
13. Baker R, Montague A, Childs J. A comparison of modified radical mastectomy to radical mastectomy in the treatment of operable breast cancer. Ann Surg 1979;189:553.
14. Turner L, Swindell R, Bell W. Radical versus modified radical mastectomy for breast cancer. Ann R Coll Surg Engl 1981;63:239.
15. Maddox W, Carpenter J, Laws H, et al. A randomized prospective trial of radical (Halsted) mastectomy versus modified radical mastectomy in 311 breast cancer patients. Ann Surg 1983;198:207.
16. Cuzick J, Stewart H, Peto R, et al. Overview of randomized trials of postoperative adjuvant radiotherapy in breast cancer. Cancer Treat Rep 1987;71:15.
17. Cuzick J, Stewart H, Rutqvist L, et al. Cause-specific mortality in long-term survivors of breast cancer who participated in trials of radiotherapy. J Clin Oncol 1994;12:447.
18. Lagios MD, Westdahl P, Rose M. The concept and implications of multicentricity in breast carcinoma. In: Sommers SG, ed. Pathology annual. New York, Appleton-Century-Crofts, 1981.
19. Qualheim R, Gall E. Breast carcinoma with multiple sites of origin. Cancer 1957;10:460.
20. Rosen P, Fracchia A, Urban J, et al. "Residual" mammary carcinoma following simulated partial mastectomy. Cancer 1975;35:739.
21. Holland R, Veling S, Mravunac M, et al. Histologic multifocality of Tis, T1-2 breast carcinomas: implication for clinical trials of breast conserving treatment. Cancer 1985;56:979.
22. Holland R, Connolly J, Gelman R, et al. The presence of an extensive intraductal component (EIC) following a limited excision correlates with prominent residual disease in the remainder of the breast. J Clin Oncol 1990;8:113.
23. Lagios M, Richards V, Rose M, et al. Segmental mastectomy without radiotherapy: short-term follow-up. Cancer 1983;52:2173.
24. Montgomery A, Greening W, Levene A. Clinical study of recurrence rate and survival time of patients with carcinoma of the breast treated by biopsy excision without any other therapy. J R Soc Med 1978;71:339.
25. Targart R. Partial mastectomy for breast cancer. Br Med J 1978;2:1268.
26. Freeman C, Belliveau N, Kim T, et al. Limited surgery with or without radiotherapy for early breast carcinoma. J Can Assoc Radiol 1981;32:125.
27. Fisher B, Redmond C, Poisson R, et al. Eight-year results of a randomized clinical trial comparing total mastectomy and lumpectomy with or without irradiation in the treatment of breast cancer. N Engl J Med 1989;320:822.
28. Fletcher G. Local results of irradiation in the primary management of localized breast cancer. Cancer 1972;29:545.
29. Kae S, Johansen H. Does simple mastectomy followed by irradiation offer survival comparable to radical procedures? Int J Radiat Oncol Biol Phys 1977;2:1163.
30. Keynes G. Conservative treatment of cancer of the breast. Br Med J 1937;2:643.
31. Peters M. Cutting the "Gordian knot" in early breast cancer. Ann R Coll Phys Surg Can 1975;8:186.
32. Hayward J. The Guy's trial of treatments on "early" breast cancer. World J Surg 1977;1:314.
33. Hayward J. The Guy's Hospital trials on breast conservation. In: Harris JR, Hellman S, Silen W, eds. Conservative management of breast cancer. Philadelphia, JB Lippincott, 1983:77.
34. Hayward J, Caleffi M. The significance of local control in the primary treatment of breast cancer. Arch Surg 1987;122:1244.
35. Veronesi U, Saccozzi R, Del Vecchio M, et al. Comparing radical mastectomy with quadrantectomy, axillary dissection, and radiotherapy in patients with small cancers of the breast. N Engl J Med 1981;305:6.
36. Veronesi U, Banfi A, Salvadori B, et al. Breast conservation is the treatment of choice in small breast cancer: long-term results of a randomized clinical trial. Eur J Cancer 1990;26:668.
37. Fisher B, Redmond C, et al. Lumpectomy for breast cancer: an

update of the NSABP experience. J Natl Cancer Inst Monogr 1992;11:7.

38. Van Dongen J, Bartelink H, Fentimen I, et al. Randomized clinical trial to assess the value of breast-conserving therapy in stage I and II breast cancer: EORTC 10801 trial. J Natl Cancer Inst Monogr 1992;11:15.

39. Blichert-Toft M, Brincker H, Andersen J, et al. A Danish randomized trial comparing breast preserving therapy with mastectomy in mammary carcinoma. Acta Oncol 1988;27:671.

40. Lichter A, Lippman M, Danforth D, et al. Mastectomy versus breast conserving therapy in the treatment of stage I and II carcinoma of the breast: a randomized trial at the National Cancer Institute. J Clin Oncol 1992;10:976.

41. Sarrazin D, Le M, Arriagada R, et al. Ten-year results of a randomized trial comparing a conservative treatment to mastectomy in early breast cancer. Radiother Oncol 1989;14:177.

42. Blichert-Toft M, Rose C, Andersen J, et al. Danish randomized trial comparing breast conservation therapy with mastectomy: six years of life-table analysis. J Natl Cancer Inst Monogr 1992;11:19.

43. Veronesi U, Salvadori B, Luini A, et al. Conservative treatment of early breast cancer: long-term results of 1232 cases treated with quadrantectomy, axillary dissection, and radiotherapy. Ann Surg 1990;211:250.

44. Haffty B, Goldberg N, Fischer D, et al. Conservative surgery and radiation therapy in breast carcinoma: local recurrence and prognostic implications. Int J Radiat Oncol Biol Phys 1989;17:727.

45. Clark R, Wilkinson R, Miceli P, et al. Breast cancer: experiences with conservation therapy. Am J Clin Oncol 1987;49:461.

46. Clarke D, Le M, Sarrazin D, et al. Analysis of local–regional relapses in patients with early breast cancers treated by excision and radiotherapy: experience of the Institut Gustave-Roussy. Int J Radiat Oncol Biol Phys 1985;11:137.

47. Fowble B, Solin L, Schultz D, et al. Ten-year results of conservative surgery and irradiation for stage I and II breast cancer. Int J Radiat Oncol Biol Phys 1991;21:269.

48. Stotter A, McNeese M, Ames F, et al. Predicting the rate and extent of locoregional failure after breast conservation therapy for early breast cancer. Cancer 1989;64:2217.

49. Fourquet A, Campana F, Zafrani B et al. Prognostic factors of breast recurrence in the conservative management of early breast cancer: a 25-year follow-up. Int J Radiat Oncol Biol Phys 1989;17:719.

50. Kurtz J, Amalric R, Brandone H, et al. Local recurrence after breast-conserving surgery and radiotherapy: frequency, time course, and prognosis. Cancer 1989;63:1912.

51. Abner A, Recht A, Eberlein T, et al. Prognosis following salvage mastectomy for recurrence in the breast after conservative surgery and radiation therapy for early-stage breast cancer. J Clin Oncol 1993;11:44.

52. Vicini F, Recht A, Abner A, et al. Recurrence in the breast following conservative surgery and radiation therapy for early-stage breast cancer. J Natl Cancer Inst Monogr 1992;11:33.

53. Fowble B, Solin L, Schultz D, et al. Breast recurrence following conservative surgery and radiation: patterns of failure, prognosis, and pathologic findings from mastectomy specimens with implications for treatment. Int J Radiat Oncol Biol Phys 1990;19:833.

54. Harris J, Recht A, Amalric R, et al. Time course and prognosis of local recurrence following primary radiation therapy for early breast cancer. J Clin Oncol 1984;2:37.

55. Recht A, Silen W, Schnitt S, et al. Time course of local recurrence following conservative surgery and radiotherapy for early stage breast cancer. Int J Radiat Oncol Biol Phys 1988;15:255.

56. Kurtz J, Spitalier J, Amalric R. Late breast recurrence after lumpectomy and irradiation. Int J Radiat Oncol Biol Phys 1983;9:1191.

57. Kurtz J, Spitalier J, Amalric R, et al. The prognostic significance

of late local recurrence after breast-conserving therapy. Int J Radiat Oncol Biol Phys 1990;18:87.

58. Gage I, Nixon A, Gelman R, et al. Long-term outcome following breast-conserving surgery and radiation therapy. Int J Radiat Oncol Biol Phys (in press).

59. Healey E, Cook E, Orav E, et al. Contralateral breast cancer: clinical characteristics and impact on prognosis. J Clin Oncol 1993;11:1545.

60. Harris J, Levene M, Svensson G, et al. Analysis of cosmetic results following primary radiation therapy for stages I and II carcinoma of the breast. Int J Radiat Oncol Biol Phys 1979;5:257.

61. Pezner R, Lipsett J, Vora N, et al. Limited usefulness of observer based cosmesis scales employed to evaluate patients treated conservatively for breast cancer. Int J Radiat Oncol Biol Phys 1985;11:1117.

62. Pezner R, Patterson M, Lipsett J, et al. Factors affecting cosmetic outcome in breast conserving cancer treatment-objective quantitative assessment. Breast Cancer Res Treat 1991;20:85.

63. Veronesi U, Volterrani F, Luini A, et al. Quadrantectomy versus lumpectomy for small size breast cancer. Eur J Cancer 1990;26:671.

64. Van Limbergen E, van der Schueren E, Van Tangelen K. Cosmetic evaluation of breast conserving treatment for breast cancer. I. Proposal of a scoring system. Radiother Oncol 1989;16:159.

65. Tsouskas L, Fentiman I. Breast compliance: a new method for evaluation of cosmetic outcome after conservative treatment of early breast cancer treatment. Breast Cancer Res Treat 1990;15:185.

66. Beadle G, Come S, Henderson I, et al. The effect of adjuvant chemotherapy on the cosmetic results after primary radiation treatment for early stage breast cancer. Int J Radiat Oncol Biol Phys 1984;10:2131.

67. Beadle G, Silver B, Botnick L, et al. Cosmetic results following primary radiation therapy for early breast cancer. Cancer 1984;54:2911.

68. Gore S, Come S, Griem K, et al. Influence of the sequencing of chemotherapy and radiation therapy in node negative breast cancer patients treated by conservative surgery and radiation therapy. In: Salmon S, Jones S, eds. Adjuvant therapy of cancer V. Orlando, Grune & Stratton, 1987;365.

69. Rose M, Olivotto I, Cady B, et al. The long-term results of conservative surgery and radiation therapy for early breast cancer. Arch Surg 1989;124:153.

70. Olivotto I, Rose M, Silver B, et al. Late cosmetic outcome after conservative surgery and radiotherapy: analysis of causes of cosmetic failure. Int J Radiat Oncol Biol Phys 1989;17:747.

71. Abner A, Recht A, Vicini F, et al. Cosmetic results after conservative surgery, chemotherapy, and radiation therapy for early breast cancer. Int J Radiat Oncol Biol Phys 1991;21:331.

72. de la Rochefordiere A, Abner A, Silver B, et al. Are cosmetic results following conservative surgery and radiation therapy for early breast cancer dependent on technique? Int J Radiat Oncol Biol Phys 1992;23:925.

73. Veronesi U, Luini A, Galimberti V, et al. Conservation approaches for the management of stage I/II carcinoma of the breast: Milan Cancer Institute Trials. World J Surg 1994;18:70.

74. Wazer D, DiPetrillo T, Schmidt-Ullrich R, et al. Factors influencing cosmetic outcome and complication risk after conservative surgery and radiotherapy for early-stage breast carcinoma. J Clin Oncol 1992;10:356.

75. Matory WJ, Mertheimer M, Fitzgerald T, et al. Aesthetic results following partial mastectomy and radiation therapy. Plast Reconst Surg 1990;85:739.

76. Clarke D, Martinez A, Cox R. Analyses of cosmetic results and complications in patients with stage I and II breast cancer treated by biopsy and irradiation. Int J Radiat Oncol Biol Phys 1983;9:1807.

77. Chin L, Cheng C, Siddon R, Three-dimensional photon dose

distributions with and without lung corrections for tangential breast intact treatments. Int J Radiat Oncol Biol Phys 1989;17:1327.

78. Gray J, McCormick B, Cox L, et al. Primary breast irradiation in large-breasted or heavy women: analysis of cosmetic outcome. Int J Radiat Oncol Biol Phys 1991;21:347.

79. Shestak K, Johnson R, Greco R, et al. Partial mastectomy and breast reduction as a valuable treatment option for patients with macromastia and carcinoma of the breast. Surg Gynecol Obstet 1993;177:54.

80. Ray G, Fish V. Biopsy and definitive radiotherapy in stage I and II adenocarcinoma of the female breast: analysis of cosmesis and the role of electron beam supplementation. Int J Radiat Oncol Biol Phys 1983;9:813.

81. Sarin R, Dinshaw K, Shirvastava S, et al. Therapeutic factors influencing the cosmetic outcome and late complications in the conservative management of early breast cancer. Int J Radiat Oncol Biol Phys 1993;27:285.

82. Fowble B, Solin L, Martz K, et al. The influence of the type of boost (electron vs implant) on local control and cosmesis in patients with stage I and II breast cancer undergoing conservative surgery and radiation. Int J Radiat Oncol Biol Phys 1986;12 (Suppl):150.

83. Siddon R, Buck B, Harris J, et al. Three-field technique for breast irradiation using tangential field corner blocks. Int J Radiat Oncol Biol Phys 1983;9:583.

84. Ray G, Fish V, Marmor J, et al. Impact of adjuvant chemotherapy on cosmesis and complications in stages I and II carcinoma of the breast treated by biopsy and radiation therapy. Int J Radiat Oncol Biol Phys 1984;10:837.

85. Gelman R, Gelber R, Henderson I, et al. Improved methodology for analyzing local and distant recurrence. J Clin Oncol 1990;8:548.

86. Vilcoq J, Calle R, Stacey P, et al. The outcome of treatment by tumorectomy and radiotherapy of patients with operable breast cancer. Int J Radiat Oncol Biol Phys 1981;7:1327.

87. Boyages J, Recht A, Connolly J, et al. Early breast cancer: predictors of breast recurrence for patients treated with conservative surgery and radiation therapy. Radiother Oncol 1990;19:29.

88. Kurtz J, Spitalier J, Amalric R, et al. Mammary recurrence in women younger than forty. Int J Radiat Oncol Biol Phys 1988;15:271.

89. Matthews R, McNeese M, Montague E, et al. Prognostic implications of age in breast cancer patients treated with tumorectomy and irradiation or with mastectomy. Int J Radiat Oncol Biol Phys 1988;14:659.

90. Haffty B, Fischer D, Rose M, et al. Prognostic factors for local recurrence in the conservatively treated breast cancer patient: a cautious interpretation of the data. J Clin Oncol 1991;9:997.

91. Nixon A, Neuberg D, Hayes D, et al. Relationship of patient age to pathologic features of the tumor and prognosis for patients with stage I or II breast cancer. J Clin Oncol 1994;12:888.

92. Kurtz J, Jacquemier J, Spitalier J, et al. Why are local recurrences (LR) after breast-conserving surgery more frequent in young patients? Proc Am Soc Clin Oncol 1989;8:19.

93. Donegan W, Perez-Mesa C, Watson F. A biostatistical study of locally recurrent breast carcinoma. Surg Gynecol Obstet 1966;122:529.

94. de la Rochefordiere A, Asselain B, Campana G, et al. Age as a prognostic factor in premenopausal breast carcinoma. Lancet 1993;341:1039.

95. Halverson K, Perez C, Taylor M, et al. Age as a prognostic factor for breast and regional nodal recurrence follow breast conserving surgery and irradiation in stage I and II breast cancer. Int J Radiat Oncol Biol Phys 1993;27:1045.

96. Eberlein T, Connolly J, Schnitt S, et al. Predictors of local recurrence following conservative breast surgery and radiation therapy: the influence of tumor size. Arch Surg 1990;125:771.

97. Fowble F, Solin L, Schultz D, et al. Breast recurrence and survival related to primary tumor location in patients undergoing conservative surgery and radiation for early-stage breast cancer. Int J Radiat Oncol Biol Phys 1992;23:933.

98. Jacquemier J, Kurtz J, Amalric R, et al. An assessment of extensive intraductal component as a risk factor for local recurrence after breast-conserving therapy. Br J Cancer 1990;61:873.

99. Borger J, Kemperman H, Hart A, et al. Risk factors in breast-conservation therapy. J Clin Oncol 1994;12:653.

100. Rosen P, Kinne D, Lesser M, et al. Are prognostic factors for local control of breast cancer treated by primary radiotherapy significant for patients treated by mastectomy? Cancer 1986;57:1415.

101. Schnitt S, Connolly J, Khettry U, et al. Pathologic findings on re-excision of the primary site in breast cancer patients considered for treatment by primary radiation therapy. Cancer 1987;59:675.

102. Healey E, Osteen R, Schnitt S, et al. Can the clinical and mammographic findings at presentation predict the presence of an extensive intraductal component in early stage breast cancer? Int J Radiat Oncol Biol Phys 1989;17:1217.

103. Noguchi S, Aihara T, Koyama H, et al. Discrimination between multicentric and multifocal carcinomas of the breast through clonal analysis. Cancer 1994;74:872.

104. Rosen P, Saigo P, Braun D, et al. Predictors of recurrence in stage I (T1N0M0) breast cancer. Ann Surg 1991;193:15.

105. Pinder S, Ellis I, Galea M, et al. Pathologic prognostic factors in breast cancer. III. Vascular invasion: relationship with recurrence and survival in a large study with long-term follow-up. Histopathology 1994;24:41.

106. Schnitt S, Connolly J, Recht A, et al. The influence of infiltrating lobular histology on local tumor control in patients treated with conservative surgery and radiotherapy. Cancer 1989;64:448.

107. Kurtz J, Jacquemier J, Terhorst J, et al. Conservation therapy for breast cancers other than infiltrating ductal carcinoma. Cancer 1989;63:1630.

108. Weiss M, Fowble B, Solin L, et al. Outcome of conservative therapy for invasive breast cancer by histologic subtype. Int J Radiat Oncol Biol Phys 1992;23:941.

109. Silverstein M, Lewinsky B, Waisman J, et al. Infiltrating lobular carcinoma: is it different from infiltrating duct carcinoma? Cancer 1994;73:1673.

110. Veronesi P, Zurrida S, Galimberti V, et al. Conservative treatment in infiltrating lobular carcinoma of the breast. (Abstract) Eur Soc Mastol, 1994.

111. Kurtz J, Jacquemier J, Amalric R, et al. Breast-conserving therapy for macroscopically multiple cancers. Ann Surg 1990;212:38.

112. Leopold K, Recht A, Schnitt S, et al. Results of conservative surgery and radiation therapy for multiple synchronous cancers of one breast. Int J Radiat Oncol Biol Phys 1989;16:11.

113. Wilson L, Beinfield M, McKhan C, et al. Conservative surgery and radiation in the treatment of synchronous ipsilateral breast cancers. Cancer 1993;72:137.

114. Schnitt S, Connolly J. Processing and evaluation of breast excision specimens: a clinically oriented approach. Am J Clin Pathol 1992;98:125.

115. Anscher M, Jones P, Prosnitz L, et al. Local failure and margin status in early-stage breast carcinoma treated with conservative surgery and radiation therapy. Ann Surg 1993;218:22.

116. Solin L, Fowble B, Schultz D, et al. The significance of the pathology margins of the tumor excision on the outcome of patients treated with definitive irradiation for early stage breast cancer. Int J Radiat Oncol Biol Phys 1991;21:279.

117. Schnitt S, Abner A, Gelman R, et al. The relationship between microscopic margins of resection and the risk of local recurrence in breast cancer patients treated with conservative surgery and radiation therapy. Cancer 1994;74:1746.

118. Van Limbergen E, van den Bogaert W, van der Schueren E, et al. Tumor excision and radiotherapy as primary treatment of breast

cancer: analysis of patient and treatment parameters and local control. Radiother Oncol 1987;8:1.

119. Chu A, Cope O, Russo R, et al. Patterns of local–regional recurrence and results in stages I and II breast cancer treated by irradiation following limited surgery. Am J Clin Oncol 1984;7:221.

120. Vicini F, Eberlein T, Connolly J, et al. The optimal extent of resection for patients with stages I or II breast cancer treated with conservative surgery and radiotherapy. Ann Surg 1992;214:200.

121. Osborne M, Ormiston N, Harmer C, et al. Breast conservation in the treatment of early breast cancer: a 20-year follow-up. Cancer 1984;53:349.

122. Slotman B, Meyer O, Njo K, et al. Importance of timing of radiotherapy in breast conserving treatment for early stage breast cancer. Radiother Oncol 1994;30:206.

123. Nixon A, Recht A, Neuberg D, et al. The relation between the surgery–radiotherapy interval and treatment outcome in patients treated with breast-conserving surgery and radiation therapy without systemic therapy. Int J Radiat Oncol Biol Phys 1994;30:17.

124. Rose M, Henderson I, Gelman R, et al. Premenopausal breast cancer patients treated with conservative surgery, radiotherapy, and adjuvant chemotherapy have a low risk of local failure. Int J Radiat Oncol Biol Phys 1989;17:711.

125. Margolese R. Surgical considerations in selecting local therapy. J Natl Cancer Inst Monogr 1992;11:41.

126. Recht A, Come S, Gelman R, et al. Integration of conservative surgery, radiotherapy, and chemotherapy for the treatment of early-stage node-positive breast cancer: sequencing, timing, and outcome. J Clin Oncol 1991;9:1662.

127. Fisher B, Anderson S, Fisher E, et al. The significance of local recurrence following lumpectomy. Lancet 1991;338:327.

128. Whelan T, Clark R, Roberts R, et al. Ipsilateral breast tumor recurrence post-lumpectomy is predictive of subsequent mortality: results from a randomized trial. Int J Radiat Oncol Biol Phys 1994;30:11.

129. Franceschi D, Osborne M, Borgen P. Survival following loco-regional recurrence of early breast cancer: a comparison between mastectomy and breast-conservation surgery. Abstracts of the 47th Annual Cancer Symposium, Society of Surgical Oncology, 1994:4.

130. Meyerowitz B. Psychological correlates of breast cancer and its treatment. Psychol Bull 1980;87:108.

131. Holmberg L, Omne-Ponte M, Burns T, et al. Psychosocial adjustment after mastectomy and breast-conserving treatment. Cancer 1989;64:969.

132. Wolberg W, Romsaas E, Tanne M, et al. Psychosexual adaptation to breast cancer surgery. Cancer 1989;63:1645.

133. Baider L, Rizel S, Kaplan De-Nour A. Comparison of couples' adjustment to lumpectomy and mastectomy. Gen Hosp Psych 1986;8:251.

134. De Haes JJ, Van Oosterom M, Welvaart K. The effect of radical and conserving surgery on the quality of life of early breast cancer patients. Eur J Surg Oncol 1986;12:337.

135. Ganz P, Schag C, Polinsky M, et al. Rehabilitation needs and breast cancer: the first month after primary therapy. Breast Cancer Res Treat 1987;10:243.

136. Schain W, Edwards B, Gorrell C, et al. Psychosocial and physical outcomes of primary breast cancer therapy: mastectomy vs excision biopsy and irradiation. Breast Cancer Res Treat 1983;3:377.

137. Fallowfield L, Baum M, Maguire G. Effects of breast conservation on psychological morbidity associated with diagnosis and treatment of early breast cancer. Br Med J 1986;293:1331.

138. Goldberg J, Scott R, Davidson P, et al. Psychological morbidity in the first year after breast surgery. Eur J Surg Oncol 1992;18:327.

139. Sanger C, Reznikoff M. A comparison of the psychological effects of breast-saving procedures and modified radical mastectomy. Cancer 1981;48:2341.

140. Levy S, Herberman R, Lee J, et al. Breast conservation versus mastectomy: distress sequelae as a function of choice. J Clin Oncol 1989;7:367.

141. Lasry J-C, Margolese R, Poisson R, et al. Depression and body image following mastectomy and lumpectomy. J Chron Dis 1987;49:529.

142. Kemeny M, Wellisch D, Schain W. Psychosocial outcome in a randomized surgical trial for treatment of primary breast cancer. Cancer 1988;62:1241.

143. Pozo C, Carver C, Noriega V, et al. Effects of mastectomy versus lumpectomy on emotional adjustment to breast cancer: a prospective study of the first year post surgery. J Clin Oncol 1992;10:1292.

144. Schain W, d'Angelo T, Dunn M, et al. Mastectomy versus conservative surgery and radiotherapy: psychosocial consequences. Cancer 1994;78:1221.

145. Beckmann J, Johnsen L, Richardt C, et al. Psychological reactions in younger women operated on for breast cancer. Dan Med Bull 1983;(Supp 2)30:10-13.

146. Ashcroft J, Leinster S, Slade P. Breast cancer-patient choice of treatment: preliminary communication. J R Soc Med 1985;78:43.

147. Bartelink M, Van Dam F, Van Dongen J. Psychological effects of breast conserving therapy in comparison with radical mastectomy. Int J Radiat Oncol Biol Phys 1985;11:381.

148. Weisman A. Early diagnosis of vulnerability in cancer patients. Am J Med Sci 1976;271:187.

149. Hughes J. Emotional reactions to the diagnosis and treatment of early breast cancer. J Psychosom Res 1982;26:277.

150. Bloom J. Social support, accommodation to stress and adjustment to breast cancer. Soc Sci Med 1982;16:1329.

151. Schonfield J. Psychological factors related to a delayed return to an earlier lifestyle in successfully treated cancer patients. J Psychosom Res 1972;16:41.

152. National Institutes of Health Consensus Development Panel Consensus Statement. Treatment of early-stage breast cancer. J Natl Cancer Inst Monogr 1992;11:11.

153. Wolberg W, Tanner M, Romsaas E, et al. Factors influencing options in primary breast cancer treatment. J Clin Oncol 1987;5:68.

154. Winchester D, Cox J. Standards for breast conservation treatment. CA Cancer J Clin 1992;42:134.

155. Boyages J, Barraclough B, Middledorp J, et al. Early breast cancer: cosmetic and functional results after treatment by conservative techniques. Aust NZ J Surg 1989;58:111.

156. Robertson J, Clarke D, Pevzner M, et al. Breast conservation therapy: severe breast fibrosis after radiation therapy in patients with collagen vascular disease. Cancer 1991;68:502.

157. Fleck R, McNeese M, Ellerbroek N, et al. Consequences of breast irradiation in patients with pre-existing collagen vascular disease. Int J Radiat Oncol Biol Phys 1989;17:829.

158. Urtasun R. A complication of the use of radiation for malignant neoplasia in chronic discoid lupus erythematosus. J Can Assoc Radiol 1971;22:168.

159. Ransoma D, Cameron F. Scleroderma: a possible contraindication to lumpectomy and radiotherapy in breast carcinoma. Australas Radiol 1987;31:317.

160. Ross J, Hussey D, Mayr N, et al. Acute and late reactions to radiation therapy in patients with collagen vascular diseases. Cancer 1993;71:3744.

161. Farrow D, Hunt W, Samet J. Geographic variation in the treatment of localized breast cancer. N Engl J Med 1992;326:1097.

162. Morrow M, Quiet C, Hellman S, et al. Treatment selection in breast cancer: are our biases correct? Proc Am Soc Clin Oncol 1994;13:99.

163. Foster R, Farwell M, Costanza M. Breast conserving surgery for invasive breast cancer: patterns of care in a geographic region and estimate of potential applicability. Ann Surg Oncol (in press).

164. Osteen R, Karnell L. Breast cancer: the National Cancer Data Base report on breast cancer. Cancer 1994;73:1994.

165. Tarbox B, Rockwood J, Abernathy C. Are modified radical mastectomies done for T1 breast cancer because of surgeon's advice or patient's choice? Am J Surg 1992;164:417.

166. Tate P, McGee E, Hopkins S, et al. Breast conservation versus mastectomy: patient preferences in a community practice in Kentucky. J Surg Oncol 1993;52:213.

167. Hrushesky W, Bluning A, Gruber S, et al. Menstrual influence on the surgical cure of breast cancer. Lancet 1989;2:949.

168. Badwe R, Gregory W, Chaudary M, et al. Timing of surgery during menstrual cycle and survival of premenopausal women with operable breast cancer. Lancet 1991;337:1261.

169. Badwe R, Richard M, Fentiman I, et al. Surgical procedures, menstrual cycle phases, and prognosis in operable breast cancer. (Letter) Lancet 1991;338:815.

170. Senie R, Rosen P, Rhodes P, et al. Timing of breast cancer excision during the menstrual cycle influences duration of disease free survival. Ann Int Med 1991;115:337.

171. Sainsbury R, Jones M, Parker D, et al. Timing of surgery for breast cancer. (Letter) Lancet 1991;338:392.

172. Spratt J, Zirnheld J, Yancey J. Breast Cancer Detection Demonstration Project data can determine whether the prognosis of breast cancer is affected by time of surgery during the menstrual cycle. J Surg Oncol 1993;53:4.

173. Sadd Z. Timing of surgery in relation to menstrual cycle in premenopausal women and its effect of survival. Can J Surg 1992;35:438.

174. Ville Y, Briere M, Lasry S, et al. Timing of surgery for breast cancer (Letter). Lancet 1991;337:1604.

175. Powles T, Ashley S, Nash A, et al. Timing of surgery for breast cancer. (Letter) Lancet 1991;337:1604.

176. Powles T, Jones A, Ashley S, Tidy A. Menstrual effect on surgical cure of breast cancer. (Letter) Lancet 1989;2:1343.

177. Gelber R, Goldhirsch A. Menstrual effect on surgical cure of breast cancer. (Letter) Lancet 1989;2:1344.

178. Low S, Galea M, Blamey R. Timing of breast cancer surgery. Lancet 1991;338:691.

179. Goldhirsch A, Gelber R, Forbes J, et al. Timing of breast cancer surgery. Lancet 1991;338:692.

180. Sigurdsson H, Baldetorp B, Borg A, et al. Timing of surgery in the menstrual cycle does not appear to be a significant determinant of outcome in primary breast cancer. Proc Am Soc Clin Oncol 1992;11:62.

181. Rageth J, Wyss P, Vorger C, et al. Timing of breast cancer surgery within the menstrual cycle: influence on lymph-node involvement, receptor status, postoperative metastatic spread and local recurrence. Ann Oncol 1991;2:269.

182. Nathan B, Bates T, Anbazhagan R, et al. Timing of surgery for breast cancer in relation to the menstrual cycle and survival of premenopausal women. Br J Surg 1993;80:43.

183. McGuire W, Hilsenbeck S, Clark G. Optimal mastectomy timing. J Natl Cancer Inst 1992;84:346.

184. Davidson N, Abeloff M. Menstrual effects on surgical treatment for breast cancer. Canc Treat Rev 1993;19:105.

185. Durkin K, Haagensen C. An improved technique for the study of lymph nodes in surgical specimens. Ann Surg 1980;191:419.

186. Morrow M, Evans J, Rosen P, et al. Does clearing of the axillary lymph nodes contribute to accurate staging of breast carcinoma? Cancer 1984;53:1329.

187. Hartveit F, Samsonsen G, Tangen M, et al. Routine histological investigation of the axillary nodes in breast cancer. Clin Oncol 1982;8:121.

188. Kingsley W, Peters G, Cheek J. What constitutes accurate study of axillary lymph nodes in breast cancer? Ann Surg 1985;201:311.

189. Fisher B, Redmond C, Fisher E, et al. Ten year result of a random-ized clinical trial comparing radical mastectomy and total mastectomy with or without irradiation. N Engl J Med 1985;312:674.

190. Harris J, Osteen R. Patients with early breast cancer benefit from effective axillary treatment. Breast Cancer Res Treat 1985;5:17.

191. Brinkley D, Haybittle J. The curability of breast cancer. Lancet 1975;2:95.

192. Fentiman I, Cuzick J, Millis R. Which patients are cured of breast cancer? Br Med J 1984;289:1108.

193. Rosen P, Groshen S, Saigo P, et al. A long-term follow-up study of survival in stage I (T1N0M0) and stage II (T1N1M0) breast carcinoma. J Clin Oncol 1989;7:355.

194. Rosen P, Martin M, Kinne D, et al. Discontinuous or "skip" metastases in breast carcinoma: analysis of 1228 axillary dissections. Ann Surg 1983;197:276.

195. Veronesi U, Rilke F, Luini A, et al. Distribution of axillary node metastases by level of invasion. Cancer 1987;59:682.

196. Smith J, Gamex A JJ, Gallager H, et al. Carcinoma of the breast: analysis of total lymph node involvement versus level of metastasis. Cancer 1977;39:527.

197. Danforth D, Findlay P, McDonald H, et al. Complete axillary lymph node dissection for stage I–II carcinoma of the breast. J Clin Oncol 1986;4:655.

198. Chevinsky A, Ferrara J, James A, et al. Prospective evaluation of clinical and pathologic detection of axillary metastases in patients with carcinoma of the breast. Surgery 1990;108:612.

199. Pigott J, Nichols R, Maddox W, et al. Metastases to the upper levels of the axillary nodes in carcinoma of the breast and its implications for nodal sampling procedures. Surg Gynecol Obstet 1984;158:255.

200. Boova R, Bonanni R, Rosato F. Patterns of axillary nodal involvement in breast cancer. Ann Surg 1982;196:642.

201. Kissin M, Thompson E, Price A, et al. The inadequacy of axillary sampling in breast cancer. Lancet 1982;1:1210.

202. Steele R, Forrest A, Gibson T, et al. The efficacy of lower axillary sampling in obtaining lymph node status in breast cancer: a controlled randomized trial. Br J Surg 1985;72:368.

203. Forrest A, Stewart H, Roberts M, et al. Simple mastectomy and axillary node sampling (pectoral node biopsy) in the management of primary breast cancer. Ann Surg 1982;196:371.

204. Haagensen C. The surgical treatment of mammary carcinoma. In: Diseases of the breast, ed 2. Philadelphia, WB Saunders, 1971:706.

205. Halverson K, Taylor M, Perez C, et al. Regional nodal management and patterns of failure following conservative surgery and radiation therapy for stage I and II breast cancer. Int J Radiat Oncol Biol Phys 1993;26:593.

206. Recht A, Pierce S, Abner A, et al. Regional node failure after conservative surgery and radiotherapy for early stage breast carcinoma. J Clin Oncol 1991;9:988.

207. Siegel B, Mayzel K, Love S. Level I and II axillary dissection in the treatment of early-stage breast cancer. Arch Surg 1990;125:1144.

208. Fowble B, Solin L, Schultz D, et al. Frequency, sites of relapse, and outcome of regional node failures following surgery and radiation for early breast cancer. Int J Radiat Oncol Biol Phys 1989;17:703.

209. Kjaergaard J, Blichert-Toft M, Andersen J, et al. Probability of false negative nodal status in conjunction with partial axillary dissection in breast cancer. Br J Surg 1985;72:365.

210. Graversen H, Blichert-Toft M, Andersen J, et al. Breast cancer: risk of axillary recurrence in node-negative patients following partial dissection of the axilla. Eur J Surg Oncol 1988;14:407.

211. Axelsson C, Mouridsen H, Zedeler K, et al. Axillary dissection of level I and II lymph nodes is important in breast cancer classification. Eur J Cancer 1992;28A:1415.

212. Somers R, Jablon L, Kaplan M, et al. The use of closed suction drainage after lumpectomy and axillary node dissection for breast cancer: a randomized trial. Ann Surg 1992;215:146.

213. Ivens D, Hoe A, Podd T, et al. Assessment of morbidity from complete axillary dissection. Br J Cancer 1992;66:136.

214. Lin P, Allison D, Wainstuck J, et al. Impact of axillary lymph node dissection on the therapy of breast cancer patients. J Clin Oncol 1993;11:1536.

215. Hladiuk M, Huchcroft S, Temple W, et al. Arm function after axillary dissection for breast cancer: a pilot study to provide parameter estimates. J Surg Oncol 1992;50:47.

216. Gutman H, Kersz T, Barzilai T, et al. Achievements of physical therapy in patients after modified radical mastectomy compared with quadrantectomy, axillary dissection, and radiation for carcinoma of the breast. Arch Surg 1990;125:389.

217. Lotze U, Duncan M, Gerber L, et al. Early versus delayed shoulder motion following axillary dissection. Ann Surg 1981;193:288.

218. Petrek J, Peters M, Nori S, et al. Axillary lymphadenectomy: a prospective, randomized trial of thirteen factors influencing drainage, including early or delayed arm mobilization. Arch Surg 1991;125:378.

219. Clarke D, Martinez A, Cox R, et al. Breast edema following staging axillary node dissection in patients with breast carcinoma treated by radical radiotherapy. Cancer 1982;49:2295.

220. Cady B, Stone M, Wayne J. New therapeutic possibilities in primary invasive breast cancer. Ann Surg 1993;183:338.

221. Silverstein M, Gierson E, Waisman J, et al. Axillary lymph node dissection for T1a breast carcinoma: is it indicated? Cancer 1994;73:664.

222. Morrow M. The role of axillary node dissection in breast cancer management. Contemp Oncol 1994;4:16.

223. Baker L. Breast Cancer Detection Demonstration Project: five-year summary report. Cancer 1982;32:194.

224. Carter C, Allen C, Henson D. Relation of tumor size, lymph node status and survival in 24,740 breast cancer cases. Cancer 1989;63:181.

225. Chadha M, Chabon A, Friedmann P, et al. Predictors of axillary lymph node metastases in patients with T1 breast cancer. Cancer 1994;73:359.

226. Dewar J, Sarrazin D, Benhamou E, et al. Management of the axilla in patients treated at Institut Gustav-Roussy. Int J Radiat Oncol Biol Phys 1987;13:475.

227. Wilson R, Donegan W, Mettlin C, et al. The 1982 national survey of carcinoma of the breast in the United States by the American College of Surgeons. Surg Gynecol Obstet 1984;159:309.

228. Silverstein M, Waisman J, Gieison E, et al. Can axillary lymph node dissection be eliminated for selected patients with invasive breast cancer by using a combination of tumor size and palpability to predict nodal positivity? Proc Am Soc Clin Oncol 1994;13:56.

229. Wilhelm M, Edge S, Cole D, et al. Nonpalpable invasive breast cancer. Ann Surg 1992;213:600.

230. Ravdin P, DeLaurentis M, Wenger C, et al. Can prognostic factors be used to predict the nodal status of breast cancer patients? (Abstract) Proc Am Soc Clin Oncol 1994;13:56.

231. Wong J, Kopald K, Morton D. The impact of microinvasion on axillary node metastases and survival in patients with intraductal breast cancer. Arch Surg 1990;125:1298.

232. Solin L, Fowble B, Yeh I-T, et al. Microinvasive ductal carcinoma of the breast treated with breast-conserving surgery and definitive irradiation. Int J Radiat Oncol Biol Phys 1992;23:961.

233. Frazier T, Copeland E, Gallagher M, et al. Prognosis and treatment in minimal breast cancer. Am J Surg 1977;133:697.

234. Nevine J, Pinzon G, Moran T, et al. Minimal breast cancer. Am J Surg 1980;139:357.

235. McDivitt R, Boyce W, Gersell D. Tubular carcinoma of the breast: clinical and pathological observations concerning 135 cases. Am J Surg Pathol 1982;6:401.

236. Peters G, Wolff M, Haagensen C. Tubular carcinoma of the breast: clinical-pathologic correlations based on 100 cases. Ann Surg 1981;193:138.

237. Glick J. Meeting highlights: adjuvant therapy for primary breast cancer. J Natl Cancer Inst 1992;84:1479.

238. Berlanger D, Moore M, Tannock I. How American oncologists treat breast cancer: an assessment of the influence of clinical trials. J Clin Oncol 1991;9:7.

239. Morton D, Wen D, Wong J, et al. Technical details of intraoperative lymphatic mapping for early stage melanoma. Arch Surg 1992;127:392.

240. Giuliano A, Kirgan D, Guenther J, et al. Lymphatic mapping and sentinel lymphadenectomy for breast cancer. Ann Surg. 1994; 220:391.

241. Amalric R, Kurtz J, Santamaria F, et al. Conservation therapy of operable breast cancer: results at five, ten and fifteen years in 2216 consecutive cases. In: Harris JR, Hellman S, Silen W, eds. Conservative management of breast cancer. Philadelphia, JB Lippincott, 1983:3.

242. Calle R, Schlienger, Vilcoq J, et al. Conservative treatment of operable breast carcinoma by irradiation with or without limited surgery: ten-year results. In: Harris JR, Hellman S, Silen W, eds. Conservative management of breast cancer. Philadelphia, JB Lippincott, 1983:3.

243. Haffty B, McKhann C, Beinfield M, et al. Breast conservation therapy without axillary dissection. Arch Surg 1993;128:1315.

244. Cabanes P, Salmon R, Vilcoq J, et al. Value of axillary dissection in addition to lumpectomy and radiotherapy in early breast cancer. Lancet 1992;339:1245.

245. Valagussa P, Bonadonna G, Veronesi U. Patterns of relapse and survival following radical mastectomy: analysis of 716 consecutive patients. Cancer 1978;41:1170.

246. Fisher B, Wolmark N, Bauer M, et al. The accuracy of clinical nodal staging and of limited axillary dissection as a determinant of histologic nodal status in carcinoma of the breast. Surg Gynecol Obstet 1981;152:765.

247. Bedwinek J, Lee J, Fineberg B, et al. Prognostic indicators in patients with isolated local–regional recurrence of breast cancer. Cancer 1981;47:2232.

248. Aberizk W, Silver B, Henderson IC, et al. The use of radiotherapy for treatment of isolated local–regional recurrence of breast cancer after mastectomy. Cancer 1986;58:1214.

249. Chen K, Montague E, Oswald M. Results of irradiation in the treatment of loco-regional breast cancer recurrence. Cancer 1985;56:1269.

250. Fletcher G, McNeese M, Oswald M. Long-range results for breast cancer patients treated by radical mastectomy and postoperative radiation without adjuvant chemotherapy: an update. Int J Radiat Oncol Biol Phys 1989;17:11.

251. Uematsu M, Bornstein B, Recht A, et al. Long-term results of post-operative radiation therapy following mastectomy with and without chemotherapy in stage I–III breast cancer. Int J Radiat Oncol Biol Phys 1993;25:765.

252. Wallgren A, Arner O, Bergstrom J, et al. Radiation therapy in operable breast cancer: results from the Stockholm trial in adjuvant radiotherapy. Int J Radiat Oncol Biol Phys 1986;12:533.

253. Rutqvist L, Wallgren A, Nilsson B. Is breast cancer a curable disease? A study of 14,731 women with breast cancer for the Cancer Registry of Norway. Cancer 1984;53:1793.

254. Rutqvist L, Pettersson D, Johansson H. Adjuvant radiation therapy versus surgery alone in operable breast cancer: long-term follow-up in a randomized clinical trial. Radiother Oncol 1993;26:104.

255. Tennvall-Nittby L, Tengrup I, Landberg T. The total incidence of loco-regional recurrence in a randomized trial of breast cancer TNM stage II: the South Sweden Breast Cancer Trial. Acta Oncol 1993;32:641.

256. Rutqvist L, Lax I, Fornander T, et al. Cardiovascular mortality in

a randomized trial of adjuvant radiation therapy versus surgery alone in primary breast cancer. Int J Radiat Oncol Biol Phys 1992;22:887.

257. Lythgoe J, Palmer M. Manchester regional breast study: 5 and 10 year results. Br J Surg 1982;69:693.

258. Haybittle J, Brinkley D, Houghton J, et al. Postoperative radiotherapy and late mortality: evidence from the Cancer Research Campaign trial for early breast cancer. Br Med J 1989;298:1611.

259. Stewart H, Jack W, Forrest A, et al. South-east Scottish trial of local therapy in node negative breast cancer. Breast 1994;3:31.

260. Bonadonna G, Valagussa P, Rossi A, et al. Ten-year experience with CMF-based adjuvant chemotherapy in resectable breast cancer. Breast Cancer Res Treat 1985;5:95.

261. Fisher B, Fisher E, Redmond C, et al. Ten year results from the NSABP clinical trial evaluating the use of L-phenylalanine mustard (L-PAM) in the management of primary cancer. J Clin Oncol 1986;4:929.

262. Howell A, George W, Crowther D, et al. Controlled trial of adjuvant chemotherapy with cyclophosphamide, methotrexate, and fluorouracil for breast cancer. Lancet 1984;2:307.

263. Rubens R, Knight R, Fentiman I, et al. Controlled trial of adjuvant chemotherapy with melphalan for breast cancer. Lancet 1983;1:839.

264. Koyama H, Wada T, Takahashi Y, et al. Surgical adjuvant chemotherapy with mitomycin-C and cyclophosphamide in Japanese patients with breast cancer. Cancer 1980;46:2372.

265. Morrison J, Howell A, Grieve R. The West Midlands Oncology Association trials of adjuvant chemotherapy for operable breast cancer. In: Salmon S, Jones S, eds. Adjuvant therapy of cancer IV. Orlando, Grune & Stratton, 1984:253.

266. Rutqvist L, Cedermark B, Fornander T, et al. The relationship between hormone receptor content and the effect of adjuvant tamoxifen in operable breast cancer. J Clin Oncol 1989;7:1474.

267. Nolvadex Adjuvant Trial Organization. Controlled trial of tamoxifen as a single adjuvant agent in management of early breast cancer: analysis at six years by the Nolvadex Adjuvant Trial Organization. Lancet 1985;1:836.

268. Breast Cancer Trials Committee of the Scottish Cancer Trials Office. Adjuvant tamoxifen in the management of operable breast cancer: the Scottish trial. Lancet 1987;2:171.

269. Stefanik D, Goldberg R, Byrne P, et al. Local–regional failure in patients treated with adjuvant chemotherapy for breast cancer. J Clin Oncol 1985;3:660.

270. Fowble B, Gray R, Gilchrist K, et al. Identification of a subgroup of patients with breast cancer and histologically positive axillary nodes receiving adjuvant chemotherapy who may benefit from postoperative radiotherapy. J Clin Oncol 1988;6:1107.

271. Goldie J, Coldman A. A mathematic model for relating the drug sensitivity of tumors to their spontaneous mutation rate. Cancer Treat Rep 1979;63:1727.

272. Ragaz J, Jackson S, Plenderleith I, et al. Can adjuvant radiotherapy improve the overall survival of breast cancer patients in the presence of adjuvant chemotherapy? 10 year analysis of the British Columbia randomized trial. (Abstract) Proc Am Soc Clin Oncol 1993;12:60.

273. Overgaard M, Christensen J, Johansen H, et al. Evaluation of radiotherapy in high-risk breast cancer patients. Int J Radiat Oncol Biol Phys 1990;19:1121.

274. Dombernowsky P, Hansen P, Mouridsen H, et al. Randomized trial of adjuvant CMF + radiotherapy (RT) vs CMF alone vs tamoxifen (TAM) in pre- and menopausal stage II breast cancer. (Abstract) Eur J Cancer 1994;30A (Suppl 2):S28.

275. Rose C, Hansen P, Dombernowsky P, et al. A randomized trial of adjuvant (ADJ) tamoxifen (TAM) + radiotherapy (RT) vs TAM alone vs TAM + CMF in postmenopausal stage II breast cancer. (Abstract) Eur J Cancer 1994;30A (Suppl 2):S28.

276. Rutqvist L, Cedermark B, Glas U, et al. Radiotherapy, chemotherapy, and tamoxifen as adjuncts to surgery in early breast cancer: a summary of three randomized trials. Int J Radiat Oncol Biol Phys 1989;16:629.

277. Nordenskjold B, Stal O, Skoog L, et al. S-phase fraction and c-erbB-2 expression related to the survival benefit from adjuvant chemotherapy of breast cancer. (Abstract) Proc Am Soc Clin Oncol 1994;13:67.

278. Glick J, Fowble B, Haller D, et al. Integration of full-dose adjuvant chemotherapy with definitive radiation for primary breast cancer. J Natl Cancer Inst Monogr 1988;6:297.

279. Come S, Botnick L, Lange R, et al. Concurrent radiation therapy and chemotherapy in the primary management of pathologic stage II breast cancer. (Abstract) Proc Am Soc Clin Oncol 1983;2:99.

280. Lippman M, Edwards B, Findlay P, et al. Influence of definitive radiation therapy for primary breast cancer on the ability to administer adjuvant chemotherapy. J Natl Cancer Inst Monogr 1986;1:99.

281. Bonadonna G, Valagussa P, Zucali R, et al. Feasibility of adjuvant chemotherapy plus radiotherapy in operable breast cancer. In: Harris JR, Hellman S, Silen W, eds. Conservative management of breast cancer. Philadelphia, JB Lippincott, 1983:329.

282. Levine J, Coleman C, Cox R, et al. The effect of postoperative and primary radiation therapy on delivered dose of adjuvant chemotherapy in breast cancer. Cancer 1984;53:237.

283. Holland J, Glidewell O, Copper R. Adverse effect of radiotherapy on adjuvant chemotherapy for carcinoma of the breast. Surg Gynecol Obstet 1980;150:817.

284. Bedwinek J. Adjuvant irradiation for early breast cancer: an ongoing controversy. Cancer 1984;53:729.

285. Griem K, Henderson I, Gelman R, et al. The 5-year results of a randomized trial of adjuvant radiation therapy after chemotherapy in breast cancer patients treated with mastectomy. J Clin Oncol 1987;5:1546.

286. Marks L, Halperin E, Prosnitz L, et al. Post-mastectomy radiotherapy following adjuvant chemotherapy and autologous bone marrow transplantation for breast cancer patients with ≥ 10 positive axillary lymph nodes. Int J Radiat Oncol Biol Phys 1992;23:1021.

287. Harris J, Hellman S. Put the "hockey stick" on ice. Int J Radiat Oncol Biol Phys 1988;15:497.

288. Ludwig Breast Cancer Study Group. Combination adjuvant chemotherapy for node-positive breast cancer: inadequacy of a single perioperative cycle. N Engl J Med 1988;319:677.

289. Kraniner M, Sevelda P, Salzer H, et al. Comparison between the application of intra- versus 3-week postoperative adjuvant chemotherapy in breast cancer. (Abstract) Eur J Cancer 1991;27(Suppl 2):39.

290. Sertoli M, Pronzato P, Querolo P, et al. Perioperative polychemotherapy for primary breast cancer. (Abstract) Gelber R, Goldhirsch A, et al, eds. Adjuvant therapy breast cancer. Berlin, Springer-Verlag, 1993:57.

291. Lara-Jimenez P, Garcia Puche J, Pedraza V. Adjuvant combined modality treatment in high risk breast cancer patients: ten-year results. (Abstract) Proceedings of the 5th EORTC Breast Cancer Working Conference, 1991:A293.

292. Glucksberg H, Rivkin S, Rasmussen S, et al. Combination chemotherapy (CMFVP) versus L-phenylalanine mustard (L-PAM) for operable breast cancer with positive axillary nodes: a Southwest Oncology Group study. Cancer 1982;50:423.

293. Buzdar A, Smith T, Powell K, et al. Effect of timing of initiation of adjuvant chemotherapy on disease-free survival in breast cancer. Breast Cancer Res Treat 1982;2:163.

294. Dalton W, Brooks R, Jones S, et al. Breast cancer adjuvant therapy trials at the Arizona Cancer Center using adriamycin and cyclophosphamide. In: Salmon S, Jones S, eds. Adjuvant therapy of cancer vol 5. Orlando, Grune & Stratton, 1987:263.

295. Brufman G, Sulkes A. A retrospective analysis of adjuvant chemo-

therapy with and without radiotherapy for stage II breast cancer: a 10-year update. (Abstract) Proceedings of the 5th European Conference on Clinical Oncology 1991:P-0882.

296. Harris J, Recht A. How to combine adjuvant chemotherapy and radiation therapy. In: Senn H-J, Gelber R, Goldhirsch A, et al, eds. Adjuvant therapy of breast cancer IV. Berlin, Springer-Verlag, 1993;129.

297. Buchholz T, Austin-Seymour M, Moe R, et al. Effect of delay in radiation in the combined modality treatment of breast cancer. Int J Radiat Oncol Biol Phys 1993;26:23.

298. Hartsell W, Recine D, Griem K, et al. Does delay in the initiation of radiation therapy adversely affect local control in treatment of the intact breast? (Abstract) Radiother Oncol 1992;24:37.

299. McCormick B, Begg C, Norton L, et al. Timing of radiotherapy in the treatment of early-stage breast cancer. (Letter) J Clin Oncol 1993;11:191.

300. Buzdar A, Kau S, Smith T, et al. The order of administration of chemotherapy and radiation and its effect on the local control of operable breast cancer. Cancer 1993;71:3680.

301. Pacini P, Cappeline M, Cardona G, et al. Conservative treatment of breast cancer: influence of boost dose and interval between surgery and radiotherapy on breast relapses. (Abstract) In: Senn H-J, Gelber R, Goldhirsch A, et al, eds. Adjuvant therapy of breast cancer. Berlin, Springer-Verlag, 1992;65.

301a. Recht A, Come SE, Silver B, et al. Sequencing of chemotherapy (CT) and radiotherapy (RT) following conservative surgery (CS) for patients with early-stage breast cancer: results of a randomized trial. (Abstract) Int J Radiat Oncol Biol Phys (in press).

302. Botnick L, Come S, Rose C, et al. Primary breast irradiation and concomitant adjuvant chemotherapy. In: Harris J, Hellman S, Silen W, eds. Conservative management of breast cancer. Philadelphia, JB Lippincott, 1983;321.

303. Hahn P, Hallberg O, Vikterlof K. Acute skin reactions in postoperative breast cancer patients receiving radiotherapy plus adjuvant chemotherapy. Am J Roentgen 1978;130:137.

304. Hansen R, Erickson B, Komaki R, et al. Concomitant adjuvant chemotherapy and radiotherapy for high risk breast cancer patients. Breast Cancer Res Treat 1990;17:171.

305. Meek A, Order S, Abeloff M, et al. Concurrent radiochemotherapy in advanced breast cancer. Cancer 1983;51:1001.

306. Sponzo R, Cunningham T, Caradonna R. Management of non-resectable (stage III) breast cancer. Int J Radiat Oncol Biol Phys 1979;5:1475.

307. Bontenbal M, Sieuwerts A, Foekens J, et al. Enhanced antitumor effects of combination chemo- and radiotherapy on the cytotoxicity in human breast cancer cells in vitro. (Abstract) Proceedings of the 5th EORTC Breast Cancer Working Conference, 1991:A196.

308. Buzzoni R, Bonadonna G, Valagussa P, et al. Adjuvant chemotherapy with doxorubicin plus cyclophosphamide, methotrexate, and fluorouracil in the treatment of resectable breast cancer with more than three positive axillary nodes. J Clin Oncol 1991;9:2134.

309. Moliterni A, Bonadonna G, Valagussa P, et al. Cyclophosphamide, methotrexate, and fluorouracil with and without doxorubicin in the adjuvant treatment of resectable breast cancer with one to three positive axillary nodes. J Clin Oncol 1991;9:1124.

310. Perez C, Presant C, Philpott G, et al. Phase I–II study of concurrent irradiation and multi-drug chemotherapy in advanced carcinoma of the breast: a pilot study by the Southeastern Cancer Study Group. Int J Radiat Oncol Biol Phys 1979;5:1329.

311. Piccart M, De Valeriola D, Paridaens R, et al. Six-year results of a multimodality treatment strategy for locally advanced breast cancer. Cancer 1988;62:2501.

312. Lingos T, Recht A, Vicini F, et al. Radiation pneumonitis in breast cancer patients treated with conservative surgery and radiation therapy. Int J Radiat Oncol Biol Phys 1991;21:355.

313. Lippman M, Lichter A, Edwards B, et al. The impact of primary

irradiation treatment of localized breast cancer on the ability to administer systemic adjuvant chemotherapy. J Clin Oncol 1984;2:21.

314. Habibollahi F, Fentiman I, Chaudary M, et al. Influence of radiotherapy on the dose of adjuvant chemotherapy in early breast cancer. Breast Cancer Res Treat 1989;13:237.

315. Ahmann D, O'Fallon J, Scanlon P, et al. A preliminary assessment of factors associated with recurrent disease in a surgical adjuvant clinical trial for patients with breast cancer with special emphasis on aggressiveness of therapy. Am J Clin Oncol 1982;5:371.

316. Cooper M, Rhyne A, Muss H, et al. A randomized comparative trial of chemotherapy and radiation therapy for stage II breast cancer. Cancer 1981;47:2833.

317. Ragaz J, Ng V. Correlation of dose intensity (DI) of individual chemotherapy agents (CA) in CMF combined with radiation therapy: a review of a randomized adjuvant study. (Abstract) Proc Am Assoc Cancer Res 1988;29:A788.

318. Sarkaria J, Miller E, Parker C, et al. 4-hydroxytamoxifen, an active metabolite of tamoxifen, does not alter the radiation sensitivity of MCF-7 breast carcinoma cells irradiated *in vitro*. Breast Cancer Res Treat 1994;30:159.

319. Wazer D, Joyce M, Chan W, et al. Effects of tamoxifen on the radiosensitivity of hormonally responsive and unresponsive breast carcinoma cells. Radiat Oncol Invest 1993;1:20.

320. Kinsella T, Gould M, Mulcahy R, et al. Keynote address: integration of cytostatic agents and radiation therapy: a different approach to "proliferating" human tumors. Int J Radiat Oncol Biol Phys 1991;20:295.

321. Gallagher H, Martin J. An orientation to the concept of minimal breast cancer. Cancer 1971;28:1501.

322. McDivitt R. Breast carcinoma. Hum Pathol 1978;9:3.

323. Silverstein M, Waisman J, Gierson E, et al. Radiation therapy for intraductal carcinoma: is it an equal alternative? Arch Surg 1991;126:424.

324. Schwartz G, Patchefsky A, Finklestein S, et al. Nonpalpable in situ ductal carcinoma of the breast: predictors of multicentricity and microinvasion and implications for treatment. Arch Surg 1989; 124:29.

325. Lagios M, Westdahl P, Margolin F, et al. Ductal carcinoma in situ: relationship of extent of noninvasive disease to the frequency of occult invasion, multicentricity, lymph node metastases, and short-term treatment failures. Cancer 1982;50:1309.

326. Kinne D, Petrek J, Osborne M, et al. Breast carcinoma in situ. Arch Surg 1989;124:33.

327. Schuh M, Nemoto T, Penetrante R, et al. Intraductal carcinoma: analysis of presentation, pathologic findings, and outcome of disease. Arch Surg 1986;121:1303.

328. Rosner D, Lane W, Penetrante R. Ductal carcinoma in situ with microinvasion: a curable entity using surgery alone without need for adjuvant therapy. Cancer 1991;67:1498.

329. The Uppsala–Orebro Breast Cancer Study Group. Sector resection with or without postoperative radiotherapy for stage I breast cancer: a randomized trial. J Natl Cancer Inst 1990;82:277.

330. Liljegren G, Holmberg L, Adami H-O, et al. Section resection with and without postoperative radiotherapy for stage I breast cancer: five–year results of a randomized trial. J Natl Cancer Inst 1994;86:717.

331. Clark R, McCulloch P, Levine M, et al. Randomized clinical trial to assess the effectiveness of breast irradiation following lumpectomy and axillary dissection for node-negative breast cancer. J Natl Cancer Inst 1992;84:683.

332. Veronesi U, Luini A, Del Vecchio M, et al. Radiotherapy after breast-preserving surgery in women with localized cancer of the breast. N Engl J Med 1993;328:1587.

333. Hayman J, Schnitt S, Gelman R, et al. A prospective trial of conservative surgery (CS) alone without radiation therapy (RT) in se-

lected patients with early-stage breast cancer. (Abstract) Int J Radiat Oncol Biol Phys (in press).

334. Sauer R, Tulusan A, Lang N, et al. Can breast irradiation be omitted in low-risk breast cancer patients after segmentectomy? first results of the Erlangen protocol. (Abstract) Int J Radiat Oncol Biol Phys 1993;(Suppl 1)27:146.

335. Moffat F, Ketcham A. Breast-conserving surgery and selective adjuvant radiation therapy for stage I and II breast cancer. Semin Surg Oncol 1992;8:172.

336. Hermann R, Esselstyn CJ, Grundjest-Broniatowski S, et al. Partial mastectomy without radiation is adequate treatment for patients with stages 0 and 1 carcinoma of the breast. Surg Gynecol Obstet 1993;177:247.

337. Stewart H, Prescott R, Forrest P. Conservative therapy of breast cancer. (Letter) Lancet 1989;2:168.

338. Levine M, Gent M, Hryniuk W, et al. A randomized trial comparing 12 weeks versus 36 weeks of adjuvant chemotherapy in stage II breast cancer. J Clin Oncol 1990;8:1217.

339. Nemoto T, Patel J, Rosner D, et al. Factors affecting recurrence in lumpectomy without irradiation for breast cancer. Cancer 1991;67:2079.

340. Cooke A, Perera F, Fisher B, et al. Tamoxifen with and without radiation after partial mastectomy in patients with involved nodes. Int J Radiat Oncol Biol Phys 1995;31:777.

341. Lee K, Plowman P, Gilmore O, et al. Breast conservation therapy: how safe is post-operative tamoxifen-only in the elderly and frail. (Abstract) Proc Am Soc Clin Oncol 1992;11:50.

342. Preece P, Wood R, Mackie C, et al. Tamoxifen as initial sole treatment of localized breast cancer in elderly women: a pilot study. Br Med J 1982;284:869.

343. Helleberg A, Lundgren B, Norin T, et al. Treatment of early localized breast cancer in elderly patients by tamoxifen. Br J Radiol 1982;55:511.

344. Allan S, Rodger A, Smyth J, et al. Tamoxifen as primary treatment of breast cancer in elderly or frail patients: a practical management. Br Med J 1985;190:358.

345. Auclerc C, Khayat D, Borel C, et al. Tamoxifen as sole treatment in patients aged 65 and over with primary breast cancer. (Abstract) Proc Am Soc Clin Oncol 1990;9:173.

346. Foudraine N, Verhoef L, Burghouts J. Tamoxifen as sole therapy for primary breast cancer in the elderly patient. Eur J Cancer Clin Oncol 1992;2894:900.

347. Gaskell D, Hawkins R, Sangsterl K, et al. Relation between immunocytochemical estimation of oestrogen receptor in elderly patients with breast cancer and response to tamoxifen. Lancet 1989;1:1044.

348. Gazet J, Ford H, Coombes R, et al. Prospective randomized trial of tamoxifen versus surgery in elderly patients with breast cancer. Eur J Surg Oncol 1994;20:207.

349. Bates T, Riley D, Houghton J, et al. Breast cancer in elderly women: a Cancer Research Campaign trial comparing treatment with tamoxifen and optimal surgery with tamoxifen alone. Br J Surg 1991;78:591.

350. Morrow M. Breast disease in elderly women. Surg Clin North Am 1994;74:145.

351. Kantorowitz D, Poulter C, Sischy B, et al. Treatment of breast cancer among elderly women with segmental mastectomy or segmental mastectomy plus postoperative radiotherapy. Int J Radiat Oncol Biol Phys 1988;15:263.

352. Toonkel L, Fix I, Jacobson L, et al. Management of elderly patients with primary breast cancer. Int J Radiat Oncol Biol Phys 1988;14:677.

353. Osteen R. Selection of patients for breast conserving therapy. Cancer 1994;74:366.

354. Margolese R, Poisson R, Shibata H, et al. The technique of segmental mastectomy (lumpectomy) and axillary dissection: a syllabus from the National Surgical Adjuvant Breast Project workshop. Surgery 1987;102:828.

355. Cox C, Ku N, Reintgen D, et al. Touch preparation cytology of breast lumpectomy margins with histologic correlation. Arch Surg 1991;126:490.

356. Ku N, Cox C, Reintgen D, et al. Cytology of lumpectomy specimens. Acta Cytol 1991;35:417.

357. Kearney T, Morrow M. Does the need for re-excision influence the success of breast conserving surgery? Ann Surg Oncol (in press).

358. Clarke D, Martinez A. Identification of patients who are at high risk for locoregional breast cancer recurrence after conservative surgery and radiotherapy: a review article for surgeons, pathologists, and radiation and medical oncologists. J Clin Oncol 1992;10:474.

359. Gwin J, Eisenberg B, Hoffman J, et al. Incidence of gross and microscopic carcinoma in specimens from patients with breast cancer after re-excision lumpectomy. Ann Surg 1993;218:729.

360. Schmidt-Ullrich R, Wazer D, DiPetrillo T, et al. Breast conservation therapy for early stage breast carcinoma with outstanding local control rates: a case for aggressive therapy to the tumor bearing quadrant. Int J Radiat Oncol Biol Phys 1993;27:545.

361. Frazier T, Wong R, Rose D. Implications of accurate pathologic margins in the treatment of primary breast cancer. Arch Surg 1989;124:37.

362. Wapnir I, Bancila E, Devereux D, et al. Residual tumor and breast biopsy margins. Breast Dis 1989;1:81.

363. Van Dongen J, Bartelink H, Fentiman I, et al. Factors influencing local relapse and survival and results of salvage treatment after breast conserving therapy in operable breast cancer: EORTC trial 10801, breast conservation compared with mastectomy in TNM stage I and II breast cancer. Eur J Cancer 1992;28A:801.

364. Fisher E, Anderson S, Redmond C, et al. Ipsilateral breast tumor recurrence and survival following lumpectomy and irradiation: pathological findings from NSAPB protocol B06. Semin Surg Oncol 1992;8:161.

365. Lesser M, Rosen P, Kinne D. Multicentricity and bilaterality in invasive breast carcinoma. Surgery 1982;91:234.

366. Fisher E, Gregorio R, Redmond C, et al. Pathologic findings from the National Surgical Adjuvant Breast Project (protocol no. 4): observations concerning the multicentricity of mammary cancer. Cancer 1975;35:247.

367. Keidan R, Hoffman J, Weese J, et al. Delayed breast abscess after lumpectomy and radiation therapy. Am Surg 1990;54:440.

368. Resigno J, McCormick B, Brown A, et al. Breast cellulitis after conservative surgery and radiotherapy. Int J Radiat Oncol Biol Phys 1994;29:163.

369. Patey D, Dysin W. The prognosis of carcinoma of the breast in relation to type of operation performed. Br J Cancer 1948;2:71.

370. Auchincloss H. Modified mastectomy. Am J Surg 1970;119:506.

371. Kodama H. Modification of muscle preserving radical mastectomy. Cancer 1979;44:1517.

372. Croce E. A neoclassical radical mastectomy. Surg Gynecol Obstet 1978;1978:147.

373. Roses D, Harris M, Gumport S. Total mastectomy with axillary dissection. Am J Surg 1977;134:674.

374. Schneiderman M, Axtell L. Deaths among female patients with carcinoma of the breast treated by a surgical procedure only. Surg Gynecol Obstet 1979;148:193.

375. Say C, Donegan W. A biostatistical evaluation of complications from mastectomy. Surg Gynecol Obstet 1974;138:370.

376. Aitken D, Minton J. Complications associated with mastectomy. Surg Clin North Am 1983;63:1331.

377. Beatty J, Robinson G, Zaia J, et al. A prospective analysis of nosocomial wound infection after mastectomy. Arch Surg 1983;118:1421.

378. Platt R, Zucker J, Zaleznik D, et al. Perioperative antibiotic pro-

phylaxis and wound infection following breast surgery. J Antimicrob Chemother 1993;(Suppl B)31:43.

379. Platt R, Zucker J, Zaleznik D, et al. Prophylaxis against wound infection following herniorrhaphy or breast surgery. J Infect Dis 1992;166:556.

380. Budd D, Cochran R, Sturtz O, et al. Surgical morbidity after mastectomy operations. Am J Surg 1978;135:218.

381. Myers M, Brock D, Cohn IJ. Prevention of skin slough after radical mastectomy by the use of a vital dye to delineate devascularized skin. Ann Surg 1971;173:920.

382. Chilson T, Chan F, Lonser R, et al. Seroma prevention after modified radical mastectomy. Ann Surg 1992;58:750.

383. Jolly P, Viar W. Reduction of morbidity after radical mastectomy. Am Surg 1981;47:377.

384. Jameson K, Wellisch D, Katz R, et al. Phantom breast syndrome. Arch Surg 1979;114:93.

385. Kroner K, Knudsen U, Lundley H, et al. Long-term phantom breast syndrome after mastectomy. Clin J Pain 1992;8:346.

386. Webster D, Manse R, Hughes L. Immediate reconstruction of the breast after mastectomy: is it safe? Cancer 1984;53:1416.

387. Johnson C, Van Heerden J, Donohue J, et al. Oncological aspects of immediate breast reconstruction following mastectomy for malignancy. Arch Surg 1989;124:819.

388. Petit J, Le M, Mouriesse H, et al. Can breast reconstruction with gel-filled silicone implants increase the risk of death and second primary cancer in patients treated by mastectomy for breast cancer? Plast Reconstr Surg 1994;94:115.

389. Kroll S, Ames F, Singletary S, et al. The oncologic risks of skin preservation at mastectomy when combined with immediate reconstruction of the breast. Surg Gynecol Obstet 1991;172:17.

390. Dao T, Nemoto T. The clinical significance of skin recurrence after radical mastectomy in women with cancer of the breast. Surg Gynecol Obstet 1963;117:447.

391. Noone R, Frazier T, Noone G, et al. Recurrence of breast carcinoma following immediate reconstruction: a 13-year review. Plast Reconstr Surg 1994;90:96.

392. Eberlein T, Crespo L, Smith B, et al. Prospective evaluation of immediate reconstruction after mastectomy. Ann Surg 1993; 218:29.

393. Noone R, Murphy J, Spear S, et al. A six-year experience with immediate reconstruction for mastectomy for cancer. Plast Reconst Surg 1985;76:258.

394. Barreau-Pouhaer L, Le M, Rietjens M, et al. Risk factors for failure of immediate breast reconstruction with prostheses after total mastectomy for breast cancer. Cancer 1992;70:1145.

396. Owen I, Yarnold J, Bliss J, et al. Randomized comparison of a 13 fraction schedule with a conventional 25 fraction schedule of radiotherapy after local excision of early breast cancer: preliminary analysis. (Abstract) Proc ESTRO 1994;S101.

397. Bentel G, Marks L. A simple device to position large/flaccid breasts during tangential breast irradiation. Int J Radiat Oncol Biol Phys 1994;29:879.

398. van Tienhoven G, Lanson J, Crabeels D, et al. Accuracy in tangential breast treatment set-up: a portal imaging study. Radiother Oncol 1991;22:317.

399. Bornstein B, Cheng C, Rhodes L, et al. Can simulation measurements be used to predict the volume of lung within the radiation therapy treatment field in breast cancer patients? Int J Radiat Oncol Biol Phys 1990;18:181.

400. Fraass B, Lichter A, McShan D, et al. The influence of lung density corrections on treatment planning for primary breast cancer. Int J Radiat Oncol Biol Phys 1988;14:179.

401. Solin L, Chu J, Sontag M, et al. Three-dimensional photon treatment planning of the intact breast. Int J Radiat Oncol Biol Phys 1991;21:193.

402. Lichter A, Fraass B, van de Geign J, et al. A technique for field matching in primary breast irradiation. Int J Radiat Oncol Biol Phys 1982;9:263.

403. Conte G, Nascimben O, Turcato G, et al. Three-field technique for breast treatment. Int J Radiat Oncol Biol Phys 1988;14:1299.

404. Hartsell W, Murthy A, Kiel K, et al. Technique for breast irradiation using custom blocks for conforming to the chest wall contour. Int J Radiat Oncol Biol Phys 1990;19:189.

405. Rosenow U, Valentine E, Davis L. A technique for treating local breast cancer using a single set-up point and asymmetric collimation. Int J Radiat Oncol Biol Phys 1990;19:183.

406. Galvin J, Powlis W, Fowble B, et al. A new technique for positioning tangential fields. Int J Radiat Oncol Biol Phys 1993;26:877.

407. Webb S, Leach M, Bentley B, et al. Clinical dosimetry for radiotherapy to the breast based on imaging with the prototype Royal Marsden Hospital CT stimulator. Phys Med Biol 1987;32:835.

408. Solin L, Danoff B, Schwartz G, et al. A practical technique for the localization of the tumor volume in definitive irradiation of the breast. Int J Radiat Oncol Biol Phys 1985;11:1215.

409. Bedwinek J. Breast conserving surgery and irradiation: the importance of demarcating the excision cavity with surgical clips. Int J Radiat Oncol Biol Phys 1993;26:675.

410. Leonard C, Harlow C, Coffin C, et al. Use of ultrasound to guide radiation boost planning following lumpectomy for carcinoma of the breast. Int J Radiat Oncol Biol Phys 1993;27:1193.

411. Gilligan D, Hendry J, Yarnold J. The use of ultrasound to measure breast thickness to select electron energies for breast boost radiotherapy. Radiother Oncol 1994;32:265.

412. Regine W, Komanduri M, Komarnicky L, et al. Computer-CT planning of the electron boost in definitive breast irradiation. Int J Radiat Oncol Biol Phys 1991;20:121.

413. Fowble B, Solin L, Schultz D. Conservative surgery and radiation for early breast cancer. In: Fowble B, Goodman R, Glick J, et al, eds. Breast cancer treatment: a comprehensive guide to management. Chicago, Mosby–Year Book, 1991:122.

414. Woudstra E, van der Werf H. Obliquely incident electron beams for irradiation of the internal mammary lymph nodes. Radiother Oncol 1987;10:209.

415. Gagliardi G, Lax I, Rutqvist L. An improved treatment technique for stage II breast cancer. (Abstract) Proc ESTRO 1994;S105.

416. Recht A, Siddon R, Kaplan W, et al. Three-dimensional internal mammary lymphoscintigraphy: implications for radiation therapy treatment planning for breast carcinoma. Int J Radiat Oncol Biol Phys 1988;14:477.

417. Marks L, Hebert M, Bentel G. To treat or not to treat the internal mammary nodes: a possible compromise. Int J Radiat Oncol Biol Phys 1994;29:903.

418. Bretton R, Nelson R. Causes and treatment of postmastectomy lymphedema of the arm. JAMA 1962;180:95.

419. Swedborg I, Wallgren A. The effect of pre- and post-mastectomy radiotherapy on the degree of edema, shoulder joint mobility, and gripping force. Cancer 1981;47:877.

420. Larson D, Weinstein M, Goldberg I, et al. Edema of the arm as a function of the extent of axillary surgery in patients with stage I and II carcinoma of the breast treated with primary radiotherapy. Int J Radiat Oncol Biol Phys 1986;12:877.

421. Dewar J, Benhamou S, Benhamou E. Cosmetic results following lumpectomy, axillary dissection and radiotherapy for small breast cancers. Radiother Oncol 1988;12:273.

422. Match R. Radiation-induced brachial plexus paralysis. Arch Surg 1975;110:384.

423. Stoll B, Andrews J. Radiation-induced peripheral neuropathy. Br Med J 1975;1:834.

424. Powell S, Cooke J, Parsons C. Radiation-induced brachial plexus injury: follow-up of two different fractionation schedules. Radiother Oncol 1990;18:213.

425. Salner A, Botnick L, Herzog A, et al. Reversible brachial plexopa-

thy following primary radiation therapy for breast cancer. Cancer Treat Rep 1981;65:797.

426. Pierce S, Recht A, Lingos T, et al. Long-term radiation complications following conservative surgery (CS) and radiation therapy (RT) in patients with early stage breast cancer. Int J Radiat Oncol Biol Phys 1992;23:915.

427. Olsen N, Pfeiffer P, Johannsen L, et al. Radiation-induced brachial plexopathy: neurological follow-up in 161 recurrence-free breast cancer patients. Int J Radiat Oncol Biol Phys 1993;26:43.

428. Ryttov N, Holm N, Qvist N, et al. Influence of adjuvant irradiation on the development of late arm lymphedema and impaired shoulder mobility after mastectomy for carcinoma of the breast. Acta Oncol 1988;27:667.

429. Bentzed S, Overgaard M, Thames H. Fractionation sensitivity of a functional endpoint: impaired shoulder movement after post-mastectomy radiotherapy. Int J Radiat Oncol Biol Phys 1989; 17:531.

430. Montague E. Experience with altered fractionation in radiation therapy for breast cancer. Radiology 1968;90:962.

431. Kim J, Chu F, Hilaris B. The influence of dose fractionation on acute and late reactions in patients with postoperative radiotherapy for carcinoma of the breast. Cancer 1975;35:1538.

432. Kimsey F, Mendenhall N, Ewald L, et al. Is radiation treatment volume a predictor for acute or late effect on pulmonary function? Cancer 1994;73:2549.

433. Hardman P, Tweeddale P, Kerr G, et al. The effect of pulmonary function of local and loco-regional irradiation for breast cancer. Radiother Oncol 1994;30:33.

434. Rothwell R, Kelly S, Joslin C. Radiation pneumonitis in patients treated for breast cancer. Radiother Oncol 1985;4:9.

435. Srinivasan G, Kurtz D, Lichter A. Pleural-based changes on chest x-ray after irradiation for primary breast cancer: correlation with findings on computerized tomography. Int J Radiat Oncol Biol Phys 1983;9:1567.

436. Committee on the Biological Effects of Ionizing Radiations, Board on Radiation Effects Research Commission on Life Sciences, National Research Council. Health effects of exposure to low levels of ionizing radiation: BEIR V. Washington, DC: National Academy, 1990.

437. Baral E, Larsson L, Mattson B. Breast cancer following irradiation of the breast. Cancer 1977;40:2905.

438. Mattsson A, Ruden B-I, Hall P, et al. Radiation-induced breast cancer: long-term follow-up of radiation for benign breast disease. J Natl Cancer Inst 1993;85:1679.

439. Gray L. Radiation biology and cancer. In: Cellular radiation biology: The M.D. Anderson Hospital and Tumor Institute 18th symposium on fundamental cancer research. Baltimore, Williams & Wilkins, 1965:7.

440. Fraass B, Roberson P, Lichter A. Dose to the contralateral breast due to primary breast irradiation. Int J Radiat Oncol Biol Phys 1985;11:485.

441. Tokunaga M, Land C, Tokuoka S, et al. Incidence of female breast cancer among atomic bomb survivors, 1950–1985. Radiat Res 1994;138:209.

442. Boice JD Jr, Harvey EB, Blettner M, et al. Cancer in the contralateral breast after radiotherapy for breast cancer. N Engl J Med 1992;326:781.

443. Storm H, Andersson M, Boice J Jr, et al. Adjuvant radiotherapy and risk of contralateral breast cancer. J Natl Cancer Inst 1992;84:1245.

444. Brady M, Garfein C, Petrek J, et al. Post-treatment sarcoma in breast cancer patients. Ann Surg Oncol 1994;1:66.

445. Taghian A, de Vathaire F, Terrier P, et al. Long-term risk of sarcoma following radiation treatment for breast cancer. Int J Radiat Oncol Biol Phys 1991;21:361.

446. Kurtz J, Amalric R, Brandone H, et al. Contralateral breast cancer and other second malignancies in patients treated by breast-conserving therapy with radiation. Int J Radiat Oncol Biol Phys 1988;15:277.

447. Zucali R, Merson M, Placucci M, et al. Soft tissue sarcoma of the breast after conservative surgery and irradiation for early mammary cancer. Radiother Oncol 1994;30:271.

448. Wijnmaalen A, van Ooijen B, van Geel B, et al. Angiosarcoma of the breast following lumpectomy, axillary lymph node dissection, and radiotherapy for primary breast cancer: three case reports and a review of the literature. Int J Radiat Oncol Biol Phys 1993;26:135.

449. Smith P, Dole R. Age and time-dependent changes in the rates of radiation-induced cancers in patients with ankylosing spondylitis. In: Late biological effects of ionizing radiation, vol 1. Vienna, International Atomic Energy Agency, 1978:203.

450. Curtis R, Boice J Jr, Stovall M, et al. Risk of leukemia risk after chemotherapy and radiation therapy for breast cancer. N Engl J Med 1992;326:1745.

451. Alderson M, Jackson S. Long-term follow-up of patients with menorrhagia treated with irradiation. Br J Radiol 1971;44:295.

452. Brinkley D, Haybittle J. The late effects of artificial menopause by x-radiation. Br J Radiol 1969;42:519.

453. Doll R, Smith P. The long-term effects of x-irradiation in patients treated for metropathia hemorrhagica. Br J Radiol 1968;41:362.

454. Curtis R, Boice J Jr, Stovall M, et al. Leukemia risk following radiotherapy for breast cancer. J Clin Oncol 1989;7:21.

455. Inskip P, Stovall M, Flannery J. Lung cancer risk and radiation dose among women treated for breast cancer. J Natl Cancer Inst 1994;86:983.

456. Neugut A, Robinson E, Lee W, et al. Lung cancer after radiation therapy for breast cancer. Cancer 1993;71:3054.

457. Neugut A, Murray T, Santos J, et al. Increased risk of lung cancer after breast cancer radiation therapy in cigarette smokers. Cancer 1994;73:1615.

458. Inskip P, Boice J Jr. Radiotherapy-induced lung cancer among women who smoke (Editorial). Cancer 1994;73:1541.

459. Fuller S, Haybittle J, Smith R, et al. Cardiac doses in post-operative breast irradiation. Radiother Oncol 1992;25:19.

460. Janjan N, Gillin M, Prows J, et al. Dose to the cardiac vascular and conduction systems in primary breast irradiation. Med Dosim 1989;14:81.

461. Valagussa P, Zambetti M, Biasi S, et al. Cardiac effects following adjuvant chemotherapy and breast irradiation in operable breast cancer. Ann Oncol 1994;5:209.

462. Jones J, Ribeiro G. Mortality patterns over 34 years of breast cancer patients in a clinical trial of post-operative radiotherapy. Clin Radiol 1989;40:204.

463. Host H, Brennhovd I, Loeb M. Postoperative radiotherapy in breast cancer: Long-term results from the Oslo study. Int J Radiat Oncol Biol Phys 1985;12:727.

464. Early Breast Cancer Trialists' Group. Treatment of early breast cancer: world-wide experience, 1985–1990, vol 1. Oxford, UK, Oxford University, 1990.

465. Velez-Garcia E, Carpenter JJ, Moore M, et al. Postsurgical adjuvant chemotherapy with and without radiotherapy in women with breast cancer and positive axillary nodes: a South-Eastern Cancer Study Group (SEG) trial. Eur J Cancer 1992;28A:1833.

466. Muss H, Cooper R, Brockschmidt J, et al. A randomized trial of adjuvant chemotherapy (CT) without radiation therapy (RT) for stage II breast cancer: 11-year follow-up of Piedmont Oncology Association (Protocol no. 74176). Breast Cancer Res Treat 1989;14:185.

467. McArdle C, Crawford D, Dykes E, et al. Adjuvant radiotherapy and chemotherapy in breast cancer. Br J Surg 1986;73:264.

468. Blomqvist C, Tiusanen K, Elomma I, et al. The combination of radiotherapy, adjuvant chemotherapy (cyclophosphamide-doxorubicin-ftorafur) and tamoxifen in stage II breast cancer: long-term results of a randomized trial. Br J Cancer 1992;66:1171.

17.2

Adjuvant Systemic Therapy of Primary Breast Cancer

C. KENT OSBORNE ▪ GARY M. CLARK ▪ PETER M. RAVDIN

Adjuvant systemic therapy is defined as the administration of cytotoxic chemotherapy or the use of ablative or additive endocrine therapy after primary surgery of breast cancer to kill or inhibit clinically occult micrometastases. Death from breast cancer results from growth of micrometastases that are present at distant sites beyond the confines of the surgically resected breast and regional lymphatics. These metastases, which are rarely evident on routine radiographs and scans at the time of diagnosis, account for the high treatment failure rate in breast cancer patients treated only with local modalities such as surgery and irradiation.

Historical Perspective and Rationale for Adjuvant Therapy

In the late 1800s, Halsted devised the radical mastectomy for breast cancer based on his belief that the disease was usually slowly spreading, metastasizing under the skin, along fascial planes, and by lymphatics, but not hematogenously. He thought that the cancer remained localized and confined for a time in the breast and in regional lymph nodes, which served as barriers to distant migration. En bloc removal of all these tissues (radical mastectomy) would then increase curability of the disease. Unfortunately, only 12% of patients treated by Halstead and his students survived 10 years, and later attempts to perform even more radical surgery failed to improve survival, leading to the conclusion that distant metastases were present in many patients by the time of the initial diagnosis.[1,2]

More recent surgical studies have provided more encouraging results from radical mastectomy, with 50% of all patients remaining disease-free at 10 years. Still, 30% of node-negative patients and 75% of node-positive patients eventually have recurrences and die of their disease when it is treated by surgery alone.[2] These observations have had two major clinical implications. First, less disfiguring breast surgical procedures may improve cosmesis and quality of life without jeopardizing survival, which is predetermined by the presence or absence of micrometastases. Second, improvements in breast cancer survival require methods to diagnose the disease in its premetastatic phase or methods of effective systemic therapy to eradicate micrometastases at the time of diagnosis of the primary tumor, when the number of metastatic foci is smallest. Forty years ago, the paradigm for adjuvant systemic therapy was established by studies in preclinical animal models demonstrating curability of cancer with a combined treatment approach of surgical resection and chemotherapy.[3,4] Later, investigators recognized that early administration of chemotherapy in animal models, when the tumor burden was low and when growth kinetics were most favorable, could eradicate cancers that became incurable when treatment was delayed.[5]

Historically, the first randomized trial of breast cancer adjuvant therapy, initiated in 1948 (in fact, one of the first randomized trials of any sort), involved ovarian ablation by irradiation.[6] This study was based on earlier observations that ovarian ablation could induce regressions of advanced breast cancer in premenopausal patients. Accrual to the first chemotherapy adjuvant study was begun in 1958. This study and other early adjuvant trials were designed on the premise that breast cancer metastases were caused by surgical manipulation of the tumor, which "seeded" the bloodstream, a hypothesis supported by experimental observations.[7–10]

Contemporary adjuvant chemotherapy trials in which prolonged postoperative treatment was used to inhibit established micrometastases were begun in the late 1960s and early 1970s. Initial studies focused on patients with axillary lymph node metastases in the mastectomy specimen; such patients have a high risk of disease recurrence, justifying the use of toxic therapy. Trials using a new endocrine therapy, the antiestrogen tamoxifen, were initiated in the mid-1970s. The 1980s brought studies of doxorubicin-based chemotherapy regimens, clinical trials of adjuvant therapy in patients without axillary nodal involvement, studies of combined chemoendocrine therapy, and a renewed interest in ovarian ablation using the new leutinizing hormone–releasing hormone (LHRH) antagonists. The 1990s will almost certainly be known as the decade for studies of chemotherapy dose intensity, including trials of extremely high-dose chemotherapy with autologous bone marrow transplantation. Clinical trials of preoperative chemotherapy designed to reduce primary tumors to a size more amenable to breast-preserving surgical procedures and designed to treat the cancer early, before the spontaneous emergence of drug-resistant cells, will soon provide additional information.

More than 100 randomized clinical trials of breast cancer adjuvant therapy have now been completed. Many of these studies have had more than 15 to 20 years of patient follow-up, and firm conclusions can be drawn about the value of treatment in different patient subsets. Although many questions remain, sufficient information is available to conclude that appropriately administered adjuvant treatment does improve survival of patients with early-stage disease.

Interpretation of Adjuvant Clinical Trial Results

An understanding by the clinician of the various methods of analysis of clinical trials of adjuvant therapy is crucial for proper data interpretation and for accurate estimation of treatment benefit. Such estimates provide critical information for the patient and physician in making clinical treatment decisions.

RANDOMIZED TRIALS

Progress in the adjuvant therapy of breast cancer is due to a large extent to randomized controlled clinical studies. Uncontrolled or historically controlled trials are acceptable only for testing the safety of new regimens and for generating hypotheses, but large randomized studies are mandatory for definitive conclusions regarding safety and efficacy of a new treatment approach, especially when the difference in treatment outcome is small. As an example, three-drug chemotherapy combined with bacillus calmette-Giérin (BCG) immunotherapy was promoted as effective adjuvant therapy for breast cancer in the late 1970s, based on a retrospective comparison of treated patients to a historical control population not receiving adjuvant therapy.[11] These data generated a series of randomized trials that eventually concluded that, not only was BCG immunotherapy ineffective, but also its addition to chemotherapy resulted in increased mortality.[12] Thus, the major contribution of randomized trials is to correct false-positive results produced by nonrandomized trials. Many randomized trials of adjuvant therapy for breast cancer are inadequate and inconclusive because of their small size, however; such trials may produce false-negative results if the study population is not large enough. Many randomized trials fail to show a statistically significant survival benefit for chemotherapy in postmenopausal patients or for tamoxifen in lymph node–negative patients. In contrast, later metaanalyses of these studies clearly demonstrate a small but worthwhile mortality reduction with these therapies.[12] The potential problems inherent in small randomized trials are magnified by the need to examine major patient subsets (eg, menopausal status, nodal status), a need that further reduces the statistical power to detect treatment differences.

Trial Endpoints

Disease-free survival (DFS), defined as the time from randomization to first evidence of treatment failure or death, and *overall survival (OS)*, defined as the time from randomization to death from any cause, are the major endpoints of interest in most randomized treatment trials. Distant DFS is the time from randomization to first evidence of treatment failure outside the primary disease site or death from any cause. Breast cancer–specific DFS or OS is used less commonly because deaths from other causes are potentially related in some way to the disease itself or its treatment. OS is probably the most important efficacy endpoint in adjuvant therapy trials; however, it is influenced not only by the impact of the adjuvant therapy, but also by treatment given after relapse, which is often not standardized in clinical trials. DFS focuses on the efficacy of the primary disease treatment, but it ignores what happens to the patient after disease recurrence, which might well be influenced by the adjuvant treatment received.

Thus, although adjuvant treatments that prolong DFS might be expected also to prolong OS, this might not occur if the adjuvant treatment jeopardizes response to treatments given after relapse resulting in shorter postrelapse survival. Similarly, prolongation of DFS or OS by adjuvant treatment does not necessarily indicate that any patients are cured or will not relapse or die during their expected lifetime. Disease recurrence or mortality may simply be delayed by some period of time that, if long enough, may still justify the toxicity and cost of treatment. Although substantial prolongations in both DFS and OS have been observed with adjuvant therapy of breast cancer, whether these treatments are curative in any patients is still uncertain.

The results from randomized clinical trials are frequently depicted by Kaplan-Meier life-table plots in which the proportion of patients remaining disease-free or remaining alive is shown as a function of the time after randomization (Fig. 17.2-1). Results are sometimes also presented as a hazard function defined as the risk of failure per unit time. In comparing two treatment groups, the

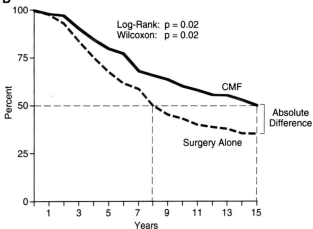

FIGURE 17.2-1 Kaplan-Meier plot of relapse-free survival (**A**) and overall survival (**B**) in premenopausal patients in the first Milan study of adjuvant CMF.[13]

hazard ratio is the ratio of the hazard function of the *control group* to that of the *experimental treatment group,* so when the ratio is close to 1, no difference in efficacy exists between the two groups. A hazard ratio greater than 1 indicates a higher relapse or death rate in the control group, whereas a ratio less than 1 indicates more untoward events in the experimental group. Although these numbers are useful in interpreting quantitative differences between two treatment groups, they provide little useful information to the physician or patient trying to make a treatment decision.

Closer examination of life-table plots can produce clinically useful information (Fig. 17.2-1). A common method of analyzing such plots is to calculate the percentage of difference between the two treatment groups at a defined point in time. To be most accurate, the chosen point in time should be equal to or shorter than the median follow-up time of all patients in the study. Figure 17.2-1 shows the long-term relapse-free survival and OS of premenopausal women enrolled in one of the first randomized trials of adjuvant combination chemotherapy in axillary lymph node–positive women.[13] At 15 years of follow-up (an appropriate time given that all the patients in the study had been followed for more than 15 years), approximately 42% of patients receiving cyclophosphamide, methotrexate, 5-fluorouracil (CMF) therapy remained relapse-free and 50% alive, compared with 28% and 35%, respectively, of control patients. Thus, the difference in relapse-free survival is 14%, and the difference in OS is 15%. This difference is defined as the *absolute benefit* or the number of recurrences or deaths avoided (in this case at 15 years) per 100 women treated. Some investigators report results in terms of the *proportional benefit* or the average annual percentage reduction in the odds of recurrence or death. In the study shown in Figure 17.2-1, 65% of the group of patients treated by surgery alone had died by 15 years, whereas only 50% of CMF-treated patients had died. These results correspond roughly to a 30% to 35% proportional reduction in mortality with adjuvant CMF therapy.

Physicians must understand the difference between absolute benefit (15% in the example above) and proportional benefit (30% to 35%) in discussing treatment options with patients. This is especially important in patients with a lower risk of recurrence. Table 17.2-1 shows the number of deaths avoided per 100 patients treated in several hypothetic subsets of patients with markedly different estimated 10-year death rates (range, 10% to 70%) without adjuvant treatment as a function of different estimates of treatment benefit shown as proportional reductions in mortality, assuming exponential death with a constant hazard ratio and not considering deaths from other causes, which can be significant in older patients. Approximately 13 of every 100 patients treated in the poorest risk group benefit at 10 years because of the treatment, given a 30% proportional reduction in mortality by the adjuvant therapy. These data are similar to the results of the Milan CMF trial in premenopausal patients described earlier. In contrast, only 3 of every 100 patients treated in the best prognostic group benefit at 10 years from the same treatment; most of the patients in this group fail to benefit because they are already cured by surgery and do not need it. The absolute benefit would be greater if treatment provided a greater proportional reduction in mortality, but reductions in the 40% to 50% range have not been observed consistently with current regimens. Proportional reductions in mortality in the 20% range, typical of the overall effects of adjuvant tamoxifen, lead to still lower absolute benefits.

Although the absolute benefit is perhaps the most important parameter and the simplest in helping patients make treatment decisions, it underestimates the true value of adjuvant therapy. In Figure 17.2-1 one might incorrectly assume that only 15 patients benefited out of every 100 patients treated with CMF. Other patients who had already died by year 15 might have had a substantial delay in their death by treatment, however. An alternative method of evaluating the benefits of therapy is to calculate the difference in median DFS or OS. In the CMF study, the median times to recurrence and median survival were about 3 and 8 years, respectively, in the control group, compared with 11 and 15 years in the group treated with chemotherapy (see Fig. 17.2-1). Thus, even though many patients eventually had recurrences and died despite receiving 1 year of CMF chemotherapy, they still benefited substantially in terms of a prolonged time to recurrence and average prolongation of life.

Two other cautions need to be considered in the interpretation of randomized trials. Randomized trials, especially small ones, can produce not only false-negative

TABLE 17.2-1

Absolute Reduction in Mortality Rate at 10 Years per 100 Patients Treated

Estimated 10-y Death Rate With No Therapy	Hypothetic Proportional Reduction in Mortality Rate Due to Treatment				
	50%	40%	30%	20%	10%
70% (several positive nodes)	25	19	13	8	4
50% (5-cm tumor, negative nodes)	21	16	12	7	4
30% (average, negative nodes)	14	11	8	5	3
10% (≤1-cm tumor, negative nodes)	5	4	3	2	1

results because of insufficient statistical power, but also false-positive results simply by chance. Trials producing positive results are more likely to be published in widely read journals, whereas negative studies may be relegated to more obscure journals or are not published at all. This publication bias may influence medical practice for years until subsequent trials fail to confirm results. As an example, the initial report of the first Milan CMF trial showed equally promising results in both premenopausal and postmenopausal patients, and these results led to widespread use of this regimen in both subsets.[14] Later analyses of this study failed to show a benefit in postmenopausal patients, and subsequent analyses of multiple studies have established that the benefit of chemotherapy in these patients is modest compared to younger patients.[12]

Another hazard in the reporting of randomized trials is multiple subset analyses. Most trials report treatment differences in numerous subsets of patients categorized by nodal status, menopausal status, receptor status, and so forth. Analysis of multiple subsets is bound to yield a misleadingly positive result simply by statistical chance even if a treatment difference does not exist. Subset analyses, unless taken into consideration in the original statistical design of a study, can only be used to generate new hypotheses, and they do not provide conclusive information.

Overview or Metaanalysis

Well over 100 different randomized prospective adjuvant therapy breast cancer trials have been reported. On the basis of chance, some of these trials are likely to be misleadingly promising, whereas others are misleadingly negative. Many individual studies are far too small to detect modest but still worthwhile treatment benefits that would have major public health implications given the high incidence of breast cancer.

One method of overcoming these pitfalls is the overview or metaanalysis technique. This approach is described previously in more detail, but, in general, it uses information from all trials addressing the same question (ie, adjuvant tamoxifen versus no adjuvant tamoxifen) by calculating the annual difference between the number of observed recurrences or deaths in the treatment group and the number expected if the events in the treatment group and control group were the same.[12] The values of observed events minus expected events from each trial can be added together to give an overall effect. Large trials with longer follow-up and more events have more weight than small trials. The large numbers of patients contributed by all individuals trials provide great statistical power and enable metaanalyses reliably to detect modest advantages for one treatment over another and thus to correct false-negative results produced by small randomized trials.

Even metaanalyses have potential problems. For instance, the metaanalysis for adjuvant chemotherapy of breast cancer is likely to be an underestimate of the actual benefit achievable in a compliant patient population given the best drug regimen, because the analysis combined the results of studies using a variety of different chemotherapy regimens with various drug doses and schedules, some of which must be more or less effective than others. Overview results of the tamoxifen or ovarian ablation trials are likely to be more accurate because compliance and differences in the treatment administered are not an issue. Nevertheless, the metaanalysis of breast cancer adjuvant therapy has contributed substantially to our current medical practice patterns by providing more certain evidence of the efficacy of adjuvant therapy, by resolving controversies originating in previously conflicting results, and by generating testable hypotheses for future studies. Data from the breast cancer metaanalysis are used extensively in this chapter to emphasize certain points.

TREATMENT TOXICITY AND QUALITY OF LIFE ESTIMATES

Treatment side effects, long-term toxicities, and their impact on patient quality of life are additional important gauges of the efficacy of adjuvant treatment. Patients' side effects recorded by a nurse or physician, while providing important information, frequently underestimate the incidence or severity of various toxicities because these parameters were not sought in a formal, prospective fashion in some trials, especially those performed many years ago. Furthermore, these estimates represent physicians' estimates of severity rather than patient's, and they tend to focus on laboratory values or purely physical parameters rather than on more subjective evidence of morbidity affecting the patient's life-style. An accurate portrayal of the adverse effects of treatment is necessary when comparing the overall efficacy of two treatments that happen to provide similar mortality reductions. An accurate toxicity profile is also mandatory for women to make an informed decision about adjuvant therapy, especially patients with a low risk of disease recurrence when the toxicity–benefit ratio may be close to 1.

Valid estimation of toxicity and its effects on quality of life have proved difficult. One approach, developed at the Ontario Cancer Treatment and Research Foundation, is the Breast Cancer Chemotherapy Questionnaire (BCCQ), which consists of 30 questions that focus on both physical and emotional or psychological issues facing patients receiving adjuvant chemotherapy.[15] BCCQ has been shown to be a valid method of estimating treatment-related morbidity in patients receiving chemotherapy, proving superior to several other methods of assessment when administered longitudinally to patients on a 2-arm adjuvant treatment trial.[15]

Another useful test, developed by the International Breast Cancer Study Group, is known as Q-TWiST (quality of life–adjusted analysis of time without symptoms and toxicity).[16,17] This modified survival analysis calculates adjusted survival time after subtracting from overall survival the time during which the patient was suffering treatment-related toxicity, the time needed to recover from treatment given for local recurrence, and the survival period after a systemic relapse of disease. Thus, Q-TWiST incorporates treatment effectiveness and morbidity into a single parameter that has been used to demonstrate an advantage for chemoendocrine therapy compared with endocrine therapy alone in postmenopausal patients,[17] and the net benefit of prolonged chemotherapy compared with a single course of perioperative treatment in patients with node-positive breast cancer.[16] Estimation of treatment effects on quality of life is an important issue in need of additional research, method development, and application to adjuvant therapy trials.

Benefits of Adjuvant Chemotherapy

POSTOPERATIVE ADJUVANT CHEMOTHERAPY IN NODE-POSITIVE PATIENTS

Randomized trials of prolonged postoperative adjuvant chemotherapy were first initiated more than 20 years ago. These early trials focused on patients with positive axillary lymph nodes; the high risk of recurrence and death (75% overall at 10 years) of these patients was thought to justify the use of potentially toxic chemotherapy. Based on estimates derived from animal studies and mathematic models, as well as a certain degree of empiricism, most early studies used 1 to 2 years of adjuvant treatment. Most trials were small, accruing fewer than 500 patients.

Studies of adjuvant chemotherapy proceeded in a logical series of experiments. First, groups receiving one-drug or multiple-drug regimens were compared with those given placebo or with a no-treatment control group. Multiple-drug regimens were then compared with single-drug regimens, and shorter durations of treatment were compared with longer durations. More recently, trials have evaluated doxorubicin-based regimens, and they have compared combination chemoendocrine therapy with each modality used alone.

Two adjuvant chemotherapy studies, begun in 1972 and 1973, respectively, had the most impact on changing the patterns of care for breast cancer patients.[14,18] A study of 349 node-positive patients performed by the National Surgical Adjuvant Breast Project (NSABP) compared 2 years of single-agent melphalan with placebo, and a similar study of 386 patients carried out at the Istituto Nazionale Tumori in Milan compared a group of patients given a regimen of CMF for 1 year with a group of patients treated with surgery alone.[13,19] Both studies showed an overall statistically significant DFS advantage for chemotherapy; a trend for improved OS was also evident in both studies, but the differences failed to reach statistical significance. Subset analyses demonstrated that the chemotherapy advantage was confined to premenopausal patients or patients younger than 50 years of age. Acute toxicity was deemed acceptable, especially with melphalan, although life-threatening or fatal reactions did occur with these treatments. Although outcomes were similar, CMF soon became the standard chemotherapy regimen for adjuvant breast cancer therapy. The shorter duration of treatment (1 year versus 2 years), the documented superiority of CMF in advanced breast cancer, and the fear of the leuke-

mogenic potential of melphalan, all contributed to the popularity of CMF, which is still used frequently today.

Numerous other studies of a variety of chemotherapy regimens compared with a no-treatment control arm have been completed in predominantly node-positive patients, and nearly all show a DFS and OS benefit confined to premenopausal patients.[12] The frequent development of amenorrhea in such patients has led some investigators to hypothesize that much of the benefit of adjuvant chemotherapy is due to a medical castration effect.[20,21] Studies of chemotherapy combined with ovarian ablation that show an additive effect,[12] studies showing an advantage for CMF in premenopausal patients regardless of menstrual irregularities or tumor estrogen receptor (ER) positivity,[22,23] and results of a study comparing ovarian ablation with chemotherapy showing a greater advantage for ablation in ER-positive patients and a greater advantage for CMF in ER-negative patients,[24] however, all suggest that the benefits of chemotherapy are mediated partly through chemical castration and partly through a cytotoxic effect.

Adjuvant Chemotherapy in Premenopausal Patients

The efficacy of adjuvant chemotherapy is illustrated best by examining the 10-year results of the overview of all trials begun before January 1, 1985.[12] The metaanalysis included 31 randomized trials of prolonged (2 months or more) combination chemotherapy versus no chemotherapy involving more than 11,000 patients.[12] Overall, adjuvant polychemotherapy given for at least 2 months caused a highly significant 28% annual reduction in the odds of recurrence and a 17% reduction in the odds of death (Table 17.2-2). When the analysis was restricted to node-positive patients, a 30% reduction in the odds of recurrence and an 18% reduction in the odds of death were

TABLE 17.2-2

Overview of Adjuvant Chemotherapy Trials: Recurrence and Mortality With Prolonged Polychemotherapy

Patient Group	Reduction (SD) in Annual Odds	
	Recurrence (%)	Death (%)
All patients	28 (3)	17 (3)
<50 y	36 (5)	24 (5)
≥50 y	24 (3)	13 (4)
<50 y, premenopausal	36 (5)	25 (6)
50–59 y, premenopausal	25 (9)	23 (9)
<50 y, postmenopausal	37 (19)	Too few patients
50–59 y, postmenopausal	29 (5)	13 (7)
60–69 y, all	20 (5)	10 (6)
70+ y	Too few patients	Too few patients

(Adapted from Early Breast Cancer Trialists' Collaborative Group. Systemic treatment of early breast cancer by hormonal, cytotoxic, or immune therapy. Lancet 1992;399:1,71)

observed. Thus, about 1 of every 3 or 4 recurrences and 1 of every 5 or 6 deaths was delayed or avoided by adjuvant chemotherapy at 10 years. Survival curves indicate that 36% of control patients remain disease-free at 10 years, compared with 44% of treated patients.[12] Forty-five percent of control patients and 51% of treated patients survived 10 years.

Consistent with results obtained in most individual trials, chemotherapy was more effective in younger patients (see Table 17.2-2). Premenopausal patients or patients younger than 50 years of age regardless of menstrual status had similar reductions in recurrence and death. One third or more of the recurrences and one fourth of the deaths were avoided or delayed at 10 years by adjuvant chemotherapy. Premenopausal patients older than 50 years of age also had significant reductions in recurrence and death. Thus, the first-generation adjuvant trials with long follow-up demonstrate a highly significant benefit in premenopausal patients with breast cancer.

Adjuvant Chemotherapy in Postmenopausal Patients

Nearly all the early controlled trials of adjuvant chemotherapy failed to find a survival benefit in patients 50 years of age or older or in patients known to be postmenopausal. Even the metaanalysis published in 1988 with 5-year follow-up could not find a statistically significant advantage in older patients.[25] The 10-year metaanalysis does show a statistically significant recurrence and mortality reduction in older women, however (Table 17.2-2).[12] The annual reduction in the odds of recurrence was 24%, and that for mortality was 13% in women 50 years of age or older. The mortality reduction was about half that seen in younger patients. The benefits were less pronounced in postmenopausal patients aged 60 to 69 years, compared with younger postmenopausal patients, and too few patients aged 70 years or older were included in these trials to provide valid estimates of the effects of adjuvant chemotherapy in elderly patients.

The reasons that postmenopausal patients seem to benefit less from adjuvant chemotherapy are not clear. Part of the difference may be attributed to the added endocrine effect of chemotherapy described earlier in premenopausal patients. Differences in tumor biology in younger and older patients may also play a role. Tumors in premenopausal women are more frequently ER-negative and tend to have higher S-phase fractions, indicating a more rapidly proliferating tumor that may be more responsive to chemotherapy.[26,27] Other investigators maintain that the arbitrarily lower chemotherapy doses given to older women because of the unjustified fear of unacceptable toxicity in this age group account for the inferior results in some studies.[28]

More recent trials raise questions about the relative ineffectiveness of adjuvant chemotherapy in older patients. Controlled trials of CMF or methotrexate and 5-fluorouracil (MF) in node-negative patients,[29,30] trials of multidrug regimens,[31] and a trial of dose intensity of doxorubicin-based therapy[32] reveal a similar magnitude of treatment benefit in premenopausal and postmenopausal patients. Whether these results represent selection of positive trials or whether they reflect greater benefits of contemporary chemotherapy administration in older patients remains to be proved. Until then, one can conclude that adjuvant chemotherapy does reduce mortality modestly in older patients, with about one in every eight deaths delayed or avoided at 10 years by treatment.

POSTOPERATIVE ADJUVANT CHEMOTHERAPY IN AXILLARY NODE–NEGATIVE PATIENTS

Many of the early controlled trials of adjuvant chemotherapy included some node-negative patients, but these trials were not designed prospectively to assess the benefit in this subgroup. Furthermore, most of these trials contained too few patients to draw definitive conclusions. Many physicians were reluctant to treat node-negative patients with chemotherapy because of the potential of life-threatening or even fatal toxicity together with the relatively favorable prognosis of this group.

Indeed, most studies report that, although 75% of all node-positive patients treated by surgery alone die within 10 years, only 25 to 30% of node-negative patients die of breast cancer in the first 10 years. Studies with extremely long-term follow-up suggest that additional recurrences and deaths, perhaps one fourth of the total, occur after 10 years, but the majority of patients with breast cancer who do not have nodal metastases do not succumb to breast cancer and are cured by surgery alone.[33] Obviously, these patients could not possibly benefit from adjuvant treatment designed to eliminate viable micrometastases that they do not have.

The node-negative breast cancer population is a heterogeneous group of patients. Other prognostic factors, reviewed in Chapter 16, can be used to distinguish node-negative patients with an extremely low risk of breast cancer recurrence and death from groups with a 10-year survival just as poor as some patients with positive lymph nodes. Patients with tumors 1 cm in diameter or smaller have only a 10% to 15% chance of ever having a recurrence, whereas those with tumors 3 cm or larger have a 50% or greater chance of disease recurrence.[29,33] Patients with ER-positive tumors have a 5% to 10% lower risk of recurrence than patients with ER-negative tumors.[34] These prognostic factors were used to identify higher risk, node-negative patients for adjuvant chemotherapy studies focusing on this subgroup that were initiated in the early 1980s.

Among the first trials to investigate the value of chemotherapy specifically in patients with negative axillary lymph nodes was the West Midlands II trial comparing chlorambucil, methotrexate, and 5-fluorouracil for 6 months with a no-treatment group of patients.[35] Nearly half the 543 patients accrued to the study, which was initiated in 1976, were premenopausal. No significant benefits in DFS or OS were observed in this study, although the regimen consisted of low oral doses of the three drugs and would be considered inappropriate by today's standards.

Interest in the adjuvant treatment of node-negative

breast cancer patients rose with the publication of the results of 5 separate trials completed in the 1980s, 1 of which examined a single course of perioperative chemotherapy, 1 of which evaluated tamoxifen for 5 years, and 3 of which evaluated postoperative chemotherapy.[29,30,36–38] The 3 postoperative trials were restricted to patients with ER-negative or large tumors because of their higher risk of early relapse and death. One of these trials accrued only 90 patients, 54 of whom were premenopausal.[38] Patients were randomized to surgery alone or to surgery and adjuvant CMF. The chemotherapy regimen was a different version from that originally studied by the Milan group, and it consisted of 9 months of intravenous therapy every 3 weeks, a regimen later proved to be inferior to standard CMF in advanced breast cancer.[39] Nevertheless, extraordinary results were obtained (Table 17.2-3). The DFS of control patients at 8 years was an exceptionally poor 39%, probably reflecting patient selection and the small size of the trial. Patients receiving CMF had an 80% DFS at 8 years, half the recurrence rate of the untreated group.[13] OS was also improved by CMF in this study.

These remarkable results were confirmed to some extent by two other trials[29,30,40,41] (see Table 17.2-3). The recurrence rates in the control groups were not as great as in the Milan trial, but sizable reductions in the rates of recurrence were observed in both studies. Postmenopausal patients benefited at least as much as younger women in both trials, and although a strong trend for improved OS was seen at the last analysis, both studies showed a statistically significant mortality reduction only in postmenopausal patients. These studies suggest that adjuvant chemotherapy is not only efficacious in node-positive patients, but also in node-negative patients.

A greater degree of certainty of the DFS and OS benefits of adjuvant chemotherapy in node-negative patients comes from the breast cancer metaanalysis[12] (Table 17.2-4). Quanti-

tatively, the improvements in DFS and in OS were similar in node-negative and node-positive patients. These data indicate that adjuvant chemotherapy provides clinically important reductions in recurrence and mortality in node-negative patients, at least those at a relatively higher risk of recurrence based on prognostic factors. Trials that have recently been completed or are in progress are addressing the value of the addition of cyclophosphamide to MF, are comparing doxorubicin-based regimens with CMF, and are comparing chemoendocrine therapy or chemotherapy alone with endocrine therapy. Whether all node-negative patients should receive some form of adjuvant therapy is discussed later in this chapter.

OPTIMAL ADJUVANT CHEMOTHERAPY REGIMEN

During the past 20 years, studies have addressed the question of what is the optimal chemotherapy regimen. Whereas these studies have not identified the optimal regimen as a standard to be used by all oncologists, they have provided important general conclusions as well as a menu of possible regimens to be considered by the practicing physician.

Single Agents Compared With Combination Chemotherapy

In 1975, the results of the NSABP trial comparing melphalan with placebo demonstrated the superiority of adjuvant chemotherapy.[18] Because combination chemotherapy was proving superior to single agents in advanced breast cancer,[42] the next logical step was to compare a multiple-drug regimen with melphalan in node-positive patients.

The Southwest Oncology Group (SWOG) began a study in 1975 comparing 2 years of single-agent melphalan with 1 year of continuous CMFVP, a regimen in which cyclophosphamide is given daily by mouth, methotrexate and 5-fluorouracil weekly intravenously, and vincristine and prednisone intravenously and orally, respectively, only

TABLE 17.2-3

Effect of Adjuvant Chemotherapy in Node-Negative Studies from Milan, the National Surgical Adjuvant Breast Project, and the Intergroup

	Milan (CMF)*		NSABP (MF)†		Intergroup (CMFP)‡	
Control	39%		67%		61%	
		P = .0002		P = .007		P < .0001
Chemotherapy	80%		76%		83%	

Milan Trial: n = 90, median follow-up 8 years; National Surgical Adjuvant Breast Project (NSABP): n = 737, median follow-up 5 years; Intergroup: n = 425, median follow-up 5 years. CMF, cyclophosphamige–methotrexate–5-fluorouracil; MF, methotrexate–5-fluorouracil; CMFP, CMF with prednisone.

* Data from Bonnadonna G. Evolving concepts in the systemic adjuvant treatment of breast cancer. Cancer Res 1992;52:2127.

† Data from Fisher B, Wickerham DL, Redmond C. Recent developments in the use of systemic adjuvant therapy for the treatment of breast cancer. Semin Oncol 1992;19:263.

‡ Data from Mansour EG, Eudey L, Tormey DC, et al. Chemotherapy versus observation in high-risk node-negative breast cancer patients. J Natl Cancer Inst Monogr 1992;11:97.

TABLE 17.2-4
Benefits of Adjuvant Chemotherapy in Node-Negative and Node-Positive Patients From the Metaanalysis

	Reduction in Annual Odds	
	Recurrence (%)	Death (%)
Node-negative	26 (7)	18 (8)
Node-positive	30 (3)	18 (3)

(Adapted from Early Breast Cancer Trialists' Collaborative Group. Systemic treatment of early breast cancer by hormonal, cytotoxic, or immune therapy. Lancet 1992;339:1,71)

for the first 10 weeks.[43] At a median follow-up of 10 years, 48% of patients treated with the combination were disease-free and 56% remained alive, compared with 35% and 43%, respectively, for patients treated with the single agent. CMFVP was superior in both premenopausal and postmenopausal patients, although the benefit in the younger subgroups was greater. Similar results were obtained in a second-generation NSABP study comparing melphalan alone with melphalan and 5-fluorouracil.[44] This study showed a greater advantage for the combination in postmenopausal patients than in premenopausal patients.

Not all studies support the conclusion that multidrug chemotherapy is superior to single agents. A large Danish study of premenopausal patients compared no treatment with cyclophosphamide alone or with CMF.[45] Both chemotherapy groups demonstrated superior DFS and OS, compared with the no-treatment group, but no significant difference was seen between the single-agent and combination regimens.

The metaanalysis included 13 studies of prolonged combination chemotherapy compared with prolonged single-agent therapy.[12] At least a trend for an advantage for combination therapy was apparent in 10 of these studies. Overall, polychemotherapy produced a 13% ± 5% and 17% ± 5% reduction in the annual odds of recurrence or death, respectively. Thus, the cumulative data suggest that combination drug therapy provides a modest advantage over single-agent therapy in both DFS and OS.

None of the single-agent versus combination studies used the single agent optimally in terms of dose. A potential problem with combination drug therapy is that doses of each of the agents in the combination often must be reduced because of overlapping toxicity. It is still plausible that a single agent given at its optimal dose and schedule would be equivalent or even superior to combination therapy. Administering each of the agents in a combination regimen sequentially and at their optimal dose is another possible strategy currently under investigation.

Longer-Duration Versus Shorter-Duration Chemotherapy

Most early trials of adjuvant chemotherapy in breast cancer empirically chose a treatment duration of 1 or 2 years. In an attempt to reduce toxicity, a series of second-generation

clinical trials compared treatment given for a shorter duration (at least several months) with the same treatment given for a longer duration. Most of these studies evaluated CMF or CMF-based regimens, and results might vary, depending on the regimens used.

Two studies beginning in the mid-1970s compared the standard, 12-month CMF regimen shown in the first Milan study to be superior to no treatment, with the same regimen given for only 6 months.[46,47] Shortening the duration of treatment to 6 cycles was not deleterious in either study; in fact, at 14 years of follow-up, a slight trend in favor of 6 cycles persists in the second Milan study.[13] Another large study done by the Eastern Cooperative Oncology Group (ECOG) in node-positive postmenopausal patients suggested that even shorter-duration therapy may be adequate, at least in that subset.[48] No significant DFS or OS benefits were observed for 12 cycles of CMF and prednisone (CMFP) plus tamoxifen, compared with only 4 cycles, although prolonging the tamoxifen to 5 years did prolong time to relapse.

The SWOG examined the question of treatment duration by testing a different strategy. This group asked whether prolonging their standard continuous CMFVP regimen from 1 to 2 years would improve DFS or OS in a poor-prognosis subset of ER-negative, node-positive patients.[49] The prolonged treatment regimen was poorly tolerated, with only 37% of patients completing the assigned full 2 years of treatment. Overall, no advantage to the more prolonged schedule was seen. Whether the apparent advantage for 2 years of CMFVP in the subset of patients with four or more positive nodes is due to multiple subset analyses and chance or whether more prolonged therapy might benefit these high-risk patients is speculative.

Two other studies suggest that extremely short durations of chemotherapy may be suboptimal.[50,51] The Ludwig Study Group compared 1 brief course of perioperative CMF plus leukovorin with perioperative chemotherapy plus 6 months of CMFP plus tamoxifen (CMFPT) with 6 months of CMFPT starting 1 month after surgery in 1229 node-positive patients. The longer treatment durations provided a sizable DFS advantage compared with a single course of perioperative treatment. A Canadian study compared only 12 weeks of adjuvant chemotherapy with 36 weeks of treatment.[51] The regimens were not identical, however, making it difficult to conclude that any difference observed was due solely to the different durations of therapy. This trial had to be closed prematurely when a significant DFS and OS advantage was observed in the group receiving 36 weeks of CMFVP compared with the group receiving 8 weeks of CMFVP followed by 4 weeks of weekly doxorubicin. Several other trials comparing different chemotherapy regimens in which duration of treatment was also a variable are reviewed later in this chapter.

The metaanalysis examined six trials in which the only variable was shorter versus longer treatment.[12] Five of the six studies used CMF-based regimens, and one used cyclophosphamide and doxorubicin (AC). Neither a significant reduction in recurrence nor a reduction in mortality was observed with longer therapy compared with shorter treatment durations.

Additional study of the optimal duration of chemotherapy is needed. For CMF-based regimens, 4 to 6 months of treatment seems to be as effective as 1 year of treatment. Possibly, however, the optimal duration of regimens composed of other drugs such as doxorubicin or strategies involving the sequential use of different regimens may well be different (see next section). Certain patient subsets might also benefit from longer treatment durations, a hypothesis that requires testing. Until the results of such studies are complete, practicing physicians should use regimens with an established record of effectiveness, which in many cases involves four to six cycles of treatment extending over 3 to 6 months.

Adjuvant Chemotherapy With Doxorubicin-Based Regimens

Modifications of the basic CMF treatment program, including the deletion, substitution, or addition of certain drugs, have been tested in randomized trials. No consistent advantages or disadvantages have emerged from these studies. The addition of methotrexate to melphalan plus 5-fluorouracil and the addition of prednisone or prednisone plus vincristine to CMF did not yield improved outcomes.[31,52–54] A small trial reported no disadvantage by deleting cyclophosphamide from CMF,[55] but definitive conclusions await the results of a similar, larger NSABP study.

An important issue that has not yet been answered definitively is the role of doxorubicin in the adjuvant treatment of breast cancer. Given the higher response rates and, in some studies, longer survivals with doxorubicin-based regimens in metastatic breast cancer, one might extrapolate that they would prove superior in the adjuvant setting. Numerous studies have now been completed, and results are inconsistent and difficult to interpret. A few studies evaluated the addition of doxorubicin to an existing regimen, whereas others used doxorubicin in one arm of a study in which not only the specific drugs, but also other variables, were modified (Table 17.2-5).

In two large trials, the NSABP (B11 and B12) randomized node-positive patients considered to be unresponsive to tamoxifen (based on age and steroid hormone receptor status) to melphalan combined with 5-fluorouracil with or without doxorubicin, whereas tamoxifen-responsive patients received phenylalanine mustard (melphalan), 5-fluorouracil and tamoxifen (PFT) with or without doxorubicin.[56] A modest albeit statistically significant improvement in DFS and OS with doxorubicin was observed only in the trial that focused on tamoxifen-unresponsive patients. The reason for this discrepancy is unknown, but it could be related to the inclusion of patients with different tumor biology. The tamoxifen-responsive group contained a relatively greater proportion of older patients with ER-positive tumors who might respond less well to chemotherapy.

Given the popularity of the CMF and cyclophosphamide, doxorubicin, and 5-fluorouracil (CAF) regimens, it is surprising that no definitive published trials have directly compared them. The Southeast Cancer Study Group (SEG) completed a study comparing versions of the two regimens, but it has not been published. Preliminary results suggest no OS difference between the arms of the trial.[57] The Intergroup recently completed a large trial of standard CMF versus CAF in high-risk, node-negative patients, but results are not yet available. Preliminary results of a European study comparing CMF with epirubicin-based 5-fluorouracil–epirubicin–cyclophosphamide (FEC) show no advantage for substituting the anthracycline for methotrexate.[58]

Several trials have compared two different regimens, one with and one without doxorubicin. Ten-year results of the Oncofrance trial in node-positive patients demonstrated a significant DFS and OS advantage for doxorubicin–vincristine–cyclophosphamide–5-fluorouracil (AVCF) compared with CMF.[59] The SWOG compared a 20-week 4-drug regimen (5-fluorouracil–doxorubicin–cyclophosphamide–methotrexate; FACM) with CMFVP given for 1 year in receptor-negative, node-positive patients.[60] At 5 years of follow-up, the study showed a nonsignificant trend in favor of CMFVP.

An important large study was reported by the NSABP after 3 years of follow-up.[61] This trial compared four cycles (about 3 months) of AC with six cycles (about 6 months) of standard CMF, both commonly used regimens. A third arm evaluated AC followed in 6 months by intravenous CMF to test the idea of interval reinduction. Although follow-up is short, no difference between the arms was apparent. If efficacy is similar, then which regimen is preferred? The AC regimen was completed in less than half the time of CMF; it was associated with one third the number of physician visits and fewer treatment days, and although alopecia was worse, days of nausea were fewer than with CMF. Cardiac toxicity was not a major problem. The investigators concluded that AC is arguably the optimal regimen, but longer follow-up is necessary for firm conclusions.

Several trials have evaluated the use of sequential or alternating regimens, one of which contains doxorubicin (see Table 17.2-5). Two studies from Milan, one in node-positive patients with one to three nodes and one in patients with four or more positive nodes, investigated variations of this theme.[64,65] In the first trial, 12 courses of intravenous CMF were compared with eight cycles of CMF followed by doxorubicin (75 mg/m^2 every 3 weeks) for 4 courses.[64] Results at 5 years demonstrated no DFS or OS advantage for the sequential doxorubicin regimen. In the second study, patients with four or more positive nodes received either doxorubicin for four cycles followed by intravenous CMF for 8 courses or CMF for two cycles followed by doxorubicin for one cycle to a total of 12 courses.[65] According to the Goldie-Coldman hypothesis, the alternating regimen would be expected to be the superior strategy.[66] Highly significant DFS and OS advantages were observed in patients treated with the sequential regimen, however. No CMF-alone arm was included in this trial, but historical comparisons with the original CMF study and with other drug regimens suggest that doxorubi-

TABLE 17.2-5
Randomized Trials Evaluating Doxorubicin or Other Anthracyclines

Trial	Regimens	Patients	Follow-Up (mo)	Disease-Free Survival %	Disease-Free Survival P	Overall Survival %	Overall Survival P
Oncofrance[59]	AVCF	137	120	54	.04	67	.01
(N+)	CMF	112		43		51	
NSABP B11[56]	PAF	344	60	51	.007	65	.08
(Tam unresponsive)	PF	353		44		59	
NSABP B12[56]	PAFT	539	60	64	.4	77	.9
(Tam responsive)	PFT	554		63		78	
ICCG[58]	FEC	319+	36	85	—	93	—
(Premen, N+)	CMF	317+		82		89	
SEG[57]	CAF	528 total	60	—	—	74	.4
(N+)	CMF					68	
SWOG 8313[60]	FAMC	267	60	50	.06	61	.27
(N+, ER−)	CMFVP	264		55		64	
NSABP B15[61]	AC	734	36	62	.5	83	.8
(N+, Tam unresponsive)	CMF	732		63		82	
	AC→CMF	728		68		81	
CALGB 8082[62]	CMFVP→VATH	945 total	—	—	.01	NA	
(N+)	CMFVP						
ECOG 5181[63]	CMFPTH/VATH	270	61	70	.04	—	NS
(Premen, N+)	CMFPT	263		63		—	
Milan[64]	CMF→A	243	61	72	.73	86	NS
(N+, 1–3)	CMF	243		74		89	
Milan[65]	A→CMF	179	60	61	.001	78	.005
(N+, 4+)	CMF/A	180		38		62	

N+, node-positive; Tam, tamoxifen; Premen, premenstrual; ER−, estrogen receptor−negative; NSABP, National Surgical Adjuvant Breast Project; ICCG, International Collaborative Cancer Group; SEG, Southeastern Cancer Study Group; SWOG, Southwest Oncology Group; CALGB, Cancer and Leukemia Group B; ECOG, Eastern Cooperative Oncology Group; AVCF, doxorubicin–vincristine–cyclophosphamide–5-fluorouracil; CMF, cyclophosphamide–methotrexate–5-fluorouracil; PAF, phenylalanine mustard–doxorubicin–5-fluorouracil; PF, phenylalanine mustard-5-fluorouracil; PAFT, PAF–tamoxifen; PFT, PF–tamoxifen; FEC, 5-fluorouracil–epirubicin–cyclophosphamide; CAF, cyclophosphamide–doxorubicin–5-fluorouracil; FAMC, 5-fluorouracil–doxorubicin–mitomycin C–cyclophosphamide; CMFVP, CMF–vincristine–prednisone; AC, doxorubicin–cyclophosphamide; VATH, vinblastine–doxorubicin–thiotepa–fluxymeterone; CMF–prednisone–tamoxifen; CMFPT–fluoxymesterone.

cin followed by CMF is a regimen to be considered for treatment of high-risk, node-positive patients.

Many physicians routinely use a doxorubicin-based regimen such as CAF or AC, especially for node-positive patients. Although these combinations are popular and arguments can be made to support their use, definitive proof of their superiority over CMF is lacking. Results of recently completed trials or other trials still in progress should help to answer this question.

Perioperative Adjuvant Chemotherapy

Chemotherapy given at the time of or just after surgery offers several theoretic advantages. The drugs may kill circulating tumor cells that conceivably are dislodged at the time of surgery. After removal of the primary tumor, DNA synthesis and proliferation of micrometastases increase almost immediately, perhaps increasing their vulnerability to cytotoxic drugs.[67] Finally, immediate treat-ment might kill metastatic cells before the spontaneous emergence of drug resistance.[66]

Several early trials of adjuvant chemotherapy used brief perioperative chemotherapy compared with a surgery-alone control group. The NSABP carried out two such trials in the 1950s and 1960s using thiotepa on the day of and 2 days after surgery in the first trial and thiotepa or 4 days of 5-fluorouracil beginning on day 7 in the second.[7] No overall difference was observed, but an advantage for thiotepa in premenopausal patients was seen in both studies.

Interest in perioperative therapy grew when the long-term results of a Scandinavian trial started in 1965 became available.[8] This trial randomized patients to 6 days of cyclophosphamide, with the first dose given immediately after surgery, or to surgery alone. One hospital in the consortium delayed chemotherapy for about 1 month to allow administration of radiation. An overall DFS and OS advantage was observed in this study, except in the institution that delayed the chemotherapy. Similar, although less impressive, results were observed in a later British study designed to confirm the Scandinavian data.[68]

The value of perioperative therapy is questionable considering the results of two large studies from the Ludwig Breast Cancer Group referred to earlier.[37,50] One cycle of perioperative CMF starting within 36 hours of surgery in node-negative patients did prolong DFS compared with no adjuvant treatment, but the results were not nearly as striking as in trials using traditional prolonged postoperative chemotherapy in this subset. More important, one cycle of perioperative CMF was inferior to six cycles of CMF begun 4 weeks postoperatively, and perioperative combined with postoperative CMF was no better than postoperative treatment alone in node-positive patients.[50] Similarly, 5-year results of an Italian study comparing perioperative chemotherapy with an epirubicin-based regimen followed by prolonged postoperative therapy versus postoperative therapy alone did not confirm early promising results.[69] The cumulative data suggest that, at present, the benefits of administering chemotherapy around the time of surgery are meager at best. Additional ongoing trials are continuing to investigate this strategy.

Preoperative, Primary, or Neoadjuvant Chemotherapy

Several theoretical advantages and disadvantages of the administration of chemotherapy immediately after the diagnosis of breast cancer, but before definitive surgery, exist. The presence of a palpable or radiographically measurable mass permits assessment of response as a direct in vivo measure of the sensitivity of the tumor cells to the particular drugs used. Early detection of a resistant tumor would enable the oncologist to discontinue a worthless therapy, thus avoiding unnecessary toxicity, or to change to a potentially more effective regimen. In addition, the earlier the disease is treated, the less likely that resistant tumor clones will have emerged spontaneously. Theoretically, even a short delay in administering systemic therapy may adversely affect outcome.[70] Finally, preoperative chemotherapy may shrink large primary tumors sufficiently to allow breast-preserving surgery, rather than mastectomy.

Disadvantages of preoperative chemotherapy include the reliance on a fine-needle aspirate or core biopsy for histologic diagnosis. Although, in experienced hands, mistakes in diagnosis using these techniques are uncommon, palpable in situ cancers may be mislabeled as invasive cancers and patients then treated with chemotherapy inappropriately. Prognostic factor analyses such as receptor status, DNA flow cytometry, and other markers that may be useful in some clinical situations are more difficult to perform (though not impossible) on these specimens. Most important, however, axillary nodal status is not known before the selection of adjuvant chemotherapy, and an accurate estimate may never be possible in some responding patients. Axillary nodal status provides important prognostic information to the physician and patient, information that may be crucial in planning for the future. Knowledge of the status of axillary lymph nodes may be-

come paramount in selecting high-risk patients (unless surrogate markers are identified) if the current generation of dose-intensive adjuvant trials brings positive results.

Preoperative chemotherapy has been used extensively in inoperable, locally advanced breast cancer to achieve tumor reduction and thus to facilitate mastectomy or irradiation. More recently, this strategy has been studied in operable primary breast cancer, most commonly in patients with tumors 3 cm or larger. A comprehensive phase II study from Milan investigating 5 different chemotherapy regimens (CMF, FAC, FEC, FNC [mitoxantrone substituting for doxorubicin], and doxorubicin alone) demonstrated partial response rates ranging from 62% (tumors larger than 5 cm) to 93% (tumors 3 to 4 cm). Overall, the response rates approached 80%, and no difference in response occurred according to the chemotherapy received.[71] Response to single-agent doxorubicin was equivalent to that of the combinations. Breast-preserving surgery (quadrantectomy) was possible in 91% of the patients. Over 73% of patients with tumors larger than 5 cm became candidates for breast preservation. At a median follow-up of 18 months, only 1 of 201 patients treated by quadrantectomy and radiation suffered a local recurrence, but it is far too early to draw conclusions about local control.

Preliminary results are now available from 2 randomized trials of preoperative chemotherapy.[72,73] A French study of 272 women with tumors larger than 3 cm randomized patients to primary chemotherapy with 3 cycles of epirubicin, vincristine, and methotrexate followed by 3 cycles of mitomycin, thiotepa, and vindesine followed by local treatment versus mastectomy and the same chemotherapy if the patients were found to be node-positive or ER-negative.[72] Sixty-three percent of patients in the preoperative-chemotherapy arm underwent breast-preserving surgery. At a median follow-up of about 3 years, local control is acceptable and survival is longer in the early-chemotherapy group.

The largest trial of this approach was recently completed by the NSABP.[73] More than 1300 patients were randomized to surgery followed by four cycles of AC or to four cycles of AC followed by surgery. The response rate to preoperative chemotherapy was 80%, including 37% complete responses (CR). The CR rate was 50% for tumors 2 cm or smaller and 18% for tumors larger than 4 cm. More than 65% of the patients in the primary-chemotherapy group underwent breast-preserving surgery, compared with 57% in the postoperative-chemotherapy group. Interestingly, 59% of the preoperative-chemotherapy patients were node-negative at the time of surgery, compared with only 42% of patients subjected to immediate surgery. Whether this downstaging of axillary nodal status and high response rates to initial chemotherapy will eventually translate into improved outcome and acceptable local control will require several more years of follow-up. In the meantime, preoperative chemotherapy remains experimental except in patients with large tumors in whom it may allow downstaging and resection of the primary tumor.

Dose-Intensive Adjuvant Chemotherapy

The results of chemotherapy for breast cancer have plateaued over the past decade. Until recently, no new active drugs have been identified for 20 years, and with few exceptions, oncologists are still using the same drug regimens today that they were using in 1980. Clearly, new treatment strategies are needed to improve on the modest efficacy of currently available approaches. One strategy now explored on a wide scale is dose intensification. The surge in popularity of dose-intensive chemotherapy is due to the recent availability of hematopoietic growth factors to reduce toxicity from myelosuppression and to the results of pilot studies and retrospective calculations of dose intensity suggesting possible advantages to this approach. Steep dose-response curves for certain drugs in preclinical models and high response rates in patients with metastatic breast cancer in whom standard therapy fails indicate that drug resistance can be overcome by raising drug dose.

Two strategies being investigated address the question of dose intensification. One method is to give a single treatment with extremely high myeloablative doses of chemotherapy that require hematopoietic reconstitution with autologous bone marrow transplantation or peripheral progenitor cell support or both. The high blood levels achieved, even for a brief time, may be sufficient to kill cells that are resistant to the same class of drugs used at standard doses. The need for supportive care and prolonged hospitalization, high cost, and relatively high morbidity and occasional mortality, are issues that complicate the widespread application of this approach.

Another method of dose intensification is to increase the amount of drug delivered per unit time (dose intensity). High dose intensity can be achieved by raising drug doses in standard regimens such as CMF or AC or by shortening the interval between drug treatments. The measure of dose intensity is frequently calculated as milligram of drug received per square meter of body surface area per week. Thus, a 50% increase in dose intensity can be achieved by administering the same doses of AC every 2 weeks instead of every 3 weeks, or by increasing the dose given every 3 weeks. Dose-intensive regimens designed in this way can be given on an outpatient basis and can be given repeatedly for prolonged periods, an attractive feature for a slowly growing, low–growth fraction tumor such as breast cancer.

The issue of dose intensity first received wide attention in 1981, when the Milan group reported a retrospective analysis of their original CMF adjuvant study suggesting that only those patients who received at least 85% of their planned CMF dose benefited significantly from adjuvant therapy, whereas those receiving less than 65% of the planned dose had the same DFS and OS as the group of control patients treated by surgery alone.[74] Unfortunately, this type of analysis has been questioned for a variety of reasons, most notably that distinguishing among several plausible explanations for a relation between DFS and chemotherapy dose received is impossible.[75] Patients may have a recurrence because they received a lower drug dose. Alternatively, patients who received a lower drug dose may have done so because they did not tolerate chemotherapy as well because of factors also associated with a greater likelihood of disease recurrence. For example, patients with subclinical bone marrow metastases who are destined to have a recurrence may tolerate chemotherapy less well and may require dose reductions. A variety of major centers performed such retrospective analyses, but no consistent results have been obtained.

Another technique to analyze dose intensity retrospectively was reported by Hryniuk.[76] An analysis of the relation between planned dose intensity of a variety of CMF-based regimens used in the adjuvant treatment of breast cancer and 3-year DFS showed that dose intensity significantly correlated with DFS independent of other factors in a multivariate analysis. These data provided additional support to the hypothesis that dose intensity might be important in the adjuvant therapy of breast cancer, but more definitive prospective studies were needed.

Early results of two prospective randomized trials evaluating dose and dose intensity in node-positive patients have been reported recently.[32,77,78] The Cancer and Leukemia Group B (CALGB) randomly assigned 1572 women to three treatment groups (Table 17.2-6). One group received high-dose CAF every 28 days for four cycles. Group 2 received lower doses but for six treatment cycles, so the total dose was the same as that of group 1. A third group received CAF for four cycles at half the doses of patients in group 1, such that both total dose and dose intensity were reduced. None of these schedules are really dose intensive by today's standard, and hematopoietic growth factors were not used.

After a short median follow-up of 3.4 years, the high and moderate dose-intensity regimens yielded superior DFS and OS, compared with the low-dose regimen. At the time of the report, 26% of group 1 patients had experienced relapse, as well as 28% of group 2 and 37% of group 3. The benefit for the more dose-intensive regimens was observed across all major patient subsets. At present, because no significant difference was seen between groups 1 and 2, one cannot distinguish between a dose-intensity effect and a total cumulative dose effect. A trend in favor of the high dose-intensity group might become more apparent with time and thus may provide more definite conclusions. The high dose-intensity schedule was the most effective regimen in the poor-prognosis subgroup of patients overexpressing the c-erbB-2 (HER-2/neu) oncogene.[77] From this study one can conclude, however, that reducing the doses of standard treatment regimens should be avoided unless severe toxicity necessitates dose reductions.

Early results from a large NSABP study investigating dose intensification and increased total dose of cyclophosphamide in their standard AC regimen have been reported.[78] This study randomly assigned 2238 node-positive patients to one of three arms (Table 17.2-7). Group 1 received standard therapy, the dose intensity of which was slightly greater while the total dose was equivalent to the dose-intensive arm of the CALGB study.[32] Group 2 received twice the dose intensity but the same total dose of cyclophosphamide, and group 3 received twice the dose

TABLE 17.2-6
Chemotherapy Doses and Schedule in the Cancer and Leukemia Group B Study of Dose Intensity

Study Group	Cyclophsophamide	Doxorubicin	5-Fluorouracil
GROUP 1			
mg/m^{2}q4wk	600	60	600 (×2)
Number of cycles	4	4	4
mg/m^2/wk	150	15	300
Cumulative dose (mg/m^2)	2400	240	4800
GROUP 2			
mg/m^2 q4wk	400	40	400 (×2)
Number of cycles	6	6	
mg/m^2/wk	100	10	200
Cumulative dose (mg/m^2)	2400	240	4800
GROUP 3			
mg/m^2 q4wk	300	30	300 (×2)
Number of cycles	4	4	4
mg/m^2/wk	75	7.5	150
Cumulative dose (mg/m^2)	1200	120	2400

(Adapted from Wood WC, Budman DR, Korzun AH, et al. Dose and dose intensity of adjuvant chemotherapy for stage II, node-positive breast carcinoma. N Engl J Med 1994;300:1253)

TABLE 17.2-7
Chemotherapy Doses and Schedule in the National Surgical Adjuvant Breast Project Study of Dose Intensity

Study Group	Cyclophosphamide	Doxorubicin
GROUP 1		
mg/m^2 q3wk	600	60
Number of cycles	4	4
mg/m^2/wk	200	20
Cumulative dose (mg/m^2)	2400	240
GROUP 2		
mg/m^2 q3wk	1200	60
Number of cycles	2	4
mg/m^2/wk	400	20
cumulative dose (mg/m^2)	2400	240
GROUP 3		
mg/m^2 q3wk	1200	60
Number of cycles	4	4
mg/m^2/wk	400	20
Cumulative dose (mg/m^2)	4800	240

(Adapted from Dimitrov N, Anderson S, Fisher B, et al. Dose intensification and increased total dose of adjuvant chemotherapy for breast cancer [BC]: findings from NSABP B22. Proc ASCO 1994;13:64)

intensity and twice the total dose of this drug. The dose of doxorubicin was held constant. Drug doses actually delivered were close to the planned doses. Disappointingly, 3-year DFS and OS estimates showed no differences in outcome for the three arms. Additional follow-up is required for definitive conclusions from this study, but thus far, doubling the total dose or dose intensity of cyclophosphamide has no proved benefit. Quadrupling the dose of cyclophosphamide in the AC regimen, feasible now with the availability of hematopoietic growth factor support, is being studied in the current-generation NSABP trial (B25). Increasing the dose or dose intensity of doxorubicin, the most active drug in the AC regimen and a drug with a relatively steep dose-response curve in advanced breast cancer, is being tested in an Intergroup trial.[79]

Studies of dose intensity, particularly those investigating extremely high-dose chemotherapy and autologous bone marrow transplantation, are being performed in patients at a high risk of disease recurrence, such as those with 10 or more positive axillary nodes. Over 90% of these patients relapse within 10 years when treated with surgery alone.[80] Over 50% of these patients relapse within 5 years and more than 70% within 10 years even when treated with the best adjuvant chemotherapy available.[80,81]

Pilot feasibility studies have been carried out by several groups in this high-risk subset. A Johns Hopkins group employed a 16-week, multiagent, dose-intense regimen in which drugs were cycled every 2 weeks.[82] Myelosuppression was the major side effect, but the regimen was reasonably well tolerated without growth factor support. Seven of the 53 patients (13%) required hospitalization for neutropenic fever, but 94% of the planned doses were administered. A provocative 80% estimated 3-year DFS was observed, an advantage compared with historic series. This regimen has now been compared with 6 months of standard CAF in an Intergroup trial focusing on ER-negative, node-positive patients. Results are not yet available.

The Duke Bone Marrow Transplant Group and the CALGB performed a feasibility study of high-dose therapy using cyclophosphamide, cisplatin, and carmustine with autologous bone marrow support as consolidation after standard-dose adjuvant chemotherapy (CAF) in a similar group of patients.[83] Actuarial event-free survival at a median follow-up of 2.5 years was 72%—again superior to historical series. Treatment-related mortality was 12%.

Given these provocative data, two randomized trials of high-dose chemotherapy with autologous bone marrow support have been initiated and are still accruing patients. Both are Intergroup studies administered by the CALGB and ECOG. The CALGB study randomizes patients with 10 or more positive axillary nodes to standard CAF followed by low-dose cyclophosphamide, cisplatin, and carmustine or to CAF followed by high doses of the same drugs combined with bone marrow support. Both groups receive tamoxifen and chest wall radiation because of the high risk of local recurrence in these patients. The ECOG study randomizes the same subset of patients to CAF followed by radiation and tamoxifen or to CAF followed by high-dose cyclophosphamide plus thiotepa along with bone marrow support, tamoxifen, and radiation. Until the results of these trials are available, high-dose therapy with bone marrow support should not be done routinely but should be restricted to well-designed peer-reviewed studies.

New Agents

Several newer agents, including navelbine, paclitaxel (Taxol), and taxotere, have shown significant activity in advanced breast cancer. These drugs have not yet been studied in the adjuvant setting, but clinical trials are in the planning stage.

Chemotherapy Summary

A variety of chemotherapy regimens have proved effectiveness in the adjuvant treatment of primary breast cancer (Table 17.2-8). The optimal regimen has not been identified, but each of the regimens in Table 17.2-8 provides an acceptable alternative. Untested alterations in drug dose or schedule should be avoided because they may significantly affect patient outcome. More important is to identify patients correctly who should be considered for chemotherapy than to choose a particular chemotherapy regimen.

Benefits of Adjuvant Endocrine Therapy

ADJUVANT THERAPY WITH TAMOXIFEN

Tamoxifen is the most commonly prescribed drug for the treatment of breast cancer. The drug is a nonsteroidal antiestrogen that binds to ER and displays both estrogen-antagonist as well as estrogen-agonist properties.[84] Tamoxifen, much like estrogen, preserves bone mineral density in postmenopausal women,[85] and it exerts a favorable effect on blood lipid profiles,[86] attractive features in patients for whom estrogen-replacement therapy is considered hazardous. Tamoxifen exerts its predominant antiestrogenic effects by competitively blocking the binding of estrogen to ER.[84] The net result is a blockade of cell cycle transit in G_1 phase, a slight increase in cell loss, and inhibition of tumor growth. Tamoxifen at high concentrations has a myriad of other cellular effects that are independent of ER and could conceivably account for the occasional response in patients with low or undetectable tumor ER. A reduction in serum insulin-like growth factor-1 (IGF-1) concentration and an increase in IGF-binding protein levels provide another mechanism for tumor growth inhibition.[87]

Because of its favorable toxicity profile and its activity in advanced breast cancer, tamoxifen entered clinical trials of adjuvant therapy in the middle to late 1970s. More than 30,000 patients in tamoxifen trials were included in the metaanalysis, and definitive conclusions are now available.

Tamoxifen in Premenopausal and Postmenopausal Patients

More than 20 trials have compared tamoxifen therapy for a year or more with a no-treatment control arm.[12,62] Many of these trials focused on postmenopausal patients, although a few included some premenopausal patients. Most of these studies included both node-positive and node-negative patients, although a large trial from the NSABP studied node-negative patients exclusively.[36] Most included ER-positive as well as ER-negative patients. Nearly all these studies found a statistically significant DFS advantage for tamoxifen, but only two large studies, the North American Treaty Organization (NATO) trial and the Scottish trial,[88,89] showed a significant OS advantage. Most of the other studies, however, found a survival trend in favor of tamoxifen.

The metaanalysis included these controlled trials as well as trials of tamoxifen combined with some form of chemotherapy compared with the same chemotherapy alone in an attempt to isolate the effects of tamoxifen.[12] When all patients are included, a significant reduction in recurrence and mortality was found for tamoxifen, which produced a 25% reduction in the odds of recurrence and a 16% reduction in the odds of death (Table 17.2-9). Although both younger and older patients received some benefit, in contrast to the chemotherapy trials, older patients tended to benefit more from adjuvant tamoxifen

TABLE 17.2-8
Popular Chemotherapy Regimens Useful in the Adjuvant Therapy of Breast Cancer

Regimen	Dose and Schedule	Cycle Interval	Cycles
CMF (STANDARD)			
Cyclophosphamide	100 mg/m^2/d PO × 14 days	28 d	6
Methotrexate	40 mg/m^2 IV d 1 & 8	28 d	6
5-Fluorouracil	600 mg/m^2 IV d 1 & 8	28 d	6
CMF (IV; TESTED IN NODE-NEGATIVE PATIENTS ONLY)			
Cyclophosphamide	600 mg/m^2 IV	21 d	12
Methotrexate	40 mg/m^2 IV	21 d	12
5-Fluorouracil	600 mg/m^2 IV	21 d	12
CMFVP			
Cyclophosphamide	60 mg/m^2/d PO	Daily	1 y
5-Fluorouracil	400 mg/m^2 IV	Weekly	1 y
Methotrexate	15 mg/m^2	Weekly	1 y
Vincristine	0.625 mg/m^2	Weekly × 10	
Prednisone	30 mg/m^2 tapering over 10 wk	—	
CAF			
Cyclophosphamide	100 mg/m^2/d PO × 14 d	28 d	6
Doxorubicin	30 mg/m^2 IV d 1 & 8	28 d	6
5-Fluorouracil	500 mg/m^2 IV d 1 & 8	28 d	6
CAF			
Cyclophosphamide	600 mg/m^2 IV d 1	21–28 d	4–6
Doxorubicin	60 mg/m^2 IV d 1	21–28 d	4–6
5-Fluorouracil	600 mg/m^2 IV d 1 & 8	21–28 d	4–6
AC			
Doxorubicin	60 mg/m^2 IV d 1	21 d	4
Cyclophosphamide	600 mg/m^2 d 1	21 d	4
A → CMF (TESTED IN NODE-POSITIVE PATIENTS ONLY)			
Doxorubicin	75 mg/m^2 IV d 1	21 d	4
Cyclophosphamide	600 mg/m^2 IV	21 d	8 (cycles 5–12)
Methotrexate	40 mg/m^2 IV	21 d	8 (cycles 5–12)
5-Fluorouracil	600 mg/m^2 IV	21 d	8 (cycles 5–12)

than patients younger than 50 years of age. The tamoxifen benefit was related more to age than to menopausal status. Patients younger than 50 years of age had a modest reduction in the annual odds of recurrence (12% ± 5%) but no significant mortality reduction (6% ± 5%). Premenopausal patients 50 to 59 years of age had a significant and sizable reduction in recurrence and mortality, however, equivalent to reductions in postmenopausal patients. Although the data are not as solid because of smaller numbers of patients, a trend exists for less tamoxifen benefit as age decreases; no statistically significant recurrence or mortality reductions were observed for patients younger than 40 years. Some evidence suggests that duration of tamoxifen treatment may influence response by menopausal status, and that prolonged treatment for 5 years or more may add to the benefit in premenopausal patients (see later).

Thus, adjuvant tamoxifen for at least 1 year clearly reduces mortality in women with primary breast cancer after 10 years of follow-up. In fact, the mortality difference between tamoxifen and control patients grew steadily bigger throughout years 1 to 10 in the metaanalysis, and we have no indication that the benefit will disappear with time.[12]

TABLE 17.2-9
Overview of Adjuvant Tamoxifen Trials

Patient Group	Reduction (SD) in Annual Odds	
	Recurrence (%)	Death (%)
All patients	25 (2)	16 (2)
<50 y	12 (4)	6 (5)
≥50 y	29 (2)	20 (2)
<50 y, premenopausal	12 (4)	6 (5)
50–59 y, premenopausal	33 (7)	23 (9)
<50 y, postmenopausal	12 (15)	Too few patients
50–59 y, postmenopausal	28 (3)	19 (4)
60–69 y, all	29 (3)	17 (4)
70+ y	28 (5)	21 (6)

(Adapted from Early Breast Cancer Trialists' Collaborative Group. Systemic treatment of early breast cancer by hormonal, cytotoxic, or immune therapy. Lancet 1992;339:1,71)

Tamoxifen in Node-Negative and Node-Positive Patients

Many trials of adjuvant tamoxifen included both node-negative and node-positive patients. Fewer recurrences and deaths in the node-negative subset make it more difficult to show significant differences between tamoxifen and no treatment, but strong trends were evident in the larger studies.[88,89] NSABP trial B14 is by far the largest trial of adjuvant tamoxifen (2644 patients), and it focused on patients with histologically negative axillary nodes.[36,40] Both patients younger than 50 years of age (820 patients) and older patients (1824 patients) were eligible, and all patients had ER-positive disease. Patients were randomly assigned to receive placebo or tamoxifen for 5 years, and patients receiving tamoxifen were reassigned at 5 years to stop therapy or to continue for 5 additional years. No data are available on the duration question, but patients randomly assigned to receive tamoxifen had a significant reduction in treatment failure at 5 years. A survival advantage has not yet emerged. In this study, the magnitude of the benefit was greater in women younger than 50 years than in older women. Tamoxifen-treated patients also had fewer ipsilateral breast, local–regional, and distant recurrences than placebo-treated patients, and a reduction in contralateral breast cancer was evident.

The metaanalysis also suggests that the benefit with adjuvant tamoxifen is similar for node-negative and node-positive patients.[12] The reduction in the annual odds of recurrence was 26% ± 4% for node-negative patients and 28% ± 2% for node-positive women. Tamoxifen also reduced the annual odds of death from any cause in both groups (17% ± 5% and 18% ± 2%, respectively). Thus, the cumulative data suggest that tamoxifen improves survival in the lower-risk, node-negative patients as well as in node-positive patients. Because of its favorable toxicity profile, tamoxifen is especially attractive for treating women at a lower risk of disease recurrence. Although the absolute benefit is modest in this group, patients who are already cured by surgery and do not need adjuvant therapy will not suffer excessive morbidity by treating them with tamoxifen.

Optimal Duration of Tamoxifen Therapy

Theoretic reasons exist for prolonged or even indefinite tamoxifen therapy, but these have not yet been confirmed by randomized clinical trials. Several trials are now in progress comparing 2 versus 5 years, 5 years versus 10 years, or 5 years versus indefinite treatment. Five randomized trials, in which duration of tamoxifen was one of the variables, have been completed and are included in the metaanalysis.[12] The largest of these trials, the ECOG trial reviewed earlier, compared 4 cycles of CMFPT with 12 cycles with 12 cycles followed by an additional 4 years of tamoxifen in postmenopausal patients. This trial found a significant reduction in the odds of recurrence but no survival benefit for 5 years compared with 1 year of tamoxifen.[48] The metaanalysis of the 5 studies comparing 3 to 5 years of tamoxifen with 1 to 2 years also showed a reduction in recurrence (22% ± 8%) but no significant reduction in mortality (7% ± 11%).[12]

Indirect comparisons of trials with different tamoxifen durations suggest that tamoxifen taken for longer than 2 years is superior to tamoxifen taken for 2 years or less in premenopausal but not postmenopausal patients[12] (Table 17.2-10). Firm conclusions await the results of ongoing randomized studies. Until then, many oncologists routinely use 5 years of adjuvant tamoxifen. Even more prolonged tamoxifen is used by some, perhaps more for its potential value as hormone-replacement therapy with its favorable effects on bone and lipids than for its potential effects on breast cancer deaths.

Benefit of Tamoxifen in Patients With ER-Poor Tumors

Many of the early tamoxifen adjuvant trials included patients with ER-negative or ER-poor as well as ER-positive tumors. These studies should enable investigators to assess the benefit of tamoxifen in both subsets. The results are difficult to interpret, however, because of varying definitions of ER-positive and ER-negative, and because only a fraction of the patients included in some of these studies had ER assays performed. Most studies of breast cancer cells grown in tissue culture or studies using animal models show little or no effects of tamoxifen in ER-negative cells at drug concentrations achieved in patients. Tamoxifen has numerous effects on cells that are not mediated through the ER, however, and the effects of the drug on the few ER-positive cells present in an ER-negative tumor could conceivably affect most cell populations lacking receptors. Finally, the drug has systemic effects that could inhibit growth of tumors regardless of ER content. An antitumor effect even in ER-negative tumors is therefore possible. The response rates observed with tamoxifen in ER-negative metastatic disease of only 5% to 10% argue

TABLE 17.2-10
*Indirect Comparison of the Optimal
Duration of Tamoxifen*

Patient Group	Reduction (SD) in Annual Odds	
	Recurrence	Death
TAMOXIFEN FOR 2 Y	28 (2%)	19 (3%)
<50 y	10 (5%)	4 (6%)
≥50 y	33 (3%)	23 (3%)
TAMOXIFEN FOR >2 Y	39 (4%)	24 (6%)
<50 y	43 (11%)★	27 (17%)★
≥50 y	38 (5%)	23 (6%)

★ Statistically unreliable; too few patients.

(Adapted from Early Breast Cancer Trialists' Collaborative Group. Systemic treatment of early breast cancer by hormonal, cytotoxic, or immune therapy. Lancet 1992;339:1,71)

that the benefit is likely to be modest in the adjuvant setting.

Nevertheless, several trials have reported some advantage for tamoxifen in ER-negative patients. The NATO trial measured ER on a proportion of their patients.[88] When 5 fmol/mg protein was used to distinguish ER-positive from ER-negative, this study found no significant prognostic significance of ER, raising questions about the validity of the assay. Using this cutoff, the effects of tamoxifen were just as great in the ER-negative as in the ER-positive group. This study did find a correlation between histologic grade, which can be thought of as a surrogate marker for ER status,[90] and tamoxifen response. Patients with grade 1 and 2 tumors, which are more likely ER-positive, benefited from tamoxifen, whereas those with grade 3 tumors did not.

The Scottish tamoxifen trial did report a relation between ER status and tamoxifen benefit.[89] The higher the ER, the greater the difference between tamoxifen and control in DFS at 3 years. Even patients with low ER had a significant benefit, however. NSABP study B09 randomized patients to chemotherapy alone or to chemotherapy and tamoxifen.[91] Overall, no significant benefit was observed for tamoxifen in patients with tumor ER less than 10 fmol/mg protein, whereas a significant improvement in DFS was observed in the ER-positive group. Multiple subset analysis by age and ER status showed that women aged 60 to 70 years received some benefit from tamoxifen even if their tumor had an ER content of 0 to 9 fmol/mg protein. The authors concluded that this result was probably related to analytic errors in receptor measurement. It might also have been related to chance, given the multiple subsets analyzed.

The metaanalysis included indirect comparisons of the effect of tamoxifen by ER status[12] (Table 17.2-11). A relation between ER level and tamoxifen benefit is clear,

with a sizable recurrence and mortality reduction evident in patients with the highest ER values. Patients with ER-poor tumors had a more modest but significant benefit with tamoxifen adjuvant therapy. Tumors categorized as poor (less than 10 fmol/mg protein) are a mixture of truly ER-negative tumors (undetectable in the assay) and borderline positive tumors with ER that is present, but at levels less than the arbitrary cutoff of 10 fmol/mg protein used in many laboratories. These low-positive tumors would be expected to benefit from adjuvant tamoxifen given the relatively frequent responses observed in this group when treated with endocrine therapy for advanced disease.[92]

Thus, whether tamoxifen reduces mortality in patients with truly ER-negative tumors is not clear. Prospective studies are underway to define the benefit in patients with different tumor ER levels. Because these studies use 10 fmol/mg as a cutoff and because most laboratories use this or even higher values to define ER status, it may never be possible to determine whether patients with undetectable ER have reduced breast cancer recurrence and prolonged survival with antiestrogen therapy. Perhaps a switch to immunohistochemical methods for ER analysis will facilitate such a study. In the meantime, the modest toxicity of tamoxifen, the ancillary benefits of the drug including its favorable effects on bone, blood lipids, and the reduction in contralateral breast cancer, provide arguments for its use in patients regardless of ER status.

Tamoxifen in Elderly Patients

Because it is generally well tolerated, tamoxifen has been used to treat elderly patients with breast cancer. The metaanalysis demonstrated a significant mortality reduction in patients older than 70 years of age treated with adjuvant tamoxifen (Table 17.2-9).[12] Some trials have specifically targeted this population. The ECOG randomized 181 patients 65 years of age or older to tamoxifen or placebo for 2 years.[93] The drug was well tolerated, and significant reductions in recurrence and borderline significant reduc-

TABLE 17.2-11
Effects of Tamoxifen by Estrogen Receptor

Patient Group	Reduction (SD) in Annual Odds	
	Recurrence	Death
ER-poor (<10 fmol/mg)	13 (4%)	11 (5%)
ER+ (10–100 fmol/mg)	29 (3%)	19 (4%)
ER+ (>100 fmol/mg)	43 (5%)	29 (7%)

ER, estrogen receptor.

(Adapted from Early Breast Cancer Trialists' Collaborative Group. Systemic treatment of early breast cancer by hormonal, cytotoxic, or immune therapy. Lancet 1992;339:1,71)

tions in mortality were observed. In addition, tamoxifen reduced the incidence of contralateral breast cancers. The majority of the patients who died in this study (61%) succumbed to breast cancer, although, as anticipated, a significant number of these older women (22%) died of illness not related to cancer, a factor that must be considered when making adjuvant therapy decisions.

Tamoxifen Summary

Tamoxifen prolongs DFS and OS in patients older than 50 years of age and should be considered for nearly all such patients, except perhaps those with a low risk of disease recurrence, in whom the absolute benefit of tamoxifen is meager. These patients might benefit from the ancillary effect of tamoxifen on bone and lipids, although the potential for occasional serious toxicity exists (see later). The NSABP study (B14) suggests that 5 years of tamoxifen may also be effective in node-negative, ER-positive younger patients,[36] a result supported by some other studies.[88,89] In view of the metaanalysis data demonstrating the lack of a survival benefit in women younger than 50 years of age, however, caution should be observed when using tamoxifen in this subset in which chemotherapy has proved survival benefits. Additional study directly comparing tamoxifen and adjuvant chemotherapy in premenopausal patients is needed. A recently reported German trial that randomly assigned ER-positive patients with one to three positive lymph nodes to receive tamoxifen for 2 years or to receive six cycles of CMF found a significant DFS and OS advantage for chemotherapy in the premenopausal subset.[94] Although this result is not definitive because it was based on subset analysis of only 119 patients, it does raise additional concern about the role of tamoxifen in younger patients.

OTHER FORMS OF ADJUVANT ENDOCRINE THERAPY

Adjuvant Ovarian Ablation

Among the first randomized trials of adjuvant therapy in breast cancer were studies of adjuvant ovarian ablation either by surgical ovariectomy or by irradiation.[12,62] Some of these trials were not properly randomized by today's standards.[6] Many were small, a few included both premenopausal and postmenopausal women, and none included ER analyses, which were not yet available. Most of these trials found a significant DFS advantage for ovarian ablation, and two reported a significant OS advantage.[95,96]

The metaanalysis included data from 10 properly randomized trials of ovarian ablation involving 3000 patients (fewer than 2000 younger than 50 years of age); 5 of these trials compared ovarian ablation with no adjuvant therapy, and 5 compared ovarian ablation and chemotherapy with the same chemotherapy alone.[12] As expected, no significant benefit was observed for ovariectomy in women older than 50 years of age, most of whom are postmenopausal. Younger women had a significant DFS and OS advantage with ovarian ablation (26% $\pm$ 6 reduction in the odds of recurrence and 25% $\pm$ 7 reduction in the odds of death).

These results are comparable to those achieved with chemotherapy in women younger than 50 years of age. Different quantitative results were noted in the studies of ovarian ablation alone compared with those studies in which the operation was combined with chemotherapy (Table 17.2-12). Yet, even in the presence of chemotherapy, which itself results in a chemical ablation in many patients, ovarian ablation still offered a significant reduction in recurrence and survival.

These results are surprising, especially considering that most of these studies did not use ER status to select patients most likely to benefit from endocrine therapy. An important question then is whether ovarian ablation or chemotherapy is the superior treatment for premenopausal patients. Although a definitive answer to this question cannot be given, the results of the first randomized trial directly comparing these two treatments were published.[24] More than 300 node-positive, premenopausal patients were randomized to intravenous CMF given every 3 weeks for six or eight cycles or to ovarian ablation, each with or without prednisolone, 7.5 mg/d for 5 years. Prednisolone offered no advantage. At a median follow-up of about 6 years, no overall difference has been noted between CMF and ovarian ablation. ER status was known for 81% of the patients in this trial, and analysis by ER status yielded interesting results. Patients with low ER (less than 20 fmol/mg protein) benefited more from chemotherapy, and those with high ER (20 fmol/mg protein or higher) benefited more from ovarian ablation. These results strongly suggest that chemotherapy works through a cytotoxic mechanism in addition to the endocrine effects achieved in those patients having chemical castration. This study also suggests that ovarian ablation is the superior treatment for ER-positive patients. Unfortunately, this report did not provide information on the incidence of amenorrhea in the patients treated with chemotherapy.

The data base from which to draw definitive conclusions on the value of ovarian ablation is much less substantial compared with that for adjuvant tamoxifen and chemother-

TABLE 17.2-12

Effects of Adjuvant Ovarian Ablation in the Presence or Absence of Chemotherapy in Women Younger Than 50 Years Old

Patient Group★	Reduction (SD) in the Annual Odds	
	Recurrence	Death
Ovarian ablation, no chemotherapy	30 (9%)	28 (9%)
Ovarian ablation, with chemotherapy	21 (9%)	19 (11%)

★ The ovarian ablation–chemotherapy group includes studies of chemotherapy alone versus the same chemotherapy combined with ovarian ablation.

(Adapted from Early Breast Cancer Trialists' Collaborative Group. Systemic treatment of early breast cancer by hormonal, cytotoxic, or immune therapy. Lancet 1992;339:1,71)

apy. Additional studies are needed comparing ovarian ablation with or without chemotherapy with chemotherapy alone. More information on the long-term consequences of inducing ovarian failure in young women is also needed. Premature coronary artery disease and osteoporosis might be expected in some patients. Studies in progress are investigating ovarian ablation induced by LHRH analogues. A large Intergroup study in ER-positive, node-positive, premenopausal patients comparing CAF chemotherapy alone with CAF followed by Zoladex versus CAF followed by Zoladex and tamoxifen has recently been completed and, together with other ongoing studies, should help to clarify the role of ovarian ablation. Until these questions are answered, it is difficult to recommend ovarian ablation as standard therapy in premenopausal breast cancer patients.

Other Trials of Adjuvant Endocrine Therapy

Individual small trials of other forms of endocrine therapy have been reported, but data are insufficient to draw conclusions or to make recommendations. High-dose diethylstilbestrol prolonged DFS similarly to tamoxifen in postmenopausal patients in a Danish study.[97] Eight-year follow-up of an English trial in which 354 postmenopausal node-positive patients were randomized to aminoglutethimide and hydrocortisone or to placebo for 2 years indicated no overall DFS or OS benefit.[98] Strong favorable trends were evident in ER-positive patients treated with aminoglutethimide, however, suggesting that a larger study may have reached statistical significance. Preliminary results of a trial using high-dose medroxyprogesterone acetate or no adjuvant therapy in 240 node-negative patients showed significant improvements in both DFS and OS.[99] All these therapies, however, are more toxic than tamoxifen, and in the absence of additional data, they cannot be recommended for adjuvant therapy, except perhaps in the rare situation when tamoxifen is not tolerated.

Benefits of Adjuvant Chemoendocrine Therapy

The benefits of adjuvant chemotherapy and endocrine therapy used as single modalities prompted investigators to consider a combined approach based on the basic oncology principle of using multiple therapies or drugs that have different mechanisms of action and nonoverlapping toxicities. Conceptually, cells in a heterogeneous tumor could be sensitive only to endocrine therapy, sensitive only to chemotherapy, sensitive to both therapies, or resistant to both. A combined approach might then provide an additive beneficial antitumor effect. In addition, cellular effects of endocrine therapy could also interact with cytotoxic agents to alter chemosensitivity. Tamoxifen and estrogen-deprivation agents are predominantly cytostatic agents that act to slow cell proliferation by blocking cell cycle transit.[100–102] These cell cycle alterations could conceivably render cells less sensitive to cell

cycle–active chemotherapeutic agents. Tamoxifen has a variety of other effects on the cell that could alter sensitivity to cytotoxic agents. It antagonizes calmodulin and is an effective Ca^{2+} channel antagonist—effects that could alter drug uptake.[103,104] Membrane lipids are altered by tamoxifen, which could alter diffusion rates of certain drugs.[105] Finally, tamoxifen and progestins inhibit *p*-glycoprotein, an effect that could enhance sensitivity to drugs such as doxorubicin.[106,107]

Preclinical studies investigating interactions between tamoxifen and various chemotherapeutic drugs have not always produced consistent results, but they do provide some evidence for both antagonistic and additive interactions, depending on the drug. Tamoxifen antagonized the cytotoxicity of melphalan and 5-fluorouracil in human breast cancer cells, an effect that perhaps explains the poorer results obtained by adding tamoxifen to these agents in premenopausal receptor-negative patients in an NSABP study.[91,108,109] On the other hand, tamoxifen demonstrated an additive effect when it was combined with doxorubicin and cyclophosphamide in vitro.[108] One of the few trials showing a significant survival advantage for chemoendocrine therapy compared with tamoxifen alone used cyclophosphamide and doxorubicin combined with tamoxifen.[110] These in vitro drug interactions were independent of ER status and were not related to the cell cycle effects of tamoxifen.

Clinical trials of chemoendocrine therapy have been designed in several ways. A few early trials compared a CMF-based chemotherapy regimen combined with tamoxifen with a no-treatment control arm in postmenopausal, node-positive patients.[111–113] These trials were small, and although all showed prolonged DFS with the adjuvant treatment, only the largest study showed a significant OS advantage. Given the proved benefit for chemotherapy in women less 50 years of age and for tamoxifen in older patients, especially those with ER-positive tumors, the two questions of greatest interest to the clinician are the following: Is it advantageous to add endocrine therapy (tamoxifen or ovarian ablation) to chemotherapy in younger women? Should chemotherapy be added to tamoxifen therapy in older women? Many studies have now been completed comparing chemotherapy alone or combined with endocrine therapy in premenopausal patients or tamoxifen with or without chemotherapy in postmenopausal patients.

CHEMOENDOCRINE THERAPY IN PREMENOPAUSAL PATIENTS

Because chemotherapy has been considered standard therapy in this subset of patients for many years, endocrine therapy by itself has not been studied widely, and insufficient data exist from trials comparing endocrine therapy alone in one arm to endocrine therapy combined with chemotherapy in the other arm, to draw any conclusions. Abundant data, however, permit more definitive conclusions from trials comparing chemotherapy with or without endocrine therapy.

Chemotherapy and Ovarian Ablation

As reviewed earlier (see Table 17.2-12), the metaanalysis suggests that DFS and OS might be improved by treating premenopausal patients with both chemotherapy and ovarian ablation instead of chemotherapy alone.[12] The added benefit of ovarian ablation might depend on the chemotherapy regimen used and the incidence of chemical ovarian ablation associated with it. ER-positive patients would be expected to receive the most benefit from ovarian ablation. Randomized trials of adjuvant surgical ovariectomy have proved difficult to perform. Patients are reluctant to undergo additional surgery immediately after lumpectomy or mastectomy, and premature menopause is frightening to some. Nevertheless, two cooperative group studies investigating the value of surgical ovariectomy in premenopausal patients with known ER status have been completed and have relatively long follow-up.[114,115]

The Ludwig Group (now called the International Breast Cancer Study Group) found, in patients who had at least four positive lymph nodes, a strong trend that did not reach statistical significance in favor of CMFP plus ovariectomy compared with CMFP alone, but only in the ER-positive subset.[113] Although menstrual history information was available in these patients, the study is too small to determine the value of permanent chemical castration in ER-positive patients treated with chemotherapy alone. Furthermore, amenorrhea, although a valuable surrogate marker, may not always indicate complete loss of ovarian function.

The SWOG has also completed a trial of 1 year of CMFVP alone versus ovariectomy and CMFVP in 314 premenopausal patients with ER-positive tumors and positive lymph nodes.[115] After 5 years of follow-up, no advantage for ovarian ablation is evident, although a trend exists in patients with at least four positive nodes. Complete menstrual cycle information is not available in this study, and a high incidence of chemotherapy-induced ovarian ablation may have precluded any significant benefit from ovariectomy. The apparent lack of benefit could also be related to the small size of the study, which had the power to detect only a major difference between the two arms. More definitive information on the value of chemotherapy and ovarian ablation will soon be available from the recently completed Intergroup trial mentioned earlier. This trial accrued more than 1500 patients and has complete hormonal profiles to determine ovarian function accurately.

Chemotherapy and Tamoxifen

Whether tamoxifen adds to the benefits achieved with chemotherapy has been addressed by numerous randomized trials.[12,62]

As described earlier, the NSABP (B09) randomly assigned 1858 patients (779 premenopausal) to receive melphalan and 5-fluorouracil (PF) therapy or PF and tamoxifen (PFT).[91] An advantage for tamoxifen was observed in postmenopausal patients, but not in premenopausal patients, who actually had worse DFS and OS. This trial raised the question of an antagonistic drug interaction, and we now know that tamoxifen inhibits cellular uptake of melphalan.[108,109] These results also caused some oncologists

to begin tamoxifen after chemotherapy is completed to avoid possible antagonisms, a strategy that has yet to be studied in clinical trials.

In another large study performed by the Danish Breast Cancer Group, 811 premenopausal patients, most of whom were ER-positive, were randomly assigned to receive CMF for 9 months or CMF and 1 year of tamoxifen.[116] The CMF–tamoxifen arm had to be closed early because of a significant survival detriment, although at 4 years of follow-up, researchers saw only a nonsignificant trend for tamoxifen-treated patients to do worse. Two smaller studies by the ECOG and the North Central Group using CMFP and CFP, respectively, also showed no advantage in DFS or OS by the addition of 1 year of tamoxifen.[117,118] Similar results were observed in an Italian study that used CMF followed by epirubicin with or without tamoxifen for 5 years in node-positive, ER-positive premenopausal patients.[119] A trend in favor of the addition of tamoxifen did not reach statistical significance in this small study.

The metaanalysis included 6362 patients younger than 50 years of age in its comparison of chemotherapy alone with chemotherapy and tamoxifen (Table 17.2-13).[12] No significant reductions in the odds of recurrence or death were observed for the addition of tamoxifen to chemotherapy in young women, confirming the individual trials. Most of the completed trials used relatively short durations of tamoxifen (2 years or less), however, and they enrolled patients regardless of ER status. The metaanalysis suggests that more prolonged tamoxifen therapy may be better in women younger than 50 years, and ER-positive patients would be expected to have the greatest benefit from endocrine therapy. No studies have analyzed the tamoxifen benefit relative to ovarian function after chemotherapy. Finally, studies have not evaluated the strategy of delaying tamoxifen until chemotherapy has been completed. This approach would avoid drug interactions, but the net result of delaying the start of endocrine therapy for 4 to 6 months is unknown. Until these questions are answered, DFS or OS data will be insufficient to recommend the addition

TABLE 17.2-13

Metaanalysis of the Effects of Chemoendocrine Therapy in Women Younger Than 50 Years of Age

Type of Study	Reduction in the Annual Odds	
	Recurrence	Death
Chemotherapy and tamoxifen versus tamoxifen	Too few patients	
Chemotherapy and tamoxifen versus chemotherapy	7 (4%)	3 (5%)

(Adapted from Early Breast Cancer Trialists' Collaborative Group. Systemic treatment of early breast cancer by hormonal, cytotoxic, or immune therapy. Lancet 1992;339:1,71)

of tamoxifen to premenopausal patients who are also receiving chemotherapy.

Chemotherapy and Tamoxifen in Postmenopausal Patients

Numerous randomized trials involving more than 12,000 patients investigated chemoendocrine therapy in older women.[12,62] Many of these trials directly compared chemotherapy alone with chemotherapy and tamoxifen. A smaller number of studies compared tamoxifen alone with tamoxifen and chemotherapy, and only a few studies compared each modality alone with the combination. A CMF-based regimen was used in most of these studies. Most of the trials assessing the addition of tamoxifen to chemotherapy found a significant benefit, not surprising considering the meager benefits of chemotherapy and the more substantial benefits of tamoxifen in this age group. A more important question is whether the addition of chemotherapy and its toxicities to tamoxifen is better than tamoxifen alone.

Several large mature trials have addressed this question. The Ludwig III study compared CMFPT versus PT for 1 year in 307 patients (ER was known to be positive in only 103 patients).[113] The chemotherapy group enjoyed a significant DFS benefit, although OS was only borderline significant. Tamoxifen was given for only 1 year in this study, a duration now considered suboptimal. A Danish study randomly assigned 1347 postmenopausal patients (only one third known to be ER-positive) to receive tamoxifen for 1 year with or without CMF.[120] A DFS, but not an OS, advantage was observed.

The two largest studies focusing on ER-positive patients reported contrasting results.[110,121] The SWOG randomly assigned 892 node-positive patients to receive tamoxifen for 1 year, aggressive chemotherapy with CMFVP for 1 year, or the combination.[121] At a median follow-up of more than 6 years, no difference among the three arms was evident for either DFS or OS. Thus, tamoxifen for a suboptimal duration of only 1 year was as good as aggressive chemotherapy, and no advantage was noted for the combination. Given the lack of toxicity of tamoxifen, this study concluded that it was superior to the chemotherapy arms. Nearly identical preliminary results were recently reported from a Canadian study that randomly assigned 705 receptor-positive postmenopausal patients to receive tamoxifen alone for 1 year versus intravenous CMF for eight cycles plus tamoxifen.[122] DFS and OS were identical in the two arms.

NSABP (B16) used a different strategy in comparing tamoxifen alone for 5 years versus AC for 4 cycles plus tamoxifen versus PAF for 17 cycles plus tamoxifen (the third arm originally was PF alone, but was modified later to include doxorubicin).[110] This trial is unique in showing a DFS benefit for AC and PAF and an OS benefit for combining AC with tamoxifen compared with tamoxifen alone. At 3 years of follow-up, OS was 85% for tamoxifen alone and 93% for AC and tamoxifen ($P = .04$). No OS difference was observed for PAFT compared with tamoxifen alone.

The metaanalysis confirmed that chemotherapy combined with tamoxifen is better than chemotherapy alone in women older than 50 years of age, and it found that chemotherapy combined with tamoxifen provides a DFS but no OS advantage compared with tamoxifen alone (Table 17.2-14). Thus, at the present time, only the NSABP trial using AC shows a statistically significant OS advantage for treating older women with a combination of chemotherapy and tamoxifen rather than tamoxifen alone. Possibly, the AC chemotherapy used in this study is superior to the CMF-based chemotherapy regimens used in most of the other chemoendocrine therapy trials, although the NSABP study showing similar results with AC or CMF does not support this explanation.[61] The trial of AC and tamoxifen did include patients who were ER-negative (about 20% of the total), which conceivably reduced the effectiveness of tamoxifen used alone. Another possibility is that tamoxifen antagonizes the cytotoxicity of CMF, while it provides an additive effect when combined with AC, an idea supported to some extent by the laboratory data reviewed earlier. Finally, chance could also explain the unique findings of the NSABP study in which AC but not PAF provided an OS advantage when combined with tamoxifen.

In conclusion, whether chemotherapy should be routinely added to tamoxifen in the treatment of ER-positive postmenopausal patients with breast cancer is not yet clear. Based on the modest DFS advantage noted in the metaanalysis and the OS advantage observed with the AC regimen in the NSABP study, an argument can be made to treat such patients with chemoendocrine therapy. The modest and unconfirmed OS benefit must be weighed against the toxicity of chemotherapy, however, especially in elderly patients. Several questions remain. Should strongly ER-positive patients who have a greater-than-average benefit with tamoxifen also receive chemotherapy? What is the optimal approach in the ER-negative subset of patients in whom tamoxifen has only a minimal impact? Should tamoxifen be given simultaneously with CMF or doxorubicin-based chemotherapy, or should it

TABLE 17.2-14

Metaanalysis of the Effects of Chemoendocrine Therapy in Women 50 Years Old or Older

Type of Study	Reduction (SD) in Annual Odds	
	Recurrence	Death
Chemotherapy and tamoxifen versus tamoxifen	26 (5%)	10 (7%)
Chemotherapy and tamoxifen versus chemotherapy	28 (3%)	20 (4%)

(Adapted from Early Breast Cancer Trialists' Collaborative Group. Systemic treatment of early breast cancer by hormonal, cytotoxic, or immune therapy. Lancet 1992;339:1,71)

be started after the completion of chemotherapy? Many of these questions will be answered by several ongoing or recently completed trials, such as the Intergroup node-negative study comparing CMF and CAF, each with or without tamoxifen, or the three-arm Intergroup trial in ER-positive, node-positive, postmenopausal patients that compares tamoxifen alone for 5 years, CAF for 6 cycles starting simultaneously with tamoxifen, and CAF followed sequentially by tamoxifen.[123]

Adjuvant Immunotherapy

More than 20 randomized trials of adjuvant immunotherapy have been completed.[12] Most of these trials included other therapies in addition to treatment with BCG, levamisole, or a variety of other nonspecific immune stimulants. None of these individual trials demonstrated a significant DFS or OS benefit for immunotherapy. Even the metaanalyses of all trials, which included more than 6000 patients, could not find a hint of benefit. In fact, the analysis of the BCG trials showed a sizable and statistically significant adverse impact on both DFS and OS (odds reduction for DFS, $-17\% \pm 8$; odds reduction for OS, $-20\% \pm 8\%$). Currently, no evidence supports the use of immunotherapy in the adjuvant treatment of breast cancer.

Toxicity of Adjuvant Treatment

TOXICITY OF ADJUVANT CHEMOTHERAPY

Acute Toxicity

In general, women with early breast cancer tolerate adjuvant chemotherapy well, better than those with metastatic disease, whose health may be compromised by the larger tumor burden. Modifications of normal life-style are required during the treatment period of usually 4 to 6 months, but most patients are able to continue working or performing their daily routines. Death due to the complications of adjuvant therapy is uncommon, but it can be devastating when an apparently healthy patient with no evidence of cancer and who has a good prognosis for cure dies of neutropenic infection. No deaths were reported in a large trial of more than 2000 node-positive patients (75% younger than 50 years old) treated with AC or CMF chemotherapy.[61] Another trial of 966 postmenopausal patients with positive lymph nodes treated with 4 or 12 cycles of CMF reported 9 treatment-related deaths (0.9%), most from neutropenic sepsis or thromboembolism, which seems to be more common in patients treated with chemotherapy, especially when combined with tamoxifen.[48,121,122,124] In another study of chemotherapy in postmenopausal patients, 4 deaths were reported in 600 patients (0.6%) receiving 1 year of CMFVP chemotherapy alone (1 death) or combined with tamoxifen (3 deaths).[121] The cumulative data suggest that lethal toxicities occur in about 1 of every 200 to 500 patients receiving adjuvant

chemotherapy, that toxic deaths may be more frequent in postmenopausal patients, and that the addition of tamoxifen to chemotherapy increases toxicity because of thromboembolism.

Although lethal toxicities are uncommon, other acute side effects are bothersome to patients (Table 17.2-15). NSABP B15 compared the toxicities of AC for four cycles and standard CMF for six cycles, both commonly used treatment regimens.[61] Cardiac toxicity was not problematic in this study with either treatment. The most common side effects were alopecia, nausea and vomiting, weight gain, and grade 3 or 4 neutropenia. Infection was uncommon. CMF was associated with slightly more neutropenia, nausea without vomiting, and weight gain. Alopecia and vomiting were more frequent with AC. Another way to evaluate toxicity is the duration of symptoms as well as the total number of physicians' or treatment visits by the patient. The AC regimen consists of only 4 intravenous drug treatments 3 weeks apart; CMF includes oral cyclophosphamide for 2 weeks and intravenous MF on days 1 and 8 of each 4-week cycle repeated 6 times for a total of 84 treatment days and 12 intravenous treatments. Thus, on average, AC was completed in 63 days, compared with 154 days for CMF. Patients given CMF required three times the number of physician visits. Finally, antiemetic medication was prescribed for a total of 84 days with CMF and only 12 days with AC. Fatigue is another side effect of chemotherapy that is difficult to quantify, and its incidence was not reported in this study.

Anxiety and psychologic distress have not been studied in detail, and separating the impact of the recent diagnosis

TABLE 17.2-15
Toxicity of AC and CMF

	Patients	
Side Effect	AC (%)	CMF (%)
WBC <2000/μL	3.7	9.7
Severe infection	2.4	1.2
Platelets <50,000/μL	0.1	0.3
Nausea only	15.5	42.8
Vomiting	75.9	38.8
Diarrhea >4 stools/d	2.9	4.8
Alopecia, severe	89.4	40.6
Thromboembolic	0.7	1.7
Cystitis	0.3	1.6
Weight gain ≥10%	3.8	14.3

AC, doxorubin and cyclophosphamide; CMF, cyclophosphamide, methotrexate, and 5-fluorouracil.

(Adapted from Kishev B, Brown AM, Dimitrov NV, et al. Two months of doxorubicin-cyclophosphamide with and without interval reinduction therapy compared with 6 months of cyclophosphamide, methotrexate, and fluorouracil in positive-node breast cancer patients with tamoxifen-nonresponsive tumor: results from the National Surgical Adjuvant Breast and Bowel Project B-15. J Clin Oncol 1990;8:1483) of a life-threatening disease from the impact of treatment is difficult. Mild symptoms of distress have been reported in patients receiving chemotherapy,[125] especially with prolonged treatment.[126] A small sample from a randomized controlled treatment trial suggested more anxiety for patients assigned to no treatment than for those assigned to chemotherapy, perhaps because of a placebo effect associated with active treatment and the hope that the intervention will improve the chance for cure.[127]

Long-Term Adverse Effects of Adjuvant Chemotherapy

Complications of adjuvant chemotherapy that may occur months to years after completion of treatment are more difficult to identify, but they can be an extremely important consideration when treating patients who have a low risk of death from breast cancer. Even serious adverse events that are uncommon can wipe out the small absolute benefits of treatment observed in node-negative patients with small tumors. The major potential toxicities to consider are cardiac dysfunction, premature menopause, and the development of second cancers.

The cardiomyopathy due to doxorubicin may occur during treatment, shortly after its completion, or many months later. The incidence of congestive heart failure in patients treated with doxorubicin-based adjuvant therapy varies according to the total cumulative dose received and perhaps according to the peak blood levels. In the NSABP trial of AC for four cycles, heart failure was not observed (maximum total dose of doxorubicin, 240 mg/m^2).[61] In two studies from Milan using sequenced CMF and doxorubicin (maximum total dose, 300 mg/m^2), congestive heart failure was observed in one patient receiving CMF and in one patient treated with doxorubicin, both of whom also were treated with irradiation to the left breast.[64,65] The incidence of cardiomyopathy was higher in two other studies (4% to 7%), but it was less than 1% when the total cumulative doxorubicin dose was less than 300 mg/m^2.[128,129] Cardiomyopathy may be less common when doxorubicin is administered by a 2- to 4-day continuous infusion, but this technique requires an indwelling venous catheter that also has a high complication rate. Whether continuous infusion has equivalent antitumor activity in the adjuvant therapy of breast cancer has not been studied definitively.

The low incidence of acute doxorubicin-induced cardiomyopathy when the cumulative dose is kept at or below 300 mg/m^2 seems acceptable for higher-risk breast cancer patients, but it may be unacceptable for patients with a low risk of disease recurrence, the majority of whom are already cured by surgery alone. CMF has equivalent efficacy and may be preferred in such patients. Another concern that will be difficult to study is the possibility that patients given doxorubicin early in life could have premature heart disease when they get older. Although no data support this worry at the present time, it emphasizes the need for long-term follow-up studies of cardiac events in randomized trials and the need for caution in

prescribing doxorubicin to patients in whom the potential benefit is small.

Another concern is premature ovarian ablation caused by chemotherapy in the majority of premenopausal women. The overall incidence of treatment-induced amenorrhea is around 70%,[130,131] although it varies according to age and the dose and type of alkylating agent. Permanent ovarian dysfunction with standard chemotherapy is less common in patients younger than 35 years old, whereas it is nearly universal in women older than 45 years of age. Chemical ovarian ablation may be a desirable side effect in higher-risk patients because it may provide an advantage in reducing the odds of breast cancer recurrence and death. In low-risk patients, however, the minimal absolute benefits of ovarian ablation may be exceeded by the discomforts related to menopausal symptoms and by the theoretic increased risk of premature osteoporosis and cardiovascular disease. Premenopausal patients treated in the first-generation adjuvant trials are just now reaching the age at which these problems may emerge, and careful study of these and other long-term effects is needed.

Many cytotoxic drugs are carcinogens, and a possible increased risk of second malignant disease is another concern. An increased risk of treatment-induced myeloproliferative disease and acute leukemia in breast cancer patients treated with adjuvant chemotherapy has been established. Data from the Surveillance, Epidemiology and End Results Program (SEER) indicate an increased risk of leukemia (cumulative incidence, 0.7% at 10 years) related to the cumulative dose and to the type of alkylating agent used.[132] Overall, a 5-fold risk of developing leukemia and an 11.5-fold risk of acute nonlymphocytic leukemia were observed. No increased risk was observed in patients treated by surgery alone. Leukemia risk was higher with more prolonged treatment regimens, and it was strongly related to the use of melphalan (relative risk [RR], 45). Similar data were reported by the NSABP.[133]

A more recent larger study of 82,700 patients from five regions of the United States provides more information on the leukemia risk associated with breast cancer treatment.[134] The risk of acute nonlymphocytic leukemia was increased after regional radiotherapy (RR, 2.4), alkylating agents alone (RR, 10), and combined chemotherapy and radiation (RR, 17.4). The risk associated with melphalan was 10 times that related to cyclophosphamide (RR, 31.4 versus 3.1). Patients who received cyclophosphamide for less than 12 months or who received less than 20 g total dose had almost no detectable increase in leukemia risk. Thus, the cumulative data suggest that the leukemia risk associated with the cyclophosphamide-containing regimens used most frequently today is modest. Regional radiation may increase this risk slightly. Whether the higher doses of alkylating agents now used experimentally or the use of hematopoietic growth factors will increase leukemia risk awaits further study.

Most treatment-induced leukemias occur within the first few years after exposure to the cytotoxic agent, but solid tumors have a much longer latency period. Thus, to draw conclusions about the risk of solid tumors in patients treated with adjuvant chemotherapy for breast cancer is premature because relatively few patients in prospective trials have been followed-up for more than 15 years.[135] The already increased risk of other tumors, such as ovarian, endometrial, and colorectal cancer, in patients with a history of breast cancer complicates estimates of risk from chemotherapy. At present, no evidence suggests an increased risk of second malignant disease in long-term follow-up studies from Milan of patients treated with CMF.[136] In any event, the slight risk of leukemia and the absence of an indication of an increased risk of solid tumors with adjuvant chemotherapy are of little concern for breast cancer patients in whom the risk of breast cancer recurrence is substantial. These small risks for second malignant disease, however, are potentially more important in treating patients at low risk of breast cancer recurrence, and they should be considered in making treatment decisions in such patients.

TOXICITY OF TAMOXIFEN ADJUVANT THERAPY

Ancillary Benefits of Tamoxifen

Certain side effects of tamoxifen contribute to its overall net benefit. The estrogen-agonist properties of tamoxifen result in reduced serum cholesterol and low-density lipoprotein and a more favorable lipid profile.[86] Long-term follow-up of controlled studies of tamoxifen adjuvant therapy suggest that these favorable changes in blood lipids translate into reduced morbidity and mortality from cardiac disease.[89,137] The estrogen-like properties of tamoxifen also affect bone mineral density.[85,138] Tamoxifen treatment for at least 2 years increased and then stabilized bone density in the axial skeleton and stabilized bone mineral content in the appendicular skeleton of postmenopausal patients. These measures decreased in control patients.

Another favorable ancillary effect of tamoxifen is a reduced incidence of contralateral breast cancer. Individual trials as well as the metaanalysis have shown a 40% reduction in risk.[12,36,139,140] These ancillary benefits of tamoxifen provide the rationale for the chemoprevention trials now ongoing worldwide in women at high risk of developing breast cancer. An argument can be made to consider the judicious use of tamoxifen in breast cancer patients with cardiovascular or osteoporosis risk factors, even if only a small benefit in reducing the odds of cancer recurrence is anticipated. Estrogen replacement therapy is still considered by many to be contraindicated in breast cancer patients.

Toxicity of Tamoxifen

Tamoxifen is well tolerated by most patients with breast cancer. The toxicity profile of tamoxifen has been assessed in placebo-controlled randomized trials.[36,141] The most frequent side effects reported in patients taking tamoxifen are menopausal symptoms. At least 50% to 60% of patients taking tamoxifen report some hot flashes, but 40% to 50% of placebo-treated patients report similar episodes. Many of these patients had hot flashes before starting tamoxifen because of natural causes or because of the withdrawal of estrogen replacement therapy when breast cancer was diagnosed. About 20% of patients report severe hot flashes while taking tamoxifen, compared with 3% of placebo patients. Vaginal discharge and irregular menses are also more common in patients taking tamoxifen. In one study, general quality-of-life scores were similar for tamoxifen and placebo.[141] Headaches were reported less frequently with tamoxifen.

Depression has not been reported to be increased in randomized, placebo-controlled trials, but this may reflect underreporting of symptoms that may be brought out by more careful and detailed questioning. Many oncologists would contend, based on their own experience, that depression is an uncommon but real side effect of tamoxifen treatment. A nonrandomized single institution study suggests that symptoms of depression can be identified in up to 10% of patients taking tamoxifen.[142] Symptoms are occasionally severe and may require dose reduction, antidepressant medication, or even discontinuation of the drug.

Ocular toxicity has been reported with high tamoxifen doses.[143] An uncontrolled study concluded that ocular toxicity in the form of retinopathy or keratopathy was a side effect of conventional doses of tamoxifen,[144] a result not confirmed in a controlled study in which complete ophthalmologic examinations were performed in a blinded fashion.[145] Although this question has not been answered definitively, clinically significant ocular toxicity must be rare, if it occurs at all. Occasional ophthalmologic examination should be sufficient monitoring for breast cancer patients receiving long-term therapy.

The most troublesome side effect of long-term tamoxifen is related to its carcinogenic potential. Although the drug is not a mutagen in the Ames assay, it is genotoxic. Electrophilic metabolites produced by rat and human liver P-450 enzymes can form covalent DNA adducts at least in the rat.[146,147] Tamoxifen is a potent hepatocarcinogen in the rat, but not in the mouse.[148,149] The presence of adducts have not yet been confirmed in human liver, but the microsomal enzymes in human liver are capable of producing reactive metabolites in vitro. Although abnormal liver function tests are occasionally observed in patients receiving tamoxifen, only a few anecdotal cases of hepatoma have thus far been reported in humans, and data on the incidence of hepatoma since the introduction of tamoxifen suggest that it does not cause a large increase in incidence.[140,150] Careful long-term follow-up studies of tamoxifen users are needed in view of the preclinical data, however, and given the long latency period usually associated with carcinogen-induced solid tumors.

Tamoxifen use, much like estrogen therapy, is clearly related to an increased incidence of endometrial cancer.[140,151,152] Even just 1 year of adjuvant tamoxifen is associated with a slightly increased incidence, but the risk rises with more prolonged treatment. Interpretation of these results is a problem because many women taking tamoxifen were treated with estrogen-replacement therapy before the diagnosis of breast cancer. Nevertheless, 8-year follow-up of NSABP B14, in which 2843 patients were randomly assigned to receive at least 5 years of tamoxifen or placebo, indicated that tamoxifen was associated with an annual hazard rate of 1.7 in 1000 an RR of 2.2 compared with population-based rates of endometrial cancer from SEER data.[151] The type of endometrial cancer in patients taking tamoxifen is similar to those in patients not exposed to tamoxifen. Eighteen of the 23 cancers were of good to moderate histologic grade, and most were stage I. Four patients died of uterine cancer, however, indicating the lethal potential of this complication and the need for regular gynecologic examinations. The role of endometrial cancer screening by vaginal ultrasound or endometrial biopsy and the role of progestins in reducing the risk of endometrial cancer are now being evaluated. The high incidence of uterine cancers with an unfavorable prognosis reported in tamoxifen-treated patients in a small retrospective study needs confirmation.[153] Data from the NSABP and the large Swedish randomized trials indicate that tamoxifen adjuvant therapy has not yet resulted in an increased incidence of other solid tumors.[140,151] Although these adverse effects of tamoxifen do not detract from the proved substantial survival benefits in patients with invasive breast cancer, they do raise caution for the use of tamoxifen in benign conditions or for breast cancer prevention. The drug should not be used for these purposes outside a clinical trial.

Cost-Effectiveness of Adjuvant Therapy

Given the high incidence of breast cancer and the moderate survival benefits of adjuvant therapy, one must evaluate both efficacy and cost-effectiveness from a public health perspective. Several such studies have been reported.[154–156] Using a decision–analysis model and reasonable assumptions of risk and benefit, adjuvant therapy increases the quality-adjusted life expectancy of an average woman at a cost similar to that of other widely accepted therapies. Treatment is more cost-effective in higher-risk patients, but even node-negative patients benefit.[154] Cost-effectiveness is greater for premenopausal than for postmenopausal patients, but even some elderly patients benefit.[156] The cost of the benefit in elderly patients is comparable to that of other reimbursed procedures until a point between 75 and 80 years old. Cost benefit ratios can be significantly improved by selection of patients at high risk of disease recurrence or by selection of patients most likely to benefit from treatment. A discussion of prognostic and predictive biomarkers is found in Chapter 16.

Making Adjuvant Treatment Decisions

Breast cancer is a heterogeneous disease. Some patients have aggressive disease that is refractory to treatment; survival may be only a few months. Many patients have more indolent disease that is responsive to hormone therapy or chemotherapy. Today, with the increasing use of mammography, the majority of patients (50% to 60%) are cured by surgery alone and do not need adjuvant treatment. Given the modest benefits of adjuvant treatment, it makes little sense to recommend therapy to all patients when many do not need it and only a few benefit. A more rational approach is to consider each patient individually and to estimate risk–benefit profiles for each patient.

Clinical decision making requires an assessment of the risk of recurrence and death, the benefits of treatment, and the costs and toxicity of treatment. Many patients overestimate or underestimate their chance of being cured by breast cancer surgery, and both physicians and patients tend to overestimate the benefits of adjuvant therapy.[157,158] An accurate estimate of both is crucial for meaningful discussions about the value of adjuvant therapy.

Estimates of the impact of the disease and the benefits of adjuvant therapy on 10-year survival can be made using patient age, natural mortality from other causes, breast cancer mortality, and mortality reductions derived from the metaanalysis data on chemotherapy and tamoxifen (Table 17.2-16). The low-risk subset in each age group might represent patients with tumors 1 cm or smaller and negative lymph nodes; the intermediate-risk group represents the average node-negative patient; and the high-risk group typifies patients with one or two positive lymph nodes. The natural mortality in patients of similar age without a diagnosis of breast cancer is nearly 10 times higher in a 65 year old than in a 40 year old. Competing causes of mortality are significant in older women and must be considered. These natural mortality rates would be even higher in women with preexisting medical illness such as diabetes or heart disease. Assuming a 25% annual reduction in the odds of death by treatment, the absolute benefit (the number of patients alive per 100 patients treated) increases as the risk of death from breast cancer increases. The total number of patients receiving some benefit from adjuvant treatment is likely to be greater than the absolute benefit, however, because some patients whose cancer recurred and who died by 10 years may have had their death delayed by therapy. Nevertheless, the benefits are modest, particularly in the subsets with a low risk of death. Given the morbidity, possible mortality, and cost of adjuvant treatment, many patients and physicians would argue that treatment is not indicated routinely in such low-risk patients. The mortality reductions (and, thus, the absolute benefit) from treatment would be even smaller than the 25% shown in the example in Table 17.2-16 for adjuvant chemotherapy in postmenopausal patients or for tamoxifen in premenopausal or ER-negative patients. Patients must also be aware that the differences in 10-year survival (absolute benefit) do not necessarily indicate that any patients are cured by treatment. At this time, without longer follow-up, one cannot differentiate between a substantial prolongation of life and a cure in some treated patients.

The real question then is at what level of benefit is adjuvant therapy indicated. This question is difficult to answer. Clinical experience suggests that some patients or physicians are willing to accept the toxicity and costs of treatment for a relatively meager potential benefit, whereas others require more substantial gains.[159] Some patients may

TABLE 17.2-16
Survival Estimates at 10 Years by Age, Risk of Breast Cancer Death,
With and Without Adjuvant Therapy

Hypothetic Risk* of Breast Cancer Death	Natural Mortality Rate Without Breast Cancer, Next 10 Years (%)	Alive at 10 Years		Absolute Benefit (%)
		No Adjuvant Therapy	Adjuvant Therapy†	
40 YEARS OLD				
10% (low risk)	2	88	90	2
28% (intermediate risk)	2	71	77	6
57% (high risk)	2	41	51	10
65 YEARS OLD				
9% (low risk)	19	73	75	2
26% (intermediate risk)	19	58	63	5
54% (high risk)	19	34	43	9

* Values shown are derived from three different risk estimates and assume exponential death with a constant hazard ratio. The differences between 40 and 65 years old reflect deaths from other causes.

† Based on a 25% annual reduction in the odds of death, a reasonable estimate of the benefits of chemotherapy in a premenopausal patient and tamoxifen in an estrogen receptor–positive postmenopausal patient.

select a less toxic therapy, such as tamoxifen, even though it may be slightly less effective than chemotherapy in certain subsets (ie, premenopausal patients). The 1990 National Institutes of Health Consensus Panel concluded that patients with node-negative tumors 1 cm or smaller in diameter "have an excellent prognosis and do not require adjuvant systemic therapy outside of clinical trials."[160] Such patients have a 10-year recurrence risk of about 10%.[161] As discussed in Chapter 16, other prognostic factors can be used to identify a group of node-negative patients with a similarly excellent prognosis. Patients with histologic or nuclear grade 1 tumors; those with a special tumor type such as tubular, mucinous, or papillary carcinoma; patients with ductal carcinoma in situ with or without microinvasion; and even patients with tumors between 1 and 2 cm in diameter with other good prognostic factors such as positive ER and a low proliferative index have 10-year recurrence rates ranging from 2% to 15%. No adjuvant therapy is an appropriate consideration in such patients. Rather than setting some arbitrary cutoff to discriminate patients who should not receive adjuvant therapy from those who should, however, a better strategy is to present an accurate risk–benefit profile to each patient and make recommendations based on a global assessment of the patient's tumor characteristics, age, and coincidental medical illness, as well as the patient's own response to the disease and the potential treatment benefits. Finally, these analyses illustrate the need for the development of additional prognostic factors to predict the risk of disease recurrence accurately and for the identification of accurate predictive factors to determine the responsiveness of a tumor to chemotherapy. A biomarker for chemotherapy sensitivity

equivalent to ER in predicting response to endocrine therapy would greatly facilitate treatment decisions.

Recommendations for the use of adjuvant therapy in clinical practice are shown in Table 17.2-17. No recipe exists with which everyone agrees, because uncertainty about the role of certain treatment approaches is still considerable. Experience and clinical judgment are required to make appropriate decisions in individual patients. Participation in clinical trials is encouraged to expedite answers to important questions. Progress would be faster if more than 4% (current rate) of patients with breast cancer were enrolled in randomized clinical trials. In the meantime, most oncologists agree that low-risk node-negative patients should not receive chemotherapy because relatively few patients stand to benefit, and the cost–benefit ratio is close to 1. Tamoxifen might be considered in some of these patients depending on the circumstances. The risk–benefit ratio in other node-negative patients favors the use of adjuvant therapy. Although some data suggest that tamoxifen may be effective in the premenopausal ER-positive subset, more substantial data support the use of chemotherapy, which definitely improves survival. Chemotherapy is optimal in the premenopausal ER-negative subset, whereas tamoxifen alone is considered standard treatment for postmenopausal ER-positive patients. Depending on the patient, no treatment at all might be considered for older women who are ER-negative. Chemotherapy or even tamoxifen (in the metaanalysis the benefit for tamoxifen in ER-negative patients was equivalent to that of chemotherapy in postmenopausal patients) might be considered in other postmenopausal, ER-negative patients. Substantial data justify the use of chemotherapy

TABLE 17.2-17
Recommendations for the Use of Adjuvant Therapy in Clinical Practice

Patient Subset	Recommended Treatment
NODE-NEGATIVE, LOW RISK*	Physician judgment; no treatment
NODE-NEGATIVE, HIGH RISK	
Premenopausal, ER+	Chemotherapy‡ or (?) tamoxifen†
Premenopausal, ER−	Chemotherapy
Postmenopausal, ER+	Tamoxifen†
Postmenopausal, ER−	Chemotherapy or tamoxifen; no treatment
NODE-POSITIVE	
Premenopausal, ER+ or −	Chemotherapy
Postmenopausal, ER+	Tamoxifen†; (?) addition of chemotherapy such as AC
Postmenopausal, ER−	Chemotherapy or tamoxifen†

ER, estrogen receptor; AC, doxorubicin−cyclophosphamide therapy.

* Low risk defined as negative axillary nodes and tumor ≤1 cm, or nuclear grade 1, or special histologic type, or 1- to 2-cm tumor along with ER+ and low proliferative index.

† Duration of 2 to 5 years.

‡ Combination chemotherapy as listed in Table 17.2-8.

alone in premenopausal node-positive patients. In the absence of significant DFS and OS benefits, it is difficult to recommend the addition of tamoxifen to chemotherapy in these patients. Although data suggest that the addition of ovarian ablation may be beneficial, additional study of the efficacy and long-term consequences of ovarian ablation are needed. Adjuvant tamoxifen should be considered in all postmenopausal ER-positive patients. Based on the NSABP data, the addition of AC chemotherapy to tamoxifen might be considered in high-risk patients. Survival is prolonged by chemotherapy or even by tamoxifen in postmenopausal, node-positive, ER-negative patients (ER-negative defined as less than 10 fmol/mg protein), but the benefits are modest, and treatment recommendations must follow careful discussions with each individual patient.

Adjuvant therapy improves long-term survival of patients with primary breast cancer. The benefits are modest but real, and given the high incidence of breast cancer, the mortality reductions achieved today with standard approaches should prevent or substantially delay hundreds of thousands of deaths worldwide in this decade.

References

1. Lewis D, Rienhoff WF Jr. A study of the results of operations for the cure of cancer of the breast. Ann Surg 1932;95:336.
2. Fisher B, Gebhardt MC. The evolution of breast cancer surgery: past, present, and future. Semin Oncol 1978;5:385.
3. Cruz EP, McDonald GO, Cole WH. Prophylactic treatment of cancer: the use of chemotherapeutic agents to prevent tumor metastasis. Surgery 1956;40:291.
4. Shapiro DM, Fugmann RA. A role of chemotherapy as an adjunct to surgery. Cancer Res 1957;17:1098.
5. Skipper HE. Kinetics of mammary tumor cell growth and implications for therapy. Cancer 1971;28:1479.
6. Cole MP. A clinical trial of an artificial menopause in carcinoma of the breast. INSERM 1975;55:143.
7. Fisher B, Ravdin RG, Ausman RK, et al. Surgical adjuvant chemotherapy in cancer of the breast: results of a decade of cooperative investigation. Ann Surg 1968;168:337.
8. Nissen-Meyer R. One short chemotherapy course in primary breast cancer: 12-year follow-up in series 1 of the Scandinavia Adjuvant Chemotherapy Study Group. In: Jones SE, Salmon SE, eds. Adjuvant therapy of cancer, vol 2. Orlando, Grune & Stratton, 1979:207.
9. Roberts S, Watne A, McGrath R, et al. Technique and results of isolation of cancer cells from the circulating blood. Arch Surg 1958;76:334.
10. Jonasson O, Long L, Roberts S, et al. Cancer cells in the circulating blood during operative management of genitourinary tumors. J Urol 1961;85:1.
11. Buzdar A, Blumenschein G, Gutterman J, et al. Adjuvant therapy with 5-flourouracil, adriamycin, cyclophosphamide and BCG (FAC-BCG) for stage II or III breast cancer. In: Jones SE, Salmon SE, eds. Adjuvant Therapy of Cancer, vol 2. New York, Grune & Stratton, 1979:277.
12. Early Breast Cancer Trialists' Collaborative Group. Systemic treatment of early breast cancer by hormonal, cytotoxic, or immune therapy. Lancet 1992;339:1,71.
13. Bonadonna G: Evolving concepts in the systemic adjuvant treatment of breast cancer. Cancer Res 1992;52:2127.
14. Bonadonna G, Brusamolino E, Valagussa P, et al. Combination chemotherapy as an adjuvant treatment in operable breast cancer. N Engl J Med 1976;294:405.

15. Levine MN, Guyatt GH, Gent M, et al. Quality of life in stage II breast cancer: an instrument for clinical trials. J Clin Oncol 1988;6:1798.

16. Gelber RD, Goldhirsch A, Cavalli F, et al. Quality-of-life-adjusted evaluation of adjuvant therapies for operable breast cancer. Ann Intern Med 1991;114:621.

17. Goldhirsch A, Gelber RD, Simes RJ, et al. Costs and benefits of adjuvant therapy in breast cancer: a quality-adjusted survival analysis. J Clin Oncol 1989;7:36.

18. Fisher B, Carbone P, Economou SG, et al. L-Phenylalanine mustard (L-PAM) in the management of primary breast cancer: a report of early findings. N Engl J Med 1975;292:117.

19. Fisher B, Fisher ER, Redmond C, and participating NSABP investigators. Ten-year results from the National Surgical Adjuvant Breast and Bowel Project (NSABP) clinical trial evaluating the use of L-phenylalanine mustard (L-PAM) in the management of primary breast cancer. J Clin Oncol 1986;4:929.

20. Padmanabhan N, Howell A, Rubens RD. Mechanism of action of adjuvant chemotherapy in early breast cancer. Lancet 1986;411.

21. Henderson IC: Adjuvant chemotherapy: a chemical oophorectomy? Breast Dis Year Book Q 1994;5:16.

22. Brincker H, Rose C, Rank F, et al. Evidence of a castration-mediated effect of adjuvant cytotoxic chemotherapy in premenopausal breast cancer. J Clin Oncol 1987;5:1771.

23. Bonadonna G, Valagussa P, Rossi A, et al. Ten year experience with CMF-based adjuvant chemotherapy in resectable breast cancer. Breast Cancer Res Treat 1985;5:95.

24. Scottish Cancer Trials Breast Group and ICFR Breast Unit, Guy's Hospital. Adjuvant ovarian ablation versus CMF chemotherapy in premenopausal women with pathological stage II breast carcinoma: the Scottish Trial. Lancet 1993;341:1293.

25. Early Breast Cancer Trialists' Collaborative Group. Effects of adjuvant tamoxifen and of cytotoxic therapy on mortality in early breast cancer: an overview of 61 randomized trials among 28,896 women. N Engl J Med 1988;319:1681.

26. Dressler LG, Seamer LC, Owens MA, et al. DNA flow cytometry and prognostic factors in 1331 frozen breast cancer specimens. Cancer 1988;61:420.

27. Osborne CK, Yochmowitz MG, Knight WA, et al. The value of estrogen and progesterone receptors in the treatment of breast cancer. Cancer 1980;46:2884.

28. Bonadonna G, Valagussa P. Dose-response effect of adjuvant chemotherapy in breast cancer. N Engl J Med 1981;304:10.

29. Mansour EG, Gray R, Shatila AH, et al. Efficacy of adjuvant chemotherapy in high-risk node-negative breast cancer: an Intergroup Study. N Engl J Med 1989;320:485.

30. Fisher B, Redmond C, Dimitrov NV, et al. A randomized clinical trial evaluating sequential methotrexate and fluorouracil in the treatment of patients with node-negative breast cancer who have estrogen-receptor–negative tumors. N Engl J Med 1989;320:473.

31. Tormey DC, Weinberg VE, Holland JF, et al. A randomized trial of five and three drug chemotherapy and chemoimmunotherapy in women with operable node positive breast cancer. J Clin Oncol 1983;1:138.

32. Wood WC, Budman DR, Korzun AH, et al. Dose and dose intensity of adjuvant chemotherapy for stage II, node-positive breast carcinoma. N Engl J Med 1994;330:1253.

33. Rosen PP, Groshen S, Saigo PE, et al. A long-term follow-up study of survival in stage 1 ($T_1N_0M_0$) and stage II ($T_1N_1M_0$) breast carcinoma. J Clin Oncol 1989;7:355.

34. McGuire WL, Clark GM. Prognostic factors for recurrence and survival in axillary node-negative breast cancer. J Steroid Biochem 1989;34:145.

35. Morrison JM, Howell A, Kelly KA, et al. West Midlands Oncology Association trials of adjuvant chemotherapy in operable breast can-

cer: results are a median follow-up of 7 years. II. Patients without involved axillary lymph nodes. Br J Cancer 1989;60:919.

36. Fisher B, Costantino J, Redmond C, et al. A randomized clinical trial evaluating tamoxifen in the treatment of patients with node-negative breast cancer who have estrogen-receptor-positive tumors. N Engl J Med 1989;320:479.

37. Ludwig Breast Cancer Study Group. Prolonged disease-free survival after one course of perioperative adjuvant chemotherapy for node-negative breast cancer. N Engl J Med 1989;320:491.

38. Bonadonna G. Conceptual and practical advances in the management of breast cancer. Karnofsky Memorial Lecture. J Clin Oncol 1989;7:1380.

39. Engelsman E, Rubens RD, Klijn JGM, et al. Comparison of "classical CMF" with a three-weekly intravenous CMF schedule in postmenopausal patients with advanced breast cancer: an EORTC study (trial 10808). Proceedings of the 4th EORTC Breast Cancer Working Conference, 1987;1.

40. Fisher B, Wickerham DL, Redmond C. Recent developments in the use of systemic adjuvant therapy for the treatment of breast cancer. Semin Oncol 1992;19:263.

41. Mansour EG, Eudey L, Tormey DC, et al. Chemotherapy versus observation in high-risk node-negative breast cancer patients. J Natl Cancer Inst Monogr 1992;11:97.

42. Taylor SG III, Canellos GP, Band P, et al. Combination chemotherapy for advanced breast cancer: randomized comparison with single drug therapy. Proc Am Soc Clin Oncol 1974;15:175.

43. Rivkin SE, Green S, Metch B, et al. Adjuvant CMFVP versus melphalan for operable breast cancer with positive axillary nodes: 10-year results of a Southwest Oncology Group Study. J Clin Oncol 1989;7:1229.

44. Wolmark N, Fisher B, and contributing NSABP investigators. Adjuvant chemotherapy in stage-II breast cancer: an overview of the NSABP clinical trials. Breast Cancer Res Treat 1983;3(Suppl 1):19.

45. Brincker H, Rose C, Rank F, et al. Evidence of a castration-mediated effect of adjuvant cytotoxic chemotherapy in premenopausal breast cancer. J Clin Oncol 1987;5:1771.

46. Tancini G, Bonadonna G, Valagussa P, et al. Adjuvant CMF in breast cancer: comparative 5-year results of 12 versus 6 cycles. J Clin Oncol 1983;1:2.

47. Velez-Garcia E, Carpenter JT Jr, Moore M, et al. Postsurgical adjuvant chemotherapy with or without radiotherapy in women with breast cancer and positive axillary nodes: progress report of a Southeastern Cancer Study Group (SEG) trial. In: Salmon SE ed. Adjuvant therapy of cancer, vol 5. Orlando, Grune & Stratton, 1987;347.

48. Falkson HC, Gray R, Wolberg WH, et al. Adjuvant trial of 12 cycles of CMFPT followed by observation or continuous tamoxifen versus four cycles of CMFPT in postmenopausal women with breast cancer: an Eastern Cooperative Oncology Group Phase III Study. J Clin Oncol 1990;8:599.

49. Rivkin SE, Green S, Metch B, et al. One versus 2 years of CMFVP adjuvant chemotherapy in axillary node-positive and estrogen receptor-negative patients: a Southwest Oncology Group Study. J Clin Oncol 1993;11:1710.

50. Ludwig Breast Cancer Study Group. Combination adjuvant chemotherapy for node-positive breast cancer: inadequacy of a single perioperative cycle. N Engl J Med 1988;319:677.

51. Levine MN, Gent M, Hryniuk WM, et al. A randomized trial comparing 12 weeks with 36 weeks of adjuvant chemotherapy in stage II breast cancer. J Clin Oncol 1990;8:1217.

52. Fisher B, Redmond CK, Wolmark N. Long-term results from NSABP trials of adjuvant therapy for breast cancer. In: Salmon SE, ed. Adjuvant therapy of cancer, vol 5. Orlando, Grune & Stratton, 1987;283.

53. Tormey DC, Gray R, Gilchrist K, et al. Adjuvant chemohormonal therapy with cyclophosphamide, methotrexate, 5-fluorouracil, and

prednisone (CMFP) or CMFP plus tamoxifen compared with CMF for premenopausal breast cancer patients: an Eastern Cooperative Oncology Group Trial. Cancer 1990;65:200.

54. Goldhirsch A, Gelber R. Adjuvant treatment for early breast cancer: the Ludwig Breast Cancer Studies. Natl Cancer Inst Monogr 1986;1:55.

55. Shapiro CL, Gelman RS, Hayes DF, et al. Comparison of adjuvant chemotherapy with methotrexate and fluorouracil with and without cyclophosphamide in breast cancer patients with one to three positive axillary lymph nodes. J Natl Cancer Inst 1993;85:812.

56. Fisher B, Redmond C, Wickerham DL, et al. Doxorubicin-containing regimens for the treatment of stage II breast cancer: the National Surgical Adjuvant Breast and Bowel Project experience. J Clin Oncol 1989;7:572.

57. Carpenter JT, Velez-Garcia E, Aron BS, et al. Five-year results of a randomized comparison of cyclophosphamide, doxorubicin (adriamcyin) and fluorouracil (CAF) vs cyclophosphamide, methotrexate and fluorouracil (CMF) for node positive breast cancer: a Southeastern Cancer Study Group Study. Proc ASCO 1994;13:66.

58. Coombes RC, Bliss JM, Marty M, et al. A randomized trial comparing adjuvant FEC with CMF in premenopausal patients with node positive resectable breast cancer. Proc ASCO 1991;10:41.

59. Misset JL, Gil-Delgado M, Chollet Ph, et al. Ten-year results of the French trial comparing adriamycin, vincristine, 5-fluorouracil and cyclophosphamide to standard CMF as adjuvant therapy for node positive breast cancer. Proc ASCO 1992;11:54.

60. Budd GT, Green S, Martino S, et al. Short course FAC-M vs 1 year of CMFVP in node-positive hormone-receptor negative breast cancer: an Intergroup Study. J Clin Oncol 1995;13:831.

61. Fisher B, Brown AM, Dimitrov NV, et al. Two months of doxorubicin-cyclophosphamide with and without interval reinduction therapy compared with 6 months of cyclophosphamide, methotrexate, and fluorouracil in positive-node breast cancer patients with tamoxifen-nonresponsive tumors: results from the National Surgical Adjuvant Breast and Bowel Project B-15. J Clin Oncol 1990;8:1483.

62. Henderson IC. Adjuvant systemic therapy of early breast cancer. In: Harris JR, Hellman SA, et al eds. Breast diseases, ed 2. Philadelphia, JB Lippincott, 1991:427.

63. Tormey DC, Gray R, Abeloff MD, et al. Adjuvant therapy with a doxorubicin regimen and long-term tamoxifen in premenopausal breast cancer patients: an Eastern Coperative Oncology Group Trial. J Clin Oncol 1992;10:1848.

64. Moliterni A, Bonadonna G, Valagussa P, et al. Cyclophosphamide, methotrexate, and fluorouracil with and without doxorubicin in the adjuvant treatment of resectable breast cancer with one to three positive axillary nodes. J Clin Oncol 1991;9:1124.

65. Buzzoni R, Bonadonna G, Valagussa P, et al. Adjuvant chemotherapy with doxorubicin plus cyclophosphamide, methotrexate, and fluorouracil in the treatment of resectable breast cancer with more than three positive axillary nodes. J Clin Oncol 1991;9:2134.

66. Goldie JH, Coldman AJ, Gudauskas GA. Rationale for the use of alternating non-cross-resistant chemotherapy. Cancer Treat Rep 1982;66:439.

67. Fisher B, Gunduz N, Saffer EA. Influence of the interval between primary tumor removal and chemotherapy on kinetics and growth of metastases. Cancer Res 1983;43:1488.

68. Preliminary Analysis by the CRC Adjuvant Breast Trial Working Party. Cyclophosphamide and tamoxifen as adjuvant therapies in the management of breast cancer. Br J Cancer 1988;57:604.

69. Sertoli MR, Pronzato P, Rubagotti A, et al. Perioperative polychemotherapy for primary breast cancer: a randomized study. Proc ASCO 1991;10:48.

70. Goldie JH. Scientific basis for adjuvant and primary (neoadjuvant) chemotherapy. Semin Oncol 1987;14:1.

71. Bonadonna G, Valagussa P, Brambilla C, et al. Adjuvant and neoadjuvant treatment of breast cancer with chemotherapy and/or endocrine therapy. Semin Oncol 1991;15:515.

72. Mauriac L, Durand M, Avril A, et al. Effects of primary chemotherapy in conservative treatment of breast cancer patients with operable tumors larger than 3 cm: results of a randomized trial in a single center. Ann Oncol 1991;2:347.

73. Fisher B, Rockette H, Ribidoux A, et al. Effect of preoperative therapy for breast cancer (BC) on local-regional disease: first report of NSABP B-18. Proc ASCO 1994;13:64.

74. Bonadonna G, Valagussa P. Dose-response effect of adjuvant chemotherapy in breast cancer. N Engl J Med 1981;304:10.

75. Redmond C, Fisher B, Wieand HS. The methodologic dilemma in retrospectively correlating the amount of chemotherapy received in adjuvant therapy protocols with disease-free survival. Cancer Treat Rep 1983;67:519.

76. Hryniuk W, Levine MN. Analysis of dose intensity for adjuvant chemotherapy trials in stage II breast cancer. J Clin Oncol 1986;4:1162.

77. Muss HB, Thor AD, Berry DA, et al. c-erbB-2 expression and response to adjuvant therapy in women with node-positive early breast cancer. N Engl J Med 1994;330:1260.

78. Dimitrov N, Anderson S, Fisher B, et al. Dose intensification and increased total dose of adjuvant chemotherapy for breast cancer (BC): findings from NSABP B22. Proc ASCO 1994;13:64.

79. Jones RB, Holland JF, Bhardwaj S, et al. A phase I–II study of intensive-dose adriamycin for advanced breast cancer. J Clin Oncol 1987;5:172.

80. Bonadonna G, Valagussa P. Dose-intense adjuvant treatment of high-risk breast cancer. J Natl Cancer Inst 1990;82:542.

81. Buzdar AU, Kau S-W, Hortobagyi GN, et al. Clinical course of patients with breast cancer with ten or more positive nodes who were treated with doxorubicin-containing adjuvant therapy. Cancer 1992;69:448.

82. Abeloff MD, Beveridge RA, Donehower RC, et al. Sixteen-week dose-intense chemotherapy in the adjuvant treatment of breast cancer. J Natl Cancer Inst 1990;82:570.

83. Peters WP, Ross M, Vrendenburgh JJ, et al. High-dose chemotherapy and autologous bone marrow support as consolidation after standard-dose adjuvant therapy for high-risk primary breast cancer. J Clin Oncol 1993;11:1132.

84. Wiebe VJ, Osborne CK, Fuqua SAW, et al. Tamoxifen resistance in breast cancer. Crit Rev Oncol Hematol 1993;14:173.

85. Love RR, Mazess RB, Barden HW, et al. Effects of tamoxifen on bone mineral density in postmenopausal women with breast cancer. N Engl J Med 1992;326:852.

86. Love RR, Newcombe PA, Wiebe DA, et al. Effects of tamoxifen therapy on lipid and lipoprotein levels in postmenopausal patients with node-negative breast cancer. J Natl Cancer Inst 1990;82:1327.

87. Lahti EI, Knip M, Laatikainen TJ. Plasma insulin-like growth factor I and its binding proteins 1 and 3 in postmenopausal patients with breast cancer receiving long-term tamoxifen. Cancer 1994;74:618.

88. NATO Steering Committee. Controlled trial of tamoxifen as a single adjuvant agent in the management of early breast cancer. Br J Cancer 1988;57:608.

89. Report from the Breast Cancer Trials Committee, Scottish Cancer Trials Office, Edinburgh. Adjuvant tamoxifen in the management of operable breast cancer: the Scottish Trial. Lancet 1987;8552.

90. Fisher ER, Osborne CK, McGuire WL, et al. Correlation of primary breast cancer histopathology and estrogen receptor content. Breast Cancer Res Treat 1981;1:37.

91. Fisher B, Redmond C, Brown A, et al. Adjuvant chemotherapy with and without tamoxifen in the treatment of primary breast cancer: 5-year results from the National Surgical Adjuvant Breast and Bowel Project Trial. J Clin Oncol 1986;4:459.

92. Knight WA, Osborne CK, McGuire WL. Hormone receptors in

primary and advanced breast cancer. Clin Endocrinol Metab 1980;9:361.

93. Cummings FJ, Gray R, Tormey DC, et al. Adjuvant tamoxifen versus placebo in elderly women with node-positive breast cancer: long-term follow-up and causes of death. J Clin Oncol 1993;11:29.

94. Kaufman M, Jonat W, Abel U, et al. Adjuvant randomized trials of doxorubicin/cyclophosphamide/tamoxifen and CMF chemotherapy versus tamoxifen in women with node-positive breast cancer. J Clin Oncol 1993;11:454.

95. Bryant AJ, Weir JA. Phrophylactic oophorectomy in operable instances of carcinoma of the breast. Surg Gynecol Obstet 1981;153:660.

96. Meakin JW, Allt WEC, Beale FA, et al. Ovarian irradiation and prednisone therapy following surgery and radiotherapy for carcinoma of the breast. Can Med Assoc J 1979;120:1221.

97. Palshof T, Carstensen B, Mouridsen HT, et al. Adjuvant endocrine therapy in pre- and postmenopausal women with operable breast cancer. Rev Endocr Rel Cancer 1985;s17:43.

98. Jones AL, Powles TJ, Law M, et al. Adjuvant aminoglutethimide for postmenopausal patients with primary breast cancer: analysis at 8 years. J Clin Oncol 1992;10:1547.

99. Focan C, Baudoux A, Beauduin M, et al. Adjuvant treatment with high dose medroxyprogesterone acetate in node-negative early breast cancer. Acta Oncol 1989;28:237.

100. Osborne CK, Boldt DH, Clark GM, et al. Effects of tamoxifen on human breast cancer cell cycle kinetics: accumulation of cells in early G_1. Cancer Res 1983;43:3583.

101. Osborne CK, Boldt DH, Estrada P. Human breast cancer cell cycle synchronization by estrogens and antiestrogens in culture. Cancer Res 1984;44:1433.

102. Osborne CK, Coronado EB, Robinson JP. Human breast cancer in the athymic nude mouse: cytostatic effects of long-term antiestrogen therapy. Eur J Cancer Clin Oncol 1987;23:1189.

103. Greenberg DA, Carpenter CL, Messing RO. Calcium channel antagonist properties of the antineoplastic antiestrogen tamoxifen in the PC12 neurosecretory cell line. Cancer Res 1987;47:70.

104. Lam H-YP. Tamoxifen is a calmodulin antagonist in the activation of cAMP phosphodiesterase. Biochem Biophys Res Commun 1984;118:27.

105. Se H-D, Mazzei GJ, Vogler WR, et al. Effect of tamoxifen, a nonsteroidal antiestrogen, on phospholipid/calcium-dependent protein kinase and phosphorylation of its endogenous substrate proteins from the rat brain and ovary. Biochem Pharmacol 1985;34:3649.

106. Berman E, Adams M, Duigou-Osterndorf R, et al. Effect of tamoxifen on cell lines displaying the multidrug-resistant phenotype. Blood 1991;77:818.

107. Naito M, Yusa K, Tsuruo T. Steroid hormones inhibit binding of *Vinca* alkaloid to multidrug resistance related p-glycoproteins. Biochem Biophys Res Commun 1989;158:1066.

108. Osborne CK, Kitten L, Arteaga CL. Antagonism of chemotherapy-induced cytotoxicity for human breast cancer by antiestrogens. J Clin Oncol 1989;7:710.

109. Goldenberg GJ, Froese EK. Antagonism of the cytocidal activity and uptake of melphalan by tamoxifen in human breast cancer cells in vitro. Biochem Pharmacol 1985;34:763.

110. Fisher B, Redmond C, Legault-Poisson S, et al. Postoperative chemotherapy and tamoxifen compared with tamoxifen alone in the treatment of positive-node breast cancer patients aged 50 years and older with tumors responsive to tamoxifen: results from the National Surgical Adjuvant Breast and Bowel Project B-16. J Clin Oncol 1990;8:1005.

111. Ingle JN, Everson LK, Wieand HS, et al. Randomized trial of observation versus adjuvant therapy with cyclophosphamide, fluorouracil, prednisone with or without tamoxifen following mastec-

tomy in postmenopausal women with node-positive breast cancer. J Clin Oncol 1988;6:1388.

112. Taylor SG, Knuiman KW, Sleeper LA, et al. Six-year results of the Eastern Cooperative Oncology Group trial of observation versus CMFP versus CMFPT in postmenopausal patients with node-positive breast cancer. J Clin Oncol 1989;7:879.

113. Goldhirsch A, Gelber RD. Adjuvant chemo-endocrine therapy or endocrine therapy alone for postmenopausal patients: Ludwig studies III and IV. In: Senn H, Goldhirsch A, Gelber RD, et al, eds. Recent results in cancer research: adjuvant therapy of primary breast cancer. Berlin, Springer-Verlag, 1989:153.

114. The International Breast Cancer Study Group. Late effects of adjuvant oophorectomy and chemotherapy upon premenopausal breast cancer patients. Ann Oncol 1990;1:30.

115. Rivkin S, Green S, Metch B, et al. Adjuvant combination chemotherapy (CMFVP) vs oophorectomy followed by CMFVP (OCMFVP) for premenopausal women with ER+ operable breast cancer with positive axillary lymph nodes: an intergroup study. Proc ASCO 1991;10:47.

116. Dombernowsky P, Brincker H, Hansen M, et al. Adjuvant therapy of premenopausal and menopausal high-risk breast cancer patients. Acta Oncol 1988;27:691.

117. Tormey DC, Gray R, Gilchrist K, et al. Adjuvant chemohormonal therapy with cyclophosphamide, methotrexate, 5-fluorouracil, and prednisone (CMFP) or CMFP plus tamoxifen compared with CMF for premenopausal breast cancer patients. Cancer 1990;65:200.

118. Ingle JN, Everson LK, Wieand HS, et al. Randomized trial to evaluate the addition of tamoxifen to cyclophosphamide, 5-fluorouracil, prednisone adjuvant therapy in premenopausal women with node-positive breast cancer. Cancer 1989;63:1257.

119. Boccardo F, Rubagotti A, Bruzzi P, et al. Chemotherapy versus tamoxifen versus chemotherapy plus tamoxifen in node-positive, estrogen receptor-positive breast cancer patients: results of a multicentric Italian study. J Clin Oncol 1990;8:1310.

120. Mouridsen HT, Rose C, Overgaard M, et al. Adjuvant treatment of postmenopausal patients with high risk primary breast cancer. Acta Oncol 1988;27:699.

121. Rivkin SE, Green S, Metch B, et al. Adjuvant CMFVP versus tamoxifen versus concurrent CMFVP and tamoxifen for postmenopausal, node-positive and estrogen receptor-positive breast cancer patients: a Southwest Oncology Group Study. J Clin Oncol 1994;12:2078.

122. Pritchard KI, Zee B, Paul N, et al. CMF added to tamoxifen as adjuvant therapy in postmenopausal women with node-positive (+VE) estrogen and/or progesterone receptor + VE breast cancer: negative results from a randomized clinical trial. Proc ASCO 1994;13:65.

123. Osborne CK. Current trials and future directions of the Southwest Oncology Group Breast Cancer Committee. Cancer, 1994; 74:1135.

124. Levine MN, Gent M, Hirsh J, et al. The thrombogenic effect of anticancer drug therapy in women with stage II breast cancer. N Engl J Med 1988;318:404.

125. Knobf MT. Physical and psychologic distress associated with adjuvant chemotherapy in women with breast cancer. J Clin Oncol 1986;4:678.

126. Hughson AVM, Cooper AF, McArdle CS, et al. Psychological impact of adjuvant chemotherapy in the first two years after mastectomy. BMJ 1986;293:1268.

127. Cassileth BR, Knuiman MW, Abeloff MD, et al. Anxiety levels in patients randomized to adjuvant therapy versus observation for early breast cancer. J Clin Oncol 1986;4:972.

128. Buzdar AU, Marcus C, Smith TL, et al. Early and delayed clinical cardiotoxicity of doxorubicin. Cancer 1985;55:2761.

129. Griem KL, Henderson IC, Gelman R, et al. The 5-year results of a randomized trial of adjuvant radiation therapy after chemother-

apy in breast cancer treated with mastectomy. J Clin Oncol 1987;5:1546.

130. Padmanabhan N, Wang DY, Moore JW, et al. Ovarian function and adjuvant chemotherapy for early breast cancer. Eur J Cancer Clin Oncol 1987;23:745.

131. Gradishar WJ, Schilsky RL. Ovarian function following radiation and chemotherapy for cancer. Semin Oncol 1989;16:425.

132. Curtis RE, Boice JD Jr, Moloney WC, et al. Leukemia following chemotherapy for breast cancer. Cancer Res 1990;50:2741.

133. Fisher B, Rockette H, Fisher ER, et al. Leukemia in breast cancer patients following adjuvant chemotherapy or postoperative radiation: the NSABP experience. J Clin Oncol 1985;3:1640.

134. Curtis RE, Boice JD, Stovall M, et al. Risk of leukemia after chemotherapy and radiation treatment for breast cancer. N Engl J Med 1992;326:1745.

135. Henderson IC, Gelman R. Second malignancies from adjuvant chemotherapy? too soon to tell. (Editorial) J Clin Oncol 1987;5:1135.

136. Valagussa P, Tancini G, Bonadonna G. Second malignancies after CMF for resectable breast cancer. J Clin Oncol 1987;5:1138.

137. Rutqvist LE, Mattsson A for the Stockholm Breast Cancer Study Group. Cardiac and thromboembolic morbidity among postmenopausal women with early-stage breast cancer in a randomized trial of adjuvant tamoxifen. J Natl Cancer Inst 1993;85:1398.

138. Kristensen B, Ejlertsen B, Dalgaard P, et al. Tamoxifen and bone metabolism in postmenopausal low-risk breast cancer patients: a randomized study. J Clin Oncol 1994;12:992.

139. Rutqvist LE, Cedermark B, Glas U, et al. Contralateral primary tumors in breast cancer patients in a randomized trial of adjuvant tamoxifen therapy. J Natl Cancer Inst 1991;83:1299.

140. Fornander T, Cedermark B, Mattsson A, et al. Adjuvant tamoxifen in early breast cancer: occurrence of new primary cancers. Lancet 1989;1:117.

141. Love RR, Cameron L, Connell BL, et al. Symptoms associated with tamoxifen treatment in postmenopausal women. Arch Intern Med 1991;151:1842.

142. Cathcart CK, Jones SE, Pumroy CS, et al. Clinical recognition and management of depression in node negative breast cancer patients treated with tamoxifen. Breast Cancer Res Treat 1993;27:277.

143. Kaiser-Kupfer MI, Lippman ME. Tamoxifen retinopathy. Cancer Treat Rep 1978;62:315.

144. Pavlidis NA, Petris C, Briassoulis E, et al. Clear evidence that long-term, low-dose tamoxifen treatment can induce ocular toxicity. Cancer 1992;69:2961.

145. Longstaff S, Siguardsson H, IO'Keeffe M, et al. A controlled study of the ocular effects of tamoxifen in conventional dosage in the treatment of breast carcinoma. Eur J Cancer Clin Oncol 1989;25:1805.

146. Potter GA, McCague R, Jarman M. A mechanistic hypothesis for DNA adduct formation by tamoxifen following hepatic oxidative metabolism. Carcinogenesis 1994;15:439.

147. Styles LA, Davies A, Lim CK, et al. Genotoxicity of tamoxifen, tamoxifen epoxide and toremifene in human lymphoblastoid cells containing human cytochrome P450s. Carcinogenesis 1994;15:5.

148. Hard GC, Iatropoulos MJ, Jordan K, et al. Major difference in the hepatocarcinogenicity and DNA adduct forming between toremifene and tamoxifen in female Crl:CD(BR) rats. Cancer Res 1993;53:4534.

149. Ahotupa M, Hirsimaki P, Rarssinen R, et al. Alterations of drug metabolizing and antioxidant enzyme activities during tamoxifen-induced hepatocarcinogenesis in the rat. Carcinogenesis 1994;15:863.

150. Muhlemann K, Cook LS, Weiss NS. The incidence of hepatocellular carcinoma in US white women with breast cancer after the introduction of tamoxifen in 1977. Breast Cancer Res Treat 1994;30:201.

151. Fisher B, Costantino JP, Redmond CK, et al. Endometrial cancer in tamoxifen-treated breast cancer patients: findings from the National Surgical Adjuvant Breast and Bowel Project (NSABP) B-14. J Natl Cancer Inst 1994;86:527.

152. Andersson M, Storm HH, Mouridsen HT. Incidence of new primary cancers after adjuvant tamoxifen therapy and radiotherapy for early breast cancer. J Natl Cancer Inst 1991;83:1013.

153. Magriples U, Naftolin F, Schwartz PE, et al. High-grade endometrial carcinoma in tamoxifen-treated breast cancer patients. J Clin Oncol 1993;11:485.

154. Hillner BE, Smith TJ. Efficacy and cost effectiveness of adjuvant chemotherapy in women with node-negative breast cancer. N Engl J Med 1991;324:160.

155. Smith TJ, Hillner BE. The efficacy and cost-effectiveness of adjuvant therapy of early breast cancer in premenopausal women. J Clin Oncol 1993;11:771.

156. Desch CE, Hillner BE, Smith TJ, et al. Should the elderly receive chemotherapy for node-negative breast cancer? a cost-effectiveness analysis examining total and active life-expectancy outcomes. J Clin Oncol 1993;11:777.

157. Siminoff LA, Fetting JH, Abeloff MD. Doctor–patient communication about breast cancer therapy. J Clin Oncol 1989;7:1192.

158. Rajagopal S, Goodman PF, Tannock IF. Adjuvant chemotherapy for breast cancer: discordance between physicians' perception of benefit and the results of clinical trials. J Clin Oncol 1994;12:1296.

159. Coates AS, Simes RJ. Patient assessment of adjuvant treatment in operable breast cancer. In: Williams CJ, ed. Introducing new treatments for cancer: practical, ethical, and legal problems. New York, John Wiley & Sons, 1992:447.

160. NIH Consensus Development Panel. Consensus statement: treatment of early-stage breast cancer: J Natl Cancer Inst Mongr 1992;11:1.

161. Rosen PP, Groshen S, Saigo PE, et al. Pathological prognostic factors in stage I ($T_1N_1M_0$) breast carcinoma: a study of 644 patients with median followup of 18 years. J Clin Oncol 1989;7:1239.

17.3

Breast Conservation Trials From the Milan National Cancer Institute

UMBERTO VERONESI ▪ BRUNO SALVADORI

A century ago, W.S. Halsted opened the so-called modern era of surgical treatment of breast cancer. His vision of the curability of breast cancer, which, like most other cancers, was considered incurable, was based on the conviction that careful surgical removal of the breast in continuity with the axillary nodes could lead to definitive cure of the disease. His concepts contain a good deal of truth, and today we can indeed cure many patients with early breast cancer by surgery alone. What Halsted overlooked was the spread of cancer cells through the circulation leading to distant dissemination. Moreover, his concept of permeation by cancer cells in the lymphatic vessels was later disproved making the en bloc removal of the axillary nodes unnecessary.

Breast cancer is seen today as a disease that spreads cancer cells in the circulation to become distant metastases or not, mainly depending on local immunologic conditions. The main objective of today's research is therefore the avoidance of distant metastases or their control, whereas local regional control may be achieved with more limited procedures than in the past. We must also take into account the considerable differences between the patients of today and those of the past. Thanks to the introduction of large-scale mammography and extensive educational and screening programs, many small breast carcinomas are seen today, and patients without palpable masses are becoming more and more common.

Early Attempts Toward Breast Conservation

Up to the 1960s, the few attempts to substitute ablative surgery of the breast with conservative methods consisted of small surgical series,[1] as well as large series of patients treated almost exclusively with radiotherapy.[2] Although these studies were encouraging, that they did not result from randomized clinical studies hindered their clinical application, and therefore, the Halsted mastectomy was the treatment of choice for breast cancer up to the 1980s.

In the first controlled clinical study conducted in London at Guy's Hospital during the 1960s, cure rates were negatively affected by breast resection and radiotherapy, with long-term survival curves significantly lower than those obtained with radical mastectomy. An accurate analysis conducted many years after termination of the study showed that the difference in cure rates in favor of the Halsted mastectomy was limited to T1 cases. Hayward and Caleffi,[3] commenting on these data in 1987, noted

that the percentage of occult metastases at the time of surgery was high in patients with tumors larger than 2 cm in diameter, so the extent of local surgery was not a determinant of the outcome. In contrast, radical surgery had an important curative role for small carcinomas limited to the breast. Another comment about Guy's Hospital study, however, is that the conservative treatment then applied cannot be considered adequate today because axillary dissection was not performed—not even in patients with clinically positive lymph nodes—and because the radiotherapy dose (30 Gy) was largely insufficient.

The results of that study did not encourage the initiation of other randomized clinical studies. When I proposed an international multicentric randomized study to the Committee of Breast Cancer Experts of the World Health Organization in 1968 and 1969, their reaction was initially unfavorable. The proposal was accepted only after much discussion at a meeting in December 1969.[4] The novelty of the proposal was a conservative technique, aggressive at the mammary level (wide surgery, defined as quadrantectomy, followed by radiotherapy), and complete axillary dissection. Radiotherapy to regional lymph nodes, which was widely used at that time, was abandoned.

Quadrantectomy was performed in Milan at the end of the 1960s as an extensive surgical excision, whose main objective was to achieve effective local control together with a good cosmetic result. The main characteristic was a radial incision, so the resection encompassed the whole ductal tree from the retroareolar region to the periphery, because we were convinced that intraductal spread was important and all branches of the involved ducts had to be removed. The main duct and its associated tree is often referred to as a breast *lobe*,[5] and the operation could have been called *lobectomy*; however, we chose the name *quadrantectomy* because the quadrant concept was simpler to explain.

After quadrantectomy, radiotherapy was given, consisting of 50 Gy administered in two tangentially opposing fields using high-energy equipment, in addition to a boost of 10 Gy on the scar with orthovoltage equipment. Total axillary lymph node dissection completed the procedure.

First Milan Study Proves the Safety of Breast Conservation

The Milan I study compared the Halsted mastectomy with quadrantectomy, axillary dissection, and radiotherapy (QUART) in 701 cases. The patients were randomly assigned to 2 groups: in the first group, the patients were treated with the Halsted mastectomy, and in the other group, quadrantectomy and axillary dissection were performed, followed by radiotherapy to the breast. Patients with invasive breast carcinoma less than 2 cm in diameter and without clinical axillary node involvement were eligible. They were randomized in the operating theatre after confirmation of the diagnosis, based on an excisional biopsy of the histologic features and size of the carcinoma. The patients were informed of both possibilities, ablative and conservative surgery, and only those who accepted both interventions were included in the study. Recruitment began in 1973, with an average of 100 patients a year entering the study. Accrual was closed in 1980 with 701 patients treated (349 by radical mastectomy and 352 by QUART). During the first years, many patients refused the conservative option and underwent mastectomy outside the study. The situation had changed toward the end of the study, when many patients insisted on having quadrantectomy.

The first results were reported in 1981[6] and were updated in 1990[7] and 1994.[8] The long-term results of the study showed identical survival curves for both groups (Fig. 17.3-1). An analysis by subgroups showed a certain advantage (not statistically significant) in patients with positive axillary lymph nodes who were treated by QUART, compared with those who underwent mastectomy. During the first 3 years of the study, patients with positive axillary lymph nodes were randomized again after surgery, and half the patients received radiotherapy to the ipsilateral supraclavicular lymph nodes. Analysis of this small series (56 cases) showed no advantage with supraclavicular radio-

therapy. The practice was abandoned in 1975, and from then on, all patients with positive axillary lymph nodes received chemotherapy (cyclophosphamide, methotrexate, 5-fluorouracil) for 12 months.

As regards local recurrences, it was difficult to distinguish real local recurrences (ie, relapses from residual tumor cell) from new ipsilateral carcinomas. Local recurrences were defined as carcinomas appearing subcutaneously on the skin or in the breast within 3 cm of the surgical scar. Nodules developing in other quadrants at more than 3 cm from the surgical scar were defined as new primary tumors. As expected, only a few recurrences were reported in patients who had undergone the Halsted mastectomy, and a limited number of local recurrences were reported in the patients who had undergone QUART. Fourteen of the patients treated conservatively showed a local recurrence (4.0%), whereas 10 patients of the same group developed a new ipsilateral tumor. Of the 14 QUART patients who had a recurrence, most of whom were treated by total mastectomy, 10 were alive without evidence of disease at 6 to 14 years after detection of the recurrences, and 4 died of metastatic disease. Of the 8 patients with local recurrences after radical mastectomy, 5 developed metastases and died. In the final analysis, the number of patients who died after local recurrence was therefore almost the same in both groups (Table 17.3-1).

TABLE 17.3-1
Milan I Trial: First Unfavorable Event

Type of Event	Halsted (N = 349)		QUART (N = 352)	
	N	%	N	%
Local recurrence	8	2.3	14	4.0
Second ipsilateral carcinoma	—	—	10	2.8
Contralateral tumor	29	8.3	22	6.3

QUART, quadrantectomy, axillary dissection, and radiotherapy.

TABLE 17.3-2
Milan II Trial: First Unfavorable Event

Type of Event	QUART (N = 360)		TART (N = 345)	
	N	%	N	%
Local recurrence	15	4.2	39	11.3
Second ipsilateral carcinoma	4	1.1	7	2.0
Contralateral tumor	15	4.2	18	5.2

QUART, quadrantectomy, axillary dissection, and radiotherapy; TART, tumorectomy, axillary dissection, and radiotherapy.

FIGURE 17.3-1 Milan Trial I. Overall survival according to the type of treatment. (Veronesi U, Costa A. In: Squartini F, Bevilacqua G, Conte PF, et al, eds. Breast cancer. 1993;698:212)

An important observation is the absence of any oncogenic effect by radiotherapy. One of the early objections to conservative therapy was the hypothesis that a substantial dose of ionizing radiation could trigger a neoplastic transformation of normal mammary cells. The long-term results of the study have removed this doubt and have absolved radiotherapy of the suspicion of oncogenicity, at least in adult women. Only 10 new primary breast cancers appeared in breasts treated by radiotherapy after surgery, and the number of contralateral breast cancers was lower in the QUART group (22 cases) than in the mastectomy, nonirradiated group (29 cases). If one considers that in the QUART group the contralateral breast received a dose of 0.5 Gy in the most lateral part and up to 10 to 15 Gy in the medial part, one could expect a considerable increase in the number of contralateral carcinoma in irradiated cases with respect to mastectomy cases. The opposite was true, however, and we thus concluded that radiotherapy had no oncogenic action on our patients.[9]

Search for an Ideal Conservative Procedure

The results of the Milan I trial were published in 1981,[6] and the data were consolidated after some time. A critical reevaluation of the experience then started. The main concern was the therapeutic efficacy of surgery and radiotherapy. Both treatments were performed with the objective of radicality, and it was therefore difficult to attribute the good results to surgery or to radiotherapy.

To remove this doubt, it was decided to start new trials to evaluate separately the efficacy of radiotherapy (after a debulking lumpectomy) and of quadrantectomy alone.

In 1985, another randomized study (Milan II) was started to compare the quadrantectomy–radiotherapy treatment, considering radiotherapy as the most important therapy. The new intervention consisted of simple excision of the primary tumor, without the scope of radicality but exclusively reductive, followed by intense radiotherapy on the breast, 45 Gy on the whole breast and about 15 Gy with iridium-192 applied interstitially in the site of the surgical resection. All patients were treated by complete axillary dissection. Eligibility criteria were similar to those of the Milan I study, except patients with tumors up to 2.5 cm in diameter were included, as well as those with clinically positive axillary nodes.

The randomized study, carried out from 1985 to 1987, recruited 705 patients: 360 treated by QUART and 345 treated by tumorectomy, axillary dissection, and radiotherapy (TART). Results were published in 1990[10] and in 1994.[8] Local relapses were again limited in the patients treated by QUART (15 recurrences and 4 new carcinomas; 5.3%), whereas in the group treated by TART there were 46 local relapses (39 recurrences and 7 new carcinomas; 13.3%) (Table 17.3-2). The incidence of contralateral carcinomas was similar in both groups (15 in the QUART group and 18 in the TART group). Actuarial survival curves were identical at 7 years, thereby confirming that differences in local recurrence do not considerably affect prognosis (Fig. 17.3-2).

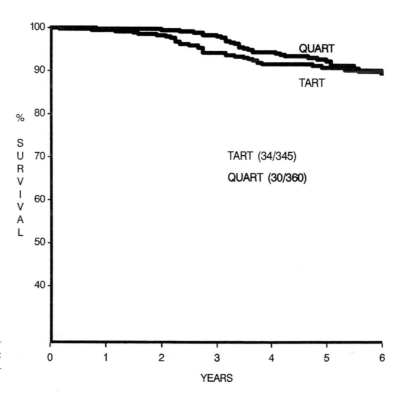

FIGURE 17.3-2 Milan Trial II. Overall survival according to the type of treatment. (Veronesi U, Costa A. In: Squartini F, Bevilacqua G, Conte PF, et al, eds. Breast cancer. 1993;698:212)

TABLE 17.3-3
Milan III Trial: First Unfavorable Event

Type of Event	QUART (N = 294)		QUAD (N = 273)	
	N	%	N	%
Local recurrence	3	1.0	24	8.8
New ipsilateral carcinoma	—	—	4	1.5
Contralateral tumor	2	0.7	5	1.8

QUART, quadrantectomy, axillary dissection, and radiotherapy; QUAD, quadrantectomy and axillary dissection.

The analysis of local recurrences in relation to the presence or absence of the histopathologic characteristic defined as *extensive intraductal component* (EIC) showed an important finding. The presence of EIC increased the risk of local recurrences in patients treated by QUART as well as in those treated by TART. The difference was much more pronounced in patients who underwent tumorectomy (11 recurrences in 38 cases; 28%) however, than in those who underwent quadrantectomy (2 recurrences in 22 cases; 9%). Whenever possible, the resection margins were accurately examined in all patients who underwent tumorectomy. When such margins were positive, the patient was given the same radiotherapy as the other patients without any further resection. Such a procedure was in line with the principles of tumorectomy—an intervention

by definition only reductive. The resection margins were also examined for positivity in the patients who underwent quadrantectomy, but given the small percentage of positive results among the first 120 patients, it was decided to suspend the examination. Among the TART group, positive margins were found in 46 of 289 patients (15.9%) in whom examination was possible. Eight patients (17.4%) had local recurrences in this subgroup, and this incidence is higher than that in patients with negative margins (21 of 243; 8.6%).

After the end of the Milan II study, another randomized study was started to evaluate the efficacy of quadrantectomy without radiotherapy. The aim of this Milan III trial was a randomized comparison between QUART and the simple intervention of quadrantectomy and axillary dissection without radiotherapy (QUAD). The QUAD regimen was administered in the case of recurrence after a second conservative treatment. The comparison was therefore between quadrantectomy and prophylactic radiotherapy and quadrantectomy and therapeutic radiotherapy (ie, limited to those patients in whom quadrantectomy had not been radical). Eligibility criteria were the same as for the Milan II study. The Milan III study was carried out from 1988 to 1989: 567 women were randomized, 294 in the QUART group and 273 in the quadrantectomy without radiotherapy group.

The results reported in 1992 demonstrated a considerable difference in the incidence of local recurrences between both treatment groups. There were 24 (8.8%) local recurrences in the 273 patients treated only by quadrantectomy, whereas only 3 local recurrences were observed among the patients treated with QUART

FIGURE 17.3-3 Milan Trial III. Overall survival according to the type of treatment. (Veronesi U, Luini A, Galimberti V, Zurrida S. Conservation approaches for the management of stage I/II carcinoma of the breast: Milan Cancer Center Trials. World J Surg 1994;18:70)

FIGURE 17.3-4 Local recurrences among patients treated with different procedures in the three Milan trials. (Veronesi U, Salvadori B, Luinia S, et al. Breast conservation is a definitely safe method in patients with small cancer of the breast: long-term results of the three randomized trials on 1,973 patients. Eur J Cancer 1995;9 [in press])

(Table 17.3-3). In patients over 55 years of age, the incidence of local recurrence was low, even in women treated only by quadrantectomy. For that reason, we concluded that a considerable difference in results exists in premenopausal and postmenopausal patients. In fact, the mammary gland atrophies during the menopause, and the breast becomes a mass of adipose tissue with scattered islands of fibroepithelial tissue. Thus, one may conceivably carry out a simple partial surgery, performed with the usual criteria of oncologic radicality, without complementary radiotherapy.

The Milan III study confirmed the predictive value of EIC for local recurrences. Patients with positive axil-

lary lymph nodes had a slightly higher (not significant) incidence of local recurrences than patients with negative axillary lymph nodes. Survival was similar in both groups (Fig. 17.3-3).

Conclusions

The most recent results of the breast conservative trials carried out at the Milan National Cancer Institute between 1973 and 1988 showed that breast conservation consisting of wide breast resection (quadrantectomy) and radiotherapy is a safe procedure, and no differences in long-term survival (up to 19 years) were noted, compared with women who had undergone the Halsted mastectomy.

The Milan randomized trials explored all the main approaches to local and regional control of breast cancer. Halsted mastectomy, wide resection with radiotherapy (QUART) and without radiotherapy (QUAD), and limited resection and radiotherapy (TART) were carefully evaluated on homogeneous groups of patients treated in a single institution by the same team, thereby avoiding the risk of misinterpretation of the protocol by investigators at different centers. A clear picture of local control of the disease and long-term survival is now available to the surgeons, the radiotherapists, and the medical oncologists, to decide the treatment of choice for their patients.

According to the data of the Milan trials, the reduction of the extent of the surgical mammary resection exposes patients to a considerable increase in local recurrences (Fig. 17.3-4). The same occurs when postoperative radiotherapy is withdrawn. An extensive resection such as quadrantectomy becomes imperative when histologic examination shows the presence of an extensive intraductal component. The age of the patient is of great importance in the choice of treatment, however, because the risk of local recurrences is much lower in postmenopausal women than in younger women,[11] and so one has the possibility to avoid radiation therapy after quadrantectomy. In regard to the value of the resection margins, the data show that the negativity of the margins is not a significant element because the number of local recurrences was high in patients with negative margins.

Finally, survival rates were similar in all groups treated with different local–regional procedures, showing that the different rates of local recurrences have no influence on the final outcome of the patients.

References

1. Crile G Jr. Results of simplified treatment of breast cancer. Surg Gynecol Obstet 1964;118:517.
2. Mustakallio S. Conservative treatment of breast carcinoma: review of 25 years follow-up. Clin Radiol 1972;23:110.
3. Hayward J, Caleffi M. The significance of local control in the primary treatment of breast cancer. Arch Surg 1987;122:1244.
4. Meeting of investigators on the evaluation of methods of diagnosis and treatment of breast cancer: final report. Geneva, WHO, 1969:8.
5. Cooper A. The anatomy and diseases of the breast. Philadelphia, Lea & Blanchard, 1845.
6. Veronesi U, Saccozzi R, Del Vecchio M, et al. Comparing radical mastectomy with quadrantectomy, axillary dissection, and radical mastectomy in patients with small cancers of the breast. N Engl J Med 1981;305:6.
7. Veronesi U, Banfi A, Salvadori B, et al. Breast conservation is the treatment of choice in small breast cancer: long-term results of a randomized trial. Eur J Cancer 1990;26:668.
8. Veronesi U, Luini A, Galimberti V, et al. Conservation approaches for the management of stage I/II carcinoma of the breast: Milan Cancer Institute Trials. World J Surg 1994;18:70.
9. Zucali R, Luini A, Del Vecchio M, et al. Contralateral breast cancer after limited surgery plus radiotherapy of early mammary tumors. Eur J Surg Oncol 1987;26:671.
10. Veronesi U, Volterrani F, Luini A, et al. Quadrantectomy versus lumpectomy for small size breast cancer. Eur J Cancer 1990;6:671.
11. Veronesi U, Luini A, Del Vecchio M, et al. Radiotherapy after breast-preserving surgery in women with localized cancer of the breast. N Engl J Med 1993;328:1587.

Diseases of the Breast, edited by Jay R. Harris,
Marc E. Lippman, Monica Morrow, and Samuel Hellman.
Lippincott-Raven Publishers, Philadelphia, © 1996.

18

Treatment of Locally Advanced and Inflammatory Breast Cancer

GABRIEL N. HORTOBAGYI · S. EVA SINGLETARY

MARSHA D. McNEESE

Definition

Locally advanced breast cancer (LABC) has been defined in many different ways. In this chapter, this designation includes all patients with stage III breast cancer and those with stage IV disease, but with metastases limited to the ipsilateral subclavicular or supraclavicular fossa.[1] Although many patients with T2 tumors that appear large in proportion to the size of the breast are treated appropriately with the same strategies recommended for patients with more advanced disease, they do not have LABC and are not discussed in this chapter. Thus, the definition includes tumors in the stage IIIA, IIIB, and IV categories of the TNM classification.

Despite its decreasing frequency, LABC remains an important and challenging problem. In mammographically screened populations, stage III breast cancer seldom amounts to 5% of those diagnosed, whereas in medically underserved areas of the United States and other countries, LABC represents 30% to 50% of newly found malignant breast neoplasms.[2-4]

The management of patients with these advanced stages has evolved substantially over the last three decades; this chapter summarizes the various therapeutic options.[5]

Historical Perspective

Adjuvant systemic treatments have become integral components of the curative management of primary breast cancer.[6] Information derived from multiple randomized clinical trials and from the Oxford metaanalysis indicates that postoperative adjuvant chemotherapy and hormone therapy decreases the odds of recurrence and death from breast cancer for patients with both node-negative and node-positive tumors. Only limited information exists

about the efficacy of postoperative adjuvant systemic therapy specifically in stage III breast cancer; however, a few randomized trials suggest that adjuvant systemic therapies also decrease the probability of recurrence and death in this group of patients.[7,8] Furthermore, most of the randomized clinical trials considered in the world overview include patients with operable stage III breast cancer, and the analyses do not identify any prognostic subgroup that has not benefited from adjuvant systemic therapy.

Historically, patients with LABC were treated with a radical mastectomy whenever possible. On the basis of this experience, Haagensen and Stout[9] defined the concepts of operable and inoperable breast cancer. Skin ulceration, edema and fixation, and fixation of the tumor to the chest wall all were correlated with almost universal treatment failure, and therefore, were markers of inoperability. Subsequent to this landmark publication, patients with operable breast cancer continued to be treated with a mastectomy, sometimes followed by radiation therapy, whereas for those with inoperable tumors, radiation therapy alone, or associated with surgical resection, became the treatment of choice.[5,10,11] However, large doses of radiation were necessary to optimize local control, and at these doses, radiation therapy often was associated with severe side effects and long-term complications, including skin and chest wall fibrosis, skin ulceration, rib necrosis or resorption, brachial plexopathy, and lymphedema of the arm.[12-14] Patients who benefitted the most from therapy and achieved long-term survival were the most likely to develop these serious late sequelae. The combination of surgery and radiation therapy improved local control rates, but no effects on overall survival duration were observed.[5]

Virtually all of the historical data are derived from open phase II studies, or even more commonly, from retrospective reviews of single-institution experiences with a treatment strategy. Today, combinations of systemic and local–regional therapies are preferred. The emphasis on the combined modality approach is based on the paradigm that successful treatment of breast cancer depends, for most patients, on the eradication of occult micrometastases.[15] With the increasing use of combinations of systemic and local therapies, the extent and timing of each treatment modality in the overall treatment strategy have become less well defined.

Diagnosis and Staging

Most LABC and inflammatory breast cancers (IBCs) are easily palpable and even visible. However, some present with diffuse infiltration of the breast, and without a dominant mass. These often require mammographic assessment and often present as large areas of calcification or parenchymal distortion; sometimes skin thickening also is present. Histologic diagnosis usually is made by obtaining a core-needle biopsy; incisional biopsies are seldom required, although a full-thickness skin biopsy often is obtained when IBC is suspected. If an experienced cytopathologist is available, diagnosis can be confirmed by fine-needle aspiration cytologic (FNAC) study. If expertly performed, this procedure is nontraumatic, and false-positive and false-negative diagnoses are in the range observed with core-needle biopsies. Flow cytometric study and tests for determining nuclear grade and estrogen and progesterone receptor status can be performed on FNAC samples, as can tests for most other proposed prognostic indicators (eg, PCNA, Ki-67, HER-2/neu). FNAC study cannot differentiate invasive and noninvasive tumors. Therefore, we aspirate both the primary tumor and palpable (or sonographically detectable) lymphadenopathies for confirmation of invasive disease; if no enlarged lymph nodes are detected, we perform a core-needle biopsy. Once the diagnosis is established and the appropriate prognostic indicators are assayed, the extent of tumor involvement is ascertained. A complete physical examination, with quantitative documentation of all palpable abnormalities, is complemented by a biochemical survey, tests for carcinoembryonic antigen and CA 15-3, chest radiograph, and bone scan. If liver function tests or tumor markers give abnormal results, imaging of the liver and abdomen (computed tomography or ultrasound) is recommended; areas of increased radionuclide uptake on bone scan are assessed by radiographs. We always perform a contralateral mammogram to rule out the presence of synchronous bilateral cancer or contralateral metastases. Other tests are indicated only by specific symptoms or are performed for investigational purposes.

Development of Combined Modality Strategies

Systemic therapy was introduced in the management of inoperable breast cancers more than 30 years ago.[16] Although both hormone therapy and chemotherapy were used for this, most of the experience in patients with LABC is based on treatment with chemotherapy, sometimes with the addition of hormone treatment. Systemic therapy was followed in these trials by surgery, radiation therapy, or both. Perhaps the most important aspect of combined-modality therapies is the conceptual framework. When patients with LABC were treated with surgical resection or radiation therapy, the surgeon or the radiation oncologist decided on the type and sequence of treatments.

For optimal use of all treatment modalities, this practice has changed, so that all interested specialists (radiologist, pathologist, surgeon, radiation and medical oncologists) review the data and examine the patient jointly to determine the optimal type and sequence of therapies. Thus, teamwork has replaced the single-specialty orientation.

Treatment strategies that include induction chemotherapy (or hormone therapy) have several potential advantages as well as several theoretic shortcomings (Table 18-1). In practice, the advantages have exceeded the disadvantages. Two of the major clinical advantages of these treatment strategies include (1) the ability to monitor response to therapy by serial measurements of the primary tumor, and (2) the achievement of downstaging, which often permits breast conservation.

Induction Chemotherapy

The first clinical trials with induction (neoadjuvant) chemotherapy started in the late 1960s, but the earliest reports were published in the 1970s.[17] Since then, the reports of the results of this strategy have multiplied, documenting

TABLE 18-1

Characteristics of Combined-Modality Therapeutic Strategies That Include Induction Chemotherapy

Advantages	Disadvantages
Early initiation of systemic treatment	Local treatment delayed for nonresponders
Inhibition of postsurgical growth spurt	Induction of drug resistance
Delivery of chemotherapy through intact tumor vasculature	Large tumor burden
In vivo assessment of response	Only clinical staging available; imprecise
Downstaging of primary tumor and lymph node metastases	May increase risk of surgical and radiotherapy-related complications
Less radical local–regional therapy needed	
Breast conservation possible	
Good biologic model to evaluate effects of chemotherapy on the tumor	

the effectiveness of primary chemotherapy in this group of patients (Table 18-2).[18-25] In almost every report, most patients (60% to 80%) achieved a major objective regression in the primary tumor volume and the enlarged regional lymph nodes.[17,18,20-22,26-34] Although a fraction of patients experience a mixed response (response in the primary tumor and no response in the regional lymph nodes, or vice versa), for most patients, response in all sites of tumor involvement is similar.[34-36] Clinical complete remissions were reported in 10% to 20% of patients so treated in most clinical trials[20,28,29,34,37,38]; one report indicates a much higher (up to 50%) complete remission rate[37]; however, these improved results remain unconfirmed, and the fact that definitions and methods for evaluating complete remissions are different from other reports may account for the improvement in therapeutic efficacy. Notice that in this trial,[37] induction chemotherapy was continued until maximal response was reached (by force a retrospective definition). Great heterogeneity existed among patients: some achieved maximal tumor reduction after only one cycle of therapy, whereas others required up to 8 months of treatment to reach that point. Although individualizing the duration of induction chemotherapy seems to improve the complete remission rate, it is puzzling that the survival rate reported in the trial reported by Lippman and others[37] was similar to that observed by others who reported much lower complete remission rates. One could hypothesize that, similar to observations in hematologic malignancies, only complete remissions that are achieved rapidly are associated with long-term survival benefit.

Clinical measurements of breast masses often are inaccurate, and substantial interindividual variation exists among examiners.[39] Therefore, other diagnostic methods often are used to achieve more reliable documentation of extent of disease.[39,40] Combining physical examination with one imaging modality (mammography or ultrasound) gives measurements that closely approach those achieved by histopathologic evaluation; this approach also prevents overestimating (or underestimating) the dimensions of the tumor and response to systemic therapy on serial monitoring. The determination of clinical complete remission requires experience and a systematic approach. No residual disease should be present by physical examination or by imaging (mammography, ultrasound, or both) in the breast or regional lymph nodes.[34] Even when following these criteria, only two thirds of patients thought to have a clinical complete remission will be found to have a pathologic complete remission (ie, no residual disease)[20,28,29,34,37] (Table 18-3). Conversely, one third of patients with no residual disease by histologic examination will have residual abnormalities detected clinically or by imaging that preclude the diagnosis of clinical complete remission. The careful determination of complete remission after induction chemotherapy is important because this group of patients has a markedly improved long-term prognosis, compared with patients who achieve less prominent or no responses.[21,45] Furthermore, these patients are excellent candidates for breast-conserving procedures, with or without surgical intervention.

Approaches to Local Therapy

For patients with operable stage III (stage IIIA) breast cancer, a modified radical mastectomy, followed by appropriate systemic adjuvant therapy, represents an established

TABLE 18-2
Locally Advanced Breast Cancer: Overall and Complete Response Rates After Induction Chemotherapy

Investigators	Induction Chemotherapy Program	Patients Treated	Patients With Objective Response	Complete Response (%)
DeLena et al[17]	AV × 3*	132	70 (53%)	15
DeLena et al[26]	AV × 4*	74	64 (86%)	15
Hortobagyi et al[27]	FAC × 3	52	43 (83%)	15
Hobar et al[28]	FAC × 3	36	26 (72%)	8
Conte et al[20]	DES-FAC × 3	39	28 (72%)	15
Lippman et al[37]	CATPMFL × (3 – 11)	51	45 (90%)	52
Coccini et al[29]	CMF(T) × 4*	49	23 (47%)	8
Perloff et al[30]	CAFVPr × 3*	113	78 (69%)	18
Jacquillat et al[21]	VbTMAFPr × (2 – 4)	98	89 (91%)	23
Rosso et al[116]	FAC × 3	113	73 (64%)	10
Poddubnaya et al[32]	AMC/CMF	503	317 (63%)	2
Touboul et al[33]	FACV × 4	82	45 (55%)	10
Hortobagyi et al[34]	FAC × 34	174	151 (87%)	10

A, Adriamycin (doxorubicin); V, vincristine; F, 5-fluorouracil; C, cyclophosphamide; DES, diethylstilbestrol; T, Tamoxifen; P, Premarin (estrogen); L, leucovorin; M, methotrexate; Pr, prednisone; Vb, Vinblastine.

* Randomized trials.

TABLE 18-3

Locally Advanced Breast Cancer: Correlation of Clinical and Pathologic Complete Remissions After Induction Chemotherapy

Investigators	Treatment Program	Patients	Complete Remission (%)	
			Clinical	Pathologic
Hobar et al[28]	CT+S±RT+CT	36	8	11
Conte et al[20]	CT+S+CT	39	15	8
Lippman et al[37]	CT±S+RT+CT	51	52	33
Cocconi et al[29]	CT+S+CT+RT	49	8	14
Hortobagyi et al[34]	CT±S+RT−CT	174	17	8

CT, chemotherapy; S, surgery; RT, radiation therapy.

and effective treatment option.[46] Selected patients with small T4 tumors also may be approached with surgery as their initial treatment modality.[47] The standard radical mastectomy has no place in the modern management of this stage of breast cancer either. An increasing number of patients with stage III breast cancer have been treated with induction chemotherapy followed by various local–regional approaches, a strategy clearly favored by Harris and coworkers.[46] Major objective responses after induction chemotherapy resulted in downstaging for approximately 70% of patients.[34,38,48] After induction chemotherapy, surgery alone,[17,28,30,49] radiation therapy alone,[17,18,21,49–52] or a combination of both[17,22,52,53] have been used in multidisciplinary management. Surgical therapy may require a total mastectomy or only a wide excision (tumorectomy or quadrantectomy), both with an axillary dissection, especially in the presence of palpable axillary lymph nodes. Total mastectomy alone has been compared, in randomized trials, to radiation therapy alone, both after primary chemotherapy[17,30,54] (Table 18-4). Early reports of these trials suggest that the two strategies are equivalent, and

indeed, no significant differences in survival have been demonstrated in these studies. However, in a retrospective analysis of the Milan Tumor Institute's experience with combined modality therapy of LABC, induction chemotherapy followed by a total mastectomy with axillary dissection appeared superior to the same chemotherapy and radiation therapy regimen in obtaining long-term local control, with a nonsignificant trend toward improved relapse-free and overall survival rates.[55] Based mostly on indirect comparisons, the highest local control rates seem to correlate with including both surgical excision and radiation therapy (after primary chemotherapy) in the treatment strategy,[17,20,21,26,28,30,33,34,56–58] compared with the local control rates achieved after only one local treatment (Table 18-5). However, the only randomized trial, in which chemotherapy followed by surgery was compared with chemotherapy followed by both surgery and radiation therapy failed to show an advantage for the triple-modality treatment, regardless of the endpoint analyzed. Therefore, this area requires additional controlled trials to establish the optimal sequence and composition of multi-

TABLE 18-4

Randomized Clinical Trials to Define Optimal Local Therapy for Locally Advanced Breast Cancer Treated With Combined Modality Approach

Investigators	Treatments Compared	Patients	CR	CR+PR (%)	Failure (%)	
					Local	Distance
DeLena et al[26]	CT→S	65	78	78	30	43
	CT→RT	67	51	85	31	26
Perloff et al[30]	CT→S	43	100	100	19	26
	CT→RT	44	52	77	27	23
Papaioannou et al[54]	CT→S→CT	57	57	57	11	11
	CT→S+RT→CT	48	48	48	8	19

CR, complete remission; PR, partial remission; CT, chemotherapy; S, surgery; RT, radiation therapy.

TABLE 18-5
Local Control Rate After Combined Modality Therapy for Locally Advanced Breast Cancer

Investigators	Treatment Program	Patients	Median Follow-Up (mo)	Local Control Rate (%)
Touboul et al[33]	CT+RT±S+CT	82	70	82
Hortobagyi et al[34]	CT±S+RT+CT	174	59	85
Cardenas et al[56]	CT+S/RT+CT	23	52	78
Jacquillat et al[21]	CT+RT+CT	98	40	87
Perloff et al[30]	CT+S/RT+CT★	113	37	63
DeLena et al[26]	CT+RT+CT★	67	36	69
	CT+S+CT	65	36	70
Hobar et al[28]	CT+S±RT+CT	36	34	81
Conte et al[20]	CT+S+CT±RT	39	24	72
Aisner et al[57]	CT+S+CT	27	24	59
Boyages et al[58]	CT+RT+CT	35	24	71
DeLena et al[17]	CT+RT±CT	110	18	54

CT, chemotherapy; RT, radiation therapy; S, surgery.

★ Randomized trials.

modality treatments. Consider that in the presence of known residual disease, higher doses of radiation therapy are required, with the consequent increase in acute and long-term complications.

For this reason, if residual disease exists after induction chemotherapy, we prefer a surgical excision followed by adjuvant chemotherapy and radiation therapy at "standard" (50- to 60-Gy) doses and conventional fractionation schedules. Although the long-term prognosis of most patients with LABC remains poor, combined-modality therapy offers excellent local control to 80% or more of those with stage IIIB or IV breast cancer, and an even higher proportion to those with stage IIIA disease.[34] Although combined-modality strategies permit the use of less radical forms of surgery and radiation therapy, optimal local–regional control remains a major goal of therapy. As is later in this chapter, if any part of the multidisciplinary treatment strategy is suboptimal, it compromises the efficacy of the entire program.

There are many possible ways to combine or sequence the therapeutic modalities used for breast cancer (Table 18-6). Because few controlled studies have been performed, only limited conclusions can be drawn. However, because of the high incidence of distant metastases in patients with LABC, the early introduction of systemic therapy seems reasonable. Whether giving simultaneous chemotherapy and radiation therapy results in improved local and distant control remains to be established.[59,60] Therefore, most combined-modality strategies for inoperable LABC start with induction chemotherapy, usually with an anthracycline-containing multidrug regimen. The subsequent sequence of local, regional, and additional systemic treatments is poorly defined. However, as shown on Table 18-2, several different sequences have been suc-

cessful, and until the optimal sequence is determined, any of the reported programs may be used. However, systemic treatment alone is insufficient in the management of LABC, and either surgical resection, radiation therapy, or both must follow induction chemotherapy. We find that induction chemotherapy followed by surgical resection, adjuvant chemotherapy, and consolidation radiation therapy is a well-tolerated, safe, effective sequence of therapies for patients with LABC.

Breast Preservation After Induction Chemotherapy

Increasing evidence from clinical trials of primary chemotherapy suggests that many patients with stage III breast cancer, including some with LABC, could be treated appropriately with breast conservation.[17,18,21,22,26,27,30,48,50,51]

TABLE 18-6
Combined-Modality Strategies for Locally Advanced Breast Cancer

Chemotherapy→surgery→chemotherapy

Chemotherapy→surgery→chemotherapy→radiation therapy

Chemotherapy→radiation therapy→chemotherapy

Chemotherapy→radiation therapy→surgery→chemotherapy

Chemotherapy + radiation therapy→chemotherapy

Chemotherapy + radiation therapy→surgery→chemotherapy

Clinical trials with induction chemotherapy and radiation therapy performed at the M.D. Anderson Cancer Center,[27] the Milan Cancer Institute,[17] the US National Cancer Institute,[22] and several european centers[21,33,50,61] demonstrate that 15% to 95% of patients with LABC were downstaged to the extent that they could be treated with radiation therapy without surgical resection. Multiple reports during the past 20 years reveal that breast conservation clearly was possible after induction chemotherapy; however, the fraction of patients offered breast conservation varied markedly between institutions because the size of the tumor was only one of several criteria used to select patients for breast conservation therapy. Table 18-7 lists the patient and tumor characteristics that must be considered in the process of selecting candidates for breast-conserving therapy. Age, histologic type, differentiation, and availability of family and social support systems are other factors variously considered for this purpose. Notice that few absolute contraindications to breast-conserving therapy exist, although each of the factors listed may moderately increase the risk of recurrence within the breast. Although these criteria are used for patients treated with induction chemotherapy, they were originally derived from patients with early (stage I and II) breast cancer. Because their application to patients with LABC has not been fully validated, selection of patients with LABC for breast-conserving therapy should be done with caution. For these reasons, patients with LABC treated with breast conservation must have close follow-up.

Also notice that different expectations of aesthetic outcome strongly influence these decisions. Because of recent technical advances in breast reconstruction, many patients with relative contraindications to breast-conserving therapy may be appropriately treated with mastectomy and immediate reconstruction. At our institution, selection of patients with LABC for breast-conserving therapy is done according to strict criteria: as a result, although the results of induction chemotherapy in our institution are similar to other centers, the average rate of breast conservation for patients with stage IIIB breast cancer is 20%. In other centers, breast-conserving therapy is offered to more than 90% of patients after induction chemotherapy or chemotherapy–radiation therapy. Only controlled trials that evaluate breast-conservation rates along with long-term aesthetic results, complications, and costs define the optimal selection criteria in this group of patients.

The use of induction chemotherapy has been extended to stage I and II breast cancer.[36,48,62–64] Clinical trials in this area have been better designed, and with additional follow-up, should provide definitive results about the relative value of this strategy compared with standard regimens that include postoperative adjuvant chemotherapy. Clinical trials in early-stage breast cancer confirm the efficacy of these regimens, suggesting that downstaging is even more likely in early stages.[36,48,65,66] Furthermore, the preliminary report of a large multicenter trial confirms that substantial downstaging after induction chemotherapy also occurred at the level of regional lymph nodes, suggesting that a similar effect might extend to distant micrometastases.[36] This latter study confirms the observation that the frequency of complete remissions after induction chemotherapy is inversely proportional to initial tumor size, which also suggests that the possibility of breast conservation is more limited for patients with LABC than for patients with earlier stage tumors.

Inflammatory Breast Cancer

Inflammatory breast cancer, perhaps the most aggressive form of breast neoplasia, represents 1% to 3% of newly diagnosed breast malignancies and is often considered together with LABC, despite specific differential features.[67] This latter entity is diagnosed on clinical grounds, based on the presence of erythema and edema (peau d'orange) of the skin of the breast, as well as wheals or ridging. Whereas a dominant mass is present in many cases, most inflammatory cancers present as diffuse infiltration of the breast without a well-defined tumor. The absence of a well-defined tumor often suggests an "inflammatory" etiology. These patients often are treated with antibiotics for

TABLE 18-7
Selection of Patients for Breast-Conserving Therapy After Induction Chemotherapy

Contraindications		Indications
Absolute	Relative	
Patient prefers mastectomy	Predicted poor cosmetic result	Patient prefers breast conservation
Extensive multifocal tumor	Extensive intraductal component	Small tumor in large breast
Extensive persistent skin changes	Extensive lymphocytic invasion	Single focus of tumor
Resection margin positive	Age	
Collagen-vascular disease	Nuclear grade	
Noncompliant patient		

several weeks before the appropriate diagnosis is made, because of the extensive inflammatory signs without the signs of a malignant neoplasm. Dermal lymphatic invasion is present in most patients, but this feature is not a necessary component of the diagnostic complex. Most IBCs are poorly differentiated ductal carcinomas and are estrogen and progesterone receptor negative. Compared with non-inflammatory LABC, the median thymidine labeling index is significantly higher for IBC than for LABC. A history of rapid onset (less than 3 months) often is used to differentiate IBC from LABC with secondary inflammatory features.[68] This differentiation is important because some of the secondary IBCs follow an indolent course and often are hormone-responsive.

Before the introduction of systemic therapy in the combined-modality treatment programs, IBC was a uniformly fatal disease.[5] Patients with IBC treated with surgery, radiation therapy, or both had an extremely poor prognosis: the local recurrence rate was high (50% to 80%), metastases developed in more than 90% of patients in less than 2 years, and 5-year survival rates were consistently less than 5%.[5,69]

With the development of induction chemotherapy-containing strategies, a dramatic change occurred in the natural history of IBC[5,17,22,23,70–80] (Table 18-8). Objective response rates after induction chemotherapy consistently reach 80% in patients with IBC, and most patients (over 95%) can be rendered disease-free after combined-modality therapy. Three-year survival rates after these treatments range from 40% to 70%, and at 5 years, up to 50% of patients remain alive. In reports with longer follow-up, 35% remain disease-free at 10 years and even longer.[80] In fact, late relapses of IBC are uncommon.

Local–regional therapy for IBC presents special challenges. Because of the diffuse nature of this type of breast cancer, determining the extent of disease preoperatively or even intraoperatively might be difficult. In addition, even after induction chemotherapy, complete normalization of cutaneous abnormalities is uncommon. Before the introduction of combined systemic and regional treatment strategies, the local–regional failure rate was 50% to 75% for this group of patients[5,69] after surgery alone, radiation therapy alone, or both. This led to the conclusion that surgical removal of the breast served no useful purpose, and surgery was considered contraindicated for IBC for the several decades that preceded the introduction of in-

TABLE 18-8
Results of Combined Modality Treatment Programs of Inflammatory Breast Carcinoma

Investigators	Treatment	Patients	Disease-Free After Treatment (%)	Median Survival (mo)	5-Year Survival Rate (%)
DeLena et al[17]	CT+RT±CT	36	73	25	NA
Chu et al[70]	RT+H	14	NA	15	NA
	RT+CT	16	NA	>26	NA
Pouillart et al[71]	CT+RT+CT	77	51	34	NA
Zylberberg et al[72]	CT+S+CT±RT	15	100	>56	70
Pawlicki et al[23]	CT±S+RT	72	NA	NA	NA
Loprinzi et al[73]	S+CT+RT+CT	9	100	>25	55
Keiling et al[74]	CT+S+CT	41	100	NR	63
Jacquillat et al[96]	CT+RT+CT+H	66	100	NR	66
Alberto et al[119]	CT+S+CT+RT	22	95	26	10
Ferriere et al[120]	CT+RT±S+CT	75	93	NR	54
Pourney et al[121]	CT+S±RT+CT	33	82	70	60
Chevallier et al[122]	CT+RT±CT±S	178	83	37	32
Rouesse et al[75]	CT+RT+CT+H	91	41	36	40
Israel et al[76]	CT+S+CT	25	96	NR	62
Krutchick et al[77]	CT+RT+CT	32	NA	24	NA
Brun et al[84]	CT+RT+S+CT	26	NA	31	NA
Thoms et al[78]	CT+S+CT+RT	61	NA	61	35
Swain et al[22]	CT+RT+S+CT+H	45	NA	36	NR
Fields et al[79]	CT+S+RT+CT	37	NA	49	44
Maloisel et al[123]	CT+S+CT+RT+H	43	NA	46	75
Koh et al[80]	CT+RT+CT	40	NA	39	37
	CT+S+CT+RT	23	NA	38	30
	CT+S+CT+RT	43	NA	31	40

CT, chemotherapy; S, surgery; RT, radiation therapy; H, hormone therapy; NA, not available; NR, not reached.

duction chemotherapy. The role of surgical resection in managing IBC remains questionable because its contribution to improved local control has been inconsistent,[78,81,82] and it has had no effect on survival. However, surgical resection provides interim local control without interrupting dose-intensive chemotherapy; provides an accurate assessment of the response to induction chemotherapy with its consequent prognostic implications; and by removing gross residual disease, permits the use of lower doses of radiation therapy.[81] This is an important consideration for responding patients with good long-term prognosis because it avoids the late complications of high-dose radiation therapy. The local control rates achieved with modern combined-modality regimens for IBC approach 70%.[75] Response to induction chemotherapy is clearly associated with long-term local control: patients who achieve a complete remission have a 90% or greater local control rate, contrasted to less than 50% local control rates observed in nonresponding patients.[78]

Accelerated fractionation schedules have been proposed for IBC, based on the biologic characteristics of this tumor.[83] Although preliminary results suggest improved local control rates for accelerated fractionation schedules,[83] this has not been confirmed on subsequent evaluation.[78] However, accelerated fractionation schedules are associated with lower rates of late complications.

Most combined-modality treatment programs for IBC consist of induction chemotherapy followed by radiation therapy to the breast and regional lymphatics and addi-

tional adjuvant chemotherapy. Others include a total mastectomy after three or four cycles of chemotherapy. By definition, programs that do not include a mastectomy offer breast-conserving therapy. However, this is done at the expense of higher doses of radiation therapy and its expected late toxicities, as well as suboptimal cosmetic results. Because skin edema, erythema, and ridging persist after chemotherapy in most patients, and because inflammatory tumors often are diffuse and poorly defined, lumpectomy or quadrantectomy are not practical options. In addition, limited data suggest that local failure rate may be higher after breast-conserving therapy.[84] Therefore, breast conservation for IBC requires higher doses of radiation because residual tumor cannot be adequately resected with less than a total mastectomy.

Tolerance and Toxicity

Combined-modality regimens have been well tolerated, and no increase in surgical complications has been reported.[85] Surgery usually is sandwiched between cycles of chemotherapy, and systemic treatment seldom needs to be interrupted. The expected acute toxic effects of combination chemotherapy are observed without apparent increase in frequency or intensity. In studies with simultaneous radiation therapy and chemotherapy, a slight increase in hematologic toxicity and enhancement of acute radia-

TABLE 18-9
Survival of Patients With Stage III Breast Cancer After Combined Modality Programs Based on Induction Chemotherapy Followed by Local Treatment: Nonrandomized Trials

Investigators	Treatment Program	Patients	Disease-Free After Treatment (%)	Median Survival (mo)	Survival Rate (%)	
					3 Years	5 Years
DeLena et al[17]	CT+RT±CT	110	83	36	50	NR
Hortobagyi et al[27]	CT+RT±S+CT	52	94	65	65	55
Bedwinek et al[86]	CT+RT+CT	22	78	28	40	NR
Pawlicki et al[23]	CT	40	NA	NA	13	NR
	CT+RT+CT	34	NA	NA	32	NR
	CT+S+RT+CT	13	NA	NA	62	NR
Valagussa et al[19]	CT+RT	72	64	30	43	20
	CT+RT+CT	126	75	42	60	36
	CT+S+CT	79	82	58	64	49
Balawajder et al[24]	CT+RT	23	NA	NA	NA	46
	CT+RT+S	30	NA	NA	NA	38
Conte et al[20]	H+CT+S+H+CT±RT	39	92	NR	60	NR
Pouillart et al[49]	CT+S+RT	82	100	NR	85	NR
Cardenas et al[56]	CT+S+RT+CT	23	100	NR	77	56
Jacquillat et al[21]	CT+RT+CT	98	100	NR	77	NR
Hortobagyi et al[34]	CT+RT+S+CT	174	96	66	65	55
Swain et al[22]	CT+RT+S+CT	75	100	39	42	NR

NR, not reached; NA, not available; S, surgery; RT, radiation therapy; CT, chemotherapy; H, hormone therapy.

tion effects (erythema, moist desquamation) have been reported.[86-89] Simultaneous administration of chemotherapy and radiation therapy impairs, to some extent, the cosmetic results of breast-conserving therapy; whereas some impairment of cosmesis also is observed with the sequential use of chemotherapy and radiation therapy, this effect is not clinically important for most patients. For patients with cancer of the left breast, synergistic cardiac toxicity is a danger when simultaneous therapy is used.[88,89] However, modifications in radiation therapy techniques and careful attention to the total dose of anthracyclines minimize this risk. Administering doxorubicin by 48- or 96-hour continuous-infusion schedules also reduces the risk of cardiac toxicity substantially.[90]

Survival Effects of Combined Modality Strategies

Most information regarding the multidisciplinary treatment of stage III LABC was obtained from open (uncontrolled) phase II trials; therefore, the effects of these treatments on survival are tentative at best, and definitive conclusions await the completion of prospective randomized trials. However, such trials are possible for patients with operable stage III breast cancer; for patients with inoperable stage III or IBC, the window of opportunity to perform such trials may have been lost many years ago. The results of phase II trials compare favorably with the outcomes of historical control series and literature controls, suggesting higher 5- and 10-year survival rates, especially in the worst prognostic subgroups: patients with IBC[5,67] (Table 18-9; see Table 18-8) patients with supraclavicular

lymph node involvement,[34] and patients with T4 primary lesions. Figure 18-1 shows the disease-free survival of patients with stage IIIA and IIIB breast cancer treated at our institution with induction chemotherapy followed by surgery, radiation therapy, and adjuvant chemotherapy, with a maximum follow-up reaching 20 years. The two curves are compared with patients with disease of similar stages (IIIA and IIIB) treated at our institution with surgery and radiation therapy, but without systemic treatment. Figure 18-2 shows the overall survival curves from the same four groups of patients. A substantial improvement is seen in both disease-free and overall survival for patients who received the combined-modality treatment, including induction chemotherapy. The median relapse-free and overall survival times for patients with stage IIIA breast cancer treated with surgery and radiation therapy were 102 and 140 months, respectively, whereas they have not been reached at 200 months by patients treated also with induction chemotherapy. The differences in both disease-free and overall survival for patients with stage IIIB breast cancer treated with these two strategies were 10 and 13 months, respectively. The 5- and 10-year disease-free and overall survival rates were about 10 points higher for patients treated with all three modalities in sequence, compared with the historical controls. These differences have persisted beyond 10 years of follow-up and are projected to continue beyond 20 years after diagnosis and treatment. It is generally accepted that patients with stage III breast cancer treated with local therapy followed by postoperative adjuvant chemotherapy have a significant relapse-free,[7,8,50,91,92] and sometimes, overall survival[7,8,92] advantage over those treated with only local therapy, although not all studies confirm this observation.[51] What remains to be determined is whether induction (or preoperative) che-

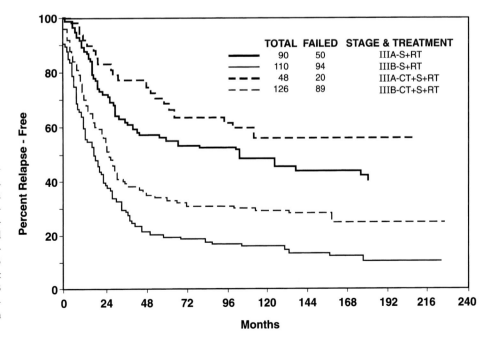

FIGURE 18-1 Relapse-free survival curves of patients with stage IIIA and IIIB breast cancer treated with induction chemotherapy (5-fluorouracil, doxorubicin, and cyclophosphamide; FAC), followed by surgical resection, radiation therapy, and adjuvant chemotherapy between 1973 and 1984. The control groups consist of patients with stage IIIA and IIIB breast cancer treated at this same institution with surgery and radiation therapy before 1974.

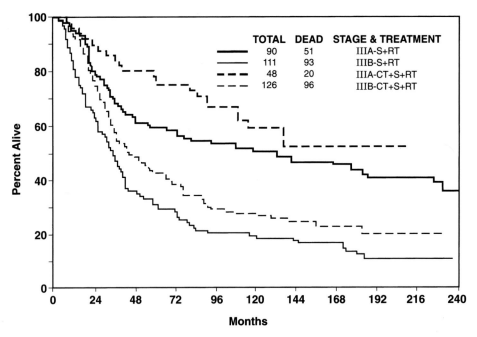

FIGURE 18-2 Overall survival curves of patients with stage IIIA and IIIB breast cancer treated with induction chemotherapy (5-fluorouracil, doxorubicin, and cyclophosphamide; FAC), followed by surgical resection, radiation therapy, and adjuvant chemotherapy between 1973 and 1984. The control groups consist of patients with stage IIIA and IIIB breast cancer treated at this same institution with surgery and radiation therapy between 1965 and 1974.

motherapy is more effective in prolonging survival than postoperative chemotherapy in the context of combined-modality treatment[18,19,51,62,63] (Table 18-10). The reported randomized trials suggest that the results obtained with induction chemotherapy are at least equivalent to those observed after postoperative chemotherapy. However, in at least two of these studies,[18,51] the dose of radiation ther-

apy administered was too low to provide appropriate local control and the dose-intensity of chemotherapy also was low. In addition, three of the five studies shown in Table 18-10 have insufficient sample size to detect even large differences in outcome. Additional well-designed trials, with adequate statistical power and sufficient follow-up, are needed to define the survival benefit obtained and the

TABLE 18-10
Survival of Patients With Stage II-III Breast Cancer After Combined Modality Programs Based on Induction Chemotherapy Followed by Local Treatment: Results of Randomized Trials

Investigators	Treatment Program	Patients	Disease-Free After Treatment (%)	Median Survival (mo)	Survival Rate (%)	
					3 Years	5 Years
Rubens et al[18]	CT→RT★→CT	12	67	36	50	NR
	RT★→CT	12	75	36	50	NR
Mauriac et al[63]†	S→CT	138	99	NR	87	NR
	CT→S	134	99	NR	94	NR
Scholl et al[62]†	RT→S→CT	190	NA	NR	87	78
	CT→RT→S	200	NA	NR	92	86
Schaake-Koning et al[51]	RT★	45	75	42	59	37
	RT★→CT	71	50	45	59	37
	CT→RT★→CT	39	71	50	61	37
Valagussa et al[19]	CT→RT★→CT	59	51	34	NA	33
	RT★→CT	60	42	24	NA	32

CT, chemotherapy; RT, radiation therapy; S, surgery; NA, not available; NR, not reached.

★ Low-dose radiation therapy, probably inadequate for optimal local control.

† Most patients in this study had stage II breast cancer.

relative benefits of induction versus postoperative adjuvant systemic therapy.

Prognostic Factors

The ability to predict outcome changes with the efficacy of the treatments used. When LABC was treated with regional therapies only, the following patient- and tumor-related factors were considered unfavorable prognostic indicators: large tumor size, involved axillary lymph nodes, involved supraclavicular lymph nodes, skin edema, IBC, diffuse primary tumor, and short duration of symptoms.[9,93] For earlier stages of breast cancer, most of these factors were predictive of decreased relapse-free and overall survival rates. Clinical axillary lymph node involvement correlated well with outcome in patients with LABC treated with radiation therapy.[94] Evaluation of the prognostic value of axillary lymph node involvement after induction chemotherapy showed that the number of involved nodes was the best predictor for both relapse and death in a multivariate analysis.[95] The pathologic nodal subgroups of 0, 1 to 3, 4 to 10, and more than 10 positive lymph nodes after induction chemotherapy predicted a prognostic distribution similar to that found in previously untreated patients. Other important and independent factors found in this study by multivariate analysis were clinical tumor stage at presentation, clinical response to induction chemotherapy, and menopausal status. Clinical response to induction chemotherapy, or its surrogate, histologically detected extent of residual disease, also have been reported by other investigators to be important prognostic indicators.[64,96]

Response (and especially complete response) to induction chemotherapy occurs significantly more often in patients with poorly differentiated tumors in some[35,64,97] reported series, but not in others.[33,98] Provocative data from pilot studies suggest that responses were more common in patients with aneuploid tumors and in those with high proliferative fraction.[99,100] Although biologically plausible, these data need additional, prospective confirmation. Other studies assess the prognostic importance of various factors in terms of relapse-free and overall survival. Initial TNM stage, clinical tumor size, clinical nodal stage, and histologic grade have been shown to correlate with both end points in univariate analyses.[21,28,33,34,64] Response to induction chemotherapy was found by all studies to predict longer disease-free and overall survival, too. In multivariate analyses, histologic and nuclear grade, both clinical and surgical nodal stage, initial tumor size, and response to induction chemotherapy were significant predictors of disease-free survival,[33,64,95] whereas tumor size, nodal status, grade, and response to induction chemotherapy correlated with overall survival.[33,64,95]

Prognostic factors for IBC are harder to detect because of the small numbers of patients included in individual studies. However, the following have been reported to correlate with lower relapse-free survival rates in univariate analyses: large tumor size,[79] diffuse tumor,[79] extent of initial erythema,[101] extent of erythema after chemotherapy,[101] extent of skin edema,[101] no systemic therapy,[79] no surgical therapy,[79,101] negative estrogen receptor status,[102] no response to chemotherapy,[101] and extent of residual disease after treatment.[101] When overall survival was the end point, large tumor size,[79] diffuse type,[79] extent of erythema and edema,[101] N2 or N3 stage,[79,101] no systemic therapy or mastectomy,[79,101] extent of residual tumor,[101] negative estrogen receptor status,[102] negative progesterone receptor status,[103] and high labeling index[103] were adverse factors. In multivariate analyses, race,[79] diffuse mass,[79] extent of erythema,[101] lymph node involvement,[101] and no chemotherapy or mastectomy[79] were the only important adverse factors.

Dose-Intensive Therapy for Locally Advanced and Inflammatory Breast Cancer

The major obstacle to long-term survival for patients with LABC is the development of distant metastases. Therefore, to improve the effectiveness of our treatments, more effective systemic therapies are required. One research approach to improve the efficacy of chemotherapy and the survival of patients with stage III and LABC is dose-intensification of induction chemotherapy, or postoperative (post–radiation therapy) consolidation treatment. Only a few, small phase II trials have been performed, and the total number of patients with stage III or IBC treated with dose-intensive chemotherapy in the five reported trials is 56. The maximum reported follow-up of any of these studies was 37 months, and the results are inconclusive.[43] Definitive studies are in progress. The risk of recurrence for appropriately treated patients with LABC or IBC is still high, and more effective treatments are needed. However, high-dose chemotherapy remains an investigational tool because it has not been demonstrated that it affects survival in any subgroup of patients with breast cancer.

Prospects for the Future

New cytotoxic agents with demonstrated antitumor efficacy against metastatic breast cancer have been developed.[104] The taxanes (paclitaxel and docetaxel), the anthrapyrazoles, and vinorelbine were reported to be highly effective, with objective responses reported in 50% to 70% of patients, including some tumors with clear-cut resistance to anthracyclines.[105,106,110–115] Amonafide, gemcitabine, lonidamine, miltefosine, CPT-11, and several elliptinium derivatives also have shown modest activity in the 20% range.[104,116,117] These exciting, new cytotoxic agents are likely to improve the efficacy of chemotherapy of breast cancer within the next several years while they are gradually integrated into multidrug regimens.

Biologic therapy, too, has exciting developments. Clinical trials are being performed using monoclonal antibodies against breast cancer–related antigens[107] and autocrine or paracrine growth factors or their receptors.[108] Although antibodies alone have not shown major antitumor efficacy, they may function as vehicles to deliver cytotoxic therapy,[109] radioisotopes, or natural toxins (immunoconjugates or immunotoxins).

The recognition of the many remaining questions about the optimal sequence of local and systemic treatments in combined-modality therapy prompted the development of clinical trials to assess the relative efficacy of various sequences of administration and to evaluate the efficacy of limited surgery, as well as several modifications of radiation therapy technique to minimize toxicity without compromising outcome.

Combined-modality therapy that includes induction chemotherapy permits optimal local control with less radical surgical and radiotherapeutic intervention. By downstaging primary and regional tumors, breast conservation becomes an option for some patients. In addition, the multidisciplinary management of stage III and LABC provides an excellent biologic model to assess the effects of systemic therapy on the primary tumor. On the clinical side, this provides in vivo assessment of response and the possibility of modifying subsequent therapy based on this evaluation of response.

Thus, this subgroup of patients, although receiving what is considered optimal therapy, provides us with clear scientific opportunities to optimize therapies for primary breast cancer.

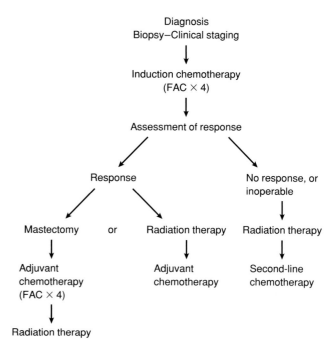

FIGURE 18-4 Flow diagram for the treatment of patients with inflammatory breast cancer.

MANAGEMENT SUMMARY

- Combined modality strategies represent the treatment of choice for patients with LABC and IBC. Effective and well-tolerated strategies are shown in Figures 18-3 and 18-4.
- Although initial prognostic evaluation is important for determining optimal therapy, treatment must be individualized during the course of treatment, depending on patient response and tolerance to therapy.
- Aggressive induction chemotherapy, careful multimodal evaluation and monitoring, and effective strategies for local and regional control are the key to the success of the overall treatment strategy.
- Close and continued interaction between all therapeutic and diagnostic specialists is needed to deliver optimal therapy.

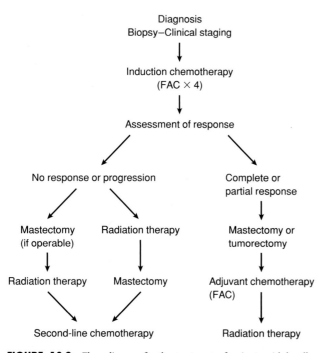

FIGURE 18-3 Flow diagram for the treatment of patients with locally advanced breast cancer.

References

1. Breast. In: Beahrs OH, Henson DE, Hutter RVP, et al, eds. Manual for Staging of Cancer, ed 3. Philadelphia, JB Lippincott, 1988:145.
2. Seidman H, Gelb SK, Silverberg E, et al. Survival experience in the Breast Cancer Detection Demonstration Project. CA Cancer J Clin 1987;37:258.
3. Zeichner GI, Mohar BA, Ramirez UMT. Epidemiologia del cancer de Mama en el Instituto Nacional de Cancerologia (1989–1990). Cancerologia 1993;39:1825.
4. Moisa FC, Lopez J, Raymundo C. Epidemiologia del carcinoma del seno mamario en Latino America. Cancerologia 1989;35:810.

5. Hortobagyi GN, Buzdar AU. Locally advanced breast cancer: a review including the MD. Anderson experience. In: Ragaz J, Ariel IM, eds. High-risk breast cancer. Berlin, Springer-Verlag, 1991:382.

6. Glick JH, Gelber RD, Goldhirsch A, et al. Meeting highlights: adjuvant therapy for primary breast cancer. J Natl Cancer Inst 1992;84:1479.

7. Grohn P, Heinonen E, Klefstrom P, et al. Adjuvant postoperative radiotherapy, chemotherapy, and immunotherapy in stage III breast cancer. Cancer 1984;54:670.

8. Rivkin SE, Green S, Metch B, et al. Adjuvant CMFVP versus melphalan for operable breast cancer with positive axillary nodes: 10-year results of a Southwest Oncology Group Study. J Clin Oncol 1989;7:1229.

9. Haagensen CD, Stout AP. Carcinoma of the breast: criteria of inoperability. Am Surg 1943;118:859.

10. Zucali R, Uslenghi C, Kenda R, et al. Natural history and survival of inoperable breast cancer treated with radiotherapy and radiotherapy followed by radical mastectomy. Cancer 1976;37:1422.

11. Harris JR, Sawicka J, Gelman R, et al. Management of locally advanced carcinoma of the breast by primary radiation therapy. Int J Radiat Oncol Biol Phys 1983;9:345.

12. Baclesse F. Roentgen therapy as the sole method of treatment of cancer of the breast. Am J Roentgenol 1949;62:311.

13. Fletcher GH, Montague ED. Radical irradiation of advanced breast cancer. Am J Roentgenology 1965;93:573.

14. Spanos WJ, Montague ED, Fletcher FH. Late complications of radiation only for advanced breast cancer. Int J Radiat Oncol Biol Phys 1980;6:1473.

15. Fisher B, Ravdin RD, Ausman RK, et al. Surgical adjuvant chemotherapy in cancer of the breast: results of a decade of cooperative investigation. Ann Surg 1968;168:337.

16. Kennedy BJ, Kelley RM, White G, et al. Surgery as an adjunct to hormone therapy of breast cancer. Cancer 1957;10:1055.

17. DeLena M, Zucali R, Viganotti G, et al. Combined chemotherapy–radiotherapy approach in locally advanced (T_{3b}–T_4) breast cancer. Cancer Chemother Pharmacol 1978;1:53.

18. Rubens RD, Sexton S, Tong D, et al. Combined chemotherapy and radiotherapy for locally advanced breast cancer. Eur J Cancer 1980;16:351.

19. Valagussa P, Zambetti M, Bignami PD, et al. T3b–T4 breast cancer: factors affecting results in combined modality treatment. Clin Exp Metastasis 1983;1:191.

20. Conte PF, Alama A, Bertelli G, et al. Chemotherapy with estrogenic recruitment and surgery in locally advanced breast cancer: clinical and cytokinetic results. Int J Cancer 1987;40:490.

21. Jacquillat C, Baillet F, Weil M, et al. Results of a conservative treatment combining induction (neoadjuvant) and consolidation chemotherapy, hormonotherapy, and external and interstitial irradiation in 98 patients with locally advanced breast cancer (IIIA–IIIB). Cancer 1988;61:1977.

22. Swain SM, Sorace RA, Bagley CS, et al. Neoadjuvant chemotherapy in the combined modality approach of locally advanced nonmetastatic breast cancer. Cancer Res 1987;47:3889.

23. Pawlicki M, Skolyszewski J, Brandys A. Results of combined treatment of patients with locally advanced breast cancer. Tumori 1983;69:249.

24. Balawajder I, Antich PP, Boland J. An analysis of the role of radiotherapy alone and in combination with chemotherapy and surgery in the management of advanced breast cancer. Cancer 1983;51:574.

25. Burn I. Primary endocrine therapy of advanced local breast cancer: reviews of endocrine-related cancer. 1985;(Suppl)16:5.

26. DeLena M, Varini M, Zucali R, et al. Multimodal treatment for locally advanced breast cancer: results of chemotherapy–radiotherapy versus chemotherapy–surgery. Cancer Clin Trials 1981;4:229.

27. Hortobagyi GN, Blumenschein GR, Spanos W, et al. Multimodal treatment of locoregionally advanced breast cancer. Cancer 1983;51:763.

28. Hobar PC, Jones RC, Schouten J, et al. Multimodality treatment of locally advanced breast carcinoma. Arch Surg 1988;123:951.

29. Cocconi G, di Blasio B, Bisagni G, et al. Neoadjuvant chemotherapy or chemotherapy and endocrine therapy in locally advanced breast carcinoma. Am J Clin Oncol 1990;13:226.

30. Perloff M, Lesnick GJ, Korzun A, et al. Combination chemotherapy with mastectomy or radiotherapy for stage III breast carcinoma: a cancer and leukemia group B study. J Clin Oncol 1988;6:261.

31. Rosso R, Gardin G, Conte PF, et al. Combined modality approach in locally advanced breast cancer. (Abstract) Ann Oncol 1990;1(Suppl):22.

32. Poddubnaya I, Letjagin V, Ognerubov N, et al. Neoadjuvant chemotherapy in the complex treatment of local-advanced mammae cancer. (Abstract) Proceedings of the Biennial Meeting of the International Association of Breast Cancer Research, Banff, Canada, April 25–28, 1993.

33. Touboul E, Lefranc JP, Blondon J, et al. Multidisciplinary treatment approach to locally advanced non-inflammatory breast cancer using chemotherapy and radiotherapy with or without surgery. Radiother Oncol 1992;25:167.

34. Hortobagyi GN, Ames FC, Buzdar AU, et al. Management of stage III primary breast cancer with primary chemotherapy, surgery, and radiation therapy. Cancer 1988;62:2507.

35. Kemeny F, Vadrot J, d'Hubert E, et al. Evaluation histologique e radioclinique de l'effet de la chimiotherapie premiere sur les cancers non inflammatoires du sein. Cahiers Cancer 1991;3:705.

36. Fisher B, Rockette H, Robidoux A, et al. Effect of preoperative therapy for breast cancer on local–regional disease: first report of NSABP B-18. (Abstract) Proc Annu Meet Am Soc Clin Oncol 1994;13:64.

37. Lippman ME, Sorace RA, Bagley CS, et al. Treatment of locally advanced breast cancer using primary induction chemotherapy with hormonal synchronization followed by radiation therapy with or without debulking surgery. Natl Cancer Inst Monogr 1986;1:153.

38. Schwartz GF, Cantor RI, Biermann WA. Neoadjuvant chemotherapy before definitive treatment for stage III carcinoma of the breast. Arch Surg 1987;122:1430.

39. Cocconi G, di Blasio B, Alberti G, et al. Problems in evaluating response of primary breast cancer to systemic therapy. Breast Cancer Res Treat 1984;4:309.

40. Fornage BD, Toubas O, Morel M. Clinical, mammographic, and sonographic determination of preoperative breast cancer size. Cancer 1987;60:765.

41. le Chevalier T, Pujol JL, Douillard JY, et al. A European multicentre randomized study comparing navelbine alone vs navelbine–cisplatin vs vindesine–cisplatin in 612 patients with advanced non-small cell lung cancer. (Abstract) Proc Amer Soc Clin Oncol 1992;11:289.

42. French Northern Oncology Group. Mitoxantrone and vinorelbine as a primary treatment of locoregional breast cancer. (Abstract) Proceedings of the IVth International Congress on Anticancer Chemotherapy 1993;223.

43. Antman KH. Dose-intensive therapy in breast cancer. In: Armitage JO, Antman KH, eds. High-dose cancer therapy. Baltimore, Williams & Wilkins, 1992:701.

44. Norton L. A Gompertzian model of human breast cancer growth. Cancer Res 1988;48:7067.

45. Feldman LD, Hortobagyi GN, Buzdar AU, et al. Pathological assessment of response to induction chemotherapy in breast cancer. Cancer Res 1986;46:2578.

46. Harris JR, Lippman ME, Veronesi U, et al. Breast cancer. N Engl J Med 1992;327:319,390,473.

47. Zucali R, Kenda R. Small size T4 breast cancer: natural history and prognosis. Tumori 1981;67:225.

48. Bonadonna G, Veronesi U, Brambilla C, et al. Primary chemotherapy to avoid mastectomy in tumors with diameters of three centimeters or more. J Natl Cancer Inst 1990;82:1539.

49. Pouillart P, Palangie T, Jouve M, et al. Essai pilote de chimiotherapie neo-adjuvante dans le cancer du sein. In: Jacquillat C, Weil M, Khayat D, eds. Neo-adjuvant chemotherapy. Paris, John Libbey, 1986:257.

50. Rubens RD, Bartelink H, Engelsman E, et al. Locally advanced breast cancer: the contribution of cytotoxic and endocrine treatment to radiotherapy. Eur J Cancer 1989;25:667.

51. Schaake-Koning C, van der Linden EH, Hart G, et al. Adjuvant chemo- and hormonal therapy in locally advanced breast cancer: a randomized clinical study. Int J Radiat Oncol Biol Phys 1985;11:1759.

52. Olson JE, Gray R, Sponzo R, et al. Primary chemotherapy for nonresectable locally advanced breast cancer: 8 yr results of an ECOG trial. (Abstract) Breast Cancer Res Treat 1990;16:148.

53. Hortobagyi GN, Kau SW, Buzdar AU, et al. Induction chemotherapy for stage III primary breast cancer. In: Salmon SE, ed. Adjuvant therapy of cancer, vol 5. Orlando, Grune & Stratton, 1987:419.

54. Papaioannou A, Lissaios B, Vasilaros S, et al. Pre- and postoperative chemoendocrine treatment with or without postoperative radiotherapy for locally advanced breast cancer. Cancer 1983;51:1284.

55. Valagussa P, Zambetti M, Bonadonna G, et al. Prognostic factors in locally advanced noninflammatory breast cancer: long-term results following primary chemotherapy. Breast Cancer Res Treat 1990;15:137.

56. Cardenas J, Ramirez T, Noriega J, et al. Multidisciplinary therapy for locally advanced breast cancer: an update. (Abstract) Proc Am Soc Clin Oncol 1987;6:67.

57. Aisner J, Morris D, Elias G, et al. Mastectomy as an adjuvant to chemotherapy for locally advanced or metastatic breast cancer. Arch Surg 1982;117:882.

58. Boyages J, Langlands AO. The efficacy of combined chemotherapy and radiotherapy in advanced non-metastatic breast cancer. Int J Radiat Oncol Biol Phys 1987;14:71.

59. Piccart MJ, de Valeriola D, Paridaens R, et al. Six-year results of a multimodality treatment strategy for locally advanced breast cancer. Cancer 1988;62:2501.

60. Bedwinek JM, Ratkin GA, Philpott GW, et al. Concurrent chemotherapy and radiotherapy for nonmetastatic, stage IV breast cancer. Am J Clin Oncol 1983;6:159.

61. Hery M, Namer M, Moro M, et al. Conservative treatment (chemotherapy/radiotherapy) of locally advanced breast cancer. Cancer 1986;57:1744.

62. Scholl SM, Fourquet A, Asselain B, et al. Neoadjuvant versus adjuvant chemotherapy in premenopausal patients with tumors considered too large for breast conserving surgery: preliminary results of a randomised trial. Eur J Cancer 1994;30A:645.

63. Mauriac L, Durand M, Avril A, et al. Effects of primary chemotherapy in conservative treatment of breast cancer patients with operative tumors larger than 3 centimeters: results of a randomized trial in a single center. Ann Oncol 1991;2:347.

64. Jacquillat C, Weil M, Baillet F, et al. Results of neoadjuvant chemotherapy and radiation therapy in the breast-conserving treatment of 250 patients with all stages of infiltrative breast cancer. Cancer 1990;66:119.

65. Mauriac L, Durand M, Dilhuydy J-M, et al. Randomized trial comparing induction chemotherapy to mastectomy for operable breast cancer larger than 3 cm. (Abstract) Breast Cancer Res Treat 1992;23:181.

66. Scholl SM, Asselain B, Beuzeboc P, et al. Improved survival rates following first line chemotherapy in operable breast cancer: 4 year results of a randomized trial. (Abstract) Proceedings of the IVth International Congress on AntiCancer Chemotherapy, 1993;64.

67. Jaiyesimi IA, Buzdar AU, Hortobagyi G. Inflammatory breast cancer: a review. J Clin Oncol 1992;10:1014.

68. Taylor GW, Metzer A. Inflammatory carcinoma of the breast. Am J Cancer 1938;33:33.

69. Singletary SE, Ames FC, Buzdar AU. Management of inflammatory breast cancer. World J Surg 1994;18:87.

70. Chu AM, Wood WC, Doucette JA. Inflammatory breast carcinoma treated by radical radiotherapy. Cancer 1980;45:2730.

71. Pouillart P, Palangie T, Jouve M, et al. Cancer inflammatoire du sein traite par une association de chimiotherapie et d'irradiation: resultats d'un essai randomise etudiant le role d'une immunotherapie par le BCG. Bull Cancer (Paris) 1981;68:171.

72. Zylberberg B, Salat-Baroux J, Ravina JH, et al. Initial chemoimmunotherapy in inflammatory carcinoma of the breast. Cancer 1982;49:1537.

73. Loprinzi CL, Carbone PP, Tormey DC, et al. Aggressive combined modality therapy for advanced local–regional breast carcinoma. J Clin Oncol 1984;2:157.

74. Keiling R, Guiochet N, Calderoli H, et al. Preoperative chemotherapy in the treatment of inflammatory breast cancer. In: Wagener DJT, Blijham GH, Smeets JBE, et al, eds. Primary chemotherapy in cancer medicine. New York, Alan R Liss, 1985:95.

75. Rouesse J, Friedman S, Sarrazin D, et al. Primary chemotherapy in the treatment of inflammatory breast carcinoma: a study of 230 cases from the Institut Gustave-Roussy. J Clin Oncol 1986;4:1765.

76. Israel L, Breau JL, Morere JF. Neo-adjuvant chemotherapy without radiation therapy in inflammatory breast carcinoma. In: Jacquillat C, Weil M, Khayat D, eds. Neo-adjuvant chemotherapy, ed 169. Paris, John Libbey, 1988:207.

77. Krutchik AN, Buzdar AU, Blumenschein GR, et al. Combined chemoimmunotherapy and radiation therapy of inflammatory breast carcinoma. J Surg Oncol 1979;11:325.

78. Thoms WW, McNeese MD, Fletcher GH, et al. Multimodal treatment for inflammatory breast cancer. Int J Radiat Oncol Biol Phys 1989;17:739.

79. Fields JN, Kuske RR, Perez CA, et al. Prognostic factors in inflammatory breast cancer. Cancer 1989;63:1225.

80. Koh EH, Buzdar AU, Ames FC, et al. Inflammatory carcinoma of the breast: results of a combined-modality approach: MD Anderson Cancer Center experience. Cancer Chemother Pharmacol 1990;27:94.

81. Schafer P, Alberto P, Forni M, et al. Surgery as part of a combined modality approach for inflammatory breast carcinoma. Cancer 1987;59:1063.

82. Fields JN, Kuske RR, Perez CA, et al. Inflammatory carcinoma of the breast: prognostic factors and results of treatment. (Abstract) Am J Clin Oncol 1987;10:110.

83. Barker JL, Montague ED, Peters LJ. Clinical experience with irradiation of inflammatory carcinoma of the breast with and without elective chemotherapy. Cancer 1980;45:625.

84. Brun B, Otmezguine Y, Feuilhade F, et al. Treatment of inflammatory breast cancer with combination chemotherapy and mastectomy versus breast conservation. Cancer 1988;61:1096.

85. Broadwater JR, Edwards MJ, Kuglen C, et al. Mastectomy following preoperative chemotherapy. Ann Surg 1991;213:126.

86. Bedwinek JM, Ratkin GA, Philpott GW, et al. Concurrent chemotherapy and radiotherapy for nonmetastatic, stage IV breast cancer: a pilot study by the Southeastern Cancer Study Group. Am J Clin Oncol 1983;6:159.

87. Recht A, Come SE. Sequencing of irradiation and chemotherapy for early-stage breast cancer. Oncology 1994;8:19.

88. Buzzoni R, Bonadonna G, Valagussa P, et al. Adjuvant chemotherapy with doxorubicin plus cyclophosphamide, methotrexate, and

fluorouracil in the treatment of resectable breast cancer with more than three positive nodes. J Clin Oncol 1991;9:2134.

89. Valagussa P, Moliterni A, Zambetti M, et al. Long-term sequelae from adjuvant chemotherapy. Recent results Cancer Res 1993; 127:248.

90. Hortobagyi GN, Frye D, Buzdar AU, et al. Decreased cardiac toxicity of doxorubicin administered by continuous intravenous infusion in combination chemotherapy for metastatic breast cancer. Cancer 1989;63:37.

91. Rainer H, Arbeitskreis fur perioperative chemotherapie. Prospective randomized clinical trial of primary therapy in breast cancer stages T3/4, N+/−, MO: chemo- vs. radiotherapy. In: Salmon SE, ed. Adjuvant therapy of cancer, vol 6. Philadelphia, WB Saunders, 1990:232.

92. Caceres E, Zaharia M, Lingan M, et al. Combined therapy of stage III adenocarcinoma of the breast. (Abstract) Proc Am Assoc Cancer Res 1980;21:199.

93. Stewart JH, King RJB, Winter PJ, et al. Oestrogen receptors, clinical features and prognosis in stage III breast cancer. Eur J Cancer Clin Oncol 1982;18:1315.

94. Fourquet A, Vilcoq JR, Julien D, et al. The prognostic significance of initial nodal involvement in patients with locally advanced breast cancer treated by radical radiotherapy. (Abstract) Am J Clin Oncol 1984;7:118.

95. McCready DR, Hortobagyi GN, Kau SW, et al. The prognostic significance of lymph node metastases after preoperative chemotherapy for locally advanced breast cancer. Arch Surg 1989;124:21.

96. Jacquillat C, Weil M, Auclerc G, et al. Neo-adjuvant chemotherapy in the conservative management of breast cancers: study on 205 patients. In: Jacquillat C, Weil M, Khayat D, eds. Neo-adjuvant chemotherapy. London, John Libbey, 1986:197.

97. Abu-Farsakh H, Sneige N, Atkinson N, et al. Tumor nuclear grade as a predictor of tumor response to preoperative chemotherapy in patients with locally advanced breast carcinoma. (Abstract) Mod Pathol 1994;7:12A.

98. Belembaogo E, Feillel V, Chollet P, et al. Neoadjuvant chemotherapy in 126 operable breast cancers. Eur J Cancer 1992;28A:896.

99. Spyratos F, Brifford M, Tubiana-Hulin M, et al. Sequential cytopunctures during preoperative chemotherapy for primary breast carcinoma. Cancer 1992;69:470.

100. Remvikos Y, Jouve M, Beuzeboc P, et al. Cell cycle modifications of breast cancers during neoadjuvant chemotherapy: a flow cytometry study on fine needle aspirates. Eur J Cancer 1995;29A:1843.

101. Chevallier B, Asselain B, Kunlin A, et al. Inflammatory breast cancer: determination of prognostic factors by univariate and multivariate analysis. Cancer 1987;60:897.

102. Delarue JC, May-Levin F, Mouriesse H, et al. Oestrogen and progesterone cytosolic receptors in clinically inflammatory tumours of the human breast. Br J Cancer 1981;44:911.

103. Paradiso A, Tommasi S, Brandi M, et al. Cell kinetics and hormonal receptor status in inflammatory breast carcinoma. Cancer 1989;64:1922.

104. Hortobagyi GN. Overview of new treatments for breast cancer. Breast Cancer Res Treat 1992;21:3.

105. Holmes FA, Walters RS, Theriault RL, et al. Phase II trial of Taxol, an active drug in the treatment of metastatic breast cancer. J Natl Cancer Inst 1991;83:1797.

106. Pazdur R, Kudelka AP, Kavanagh JJ, et al. The taxoids: paclitaxel (Taxol) and docetaxel (Taxotere). Cancer Treat Rev 1993;19:351.

107. Goodman GE, Hellstrom I, Brodzinsky L, et al. Phase I trial of murine monoclonal antibody L6 in breast, colon, ovarian, and lung cancer. J Clin Oncol 1990;8:1083.

108. Baselga J, Norton L, Masui H, et al. Antitumor effects of doxorubicin in combination with anti-epidermal growth factor receptor monoclonal antibodies. J Natl Cancer Inst 1993;85:1327.

109. Trail PA, Willner SJ, Lasch AJ, et al. Cure of xenografted human carcinomas by BR96–doxorubicin immunoconjugates. Science 1993;261:212.

110. Platini C, Weber B, Luporsi E. Low efficiency of vinorelbine/ 5-fluorouracil combination in previously treated metastatic breast cancer patients. (Abstract) Proc IVth International Congress on Anticancer Chemotherapy, 1993;145.

111. Cigolari S, Lucariello A, Albore S, et al. Navelbine and 5-fluorouracil combination in metastatic breast cancer failed to prior chemotherapy. (Abstract) Proceedings of the IVth International Congress on Anticancer Chemotherapy, 1993;148.

112. Spielmann M, Dorval T, Turpin F, et al. Phase II study with navelbine–adriamycin combination in advanced breast cancer. (Abstract) Proc Am Soc Clin Oncol 1991;10:66.

113. Galvez CA, Botto HG, Botto I, et al. Chemotherapy with mitoxantrone, ifosfamide and navelbine as third line chemotherapy in advanced breast cancer. (Abstract) Ann Oncol 1992;(Suppl 5)3:84.

114. Turpin F, Namer M, Spielmann M, et al. Phase II trial of datelliptium chloride hydrochloride in metastatic breast cancer. (Abstract) Proc Am Assoc Cancer Res 1992;33:214.

115. Ferrero JM, Wendling JL, Hoch M, et al. Mitoxantrone–vinorelbine as first line chemotherapy in metastatic breast cancer: a pilot study. (Abstract) Proceedings of the IVth International Congress on Anticancer Chemotherapy, 1993;222.

116. Rosso R, Amoroso D, Gardin G, et al. Lonidamine in metastatic breast cancer. Semin Oncol 1991;(Suppl 4)18:62.

117. ten Bokkel Huinink WW, Hilton A, Somers R. Topical application of miltefosine against skin metastases of breast cancer. (Abstract) Ann Oncol 1992;(Suppl 1)3:65.

118. Hansen R, Quebbeman E, Beatty P, et al. Continuous 5-fluorouracil infusion in refractory carcinoma of the breast. Breast Cancer Res Treat 1987;10:145.

119. Alberto P, Schafer P, Mermillod B, et al. Traitement combine des cancers inflammatoires du sein par chimiotherapie suivie de chirurgie et de radiotherapie. In: Jacquillat C, Weil M, Khayat D, eds. Neo-adjuvant chemotherapy. London, John Libbey, 1986:237.

120. Ferriere JP, Bignon YJ, Legros M, et al. Resultats du traitement des cancers inflammatoires du sein par une association therapeutique comportant une chimiotherapie initiale. In: Jacquillat C, Weil M, Khayat D, eds. Neo-adjuvant chemotherapy. London, John Libbey, 1986:271.

121. Pourny C, Nguyen TD, Nzengu B, et al. Traitements par chimiotherapie premiere de cancers du sein MO, localement avances (T3–T4) ou s'accompagnant de signes inflammatoires locaux. In: Jacquillat C, Weil M, Khayat D, eds. Neo-adjuvant chemotherapy. London, John Libbey, 1986:293.

122. Chevallier B, Bastit P, Graic Y, et al. The Centre H. Becquerel studies in inflammatory non metastatic breast cancer: combined modality approach in 178 patients. Br J Cancer 1993;67:594.

123. Maloisel F, Dufour P, Bergerat JP, et al. Results of initial doxorubicin, 5-fluorouracil, and cyclophosphamide combination chemotherapy for inflammatory carcinoma of the breast. Cancer 1990;65:851.

Diseases of the Breast, edited by Jay R. Harris, Marc E. Lippman, Monica Morrow, and Samuel Hellman. Lippincott-Raven Publishers, Philadelphia, © 1996.

19

Breast Reconstruction

19.1
Reconstructive Breast Surgery

GREG J. MACKAY ▪ JOHN BOSTWICK III

During the past two decades, breast reconstruction has become an integral part of the treatment plan and management of breast cancer. Women now expect the treatment of breast cancer to include either breast preservation or breast reconstruction. Recent advances in devices to expand skin, materials for reconstruction, endoscopic surgery, and sources of autogenous tissues, together with advances in microsurgery, have improved the aesthetic and functional outcome of breast reconstruction. Several studies have provided reassurance that well-planned breast reconstruction does not affect the detection of local recurrent disease.[1,2]

Psychologic Aspects

Any change in body image requires psychologic adjustment, but the importance of breasts as a primary symbol of femininity makes the loss of a breast especially difficult.[3-5] The emotional devastation that can accompany mastectomy has only recently been fully recognized. Researchers now have documented in the aggregate what most of our patients have told us individually: the breast is a symbol of femininity, and for many women, its loss brings about depression and lowered self-esteem that may last for years. This is illustrated poignantly by the return to reconstructive surgeons' offices of women in their sixth or sometimes seventh decade who had lost a breast 20 or 30 years earlier and who wonder whether the new procedures in the field might ease the loss they still feel.[6] Many women, perhaps *most* women, equate their breasts, not their reproductive organs, with the male genitalia; to these women, breast loss has nothing to do with whether they are past their childbearing years. They mourn the destruction of their body image—the image we have of ourselves as whole and valuable.[7]

For many women, the threat to femininity is a more psychologically damaging aspect of breast cancer than is the fear of death. One psychiatric study reported that one in four women considered suicide after mastectomy.[6] External prostheses do little if anything to improve a woman's body image or to diminish the sense of deformity after mastectomy. Breast reconstruction does both, especially if the reconstruction is part of the initial planning and begins as soon as possible after the mastectomy.

Breast Management Team

The goal of modern breast reconstruction is to alleviate the deformity of the breast and chest wall that results from virtually all local treatments of breast cancer; to construct breasts that meet the patient's expectations, both aesthetically and psychologically; and to adhere faithfully to sound oncologic management. Central to the numerous decisions about the timing, type, and extent of breast reconstruction is the primary goal of the best possible management of the cancer itself. Under ideal circumstances and, indeed, under what increasingly is the usual circumstance, the reconstructive surgeon is part of a team of medical specialists who focus on the optimal management of the breast cancer patient.[8,9] This team includes the oncologic surgeon, medical oncologist, and radiation oncologist, as well as adjunctive members, such as the family physician, pathologist, psychiatrist, social worker, and nurse. It is essential that the reconstructive surgeon be brought into this team from the beginning, especially during the initial treatment planning, because the patient's clinical status and the type of local treatment are significant determinants of the reconstructive options. Furthermore, awareness of the possibility of breast reconstruction may influence the patient's choice of local treatment for breast cancer as well as lessen the psychologic trauma of the diagnosis.

Timing of Breast Reconstruction

Breast reconstruction must be integrated into the initial treatment plan for the patient. The psychologic effects on the patient, in both facing deformity and willingness to consider more conservative approaches to treatment, have already been described.

Central to the numerous decisions about the timing, type, and extent of breast reconstruction is place of reconstruction in the primary goal of the entire breast cancer management team—to provide the best management possible of the breast cancer itself. Earlier in the history of breast reconstruction, physicians urged women to "live with" their mastectomies for a time, believing this period offered a chance for some emotional recuperation from and adjustment to the loss of the breast and gave the women a perspective from which they would better appreciate the reconstruction as reconstruction, rather than expect it to restore their original breasts as if by magic.[10,11] This is no longer the assumption.[12] Depending on the patient's wishes and clinical status, as well as the treatment plan of the team, breast reconstruction can be delayed indefinitely or can begin at the time of the local surgical treatment.

IMMEDIATE RECONSTRUCTION

Since its introduction in the late 1970s, breast reconstruction immediately after mastectomy has generated many concerns about follow-up and primary treatment of the breast cancer. Implantation of a silicone implant had been feared as a potential promoter of tumor recurrence and as a link to autoimmune disease. No evidence has been found to uphold these concerns.[13,14] Seeding of tumor cells in surgical planes, alteration of mastectomy technique to accommodate immediate reconstruction, and the ability to detect and treat locally recurrent breast cancer when a breast prosthesis is in place are concerns that have been addressed in numerous studies.[15,16] It has become increasingly clear that the biology of breast cancer is not altered by breast reconstruction, nor is the ability to detect or treat local recurrences altered by reconstruction. The recognition that the presence of axillary node metastases is the greatest risk factor for both local and distant treatment

failure allows the selection of some women who can be presumed to be at a higher risk for local failure postoperatively, however. Women at higher risk for local failure, particularly those with stage III disease, may benefit from postoperative radiation therapy of the chest wall. Because a significant rate of capsular contracture is seen in women with implants or expanders placed after radiation therapy, this group of patients should be considered for either flap reconstruction or delayed reconstruction (Fig. 19.1-1).

Immediate reconstruction has become the standard of care during the past 10 years not only because of the beneficial psychologic aspects for women but also because of the advanced surgical techniques, the improved aesthetic result, and the reduced cost and hospitalization.[17]

DELAYED RECONSTRUCTION

Delayed reconstruction can be performed anytime after the initial mastectomy or lumpectomy, even up to 40 years later. We advocate immediate reconstruction in most patients, but delayed reconstruction has certain benefits. Delaying reconstruction affords the woman the time to recover from mastectomy, to recover from adjunctive therapy, to get acquainted with her plastic surgeon, and to make an informed decision. The downside to delayed reconstruction is manifold:

1. It gives the patient more time to dwell on the cancer.
2. The patient may experience depression from the mastectomy status.

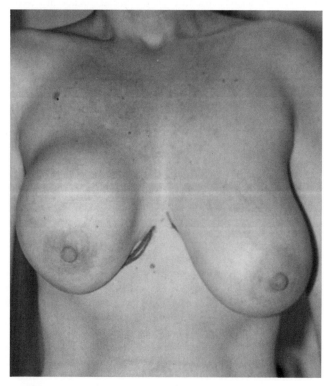

FIGURE 19.1-1 Lumpectomy and radiation therapy have been performed on the right breast in a patient with silicone implants.

3. The patient may never "get around" to having reconstruction.
4. Two surgeries and two anesthetics are associated with additional time and cost.

As discussed earlier, certain patients with advanced breast cancer may require extensive postoperative radiation therapy or chemotherapy and might benefit from a delay in reconstruction.

Techniques of Reconstruction

A main reason to involve the reconstructive surgeon in the treatment planning of a breast cancer patient is that the mastectomy technique selected by the oncologic surgeon affects the mastectomy deformity and consequently the technique of breast reconstruction.[18-20] The position of the surgical incision and amount of skin preserved during the mastectomy can facilitate the aesthetic outcome of immediate breast reconstruction, thereby obviating the need for surgery on the opposite breast to achieve symmetry (Fig. 19.1-2).

Until the mid-1970s, the most common technique of breast reconstruction was implant placement.[21,22] With the development of tissue expanders and their placement at the mastectomy site, implants could readily be used in almost any postmastectomy patient after expansion. Breast reconstruction using the tissues that remain after mastectomy, together with a breast implant beneath the musculofascial layer, is the preferred method of reconstruction after

FIGURE 19.1-2 **A** and **B.** Modified radical mastectomy with reconstruction. **C** and **D.** Skin-preserving mastectomy with reconstruction.

both total mastectomy and modified radical mastectomy. A decision should be made during the initial planning of whether the available tissues are suitable or whether distant tissue in the form of a flap is necessary.

Breast implants have recently undergone evaluation by the US Food and Drug Administration (FDA). Consequently, only implants filled with saline solution are generally available for breast reconstruction. Implants filled with silicone gel are no longer available for implantation except under strict FDA study guidelines. No scientific evidence shows that silicone implants increase the incidence of breast cancer, but they may create difficulty for interpretation of mammograms, especially if a capsular contracture is present. Some concern has been raised about the possibility of an association between silicone breast implants and autoimmune conditions, but several studies have failed to show any link.[23]

After mastectomy, most patients either request autogenous tissue or require autogenous tissue for reconstruction because of a severe tissue deficit. Other women have one large and ptotic breast, which must be matched to create symmetry and aesthetic effect, and this requires larger amounts of tissue than are available at the treated site. For such patients, the surgeon can use additional skin or muscle from elsewhere on the body. The choice of distant tissue usually depends on the amount of muscle and tissue fill needed to create the appropriate breast mound, as well as the amount of fat, muscle, and skin available in various areas of the woman's body. The different amounts of blood flow needed by various flaps for adequate microcirculation are sometimes a factor, particularly for women who smoke (thereby compromising the needed circulation) and for those with health problems that can damage the microcirculation, such as diabetes mellitus. The three

FIGURE 19.1-3 A. Saline implant. **B.** Implant placed in submuscular pocket.

types of flaps most commonly used, in descending order, are the latissimus dorsi flap from the back, the transverse rectus abdominis musculocutaneous (TRAM) flap from the lower abdomen, and the gluteus maximus musculocutaneous flap from the buttocks.

BREAST RECONSTRUCTION WITH AVAILABLE TISSUE AND SALINE IMPLANTS

The simplest procedure for breast reconstruction involves the use of available tissue and the placement of an implant. This method requires only that the tissues be of good quantity and quality after mastectomy. It works best when the patient's opposite breast is small to moderate with minimal ptosis.

The reconstructive surgeon positions the breast implant beneath the musculofascial layer of the chest wall.[24,25] A pocket beneath the pectoral muscles is created, and the implant is secured into the desired position (Fig. 19.1-3). This procedure can be done immediately or at any time after the mastectomy. Generally, it adds only 1 hour to the operative time after the mastectomy. Because the tight tissues of the mastectomy site are gradually stretched by the implant, the final result is not achieved until several months after the implant is placed (Fig. 19.1-4).

The most common problem of breast reconstruction with implant placement is the development of a capsular contracture about the implant, resulting in a spherical contour.[26] Placement of the implant beneath the pectoral muscle, rather than in the subcutaneous tissues, lessens the likelihood of contracture development.[27] Saline-filled implants and textured implants, when compared with gel-filled silicone implants, reduce the incidence of capsular contracture.[28–30] Inflatable saline implants have their own set of associated problems, however, including their liquid feel, their higher deflation rate, and their palpable folds and valves, which can occasionally produce a visible rippling effect across the breast, especially when the textured devices are used.

TISSUE EXPANSION

Reconstruction of the breast by tissue expansion was introduced by Radovan in 1982.[31] This technique allowed for creation of a breast mound in women using local tissues and decreased the need for musculocutaneous flaps. Creation of a breast that required an implant larger than 250 cc was often associated with an increased rate of breakdown of overlying tissue, exposure and extrusion of the implant, or significant capsular contracture. Using the principles of tissue expansion, a larger and more ptotic breast could be produced to more closely match the opposite breast in women who required this.

This relatively simple technique involves gradually stretching the tissues of the chest wall to recruit sufficient cover for an implant that is larger than the one that could be positioned during an initial operation. This reduces the tightness and subsequent firmness of the chest wall against the implant. The expander consists of an outer envelope made of silicone, which is connected to a fill valve that is injected with saline. The tissue expander is generally placed under the pectoral muscle in the musculofascial layer immediately after the mastectomy. After the mastectomy wound has healed, the tissue expander is gradually inflated with saline during a period of 6 to 8 weeks (Fig. 19.1-5). The expander is overfilled about 200 cc beyond the volume of the opposite breast and is kept overfilled for several months so the tissues can accommodate the expanded condition. During a second operation, the tissue expander is replaced with a permanent breast implant that is symmetric to the opposite breast.

An expansion device that can be converted to a permanent implant without a second operation has been used for several years with good success.[32] This biluminal device

FIGURE 19.1-4   Postmastectomy of the left breast with submuscular implant reconstruction.

FIGURE 19.1-5 A and **B.** Submuscular expander. **C.** Filling the expander.

has saline and silicone gel reservoirs. After satisfactory size and position are obtained, the fill valve of the implant is removed, and the device becomes a permanent double-lumen breast implant.

The great advantage of tissue expansion is that it permits breast reconstruction without the use of distant flaps, simplifying reconstruction and minimizing scarring. The slight disadvantages are the time involved and the possible complications. Patient selection is important. Even with maximal expansion, it is difficult to produce a large, ptotic breast. As with all implants, complications include expander extrusion, infection, and expander deflation. Obese patients and those who have received chest wall radiation therapy are especially prone to failure.[33]

FLAP PROCEDURES

The options of placement of a simple saline breast implant under the musculofascial layer and tissue expansion are not available to some women who have a large and ptotic opposite breast that necessitates construction of a larger matching breast. Many women with one full breast prefer a flap transfer—with the scars hidden on the back, abdomen, or buttocks—to reduction surgery on the opposite, unscarred breast. If the tissues of the mastectomy are relatively tight, tissue expansion techniques will not provide a satisfactory breast reconstruction. For these women, it is necessary to use a flap of distant tissue for reconstruction. Transfer of tissue with its own blood supply is also necessary when the patient's own tissue is damaged, which occurs with radiation ulcers of radionecrosis involving bone.

The choice of distant tissue usually depends on two factors: (1) the amount of muscle and tissue fill needed for the chest, and (2) the amount of fat, muscle, and skin available in various other areas of the body. Although the success of all flaps depends on good microcirculation, some flaps require a larger blood flow for survival than do others. Women are told explicitly that cigarette smoking can compromise the needed circulation, as can other factors, especially diabetes mellitus.

LATISSIMUS DORSI MUSCULOCUTANEOUS FLAP

The latissimus dorsi musculocutaneous flap was first reported for chest wall reconstruction by d'Este in 1912.[34] It was introduced for breast reconstruction in 1977 by Schnieder and associates.[35] This flap of skin, fat, and muscle from the upper back is the flap of choice when it is necessary to replace the missing pectoralis major muscle from the upper breast area and axilla.[36] It also is useful as a supplement to the skin and for additional muscle cover for the breast implant when the breast reconstruction must be fuller and have some ptosis. Thin women who are not candidates for the TRAM flap are the most frequent candidates for this particular flap. Tight or irradiated skin is another good indication for this procedure.

The anatomy of the latissimus dorsi muscle contributes to its usefulness in breast reconstruction. It is a large triangular muscle of the back whose origin is from the lower six thoracic vertebrae and whose insertion is by a short tendon into the humerus. The thoracodorsal pedicle is its main blood supply. The muscle can be completely freed from its origin and insertion, remaining attached only by its thoracodorsal pedicle, and can be swung around from the back to fill a breast defect. The muscle is then sutured to the lower margin of the pectoralis major muscle and along the inframammary fold (Fig. 19.1-6).

The flap is planned on the back to replace the missing tissue and to permit the introduction of a breast implant beneath it to give the proper size and shape to the reconstructed breast. The design of the flap and its accompanying skin island is tailored to meet the type of mastectomy defect[22] (Fig. 19.1-7). If a large skin island is necessary, the skin of the back can be expanded before the latissimus dorsi reconstruction, allowing for a larger transfer of tissue.[37]

The latissimus dorsi flap is one of the safest and most reliable flaps used in reconstructive surgery. The incidence of total flap necrosis is less than 1% and of partial necrosis is below 5%.[38] Seroma at the donor site is the most common complication, with an incidence of 10% to 30%.[39,40] Capsular contracture around the implant remains a problem and has been reported in 20% to 50% of patients.[41] The transfer of this muscle does not cause a functional loss of shoulder strength. Although it is one of the safest and most reliable flaps, it has the disadvantage of a temporary loss of muscle or skin on the back and the resultant scarring in a part of the body that may be more visible than the sites of other potential flaps.

Thin women are the most frequent candidates for the latissimus dorsi musculocutaneous flap. Women who have extra lower abdominal tissue should be considered for TRAM flaps as the first-line option for reconstruction.

EXTENDED LATISSIMUS DORSI FLAP

The standard latissimus dorsi flap does not provide enough tissue or bulk to create a breast without the use of an accompanying implant. A modification of the latissimus dorsi ellipse, in which additional subcutaneous tissue is taken with the elevated flap, provides extra autogenous tissue for breast reconstruction. During harvest of the flap, subcutaneous tissue is preserved on the underlying latissimus dorsi muscle. This gives considerably more autogenous tissue but leaves a more significant donor scar and flattening of the back; the propensity for seroma formation is also greater. The extended latissimus flap often obviates the need for an accompanying implant in selected patients.[42,43]

TRAM FLAP

The TRAM flap is an ellipse of skin and fat from the lower abdomen that is attached to the rectus abdominis muscle. It was introduced in 1982 by Hartrampf and colleagues[44] and has become the flap of choice for breast reconstruction. The skin island is moved to the chest area and pedicled as a musculocutaneous flap on the upper rectus abdominis muscle (Figs. 19.1-8 to 19.1-10). When the amount of tissue required is relatively great, the TRAM flap can be moved to the breast area on two pedicles of rectus abdominis muscle. The blood supply is based on the superior epigastric artery, a terminal branch of the internal mammary artery. The vessels through the chest and the upper rectus abdominis muscle join the vessels of the deep inferior epigastric artery and then perforate up through the fascia around the umbilicus to supply blood to the fat and skin of the flap.

TRAM flaps have certain advantages:

1. Many women with large lower abdomens are pleased to have the extra tissue removed.
2. The donor scar is transverse and in the lower abdomen rather than on the back or side.
3. It is usually possible to give the proper breast contour without a breast implant.

When the amount of skin of the mastectomy is satisfactory, the outer covering of the skin of the flap can be deepithelialized and the flap positioned to provide the proper breast contour, which ordinarily depends on the use of an implant.

Breast reconstruction using a TRAM flap is a complex surgical procedure, and the need for an adequate blood supply is extremely important. Poor microcirculation in the flap can lead to fat necrosis in the flap, resulting in loss of portions of the flap and the subsequent development of hard, fibrotic areas in the reconstructed breast. Candidates for the TRAM flap must be selected carefully and critically to avoid serious complications. Long-term ciga-

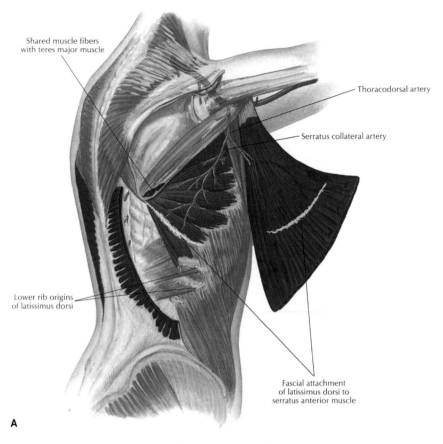

Shared muscle fibers
with teres major muscle

Thoracodorsal artery

Serratus collateral artery

Lower rib origins
of latissimus dorsi

Fascial attachment
of latissimus dorsi to
serratus anterior muscle

A

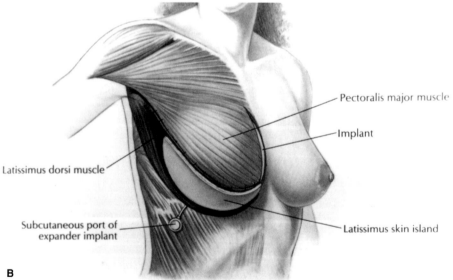

Pectoralis major muscle

Implant

Latissimus dorsi muscle

Subcutaneous port of
expander implant

Latissimus skin island

B

FIGURE 19.1-6 A. Latissimus muscle freed from posterior attachment. **B.** Latissimus muscle as used to reconstruct breast with expander.

FIGURE 19.1-7 **A.** Skin paddle to be used with latissimus muscle. **B.** Postoperative latissimus donor site scar.

rette smoking (more than 20 pack-years) has an acute and chronic effect on microcirculation and, in many centers, is a contraindication to the operation. Patients who are morbidly obese[45] and persons with diabetes mellitus or other diseases that cause microcirculatory problems also are likely to have compromised microcirculation of the TRAM flap. Flap compromise and necrosis also can result from heavy irradiation of the base of the flap or of the mediastinum, or from the surgical division of the superior epigastric pedicle, as might occur with a subcostal incision.

TRAM flap reconstruction is a highly technical procedure that generally requires a 5- to 7-day hospitalization and a 2- to 3-month recovery period. Complications involving the protrusion of the lower abdominal wall can usually be obviated with accurate abdominal closure and securing of the closure with Prolene mesh when indicated. The incidence of abdominal wall hernia is reported to be between 2% and 5%.[46-48] Results can be excellent and complications minimal if patients are well selected and the surgeon has the proper technical skills.[49,50]

FIGURE 19.1-8 TRAM flap elevated on rectus muscle to reconstruct left breast.

FIGURE 19.1-9 TRAM flap undergoing final reshaping and position of new umbilicus.

MICROVASCULAR TISSUE TRANSFER

When there is no local tissue or a pedicled flap is unavailable, microvascular tissue transfer, or a free flap, is sometimes the only means for breast reconstruction. Other candidates for free tissue transfer include patients who have several risk factors for pedicled tissue transfer, such as smoking, obesity, multiple abdominal scars, or a failed previous pedicle flap. The gluteus maximus musculocutaneous flap, based on either the superior or inferior gluteal artery, and the TRAM flap, based on the inferior epigastric pedicle, are the most popular flaps. Although more technically demanding and usually requiring somewhat more operative time, these flaps offer significant tissue for breast reconstruction and therefore superb results.

The free TRAM flap has better vascularity than the pedicled TRAM flap and requires less muscle dissection, while reducing abdominal wall morbidity. The inferior epigastric vessel has satisfactory pedicle length and is usually anastomosed to the thoracodorsal vessels (Fig. 19.1-11). In two reported series, the data have shown that the free TRAM flap is associated with a lower incidence of complications, a shorter hospitalization, and probably a faster recovery than the conventional TRAM flap[50] (Fig. 19.1-12). The major disadvantage of the free TRAM flap is that its viability depends entirely on the success of the microvascular anastomosis (Fig. 19.1-13). Failure of nour-

FIGURE 19.1-10 Final result of TRAM flap reconstruction of the left breast.

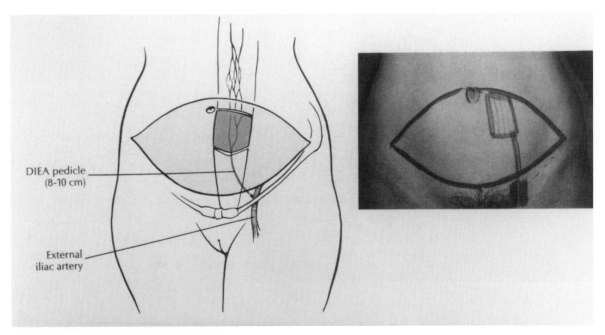

FIGURE 19.1-11   Free TRAM flap based on interior epigastric vessels.

ishing blood flow can result in tissue death within 6 hours and complete flap loss.

The gluteus maximus flap is another good option for a free muscle tissue transfer, since most women, even when thin, have adequate tissue in the buttocks for use in breast reconstruction (Fig. 19.1-14). The gluteus maximus has the added advantage that the donor scar can be hidden at the fold of the buttocks area (Fig. 19.1-15). The procedure is less painful and the recovery less prolonged than with the TRAM flap procedure.

The tissue needed for breast reconstruction, along with a segment of the gluteus maximus muscle, is elevated on its vascular pedicle.[51,52] The internal mammary artery or

axillary vessels are prepared, and the buttocks tissue is transferred with microvascular technique and anastomosed to the internal mammary artery. Gluteal flaps are used when other options are not available, since they are generally technically more demanding than the free TRAM flap (Fig. 19.1-16).

Endoscopically Assisted Breast Reconstruction

The increasing acceptance of wide excision and radiation therapy as the treatment of choice for early-stage breast cancer has presented the reconstructive breast surgeon with smaller breast incisions and smaller defects to reconstruct.[53] Lumpectomy allows a woman to maintain most of her natural breast tissue, but a significant cosmetic defect can remain after the surgery and subsequent radiation therapy[54] (Fig. 19.1-17). The recent introduction of the endoscope into plastic surgery has allowed the latissimus muscle to be harvested through small incisions placed in the axillary line[55] (Fig. 19.1-18). Harvested endoscopically, a portion of the latissimus muscle can be rotated around to fill the lumpectomy defect with the advantage of no additional scar on the back.

Reconstruction of the lumpectomy defect has improved, but the best timing of breast reconstruction in a patient that has undergone radiation therapy and lumpectomy has not yet been determined. Many questions remain about exactly when the breast appearance stabilizes and when the fibrosis and retraction from radiation subside. Cancer surveillance in a patient who undergoes breast

FIGURE 19.1-12   Free TRAM flap reconstruction of left breast. (Courtesy of G.W. Carlson, Emory University)

FIGURE 19.1-13   Microvascular anastomosis of inferior epigastric vessels to thoracodorsal vessels.

reconstruction after radiation therapy and lumpectomy may prove to be more difficult, because the differentiation of new cancerous lesions from microcalcifications, fibroadenomas, and fat necrosis by physical examination and mammography is complicated by the reconstruction. It is hoped that long-term studies involving large patient populations will resolve many of these issues.

Chest Wall Reconstruction After Radiation Therapy

Complications of radiation therapy after adjunctive or therapeutic management are rare but often devastating. These are usually major sequelae such as osteoradionecrosis

of the chest wall, chest wall ulceration, induction of second primary carcinomas, and complications from the reduced blood supply in the irradiated area. Reconstructive techniques for these problems usually require the excision of the damaged tissue and reconstruction with large flaps that have their own blood supply.

Characteristically painful and malodorous, radionecrotic wounds of the chest wall pose a threat to the patient's life. They often involve the full thickness of the chest wall and threaten mediastinal vessels, the heart, and intrathoracic organs.

The method of closure of these wounds is influenced by the site of the radiation damage and possible compromise of the vascular pedicle of the proposed flaps. Excision of the affected irradiated tissue creates a large chest

FIGURE 19.1-14   Postoperative left breast reconstruction with gluteus maximus musculocutaneous flap.

FIGURE 19.1-15 Postoperative scar on right buttock after harvest of gluteus maximus flap.

wall defect. The TRAM flap is usually the preferred flap for closure of the wound, because it brings in a well-vascularized muscle with a large associated skin paddle for closure. If the radiation injury is centered over the inframammary vessels, a double-pedicle TRAM flap, vertical TRAM flap, or free TRAM flap is indicated (Fig. 19.1-19).

The latissimus dorsi musculocutaneous flap is another option. It can provide muscle for filling the defect and an associated skin paddle for wound closure. The latissimus dorsi flap is not the primary choice, however, when radiation damage is heavy in the lower axilla over the thoracodorsal pedicle (Table 19.1-1).

Reconstruction of the Nipple and Areola

Nipple–areolar reconstruction provides the finishing touch that contributes to a natural and realistic breast appearance. This is almost always performed as a separate procedure after satisfactory breast symmetry has been achieved.

Earlier nipple reconstruction often used tissue taken from an opposite large nipple. Nipple–areolar reconstruc-

FIGURE 19.1-16 Inferior gluteus maximus flap markings drawn before surgery.

FIGURE 19.1-17 Patient after lumpectomy and radiation therapy of the left breast.

FIGURE 19.1-18 Endoscopic harvest of the latissimus muscle minimizes the scar.

tions are optimal when donor material closely matches the opposite side. New procedures enable the reconstruction of the nipple with tissues available at the skin site of the new nipple. Two primary methods of nipple reconstruction use local tissue at the site of the future nipple and areola to build the new nipple—the skate flap (Fig. 19.1-20) and the C-V flap[56,57] (Fig. 19.1-21). With these techniques, a layer of skin and fat on the reconstructed breast is shifted to the center of what will be the future nipple–areolar area and formed into a nipple. The skin is used to create the nipple, and the underlying fat is used to add bulk, fullness, and permanent shape.

Areolar reconstruction should produce an areola that is symmetric and of proper diameter and color to match the areola of the opposite breast. Methods for recreating the areola range from simple tattooing to the more complex graft techniques. When local breast tissue is used for the nipple reconstruction, the tissue for the areolar graft is usually taken from the lateral portion of the mastectomy scar or the lateral portion of the abdominal scar if the patient had a TRAM flap (Fig. 19.1-22). After the nipple–areolar reconstruction is healed, the pigment can be refined with the use of intradermal tattoo[58] (Fig. 19.1-23).

FIGURE 19.1-19 A. Necrosis of the chest wall after lumpectomy and radiation therapy. **B.** Chest wall and breast reconstruction with TRAM flap. Mastopexyaugmentation was performed on the right breast.

TABLE 19-1
Comparison of Breast Reconstruction Procedures

Type	Advantages	Disadvantages	Indications	Contradications
Implant	Short operative time One-stage procedure Low cost	Capsular contracture Rupture of implant Implant leakage Autoimmune disease (<0.5%)	Small breast (400–600 cc)	Thin flaps Radiation therapy
Tissue expander and implant	Short operative time Low cost	Multiple expansions Capsular contracture Rupture of implant Implant leakage	Medium size breast (400–800 cc) Mild to moderate ptosis	Thin flaps Radiation therapy
Latissimus dorsi flap Muscle only	Autogenous tissue Small donor scar	Minor muscle dysfunction Seroma formation Flap necrosis	Small to medium size breast Lumpectomy defect Tight irradiated skin	None
Skin paddle	Autogenous tissue	Moderate donor scar Seroma formation Minor muscle dysfunction Flap necrosis	All breast defects	None
TRAM flap Unipedicle	Autogenous tissue Abdominoplasty scar	Added donor scar Minor muscle dysfunction Extended operative time 2- to 3-month recovery time Abdominal wall hernia Fat necrosis	All breast defects	Previous abdominal surgery
Bipedicle	Autogenous tissue Abdominoplasty	Added donor scar Seroma formation Minor muscle dysfunction 2- to 3-month recovery time Abdominal wall hernia Fat necrosis	Cigarette smokers Moderate obesity Previous abdominal surgery	None
Free tissue transfer (gluteal TRAM flap)	Autogenous tissue	Donor site scar 2- to 3-month recovery time Extended operative time Flap failure	Cigarette smokers Previous adbominal surgery	None

The upper inner thigh is a source of skin with a color match most approximating the areola and can be used for areola reconstruction. This technique, however, involves a painful donor site and scar and is rarely used.

Management of the Opposite Breast

The goal of breast reconstruction is to provide the patient with aesthetically pleasing, symmetric breasts. Some women resist any procedure on the unscarred breast, but many are open to the surgeon's suggestions for making the opposite breast more attractive and easier to match in reconstruction.

When the opposite breast is small and flat, it may need a breast implant. Any enlargement of the opposite breast must be planned to match the reconstructed breast. The breast implant is placed in the submusculofascial position behind the breast tissue, where it will not interfere with future breast observation, imaging, and treatment.

When the opposite breast is hypoplastic and ptotic, it can be corrected with a submusculofascial breast implant and a mastopexy to elevate with nipple and areola and to remove excess skin vertically beneath the nipple and areola and, if necessary, horizontally in the inframammary crease.

When the opposite breast is enlarged and heavy, a reduction mammaplasty can usually be performed at the time of the breast reconstruction, so that the breast reconstruction (often with a lower TRAM flap) can be performed to match the reduced breast[59] (Fig. 19.1-24).

Prophylactic Mastectomy

Prophylactic mastectomy is a controversial operation sometimes performed for women who are considered at high risk of developing breast cancer. Prophylactic mastec-

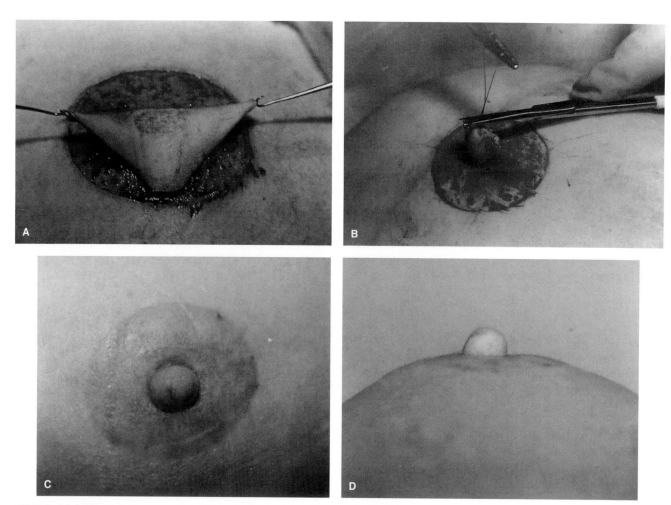

FIGURE 19.1-20 The skate flap. **A.** Elevating the flap at the determined nipple site. **B.** Forming the nipple. **C** and **D.** The final result.

FIGURE 19.1-21 The C-V flap for nipple reconstruction.

FIGURE 19.1-22 Reconstruction of the areola using skin from the mastectomy scar.

tomy can cause serious aesthetic and psychologic problems, as well as operative complications.[60] It is associated with complications such as infection and hematoma. Perhaps most significantly, it is not an absolute guarantee of breast cancer prevention. In short, women considering prophylactic mastectomy should obtain several professional opinions and weigh the risks and benefits of the operation before making a decision.

For women who elect to undergo prophylactic mastectomy, it should be a total mastectomy that removes most of the breast tissue at risk. The subcutaneous mastectomy incisions at the inframammary crease or that extend laterally around the areola provide good access for the mastectomy. If no significant breast ptosis is present, the nipple and areola can be preserved with the breast skin. With mammary ptosis, excess skin is removed and the nipple–areolar complex is moved to its new position with a skin-grafting technique. Breast reconstruction is now done at the time of the prophylactic mastectomy as an immediate procedure. A breast implant is placed beneath the muscular layer if desired. If the tissues are tight, a tissue expander is placed beneath the musculofascial layer and inflated a few weeks after the tissues have healed.

Summary

Advances in breast reconstruction, especially those involving transposition of muscle and skin flaps, have improved the quality and aesthetic outcome of breast reconstruction. For many women, the availability of procedures to restore realistic and natural breast shape after mastectomy or lumpectomy has significant impact on their emotional stability and social adjustment after breast cancer surgery. Furthermore, knowledge and consideration of breast reconstruction can be an important part of a woman's decision to seek screening in the first place and to choose among treatment alternatives if breast cancer is found.

FIGURE 19.1-23 Pigments used to produce the proper color match for the new areola.

FIGURE 19.1-24 A. Patient postmastectomy with a large ptotic right breast. **B.** Postoperative result after reduction mammaplasty of the right breast and TRAM reconstruction of the left breast.

It is essential that the reconstructive surgeon be part of the breast cancer management team from the beginning of treatment planning and that he or she work closely with the general surgeon, medical oncologist, radiation therapist, and adjunctive treatment team members. The patient's clinical status and the type of local treatment are significant determinants of the reconstructive options.

In the past decade, the use of the modified radical mastectomy has decreased significantly in the treatment of stage I and II breast cancer, whereas the use of conservative breast surgery with adjunctive radiation therapy has steadily increased. Lumpectomy and skin-preserving mastectomy have allowed for reconstruction of more natural-looking, aesthetically pleasing breasts. The promise of attractive, symmetric, and natural-appearing breasts, complete with a nipple–areolar complex, has somewhat eased the diminishment of self-esteem and the threat to feminity that often accompany the loss of a breast. Wide recognition of the availability of breast reconstruction may encourage more women to monitor their breasts and to seek diagnosis of changes, and it may influence selection of the type of local treatment if cancer is detected.

References

1. Noone RB, Frazier TG, Noone GC, et al. Recurrence of breast carcinoma following immediate reconstruction: a 13-year review. Plast Reconstr Surg 1994;93:96.
2. Webster DJT, Mansel RE, Hughes LE. Immediate reconstruction of the breast after mastectomy. Is it safe? Cancer 1984;53:1416.
3. Berger K, Bostwick J. A woman's decision: breast care, treatment, and reconstruction, ed 2. St Louis, Quality Medical, 1994.
4. Bostwick J. Plastic and reconstructive breast surgery. St Louis, Quality Medical, 1990.
5. Schain WS, Jacobs E, Wellisch DK. Psychosocial issues in breast reconstruction: intrapsychic, intrapersonal, and practical concerns. Clin Plast Surg 1984;11:237.
6. Goin JM, Goin MK. Changing the body: psychological effects of plastic surgery. Baltimore, Williams & Wilkins, 1981.
7. Graham J. In the company of others: understanding the human needs of cancer patients. New York, Harcourt Brace Jovanovich, 1982.
8. Bostwick J. Breast cancer: strategies for the 1990s. II. Reconstruction after mastectomy. Surg Clin North Am. 1990;70:5;1125.
9. Bostwick J. Breast reconstruction after mastectomy: an update. In: Wise L, Johnson H Jr, eds. Breast cancer: controversies in management. New York, Futura, 1994:259.
10. Teimourian B, Adham MN. Survey of patients' responses to breast reconstruction. Ann Plast Surg 1982;9:321.
11. Klein R. A crisis to grow on. Cancer 1971;28:1660.
12. Wellisch KD, Schain WS, Noone RB, et al. Psychosocial correlates of immediate versus delayed reconstruction of the breast. Plast Reconstr Surg 1985;76:713.
13. Park AJ, Black KRJ, Watson A. Silicone gel breast implants, breast cancer and connective tissue disorders. Br J Surg 1993;80:1097.
14. Schusterman MA, Kroll SS, Reece GP, et al. Incidence of autoimmune disease in patients after breast reconstruction with silicone gel implants versus autogenous tissue: a preliminary report. Ann Plast Surg 1993;31:1.
15. Kroll SS, Ames F, Singletary SE, et al. The oncologic risks of skin preservation at mastectomy when combined with immediate reconstruction of the breast. Surg Gynecol Obstet 1991;172:17.
16. Johnson CH, vanHeerden JA, Donohue JH, et al. Oncological aspects of immediate breast reconstruction following mastectomy for malignancy. Arch Surg 1989;124:819.
17. Trabulsy PP, Anthony JP, Mathes SJ. Changing trends in postmastec-

tomy breast reconstruction: a 13-year experience. Plast Reconstr Surg 1994;93:1418.

18. Farley DR, Meland NB. Importance of breast biopsy in final outcome of breast reconstruction. Mayo Clin Proc 1992;67:1050.

19. Silverstein MJ, Murphy GP, Bostwick J, et al. Breast reconstruction: state of the art for the 1990s. Cancer 1991;68:1180.

20. Kroll SS, Ames F, Singletary SE, et al. The oncologic risks of skin preservation at mastectomy when combined with immediate reconstruction of the breast. Surg Gynecol Obstet 1991;172:17.

21. Bostwick J, Vasconez LO, Jurkiewicz MJ. Breast reconstruction after a radical mastectomy. Plast Reconstr Surg 1978;61:682.

22. Woods JE, Irons GB, Arnold PG. The case for submuscular implantation of prostheses in reconstructive breast surgery. Ann Plast Surg 1980;5:115.

23. Gabriel SE, O'Fallon WM, Kurland LT, et al. Risk of connective-tissue diseases and other disorders after breast implantation. N Engl J Med 1994;330:1697.

24. Little JW III, Golembe EV, Fischer JB. The "living bra" in immediate and delayed reconstruction of the breast following mastectomy for malignant and nonmalignant disease. Plast Reconstr Surg 1981;68:392.

25. Woods JE, Irons GB Jr, Arnold PG. The case for submuscular implantation of prostheses in reconstructive breast surgery. Ann Plast Surg 1980;5:115.

26. Asplund O. Capsular contracture and silicone gel and saline-filled breast implants after reconstruction. Plast Reconstr Surg 1984;73:270.

27. Gruber RP, Kahn RA, Lash H. Breast reconstruction following mastectomy: a comparison of submuscular and subcutaneous techniques. Plast Reconstr Surg 1981;67:312.

28. Burkhardt BR. Capsular contracture: hard breasts, soft data. Clin Plast Surg 1988;15:521.

29. McKinney P, Tresley G. Long-term comparison of patients with gel and saline mammary implants. Plast Reconstr Surg 1983;72:27.

30. Maxwell GP, Falcone PA. Eighty four consecutive breast reconstructions using a textured silicone expander. Plast Reconstr Surg 1992;89:1022.

31. Radovan C. Tissue expansion in soft-tissue reconstruction. Plast Reconstr Surg 1983;74:482.

32. Becker H. The expandable mammary implant. Plast Reconstr Surg. 1985;79:631.

33. Carlson GW. Breast reconstruction: surgical options and patient selection. Cancer 1994;74:436.

34. d'Este S. La technique de l'amputation de la mammelle pour carcinome mammaire. Rev Chir 1912;45:164.

35. Schneider WJ, Hill LH, Brown RG. Latissimus dorsi myocutaneous flap for breast reconstruction. Br J Plast Surg 1981;30:286.

36. Bostwick J, Vasconez LO, Jurkiewicz MJ. Breast reconstruction after a radical mastectomy. Plast Reconstr Surg 1978;61:381.

37. Slavin SA. Improving the latissimus dorsi myocutaneous flap with tissue expansion. Plast Reconstr Surg 1994;93:811.

38. Moore TS, Farrell LD. Latissimus dorsi myocutaneous flap for breast reconstruction: long-term results. Plast Reconstr Surg 1992;89:666.

39. Bostwick J, Scheflan M. The latissimus dorsi musculocutaneous flap: one-stage breast reconstruction. Clin Plast Surg 1980;7:71.

40. Kroll SS, Baldwin B. A comparison of outcomes using three different methods of breast reconstruction. Plast Reconstr Surg 1992;90:455.

41. McGraw JB, Maxwell GP. Early and late capsular "deformation" as a cause of unsatisfactory results in the latissimus dorsi breast reconstruction. Clin Plast Surg 1988;15:717.

42. Bostwick J. Latissimus dorsi flap reconstruction. In: Plastic and reconstructive breast surgery. St Louis, Quality Medical, 1990:700.

43. Hokin JAB, Silverkiold KL. Breast reconstruction without an implant: results and complications using an extended latissimus dorsi flap. Plast Reconstr Surg 1987;79:58.

44. Hartrampf CR, Scheflan M, Black PW. Breast reconstruction with a transverse abdominal island flap. Plast Reconstr Surg 1982;69:216.

45. Kroll SS, Netscher DT. Complications of TRAM flap breast reconstruction in obese patients. Plast Reconstr Surg 1989;84:886.

46. Mizgala CL, Hartrampf CR, Bennett GK. Assessment of the abdominal wall after pedicled TRAM flap surgery: 5 to 7 year follow-up of 150 consecutive patients. Plast Reconstr Surg 1994;93:988.

47. Kroll SS, Marchi M. Comparison of strategies for preventing abdominal wall weakness after TRAM flap breast reconstruction. Plast Reconstr Surg 1992;89:1045.

48. Lejour M, Dome M. Abdominal wall function after rectus abdominis transfer. Plast Reconstr Surg 1991;87:1054.

49. Hartrampf CR, Bennett GK. Autogenous tissue reconstruction in the mastectomy patient: a critical review of 300 patients. Ann Surg 1987;205:508.

50. Elliot LF, Eskenazi L, Beegle PH, et al. Immediate TRAM flap breast reconstruction: 128 consecutive cases. Plast Reconstr Surg 1992;92:217.

51. Shaw WW. Breast reconstruction by superior gluteal microvascular free flaps without silicone implants. Plast Reconstr Surg 1983;72:490.

52. Paletta CE, Bostwick J, Nahai F. The inferior gluteal free flap in breast reconstruction. Plast Reconstr Surg 1989;84:875.

53. Fischer B, Redmond C, Poisson R, et al. Eight year results of a randomized clinical trial comparing total mastectomy and lumpectomy with or without irradiation in the treatment of breast cancer. N Engl J Med 1989;320:822.

54. Matory WE Jr, Wertheimer M, Fitzgerald TJ, et al. Aesthetic results following partial mastectomy and radiation therapy. Plast Reconstr Surg 1990;85:739.

55. Eaves FF, Price CI, Bostwick J III, et al. Subcutaneous endoscopic plastic surgery using a retractor mounted endoscopic system. Perspect Plast Surg 1993;7:1.

56. Little JW, Spear S. Nipple-areola reconstruction. Perspect Plast Surg 1988;2:1.

57. Eskenazi L. A one stage nipple reconstruction with the modified star flap and immediate tattoo: a review of 100 cases. Plast Reconstr Surg 1993;92:671.

58. Becker H. The use of intradermal tattoo to enhance the final result of nipple–areola reconstruction. Plast Reconstr Surg 1986;77:673.

59. Stevenson TR, Goldstein JA. TRAM flap breast reconstruction and contralateral reduction or mastopexy. Plast Reconstr Surg 1993;92:228.

60. Slade CL. Subcutaneous mastectomy: acute complications and long-term follow up. Plast Reconstr Surg 1984;73:84.

19.2

Silicone Autoimmune Disease

GAIL S. LEBOVIC ▪ DONALD R. LAUB

Silicone, once touted as the most biologically inert substance known to humans, has become the center of widespread debate. Laboratory and clinical data accumulated during the past 20 to 30 years suggest that silicone and its related chemical compounds cause a local inflammatory response, which can be severe.[1-6] But the question remains of whether silicone can activate a systemic immunologic response and whether this may manifest as a clinically significant disease entity. Retrospective epidemiologic studies both support and reject this hypothesis. Clinical studies supporting a direct link between silicone and autoimmune disorders remain sparse.

Despite the controversy, enough suspicion exists to have prompted the US Food and Drug Administration (FDA) to prohibit the use of silicone gel implants until sufficient evidence to prove their safety is obtained.[1] Presentation of anecdotal case reports and sensational news coverage relating to this topic have caused many women with silicone breast prostheses to request explantation (surgical removal of the implants) and financial remuneration. Because over 2 million women in the United States have breast implants, physicians specializing in breast diseases must become familiar with the clinical presentation, evaluation, and options for treating these women.

Historical Background

Before the advent of implants, breast enlargement was performed by direct injection of paraffin or liquid silicone into the breast. In many parts of the world, this type of breast augmentation still is common practice. In 1964, Miyoshi raised the first questions about the possible dangers of injecting various substances into the breast.[2-4] Subsequent reports described local inflammatory skin changes and subcutaneous reactions after these procedures. At the time, these problems were ascribed to impurities in the liquid silicone; however, it has since become apparent that even highly purified medical-grade silicone can cause an intense inflammatory tissue reaction.[2,4-8] The body of anecdotal literature supporting clinical complications has continued to grow; in 1984, Kumagai reviewed 46 patients with a variety of unusual symptoms after silicone injection. He also suggested a possible link to various systemic connective tissue disorders, because a number of women had developed problems such as scleroderma.[1,4,5,9,10]

The quest to devise a technique for breast enlargement that was safer than silicone injection continued. The article introducing the new natural-feel breast implant by Cronin and others[9] recommended augmentation as the solution to wearing prosthetic breasts. The first breast implants consisted of a Silastic bag filled with Siloxane, an "inert and stable" synthetic compound created at the Dow Corning Center for Medical Research.

At the time, Dow Corning was producing a Silastic gel that was used as an insulating and protective medium for electrical devices. Later, this gel was transformed into an even softer material, which became the filling for the new breast implants. This material was extremely tenacious, and scientists believed that the gel would stay in place by sticking to itself, precluding its migrating throughout the body. In their opinion, this would protect patients if rupture or leakage of the implants occurred. Furthermore, the body formed a fibrous tissue capsule around the implants that scientists believed would act as a built-in protective mechanism should the implants rupture.[9] At the time, there were no requirements mandating clinical testing of these products before widespread use. So, in 1962, the first breast implants were placed into women in this country.[10]

In 1976, the Medical Device Amendment Act was introduced through Congress. This act granted the FDA the power to regulate all medical devices. Because breast implants had endured many years of clinical use, the FDA accepted their track record as a reflection of their clinical safety, and the implants were "grandfathered" in as class II medical devices. This class rating included products temporarily inserted into the body, such as pacemakers and cardiac valves. As concern began to surface about the possible dangers of silicone, however, the FDA reclassified breast implants as class III medical devices and in 1982 requested that all implant manufacturers submit formal documentation establishing their safety. After a lengthy review process lasting almost 10 years, the consensus committee believed that adequate data demonstrating the safety and effectiveness of silicone gel breast implants did not exist. In April 1992, the FDA announced a voluntary moratorium on the use of silicone gel breast implants. Furthermore, it recommended stringent controls limiting their use to cases of special need.[1,10-12] Thus, these gel implants have become unavailable for clinical use in the United States.

Chemical Properties of Silicone

A brief overview of the biochemical and physical properties of organosilicones is essential to understand the possible role they may have in the pathogenesis of disease. Silicon is an element, adjacent to carbon on the periodic table, and is the second most abundant substance on earth after oxygen. Silicone is the generic name that was given to a family of silicon-based polymers, selected for use in medical devices because of their presumed biologic inertness. Medical-grade silicone is processed into three forms—oils, gels, and rubbers (elastomers). Oils are used for coating needles and syringes and for lubricating surgical instruments. Silicone gels, used in breast and testicular implants, are branching polymers of dimethlysilaxone. The viscosity of the gel is determined by the number of side branches on the polymer. Long chains of the polymers can be joined together by a process known as high-temperature vulcanization. Using this technique, silicone rubbers are produced and used to coat pacemakers, heart valves, and shunts. These silicone rubbers also are used to form the outer shell of all breast implants.[9,11,13–17]

Over the years silicone breast implants have evolved, and there have been substantial changes in their design and chemical composition. The basic structure, however, remains the same and consists of a silicone elastomer shell filled with silicone gel. The outer shell is, for the most part, a cross-linked polymer compounded with fumed silica (SiO_2).[18–20] The gel consists of approximately 10% silicone oil and 90% polymerized gel.

Silicone breast implants contain a number of chemical impurities (produced during the manufacturing process), including crystalline silica and other organic and inorganic compounds.[21] As mentioned earlier, silica is used in the production of the elastomer shells, and numerous studies have shown that microscopic pieces of the shell can break off and become engulfed by macrophages, exposing body tissues to fumed silica. In addition, some authors have suggested that silicone gel may be converted to silica in surrounding tissues.[23–25] These findings may be important, because diseases occurring after exposure to silica, such as silicosis, represent a possible link between this form of silicone and immune diseases.

Exposure to Silicone Gel

To determine the possible risks associated with silicone breast implants, the mechanisms by which the immune system may become exposed to free silicone gel must be examined. Relevant issues include the following:

1. What is the risk (incidence) of rupture of silicone implants over time?
2. Does significant bleed or leakage of silicone occur across the intact elastomer shell, and if so, what are the consequences?
3. When rupture occurs, does exposure of body tissues to silicone induce local or systemic reactions?

Questions about the risk of rupture or leakage of silicone gel from implants is a concern for many women who have these devices. Findings presented at the FDA's advisory panel estimated that rupture of modern silicone implants occurs in about 4% to 6% of women with no symptoms.[22] In contrast, another study reported that 90% of implants show evidence of severe leakage or rupture

after 10 years.[1,23–26] In any event, the two accepted mechanisms by which silicone can escape from within the implant are overt breakage or rupture, and gel bleed, which occurs by seepage of silicone gel through the semipermeable outer membrane, the end result being free silicone particles in the surrounding tissues.

Many authors have observed this phenomenon, and we confirmed it through histologic examination of more than 50 fibrous capsules surrounding *intact* silicone implants that showed that all of them contained silicone particles within foamy macrophages.[27] The degree of bleed depends on several factors, including the type of implant and the time since implantation.[16,28,29] Silicone gel remains the primary agent of concern because data suggest that the small particles of silicone (60 to 80 μm) that bleed through the implant are engulfed by macrophages, which may then trigger an antigenic response.[4,18,30–36]

Biologic Effects of Silicone

The biologic effects of silicone remain poorly understood, but the original notion that silicone is an inert substance deserves reconsideration. Fundamental questions about silicone, such as the degree of biologic activity and the long-term significance of this activity on the human body, remain unanswered.

Some scientists suggest that silicone may act as an adjuvant, rather than as a direct antigen, whereas others believe that it causes a reaction after being converted to chemically related substances such as silica.[3,14,28,37–40] Both of these theories take into account the chemical structure of silicone, because it is similar to many natural and synthetic adjuvants and immunogens.[40]

Whatever the mechanisms or exact chemical agent, silicone does stimulate a local inflammatory response of variable degree when in contact with body tissues. This is characterized by infiltration of the area with polymorphonuclear cells, followed by recruitment of fibroblasts, lymphocytes, and plasma cells (Fig. 19.2-1). Macrophages are plentiful and become surrounded by extracellular deposits of connective tissue, foreign body giant cells, and ultimately granulomas.[5,10,21,43] These histologic features have been documented in animal models and human specimens after direct injection or passive exposure to silicone.[2,4–8,16,41–43] Similar tissue reactions have also been reported around the breasts and in regional axillary lymph nodes of women with implants.[44–46]

Whether this local inflammatory response can progress to a systemic disorder remains hypothetical. Some authors suggest this as a reasonable hypothesis, because they have documented specific alterations in the immune system (changes in lymphocyte subsets and serum immunoglobulin levels) after exposure to silicates.[20,50]

A number of laboratory studies support the theory that the immunogenic response to silicone is directed against specific proteins rather than to the silicone itself. Newly identified proteins seem to become adherent to the surface of silicone molecules. It is hypothesized that further reac-

FIGURE 19.2-1 Photomicrograph of fibrous tissue capsule surrounding intact silicone implant. Foamy macrophages contain silicone debris, and surrounding area shows infiltration with lymphocytes and plasma cells.

tion to these proteins may stimulate production of autoantibodies in the circulation. This has been demonstrated in a number of animal models and in tissue cell cultures of human mononuclear cells.[17,44,47,48]

Cytokines may also play a role. Large quantities of interleukin-2 (IL-2) are found in the fibrous capsules surrounding silicone implants.[35] Under normal circumstances, IL-2 is produced and released by activated lymphocytes and can stimulate T-cell growth, differentiation, and activation, as well as immunoglobulin production. The authors studying the role of cytokines in this process propose this as an important link between local inflammatory changes and systemic disease. This same study, however, was unable to demonstrate elevated antibody titers or IL-2 levels in the sera of these patients.

Numerous clinical studies also have tried to identify bioactive substances in the sera of women with breast implants. Most of these studies were unable to show consistently elevated antibody production even in women with symptoms. However, two recent studies did identify specific antibodies to silicone in the sera of patients.[2,38] Furthermore, Kossovsky and coworkers[44] demonstrated silicone-associated antibodies in a group of 250 women with breast implants. These antibodies were not present in either of the control groups (healthy women and women with rheumatoid arthritis). Studies that have demonstrated similar findings suggest that standard serologic screening tests may not be able to detect these specific antibodies to silicone.[17,44,47,48] If they indeed exist, some authors believe that these antibodies may help to define a mechanism by which the local inflammatory response to silicone becomes systemic. Most results have been highly variable, difficult to reproduce, and often difficult to interpret.[4,31,32,49]

Some scientists have taken things one step further and have postulated that a genetic predisposition for silicone sensitivity exists in some women, thereby accounting for the degree of variability seen in the local tissue response

and explaining the fact that a relatively small group of women with implants seem to have systemic complaints. This hypothesis, initially presented in 1986, suggests that some patients, perhaps with a specific HLA phenotype, are sensitive to silicone as an antigen.[11,39,50] They believe that these women are at a greater risk of developing a systemic autoimmune reaction to silicone.

Obviously, an understanding of how silicone interacts with the immune system is far from complete and remains, for the most part, hypothetical. Proof of a causal relation between silicone breast implants and silicone autoimmune disease does not exist. This question offers many opportunities for clinical and basic scientific research and certainly warrants further investigation.

Clinical Implications

Silicone implants, like all medical devices, have certain benefits as well as risks. Surveys have shown that over 80% of women with breast implants are pleased with their results.[47] Excluding capsular contracture, complications associated with breast implantation, such as the occurrence of systemic symptoms, are relatively uncommon. Data regarding the incidence of systemic complaints in women with silicone implants are not available, and given the lack of reliable, objective laboratory tests and clinical observations, it is difficult at this point to estimate.

For the most part, studies attempting to define a systemic disease entity related to silicone exposure have used definitions for classic rheumatoid arthritis, autoimmune, and connective tissue disorders. A number of authors have recently pointed out, however, that silicone autoimmune disease may represent a new, unrelated disease entity characterized by vague symptoms such as chronic fatigue, cognitive dysfunction, neurologic symptoms, sicca syndrome, and arthralgias.[17,47,51–55] Information presented at a recent symposium at George Washington University Medical Center in Washington, DC, supports the theory that newly identified antibodies, not tested in previous studies, may account for some of the difficulties previous studies have had in detecting or quantifying antibody titers using standard methods.[47,48]

Strong opinions have formed on both sides of the controversy using data obtained from epidemiologic studies. Many of these studies report no association of connective tissue diseases with silicone implants.[22,56–58] For example, a widely quoted study by Gabriel and associates[57] presented a retrospective population-based study to examine the risk of these disorders after breast implant surgery. The authors used meticulous chart review and analysis of medical records spanning an 8-year period. They found no significant increase in the relative risk of a number of specified connective tissue diseases or autoimmune disorders. The authors caution, however, that these results are limited in their conclusive power because of flaws in study design. For example, in this article, the authors[57] state that they would have needed a sample size of 62,000 women and a control group of 124,000 women, monitored for 10 years, to detect a causal relation between silicone and these disorders (their study included 749 patients with implants and 1498 subjects in the control group).

Although this important study has received much attention, editorial review concurred with the authors and stated that "these results cannot conclusively rule out some association of breast implants with the disorders studied." Other epidemiologic studies have been cited in the literature as evidence refuting a relation between silicone and systemic diseases. Here again, as Swan[55] points out, many of these published studies are plagued with limitations, most commonly: inadequate sample size, inappropriate control groups, lack of stratification of patients (ie, by implant type), lack of disease definition, inadequate patient follow-up, and confounding variables.[61] Clearly, determination of whether silicone causes a clinically significant disease "must await further studies which present sufficient amounts of carefully gathered and critically analyzed data."[59]

TABLE 19.2-2

Common Clinical Symptoms That May Indicate Silicone Autoimmune Disease

LOCAL SYMPTOMS

Breast pain (eg, sharp, burning)
Changes in sensation
Firmness or hardening (capsular contracture)
Masses, nodules
Lymphadenopathy
Inflammation (mastitis)
Infection
Nipple changes/discharge

SYSTEMIC SYMPTOMS

Chronic fatigue
Migratory joint or muscle pains
Migraine headaches
Neurologic symptoms (eg, muscle weakness)
Cognitive dysfunction (eg, memory loss)
Skin rashes
Hair loss
Sicca (dry mouth, eyes)
Rheumatoid arthritis
Raynaud's phenomenon
Sjögren syndrome
Atypical connective tissue disease
Lupus erythematosus
Thyroiditis
Fibromyalgia or fibromyositis
Flulike symptoms

Clinical Assessment

To classify and collect data from patients with clinically significant symptoms, we have developed a clinical staging system (Table 19.2-1) as well as an algorithm to guide patient evaluation. The spectrum of clinical symptoms suspected of being related to silicone autoimmune disease is a collection of poorly defined, vague complaints that can be associated with a multitude of different diseases; however, the most common clinical symptoms have been observed in several large epidemiologic studies[37,39,48,51,52,60] (Table 19.2-2).

In general, symptomatic patients fall into two broad categories: those with local signs and symptoms of an inflammatory reaction, and those with systemic complaints. The group of patients with systemic symptoms can be further subdivided into two broad categories: those pa-

TABLE 19.2-1

Clinical Staging System for Silicone Autoimmune Disease

Stage	Description
0	Asymptomatic
I	Capsular contracture
Ia	Contour abnormality (mild to moderate)
Ib	Painful, calcified
II	Breast abnormalities
IIa	Mammographic abnormality
IIb	Palpable or painful mass
III	Evidence for systemic involvement
IIIa	Serologies, antibody titers
IIIb	Rheumatoid arthritis, other symptoms
IV	Debilatating systemic disease

Silicone breast implants

↓

Complete history and physical examination

No symptoms · Symptoms

Negative family history Immune disease · Positive family history Immune disease → Laboratory and radiologic studies

Observe

Serologic studies
Xeromammography
Ultrasound
Magnetic resonance imaging

FIGURE 19.2-2 Organized approach for clinical work-up.

tients exibiting features recognized as classic connective tissue diseases (such as lupus, scleroderma, and rheumatoid arthritis); and those with clinical or laboratory evidence suggestive of connective tissue disease but with an atypical diagnostic pattern.[47,48,51]

Clinical evaluation begins with an extensive history and physical examination focusing on local breast problems and systemic symptoms. Gathering information regarding specific symptoms and family history of rheumatoid arthritis, lupus, scleroderma, and other autoimmune disorders is important. The onset and progression of clinical symptoms, as well as the degree of disability resulting from these symptoms, should be clearly delineated if possible. Further work-up, including laboratory and radiologic tests, follows an organized pathway as needed for each patient (Fig. 19.2-2).

Breast cancer risk is assessed by clinical history, physical examination, and review of mammograms. The literature suggests that women with silicone breast implants may face a delay in the detection of early breast cancers. In fact, a number of studies have suggested that patients with

FIGURE 19.2-3 A. Conventional mammogram with silicone implant. **B.** Conventional mammogram with radiolucent implant (Trilucent). Additional areas of breast tissue previously obscured by silicone implant are seen clearly.

silicone breast implants are diagnosed at a later stage of disease (with palpable versus nonpalpable lesions) and therefore face a worse prognosis.[10,61,62] As seen in Figure 19.2-3*A*, adequate mammography is hindered by a submammary silicone implant, which shadows a large portion of breast tissue. Concern about this problem has stimulated the development of a new implant prototype. The (Trilucent) implant is filled with triglyceride oil (which has the same density as breast tissue), thereby making the implant radiolucent (see Fig. 19.2-3*B*). Alternatively, placement of the implant in the subpectoral position allows for use of displacement techniques to improve visualization of the breast parenchyma.

Physical examination includes assessment of local symptoms and evaluation of lymph nodes, skin, soft tissue, joints, and neuromusclar systems. The breasts are carefully examined for nodules and evidence of implant problems, including possible rupture, inflammation, and severe capsular contracture (Fig. 19.2-4). If clinical evidence of systemic involvement exists, further work-up, including consultation by a physician in the appropriate specialty area (ie, neurologist, rheumatologist, immunologist), can be helpful.

Objective, noninvasive methods available to determine implant rupture include mammography, ultrasonography,

FIGURE 19.2-5 Ultrasound scan of breast implant showing intracapsular rupture. The thinner arrow indicates the fibrous capsule. The "snowstorm" (*thicker arrow*) indicates silicone gel floating free within the capsule.

FIGURE 19.2-4 A. Patient with severe capsular contracture (calcified) and painful breasts. **B.** Calcified capsules after removal with intact silicone implant inside.

and magnetic resonance imaging (MRI). For the most part, these studies are helpful, but each test alone remains limited in its accuracy. Conventional mammography is limited in its usefulness for detection of rupture; however, ultrasound and MRI have proved helpful. Figure 19.2-5 shows an ultrasonographic examination illustrating features of a classic implant rupture (snowstorm). Advantages to ultrasonographic examination include accessibility and cost efficiency.[63,64]

MRI also has been studied as a tool in assessing the integrity of silicone implants.[63–65] Findings have been identified that can delineate intracapsular versus extracapsular rupture (silicone outside the fibrous capsule). The echogenicity of silicone makes it appear very different from the surrounding tissue and thus, obvious when it has been extruded outside the capsule or is contained in adjacent lymphatic tissue. MRI can further delineate details of the implant, such as the elastomer shell, which becomes clearly visible when it has collapsed (Fig. 19.2-6). Complex reconstructive implants are more difficult to assess by radiologic techniques, because many of them contain multiple chambers, which can simulate intracapsular rupture. As seen in these examples, documenting implant integrity using ultrasonography or MRI provides useful information that can significantly aid in the clinical evaluation of these women. A study compared the accuracy of mammography, ultrasonography, and MRI for detection of implant integrity. Sensitivity was 11%, 70%, and 81%, and specificity was 89%, 92%, and 92% for mammography, ultrasonography, and MRI, respectively.[66] This study supports the diagnostic value of ultrasonography and MRI in evaluating symptomatic patients; in most institutions, however, MRI remains prohibitively expensive, so ultrasonography can be used as a reliable option.

As discussed earlier, serologic studies can be employed to screen for antinuclear antibodies (ANAs), rheumatoid factors, and specific silicone antibodies. Again, it has been

FIGURE 19.2-6 MRI showing ruptured implant with collapsed elastomer shell (*short arrow*) and free silicone in adjacent tissue (*long arrow*).

it is helpful to follow an organized approach in the clinical assessment of these women.

Clinical Treatment Options

After sufficient clinical information is obtained, treatment options can be reviewed with the patient. Patients who have no symptoms and no evidence of implant rupture, local disease, or systemic complaints are monitored clinically. If they notice any changes in the breast or develop significant symptoms, they are instructed to return for reevaluation. Most women with implants are asymptomatic and remain pleased after augmentation. For women who are symptomatic, most complain of local rather than systemic problems.

Localized symptoms of the breast, such as pain and hardening, with or without inflammation, are often related to capsular contracture. Although this phenomenon has been studied and reported on extensively in the literature on plastic surgery, the mechanism by which it occurs remains elusive. In many earlier series (when the implants were placed directly underneath the breast tissue), the incidence of capsular contracture was unusually high, between 34% and 70%.[26,56,67] Surgical placement of implants in the subpectoral position (behind the muscle), markedly reduces the incidence of capsular contracture (5% to 10%). When severe, capsular contracture is best treated by open capsulectomy.

If the patient has symptoms that suggest autoimmune disease (or atypical connective tissue disorder) or if there is local or radiographic evidence of rupture, explantation should be considered. When planning the surgical approach, mammograms should be reviewed carefully so that biopsy can be performed on suspect lesions at the time of explantation. During this initial planning phase, the desired

difficult to identify populations of women with silicone implants that show consistent elevation of antibody titers. Although several studies have documented high titers of antinuclear antibodies, other reports cannot claim these same findings. As some suggest, it is possible that unknown serologic markers exist that we are unable to detect. Therefore, although standard serologic tests may be helpful, they cannot be considered as conclusive evidence in evaluating these patients and must be considered in the context of other clinical findings.

While the theory of silicone autoimmune disease remains neither proved nor disproved by scientific process,

FIGURE 19.2-7 A. Symptomatic patient before explantation. Photograph demonstrates moderate capsular contractures and ptosis. Surgical markings for restructuring of the breast after implant removal are illustrated. **B.** Same patient 5 days after surgery. Procedure included bilateral capsulectomies, implant removal, and restructuring of the breast.

approach for breast restoration must also be addressed. This can be done using saline implants or myocutaneous flaps, or by restructuring the remaining breast tissue using a combination of surgical techniques. Patients who have evidence of possible systemic disease (atypical connective tissue disorder) should be advised that replacement with another implant, even a saline-filled implant, may not be prudent. Although unlikely, some authors have suggested that over time, the presence of the silicone elastomer shell itself may pose an unknown degree of risk in some women.[67] Clinical improvement of systemic symptoms occurs in up to 60% of women after implant removal.[27,29,32,38]

Many women who request or are recommended for explantation require restructuring of the breast because the skin and overlying breast tissue have become stretched and ptotic (Fig. 19.2-7). The surgical approach to this problem is addressed by using modifications of the standard mastopexy procedure after implant removal. In addition, the fibrous capsule around the implant should be removed since most of them contain particles of silicone (even when surrounding an intact implant) and can later create clinical problems such as seroma formation and abnormalities on mammography.[10,12,23–25,27,29]

The surgical management of these patients can be challenging and often requires that patients accept a new body image. Implant removal should not be performed without careful consideration to the aesthetic outcome, since simple explantation rarely results in an acceptable cosmetic outcome (Fig. 19.2-8). When considering explantation, both the physical and psychologic needs of these patients must be met.

Summary

The debate about silicone implants is likely to continue until adequate scientific information can either prove or disprove an association between silicone and various systemic disorders. Many questions remain unanswered. With the recognition that the multitude of women who have implants are simply concerned but that others feel strongly that their implants are related to their medical problems, the answers to these questions must be pursued. Given the highly controversial and emotionally charged opinions surrounding this debate, clinicians should approach these patients by realizing that the truly objective tests that are needed are not yet available. Appropriate recommendations for therapy logically follows thorough clinical evaluation of these patients.

References

1. Kessler D. The basis of the FDA's decision on breast implants. N Engl J Med 1992;326:1713.
2. Symmers W. Silicone mastitis in topless waitresses and some other varieties of foreign body mastitis. BMJ 1968;3:19.
3. Miyoshi K, TM, Kobayashi Y, et al. Hypergammaglobulinemia by prolonged adjuvanticity in man: disorders developed after augmentation mammoplasty. Jpn J Med, 1964;2122:9.
4. Endo L, Edwards NL, Longley S, et al. Silicone and rheumatic diseases. Semin Arthr Rheum 1987;17:112.
5. Ashley F, Braley S, Reese T. The present status of silicone fluid and soft tissue augmentation. Plast Reconstr Surg 1967;39:411.
6. Ortiz-Monsantario F, Trigus I. Management of patients with complications from injection of foreign materials into the breasts. Plast Reconstr Surg 1972;50:42.
7. Parsons R, Thering HR. Management of the silicone injected breast. Plast Reconstr Surg 1978;60:534.
8. Picha G, Goldstein JA. Analysis of the soft-tissue response to components used in the manufacture of breast implants: rat animal model. Plast Reconstr Surg 1990;87:490.
9. Cronin T, Gerow FJ. Augmentation mammaplasty: a new "natural feel" prosthesis. In: Transactions of the Third International Congress of Plastic Surgery. Amsterdam, Excerpta Medica, 1964:41.
10. Riolo-Nemecek J, Young VL. How safe are silicone breast implants? South Med J 1993;86:932.
11. Spiera R, Giborsky A, Spiera H. Silicone gel filled breast implants and connective tissue disease: an overview. J Rheumatol 1994;21:239.
12. Independent Advisory Committee. Summary of the report on silicone-gel-filled breast implants. Can Med Assoc J 1992;147:1141.
13. Speirs A, Blocksma R. New implantable silicone rubbers. Plast Reconstr Surg 1963;31:166.
14. Yoshida S, Gershwin ME. Autoimmunity and selected environmental factors of disease induction. Semin Arthritis Rheum 1993;22:399.
15. Blocksma R, Braley S. The silicones in plastic surgery. Plast Reconstr Surg 1965;35:366.
16. Dunn K, Hall PN, Khoo CTK. Breast implant materials: sense and safety. Br J Plast Surg 1992;45:315.
17. Kossovsky N, Stassi J. A pathophysiological examination of the biophysics and bioreactivity of silicone breast implants. Semin Arthritis Rheum 1994;24:18.
18. Shons A, Schubert W. Silicone breast implants and immune disease. Ann Plast Surg 1992;28:491.
19. Heggers J, Kossovsky N, Parsons RW, et al. Biocompatibility of silicone implants. Ann Plast Surg 1983;11:38.
20. Wilkerson P. General silicone chemistry. Distributed communication to FDA Advisory Panel, February 1992.
21. Busch H. Silicone toxicology. Semin Arthritis Rheum 1994;24:11.
22. Fisher J. The silicone controversy: when will science prevail? N Engl J Med 1992;326:1696.

FIGURE 19.2-8 Unacceptable cosmetic results after explantation (removal of implants only).

23. Peters W, Keystone E, Smith D. Factors affecting the rupture of silicone-gel breast implants. Ann Plast Surg 1994;32:449.

24. Peters W. The mechanical properties of breast prostheses. Ann Plast Surg 1981;6:179.

25. de Camara JS, Kammer BA. Rupture and aging of silicone gel breast implants. Plast Reconstr Surg 1993;91:829.

26. McGrath M, Burkhardt BR. The safety and efficacy of breast implants for augmentation mammaplasty. Plast Reconstr Surg 1984;74:550.

27. Lebovic G, Laub DR, Hadler K. Silicone autoimmune disease: clinical and histologic findings 1995 (in press).

28. Vargas A. Shedding of silicone particles from inflated breast implants. Plast Reconstr Surg 1979;64:252.

29. Barker D, Retsky MI, Schultz S. "Bleeding" of silicone from bag-gel breast implants, and its clinical relation to fibrous capsule reaction. Plast Reconstr Surg 1978;61:836.

30. Smith D, Sazy JA, Crissman JD, et al. Immunogenic potential of carpal implants. J Surg Res 1990;48:13.

31. Claman H, Robertson AD. Antinuclear antibodies and breast implants. West J Med 1993;160:225.

32. Press R, Peebles CL, Kumagai Y, et al. Antinuclear autoantibodies in women with silicone breast implants. Lancet 1992;340:1304.

33. Goldblum R, Pelley RP, O'Donell AA, et al. Antibodies to silicone elastomers and reactions to ventriculoperitoneal shunts. Lancet 1992;340:510.

34. Stone O. Autoimmunity as a secondary phenomenon in scleroderma (and so-called human adjuvant disease). Med Hypotheses 1991;34:127.

35. Wells A, Daniels S, Gunasekaran S, et al. Local increase in hyaluronic acid and interleukin-2 in the capsules surrounding silicone breast implants. Ann Plast Surg 1994;33:1.

36. Jacobs J, Imundo L. Silicone implants and autoimmune disease. Lancet 1994;343:354.

37. Kumagai Y, Abe C, Shiokawa Y. Clinical spectrum of connective tissue disease after cosmetic surgery: observations on 18 patients and a review of the Japanese literature. Semin Arthritis Rheum 1984;27:1.

38. Kaiser W, Biesenbacvk G, Stuby U, et al. Human adjuvant disease: remission of silicone induced autoimmune disease after explantation of breast augmentation. Ann Rheum Dis 1990;49:937.

39. Sergott T, Limoli JP, Baldwin CM, et al. Human adjuvant disease, possible autoimmune disease after silicone implantation: a review of the literature, case studies and speculation for the future. Plast Reconstr Surg 1986;78:104.

40. Naim J, Lanzafame RJ, van Oss CJ. The adjuvant effect of silicone-gel on antibody formation in rats. Immunol Invest 1993;22:151.

41. Chastre J, Basset F, Viau F, et al. Acute pneumonitis after subcutaneous injections of silicone in transsexual men. N Engl J Med 1983;308:764.

42. Sank A, Chalabian-Baliozian J, Ertl D, et al. Cellular responses to silicone and polyurethane prosthetic surfaces. J Surg Res 1993;54:12.

43. Brautbar N, Vojdani A, Campbell A. Silicone breast implants and autoimmunity: causation or myth? Arch Environ Health 1994;3:151.

44. Kossovsky N, Heggers JP, Robson MC. Experimental demonstration of the immunogenicity of silicone-protein complexes. J Biomed Mater Res 1987;21:1125.

45. Corrin B. Silicone lymphadenopathy. J Clin Pathol 1982;35:901.

46. Truong L, Cartwright J, Goodman MD, et al. Silicone lymphadenopathy associated with augmentation mammaplasty: morphologic features of nine cases. Am J Surg Pathol 1988;12:484.

47. Kossovsky N. Silicone breast implant pathology. Arch Pathol Lab Med 1994;118:686.

48. Bridges A. Autoantibodies in patients with silicone implants. Semin Arthritis Rheum 1994;24.

49. Peters W, Keystone E, Snow K, et al. Is there a relationship between autoantibodies and silicone-gel implants. Ann Plast Surg 1994;32:1.

50. Young V, Nemecek JR, Gilliam C, et al. Human leukocyte antigen (HLA) typing in women with silicone gel-filled implants. Aesthetic Society's 26th Annual Meeting, 1993.

51. Solomon G. A clinical and laboratory profile of symptomatic women with silicone breast implants. Semin Arthritis Rheum 1994;24:29.

52. Vasey F, Havice DL, Bocanegra TS, et al. Clinical and immunologic findings in fifty consecutive women with silicone breast implants and connective tissue disease. Semin Arthritis Rheum 1994;24:22.

53. Lappe M. Silicone-reactive disorder: a new autoimmune disease caused by immunostimulation and superantigens. Med Hypotheses 1993;41:348.

54. Hirmand H, LaTrenta GS, Hoffman LA. Autoimmune disease and silicone breast implants. Oncology 1993;7:17.

55. Swan S. Epidemiology of silicone-related diseases. Semin Arthritis Rheum 1994;24:38.

56. Fiala T, Lee WPA, May Jr JW. Augmentation mammoplasty: results of a patient survey. Ann Plast Surg 1993;30:503.

57. Gabriel S, O'Fallon WM, Kurland LT, et al. Risk of connective-tissue disease and other disorders after breast implantation. N Engl J Med 1994;330:1697.

58. Schusterman M, Kroll SS, Reece GP, et al. Incidence of autoimmune disease in patients after breast reconstruction with silicone gel implants versus autogenous tissue: a preliminary report. Ann Plast Surg 1993;31:1.

59. Angell M. Do breast implants cause systemic disease? N Engl J Med 1994;330:1748.

60. Silverstein M. Oncologic aspects of augmentation mammaplasty. Plast Reconstr Surg 1994;93:1523.

61. Birdsell D, Berkel J, Lindsay RL, et al. The relationship of mammary augmentation and breast cancer: an epidemiologic study. (Abstract) Plast Reconstr Surg 1993;92:795.

62. Peters W, Pugash R. Ultrasound analysis of 150 patients with silicone gel breast implants. Ann Plast Surg 1993;31:7.

63. Levine R, Collins TL. Definitive diagnosis of breast implant rupture by ultrasonography. Plast Reconstr Surg 1990;87:1126.

64. Ahn C, Shaw W, Narayanan K, et al. Definitive diagnosis of breast implant rupture using MRI: experience with 90 patients. (Abstract) Plast Reconstr Surg 1993;92:681.

65. Ahn C, DeBruhl ND, Gorczya DP, et al. Comparative silicone breast implant evaluation using mammography, sonography, and magnetic resonance imaging: experience with 59 implants. Plast Reconstr Surg 1994;94:620.

66. Kossovsky N, Stassi J. Biophysical, inflammatory and immunological phenomena associated with silicone breast implants: a pathophysiological approach. Semin Arthritis Rheum 1994;24:18.

67. Copeland M, Choi M, Bleiweiss IJ. Silicone breakdown and capsular synovial metaplasia in textured-wall saline breast prostheses. Plast Reconstr Surg 1994;94:628.

Diseases of the Breast, edited by Jay R. Harris,
Marc E. Lippman, Monica Morrow, and Samuel Hellman.
Lippincott-Raven Publishers, Philadelphia, © 1996.

20

Evaluation of Patients After Primary Therapy

DANIEL F. HAYES ▪ WILLIAM KAPLAN

In the past 20 years, technologic advances have enabled the detection of metastatic breast cancer earlier in the course of the disease than was previously possible. The clinical utility of screening for early relapse, and the precise strategies to do so, remain controversial, however. In this chapter, the utility of early detection in patient care is discussed, with recommendations for the most appropriate means of follow-up of patients after primary therapy.

Clinical Significance of Early Detection of Cancer

In general, it has been widely assumed by both patients and caregivers that early detection of any cancer, whether as a new primary malignant tumor or as a recurrence, leads to more effective therapy. Thus, many studies have addressed methods to improve diagnostic techniques (see later in this chapter). Moreover, investigations of the natural history of patients with breast cancer have generated data regarding risk, timing, and sites of recurrence. These data are reviewed in greater detail in Chapters 12 and 16. Studies evaluating the clinical utility of ongoing routine follow-up after primary therapy have only recently been reported, however. In this regard, potential benefits of routine follow-up might include detection of new primary cancers or improved treatment of metastatic disease. These two issues are fundamentally different and are discussed separately.

SCREENING FOR NEW PRIMARY CANCERS

The detection of new intraparenchymal malignant breast tumors may be the most important indication for careful follow-up of patients with breast cancer after primary treatment. Large screening trials of the general population have demonstrated that mortality from breast cancer can be reduced as a function of early detection and therapy of new primary breast cancers. The risk of a subsequent second primary breast cancer is elevated relative to the general population in women who have had a prior breast cancer. Although no randomized screening trials have been performed in patients who have had previous malignant tumors, several studies in which patients were monitored after primary therapy for the detection of recurrent breast cancer have demonstrated that approximately 0.5% to 1% patients per year develop contralateral breast cancer.[1–7] Screening patients after primary therapy of a first breast cancer for the occurrence of a second breast cancer, using criteria at least as stringent as current recommendations for the general population, is indicated. Patients with an ipsilateral breast recurrence after breast-conserving therapy may have the same prognosis as patients with a new primary breast cancer, and follow-up and therapy of patients treated with breast-conserving therapy to detect such recurrences at an early stage is important[8,9] (see Chap. 21).

The incidence of colon and ovarian cancers may also be *statistically* elevated in patients with a previous history of breast cancer, although this risk is not dramatically higher than in the general population.[10–12] Thus, because screening programs for these diseases are already reasonably widespread, more aggressive follow-up beyond what is recommended for the routine population is not indicated in patients who have had a primary breast cancer.[10] Moreover, patients treated with adjuvant therapies may be at risk for treatment-related induction of second malignant diseases.[13] For example, uterine carcinoma is increased two- to three-fold in patients taking adjuvant tamoxifen, compared with untreated controls.[14,15] The absolute incidence of such malignant tumors is still low (under 1% per 5-year follow-up period), however. Routine screening should include yearly pelvic examination and Papanicolaou smears and careful evaluation of any reported abnormal vaginal bleeding or pelvic symptoms.

629

IS EARLY DETECTION OF EXTRAMAMMARY RECURRENCES BENEFICIAL?

Although technologic advances may permit early detection of metastases (see later), controversy remains regarding whether such detection is clinically relevant.[16–23] Several reasons might justify early detection of metastases:

1. Metastases might be more effectively treated if detected earlier than if found at a more advanced stage. More effective treatment of patients with recurrent disease implies that these patients can be cured, that their survival can be prolonged, or that their physical quality of life is improved (palliation).
2. Early detection, or the lack of it, may be of emotional value to either the patient or the treating physician.
3. Delay of recurrence after primary therapy is frequently used as an endpoint for many investigative therapies. Therefore, detection of recurrence on a consistent basis is important for research purposes.

In contrast, routine screening has at least three potential disadvantages:

1. Inappropriate application of therapy with associated morbidity and, occasionally, mortality in a setting in which the benefits of early treatment have not been demonstrated.
2. Increased emotional trauma for patients whose lives may be shattered by finding an asymptomatic recurrence months to years before the onset of symptoms.
3. Increased direct expense due to the costs of the screening diagnostic tests, and increased indirect costs incurred by any further testing required to confirm suspicious findings and by early application of therapy.

ROUTINE SCREENING FOR METASTASES AS A MEANS OF PROVIDING MORE EFFECTIVE TREATMENT

Cure or Prolongation of Survival

Most studies of long-term follow-up of patients with recurrent breast cancer suggest that few women are ever cured, regardless of whether or not they receive therapy.[24–27] The success of adjuvant systemic therapy in certain subgroups of patients after primary therapy suggests that treatment of breast cancer might be more successful if administered relatively early in the clinical course.[28] The survival benefits of treatment of patients with metastatic disease remain unproved, however (see Chap. 22.1). Studies with historic controls suggest that certain subgroups of patients with metastatic disease benefit from aggressive treatment, but these studies are limited by their retrospective design. Survival benefits observed in prospectively randomized trials in which more effective treatments are compared with less effective regimens suggest that treatment of patients with metastases might prolong survival. Such survival differences have been modest, however.[29,30]

The studies discussed in the previous paragraph pertained to patients with documented, evaluable metastatic disease. Treatment of patients with metastases at an earlier stage might be more beneficial than when treatment is given when the disease is more widespread. No study has been reported in which routinely screened patients with asymptomatic recurrences have been randomly assigned to immediate treatment versus observation until symptoms occur. Several retrospective studies have addressed this issue, however. For example, in a study in which more than 400 patients were monitored for a minimum of 4 years, recurrences were detected earlier in screened patients than in patients who had presented to their physicians with symptoms.[31] In this study, 50 patients were selected for further evaluation. Half presented with symptoms, and the other half were asymptomatic when metastases were detected. Response to therapy and survival after recurrence were identical in both groups. In a retrospective study of more than 250 patients in Norway, the time to death after detection of metastases was slightly longer for patients who presented with symptoms (36 months compared with 32 months).[32] This difference was not significant, and the overall survival of both groups was identical. Other retrospective studies have confirmed these findings[2,3] (Fig. 20-1).

In contrast, in a different study, patients who presented with asymptomatic metastases had a substantially longer survival from the time of recurrence than those who presented with symptomatic recurrences (29 months versus 17 months, respectively, $P = .0017$).[33] These authors did not provide a comparison of overall survival from the time of primary therapy for these two groups of patients. Because routine screening might provide a lead time for patients whose metastases are detected asymptomatically, the improved survival for patients whose metastases are detected when asymptomatic may reflect *lead-time bias,* rather than the effects of early treatment.

Survival from time of first recurrence also depends on the site of the first recurrence. For example, median survival after relapse of patients with local chest wall recurrence after mastectomy is superior to that in patients with visceral metastases[33–35] (Fig. 20-2). In this regard, in one retrospective study, those patients who had asymptomatic recurrences had a prolonged overall survival compared with those with symptomatic recurrences if their first site of recurrence was on the chest wall or in bone. Patients with visceral metastases, however, had a similar survival from first recurrence, regardless of whether they had presenting symptoms or not.[33]

Two large randomized trials have addressed overall survival in patients diagnosed and treated earlier as a result of more intense follow-up.[36,37] In these Italian studies, women with early (nonmetastatic) newly diagnosed breast cancer were randomly assigned to undergo intensive follow-up (consisting of physician's visits, bone scans, and chest radiographs) or to be followed-up less rigorously (routine physician's visits, other tests performed only as indicated). In one study, the intensive follow-up arm of the trial also included non–tumor-marker blood tests (eg, alkaline phosphatase [AP], transaminases) and liver echography.[37] Both studies included mammography in each arm of the trial. Therapy for patients with metastases was pro-

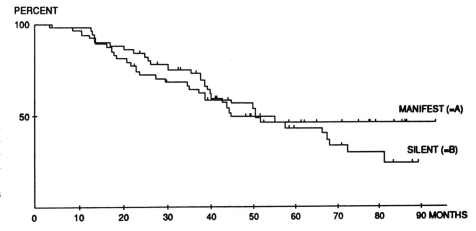

FIGURE 20-1 Overall survival in patients with breast cancer according to whether patients presented with symptomatic (manifest) or asymptomatic (silent) metastases: ($P = .1105$). (Stierer M, Rosen HR. Influence of early diagnosis on prognosis of recurrent breast cancer. Cancer 1989;64:1128)

vided according to standard practice and was generally initiated at the time of documented recurrence.

The results of these studies are remarkably similar. Intensive follow-up resulted in slightly increased frequency of detection of recurrence in one study,[36] but not in the other.[37] In both studies, however, overall survival from time of randomization was identical for patients followed intensively or with physicians' visits only (Fig. 20-3).

In both studies, the percentage of patients who relapsed accounted for less than 40% of the total patients enrolled. Therefore, it is possible that a small difference in survival of those who relapsed could have been missed. Both studies are large (more than 1200 patients in each), and each has more than 100 relapsed patients per arm of the trial, however. Neither has even a trend toward overall survival benefit for the intensively screened (and therefore early-treated) patients. Thus, the results of these studies suggest that intensive follow-up with frequent radiographic evaluation is not indicated after primary and adjuvant therapy.

In a small group of patients with breast cancer, surgical excision of isolated metastases has possibly resulted in prolonged disease-free survival (3 to 5 years).[38-40] No randomized trial of the effects of metastatectomy has ever been performed, however, nor is one likely to be. In general, patients are selected for metastatectomy if they have a long disease-free interval from primary treatment to first relapse, a good performance status, and relatively good prognostic factors.[41] Such patients are likely to have a prolonged survival regardless of the type of treatment they receive.[42] Although these patients may be rendered disease-free, their overall survival may not be altered. Therefore, routine screening with hopes of performing metastatectomy cannot be routinely recommended and should, in general, be considered investigational (see Chap. 23).

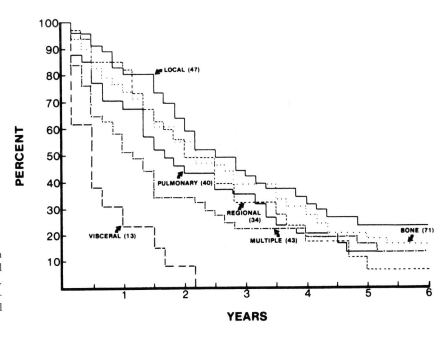

FIGURE 20-2 Survival after recurrence in patient with breast cancer according to initial site of recurrence. (Tomin R, Donegan WL. Screening for recurrent breast cancer: its effectiveness and prognostic value. J Clin Oncol 1987;5:62)

FIGURE 20-3   Relapse-free survival (DFS) and overall survival (OS) of patients in two different trials who were randomly assigned to intensive follow-up or to physician visits only after primary and adjuvant therapy for carcinoma of the breast. **A.** GIVIO study. **B.** National Research Council Project on Breast Cancer Follow-Up Study. (Rosselli Del Turco M, Palli D, Cariddi A, et al. Intensive diagnostic follow-up after treatment of primary breast cancer: a randomized trial. JAMA 1994;271:1593)

Improved Physical Palliation

In lieu of curing or prolonging survival of patients with recurrent breast cancer, improved palliation might result from earlier detection and treatment of recurrence. Evaluation of palliation as an endpoint is difficult because of the subjective nature of this treatment result. Nonetheless, many clinicians and patients believe that the use of systemic therapy at the time of first relapse to delay the time at which symptoms occur is justified, even though improved palliation due to early treatment of asymptomatic metastatic disease has not been demonstrated in a randomized trial.[20,43] In one survey, nearly 43% of physicians who belonged to the American Society of Clinical Oncology reported that they believed that early detection of metastatic disease would have a positive impact on patients' quality of life.[43]

Detection of asymptomatic recurrences in certain sites might lead to therapy to prevent a catastrophic result of untreated tumor. For example, detection of large lytic lesions in major weight-bearing bones might allow prophylactic orthopedic stabilization to prevent a disabling fracture (see Chap. 23.6). The incidence of asymptomatic lesions that result in catastrophic fractures is small (probably less than 10%), however, and the value of prophylactic

therapy of isolated lytic metastases is unknown.[44] Similarly, although patients may present with the neurologic complications of spinal cord compression without preceding symptoms, over 90% of patients with epidural involvement have had antecedent episodes of back pain.[45–47]

In summary, the usefulness of early detection of recurrent disease for improving palliative care is not defined. As a result, the physician and patient must assess whether treatment of asymptomatic metastases may result in improved palliation, weighing the toxicity of whatever therapy is administered against the benefits of delaying or preventing future symptoms. Few data offer guidelines in patients with metastatic disease, although several ongoing trials of patients with metastatic disease have incorporated quality-of-life assessments to quantify more objectively any symptomatic benefits accrued from therapy.

ROUTINE SCREENING FOR METASTASES AS A MEANS OF PROVIDING EMOTIONAL SUPPORT

Regular evaluation of breast cancer patients after primary therapy might provide additional emotional support to women at a time when they have suffered considerable psychologic stress related to the diagnosis and treatment of their tumor. The knowledge that she remains disease-free might be an important aid in returning the patient to a normal role in society. In contrast, if the treatment of asymptomatic metastases cannot be justified, then routine screenings may, in fact, have the opposite effect. The knowledge of an asymptomatic recurrence may substantially diminish the patient's quality of life during a period when she might otherwise be emotionally secure.[48] In a survey of breast cancer patients in North Carolina, however, over half preferred frequent (every 3 to 12 months) physicians' visits.[22] In a similar survey of patients followed-up after primary and adjuvant therapy in England, 81% felt "reassured and less anxious" when they had their follow-up visit, and over 75% preferred to visit a specialty clinic rather than a general practitioner.[16]

In one of the two Italian randomized trials of intensive follow-up versus physicians' visits only, prospective analysis of quality of life was performed.[37] Over 70% of all patients in both arms of this trial stated that they wished to have regular and frequent physicians' visits, even if they had no symptoms. Overall quality-of-life perceptions, overall health perceptions, and specific measures of body image, emotional well-being, social functioning, symptoms, and satisfaction with health care were nearly identical in the two follow-up groups, however. In a selected group of women in this study, quality of life was shown to decline after relapse. Thus, if early detection of asymptomatic recurrence does not lead to prolonged survival or improved palliation, it may decrease quality of life. These results suggest that although a follow-up schedule does appear to be reassuring and worthwhile, the less intense, and therefore less expensive, program may be more satisfactory.

DETECTION OF METASTASES AS AN INVESTIGATIONAL ENDPOINT

An important indication for systematic follow-up is to compare the time to recurrence between patients on different arms of investigational studies. Such an endpoint (ie, disease-free interval) is important for many studies in which different forms of either primary or adjuvant systemic therapy are compared. Evaluation of disease-free interval may allow analysis of trials earlier than when either overall survival or cure is used as an endpoint, and differences in disease-free intervals (in lieu of overall survival differences) have served as valid criteria for early stoppage of trials and alterations in general health care policies.[49–53] Most patients are unlikely to consider this endpoint sufficient to justify the more costly and potentially hazardous intensive follow-up if they derive no direct benefit, however.[16]

EXPENSE OF ROUTINE SCREENING

As discussed, potential disadvantages of early detection of metastatic disease include inappropriate application of toxic therapy for which no benefit is established and decreased emotional well-being for patients who were otherwise doing well. A third disadvantage is the additional cost of performing diagnostic tests.

The direct cost of any follow-up strategy depends on the frequency of follow-up, the precise tests performed, and the costs of the tests in that particular institution. Indirectly, more intense follow-up may also generate expenses related to more extensive work-up of suspicious but nondiagnostic test results. Finally, therapy-related costs may be escalated in patients who are diagnosed earlier and therefore are treated for a longer period than they would be if their recurrence were detected when they developed symptoms.

One analysis estimated that direct costs in an intensive follow-up program in the United States in 1990 would be nearly five times higher than for a "minimalist" (physical examination and mammography) schedule ($5375 versus $1025 per 5-year follow-up period).[19] The same author projected that a universal minimalist surveillance policy in the United States would save nearly $812 million in 1995. Therefore, intensive follow-up programs are expensive, especially in light of the relative lack of improved benefit.

In summary, to justify intense follow-up of patients after primary or adjuvant therapy for newly diagnosed breast cancer is difficult. Some follow-up does appear to be both beneficial and indicated, however, as reflected in the Management Summary at the conclusion of this chapter.

Incidence, Sites, and Timing of Metastases

Although intensive screening for metastases may not be indicated currently, it is worthwhile to review available technology to do so. Screening for metastatic disease would be most efficiently performed with a test that has 100% sensitivity and specificity for breast cancer. Currently, no such test exists. The development of monoclonal antibody technology generated optimism that a specific scintigraphic or serologic test for cancer might be available. Unfortunately, the results of radiolabeled antibody imaging have been disappointing.[54] Moreover, available serologic assays may suggest recurrent cancer, but they are not site-specific.[55,56] Thus, the clinician must rely on organ-specific radiographic and scintigraphic techniques.

CANDIDATES AND TIME FRAME

Screening is most efficiently applied to those patients most likely to suffer a relapse. The risk of subsequent systemic relapse following primary therapy is related to certain prognostic factors (see Chap. 16). Of these, the presence of histologic invasion beyond the basement membrane, the clinical stage, and the presence and number of axillary lymph node metastases are the most important determinants.[25,57,58] Other prognostic factors have been identified, but they are less powerful in predicting subsequent distant recurrence (see Chap. 16). Nonetheless, the likelihood of detecting recurrent disease is greater in patients with more advanced disease at presentation than in patients with favorable clinical and pathologic prognostic factors.

Screening might be focused during a time when cancer is most likely to recur. Although the risks of relapse in patients in different clinical prognostic categories differs, the risk of relapse within a given category varies according to the follow-up time after primary therapy. The rate of recurrences after primary therapy rises to a peak during the second to fifth year of follow-up.[25,59] Although the yearly risk of relapse in the remaining patients decreases after the fifth year, the risk of recurrence continues for as long as 15 or more years.[25,26,60] Thus, patients with breast cancer may never be free from risk of relapse, even if their original prognostic factors are favorable. Although frequent follow-up during the first 1 to 5 years of high-risk patients may be justified after primary therapy, the current practice of gradually increasing the interval between evaluations may not be consistent with the ongoing hazard of relapse following primary therapy.

The beneficial effect of adjuvant systemic therapy on the risk of relapse in certain subgroups of patients has been well documented (see Chap. 17.2). Nonetheless, disease-free survival curves for both treated and control patients in large randomized adjuvant trials continue to decline for as long as follow-up continues.[28,61,62] Although treated populations relapse at a lower rate, the survival curves have not yet begun to plateau, even in the more mature

studies, suggesting that even those patients who benefit from adjuvant systemic therapy remain at risk for recurrence throughout their lives. Thus, follow-up practices in groups treated with adjuvant systemic therapy should probably not differ from those in other groups with similar initial risks of relapse.

ORGAN SCREENING

Breast cancer metastasizes to almost all organs of the body. Autopsy studies have demonstrated that, in patients who ultimately die of breast cancer, the disease is usually widespread, involving bone, lungs, and liver in roughly 50% to 75% of patients[63–65] (see Chap. 12).

Several studies, however, have demonstrated that distribution of metastases in patients at first recurrence differs from that in patients studied at autopsy (Table 20-1). Between 50% and 75% patients relapse first in a single organ, whereas the remaining patients suffer recurrence in multiple organs simultaneously. Between 15% and 40% of first recurrences are local or regional, involving chest wall or axillary–supraclavicular lymph nodes. An additional 30% to 60% of first recurrences are in bone, with another 10% to 15% involving bone in combination with other sites. Patients less commonly manifest pulmonary, hepatic, or central nervous system (CNS) disease as their first site of metastasis. In most studies, only 5% to 15% of all first recurrences are in the lung or thorax, only 3% to 10% are

TABLE 20-1

Distribution of Sites of First Recurrence After Primary Therapy for Carcinoma of the Breast

Investigators	Bone Scan*	Local–Regional	Recurrence Site as Percentage of All Recurrences† Distant			
			All	Bone	Lung	Liver
Rutgers et al[2]	No	23	76	62	26	22
Stierer & Rosen[3]	NA	30	70	44	32	NA
Tomin & Donegan[33]	NA	32	68	28	16	5
Pedrazzini et al[82]	Yes	29	71	16	NA	NA
Pandya et al[71]	Yes	39	NA	37	—	25 —
Winchester et al[83]	No	19	NA	38	NA	NA
Zwaveling et al[31]	No	19	NA	63	29	21
Broyn & Froyen[32]	As needed	32	NA	20	<1	NA
Kamby & Rose[193]	Yes × 1 y	38	62	35	23	6–10
Hatschek et al[194]	Yes	36	63	30	22	11
Pisansky et al[195]	No	37	63	—	—	—
Zedeler et al[66]	No	31	69	45	25	18
Crippa et al[67]	Yes	24	76	42	—	29 —
Hannisdal et al[59]	Yes	29	71	44	23	10

NA, not available.

* If yes, bone scans were performed routinely. If no, bone scans performed as needed or not performed.

† Site of first relapse either singly or in combination with all sites.

in the liver, and fewer than 5% are in the CNS (see Table 20–1).[2,31–33,59,66,67]

FACTORS PREDICTIVE OF THE FIRST SITE OF RELAPSE

Although many prognostic factors have been identified to predict whether and when a patient will suffer a relapse, few factors provide clues regarding where the relapse will occur. As discussed in Chapter 21, the risk of local–regional relapse after mastectomy is higher in certain subgroups of patients. These include patients with positive lymph nodes and patients with large or locally advanced primary tumors.[68] Estrogen receptor (ER)-negative patients are more likely to have a recurrence in visceral organs than are ER-positive patients, although overlap is considerable.[31,32,68–77] Lobular carcinomas may recur more commonly on serosal surfaces than ductal carcinomas, particularly in the peritoneum and meninges.[78,79]

The effect of adjuvant systemic therapy on the site of recurrence is not well established. Scant data have been reported about the effect of adjuvant systemic therapy on the distribution of distant metastases. Patients receiving adjuvant chemotherapy may be slightly more likely to have liver metastases as the first site of recurrence.[6,80] In one study, of patients who did not receive adjuvant therapy and who experienced relapse, only 2.2% had initial liver metastases.[6] In contrast, 12.5% of those who received cyclophosphamide–methotrexate–5-fluorouracil (CMF) for 6 months and 6.9% of those who received CMF for 12 months and who relapsed had initial hepatic recurrence.

The incidence of CNS metastases may be higher in patients who have received cytotoxic chemotherapy and hormonal therapy.[63,81] Moreover, the Milan group reported that the incidence of CNS metastases after 12 months of adjuvant therapy appeared to be higher than in untreated control patients or in patients who received 6 months of CMF, although the percentage of patients with CNS as the first site of recurrence was still less than 5%.[6] In a more recent study, investigators from the Netherlands reported that the brain was the first site of metastases in 30% of all patients with relapse, and this incidence was twice as high in patients who received adjuvant chemotherapy than in those who did not (50% versus 26%).[81]

In summary, the incidence and sites of local–regional and distant relapse may be altered by various primary and adjuvant treatments. Although the time to recurrence (and ultimately survival) may be affected by the use of adjuvant therapy, the ratio of local recurrence to distant recurrence as initial sites of relapse is not substantially affected. Therefore, screening recommendations for follow-up should be based on likelihood of recurrence and the clinical utility of early detection.

Detection of Early Metastases

ASSOCIATION OF METASTASES WITH SYMPTOMS

Several retrospective studies indicate that well over 50%, and perhaps as many as 75%, of all patients with recurrent breast cancer present with symptomatic metastases (Table 20–2). Most of these studies were retrospective and were not designed specifically to evaluate the detection of metastases before the onset of symptoms.[2,3,5,31–33,71,80,82,83] In studies in which patients were carefully and routinely monitored, however, only 20% to 30% of recurrences were detected before the onset of symptoms[2,31,36,37,59,66–68,71,80,82] (Table 20–2). Those patients who had asymptomatic metastases detected by routine scanning appeared to represent 5% to 30% of all patients who had undergone primary and adjuvant therapy for breast cancer.[82,84] In one randomized trial, 31% of patients screened intensively were found to have asymptomatic recurrence, compared with 31% of those followed by physicians' visits only.[37]

The detection of asymptomatic metastases might be related to the first site of metastasis. For example, although local recurrences may cause pain, itching, or bleeding, more commonly they are discovered by the patient or her physician as asymptomatic masses on the chest wall or in the regional lymph nodes (Table 20–2). Indeed, in one study with routine follow-up, only 8% of all metastases were detected clinically while the patient was asymptomatic.[59] Of those whose first recurrences were local–regional, however, 60% were detected by the physician in asymptomatic patients. Patients with visceral metastases as their first site of recurrence more commonly present with symptoms.[3,59] Of patients with bone as first site of metastasis, between 35% and 70% present with bone pain as an indication of their relapse. Patients with first recurrence in other organs manifest symptoms appropriate to the specific organ system, but the percentage of asymptomatic first recurrences in these patients is not substantially different than in patients with local or bone relapses (see Table 20–2). Patients with intrathoracic or pulmonary metastases may present with cough, shortness of breath, or chest pain.[4,85] Patients with liver metastases as their first recurrence most commonly present with anorexia, weight loss, malaise, and, occasionally, right upper quadrant pain. Jaundice is usually an indication of far advanced disease and is extremely uncommon as a sign of first relapse.[86] In the occasional patient who presents with CNS metastases as the first site of recurrence, symptoms are normally related to the specific site of involvement. These may include such nonspecific findings as headache, nausea, vomiting, or mental status changes, or they may be the result of specific neurologic damage such as cranial nerve palsies, motor dysfunction, or spinal cord compression[87] (see Chaps. 23.1 and 23.4).

Symptoms are not always a reliable indicator of recurrent disease and frequently may result in further evaluations that do not demonstrate metastatic cancer. For example, in one study, of all patients who presented with a symptom that was believed to be suggestive of recurrent disease, further evaluation indicated metastases in only 35%.[74] Investigators from The Netherlands reported that as many as 40% of patients believed to be free of disease who presented with perceived bone pain had normal bone scans and did not develop malignant disease during the subsequent year of follow-up.[88]

Thus, about 70% of all patients whose cancer recurs bring their relapse to the attention of the physician with

TABLE 20-2
Association of Symptoms With First Recurrence

Investigators	Symptoms at Recurrence (% of All Recurrences)	Bone Symptoms if Positive Bone Scan (%)	Lung Symptoms if Positive Check Radiograph (%)	Lead Time*
Rutgers et al[2]	77	59	NA	None
Stierer & Rosen[3]	60	36	82	None
Tomin & Donegan[33]	64	69	66	12 mo
Pandya et al[71]	NA	69	50 ("Visc.")	NA
Scanlon et al[5]	79	NA	NA	NA
Winchester et al[83]	91 (if not on a routine) 65 (if on protocol)	NA	NA	NA
Zwaveling et al[31]	73	57	46	NA
Broyn & Froyen[32]	64	NA	NA	None
Crippa et al[67]	NA	41	NA	NA
Hannisdal et al[59]	66	63	84	19 mo
GIVIO[37]	69 (intensive)† 79 (control)	NA	NA	NA

NA, not available.

* Median time from diagnosis by diagnostic test to onset of symptoms.

† Patients were randomly assigned to intensive or control follow-up schedules. See text for details.

specific symptoms. With the exception of local–regional relapse, which is more commonly asymptomatic, no common site of relapse appears more likely to produce symptoms than another. Of the 20% to 25% of patients found to have asymptomatic recurrences by routine evaluation, the lead time from diagnosis to time of symptoms has been estimated to be about 12 months.[33] This figure depends on the criteria and intervals specified for obtaining scans, however, and may be much shorter or longer.[3,31,72]

EVALUATION OF SPECIFIC SITES OF METASTASIS

The performance characteristics of any diagnostic tool determine how useful it will be to detect early recurrences. For any screening test to be of value, it must be sufficiently sensitive to detect the event in question commonly, yet it must be sufficiently specific that a positive test result reliably predicts that event. The most frequently used tests, other than symptoms and physical examination, are bone scans, chest radiographs, liver–spleen scans, computed tomography (CT) scans, and serologic tests.

Bone Metastases

Approximately 40% to 50% of all first recurrences are in bone (see Table 20-1). Of the available imaging modalities, bone scintigraphy is the most sensitive method of detecting skeletal metastases. Bone scan results can vary, depending on technical details, such as the type of radiotracer and equipment used, and the radiologist's interpretation.

Bone scintigraphy is abnormal if increased uptake is detected when compared with adjacent bone. New scintigraphic lesions in a patient who has otherwise not had a recurrence must be interpreted carefully to distinguish bone metastases from benign disorders. If such foci are changed in relation to a baseline scintigraphic study, the nature of the abnormalities will require further evaluation. Several features have been identified that help to predict whether new foci of uptake represent malignancy. These include the appearance of new lesions when compared with a baseline scintigraphic image and the appearance of more than one new lesion (Table 20-3).[89,90] The annual hazard rate of bone scan conversion from negative to positive parallels that of the risk of metastases in general.[67] Thus, the timing of new lesions may also be helpful in interpreting the bone scan.

The site of a new lesion is also helpful in distinguishing benign from malignant findings. Abnormal radiotracer uptake in the axial skeleton (pelvis, spine, sternum) is more likely to represent metastases than is a "hotspot" in ribs, skull, or long bones.[90,91] Radiographic evaluation of new foci of scintigraphic uptake can be critical in diagnosis of bone metastasis. In one study, plain radiographs were helpful in determining the cause of uptake in nearly half the cases (Table 20-4).[92] Lytic or blastic lesions that correlate with the scintigraphic abnormality are highly suggestive of a malignant cause. Moreover, benign causes of uptake, such as degenerative joint disease, trauma, or bone infarcts, can also be well defined.

In summary, new scintigraphic findings due to bone metastases can usually be distinguished from those caused by benign processes by careful interpretation and judicious

TABLE 20-3
Occurrence of Metastases as a Function of Number of New Abnormalities on Bone Scintigraphy

New Abnormalities	Occurrences	With Metastases
1	182	20 (11%)
2	26	9 (35%)
3	9	4 (45%)
4	2	1 (50%)
5	4	4 (100%)
6	2	2 (100%)
>6	14	14 (100%)
TOTAL	239	54 (23%)

(Modified from Jacobson A, Cronin E, Stomper P, et al. Bone scans with one or two new abnormalities in cancer patients with no known metastases: frequency and serial scintigraphic behavior of benign and malignant lesions. Radiology 1990;175:229.)

use of plain bone radiography. If indicated, CT or magnetic resonance imaging (MRI) can help to further evaluate such lesions. Indeed, MRI may be more sensitive and specific than bone scintigraphy in detecting bone metastases.[93–95] Therefore, in symptomatic patients with normal skeletal scintigraphy and plain radiographs, MRI evaluation is indicated. MRI may be especially helpful in distinguishing patients with vertebral body wedge collapse due to extraosseous metastases from patients with osteoporotic compression fractures, which of course would be treated much differently.[93]

Routine bone scanning can also be used to monitor patients with known metastatic disease who are receiving palliative therapy. Response of bone lesions may be documented by decrease or disappearance of tracer uptake in areas of previously demonstrated metastases. Complete normalization of abnormal bone scans is unusual, however.[96] Responses can be further confirmed by radiographic demonstration of conversion of a lytic lesion to a blastic lesion. A more subtle finding is the appearance of a sclerotic rim around a previously defined lytic lesion, suggesting incomplete healing.

Serial bone scans obtained during therapy may actually worsen in association with a clinical response.[96–99] This so-called scintigraphic flare is manifested by increased uptake in previously observed metastatic sites and even by the appearance of new abnormal uptake in previously normal sites. Flare can be distinguished from disease progression by clinical history and by the appearance of obvious healing (sclerosis) on correlative bone radiographs. Scintigraphic flare can be observed in 30% to 50% of patients experiencing a response to systemic therapy (hormone or chemotherapy). It is detectable within 1 or 2 months of initiation of therapy and may last as long as 6 or more months.[96] One study demonstrated that scintigraphic flare is frequently misinterpreted as disease progression, re-

sulting in inappropriate clinical changes to an alternative regimen.[99]

The mechanism of flare is not certain, but it probably occurs from preferential adsorption of the technetium-99m (^{99m}Tc)-phosphonate compound in foci of new hydroxyapatite crystal formation at a time of bone repair, mediated by osteoblastic activity. Scintigraphic flare should be distinguished from clinical flare, which is manifested by increased bone pain or transient hypercalcemia, often in association with initiation of a new endocrine regimen. Whether those patients who experience scintigraphic flare with response have a more prolonged time to treatment failure or overall survival is not clear.[96,97,100]

Liver Metastases

Liver is an unusual site for first metastases, especially in the absence of disease elsewhere (see Table 20-1). Therefore, routine liver scanning is less likely to be diagnostic for recurrence than routine bone scintigraphy. As discussed later, hepatic enzyme elevations or elevations of tumor markers may serve a indications for further evaluation of the liver. CT scanning detects more than 90% of hepatic lesions and is generally considered the method of choice.[101–104] Certain benign diseases of the liver may cause misinterpretation of a hepatic CT scan, however. For example, fatty liver involvement may create focal alterations of hepatic density on CT scan that mimic metastases. In patients with minor degrees of fatty infiltration, liver scanning with ^{99m}Tc–sulfur colloid is normal, because the hepatic reticuloendothelial system is not affected by this benign condition. With extensive fatty infiltration, hepatomegaly and redistribution to the spleen and bone can

TABLE 20-4
Initial Radiographic Characterization and Diagnosis at Follow-Up for 236 New Bone Scan Abnormalities in 183 Patients With Breast Cancer

Initial Radiographic Interpretation	Diagnosis at Follow-Up	
	Benign	Malignant*
Normal	92	13 (12%)
Degenerative disease	58	1 (2%)
Fracture	19	0
Other benign process	14	0
Equivocal abnormality	15	1 (6%)
Abnormality suggestive of metastasis	11	2 (15%)
Consistent with metastasis	5	5 (50%)
TOTAL	214	22 (9%)

* Values in parentheses are percentages of patients with that condition who developed bone metastases.

(Modified from Jacobson A, Stomper P, Cronin E, et al. Bone scans with one or two new abnormalities in cancer patients with no known metastases: reliability of interpretation of initial correlative radiographs. Radiology 1990;174:503.)

occur, but focal photopenic abnormalities on the radiocolloid scan have not been reported.

Hepatic hemangiomas are relatively common causes of false-positive CT scans. These lesions can be solitary or multiple, and they can be distinguished from malignant lesions by several modalities, including real-time sonography, MRI, and contrast-enhanced CT.[105–107] Hepatic hemangiomas can also be distinguished by the observation of diminished initial flow followed by intense focal uptake in delayed images during scintigraphy after intravenous injection with ^{99m}Tc-labeled autologous red blood cells.[108–111] Single photon emission CT (SPECT) images may also provide high-resolution evaluation of suspicious lesions, especially if these lesions are deep-seated.[112] Ultimately, fine-needle biopsy may be required for a definitive diagnosis. On occasion, patients may have physical or biochemical evidence of hepatic metastases in the presence of a normal CT scan. These patients may have microscopic malignant infiltration of the liver sinusoid, as opposed to focal deposits of parenchymal disease. In such cases, radiocolloid liver–spleen scintigraphy may be more sensitive than CT.[113] Although not absolutely diagnostic, heterogeneous tracer uptake strongly suggests metastasis.

Pulmonary Metastases

Like the liver, the thorax is an uncommon site of first recurrence, accounting for 5% to 20% of all initial relapses (see Table 20-1). Intrathoracic metastases can be identified with the use of routine chest radiography, which may demonstrate hilar or mediastinal lymphadenopathy, pulmonary nodules, pleural-based nodules, or a pleural effusion. In less than 1% of patients, breast cancer metastases present as lymphangitic spread, manifested on chest radiograph as diffuse reticular nodular infiltrates that are usually bilateral.[34,114–116] Thoracic CT scanning is more sensitive than routine chest radiograph for defining metastases. Because the incidence of intrathoracic metastases as a site of first recurrence is low and routine plain radiography is reasonably sensitive, however, CT scanning should be reserved for further evaluation of suspicious findings.[117–119] Similarly, MRI should be limited to evaluating patients with particularly difficult diagnostic problems.

Pleural effusions have several causes, many of which are benign. Therefore, the appearance of a new pleural effusion in a patient without prior or concurrent evidence of metastatic breast cancer should be further evaluated by thoracentesis and cytologic examination (see Chap. 23.9). The presence of elevated tumor markers within a pleural effusion or staining of suspicious cells with monoclonal antibodies directed against tumor-associated antigens (TAAs) may suggest a malignant origin. These assays are not sufficiently specific to be an absolute indicator of metastases, however.[120–125] In the absence of positive cytologic findings or evidence of recurrence elsewhere, especially in a patient with a relatively low risk of relapse, a benign cause of a new pleural effusion should be considered.

Of particular interest is the development of pleural or pulmonary changes in patients who have undergone excisional biopsy and breast irradiation. Up to 15% of patients who receive tangential field irradiation for breast conservation develop pleural-based changes in the anterior upper thorax during the first 2 to 24 months after treatment.[126–128] This occurrence may be less frequent in patients treated with modern techniques.[128] These changes may mimic pulmonary metastases, and thoracic CT scanning may be helpful in distinguishing benign from malignant causes. The risk of secondary lung cancer may be increased in patients who had been previously treated with radiation to the chest wall.[129] Thus, it is important to evaluate a patient with new pulmonary changes fully to rule out a curable, new primary lung cancer.

CNS Metastases

Because the incidence of the nervous system as a site of first recurrence is extremely low (see Table 20-1), routine screening for recurrence in these sites is not recommended for breast cancer patients. Evaluation of the central or peripheral nervous systems should be reserved for patients in whom symptoms are suggestive of recurrent breast cancer. In one autopsy series, about 60% of CNS metastases were parenchymal, whereas the remainder were dural (about 25%) or leptomeningeal (about 15%).[79]

CT scanning provides an accurate evaluation of the brain in such patients. The classic finding is an enhancing ring lesion or a lesion within the parenchyma with most metastases located in the supratentorial gray–white matter junction, although cerebellar lesions are not uncommon.[81,130] Brain metastases are solitary in about 40% to 50% of patients with CNS parenchymal disease.[81,87,131] Other CT findings include osteolytic skull metastases with contiguous extension into the extradural and dural mater.

In patients with highly suggestive clinical symptoms and normal CT scans, the use of MRI, especially with gadolinium (Gd) enhancement, provides a more sensitive test.[130,132–134] In one study of patients with small cell lung cancer, both methods detected all CNS lesions 2 cm or larger.[132] Gd-enhanced T1-weighted images were superior in detecting smaller metastases, however.[132] Short repetition time, Gd-enhanced scans may be particularly helpful in detecting posterior fossa lesions.[133]

As with the evaluation of suspicious effusions, investigators have assayed cerebrospinal fluid (CSF) for the presence of tumor markers such as carcinoembryonic antigen (CEA).[135] Although CEA may be elevated in patients with carcinomatous meningitis, elevated CEA in CSF does not definitively indicate leptomeningeal involvement, because elevated peripheral CEA levels may produce high CSF levels as well.[135] The lack of 100% specificity for neoplastic cells prevents complete reliance on positive monoclonal antibody staining as an indication of malignant involvement.[136–138]

Intracranial findings may not necessarily represent metastases. For example, patients with a history of breast cancer have a slightly higher than expected incidence of meningiomas.[139–142] Differentiation of meningioma from metastases is not always easily performed by noninvasive techniques and may require biopsy. Furthermore, other benign diseases, such as cerebrovascular accidents and intracranial infections, must also be considered. In one study, all patients with a history of cancer who had CT or MRI findings suggestive of metastases underwent biopsy to determine eligibility for a prospectively randomized therapeutic trial. Eleven percent (6 of 54) were found to have benign conditions, and half of these conditions were reversible.[40]

USE OF SEROLOGIC ASSAYS FOR SCREENING AND EVALUATION OF PATIENTS WITH BREAST CANCER

An inexpensive and accurate blood test that indicates metastases would be of great utility in screening asymptomatic patients for recurrence. As with all screening modalities, such a test would be valuable only if it were both sensitive and specific, and if the incidence of the event for which it predicts were high. Several such markers have been proposed. These include molecules that are elevated nonspecifically with any inflammatory process (so-called acute-phase reactants), substances that are elevated in the setting of abnormalities of specific organs (such as liver function enzymes or enzymes and proteins contained within bone), or specific tumor markers such as CEA and CA15-3.

Nonspecific Circulating Markers

Although acute-phase reactants are frequently elevated in patients with metastatic breast cancer, they are also elevated in association with many other nonmalignant processes. The poor specificity of acute-phase reactants precludes reliable clinical utility. In contrast, elevations of bone-related enzymes, such as AP, and liver function tests, such as AP or serum glutamic oxaloacetic transaminase (SGOT), may be predictive of recurrent metastases. Of those patients who have suffered a relapse, few patients with local or regional relapse have elevated AP or transaminase levels.[59] Therefore, a rising level of either of these two enzymes (or similar bone- or liver-based enzymes), if associated with recurrence, is most likely predictive of distant metastases.

Between 30% and 60% of patients with true positive bone scans have elevated AP levels.[59,82,86,143,144] Unfortunately, many patients with bone metastases have normal AP levels. Furthermore, an elevated AP may be secondary to causes other than bone metastases, including liver metastases (see later in this chapter) and many benign liver and bone conditions. For example, the Ludwig Breast Cancer Study Group observed that only 34% of 290 patients with elevated AP levels had bone metastases when these patients were scintigraphically or radiographically evaluated.[82] Other investigators have reported that almost 20% of patients with an elevated AP remained free of detectable metastatic disease.[143] In summary, the negative predictive value of AP for bone metastases (ie, a negative test implies the absence of diseases) is relatively low. Moreover, many elevated AP levels represent false-positives. Nonetheless, rising serial AP levels do provide an indication for bone scintigraphy in patients with a history of breast cancer, especially in the setting of suspicious symp-

toms, because 40% to 80% of these patients have detectable bone metastases.

As with AP levels for bone recurrence, serial liver function tests (LFTs) may be valuable for monitoring for liver metastases, although again, these tests are relatively insensitive and nonspecific. Furthermore, the low incidence of liver as a first site of recurrence further reduces the predictive value of AP for liver metastases (see Table 20-1). The frequency of LFT elevations in patients with liver metastases ranges from 32% to 95%[143,145–152] (Table 20-5). Unfortunately, as is the case in using AP to screen for bone recurrence, LFTs may be falsely elevated in 60% to 80% of patients[143,146,148,149] (Table 20-5). Persistently rising AP levels, in the absence of known benign liver disease, are more predictive of recurrent breast cancer than are isolated elevations.[143] Likewise, SGOT is elevated in many nonmalignant conditions of the liver, but abnormal levels associated with elevations in other markers and LFTs may indicate hepatic metastases. Thus, serial AP and SGOT levels may, by themselves, be unreliable indicators of relapse. Their use in combination with clinical evaluation and specific tumor markers, however, serves to indicate the necessity for further radiographic evaluation.

TUMOR-ASSOCIATED ANTIGENS

Ideally, monitoring of a substance produced specifically by the cancer for which the patient is being followed-up would provide a sensitive and reliable means of detecting early recurrence. Although many such tumor markers have been proposed for patients with breast cancer, CEA is the most commonly used and is the marker for which the greatest clinical experience is available. Although several reports suggest that CEA might be useful to monitor patients for relapse, others suggest that it is not sufficiently sensitive or specific for this indication.[56] CEA levels are

TABLE 20-5
Alkaline Phosphatase as an Indicator of Recurrent Breast Cancer in Liver

Study	Patients	Sensitivity*	Specificity†
Royal Marsden[145]	287	8/51 (35%)	NA
Brigham[146]	55	35/51 (71%)	60%
Naval[147]	NA	5/8 (63%)	NA
Surrey[196]	152	15/46 (44%)	77/94 (82%)
Case[148]	192	18/19 (95%)	80%
Bowman-Gray[143]	146	45/91 (49%)	37/39 (95%)
UCLA[149]	109	29/50 (95%)	29/35 (83%)
Guys[150]	730	NA	45/106 (42%)

NA, not available.

* Number of patients with positive liver–spleen scan (denominator) who had elevated alkaline phosphatase level (numerator).

† Number of patients with elevated alkaline phosphatase level (denominator) who had positive liver–spleen scan (numerator).

elevated in 40% to 50% of patients with metastatic breast cancer.[153-157] Elevations in patients destined to have a relapse but who have not yet done so are lower (Table 20-6). Nonetheless, lead times between elevation of CEA levels and detection of recurrence in these patients ranges from 0 to 20 months (Table 20-6). Furthermore, as many as 30% of elevated CEA levels in patients who are free of detectable disease represent false-positive results. Several benign conditions may cause low-level CEA elevation.[55,158-160] These include cigarette smoking and benign inflammatory diseases of the liver, gastrointestinal tract, or breasts. The pattern of serial CEA levels is highly predictive of relapse, however. Serial CEA levels that are consistently increasing above normal levels, especially levels higher than 10 ng/mL, are highly suggestive of current or subsequent metastases.[161] Unfortunately, the time required to determine such a pattern, by definition, decreases the lead time before documentation of metastatic disease.

Data for the use of other TAAs to monitor patients for recurrent breast cancer are more limited. One group of authors suggested that the use of gross cystic disease protein in combination with CEA provided lead times of 1 to 7 months in approximately 25% of patients who experienced relapse.[162] These data are not substantially better than those with CEA alone.

Over the last 15 years, specific and reproducible assays have been constructed using monoclonal antibodies that detect a high-molecular-weight, mucin-like glycoprotein in the serum of patients with breast cancer. Designations for these assays include CA15-3, CA549, mammary cancer antigen (MCA), mammary serum antigen (MSA), and breast mucin antigen (BCM).[154,163-166] Studies with these assays have demonstrated that monitoring of these circulating mucins in patients with metastatic breast cancer is superior to that for CEA or other TAAs (Table 20-7).[55] In general, the superior utility of these circulating mucins

when compared with CEA in patients with breast cancer stems from an increased sensitivity, although specificity is usually equivalent or superior as well.[55] CA15-3 is elevated in 75% to 80% of patients with metastatic breast cancer and in 20% to 50% of patients with newly diagnosed primary breast cancer.

CA15-3 levels may be elevated in patients with certain benign conditions.[55] Of patients with benign breast conditions, 20% have elevated CA15-3 levels. Furthermore, inflammatory diseases of the liver, gastrointestinal tract, and lungs can elevate CA15-3 levels, although cigarette smoking has not been reported to cause elevated CA15-3 levels. Neither pregnancy nor lactation appears to be associated with elevated CA15-3 levels. As with CEA, none of the mucin assays is specific for breast cancer. Although these assays differ slightly in their detection of circulating antigen in patients with nonbreast malignant disease, up to 70% of patients with advanced epithelial cancers of the lung, colon, ovary, or prostate have elevated circulating levels (see Table 20-7). The sensitivity, specificity, and predictive values for relapse of these markers in patients who are free of disease have not yet been determined. As with CEA, CA15-3 levels may commonly be elevated before relapse, and preliminary reports suggest that elevated CA15-3 levels are predictive of recurrent cancer in 40% to 60% of patients.[167-169] In one study, when CA15-3 levels were elevated in two consecutive visits, the positive predictive value of a rising CA15-3 level for subsequent metastases was 58%.[168] The specificity of CA15-3 in these studies was greater than 99%,[167,168,170] and in at least one study, CA15-3 was more sensitive than CEA in detecting metastases.[169] Unlike AP or the transaminases (see earlier), rising tumor-associated markers may be likely to reflect local or regional relapse as well as distant metastases.[170] A higher percentage of patients with distant metastases have elevated levels, however.[154] Finally, cutoffs

TABLE 20-6
Carcinoembryonic Antigen as an Indicator of Recurrent Breast Cancer

| Investigators | Patients | Patients With Relapse | Patients With Elevations in CEA (%) | | Median Lead Time (mo) |
			True-Positive (%)	False-Positive (%)	
Lamerz et al[197]	2095	285	22	NA	NA (0–7)
Lee[158]	243	50	68	27	NA
Staab et al[198]	229	65	80	NA	4.8 (0–12)
Haagensen et al[162]	235	58	26	NA	4.8 (0–12)
DeJong-Balcker et al[182]	206	NA	38	NA	6.5 (NA)
Falkson et al[161]	114	17	45	NA	6 (0–10)
Bezwoda et al[181]	107	57	23	27	NA
Chatal et al[199]	76	27	15	10	NA
Nicolini et al[200]	224	33	58	11	5.1 (0–20)

CEA, carcinoembryonic antigen; NA, not available.

TABLE 20-7
Sensitivity and Specificity of Circulating Breast Cancer Tumor–Associated Antigens

| Antigen | Reference | Cutoff | Controls | Breast Cancer Stage | | | | Benign | | Other Malignancies | | |
				I	II	III	IV/Met	Breast	Liver	RT	GI	Other
CEA	201	5 ng/mL	5	10	15	35	60	20	60	55	85	50
TPA	202	90 U/mL	—	27	37	57	—	30	—	—	—	—
GCDP	203	50 ng/mL	15	20	30	12	50	30	—	16	11	—
CA15-3	154	22 U/mL	9	—	36	—	73	20	50	71	61	66
DF3	204	25 U/mL	9	17	—	—	68	—	25	7	9	58
CA549	163	10 U/mL	2	1	—	53	88	4	26	32	18	50
MCA	205	11 U/mL	5	20	21	35	—	—	—	—	—	—
MSA	165	300 U/mL	2	72	82	75	87	18	—	71	60	70

RT, carcinomas of the respiratory tract; GI, carcinomas of the gastrointestinal tract; CEA, carcinoembryonic antigen; TPA, tissue plasminogen activator; GCDP, gross cystic disease protein; MCA, mammary cancer antigen; MSA, mammary serum antigen.

for determining a positive tumor marker to predict recurrence may need to include both absolute marker levels and relative changes in levels over time. The latter evaluation must take into account biologic variations that frequently occur at levels at or below the absolute cutoff used to distinguish normal from abnormal. These variations may range as high as 23% from one time-point to another.[171]

In summary, the usefulness of monitoring TAAs for the detection of relapse has not been entirely established. Few of the trials to determine potential lead times of these markers have been performed in a carefully controlled prospective manner, and, therefore, the reported lead times, estimated to be 2 to 12 months, may represent artifacts of the trial design. Studies remain to be performed to determine whether elevated tumor markers provide substantial lead times over routine clinical follow-up and to determine whether such lead times are clinically important. These markers may well be useful in increasing or decreasing the clinician's suspicion of the presence of metastases and the need for more extensive evaluation, however, because consistently rising levels of CEA or CA15-3 are frequent harbingers of recurrent disease.[153,161]

Although the use of TAAs for screening for cancer recurrence is not established, determination of serial levels of these markers can aid in monitoring the clinical response of patients with metastatic breast cancer who are receiving palliative therapy (Fig. 20-4). In this setting, CA15-3 has been shown to be superior to CEA, because substantially more patients have elevated levels, and yet the specificity of changes in serial CA15-3 levels is as good as or better than that for CEA.[55,153] Serial CA15-3 levels correlate with disease course in 60% to 70% of patients with metastatic cancer during therapy, compared with only an approximately 40% correlation for CEA.[153] Serial CA15-3 levels can be particularly helpful in increasing or decreasing the clinical suggestion of a change in clinical course. For example, if a patient receiving therapy is believed to have a 30% chance of disease progression, but the CA15-3 level increases by at least 25%, the probability of true progression (assuming that the elevation is not a spike, discussed later) is raised to 75%. Thus, serial CA15-3 levels can be particularly helpful as an adjunct to other clinical evaluations in patients whose disease course is difficult to determine.

Investigators have reported the occurrence of temporary antigen-level spikes in patients who have recently begun effective therapies and in whom clinical responses eventually occur.[172,173] Spikes in CEA levels have been reported 1 to 4 months after the initiation of effective

FIGURE 20-4 Changes in CA15-3 levels with clinical course. Serial changes in CA15-3 levels were determined during 57 clinical courses in patients with progressive, stable, or regressive breast cancer. (Hayes DF, Zurawski Jr VR, Kufe DW. Comparison of circulating CA15-3 and carcinoembryonic antigen levels in patients with breast cancer. J Clin Oncol 1986;4:1542)

therapy in up to 48% of responding patients. Similarly, spikes in CA15-3 levels have also been observed (Fig. 20-5). The clinician must be careful not to interpret a rising TAA level during an early period of a new therapeutic modality as representing disease progression. Rather, such a spike may predict ultimate response. Unfortunately, distinguishing between a spike and true disease progression may be difficult and may be possible only with longer follow-up of the patient.

Other potential uses for monitoring circulating tumor markers include screening the general population for the presence of new primary breast cancers and determining prognosis for patients with newly diagnosed cancers. In general, none of the currently available assays for any of the TAAs is sufficiently sensitive or specific to be used for screening the general population. For example, CA15-3 is elevated in only 30% of patients with new primary breast cancers.[154,174–178] With a specificity of about 90% in a normal population, the predictive value of a positive test would be only approximately 1.8%. Another assay that detects a member of the sialomucin family, MSA, has been reported to have a sensitivity of 76% in patients with new primary breast cancers. In one study, the specificity of this assay was 82%, and the predictive value for a positive test in this study was 72%.[179] Although intriguing, these preliminary data were not derived from a general, normal population. None of these tests should yet be considered adequate for screening.

Likewise, circulating markers are of little value in the determination of the differential diagnosis of newly discovered suspicious lesions of the breast. Because up to 20% of patients with benign mammary diseases have elevated CA15-3 or CEA levels, the predictive value of either of these tests in this setting is unacceptably low. Moreover, none of these assays is tissue-specific, although gross cystic disease protein may be restricted to only a few malignant diseases other than breast cancer.[180] Therefore, in general, circulating markers are unreliable indicators of the primary site in patients with tumors of unknown origin. The mucin assays are relatively specific for epithelial tissues, however, and may be useful in distinguishing poorly differentiated carcinomas from mesenchymal or hematologic malignant diseases.

Circulating tumor markers could be useful as prognostic indicators in breast cancer. Although some authors have reported that patients with primary or metastatic disease with elevated CEA levels may have a worse prognosis, other studies have failed to show a correlation between perioperative CEA levels and clinical outcome.[172,181–187] Immunoperoxidase and immunoblot studies have suggested that expression of the mucin antigens in primary breast tissues may be associated with prolonged disease-free intervals.[188] No study has been published in which circulating mucin levels have been investigated for prediction of prognosis, however. A monoclonal antibody enzyme-linked immunosorbent assay (ELISA) has been used to detect a circulating protein related to the *c-neu* oncogene.[189–191] Because overproduction of *c-neu* in primary tumors predicts for a worse-prognosis in patients with lymph node–positive breast cancer, monitoring levels of circulating *neu*-related protein might also have prognostic significance. Such studies have not yet been performed, however.

Current Screening Practices After Primary Therapy

Two surveys have documented patterns of care among two sets of oncologists: those who practiced in the southeastern United States during the late 1980s[192] and those who belonged to the American Society of Clinical Oncology (ASCO) in the early 1990s.[43] In both studies, history and physical examinations were recommended by most physicians every 3 to 6 months for the first 5 years, with decreasing frequency afterward. Furthermore, complete blood counts and liver function tests were ordered on a similar frequency. Approximately 25% of physicians ordered specific tumor-marker assays (CEA or CA15-3). Chest radiographs were ordered every 9 to 12 months by over 50% of respondents in one study and by over 80% in the other. Routine bone scintigraphy was obtained by 50% of the southeastern oncologists and by 25% of the ASCO respondents. Other radiographs and scans were much less commonly ordered. These results suggest the absence of consensus regarding follow-up schedules, with heterogeneous practice patterns.

FIGURE 20-5 Spike in serial circulating CA15-3 levels during treatment. Patient A progressed while receiving chemotherapy (*hatched area*) and was then treated by oophorectomy (*arrow*). During the 2 months postoperatively, the CA15-3 (*closed circles*) rose to three times the baseline value and then returned to baseline. The patient ultimately responded to the oophorectomy, and CA15-3 levels declined in correlation. Patient B was treated with chemotherapy (*hatched area*), to which she responded. In this patient, serial CA15-3 levels declined in correlation, without a spike. (Hayes DF, Zurawski Jr VR, Kufe DW. Comparison of circulating CA15-3 and carcinoembryonic antigen levels in patients with breast cancer. J Clin Oncol 1986; 4:1542)

MANAGEMENT SUMMARY

Intensive follow-up may be indicated for patients who participate in clinical research protocols in which disease-free survival is an endpoint. Furthermore, clinical trials testing innovative therapies might best be performed in patients with asymptomatic recurrence, so effective palliative therapy is not required immediately. Studies of newer tumor markers may provide longer lead times between evidence of occult recurrence and detectable metastases, although further studies are required to determine whether treatment of such patients is advantageous. In the meantime, the following recommendations are suggested for routine follow-up of patients after primary therapy for breast cancer:

- No specific follow-up measures for detection of recurrence should be performed while patients are receiving adjuvant chemotherapy.
- Mammography (and other screening for *new* malignancies such as colorectal, ovarian, cervical, and uterine cancers) should be performed yearly.
- Routine clinic visits, including history and physical examination, are reasonably performed every 3 to 4 months during the first 3 years following primary therapy, every 6 months for the next 2 to 3 years, and then perhaps yearly thereafter. Routine monitoring of LFTs and tumor markers may provide inexpensive indications of recurrence, but the clinical advantage of such information is uncertain. The use of bone scans, chest radiographs, or liver imaging modalities does not appear to be indicated on a routine basis unless the patient has symptoms that warrant further evaluation or unless serologic tests are rising in a manner strongly indicative of recurrent disease.

ACKNOWLEDGMENT

Dr. Hayes would like to acknowledge the contributions, to this chapter and to the field, of his coauthor and good friend Dr. William Kaplan, who passed away during the preparation of this book.

References

1. Umbach GE. Screening for recurrent breast cancer. (Letter) J Clin Oncol 1987;5:1127

2. Rutgers EJ, van Slooten EA, Kluck HM. Follow-up after treatment of primary breast cancer. Br J Surg 1989;76:187.

3. Stierer M, Rosen HR. Influence of early diagnosis on prognosis of recurrent breast cancer. Cancer 1989;64:1128.

4. Chaudary MA, Maisey MN, Shaw PJ, et al. Sequential bone scans and chest radiographs in the postoperative management of early breast cancer. Br J Surg 1983;70:517.

5. Scanlon EF, Oviedo MA, Cunningham MP, et al. Preoperative and follow-up procedures on patients with breast cancer. Cancer 1980 46:977.

6. Valagussa P, Tesoro Tess JD, Rossi A, et al. Adjuvant CMF effect on site of first recurrence and appropriate follow-up intervals, in operable breast cancer with positive axillary nodes. Breast Cancer Res Treat 1982;1:349.

7. Adair F, Berg J, Joubert L, et al. Long-term follow-up of breast cancer patients: the 30-year report. Cancer 1974;33:1145.

8. Fisher B, Anderson S, Fisher E, et al. Significance of ipsilateral breast tumor recurrence after lumpectomy. Lancet 1991;338:327.

9. Harris JR, Connolly JL, Schnitt SJ, et al. The use of pathologic features in selecting the extent of surgical resection necessary for breast cancer patients treated by primary radiation therapy. Ann Surg 1985;201:164.

10. Rozen P, Fireman Z, Figer A, et al. Colorectal tumor screening in women with a past history of breast, uterine, or ovarian malignancies. Cancer 1986;57:1235.

11. Fraumeni J, Grundy G, Creagan E, et al. Six families prone to ovarian cancer. Cancer 1975;36:364.

12. Lynch H, Harris R, Guirgis H, et al. Familial association of breast/ovarian carcinoma. Cancer 1978;41:1543.

13. Shapiro CL, Henderson IC. Late cardiac effects of adjuvant therapy: too soon to tell? Ann Oncol 1994;5:196.

14. Fornander T, Cedermark B, Mattsson A, et al. Adjuvant tamoxifen in early breast cancer: occurrence of new primary cancers. Lancet 1989;1:117.

15. Fisher B, Costantino JP, Redmond CK, et al. Endometrial cancer in tamoxifen-treated breast cancer patients: findings from the National Surgical Adjuvant Breast and Bowel Project (NSABP) B-14. J Natl Cancer Inst 1994;86:527.

16. Morris S, Corder AP, Taylor I. What are the benefits of routine breast cancer follow-up? Postgrad Med J 1992;68:904.

17. Tomiak EM, Piccart MJ. Routine follow-up of patients following primary therapy for early breast cancer: what is useful? Acta Clin Belg Suppl 1993;15:38.

18. Tomiak E, Piccart M. Routine follow-up of patients after primary therapy for early breast cancer: changing concepts and challenges for the future. Ann Oncol 1993;4:199.

19. Schapira DV. A minimalist policy for breast cancer surveillance. JAMA 1991;265:380.

20. Wertheimer MD. Against minimalism in breast cancer follow-up (Editorial). JAMA 1991;265:396.

21. Holli K, Hakama M. Effectiveness of routine and spontaneous follow-up visits for breast cancer. Eur J Cancer Clin Oncol 1989;25:251.

22. Muss HB, Tell GS, Case LD, et al. Perceptions of follow-up care in women with breast cancer. Am J Clin Oncol 1991;14:55.

23. Kagan AR, Steckel RJ. Routine imaging studies for the posttreatment surveillance of breast and colorectal carcinoma. J Clin Oncol 1991;9:837.

24. Langlands A, Pocock S, Kerr G, et al. Long-term survival of patients with breast cancer: a study of the curability of the disease. BMJ 1979;2:1247.

25. Rosen P, Groshen W, Saigo P, et al. A long-term follow-up study of survival in stage I (T1N0M0) and stage II (T1N1M0) breast carcinoma. J Clin Oncol 1989;7:355.

26. Rutqvist LE. Increasing incidence and constant mortality rates of breast cancer: time trends in Stockholm County 1961–1973. Breast Cancer Res Treat 1984;4:233.

27. Harris J, Hellman S. Observations on survival curve analysis with particular reference to breast cancer treatment. Cancer 1986;57:925.

28. Early Breast Cancer Trialists' Collaborative Group T. Systemic treatment of early breast cancer by hormonal, cytotoxic, or immune therapy: 133 randomised trials involving 31,000 recurrences and 24,000 deaths among 75,000 women. Lancet 1992;339:1,71.

29. Hayes DF, Henderson IC. CAF in metastatic breast cancer: standard therapy or another effective regimen. J Clin Oncol 1987;5:1497.

30. Hayes DF, Henderson IC, Shapiro CL. Treatment of metastatic

breast cancer: present and future prospects. Semin Oncol 1995;22:5.

31. Zwaveling A, Albers GHR, Felthuis W, et al. An evaluation of routine follow-up for detection of breast cancer recurrences. J Surg Oncol 1987;34:194.

32. Broyn T, Froyen J. Evaluation of routine follow-up after surgery for breast carcinoma. Acta Chir Scand 1982;148:401.

33. Tomin R, Donegan WL. Screening for recurrent breast cancer. Its effectiveness and prognostic value. J Clin Oncol 1987;5:62.

34. Hietanen P. Chest radiography in the follow-up of breast cancer. Acta Rad Oncol 1986;25:15.

35. Karabali-Dalagama S, Souhami RL, O'Higgins NJ, et al. Natural history and prognosis of recurrent breast cancer. Br Med J 1978;2:730.

36. Rosselli Del Turco M, Palli D, Cariddi A, et al. Intensive diagnostic follow-up after treatment of primary breast cancer: a randomized trial. JAMA 1994;271:1593.

37. GIVIO Investigators. Impact of follow-up and testing on survival and health-related quality of life in breast cancer patients: a multicenter randomized controlled trial. JAMA 1994;271:1587.

38. Martin EWJ, Minton JP, Carey LC. CEA-directed second-look surgery in the asymptomatic patient after primary resection of colorectal carcinoma. Ann Surg 1985;202:310.

39. Wilkins E, Head J, Burke J. Pulmonary resection for metastatic neoplasms in the lung. Am J Surg 1978;135:480.

40. Patchell R, Tibbs P, Walsh J, et al. A randomized trial of surgery in the treatment of single metastases to the brain. N Engl J Med 1990;322:494.

41. Hayes DF. Is there a role for pulmonary nodulectomy in urologic cancers? In: Garnick M, eds. Genitourinary cancer. New York, Churchill Livingstone, 1985:243.

42. Anderson J, Cain K, Gelber R. Analysis of survival by tumor response. J Clin Oncol 1983;1:710.

43. Simon MS, Hoff M, Hussein M, et al. An evaluation of clinical follow-up in women with early stage breast cancer among physician members of the American Society of Clinical Oncology. Breast Cancer Res Treat 1993;27:211.

44. Ryan J, Rowe D, Salcicuolio G. Prophylactic internal fixation of the femur for neoplastic lesions. J Bone Joint Surg 1976;58:1071a.

45. Harrison K, Muss H, Ball M, et al. Spinal cord compression in breast cancer. Cancer 1985.

46. Boogerd W, van der Sande JJ, Kröger R. Early diagnosis and treatment of spinal epidural metastasis in breast cancer: a prospective study. J Neurol Neurosurg Psychiatry 1992;55:1188.

47. Maranzano E, Latini P, Checcaglini F, et al. Radiation therapy of spinal cord compression caused by breast cancer: report of a prospective trial. Int J Radiat Oncol Biol Phys 1992;24:301.

48. Mueller CB. Asymptomatic metastases: to treat or not to treat? Surg 1983;93:328.

49. Fisher B, Redmond C, Dimitrov N, et al. A randomized clinical trial evaluating sequential methotrexate and fluorouracil in the treatment of patients with node-negative breast cancer who have estrogen-receptor-negative tumors. N Engl J Med 1989;320:473.

50. Fisher B, Costantino J, Redmond C, et al. A randomized clinical trial evaluating tamoxifen in the treatment of patients with node-negative breast cancer who have estrogen-receptor-positive tumors. N Engl J Med 1989;320:479.

51. Mansour E, Gray R, Shatila A, et al. Efficacy of adjuvant chemotherapy in high-risk node-negative breast cancer. N Engl J Med 1989;320:485.

52. Ludwig Breast Cancer Study Group. Prolonged disease-free survival after one course of perioperative adjuvant chemotherapy for node-negative breast cancer. N Engl J Med 1989;320:491.

53. DeVita V. Breast cancer therapy: exercising all our options. (Editorial) N Engl J Med 1989;320:527.

54. Dillman RO. Monoclonal antibodies for treating cancer. Ann Intern Med 1989;111:592.

55. Hayes DF, Tondini C, Kufe DW. Clinical applications of CA15-3. In: Sell S, eds. Serological cancer markers. Totowa, NJ, Humana, 1992:281.

56. Hayes DF. Tumor markers for breast cancer. Ann Oncol 1993;4:807.

57. Fisher E, Sass R, Fisher B. Pathologic findings from the National Surgical Adjuvant Project for breast cancers (protocol no. 4). Cancer 1984;53:712.

58. Osborne CK. Prognostic factors for breast cancer: have they met their promise? (Editorial) J Clin Oncol 1992;10:679.

59. Hannisdal E, Gundersen S, Kvaloy S, et al. Follow-up of breast cancer patients stage I–II: a baseline strategy. Eur J Cancer 1993;29A:992.

60. Brinkley D, Haybittle J. The curability of breast cancer. Lancet 1975;2:95.

61. Bonadonna G, Valagussa P. Systemic therapy in resectable breast cancer. Hematol Oncol Clin North Am 1989;3:727.

62. Fisher B, Fisher ER, Redmond C. Ten-year results from the National Surgical Adjuvant Breast and Bowel Project (NSABP) clinical trial evaluating the use of L-phenylalanine mustard (L-PAM) in the management of primary breast cancer. J Clin Oncol 1986;4:929.

63. Amer MH. Chemotherapy and pattern of metastases in breast cancer patients. J Surg Oncol 1982;19:101.

64. Cho S, Choi H. Causes of death and metastatic patterns in patients with mammary cancer. Am J Clin Pathol 1980;73:232.

65. Hagemeister FBJ, Buzdar AU, Luna MA, et al. Causes of death in breast cancer: a clinicopathologic study. Cancer 1980;46:162.

66. Zedeler K, Keiding N, Kamby C. Differential influence of prognostic factors on the occurrence of metastases at various anatomical sites in human breast cancer. Stat Med 1992;11:281.

67. Crippa F, Seregni E, Agresti R, et al. Bone scintigraphy in breast cancer: a ten-year follow-up study. J Nucl Biol Medicine 1993;37:57.

68. Pisansky TM, Ingle JM, Schaid DJ, et al. Patterns of tumor relapse following mastectomy and adjuvant systemic therapy in patients with axillary lymph node-positive breast cancer: influence of clinical, histopathologic, and flow cytometric factors. Cancer 1993;72:1247.

69. Campbell FC, Blamey RW, Elston CW, et al. Oestrogen-receptor status and sites of metastasis in breast cancer. Br J Cancer 1981;44:456.

70. Qazi R, Chuang J-L, Drobyski W. Estrogen receptors and the pattern of relapse in breast cancer. Arch Intern Med 1984;144:2365.

71. Pandya KJ, McFadden ET, Kalish LA, et al. A retrospective study of earliest indicators of recurrence in patients on Eastern Cooperative Group adjuvant chemotherapy trials for breast cancer: a preliminary report. Cancer 1985;55:202.

72. Kamby C, Dirksen H, Vejborg I, et al. Incidence and methodologic aspects of the occurrence of liver metastases in recurrent breast cancer. Cancer 1987;59:1524.

73. Powles TJ, Smith IE, Ford HT, et al. Failure of chemotherapy to prolong survival in a group of patients with metastatic breast cancer. Lancet 1980;580.

74. Ormiston MC, Timoney AG, Qureshi AR. Is follow-up of patients after surgery for breast cancer worthwhile? J R Soc Med 1985;78:920.

75. Horton J. Follow-up of breast cancer patients. Cancer 1984;53:790.

76. Forrest APM, Cant ELM, Roberts MM, et al. The computed tomographic findings in intracranial metastases due to breast carcinoma. Br J Surg 1979;66:749.

77. Kamby C, Rose C, Ejlertsen B, et al. Stage and pattern of metastases

in patients with breast cancer. Eur J Cancer Clin Oncol 1987; 23:1925.

78. Harris M, Howell A, Chrissohou M, et al. A comparison of the metastatic pattern of infiltrating lobular carcinoma and infiltrating duct carcinoma of the breast. Br J Cancer 1984;50:23.

79. Lamovec J, Zidar A. Association of leptomeningeal carcinomatosis in carcinoma of the breast with infiltrating lobular carcinoma: an autopsy study. Arch Pathol Lab Med 1991;115:507.

80. Kamby C, Rose C, Ejlertsen J, et al. Adjuvant systemic treatment and the pattern of recurrences in patients with breast cancer. Eur J Cancer Clin Oncol 1988;24:439.

81. Boogerd W, Vos VW, Hart AAM, et al. Brain metastases in breast cancer: natural history, prognostic factors and outcome. J Neurol Oncol 1993;15.

82. Pedrazzini A, Gelber R, Isley M, et al. First repeated bone scan in the observation of patients with operable breast cancer. J Clin Oncol 1986;4:389.

83. Winchester DP, Sener SF, Khandekar JD, et al. Symptomatology as an indicator of recurrent or metastatic breast cancer. Cancer 1979;43:956.

84. Wickerham L, Fisher B, Cronin W. The efficacy of bone scanning in the follow-up of patients with operable breast cancer. Breast Cancer Res Treat 1984;4:303.

85. Heitanen P, Miettenen M, Makinen J. Survival after first recurrence in breast cancer. Eur J Cancer Clin Oncol 1986;22:913.

86. Arnstein NB, Harbert JC, Byrne PJ. Efficacy of bone and liver scanning in breast cancer patients treated with adjuvant chemotherapy. Cancer 1984;54:2243.

87. Weisberg L. The computed tomographic findings in intracranial metastases due to breast carcinoma. Comput Radiol 1986;6:297.

88. Schutte HF. The influence of bone pain on the results of bone scans. Cancer 1979;44:2039.

89. Jacobson A, Cronin E, Stomper P, et al. Bone scans with one or two new abnormalities in cancer patients with no known metastases: frequency and serial scintigraphic behavior of benign and malignant lesions. Radiology 1990;175:229.

90. Jacobson A, Stomper P, Jochelson M, et al. Association between number and sites of new bone scan abnormalities and presence of skeletal metastases in patients with breast cancer. J Nucl Med 1990;31.

91. Corcoran RJ, Thrall JH, Kyle RW, et al. Solitary abnormalities in bone scans patients with extraosseous malignancies. Radiology 1976;121:663.

92. Jacobson A, Stomper P, Cronin E, et al. Bone scans with one or two new abnormalities in cancer patients with no known metastases: reliability of interpretation of initial correlative radiographs. Radiology 1990;174:503.

93. Jones AL, Williams MP, Powles TJ, et al. Magnetic resonance imaging in the detection of skeletal metastases in patients with breast cancer. Br J Cancer 1990;62:296.

94. Algra PR, BLoem JL, Tissing H, et al. Detection of vertebral metastases: comparison between MR imaging and bone scintigraphy. Radiographics 1991;11:219.

95. Petren MM, ANdreasson I, Nyman R, et al. Detection of breast cancer metastases in the cervical spine. Acta Radiol 1993;34:543.

96. Janicek MJ, Hayes DF, Kaplan WD. Healing flare in skeletal metastases from breast cancer. Radiology 1994;192:201.

97. Alexander JL, Gillespie PJ, Edelstyn GA. Serial bone scanning using technetium 99m diphosphonate in patients undergoing cyclical combination chemotherapy for advanced breast cancer. Clin Nucl Med 1976;1:13.

98. Rossleigh M, Lovegrove F, Reynolds P, et al. The assessment of response to therapy of bone metastases in breast cancer. Aust NZ J Med 1984;14:19.

99. Vogel CL, Shemano I, Reynolds R, et al. The "worsening" bone scan in breast cancer clinical trials: a potentially significant source of error in response evaluation. Proc Am Soc Clin Oncol 1992;11:50.

100. Coleman R, Mashiter G, Whitaker K, et al. Bone scan flare predicts successful systemic therapy for bone metastases. J Nucl Med 1988;29:1354.

101. Snow J, Goldstein H, Wallace S. Comparison of scintigraphy, sonography, and computed tomography in the evaluation of hepatic neoplasms. Am J Radiol 1979;132:915.

102. Knopf D, Torres W, Fajman W, et al. Liver lesions: comparative accuracy of scintigraphy and computed tomography. Am J Radiol 1982;138:623.

103. Alderson P, Adams D, McNeil B, et al. Computed tomography, ultrasound, and scintigraphy of the liver in patients with colon or breast carcinoma: a prospective comparison. Radiology 1983; 149:225.

104. Bronskill M, Henkelman M, Poon P, et al. Magnetic resonance imaging, computed tomography, and radionuclide scintigraphy in detection of liver metastases. J Can Assoc Radiol 1988;39:3.

105. Bree R, Schwab R, Neiman H. Solitary echogenic spot in the liver: is it diagnostic of a hemangioma? Am J Radiol 1982;140:41.

106. Itai Y, Ohtomo K, Furui S, et al. Noninvasive diagnosis of small cavernous hemangioma of the liver: advantage of MRI. Am J Radiol 1985;145:1195.

107. Freeny P, Marks W. Patterns of contrast enhancement of benign and malignant hepatic neoplasms during bolus dynamic and delayed CT. Radiology 1986;160:613.

108. Front D, Royal H, Israel O, et al. Scintigraphy of hepatic hemangiomas: the value of Tc-99m–labeled red blood cells: concise communication. J Nucl Med 1981;22:684.

109. Rabinowitz S, McKusick K, Strauss H. 99mTc red blood cell scintigraphy in evaluating focal liver lesions. Am J Radiol 1984; 143:63.

110. Moinuddin M, Allison J, Montgomery J, et al. Scintigraphic diagnosis of hepatic hemangioma: its role in the management of hepatic mass lesions. Am J Radiol 1985;145:223.

111. Watson A. Diffuse intra-sinusoidal metastatic carcinoma of the liver. J Pathol Bacteriol 1955;69:207.

112. Tumeh S, Benson C, Nagel J, et al. Cavernous hemangioma of the liver: detection with single-photon emission computed tomography. Radiology 1987;164:353.

113. Drum D, Beard J. Scintigraphic criteria for hepatic metastases from cancer of the colon and breast. J Nucl Med 1976;17:677.

114. Vestergaard A, Herrstedt J, Thomsen HS, et al. The value of yearly chest x-ray in patients with stage I breast cancer. Eur J Cancer Clin Oncol 1989;25:687.

115. Logager VB, Vestergaard A, Herrstedt J, et al. The limited value of routine chest x-ray in the follow-up of stage II breast cancer. Eur J Cancer 1990;26:553.

116. Ciatto S, Pacini P, Andreoli C, et al. Chest x-ray survey in the follow-up of breast cancer patients. Br J Cancer 1989;60:102.

117. Libshitz H, North L. Pulmonary metastases. Radiol Clin North Am 1982;20:437.

118. Chang A, Schaner E, Conkle D, et al. Evaluation of computed tomography in the detection of pulmonary metastases. Cancer 1979;43:913.

119. Mintzer R, Malave S, Nelman H, et al. Computed vs. conventional tomography in evaluation of primary and secondary pulmonary neoplasms. Radiology 1979;132:653.

120. Pinto M, Bernstein L, Brogan D, et al. Immunoradiometric assay of CA 125 in effusions: comparison with carcinoembryonic antigen. Cancer 1987;59:218.

121. Ghosh A, Spriggs A, Taylor-Papadimitriou J, et al. Immunocytochemical staining of cells in pleural and peritoneal effusions with a panel of monoclonal antibodies. J Clin Pathol 1983;36:1154.

122. Epenetos A, Canti G, Taylor-Papadimitriou J, et al. Use of two

epithelium-specific monoclonal antibodies for diagnosis of malignancy in serous effusions. Lancet 1982;2:1004.

123. Menard S, Rilke F, Della Torre G, et al. Sensitivity enhancement of the cytologic detection of cancer cells in effusions by monoclonal antibodies. Am J Clin Pathol 1985;83:571.

124. Martin S, Moshiri S, Thor A, et al. Identification of adenocarcinoma in cytospin preparations of effusions using monoclonal antibody B72.3. Am J Clin Pathol 1986;86:10.

125. Johnston W, Szpak C, Lottich S, et al. Use of a monoclonal antibody (B72.3) as an immunocytochemical adjunct to diagnosis of adenocarcinoma in human effusions. Cancer Res 1985;45:1894.

126. Srinivasan G, Kurtz DW, Lichter AS. Pleural-based changes on chest x-ray after irradiation for primary breast cancer: correlation with findings on computerized tomography. Int J Radiat Oncol Biol Phys 1983;9:1567.

127. Polansky S, Ravin C, Prosnitz L. Pulmonary changes after primary irradiation to rearly breast cancer. Am J Roentgenol 1980;134:101.

128. Lingos TI, Recht A, Vicini F, et al. Radiation pneumonitis in breast cancer patients treated with conservative surgery and radiation therapy. Int J Radiat Oncol Biol Phys 1991;21:355.

129. Neugut AI, Robinson E, Lee WC, et al. Lung cancer after radiation therapy for breast cancer. Cancer 1993;71:3054.

130. Peretti-Viton P, Margain D, Murayama N, et al. Brain metastases. (Review) J Neuroradiol 1991;18:161.

131. Khansur T, Haick A, Patel B, et al. Preoperative evaluation with radionuclide brain scanning and computerized axial tomography of the brain in patients with breast cancer. Am J Surg 1988;155:232.

132. Golfieri R, Cherryman GR, Olliff JF, et al. Comparative evaluation of computerized tomography/magnetic resonance (1.5 T) in the detection of brain metastasis. Radiol Med 1991;82:27.

133. Sze G, Milano E, Johnson C, et al. Detection of brain metastases: comparison of contrast-enhanced MR with unenhanced MR and enhanced CT. Am J Neuroradiol 1990;11:785.

134. Davis PC, Hudgins PA, Peterman SB, et al. Diagnosis of cerebral metastases: double-dose delayed CT vs contrast-enhanced MR imaging. Am J Neuroradiol 1991;12:293.

135. Klee G, Tallman R, Goellner J, et al. Elevation of carcinoembryonic antigen in cerebrospinal fluid among patients with meningeal carcinomatosis. Mayo Clin Proc 1986;61:9.

136. Garson J, Coakham H, Kemshead J, et al. The role of monoclonal antibodies in brain tumor diagnosis and CSF cytology. J Neurol Oncol 1985;3:165.

137. Coakham H, Brownell B, Harper E, et al. Use of monoclonal antibody panel to identify malignant cells in cerebrospinal fluid. Lancet 1984;1:1095.

138. Hancock W, Medley G. Monoclonal antibodies to identify tumor cells in CSF. Lancet 1983;2:739.

139. Schoenberg B, Christine B, Whisnant J. Nervous system neoplasms and primary malignancies of other sites: the unique association between meningiomas and breast cancer. Neurology 1975;25:7105.

140. Smith F, Slavik M, MacDonald J. Association of breast cancer with meningioma: report of two cases and review of the literature. Cancer 1978;42:1992.

141. Burns P, Naresh J, Bain G. Association of breast cancer with meningioma: a report of five cases. Cancer 1986;58:1537.

142. Zon L, Johns W, Stomper P, et al. Breast carcinoma metastatic to a meningioma. Arch Intern Med 1989;149:959.

143. White DR, Maloney III JJ, Muss HB, et al. Serum alkaline phosphatase determination: value in the staging of advanced breast cancer. JAMA 1979;242:1147.

144. Khansur T, Haick A, Patel B, et al. Evaluation of bone scan as a screening work-up in primary and local-regional recurrence of breast cancer. Am J Clin Oncol 1987;10:167.

145. DeRivas L, Coombes RC, Mccready VR, et al. Tests for liver

metastases in breast cancer: evaluation of liver scan and liver ultrasound. Clin Oncol 1980;6:225.

146. Sugarbaker PH, Beard JO, Drum DE. Detection of hepatic metastases from cancer of the breast. Am J Surg 1977;133:531.

147. Sears HF, Gerber FH, Strurtz DL, et al. Liver scan and carcinoma of the breast. Surg Gynecol Obstet 1975;140:409.

148. Wiener SN, Sachs SH. An assessment of routine liver scanning in patients with breast cancer. Arch Surg 1978;113:126.

149. Castagna J, Benfield JR, Yamada H, et al. The reliability of liver scans and function tests in detecting metastases. Surg Gynecol Obstet 1972;134:463.

150. Wang DY, Knyba RE, Bulbrook RD, et al. Serum carcinoembryonic antigen in the diagnosis and prognosis of women with breast cancer. Eur J Cancer Clin Oncol 1984;20:25.

151. Schreve R, Terpstra O, Ausema L, et al. Detection of liver metastases: a prospective study comparing liver enzymes, scintigraphy, ultrasonography and computed tomography. Br J Surg 1984;71:947.

152. Kemeny M, Sugarbaker P, Smith T, et al. A prospective analysis of laboratory tests and imaging to detect hepatic lesions. Ann Surg 1982;195:163.

153. Tondini C, Hayes DF, Gelman R, et al. Comparison of CA15-3 and carcinoembryonic antigen in monitoring the clinical course of patients with metastatic breast cancer. Cancer Res 1988;48:4107.

154. Hayes DF, Zurawski Jr VR, Kufe DW. Comparison of circulating CA15-3 and carcinoembryonic antigen levels in patients with breast cancer. J Clin Oncol 1986;4:1542.

155. Tormey D, Waalkes T, Snyder J, et al. Biological markers in breast carcinoma. Cancer 1977;39:2397.

156. Tormey D, Waalkes T. Clinical correlation between CEA and breast cancer. Cancer 1978;42:1507.

157. Lokich J, Zamcheck N, Lowenstein M. Sequential carcinoembryonic antigen levels in the therapy of metastatic breast cancer. Ann Intern Med 1978;89:902.

158. Lee YN. Carcinoembryonic antigen as a monitor of recurrent breast cancer. J Surg Oncol 1982;20:109.

159. Ashman L, Ludbrook J, Marshall V. Probabilistic application of plasma carcinoembryonic antigen assay in cancer patients. Br Med J 1975;2:721.

160. Moore T, Kantrowitz P, Zamcheck N. Carcinoembryonic antigen (CEA) in inflammatory bowel disease. JAMA 1972;222:944.

161. Falkson HC, Flakson G, Portugal MA, et al. Carcinoembryonic antigen as a marker in patients with breast cancer receiving postsurgical adjuvant chemotherapy. Cancer 1982;49:1859.

162. Haagensen D, Ammirata S, Dilley W, et al. Tumor markers for detection of occult metastasis during the disease-free interval after mastectomy. Surg Forum 1980;31:433.

163. Beveridge R, Chan D, Bruzek D, et al. A new biomaker in monitoring breast cancer: CA 549. J Clin Oncol 1988;6:1815.

164. Bombardieri E, Gion M, Mione R, et al. A mucinous-like carcinoma-associated antigen (MCA) in the tissue and blood of patients with primary breast cancer. Cancer 1989;63:490.

165. Stacker SA, Sacks NP, Golder J, et al. Evaluation of MSA as a serum marker in breast cancer: a comparison with CEA. Br J Cancer 1988;57:298.

166. Xu F-J, Yu Y-H, Daly L, et al. OVX1 radioimmunoassay complements CA-125 for predicting the presence of residual ovarian carcinoma at second-look surgical surveillance procedures. J Clin Oncol 1993;11:1506.

167. Molina R, Prats M, Zanon G, et al. Use of serial determinations of tumor markers (CEA, CA 15-3) in the early diagnosis of relapse in breast cancer patients. Breast Cancer Res Treat 1989;14:169a.

168. Ruibal A, Colomer R, Genolla J. Prognostic value of CA15-3 serum levels in patients having breast cancer. Horm Metab 1987;1:11.

169. Thirion B, Ricolleau G, Fumoleau P. Result of a prospective

study of the CA15-3 reliability in early detection of breast cancer recurrence. Third International Workshop on Monoclonal Antibodies and Breast Cancer, San Francisco, 1988.

170. Al-Jarallah MA, Behbehani AE, El-Nass SA, et al. Serum CA-15.3 and CEA patterns in postsurgical follow-up, and in monitoring clinical course of metastatic cancer in patients with breast carcinoma. Eur J Surg Oncol 1993;19:74.

171. Gion M, Cappelli G, Mione R, et al. Variability of tumor markers in the follow-up of patients radically resected for breast cancer. Tumour Biol 1993;14:325.

172. Loprinzi CL, Tormey DC, Rasmussen P, et al. Prospective evaluation of carcinoembryonic antigen levels and alternating chemotherapeutic regimens in metastatic breast cancer. J Clin Oncol 1986; 4:46.

173. Hayes DF, Kiang DT, Korzun A, et al. CA15-3 and CEA spikes during chemotherapy for metastatic breast cancer. Proc Am Soc Clin Oncol 1988;7:38a.

174. Colomer R, Ruibal A, Navarro M, et al. Circulating CA 15.3 levels in breast cancer: our present experience. Int J Biol Markers 1986;1:89.

175. Gion M, Mione R, Dittadi R, et al. Evaluation of CA15/3 serum levels in breast cancer patients. J Nucl Med Allied Sci 1986;30:29.

176. Pons-Anicet DM, Krebs BP, Mira R, et al. Value of CA 15:3 in the follow-up of breast cancer patients. Br J Cancer 1987;55:567.

177. Fujino N, Haga Y, Sakamoto K, et al. Clinical evaluation of an immunoradiometric assay for CA15-3 antigen associated with human mammary carcinomas: comparison with carcinoembryonic antigen. Jpn J Clin Oncol 1986;16:335.

178. Kallioniemi O, Oksa H, Aaran R, et al. Serum CA15-3 assay in the diagnosis and follow-up of breast cancer. Br J Cancer 1988;58:213.

179. Hare WS, Tjandra JJ, Russell IS, et al. Comparison of mammary serum antigen assay with mammography in patients with breast cancer. Med J Aust 1988;149:402.

180. Mazoujian G, Pinkus GS, Davis S, et al. Immunohistochemistry of a gross cystic disease fluid protein (GCDFP-15) of the breast: a marker of apocrine epithelium and breast carcinomas with apocrine features. Am J Pathol 1983;110:105.

181. Bezwoda W, Derman D, Bothwell T. Significance of serum concentrations of carcinoembryonic antigen, ferritin and calcitonin in breast cancer. Cancer 1981;48:1623.

182. DeJong-Bakker M, Hart A, Persijn J. Prognostic significance of CEA in breast cancer: a statistical study. Eur J Cancer Clin Oncol 1981;17:1307.

183. Krebs B, Lupo R, Namer M. CEA associated with hormonotherapy in metastatic breast cancer. Bull Cancer 1976;63:485.

184. Doyle P, Nicholson R, Groome G. Carcinoembryonic antigen: its role as tumor marker in breast cancer. Clin Oncol 1981;7:53.

185. Koch M, Paterson A, McPherson T. Slope analysis of plasma carcinoembryonic antigen levels in monitoring response to treatment in patients with metastatic carcinoma of the breast. Clin Oncol 1980;6:323.

186. Mughal AW, Hortobagyi GN, Fritsche HA, et al. Serial plasma carcinoembryonic antigen measurements during treatment of metastatic breast cancer. JAMA 1983;249:1881.

187. Theriault RL, Hortobagyi GN, Fritsche HA, et al. The role of serum CEA as a prognostic indicator in stage II and III breast cancer patients treated with adjuvant chemotherapy. Cancer 1989;63:828.

188. Wilkinson M, Howell A, Harris M, et al. The prognostic significance of two epithelial membrane antigens expressed by human mammary carcinomas. Int J Cancer 1984;33:299.

189. Hayes DF, Carney W, Tondini C, et al. Elevated circulating c-neu oncogene product in patients with breast cancer. Breast Cancer Res Treat 1989;14:135a.

190. Carney W, Hamer P, Petit D, et al. Detection and quantitation of the neu oncoprotein. J Tumor Marker Oncol 1991;6:53.

191. Hayes DF, Cirrincione C, Carney W, et al. Elevated circulating HER-2/neu related protein (NRP) is associated with poor survival in patients with metastatic breast cancer. Proc Am Soc Clin Oncol 1993;58.

192. Loomer L, Brockschmidt JK, Muss HB, et al. Postoperative follow-up of patients with early breast cancer. Cancer 1991;67:55.

193. Kamby C, Rose C. Metastatic pattern response to endocrine therapy in human breast cancer. Br Cancer Res Treat 1986;8:197.

194. Hatschek T, Carstensen J, Fagerber G, et al. Influence of s-phase fraction on metastatic pattern and post-recurrence survival in a randomized mammography screening trial. Br Cancer Res Treat 1989;14:321.

195. Pisansky TM, Cha SS, Earle JD, et al. Prostate-specific antigen as a pretherapy prognostic factor in patients treated with radiation therapy for clinically localized prostate cancer. J Clin Oncol 1993; 11:2158.

196. Coombes RC, Powels TJ, Gazet JC, et al. Assessment of biochemical tests to screen for metastases in patients with breast cancer. Lancet 1980;1:296.

197. Lamerz R, Leonhardt A, Ehrhart H. Serial carcinoembryonic antigen determination in the management of metastatic breast cancer. Oncodev Biol Med 1980;1:123.

198. Staab HJ, Ahlemann LM, Anderer FA, et al. Optimizing tumor markers in breast cancer: monitoring, prognosis, and therapy control. Cancer Detect Prev 1985;8:35.

199. Chatal J, Chupin F, Ricolleau G. Use of serial carcinoembryonic antigen assays in detecting relapse in breast cancer involving high risk of metastasis. Eur J Cancer 1981;17:233.

200. Nicolini A, Carpi A, Di MG, et al. A rational postoperative follow-up with carcinoembryonic antigen, tissue polypeptide antigen, and urinary hydroxyproline in breast cancer patients. Cancer 1989; 63:2037.

201. Beard D, Haskell C. Carcinoembryonic antigen in breast cancer. Am J Med 1986;80:241.

202. Lepera P, Valtolina M, Cocciolo M. A preliminary evaluation of CEA and TPA clinical value in an ongoing trial on patients with operable breast cancer. J Nucl Med Allied Sci 1985;29:97.

203. Haagensen D, Mazoujian G, Holder W, et al. Evaluation of a breast cyst fluid protein detectable in the plasma of breast carcinoma patients. Ann Surg 1977;185:279.

204. Hayes DF, Sekine H, Ohno T, et al. Use of a murine monoclonal antibody for detection of circulating plasma DF3 antigen levels in breast cancer patients. J Clin Invest 1985;75:1671.

205. Kerin MJ, McAnena OJ, OMalley VP, et al. CA15-3: its relationship to clinical stage and progression to metastatic disease in breast cancer. Br J Surg 1989;76:838.

Diseases of the Breast, edited by Jay R. Harris,
Marc E. Lippman, Monica Morrow, and Samuel Hellman.
Lippincott-Raven Publishers, Philadelphia, © 1996.

21

Local–Regional Recurrence After Mastectomy or Breast-Conserving Therapy

ABRAM RECHT ▪ DANIEL F. HAYES

TIMOTHY J. EBERLEIN ▪ NORMAN L. SADOWSKY

We define *local recurrence* as any reappearance of cancer in the ipsilateral breast, chest wall, or skin overlying the chest wall after initial therapy. *Regional recurrence* refers to tumor involving the ipsilateral axillary lymph nodes, supraclavicular lymph nodes, infraclavicular lymph nodes, or internal mammary lymph nodes. An *isolated* (or *solitary*) *recurrence* refers to the reappearance of breast cancer in one of these areas in the absence of other disease on routine evaluation.

In this chapter, we discuss the detection of local and regional recurrence, patient evaluation after its discovery, management, and subsequent prognosis. Although we have tried to separate local from regional treatment failures, many authors have not made sharp distinctions between them, especially with regard to patients treated initially with mastectomy. Therefore, some overlap among the sections is inevitable.

Local Disease Recurrence After Mastectomy

PRESENTING SYMPTOMS AND SIGNS

Local recurrence after mastectomy usually appears as one or more asymptomatic nodules in or under the skin of the chest wall. In a series of 60 patients, 62% had only a single nodule, 15% had two skin nodules, 13% had three or four nodules, and 10% had five or more nodules.[1] Multiple nodules occur more frequently among patients who originally had axillary node involvement.[2] These nodules are usually located in or near the scar of the mastectomy or skin graft, with most others in the skin flaps.[1,3] A few patients present with diffuse chest wall involvement with multiple nodules; this, however, seems most common in patients who had locally advanced tumors originally.[4] The development of multiple nodules or diffuse disease of the chest wall appears to be less common in patients whose cancer recurs more than 5 years after mastectomy.[2] Occa-

sionally, local recurrence takes the form of an erythematous, often pruritic skin rash. Recurrences in the pectoralis muscles alone have been described, but they appear to be rare.[5] Asymptomatic gross and microscopic recurrences are rarely discovered at the time of delayed reconstruction.[6] Recurrences may develop at the suture lines or remaining skin of the chest wall after reconstruction with a myocutaneous flap, but recurrences have not been described under or on the flap itself. Simultaneous recurrence in the chest wall and in regional nodal sites occurs in about 30% of patients.[1,3,7–9]

Carcinoma en cuirasse is a distinct form of diffuse infiltration of the skin or subcutaneous tissues of the chest wall, with woody induration and spread of tumor well beyond the boundaries of standard surgery or radiation therapy. Nodules and ulceration are often present (Fig. 21-1). The disease is generally resistant to both local and systemic therapy.

Some 80% to 90% of local recurrences appear by 5 years after mastectomy; nearly all occur by 10 years.[3,8,10–18] Local recurrences occurring 15 to 50 years after initial surgery have been reported.[12,19–21]

About 25% to 30% of patients with local or regional recurrence have preceding distant metastases.[18,22–25] Another 25% of patients are diagnosed as having simultaneous local and distant treatment failure or develop distant metastases within a few months of the discovery of local recurrence.[1,9,24] This pattern appears to hold true regardless of the interval from initial surgery to recurrence.[26]

SUBSEQUENT MORBIDITY AND SPREAD

Only 25% to 30% of patients with chest wall failure suffer significant morbidity from their local recurrence.[18,24] To what extent this favorable outcome is the result of the treatments received, rather than the natural history of their illness, is not clear. In a series of 100 patients with uncontrolled local–regional disease, however, 62 had one or

FIGURE 21-1 Carcinoma en cuirasse. (Courtesy of Arthur Skarin, MD, Dana-Farber Cancer Institute, Boston)

more significant symptoms before death: 47 patients had bleeding or ulceration that required a daily dressing change; 17 patients had pain requiring narcotics; 7 patients had arm edema; and 3 patients had brachial plexus paralysis.[22] Patients with carcinoma en cuirasse may also have restrictive pulmonary deficits related to the bandlike subcutaneous infiltration that may circumscribe chest expansion. Local recurrence in itself may rarely be a cause of death due to infection or pneumothorax.[9,24,27,28]

PROGNOSIS

Despite aggressive local treatment, almost all patients with an isolated local recurrence after mastectomy eventually develop distant metastases. For example, in a series of patients with local–regional recurrence treated from 1968

to 1978 at the Joint Center for Radiation Therapy (JCRT), the 5- and 10-year actuarial rates of freedom from distant metastases were 30% and 7%, respectively[29] (Fig. 21-2). The corresponding rates of overall survival were 50% and 26%. Patients surviving without disease 15 years and 21 years[30] after treatment with radiotherapy have been described, however, and two patients were reported alive and without disease at 13 years[31] and 24 years[16] after radical surgical procedures. Even these patients may ultimately succumb to breast cancer. Morton and Morton[20] described a patient who had a further local recurrence 16 years after initial treatment of a chest wall recurrence.

Numerous factors have been proposed as influencing the disease-free interval and length of survival after the discovery and treatment of an isolated local–regional recurrence. These different types of recurrence have not

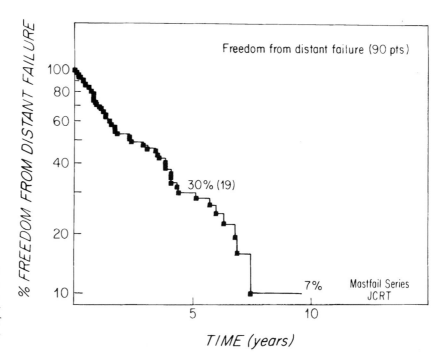

FIGURE 21-2 Freedom from distant failure after radiotherapy for isolated local recurrence, JCRT 1968 to 1978. (Aberizk WJ, Silver B, Henderson IC, et al. The use of radiotherapy for treatment of isolated locoregional recurrence of breast carcinoma after mastectomy. Cancer 1986;58:1214)

usually been separately examined, unfortunately. Multivariate statistical tests have rarely been used to separate the impact of these factors from one another; when these tests have been used, usually only a few factors have been examined because of the limitations of patient numbers and available information.

The largest patient group subjected to a multivariate analysis was 230 patients with isolated local–regional recurrence treated at the Mallinckrodt Institute of Radiology in St Louis.[32] Both site of recurrence and disease-free interval were statistically significant predictors for overall survival; the number of positive lymph nodes at mastectomy, the period when the patient was treated, and the age and menopausal status of the patient at the time of recurrence were not. When 116 patients with disease found only on the chest wall were examined, the size and extent of the recurrent disease was the only significant factor predicting the subsequent length of disease-free survival, but the only significant predictor of overall survival was the disease-free interval.

In the JCRT series of patients with local–regional recurrence, the disease-free interval after mastectomy was significantly associated with the length of subsequent survival ($P = .002$, Cox regression analysis), but age, prior local recurrence, the type of mastectomy, and whether the recurrence could be completely excised were not (JCRT, unpublished data). In a group of 225 patients from Switzerland, the time to development of distant metastases depended on the disease-free interval, initial nodal status, and extent of disease at the time of recurrence, but the disease-free interval was not a statistically significant factor in predicting overall survival.[33] A disease-free interval of 24 months or longer, the ability to excise the recurrence, and the initial axillary nodal status were predictive of

disease-free survival among 128 patients treated at the University of Pennsylvania in Philadelphia; prolonged disease-free interval, tumor excision, and local tumor control were statistically significant predictors of overall survival.[34] When all three factors were favorable (as occurred in 18% of their patient population), the 5-year rates of relapse-free and overall survival were 59% and 61%, respectively.

The interval between mastectomy and local recurrence is thus probably the most reliable indicator of the length of time to distant treatment failure and subsequent survival time, as is true for patients with distant metastases. This may simply reflect the intrinsic growth rate of the tumor cells. For example, patients treated at the University of California at San Francisco from 1918 to 1947 (ie, before truly effective local or systemic therapy) who had a recurrence less than 2 years after mastectomy had a median survival of 13 months, compared with 31 months for those patients who had a recurrence from 2 to 5 years after surgery and 57.5 months (average, 64 months) for patients who had a recurrence more than 5 years after surgery.[16] At the JCRT, the relapse-free survival at 3 years was 20% for patients treated with aggressive radiation therapy who had isolated local recurrence less than 24 months after initial surgery, compared with 36% in patients who had isolated local recurrence 24 months or longer after surgery. The respective 5-year survival rates were 33% and 58%, and 10-year survival rates were 7% and 36%.[29] Similar results have been found in nearly all radiation therapy series,[15,30,32,34–41] with one exception.[42]

Lymph node status at the time of mastectomy also appears to influence prognosis.[32,34,43] For example, among a group of 208 patients with chest wall recurrence treated with excision and radiation therapy in Milan, the 5-year rate of freedom from disease progression was 37% for patients with negative axillary nodes, compared with 19% for node-positive patients.[43] A similar trend was seen for patients whose recurrence could not be grossly excised, but the results were much worse in both groups (rates of 13% and 6%, respectively).

The number of sites of recurrence may be prognostically significant, with superior 5- and 10-year survivals seen in patients who have only a single site of recurrence.[25,30,32,34,35,37,40,41,44] Whether the particular site of recurrence (ie, in lymph nodes alone, in the chest wall alone, in a combination of these, or in specific lymph nodes), rather than the total volume of disease, plays a substantial role in prognosis is unclear.

Tumor grade was one factor not included in any of the foregoing multivariate analyses. Retrospective univariate analyses have had contradictory results about its importance.[25,37] Contradictory retrospective data also exist on the following: the initial surgical stage of the patient,[1,25,34,36–38,41,42] survival of patients with only chest wall disease compared with survival in patients with isolated or concurrent involvement of the regional lymph nodes,[29,30,32,34,35,39,40,42] patient age,[29,32,39] and menopausal status.[15,25,32] The estrogen and progesterone receptor status of the recurrent tumor and the estrogen receptor status of the initial tumor influenced outcome in one series on univariate analysis but were not examined in multivariate analyses.[34]

Little information exists about whether patients who develop a local recurrence despite postmastectomy radiation have a different prognosis after local recurrence than patients who never underwent radiotherapy; results from two randomized trials were contradictory.[18,45] Prior systemic therapy did not seem to affect outcome adversely subsequent to local treatment failure in a randomized trial[18] or in several nonrandomized series.[32,34,39,46,47] In another nonrandomized series, however, only 4% (1 of 23) of such patients survived 5 years or more after local treatment failure;[40] this may have reflected patient selection for such adjuvant therapy, rather than the treatment itself.

PRETREATMENT EVALUATION

Occasionally, other benign or malignant conditions may mimic a local recurrence. The most common of these is a foreign body cyst around suture material. Sometimes, a bony nodule develops on a rib or costal cartilage as a result of surgical trauma.[48] Patients who undergo surgical reconstruction with a myocutaneous flap can develop areas of fat necrosis that may clinically or radiologically mimic recurrent disease.[49] Radiation-induced sarcomas of the bones or soft tissues of the chest wall appear at a median of 10 years after postoperative treatment, but this latency period is variable.[50] Although rare, this diagnosis must be considered in irradiated patients. Therefore, a biopsy should be obtained in all cases of suspected local recurrence, both to establish the diagnosis and to obtain tissue for estrogen and progesterone receptor assays. The estrogen receptor status of the primary tumor and that of subse-

quent metastases are the same in only 75% to 85% of patients.[51]

The patient should have a complete restaging to find distant metastases, as outlined in Chapter 22.1. In addition, as many as 25% to 67% of patients with chest wall or nodal recurrences may have additional sites of involvement discovered only on a computed tomographic (CT) scan of the chest.[52–55] The most common site of unsuspected disease (in 20% to 33% of patients) is in the internal mammary lymph nodes. Multiple involved nodes are frequently seen, most commonly under or near the second and third intercostal spaces.[54] Other evidence of disease sometimes detected only on CT scan includes sternal erosion, mediastinal adenopathy, ipsilateral and contralateral axillary adenopathy, rib metastasis, involvement of the brachial plexus, nonpalpable tumor in the chest wall, and lung metastases. As yet, no studies have compared the effectiveness of magnetic resonance imaging (MRI) with that of CT in this context; in practice, the two may be used interchangeably.

TREATMENT RESULTS

Radiation Therapy

Most patients treated for local recurrence with radiation therapy initially have complete regression of disease (see later). Despite this result, a disappointingly large proportion of those treated in published series have suffered further appearance of local–regional disease. These results may be partly due to deficiencies in prescribing adequate radiation therapy target volumes and doses, however.

Patients with a recurrence in one portion of the chest wall or draining lymph node area may develop a further local recurrence if treatment is not given to the entire chest wall. In the Mallinckrodt series, the 5-year chest wall treatment failure rate was 25% when apparently adequate volumes were treated, compared with 64% when small fields were treated; the respective 10-year actuarial rates were 37% and 82% (Table 21-1).[56] In the groups treated

TABLE 21-1
Sites of Further Local Disease Recurrence

Site	No Radiation Therapy	Elective Radiation Therapy
Chest wall	7/26 (27%)	3/24* (12%)
Supraclavicular nodes†	5/31 (16%)	2/28 (6%)
Axillary nodes	3/108 (3%)	1/75 (1%)
Internal mammary nodes‡	2/68 (3%)	0/118 (0%)

* Includes only patients receiving a dose of 50 Gy or greater.
† P < .05
‡ P = .06

(Data from Halverson KJ, et al. Isolated local–regional recurrence of breast cancer following mastectomy: radiotherapeutic management. Int J Radiat Oncol Biol Phys 1990;19:851) with small fields, two thirds of the subsequent treatment failures occurred outside the field margins. Doses of 50 Gy or higher prevented new lesions from appearing in the uninvolved chest wall in about 90% of patients in this series. In the Milan experience, the 5-year local recurrence rate among patients undergoing tumor excision was 15% when the entire chest wall was irradiated, compared with 36% when limited fields were used.[43] The rates among patients irradiated without tumor excision were 37% and 56%, respectively.

Similarly, patients with chest wall lesions may have subsequent recurrences in regional lymph nodes when only the chest wall is irradiated. The risk of recurrence in untreated supraclavicular nodes was substantial (16%) in one series[56] (see Table 21-1), but it was much lower (5%) in another.[34] The risks of clinically evident recurrences in untreated axillary or internal mammary nodes appear to be small.[34,56]

When large chest wall fields and appropriate nodal irradiation are used, most subsequent local failures are at the original site of disease.[29] In general, the higher the dose of radiation delivered, the less likely is such in-field failure.[30,35,56,57] The volume of disease remaining at the time of irradiation is a critical determinant of the likelihood of achieving long-term local control (Table 21-2). If excision can be performed, then the size of lesion has little impact on the likelihood of achieving local control.[34] Gross tumor excision was possible, however, in only one third to two thirds of patients treated in several series.[29,34,56] When gross residual disease is present, giving a boost dose to achieve a total of more than 60 Gy is needed. Such doses achieve long-term local disease control in perhaps half of such patients.[34,56] Even when large fields are used, failures in the adjacent chest wall or other areas at the edges of the fields can occur. These marginal misses appear to be more likely in patients with larger or more numerous recurrences. In the JCRT series, the incidence of marginal misses was 3% (1 of 29 patients) among patients undergoing complete tumor excision (ie, who had small amounts

of disease); the incidence was 16% (9 of 58) among the remaining patients.[29] Other investigators have found similar results.[44]

The ability to achieve local disease control with radiation therapy also appears to be related to the specific sites involved. Most series show higher local disease control rates when the chest wall or the lymph nodes are involved, rather than both.[29,37,41,42] Recurrences in the mastectomy scar itself may be more difficult to eradicate than other chest wall recurrences.[36] Control of inflammatory-type skin recurrences may be especially difficult. To what degree these findings are governed by the volume or resectability of disease, rather than the specific site, is not clear, however. Patients who suffer a local treatment failure after mastectomy and reconstruction appear to have local disease control rates and outcome that are similar to those of patients who had not had a reconstruction.[58]

No clear differences are seen in local disease control between the different megavoltage photon or electron treatment techniques, and the selection of these techniques is dictated by individual preference and facilities. At the JCRT, we generally use the same techniques as for treatment of the intact breast (see Chap. 17.1). To treat the internal mammary nodes adequately, one must usually include larger volumes of the lung and (for left-sided lesions) heart than are needed to treat the chest wall and supraclavicular nodes. Given the rarity of subsequent recurrence there, the value of treating the internal mammary nodes is uncertain; hence, one must carefully weigh the increased potential morbidity, especially in patients who may have received high doses of doxorubicin. When the internal mammary nodes are included, we use CT scan or radionuclide lymphoscintgraphy to localize them; if these means are not available, the fields are generally extended empirically 3 cm across the midline. The lateral border of the tangential fields is usually placed at the midaxillary line, unless tumor is located close to this edge. Sometimes, one must use supplementary electron-beam fields matched to the edge of the photon fields to cover the extent of the tumor laterally or inferiorly adequately. The placement of the matchline between the tangential and supraclavicular fields must also be done carefully, because one should avoid putting this in an area of gross disease. Because of the potential complications, the previously dissected axilla is not irradiated unless clinically involved or unless only a minimal dissection had been performed initially, but a supraclavicular field is always used. The optimal frequency with which to use bolus therapy is not known. At a minimum, gross lesions and biopsy scars should be covered with bolus daily, and the remainder of the chest wall treated with bolus in place at least every other day. When patients have had prior reconstruction with a myocutaneous flap, bolus needs to be applied only to the native skin. Boosts are usually done with electrons, making sure to cover the entire depth of the chest wall.

Many patients at the JCRT were treated in past years with 2.25-Gy fractions given four times weekly; these patients often developed significant telangiectasia and skin fibrosis.[29] Therefore, we now recommend 1.8- to 2-Gy fractions given five times weekly. Initial doses of 45 to 50

TABLE 21-2
*Radiation Dose, Extent of Surgery, and Chance of In-Field Tumor Recurrence**

Dose (Gy)	Complete Excision	Residual Tumor ≤3 cm	>3 cm or Diffuse or Multiple Tumors
≤49.99	1/9 (11%)	2/7 (29%)	7/8 (88%)
50–54.99	1/26 (4%)	1/5 (20%)	7/15 (47%)
55–59.99	1/21 (5%)	2/9 (22%)	2/11 (18%)
60–64.99	4/22 (18%)	0/9 (0%)	10/20 (50%)
≥65	0/2 (0%)	0/6 (0%)	7/15 (47%)

* Patients treated to small fields excluded.

(Data from Halverson KJ, et al. Isolated local-regional recurrence of breast cancer following mastectomy: radiotherapeutic management. Int J Radiat Oncol Biol Phys 1990;19:851)

Gy are used, with a boost of 10 to 20 Gy to areas of gross disease and biopsy scars, yielding a minimum total dose of 60 Gy or higher.

Treatment can also be given with electron beams alone or with mixed photon—electron beams. At the M.D. Anderson Hospital, several large fields are matched to one another and are irradiated with 7- or 9-MeV electrons.[59] The use of lower-energy electrons has sometimes resulted in avoidable parasternal recurrences.[42] CT scans can therefore be helpful in planning such treatment.[60] Such patients are treated with conventional once-daily fractionation. In the past, twice-daily fractions of 1.5 Gy to a dose of 45 Gy in 3 weeks were given at M.D. Anderson, with a boost of 15 Gy, also given with twice-daily fractionation.[59] Techniques using electron arcs or rotational motions have also been described.[57,61] Other radiotherapy techniques have also been used, either in conjunction with conventional external-beam treatments or by themselves, such as surface molds,[62] interstitial implantation,[63] and neutron beams.[64] The advantages and disadvantages of these modalities have not been rigorously compared, however.

Complication rates from properly performed radiation therapy are low. Acute erythema and skin desquamation are nearly universal but self-limited. Telangectasias and mild subcutaneous fibrosis commonly develop in time, but serious subacute or chronic complications are rare. In a series of 224 patients (all of whom previously had undergone axillary dissection), 3% developed radiation pneumonitis, 4% had soft tissue necrosis or ulceration, 3% had bone necrosis, and 1% had neuropathy.[56] The risk of arm edema was 11% (8 of 75 patients) when elective irradiation was given, compared with 1% (1 of 109) when it was not used. All soft tissue complications occurred among patients who received a dose of 60 Gy or higher, except 1 patient, who received 50 Gy and in whom doxorubicin was given concurrently with radiation therapy. Bone complications occurred only among patients receiving doses of 54 Gy or higher. Chest wall ulceration or soft tissue necrosis occurred in about 5% of patients treated with doses higher than 60 Gy in 2 other series.[57,65] Concurrent administration of chemotherapy may also increase the risk of pneumonitis, pericarditis, or brachial plexopathy,[41] as well as acute skin and hematologic reactions.

Most investigators have reported a high incidence of capsular fibrosis and worsening of the cosmetic results in patients who have had breast augmentation or reconstruction with silicone prostheses and are then treated with radiation therapy,[66–71] although other clinicians have not.[58,72,73] Myocutaneous flaps tolerate irradiation without difficulty, however.[69,70]

Finally, does aggressive radiation therapy change the outcome in these patients? Most series suggest that patients who achieve a complete response or who maintain local disease control after aggressive radiation therapy for an isolated local recurrence have longer survival times than patients who do not.[30,34,38,39,41,42,56] Whether this result reflects the effects of therapy or a correlation of the likelihood of response with a less aggressive natural history is unclear. Nonetheless, all but a few patients who achieved local control in past series eventually developed distant metastases and died of breast cancer. Even if it is only rarely curative, however, effective local treatment may have an important impact on the overall quality of a patient's life.

Reirradiation

Little information exists on retreating patients after postoperative chest wall irradiation or previous radiation therapy given for recurrence. In 1 series, 36 previously irradiated patients had lower rates of local control (36% versus 68%) and survival at 10 years (20% versus 35%) than 88 previously untreated patients.[36] Chen and colleagues[42] reported similar findings. Patients in these two series did not, however, undergo reirradiation of all previously treated areas for fear of complications. In another series, no evidence of soft tissue necrosis was seen in 13 patients receiving an additional 40 to 60 Gy in 4 to 6 weeks using electrons, after previous treatment with 40 to 50 Gy to the entire chest wall.[74] The sizes of the electron fields were not reported, however. Although 9 of 13 patients were described as having local disease control for their remaining lifetimes or follow-up, 3 of these patients had further chest wall recurrences outside the retreated volume. Another group of 7 patients who had previous postoperative radiation therapy were retreated with electrons to small fields, giving a dose of 40 to 50 Gy, sometimes with a 10- to 15-Gy boost.[75] At death or last follow-up, 5 of 9 patients had a complete response to treatment with full healing of the chest wall, and 8 of 9 patients had stable or controlled disease. One patient suffered osteomyelitis; most patients had milder complications, which were slow to resolve, however. In-field local disease control was achieved among 9 of 11 patients retreated with a surface mold to doses of 60 Gy in two or three applications.[62] One patient developed a superficial necrosis, which healed after 8 weeks. Thus, retreatment of limited volumes with limited radiation doses can result in meaningful palliation in selected patients.

Surgery

Limited local excision has been used in only a few patients.[10,38,76–78] Further local treatment failure occurs in 60% to 75% of patients so treated. For selected patients, local disease control rates in excess of 75% have been obtained with wide local excision of skin and subcutaneous tissue[79] or partial or full-thickness chest wall resection,[31,80–85] with some patients surviving 5 years or more. (Technical aspects of radical resection for chest wall recurrence or necrosis are discussed in Chapter 19.1.) The likelihood of further local recurrence appears higher for patients presenting with multiple nodules on the chest wall than for those with a single nodule.[86]

Some authors have advocated using chest wall resection as the initial treatment of isolated local failure. The local and distant relapse rates after this approach are high, however, and treated-related morbidity may be substantial. In a series of 69 patients from Copenhagen treated in this manner, the 5-year actuarial local control rate was 50%, with a 62% rate of overall survival.[87] Among 23 such patients in Osaka, 48% had further local–regional recurrences. The 5-year relapse-free and overall survival rates were 26% and 48%, respectively.[88] (These patients also received chemotherapy and tamoxifen, but apparently not radiation therapy, after resection.) Thirty percent of patients were found to have unsuspected mediastinal nodal involvement at the time of surgery; none of these 7 patients lived 5 years, compared with 4 of 16 patients with negative mediastinal lymph nodes.

About 40% of patients with breast cancer who underwent partial or full-thickness chest wall resection from 1979 to 1988 at the M.D. Anderson Hospital developed significant complications, although most of these did not require major interventions.[84] In a series of 18 patients treated in Milan from 1977 to 1988, only 1 patient required reoperation (for repair of flap necrosis).[85]

Clearly, patients who undergo radical chest wall resections must be carefully selected from the entire group of patients with local recurrence. Few patients are best served by such surgery as the initial form of treatment, because radiation therapy gives similar results but with less morbidity. Nonetheless, chest wall resection may be a useful form of treatment and palliation for patients in whom other measures have failed. Most authors recommend that only patients with a life expectancy of 1 year or more be submitted for operation. The presence of distant metastases in itself is not an absolute contraindication to surgery, however. Such operations should be performed only by skilled, experienced surgical teams.

Hyperthermia

Excellent results have been achieved in some studies combining hyperthermia with radiation therapy in previously unirradiated patients who had local treatment failure after mastectomy. For example, a nonrandomized study by the Radiation Therapy Oncology Group (RTOG) of the combination of twice-weekly hyperthermia and radiation (given in conventional fractionation to 60 to 66 Gy) resulted in complete tumor regression in 85% of 54 patients; the regression was maintained at 2 years follow-up in nearly all evaluable patients.[89] Similar results have been reported by other groups,[90] although response rates and duration have been lower in some studies.[91] Hyperthermia has also been used as an adjunct to high-dose radiation therapy in treating clinically uninvolved areas of the chest wall.[92] Hyperthermia may be most useful as an adjunct to radiation therapy when patients have been previously irradiated. Many or most patients treated with low-dose radiation therapy and hyperthermia achieve complete response with acceptable complication rates.[90,91,93,94] Many of these responses are transient, however.

Whether the addition of hyperthermia improves local control rates over those achieved solely with modern radiation therapy techniques and doses is unclear. Only one randomized trial has been published fully.[95] Complete responses were obtained in 62% of patients (8 of 13) with breast or chest wall lesions smaller than 3 cm, who received hyperthermia, compared with 40% of patients (4 of 10)

treated only with irradiation; the respective rates were 21% (6 of 29) and 28% (8 of 29) among patients with larger lesions. This study used an unusual radiation therapy schedule and low total dose (4 Gy given twice weekly to a total of 32 Gy), however. This study has also been criticized for inadequate assessment of thermal doses and an inability to achieve sufficient heating in many tumors (especially the larger ones). In a study from Amsterdam, the complete response rate was much higher when a minimum temperature of 41°C was achieved or when the duration of increased temperature was longer than 20 minutes.[96] Achieving the desired thermal parameters had only a limited beneficial effect in a large series from Stanford University, however.[91]

Hyperthermia may increase the risk of complications after radiation therapy. Severe thermal blisters and necrosis or poorly healing skin ulcers were observed in 16% of patients in the RTOG study[89] and in 35% of patients treated at Stanford.[91] Many of these patients had previously received radiation therapy, however. Most of these complications heal slowly with conservative management, although rarely surgery may be needed. Concomitant chemotherapy, radiation therapy, and hyperthermia were used in a study conducted at the JCRT.[97] No improvement in response rate was obtained, compared with studies using radiation therapy alone or radiation therapy and hyperthermia. Toxicity was substantial, however, particularly among previously irradiated patients.

Thus, the value of hyperthermia in combination with radiation therapy in the management of patients with locally recurrent breast cancer remains unsettled. At the end of 1993, a consortium of European institutions, the British Medical Research Council, and the Princess Margaret Hospital in Toronto completed a phase III trial comparing the results obtained with radiation therapy alone or with radiation therapy combined with hyperthermia in these patients. The detailed publication of their results may help to resolve these issues. Substantial technical problems also remain to be solved in administering hyperthermia and in measuring its effects.

Photodynamic and Other Local Therapies

Photodynamic therapy (using hematoporphyrin derivatives as a photosensitizing agent for treatment with high-intensity xenon arc lamps or lasers) has resulted in only a minority of patients' having a complete response, which is usually transient.[98–100] Nearly all patients included in these series were heavily pretreated and also often had extensive disease, however. The long-term benefits of photodynamic therapy in untreated patients with less extensive disease are thus unknown. Photodynamic therapy can cause considerable pain. Superficial skin necrosis is also common, although surgical repair is rarely needed.[99]

Intraarterial regional chemotherapy was used in a small series of patients with previously treated local recurrences in Bobigny, France.[101] Two groups reported using anticancer drugs topically in patients with ulcerating breast tumors or subcutaneous metastases.[102,103] Some responses have been produced by these approaches, and toxicities were limited, but detailed long-term data are not available.

Although feasible in principle, direct injection of chemotherapeutic drugs or biologic response modifiers into chest wall recurrences has not been frequently used. In one series, giving intralesional interferon-β simultaneously with further external-beam radiation therapy resulted in four complete responses in previously irradiated patients.[104]

Meticulous topical treatments may provide adequate control of local infections and pain. The use of 0.5% silver nitrate–soaked dressing with local debridement and skin grafts may substantially reduce bleeding and infection.[75] Such aggressive local management, similar to treatment of burn patients, may palliate symptoms in many patients for their remaining life. Local infections can also be vigorously treated with frequent changes of povidine or saline-wetted gauze bandages. Other aspects of the nursing care of breast cancer patients with compromise of the skin can be found in Chapter 25.4. Broad-spectrum oral antibiotics may be helpful. Metronidazole has been effective in treating foul-smelling ulcerated lesions.[105]

Systemic Therapy

Whether using adjuvant systemic therapy in conjunction with other treatment at the time of local recurrence can prolong disease-free or overall survival time is not clear. Because so many variables can influence outcome in these patients, this question is best answered by a large, randomized trial with a control arm of no systemic treatment. The only randomized trial addressing this issue began in Switzerland in 1982 and was completed in 1991.[106] The 167 patients had positive or undetermined estrogen receptor assays, disease-free intervals longer than 1 year, and three or fewer nodules, each 3 cm or smaller in diameter, without fixation; these patients underwent complete gross tumor resection and radiation therapy. A total dose of 50 Gy in 25 fractions was given to the involved region; whether the entire chest wall or nodal regions were irradiated is not stated. These patients were then were randomly allocated to receive either tamoxifen until relapse or observation. (An attempt was made to treat a high-risk group that did not meet these entry criteria with doxorubicin, cyclophosphamide, and vincristine; however, only 50 patients could be accrued to that portion of the study, which was not further analyzed.) With a median follow-up of 6.3 years, the 5-year relapse free survival rates were 59% and 36% in the tamoxifen and observation arms, respectively, which was a statistically significant difference. This difference had nearly disappeared by 8 to 9 years after randomization, however. Tamoxifen seemed to reduce the risk of local treatment failure substantially (from 33% to 12% as a first site of failure by 5 years), but it had no impact on the risk of developing distant metastases. Whether such recurrences were within or outside the radiation therapy fields was not analyzed. Overall survival rates were the same in both groups.

The same authors described a larger retrospective series in which no apparent improvement in outcome was found for those patients who received systemic therapy compared with those who did not.[33] Another retrospective series was performed by investigators at the Mallinckrodt Institute of Radiology in which a matched-pair analysis was used to compare the results in patients treated with and without systemic therapy.[32] Differences between the chemotherapy-treated group (53 patients) and its control group with regard to local control, freedom from distant metastases, disease-free survival, and overall survival were small and did not reach statistical significance. These differences were statistically significant (except for local disease control) when comparing 59 patients treated with hormonal therapy and irradiation with those treated with radiation therapy alone, however. Other investigators using retrospective reviews have also shown some benefit to the use of systemic therapy,[34,38,107–109] but the validity of these reviews is difficult to assess.

Few data exist about the results of extremely high-dose chemotherapy with autologous bone marrow or peripheral stem cell support in patients with local disease recurrence after mastectomy. A recent report from the University of Chicago included nine patients who had isolated local–regional disease (including one patient with disease in an intact breast and lymph nodes).[110] Only one of these patients did not relapse after bone marrow transplantation therapy, however. Five patients did not receive radiation to the sites of initial recurrence, and three had treatment failures in these sites; only one of four patients who were irradiated had a relapse at a previous site of disease. No additional toxicity resulted from consolidation radiotherapy.

Most investigators have not found that the addition of chemotherapy or hormonal therapy markedly improves local control when compared with technically adequate radiation therapy alone.[32,107,109] In one study, 18 patients who had gross total excision of tumor and who received chemotherapy had an actuarial 5-year local disease control rate of 78%, compared with 38% among 58 such patients treated with radiation therapy only.[34] No difference in local disease control rates for patients with gross residual disease or for any patients treated with hormonal therapy existed, however. One small randomized study observed improved local disease control with the concurrent use of actinomycin D and irradiation.[111] Local disease control was 80% (12 of 15) when chemotherapy was given, as opposed to 59% (10 of 17) when it was not. The median follow-up in this series was only 15 to 18 months, however, and important details of radiation therapy (such as field sizes) were not described.

Little information is available on the ability of systemic chemotherapy or hormonal therapy to control local disease without the use of radiation therapy or surgery. The Southwest Oncology Group treated 53 patients with local recurrence with doxorubicin or cyclosphosphamide, doxorubicin, and 5-fluorouracil combinations, without irradiation.[112] Complete response was obtained in 34%, and a partial response was noted in 28% of patients. The duration of these responses was not given. Another series found a local disease control rate of 46% (23 of 50) in patients treated with surgical excision and similar chemotherapy.[107]

Nine of 11 patients with local—regional disease treated in Edinburgh with continuous-infusion 5-fluorouracil had a symptomatic response to therapy, but an objective response was seen only in 3 patients.[113] Response rates (complete and partial) of local disease to various hormonal manipulations have been reported in 30% to 40% of patients in older series, in which hormone receptor levels were not known.[1,10,13] The median duration of response ranges from 8 to 19 months.[10,13,38] Bedwinek and colleagues[22] found that 4 of 11 patients had lifetime local disease control. One study showed a surprisingly high complete response rate of 64% and a partial response rate of 21% in 42 patients treated with either chemotherapy (12 patients) or hormonal therapy (30 patients), with 6 patients still in complete response at 3 years.[38] In general, however, systemic treatment alone is unlikely to cause local disease to regress permanently.[18]

Several other considerations are important in deciding whether systemic treatment should be used at the time of local recurrence, either as the sole therapy or as part of a combined-modality program. Adjuvant systemic therapy is now commonly used following initial diagnosis of the primary tumor. Therefore, for many patients who suffer local recurrence, questions of drug resistance and tolerance to further treatment must be addressed.[114,115]

MANAGEMENT

Most patients who suffer local disease recurrence after mastectomy ultimately develop distant metastases. Many patients may live for years after local recurrence, however, especially if they have favorable prognostic factors. The side effects of uncontrolled local recurrence may be highly distressing, although only rarely do they lead directly to the death of the patient.

No agreement exists on which patients benefit from the different available treatments or at what point in the course of the disease should treatment be instituted. Whether local or systemic therapy (or combined-modality treatment) can improve disease-free or overall survival is uncertain, nor is it clear that immediate local therapy given to all patients at presentation is more effective in preventing uncontrollable local morbidity than timely selective treatment of patients who develop significant local disease progression later in their course. Hence, one reasonable treatment option is to defer all treatment until warranted by symptoms.

Local treatment of patients with no evidence of distant metastases reduces morbidity for many patients and, possibly, may increase survival time for a few individuals. To offer such treatment is reasonable if the patient understands its potential limitations and complications. Local therapy may yield the greatest benefits for patients with a prolonged initial disease-free interval or other relatively favorable prognostic factors, such as a small number of resectable lesions.

Available data do not clearly support the routine use of adjuvant systemic therapy in the setting of an isolated local recurrence. To use hormonal therapy in selected individuals appears reasonable, however, given the sugges-

tion of benefit in some studies and the limited toxicities associated with such treatment. The use of chemotherapy is a problem, because it is likely to be associated with more side effects. Nonetheless, in many similar situations, patients at high risk of distant treatment failure (eg, those who present with stage III disease) are treated with chemotherapy in addition to local—regional therapy. In particular, it seems reasonable to use neoadjuvant chemotherapy or hormone therapy before local treatments in patients with inoperable recurrences. No information is available regarding the benefits of treating patients who received systemic therapy before local relapse of the disease.

Patients who are treated only with systemic chemotherapy or hormonal therapy (or with observation alone) should be carefully observed for progression of local disease, because local disease control with radiation therapy is probably easier when the local tumor burden is minimal.

In patients with concurrent or prior distant metastases, appropriate systemic therapy should be used. Radiation therapy should be used only for patients with progressive local symptoms.

The value of irradiating patients who previously received prophylactic postoperative radiation therapy is not well established. For selected patients with significant local symptoms, however, retreatment with moderate to high doses using small fields may be warranted. Concomitant hyperthermia or other experimental treatments may be appropriate options in such situations. Only individuals with relatively circumscribed lesions can be considered for radical surgical procedures, but some patients may benefit from these procedures when other options have failed.

Local Disease Recurrence After Conservative Surgery

PRESENTING SYMPTOMS AND SIGNS

Roughly 30% to 50% of local recurrences after initial treatment with conservative surgery and radiation therapy are detected solely by follow-up mammography, with the rest divided nearly equally between those found on physical examination without any suspicious radiologic signs and those detected both by examination and mammography.[116–122] The physical and radiologic characteristics of recurrent lesions are the same in general as those of tumors that are discovered initially.

In general, the physical examination after treatment shows only mild thickening without a mass effect. Either surgery or radiation therapy may cause changes in physical examination, however, such as masslike regions of fibrosis, which may occasionally be difficult clinically to distinguish from a local recurrence.[123,124] The findings associated with disease recurrence may be subtle, especially when the primary tumor was of the infiltrating lobular histologic type. Recurrences of these lesions often produce only minimal thickening or retraction at the biopsy site without a mass.[125] In rare patients, the only sign of recurrence may be diffuse breast retraction.[120] Hence, changes in the physical examination that occur more than 1 to 2 years after the completion of radiation therapy must be viewed as suspicious. Recurrence in the nipple alone, presenting as Paget disease, has been reported but seems rare.[126,127]

The anticipated radiologic changes in the treated breast are highly variable but usually include skin thickening, increased density of the fibroglandular and suspensory apparatus of the breast, the appearance of coarse calcifications, and mass or distortion in the tumor bed.[124,128] Scarring in the tumor bed is particularly frequent in patients who had postoperative hematomas.[129] One can see substantial overlap in radiologic appearance between benign and malignant lesions.[116,120,130–134] Some authors have suggested that the presence of a central lucency in a mass occurring in the tumor bed is indicative of surgical scarring rather than a recurrence.[135] Suspicious microcalcifications that develop after treatment may be either benign or malignant histologically, although ones that develop in a different quadrant from the initial tumor have a high likelihood of malignancy.[136] If the original lesion was noted by the detection of microcalcifications only, a recurrence is likely to appear in the same way, whereas when the first presentation radiologically was a mass, recurrence is just as likely to appear as a mass (with or without calcifications) or as calcifications alone.[128] Benign and malignant radiologic changes may coexist (Fig. 21-3). Recurrences of infiltrating lobular carcinomas are particularly likely to be radiographically occult.[117] In 1 series, two of six recurrences among 55 patients who had tumors that originally could not be detected radiologically were detected solely by mammograms[137]; hence, mammography is an important part of the follow-up of all patients, regardless of the original presentation of the tumor.

PROGNOSIS

In most institutions' experiences, local disease recurrence after conservative surgery and radiation therapy has a better prognosis than local recurrence after mastectomy. The 5-year actuarial rate of distant or further local recurrence in a group of 90 patients from the JCRT with breast treatment failure (either before or simultaneous with the appearance of distant metastases) was 46%.[138] In other series, 45% to 70% of all patients with local recurrences were alive at 5 years, with long-term disease-free survival in about 30% to 50% of patients.[121,122,139–146] In one randomized trial comparing breast-conserving therapy with mastectomy, however, prognosis following local disease relapse was similar in both groups.[147] Patients often received doses of 75 Gy to the tumor bed, making early detection of recurrences difficult, according to the investigators.

Of patients with local disease recurrence, 5% to 10% present with concurrent distant metastases.[121,122,138–142] A similar proportion will have locally extensive recurrences that preclude surgery or concomitant inoperable regional nodal recurrences.[121,138,142,148,149] Patients whose disease recurs in the skin alone or who have an inflammatory-type picture have a poor prognosis, more similar to the prognosis in patients with extensive and rapid chest wall

FIGURE 21-3 Spot compression mammogram showing fibrous distortion and coarse calcifications of fat necrosis (*single arrow*) after conservative surgery and radiation therapy, with new casting-type intraductal calcifications (*double arrows*) representing recurrent carcinoma.

recurrence after mastectomy than patients with breast parenchymal treatment failures.[138,149]

Factors that influence prognosis in operable patients (discussed further later) are not well established. The most important variable affecting subsequent outcome in patients undergoing mastectomy in the JCRT experience was the histologic features of the recurrence.[150] One hundred twenty-three patients had salvage mastectomy. The median subsequent follow-up in patients without further disease was 39 months (range, 0 to 144 months). The 5-year actuarial rate of further recurrence in this group was 37%, and the 5-year cause-specific survival rate was 79% (Fig. 21-4). No further recurrences were noted among 14 patients with only noninvasive cancer or among 10 patients with predominantly noninvasive disease with only focal areas of invasion. In contrast, 38% of patients (38 of 99) with predominantly infiltrating tumors suffered a further recurrence. The first sites of further recurrence were the chest wall (7 patients), regional nodes (1 patient), dis-

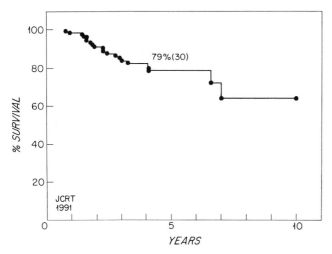

FIGURE 21-4 Actuarial cause-specific survival rate in patients undergoing salvage mastectomy. (Abner AL, Recht A, Eberlein T, et al. Prognosis following salvage mastectomy for recurrence in the breast after conservative surgery and radiation therapy for early-stage breast cancer. J Clin Oncol 1993;11:44)

tant metastases only (25 patients), or both local–regional and distant sites simultaneously (5 patients). The 5-year actuarial rate of further relapse in this subgroup was therefore 52%. Similar results have been reported from the University of Pennsylvania[119] but not in a series from Memorial Sloan-Kettering Cancer Center.[146]

Considerable controversy exists about the prognostic significance of other factors. Tumor size greater than 2 cm at recurrence[141] and diffuse involvement of the breast or dermal lymphatic involvement[121,122] have been reported to be poor prognostic signs. Axillary nodal involvement at recurrence was a prognostic factor in two series in which the effect of histologic features was not separately examined[141,146,151] but was not in the JCRT experience, in which histologic features were examined. Axillary nodal status at the time of recurrence often cannot be assessed adequately, however, because axillary dissection is frequently performed as part of the patient's initial treatment. In most,[119,121,139,141,146,151,152] but not all,[122,143,150] series, the longer the time to treatment failure after initial therapy, the better the prognosis. Time to recurrence was not a significant prognostic factor in a multivariate analysis performed on a small series.[153] The clinical size of the original primary tumor[121] and the original clinical stage[141,151] had an impact on prognosis at recurrence in some series but not in others.[150] Patients who originally had pathologically positive lymph nodes who undergo salvage mastectomy do not appear to do worse than node-negative patients.[121] In the JCRT experience, the location of the tumor with regard to the original lesion was not a significant prognostic factor.[150] In a report from Yale University, patients with new primary tumors had better prognoses than patients with a true recurrence[144]; the results were not subdivided by the histologic type of the lesion at relapse, however. No information is available about the implications of hormone receptor assays performed on the recurrence,

nor are many data available for interpreting more recently used prognostic markers in this setting. Among patients in a series with operable, localized recurrences studied with flow cytometry, none of 13 patients who had favorable profiles at relapse (ie, diploid with low S-phase fraction), had recurrences, compared with 10 of 15 patients with a poor profile.[153] This was statistically significant on multivariate analysis.

Whether overall outcome or prognostic factors are different for patients who suffer local disease relapse after initial treatment with breast-conserving surgery without radiation therapy is not known. In a series from Roswell Park Memorial Institute in Buffalo, the median follow-up after salvage mastectomy was 52 months. All 10 patients with pathologic nodal involvement at the time of salvage surgery subsequently developed further local–regional or systemic recurrence. Thirteen of 15 patients with negative lymph nodes were without evidence of disease at last follow-up.

PRETREATMENT EVALUATION

Even highly suspicious findings may be due to benign causes. For example, in one series, 28% of patients who had suspicious radiologic masses that could also be palpated had no evidence of recurrence on biopsy.[132] The differential diagnosis includes several entities as well as treatment-related changes and benign breast diseases. The most common of these other benign causes of suspicious findings is probably fat necrosis. This may create a mass on palpation,[154–156] or it may mimic a carcinoma radiologically.[156] Occasionally, breast abscesses or cellulitis developing after treatment may mimic an inflammatory-type recurrence.[157,158] Although the presence of pain, possible systemic symptoms of infection, and the time course of development usually make the distinction clear, biopsy is sometimes required to distinguish among them. Rarely, patients develop patches of white or yellowish well-circumscribed sclerosis and induration following radiotherapy. These may be surrounded by a more highly pigmented, bruiselike area and are sometimes preceded by the development of erythema. This phenomenon has been termed *postirradiation morphea* or *circumscribed scleroderma*. Such lesions may appear weeks[159] to years[160] after treatment. Again, biopsy is required to confirm the clinical impression.

Sarcomas are the most dangerous of the alternative diagnoses, but fortunately they are rare in this patient population (see Chap. 17.1). These lesions tend to occur 8 to 10 years or longer after treatment, but the shortest reported interval is 16 months.[161]

Other imaging studies may be useful in evaluating patients with abnormal findings on physical examination or mammography. Ultrasound may sometimes be helpful in distinguishing benign from malignant lesions.[133,134,162] Color Doppler ultrasound is not useful, however, because five of seven recurrent lesions in one series did not display increased flow.[163] On spin-echo T1-weighted MRI scans, significant early contrast enhancement with gadolinium has been reported in nearly all patients with suspicious findings in whom biopsy reveals recurrent cancer, but enhancement is rare in patients with benign findings at biopsy or on follow-up.[164–166] Contrast-enhanced CT scans[167] and positron emission tomography[168] have also demonstrated excellent accuracy in small series. More experience with these modalities is needed before they can be relied on in place of biopsy, however.

In a previous study, we found that open biopsy specimens larger than 1 cc in volume had a false-negative rate of 3% (1 of 31 cases), as opposed to 14% (2 of 14) for smaller specimens (mostly needle biopsies).[169] Other investigators have reported high accuracy for fine-needle aspiration cytology,[170] especially in patients with new microcalcifications on follow-up mammograms.[171] Mammogram- or ultrasound-directed core-needle biopsy is an increasingly popular alternative to aspiration cytology, which has the advantage of producing a larger specimen for evaluation. It is sometimes difficult to distinguish between radiation-induced cellular atypia and malignant disease.[172–175] Hence, consultation with expert pathologists may be helpful in deciding on the management of a patient with an equivocal tissue or cytologic specimen.

Complications were rare in two series when the volume of removed tissue was less than 10 cc,[132,169] although in another series, 4 of 16 such biopsies resulted in a wound infection.[176] Complication rates were higher when larger biopsies were performed or, in one series, in patients with larger breasts or when skin was removed.[176] Patients with wound-healing complications may have substantial worsening of the cosmetic results of therapy.[176]

Some patients present with simultaneous breast and distant treatment failure. Hence, appropriate staging for distant metastases should be performed before definitive therapy is undertaken.

TREATMENT RESULTS

Mastectomy

Five-year relapse-free survival rates for patients with an isolated operable breast cancer relapse treated with mastectomy are 60% to 75%. Overall or cause-specific survival rates are 80% to 85%.[121,150,151,177,178] Subsequent chest wall recurrences occur in less than 10% of patients treated with mastectomy in most series.[150,151,179] In one series, however, 4 of 25 patients suffered chest wall treatment failures, and 1 patient had an axillary treatment failure.[127] Most such patients have progressive local disease despite further treatment.[179] In our experience, patients with skin involvement usually have a rapid recurrence of cancer on the chest wall following mastectomy.

In an earlier review of the JCRT experience,[138] 37 patients underwent ipsilateral axillary sampling or dissection at the time of their breast recurrence. In 9 cases (24%), metastatic carcinoma was found; no nodal involvement was seen in 19 patients (51%), and no nodal tissue was recovered in 9 patients (24%). Axillary exploration was more likely to reveal some nodal tissue in patients who had not had prior dissection (10 of 11) than in patients who did (3 of 14). Although in this series no complications

were related to the exploration, such complications have been reported by others.[179] Hence, reexploration of the previously dissected axilla does not seem warranted in the absence of suspicious adenopathy. In 1 series, 3 of 19 patients treated initially with axillary irradiation only developed a lymphocele after complete axillary dissection performed at the time of mastectomy.[127]

Postoperative complications following mastectomy were rare in two series.[138,146] Slow wound healing, wound breakdown, and infections have been more common in other series, however.[127,179]

Patients suffering breast cancer treatment failure after initial treatment with conservative surgery without radiation therapy for invasive cancer may develop further local–regional treatment failure despite treatment with salvage mastectomy. In a series of 25 such operations performed at Roswell Park Memorial Institute, chest wall treatment failure developed in 8 patients (32%). The 5-year actuarial rate of freedom from second local recurrence was 51%.[180] In a series from Women's College Hospital in Toronto, the 5-year actuarial incidence of chest wall failure among 25 patients treated with mastectomy was 55%.[181] Two of 4 patients who received postmastectomy radiation therapy also had local treatment failures. Details of patient presentation and histologic features at recurrence were not reported for either series, however.

Many patients treated with mastectomy for local treatment failure desire breast reconstruction. Immediate reconstruction with a myocutaneous flap at the time of mastectomy is psychologically advantageous and also promotes tissue healing.[182–184] The risk of complications is slightly higher than in patients who have not had prior radiation therapy, and overall cosmetic results may not be as favorable.[185] Complication rates in one series were higher when latissimus flaps were used (47%) than when rectus abdominis flaps were used (25%),[185] but many of these complications were minor. Complete flap loss has not been reported.[185,186] Submuscularly placed tissue expanders have been poorly tolerated by previously irradiated patients.[187,188] One such patient developed a concave deformity of the chest wall.[189] Other types of subpectoral prostheses appear less subject to complications, at least in carefully selected individuals.[121,190,191]

Breast-Conserving Surgery

Whether salvage mastectomy results in superior long-term survival rates for patients with local treatment failure following initial breast-conserving therapy compared with treatment with lesser procedures is unclear. Mastectomy specimens frequently reveal substantial residual disease outside the biopsy cavity, however. In two series, 22% and 29% of evaluated specimens had residual tumor located in two or more quadrants of the breast.[121,173]

Little published experience has been reported using breast-conserving surgery for the treatment of local disease recurrence. Ninety-one patients were treated with wedge excisions for breast cancer recurrence after lumpectomy and radiotherapy at the Marseilles Cancer Institute.[192] This group constituted 52% of their patients undergoing salvage procedures between 1963 and 1982. In earlier reports, these patients were described as having mobile lesions smaller than 2 cm without skin involvement.[177,178] The actuarial 10-year survival rate was 65%. One third of these patients had further local treatment failure by 5 years. The use of further salvage therapy resulted in an ultimate local failure rate of 9% (8 of 91 patients), however, compared with 9% (8 of 85) among patients whose initial salvage surgery was mastectomy. In the JCRT series, 16 patients refused mastectomy for a biopsy-proved recurrence and were treated with excision only.[150] Two of 10 patients with noninvasive recurrences and 3 of 6 patients with invasive recurrences had local treatment failures 20 to 78 months later. In another series, 2 of 6 patients treated with wide excision had further local failure.[179] Morbidity from wide local excision as a salvage procedure has been reported as low.[177,178]

Few data are available about the use of further conservative surgery (with or without radiation therapy) in patients whose initial treatment with conservative surgery without radiation therapy for invasive cancer fails. In a study from Toronto with a median follow-up of 64 months after disease recurrence, the 5-year actuarial rate of second local disease recurrence was 70% for 21 patients treated again with breast-conserving surgery alone, compared with 23% for 14 patients treated conservative surgery and radiation therapy.[181] In a study performed in Milan, 64% of such patients (18 of 28) were treated with further breast-conserving surgery and radiation. Two of these patients have had further local recurrence.[193]

Reirradiation

Some patients have been retreated with wide excision and interstitial implantation or external irradiation to a small part of the breast. In the largest such series, 25 patients in Marseilles whose disease recurred after treatment to a dose of 70 Gy (including a boost) were retreated with reexcision and brachytherapy between 1974 and 1992; 6 patients were treated with brachytherapy alone.[194] A dose of 40 to 60 Gy was given. With a mean follow-up of 4 years, 7 patients (23%) suffered further local treatment failure (4 in the same quadrant as the recurrence and 3 in another quadrant). One patient had necrosis in the tumor bed. Cosmetic results were considered fair in 24 of the 25 patients.

At the University of Pittsburgh, 19 patients who had received initial doses of 50 Gy to the breast (without a boost) were treated with repeat lumpectomy and reirradiation of the operative site to 50 Gy in 25 fractions with electrons.[195] With a median follow-up of 31 months, there were 2 further local treatment failures, both in the skin of the breast. The projected 5-year actuarial rate of second local treatment failure was 20%. No complications were seen at this short follow-up. Other groups have treated only a handful of patients in this manner.[138,179]

Systemic Therapy

Assessing the roles of adjuvant chemotherapy or hormonal therapy after local disease recurrence after initial breast-conserving management poses the same problems as does assessing the roles of these methods following chest wall recurrence after mastectomy. No improvement occurred in outcome in patients so treated in the JCRT experience, but the patients selected were thought to have poor prognoses.[150] Some individuals with chest wall fixation of tumor may respond sufficiently to chemotherapy or hormonal therapy to allow mastectomy.[140,179] Systemic therapy alone is not effective in obtaining permanent local control of inoperable disease, however.[179]

MANAGEMENT

Breast cancer recurrence after conservative surgery and radiation therapy has a better prognosis than chest wall treatment failure after mastectomy. Because early detection of a recurrence might lead to improved salvage results, biopsy should be used when recurrence cannot be easily excluded. We prefer a small open biopsy or an ultrasound- or stereotactically guided core-needle biopsy to aspiration cytology; if these latter procedures are performed, a negative result should be interpreted cautiously. If a recurrence is detected and there is no evidence of dissemination on appropriate restaging, mastectomy is generally viewed as the standard therapy. If desired, reconstruction should be performed using a myocutaneous flap. Treatment by wide local excision alone is associated with a substantial risk of further breast treatment failure. Whether such an approach decreases long-term survival is not known, however. Such an approach should probably only be used rarely (eg, for patients who refuse mastectomy).

The role of adjuvant systemic therapy after breast cancer recurrence has not established. If patients have not previously been treated with systemic therapy, we tend to recommend such treatment based on our current policy in patients presenting with the same clinicopathologic features who have not had a prior diagnosis of breast cancer (see Chap. 17.2). The value of retreating patients who received prior systemic therapy is unknown.

Regional Lymph Node Recurrence of Cancer

PRESENTING SIGNS AND SYMPTOMS

The first manifestation of nodal recurrence is usually an asymptomatic mass in the axilla or in the supraclavicular fossa. Some solitary sternal metastases may result from direct extension of involved internal mammary lymph nodes.[196] Nodal treatment failures may occur more than 5 years after primary treatment.[197]

Only a minority of patients present with symptoms referable to regional treatment failure (eg, arm edema, neurologic impairment, or pain) in addition to lymphadenopathy. In the JCRT series of patients with nodal disease recurrence without simultaneous breast treatment failure,[197] such symptoms were found at presentation in 31% of patients (12 of 38). These totals included 23% of patients (5 of 22) with (initially) isolated axillary treatment failure and 44% of patients (7 of 16) with other sites of nodal treatment failure.

SUBSEQUENT MORBIDITY AND SPREAD

Significant pain or other distressing symptoms at last follow-up or during the patients' lifetimes were present in 32% of patients with regional treatment failure (12 of 38) in the JCRT experience.[197] Sixteen percent of patients (3 of 19) with isolated axillary treatment failure and 25% of patients (3 of 12) with other nodal disease sites who did not have such symptoms on presentation developed them despite treatment. In another series, 24% of patients who developed regional nodal treatment failure following mastectomy had at least 1 significant symptom during follow-up.[18] Pain or arm edema may be more common among patients with supraclavicular disease recurrence; in a series from Vienna, 38% of patients (15 of 39) with isolated supraclavicular disease recurrences suffered such symptoms at diagnosis or during their lifetimes.[198]

In 1 series, recurrence of tumor on the chest wall occurred in 27% of patients (7 of 26) with nodal treatment failure who did not undergo elective chest wall irradiation.[56] The risk of such subclinical involvement at other nodal sites is unknown.

PROGNOSIS

Prognosis after nodal tumor recurrence may be related to the site involved. In the JCRT series, with a median follow-up of 45 months, 61% (11 of 18) of patients with isolated axillary failure were alive without disease, compared with 38% (3 of 8) for patients with other involved nodal sites.[197] Median and long-term survival rates after disease recurrence in the supraclavicular lymph nodes after mastectomy are similar to those of patients with isolated chest wall recurrence in most series,[29,199,200] but some suggest a worse prognosis.[32,198] A few long-term survivors have been reported.[201] In one series, 19 patients with isolated internal mammary node tumor recurrences had a better prognosis than other patients with local disease recurrence (median disease-free interval, 60 months)[29]; others have reported similar findings.[32] In other series, however, such patients had a worse prognosis.[40,198]

PRETREATMENT EVALUATION

Careful evaluation for other nodal and distant sites of treatment failure should be conducted before therapy is instituted. In patients with symptoms suggestive of brachial plexopathy, it may be difficult to distinguish clinically between tumor recurrence in the axilla and the effects of postoperative radiation therapy. The use of MRI may be helpful in this regard; focal enhancement with gadolinium suggests the presence of tumor rather than radiation-related fibrosis.[202] In patients with axillary treatment failure after breast-conservation therapy, the presence of a simultaneous breast tumor recurrence should be ruled out by careful physical examination and mammography.

TREATMENT RESULTS

Surgery and Radiation Therapy

Radiation therapy has been roughly as effective in controlling nodal treatment failures after mastectomy as it has for chest wall tumor recurrences in most series.[29,41,42,65,201,203] For example, in a series from the JCRT, the 5-year actuarial control rate among 21 such patients was 78%.[29] Nodal disease control was 82% among 28 patients treated with complete gross excision at the Mallinckrodt Institute of Radiology, compared with 66% among 62 patients who did not undergo excision.[56]

The results of salvage treatment in patients with nodal treatment failure after initial breast-conserving therapy appear similar. Regional disease control was achieved in 78% of patients (18 of 23) in the JCRT series when gross total excision or radiation therapy was used;[197] no differences were noted between among nodal sites in this regard (JCRT, unpublished data). Similar results have been reported by others.[203,204]

The risks of complications after salvage therapy for regional treatment failure alone have not been reported in these series.

Systemic Therapy

Adjuvant chemotherapy or hormonal therapy was frequently given to patients after regional nodal tumor recurrence after breast-conserving therapy in the JCRT series. Its impact on the subsequent course was difficult to assess because of the heterogeneity of the population.[197] When used alone, systemic therapy was unable to control regional disease,[197] although better success has been reported by other investigators.[203]

Extremely high-dose chemotherapy has also been used in patients with regional treatment failure alone. In one series, 4 of the 13 long-term disease-free survivors (of 80 patients undergoing bone marrow transplantation) had nodal relapses only, but the total number of patients with isolated regional tumor recurrence was not reported.[205]

MANAGEMENT

Patients with isolated axillary tumor recurrences can often be successfully treated with surgery or radiation therapy, with some long-term survivors. Patients with other regional nodal treatment failure sites fare much worse. The risk of subsequent relapse in the clinically uninvolved chest wall in patients treated initially with mastectomy is sufficiently high to justify the use of comprehensive radiation therapy fields in patients not previously irradiated. No evidence, however, requires the use of mastectomy in patients initially treated with breast-conserving surgery who do not have a clinically apparent simultaneous local treatment failure. Systemic therapy alone cannot control gross nodal disease; its value in this setting in conjunction with surgery or radiation therapy is unclear.

References

1. Gilliland MD, Barton RM, Copeland EM. The implications of local recurrence of breast cancer as the first site of therapeutic failure. Ann Surg 1983;197:284.
2. Greco M, Cascinelli N, Galluzo D, et al. Locally recurrent breast cancer after "radical" surgery. Eur J Surg Oncol 1992;18:209.
3. Pawlias KT, Dockerty MB, Ellis FH. Late local recurrent carcinoma of the breast. Ann Surg 1958;148:192.
4. Auchincloss H. The nature of local recurrence following radical mastectomy. Cancer 1958;11:611.
5. Scanlon EF. Local recurrence in the pectoralis muscles following modified radical mastectomy for carcinoma. J Surg Oncol 1985;30:149.
6. Granik MS, Bragdon RW, Hanna DC. Recurrent breast cancer at the time of breast reconstruction. Ann Plast Surg 1987;18:69.
7. Donegan WL. The influence of untreated internal mammary metastases upon the course of mammary cancer. Cancer 1977;39:533.
8. Zimmerman K, Montague E, Fletcher G. Frequency, anatomical distribution and management of local recurrences after definitive therapy for breast cancer. Cancer 1966;19:67.
9. Andry G, Suciu S, Vico P, et al. Locoregional recurrences after 649 modified radical mastectomies: incidence and significance. Eur J Surg Oncol 1989;15:476.
10. Donegan WL, Perez-Mesa CM, Watson FR. A biostatistical study of locally recurrent breast carcinoma. Surg Gynecol Obstet 1966;122:529.
11. Oliver DR, Sugarbaker ED. The significance of skin recurrence following radical mastectomy. Surg Gynecol Obstet 1947;85:360.
12. Demaree EW. Local recurrence following surgery for cancer of the breast. Ann Surg 1951;134:863.
13. Helman P. Breast cancer: aspects of local recurrence. South Afr Med J 1961;35:197.
14. Karabali-Dalamaga S, Souhami RL, O'Higgins NJ, et al. Natural history and prognosis of recurrent breast cancer. Br Med J 1978;2:730.
15. Di Pietro S, Bertario L, Piva L. Prognosis and treatment of locoregional breast cancer recurrences: critical considerations on 120 cases. Tumori 1980;66:331.
16. Shimkin MB, Lucia EL, Low-Beer VA, et al. Recurrent cancer of the breast: analysis of frequency, distribution, and mortality at the University of California Hospital, 1918 to 1947, inclusive. Cancer 1954;7:29.
17. Spratt JS, Donegan WL. Cancer of the breast. Philadelphia, WB Saunders, 1967.
18. Tennvall-Nittby L, Tenegrup I, Landberg T. The total incidence of loco-regional recurrence in a randomized trial of breast cancer TNM stage II: the South Sweden Breast Cancer Trial. Acta Oncol 1993;32:641.
19. Danckers UF, Hamann A, Savage JL. Postoperative recurrence of breast cancer after thirty-two years: a case report and review of the literature. Surgery 1960;47:656.
20. Morton JJ, Morton JH. Cancer as a chronic disease. Ann Surg 1953;137:683.
21. LaRaja RD, Meo MA, Alcindor F. Local chest wall recurrence of breast cancer forty years after radical mastectomy: a case report. Breast 1994;7:203.
22. Bedwinek JM, Fineberg B, Lee J, et al. Analysis of failures following local treatment of isolated local–regional recurrence of breast cancer. Int J Radiat Oncol Biol Phys 1981;7:581.
23. Bedwinek JM, Munro D, Fineberg B. Local–regional treatment of patients with simultaneous local–regional recurrence and distant metastases following mastectomy. Am J Clin Oncol 1983;6:295.
24. Marshall K, Redfern A, Cady B. Local recurrences of carcinoma of the breast. Surg Gynecol Obstet 1974;139:406.
25. Fentiman IS, Matthews PN, Davison OW, et al. Survival following local skin recurrence after mastectomy. Br J Surg 1985;72:14.
26. Papaioannou AN, Tanz FJ, Volk H. Fate of patients with recurrent carcinoma of the breast: recurrence five years or more after initial treatment. Cancer 1967;20:371.
27. Cho SY, Choi HY. Causes of death and metastatic patterns in patients with mammary cancer: ten-year autopsy study. Am J Clin Pathol 1980;73:232.
28. Hagemeister FB, Buzdar AU, Luna MA, et al. Causes of death in breast cancer: a clinicopathologic study. Cancer 1980;46:162.
29. Aberizk WJ, Silver B, Henderson IC, et al. The use of radiotherapy for treatment of isolated locoregional recurrence of breast carcinoma after mastectomy. Cancer 1986;58:1214.
30. Chu FCH, Lin FJ, Kim JH, et al. Locally recurrent carcinoma of the breast: results of radiation therapy. Cancer 1976;37:2677.
31. Snyder AF, Farrow GM, Masson JK, et al. Chest-wall resection for locally recurrent breast cancer. Arch Surg 1968;97:246.
32. Halverson KJ, Perez CA, Kuske RR, et al. Locoregional recurrence of breast cancer: a retrospective comparison of irradiation alone versus irradiation and systemic therapy. Am J Clin Oncol 1992;15:93.
33. Brunner KW, Harder F, Greiner R, et al. Das loko–regionale Rezidiv nach operiertem Mammakarzinom: prognostische Faktoren und therapeutische Konsequenzen. Schweiz Med Wochenschr 1988;118:1976.
34. Schwaibold F, Fowble BL, Solin LJ, et al. The results of radiation therapy for isolated local regional recurrence after mastectomy. Int J Radiat Oncol Biol Phys 1991;21:299.
35. Patanaphan V, Salazar OM, Poussin-Rosillo H. Prognosticators in recurrent breast cancer: a 15-year experience with irradiation. Cancer 1984;54:228.
36. Toonkel LM, Fix I, Jacobson LH, et al. The significance of local recurrence of carcinoma of the breast. Int J Radiat Oncol Biol Phys 1983;9:33.
37. Magno L, Bignardi M, Micheletti E, et al. Analysis of prognostic factors in patients with isolated chest wall recurrence of breast cancer. Cancer 1987;60:240.
38. Beck TM, Hart NE, Woodard DA, et al. Local or regionally recurrent carcinoma of the breast: results of therapy in 121 patients. J Clin Oncol 1983;1:400.
39. Danoff BF, Coia LR, Cantor RI, et al. Locally recurrent breast carcinoma: the effect of adjuvant chemotherapy on prognosis. Radiology 1983;147:849.
40. Deutsch M, Parsons J, Mittal BB. Radiation therapy for local–regional recurrent breast cancer. Int J Radiat Oncol Biol Phys 1986;12:2061.
41. Mendenhall NP, Devine JW, Mendenhall WM, et al. Isolated local–regional recurrence following mastectomy for adenocarcinoma of the breast treated with radiation therapy alone or combined with surgery and/or chemotherapy. Radiother Oncol 1988;12:177.
42. Chen KK-Y, Montague E, Oswald M. Results of irradiation in the treatment of locoregional breast cancer recurrence. Cancer 1985;56:1269.
43. Kenda R, Lozza L, Zucali R. Results of irradiation in the treatment of chest wall recurrent breast cancer. (Abstract) Radiother Oncol 1992;24 (Suppl):S41.
44. Stadler B, Kogelnik HD. Local control and outcome of patients irradiated for isolated chest wall recurrences of breast cancer. Radiother Oncol 1987;8:105.
45. Baral E, Ogenstad S, Wallgren A. The effect of adjuvant radiotherapy on the time of occurrence and prognosis of local recurrence in primary operable breast cancer. Cancer 1985;56:2779.
46. Valagussa P, Rossi A, Tancini G, et al. Is there any effective salvage

treatment for relapsing operable breast cancer with N+? (Abstract) Proc Am Soc Clin Oncol 1985;4:56.

47. Buzdar A, McNeese MD, Hortobagyi GN, et al. Is chemotherapy effective in reducing the local failure rate in patients with operable breast cancer? Cancer 1990;65:394.

48. Haagensen CD. Diseases of the breast, ed 3. Philadelphia, WB Saunders, 1986.

49. Lee CH, Poplack SP, Stahl RS. Mammographic appearance of the transverse rectus abdominus musculocutaneous (TRAM) flap. Breast Dis 1994;7:99.

50. Brady MS, Gaynor JJ, Brennan MF. Radiation-associated sarcoma of bone and soft tissue. Arch Surg 1992;127:1379.

51. Allegra JC, Barlock A, Huff KK, et al. Changes in multiple or sequential estrogen receptor determinations in breast cancer. Cancer 1980;45:792.

52. Lindfors KK, Meyer JE, Busse PM, et al. CT evaluation of local and regional breast cancer recurrence. AJR 1985;145:833.

53. Rosenman J, Churchill CA, Mauro MA, et al. The role of computed tomography in the evaluation of post-mastectomy locally recurrent breast cancer. Int J Radiat Oncol Oncol Biol Phys 1988;14:57.

54. Scatarige JC, Fishman EK, Zinreich ES, et al. Internal mammary lymphadenopathy in breast carcinoma: CT appraisal of anatomic distribution. Radiology 1988;167:89.

55. Jacobs CG, Zinreich ES, Fishman EK, et al. Computed tomography in radiotherapy planning of the axillary region. J Comput Tomogr 1986;10:221.

56. Halverson KJ, Perez CA, Kuske RR, et al. Isolated local–regional recurrence of breast cancer following mastectomy: radiotherapeutic management. Int J Radiat Oncol Biol Phys 1990;19:851.

57. Lo TCM, Salzman FA, Wright KA, et al. Megavolt electron irradiation in the treatment of recurrent carcinoma of the breast on the chest wall. Acta Radiol Oncol 1983;22:97.

58. Chu FCH, Kaufmann TP, Dawson GA, et al. Radiation therapy of cancer in prosthetically augmented or reconstructed breasts. Radiology 1992;185:429.

59. McNeese MD, Fletcher GH, Levitt SH, et al. Breast cancer. In: Levitt SH, Khan FM, Potish RA, eds. Levitt and Tapley's technological basis of radiation therapy: practical clinical applications, ed 2. Philadelphia, Lea & Febiger, 1992:232.

60. Badcock PC. CT scanning: its value in the planning of radiotherapy of the chest wall. Strahlenther Onkol 1982;158:558.

61. McNeely LK, Jacobson GM, Leavitt DD, et al. Electron arc therapy: chest wall irradiation of breast cancer patients. Int J Radiat Oncol Biol Phys 1988;14:1287.

62. Delanian S, Housset M, Brunel P, et al. Iridium 192 plesiocurietherapy using silicone elastomer plates for extensive locally recurrent breast cancer following chest wall irradiation. Int J Radiat Oncol Biol Phys 1992;22:1099.

63. Weshler Z, Wygoda A, Newman R, et al. The role of brachytherapy in the treatment of chest-wall recurrences of breast carcinoma. (Abstract) Eur J Cancer 1993;29A(Suppl. 6):S70.

64. Musabaeva LI, Slonimskaya YM. 6.3 MeV fast neutron therapy of local recurrences and metastases from breast cancer. Venice, European Society of Mastology, 1994:153.

65. Madoc-Jones H, Nelson AJ, Montague ED. Evaluation of the effectiveness of radiotherapy in the management of early nodal recurrences from adenocarcinoma of the breast. Breast 1976;2:31.

66. Halpern J, McNeese MD, Kroll SS, et al. Irradiation of prosthetically augmented breasts: a retrospective study on toxicity and cosmetic results. Int J Radiat Oncol Biol Phys 1990;18:189.

67. Handel N, Lewinsky B, Siverstein MJ, et al. Conservation therapy for breast cancer following augmentation mammoplasty. Plast Reconstr Surg 1991;87:873.

68. Ryu J, Yahalom J, Shank B, et al. Radiation therapy after breast augmentation or reconstruction in early or recurrent breast cancer. Cancer 1990;66:844.

69. Schuster RH, Kuske RR, Young VL. Breast reconstruction in women treated with radiation therapy for breast cancer: cosmesis, complications, and tumor control. Plast Reconstr Surg 1992;90:445.

70. Kuske RR, Schuster R, Klein E, et al. Radiotherapy and breast reconstruction: clinical results and dosimetry. Int J Radiat Oncol Biol Phys 1991;21:339.

71. Rosato RM, Dowden RV. Radiation therapy as a cause of capsular contracture. Ann Plast Surg 1994;32:342.

72. Jacobson GM, Sause WT, Thomson JW, et al. Breast irradiation following silicone gel implants. Int J Radiat Oncol Biol Phys 1986;12:835.

73. Halpern J, McNeese M, Kroll S. Cosmesis after irradiation of subcutaneous breast prosthetic implants: long-term follow-up in six patients. (Abstract) Proc Am Soc Clin Oncol 1988;7:28.

74. Laramore GE, Griffin TW, Parker RG, et al. The use of electron beams in treating local recurrence of breast cancer in previously irradiated fields. Cancer 1978;41:991.

75. Elkort RJ, Kelly W, Mozden PJ, et al. A combined treatment program for the management of locally recurrent breast cancer following chest wall irradiation. Cancer 1980;46:647.

76. Tough ICK. The significance of recurrence in breast cancer. Br J Surg 1966;53:897.

77. Bedwinek JM, Lee J, Fineberg B, et al. Prognostic indicators in patients with isolated local–regional recurrence of breast cancer. Cancer 1981;47:2232.

78. Probstfeld MR, O'Connell TX. Treatment of locally recurrent breast carcinoma. Arch Surg 1989;124:1127.

79. Salvadori B, Rovini D, Squicciarini P, et al. Surgery for local recurrences following deficient radical mastectomy for breast cancer: a selected series of 39 cases. Eur J Surg Oncol 1992;18:438.

80. Shah JP, Urban JA. Full thickness chest wall resection for recurrent breast carcinoma involving the bony chest wall. Cancer 1975;35:567.

81. McCormack PM, Bains MS, Burt ME, et al. Local recurrent mammary carcinoma failing multimodality therapy: a solution. Arch Surg 1989;124:158.

82. Zoetmulder FAN, van Dongen JA. Chest wall resection in the treatment of local recurrence of breast cancer. Eur J Surg Oncol 1988;14:127.

83. McKenna RJ, McMurtrey MJ, Larson DL, et al. A perspective on chest wall resection in patients with breast cancer. Ann Thorac Surg 1984;38:482.

84. Kroll SS, Schusterman MA, Larson DL, et al. Long-term survival after chest-wall reconstruction with musculocutaneous flaps. Plast Reconstr Surg 1990;86:697.

85. Muscolino G, Valente M, Lequaglie C, et al. Correlation between first disease-free interval from mastectomy to second disease-free interval from chest wall resection. Eur J Surg Oncol 1992;18:49.

86. Flook D, Webster DJT, Hughes LE, et al. Salvage surgery for advanced local recurrence of breast cancer. Br J Surg 1988;76:512.

87. Dahlstrom KK, Andersson AP, Andersen M, et al. Wide local excision of recurrent breast cancer in the thoracic wall. Cancer 1993;72:774.

88. Miyauchi K, Koyama H, Noguchi S, et al. Surgical treatment for chest wall recurrence of breast cancer. Eur J Cancer 1992;28A:1059.

89. Scott R, Gillespie B, Perez CA, et al. Hyperthermia in combination with definitive radiation therapy: results of a phase I/II RTOG study. Int J Radiat Oncol Biol Phys 1988;15:711.

90. Amicheti M, Valdagni R, Graiff C, et al. Local–regional recurrences of breast cancer: treatment with radiation therapy and local microwave hyperthermia. Am J Clin Oncol 1991;14:60.

91. Kapp DS, Barnett TA, Cox RS, et al. Hyperthermia and radiation

therapy of local—regional recurrent breast cancer: prognostic factors for response and local control of diffuse or nodular tumors. Int J Radiat Oncol Biol Phys 1991;20:1147.

92. Kapp DS, Cox RS, Barnett TA, et al. Thermoradiotherapy for residual microscopic cancer: elective or post-excisional hyperthermia and radiation therapy in the management of local—regional recurrent breast cancer. Int J Radiat Oncol Biol Phys 1992;24:261.

93. Van der Zee J, Treurniet-Donker AD, The SK, et al. Low dose irradiation in combination with hyperthermia: a palliative treatment for patients with breast cancer recurring in previously irradiated areas. Int J Radiat Oncol Biol Phys 1988;15:1407.

94. Dragovic J, Seydel HG, Sandhu T, et al. Local superficial hyperthermia in combination with low-dose radiation therapy for palliation of locally recurrent breast carcinoma. J Clin Oncol 1989;7:30.

95. Perez CA, Pajak T, Emami B, et al. Randomized phase III study comparing irradiation and hyperthermia with irradiation alone in superficial measurable tumors. Am J Clin Oncol 1991;14:133.

96. Gonzalez DG, van Dijk JDP, Blank LECM. Chest wall recurrences of breast cancer: results of combined treatment with radiation and hyperthermia. Radiother Oncol 1988;12:95.

97. Bornstein BA, Zouranjian PS, Hansen JL, et al. Local hyperthermia, radiation therapy, and chemotherapy in patients with local—regional recurrence of breast carcinoma. Int J Radiat Oncol Biol Phys 1992;25:79.

98. Schuh M, Nseyo UO, Potter WR, et al. Photodynamic therapy for palliation of locally recurrent breast carcinoma. J Clin Oncol 1987;5:1766.

99. Sperduto PW, DeLaney TF, Thomas G, et al. Photodynamic therapy for chest wall recurrence in breast cancer. Int J Radiat Oncol Biol Phys 1991;21:441.

100. Khan SA, Dougherty TJ, Mang TS. An evaluation of photodynamic therapy in the management of cutaneous metastases of breast cancer. Eur J Cancer 1993;29A:1686.

101. Morere JF, Boaziz C, Breau JL, et al. Continuous intraarterial (IA) chemotherapy in locally recurrent breast carcinoma. (Abstract) Proc Am Soc Clin Oncol 1991;10:50.

102. Ban T, Nistor C, Nistor V, et al. Ointments with 5-fluorouracile, used in care of patients with breast exulcerative cancers. (Abstract) Ann Oncol 1990;1(Suppl):20.

103. Khayat D, Breau JL, Pouillart P, et al. Miltefosine 6% solution (MIL) as a local treatment in cutaneous metastases of breast cancer in patients receiving a concomitant systemic therapy: preliminary results. (Abstract) Proc Am Soc Clin Oncol 1993;12:62.

104. Szepesi S, Schopohl B, Böttcher HD. Combined treatment with radiation therapy and IFN-β intralesional: clinical results. (Abstract) Eur J Cancer 1991;27(Suppl 2):S220.

105. Ashford R, Plant G, Maher J, et al. Double blind trial of metronidazole in malodorous ulcerating tumors. (Letter) Lancet 1984;1:1232.

106. Borner M, Bacchi M, Goldhirsch A, et al. First isolated locoregional recurrence following mastectomy for breast cancer: results of a phase III multicenter trial comparing systemic treatment with observation after excision and radiation. J Clin Oncol 1994;12:2071.

107. Janjan NA, McNeese MD, Buzdar AU, et al. Management of locoregional recurrent breast cancer. Cancer 1986;58:1552.

108. Holmes FA, Buzdar AU, Kau S-W, et al. Combined-modality approach for patients with isolated recurrences of breast cancer (IV-NED). Breast Dis 1994;7:7.

109. Renner K, Renner H. Simultaneous combined radio-chemotherapy of locally recurrent or haematogeneous metastatic breast carcinoma. (Abstract) Strahlenther Onkol 1988;164:20.

110. Mundt AJ, Sibley GS, Williams S, et al. Patterns of failure of complete responders following high dose chemotherapy and autologous bone marrow transplantation for metastatic breast cancer: implications for the use of adjuvant radiation therapy. Int J Radiat Oncol Biol Phys 1994;151.

111. Olson CE, Ansfield F, Richards M, et al. Review of soft tissue recurrence of breast cancer irradiated with and without actinomycin D. Cancer 1977;39:1981.

112. Hoogstraten B, Gad-el-Mawla N, Maloney TR, et al. Combined modality therapy for first recurrence of breast cancer: a Southwest Oncology Group study. Cancer 1984;54:2248.

113. Ng JSY, Cameron DA, Lee L, et al. Infusional 5 fluorouracil given as a single agent in relapsed breast cancer: its activity and toxicity. Breast 1994;3:87.

114. Rubens RD, Bajetta E, Bonneterre J, et al. Treatment of relapse in breast cancer after adjuvant systemic therapy: review and guidelines for future research. Eur J Cancer 1994;30A:106.

115. Kennedy MJ, Abeloff MD. Management of locally recurrent breast cancer. Cancer 1993;71:2395.

116. Stomper PC, Recht A, Berenberg AL, et al. Mammographic detection of recurrent cancer in the irradiated breast. AJR 1987;148:39.

117. Dershaw DD, McCormick B, Osborne MP. Detection of local recurrence after conservative therapy for breast carcinoma. Cancer 1992;70:493.

118. Orel SG, Troupin RH, Patterson EA, et al. Breast cancer recurrence after lumpectomy and irradiation: role of mammography in detection. Radiology 1992;183:201.

119. Orel SG, Fowble BL, Solin LJ, et al. Breast cancer recurrence after lumpectomy and radiation therapy for early-stage disease: prognostic significance of detection method. Radiology 1993;188:189.

120. Hassell PR, Olivotto IA, Mueller HA. Early breast cancer: detection of recurrence after conservative surgery and radiation therapy. Radiology 1990;176:731.

121. Fowble B, Solin L, Schultz D, et al. Breast recurrence following conservative surgery and radiation: patterns of failure, prognosis, and pathologic findings from mastectomy specimens with implications for treatment. Int J Radiat Oncol Biol Phys 1990;19:833.

122. Haffty BG, Fischer D, Beinfield M, et al. Prognosis following local recurrence in the conservatively treated breast cancer patient. Int J Radiat Oncol Biol Phys 1991;21:293.

123. Silen W, Botnick LE. Physical examination of the treated breast. In: Harris JR, Hellman S, Silen W, eds. Conservative management of breast cancer. Philadelphia, JB Lippincott, 1983:261.

124. Recht A, Sadowsky NL, Cady B. Clinical problems in follow-up of patients following conservative surgery and radiotherapy. Surg Clin North Am 1990;70:1179.

125. Schnitt SJ, Connolly JL, Recht A, et al. The influence of infiltrating lobular histology on local tumor control in breast cancer patients treated with conservative surgery and radiotherapy. Cancer 1989;64:448.

126. Markopoulos C, Gazet JC. Paget's disease of the nipple occurring after conservative management of early breast cancer. Eur J Surg Oncol 1988;14:77.

127. Barr LC, Phillips RH, Brunt AM. Salvage mastectomy after failed breast-conserving therapy for carcinoma of the breast. Ann R Coll Surg 1991;73:126.

128. Sadowsky NL, Semine A, Harris JR. Breast imaging: a critical aspect of breast conserving treatment. Cancer 1990;65:2113.

129. Orford JE, Ingram DM, Kaard AO, et al. Scar formation after breast-conserving surgery for cancer. Br J Surg 1993;80:1003.

130. Dershaw DD, McCormick B, Cox L, et al. Differentiation of benign and malignant local tumor recurrence after lumpectomy. Radiology 1990;155:35.

131. Stigers KB, King JG, Davey DD, et al. Abnormalities of the breast caused by biopsy: spectrum of mammographic findings. AJR 1991;156:287.

132. Solin LJ, Fowble BL, Schultz DJ, et al. The detection of local recurrence after definitive irradiation for early stage carcinoma of the breast: an analysis of the results of breast biopsies performed in previously irradiated breasts. Cancer 1990;65:2497.

133. Mendelson EB. Evaluation of the postoperative breast. Radiol Clin North Am 1992;30:107.

134. Mendelson EB. Radiation changes in the breast. Semin Roentgenol 1993;28:344.

135. Mitnick J, Roses DF, Harris MN. Differentiation of postsurgical changes from carcinoma of the breast. Surg Gynecol Obstet 1988;166:549.

136. Solin LJ, Fowble BL, Troupin RH, et al. Biopsy results of new calcifications in the postirradiated breast. Cancer 1989;63:1956.

137. Samuels JL, Haffty BG, Lee CH, et al. Breast conservation therapy in patients with mammographically undetected breast cancer. Radiology 1992;185:425.

138. Recht A, Schnitt SJ, Connolly JL, et al. Prognosis following local or regional recurrence after conservative surgery and radiotherapy for early stage breast carcinoma. Int J Radiat Oncol Biol Phys 1989;16:3.

139. Fourquet A, Campana F, Zafrani B, et al. Prognostic factors of breast recurrence in the conservative management of early breast cancer: a 25-year follow-up. Int J Radiat Oncol Biol Phys 1989;17:719.

140. Stotter AT, McNeese MD, Ames FC, et al. Predicting the rate and extent of locoregional failure after breast conservation therapy for early breast cancer. Cancer 1989;64:2217.

141. Kurtz JM, Amalric R, Brandone H, et al. Local recurrence after breast-conserving surgery and radiotherapy: frequency, time course, and prognosis. Cancer 1989;63:1912.

142. Leung S, Otmezguine Y, Calitchi E, et al. Locoregional recurrences following radical external beam irradiation and interstitial implantation for operable breast cancer: a twenty three year experience. Radiother Oncol 1986;5:1.

143. Harris JR, Recht A, Amalric R, et al. Time course and prognosis of local recurrence following primary radiation therapy for early breast cancer. J Clin Oncol 1984;2:37.

144. Haffty BG, Carter D, Flynn SD, et al. Local recurrence versus new primary: clinical analysis of 82 breast relapses and potential applications for genetic fingerprinting. Int J Radiat Oncol Biol Phys 1993;27:575.

145. Stotter A, Atkinson EN, Fairston BA, et al. Survival following locoregional recurrence after breast conservation therapy for cancer. Ann Surg 1990;212:166.

146. Osborne MP, Borgen PI, Wong GY, et al. Salvage mastectomy for local and regional recurrence after breast-conserving operation and radiation therapy. Surg Gynecol Obstet 1992;174:189.

147. Van Dongen JA, Bartelink H, Fentiman IS, et al. Factors influencing local relapse and survival and results of salvage treatment after breast-conserving therapy in operable breast cancer: EORTC Trial 10801, breast conservation compared with mastectomy in TNM stage I and II breast cancer. Eur J Cancer 1992;28A:801.

148. Delouche G, Bachelot F, Premont M, et al. Conservation treatment of early breast cancer: long term results and complications. Int J Radiat Oncol Biol Phys 1987;13:29.

149. Kurtz JM, Jacquemier J, Brandone H, et al. Inoperable recurrence after breast-conserving surgical treatment and radiotherapy. Surg Gynecol Obstet 1991;172:357.

150. Abner AL, Recht A, Eberlein T, et al. Prognosis following salvage mastectomy for recurrence in the breast after conservative surgery and radiation therapy for early-stage breast cancer. J Clin Oncol 1993;11:44.

151. Kurtz JM, Spitalier J-M, Amalric R, et al. The prognostic significance of late local recurrence after breast-conserving therapy. Int J Radiat Oncol Biol Phys 1990;18:87.

152. Chauvet B, Lemseffer A, Fetissoff F, et al. Disappearance of the in situ component: a criterion predictive of metastasis in breast cancer after local relapse. Radiother Oncol 1992;25:181.

153. Haffty BG, Toth M, Flynn S, et al. Prognostic value of DNA flow cytometry in the locally recurrent, conservatively treated breast cancer patient. J Clin Oncol 1992;10:1839.

154. Stefanik DF, Brereton HD, Lee TC, et al. Fat necrosis following

155. Rostom AY, El-Sayed ME. Fat necrosis of the breast: an unusual complication of lumpectomy and radiotherapy in breast cancer. Clin Radiol 1987;38:31.

156. Boyages J, Bilous M, Barraclough B, et al. Fat necrosis of the breast following lumpectomy and radiation therapy for early breast cancer. Radiother Oncol 1988;13:69.

157. Keidan RD, Hoffman JP, Weese JL, et al. Delayed breast abscesses after lumpectomy and radiation therapy. Ann Surg 1990;56:440.

158. Staren E, Klepek S, Hartsell B, et al. The dilemma of breast cellulitis after conservation surgery and radiation therapy. (Abstract) Breast Cancer Res Treat 1993;27:188.

159. Trattner A, Figer A, David M, et al. Circumscribed scleroderma induced by postlumpectomy radiation therapy. Cancer 1991;68:2131.

160. Colver GB, Rodger A, Mortimer PS, et al. Post-irradiation morphoea. Br J Derm 1989;120:831.

161. Zucali R, Merson M, Placucci M, et al. Soft tissue sarcoma of the breast after conservative surgery and irradiation for early mammary carcinoma. Radiother Oncol 1994;30:271.

162. Frazier TG, Furnay AP, Rose D, et al. Ultrasound mammography in the follow-up of the post irradiated breast. (Abstract) Breast Cancer Res Treat 1988;12:113.

163. Cosgrove DO, Bamber JC, Davey JB, et al. Color Doppler signals from breast tumors: work in progress. Radiology 1990;176:175.

164. Dao TH, Rahmouni A, Campana F, et al. Tumor recurrence versus fibrosis in the irradiated breast: differentiation with dynamic gadolinium-enhanced MR imaging. Radiology 1993;187:751.

165. Gilles R, Guinebretière J-M, Shapeero LG, et al. Assessment of breast cancer recurrence with contrast-enhanced subtraction MR imaging: preliminary results in 26 patients. Radiology 1993;188:473.

166. Lewis-Jones HG, Whitehouse GH, Leinster SJ. The role of magnetic resonance imaging in the assessment of local recurrent breast cancer. Clin Radiol 1991;43:197.

167. Hagay C, Cherel P, De Maulmont C, et al. Contrast-enhanced CT mammography: evaluation in local breast recurrence. (Abstract) Radiology 1993;189(P):406.

168. Chaiken L, Rege S, Hoh C, et al. Positron emission tomography with fluorodeoxyglucose to evaluate tumor response and control after radiation therapy. Int J Radiat Oncol Biol Phys 1993;27:455.

169. Recht A, Harris JR. Negative breast biopsies after primary radiation therapy: safety and accuracy. (Abstract) Int J Radiat Oncol Biol Phys 1985;11(Suppl 1):131.

170. Ciatto S. Letter to the editor. Breast 1994;3:130.

171. Mitnick JS, Vasquez MF, Roses DF, et al. Recurrent breast cancer: stereotaxic localization for fine-needle aspiration biopsy: work in progress. Radiology 1992;182:103.

172. Schnitt SJ, Connolly JL, Harris JR. Radiation-induced changes in the breast. Hum Pathol 1984;15:545.

173. Schnitt SJ, Connolly JL, Recht A, et al. Breast relapse following primary radiation therapy for early breast cancer. II. Detection, pathologic features and prognostic significance. Int J Radiat Oncol Biol Phys 1985;11:1277.

174. Connolly JL, Schnitt SJ. Evaluation of breast biopsy specimens in patients considered for treatment by conservative surgery and radiation therapy for early breast cancer. Pathol Annu 1988;23:1.

175. Petersen JL, Van Heerde P. Fine needle cytology of breast lesions after breast conserving treatment: cytology of radiation induced changes in normal breast epithelium. Fourth EORTC Breast Cancer Working Conference, London, 1987.

176. Pezner RD, Lorant JA, Terz J, et al. Wound-healing complications following biopsy of the irradiated breast. Arch Surg 1992;127:321.

breast irradiation for carcinoma: clinical presentation and diagnosis. Breast 1982;8:4.

177. Kurtz JM, Amalric R, Brandone H, et al. Results of salvage surgery for mammary recurrence following breast-conserving therapy. Ann Surg 1988;207:347.

178. Kurtz JM, Amalric R, Brandone H, et al. Results of wide excision for mammary recurrence after breast conserving therapy. Cancer 1988;61:1969.

179. Stotter A, Kroll S, McNeese M, et al. Salvage treatment of loco-regional recurrence following breast conservation therapy for early breast cancer. Eur J Surg Oncol 1991;17:231.

180. Cajucom CC, Tsangaris TN, Nemoto T, et al. Results of salvage mastectomy for local recurrence after breast-conserving surgery without radiation therapy. Cancer 1993;71:1774.

181. McCready D, Fish E, Hiraki G, et al. Total mastectomy is not mandatory treatment for breast recurrence following lumpectomy. (Abstract) Breast Cancer Res Treat 1990;16:173.

182. Bostwick J, Paletta C, Hartrampf CR. Conservative treatment for breast cancer: complications requiring reconstructive surgery. Ann Surg 1986;203:481.

183. Salmon RJ, Razaboni R, Soussaline M. The use of the latissimus dorsi musculocutaneous flap following recurrence of cancer in irradiated breasts. Br J Plast Surg 1988;41:41.

184. Bostwick J. Reconstruction after mastectomy. Surg Clin North Am 1990;70:1125.

185. Kroll SS, Schusterman MA, Reece GP, et al. Breast reconstruction with myocutaneous flaps in previously irradiated patients. Plast Reconstr Surg 1994;93:460.

186. Howrigan P, Slavin SA. Salvage mastectomy and chest wall reconstruction using myocutaneous flaps. (Abstract) Breast Dis 1991; 4:39.

187. Dickson MG, Sharpe DT. The complications of tissue expansion in breast reconstruction: a review of 75 cases. Br J Plast Surg 1987;40:629.

188. Olenius M, Jurell G. Breast reconstruction using tissue expansion. Scand J Plast Reconstr Hand Surg 1992;26:83.

189. Fodor PB, Swistel AJ. Chest wall deformity following expansion of irradiated soft tissue for breast reconstruction. NY State J Med 1989;89:419.

190. Barreau-Pouhaer L, Lê MG, Rietjens M, et al. Risk factors for failure of immediate breast reconstruction with prosthesis after total mastectomy for breast cancer. Cancer 1992;70:1145.

191. LaRossa D. Reconstructive surgery. In: Fowble B, Goodman RL, Glick JH, et al, eds. Breast cancer treatment: a comprehensive guide to management. St Louis, Mosby—Year Book, 1991:311.

192. Spitalier J-M, Ayme Y, Brandone H, et al. Treatment of mammary recurrences after breast conservation. (Abstract) Breast Dis 1991; 4:20.

193. Veronesi U, Luini A, Del Vecchio M, et al. Radiotherapy after breast-preserving surgery in women with localized cancer of the breast. N Engl J Med 1993;328:1587.

194. Cowen D, Altschuler C, Blanc B, et al. Second conservative surgery and brachytherapy for isolated breast carcinoma recurrence. (Abstract) Venice, European Society of Mastology, 1994: 146.

195. Mullen E, Deutsch M, Bloomer W. Re-excision and reirradiation of local recurrence for salvage of lumpectomy failures. (Abstract) Proc Am Soc Clin Oncol 1992;11:60.

196. Kwai AH, Stomper PC, Kaplan WD. Clinical significance of isolated scintigraphic sternal lesions in patients with breast cancer. J Nucl Med 1988;29:324.

197. Recht A, Pierce SM, Abner A, et al. Regional nodal failure after conservative surgery and radiotherapy for early-stage breast carcinoma. J Clin Oncol 1991;9:988.

198. Hirn-Stadler B. Das Supraklavikularrezidiv des Mammakarzinoms. Strahlenther Onkol 1990;166:774.

199. Fentiman IA, Lavelle MA, Caplan D, et al. The significance of supraclavicular fossa node recurrence after radical mastectomy. Cancer 1986;57:908.

200. Kiricuta IC, Willner J, Kölbl O, et al. The prognostic significance of the supraclavicular lymph node metastases in breast cancer patients. Int J Radiat Oncol Biol Phys 1993;28:387.

201. Jackson SM. Carcinoma of the breast: the significance of supraclavicular lymph node metastases. Clin Radiol 1966;17:107.

202. Bonnerot V, Dao T, Campana F, et al. Evaluation of MR imaging for detecting recurrent tumor within irradiated brachial plexus. (Abstract) Radiology 1993;189:151.

203. Gateley CA, Mansel RE, Owen A, et al. Treatment of the axilla in operable breast cancer. (Abstract) Br J Surg 1991;78:750.

204. Fowble B, Solin LJ, Schultz DJ, et al. Frequency, sites of relapse, and outcome of regional node failures following conservative surgery and radiation for early breast cancer. Int J Radiat Oncol Biol Phys 1989;17:703.

205. Dunphy FR, Spitzer G, Rossiter Fornoff JE, et al. Factors predicting long-term survival for metastatic breast cancer patients treated with high-dose chemotherapy and bone marrow support. Cancer 1994;73:2157.

Diseases of the Breast, edited by Jay R. Harris,
Marc E. Lippman, Monica Morrow, and Samuel Hellman.
Lippincott-Raven Publishers, Philadelphia, © 1996.

22

Treatment of Metastatic Disease

22.1
Hormonal Therapy and Chemotherapy
SUSAN FLAMM HONIG

Metastatic breast cancer is a significant and growing problem in the United States. Despite improved techniques for breast cancer screening, many women continue to be diagnosed at presentation with metastatic disease, either because of lack of access to diagnostic studies or because of early spread of small tumors. Between 1983 and 1987, 7% of women newly diagnosed with breast cancer presented with distant metastases.[1] Despite improvements in adjuvant therapy, a percentage of women initially diagnosed with early-stage disease experience recurrence. Twenty-four to 30% of women with node-negative disease and at least 50% to 60% of women with positive nodes at diagnosis will experience relapse despite adjuvant therapy if they do not die of other causes.[2] The Surveillance, Epidemiology and End Results (SEER) data projected 182,000 new cases of breast cancer during 1995.[1] Using these data, one would expect 12,740 women to present yearly with advanced disease; 22,750 node-negative women and 46,956 women with stage II or III disease would have recurrences, averaged over 25 years. Thus, nearly 83,000 women yearly would develop metastatic disease, and 46,000 women yearly would die of metastatic breast cancer. The death rate for breast cancer has remained essentially stable since 1930, suggesting that therapy in advanced disease has not improved substantially[1] (Fig. 22.1-1).

There is no curative treatment for metastatic disease, but effective measures to provide palliation and probably some prolongation of life exist. In addition, active research to identify new agents and techniques to improve outcome

for these patients is ongoing. Combinations of systemic therapy, radiation therapy, and surgery may be beneficial. Investigational drugs and continued phase I evaluation of chemotherapeutic and biologic agents may lead to more effective therapies. This chapter focuses on systemic treatments, side effects, and response rates, and reviews new treatments. Biologic treatment, immunologic approaches, high-dose chemotherapy with transplant support, and hormonal kinetic approaches are discussed in detail in other chapters. This chapter is intended to provide a framework for the principles of therapy rather than to serve as an encyclopedic compendium of all available regimens.

Natural History

Breast cancer is most likely to recur in the liver, the lungs, or the bone, as described in detail by Valagussa and colleagues.[2] The site of relapse appears to be affected by disease-free survival. In the Italian series, bone lesions appeared after a median of 2.4 years, but visceral disease occurred 1.1 years after initial diagnosis.

The most common sites of distant involvement have already been mentioned, but breast cancer can frequently involve other organs, particularly endocrine organs. Saphir and Parker[3] reported on the frequency of involvement of the adrenal glands (2% to 44% in various autopsy series) and ovaries (15% on average) and also noted occasional metastases to the thyroid.

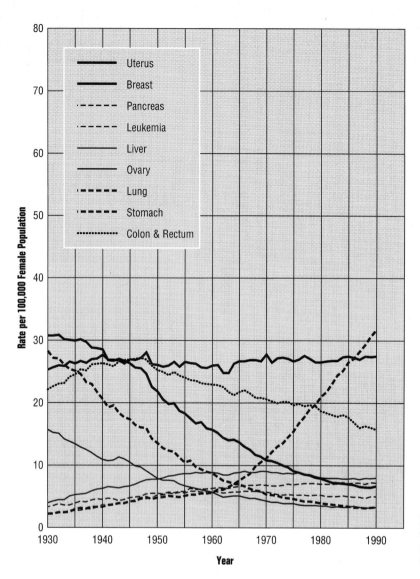

FIGURE 22.1-1 Age-adjusted cancer death rates in women by site, United States, 1930 to 1990. (Boring CC, Squires TS, Tong T, et al. Cancer statistics 1994. CA Cancer J Clin 1994;44:7)

Authors have attempted to delineate differential patterns of relapse based on histology (Table 22.1-1). Borst and Ingold[4] reviewed 2605 cases of breast cancer and identified 359 cases of infiltrating lobular carcinoma. Lobular tumors were more likely to metastasize to the peritoneum, the adrenal glands, the uterus and ovaries, and the pleural surface. Other authors have also reported on an association between infiltrating lobular carcinoma and metastasis to the peritoneum and other unusual sites.[5-8]

A recent publication suggests that adjuvant therapy may affect the pattern of relapse.[9] The International Breast Cancer Study Group (IBCSG; formerly the Ludwig Group) conducted a series of adjuvant therapy trials that enrolled 2108 patients treated with (1) cyclophosphamide, methotrexate, 5-fluorouracil (5-FU), and prednisone (CMFp) chemotherapy with or without tamoxifen, or (2) tamoxifen and prednisone. This group of patients was considered to have had "more effective" therapy. An addi-

tional 722 patients were treated with only one perioperative cycle of chemotherapy or with observation alone, considered "less effective" therapy based on long-term trial results. These patients were monitored for site of first relapse. For both groups, the incidence of recurrence in bone or visceral sites was the same: 18% of patients on more effective therapy versus 17% on less effective therapy had bone metastases; 17% versus 19% of these patients, respectively, developed visceral metastases. A significant difference, however, existed for local–regional and soft tissue relapses, for which more effective therapy resulted in an 18% relapse rate compared with a 36% relapse rate with less effective treatment. These values are significantly different at 10 years of follow-up. These data are intriguing but not conclusive. They suggest that adjuvant chemotherapy affects primarily soft tissue recurrence but not bone or visceral metastases. Whereas any metastatic recurrence is incurable, visceral disease is more immediately life-

TABLE 22.1-1
Sites of Breast Cancer Relapse by Histologic Type

Investigators	Site	ILC	IDC	*P* Value
Borst & Ingold[4]	Gastrointestinal	16 (4.5%)	5 (0.2%)	<.001
	Gynecologic	16 (4.5%)	18 (0.8%)	<.001
	Peritoneum	11 (3.1%)	13 (0.6%)	<.001
	Adrenal	2 (0.6%)	0 (0%)	.019
	Bone marrow	76 (21.2%)	324 (14.4%)	.001
	Lung pleura	9 (2.5%)	230 (10.2%)	<.001
Harris et al[5]	Lung	7 (13.7%)	98 (33.3%)	.0082
	Bone marrow	13 (72.2%)	33 (27.3%)	.0004
	Meninges	9 (16.1%)	1 (0.3%)	<.0001
Dixon et al[6]	Liver	27 (35%)	13 (18%)	.01
	Peritoneum	14 (18%)	1 (1%)	.0003
Lamovec et al[7]	Lung	10 (40%)	137 (70.3%)	<.006
	Myocardium	7 (28%)	2 (1%)	<.000001
	Meninges	3 (12%)	2 (1%)	<.006
	Stomach	5 (20%)	7 (3.6%)	<.004
	Intestine	10 (40%)	4 (2%)	<.004
	Ureter	8 (32%)	7 (3.6%)	<.00001
	Bladder	3 (12.9%)	3 (1.5%)	<.002
	Uterus	13 (52.2%)	0 (0%)	<.000001
	Ovary	13 (52.2%)	22 (11.3%)	<.000001
	Fallopian tube	2 (8%)	0 (0%)	<.004
	Peritoneum	15 (60%)	30 (15.4%)	<.000001
Jain et al[8]	Bone marrow	9 (15%)	20 (5%)	.009
	Lung	10 (16%)	123 (31%)	.02
	Pleura	13 (21%)	136 (34%)	.04
	Brain	1 (2%)	44 (11%)	.02
	Peritoneum	7 (11%)	11 (3%)	.006

ILC, infiltrating lobular carcinoma; IDC, infiltrating ductal carcinoma.

threatening. These data are at odds with the survival benefit reported in many adjuvant trials; they require confirmation in independent trials.

Site of relapse also affects subsequent survival. Recurrence in bony sites alone has been associated with a better prognosis by a number of authors. Perez and coworkers[10] retrospectively reviewed the records of 510 patients treated for metastatic breast cancer. Of these patients, 77 had visceral disease alone and 80 had bone-only disease. Patients were treated with a variety of chemotherapy and hormonal therapies; no significant differences in response rates were noted by location of disease. However, patients with bony disease had a median survival of 28 months compared with 13 months for those with visceral disease, a difference that was statistically significant. Postmenopausal women were more likely to have a longer disease-free interval (41 months versus 21 months for premenopausal women), but, overall, menopausal status and disease-free interval were not independent prognostic variables for survival.

A prospective study has also validated these findings. Chiedozi[11] reported the results of a trial of 60 Nigerian women. Thirty had bone-only metastatic disease, and 30 had nonskeletal metastases; all had untreated breast primary tumors. Both groups were treated with mastectomy and CMFp chemotherapy. Patients with visceral disease had a median survival of 6 months; tumors were present for a median of 6 months before the patients sought medical attention. In contrast, women with skeletal disease had a median survival of 12 months, with a 12-month median history of tumor presence before seeking medical attention.

Sherry and others[12] retrospectively reviewed the records of 86 patients with bone-only metastatic breast cancer treated at Vanderbilt. Seventy-five percent had tumors that were estrogen receptor (ER) positive; 55% were postmenopausal women. Median survival was 48 months, and 33% lived longer than 5 years (Fig. 22.1-2). At the authors' institution, median survival with extraskeletal metastases was 17 months, and the 5-year survival rate was only 13%. In this group of bone-only metastatic patients, the development of nonskeletal metastases was a poor prognostic sign, with a subsequent median survival of only 9 months. Similar findings have been reported by other authors.[13,14]

FIGURE 22.1-2 Actuarial 5-year survival curves comparing patients with skeletal versus extraskeletal metastases. (Sherry MM, Greco FA, Johnson DH, et al. Metastatic breast cancer confined to the skeletal system: an indolent disease. Am J Med 1986;81:383)

Although site of disease is associated with survival, a wide range of survival times exists within the subsets. For example, Sherry and associates[15] found survival times that ranged from 1 to 24 months in patients with visceral disease. For patients with bone-only disease, survival ranged from 8 to 97 months.[12] Breast cancer is a heterogeneous disease, and the prognosis of individual patients frequently does not conform to published predictions.

Attention has also been directed toward the influence of race on survival. The SEER data from 1955 to 1987 show a 29% increase in the death rate from breast cancer in African American women, but essentially no change in the death rate when women of all races are considered.[16] Some of this difference may be attributed to stage of diagnosis. Fifty-two percent of white women diagnosed with breast cancer between 1981 and 1987 were found to have early-stage disease, compared with 43% of African American women.[16] This disparity has been attributed to differences in socioeconomic status, access to medical care, educational level, awareness of recommended screening procedures, and compliance with medical recommendations.[17,18] Several investigators have reported poorer survival in African American patients with breast cancer even when matched groups received similar therapy. The Piedmont Oncology Association (POA) reviewed the outcome of 74 African American patients treated in five studies of doxorubicin-based chemotherapy for metastatic disease.[19] These patients were matched with 74 randomly selected white patients treated in the same studies. No significant difference in performance status, disease-free interval, or receptor status was found. African American patients were more likely to have skin metastases, and white patients were more likely to have bone metastases. No differences in response rates to therapy or in time to progression were observed. However, the median survival for white patients was 20.3 months compared with 14.3 months for Afri-

can American women ($P = .0059$). African American women were estimated to have a relative risk (RR) of death of 1.7 compared with white women. The authors suggested that unidentified biologic factors may account for the difference in survival.

The National Cancer Institute (NCI) published results of the Black/White Cancer Survival Study, which evaluated 1130 women from three geographic regions of the United States.[20] It included 612 African American women and 518 white women. African American women were more likely to have comorbid illnesses and to have their cancer diagnosed at a later stage. Chemotherapy was administered more often to African American women. African American women were more likely to have ER-negative and poorly differentiated tumors. After controlling for stage, tumor pathology, treatment, comorbid illnesses, and sociodemographic factors, African American women were still more likely to die of breast cancer than white women (RR, 1.3; Fig. 22.1-3).

Elledge and colleagues[21] evaluated breast tumor specimens and accompanying clinical data from the San Antonio Tumor Bank for biologic factors related to race. The study included 4885 white patients, 1016 African American patients, and 777 Hispanic patients. Five-year survival rates were 75%, 65%, and 70%, respectively. Although African American and Hispanic women were more likely to present with advanced disease than were white women, differences in survival remained even after adjustment for stage. No difference in systemic therapy was observed between the three groups, although dose-intensity and compliance data were not available. African American women and Hispanic women were more likely to have ER-or progesterone receptor (PR)-negative tumors and to have a high S-phase fraction. Black race was found to be an independent prognostic variable of survival compared with white race and Hispanic race. Hispanic race was not an independent prognostic variable when compared with white race. These data suggest that African American and Hispanic women are more likely to have tumors with poor prognostic variables such as receptor negativity and high growth fraction accounting for survival differences. The molecular basis of these differences is unknown.

Thus, breast cancer has a recognizable metastatic pattern. The development of visceral metastases is usually associated with a shorter disease-free interval and a subsequent decreased survival. Patients with disease confined to the bone frequently have indolent disease and can survive, on average, 4 years with therapy. African American and Hispanic women are likely to have a shorter survival, in part because of differences in stage at presentation but largely because of poor prognostic factors. However, a wide range of survival times is observed in all groups of patients, and individual patient factors should be taken into account when planning therapy and discussing prognosis.

Evaluation of a Patient With Newly Diagnosed Metastases

The accepted evaluation for newly diagnosed metastatic breast cancer includes a chest radiograph, a bone scan, and an abdominal computed tomographic (CT) scan in

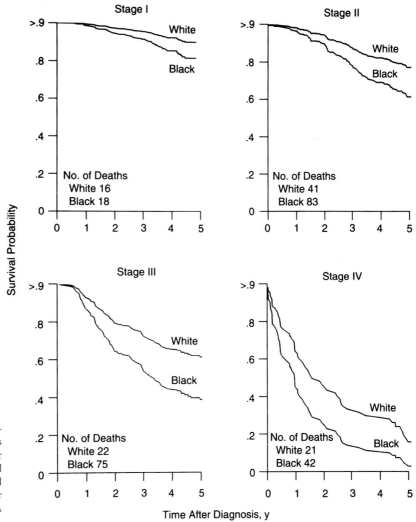

FIGURE 22.1-3 Survival experience by race, stratified by stage. Five-year all-cause mortality rates among women diagnosed with invasive breast cancer in the Black/White Survival Study. (Eley JW, Hill HA, Chen VN, et al. Racial differences in survival from breast cancer: results of the National Cancer Institute Black/White Cancer Survival Study. JAMA 1994;272:953)

addition to a routine complete blood count and blood chemistry tests. Additional testing should be dictated by physical examination findings and patient symptoms, by any abnormalities detected in the usual studies that require additional work-up, or by prechemotherapy testing:

- Complete history and physical examination
- Complete blood count
- Routine chemistries, including transaminases and alkaline phosphatase
- Chest radiograph
- Bone scan
- CT scan of the abdomen
- Other testing as indicated by history, physical examination findings, or laboratory abnormalities
- Prechemotherapy testing (cardiac evaluation for anthracyclines, creatinine clearance for platin analogues)

The results of these studies are used to make optimal treatment decisions, to help assess response to treatment, and to anticipate and prevent potential complications.

Histologic Documentation of Recurrence

The importance of biopsy confirmation of newly diagnosed metastatic disease cannot be overemphasized. Benign lesions are frequently mistaken for recurrent cancer, leading to unnecessary and toxic therapies. If clinical or radiologic findings are malignant, they may represent a new primary or metastases from a new primary and not recurrent breast cancer. In my own institution, for example, patients clinically diagnosed with pulmonary metastases from breast cancer at outside institutions have been found to have bronchoalveolar carcinoma, squamous cell lung cancer, primary pulmonary carcinoid tumor, hamartoma, tuberculosis, and cryptococcosis after lung biopsy. The site of biopsy should be determined by the physical examination and radiographic results. The site that is most accessible and can therefore undergo biopsy with the least chance of complication is preferred, such as a palpable chest wall nodule rather than a liver lesion. In most cases, one should not administer toxic therapies or present a diagnosis of an incurable disease without validating recurrence pathologically. Even if the diagnosis is one of a nonbreast carcinoma, therapeutic implications, potential sites and types of complications, and overall prognosis are altered by this information.

Tumor Markers

Tumor markers can aid the clinician in assessing response to therapy in the metastatic setting. The reader is referred to Chapter 20, where tumor markers are discussed in detail.

Treatment

Because metastatic breast cancer is incurable with the available standard therapies, the goal of therapy is effective palliation with minimal toxicity. The assessment of which therapy best fits this description depends on patient factors as well as sites of disease. In addition, consideration must be given to incorporation of surgery and radiation therapy in an effort to improve quality of life. This chapter addresses available and new hormonal and chemotherapy agents, principles of therapy, and investigational approaches to treatment. The use of other modalities, such as surgery and radiation, is addressed elsewhere in this volume.

Hormonal Therapy

HISTORICAL BACKGROUND

Antihormonal therapy for breast cancer was first described by Beatson in 1896, when he treated women with metastatic breast cancer with oophorectomy and documented regression of skin nodules.[22] DeCourmelles described the use of irradiation of the ovary as a therapy in 1905.[22] Subsequent modern trials have shown a benefit for oophorectomy primarily in ER-positive premenopausal women.[23] As expected, however, this procedure is ineffective in postmenopausal women, in whom the predominant form of estrogen is estrone, synthesized by the adrenal from androstenedione. Thus, adrenalectomy was used as a means of interrupting hormone synthesis in postmenopausal women.[24] Hypophysectomy was also used to produce total endocrine blockade.[24,25] Because these procedures require major surgery and interrupt other endocrine functions, medical agents were developed to achieve these goals instead. In addition, while associated with a response rate of 30% to 40%, these operations are also associated with a mortality rate of 1% to 5%.[23] Thus, use of these operations is generally no longer indicated. The exception may be the use of oophorectomy in appropriately selected patients, although the use of luteinizing hormone–releasing hormone (LHRH) agonists may be preferable to surgical intervention.

A number of estrogen preparations have been used for breast cancer treatment, including diethylstilbestrol (DES), ethinyl estradiol, and conjugated estrogens.[23] The mechanism by which pharmacologic increases in estrogen concentration suppress breast cancer growth is unknown. Overall, these agents are associated with a 20% to 40% response rate.[23] However, about 30% of patients also experience toxicity, including nausea, vomiting, uterine bleeding, breast pain, and edema.[23] Other risks include thromboembolic events and congestive heart failure. Because of these side effects and the risk of stimulating breast cancer growth, the development of antihormonal agents has supplanted the use of estrogens as a breast cancer therapy.

Overall, hormonal therapies result in a 30% to 35% response rate in unselected patients[23,24] (Table 22.1-2). The development of easily used assays for ER and PR content in breast tumors and demonstration that these receptor levels correlate with response have allowed selective prescription of these agents.[26–42] Initial response rate to therapy in ER- and PR-positive patients is 60% to 75%, whereas in ER- and PR-negative patients, the response rate is less than 10%.[29,30,32,33,35,37,40–43] Responses are seen in patients with mixed receptor results. Tumors that are ER-positive and PR-negative have a response rate of 25% to 30%; tumors that are ER-negative and PR-positive have a response rate of 40% to 45%[29,30,32,33,35,37,40–43] (Table 22.1-3). An intact ER is required to produce PR protein.[35] ER-negative, PR-positive tumors may reflect a false-negative assay of the ER or mutations in the receptor that differentially affect estrogen and tamoxifen binding.[44]

TABLE 22.1-2
Response Rates of Unselected Patients to Endocrine Therapies

Therapy	Response Rate (%)	References
Tamoxifen	6–53	24, 43, 45, 48, 50
Oophorectomy	21–37	24, 142, 143
Progestins	10–67	23, 24, 157, 159, 161–165, 169, 171
Aminoglutethimide	16–54	23–25, 178, 180–182
LHRH analogues	11–45	23, 24, 186, 189, 191–194
Estrogens	20–41	23, 24, 201
Androgens	5–21	23, 24, 195
Adrenalectomy	30–45	23, 24, 180
Hypophysectomy	21–40	23–25
Corticosteroids	20–25	23, 24, 181
Antiprogestins	9–18★	175, 176

LHRH, luteinizing hormone–releasing hormone.

★ Included partial response and disease stabilization.

TABLE 22.1-3
*Relation Between Steroid Receptor Status of Breast Tumor
and Patient's Objective Response to Endocrine Therapy*

Investigators	Steroid Receptor Status*			
	ER+/PR+	ER+/PR−	ER−/PR−	ER−/PR+
Brooks et al[29]	4/6	2/7	—	—
Dao & Nemoto[30]	10/13	18/31	2/28	—
Degenshein et al[32]	26/33	3/14	0/14	1/1
King[32a]	10/11	3/15	2/9	0/2
McCarty et al[32b]	33/40	2/20	3/35	1/3
Nomura et al[34]	7/10	8/12	2/20	0/1
Osborne et al[35]	16/20	14/45	3/20	—
Skinner et al[40]	9/12	2/6	3/30	2/3
Young et al[41]	20/29	3/14	2/9	1/1
TOTAL	135/174 (78%)	55/164 (34%)	17/165 (10%)	5/11 (45%)

ER, estrogen receptor; PR, progesterone receptor.

* Number of patients responding to treatment/number with receptor status designated.

(Wittliff JL. Steroid-hormone receptors in breast cancer. Cancer 1984;53:638; adapted from the collective papers presented at the NIH Consensus Development Conference on Steroid Receptors in Breast Cancer. Cancer 1980;46:2759)

Thus, hormonal therapy should be strongly considered for any patient with positive results for either ER or PR. Because the objective response rate is 10% even in receptor-negative patients, a trial of hormonal therapy should be considered at some point in this metastatic patient population as well.

HORMONAL AGENTS

Tamoxifen

PHARMACOLOGY. Tamoxifen is a synthetic antiestrogen that acts primarily by binding to the ER. First described in 1971, it is the most widely used hormonal therapy.[45] Numerous clinical trials have shown it to be a safe and effective therapy for advanced breast cancer, with response rates ranging from 16% to 52%.[43,46–50] Higher response rates are observed when patients are selected for ER or PR positivity.[43,46–50]

Tamoxifen has a half-life of 7 days.[50] Thus, it takes 4 weeks to reach a steady-state drug concentration and at least that long to completely clear tamoxifen and its metabolites after the drug is discontinued. There is wide variation in intrapatient and interpatient serum concentrations, and concentrations do not correlate well with response.[51] Because of the long half-life of tamoxifen, only once daily dose is required, rather than the widely used twice-daily administration, simplifying the regimen.[52] A new 20-mg tablet is under development, which may further facilitate compliance with therapy.[53]

Tamoxifen is metabolized by a number of pathways (Fig. 22.1-4). Its primary metabolite is N–desmethyltamoxifen (N–dMT), which functions as a weak antiestrogen.[54] Its binding affinity for the ER is similar to that of tamoxifen.[55] N–dMT can be further metabolized to N–desdimethyltamoxifen and subsequently to metabolite Y, a primary alcohol.[56] A secondary pathway converts tamoxifen to 4-hydroxytamoxifen (4–OH–T), a potent antiestrogen.[54] This compound exists as two isomers, the Z and the E form. The E form is a weak antiestrogen, but the Z form is an extremely potent antiestrogen. Workers have theorized that a third metabolism pathway exists, resulting in metabolite E, which also exists as two isomers, Z and E.[54] Both are primarily estrogen agonists, and the E form is more potent than the Z form.

NON–RECEPTOR-MEDIATED MECHANISMS OF ACTION. Responses to tamoxifen therapy have been observed in patients with ER-negative tumors at a rate of about 10%.[43] It has therefore been postulated that tamoxifen may have non–receptor-mediated mechanisms of action that may also be important therapeutically.

Tamoxifen has positive effects on the immune system and has been demonstrated to increase antibody production and to increase natural killer cell activity and inhibit suppressor T cells.[57–60] However, similar results have been obtained with estrogen administration, suggesting that these effects occur through an ER pathway.[58,59]

Insulin-like growth factor 1 (IGF-1) is a known mitogen for breast cancer cells in culture.[61,62] Tamoxifen decreases levels of IGF-1 and was initially thought

A

B

Fixed Ring Analog	R1	R2	Activity
(Z) TAM*	H	OCH2CH2N(CH3)2	weak antiestrogen
(E) TAM	OCH2CH2N(CH3)	H	weak estrogen
(Z) 4-OHT*	OH	OCH2CH2N(CH3)2	potent antiestrogen
(E) 4-OHT	OCH2CH2N(CH3)2	OH	weak antiestrogen
(Z) met E*	H	OH	weak estrogen
(E) met E	OH	H	potent estrogen

* Potential products of the metabolism of (Z) fixed ring TAM

FIGURE 22.1-4   A. Potential pathways of tamoxifen metabolism. **B.** Structure of fixed-ring analogues of tamoxifen and its metabolites. (Wolf DM, Langan-Fahey SM, Parker CJ, et al. Investigation of the mechanism of tamoxifen-stimulated breast tumor growth with nonisomerizable analogues of tamoxifen and metabolites. J Natl Cancer Inst 1993;85:808)

to act through a growth hormone–mediated pathway or through direct interaction with IGF-1 receptors.[61,62] Estrogen administration in normal postmenopausal women also results in a decrease in IGF-1 levels, suggesting that the observed effect is hormone mediated.[63] The decrease is accompanied by an increase in growth hormone levels.

Tamoxifen lowers IGF-1 and possibly growth hormone levels, suggesting that its effect may be mediated through interactions with pituitary estrogen receptors.[62]

Tamoxifen also increases transforming growth factor β (TGF-β) production, an inhibitory growth factor for breast cancer cells.[64–66] Knabbe and colleagues,[67] however, showed that the effects of TGF-β are hormonally controlled and thus are not ER independent.

Tamoxifen has been reported to inhibit protein kinase C, thought to be a novel mechanism of action related to cell cycle regulation.[68–71] Initial experiments demonstrated inhibition of protein kinase C by tamoxifen, but not by estradiol or DES.[68] These results were replicated by O'Brian and colleagues.[69] However, different results were obtained by Issandou and colleagues.[71] Although previous investigators' results were replicated in vitro, experiments in intact living cell systems showed no inhibition of protein kinase C by tamoxifen, suggesting a significant role for the phospholipid environment. Thus, protein kinase C inhibition is unlikely to be important in vivo.

Calmodulin antagonism has been proposed as a non–receptor-mediated mechanism of action.[68,72,73] Calcium channel antagonists have been proposed as potential reversers of multidrug resistance, and high-dose tamoxifen in other cancers, such as melanoma, has been found to increase response rates.[74] However, the effect of tamoxifen in this regimen has been found to be unrelated to calmodulin effects.[75] The effect in one laboratory is receptor independent, as tamoxifen–platinum synergy can be demonstrated in ER-negative melanoma cell lines.[75] This interaction appears to be one of the few examples of a hormone-independent mechanism of action for tamoxifen.

Many of these findings have therefore been found to be related to an ER effect. The primary action of tamoxifen appears to be receptor mediated, and these additional functions probably make a minor contribution to the observed therapeutic effects.

MECHANISMS OF RESISTANCE. Despite initial high response rates with tamoxifen for receptor-positive tumors, tamoxifen resistance eventually develops. Many investigators have examined this phenomenon, since delineation of the cause could lead to new therapies or means of preventing or overcoming drug resistance.

Jordan's laboratory reported the development of an MCF-7 cell line that is tamoxifen stimulated rather than inhibited.[76] This cell line is an excellent model for examining molecular changes that may be relevant in human tamoxifen resistance. Osborne and colleagues[54,77,78] suggested that resistance is mediated by active transport of tamoxifen out of the cell, but other authors have not found this to be significant. Fendl and Zimniski[79] observed that rats treated with dimethylbenzanthracene (DMBA) placed on suppressive tamoxifen can develop mammary tumors; these tumors are exclusively hormone independent with a faster growth rate than tumors seen with DMBA exposure alone. This phenomenon suggests a selective pressure in favor of hormone-independent tumor cells.

Alterations in the normal metabolism of tamoxifen have

also been cited. Osborne and colleagues[78] measured levels of tamoxifen and its major metabolites in 14 tumors from patients with metastatic breast cancer treated with tamoxifen. High levels of the *cis* isomer of 4-hydroxytamoxifen, an estrogen agonist form, were found in nonresponding patients. These results could explain the reported phenomenon of "withdrawal" responses.[80] These assays were performed in only a small number of tumors, and the results require replication in a larger series. Opposite results were found in an animal model system by Wolf and colleagues.[81] They treated MCF-7 tumors in nude mice with both tamoxifen and a nonisomerizable fixed-ring structure of tamoxifen. Both compounds were able to stimulate tumor growth equally, suggesting that differential metabolism is not responsible for the observed phenomena.

Pommier and colleagues[82] found elevated levels of dihydroepiandrosterone (DHEA) in 15 postmenopausal patients with progressive disease on tamoxifen. Levels of DHEA decreased in 8 of 9 patients evaluated after discontinuation of tamoxifen. In 1 patient who then underwent hypophysectomy, rechallenge with tamoxifen resulted in increased DHEA levels. In 2 patients who underwent adrenalectomy, rechallenge with tamoxifen did not change the minimal detectable levels of DHEA. The researchers postulated that tamoxifen stimulates DHEA production, leading to increased conversion to 4-androstenedione. This compound in turn can be aromatized to estrone in peripheral tissue or, alternatively, converted to testosterone and in turn to estradiol. Increased circulating estrogen would then preferentially compete for ERs and result in growth stimulation of tumors.

McGuire and colleagues[44] examined ER variants in breast tumors (see Chap. 3). Briefly, they identified several mutations, including deletion of exon 5 found in half of the examined ER-negative, PR-positive tumors; deletions of exons 3 and 7; several amino acid substitutions and insertions; and base-pair substitutions. The exon 5 deletion functionally resulted in a dominantly positive receptor, one transcriptionally active in the absence of estrogen, suggesting potential continued tumor growth stimulation. The exon 7 deletion resulted in a dominantly negative receptor, one that is transcriptionally inactive but prevents the function of normal ER. These mutated receptors may therefore play a role in either stimulation or suppression of tumor growth.

Horwitz[83] investigated heterogeneity in PRs; her research suggests that alterations in PR structure may also account for tamoxifen stimulation. This selective pressure may result in the appearance of subclones that are hormone-independent, leading to a change in the tumor phenotype and escape from the inhibitory actions of tamoxifen.[84]

Thus, although many candidate hypotheses for tamoxifen resistance exist, their quantitative contribution remains unknown.

TOXICITY OF TAMOXIFEN THERAPY. While primarily an estrogen antagonist, tamoxifen also has estrogen-agonist properties that account for both secondary benefits of this agent and toxicities (Table 22.1-4). In addition to an antitumor effect, benefits of tamoxifen therapy include preservation of bone density, decreased cholesterol levels with a reduction in cardiovascular morbidity, and a decrease in second breast primary tumors.[85–94] These benefits are relevant in the adjuvant setting and are discussed in Chapter 17.

Despite these benefits, tamoxifen has a wide range of side effects and toxicities, also discussed in greater detail in Chapter 17. The best documentation of tamoxifen side effects comes from an adjuvant tamoxifen trial conducted by the National Surgical Adjuvant Breast Project (NSABP), NSABP B-14.[95] Hot flashes were reported significantly more often in women treated with tamoxifen (57%) than in women on placebo (41%). About 24% of women on tamoxifen therapy reported increased vaginal secretions.[96] For many women, this side effect was not distressing, and some even considered it beneficial because it relieved postmenopausal vaginal dryness. Many other

TABLE 22.1-4
Toxicity of Tamoxifen

Study	Adverse Effect	Incidence (%)		Dose (mg)
		Treated	Controls	
B-14[95]	Hot flashes	57	41	20
B-14[95]	Vaginal discharge	24	12	20
B-14[95]	Thromboembolic events	1	<1	20
ECOG[97]		2.3	0.3	20
Lipton et al[98]		3.2	—	NS
Uziely et al[104]	Uterine cancer	3	—	20
Fornander et al[108]		1.5	0.4	40
Fornander et al[108]	Liver cancer	0.2	0	40
Kaiser-Kupfer et al[116]	Retinopathy	3.7	—	240–320
Vinding & Nielson[117]		11.8	—	30
Pavlidis et al[118]		6.3	—	20

side effects, traditionally attributed to tamoxifen, were not significantly different between the two arms.[96]

Tamoxifen is a partial estrogen agonist, resulting in additional serious side effects. Overall, tamoxifen causes a 1.5% incidence of thromboembolic events when a number of adjuvant trials are examined.[93,95–97] Lipton and colleagues[98] reported a 3.2% incidence of both phlebitis and thrombosis in patients with metastatic breast cancer, with no fatal events. It is important to also report the incidence of thromboembolic events in metastatic trials, since patients with advanced cancer are historically reported to be at higher risk of thromboembolic events.[98] No mechanism for the increased clotting rate has been determined. Some investigators have reported lowered levels of antithrombin III in patients with metastatic breast cancer receiving tamoxifen, but these findings have not been correlated in a cause-and-effect manner with thrombosis.[99]

The risk of uterine cancer associated with tamoxifen has received extensive attention in peer-reviewed journals and the media.[100–108] Further studies are required to determine accurately the risk of endometrial cancer with tamoxifen use and to correlate risk with duration of therapy. In addition, optimal surveillance methods must be developed, and care must be taken to watch for additional endometrial abnormalities reported to be associated with tamoxifen, such as the development of polyps and fibroid tumors.[109–112]

A third concern is the possible development of liver cancer. Tamoxifen can cause liver cancer in rats.[113,114] Unopposed estrogen in patients results in a low but measurable rate of liver tumors. Fornander and colleagues[108] also reported the finding of two cases of liver cancer on the tamoxifen arm of the study described earlier. However, this incidence is too small to draw meaningful conclusions about the RR of disease in patients taking tamoxifen. Animal studies have indicated that tamoxifen does not act as an initiator for hepatocellular carcinoma but acts as an effective promoting agent.[115] This problem requires further study and is a more critical question in the setting of adjuvant therapy rather than treatment of metastatic disease.

Ophthamologic side effects have also been reported, more frequently in doses exceeding 20 mg/d. Kaiser-Kupfer and Lippman[116] reported corneal and retinal changes in four women treated on a dose-intensification trial of tamoxifen at the NCI. Additional studies, in addition to many case reports, have also confirmed this rare finding.[117–124]

Despite these side effects, tamoxifen is generally a safe and well-tolerated therapy, especially compared with cytotoxic drugs. Many of the more serious long-term complications are not relevant in the metastatic setting, making tamoxifen an excellent choice for palliative treatment of appropriate patients.

DOSE INTENSITY CONSIDERATIONS. In the United States, the current recommended dosage of tamoxifen is 20 mg orally (PO) daily. Several trials reported the dose-response effect for this drug (Table 22.1-5). Tormey and colleagues[125] at the NCI looked at the effect of increasing tamoxifen doses in the context of a trial that randomly assigned patients to receive tamoxifen or tamoxifen plus fluoxymesterone. One hundred eight patients with metastatic breast cancer were enrolled. Tamoxifen was administered as 2 mg/m² PO twice a day (BID). Every fourth patient had the tamoxifen dose increased; the dose levels were 4, 8, 16, 32, 50, 60, 80, and 100 mg/m² PO BID. The increased dose of tamoxifen was associated with an increased likelihood of objective response to therapy, but there was no association with time to treatment failure. The higher dose of tamoxifen was associated with an increased incidence of ocular toxicity.[116] Thus, an increase in tamoxifen dose was not associated with a clear benefit in outcome but was associated with increased toxicity.

Ward[126] reported on a randomized trial of metastatic breast cancer patients who received tamoxifen either 10 or 20 mg PO BID. Sixty-eight patients were enrolled. Objective response rates were 51% and 60%, respectively. No difference in side effect profile was noted. No survival data were provided, nor was a statistical analysis of the difference between these response rates performed. Bratherton and colleagues[127] performed a randomized, double-

TABLE 22.1-5
Dose-Response Trials of Tamoxifen in Postmenopausal Patients With Metastatic Breast Cancer

		Response Rate (%)			Median Duration (mo)		
Dose (mg/d)	Patients	Low Dose	Medium Dose	High Dose	Low Dose	High Dose	Reference
20 vs 40	68	61	—	77	—	—	126
<12 vs 12–32 vs >32	108	41	31	46	—	—	125
30 vs 90	143	37	—	35	13+	11+	129
20 vs 40	237	34	—	31	18	12	127
30 or 40★	23	4	—	6	—	—	128

★ Nonrandomized study.

blind trial of tamoxifen, 10 versus 20 mg PO BID. No difference in response rate or duration of response was found. Goldhirsch and associates[128] reported similar results. Rose and colleagues[129] randomly assigned patients to receive 30 or 90 mg/d and observed no difference in response rates.

Overall, these studies have not suggested a clear increase in response with higher doses of tamoxifen, but a higher incidence of side effects can be elicited. Therefore, the standard recommended dose is 20 mg PO daily.

ROLE IN PREMENOPAUSAL WOMEN. The role of tamoxifen in premenopausal women continues to be debated. Few premenopausal women have been included in randomized trials of tamoxifen, either in the adjuvant or metastatic setting.[23,24,130] There are several reasons for this exclusion. First, younger women more frequently have ER-negative tumors, making it less likely that tamoxifen will be of benefit to them.[24] Secondly, in ER-positive women, endocrine blockade with an LHRH agonist or ovarian ablation with either surgery or radiation therapy has been an acceptable alternative to prolonged oral medication.[23,24] Although ovarian ablation has been used less frequently since the development of tamoxifen, there has been renewed interest in this approach, sparked by a recently published metaanalysis in the adjuvant setting.[130] Third, there is concern by many breast oncologists that tamoxifen may have different and possibly more significant toxicities in premenopausal women than in postmenopausal women. A number of hormonal effects and side effects have been described in premenopausal but not postmenopausal women on tamoxifen. Jordan and colleagues[131] evaluated eight premenopausal patients on adjuvant tamoxifen therapy. All maintained regular menses. Tamoxifen had no clear-cut effect on levels of follicle-stimulating hormone (FSH) or luteinizing hormone (LH). Both estradiol and estrone levels were significantly increased by tamoxifen administration. In contrast, in postmenopausal women, tamoxifen does not change estradiol levels.[55] Only small reductions in FSH and LH are observed, and the rate and degree of decrease do not correlate with response.[24,50,55] These results indicate that, in premenopausal women, tamoxifen causes stimulation of ovarian steroidogenesis directly or results in more efficient steroidogenesis. These findings are in accord with descriptions of the efficacy of tamoxifen in increasing the ovulation rate in infertile women without breast cancer.[132-134] Thus, premenopausal women on tamoxifen therapy can still become pregnant; amenorrhea is unlikely to be a result of tamoxifen administration and should prompt a β-human chorionic gonadotropin test or a menopausal work-up. Premenopausal women on tamoxifen should be counseled about contraceptive use, since the risk of pregnancy may be increased. This evidence of a direct ovarian effect is also consistent with a case report of cystic ovarian necrosis thought to be secondary to tamoxifen.[135]

Investigators have also hypothesized that the increased levels of circulating estradiol induced by tamoxifen might stimulate tumor growth.[131] Alternatively, high circulating estrogen levels in premenopausal women might provide competitive inhibition of tamoxifen's effects, because estradiol has a higher binding affinity for the ER than does tamoxifen.[50,136] Thus far, there is no clinical evidence to support this hypothesis.

Despite these concerns, tamoxifen therapy has been used in premenopausal women with metastatic breast cancer. Pritchard and colleagues[137] treated 42 patients with a 31% response rate. Side effects were mild. Five patients developed ovarian cysts, a side effect reported in premenopausal but not postmenopausal women. Manni and Pearson[138] treated 11 premenopausal women with tamoxifen and reported a 45% response rate. In addition, tamoxifen caused increased serum levels of estrone and estradiol, although FSH and LH were unaffected. No adverse events were reported. Similar results were reported by Margreiter, Planting, and Sawka and in trials cited by Sunderland and Osborne.[55,139-141]

COMPARISON WITH OOPHORECTOMY. Tamoxifen is equivalent in efficacy to ovarian ablation. Studies from the Mayo Clinic and from Britain compared tamoxifen at 20 and 40 mg/d, respectively, with oophorectomy.[142,143] Response rates were similar for both arms in both trials: 27% for tamoxifen versus 37% for oophorectomy, and 24% versus 21%, respectively. However, both trials had small numbers of patients—122 in the British study, and 53 in the Mayo Clinic study, which was closed early because of poor accrual. Thus, although there does not appear to be any difference between these two studies, there may have been insufficient statistical power to detect a difference.

There have been varying reports about the likelihood of response to ovarian ablation after use of tamoxifen. Pritchard and colleagues[137] treated 42 evaluable premenopausal women with tamoxifen, 40 mg/d. Patients who failed to respond or subsequently progressed on therapy were treated with ovarian ablation with radiation or surgery. Twenty-five patients did not respond to tamoxifen; 13 underwent ovarian ablation with no observed responses. At the time of publication, 9 patients progressed after an initial response to tamoxifen, and 8 received ovarian ablation. Five patients had a partial response; 1 had therapy too close to the time of publication to evaluate. The authors concluded that initial response to tamoxifen predicted a high likelihood of response to subsequent ovarian ablation. Planting and colleagues[140] reported additional responses after oophorectomy in 4 of 8 women who had previously responded to tamoxifen. One patient with stable disease responded to ovarian ablation, and 2 of 12 patients who had not responded to tamoxifen responded to oophorectomy. The Southwest Oncology Group (SWOG) found similar results.[144] Premenopausal patients treated with tamoxifen who subsequently developed progressive disease or did not respond were then treated with oophorectomy. All patients continued on tamoxifen therapy. Of 14 patients who initially responded to tamoxifen, none responded to the addition of oophorectomy. For the 22 patients who failed with tamoxifen therapy, 5 subsequently responded to oophorectomy. It is possible that tamoxifen may not induce a total endocrine blockade, demonstrated by the fact that many women continue to menstruate during tamoxifen therapy. These results suggest that some premenopausal women may respond to oophorectomy after progression on tamoxifen therapy. However, data compiled by Sunderland and Osborne[55] suggest that the likelihood of response in patients with stable or progressive disease on tamoxifen is 13% to 19% (Table 22.1-6). With the availability of additional antihormonal agents, this small degree of benefit probably does not warrant the risks of an ovarian ablation procedure.

Other Antiestrogens

Toremifene is a triphenylethylene derivative of tamoxifen, developed in Finland as a more potent and specific blocker of the ER.[145] Initial reports indicated that toremifene had fewer estrogen-agonist properties than tamoxifen and might therefore provide increased efficacy and fewer side effects in the treatment of breast cancer.[146] Phase II trials of this agent at doses of 60 mg or more demonstrated response rates of 48% to 68%.[147] Several phase III trials were conducted in a direct comparison of this drug to tamoxifen. Stenbygaard and colleagues[145] treated 66 postmenopausal women with measurable or evaluable metastatic disease; tumors were required to be ER-positive or of unknown receptor status. Women were randomly assigned to receive either tamoxifen, 40 mg PO daily, or toremifene, 120 mg PO BID, in a double-blind fashion. Patients remained on therapy until progressive disease was documented and were then crossed over to the other treatment. Sixty-two women were evaluable. About half had received prior treatment for metastatic disease; 18 had received tamoxifen in the adjuvant setting. Front-line response rates were 29% for toremifene and 42% for tamoxifen. A higher complete response rate was seen with tamoxifen (16%) than with toremifene (3%). At the time of publi-

cation, only 44 women had crossed over to the other therapy. Twenty-one were initially treated with toremifene and 23 initially with tamoxifen. No responses were seen in this phase of the study. Overall survival for the two groups was not statistically different. This study suggests that response rates may be higher with tamoxifen, but survival is not affected. More importantly, this study suggests cross-resistance between these two agents.

A larger phase II trial of toremifene to further examine this question was performed by Vogel and colleagues[148] in 102 perimenopausal or postmenopausal women with measurable ER- and PR-positive or unknown metastatic breast cancer. All patients had failed to respond or had progressed through prior tamoxifen therapy. Patients were treated with 200 mg toremifene daily. Only a 5% response rate was observed. One response was seen in a patient who had failed to respond to tamoxifen; four responses were seen in patients who had initially responded to tamoxifen but who had later progressed. Toxicity was generally mild and similar to side effects reported for tamoxifen, including hot flashes, nausea, and vaginal discharge. No liver function test elevation was observed; no thromboembolic events were noted. Although eight cases of ophthalmologic changes were reported, only one (dry eyes) was judged to be drug related. These data also support the likelihood that there is clinical cross-resistance between these two agents.

No large trials comparing the frontline efficacy of tamoxifen to toremifene have been published, although at least five studies have completed accrual.[149] Both agents appear to be effective and well tolerated. However, many patients receive tamoxifen as long-term adjuvant therapy, and toremifene is unlikely to be effective at time of relapse. Thus, a clear niche for this agent does not exist.

Other antiestrogens in clinical development include droloxifene (3-OH-tamoxifen), ICI 182,780, ZK119010,

TABLE 22.1-6
Response to Oophorectomy After Tamoxifen

Response to Tamoxifen	Patients	Response to Ovarian Ablation			
		CR, PR	SD	PD	NA
CR, PR	54	19 (35%)	8 (15%)	26 (48%)	1 (2%)
SD	27	5 (19%)	7 (26%)	11 (41%)	4 (15%)
PD	71	9 (13%)	6 (8%)	55 (77%)	1 (1%)

CR, complete response; PR, partial response; PD, progressive disease; SD, stable disease; NA, nonassessable.

(Sunderland MC, Osborne CK. J Clin Oncol 1991;9:591; data compiled from references 139–142 and 144, and from Pearson OH, Manni A, Arafah BM. Antiestrogen treatment of breast cancer: an overview. Cancer Res 1982;42[Suppl]:3424S; Kalham AM, Thompson T, Vogel CL. Response to oophorectomy after tamoxifen failure in a premenopausal patient. Cancer Treat Rep 1982;66:1867) pyrrolidino-4-iodotamoxifen, and 4-iodotamoxifen.[150–156] All have been developed as pure antiestrogens, increasing the specificity of response. Drolixifene has a greater affinity for the ER in vitro than tamoxifen, and has been shown in rat systems to have fewer estrogen-agonist properties.[150] This agent has been in clinical trial in Europe, and phase III studies comparing it to tamoxifen are planned. ICI 182,780 is reported to be a pure antiestrogen, with no uterotropic effect documented in the laboratory.[151] This compound inhibits the growth of ER-positive breast cancer cells to a greater extent than tamoxifen.[151] ICI 182,780 can inhibit the growth of a subline of MCF-7 breast cancer cells that are resistant to tamoxifen, suggesting that its pure antiestrogen effect is maintained and might produce responses in patients who have progressed through tamoxifen.[152,153] This compound has been tested for short-term administration in postmenopausal women with breast cancer diagnosed by core biopsy.[154] Fifty-six women were randomly assigned to receive daily intramuscular injections of ICI 182,780 at two dose levels (6 or 18 mg) for 1 week before surgery or to a control group. The drug was well tolerated. Treatment with ICI 182,780 caused a decrease in ER and PR expression in tumors that were initially ER- and PR-positive; a decrease in Ki67-labeling index was also observed. These findings suggest biologic activity as an estrogen antagonist. Phase II studies with this agent are in progress. All of these agents remain under investiga-

tion and are not approved agents for the treatment of breast cancer.

Progestational Agents

Progestins have been shown to induce response rates in metastatic breast cancer, although their mechanism of action is unknown.[23,24] Suggested mechanisms of action have included interaction with the PR with direct growth inhibition, or indirect action by decreasing ER content through negative inhibition.[24] These agents also bind to androgen and glucocorticoid receptors, with possible secondary mechanisms.[24] Medroxyprogesterone acetate (MPA) and megestrol acetate are the best known agents.

MPA is widely used outside the United States. It has been most commonly studied as an intramuscular injection. Doses of 500 to 1000 mg/d IM for 30 days followed by a maintenance dose given weekly have resulted in response rates of 40%.[157] Pannuti and colleagues[158] demonstrated no difference in response or survival between doses of 1500 mg/d compared with 500 mg/d, suggesting no advantage for dose escalation. Although it has been given orally, it has poor bioavailability at low doses.[24] More consistent blood levels are obtained with intramuscular injections, which result in more patient discomfort and side effects such as gluteal abscesses.[157] Ten to 15% of patients on MPA develop cushingoid features.[157] Weight

TABLE 22.1-7
Toxicities Associated With Progestin Treatment in Metastatic Breast Cancer Patients

		Frequency			
		Megestrol Acetate		Medroxyprogesterone Acetate	
Sympton	References	Standard Dose	High Dose	Standard Dose	High Dose
Vaginal bleeding	158, 160, 163, 164, 171	2%–5%	8%	0%	6%
Hot flashes	159		Occasional		
Cushingoid facies	158		Rare	4%	11%
Fluid retention	163, 171	2%–9%	29%–34%		
Hypertension	159, 169, 170	Rare	19%–61%	Rare	
Diabetes	159, 169, 170	Rare	8%–13%	Rare	
Weight gain (≥2 kg)	159, 163–165, 169, 170	14.5%–36%	71%–81%	75%	75%
Increased appetite	164, 169, 170	Frequent	56%	Frequent	Frequent
Nausea, vomiting	159		Occasional		
Tremor	158			2%	19%
Depression	159		Occasional		
Rash	159		Rare		
Abscesses	158			2%	15%
Infiltration	158			9%	6%
Thrombophlebitis	158, 164, 165, 169, 170	4%	4%	0%	0%
Deep venous thrombosis	158, 171	1.2%	2.5%	2%	19%
Pulmonary embolus	172	0.8%	4%		
Congestive heart failure	164, 169, 170	—	2%–4%		

gain, edema, uterine bleeding, hot flashes, and thromboembolic phenomena have been observed[159] (Table 22.1-7).

For this reason, megestrol acetate is the most commonly used progestin in the United States. Its mechanism of action is unknown, although a variety of hypotheses have been proposed. Megestrol acetate may interfere with binding to the ER, may accelerate estrogen catabolism, or may interfere with aromatization of androgens to estrogens.[157] It may also have direct actions through the progesterone, androgen, and glucocorticoid receptors.[160] When administered orally to women with metastatic breast cancer, megestrol acetate caused increased prolactin and insulin levels as well as decreased levels of LH, FSH, estradiol and sex hormone–binding globulin, and basal glucose levels.[160] No differences in growth hormone or thyroid-stimulating hormone were observed.[160] These results indicate some sort of suppression of the pituitary–adrenal axis. Other authors have demonstrated a direct cytotoxic effect on breast cancer cells.[159] Many trials have documented its effectiveness with response rates of 25% to 45% in pretreated patients.[159-164] Toxicities include weight gain, vaginal bleeding, fluid retention, and thromboembolic events. Weight gain is perhaps the most distressing side effect for patients. Whereas some studies have reported that weight gain of over 10% of body weight occurs in only 10% to 15%, others have reported a median weight gain of 2 kg in 70% of treated patients.[159,160,162,163]

Megestrol acetate is as effective as tamoxifen as a first-line agent but is usually used in patients who have failed on tamoxifen therapy for several reasons. First, it has more side effects than tamoxifen. Second, it is usually given on a four-times-daily basis, which is less convenient than the daily dosing of tamoxifen. Recent studies have demonstrated the efficacy of daily dosing of megestrol acetate. Pronzato and colleagues[165] tested a new megestrol acetate formulation of a 160-mg tablet. Sixty-nine patients were entered on the study and treated with the new formulation. Sixty-five patients had received previous therapy for metastatic disease, and 5 had previously received megestrol acetate. The response rate was 21.5%, with a median duration of response of 7 months. Thirty-six percent experienced a median weight gain of 2 kg. Three patients experienced lower extremity thrombophlebitis. These results are comparable to other hormonal agents used in pretreated patients. Gaver and colleagues[166] also tested new investigational preparations of megestrol acetate. The 160-mg tablet was shown to have the same absorption rate constant and the same extent of absorption as the 40-mg tablet administered four times a day. Half-lives and bioavailability were similar. The second preparation was a micronized form of megestrol acetate administered as a 160-mg tablet. This preparation has a higher absorption rate constant, a greater extent of absorption, and increased bioavailability. It has been marketed in the United States only as an oral suspension approved for treatment of cachexia. It is not available for treatment of breast cancer.

Carpenter and Peterson[167] used standard 40-mg tablets and administered 160 mg as a once-daily dose in 20 patients. No difference in toxicity profile was reported, and the partial response rate of 30% is similar to results reported in other studies with pretreated patients. It appears that once-a-day dosing is safe and effective. Daily drug administration may increase compliance and thus improve efficacy. The only inconvenience is the need to take four pills until the newer formulations are available in the United States.

DOSE INTENSITY CONSIDERATIONS. The standard dose of megestrol acetate in the United States is 40 mg PO four times a day. Alexieva-Figusch and colleagues[168] recommended 180 mg/d as the optimal dose of megestrol acetate based on serial hormonal assays. In their work, lower doses did not completely suppress the pituitary–adrenal axis, and higher doses resulted in higher levels of circulating insulin with concern about hypoglycemia. Despite these findings, other investigators have found evidence of a dose-response relation (Table 22.1-8). Parnes and colleagues[164,169,170] administered megestrol acetate in a phase I trial to 57 patients with metastatic breast cancer. The initial starting dose was 480 mg/d, and subsequent elevations included 800, 1280, and 1600 mg/d. Because of expense of therapy and number of tablets required at this level, no further escalations were performed. Three patients were treated at each dose level in a classic phase I design, and a total of 48 patients were treated at the 1600-mg/d dose to further evaluate toxicity. Almost all patients (98%) had received prior therapy, and 88% had progressed during a prior hormonal therapy. Thirty-seven patients had measurable disease. Among these patients, the overall response rate was 33%, with a median duration of response of 8.25 months. Responses were seen at all dose levels, and the number of patients treated at each dose level was too small to allow a statistical comparison of a dose-response effect. The primary side effects included a median weight gain of 5.2 kg, ranging from a loss of 1 kg to a gain of 44 kg (81% of patients), increases in blood pressure of greater than 10 mmHg (17%), and edema (34%). Two

TABLE 22.1-8

Trials Evaluating Response to High-Dose Megestrol Acetate

Study	Dose (mg)	Patients	Response Rate (%)
Piedmont Oncology Association[171]	160	81	10
	800	80	27
University of Maryland[164,169,170]	480	3	
	800	3	32 (overall)
	1280	3	
	1600	48	
Cancer and Leukemia Group B[172]	160	117	24
	800	116	24
	1600	108	28

patients developed congestive heart failure, and 2 patients developed thrombotic complications. The authors concluded that high-dose therapy appeared to be safe and effective.

Based on this small study, which suggested benefit, a randomized comparison of two dose levels of megestrol acetate was performed. The POA compared 160 mg/d with 800 mg/d in 170 evaluable women with metastatic breast cancer.[171] All had received prior hormonal therapy, primarily tamoxifen, either as adjuvant therapy (45 patients) or treatment for metastatic disease. On the standard-dose arm, a 10% response rate was observed compared with 28% on the high-dose arm. Patients with Eastern Cooperative Oncology Group (ECOG) performance status 3 were all treated on the standard-dose arm, and the standard-dose arm contained more patients who were ER-positive but PR-negative. Time to treatment failure was 3.2 months for patients treated with standard doses and 8 months for patients treated with the high-dose regimen. Survival was also significantly different, 16.5 months on the standard-dose arm and 22.4 months on the high-dose arm. Patients on the high-dose arm experienced more edema (31% versus 9%). In addition, 15% of patients on the high-dose arm had the dose of megestrol acetate modified because of weight gain. Deep venous thrombosis was observed in 2 patients on the high-dose arm and 1 on the standard-dose arm. One patient on the high-dose arm suffered a fatal myocardial infarction, and one had a thrombotic stroke. No significant differences in the occurrence of vaginal bleeding were reported. The response on the standard-dose arm in this trial is lower than that reported by other investigators, as is the response duration for a second-line agent.[23,159–163,165] The side effect of weight gain was significant and particularly striking in that 15% of patients had dose modifications made on the basis of this side effect. The authors report that this side effect was distressing to patients, although no formal quality-of-life study was performed. Thus, while high-dose megestrol acetate therapy may improve response rates, this benefit must be weighed against the increased toxicity and decreased quality of life.

The findings of improved response rates with higher doses of megestrol acetate were not replicated by the Cancer and Leukemia Group B (CALGB) in a larger study.[172] This trial randomly assigned 368 women to receive 160, 800, or 1600 mg/d of megestrol acetate. At 26 months of follow-up, no difference in response rate was observed for the three arms (24%, 24%, and 28%, respectively). Median duration of response was 13.9, 14.2, and 7.8 months, respectively. Again, significant weight gain was observed. Vascular complications were observed more frequently at higher doses: one pulmonary embolus at 160 mg, one arterial thrombosis and one pulmonary embolus at 800 mg, and two deep venous thromboses, one arterial thrombosis, and four pulmonary emboli at 1600 mg. These data therefore do not support the use of high-dose megestrol acetate.

The CALGB also measured quality of life in this trial.[173] One hundred thirty-one patients completed the compan-

ion study. With increasing dose, weight gain, fatigue, and bloating increased significantly based on subjective patient evaluations. Within 1 month of beginning the drug therapy, a significant difference in quality of life existed between the low-dose and highest-dose arms. Within 3 months, a significant difference existed between all three arms. Measures such as the Rand Functional Limitations score, the Rand Global Psychologic Distress scale, and Functional Living Index—Cancer indicated decreased level of functioning and increased distress within 1 to 3 months. Interestingly enough, the Body Image subscale showed no differences and thus did not account for the decreased level of functioning perceived by the patients. Most significant were complaints of fatigue and bloating. Because studies have shown no survival difference between the three doses, it appears that quality of life is worsened by higher doses of megestrol acetate, so 160 mg/d should be considered standard dose.

Antiprogestins

RU 486 (mifepristone) is a synthetic antiprogestin and antiglucocorticoid. It binds to both PR and to the glucocorticoid receptor more potently than natural ligands.[174] In the laboratory, RU 486 has an antiproliferative effect on PR-positive breast cancer cell lines.[174] Two clinical trials using RU 486 for the treatment of breast cancer have been described. Romieu and colleagues[175] administered 200 mg/d of RU 486 to 22 postmenopausal or oophorectomized women with metastatic breast cancer. RU 486 was administered in divided doses—100 mg in the morning, 50 mg at midday, and 50 mg in the evening. Most women had been heavily pretreated (7 with chemotherapy; 9 with two or more hormonal therapies); results were confounded by the fact that most women received concomitant tamoxifen therapy. The drug was in general well tolerated: nausea, hot flashes, and dizziness were reported by 4 patients (18%). An increase in baseline cortisol levels was noted from 236 to 417 ng/mL. This increase was evident during the first 5 days of therapy and remained constant for the 3-month duration of the trial. Only morning values were affected. No significant changes in adrenocorticotropic hormone (ACTH) levels, heart rate, or blood pressure were noted. Four of 22 patients (18%) had partial responses. Two mixed responses were reported. Only 8 patients had known receptor status.

A second study, by Klijn and colleagues[176] administered RU 486 at doses of 200 to 400 mg/d to 11 postmenopausal women with metastatic breast cancer. All patients had previously received tamoxifen. One of 11 patients had an objective partial response of 5 months duration. Seven patients had known receptor status: 5 patients were ER-positive but PR-negative and 2 had tumors that were strongly ER- and PR-positive. This study confirmed an increase in cortisol levels and also documented an increase in ACTH levels. The drug was well tolerated. Although these studies suggest RU 486 may be an active agent in the treatment of breast cancer, further studies have been slowed by the political implications of its use as an abortifacient in Europe.

Onapristone is a second antiprogestin that inhibits the growth of breast cancer cells in vitro.[177] It has shown activity in early unpublished trials and is under investigation in active clinical trials in the United States. Antiprogestins remain investigational agents at present.

Aromatase Inhibitors

AMINOGLUTETHIMIDE. Aminoglutethimide is an aromatase inhibitor that blocks the peripheral conversion of androstenedione to estrone[24] (Fig. 22.1-5). This process occurs in multiple tissues in the body, including the ovary (the primary site in premenopausal women) and extraovarian sites (important in postmenopausal women), such as adipose tissue, skin, muscle, and liver.[24] In the adrenal gland itself, it blocks the conversion of cholesterol to pregnenolene, the direct precursor of androstenedione.[178] It is not a pure aromatase inhibitor, however, and also blocks 20,22-desmolase, 21-hydroxylase, and 11-β-hydroxylase.[179] To prevent stimulatory feedback to the hypothalamic–pituitary axis that increases ACTH and overcomes this blockade, aminoglutethimide must be administered with hydrocortisone[24] (Fig. 22.1-6). This drug was developed as an alternative to adrenalectomy, and randomized clinical trials have demonstrated similar response rates.[180] Numerous studies have documented the efficacy of aminoglutethimide in the treatment of metastatic breast cancer. Brufman and Biran[178] published one such study, in which 120 postmenopausal patients, 98% of whom had received tamoxifen, were treated with an initial dose of 250 mg/d, with escalation to 250 mg PO four times a day. Hydrocortisone was administered at 100 mg/d and was subsequently decreased to 10 mg PO four times a day. A response rate of 34% was observed, with a median duration of response of 9 months for complete responders and 10 months for partial responders. Because ER or PR positivity was not a requirement for study entry, response was reported separately in this subset of patients. ER-positive patients had a response rate of 57%, whereas ER-negative patients had a response rate of 12%. Side effects and toxicity were significant in this trial. Forty percent complained of dizziness, and 35% experienced a skin rash. Seventeen percent of patients could not have the dose of aminoglutethimide escalated because of toxicity. Four patients required discontinuation of therapy because of severe side effects, including reversible agranulocytosis, skin rash, unspecified electrolyte disturbances, and ataxia. Thus, although aminoglutethimide produces meaningful response rates in patients with metastatic hormone receptor positive disease, it is associated with significant side effects that can interfere with patient compliance and decrease quality of life (Table 22.1-9).

Overall, the response rate for this drug is between 20% and 40%, with a median duration of response of 11 months, similar to other endocrine therapies.[178,179,181] In examining a series of studies, toxicities include lethargy in 36% of patients, rash in 22%, nausea and vomiting in 14%, dizziness in 16%, and ataxia in 9%.[181] The rash may remit spontaneously or may respond to drug discontinuation, followed by rechallenge at gradually increasing doses with an initially higher dose of steroids.

The necessity of hydrocortisone use with aminoglutethimide has been debated. Several studies used doses of 250 mg/d of aminoglutethimide without hydrocortisone and observed lower response rates of 16% to 19%.[24] An Italian study[182] showed similar response rates with and without hydrocortisone if 500 mg/d aminoglutethimide was used (44% compared with 41%, respectively). The need for hydrocortisone is therefore likely to depend on the dose of aminoglutethimide used, and one must consider the trade-off between dose-related side effects with aminoglutethimide and the inconvenience of two-drug administration for one purpose.

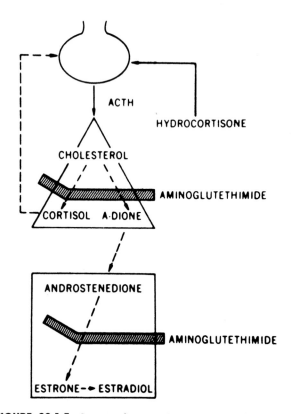

FIGURE 22.1-5 Sources of estrogen in postmenopausal women and possible sites of aminoglutethimide action. ACTH, adrenocorticotropic hormone; A-DIONE, androstenedione. (Santen RJ, Samojlik E, Worgul TJ, et al. Aminoglutethimide. In: Santen RJ, Henderson IC, eds. A comprehensive guide to the therapeutic use of aminoglutethimide. Basel, Karger, 1982:101)

DOSE-INTENSITY CONSIDERATIONS. A dose-response relation has been investigated for aminoglutethimide. Unlike for tamoxifen and the progestins, investigators sought the lowest effective dose in an attempt to decrease side effects. Daily doses of 125 mg can block aromatase activity; blockade is maximized at doses of 250 to 500 mg/d.[24] Individual

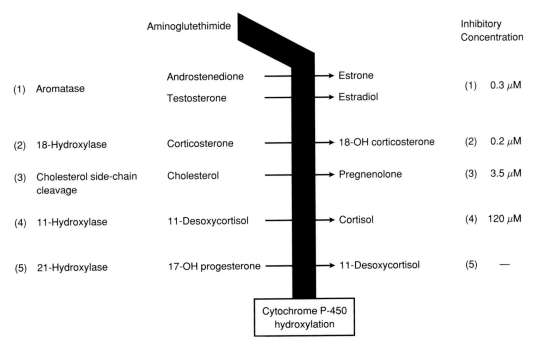

FIGURE 22.1-6 Enzymatic reactions blocked by aminoglutethimide and inhibitory concentrations of aminoglutethimide necessary to block each reaction. (Santen RJ, Samojlik E, Worgul TJ, et al. Aminoglutethimide. In: Santen RJ, Henderson IC, eds. A comprehensive guide to the therapeutic use of aminoglutethimide. Basel, Karger, 1982:101)

TABLE 22.1-9
Toxicities Associated With Administration of Aminoglutethimide to Postmenopausal Women With Metastatic Breast Cancer

Symptoms and Signs	Frequency (%)	References
Lethargy	9	23, 25, 181
Dizziness	15–20	23, 180, 181
Ataxia	5–10	178, 180
Depression	1	181
Confusion	Rare	181, 182
Cushingoid symptoms	2.8	181
Hypotension	<1	181
Edema	<1	181
Inappropriate antidiuretic hormone secretion	Rare	181
Nausea, vomiting	10–14	23, 181
Weight gain or loss	<1	181
Rash	10–35	23, 25, 178, 180–182
Stevens-Johnson syndrome	Rare	181
Thrombocytopenia	Rare	181
Leukopenia	<1	23
Elevated thyroid-stimulating hormone	10	25

nonrandomized studies have examined response rates in metastatic breast cancer patients at doses of 250, 375, 500, and 1000 mg/d.[24] The response rates have ranged from 13% to 45% without a clear dose-response relation.[24] Side effects such as rash occurred with equal frequency at all dose levels. The sedating properties of the drug were somewhat less frequent at lower doses.[24] Thus, doses of greater than 250 mg/d are unlikely to have additional benefit, and like the other agents mentioned earlier, are more likely to add additional toxicity.

OTHER AROMATASE INHIBITORS. Aminogluthethimide, although an effective agent for the treatment of breast cancer, is not a pure aromatase inhibitor and thus frequently requires concomitant administration of hydrocortisone. Taking two drugs daily with the possibility of additional side effects is less attractive to patients. Thus, efforts have been directed at developing more specific aromatase inhibitors. Several classes have been developed, including the steroids and the imidazoles.

The best-known member of the steroidal inhibitors is formestane. Formestane, 4-hydroxy-androstenedione, provides competitive inhibition of aromatase.[183] Some work indicates that this drug is oxygenated by aromatase to produce an activated intermediate that then binds covalently to the active site of aromatase, leading to inhibition of the enzyme.[183] It is 30 to 60 times more potent than aminoglutethimide[183] (Table 22.1-10). Several studies indicate that this drug inhibits circulating estradiol levels in postmenopausal women by 60%, but it has little effect on estradiol level suppression in premenopausal women.[183]

TABLE 22.1-10
Relative Potencies of Aromatase Inhibitors

Aromatase Inhibitor	Potency*	Reference
Aminoglutethimide	1	—
Formestane	30–60	183
Testololactone	0.1	179
Atamestane	7	79
6-Methylene-androstadienedione	20	179
Fadrazole	100–3000	179, 184
CGS 20267	900	179

* 1 = 600 nM/L.
(Modified from Hoffken K. Experience with aromatase inhibitors in the treatment of advanced breast cancer. Cancer Treat Rev 1993;19[Suppl B]:38)

These results suggest that negative feedback to the ovary by FSH and LH can overcome the efficacy of this drug. Formestane does not alter levels of testosterone, androstenedione, 5-α-dihydrotestosterone, sex hormone–binding globulins, or thyroxine.[183] The drug is administered intramuscularly every 2 weeks.

The overall response rate in phase II trials, usually in patients who had received one to three previous hormonal therapies, was 7% to 39%.[183] Only five premenopausal women have been tested and none responded. No suppression of estradiol levels was observed.

Few side effects are associated with formestane.[183] The most common are injection site reactions (13%). Less common are hot flashes, lethargy, rash, dizziness, all reported at an incidence of less than 7%. No androgenic effects have been observed. Overall, less than 5% of patients treated on clinical trials have discontinued the drug therapy because of side effects.

Other members of the steroid class include testololactone, atamestane (1-methyl-androstenedione), and MAD (6-methylene-androstadienedione). Similar response rates with fewer side effects than aminoglutethimide have been observed.[179]

The imidazole class of drugs was targeted for breast cancer development by observations made in patients taking ketoconazole for fungal infections.[179] Ketoconazole inhibits cleavage of cholesterol and thus inhibits adrenal function. Derivatives have been synthesized that inhibit aromatase and that have shown activity in breast cancer. Fadrazole (CGS 16949A) is a nonsteroidal azole imidazole that is 100 to 3000 times more potent in aromatase inhibition than aminoglutethimide[179,184] (see Table 22.1-10). Response rates have been reported to be between 20% and 30% in pretreated patients.[184,185] Toxicity was mild and consisted of hot flashes, nausea, fatigue, and anorexia.[184] A newer agent, CGS 20267, has been developed with a more favorable pharmacokinetic profile that will permit daily dosing.[179] A third agent in current clinical trials is exemus-

tane. This drug also has demonstrated activity in unpublished trials.

Luteinizing Hormone–Releasing Hormone Agonists

Luteinizing hormone–releasing hormone agonists are medications that suppress ovarian production of estradiol by desensitizing pituitary LHRH receptors.[24] The administration of these agents initially stimulates gonadotropin production but subsequently blocks release of FSH and LH with a net decrease of ovarian production of both estrogen and progesterone.[24] A complete endocrine blockade is produced, with cessation of menses in all treated women. These drugs have optimal activity in premenopausal women but little efficacy in postmenopausal women, in whom ovarian estrogen production is minimal.[186] In addition, LHRH receptors have been demonstrated on the surface of human breast cancer cell lines and on human breast tumors, suggesting an additional mechanism for the observed antitumor effect.[187,188]

Goserelin is perhaps the best-known agent in this class of drugs. It is 10 amino acids long and has a D-serine substituted for an L-glycine at position 6 that distinguishes it from natural LHRH.[189] It is 50 to 100 times more potent than the natural hormone.[190] It comes in pellet form and is administered by subcutaneous implantation on a monthly basis. It initially causes increased estrogen levels, but subsequently results in suppression due to down-regulation of LHRH receptors in the pituitary.[191] Brambilla and colleagues[191] administered this drug to 23 premenopausal patients with ER-positive metastatic breast cancer. Seventy-three percent had received prior chemotherapy for advanced disease. A 32% response rate was observed. Toxicity included hot flashes in 82% as a result of medical menopause. Forty-five percent had injection site reactions. Twelve patients experienced an average weight gain of 3 kg. The drug was shown to reduce 17-β-estradiol levels to postmenopausal values. As expected, FSH and LH values were affected to a lesser extent.

A larger trial was conducted in 118 evaluable premenopausal women previously untreated for metastatic disease by the German Zoladex Trial Group.[192] A 45% response rate was observed with documented suppression of serum levels of estradiol, LH, and FSH. Toxicity was limited to injection site reactions and hot flashes (63%).

A study conducted by ECOG evaluated the activity of goserelin in postmenopausal ER-positive patients.[189] Some reports had documented effectiveness of LHRH agonists in postmenopausal patients, suggesting the possibility of alternative mechanisms of action.[186,189] Because goserelin decreases FSH and LH secretion, it was suggested that, in postmenopausal women, this reduction results in decreased androgen production by the ovaries and thus decreased conversion to estrone in peripheral tissues. In addition, as mentioned, the presence of cell surface receptors for LHRH might also account for activity.[187,188] To investigate these possibilities, ECOG initiated a trial of goserelin in postmenopausal patients.[189] Fifty-two evaluable patients were entered. Thirty-six had ER-positive tumors, and in this group, the response rate was 11% with durations of response of 2 to 6 months. None of the ER-negative patients had an objective response to therapy. Thus, activity of this agent in postmenopausal women appears to be low. Additional studies have shown that responses are also low in ER-negative patients.[192]

Leuprolide (D-leu6-desgly 10-pro9-NHEt-LHRH) has been shown to induce tumor regression in DMBA-induced tumors in rats.[193] One published study[193] demonstrated a 44% response rate to this agent in 26 premenopausal women with metastatic breast cancer. Side effects were limited primarily to hot flashes. Its activity profile is similar to that of goserelin.

It is not known whether LHRH agonists effectively replace oophorectomy. Case reports of responses to oophorectomy after progression on LHRH agonists have been reported.[194] Further trials are needed to address this issue.

Androgens

Androgens have also been used in the treatment of metastatic breast cancer. Danazol, one of the most widely used agents, is a synthetic steroid with partial androgen action that blocks pituitary gonadotropin secretion.[195] It has been hypothesized that it may have antiprogestational activity. It has been used in advanced breast cancer with an average response rate of 20%. Side effects include edema and hot flashes.

Virilizing androgens—including testosterone, fluoxymesterone, testolactone, and calusterone—have also been used, with response rates of about 20%.[23] These drugs are less commonly used because of their virilizing side effects. They include hirsutism and deepening of the voice in 60% to 70% of patients and a 20% to 40% incidence of hair loss, acne, and increased libido.[23] Jaundice has also been reported.

Overall, there are many effective endocrine therapies available for the treatment of metastatic breast cancer that have fewer or less undesirable side effects. Androgens are therefore primarily used as a fourth- or fifth-line agent for patients who remain hormone responsive.

Other Agents

The somatostatins are a series of somatostatin-related peptides that act as regulatory hormones in the gut as well as in exocrine and endocrine systems through the body. They also have antiproliferative properties.[196] The best-known peptide is octreotide, which is 45 times more potent than natural somatostatin in inhibition of growth hormone.[197] It preferentially inhibits growth hormone secretion rather than insulin release, making it more attractive for clinical trials.[197] It is given subcutaneously three times a day. The best evidence for its mechanism of action supports a direct interaction with a cell surface receptor, as evidenced by its in vitro activity.[196,197] Potential antipituitary effects are less well established.

A dose-escalation study of octreotide was conducted in patients with metastatic breast cancer.[198] Twenty patients were entered on study; all had failed prior therapy. At a dose of 2000 μg SQ every 8 hours, no significant toxicities were observed. One patient had stable disease for 24 weeks; a second had a partial response in liver but stable bony disease. Because of dose and volume considerations, phase II studies at this dose level are underway.

Additional work has suggested that octreotid may be best used in combination. Hung and Pollak[199] found that tamoxifen decreased serum levels of IGF-1 in rats to 78% of control levels. An isolated injection of somatostatin had no effect, but administration of this drug to animals pretreated with tamoxifen decreased serum levels to 54% of control values. Combined trials of somatostatin and tamoxifen are planned.

A number of investigators have reported that 20% to 50% of breast cancer tumors contain prolactin receptors, and prolactin has been reported to be mitogenic for breast cancer cell lines.[24] However, studies of bromocriptine and other dopaminergic drugs have shown these agents to have little effect in the treatment of breast cancer. Manni and associates[200] have hypothesized that these agents are ineffective because they cannot overcome the lactogenic effects of growth hormone. Therefore, these investigators treated 10 pretreated postmenopausal women with metastatic breast cancer with a combination of octreotide and bromocriptine. The drugs were given at twice-daily doses of 100 to 200 μg SQ and 2.5 mg PO, respectively. The investigators demonstrated decreased growth hormone release with this regimen, although the degree of suppression showed significant interindividual variation. No clinical responses were seen. The researchers concluded that this combination warrants testing in less heavily pretreated patients. It is also possible that optimal use of these agents involves appropriate sequencing and the use of biologic endpoints to accurately guide dosing.

OPTIMAL SEQUENCING OF HORMONAL AGENTS

Studies have also investigated the optimal sequence of hormonal agents. Tamoxifen became the most widely used first-line agent after Ingle and colleagues[201] reported equivalent efficacy with DES but significantly decreased toxicity with tamoxifen in a prospective randomized trial. While tamoxifen has been the most commonly used initial hormonal therapy, several studies have examined response rates in previously untreated patients with a variety of endocrine agents (Table 22.1-11).

The POA randomly assigned 124 women with metastatic breast cancer to treatment with tamoxifen, 10 mg PO twice a day, or with megestrol acetate, 40 mg PO four times a day.[202] Response rates on each arm were similar (31% and 29%, respectively). At the time of publication, a survival advantage for tamoxifen was projected, but longer follow-up was needed to validate this assertion. A similar study was reported by Ettinger and colleagues.[203] Response rates were similar between the two treatment arms. Morgan[204] also reported response rates of 31% versus

TABLE 22.1-11
Trials Comparing the Efficacy of Various Hormonal Agents

Investigators	Evaluable Patients	Therapy	Response Rate (%)	P Value
Ingle et al[201]	74	Diethylstilbestrol vs	41	
	69	tamoxifen	33	.37
POA[202]	63	Megestrol acetate vs	29	
	61	tamoxifen	31	NS
Ettinger et al[203]	91	Megestrol acetate vs	35	
	99	tamoxifen	42	NS
Morgan[204]	46	Megestrol acetate vs	31	
	48	tamoxifen	36	NS
SAKK[205]	55	MPA vs	50	
	64	tamoxifen	30	.023
POA[206]	82	MPA vs	34	
	84	tamoxifen	17	.01
Smith et al[207]	57	Aminoglutethimide vs	30	
	60	tamoxifen	30	NS
ECOG[208]	108	Aminoglutethimide vs	45	
	108	tamoxifen	27	Not done

POA, Piedmont Oncology Association; NS, not significant; SAKK, Swiss Group for Clinical Cancer Research; MPA, medroxyprogesterone acetate; ECOG, Eastern Cooperative Oncology Group.

36% for tamoxifen, with no difference in duration of response.

The Swiss Group for Clinical Cancer Research (SAKK) randomly assigned 119 evaluable postmenopausal women with metastatic breast cancer to receive either tamoxifen, 20 mg/d, or MPA, 500 mg/wk, intramuscularly after a loading period of intramuscular administration at the dose of 1 g/d Monday through Friday for a 28-day period.[205] No patient had received prior hormonal therapy, although 23 had received chemotherapy for metastatic disease. Second-line therapy was defined by the protocol. Patients with progression after tamoxifen were randomly assigned to receive either MPA or aminoglutethimide; patients with progression after MPA were assigned to receive either tamoxifen or aminoglutethimide. Response rates were 50% with MPA compared with 30% for tamoxifen. The POA randomly assigned 166 eligible patients with metastatic breast cancer to receive tamoxifen, 20 mg/d, or MPA, 1 g/d PO.[206] A response rate of 17% was observed with tamoxifen therapy, compared with 34% for MPA. However, no difference in time to treatment failure or in survival was seen. Despite the evidence of a higher response rate with MPA in these studies, this agent has not been widely used in the United States. Its toxicities were outlined earlier. The need for a loading dose program and for continued intramuscular injections, as well as its variable bioavailability when given orally, has limited its usefulness, particularly because it is not a curative agent.

Smith and colleagues[207] randomly assigned 117 patients with metastatic breast cancer to receive tamoxifen versus aminoglutethimide as first-line therapy. After disease progression, patients crossed over to the other arm. Response rates were similar on both arms, as was median duration of response. Toxicity was greater in patients receiving aminoglutethimide, with lethargy, drowsiness, and rash as the most commonly reported side effects. Seven patients on aminoglutethimide therapy stopped treatment because of toxicity. No patient on the tamoxifen arm stopped treatment. A larger trial performed by ECOG randomly assigned 216 evaluable postmenopausal women to receive aminoglutethimide or tamoxifen.[208] Overall, no significant differences in response rates or survival were reported.

Thus, in general, all hormonal therapies have about the same response rates when used in patients previously untreated for metastatic disease. However, toxicity profiles differ, and tamoxifen has fewer side effects than the other agents mentioned in this chapter. Because the goal of treatment of metastatic disease remains effective palliation with minimal toxicity, tamoxifen remains the first-line agent of choice.

HORMONE-INDUCED TUMOR FLARE

Hormone-induced tumor flare is a well-described phenomenon in the literature.[209-213] It is characterized by bone pain, diffuse increase in uptake on bone scan, and increased size and number of metastatic skin nodules with erythema.[209-213] Hypercalcemia has also been associated as part of this syndrome,[210] but it is more commonly observed in patients with skeletal metastases. Symptoms occur 2 to 21 days after hormonal therapy has begun.[210,211] Tumor flare is usually associated with estrogen, tamoxifen, or androgen therapy, with an incidence rate of 1% to 3%[210]

(Table 22.1-12). It has been reported less commonly with the use of progestins and aminoglutethimide.

The mechanism of the flare response was examined by Tormey and colleagues.[212] Flare appears to reflect rapid tumor growth that was present before the initiation of therapy. The researchers found no increase in the rate of growth of these lesions. It is likely that flare represents a reactive process, terminated by achieving therapeutic blood levels of the hormonal agent with subsequent cell death. Alternatively, in skeletal disease, it may represent increased osteoblastic activity with early healing.[213] Coleman and colleagues[213] reported increased osteocalcin and bone-specific alkaline phosphatase levels associated with flare symptoms, with falling levels as symptoms abated.

It is important to recognize tumor flare in order to avoid misinterpreting the patient's signs and symptoms as progressive disease. Therapy should be continued, with supportive measures to control bone pain and hypercalcemia. The symptoms resolve spontaneously within 2 to 3 weeks. The occurrence of tumor flare actually predicts an excellent response to the hormonal therapy, and patients should not be prematurely taken off an effective therapy.

COMBINATION ENDOCRINE THERAPY

In the early development of successful chemotherapy combinations for the treatment of Hodgkin disease, the use of active agents with differing spectra of activity was emphasized. Many researchers have questioned whether using hormonal agents with different mechanisms of action in combination could improve response rates and improve survival. A number of studies addressing this issue have been published (Table 22.1-13).

Bishop and colleagues[214] enrolled 183 patients with stage III or IV disease to receive tamoxifen, 20 mg/d, or tamoxifen with danazol, 200 mg/d. The study was randomized and double-blind. The combination-therapy arm yielded a 27% response rate compared with a 24% response rate on the tamoxifen-alone arm. No significant differences were seen in time to progression (6.4 and 6.2 months, respectively) or in survival (22.6 and 23.5 months, respectively). No difference in toxicity was observed between the two arms. Only 3% of patients on the danazol arm developed hirsutism, a lower percentage than usually

reported. Thus, combination therapy did not offer any advantage over monotherapy.

The North Central Cancer Treatment Group (NCCTG) examined the value of combination therapy with tamoxifen and fluoxymesterone compared with tamoxifen alone in 238 eligible postmenopausal, predominantly ER-positive patients who had received no previous hormonal therapy for metastatic disease.[215] Patients may have received up to one prior chemotherapeutic regimen for metastatic disease. Updated findings were recently published.[215] Reported response rates were 54% for combination therapy and 42% for tamoxifen alone, a difference that was not statistically significant. Both regimens provided a median duration of response of 15.6 months. Patients who received combination therapy had a longer time to progression (11.6 months) than patients in the tamoxifen arm (6.5 months), but the difference was not statistically significant. No statistically significant difference in survival was observed. Patients who received fluoxymesterone in addition to tamoxifen had a significant increase in alopecia (2% for tamoxifen; 14% for combination therapy). Although no skin or voice changes were reported on the tamoxifen arm, there was a 24% incidence of skin changes (oiliness, erythema) and a 43% incidence of hoarseness with the addition of fluoxymesterone. These findings are similar to those published by Tormey and coworkers in an NCI study.[125]

Powles and colleagues[216] treated patients with tamoxifen, aminoglutethimide, and danazol versus tamoxifen alone. Hydrocortisone was used in the combined arm not as a primary endocrine therapy but as adjunct therapy for aminoglutethimide. Two hundred twenty-two patients were entered in the study. Patients treated with the combination therapy had a 43% response to therapy compared with a 31% response in the tamoxifen-alone arm. This difference just reached statistical significance ($P = .05$). However, remission duration and survival were equal in both groups. Although both regimens were generally well tolerated, the incidence of side effects was higher in the combination therapy arm because of the additive side effects of each component.

In a follow-up study, Powles and Hardy,[217] in association with other investigators, looked at combination therapy with tamoxifen, aminoglutethimide, danazol, and

TABLE 22.1-12
Incidence of Flare With Hormonal Therapy

Therapy	Incidence (%)	Hypercalcemia (%)	References
Estrogens	1	5	210
Androgens	3	11	210
Tamoxifen	2.2–20	1.2	210–212
Aminogluthethimide	0	—	210
Tamoxifen plus fluoxymesterone	20		212

TABLE 22.1-13
Trials of Combination Endocrine Therapy

Investigators	Therapy	Evaluable Patients	Response Rate (%)	P Value
Bishop et al[214]	Tam + placebo vs	91	24	NS
	Tam + danazol	92	27	
NCCTG[215]	Tam vs	119	42	.07
	Tam + Flu	119	54	
NCI[125]	Tamoxifen vs	52	15	.016
	Tam + Flu	56	38	
Powles et al[216]	Tam vs	111	31	.05
	TAD	111	43	
Hardy et al[217]	POND	74	44	—
DBCG I[218]	Tam vs	46	44	>.2
	Tam + MPA	55	26	
DBCG II[218]	Tam vs	38	42	>.8
	Tam + DES	32	38	
DBCG[219]	Tam vs	91	34	.35
	Tam + AG	75	28	
Smith et al[220]	Tam vs	60	30	NS
	AG vs	57	30	
	TAM + AG	62	28	
Corkery et al[221]	Tam vs	9	33	NS
	Tam + AG	11	36	
Ingle et al[222]	Tam vs	49	43	.54
	Tam + AG	51	49	

Tam, tamoxifen; NS, not significant; NCCTG, North Central Cancer Treatment Group; Flu, fluoxymesterone; NCI, National Cancer Institute; TAD, tamoxifen, aminoglutethimide, and danazol; POND, tamoxifen, aminoglutethimide, danazol, and medroxyprogesterone acetate; DBCG, Danish Breast Cancer Group; MPA, medroxyprogesterone acetate; DES diethylstilbestrol; AG, aminoglutethimide.

MPA. Hydrocortisone was not required, since MPA provided adequate pituitary feedback. Seventy-four patients were treated; 72% had not received previous therapy for metastatic disease. An overall response rate of 43% was observed, with a 14% rate of complete remission. The median duration of response was 19 months, with a median time to progression of 8 months. Overall survival was 27 months. Toxicity was significant; the most frequently reported side effects were nausea, lethargy, constipation, and rash. Forty-one percent of patients required a dose reduction or discontinuation of one or several drugs because of weight gain, hirsutism, voice change, rash, or lethargy.

Mouridsen, Palshof, and Rose[49,218] found no difference between tamoxifen versus tamoxifen plus MPA, or between tamoxifen and tamoxifen plus DES. In addition, the Danish Breast Cancer Group[219] evaluated patients treated with tamoxifen alone versus tamoxifen plus aminoglutethimide and hydrocortisone. No significant difference in response rates, remission duration, and time to treatment failure were seen. Smith and colleagues[220] found no difference in either tamoxifen or aminoglutethimide administered alone versus combination administration.

Similar data were reported by Corkery and colleagues[221] and by Ingle and coworkers.[222]

These studies suggest that although combination therapy may initially induce higher response rates, it offers no survival advantage over sequential single-agent therapy. In one instance, the combination was associated with shorter survival, suggesting that resistance is acquired more quickly than with single-agent therapy.[216] In addition, combination therapy is associated with additive toxicity. It may be that combination hormonal therapy depends on developing a rational sequence of administration, with adequate time to achieve a molecular biologic effect before the next agent is added. For example, tamoxifen is administered first, allowing an increase in PR synthesis, followed by megestrol acetate after an appropriate delay.[35] Alternatively, some investigators have reported antagonism with combined endocrine strategies. In one study,[56] six postmenopausal women with breast cancer were treated with tamoxifen alone, followed by tamoxifen plus aminoglutethimide for 6 weeks, followed by discontinuation of tamoxifen with repeated pharmacokinetic studies performed in patients treated with aminoglutethimide alone after a 6-week washout period for tamoxifen. The concentration of tamoxifen and its metabolites was decreased by coadministration of aminoglutethimide, suggesting an induction effect. Tamoxifen had no effect on aminoglutethimide pharmacokinetics. Thus, the success of these strategies will depend on significantly more basic science input and an appreciation of the time course and relevance of these events in human tumors.

Although combined endocrine therapy has not been shown to increase response rates, sequential single agents can be used effectively. Once a patient has progressed through single-agent therapy, continued responsiveness to subsequent endocrine therapies is frequently observed, although the likelihood of response decreases somewhat with each successive treatment. Thus, current recommendations are sequential use of single-agent hormonal therapies.

PREDICTIVE MARKERS AND VARIABLES FOR RESPONSE TO ENDOCRINE THERAPY

Predictive markers of response to endocrine therapy include the following:

Proven
ER positivity
PR positivity
Noncritical disease: isolated, osseous, or soft tissue metastases
Prior response to endocrine therapy
Prolonged disease-free interval
Postmenopausal status

Potential
pS2 positivity
c-*erb*B-2 positivity

The best-established marker for response to hormonal therapy is the presence of ER protein in the tumor. As discussed earlier, patients with ER-positive tumors have a 50% to 75% response rate to hormonal therapy, whereas patients with ER-negative tumors have less than a 10% chance of response.[43] These response rates for ER-positive patients treated with endocrine therapy are similar to those for a similar patient group treated with chemotherapy.[223,224] Thus, in a patient with receptor-positive disease and disease in a so-called noncritical site, hormonal therapy provides optimal palliation with minimal toxicity. Such noncritical sites of disease include isolated metastases, bone-only disease, and disease in soft tissue sites.

Because ER-negative patients have a 10% response to hormonal therapies, a trial of endocrine therapy should be considered at some point in the patient's course. An asymptomatic ER-negative patient with bone-only disease may be treated initially with tamoxifen. In patients with visceral or symptomatic disease, tamoxifen or other agents can be reserved until the patient has progressed through several chemotherapy regimens but can then be valuable in providing a chance of response with minimal toxicity.

The PR is considered to be a more sensitive marker of endocrine response, since a functional, rather than merely

detectable, ER is required to induce synthesis of PR protein.[225] Several trials have shown a significant association between the level of PR protein and response to endocrine therapy.[43,163,226,227]

The site of metastasis is also important in predicting response to hormonal therapy. Soft tissue and bony lesions have been reported to respond better than visceral lesions.[23,24,203,228] Investigators have also reported that visceral metastases are less likely to contain ER-positive tumor, accounting for the difference in response rates.[27] Parnes and colleagues[164] reported a 33% response rate to megestrol acetate in patients with soft tissue sites of disease, 70% response or stabilization with bony disease, and only a 21% response in visceral sites. Similar data have been reported by others.[161,162]

Brufman[229] found that the most significant factors in predicting a response to hormonal therapy were prior response to tamoxifen and a disease-free interval of more than 36 months before recurrence. Other authors[23] also reported on the important of disease-free interval and prior response to endocrine therapy. Age and menopausal status have also been associated with response to hormonal therapy, probably because older, postmenopausal women are more likely to have receptor-positive tumors than premenopausal women.

Authors have also evaluated whether prior chemotherapy affects the response rate to subsequent hormonal therapy. Lippman and Allegra[230] reported retrospectively on 40 patients who had received chemotherapy then hormonal therapy. Twenty-one of these 40 patients (53%) had ER-positive tumors and 14 of the 21 (67%) had an objective response to endocrine therapy. Thirty-one ER-positive patients had not received prior chemotherapy and had a reported 64% response rate to hormonal therapy, a difference that was not significant. For ER-negative patients, response to endocrine therapy was low regardless of pretreatment with chemotherapy. Thus, the sequence of therapy type does not affect response rates, and the treatment likely to provide the greatest benefit with the least toxicity should be chosen.

Investigators have examined the value of molecular biologic markers of prognosis and therapeutic response. Schwartz and colleagues[231] analyzed pS2 expression in the tumors of 72 women with metastatic breast cancer. This protein is estrogen-regulated and may therefore act as a surrogate marker of ER function. Sixty-four percent of the tumors were ER-positive, 29% were PR-positive, and 29% were pS2-positive. In the pS2-positive tumors, 52% had an objective response to hormonal therapy, compared with 27% of pS2-negative patients. Forty percent of the ER-positive patients had a response to hormonal therapy. These results suggest that pS2 may further identify a subset of ER-positive tumors most likely to respond to endocrine treatment. Wright and coworkers[232] looked at c-*erb*B-2 protein expression and response to hormonal therapy in 221 patients. The assays were performed on the primary breast tumor. Patients did not receive any adjuvant therapy. At relapse, postmenopausal women received tamoxifen; aminoglutethimide and hydrocortisone were used as second-line therapy. Premenopausal women were treated with ovarian ablation; tamoxifen was used as second-line therapy. Expression of c-*erb*B-2 was associated with a decreased likelihood

TABLE 22.1-14
Single-Agent Activity of Drugs Tested in Metastatic Breast Cancer

Drug Name	Patients Studied		Response Rate (%)	References
	Total	Previously Untreated		
Actinomycin D	59	—	0–20	498, 499
Amonafide	26	26	23	500
Amsacrine	235	1	3–15	501–505
Azacytidine	27	6	—	506
BCNU (carmustine)	155	5	7–29	507
Bisantrene	306	0	5–23	508–514
Bleomycin	39	3	0–5	515–517
Carboplatin	122	47	0–20	518–524
CCNU (lomustine)	103	21	0–14	506, 525–527
Chlorambucil	58	—	0–19	498, 528
Cisplatin	191	54	0–54	529–535
Cyclophosphamide	887	594	11–59	307, 536–550
Cytosine arabinoside (cytarabine)	64	—	0–15	551
Dacarbazine	51	—	0–14	552
Docetaxel (Taxotere)	106	79	50–72	387, 388
Doxorubicin (Adrimycin)	1122	182	0–87	234–236, 254, 508, 525,551, 553–569
Elliptinium	228	66	0–33	570–574
Epirubicin	390	67	16–71	561–564, 575–584
Esorubicin	82	69	0–35	284, 285, 564, 585, 586
Estradiol mustard	17	—	—	587
Estramustine (Estracyt)	97	12	5–39	588
Etoposide	319	20	0–15	589–597
Fenretinide	30	16	0–33	598, 599
Floxuridine (5-fluoro-2′-deoxyuridine)	152	7	12–48	600–605
Fludarabine	14	0	0	606
Fluorouracil	1921	667	0–68	536, 537, 539–541, 549, 550, 600, 604, 607–622
Ftorafur	29	—	—	623
Gallium nitrate	—	—	0–9	624
Hexamethylmelamine	151	0	0–31	625–630
Hydroxyurea	21	—	13–14	551
Idarubicin	342	173	11–46	292, 564, 631–638
Ifosfamide	48	20	15–40	639, 640
Lonidamine	74	11	5–20	641–643
Losoxantrone	31	—	63	299
Melphalan	222	91	0–23	311, 551, 621, 644, 645
Menogaril	71	13	8–18	646–648
6-Mercaptopurine	44	—	14	649
Methotrexate	547	76	4–54	444, 498, 549–551, 600, 650–658
Methyl-6-CCNU (semustine)	61	22	3–3	525, 659
Mithramycin (Plicamycin)	48	—	0–19	499, 507
Mitolactol	142	17	0–44	660–664
Mitomycin	307	0	5–35	420, 559, 665–668

(continued)

TABLE 22.1-14
Single-Agent Activity of Drugs Tested in Metastatic Breast Cancer (continued)

Drug Name	Patients Studied		Response Rate (%)	References
	Total	Previously Untreated		
Mitoxantrone (Novantrone)	848	266	3–36	262, 669–677
Nitrogen mustard	95	39	8–25	540, 678
Paclitaxel (Taxol)	568	202	20–62	361, 366–368, 372
PALA (N-phosphonacetyl-L-aspartate)	49	1	5–10	679
Pirarubicin	364	61	17–53	680–685
Prednimustine	166	35	22–40	686, 687
Procarbazine	21	—	—	551
Spirogermanium	75	0	0–11	688–690
Streptozocin	24	0	0	515, 691
Teniposide	—	—	3–9	624
Thioguanine	23	0	—	692
Thiotepa	266	139	8–37	498, 540, 545, 621, 622, 678
Trimetrexate	20	20	0	693
Vinblastine	119	—	0–45	551, 694–698
Vincristine	251	12	0–40	539, 550, 551, 621, 699–701
Vindesine	218	24	4–31	346, 347, 702–708
Vinorelbine (Navelbine)	88	70	20–52	349–353, 709, 710, 711
VM-26 (teniposide)	20	0		712

of response to endocrine therapy. For ER-positive patients, response was 48% in those with a negative c-*erb*B-2 stain but dropped to 20% for patients with a positive c-*erb*B-2 stain. For ER-negative patients, the response rate was 27% with c-*erb*B-2 negative tumors but 0% with c-*erb*B-2 expression. Thus, evaluation of additional markers may allow further refinement of therapeutic options and decrease the likelihood of administering an ineffective therapy. As research continues, better molecular biologic markers will be identified.

Chemotherapy

Many active agents are available for the treatment of metastatic breast cancer, and numerous regimens have been reported. This section highlights selected drugs that form the cornerstone of treatment and is not intended to be an exhaustive review of all agents or all regimens. This section also discusses the principles of chemotherapy administration with these agents and describes prognostic markers for predicting response to therapy.

CHEMOTHERAPEUTIC AGENTS AND REGIMENS

Chemotherapeutic agents for breast cancer were first tested in the metastatic setting as single agents. Table 22.1-14 lists the individual response rates of these drugs, which

range from 0% to 71%. Nearly all drugs have been tested in breast cancer, and the agents with the greatest activity historically are anthracyclines, cyclophosphamide, methotrexate, and 5-FU. In addition, the vinca alkaloids, etoposide, platinum, ifosfamide, and mitomycin are also active. More recently, paclitaxel (Taxol) has become widely used as an agent particularly effective in anthracycline-resistant tumors. Newer promising agents include other taxanes (such as taxotere), the camptothecins, the anthrapyrazones, and navelbine. These drugs are discussed as single agents and in combination.

Anthracyclines

DOXORUBICIN. The anthracyclines have long been considered the most active agents in the treatment of breast cancer. An antitumor antibiotic, doxorubicin (Adriamycin) is the most widely used of these agents. Its mechanism of action is probably due to intercalation within DNA and inhibition of topoisomerase II.[233] When doxorubicin is used as a single agent in untreated patients with metastatic breast cancer, response rates range from 40% to 50%.[234–236] Combination regimens with doxorubicin increase the response rate somewhat. Such combinations include doxorubicin with cyclophosphamide (CA); with cyclophosphamide, methotrexate, and 5-FU (CAMF), with cyclophosphamide and vincristine (VAC); with cyclophosphamide, methotrexate, 5-FU, and prednisone

(CAMFp); with cyclophosphamide and 5-FU (FAC); and with vincristine added to CAMFp (CAMFVp).[237-240] Response rates range from 44% to 72%.

A number of studies have also compared doxorubicin-containing regimens with non–doxorubicin-containing regimens in metastatic settings to evaluate the contribution of anthracyclines.[241-249] A'Hern and colleagues[250] added doxorubicin to Cooper-like regimens in randomized clinical trials (Fig. 22.1-7). Five trials with 1088 patients were identified. Overall, the addition of doxorubicin increased the odds of response. The risk of dying was decreased by 22%, and the risk of treatment failure was decreased by 31%. These results translated into an increase in median survival from 14 to 18 months and an increase in the median time to treatment failure from 5 to 7 months. These gains are modest. In this analysis, significant nausea and vomiting was associated with anthracycline administration, leading to presumed decreased quality of life. With the advent of new serotonin-antagonist antiemetic agents, this toxicity will be decreased. Thus, treatment with doxorubicin may increase the likelihood of response and may improve survival by a few months without sacrifice of quality of life in patients with metastatic disease.

Further efforts to improve the cytotoxicity of doxorubicin are under active investigation. One area of investigation has centered on the optimal schedule of administration. Large bolus doses given every 3 weeks and weekly low-dose administration have both been shown to be effective.[233-236] In the laboratory, prolonged infusion of doxorubicin has been shown to have greater activity against slowly proliferating cells, thus possibly increasing efficacy

in established metastatic tumors with a proportionately slower growth fraction.[251] A subsequent clinical study documented residual doxorubicin drug levels of 1 to 20 nmol/L at day 7 of a weekly administration schedule in half the patients assayed.[252] The investigators replicated these exposures in the laboratory and found that the combination of a low-level continuous doxorubicin exposure coupled with intermittent pulse doses, similar to the pharmacokinetic results produced in patients with a weekly doxorubicin schedule, resulted in greater toxicity than continuous exposure alone.

In addition to duration of exposure, a dose-response relation exists for doxorubicin that has been well-described in animal model systems as well as in nonbreast malignant diseases.[253,254] The hypothesis that increased dose rate of doxorubicin will result in improved response has been tested in a number of breast cancer studies. Jones and colleagues[254] treated 26 women with metastatic breast cancer with single-agent doxorubicin therapy. Patients received either 25 or 30 mg/m²/d for 3 days. Cycles were repeated monthly, and doses were escalated by 5 mg/m²/d each month. Eighteen patients were treated at 35 mg/m²/d for 23 cycles; 11 patients received 40 mg/m²/d for 11 cycles; and 5 patients received a total of 7 cycles at 45 mg/m²/d. The response rate was 85%, with a 38% complete response rate. Dose-limiting toxicity consisted of leukopenia and febrile neutropenia or mucositis. The hospitalization rate increased as the dose increased. In addition, 16 of 26 patients (62%) were removed from the study because of a decline in ejection fraction. Three of these patients experienced symptomatic congestive heart

FIGURE 22.1-7 Diagrams showing odds ratios for response rates and estimates of failure-free survival and survival in randomized trials examining the substitution with doxorubicin in Cooper-type regimens. The overall estimates are shown as diamonds, the width of the diamonds denoting a 95% confidence limit. For the individual trials, the area of the boxes is proportional to the weight given to each trial; the horizontal lines denote 95% confidence intervals. (A'Hern RP, Smith IE, Ebbs SR. Chemotherapy and survival in advanced breast cancer: the inclusion of doxorubicin in Cooper type regimens. Br J Cancer 1993;67:802)

failure. This trial suggests an important dose-response relation for doxorubicin in metastatic breast cancer, although the 3-day schedule may also have contributed to increased efficacy. However, the toxicity was substantial. Survival data by dose level were not recorded by the authors, but overall survival was 18 months, not significantly different from schedules of doxorubicin administration that were less dose intense and less toxic.

This high response rate was replicated by Bronchud and colleagues,[255] who treated 15 metastatic breast cancer patients with doxorubicin at doses of 75, 100, 125, and 150 mg/m^2 intravenously every 2 weeks for a maximum of three cycles. This therapy was supported by granulocyte colony-stimulating factor (G-CSF). Twelve of the 15 patients (80%) responded to treatment, with a 33% complete response rate. At doses of 125 and 150 mg/m^2, half of the patients required platelet transfusions and most required blood transfusions. Seven of the eight patients treated at the two higher dose levels were admitted for febrile neutropenia. Mucositis was also a dose-limiting toxicity. No patients developed symptomatic congestive heart failure, although the mean ejection fraction for the group decreased with progressive therapy. These two trials suggest a clinical advantage in dose intensification of doxorubicin regimens. Means to overcome toxicity, however, such as the use of colony stimulating factors, the development of cardioprotective and mucoprotective agents, the use of liposomes to decrease cardiac uptake, will be necessary to implement this schedule safely into clinical practice.

The cardioprotective agent that has been most widely tested is ADR-529 (ICRF-187), a bisdioxpiperazine compound that is subsequently metabolized to an effective chelating agent. A randomized clinical trial enrolled 150 women with metastatic breast cancer.[256] These patients were treated with FAC, with or without prior treatment with 1000 mg/m^2 of ADR-529. Patients who received the cardioprotective agent received more cycles of therapy than did the control group (11 compared with 9) and a higher median cumulative dose of doxorubicin (500 mg/m^2 compared with 441 mg/m^2). In addition, individual patients treated with ADR-529 were more likely to tolerate higher cumulative doses of doxorubicin than patients treated without this agent. For example, 26 patients in the experimental arm received 700 mg/m^2 and 11 received 1000 mg/m^2; 3 patients in the control arm received 700 mg/m^2, and only 1 patient received a maximum dose of 950 mg/m^2. A significant reduction in decreases in ejection fraction and in clinical congestive heart failure was observed in patients in the experimental arm. However, additional studies have suggested that the primary toxicity of ADR-529 is neutropenia; in addition, antagonism between doxorubicin and ADR-529 with regard to topoisomerase II–induced DNA strand breaks has been observed in the laboratory.[257,258] Although ADR-529 offers significant cardioprotection, these additional findings may limit the ability to administer large doses of drug or may decrease the effectiveness of doxorubicin. Therefore, doses of doxorubicin of 30 mg/m^2 in weekly schedules and 60 mg/m^2 in combination therapy every 3 weeks are most common in clinical practice.

Novel methods of improving cytotoxicity of doxorubicin include hormonal modulation. In the laboratory, preincubation of breast cancer cells with MPA synergistically increases the cytotoxicity of doxorubicin in MCF-7 cells.[259] Incubation with doxorubicin followed by MPA resulted in additive, but not synergistic, cytotoxicity, suggesting that the effect is not due purely to antihormonal therapy of this ER-positive cell line. In the clinical setting, investigators at the University of California at San Diego[260] conducted a phase I trial of high-dose progesterone administered over 24 hours, followed by 60 mg/m^2 doxorubicin. Dose-limiting toxicity was myelosuppression. Progesterone did not alter doxorubicin pharmacokinetics but appeared to modulate doxorubicin cytotoxicity using leukopenia as a surrogate endpoint. The authors surmised that the mechanism of action is related to modulation of *mdr* P-glycoprotein expressed by myeloid cells. These data provide interesting possibilities for the combination of chemotherapy and hormonal therapy.

MITOXANTRONE. Because the cumulative dose and dose rate of doxorubicin are limited by the cardiotoxicity of this agent, many anthracycline analogues have been developed in an attempt to decrease the likelihood of this significant side effect. Mitoxantrone (Novantrone) is the best known and most widely clinically used of these agents in breast cancer. It is an anthraquinone derivative of doxorubicin.[261] Mitoxantrone is reported to have less cardiotoxicity than doxorubicin, but clinical trials have continued to demonstrate cardiac effects with cumulative dosing.[233] In addition, the cardiotoxicity of mitoxantrone is additive to the cardiotoxicity seen with doxorubicin, limiting its effectiveness in patients previously treated with the parent compound.[233] Response rates as a single agent at doses of 12 to 14 mg/m^2 given every 3 weeks range from 17% to 35%.[261–265] All of these studies except one reported cardiotoxicity in patients receiving mitoxantrone, including patients who had not received prior anthracyclines.[261] Responses were seen in patients who had failed prior anthracycline therapy and in patients who had failed mitoxantrone first and received subsequent doxorubicin.[261,262,264,265] Acute side effects, such as nausea, vomiting, mucositis, and alopecia, are reported to be less with mitoxantrone than with doxorubicin.

In combination, response rates are higher—40% to 45%.[266–268] The highest response rates have been reported for mitoxantrone given with 5-FU and leucovorin. Hainsworth and colleagues[269] and Jones and coworkers[270] have each published results with this drug combination and have reported 65% and 45% response rates, respectively. The recommended usage of mitoxantrone in comparison to doxorubicin is discussed later in this section.

EPIRUBICIN. Epirubicin is a semisynthetic doxorubicin stereoisomer used extensively in Europe, although not approved in the United States. Its single-agent response rate is comparable to that of doxorubicin, ranging from

25% in previously treated patients to 62% in untreated patients.[271] It has been reported to be associated with less cardiotoxicity, although this side effect may still occur.[272] It has most frequently been used in combination regimens with ifosfamide, cyclophosphamide and 5-FU, or with 5-FU and leucovorin, with reported response rates of 40% to 64%.[273-277]

As for doxorubicin, the efficacy of epirubicin is schedule dependent and shows a dose-intensity relationship. Marschner and colleagues[278] treated 26 women with metastatic breast cancer with a combination of cyclophosphamide and epirubicin. The cyclophosphamide dose was fixed at 600 mg/m²; epirubicin was administered in increments of 20 mg/m² beginning at 60 mg/m². The maximum tolerated dose of epirubicin in this combination was 120 mg/m². At this dose, 17 of 18 patients had objective tumor responses after one cycle. The predominant toxicity was myelosuppression. Overall, 15% of patients had a 20% decrease in ejection fraction, although only 1 patient had clinical cardiotoxicity. A follow-up study randomly assigned 197 evaluable patients to receive either high-dose EC (epirubicin, 120 mg/m², cyclophosphamide, 600 mg/m²) or standard-dose therapy (epirubicin, 60 mg/m², cyclophosphamide, 600 mg/m²), both given intravenously every 3 weeks.[279] The response rates were 63% and 47%, respectively. Again, the predominant toxicity was myelosuppression. In addition, 10% of patients in the high-dose arm experienced cardiotoxicity compared with 5% in the standard-dose arm. None had signs of congestive heart failure. No difference in time to progression or in survival was observed.

Focan and colleagues[280] compared two doses of epirubicin in the FEC regimen (5-FU, epirubicin, and cyclophosphamide). 5-FU and cyclophosphamide were each given at doses of 500 mg/m² IV on day 1. Epirubicin was given at 50 mg/m² either days 1 and 8 or only on day 1. Cycles were repeated every 21 days. The response rate in the dose-intensified regimen was 69% compared with 41% in the day-one regimen, a statistically significant difference. Myelosuppression, anemia, and stomatitis were more pronounced in the patients who received the dose-intense regimen. No cardiac abnormalities were reported. The French Epirubicin Study Group[281] randomly assigned patients to receive FEC with the doses of 5-FU and cyclophosphamide as above in three different regimens. Epirubicin was administered in regimen A at 75 mg/m² for 11 cycles, in regimen B at 100 mg/m² for 4 cycles followed by a dose reduction to 50 mg/m², and in regimen C at 100 mg/m² for 4 cycles followed by cessation of chemotherapy. The response rates were 54%, 71%, and 55%, respectively; regimen B was superior. However, no difference in time to progression or in survival was noted.

Although these studies have shown an impressive response rate for high-dose epirubicin, a high response rate has been reported for single-agent epirubicin therapy administered at 120 mg/m² every 3 weeks or at 25 mg/m² weekly.[282,283] Thus, doses of epirubicin of 100 mg/m² or greater appear to be optimal in inducing tumor regression. The addition of additional chemotherapeutic agents may

decrease the time to response but does not appear to affect survival.

OTHER ANTHRACYCLINE AND ANTHRACYCLINE-LIKE DRUGS. Additional investigational anthracycline-like agents include esorubicin (4'-deoxydoxorubicin); pirarubicin (4'-O-tetrahydropyranyladriamycin); idarubicin (4-demethoxydaunorubicin); bisantrene, an anthracene derivative; and menogaril, a structural analogue of doxorubicin.[284-298] All of these agents have been reported to cause cardiac toxicity despite the hope of structural modification to avoid this side effect. Response rates range from 12% to 73% in these reports, and response appears to be related to degree of pretreatment and to dose of anthracycline used.[284-298]

ANTHRAPYRAZOLES. The anthrapyrazoles are a novel class of chemotherapeutic agents that also inhibit topoisomerase II. They differ from anthracyclines in the presence of the anthrapyrazole ring structure.[299] Because of this structure, they are less susceptible to metabolism to free radicals, thought to be a potential mechanism of anthracycline-induced cardiac toxicity.[299] Three drugs are in clinical development: DuP937, losoxantrone (DuP941), and piroxantrone (DuP942). DuP937 has been evaluated in a number of tumor types; preliminary data suggest it has less activity against breast cancer than other members of this family.[299] Losoxantrone, 50 mg/m² every 3 weeks, was administered to metastatic breast cancer patients, none of whom had received prior anthracycline-like therapy, with a response rate of 63%. Myelosuppression was the primary toxicity observed. No significant cardiotoxicity was reported, and alopecia was reported as grade 1 or 2.[299] Studies are underway with piroxantrone.

COMPARISON WITH DOXORUBICIN. Direct comparisons to doxorubicin have been made for many of these agents. One representative study performed by the SWOG randomly assigned 411 women with previously treated (one chemotherapy regimen) metastatic breast cancer to receive doxorubicin, 60 mg/m², mitoxantrone, 14 mg/m², or bisantrene, 320 mg/m², IV every 3 weeks.[296] The response rates were 28%, 14%, and 13%, respectively, with a statistically significant difference between doxorubicin and the other two agents. Toxicity was greater in the doxorubicin arm, with increased nausea, vomiting, and mucositis, and more complete alopecia. Seven percent of doxorubicin-treated patients developed congestive heart failure compared with 2% of those treated with mitoxantrone and none treated with bisantrene. No difference in survival was found. In combination therapy, cyclophosphamide, mitoxantrone, and 5-FU yielded a response rate of 29% compared with a rate of 37% for patients who received cyclophosphamide, doxorubicin, and 5-FU.[300] Thus, doxorubicin appears to have more activity than other anthracycline analogues. This efficacy does not translate into improved survival, however, and must be weighed against the additional toxicity of this agent. As mentioned, with the development of better antiemetic agents and additional supportive measures, the risk/benefit ratio is constantly altering and should be carefully evaluated for each patient. Doxorubicin appears to be the anthracycline of choice. Mitoxantrone is usually reserved for patients with an increased potential for cardiac or other toxicity, such as elderly patients. Overall, anthracycline-based regimens should be considered the first-line chemotherapy of choice in patients who did not receive these drugs in the adjuvant setting.

Cyclophosphamide-Based Combinations

Although cyclophosphamide is an active single agent in the treatment of breast cancer, it is conventionally used in combination with other agents. Cyclophosphamide-based regimens are some of the earliest multidrug therapies designed for breast cancer treatment. Cooper treated women with metastatic breast cancer with cyclophosphamide, methotrexate, 5-FU, vincristine, and prednisone weekly and had a reported response rate of 90%, leading to the development of so-called Cooper regimens.[301] Based on the success of multidrug combinations in Hodgkin disease and leukemia and on this report, one of the earliest reported regimens for breast cancer was cyclophosphamide, 5-FU, and methotrexate (CMF). Canellos and colleagues[302] treated 25 women with metastatic breast cancer with this combination. Cyclophosphamide was given orally for 14 days at a dose of 100 mg/m²/d with prednisone at 40 mg/m²/d; methotrexate and 5-FU were given intravenously on days 1 and 8 at doses of 60 and 700 mg/m², respectively. A 68% response rate was observed, with a median remission duration of 9 months. Further investigation has suggested that prednisone and vincristine add little to the efficacy of this regimen but can increase toxicity.[303,304] The CMF regimen was later modified for patient convenience and to ensure compliance by administering all three drugs intravenously on day 1. The European Organization for Research and Treatment of Cancer (EORTC) investigated the relative efficacy of these regimens in the metastatic setting.[305] Because cyclophosphamide is a cell cycle–dependent drug, an alteration in schedule might alter its efficacy. Two hundred fifty-four eligible patients were randomly assigned to receive classic CMF (cyclophosphamide, 100 mg/m² PO on days 1 to 14; methotrexate, 40 mg/m² IV on days 1 and 8; 5-FU, 600 mg/m² IV on days 1 and 8 repeated every 28 days) or bolus therapy (cyclophosphamide, 600 mg/m², methotrexate, 40 mg/m², and 5-FU, 600 mg/m², all IV on day 1, repeated every 21 days). The response on the classic arm was 48% compared with 29% on the bolus arm. Time to progression was significantly longer in patients treated with the classic schedule, and median survival was 17 months in the classic arm compared with 12 months in the bolus group ($P=.016$) Thus, this regimen appears to be schedule dependent, and use of the classic format maximizes response.

Multiple trials have been performed with the Cooper regimen and its variations.[235,241,250,274,275,280,301–304,306–313] Response rates range from 32% to 63%, with no significant difference in duration of response or overall survival. As mentioned earlier, the substitution of doxorubicin and potentially epirubicin for methotrexate appears to increase the efficacy of this combination. Therefore, the traditional CMF regimen is usually reserved for patients at risk for cardiotoxicity.

5-Fluorouracil

5-Fluorouracil is a pyrimidine analogue that has been used in cancer chemotherapy for more than 30 years. The drug is metabolized to FdUMP (5-fluoro-2′-deoxyuridine monophosphate), which binds to thymidylate synthase (TS), preventing DNA synthesis.[314] The TS–FdUMP complex depends on the concentration of 5,10-methylene-tetrahydrofolate for stability.[314] Thus, the TS–FdUMP complex can be further stabilized by coadministration of leucovorin.[314] 5-FU can also be metabolized to 5-fluorouridine-5′-triphosphate (FUTP), which is incorporated into RNA as a false substrate.[314] Resistance to 5-FU can occur through alteration of cellular metabolism, alteration or overexpression of thymidylate synthase, and other mechanisms.[314]

The activity of 5-FU depends on peak concentrations and on duration of exposure.[314] It is poorly bioavailable and is therefore used exclusively as an intravenous preparation.[314] These features have led to a number of different schedules of administration. In early trials in breast cancer, 5-FU was administered in bolus form as described in the CMF studies.[301–305]

Swain and colleagues[315] tested a 5-day schedule, wherein leucovorin, 500 mg/m²/d, was administered on days 1 to 5. One hour after completion of the leucovorin administration, 5-FU was given at a dose of 375 mg/m²/d. Cycles were repeated every 4 weeks. Fifty evaluable patients were entered on the study; all had received prior chemotherapy, and 61% had received prior 5-FU. The response rate was 24%, and responses were seen in patients who had received prior 5-FU. Toxicities included a 33% incidence of grade 3 or 4 mucositis, a 13% incidence of grade 3 diarrhea, and a 15% incidence of neutropenic sepsis. Patients with accessible tumors received the first cycle with 5-FU alone, with biopsies performed before and after therapy; the second cycle included 5-FU and leucovorin, again with paired biopsies. Seventy-six biopsy specimens were obtained from 17 patients. Increased binding of 5-FU to TS was demonstrated with the addition of leucovorin with increased stability of the complex. However, at least two patients failed to saturate TS with FdUMP, and neither responded to therapy. Patients who responded were found to have a higher level of enzyme inactivation than patients with progressive disease. These data provide intriguing information about the use of biochemical assays to determine optimal drug dose and scheduling. These results were corroborated by a Mayo Clinic study.[316]

Because the effectiveness of 5-FU is related to duration of exposure in the laboratory, continuous infusion of 5-FU has been evaluated in the clinical setting. Chang and colleagues[317] administered 200 to 300 mg/m²/d to patients who had failed at least two prior chemotherapy regimens; infusions were continued until signs of toxicity developed. Ten patients were enrolled in this study and were treated for 17 to 396 days. Toxicity included diarrhea and mucositis. One patient developed cerebellar ataxia and one developed hand–foot syndrome. Three partial responses were observed, suggesting that continuous infusion may be beneficial. Jabboury and colleagues[318] at M.D. Anderson Cancer Center studied 36 women with metastatic breast cancer who had received multiple prior chemotherapy regimens (a median of four); all had received prior 5-FU therapy. Patients received 250 mg/m^2/d infusional 5-FU until toxicity necessitated an interruption in treatment. The median duration of therapy was 65 days. A 16% response rate was observed, significant in this heavily pretreated patient population with a median performance status of 3. These data suggest that prolonged infusion may overcome resistance from previous 5-FU exposure. Current studies focus on the use of infusional 5-FU with additional chemotherapeutic agents, such as epirubicin and cisplatin, cisplatin and etoposide, and cyclophosphamide and doxorubicin.[319–321]

Other efforts to extend the clinical efficacy of 5-FU–based regimens have included weekly 24-hour infusions and biochemical modulation by additional agents such as N-phosphonacetyl-L-aspartic acid (PALA), 3′-azido-2′,3′-dideoxythymidine (AZT), and iododeoxyuridine.[322–329] These efforts, although biochemically based, have thus far met with limited success in the clinic. At present, the optimal use of 5-FU appears to be either by prolonged infusion or with 24-hour weekly infusion with the addition of leucovorin.

Methotrexate

Methotrexate is the 4-NH2, N-10-methyl analogue of folic acid and has been extensively used in chemotherapeutic regimens for various malignant conditions. This agent inhibits dihydrofolate reductase, which blocks thymidylate synthesis.[330] At low doses, it can be used alone; in high doses (1 to 30 g/m^2), it requires leucovorin as a rescue agent to restore a pool of reduced folates to normal cells. Activity is related to concentration and to duration of exposure. Many molecular mechanisms of resistance have been outlined.[330]

In breast cancer, it has been primarily used in the CMF regimens outlined earlier. However, methotrexate interacts synergistically with other chemotherapeutic agents, including fluoropyrimidines. These positive interactions have led to other combination therapies. Several trials have examined the efficacy of methotrexate in combination with 5-FU.[331–333] Methotrexate increases the levels of phosphoribosylpyrophosphate (PRPP) levels, increasing the phosphorylation of 5-FU and enhancing intracellular accumulation. In pretreated patients with metastatic breast cancer, studies of sequential methotrexate (in doses of 50 to 300 mg/m^2) and 5-FU (in doses of 600 to 900 mg/m^2) yielded response rates of 20% to 28%.[331,332] One study reported a response rate of 53%, although only 17

patients were entered in this trial.[333] Toxicity was mild, suggesting that these regimens are well tolerated.

Plant Alkaloids

VINCA ALKALOIDS. Vincristine, vinblastine, and vindesine have been used extensively in the treatment of breast cancer. Vincristine has been used primarily in the Cooper regimen and, as described earlier, was found to add little in terms of efficacy to CMF.[303,304] Its primary side effect is neurotoxicity, which can be dose limiting. It has been used in other combination therapies, but, because of its neurotoxicity and the availability of other less toxic and more effective vinca alkaloids, vincristine does not have a clear role in the treatment of breast cancer.[334]

Vinblastine (Velban) has been used as a single agent administered by continuous infusion. One study used vinblastine at a dose of 1.4 to 2 mg/m^2/d for 5 days.[335] One hundred six patients were entered on study with an overall response rate of 37%. The response rate increased to 48% in patients who received 1.7 mg/m^2 or more. The primary observed toxicity was myelosuppression. A recent study demonstrated that the use of granulocyte-macrophage colony-stimulating factor (GM-CSF) could ameliorate the myelosuppression but did not allow for dose escalation.[336] Bolus dosing of vinblastine has resulted in negligible response rates.[337] Vinblastine has also been used in combination, such as vinblastine, doxorubicin, thiotepa, and halotestin (VATH), and methotrexate, vinblastine, doxorubicin, and cisplatin (MVAC), and with mitomycin C or mitoxantrone.[338–345] Response rates in these trials ranged from 11.5% to 64%. The relative contribution of vinblastine to combination regimens when administered in bolus form is unclear. Although it is an active agent, its clinical utility may be limited by patient acceptance of the need for prolonged infusion.

Vindesine is a third vinca alkaloid with activity in breast cancer. As a single agent administered in weekly bolus fashion at a dose of 3 mg/m^2, its reported response rate is 20% to 28%; it is not clear that combination therapy with this agent improves the response rate.[344,346–348]

Vinorelbine (Navelbine) is the newest and most active vinca alkaloid in breast cancer (Table 22.1-15). It differs from the classic vinca alkaloids by modification of the catharanthine moiety of the molecule.[349] This modification has led to an increase in clinical activity and an alteration in the typical pattern of toxicity.[349] Gasparini and colleagues[350] reported on the use of vinorelbine at doses of 20 to 25 mg/m^2 given weekly in 67 evaluable women with pretreated metastatic breast cancer. A 36% response rate was observed. Myelosuppression of all three hematopoietic lineages was observed, limiting the ability to escalate the drug dose. Additional toxicities included phlebitis, gastrointestinal symptoms, and peripheral neuropathy. Two trials of vinorelbine administered as first-line therapy for metastatic breast cancer have been reported. Fumoleau and colleagues[351] treated 157 women with metastatic disease with vinorelbine at a dose of 30 mg/m^2 given weekly as a 20-minute infusion. The response rate was 41%. The

TABLE 22.1-15
Activity of Vinorelbine in Metastatic Breast Cancer Patients

Study	Reference	Dosing Schedule	Patients	Response Rate PR + CR (%)	CR (%)	Median Duration of Response (wk)
France	349	30 mg/m^2/wk over 20 min	33	30	6	21
Italy	350	20–25 mg/m^2/wk over 60 min	67	36	4.5	29
France	351	30 mg/m^2/wk over 20 min	157	41	7	34
Argentina	352	30 mg/m^2/wk over 1 h	45	41	7	36
France	353	8 mg/m^2 bolus day 1, then 5.5–10 mg/m^2/d days 1–4, continuous infusion	64	36	3	24

PR, partial response; CR, complete response.

primary toxicity was myelosuppression; a 3% incidence of peripheral neuropathy was observed. Romero and co-workers[352] replicated these findings with the same schedule but noted additional toxicities. A high rate of phlebitis occurred in patients without central venous access devices. Thirty-three percent developed peripheral neuropathy, and 44% experienced myalgias, a significantly higher incidence than that reported in the French trial. This difference in toxicity may be related to the mean number of cycles administered, 9 in the French study compared with 12 in the trial of Romero and associates. A continuous infusion schedule has also been investigated. Toussaint and colleagues[353] treated 64 patients with vinorelbine given as an initial intravenous bolus of 8 mg/m^2 followed by 5.5 to 10 mg/m^2/d for 4 days in a dose-escalation evaluation. A dose of 10 mg/m^2/d produced dose-limiting toxicity of neutropenia. Mucositis was also observed; neurotoxicity was minimal. An overall 36% response rate was observed. Response was related to the achieved dose intensity, both in terms of dose and ability to treat every 3 weeks instead of every 4 weeks. The recommended dose in this schedule is an 8-mg/m^2 IV bolus, followed by an infusion of 9 mg/m^2/d for 4 days. Current trials are focusing on the use of this agent in combination. The significant activity of vinorelbine will make it the vinca alkaloid of choice when approved for use in breast cancer.

EPIPODOPHYLLOTOXIN. Etoposide (VP-16) is a semisynthetic podophyllotoxin that has antimicrotubule activity.[354] It has been used extensively in the treatment of lung cancer and germ cell malignancies but has only recently been investigated in metastatic breast cancer patients. Etoposide is schedule dependent, suggesting that the traditional administration of this drug as a bolus agent may not provide maximal efficacy.[354] Laboratory findings have shown it to be more effective when administered repetitively rather than in bolus fashion.[355] In addition, VP-16 has excellent bioavailability when taken by mouth. These findings have led to trials of prolonged oral daily administration.

At least 16 trials of VP-16 as a single agent in previously treated patients with metastatic disease have been published[354,356,357] (Table 22.1-16). Most of these trials used VP-16 on days 1 to 5 on a cyclic basis and found overall response rates of 6% to 7%. Martin and colleagues,[354] however, administered VP-16 at a dose of 50 mg/m^2/d for 21 days, given every 4 weeks. Forty-three patients with metastatic disease were treated; half had received chemotherapy adjuvantly and all but two had received prior chemotherapy for metastatic disease. The reported response rate was 35%. The toxicities included nausea, vomiting, alopecia, and myelosuppression. Calvert and co-workers[357] reported similar results using either 50 or 100 mg/d for 14 days. These data suggest that optimal scheduling of this drug may have greater impact on activity than the extent of pretreatment.

Etoposide has been shown in the laboratory to have synergistic clinical activity with cisplatin and cyclophosphamide.[358,359] Platinum-based combinations are discussed later in this chapter. Because of this synergy, one study examined the efficacy of VP-16 with cyclophosphamide in patients with metastatic breast cancer.[359] These investigators gave VP-16, 120 mg/m^2/d PO on days 1 to 5, with cyclophosphamide, 120 mg/m^2 IV every 3 weeks. Sixteen patients were enrolled in this trial. All had documented liver metastases. Eight were previously untreated either adjuvantly or for metastatic disease, two had not responded to a prior chemotherapeutic regimen, and six had had CMF as adjuvant therapy but no chemotherapy for metastatic disease. The response rate was 50%, with a median duration of response of 13 months and median survival of 16 months. Toxicity consisted primarily of leukopenia, with an average nadir of 2400 cells/μL. Thus, VP-16 may be better used in drug combinations to exploit synergistic interactions than as a single agent, and it may be more effective with prolonged oral administration.

TAXANES. Paclitaxel (Taxol) is a novel chemotherapeutic agent derived from the western yew tree, *Taxus brevifolia,* and the most widely used taxane at present (Fig.

TABLE 22.1-16
Trials of Single-Agent Etoposide in Metastatic Breast Cancer

Investigtors	Patients*	Dosing Schedule	Response Rate (%)
Holmes et al[713]	37	70 mg/m² d × 5 d q 3 wk IV	2.7
Vaughn et al[714]	60	45 mg/m²/d × 5 d q 3 wk IV	5
	59	75 mg/m²/d × 5 d q 3 wk IV	8.5
Eagan et al[592]	19	100–125 mg/m²/d × 3 d q 4–5 wk IV	10.5
Ahmann et al[590]	15	125 mg/m²/d × 3 d q 3 wk IV	0
Schell et al[594]	77	70 mg/m²/d × 5 d q 3 wk IV	12
EORTC[715]	41†	50 mg/m²/d × 5 d q 3 wk IV *or* 100 mg/m²/d × 5 d q 3 wk PO	7
Nissen et al[716]	24	60–135 mg/m² 2×/wk IV	4
Fraschini et al[717]	15	300–450 mg/m²/d × 3 d q 4 wk IV	7
Bezwoda et al[718]	23	1500–2500 mg/m²/d × 1 d q 3 wk IV	26
Wander et al[596]	20‡	230 mg/m²d × 3 d q 4 wk IV	15
Palombo et al[719]	18	50 mg/m²/d × 21 d q 4 wk PO	22
Cerar et al[720]	21	100 mg × 10 d q 3 wk PO	52
Martin et al[354]	43	50 mg/m²/d × 21 d q 4 wk PO	35
Cavalli et al[589]	15	150 mg/m²/d × 5 d q 3 wk PO	0
	15	150 mg/m² × 1 d q wk IV	0
Falkson et al[591]	20	200 mg/m²/d × 5 d q 3 wk PO *or* 300–400 mg/m²/d × 5 d q 2 wk PO	0
Calvert et al[357]	38	50 mg/d × 2 wk q 4 wk PO	9
		100 mg/d × 2 wk q 4 wk PO	26

★ All patients with prior therapy except as noted.

† Prior therapy not specified.

‡ Untreated patients.

(Modified from Martin M, Lluch A, Casado A, et al. J Clin Oncol 1994;12:990; and Nichols CR. Semin Oncol 1992;19:68)

22.1-8). It has a unique mechanism of action and promotes microtubule assembly, in contrast to the vinca alkaloids, which prevent microtubule assembly.[360] Paclitaxel also shifts the equilibrium to stabilize the polymerized assembled form and thus prevents cell division.[360] Its taxane ring has only been isolated from natural products and has evaded synthesis in the laboratory. Paclitaxel has therefore been extracted from the bark of the yew tree. Because this process kills the trees, which take 60 years or so to reach maturity, investigation has centered on a renewable source of the drug. A technique to extract paclitaxel from the needles of the yew tree has been developed, and chemists continue to work on synthetic or semisynthetic methods of production.

Paclitaxel was initially discovered in the 1960s in an NCI screening project but was abandoned because of toxicity and solubility problems.[360] New advances have overcome these problems, although this drug is still associated with significant side effects. The dose-limiting toxicity of paclitaxel is neutropenia.[360] Nadir counts are usually reached at about day 8 rather than day 14 as with most other chemotherapeutic agents.[360]

Because of solubility problems, paclitaxel must be dissolved in polyoxyethylated castor oil and alcohol (Cremophor EL; BASF Aktiengesellschaft).[360] It also must be infused in non–polyvinyl chloride tubing, since it will leach out di-(2-ethylhexyl)phthalate (DEHP) and expose the patient to this toxic plastic derivative.[360]

Hypersensitivity reactions were observed in the initial trials of paclitaxel, which were attributed initially to bolus infusion schedules. These reactions were type I hypersensitivity reactions, with hypotension, dyspnea, bronchospasm, and urticaria.[360] It is also possible that they are caused by the Cremophor vehicle. Premedication with dexamethasone, 20 mg PO or IV 14 and 7 hours before therapy, diphenhydramine, 50 mg IV 30 minutes before therapy, and cimetidine, 300 mg, or ranitidine, 50 mg, IV 30 minutes before therapy, has significantly decreased the occurrence of hypersensitivity reactions.[360]

Neuropathy has also been seen, which is not unex-

FIGURE 22.1-8 Structure of taxol. (Rowinsky EK, Cazenave LA, Donehower RC. Taxol: a novel investigational antimicrotubule agent. J Natl Cancer Inst 1990;82:1248)

pected for an agent that affects microtubules. This side effect has occurred as initial subjective complaints of numbness and tingling; with continued drug use, it can progress to a stocking–glove neuropathy with loss of distal deep tendon reflexes.[361] It is a cumulative, dose-related toxicity that resolves slowly after discontinuing the drug.[360]

Many patients also experience myalgia and arthralgia 2 to 4 days after drug infusion that lasts 2 to 4 days.[360] These symptoms can be relieved or prevented with nonsteroidal antiinflammatory drugs. In rare cases, patients may require short-term oral narcotics to alleviate symptoms. Paclitaxel also has cardiac side effects. The best-known is sinus bradycardia, which is frequently asymptomatic. In rare cases, progression to heart block has been reported.[360,362]

As experience with paclitaxel grows, so do reports of side effects and toxicity. Paclitaxel appears to act as a radiation sensitizer. Several letters have been published reporting radiation-recall dermatitis.[363,364] Recent reports have centered on the association of paclitaxel with typhlitis, probably because of the profound although short-lived neutropenia induced by this drug.[365]

Despite these side effects, the significant activity of this drug has warranted continued clinical evaluation. Paclitaxel was first used in the treatment of ovarian cancer and showed high activity.[360] It has also been used in breast cancer patients with good results. The first phase II trial of paclitaxel in patients with metastatic breast cancer was performed by Holmes and colleagues[361] with a dose of 250 mg/m² and an infusion duration of 24 hours. Twenty-five patients were enrolled. Sixty percent had visceral disease. Patients could have had one prior course of chemotherapy, either adjuvant or for metastatic disease. Twenty-three patients had received prior doxorubicin, and six were doxorubicin resistant, defined by the investigators as having experienced relapse within 6 months of an adjuvant doxorubicin-containing regimen or progressive

disease while receiving doxorubicin for metastatic disease. The overall response rate was 56%, with a complete response rate of 12%. The median time to disease progression was 9 months. In the six patients with doxorubicin-resistant disease, two partial responses were observed. Seven patients required no dose reductions; the rest required dose reductions as a result of neutropenia, infection, or neurotoxicity. These results are particularly impressive given the response in doxorubicin-resistant patients, for whom subsequent response rates are expected to be 20% to 30% at best.

Because the dose-limiting toxicity of paclitaxel is neutropenia, some investigators looked at the ability of G-CSF to prevent or ameliorate the myelosuppression associated with this agent.[366] This trial accrued 28 patients with previously untreated metastatic breast cancer. Patients received 250 mg/m² of paclitaxel over 24 hours. Dose reductions were planned for an absolute neutrophil count (ANC) of less than 250, thrombocytopenia defined as a platelet count less than 50,000/μL, infection, or bleeding. In patients without these toxicities, the dose was escalated to 275 or 300 mg/m² based on nadir counts. G-CSF was given at 5 μg/kg/d for each course on days 3 to 10 or until the ANC was higher than 2000 for 3 consecutive days. Eight patients had received doxorubicin as adjuvant chemotherapy. A 62% response rate was observed, with a 12% complete response rate. Despite the use of G-CSF, only one patient was able to undergo a dose escalation to 300 mg/m². Again, despite the use of G-CSF, 12 of 26 patients (46%) required a dose reduction by cycle 2. By cycle 9, with 6 patients still under study, none was treated at the initial dose level, and doses for all had been reduced. Six of the 28 patients (21%) required hospitalization for febrile neutropenia, although only 4% of all administered cycles resulted in hospitalizations. Thus, G-CSF can decrease the morbidity associated with taxol-induced neutropenia, but it is unlikely that the use of this agent will allow further dose escalation.

Schiller and colleagues[367] looked at the ability of G-CSF to modulate the maximum tolerated dose of paclitaxel when administered as a 3-hour infusion. Thirty-five patients with a variety of cancer diagnoses were entered on study; two prior therapies for metastatic disease were allowed. No difference in the reported rate of hypersensitivity reactions was noted in this study (2.8%; similar to published values for a 24-hour infusion). Dose-limiting toxicity without the administration of G-CSF was myelosuppression, and the recommended phase II dose was 210 mg/m². With G-CSF, the maximum tolerated dose was 250 mg/m² and dose-limiting toxicity was peripheral neuropathy. Thus, the 3-hour infusion is safe and well tolerated. However, even with a shorter infusion duration, the dose of paclitaxel could be escalated by only about 20%.

The optimal dose of paclitaxel has yet to be determined. Nabholtz and colleagues[368] looked at 135 versus 175 mg/m², each given over 3 hours. Four hundred seventy-one patients with metastatic breast cancer were entered in the study. Fifty-eight percent of the patients had experienced relapse within 6 months of adjuvant therapy. One or two prior therapies, for either adjuvant or metastatic disease, were allowed. Sixty-six percent of patients had received anthracyclines. A 29% response rate was observed in the 175-mg/m^2 arm, and a 22% response rate was seen in the 135-mg/m^2 arm. These values are not significantly different, although a trend toward a higher percentage of complete responses was observed with the higher dose (5% versus 2%). No difference in survival was observed. Based on these results and on data from the National Cancer Institute of Canada study discussed later, most investigators have accepted that doses below 175 mg/m^2 are probably less effective.[368,369] It is unclear, however, whether doses of 250 mg/m^2 offer an advantage over doses of 175 mg/m^2.[367,370] The CALGB has opened a trial of 175 versus 210 versus 250 mg/m^2 with G-CSF support to look for a dose-response effect.

The optimal infusion duration of paclitaxel is also unknown. Many authors have reported on the efficacy of a 3-hour infusion. This schedule has the convenience of outpatient administration without the monitoring required for 24-hour infusion, even in the outpatient setting. The National Cancer Institute of Canada Clinical Trials Group reported on a 2 × 2 factorial design that randomly assigned patients with ovarian cancer to receive either 175 or 135 mg/m^2 of paclitaxel and to receive it either over 3 hours or over 24 hours.[369] Their results showed a 24% response rate in patients who received 175 mg/m^2, compared with a 13% response rate in patients who received 135 mg/m^2, supporting other work that suggests that 135 mg/m^2 is a less effective dose. Patients who received taxol as a 24-hour infusion, regardless of dose, had a 20% response rate, whereas those who received the drug over 3 hours had a 17% response rate. Patients on the 24-hour arm had a 74% incidence of grade IV neutropenia, with a 12% incidence of admission for febrile neutropenia, compared with a 17% incidence of grade IV neutropenia and no admissions for febrile neutropenia on the 3-hour arm. These data suggest that longer administration conveys increased toxicity without increased benefit. However, this study did not use G-CSF. Thus, it remains unanswered whether G-CSF would ameliorate this toxicity and, if so, whether the maintenance of dose intensity with a prolonged infusion schedule would make any difference in response rates and, ultimately, survival. These are important questions, especially as paclitaxel moves into use in the adjuvant setting.

Based on these trial results, studies are underway by the NSABP to compare 3- versus 24-hour infusions of paclitaxel at 250 mg/m^2 with G-CSF and by Bristol-Meyers Squibb to compare 3- versus 24-hour infusions of paclitaxel at a dose of 175 mg/m^2.

Others have suggested that prolonged infusion may be more beneficial. Paclitaxel is schedule dependent in vitro.[371] Wilson and coinvestigators[372] therefore looked at 96-hour infusional paclitaxel at a dose of 140 mg/m^2, a dose determined in a phase I study. Thirty-six patients with metastatic breast cancer were treated; all had received prior therapy, and progression after treatment with an anthracycline was a study eligibility requirement. A 48%

partial response rate was seen, with no complete responses. Toxicity was not significantly different from other reported studies. No hypersensitivity reactions were observed, however, despite the omission of the traditional premedication regimens. Thus, longer infusion times did not increase the response rate. However, longer infusion is related to additional factors, such as pump management and patient inconvenience. Because hypersensitivity is adequately managed with a simple premedication regimen there is no clear evidence to support 96-hour paclitaxel over 24-hour paclitaxel in terms of either improved response or reduced toxicity.

In addition to dose and infusion schedule (Table 22.1-17), other unanswered questions include how best to use paclitaxel—as a single agent or in combination with doxorubicin, cisplatin, or cyclophosphamide.[372-380] The optimal use of paclitaxel remains an area of active investigation. At present, it is the agent of choice in patients with metastatic breast cancer who have progressed through prior anthracycline-based chemotherapy.

Other taxanes have also become of interest in the treatment of breast cancer, such as docetaxel (Taxotere). This drug is derived from the European yew tree and can be extracted from the needles, a renewable source.[381] Docetaxel also blocks microtubule depolymerization and is 2.5 times more potent than taxol.[381] It is also slightly more water-soluble than taxol.[381] Five phase I trials have been performed with this agent and have included more than 36 breast cancer patients[382-386] (Table 22.1-18). These studies evaluated different administration schedules, including 24-, 6-, and 2-hour infusions and 1-hour infusions, given once, given on days 1 and 8 or daily for 5 days.[382-386] Each cycle was repeated every 3 weeks. Dose-limiting toxicity was myelosuppression in all these trials. The highest dose administered per cycle was 90, 100, 115, 115, 110, and 80 mg/m^2, respectively. These data suggest that the myelosuppression associated with docetaxel is dose but not schedule dependent, a finding different from that for paclitaxel.[381] Mucositis was observed in the 24-hour, daily for 5 days, and 6-hour infusion schedules.[383,384,386] No pre-

TABLE 22.1-17
Dosing Schedule Studies of Paclitaxel

Investigators	Patients	Dosing Schedule	Response Rate (%)
Holmes et al[361]	25	250 mg/m^2 over 24 h	56
Reichman et al[366]	28	250 mg/m^2 over 24 h	62
Nabholtz et al[368]	471	135 mg/m^2 over 3 h vs	22
		175 mg/m^2 over 3 h	29
NCI/Canada[369]	407	175 mg/m^2 vs	24
		135 mg/m^2	13
		24 h vs	20
		3 h	17
Wilson et al[372]	36	140 mg/m^2 over 96 h	48

TABLE 22.1-18
Phase I Trials of Docetaxel

Investigators	Dosing Schedule	Total Maximum Tolerated Dose (mg/m²)
de Valeriola et al[382]	1-h infusion days 1 and 8 q 3 wk	110
Pazdur et al[383]	1-h infusion days 1–5 q 3 wk	80
Bissett et al[384]	24-h infusion q 3 wk	90
Extra et al[385]	1– to 2-h infusion q 2–3 wk	115
Burris et al[389]	6-h infusion q 3 wk	100
	2-h infusion q 3 wk	115

medication to prevent hypersensitivity reactions was used, with an observed rate of such reactions of 18%.[381] Cutaneous toxicity was reported in the trials of 1-, 2-, or 6-hour infusion.[385,386] Occasional neurotoxicity was observed; no patient experienced cardiotoxicity.[381] A few responses were seen in the pretreated patients.[381–386] Based on these results, a 1-hour infusion of docetaxel given every 3 weeks was recommended for phase II trials.[381]

Valero and colleagues[387] treated 35 patients with anthracycline-resistant metastatic breast cancer with 100 mg/m² of docetaxel every 3 weeks. A 55% response rate was observed. Toxicities consisted of myelosuppression, fatigue, skin toxicity, and fluid retention. Dieras and colleagues[388] treated patients with untreated metastatic breast cancer with docetaxel, 100 mg/m² as a 1-hour infusion every 3 weeks, with a response rate of 72%. The number of cycles administered was limited by severe fluid retention. A follow-up trial used 75 mg/m² every 3 weeks in 38 evaluable patients.[388] The response rate was 50%, but fluid retention occurred in 70% of the patients. These authors recommended continued use of 100 mg/m² of docetaxel with the addition of premedication in an attempt to reduce fluid retention. This agent appears to be highly active in breast cancer, with perhaps the highest observed rate of activity in anthracycline-resistant patients. Continued trials of this unapproved agent will define its role in breast cancer and will attempt to decrease the observed side effects.

CAMPTOTHECINS. The camptothecins are heterocyclic alkaloids isolated from the bark and wood of the *Camptotheca acuminata* tree. These agents are the only known inhibitors of topoisomerase I. These drugs were identified in the 1960s and 1970s, but clinical trials were discontinued because of hemorrhagic cystitis and myelosuppression.[389] Later studies of structure–function relations allowed the development of more soluble, less toxic compounds for clinical development. The investigational agents in current clinical trials include topotecan, irinotecan (CPT-11),

9-amino-camptothecin, and 9-nitro-camptothecin.[390] Topotecan has been tested in phase I settings, with a recommended phase II dose of 1.5 to 2 mg/m² given as a 30-minute infusion daily for 5 days and repeated every 3 weeks.[391] Dose-limiting toxicity was myelosuppression. In an attempt to deliver higher drug doses, G-CSF was coadministered with topotecan.[391,392] However, only small increases in drug dose (from 1.5 to 1.75 mg/m²/d) occurred before dose-limiting thrombocytopenia developed. Thus, the available growth factors will not permit dose escalation; this issue needs to be reevaluated when platelet-stimulating factors become available. Dose intensity can be increased using a continuous 21-day infusion. With this schedule, the maximum tolerated dose intensity was reported as 2.8 mg/m²/wk.[393] Studies are examining combination therapy with taxol, VP-16, cisplatin, and doxorubicin.[394–397] Irinotecan has been evaluated in patients with previously treated metastatic breast cancer at a dose of 350 mg/m² as a 30-minute infusion once every 3 weeks.[398] No response data are available yet, but toxicity has been acceptable.[398] Animal data suggest that 9-nitro-camptothecin can be administered orally; if effective antitumor activity is observed clinically, this drug may become the camptothecin of choice.[399]

Other Active Agents

PLATINUM COMPOUNDS. Platinum compounds were first widely used in the treatment of germ cell tumors, followed by use in lung and ovarian cancer. These compounds appear to work by forming adducts with DNA that inhibit replication.[400] In metastatic breast cancer, cisplatin has been used primarily in combination, most frequently with VP-16, based on the activity seen clinically and in the laboratory. The NCCTG treated 44 women with metastatic breast cancer with infusional VP-16 and infusional cisplatin.[401] They could have only had one prior therapy for metastatic disease. The initial VP-16 dose was 130 mg/m²/d over 3 days with cisplatin, 45 mg/m²/d, given as a 48-hour continuous infusion beginning on day 2 of VP-16 use. The dose of VP-16 was decreased to 100 mg/m²/d because of toxicity. An overall 25% response rate was observed, with no complete responses. The response rate was higher (30%) in the patients who received the higher VP-16 dose than in the those on the lower dose (19%). Significant toxicity was associated with this treatment, however, including two treatment-related deaths from sepsis and renal failure. Twenty percent of patients had serum creatinine levels over 2 mg/dL, and 11% developed paresthesias. Other investigators observed a higher response rate in previously untreated patients with this combination (Table 22.1-19). The Italian Oncology Group for Clinical Research compared cisplatin and etoposide with CMF as first-line therapy for metastatic breast cancer.[402] One hundred forty patients were enrolled; they could have received prior hormonal therapy, but prior chemotherapy was not allowed. CMF was administered as cyclophosphamide, 100 mg/m² PO on days 1 to 14, methotrexate, 40 mg/m² IV on days 1 and 8, and 5-FU,

TABLE 22.1-19
Response Rates to Platinum Analogues in Treated and Untreated Metastatic Breast Cancer Patients

Investigators	Patients	Extent of Pretreatment for Metastatic Disease	Regimen	Response Rate (%)
NCCTG[401]	44	One regimen	Cisplatin/VP-16	25
Cocconi et al[402]	140	None	Cisplatin/VP-16	63
Kochupillai et al[403]	12	None	CAP	83
	13	One	CAP	23
Crown et al[404]	31	None	Carboplatin/VP-16	29
	14	One	Carboplatin/VP-16	0
Kolaric & Vukas[405]	20	None	Carboplatin	20
Martin et al[406]	14	Adjuvant, neoadjuvant chemotherapy, or metastatic	Carboplatin	0
	21	None	Carboplatin	32
O'Brien et al[407]	40	Adjuvant or metastatic	Carboplatin	25

NCCTG, North Central Cancer Treatment Group; CAP, cisplatin, doxorubicin, cyclophosphamide.

600 mg/m² IV on days 1 and 8, repeated every 4 weeks. Cisplatin was given at 100 mg/m² IV on day 1 with VP-16 100 mg/m² IV on days 1, 3, and 5. The response rate was 63% with the cisplatin and VP-16 combination but was not statistically different from the response rate of 48% with CMF. There was no difference in time to progression, response duration, or survival. Toxicity on the cisplatin and VP-16 arm was significantly greater, both for hematologic and nonhematologic side effects.

Kochupillai and coworkers[403] combined platinum with two other active agents for breast cancer, doxorubicin and cyclophosphamide. Even with the addition of the "best" drugs for breast cancer, a 52% response rate was observed. This number is not significantly different than that for treatment with cyclophosphamide and doxorubicin alone in untreated patients. The study regimen was more toxic, however, with anemia in 50% of patients, leukopenia in 80%, ototoxicity in 12%, and peripheral neuropathy in 8%.

Investigators at Memorial Sloan-Kettering Cancer Center substituted carboplatin at 350 mg/m² IV on day 1 with VP-16 at 100 mg/m² IV on days 1 to 3.[404] Forty-six patients were entered, including 32 with no prior therapy for metastatic disease. The overall response rate was 20%, but this rate was 29% for patients without prior therapy for metastatic disease and increased to 42% for patients who had never received chemotherapy, even in the adjuvant setting. Primary toxicity was hematologic, with two treatment-related deaths. These results are lower than those reported for cisplatin, suggesting a different activity level between these two drugs. This decreased activity was confirmed in a trial of single-agent carboplatin, which reported a response rate of 20%.[405]

The lack of response to cisplatin in previously treated patients has been observed with carboplatin also. Martin and colleagues[406] conducted two trials of carboplatin at 400 mg/m² IV every 4 weeks, one in untreated patients and one in patients who had received prior chemotherapy for metastatic disease. The previously treated patients showed no objective responses. In untreated patients, a response rate of 32% was observed. Similar results were seen in a study performed by O'Brien and colleagues,[407] in which carboplatin was used as a single agent with a schedule designed pharmacokinetically to maximize the area under the concentration-versus-time curve. Previously treated patients had an 8% response rate; untreated patients had a 33% response rate.

Although platinum and carboplatin combinations are effective in untreated patients with metastatic breast cancer, their efficacy is low in patients who have previously received chemotherapeutic agents. Given the generally long response durations in patients with metastatic breast cancer and the current treatment recommendations to give continuous chemotherapy to patients with advanced disease, patients are at increased risk not only from acute toxicities of this regimen but also from the long-term risks. Thus, peripheral neuropathy, renal toxicity, and ototoxicity pose major risks to quality of life without a compensatory improvement in survival. In addition, first-line therapy with anthracyclines is likely to provide equivalent or better response rates without the excess toxicity. The usefulness of platinum analogues in routine outpatient chemotherapy of metastatic disease is therefore limited.

IFOSFAMIDE. Ifosfamide is an alkylating agent that is a cyclophosphamide analogue. It differs from the parent compound in the placement of a chloroethyl group on the cyclic nitrogen.[408] Like cyclophosphamide, it requires hepatic activation. Because it is activated more slowly than cyclophosphamide and because 10 times as many inactive metabolites are produced, the effective dose of ifosfamide is 4 times that of cyclophosphamide.[409] Its dose-limiting toxicity of hemorrhagic cystitis is due to metabolism to acrolein. In addition, it can cause direct tubular toxicity through its prolonged half-life and slow renal clearance.[409] The development of 2-mercaptoethene sulfonate (MESNA), a urothelial protective agent, has allowed continued clinical trials with ifosfamide. In addition, ifosfamide can cause neurotoxicity, probably as a result of accumulation of chloroacetaldehyde, one of its metabolites.

Ifosfamide has been used in place of cyclophosphamide in established regimens in patients with metastatic breast cancer at doses of 1.2 to 5 g/m^2. A regimen of ifosfamide, methotrexate, and 5-FU in pretreated patients has a reported response rate of 20% to 25%.[410,411] Trials of ifosfamide with doxorubicin, with epirubicin alone or with mitoxantrone, have been conducted with response rates of 40% to 79%.[412–415] The highest response rates were seen in previously untreated patients, which is consistent with results from other regimens. High-dose ifosfamide, with doses of 6 to 9 g/m^2/cycle, has shown activity in metastatic breast cancer.[416–418]

Despite these results, there is not much impetus to substitute ifosfamide for cyclophosphamide in the treatment of breast cancer, where the two agents appear to have similar efficacy. Cyclophosphamide has fewer side effects, including no incidence of neurotoxicity or nephrotoxicity and a significantly lower incidence of hemorrhagic cystitis. Cyclophosphamide also does not require coadministration of MESNA in usual outpatient regimens, and hospitalization for treatment or long stays in the outpatient chemotherapy department can be avoided. Thus, ifosfamide, although active, is not widely used in conventional outpatient therapy of metastatic breast cancer.

MITOMYCIN. Mitomycin is an antitumor antibiotic that forms covalent cross-links with DNA and also binds to DNA through monofunctional alkylation.[419] It also directly inhibits DNA, RNA, and protein synthesis. Mitomycin as a single agent at a dose of 20 mg/m^2 in pretreated metastatic breast cancer patients has been reported to produce a 12% response rate.[420] Higher response rates have been reported from the United Kingdom for the MMM regimen, which consists of mitomycin C, 8 mg/m^2 IV every 6 weeks, in combination with mitoxantrone, 8 mg/m^2 and methotrexate, 35 mg/m^2, both given every 3 weeks.[421] This regimen has a reported response rate of 51%. However, mitomycin C causes cumulative myelotoxicity, and 43% of patients treated with MMM require dose reduction or treatment delays. In addition to neutropenia, thrombocytopenia was seen in 34% to 54% of patients in these two studies. Pulmonary and cardiotoxicity have been reported in 7% of patients and hemolytic-uremic syndrome also has been seen, although rarely. Again, because many active agents with less toxicity are available for the treatment of breast cancer, mitomycin is not used extensively in the United States.

PRINCIPLES OF CHEMOTHERAPY IN METASTATIC DISEASE

The rational use of the described agents in the treatment of metastatic breast cancer is based on the clinical observation of drug resistance in this setting. A number of principles of therapy have been described by early investigators and remain the cornerstones of treatment. Drug resistance is discussed first, followed by a number of strategies to overcome this problem in an attempt to improve outcome and survival in patients with metastatic disease who undergo chemotherapy.

Drug Resistance

Despite the availability of many effective chemotherapeutic agents, metastatic disease is incurable. Although a partial response can offer significant palliation, it does not lead to cure. Even a complete response is rarely durable, since relapse tends to occur in sites of prior disease. These clinical data support basic science work published by Skipper and associates,[422] whose experiments demonstrated that a single malignant clone can grow large enough to kill the host animal; thus, all malignant cells must be eradicated in order to produce a cure. Many reasons have been postulated for the failure of chemotherapeutic drugs to produce a cure. Tumor cells grow in a gompertzian fashion and eventually demonstrate slowed growth as mass increases.[423] Chemotherapy works best in rapidly dividing cells.[424] In addition, cell kill by chemotherapy is a logarithmic function—a given drug dose kills a constant fraction of cells, not a given number of cells.[425] Thus, the greatest benefit is achieved early in the course of treatment, with diminishing benefit with each successive course. The ability of chemotherapy to achieve complete eradication of cells diminishes as tumor size increases.

The inability of chemotherapy to cure advanced disease has been compared with the development of antibiotic resistance observed by Luria and Delbruck in bacterial systems.[426] The development of chemotherapeutic drug resistance is perhaps the primary reason that metastatic breast cancer cannot be cured, although the universal molecular mechanism of this phenomenon is unknown. Resistance can be considered in several categories. First, there may be a physiologic barrier that prevents delivery of chemotherapeutic drugs to the site of disease. The blood–brain barrier has often been cited as the reason for the late development of central nervous system metastases in a sanctuary site. Similarly, as the tumor mass outgrows its blood supply, necrosis and decreased oxygenation occur in the center of the tumor. Decreased oxygenation results in slowed proliferation and decreased efficacy of chemotherapeutic drugs.[427] Because intact blood vessels must be present to deliver the drug to the site of interest, delivery may be impaired. Patients who have undergone surgery or radiation therapy may have altered vascular and lymphatic drainage as well. Most important, however, are random mutations in tumor cells that produce drug resistance. Goldie and Coldman[428,429] hypothesized that the mutation rate is 1 in 100,000 to 1,000,000. This model assumes that resistant cells arise from random mutations, that resistant cells have the same growth kinetics as sensitive cells, and that all tumor cells are stem cells with unlimited proliferation. The first assumption is borne out by clinical observation. If no resistance occurred, one would expect all patients to be cured with chemotherapy. The randomness of the mutations fits in with the clinical observation that patients with similar tumor burdens treated with the same regimens respond at varying rates and to varying extents. The second assumption is unproved; one might suspect that resistant cells grow at a different rate, for example, than responsive cells. The last assumption is unlikely to be valid. Studies of cell kinetic data, in vitro cloning experiments, and bioassays of spontaneous murine lymphomas all suggest that only a small portion of the tumor cell population is proliferating.[429] One could overcome this resistance by using multiple chemotherapeutic drugs, since the cells would need to become resistant to all agents to prevent a cure. Based on these theories, Skipper[430] suggested that tumors of 1000 cells or less could be cured with one drug, that tumors of 100,000 cells would require two-drug treatment, and that tumors of more than a billion cells would need three or more drugs to produce a cure.

The limited sensitivity of tumor cells to chemotherapeutic agents has been documented in the laboratory, substantiating this hypothesis. When in vitro sensitivity was examined, some investigators found that 40% to 44% of human breast tumors tested in a subrenal capsule assay were sensitive to only one or two of the drugs in standard three-drug treatment regimens.[431]

Recent work has also investigated the opposite hypothesis, screening cells not for sensitivity but for the likelihood of drug resistance. Kern and Weisenthal[432] reported that, in an unselected group of patients with a variety of malignancies, 18% to 42% (depending on tumor type) failed to respond in vitro to high concentrations of accepted chemotherapy drugs. This assay evaluates thymidine incorporation and uses a long drug exposure time. Although its predictive accuracy is only 72%, its ability to predict drug resistance in the clinical setting is 92%.[433] These data also provide support for the development of random resistance but do not provide a mechanism that could be exploited to overcome this problem.

Clinical efforts to circumvent drug resistance have included evaluation of multidrug regimens, non–cross-resistant regimens, and dose intensification in both the outpatient and the transplant setting. These areas are discussed in the following sections.

Number of Drugs

The data discussed suggest that, in metastatic disease, the potential for cure exists if multidrug regimens are used. This assumption has not been borne out in clinical practice, however. Greenspan and coworkers[434] were the first to use combination chemotherapy for metastatic disease. Forty patients received thiotepa and oral methotrexate, with a 25% response rate and a 30% 1-year survival rate. Cooper[301] used a combination of cyclophosphamide, methotrexate, 5-FU, vincristine, and prednisone given

weekly with a reported response rate of 90%.[301] However, many follow-up studies have been unable to reproduce this response rate.[243] In addition, studies comparing CMF with CMFVp (CMF plus vincristine and prednisone) and CMFp with CMFVp have shown no difference in response or survival.[303,304] The addition of doxorubicin to these regimens has not improved outcome either. Single-arm studies of CA, CAMF, and VAC, as well as comparative studies of CA versus CAMF and FAC versus AC versus CAMFVp, have showed no difference in response or survival rates between the study arms.[237–239] Response rates in doxorubicin-based regimens have been between 50% and 60%, a value not significantly different from the reported single-agent response rate for doxorubicin of 40% to 50%.[234–236] Thus, the concept that multiple drugs should be used may not be accurate. It appears that effective palliation without excessive toxicity can be achieved in metastatic breast cancer patients by using active agents in full doses at scheduled intervals. Unlike adjuvant therapy, single-agent treatment in selected patients with metastatic disease may be appropriate and effective.

Non–Cross-Resistant Regimens

The Goldie-Coldman hypothesis suggests that giving multiple drugs in a short time may cure patients, since the likelihood that all cells have acquired resistance to all drugs diminishes as the number of drugs given increases.[429] These authors thus postulated that the use of non–cross-resistant therapy could increase cure rate.[435] For example, let us assume that two effective regimens for the treatment of breast cancer exist. They cannot be given simultaneously without incurring substantial toxicity. However, alternating therapy would treat cells sensitive to both treatments as well as cells with selective resistance. The therapies will be effective until the cells develop resistance to all drugs in the regimen. If one assumes that the two resistant populations are of equal size with similar kinetics, the maximal probability of cure with this approach is only 64%, still not as effective as one would hope.[435] Nonetheless, this theory has been tested in clinical practice (Table 22.1-20). Nemoto and coworkers[245] randomly assigned patients with metastatic disease to receive cyclophosphamide, 5-FU, and prednisone (CFP) versus cyclophosphamide, doxorubicin, and 5-FU (CAF) versus CA versus CFP-CA given in an alternating fashion. The highest response rate, 63%, was observed in the alternating-regimen arm compared with response rates of 17%, 25%, and 42%, respectively. However, no difference in remission duration or survival was seen.

Ransom and colleagues,[436] attempting to maximize numbers of drugs and regimens, treated 27 eligible patients with metastatic disease with three alternating regimens. Patients first received CAF, then a combination of dibromodulcitol, mitoxantrone, and vincristine. The third regimen consisted of thiotepa, doxorubicin, and vinblastine. Patients were treated with the three regimens in sequence. The response rate was 61%. Median survival was 77 weeks, not significantly different from that reported with CAF

TABLE 22.1-20
Response Rates to Selected Trials of Non–Cross-Resistant Regimens

Investigators	Regimen	Response Rate (%)	Median Survival
Nemoto et al[245]	CFp vs CAF vs CA vs CFp-CA	17 24 42 63	Not significantly different ~72 wk★
Ransom et al[436]	CAF → DMiV → TsAVb	61	77 wk
Kolaric & Tomek[437]	CMFVp-CAP	82	60+ wk

C, cyclophosphamide, F, 5-fluorouracil, p, prednisone; A, doxorubicin; D, dibromodulcitol, Mi, mitoxantrone, V, vincristine; Ts, thiotepa; Vb, vinblastine; M, methotrexate; P, cisplatin.

★ Estimated from survival curves.

alone. Nearly all patients required treatment delays or dose reductions. Eight patients had life-threatening neutropenia. Thus, these regimens added toxicity without prolongation of survival. Kolaric and Tomek[437] treated 45 patients with previously untreated metastatic breast cancer with CMFVp alternating with cyclophosphamide, doxorubicin, and cisplatin (CAP). The CMFVp regimen consisted of cyclophosphamide, 200 mg/m^2 IV on days 1 to 5; methotrexate, 30 mg/m^2 IV on days 2 and 4; 5-FU, 500 mg/m^2 IV on days 1, 3, and 5; vincristine, 1.4 mg/m^2 IV on days 1 and 5; and prednisolone, 40 mg PO daily on days 1 to 5. The CAP regimen consisted of cyclophosphamide, 300 mg/m^2 IV on days 1, 3, and 5; doxorubicin, 50 mg/m^2 IV on day 1; and cisplatin, 30 mg/m^2 IV on days 1, 3, and 5. Treatment cycles were repeated every 3 to 4 weeks. An overall response rate of 82% was noted, with a median duration of remission of 12 months. Median survival was 15 months. One patient died of marrow aplasia; 51% of patients experienced hematologic toxicity. Despite this high response rate, survival was not affected.

A modification of this principle has consisted of giving all drugs, not in two separate alternating regimens, but in a single monthly cycle. This approach is similar to the schedule in the original Cooper regimen and might have accounted for its success. Tormey and colleagues[438] performed this study in 23 patients with metastatic breast cancer. The regimen used doxorubicin, vincristine, dibromodulcitol, prednisone, methotrexate, leucovorin, hexamethylmelamine, tamoxifen, fluoxymesterone, and bleomycin within a 28-day period. Patients received three to six cycles of therapy and were observed. Overall, a 78% complete response rate and a 13% partial response rate was observed. The time to treatment failure was 12 months with a 20-month median survival. Although survival did not differ from historical controls, the time to treatment failure was unmaintained, allowing patients to remain off therapy for about 1 year. Significant toxicity was incurred, however, including three treatment-related deaths. This multidrug approach to therapy appears not to prolong survival.

Blomqvist and colleagues[439] conducted a randomized trial that examined the issue of schedule dependence. One hundred forty-eight evaluable women with metastatic breast cancer were randomly assigned to receive cyclophosphamide, 500 mg/m^2, 5-FU, 500 mg/m^2, and epirubicin, 60 mg/m^2 in two schedules. One group received all drugs intravenously on day 1 every 4 weeks; the other received drugs weekly, with identical total monthly dose. The response rate in patients treated monthly was 47% compared with 30% in the weekly therapy group. Calculated dose intensity was similar in both arms. Patients in the monthly therapy arm had better survival (21.2 months compared with 11.8 months). These results may be attributable to the fact that only 62 patients had measurable disease, thus affecting the statistical significance.

These studies do not show additional benefit for complex, multidrug, alternating regimens. Equivalent results with less toxicity can be obtained with simpler regimens.

Dose Intensity

Many investigators have explored the role of dose intensity in overcoming drug resistance, hypothesizing that higher doses of active drugs may be more important than the number of drugs used. Bruce and colleagues[440] noted in the laboratory that most chemotherapy drugs showed a linear or logarithmic relation between dose and cell kill. Bross and coworkers[441] explored this issue in 1966, examining the assumption that tumor response was linked to "host toxicity." They examined the ratio of tumor response to toxicity in 956 patients with metastatic breast cancer treated with 5-FU, 6-mercaptopurine, chlorambucil, or mitomycin C in phase II trials. Tumor response was defined as a 50% or higher regression in tumor size. Patients with white blood cell nadirs of 3000 cells/μL or less had a 28% response rate, and patients with nadirs above 5000 cells/μL had a 23% response rate, not significantly different. Patients who required treatment delays or interruptions for toxicity also had different response rates. It can now be argued that none of these agents are the most effective agents for the treatment of breast cancer and that current definitions of acceptable patient toxicity have changed.

Hryniuk and Bush[442] subsequently published extensively on the concept of dose intensity, with results based on clinical cancer trials. They defined *dose intensity* as the amount of drug administered per unit time, reported as $mg/m^2/wk$. This definition examines actual delivered drug dose rather than planned drug dose. They published a retrospective study of dose intensity in chemotherapy for metastatic breast cancer.[442] Only published trials using a Cooper-like regimen with cyclophosphamide, methotrexate, and 5-FU, with or without vincristine and prednisone, were examined. The investigators found a higher likelihood of response with increasing delivered drug doses. This analysis also suggested that the addition of prednisone to a Cooper regimen allowed higher drug dose delivery and that vincristine added little to outcome. No survival data were included in this analysis. When cyclophosphamide, doxorubicin, and 5-FU combinations were examined, a similar relation was observed, with response rate linked to dose intensity. No clear benefit in terms of survival was seen, however. An association between dose intensity and survival is suggested by the finding that a dose intensity of 0.56 in one trial resulted in a lower median survival time (10 months) compared with higher dose intensities (average, 0.96) in other trials with better reported survival time (20 months). These analyses assume equal activity of all drugs in a regimen, an assumption that clinically is probably not justified. In addition, the importance of drug scheduling and drug sequencing is not considered.

As described earlier, doxorubicin has been shown to have a dose-response curve in the laboratory and in the clinic. The impact of dose intensity on the efficacy of this agent has also been studied. Carmo-Pereira and associates[443] randomly assigned 48 women with metastatic breast cancer to receive doxorubicin, $70 \ mg/m^2$ every 3 weeks for 8 cycles, or $35 \ mg/m^2$ every 3 weeks for 16 cycles. Although the total dose was the same in both arms, the first treatment was more dose intense according to the definition of Hryniuk and Bush. Patients on the dose-intense arm had a response rate of 58% compared with 25% on the less dose-intense arm. The dose-intense arm also resulted in improved duration of response and survival.

Henderson and colleagues[444] looked at the value of "super-CMF" in 66 patients with metastatic breast cancer. The treatment regimen consisted of cyclophosphamide, 100 mg/m^2 PO on days 1 to 14; methotrexate, 3 g/m^2 IV on days 1 and 8; 5-FU, 600 mg/m^2 IV on days 1 and 8; leucovorin, 10 mg/m^2 IV on days 2 and 9; then 10 mg/m^2 PO every 6 hours on days 2 to 4 and 9 to 11; and doxorubicin, 70 to 100 mg/m^2 IV on day 29 (doxorubicin was begun at 70 mg/m^2 but was escalated to 100 mg/m^2). The response rate was 78%, with a 27% complete response rate. The median time to treatment failure was 21.6 months. Median survival figures were not provided, although at the

time of publication, 17 patients had died. This study suggests that this regimen is effective but not necessarily superior to conventional chemotherapy regimens.

Investigators at M.D. Anderson Cancer Center used a high-dose FAC regimen that required treatment in a protected environment, similar to those in use for bone marrow transplantation.[445] Thirty-three premenopausal or perimenopausal patients were entered on this trial. The treatment regimen consisted of 5-FU, 500 mg/m^2 IV on days 1 to 5 in a continuous infusion, doxorubicin, 60 mg/m^2 IV on day 1, and cyclophosphamide, 1 g/m^2 IV on day 1. Subsequent cycles used dose escalation of doxorubicin to 70 and then 80 mg/m^2 on cycles 2 and 3, and escalation of cyclophosphamide to 1200 and then 1500 mg/m^2 on cycles 2 and 3. All patients received the first three cycles in the hospital; subsequent cycles were administered in the protected environment at these doses or as an outpatient with a standard FAC regimen based on randomization at study entry. An 84% response rate was observed, with a 34% complete response rate. About 70% of patients who remained on the dose-intense arm required dose reductions; thus, the dose intensity over time between the two arms was not significantly different. Not surprisingly, no difference in duration of response or survival was observed.

Tannock and colleagues[446] compared two dose levels of CMF in 133 patients with previously untreated metastatic breast cancer. Low-dose CMF consisted of cyclophosphamide, 300 mg/m^2, methotrexate, 20 mg/m^2, and 5-FU, 300 mg/m^2 all IV on day 1. The high-dose arm used double these doses (600, 40, and 600 mg/m^2, respectively). Response to the higher dose chemotherapy was 26%; an 11% response was reported in the low-dose arm. Median survival on the high-dose arm was 15.6 months, compared with 12.8 months on the low-dose arm. When adjusted for the imbalance in pretreatment characteristics, however, no survival difference was observed. These response rates are lower than those observed in the other trials described here and are likely to be due to the relatively low doses of chemotherapy administered, even on the so-called high-dose arm. One can conclude that although high-intensity therapy with conventional means is not proved to be of benefit, it is important to use conventional therapy in adequate doses in a dose-intense fashion.

These studies demonstrate that survival in metastatic patients has not been improved by dose-intense chemotherapy, although response rates are increased (Table 22.1-21). Inadequate data exist to support the use of colony-stimulating factors to increase dose intensity of therapy not requiring progenitor cell support. It is therefore recommended that, in metastatic disease, effective doses of active agents be used without attempts at dose escalation in the conventional outpatient setting. The use of colony-stimulating factors should be reserved for patients who have experienced febrile neutropenia; physicians should also consider dose reduction.[447]

Bone Marrow Transplant

Because the dose-limiting toxicity of conventionally administered chemotherapy is bone marrow suppression, investigation during the past decade has centered on autolo-

TABLE 22.1-21
Selected Trials of Dose Intensity in Metastatic Breast Cancer

Investigators	Regimen*	Response Rate (%)	Median Duration of Response (mo)	Median Survival (mo)
Henderson et al[444]	Super CMF	78	24.5	—
Hortobagyi et al[445]	High-dose FAC	84	15	43†
Tannock et al[446]	Low-dose vs	11	—	12.8
	high-dose CMF	26		15.6

CMF, cyclophosphamide, methotrexate, and 5-fluorouracil; FAC, 5-fluorouracil, doxorubicin, and cyclophosphamide.

* For doses, see text.

† For patients with a complete response.

gous bone marrow and subsequently peripheral stem cell collections as supportive therapy for further increases in chemotherapy dose. With these procedures, the use of marrow-ablative doses of chemotherapy is possible. It is possible that quantum increases in drug dose may help to overcome drug resistance. High-dose chemotherapy with transplantation is outlined in detail in Chapter 22.2. Overall, results from multiple centers in metastatic disease have suggested a 25% 5-year disease-free survival rate.[448] These results are better than historical controls, but it is important to remember that patients eligible for transplantation at most centers are those under the age of 55 years who have a good performance status, documented partial or complete response to conventionally administered chemotherapy, and no evidence of cardiac, pulmonary, renal, or hepatic toxicity. Thus, this highly selected patient population might be expected to do better than historical controls, who include patients with a variety of performance statuses and tumor responsiveness. In addition, survival rates frequently are reported from past decades, when modern diagnostic, therapeutic, and supportive techniques were unavailable. Randomized studies comparing high-dose therapy with transplantation to conventional chemotherapy are ongoing; their results are eagerly awaited.

If high-dose therapy and transplantation are beneficial, many questions remain about optimal use of these techniques. In the laboratory, repeated chemotherapy doses have been shown to be more effective than one-time administration.[440] Should high-dose therapy be repeated more than once? With the wide availability of G-CSF and GM-CSF, the use of erythropoietin, and the impending availability of platelet support factors, autologous transplantation is likely to become safer and less expensive, and should be able to be performed in the outpatient setting. In addition, it is possible that these growth factors will make the use of marrow or stem cells unnecessary. Thus, high-dose chemotherapy with transplantation will remain an active area of investigation.

DURATION OF THERAPY

In the adjuvant setting, a set number of cycles is administered, and there is no evidence that prolonged maintenance therapy is of benefit to the patient. In the metastatic setting, however, therapy is commonly continued as long as disease is present. The rationale for this recommendation comes from a series of trials that examined both quality of life and survival.

The POA treated 250 women with metastatic disease who had undergone no prior chemotherapy either in the adjuvant or advanced setting with CAF for six cycles.[449] After six cycles, patients without progressive disease were randomly assigned to receive CMF maintenance chemotherapy or to undergo observation. Patients on the observation arm received CMF when disease progression was documented. Seventeen patients were unable to be evaluated for response to CAF. Among the remaining patients, there was a 24% partial response rate and a 6% complete response rate to the initial treatment. One hundred forty-five patients remained to be randomly assigned to receive maintenance therapy or to undergo observation. The patients on the observation arm had a median time to progression of 3.2 months compared with 9.4 months on the continuous treatment arm. Median survival times were 19.6 months and 21.1 months, respectively. Thus, no clear differences in survival were found, although these results suggest a benefit to continuous therapy.

The Australian–New Zealand Breast Cancer Trials Group entered 30 evaluable women on a study examining the benefit of continuous versus intermittent therapy.[450] Patients were randomly assigned to receive either AC or CMFp; they were reassigned to either receive continuous chemotherapy or intermittent therapy. Intermittent therapy consisted of three cycles of therapy; if patients did not have progressive disease, treatment was stopped and they were observed until progression occurred. At that point, three more cycles of chemotherapy were administered, with the same endpoints. Quality-of-life measurements were made for both patient groups. The response rate was higher (48%) in patients who received continuous therapy than in those undergoing intermittent therapy (33%). Although no survival differences were seen between the two groups, time to treatment failure was significantly increased in the patients on continuous therapy (6 versus 4 months). More importantly, quality-of-life scores showed a significant benefit for patients on continuous therapy, with improvements in mood, sense of well-being, appetite, and overall quality-of-life rating (Fig. 22.1-9). This study provides a strong rationale for the recommendation of continuous therapy in metastatic breast cancer patients.

A small study in England replicated these results. Dixon and coworkers[451] considered 26 patients who had achieved an objective response after 6 months of first-line chemotherapy for metastatic disease. Patients were then randomly assigned to discontinue therapy and to begin tamoxifen therapy until there was evidence of disease progression or to continue the same chemotherapeutic regimen. All of these patients had failed to respond to tamoxifen or their disease had progressed while they were on tamoxifen or they had been judged to have sufficiently serious disease to begin chemotherapy as the first therapy for recurrent

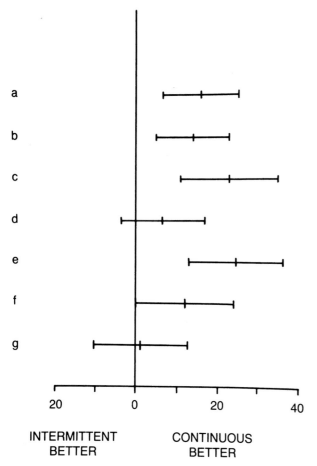

FIGURE 22.1-9 Changes in quality-of-life scores after intermittent treatment diverged from continuous treatment and before disease progression. Bars show 95 percent confidence intervals and means. The scale is expressed as a percentage of the possible range, corresponding to millimeters for linear-analogue scores. A, quality-of-life index; b, uniscale score; c, score for physical well-being; d, pain; e, mood; f, appetite; g, nausea and vomiting. (Coates A, Gebski V, Stat M, et al. Improving the quality of life during chemotherapy for advanced breast cancer: a comparison of intermittent and continuous treatment strategies. N Engl J Med 1987;317:1494)

disease. On initial study entry and after 6 months of chemotherapy, quality-of-life indicators were similar for both groups. At 3 months after randomization, the control group taking tamoxifen was recorded to have significantly worse quality of life than patients on continuous therapy. The patients on continuous therapy continued to have improving quality-of-life scores, even at 15 months after randomization. All but 2 patients in the continuous therapy group rated their quality of life as normal. Only three patients in the control group rated their quality of life as normal. These studies suggest that patients feel better on continuous therapy. It is possible that continuous therapy provides slower progression of disease, that more frequent office visits detects problems that can be palliated before they cause significant complications, or that continuous therapy provides a significant benefit in terms of emotional and psychiatric support.

Tannock and colleagues[446] also examined the effect of chemotherapy dose on quality of life. Their trial randomly assigned 133 patients with metastatic breast cancer to receive CMF at doses of 600, 40, and 600 mg/m^2, respectively, or at half these doses. Quality-of-life scales were completed in 26 patients immediately before or after chemotherapy; 35 patients completed quality-of-life scales at 24 hours after the second or additional cycles. The first set of data indicated more emesis and alopecia related to chemotherapy. Patients reported less pain, anxiety, and difficulty sleeping after chemotherapy, however, suggesting that anticipation of therapy created emotional anxiety but that this anxiety was relieved with treatment. When low- and high-dose chemotherapy were compared, a trend to increase nausea and alopecia was observed for the high-dose arm. Measures of general health, however, such as pain, body image, mobility, energy, and ability to perform activities of daily living, showed a trend to improved functioning on the high-dose arm. Although the researchers referred to these arms as high dose and low dose, they may be better described as standard dose and low dose. It appears from this study that low doses of chemotherapy may add toxicity without providing adequate antitumor effect to improve quality of life.

Treatment for advanced disease has been shown to improve quality of life, but whether it increases survival is a controversial topic. It has been difficult to prove a survival benefit, since it is generally considered unethical to randomly assign patients with disease to receive a placebo or no treatment. Thus, many studies have been performed as nonrandomized trials and compared with historical controls. These results must be viewed cautiously, because better diagnostic techniques, closer follow-up, and better access to medical care may create a lead-time bias, with earlier detection of metastatic disease and thus a false increase in survival time. The studies of intensive follow-up compared with clinical evaluation cited earlier refute this argument. In addition, prompt recognition of complications of malignancy and palliative measures may also increase survival. Henderson and colleagues[452] provided an extensive review of trials for metastatic disease and concluded that treatment conveys, on average, a 6-month improvement in survival. A population-based study from Denmark, using the comprehensive Danish Cancer Registry, concluded that chemotherapy for metastatic disease prolongs survival by 9.5 months.[453] Thus, it appears that chemotherapy has a modest impact on survival. This improvement, however, coupled with the replicated findings of improved quality of life on continuous treatment, forms the basis for recommending that all patients remain on treatment as long as objective evidence of disease persists.

PREDICTIVE FACTORS FOR RESPONSE TO CHEMOTHERAPY

Investigators have reported on factors associated with an increased likelihood of response to and survival with chemotherapy, which include the following:

- High proliferative rate
- Premenopausal status
- Presence of visceral involvement
- Presence of two or more metastatic sites
- Disease-free interval
- Good performance status

A recent report suggested that evaluation of the proliferative activity of a metastatic tumor by using the Ki67 monoclonal antibody could predict response.[454] In patients with tumors with a low proliferative rate (staining of 25% of cells or less), a 24% response rate was observed compared with 48% in patients with tumors with a high proliferative rate. These data fit with the laboratory and clinical data demonstrating the cell cycle dependence of many chemotherapeutic agents and the observation that rapidly growing tumors usually show the greatest response to therapy. Ploidy, however, does not appear to be related to response or survival. De Lena and coinvestigators[455] evaluated with flow cytometry the tumors of 55 patients who presented with de novo metastatic disease. Thirty-five women had aneuploid tumors, and this finding was distributed evenly between the category of bone-only and visceral-only disease. Ploidy had no relation to the likelihood of response or to survival, a finding replicated in a follow-up study reported by these authors.[456]

Another potential molecular marker may be the use of c-*erb*B-2 overexpression. In the adjuvant setting, a CALGB study reported that the effectiveness of CAF chemotherapy was related to overexpression of c-*erb*B-2.[457] Overexpression of this marker may also correlate with response in the metastatic setting. It is hoped that additional molecular markers will be identified to guide therapeutic decisions.

Ziegler and colleagues[458] reported no difference in response to chemotherapy or hormonal therapy, time to treatment failure, or survival based on histology. Thus, infiltrating lobular and infiltrating ductal carcinoma do not behave in biologically different manners.

Findings from the University of Arizona identified age under 40 years as an adverse prognostic sign.[459] The presence of liver involvement, more than two metastatic sites, and a performance status below 40 in the Karnofsky scoring system were also adverse signs and predicted both the likelihood of response and the likelihood of survival.

Rouesse and colleagues[460] examined the outcome of 760 patients who had initially had with localized disease but subsequently experienced relapse. Statistically significant factors in predicting survival were time to relapse, the factors that influenced initial adjuvant chemotherapy, the presence of inflammatory breast cancer at relapse, and systemic therapy for metastatic disease. A shorter time to relapse (not defined by the investigators) and poor prognostic factors present at initial diagnosis predicted a shorter survival in this model. Inflammatory breast cancer was a poor prognostic feature. Patients who received systemic therapy for metastatic disease had better survival times than those who were not treated. This study, however, included a large number of patients with initially locally advanced or inoperable disease and may not be reflective of the general population of breast cancer patients.

Inoue and associates[461] examined prognostic factors in a series of 205 patients with metastatic breast cancer treated with doxorubicin, cyclophosphamide, and ftorafur. Survival was significantly associated with a complete response to therapy, with a median survival of 50.2 months for complete responders compared with 20.3 months for partial responders and 5.5 months for patients with progressive disease. Survival was also positively correlated with a Karnofsky performance status of 80 to 100 and a disease-free interval of 2 years or more. The presence of liver metastases was associated with poorer survival.

Complete responders to chemotherapy have a better outcome but are not cured. Legha and associates[462] reported that 116 of 619 women with metastatic breast cancer achieved a complete response with chemotherapy. Most of these patients had only one or two metastatic sites at presentation. Chemotherapy was usually continued for a total of 2 years. The median duration of complete response was 17 months; ultimately, however, 70% of patients experienced relapse within 3 to 44 months. Most of these relapses were in sites of previous disease, suggesting the persistence of resistant cells. In addition, 24% of patients had relapses in the central nervous system, a sanctuary site for chemotherapy. The median duration of follow-up was 48 months, and at this point, there was no suggestion that the rate of relapse was stabilizing, suggesting that all patients might be expected to experience relapse over time.

The effect of prior adjuvant therapy on response to chemotherapy for metastatic disease has been investigated. Buzdar and colleagues[463] looked at the outcome of 62 patients who had relapses after adjuvant therapy with doxorubicin-based chemotherapy. Four patients had relapses with brain involvement. These patients were treated with FAC-CMF, tamoxifen, or other chemotherapeutic agents. Overall, a 57% response rate was noted. Response rate was 40% for both patients treated with hormonal therapy and for those treated with chemotherapy. Median survival was 15 months for all patients and 25.7 months for responding patients. These numbers are not significantly different than those reported for untreated patients, making it unlikely that adjuvant therapy compromises future therapy.

Bitran and coworkers[464] reviewed their experience in 26 patients who experienced relapse after adjuvant therapy with either CMF or doxorubicin and vincristine. Overall, a 30% response rate was observed, with a median survival of 9.6 months. The disease-free interval ranged from 2 to 40 months, and 18 patients had relapses during adjuvant therapy. Given the heterogeneity of these patient populations, it does not appear that adjuvant therapy itself adversely affects subsequent response to systemic treatment.

In an ECOG trial,[465] 501 eligible patients were treated with mitolactol, doxorubicin, and vincristine with tamoxifen and fluoxymesterone. In this study, adverse prognostic factors included ER-negative tumors, the presence of liver metastases, involvement in three or more sites, and any form of adjuvant therapy, regardless of disease-free interval. These results differ from those of other investigators with regard to the influence of adjuvant therapy. The researchers reported a wide overlap in survival curves among good-risk and poor-risk patients. In addition, attempts to fit a multivariate model with linear regression yielded limited results. These authors produced a model with 67% sensitivity, 62% specificity, a positive predictive value of 66%, and a negative predictive value of 63% in order to predict a response rate of 50% or greater to chemotherapy. Attempts to derive a model that predicted response rates of 80% or less than 20% were unsuccessful. These results suggest that many factors are involved in both response and survival. Although some general disease factors are important, individual patient factors must be taken into account as well.

Based on these data, the presence of poor prognostic signs such as multiple disease sites, visceral lesions, and negative receptors predicts for shorter survival but is not particularly reliable for an individual patient. These patients, however, have a high likelihood of response to chemotherapy and should be treated aggressively.

CHEMOTHERAPY IN THE ELDERLY

Treatment of postmenopausal women with breast cancer and patients over the age of 70 years is an issue of increasing importance in oncology. The incidence of breast cancer has steadily increased in women over age 50, and the age-specific incidence of breast cancer increases with increasing age.[466] Age is a known risk factor for breast cancer, and as the population continues to live longer, additional breast cancer cases are expected. Increased longevity of the population makes it essential to provide optimal therapy for older women, since many of these patients will otherwise be in good health. Postmenopausal breast cancer patients are more likely to have ER-positive tumors than premenopausal women, but these tumors are not necessarily associated with a relatively indolent growth pattern. It is not clear that age itself is an independent prognostic factor for survival from breast cancer or for the likelihood of response to chemotherapy. Nonetheless, many physicians are reluctant to prescribe chemotherapy

for older women with metastatic disease, even for those who have tumor characteristics that suggest greater benefit from cytotoxic rather than hormonal therapy. A study of the patterns of care for breast cancer performed at seven California hospitals identified patients stratified by three levels of comorbid illness (none, mild controlled comorbid illness, and moderate to severe comorbid illness) and by two age groups (50 to 69 years and aged 70 years or older).[467] A total of 420 patients was studied and their treatment was compared with optimal breast cancer management strategies derived from standard oncology reference texts. In patients 70 years of age and older, 67% received optimal therapy compared with 83% in the younger patients. These values improved somewhat after adjusting for comorbid illnesses, but they did not equalize. Stage III and IV breast cancer was associated with only a 34% likelihood of receiving optimal therapy. These data suggest that physicians are more likely to treat based on chronologic age rather than physiologic age. Similar results have been reported by other authors, with only 10% to 22% of women over 75 years of age treated with chemotherapy for metastatic disease compared with 49% to 73% of women aged 66 to 74 years.[468–471] When chemotherapy is prescribed, physicians are likely to inappropriately reduce the dose of chemotherapy based on age alone rather than factors such as nadir count or development of febrile neutropenia.[472]

Several cooperative groups have published studies on differential toxicity in older patients. The ECOG reviewed data from EST 2173, a trial of induction chemotherapy followed by maintenance chemohormonal therapy, and from EST 3175, in which CMFp was compared with CMFp followed by doxorubicin and vincristine.[473] These trials excluded women over the age of 65 years. No difference in toxicity was seen between women aged 60 to 65 years and younger women. The POA reviewed response and toxicity in women over the age of 70 years entered in five breast cancer protocols for metastatic disease.[474] All of these trials included doxorubicin. A randomly selected group of younger women from these same trials was used for comparison. Age groups were defined as less than age 50 (44 patients), age 50 to 69 years (47 patients), and age 70 years and older (70 patients). The response rates by age group were 40%, 31%, and 29%, which was not statistically different. This finding is particularly important in light of the requirement in three of the five protocols to reduce all drug doses by 25% for patients over age 65 years. Performance status was the best indicator of response; age was not an independent prognostic variable. No difference in time to progression or in survival was observed among the three groups. Therapeutic delays because of toxicity occurred in 17%, 14%, and 19% of the groups, respectively. Nonhematologic toxicity was evenly distributed between all groups. Patients younger than 50 years were more likely to have gastrointestinal side effects (55% compared with 47% in women aged 50 to 69 years and 46% in women aged 70 years or older). Women over 70 years of age were as likely as younger women to experience moderate leukopenia, but they had a significantly higher incidence of severe neutropenia, defined as a white blood cell count below 1000 cells/μL (13% versus 4% to 5% for younger women).

These studies suggest that chemotherapy can be administered safely to elderly women if it is warranted by the stage of presentation, tumor characteristics, and general state of health. Toxicity may be ameliorated by dose modification or by the use of colony-stimulating factors to prevent profound neutropenia and by avoidance of potentially cardiotoxic agents.

Choice of Hormonal Therapy Compared With Chemotherapy

In selected patients, response rates to chemotherapy and hormonal therapy are similar. As mentioned, the goal of treatment of metastatic disease is effective palliation with minimal toxicity. Hormonal therapy should therefore be considered as the treatment of choice for patients with receptor-positive disease, with relatively small volume, or with slowly progressing disease. The choice of chemotherapy as initial therapy over hormonal therapy for metastatic disease should be reserved for patients with ER-negative tumors or critical lesions. Critical disease includes lymphangitic lung disease, the presence of significant liver metastases, or bone marrow involvement. In other cases in which a rapid response is needed, chemotherapy offers an advantage over endocrine therapy, for which responses may not be observed for several months. Patients who have progressed within a short period (3 months) despite endocrine therapy should also be treated with chemotherapy.

Chemohormonal Therapy

Most breast cancers are heterogeneous by microscopic, biochemical, or molecular characterization. When hormone receptor assays are performed by immunohistochemistry, it is typical to see a percentage of cells that express receptor but rare to observe uniform and complete staining. It is therefore likely that tumors consist of mosaics of hormone-dependent and hormone-independent cells. These observations led to a series of trials examining the value of combined chemotherapy and hormonal therapy in an attempt to increase cure rates (Table 22.1-22).

The Australian and New Zealand Breast Cancer Trials Group randomly assigned postmenopausal patients to receive tamoxifen followed by AC at relapse, initial AC followed by tamoxifen at progression, or combined treatment with tamoxifen and AC.[475] No difference in response rates or survival was observed. Thus, the researchers recommended initial therapy with hormonal agents if appropriate and found no advantage to combined-modality treatment.

Cocconi and colleagues[476] investigated the value of adding tamoxifen to a chemotherapy regimen. They randomly assigned 143 evaluable postmenopausal receptor-positive women to receive CMF or CMF with tamoxifen. The response rate with combined therapy was 74% compared with 51% on the chemotherapy-alone arm. However, median duration of remission and survival were not significantly different. These investigators concluded that unless a rapid response to therapy was required, there was no advantage to combined therapy and that single-modality sequential treatment should be considered standard. A similar study performed by the CALGB showed no difference in response rates in women with metastatic breast cancer treated with CAF versus CAF plus tamoxifen.[477] The EORTC study of CMF versus CMF plus tamoxifen showed a 75% response rate with combined therapy compared with 49% for chemotherapy alone, but there was no difference in remission duration or survival.[478] The multidrug dose-intense study by Tormey and colleagues[438] described earlier was nonrandomized, but its single arm included both chemotherapy and hormonal therapy. No improved survival was seen relative to historical controls.

In one of the few positive trials of combined therapy, Kiang and colleagues[479] randomly assigned 81 postmenopausal women with metastatic breast cancer to receive DES or cyclophosphamide and 5-FU with DES if their tumors were ER-positive, or to receive chemotherapy versus the combined regimen if their tumors were ER-negative. These investigators found a significantly higher response rate (85%) and survival (72 versus 29 months) in ER-positive patients who received combined therapy compared with ER-positive patients who received hormonal therapy alone (53% and 29 months). In ER-negative patients, no differences were observed between the two treatment arms. These data suggest no additional benefit of hormonal therapy in ER-negative patients but suggest a potential benefit to combined-modality therapy in ER-positive patients. These results may be due to a kinetic interaction, which is addressed in the next section.

Nearly all these studies were performed in postmenopausal women, who are more frequently ER-positive than premenopausal women. An Intergroup trial, however, entered 130 premenopausal women;[480] accrual was completed in 1983. If ER-positive (80 women), patients were randomly assigned to receive CAF or the same chemotherapy with oophorectomy. ER-negative patients were assigned to receive CAF. In the ER-positive group, median survival in patients treated with chemotherapy and oophorectomy was 59 months compared with 26 months in patients who received only chemotherapy. These results suggest that ovarian ablation coupled with chemotherapy may offer improved outcome in a selected patient population. This study does not address the value of combining other hormonal modalities with chemotherapy.

Laboratory-based work in vitro suggests that combination therapy may be detrimental. Tamoxifen can decrease the cytotoxicity of both 5-FU and doxorubicin in both ER-positive and ER-negative breast cancer cells.[481] Tamoxifen slows cellular proliferation and thus interferes with the activity of chemo-

TABLE 22.1-22
Trials Testing Chemohormonal Therapy of Postmenopausal Metastatic Breast Cancer Patients

Investigators	Regimen	Response Rate (%)	Survival (mo)	P Value
ANZBCTG[475]	AC → tam at PD vs	45.1	18	NS
	tam → AC at PD vs	22.1 → 42.5	21	
	AC + tam	51.3	20	
Cocconi et al[476]	CMF vs	51	28	0.25
	CMF + tam	74	20	
CALGB[477]	CAF vs	55	20	0.76
	CAF + tam	61	21	
EORTC[478]	CMF vs	49	19	0.07
	CMF + tam	75	24	
Kiang et al[479]	DES vs	53	29	0.05
	DES + CF if ER+	85	72	
	CF vs CF	29	Not given	0.48
	+ DES if ER−	53	Not given	

ANZBCTG, Australian and New Zealand Breast Cancer Trials Group; A, doxorubicin; C, cyclophosphamide; PD, progressive disease; tam, tamoxifen; NS, not significant; MF, methotrexate; F, 5-fluorouracil; DES, diethylstilbestrol; ER, estrogen receptor.

therapeutic agents, which work best in rapidly dividing cells. Thus, current recommendations are to use hormonal agents or chemotherapy regimens sequentially. While there is no clear therapeutic advantage for simultaneous use, there is an in vitro suggestion of antagonism and an increased incidence of side effects with combination therapy.

Hormonal Recruitment Strategies

Another use of hormone therapy in the treatment of metastatic breast cancer has been in the form of estrogen recruitment. It has been shown in the laboratory that estrogen induces rapid division of both ER-positive and ER-negative breast cancer cells and also synchronizes cell division.[482,483] Because chemotherapy works best in rapidly dividing cells, investigators have hypothesized that the use of estrogen in breast cancer patients would result in improved response rates. This synergy has been demonstrated in nude mice tumor model systems.[484,485] Additional work has suggested that improvement of tumor cell kill may be due to direct effects on chemotherapeutic drugs as well. For example, Bontenbal and colleagues[486] reported increased uptake of doxorubicin into MCF-7 cells and enhanced sensitivity to drug after pretreatment with estradiol.

Conte and associates[487] recently reported the results of two trials in metastatic breast cancer patients. One hundred seventeen patients were randomly assigned to receive cyclophosphamide, 600 mg/m^2, epirubicin, 60 mg/m^2, and 5-

FU, 600 mg/m^2 given on day 1 every 21 days, versus cyclophosphamide, 600 mg/m^2 on day 1, DES, 1 mg PO on days 5 to 7, and epirubicin, 60 mg/m^2, and 5-FU, 600 mg/m^2 on day 8, also given every 21 days. Patients were treated with at least 11 cycles or until documentation of progressive disease. All patients were required to have measurable disease and no prior therapy for metastatic disease. The response rates were not significantly different between the two arms (57.2% versus 53.7%) nor were the survival rates (15 versus 22 months). The DES arm was significantly more toxic, however, with a 77.2% incidence of leukopenia on day 1 compared with 42.4% in the control arm. The investigators hypothesized that this toxicity, attributable to the schedule, might have compromised dose intensity and thus masked a true difference in response rates between the two arms.

A follow-up study was designed with a different schedule.[487] This study enrolled 258 patients, who were randomly assigned to receive either the control regimen as described earlier or DES 1 mg PO on days 1 to 3, with cyclophosphamide, epirubicin, and 5-FU, all IV on day 4 at the same doses as the first study. Again, no difference in response was noted (47.3% versus 50.9% for the DES arm). Median survival times were 17 and 20 months, respectively. Again, the DES-containing arm produced grade I or greater leukopenia in 52.4% of patients, compared with 31.7% in the chemotherapy-alone arm. These data suggest that DES may recruit bone marrow cells and thus offset any potential benefit in tumor cell kill with increased myelotoxicity.

The EORTC performed a study designed to maximize

any potential benefit of estrogen recruitment.[488] Only patients with ER- or PR-positive metastatic breast cancer were eligible. No patient had received previous therapy for metastatic disease. Adjuvant therapy was permitted if it had not contained anthracyclines and if patients had had disease-free intervals of at least 1 year. One hundred fifty-four patients were evaluable. Patients received aminoglutethimide, 1 g/d, with hydrocortisone, 40 mg/d. Premenopausal women were required to undergo ovarian ablation with oophorectomy as well. This segment of the trial was designed to produce deep and prolonged estrogenic suppression. Two weeks later, patients were treated with 5-FU, 500 mg/m^2, doxorubicin, 50 mg/m^2, and cyclophosphamide, 500 mg/m^2 IV day 1 every 21 days. In addition, patients were randomly assigned to receive either ethinyl estradiol, 50 μg, or placebo, administered 24 hours before each cycle of chemotherapy. No difference in response rates was observed (64% in the ethinyl estradiol arm and 63% in the placebo arm). No significant difference in survival was observed (106 versus 127 weeks, respectively).

At the NCI, 110 women with metastatic breast cancer were randomly assigned to receive cyclophosphamide, 750 mg/m^2, and doxorubicin, 30 mg/m^2 IV on day 1, with 5-FU, 500 mg/m^2, and methotrexate, 40 mg/m^2 IV on day 8, versus the same regimen with tamoxifen, 20 mg/ m^2 PO on days 2 to 6, and premarin, 0.625 mg PO every 12 hours for 3 days beginning on day 7.[489] Therapy was repeated every 21 days. Although response rates were similar on the two arms (65%), time to progression was longer on the hormonally synchronized arm (17.5 versus 11.1 months). Survival, however, was not statistically different (17 versus 19 months for hormonal synchronization).

All of these studies and several other published trials suggest either no benefit or a modest advantage for the use of hormonal priming[490–492] (Table 22.1-23). It is possible that this technique does not increase response. It is also likely that the optimal technology for hormonal synchronization or recruitment has not been used and varies greatly among patients. These strategies cannot yet be considered to be standard practice and should be used only in the context of a clinical trial, preferably one that involves direct measures of tumor kinetics.

Chemoimmunotherapy

In an effort to maximize the effects of chemotherapy, chemoimmunotherapy has been attempted. Initial results from pathologic examinations of mastectomy specimens suggested that a histiocytic response in the lymph nodes conveyed a better prognosis. This finding was interpreted to mean that host immune resources were being recruited to fight cancer cells. Subsequent analysis by the NSABP, however, suggested that no prognostic implication was conveyed by nodal reactivity.[493] Nonetheless, a number of trials added bacillus Calmette-Guerin (BCG) or levamisole to accepted regimens in an attempt to stimulate the immune system. Patients who received BCG did significantly worse than patients treated with chemotherapy alone; levamisole was ineffective.[312,494] One criticism of these studies has been that these are nonspecific immunostimulatory agents, and that agents targeted to produce a specific cellular response might show improved activity. Strategies to explore these possibilities, such as tumor vaccines, are in clinical trial and are discussed more extensively in a later section.

TABLE 22.1-23
Trials Testing Hormonal Recruitment Strategies in Metastatic Breast Cancer

Investigators	Regimen	Response Rates (%)
Conte et al[487]	CEF vs	57.2
	C → DES → EF	53.7
EORTC[488]	AG (and oophorectomy if premenopausal) → placebo → CAF vs	
	AG (and oophorectomy if premenopausal) →	63
	E2 → CAF	64
NCI[489]	CAMF vs	65
	CA → tam → E2 → MF	65
Allegra et al[490]	Tam → E2 → MFL	72
Benz et al[491]	Tam alternating with E2 monthly + MFL days 6 and 20	39
Lipton et al[492]	AG → CAF/CMFL vs	29
	AG → E2 → CAF/CMFL	61

C, cyclophosphamide; E, epirubicin; F, 5-fluorouracil; DES, diethylstilbestrol; AG, aminoglutethimide; E2, estradiol; A, doxorubicin; M, methotrexate; tam, tamoxifen; L, leucovorin.

Stage IV, No Evidence of Disease

A special group of patients with metastatic breast cancer deserves comment. Some breast cancer patients experience relapse with a solitary site of disease that is amenable to treatment with surgical resection or radiation therapy, and they are then rendered disease-free. Examples of such patients include those who experience relapse with chest wall nodules that are excised and irradiated and those who develop solitary bony metastases that can undergo radiation therapy. These patients are classified as stage IV, no evidence of disease (NED). Their optimal treatment has long been debated, particularly in patients with ER-negative tumors. Many have advocated watchful waiting or treatment with a nontoxic hormonal manipulation.

Some clinicians advocate treatment with six cycles of chemotherapy, extrapolated from outcomes in the adjuvant setting. About 80% of stage IV NED patients die of metastatic breast cancer within 5 years, however, suggesting the presence of micrometastates despite the inability of scans to demonstrate residual disease. These survival figures are not altered by initial site of relapse. The only exception may be for patients who have a local–regional relapse within lymph nodes, for whom 5-year survival rates in some studies approach 50%.[495] One might expect that treatment with chemotherapy when tumor burden is small would eradicate disease and delay or prevent recurrence. No prospective randomized trials have addressed this issue. Blumenschein and colleagues[496] published a retrospective study that reviewed outcomes of 136 stage IV NED patients treated with several different doxorubicin-

FIGURE 22.1-10 Recommendations for treatment of metastatic breast cancer. *Visceral crisis: lymphangitic lung disease, multiple hepatic metastases, bone marrow involvement, and significant symptoms or functional impairment that warrant rapid response to therapy. ER, estrogen receptor; PR, progesterone receptor; LHRH, luteinizing hormone–releasing hormone.

based regimens. These patients were compared with 62 historical control patients who had not received systemic therapy for stage IV NED status. The control group had a disease-free survival of 9 months compared with 38 months for the patients treated with FAC. Although the authors conclude that adjuvant chemotherapy in this setting is warranted, this study is flawed by its retrospective nature and the fact that most of the control patients (65%) were over the age of 50 years, raising the question of intercurrent medical problems, performance status differences, and other factors that bias the decision to treat with chemotherapy and thus bias the outcome of these patients. Lippman and colleagues attempted to perform a prospective randomized trial in stage IV NED patients at the NCI (written communication). Only 12 patients were accrued to this trial, however, and no conclusions can be drawn about outcome.

A recently published study evaluated the efficacy of tamoxifen therapy in a select group of stage IV NED patients.[497] One hundred sixty-seven patients with local–regional recurrence amenable to complete surgical excision followed by radiation therapy were then randomly assigned to receive tamoxifen, 20 mg/d, until progression or to undergo observation. Local recurrence was defined as initial relapse in the ipsilateral chest wall, shoulder, neck, or upper arm; or the axillary, infraclavicular, supraclavicular, or cervical lymph nodes on either side. In the good-risk patients, the median disease-free survival was 26 months in the observation group and 82 months in the tamoxifen treated patients. No overall survival difference was observed, although median survival in the tamoxifen-treated group has not yet been reached. Tamoxifen, therefore, significantly increases disease-free survival in this selected group of ER-positive women. Poor-risk patients were also included in this study, with features of ER negativity, a disease-free interval of less than 12 months, or more than four tumor nodules with a diameter larger than 3 cm. These patients were randomly assigned to undergo chemotherapy with vincristine, doxorubicin, and cyclophosphamide versus observation. Despite an accrual time of 9 years, only 50 patients were entered on the poor-risk arm and were therefore inevaluable because of small numbers. The value of chemotherapy in this setting therefore remains unproved.

Another approach has been to offer these patients high-dose chemotherapy with either autologous bone marrow transplant or peripheral stem cell transplant support. These patients have not been reported on as a separate group nor has a metaanalysis of outcome in these patients been published. Outcome for high-dose chemotherapy, however, appears to depend on the amount of tumor bulk at the time of therapy. Thus, these patients are likely to be good candidates for this investigational procedure and should be offered participation in an appropriate clinical trial.

Based on the available literature, there is no evidence that another course of chemotherapy improves disease-free survival or overall survival. Therapy with tamoxifen or megestrol acetate for patients who fail while receiving tamoxifen offers a chance at palliation with less toxicity and significantly prolongs disease-free interval. High-dose chemotherapy regimens with transplant support need to be validated in terms of efficacy.

Summary

Metastatic breast cancer is an incurable disease that affects a significant number women on a yearly basis. Despite the poor prognosis associated with this diagnosis, many patients survive 2 to 4 years, and prolonged survival has been observed in some patients by nearly every practicing oncologist. Many therapeutic alternatives offer meaningful palliation, a modest prolongation of survival, and good quality of life. Single-agent hormonal therapy should be considered as the treatment of choice, with sequential administration of other active agents in responding patients. For patients with rapidly progressive or receptor-negative disease, chemotherapy should be administered. These recommendations are summarized in Figures 22.1-10 and 22.1-11. Combination regimens are associated with a higher response rate, although single-agent therapy can be effective. Dose-intense outpatient regimens offer no therapeutic advantage, although high-dose transplant regimens are promising and require continued evaluation. There is no advantage to combined chemotherapy and hormonal therapy regimens. Active investigation into new treatments continues and may offer advances in outcome for patients within the next decade.

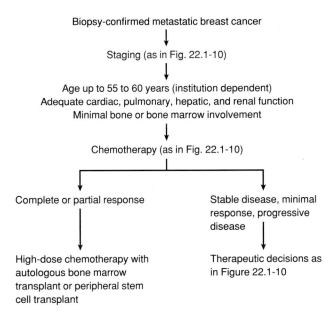

FIGURE 22.1-11 Special considerations for treatment of metastatic breast cancer.

References

1. Wingo PA, Tong T, Bolden S. Cancer statistics, 1995. CA Cancer J Clin 1995;45:12.
2. Valagussa P, Bonadonna G, Veronesi U. Patterns of relapse and survival following radical mastectomy. Cancer 1978;41:1170.
3. Saphir O, Parker ML. Metastasis of primary carcinoma of the breast. Arch Surg 1941;42:1003.
4. Borst MJ, Ingold JA. Metastatic patterns of invasive lobular versus invasive ductal carcinoma of the breast. Surgery 1993;114:637.
5. Harris M, Howell A, Chrissohou M, et al. A comparison of the metastatic pattern of infiltrating lobular carcinoma and infiltrating duct carcinoma of the breast. Br J Cancer 1984;50:23.
6. Dixon AR, Ellis IO, Elston CW, et al. A comparison of the clinical metastatic patterns of invasive lobular and ductal carcinomas of the breast. Br J Cancer 1991;63:634.
7. Lamovec J. Metastatic pattern of infiltrating lobular carcinoma of the breast: an autopsy study. J Surg Oncol 1991;48:28.
8. Jain S, Fisher C, Smith P, et al. Patterns of metastatic breast cancer in relation to histological type. Eur J Cancer 1993;29A:2155.
9. Goldhirsch A, Gelber RD, Price KN, et al. Effect of systemic adjuvant treatment on first sites of breast cancer relapse. Lancet 1994;343:377.
10. Perez JE, Machiavelli M, Leone BA, et al. Bone-only versus visceral-only metastatic pattern in breast cancer: analysis of 150 patients. Am J Clin Oncol 1990;13:294.
11. Chiedozi LC. Prognostic significance of exclusive skeletal metastases in stage IV primary carcinoma of the breast. Surg Gynecol Obstet 1988;167:303.
12. Sherry MM, Greco FA, Johnson DH, et al. Metastatic breast cancer confined to the skeletal system. Am J Med 1986;81:381.
13. Leone BA, Romero A, Rabinovich MG, et al. Stage IV breast cancer: clinical course and survival of patients with osseous versus extraosseous metastases at initial diagnosis. Am J Clin Oncol 1988;11:618.
14. Scheid V, Buzdar AU, Smith TL, et al. Clinical course of breast cancer patients with osseous metastasis treated with combination chemotherapy. Cancer 1986;58:2589.
15. Sherry MM, Greco FA, Johnson DH, et al. Breast cancer with skeletal metastases at initial diagnosis. Cancer 1986;58:178.
16. Boring CC, Squires TS, Heath CW. Cancer statistics for African-Americans. CA Cancer J Clin 1992;42:7.
17. Gordon NH, Crowe JP, Brumberg DJ, et al. Socioeconomic factors and race in breast cancer recurrence and survival. Am J Epidemiol 1992;135:609.
18. Chen F, Trapido E, Davis K. Differences in stage at presentation of breast and gynecologic cancers among whites, blacks, and Hispanics. Cancer 1994;73:2838.
19. Kimmick G, Muss HB, Case LD, Stanley V. A comparison of treatment outcomes for black patients and white patients with metastatic breast cancer: the Piedmont Oncology Association experience. Cancer 1991;67:2850.
20. Eley JW, Hill HA, Chen VW, et al. Racial differences in survival from breast cancer. JAMA 1994;272:947.
21. Elledge RM, Clark GM, Chamness GC, et al. Tumor biologic factors and breast cancer prognosis among white, hispanic, and black women in the United States. J Natl Cancer Inst 1994;86:705.
22. Ravdin RG, Lewison EF, Slack NH, et al. Results of a clinical trial concerning the worth of prophylactic oophorectomy for breast carcinoma. Surg Gynecol Obstet 1970;31:1055.
23. Muss HB. Endocrine therapy for advanced breast cancer: a review. Breast Cancer Res Treat 1992;21:15.
24. Santen RJ, Manni A, Harvey H, et al. Endocrine treatment of breast cancer in women. Endocr Rev 1990;11:221.
25. Harvey HA, Santen RJ, Osterman J, et al. A comparative trial of transsphenoidal hypophysectomy and estrogen suppression with aminoglutethimide in advanced breast cancer. Cancer 1979;43:2207.
26. Byar DP, Sears ME, McGuire WL. Relationship between estrogen receptor values and clinical data in predicting the response to endocrine therapy for patients with advanced breast cancer. Eur J Cancer 1979;15:299.
27. Allegra JC, Lippman ME, Thompson EB, et al. Distribution, frequency and quantitative analysis of estrogen, progesterone, androgen and glucocorticoid receptors in human breast cancer. Cancer Res 1979;39:1447.
28. Blamey RW, Bishop HM, Blake JRS, et al. Relationship between primary breast tumor receptor status and patient survival. Cancer 1980;46:2765.
29. Brooks SC, Saunders DE, Singhakowinta A, et al. Relation of tumor content of estrogen and progesterone receptors with response of patient to endocrine therapy. Cancer 1980;46:2775.
30. Dao TL, Nemoto T. Steroid receptors and response to endocrine ablations in women with metastatic cancer of the breast. Cancer 1980;46:2779.
31. DeSombre ER, Jensen EV. Estrophilin assays in breast cancer: quantitative features and application to the mastectomy specimen. Cancer 1980;46:2783.
32. Degenshein GA, Bloom N, Tobin E. The value of progesterone receptor assays in the management of advanced breast cancer. Cancer 1980;46:2789.
32a. King RJB. Analysis of estradiol and progesterone receptors in early and advanced breast tumors. Cancer 1980;46:2818.
32b. McCarty KS, Cox C, Silva JS, et al. Comparison of sex steroid receptor analysis and carcinoembryonic antigen with clincial response to hormone therapy. Cancer 1980;46:2846.
33. Manni A, Arafah BU, Pearson OH. Estrogen and progesterone receptors in the prediction of response of breast cancer to endocrine therapy. Cancer 1980;46:2838.
34. Nomura Y, Yamagata J, Takenaka K, et al. Steroid hormone receptors and clinical usefulness in human breast cancer. Cancer 1980;46:2880.
35. Osborne CK, Yochmowitz MG, Knight WA, et al. The value of estrogen and progesterone receptors in the treatment of breast cancer. Cancer 1980;46:2884.
36. Paridaens R, Sylvester RJ, Ferrazzi E, et al. Clinical significance of the quantitative assessment of estrogen receptors in advanced breast cancer. Cancer 1980;46:2889.
37. Pertschuk LP, Tobin EH, Gaetjens E, et al. Histochemical assay of estrogen and progesterone receptors in breast cancer: correlation with biochemical assays and patients' response to endocrine therapies. Cancer 1980;46:2896.
38. Rubens RD, Hayward JL. Estrogen receptors and response to endocrine therapy and cytotoxic chemotherapy in advanced breast cancer. Cancer 1980;46:2922.
39. Singhakowinta A, Saunders DE, Brooks SC, et al. Clinical application of estrogen receptor in breast cancer. Cancer 1980;46:2932.
40. Skinner LG, Barnes DM, Ribeiro GG. The clinical value of multiple steroid receptor assays in breast cancer management. Cancer 1980;46:2939.
41. Young PC, Ehrlich CE, Einhorn LH. Relationship between steroid receptors and response to endocrine therapy and cytotoxic chemotherapy in metastatic breast cancer. Cancer 1980;46:2961.
42. Bezwoda WR, Esser JD, Dansey R, et al. The value of estrogen and progesterone receptor determinations in advanced breast cancer. Cancer 1991;68:867.

43. Wittliff JL. Steroid-hormone receptors in breast cancer. Cancer 1984;53:630.

44. McGuire WL, Chamness GC, Fuqua SAW. Estrogen receptor variants in clinical breast cancer. Molec Endocrinol 1991;5:1571.

45. Cole MP, Jones CTA, Todd IDH. A new antioestrogenic agent in late breast cancer: an early clinical appraisal with ICI 46474. Br J Cancer 1971;25:270.

46. Westerberg H, Nordenskjold B, De Schryver A, et al. Anti-oestrogen therapy of advanced mammary carcinoma. Acta Radiol Ther Phys Biol 1976;15:513.

47. Morgan LR, Schein PS, Woolley PV, et al. Therapeutic use of tamoxifen in advanced breast cancer: correlation with biochemical parameters. Cancer Treat Rep 1976;60:1437.

48. Manni A, Trujillo JE, Marshall JS, et al. Antihormone treatment of stage IV breast cancer. Cancer 1979;43:444.

49. Rose C, Mouridsen HT. Treatment of advanced breast cancer with tamoxifen. Cancer Res 1984;91:230.

50. Furr JA, Jordan VC. The pharmacology and clinical uses of tamoxifen. Pharmacol Ther 1984;25:127.

51. Langan-Fahey SM, Tormey DC, Jordan VC. Tamoxifen metabolites in patients on long-term adjuvant therapy for breast cancer. Eur J Cancer 1990;26:883.

52. Fabian C, Sternson L, El-Serafi M, et al. Clinical pharmacology of tamoxifen in patients with breast cancer. Cancer 1981;48:876.

53. Buzdar AU, Hortobagyi GN, Frye D, et al. Bioequivalence of 20-mg once-daily tamoxifen relative to 10-mg twice-daily tamoxifen regimens for breast cancer. J Clin Oncol 1994;12:50.

54. Wolf DM, Langan-Fahey SM, Parker CJ, et al. Investigation of the mechanism of tamoxifen-stimulated breast tumor growth with nonisomerizable analogues of tamoxifen and metabolites. J Natl Cancer Inst 1993;85:806.

55. Sunderland MC, Osborne CK. Tamoxifen in premenopausal patients with metastatic breast cancer: a review. J Clin Oncol 1991;9:1283.

56. Lien EA, Anker G, Lonning PE, et al. Decreased serum concentrations of tamoxifen and its metabolites induced by aminoglutethimide. Cancer Res 1990;50:5851.

57. Nagy E, Berczi I. Immunomodulation by tamoxifen and pergolide. Immunopharmacology 1987;12:541.

58. Gulino A, Santoni A, Screpanti I, et al. Antitumoral antiestrogen stimulates natural killer (NK) activity in C3H mouse. J Leukoc Biol 1985;38:159.

59. Paavonen T, Andersson LC. The oestrogen antagonists, tamoxifen and FC-1157a, display oestrogen-like effects on human lymphocyte functions in vitro. Clin Exp Immunol 1985;61:467.

60. Paavonen T, Aronen H, Pyrhonen S, et al. The effects of antiestrogen therapy on lymphocyte functions in breast cancer patients. APMIS 1991;99:163.

61. Colletti RB, Roberts JD, Devlin JT, et al. Effect of tamoxifen on plasma insulin-like growth factor I in patients with breast cancer. Cancer Res 1989;49:1882.

62. Pollak M, Costantino J, Polychronakos C, et al. Effect of tamoxifen on serum insulin-like growth factor I levels in stage I breast cancer patients. J Natl Canc Inst 1990;82:1693.

63. Dawson-Hughes B, Stern D, Goldman J, et al. Regulation of growth hormone and somatomedin-C secretion in postmenopausal women: effect of physiological estrogen replacement. J Clin Endocrinol Metab 1986;63:424.

64. Thompson AM, Kerr DJ, Steel CM. Transforming growth factor beta-1 is implicated in the failure of tamoxifen therapy in breast cancer. Br J Cancer 1991;63:609.

65. Knabbe C, Zugmaier G, Schmahl M, et al. Induction of transforming growth factor beta by the antiestrogens droloxifene, tamoxifen, and toremifene in MCF-7 cells. Am J Clin Oncol 1991;14:S15.

66. Butta A, MacLennan K, Flanders KC, et al. Induction of transforming growth factor beta-1 in human breast cancer in vivo following tamoxifen treatment. Cancer Res 1992;52:4261.

67. Knabbe C, Lippman ME, Wakefield L, et al. Evidence that transforming growth factor beta is a hormonally regulated negative growth factor in human breast cancer cells. Cell 1987;48:417.

68. Su HD, Mazzei GJ, Vogler WR, et al. Effect of tamoxifen, a nonsteroidal antiestrogen, on phospholipid/calcium-dependent protein kinase and phosphorylation of its endogenous substrate proteins from the rat brain and ovary. Biochem Pharmacol 1985;34:3649.

69. O'Brian CA, Liskamp RM, Solomon DH, et al. Inhibition of protein kinase C by tamoxifen. Cancer Res 1985;45:2462.

70. O'Brian CA, Housey GM, Weinstein IB. Specific and direct binding of protein kinase C to an immobilized tamoxifen analogue. Cancer Res 1988;48:3626.

71. Issandou M, Faucher C, Bayard F, et al. Opposite effects of tamoxifen on in vitro protein kinase C activity and endogenous protein phosphorylation in intact MCF-7 cells. Cancer Res 1990;50:5845.

72. Gulino A, Barrera G, Vacca A, et al. Calmodulin antagonism and growth-inhibiting activity of triphenylethylene antiestrogens in MCF-7 human breast cancer cells. Cancer Res 1986;46:6274.

73. Greenberg DA, Carpenter CL, Messing RO. Calcium channel antagonist properties of the antineoplastic antiestrogen tamoxifen in the PC12 neurosecretory cell line. Cancer Res 1987;47:70.

74. McCaly EF, Mastrangelo MJ, Sprandio JD, et al. The importance of tamoxifen to a cisplatin-containing regimen in the treatment of metastatic melanoma. Cancer 1989;63:1292.

75. McClay EF, Albright KD, Jones JA, et al. Tamoxifen modulation of cisplatin sensitivity in human malignant melanoma cells. Cancer Res 1993;53:1571.

76. Jordan VC. Long-term adjuvant tamoxifen therapy for breast cancer. Breast Cancer Res Treat 1990;15:125.

77. Osborne CK, Coronado E, Allred DC, et al. Acquired tamoxifen resistance: correlation with reduced breast tumor levels of tamoxifen and isomerization of trans-4-hydroxytamoxifen. J Natl Cancer Inst 1991;83:1477.

78. Osborne CK, Wiebe VJ, McGuire WL, et al. Tamoxifen and the isomers of 4-hydroxytamoxifen in tamoxifen-resistant tumors from breast cancer patients. J Clin Oncol 1992;10:304.

79. Fendl KC, Zimniski SJ. Role of tamoxifen in the induction of hormone-independent rat mammary tumors. Cancer Res 1992;52:235.

80. Kaufman RJ, Escher GC. Rebound regression in advanced mammary carcinoma. Surg Gynecol Obstet 1961;635.

81. Wolf DM, Parker CJ, Langan-Fahey SM, et al. Investigation of the mechanism of tamoxifen stimulated breast tumor growth using non-isomerizable (fixed-ring) analogs of tamoxifen and its metabolites. Proc ASCO 1992;33:463.

82. Pommier RF, Woltering EA, Keenan EJ, et al. The mechanism of hormone-sensitive breast cancer progression on antiestrogen therapy. Arch Surg 1987;122:1311.

83. Horwitz KB. Mechanisms of hormone resistance in breast cancer. Breast Cancer Res Treat 1993;26:119.

84. Graham ML, Smith JA, Jewett PB, et al. Heterogeneity of progesterone receptor content and remodeling by tamoxifen characterize subpopulations of cultured human breast cancer cells: analysis by quantitative dual parameter flow cytometry. Cancer Res 1992;52:593.

85. Turken S, Siris E, Seldin D, et al. Effects of tamoxifen on spinal bone density in women with breast cancer. J Natl Cancer Inst 1989;81:1086.

86. Fornander T, Rutqvist LE, Sjoberg HE, et al. Long-term adjuvant tamoxifen in early breast cancer: effect on bone mineral density in postmenopausal women. J Clin Oncol 1990;8:1019.

87. Love RR, Mazess RB, Barden HS, et al. Effects of tamoxifen on bone mineral density in postmenopausal women with breast cancer. N Engl J Med 1992;326:852.

88. Fornander T, Rutzvist LE, Wilking N, et al. Oestrogenic effects of adjuvant tamoxifen in postmenopausal breast cancer. Eur J Cancer 1993;29A:497.

89. Kristensen B, Ejlertsen B, Dalgaard P, et al. Tamoxifen and bone metabolism in postmenopausal low-risk breast cancer patients: a randomized study. J Clin Oncol 1994;12:992.

90. Schapira DV, Kumar NB, Lyman GH. Serum cholesterol reduction with tamoxifen. Breast Cancer Res Treat 1990;17:3.

91. Love RR, Newcomb PA, Wiebe DA, et al. Effects of tamoxifen therapy on lipid and lipoprotein levels in postmenopausal patients with node-negative breast cancer. J Natl Cancer Inst 1990;92:1327.

92. McDonald CC, Stewart HJ. Fatal myocardial infarction in the Scottish adjuvant tamoxifen trial. BMJ 1991;303:435.

93. Rutqvist LE, Mattsson A. Cardiac and thromboembolic morbidity among postmenopausal women with early-stage breast cancer in a randomized trial of adjuvant tamoxifen. J Natl Cancer Inst 1993;85:1398.

94. Nayfield SG, Karp JE, Ford LG, et al. Potential role of tamoxifen in prevention of breast cancer. J Natl Cancer Inst 1991;83:1450.

95. Fisher B, Costantino J, Redmond C, et al. A randomized clinical trial evaluating tamoxifen in the treatment of patients with node-negative breast cancer who have estrogen-receptor-positive tumors. N Engl J Med 1989;320:479.

96. Professional Information Brochure. Nolvadex. NSABP, SIC 64033-01 1992:1.

97. Saphner T, Tormey DC, Gray R. Venous and arterial thrombosis in patients who received adjuvant therapy for breast cancer. J Clin Oncol 1991;9:286.

98. Lipton A, Harvey HA, Hamilton RW. Venous thrombosis as a side effect of tamoxifen treatment. Cancer Treat Rep 1984;68:887.

99. Enck RE, Rios CN. Tamoxifen treatment of metastatic breast cancer and antithrombin III levels. Cancer 1984;53:2607.

100. Friedl A, Gottardis MM, Pink J, et al. Enhanced growth of an estrogen receptor-negative endometrial adenocarcinoma by estradiol in athymic mice. Cancer Res 1989;49:4758.

101. Gottardis MM, Robinson SP, Satyaswaroop PG, et al. Contrasting actions of tamoxifen on endometrial and breast tumor growth in the athymic mouse. Cancer Res 1988;48:812.

102. Anzai Y, Holinka CF, Kuramoto H, et al. Stimulatory effects of 4-hydroxytamoxifen on proliferation of human endometrial adenocarcinoma cells (Ishikawa line). Cancer Res 1989;49:2362.

103. Gorodeski GI, Beery R, Lunenfield B, et al. Tamoxifen increases plasma estrogen-binding equivalents and has an estradiol agonistic effect on histologically normal premenopausal and postmenopausal endometrium. Fertil Steril 1992;67:320.

104. Uziely B, Lewin A, Brufman G, et al. The effect of tamoxifen on the endometrium. Breast Cancer Res Treat 1993;26:101.

105. Killackey MA, Hakes TB, Pierce VK. Endometrial adenocarcinoma in breast cancer patients receiving antiestrogens. Cancer Treat Rep 1985;69:237.

106. Mathew A, Chabon AB, Kabakow B, et al. Endometrial carcinoma in five patients with breast cancer on tamoxifen therapy. N Y State J Med 1990;April:207.

107. Atlante G, Pozzi M, Vincenzoni C, et al. Four case reports presenting new acquisitions on the association between breast and endometrial carcinoma. Gynecol Oncol 1990;37:378.

108. Fornander T, Cedermark B, Mattsson A, et al. Adjuvant tamoxifen in early breast cancer: occurrence of new primary cancers. Lancet 1989;Jan:117.

109. Nuovo MA, Nuovo GJ, McCaffrey RM, et al. Endometrial polyps in postmenopausal patients receiving tamoxifen. Int J Gynecol Pathol 1989;8:125.

110. De Muylder X, Neven P, De Somer M, et al. Endometrial lesions in patients undergoing tamoxifen therapy. Int J Gynecol Obstet 1991;36:127.

111. Corley D, Rowe J, Curtis MT, et al. Postmenopausal bleeding from unusual endometrial polyps in women on chronic tamoxifen therapy. Obstet Gynecol 1992;79:111.

112. Dilts PV, Hopkins MP, Chang AE, et al. Rapid growth of leiomyoma in patient receiving tamoxifen. Am J Obstet Gynecol 1992;166:167.

113. Diver JMJ, Jackson IM, Fitzgerald JD. Tamoxifen and non-malignant indications. Lancet 1986;1:833.

114. Fentiman IS, Powles TJ. Tamoxifen and benign breast problems. Lancet 1987;2:1070.

115. Dragan YP, Xu YD, Pitot HC. Tumor promotion as a target for estrogen/antiestrogen effects in rat hepatocarcinogenesis. Prev Med 1991;20:15.

116. Kaiser-Kupfer MI, Lippman ME. Tamoxifen retinopathy. Cancer Treat Rep 1978;62:315.

117. Vinding T, Nielsen NV. Retinopathy caused by treatment with tamoxifen in low dosage. Acta Ophthalmol 1983;61:45.

118. Pavlidis NA, Petris C, Briassoulis E, et al. Clear evidence that long-term, low-dose tamoxifen treatment can induce ocular toxicity. Cancer 1992;69:2961.

119. Kaiser-Kupfer MI, Kupfer C, Rodrigues MM. Tamoxifen retinopathy. Ophthalmology 1981;88:89.

120. McKeown CA, Swartz M, Blom J, et al. Tamoxifen retinopathy. Br J Ophthalmol 1981;65:177.

121. Pugesgaard T, Edler Von Eyben F. Bilateral optic neuritis evolved during tamoxifen treatment. Cancer 1986;58:383.

122. Griffiths MFP. Tamoxifen retinopathy at low dosage. Am J Ophthalmol 1987;104:185.

123. Ashford AR, Doney I, Tiwari RP, et al. Reversible ocular toxicity related to tamoxifen. Cancer 1988;61:33.

124. Gerner EW. Ocular toxicity of tamoxifen. Ann Ophthalmol 1989;21:420.

125. Tormey DC, Lippman ME, Edwards BK, et al. Evaluation of tamoxifen doses with and without fluoxymesterone in advanced breast cancer. Ann Intern Med 1983;98:139.

126. Ward HWC. Anti-oestrogen therapy for breast cancer: a trial of tamoxifen at two dose levels. BMJ 1973;1:13.

127. Bratherton DG, Brown CH, Buchanan R, et al. A comparison of two doses of tamoxifen (Nolvadex) in postmenopausal women with advanced breast cancer: 10 mg bd versus 20 mg bd. Br J Cancer 1984;50:199.

128. Goldhirsch A, Joss RA, Leuenberger U, et al. An evaluation of tamoxifen dose escalation in advanced breast cancer. Am J Clin Oncol 1982;5:501.

129. Rose C, Theilade K, Boesen E, et al. Treatment of advanced breast cancer with tamoxifen. Breast Cancer Res Treat 1982;2:395.

130. Early Breast Cancer Trialists' Collaborative Group. Systemic treatment of early breast cancer by hormonal, cytotoxic or immune therapy. Lancet 1992;339:1.

131. Jordan VC, Fritz NF, Langan-Fahey S, et al. Alteration of endocrine parameters in premenopausal women with breast cancer during long-term adjuvant therapy with tamoxifen as the single agent. J Natl Cancer Inst 1991;83:1488.

132. Ruiz-Velasco V, Rosas-Arceo J, Matute MM. Chemical inducers of ovulation: comparative results. Int J Fertil 1979;24:61.

133. Gerhard I, Runnebaum B. Comparison between tamoxifen and

clomiphene therapy in women with anovulation. Arch Gynecol 1979;227:279.

134. Tajima C. Luteotropic effects of tamoxifen in infertile women. Fertil Steril 1984;42:223.

135. Jolles CJ, Smotkin D, Ford KL, et al. Cystic ovarian necrosis complicating tamoxifen therapy for breast cancer in a premenopausal woman. J Reprod Med 1990;35:299.

136. Darbre PD, Curtis S, King RJB. Effects of estradiol and tamoxifen on human breast cancer cells in serum-free culture. Cancer Res 1984;44:2790.

137. Pritchard KI, Thomson DB, Myers RE, et al. Tamoxifen therapy in premenopausal patients with metastatic breast cancer. Cancer Treat Rep 1980;64:787.

138. Manni A, Pearson OH. Antiestrogen-induced remissions in premenopausal women with stage IV breast cancer: effects on ovarian function. Cancer Treat Rep 1980;64:779.

139. Margreiter R, Wiegele J. Tamoxifen (Nolvadex) for premenopausal patients with advanced breast cancer. Breast Cancer Res Treat 1984;4:45.

140. Planting AST, Alexieva-Figusch J, Blonk-VD, et al. Tamoxifen therapy in premenopausal women with metastatic breast cancer. Cancer Treat Rep 1985;69:363.

141. Sawka CA, Pritchard KI, Paterson AHG, et al. Role and mechanism of action of tamoxifen in premenopausal women with metastatic breast carcinoma. Cancer Res 1986;46:3152.

142. Ingle JN, Krook JE, Green SJ, et al. Randomized trial of bilateral oophorectomy versus tamoxifen in premenopausal women with metastatic breast cancer. J Clin Oncol 1986;4:178.

143. Buchanan RB, Blamey RW, Durrant KR, et al. A randomized comparison of tamoxifen with surgical oophorectomy in premenopausal patients with advanced breast cancer. J Clin Oncol 1986; 4:1326.

144. Hoogstraten B, Fletcher WAS, Gad-el-Mawla N, et al. Tamoxifen and oophorectomy in the treatment of recurrent breast cancer. Cancer Res 1982;42:4788.

145. Stenbygaard LE, Herrstedt J, Thomsen JF, et al. Toremifene and tamoxifen in advanced breast cancer: a double-blind cross-over trial. Breast Cancer Res Treat 1993;25:57.

146. Kallio S, Kangas L, Blanco G, et al. A new triphenyethylene compound, FC-1157a. I. Hormonal effects. Cancer Chemother Pharmacol 1986;17:103.

147. Valavaara R. Phase II trials with toremifene in advanced breast cancer: a review. Breast Cancer Res Treat 1990;16:S31.

148. Vogel CL, Shemano I, Schoenfelder J, et al. Multicenter phase II efficacy trial of toremifene in tamoxifen-refractory patients with advanced breast cancer. J Clin Oncol 1993;11:345.

149. Pyrhonen SO. Phase III studies of toremifene in metastatic breast cancer. Breast Cancer Res Treat 1990;16:S41.

150. Eppenberger U, Wosikowski K, Kung W. Pharmacologic and biologic properties of droloxifene, a new antiestrogen. Am J Clin Oncol 1991;14:S5.

151. Wakeling AE, Dukes M, Bowler J. A potent specific pure antiestrogen with clinical potential. Cancer Res 1991;51:3867.

152. Lykkesfeldt AE, Madsen MW, Briand P. Altered expression of estrogen-related genes in a tamoxifen-resistant and ICI 164,384 and ICI 182,780 sensitive human breast cancer cell line, MCF-7/TAMR-1. Cancer Res 1994;54:1587.

153. Coopman P, Garcia M, Brunner N, et al. Anti-proliferative and anti-estrogenic effects of ICI 164,384 and ICI 182,780 in 4-OH-tamoxifen-resistant human breast-cancer cells. Int J Cancer 1994;56:295.

154. DeFriend DJ, Howell A, Nicholson RI, et al. Investigation of a new pure antiestrogen (ICI 182780) in women with primary breast cancer. Cancer Res 1994;54:408.

155. Nishino Y, Schneider MR, Michna H, et al. Pharmacological characterization of a novel oestrogen antagonist, ZK 119010, in rats and mice. J Endocrinol 1991;130:409.

156. Chander SK, McCague R, Luqmani Y, et al. Pyrrolidino-4-iodotamoxifen and 4-iodotamoxifen, new analogues of the antiestrogen tamoxifen for the treatment of breast cancer. Cancer Res 1991;51:5851.

157. Mattsson W. Current status of high dose progestin treatment in advanced breast cancer. Breast Cancer Res Treat 1983;3:231.

158. Pannuti F, Martoni A, Di Marco AR, et al. Prospective, randomized clinical trial of two different high dosages of medroxyprogesterone acetate (MAP) in the treatment of metastatic breast cancer. Eur J Cancer 1979;15:593.

159. Haller DG, Glick JH. Progestational agents in advanced breast cancer: an overview. Semin Oncol 1986;13:2.

160. Alexieva-Figusch J, Van Gilse HA, Hop WCJ, et al. Progestin therapy in advanced breast cancer. Cancer 1980;46:2369.

161. Ansfield FJ, Kallas GJ, Singson JP. Clinical results with megestrol acetate in patients with advanced carcinoma of the breast. Surg Gynecol Obstet 1982;155:888.

162. Ross MB, Buzdar AU, Blumenschien GR. Treatment of advanced breast cancer with megestrol acetate after therapy with tamoxifen. Cancer 1982;49:413.

163. Gregory EJ, Cohen SC, Oines DW, et al. Megestrol acetate therapy for advanced breast cancer. J Clin Oncol 1985;3:155.

164. Parnes HL, Abrams JS, Tchekmedyian NS, et al. A phase I/II study of high-dose megestrol acetate in the treatment of metastatic breast cancer. Breast Cancer Res Treat 1991;18:171.

165. Pronzato P, Brema F, Amoroso D, et al. Megestrol acetate: phase II study of a single daily administration in advanced breast cancer. Breast Cancer Res Treat 1990;17:51.

166. Gaver RC, Pittman KA, Reilly CM, et al. Bioequivalence evaluation of new megestrol acetate formulations in humans. Semin Oncol 1985;12:17.

167. Carpenter JT, Peterson L. Use of megestrol acetate in advanced breast cancer on a single-daily-dose schedule. Semin Oncol 1985; 12:40.

168. Alexieva-Figusch J, Blankenstein MA, Hop WCJ, et al. Treatment of metastatic breast cancer patients with different dosages of megestrol acetate: dose relations, metabolic and endocrine effects. Eur J Cancer Clin Oncol 1984;20:33.

169. Aisner J, Tchekmedyian S, Moody M, et al. High-dose megestrol acetate for the treatment of advanced breast cancer: dose and toxicities. Semin Hematol 1987;24:48.

170. Tchekmedyian NS, Tait N, Abrams J, et al. High-dose megestrol acetate in the treatment of advanced breast cancer. Semin Oncol 1988;15:44.

171. Muss HB, Case D, Capizzi RL, et al. High-versus standard-dose megestrol acetate in women with advanced breast cancer: a phase III trial of the Piedmont Oncology Association. J Clin Oncol 1990;8:1797.

172. Abrams JS, Cirrincione C, Aisner J, et al. A phase III dose-response trial of megestrol acetate (MA) in metastatic breast cancer. Proc ASCO 1992;11.

173. Kornblith AB, Hollis DR, Zuckerman E, et al. Effect of megestrol acetate on quality of life in a dose-response trial in women with advanced breast cancer. J Clin Oncol 1993;11:2081.

174. Bardon S, Vignon F, Chalbos D, et al. RU486, a progestin and glucocorticoid antagonist, inhibits the growth of breast cancer cells via the progesterone receptor. J Clin Endocrinol Metab 1985; 60:692.

175. Romieu G, Maudelonde T, Ulmann A, et al. The antiprogestin RU486 in advanced breast cancer: preliminary clinical trial. Bull Cancer 1987;74:455.

176. Klijn JGM, De Jong FH, Bakker GH, et al. Antiprogestins, a new form of endocrine therapy for human breast cancer. Cancer Res 1989;49:2851.

177. Mincha H, Nishino Y, Neef G, et al. Progesterone antagonists: tumor-inhibiting potential and mechanism of action. J Steroid Biochem Mol Biol 1992;41:339.

178. Brufman G, Biran S. Second line hormonal therapy with aminoglutethimide in metastatic breast cancer. Acta Oncol 1990;29:717.

179. Hoffken K. Experience with aromatase inhibitors in the treatment of advanced breast cancer. Cancer Treat Rev 1993;19:37.

180. Santen RJ, Worgul TJ, Samojlik E, et al. A randomized trial comparing surgical adrenalectomy with aminoglutethimide plus hydrocortisone in women with advanced breast cancer. N Engl J Med 1981;305:545.

181. Stuart-Harris RC, Smith IE. Aminoglutethimide in the treatment of advanced breast cancer. Cancer Treat Rev 1984;11:189.

182. Cocconi G, Bisagni G, Ceci G, et al. Low-dose aminoglutethimide with and without hydrocortisone replacement as a first-line endocrine treatment in advanced breast cancer: a prospective randomized trial of the Italian Oncology Group for clinical research. J Clin Oncol 1992;10:984.

183. Wiseman LR, McTavish D. Formestane: a review of its pharmacodynamic and pharmacokinetic properties and therapeutic potential in the management of breast cancer and prostatic cancer. Drugs 1993;45:66.

184. Beretta KR, Hoeffken K, Kvinnsland S, et al. CGS 16949A, a new aromatase inhibitor in the treatment of breast cancer: a phase I study. Ann Oncol 1990;1:421.

185. Raats JI, Falkson G, Falkson HC. A study of fadrozole, a new aromatase inhibitor, in postmenopausal women with advanced metastatic breast cancer. J Clin Oncol 1992;10:111.

186. Harris AL, Carmichael J, Cantwell BMJ, et al. Zoladex: endocrine and therapeutic effects in post-menopausal breast cancer. Br J Cancer 1989;59:97.

187. Miller WR, Scott WN, Morris R, et al. Growth of human breast cancer cells inhibited by a luteinizing hormone-releasing hormone agonist. Nature 1985;313:231.

188. Fekete M, Wittliff JL, Schally AV. Characteristics and distribution of receptors for (D-trp6)-luteinizing hormone-releasing hormone, somatostatin, epidermal growth factor, and sex steroids in 500 biopsy samples of human breast cancer. J Clin Lab Anal 1989;3:137.

189. Saphner T, Troxel AB, Tormey DC, et al. Phase II study of goserelin for patients with postmenopausal metastatic breast cancer. J Clin Oncol 1993;11:1529.

190. Nicholson RI, Walker KJ, Davies P. Hormone agonists and antagonists in the treatment of hormone sensitive breast and prostate cancer. Cancer Surv 1986;5:463.

191. Brambilla C, Escobedo A, Artioli R, et al. Medical castration with Zoladex: a conservative approach to premenopausal breast cancer. Tumori 1991;77:145.

192. Kaufmann M, Jonat W, Kleeberg U, et al. A depot gonadotropin-releasing hormone agonist in the treatment of premenopausal patients with metastatic breast cancer. J Clin Oncol 1989;7:1113.

193. Harvey HA, Lipton A, Max DT, et al. Medical castration produced by the GnRH analogue leuprolide to treat metastatic breast cancer. J Clin Oncol 1985;3:1068.

194. Williams MR, Waler KJ, Turkes A, et al. The use of an LHRH agonist (ICI 118630, Zoladex) in advanced premenopausal breast cancer. Br J Cancer 1986;53:629.

195. Coombes RC, Dearnaley D, Humphreys J, et al. Danazol treatment of advanced breast cancer. Cancer Treat Rep 1980;64:1073.

196. Parmar H, Bogden A, Mollard M, et al. Somatostatin and somatostatin analogues in oncology. Cancer Treat Rev 1989;16:95.

197. Lamberts SWJ. A guide to the clinical use of the somatostatin analogue SMS 201-995 (Sandostatin). Acta Endocrinol 1987; 286:54.

198. Somlo G, Vogel C, Honig SF, et al. A phase I study of octreotide (SMS) in patients with advanced breast cancer. Proc ASCO 1993;12:93.

199. Hung H, Pollak M. Synergistic reduction of expression of the IGF-I gene by the combination of somatostatin and tamoxifen. Proc ASCO 1993;12:121.

200. Manni A, Boucher AE, Demers LM, et al. Endocrine effects of combined somatostatin analog and bromocriptine therapy in women with advanced breast cancer. Breast Cancer Res Treat 1989;14:289.

201. Ingle JN, Ahmann DL, Green SJ, et al. Randomized clinical trial of diethystilbestrol versus tamoxifen in postmenopausal women with advanced breast cancer. N Engl J Med 1981;304:16.

202. Muss HB, Paschold EH, Black WR, et al. Megestrol acetate v. tamoxifen in advanced breast cancer: a phase III trial of the Piedmont Oncology Association (POA). Semin Oncol 1985;12:55.

203. Ettinger DS, Allegra J, Bertino JR, et al. Megestrol acetate versus tamoxifen in advanced breast cancer: correlation of hormone receptors and response. Semin Oncol 1986;13:9.

204. Morgan LR. Megestrol acetate v. tamoxifen in advanced breast cancer in postmenopausal patients. Semin Oncol 1985;12:43.

205. Castiglione-Gertsch M, Pampallona S, Varini M, et al. Primary endocrine therapy for advanced breast cancer: to start with tamoxifen or with medroxyprogesterone acetate? Ann Oncol 1993;4:735.

206. Muss HB, Case LD, Atkins JN, et al. Tamoxifen versus high-dose oral medroxyprogesterone acetate as initial endocrine therapy for patients with metastatic breast cancer: a Piedmont Oncology Association study. J Clin Oncol 1994;12:1630.

207. Smith IE, Harris AL, Morgan M, et al. Tamoxifen versus aminoglutethimide in advanced breast carcinoma: a randomised cross-over trial. BMJ 1981;283:1432.

208. Gale KE, Anderson JW, Tormey DC, et al. Hormonal treatment for metastatic breast cancer. Cancer 1994;73:354.

209. McIntosh IH, Thynne GS. Tumour stimulation by anti-oestrogens. Br J Surg 1977;64:900.

210. Clarysse A. Hormone-induced tumor flare. Eur J Cancer Clin Oncol 1985;21:545.

211. Plotkin D, Lechner JJ, Jung WE, et al. Tamoxifen flare in advanced breast cancer. JAMA 1978;240:2644.

212. Tormey DC, Simon RM, Lippman ME, et al. Evaluation of tamoxifen dose in advanced breast cancer: a progress report. Cancer Treat Rep 1976;60:1451.

213. Coleman RE, Mashiter G, Whitaker KB, et al. Bone scan flare predicts successful system therapy for bone metastases. J Nucl Med 1988;29:1354.

214. Bishop JF, Smith JG, Jeal PN, et al. The effect of danazol on tumour control and weight loss in patients on tamoxifen therapy for advanced breast cancer: a randomised double-blind placebo controlled trial. Eur J Cancer 1993;29A:814.

215. Ingle JN, Twito DI, Schaid DJ, et al. Combination hormonal therapy with tamoxifen plus fluoxymesterone versus tamoxifen alone in postmenopausal women with metastatic breast cancer. Cancer 1991;67:886.

216. Powles TJ, Ford HT, Nash AG, et al. Treatment of disseminated breast cancer with tamoxifen, aminoglutethimide, hydrocortisone, and danazol, used in combination or sequentially. Lancet 1984;June:1369.

217. Hardy JR, Powles TJ, Judson IR, et al. Combination of tamoxifen, aminoglutethimide, danazol and medroxyprogesterone acetate in advanced breast cancer. Eur J Cancer 1990;26:824.

218. Mouridsen HT, Palshof T, Rose C. Therapeutic effect of tamoxifen alone versus tamoxifen in combination with gestagen and oes-

trogen in advanced breast cancer. In: Hennigen B, Linder L, Steichele C, eds. Endocrine treatment of breast cancer: a new approach. 1980:169.

219. Rose C, Kamby C, Mouridsen HT, et al. Combined endocrine treatment of postmenopausal patients with advanced breast cancer. Breast Cancer Res Treat 1986;7:45.

220. Smith IE, Harris AL, Morgan M, et al. Tamoxifen versus aminoglutethimide versus combined tamoxifen and aminoglutethimide in the treatment of advanced breast carcinoma. Cancer Res (Suppl) 1982;42:3430s.

221. Corkery J, Leonard RCF, Henderson IC, et al. Tamoxifen and aminoglutethimide in advanced breast cancer. Cancer Res 1982;42:3409S.

222. Ingle JN, Green SJ, Ahmann DL, et al. Randomized trial of tamoxifen alone or combined with aminoglutethimide and hydrocortisone in women with metastatic breast cancer. J Clin Oncol 1986;4:958.

223. Hilf R, Feldstein ML, Savlov ED, et al. The lack of relationship between estrogen receptor status and response to chemotherapy. Cancer 1980;46:2797.

224. Jonat W, Maass H, Stolzenbach G, et al. Estrogen receptor status and response to polychemotherapy in advanced breast cancer. Cancer 1980;46:2809.

225. Horwitz KB, McGuire WL, Pearson OH. Predicting response to endocrine therapy in human breast cancer: a hypothesis. Science 1975;189:726.

226. Bloom ND, Tobin EH, Schreibman B, et al. The role of progesterone receptors in the management of advanced breast cancer. Cancer 1980;45:2992.

227. Bonomi P, Johnson P, Anderson K, et al. Primary hormonal therapy of advanced breast cancer with megestrol acetate: predictive value of estrogen receptor and progesterone receptor levels. Semin Oncol 1985;12:48.

228. Epstein RJ. The clinical biology of hormone-responsive breast cancer. Cancer Treat Rev 1988;15:33.

229. Brufman G. Prognostic factors affecting response to aminoglutethimide in advanced breast cancer. Anticancer Res 1993;13:1235.

230. Lippman ME, Allegra JC. The response to endocrine and cytotoxic chemotherapy in human breast cancer and the disease-free interval. Cancer 1980;46:2829.

231. Schwartz LH, Koerner FC, Edgerton SM, et al. pS2 expression and response to hormonal therapy in patients with advanced breast cancer. Cancer Res 1991;51:624.

232. Wright C, Nicholson S, Angus B, et al. Relationship between c-erbB-2 protein product expression and response to endocrine therapy in advanced breast cancer. Br J Cancer 1992;65:118.

233. Myers CE, Chabner BA. Anthracyclines. In: Chabner B, Collins JM, eds. Cancer chemotherapy: principles and practice. Philadelphia, JB Lippincott, 1990:356.

234. Ahmann DL, Bisel HF, Eagan RT, et al. Controlled evaluation of adriamycin (NSC-123127) in patients with disseminated breast cancer. Cancer Chemother Rep 1974;58:877.

235. Hoogstraten B, George SL, Samal B, et al. Combination chemotherapy and adriamycin in patients with advanced breast cancer. Cancer 1976;38:13.

236. Taylor SG, Gelber RD. Experience of the Eastern Cooperative Oncology Group with doxorubicin as a single agent in patients with previously untreated breast cancer. Cancer Treat Rep 1982;66:1594.

237. Kennealey GT, Boston B, Mitchell MS, et al. Combination chemotherapy for advanced breast cancer: two regimens containing adriamycin. Cancer 1978;42:27.

238. Tranum BL, McDonald B, Thigpen T, et al. Adriamycin combinations in advanced breast cancer. Cancer 1982;49:835.

239. Rainey JM, Jones SE, Salmon SE. Combination chemotherapy for advanced breast cancer utilizing vincristine, adriamycin, and cyclophosphamide (VAC). Cancer 1979;43:66.

240. Irwin LE, Chlebowski RT, Weiner JM, et al. Randomized comparison of two combination chemotherapy regimens containing doxorubicin in patients with metastatic breast cancer: a Western Cancer Study Group trial. Cancer Treat Rep 1980;64:981.

241. Smalley RV, Carpenter J, Bartolucci A, et al. A comparison of cyclophosphamide, adriamycin, 5-fluorouracil (CAF) and cyclophosphamide, methotrexate, 5-fluorouracil, vincristine, prednisone (CMFVP) in patients with metastatic breast cancer. Cancer 1977;40:625.

242. Muss HB, White DR, Richard SF, et al. Adriamycin versus methotrexate in five-drug combination chemotherapy for advanced breast cancer: a randomized trial. Cancer 1978;42:2141.

243. Bull JM, Tormey DC, Lis H, et al. A randomized comparative trial of adriamycin versus methotrexate in combination drug therapy. Cancer 1978;41:1649.

244. Bezwoda WR, De Moor NG, Derman D, et al. Combination chemotherapy of metastatic breast cancer. Cancer 1979;44:392.

245. Nemoto T, Horton J, Simon R, et al. Comparison of four-combination chemotherapy programs in metastatic breast cancer. Cancer 1982;49:1988.

246. Tormey DC, Gelman R, Band PR, et al. Comparison of induction chemotherapies for metastatic breast cancer. Cancer 1982;50:1235.

247. Kolaric K, Roth A, Vukas D, et al. CAP (cyclophosphamide, adriamycin, platinum) vs CMFVP (cyclophosphamide, methotrexate, 5-fluorouracil, vincristine, prednisolone) combination chemotherapy in untreated metastatic breast cancer. Cancer Chemother Pharmacol 1984;13:142.

248. Tormey DC, Weinberg VE, Leone LA, et al. A comparison of intermittent vs continuous and of adriamycin vs methotrexate 5-drug chemotherapy for advanced breast cancer. Am J Clin Oncol 1984;7:231.

249. Falkson G, Tormey DC, Carey P, et al. Long-term survival of patients treated with combination chemotherapy for metastatic breast cancer. Eur J Cancer 1991;27:973.

250. A'Hern RPA, Smith IE, Ebbs SR. Chemotherapy and survival in advanced breast cancer: the inclusion of doxorubicin in Cooper type regimens. Br J Cancer 1993;67:801.

251. Ritch PS, Occhipinti SJ, Skramstad KS, et al. Increased relative effectiveness of doxorubicin against slowly proliferating sarcoma 180 cells after prolonged drug exposure. Cancer Treat Rep 1982;66:1159.

252. Milano G, Cassuto-Viguier E, Fischel JL, et al. Doxorubicin weekly low dose administration: in vitro cytotoxicity generated by the typical pharmacokinetic profile. Eur J Cancer 1992;28A:1881.

253. Frei E, Canellos GP. Dose: a critical factor in cancer chemotherapy. Am J Med 1980;69:585.

254. Jones RB, Holland JF, Bhardwaj S, et al. A phase I–II study of intensive-dose adriamycin for advanced breast cancer. J Clin Oncol 1987;5:172.

255. Bronchud MH, Howell A, Crowther D, et al. The use of granulocyte colony-stimulating factor to increase the intensity of treatment with doxorubicin in patients with advanced breast and ovarian cancer. Br J Cancer 1989;60:121.

256. Speyer JL, Green MD, Zeleniuch-Jacquotte A, et al. ICRF-187 permits longer treatment with doxorubicin in women with breast cancer. J Clin Oncol 1992;10:117.

257. Hochster H, Liebes L, Wadler S, et al. Pharmacokinetics of the cardioprotector ADR-529 (ICRF-187) in escalating doses combined with fixed-dose doxorubicin. J Natl Cancer Inst 1992;84:1725.

258. Sehested M, Buhl Jensen P, Sandahl Sorensen B, et al. Antagonistic

effect of the cardioprotector (+)-1,2-Bis(3,5-dioxopiperazinyl-1-yl) propane (ICRF-187) on DNA breaks and cytotoxicity induced by the topoisomerase II directed drugs daunorubicin and etoposide (VP-16). Biochem Pharmacol 1993;46:389.

259. Shaikh NA, Owen AM, Ghilchik MW, et al. Adriamycin action of human breast cancer cells: enhancement by medroxyprogesterone acetate. Int J Cancer 1989;43:733.

260. Christen RD, McClay EF, Plaxe SC, et al. Phase I/pharmacokinetic study of high-dose progesterone and doxorubicin. J Clin Oncol 1993;11:2417.

261. Stuart-Harris RC, Smith IE. Mitoxantrone: a phase II study in the treatment of patients with advanced breast carcinoma and other solid tumors. Cancer Chemother Pharmacol 1982;8:179.

262. Stuart-Harris RC, Bozek T, Pavlidis NA, et al. Mitoxantrone: an active new agent in the treatment of advanced breast cancer. Cancer Chemother Pharmacol 1984;12:1.

263. Brambilla C, Moliterni A, Codazzi D, et al. Mitoxantrone as first-salvage chemotherapy in relapsed breast cancer. Tumori 1989;75:145.

264. Harris AL, Cantwell BMJ, Carmichael J, et al. Comparison of short-term and continuous chemotherapy (mitoxantrone) for advanced breast cancer. Lancet 1990;335:186.

265. Stein M, Borovik R, Robinson E. Mitoxantrone as second-line single agent in metastatic breast cancer. Oncology 1991;48:265.

266. Burghouts JTM. Mitoxantrone, methotrexate and chlorambucil in metastatic breast cancer, a combination with relatively low subjective toxicity. Neth J Med 1990;36:43.

267. Bhardwaj S, Holland JF. A pilot trial of TMM (thiotepa, mitoxantrone and methotrexate) chemotherapy for metastatic breast cancer. Ann Oncol 1990;1:443.

268. Samonigg H, Stoger H, Kasparek AK, et al. Prednimustine combined with mitoxantrone and 5-fluorouracil for first and second-line chemotherapy in advanced breast cancer. Cancer Chemother Pharmacol 1991;27:477.

269. Hainsworth JD, Andrews MB, Johnson DH, et al. Mitoxantrone, fluorouracil, and high-dose leucovorin: an effective, well-tolerated regimen for metastatic breast cancer. J Clin Oncol 1991;9:1731.

270. Jones SE, Mennel RG, Brooks B, et al. Phase II study of mitoxantrone, leucovorin, and infusional fluorouracil for treatment of metastatic breast cancer. J Clin Oncol 1991;9:1736.

271. Robert J. Epirubicin: clinical pharmacology and dose–effect relationship. Drugs 1993;45:20.

272. Brambilla C, Rossi A, Bonfante V, et al. Phase II study of doxorubicin versus epirubicin in advanced breast cancer. Cancer Treat Rep 1986;70:261.

273. Ghavamzadeh A. Treatment of metastatic breast cancer with the combination of ifosfamide, epirubicin and 5-fluorouracil. Cancer Chemother Pharmacol 1990;26:S66.

274. Heidemann E, Steinke B, Hartlapp J, et al. Randomized clinical trial comparing mitoxantrone with epirubicin and with doxorubicin, each combined with cyclophosphamide in the first-line treatment of patients with metastatic breast cancer. Onkologie 1990;13:24.

275. Periti P, Pannuti F, Della Cuna GR, et al. Combination chemotherapy with cyclophosphamide, fluorouracil, and either epirubicin or mitoxantrone: a comparative randomized multicenter study in metastatic breast cancer. Cancer Invest 1991;9:249.

276. Gebbia V, Testa A, Valenza R, et al. Levo folinic acid and 5-fluorouracil plus high dose epidoxorubicin as first line treatment for metastatic breast carcinoma. Anticancer Res 1993;13:141.

277. Stoger H, Bauerhofer T, Kasparek AK, et al. Weekly 5-fluorouracil and high-dose folinic acid in combination with epidoxorubicin as first-line therapy in advanced breast cancer: a phase II study. Cancer Chemother Pharmacol 1994;34:75.

278. Marschner N, Nagel GA, Beyer JH, et al. High-dose epirubicin in combination with cyclophosphamide (HD-EC) in advanced breast cancer: final results of a dose finding study and phase II trial. Onkologie 1990;13:272.

279. Marschner N, Kreienberg R, Souchon R, et al. Evaluation of the importance and relevance of dose intensity using epirubicin and cyclophosphamide in metastatic breast cancer: interim analysis of a prospective randomized trial. Semin Oncol 1994;21:10.

280. Focan C, Andrien JM, Closon MT, et al. Dose-response relationship of epirubicin-based first-line chemotherapy for advanced breast cancer: a prospective randomized trial. J Clin Oncol 1993;11:1253.

281. Bastit PH, Chevallier B, Roche H, et al. Epirubicin dose and schedule dependency in 3 FEC regimens (reg) first line in metastatic breast cancer: early report. Proc ASCO 1994;13:67.

282. Carmo-Pereira J, Costa FO, Miles DW, et al. High-dose epirubicin as primary chemotherapy in advanced breast carcinoma: a phase II study. Cancer Chemother Pharmacol 1991;27:394.

283. Barni S, Archilli C, Lissoni P, et al. A weekly schedule of epirubicin in pretreated advanced breast cancer. Tumori 1993;79:45.

284. Carlson RW, Billingham ME, Kohler M, et al. Esorubicin in refractory metastatic carcinoma of the breast: a Northern California Oncology Group study. Cancer Treat Rep 1987;71:427.

285. Muss HB, Van Echo D, Korzun AH, et al. Esorubicin (4'-deoxy-doxorubicin, NSC 267469) in advanced breast cancer. Am J Clin Oncol 1990;13:233.

286. Gianni L, Vigano L, Surbone A, et al. Pharmacology and clinical toxicity of 4'-iodo-4'-deoxydoxorubicin: an example of successful application of pharmacokinetics to dose escalation in phase I trials. J Natl Canc Inst 1990;82:469.

287. Martino S, Samal BA, Redman B, et al. Phase II study of deoxy-doxorubicin in previously untreated metastatic breast cancer. Breast Cancer Res Treat 1990;17:139.

288. Hortobagyi GN, Theriault RL, Frye D, et al. Pirarubicin in combination chemotherapy for metastatic breast cancer. Am J Clin Oncol 1900;13:S54.

289. Lenk H, Tanneberge RS, Wiener N, et al. Phase II study of pirarubicin (THP-adriamycin) in metastatic breast cancer patients. Oncology 1990;47:97.

290. Dittrich C, Baur M, Mader R, et al. Phase I–II study on weekly administration of pirarubicin in patients with metastatic breast cancer. Am J Clin Oncol 1990;13:S29.

291. Scheithauer W, Samonigg H, Depisch D, et al. Pirarubicin (4'-o-tetrahydropyranil–adriamycin) for treatment of advanced breast cancer. Invest New Drugs 1990;8:207.

292. Bastholt L, Dalmark M. Phase II study of idarubicin given orally in the treatment of anthracycline-naive advanced breast cancer patients. Cancer Treat Rep 1987;71:451.

293. Pronzato P, Bertelli G, Amoroso D, et al. Oral chemotherapy with idarubicin plus cyclophosphamide in advanced breast cancer. Chemotherapy 1991;37:449.

294. Possinger K, Wagner H, Worst P, et al. Oral administration of idarubicin as first line cystostatic therapy in patients with metastasized breast cancer and favourable prognosis. Onkologie 1991;14:31.

295. Lopez M, Vici P, Carpano S, et al. Combination chemotherapy with oral idarubicin and cyclophosphamide for metastatic breast cancer. J Cancer Res Clin Oncol 1991;117:61.

296. Cowan JD, Neidhart J, McClure S, et al. Randomized trial of doxorubicin, bisantrene, and mitoxantrone in advanced breast cancer: a Southwest Oncology Group study. J Natl Cancer Inst 1991;83:1077.

297. Chandrasekaran B, Dimling J, Capizzi RL. Cross-resistance of menogaril and mitoxantrone in a subline of P388 leukemia resistant to doxorubicin. Cancer Treat Rep 1987;71:195.

298. Kennedy MJ, Donehower RC, Grochow LB, et al. Phase II trial of menogaril as initial chemotherapy for metastatic breast cancer. Invest New Drugs 1990;8:289.

299. Judson IR. The anthrapyrazoles: a new class of compounds with clinical activity in breast cancer. Semin Oncol 1992;19:687.

300. Bennett JM, Muss HB, Doroshow JH, et al. A randomized multicenter trial comparing mitoxantrone, cyclophosphamide, and fluorouracil with doxorubicin, cyclophosphamide, and fluorouracil in the therapy of metastatic breast carcinoma. J Clin Oncol 1988;6:1611.

301. Cooper RG. Combination chemotherapy in hormone resistant breast cancer. Proc Am Assoc Cancer Res 1963;10:15.

302. Canellos GP, Devita VT, Gold GL, et al. Cyclical combination chemotherapy for advanced breast carcinoma. Br Med J 1974;1:218.

303. Muss HB, White DR, Cooper R, et al. Combination chemotherapy in advanced breast cancer: a randomized trial comparing a three- vs. a five-drug program. Arch Intern Med 1977;137:1711.

304. Segaloff A, Hankey BF, Carter AC, et al. An evaluation of the effect of vincristine added to cyclophosphamide, 5-fluorouracil, methotrexate, and prednisone in advanced breast cancer. Breast Cancer Res Treat 1985;5:311.

305. Englesman E, Klijn JCM, Rubens RD, et al. "Classical" CME versus a 3-weekly intravenous CMF schedule in postmenopausal patients with advanced breast cancer. Eur J Cancer 1991;27:966.

306. Ramirez G, Klotz J, Strawitz JG. Combination chemotherapy in breast cancer: a randomized study of 4 versus 5 drugs. Oncology 1975;32:101.

307. Mouridsen HT, Palshof T, Brahm M, et al. Evaluation of single-drug versus multiple-drug chemotherapy in the treatment of advanced breast cancer. Cancer Treat Rep 1977;61:47.

308. Cummings FJ, Gelman R, Horton J. Comparison of CAF versus CMFP in metastatic breast cancer: analysis of prognostic factors. J Clin Oncol 1985;3:932.

309. Brambilla C, DeLena M, Rossi A. Response and survival in advanced breast cancer after two non-cross-resistant combinations. Br Med J 1976;1:801.

310. Valagussa P, Brambilla C, Bonadonna G. Interim vs final analysis: comparability of results in advanced breast cancer trials. Proc Am Soc Clin Oncol 1983;2:111.

311. Canellos GP, Pocock S, Taylor S. Combination chemotherapy for metastatic breast carcinoma. Cancer 1976;38:1882.

312. Aisner J, Weinberg V, Perloff M, et al. Chemotherapy versus chemoimmunotherapy (CAF v CAFVP v CMF each +/− MER) for metastatic carcinoma of the breast: a CALBG study. J Clin Oncol 1987;5:1523.

313. Creech RH, Catalano R, Mastrangelo MJ, et al. An effective low-dose intermittent cyclophosphamide, methotrexate and 5-fluorouracil treatment regimen for metastatic breast cancer. Cancer 1975;35:1101.

314. Diasio RB, Harris BE. Clinical pharmacology of 5-fluorouracil. Clin Pharmacokinet 1989;16:215.

315. Swain SM, Lippman ME, Egan EF, et al. Fluorouracil and high-dose leucovorin in previously treated patients with metastatic breast cancer. J Clin Oncol 1989;7:890.

316. Loprinzi CL, Ingle JN, Schaid DJ, et al. 5-Fluorouracil plus leucovorin in women with metastatic breast cancer. Am J Clin Oncol 1991;14:30.

317. Chang AYC, Most C, Pandya KJ. Continuous intravenous infusion of 5-fluorouracil in the treatment of refractory breast cancer. Am J Clin Oncol 1989;12:453.

318. Jabboury K, Holmes FA, Hortobagyi G. 5-Fluorouracil rechallenge by protracted infusion in refractory breast cancer. Cancer 1989;64:793.

319. Jones AL, Smith IE, O'Brien MER, et al. Phase II study of continuous infusion fluorouracil with epirubicin and cisplatin in patients with metastatic and locally advanced breast cancer: an active new regimen. J Clin Oncol 1994;12:1259.

320. Saphner T, Tormey DC, Albertini M. Continuous infusion 5-fluorouracil with escalating doses of intermittent cisplatin and etoposide. Cancer 1991;68:2359.

321. Saphner T, Tormey DC, Carey P. Continuous-infusion 5-fluorouracil combined with doxorubicin and cyclophosphamide: feasibility study. Med Pediatr Oncol 1992;20:321.

322. Delap RJ, Marshall JL, Woolley P, et al. Leucovorin, fluorouracil, and iododeoxyuridine (LIF): a phase I study in patients with advanced cancer. Proc ASCO 1993;12:221.

323. Muggia FM, Camacho FJ, Kaplan BH, et al. Weekly 5-fluorouracil combined with PALA: toxic and therapeutic effects in colorectal cancer. Cancer Treat Rep 1987;71:253.

324. Scher RM, Goldstein LJ, Kosierowski R, et al. Phase II study of high dose weekly 5-fluorouracil (5-FU) and phosphonacetyl-l-acid (PALA) in metastatic breast cancer. Proc ASCO 1994;13:112.

325. Brunetti I, Darnowski J, Falcone A. Azidothymidine enhances fluorouracil and methotrexate antitumor and therapeutic activity. Proc Am Assoc Ca Res 1989;30:595.

326. Posner M, Darnowski J, Weitberg A. A phase I trial of azidothymidine and 5-fluorouracil with phosphonacetyl-L-aspartic acid (PALA) and leucovorin: a phase I study. Proc Am Assoc Cancer Res 1990;9:104.

327. Papac R, Jacobs E, Wong F. Clinical evaluation of the pyrimidine nucleosides 5-fluoro-2'-deoxyuridine and 5-iodo-2'-deoxyuridine. Cancer Chemother Rep 1963;20:143.

328. Speth P, Kinsella T, Belanger K. Fluorodeoxyuridine modulation of the incorporation of iododeoxyuridine into DNA of granulocytes: a phase I and clinical pharmacological study. Cancer Res 1988;48:2933.

329. Remick S, Benson A, Weese J. Phase I trial of 5-iodo-2'-deoxyuridine and 5-fluorouracil in patients with advanced hepatic malignancy: biochemically based combination chemotherapy. Cancer Res 1989;49:6437.

330. Jolivet J, Cowan KH, Curt GA, et al. The pharmacological and clinical use of methotrexate. N Engl J Med 1983;309:1094.

331. Kaye SB, Sangster G, Hutcheon A, et al. Sequential methotrexate plus 5-FU in advanced breast and colorectal cancers: a phase II study. Cancer Treat Rep 1984;68:547.

332. Herrmann R, Manegold C, Schroeder M, et al. Sequential methotrexate and 5-FU in breast cancer resistant to the conventional application of these drugs. Cancer Treat Rep 1984;68:1279.

333. Gewirtz AM, Cadman E. Preliminary report on the efficacy of sequential methotrexate and 5-fluorouracil in advanced breast cancer. Cancer 1981;47:2552.

334. Friedman MA, Marcus FS, Cassidy MJ, et al. 5-Fluorouracil + oncovin + adriamycin + mitomycin C (FOAM): an effective program for breast cancer, even for disease refractory to previous chemotherapy: a Northern California Oncology Group (NCOG) Study. Cancer 1983;52:193.

335. Fraschini G, Yap HY, Hortobagyi G, et al. Five-day continuous-infusion vinblastine in the treatment of breast cancer. Cancer 1985;56:225.

336. Theriault RL, Fraschini G, Holmes FA, et al. The myeloprotective effect of recombinant human granulocyte-macrophage colony-stimulating factor given sequentially with continuous infusion vinblastine in metastatic breast cancer patients. Am J Clin Oncol 1993;16:132.

337. Giaccone G, Bagatella M, Donadio M, et al. Phase II study of divided-dose vinblastine in advanced cancer patients. Tumori 1989;75:248.

338. Hart RD, Perloff M, Holland JF. One-day VATH (vinblastine, adriamycin, thiotepa, and halotestin) therapy for advanced breast cancer refractory to chemotherapy. Cancer 1981;48:1522.

339. Roth BJ, Sledge GW, Williams SD, et al. Methotrexate, vinblastine, doxorubicin, and cisplatin in metastatic breast cancer. Cancer 1991;68:248.

340. Bisagni G, Cocconi G, Ceci G, et al. M-VAC combination in locally advanced, locally recurrent or metastatic breast carcinoma: a phase II study. Ann Oncol 1994;5:93.

341. Perrone F, De Placido S, Carlomagno C, et al. Chemotherapy with mitomycin C and vinblastine in pretreated metastatic breast cancer. Tumori 1993;79:254.

342. Sedlacek SM. First-line and salvage therapy of metastatic breast cancer with mitomycin/vinblastine. Oncology 1993;50(Suppl):16.

343. Brambilla C, Zambetti M, Ferrari L, et al. Mitomycin C and vinblastine in advanced refractory breast cancer. Tumori 1989;75:141.

344. Garewal HS, Brooks RJ, Jones SE, et al. Treatment of advanced breast cancer with mitomycin C combined with vinblastine or vindesine. J Clin Oncol 1983;1:772.

345. Cruciani G, Tienghi A, Florentini G, et al. Mitoxantrone (M) and vinblastine (V) in the treatment of advanced breast cancer. Tumori 1990;76:196.

346. Robins HI, Tormey DC, Skelley MJ, et al. Vindesine: a phase II trial in advanced breast cancer patients. Cancer Clin Trials 1981;4:371.

347. Cobleigh MA, Williams SD, Einhorn LH. Phase II study of vindesine in patients with metastatic breast cancer. Cancer Treat Rep 1981;65:659.

348. Rausa L, Russo A, Gebbia V, et al. Combination chemotherapy with mitomycin C, vindesine and melphalan for refractory metastatic breast cancer. J Cancer Res Clin Oncol 1991;117:266.

349. Marty M, Extra JM, Dieras V, et al. A review of the antitumour activity of vinorelbine in breast cancer. Drugs 1992;44:29.

350. Gasparini G, Caffo O, Barni S, et al. Vinorelbine is an active antiproliferative agent in pretreated advanced breast cancer patients: a phase II study. J Clin Oncol 1994;12:2094.

351. Fumoleau P, Delgado FM, Delozier T, et al. Phase II trial of weekly intravenous vinorelbine in first-line advanced breast cancer chemotherapy. J Clin Oncol 1993;11:1245.

352. Romero A, Rabinovich MG, Vallejo CT, et al. Vinorelbine as first-line chemotherapy for metastatic breast carcinoma. J Clin Oncol 1994;12:336.

353. Toussaint C, Izzo J, Spielman M, et al. Phase I/II trial of continuous infusion vinorelbine for advanced breast cancer. J Clin Oncol 1994;12:2102.

354. Martin M, Lluch A, Casado A, et al. Clinical activity of chronic oral etoposide in previously treated metastatic breast cancer. J Clin Oncol 1994;12:986.

355. Dombernowsky P, Nissen NI. Schedule dependency of the antileukemic activity of the podophyllotoxin-derivative VP 16-213 (NSC-141540) in L1210 leukemia. APMIS 1973;715.

356. Nichols CR. Role of etoposide in treatment of breast cancer. Semin Oncol 1992;19:67.

357. Calvert AH, Lind MJ, Millward MM, et al. Long-term oral etoposide in metastatic breast cancer: clinical and pharmacokinetic results. Cancer Treat Rev 1993;19:27.

358. Schabel FM Jr, Trader MW, Laster WR, et al. cis-Dichlorodiammineplatinum(II): combination chemotherapy and cross-resistance studies with tumor of mice. Cancer Treat Rep 1979;63:1459.

359. Estape J, Daniels M, Vinolas N, et al. Combination chemotherapy with oral etoposide plus intravenous cyclophosphamide in liver metastases of breast cancer. Am J Clin Oncol 1990;13:98.

360. Rowinsky EK, Cazenave LA, Donehower RC. Taxol: a novel investigational antimicrobule agent. J Natl Cancer Inst 1990;82:1247.

361. Holmes FA, Walters RS, Theriault RL, et al. Phase II trial of taxol, an active drug in the treatment of metastatic breast cancer. J Natl Cancer Inst 1991;83:1797.

362. McGuire WP, Rowinsky EK, Rosenshein NB, et al. Taxol: a unique antineoplastic agent with significant activity in advanced ovarian epithelial neoplasms. Ann Intern Med 1989;111:273.

363. Raghavan VT, Bloomer WD, Merkel DE. Taxol and radiation recall dermatitis. Lancet 1993;341:1354.

364. Shenkier T, Gelmon K. Paclitaxel and radiation-recall dermatitis. J Clin Oncol 1994;12:439.

365. Pestalozzi BC, Sotos GA, Choyke PL, et al. Typhlitis resulting from treatment with taxol and doxorubicin in patients with metastatic breast cancer. Cancer 1993;71:1797.

366. Reichman BS, Seidman AD, Crown JPA, et al. Paclitaxel and recombinant human granulocyte colony-stimulating factor as initial chemotherapy for metastatic breast cancer. J Clin Oncol 1993;11:1943.

367. Schiller JH, Storer B, Tutsch K, et al. Phase I trial of 3-hour infusion of paclitaxel with or without granulocyte colony-stimulating factor in patients with advanced cancer. J Clin Oncol 1994;12:241.

368. Nabholtz JM, Gelmon K, Bontenbal M, et al. Randomized trial of two doses of taxol in metastatic breast cancer: an interim analysis. Proc ASCO 1993;12:60.

369. Swenerton K, Eisenhauer E, ten Bokkel Huinink W, et al. Taxol in relapsed ovarian cancer: high *vs* low dose and short *vs* long infusion: a European-Canadian study coordinated by the NCI Canada Clinical Trials Group. Proc ASCO 1993;12:256.

370. Arbuck SG. Paclitaxel: what schedule? what dose? J Clin Oncol 1994;12:233.

371. Lopes NM, Adams EG, Pitts TW. Cell kill kinetics and cell cycle effects of taxol on human and hamster ovarian cell lines. Cancer Chemother Pharmacol 1993;32:235.

372. Wilson WH, Berg SL, Bryant G, et al. Paclitaxel in doxorubicin-refractory or mitoxantrone-refractory breast cancer: a phase II trial of 96-hour infusion. J Clin Oncol 1994;12:1621.

373. Koechli OR, Sevin BU, Perras JP, et al. Characteristics of the combination paclitaxel plus doxorubicin in breast cancer cell lines analyzed with the ATP-cell viability assay. Breast Cancer Res Treat 1993;28:21.

374. Berg SL, Cowen KH, Balis FM, et al. Pharmacokinetics of taxol and doxorubicin administered alone and in combination by continuous 72-hour infusion. J Natl Cancer Inst 1994;86:143.

375. Gianni L, Straneo M, Capri G, et al. Optimal dose and sequence finding study of paclitaxel (P) by 3 H infusion combined with bolus doxorubicin (D) in untreated metastatic breast cancer patients (PTS). Proc ASCO 1994;13:74.

376. Rowinsky EK, Gilbert MR, McGuire WP, et al. Sequences of taxol and cisplatin: a phase I and pharmacologic study. J Clin Oncol 1991;9:1692.

377. Gelmon KA, O'Reilly S, Plenderleith IH, et al. Bi-weekly paclitaxel and cisplatin in the treatment of metastatic breast cancer. Proc ASCO 1994;13:71.

378. Wasserheit C, Alter R, Speyer J, et al. Phase II trial of paclitaxel and cisplatin (DDP) in women with metastatic breast cancer. Proc ASCO 1994;13:100.

379. Pagani O, Sessa C, Goldhirsch A, et al. Taxol (T) and cyclophosphamide (C) in patients (PTS) with advanced breast cancer (ABC): a dose-finding study with the addition of G-CSF. Proc ASCO 1994;13:61.

380. Tolcher A, Cowan K, Riley J, et al. Phase I study of paclitaxel

(T) and cyclophosphamide (CTX) and G-CSF in metastatic breast cancer. Proc ASCO 1994;13:73.

381. Pazdur R, Kudelka AP, Kavanagh JJ, et al. The taxoids: paclitaxel (Taxol) and docetaxel (Taxotere). Cancer Treat Rev 1993;19:351.

382. de Valeriola D, Brassine C, Piccart M, et al. Phase I pharmacokinetic (PK) study of taxotere (T) (RP56976, NSC628503) administered as a weekly infusion. Proc Am Assoc Cancer Res 1992;33:261.

383. Pazdur R, Newman RA, Newman BM, et al. Phase I trial of taxotere: five-day schedule. J Natl Cancer Inst 1992;84:1781.

384. Bissett D, Setanoians A, Cassidy J, et al. Phase I and pharmacokinetic study of taxotere (RP#56976) administered as a 24-hour infusion. Cancer Res 1993;53:523.

385. Extra JM, Rousseau F, Bruno R, et al. Phase I and pharmacokinetic study of taxotere (RP 56976; NSC 628503) given as a short intravenous infusion. Cancer Res 1993;53:1037.

386. Burris H, Irvin J, Kalter S, et al. Phase I clinical trial of taxotere administered as either a 2-hour or 6-hour intravenous infusion. J Clin Oncol 1993;11:950.

387. Valero V, Walters R, Theriault R, et al. Phase II study of docetaxel (taxotere) in anthracycline-refractory metastatic breast cancer (armbc). Proc ASCO 1994;13:470.

388. Dieras Y, Furnoleau P, Chevallier B, et al. Second EORTC-clinical screening group (CSG) phase II trial of taxotere (docetaxel) as first line chemotherapy (CT) in advanced breast cancer. Proc ASCO 1994;13:78.

389. Rothenberg ML, Kuhn JG, Burris H, et al. Phase I clinical trial of taxotere administered as either a 2-hour or 6-hour intravenous infusion. J Clin Oncol 1993;11:950.

390. Hawkins MJ. New anticancer agents: taxol, camptothecin analogs and anthrapyrazoles. Oncology 1992;6:17.

391. Rowinsky E, Sartorius S, Grochow L, et al. Phase I and pharmacologic study of topotecan, an inhibitor of topoisomerase I, with granulocyte colony-stimulating factor (G-CSF): toxicologic differences between concurrent and posttreatment G-CSF administration. Proc ASCO 1992;11:116.

392. Murphy B, Saltz L, Sirott M, et al. Granulocyte-colony stimulating factor (G-CSF) does not increase the maximum tolerated dose (MTD) in a phase I study of topotecan. Proc ASCO 1992;11:139.

393. Hochster H, Speyer J, Oratz R, et al. Topotecan 21 day continuous infusion: excellent tolerance of a novel schedule. Proc ASCO 1993;12:139.

394. Lilenbaum RC, Rosner GL, Ratain MJ, et al. Phase I study of taxol and topotecan in patients with advanced solid tumors (calgb 9362). Proc ASCO 1994;13:131.

395. Eckhardt JR, Burris JA, Von Hoff DD, et al. Measurement of tumor topoisomerase I and II levels during the sequential administration of topotecan and etoposide. Proc ASCO 1994;13:141.

396. Rowinsky E, Grochow L, Kaufmann S, et al. Sequence-dependent effects of topotecan (T) and cisplatin (C) in a phase I and pharmacokinetic (PR) study. Proc ASCO 1994;13:142.

397. Tolcher AW, O'Shaughnessy JA, Weiss RB, et al. A phase II study of topotecan (a topoisomerase I inhibitor) in combination with doxorubicin (a topoisomerase II inhibitor). Proc ASCO 1994; 13:157.

398. Bonneterre J, Pion JM, Adenis A, et al. A phase II study of a new camptothecin analogue CPT-11 in previously treated advanced breast cancer patients. Proc ASCO 1993;12:94.

399. Pantazis P, Kozielski AJ, Vardeman DM, et al. Efficacy of camptothecin congeners in the treatment of human breast carcinoma xenografts. Oncol Res 1993;5:273.

400. Reed E, Kohn KW. Platinum analogues. In: Chabner B, Collins JM, eds. Cancer chemotherapy: principles and practice. Philadelphia, JB Lippincott, 1990:465.

401. Krook JE, Loprinzi CL, Schaid DJ, et al. Evaluation of the continuous infusion of etoposide plus cisplatin in metastatic breast cancer. Cancer 1990;65:418.

402. Cocconi G, Bisagni G, Bacchi M, et al. Cisplatin and etoposide as first-line chemotherapy for metastatic breast carcinoma: a prospective randomized trial of the Italian Oncology Group for clinical research. J Clin Oncol 1991;9:664.

403. Kochupillai V, Gupta P, Misra A. A phase II trial of cyclophosphamide, doxorubicin, and cisplatin in advanced breast cancer. Am J Clin Oncol 1992;15:388.

404. Crown J, Hakes T, Reichman B, et al. Phase II trial of carboplatin and etoposide in metastatic breast cancer. Cancer 1993;71:1254.

405. Kolaric K, Vukas D. Carboplatin activity in untreated metastatic breast cancer patients: results of a phase II study. Cancer Chemother Pharmacol 1991;27:409.

406. Martin M, Diaz-Rubio E, Casado A, et al. Phase II study of carboplatin in advanced breast cancer: preliminary results. Semin Oncol 1991;18:23.

407. O'Brien MER, Talbot DC, Smith IE. Carboplatin in the treatment of advanced breast cancer: a phase II study using a pharmacokinetically guided dose schedule. J Clin Oncol 1993;11:2112.

408. Zalupski M, Baker LH. Ifosfamide. J Natl Cancer Inst 1988;80:556.

409. Weiss RB. Ifosfamide vs cyclophosphamide in cancer therapy. Oncology 1991;5:67.

410. Gad-El-Mawla N, Hamza MR, Zikri ZK, et al. Ifosfamide, methotrexate, and 5-fluorouracil: effective combination in resistant breast cancer. Cancer Chemother Pharmacol 1990;26:S85.

411. Becher R, Hofeler H, Kloke O, et al. Ifosfamide, methotrexate and 5-fluorouracil for pretreated advanced breast cancer. Oncology 1991;48:459.

412. Millward MJ, Harris AL, Cantwell BM. Phase II study of doxorubicin plus ifosfamide/mesna in patients with advanced breast cancer. Cancer 1990;65:2421.

413. Lange OF, Scheef W, Haase KD, et al. Palliative chemo-radiotherapy with ifosfamide and epirubicin as first-line treatment for high-risk metastatic breast cancer. Cancer Chemother Pharmacol 1990;26:S74.

414. Perez JE, Machiavelli M, Leone BA, et al. Ifosfamide and mitoxantrone as first-line chemotherapy for metastatic breast cancer. J Clin Oncol 1993;11:461.

415. Bellmunt J, Morales S, Navarro M, et al. Ifosfamide + mitoxantrone in advanced breast cancer previously treated with anthracyclines. Cancer Chemother Pharmacol 1990;26:S81.

416. Langenbuch T, Mross K, Jonat W, et al. A phase II study of intensive-dose epirubicin/verapamil as induction therapy followed by intensive-dose ifosfamide for advanced breast cancer. Cancer Chemother Pharmacol 1990;26:S93.

417. Sanchiz F, Milla A. High-dose ifosfamide and mesna in advanced breast cancer. Cancer Chemother Pharmacol 1990;26:S91.

418. Bitran JD, Samuels BL, Stone LA, et al. A phase I/II trial of ifosfamide (I) and doxorubicin (D) in stage IV breast cancer. Proc ASCO 1994;13:82.

419. Verweij J, Den Hartigh J, Pinedo HM. Antitumor antibiotics. In: Chabner B, Collins JM, eds. Cancer chemotherapy: principles and practice. Philadelphia, JB Lippincott, 1990:382.

420. Pasterz RB, Buzdar AU, Hortobagyi GN, et al. Mitomycin in metastatic breast cancer refractory to hormonal and combination chemotherapy. Cancer 1985;56:2381.

421. Jodrell DI, Smith IE, Mansi JL, et al. A randomised comparative trial of mitozantrone/methotrexate/mitomycin C (MMM) and cyclophosphamide/methotrexate/5 FU (CMF) in the treatment of advanced breast cancer. Br J Cancer 1991;63:794.

422. Skipper HE, Schable FMJR, Wilcox WAS. Experimental evaluation of potential anti-cancer agents. XII: On the criteria and kinet-

ics associated with "curability" of experimental leukemia. Cancer Chemother Rep 1964;35:1.

423. Norton L. A Gompertzian model of human breast cancer growth. Cancer Res 1988;48:7067.

424. Skipper HE. Kinetics of mammary tumor cell growth and implications for therapy. Cancer 1971;28:1479.

425. Skipper HE, Schabel FMJR. Tumor stem cell heterogeneity: implications with respect to classification of cancer by chemotherapeutic effect. Cancer Treat Rep 1984;68:43.

426. Luria SE, Delbruck M. Mutations of bacteria from virus sensitivity to virus resistance. Genetics 1943;28:491.

427. Luk CK, Veinot-Drebot L, Tjan E, et al. Effect of transient hypoxia on sensitivity to doxorubicin in human and murine cell lines. J Natl Cancer Inst 1990;92:684.

428. Goldie JH, Coldman AJ. A mathematic model for relating the drug sensitivity of tumors to their spontaneous mutation rate. Cancer Treat Rep 1979;63:1727.

429. Goldie JH, Coldman AJ. Quantitative model for multiple levels of drug resistance in clinical tumors. Cancer Treat Rep 1983;67:923.

430. Skipper HE. Stepwise progress in the treatment of disseminated cancers. Cancer 1983;51:1773.

431. Bogden AE, Costanza ME, Reich SD, et al. Chemotherapy responsiveness of human breast tumors in the 6-day subrenal capsule assay: an update. Breast Cancer Res Treat 1983;3:33.

432. Kern DH, Weisenthal DH. Highly specific prediction of antineoplastic drug resistance with an in vitro assay using suprapharmacologic drug exposures. J Natl Cancer Inst 1990;82:582.

433. Fruehof JP, Bosanquet AG. In vitro determination of drug response: a discussion of clinical applications. Princ Pract Oncol 1993;7:1.

434. Greenspan EM, Fieber M, Lesnick G, et al. Response of advanced breast carcinoma to the combination of the antimetabolite, methotrexate, and the alkylating agent, thio-TEPA. J Mt Sinai Hosp 1963;30:246.

435. Goldie JH, Coldman AJ, Gudauskas GA. Rationale for the use of alternating non-cross-resistant chemotherapy. Cancer Treat Rep 1982;66:439.

436. Ransom DT, Neuberg D, Loprinzi CL, et al. A pilot study of three sequential chemotherapeutic regimens in metastatic breast cancer. Am J Clin Oncol 1991;14:45.

437. Kolaric K, Tomek R. Cis-platinum–based alternating non–cross-resistant chemotherapy as a first-line treatment in metastatic breast cancer: a phase II study. Tumori 1990;76:472.

438. Tormey DC, Kline JC, Palta M, et al. Short-term high-density systemic therapy for metastatic breast cancer. Breast Cancer Res Treat 1985;5:177.

439. Blomqvist C, Elomaa I, Rissanen P, et al. Influence of treatment schedule on toxicity and efficacy of cyclophosphamide, epirubicin and fluorouracil in metastatic breast cancer: a randomized trial comparing weekly and every-4-week administration. J Clin Oncol 1993;11:467.

440. Bruce WR, Meeker BE, Valeriote FA. Comparison of the sensitivity of normal hematopoietic and transplanted lymphoma colony-forming cells to chemotherapeutic agents administered in vivo. J Natl Canc Inst 1966;37:233.

441. Bross ID, Rimm AA, Slack NH, et al. Is toxicity really necessary? Cancer 1966;1:1780.

442. Hryniuk W, Bush H. The importance of dose intensity in chemotherapy of metastatic breast cancer. J Clin Oncol 1984;2:1281.

443. Carmo-Pereira J, Oliveira Costa F, Henriques E, et al. A comparison of two doses of adriamycin in the primary chemotherapy of disseminated breast carcinoma. Br J Cancer 1987;56:471.

444. Henderson IC, Gelman R, Canellos GP, et al. Prolonged disease-free survival in advanced breast cancer treated with "super-CMF"

adriamycin: an alternating regimen employing high-dose methotrexate with citrovorum factor rescue. Cancer Treat Rep 1981;65:67.

445. Hortobagyi GN, Buzdar AU, Bodey GP, et al. High-dose induction chemotherapy of metastatic breast cancer in protected environment: a prospective randomized study. J Clin Oncol 1987;5:178.

446. Tannock IF, Boyd NF, DeBoer G, et al. A randomized trial of two dose levels of cyclophosphamide, methotrexate, and fluorouracil chemotherapy for patients with metastatic breast cancer. J Clin Oncol 1988;6:1377.

447. ASCO Ad Hoc Colony-Stimulating Factor Guideline Expert Panel. American Society of Clinical Oncology recommendations for the use of hematopoietic colony-stimulating factors: evidence-based, clinical practice guidelines. J Clin Oncol 1994;12:2471.

448. Myers SE, Williams SF. Role of high-dose chemotherapy and autologous stem cell support in treatment of breast cancer. Hematol Oncol Clin North Am 1993;7:631.

449. Muss HB, Case LD, Richards F, et al. Interrupted versus continuous chemotherapy in patients with metastatic breast cancer. N Engl J Med 1991;325:1342.

450. Coates A, Gebski V, Stat M, et al. Improving the quality of life during chemotherapy for advanced breast cancer: a comparison of intermittent and continuous treatment strategies. N Engl J Med 1987;317:1490.

451. Dixon AR, Jackson L, Chan SY, et al. Continuous chemotherapy in responsive metastatic breast cancer: a role for tumour markers. Br J Cancer 1993;68:181.

452. Henderson IC, Garber JE, Breitmeyer JB, et al. Comprehensive management of disseminated breast cancer. Cancer 1990;66:1439.

453. Cold S, Jensen NV, Brincker H, et al. The influence of chemotherapy on survival after recurrence in breast cancer: a population-based study of patients treated in the 1950s, 1960s and 1970s. Eur J Cancer 1993;29A:1146.

454. Bonetti A, Sperotto L, Turazza M, et al. Tumor proliferative activity and response to first-line chemotherapy in advanced breast cancer. Proc ASCO 1994;13:77.

455. De Lena M, Romero A, Rabinovich M, et al. Metastatic pattern and DNA ploidy in stage IV breast cancer at initial diagnosis. Am J Clin Oncol 1993;16:245.

456. De Lena M, Barletta A, Lorusso V, et al. Visceral metastatic pattern and DNA ploidy in stage IV breast cancer at initial diagnosis. Proc ASCO 1994;13:83.

457. Muss HB, Thor AD, Berry DA, et al. c-erbB-2 expression and response to adjuvant therapy in women with node-positive early breast cancer. N Engl J Med 1994;330:1260.

458. Ziegler LD, Connelly JH, Frye D, et al. Lack of correlation between histologic findings and response to chemotherapy in metastatic breast cancer. Cancer 1991;68:628.

459. Nash CH, Jones SE, Moon TE, et al. Prediction of outcome in metastatic breast cancer treated with adriamycin combination chemotherapy. Cancer 1980;46:2380.

460. Rouesse J, Friedman S, Guash-Jordan I, et al. Survival effect of systemic therapy on patients developing metastatic breast carcinoma. Breast Cancer Treat Res 1990;15:13.

461. Inoue K, Ogawa M, Horikoshi N, et al. Evaluation of prognostic factors for 233 patients with recurrent advanced breast cancer. Jpn J Clin Oncol 1991;21:334.

462. Legha SS, Buzdar AU, Smith TL, et al. Complete remissions in metastatic breast cancer treated with combination drug therapy. Ann Int Med 1979;91:847.

463. Buzdar AU, Legha SS, Hortobagyi GN, et al. Management of breast cancer patients failing adjuvant chemotherapy with adriamycin-containing regimens. Cancer 1981;47:2798.

464. Bitran JD, Desser RK, Shapiro CM, et al. Response to secondary

therapy in patients with adenocarcinoma of the breast previously treated with adjuvant chemotherapy. Cancer 1983;58:381.

465. Falkson G, Gelman R, Falkson CI, et al. Factors predicting for response, time to treatment failure, and survival in women with metastatic breast cancer treated with DAVTH: a prospective eastern cooperative oncology study group. J Clin Oncol 1991;9:2153.

466. Miller BA, Feuer EJ, Hankey BF. Recent incidence trends for breast cancer in women and the relevance of early detection: an update. CA Cancer J Clin 1993;43:27.

467. Greenfield S, Blanco DM, Elashoff RM, et al. Patterns of care related to age of breast cancer patients. JAMA 1987;257:2766.

468. Mor V, Masterson-Allen S, Goldberg RJ, et al. Relationship between age at diagnosis and treatments received by cancer patients. J Am Geriatr Soc 1985;33:585.

469. Allen C, Cox EB, Manton KG, et al. Breast cancer in the elderly: current patterns of care. Am Geriatr Soc 1986;34:637.

470. Chu J, Diehr P, Feigl P, et al. The effect of age on the care of women with breast cancer in community hospitals. J Gerontol 1987;42:185.

471. Silliman RA, Guadagnoli E, Weitberg AB, et al. Age as a predictor of diagnostic and initial treatment intensity in newly diagnosed breast cancer patients. J Gerontol 1989;44:M46.

472. Schleifer SJ, Bhardwaj S, Lebovits A, et al. Predictors of physician nonadherence to chemotherapy regimens. Cancer 1991;67:945.

473. Begg CB, Cohen JL, Ellerton J. Are the elderly predisposed to toxicity from cancer chemotherapy? Cancer Clin Trials 1980;3:369.

474. Christman K, Muss HB, Case LD, et al. Chemotherapy of metastatic breast cancer in the elderly. JAMA 1992;268:57.

475. Australian and New Zealand Breast Cancer Trials Group, Clinical Oncological Society of Australia. A randomized trial in postmenopausal patients with advanced breast cancer comparing endocrine and cytotoxic therapy given sequentially or in combination. J Clin Oncol 1986;4:186.

476. Cocconi G, De Lisi V, Boni C, et al. Chemotherapy versus combination of chemotherapy and endocrine therapy in advanced breast cancer. Cancer 1983;51:581.

477. Perry MC, Kardinal CG, Korzun AH, et al. Chemohormonal therapy in advanced carcinoma of the breast: Cancer and Leukemia Group B Protocol 8081. J Clin Oncol 1987;5:1534.

478. Mouridsen HT, Rose C, Engelsman E, et al. Combined cytotoxic and endocrine therapy in postmenopausal patients with advanced breast cancer: a randomized study of CMF vs. CMF plus tamoxifen. Eur J Cancer Clin Oncol 1985;21:291.

479. Kiang DT, Gay J, Goldman A, et al. A randomized trial of chemotherapy and hormonal therapy in advanced breast cancer. N Engl J Med 1985;313:1241.

480. Falkson G, Gelman RS, Tormey DC, et al. Median survival of 59 months for premenopausal women with ER-positive metastatic breast cancer. Proc ASCO 1994;13:57.

481. Hug V, Hortobagyi GN, Drewinko B, et al. Tamoxifen-citrate counteracts the antitumor effects of cytotoxic drugs in vitro. J Clin Oncol 1985;3:1672.

482. Dao TL, Sinha DK, Nemoto T, et al. Effect of estrogen and progesterone on cellular replication of human breast tumors. Cancer Res 1982;42:359.

483. Brunner N, Bronzert D, Vindelov LL, et al. Effect on growth and cell cycle kinetics of estradiol and tamoxifen on MCF-7 human breast cancer cells grown in vitro and in nude mice. Cancer Res 1989;49:1515.

484. Markaverich BM, Medina D, Clark JH. Effects of combination estrogen: cyclophosphamide treatment on the growth of the MXT transplantable mammary tumor in the mouse. Cancer Res 1983;43:3208.

485. Hug V, Johnston D, Finders M, et al. Use of growth-stimulatory hormones to improve the in vitro therapeutic index of doxorubicin for human breast tissues. Cancer Res 1986;46:147.

486. Bontenbal M, Sonneveld P, Foekens JA, et al. Oestradiol enhances doxorubicin uptake and cytotoxicity in human breast cancer cells. Eur J Cancer Clin Oncol 1988;24:1409.

487. Conte PF, Gardin G, Pronzato P, et al. In vivo manipulation of human breast cancer growth by estrogens and growth hormone: kinetic and clinical results. J Steroid Biochem Mol Biol 1990;37:1103.

488. Paridaens R, Heuson JC, Julien JP, et al. Assessment of estrogenic recruitment before chemotherapy in advanced breast cancer: a double-blind randomized study. J Clin Oncol 1993;11:1723.

489. Lippman ME, Cassidy J, Wesley M, et al. A randomized attempt to increase the efficacy of cytotoxic chemotherapy in metastatic breast cancer by hormonal synchronization. J Clin Oncol 1984;2:28.

490. Allegra JC, Woodcock TM, Richman SP, et al. A phase II trial of tamoxifen, premarin, methotrexate and 5-fluorouracil in metastatic breast cancer. Breast Cancer Res Treat 1982;2:93.

491. Benz C, Gandara D, Miller B, et al. Chemoendocrine therapy with prolonged estrogen priming in advanced breast cancer: endocrine pharmacokinetics and toxicity. Cancer Treat Rep 1987;71:283.

492. Lipton A, Santen RJ, Harvey HA, et al. A randomized trial of aminoglutethimide +/− estrogen before chemotherapy in advanced breast cancer. Am J Clin Oncol 1987;10:65.

493. Fisher ER, Sass R, Fisher B. Pathologic findings from the National Surgical Adjuvant Project for Breast Cancers (Protocol No. 4). X. Discriminants for tenth year treatment failure. Cancer 1984;53:712.

494. Carpenter JT, Smalley RV, Raney M, et al. Ineffectiveness of levamisole in prolonging remission or survival of women treated with cyclophosphamide, doxorubicin, and 5-fluorouracil for good-risk metastatic breast carcinoma: a Southeastern Cancer Study Group trial. Cancer Treat Rep 1986;70:1073.

495. Aberizk WJ, Silver B, Henderson IC. The use of radiotherapy for treatment of isolated locoregional recurrence of breast carcinoma after mastectomy. Cancer 1986;58:1214.

496. Blumenschein GR, Pinnamaneni K, Buzdar AU, et al. Combined regional and systemic therapy in breast cancer patients with an isolated metastasis with or without prior chemotherapy. In: Jones SE, Salmon SE, eds. Adjuvant therapy of cancer IV. Orlando, Grune & Stratton, 1984:311.

497. Borner M, Bacchi M, Goldhirsch A, et al. First isolated locoregional recurrence following mastectomy for breast cancer: results of a phase III multicenter study comparing systemic treatment with observation after excision and radiation. J Clin Oncol 1994;12:2071.

498. Wright JC, Cobb JP, Golomb FM. Chemotherapy of disseminated carcinoma of the breast. Ann Surg 1959;150:221.

499. Livingston RB, Carter SK. Single agents in cancer chemotherapy. New York, Plenum, 1970.

500. Constanza ME, Korzun AH, Henderson IC. Amonafide: an active agent in metastatic breast cancer (CALGB 8642). Proc Am Soc Clin Oncol 1990;9:31.

501. Legha SS, Blumenschein GR, Budzar AU. Phase II study of 4′-(9-acridinylamino)methanesulfon-m-anisidide (AMSA) in metastatic breast carcinoma. Cancer Treat Rep 1979;63:1961.

502. De Lena M, Rossi A, Bonadonna G. Phase II trial of AMSA in refractory breast cancer. Cancer Treat Rep 1982;66:403.

503. Currie VE, Howard J, Wittes R. A phase II evaluation of m-AMSA, 4′-(9-acridinylamino)methanesulfon-m-anisid, in patients with breast cancer. Cancer Clin Trials 1981;4:249.

504. Amrein PC, Coleman M, Richards FII. Phase II study of AMSA

in patients with metastatic breast cancer: a Cancer and Leukemia Group B study. Cancer Treat Rep 1982;66:1211.

505. Ahmann FR, Meyskens FL, Jones SE. Phase II evaluation of amsacrine (m-AMSA) in solid tumors, myeloma, and lymphoma: a University of Arizona and Southwest Oncology Group study. Cancer Treat Rep 1983;67:697.

506. Cunningham TJ, Nemoto T, Rosner D. Comparison of 5-azacytidine (NSC-102816) with CCNU (NSC-79037) in the treatment of patients with breast cancer and evaluation of the subsequent use of cyclophosphamide (NSC-26271). Cancer Chemother Rep 1974;58:677.

507. Hoogstraten B, Fabian C. A reappraisal of single drugs in advanced breast cancer. Cancer Clin Trials 1979;2:101.

508. Osborne CK, Cowan JD, Neidhart JA. The Southwest Oncology Group randomized trial of novantrone, adriamycin, and bisantrene in advanced breast cancer. In: Coltman CA Jr, ed. The current status of novantrone. 1985:55.

509. Forastiere AA, Budman DR, Perry MC. Phase II trials of aclacinomycin-A (A) and bisantrene (B) in advanced breast cancer: CALGB studies. Proc Am Assoc Cancer Res 1983;24:152.

510. Osborne CK, Von Hoff DD, Cowan JD, et al. Bisantrene, an active drug in patients with advanced breast cancer. Cancer Treat Rep 1984;68:357.

511. Cavalli F, Gerard B, Ten Bokkel HW. Phase II evaluation of bisantrene in metastatic breast cancer. Cancer Treat Rep 1985;69:337.

512. Pandya KJ, Muggia FM, Skeel RT. A phase II study of bisantrene in advanced refractory breast cancer. Am J Clin Oncol 1985;8:353.

513. Holmes F, Esparza L, Yap H. A comparative study of bisantrene (B) given by single iv dose (S) vs daily for five days (DX5) in patients (pts) with metastatic breast cancer (MBC). Breast Cancer Res Treat 1985;6:170.

514. Yap HY, Yap BS, Blumenschein GR. Bisantrene, an active new drug in the treatment of metastatic breast cancer. Cancer Res 1983;43:1402.

515. Cummings FJ, Gelman R, Skeel RT. Phase II trials of Baker's Antifol, bleomycin, CCNU, streptozotocin, tilorone, and 5-fluorodeoxyuridine plus arabinosyl cytosine in metastatic breast cancer. Cancer 1981;48:681.

516. Bonadonna G, De Lena M, Monfardini S. Clinical trials with bleomycin in lymphomas and in solid tumors. Eur J Cancer 1972;8:205.

517. Haas CD, Coltman CA Jr, Gottlieb JA. Phase II evaluation of bleomycin. Cancer 1976;38:8.

518. Booth BW, Weiss RB, Korzun AH. Phase II trial of carboplatin in advanced breast carcinoma: a Cancer and Leukemia Group B study. Cancer Treat Rep 1985;69:919.

519. Carmo-Pereira J, Oliveira C, Henriques E, et al. Carboplatin (C) as primary chemotherapy for disseminated breast carcinoma: a Phase II study [abstr P-0971]. London, Proc ECC05, 1989.

520. Martin M, Diaz-Rubio E, Gonzales JL. Phase II study of carboplatin (CB) in breast cancer: preliminary results (Abstract P-0998). London, Proc ECC05, 1989.

521. Kolaric K, Vukas D. Carboplatin activity in untreated metastatic breast cancer: a phase II trial. Proc Am Soc Clin Oncol 1990;9:26.

522. Wander HE, Nagel GA. Carboplatinum in advanced breast cancer. J Cancer Res Clin Oncol 1988;114:S60.

523. Franks CR, Nys G, Schultz HP. Randomized phase II trial of carboplatin vs iproplatin in solid tumors. Proc Am Soc Clin Oncol 1986;5:129.

524. Curt GA, Grygiel JJ, Corden BJ. A phase I and pharmacokinetic study of diamminecyclobutane-dicarboxylato-platinum (NSC-241240). Cancer Res 1983;43:4470.

525. Gottlieb JA, Rivkin SF, Spigel SC. Superiority of adriamycin over oral nitrosoureas in patients with advanced breast carcinoma. Cancer 1974;33:519.

526. Hoogstraten B, Haas CD, Haut A, et al. CCNU and bleomycin in the treatment of cancer: a Southwest Oncology Group study. Med Pediatr Oncol 1975;1:95.

527. Ahmann DL, Bisel HF, Hahn RG. Difficulties designing clinical trials as exemplified by a phase 2 drug evaluation of 5[3,3-bis(2-chloroethyl)-1-triazenol]-imidazole-4-carboxamide and 1-(2-chloroethyl)-3-cyclohexyl-1-nitrosourea in patients with disseminated breast cancer. Cancer Res 1973;33:1707.

528. Moore GE, Bross IDJ, Ausman R. Effects of chlorambucil (NSC-3088) in 374 patients with advanced cancer. Cancer Chemother Rep 1968;52:661.

529. Bull JM, Anderson T, Lippman ME. A phase II trial of cis-dichlorodiammine platinum II (CIS-DDP) in breast and ovarian carcinomas. Proc Am Soc Clin Oncol 1978;19:87.

530. Forastiere AA, Hakes TB, Wittes JT, et al. Cisplatin in the treatment of metastatic breast cancer: a prospective randomized trial of two dosage schedules. Am J Clin Oncol 1982;5:243.

531. Ostrow S, Egorin M, Aisner J. High-dose cis-diamminedichloroplatinum therapy in patients with advanced breast cancer: pharmacokinetics, toxicity, and therapeutic efficacy. Cancer Clin Trials 1980;3:23.

532. Martino S, Samal BA, Singhakowinta Z. A phase II study of cis-diamminedichlorophatinum II for advanced breast cancer: two-dose schedules. J Cancer Res Clin Oncol 1984;108:354.

533. Yap HY, Salem P, Hortobagyi GN, et al. Phase II study of cis-dichlorodiammineplatinum (II) in advanced breast cancer. Cancer Treat Rep 1978;62:405.

534. Abe O, Enomoto K, Nomura Y. cis-Dichlorodiammineplatinum (II) in advanced breast cancer. Jpn Pharmacol Ther 1986;14:233.

535. Sledge J, Loehrer PJ, Roth BJ, et al. Cisplatin as first-line therapy for metastatic breast cancer. J Clin Oncol 1988;6:1811.

536. Talley RW, Vaitkevicius VK, Leighton GA. Comparison of cyclophosphamide and 5-fluorouracil in the treatment of patients with metastatic breast cancer. Clin Pharmacol Ther 1965;6:740.

537. Nemoto T, Dao TL. 5-Fluorouracil and cyclophosphamide in disseminated breast cancer. NY State J Med 1971;71:554.

538. Rubens RD, Knight R, Hayward JL. Chemotherapy of advanced breast cancer: a controlled randomized trial of cyclophosphamide versus a four-drug combination. Br J Cancer 1975;32:730.

539. Baker LH, Vaughn CB, Al-Sarraf M. Evaluation of combination versus sequential cytotoxic chemotherapy in the treatment of advanced breast cancer. Cancer 1974;33:513.

540. Hurley JD, Trump DS, Flatley TJ, et al. A method of selecting patients for cancer chemotherapy. Arch Surg 1961;83:611.

541. Firat D, Olshin S. Treatment of metastatic carcinoma of the female breast with combination of hormones and other chemotherapy. Cancer Chemother Rep 1968;52:743.

542. Rundles RW, Laszlo J, Garrison FE, et al. The antitumor spectrum of cyclophosphamide. Cancer Chemother Rep 1962;16:407.

543. Wall RL, Conrad FG. Cyclophosphamide therapy. Arch Intern Med 1961;108:456.

544. Atkins HL, Gregg HG, Hyman GA. Clinical appraisal of cyclophosphamide in malignant neoplasms. Cancer 1962;15:1076.

545. Edelstyn G, Gleadhill C, Lyons A. Total hypophysectomy for advanced breast cancer. Clin Radiol 1968;19:426.

546. Kunkler PB, Evans IH, Jones V, et al. Cyclophosphamide in the management of breast cancer. In: Forrest APM, Kunkler RB, eds. Prognostic factors in breast cancer. Edinburgh, E & S Livingstone, 1968;211.

547. Coggins P, Eisman SH, Elkins W, et al. Cyclophosphamide therapy in carcinoma of the breast and ovary: a comparative study of inter-

mittent massive versus continuous maintenance dosage regimens. Cancer Chemother Rep 1961;15:3.

548. Piro AJ, Wilson RE, Nevinny HB. Cyclophosphamide therapy in patients with advancing breast cancer following adrenalectomy and 5-fluorouracil. Cancer 1971;27:1342.

549. Chlebowski R, Irwin LE, Pugh RP. Survival of patients with metastatic breast cancer treated with either combination or sequential chemotherapy. Cancer Res 1979;39:4503.

550. Smalley RV, Murphy S, Huguley CM, et al. Combination versus sequential five-drug chemotherapy in metastatic carcinoma of the breast. Cancer Res 1976;36:3911.

551. Carter SK. Single and combination nonhormonal chemotherapy in breast cancer. Cancer 1972;30:1543.

552. Slavik M. Clinical studies with DTIC (NSC-45388) in various malignancies. Cancer Treat Rep 1976;60:213.

553. Tormey DC. Adriamycin (NSC-123127) in breast cancer: an overview of studies. Cancer Chemother Rep 1975;6:319.

554. O'Bryan RM, Baker LH, Gottlieb JE. Dose response evaluation of adriamycin in human neoplasia. Cancer 1977;39:1940.

555. Ingle J, Ahmann D, O'Fallon J. Randomized phase II trial of rubidazone and adriamycin in women with advanced breast cancer. Cancer Treat Rep 1979;63:1701.

556. Frederiksen PL, Joergensen ST, Roesdahl K. Activity of adriamycin in metastatic breast cancer resistant to a combination regimen with cyclophosphamide, methotrexate, 5-fluorouracil, vincristine, and prednisone. Cancer Treat Rep 1978;62:449.

557. Bonadonna G, Beretta G, Tancini G. Adriamycin (NSC-123127) studies at the Instituto Nazionale Tumori, Milan. Cancer Chemother Rep 1975;6:231.

558. Creech RH, Catalano RB, Shah MK. An effective low-dose adriamycin regimen as secondary chemotherapy for metastatic breast cancer patients. Cancer 1980;46:433.

559. Creech RH, Catalano RB, Shah MK, et al. A randomized trial of adriamycin versus mitomycin at low doses in CMF-refractory metastatic breast cancer patients. Proc Am Soc Clin Oncol 1982;1:88.

560. Vaughn CB, O'Bryan R, Reed M. Adriamycin + VP-16 versus adriamycin alone in advanced adenocarcinoma of the breast, phase II: a Southwest Oncology Group study. Proc Am Assoc Cancer Res 1984;25:184.

561. Dean JC, Griffith KS, Cetas TC. Scalp hypothermia: a comparison of ice packs and Kold Kap in the prevention of doxorubicin-induced alopecia. J Clin Oncol 1983;1:33.

562. Jain KK, Casper ES, Geller NL. A prospective randomized comparison of epirubicin and doxorubicin in patients with advanced breast cancer. J Clin Oncol 1985;3:818.

563. van Oosterom AT, Mouridsen HT, Wildiers J. Doxorubicin (ADM) versus 4'epidoxorubicin(4'EPI), a preliminary report: report of a randomized phase II–III study in pretreated breast cancer patients. Proceedings of the International Symposium on Advances in Anthracycline Chemotherapy: Epirubicin. Milan, Farmitalia Carlo Erba, 1984;23.

564. Bonfante V, Ferrari L, Brambilla C. New anthracycline analogs in advanced breast cancer. Eur J Cancer Clin Oncol 1986;22:1379.

565. Henderson IC, Wolff S, Allegra J, et al. A randomized trial comparing mitoxantrone and doxorubicin in patients with metastatic breast cancer. In: Coltman CA Jr., ed. The current status of novantrone. New York, John Wiley & Sons, 1985:45.

566. Neidhart JA, Gochnour D, Roach R, et al. Comparable efficacy of novantrone and adriamycin in breast cancer. In: Coltman CA Jr, ed. The current status of novantrone, New York, John Wiley & Sons, 1985:45.

567. Nemoto T, Rosner D, Diaz R, et al. Combination chemotherapy for metastatic breast cancer. Cancer 1978;41:2073.

568. Manni A, Trujillo JE, Pearson OH. Sequential use of endocrine therapy and chemotherapy for metastatic breast cancer: effects on survival. Cancer Treat Rep 1980;64:111.

569. Stoll BA. Evaluation of cyclophosphamide dosage schedules in breast cancer. Br J Cancer 1970;24:475.

570. Buzdar AU, Goodman A, Chou I. Elliptinium acetate in advanced breast cancer refractory to combination chemotherapy (CHEMO): results of phase I–II studies. Breast Cancer Res Treat 1984;4:346.

571. Byrne P, Grady K, Smith F. Phase II clinical trial of 2-N-methyl-9-hydroxy-ellipticium (elliptinium) in patients with advanced breast cancer. Proc Am Soc Clin Oncol 1984;3:127.

572. Einzig AI, Gralla RJ, Leyland-Jones BR. Phase I trial of elliptinium (2-methyl-9-hydroxyellipticinium). Proc Am Assoc Cancer Res 1983;24:166.

573. Juret P, Heron JF, Couette JE. Hydroxy-9-methyl-2-elliptinium for osseous metastases from breast cancer: a 5-year experience. Cancer Treat Rep 1982;66:1909.

574. Rouesse JG, Le Chevalier T, Caille P. Phase II study of elliptium in advanced breast cancer. Cancer Treat Rep 1985;69:707.

575. Twelves CJ, O'Reilly S, Coleman RE. Weekly epirubicin for liver metastases in breast cancer. Proc Am Soc Clin Oncol 1989;8:32.

576. Jones WG, Mattsson W. Phase II study of weekly low-dose 4'-epi-doxorubicin in advanced postmenopausal breast cancer. Cancer Treat Rep 1984;68:675.

577. Campora E, Nobile MT, Sertoli MR, et al. Phase II study of 4'-epi-doxorubicin in advanced breast cancer. Cancer Treat Rep 1984;68:1285.

578. Hurteloup P, Cappelaere P, Armand JP, et al. Phase II clinical evaluation of 4'-epi-doxorubicin. Cancer Treat Rep 1983;67:337.

579. Gasparini G, Pozza F, Panizzoni GA. Weekly low-dose epirubicin versus doxorubicin: a randomized phase II study, as second-line therapy, in advanced breast cancer (ABC). Proc Am Soc Clin Oncol 1990;9:29.

580. Barni S, Lissoni P, Archili C. Immunomodulating effects of weekly epirubicin (EPI) in breast cancer and their relation to tumor objective regression. Proc Am Soc Clin Oncol 1990;9:30.

581. Pacini P, Neri B, Algeri R. Epirubicin high dose chemotherapy in liver metastases from breast cancer: preliminary results (Abstract P-1041). London, Proc ECC05, 1989.

582. Blackstein M, Wilson K, Meharchand J. Phase I study of epirubicin in metastatic breast cancer. Proc Am Soc Clin Oncol 1988;7:23.

583. Carmo-Pereira J, Henriques E, Costa FO, et al. Epirubicin (E) as first-line chemotherapy in disseminated breast carcinoma: a Phase II study: preliminary results. Proc Am Soc Clin Oncol 1989;8:31.

584. Barni G, Tancini G, Paolorossi F. A weekly schedule of epirubicin (EPI) in pretreated metastatic breast cancer. Proc Am Soc Clin Oncol 1989;8:29.

585. Martino S, Samal BA, Vaitkevicius VK. 4'-Deoxydoxorubicin (DXDX) as first line therapy for metastatic breast cancer. Breast Cancer Res Treat 1985;6:171.

586. Leitner SP, Casper ES, Hakes TB. Phase II trial of 4'-deoxydoxorubicin in patients with advanced breast cancer. Cancer Treat Rep 1985;69:1319.

587. Schapira D, Hall TC, Bennett JM. A phase II study of estradiol mustard (NSC-112259) by the Eastern Cooperative Oncology Group. Cancer Clin Trials 1978;1:5.

588. Dawes PJDK. A pilot study of estracyt in advanced breast cancer. Cancer Treat Rep 1982;66:581.

589. Cavalli F, Jungi WF, Brunner KW. Randomisierte phase-II studie mit VP-16-213 (Etoposide) in der behandlung vom fortgeschrittenen Mammakarzinom. Onkologie. 1981;4:80.

590. Ahmann DL, Bisel HF, Eagan RT. Phase II evaluation of VP-16-213 (NSC-141540) and cytembena (NSC-104801) in patients with advanced breast cancer. Cancer Treat Rep 1976;60:633.

591. Falkson G, van Dyk JJ, van Eden EB. A clinical trial of the oral form of 4'-demethyl-epipodophyllotoxin-beta-D ethylidene glucoside (NSC-141540) VP 16-213. Cancer 1975;35:1141.

592. Eagan RT, Ahmann DL, Bisel HF. Evaluation of VP-16 and the combination of adriamycin and vincristine in advanced breast cancer. Oncology 1976;33:146.

593. Nissen NI, Hansen HH, Pedersen H. Clinical trial of the oral form of a new podophyllotoxin derivative, VP-16-213 (NSC-141540) in patients with advanced neoplastic disease. Cancer Chemother Rep 1975;59:1027.

594. Schell FC, Yap HY, Hortobagyi GN. Phase II study of VP16-213 (etoposide) in refractory metastatic breast carcinoma. Cancer Chemother Pharmacol 1982;7:223.

595. Marques LA, Franco EL, Torloni H. Independent prognostic value of laminin receptor expression in breast cancer survival. Cancer Res 1990;50:1479.

596. Wander HE, Rauschning W, Meyer D. Phase II study with etoposide in previously untreated advanced breast cancer. Cancer Chemother Pharmacol 1989;24:261.

597. Wolff SN, Fer MF, McKay CM. High-dose VP-16-213 and autologous bone marrow transplantation for refractory malignancies: a phase I study. J Clin Oncol 1983;1:701.

598. Modiano MR, Dalton WS, Lippman SM, et al. Phase II study of fenretinide (N-[4-hydroxyphenyl]retinamide) in advanced breast cancer and melanoma. Invest New Drugs 1990;8:317.

599. Cobleigh MA, Dowlatshahi K, Deutsch TA, et al. Phase I/II trial of tamoxifen with or without fenretinide, an analog of vitamin A, in women with metastatic breast cancer. J Clin Oncol 1993;11:474.

600. Eastern Cooperative Group. Comparison of antimetabolites in the treatment of breast and colon cancer. JAMA 1967;200:110.

601. Sullivan RD, Miller E. The clinical effects of prolonged intravenous infusion of 5-fluoro-2'-deoxyuridine. Cancer Res 1965;25:1025.

602. DeConti RC, Kaplan SR, Papac RJ, et al. Continuous intravenous infusions of 5-fluoro-2'-deoxyuridine in the treatment on solid tumors. Cancer 1973;31:894.

603. Wilson WL, Bisel HF, Krementz ET. Further clinical evaluation of 2'-deoxy-5-fluorouridine. Cancer Chemother Rep 1967;51:85.

604. Dao TL, Grinberg R. Fluorinated pyrimidines in treatment of breast cancer patients with liver metastases. Cancer Chemother Rep 1963;27:71.

605. Ansfield FJ, Curreri AR. Further clinical comparison between 5-fluorouracil (5-FU) and 5-fluoro-2'-deoxyuridine. Cancer Chemother Rep 1963;32:101.

606. Carpenter JT Jr, Vogel CL, Wang G, et al. Phase II evaluation of fludarabine in patients with metastatic breast cancer: a Southeastern Cancer Study Group trial. Cancer Treat Rep 1986;70:123.

607. Carbone PP, Bauer M, Band P, et al. Chemotherapy of disseminated breast cancer. Cancer 1977;39:2916.

608. Ansfield FJ, Ramirez G, Mackman S. A ten-year study of 5-fluorouracil in disseminated breast cancer with clinical results and survival times. Cancer Res 1969;29:1062.

609. Chlebowski RT, Pugh RP, Weiner JM, et al. Treatment of advanced breast carcinoma with 5-fluorouracil: a randomized comparison of two routes of delivery. Cancer 1981;48:1711.

610. Lemkin SR, Dollinger MR. Combination vs. single drug therapy in advanced breast cancer. Proc Am Assoc Ca Res 1973;14:37.

611. Ansfield F, Klotz J, Nealon T. A phase III study comparing the clinical utility of four regimens of 5-fluorouracil. Cancer 1977;39:34.

612. Mackman S, Ramirez G, Ansfield FJ. Results of 5-fluorouracil (NSC-19893) given by the multiple daily dose method in disseminated breast cancer. Cancer Chemother Rep 1967;51:483.

613. Moore GE, Bross IDJ, Ausman R, et al. Effects of 5-fluorouracil (NSC-19893) in 389 patients with cancer. Cancer Chemother Rep 1968;52:641.

614. Field JB. 5-fluorouracil (NSC-19893) treatment of advanced cancer in ambulatory patients. Cancer Chemother Rep 1963;33:45.

615. Kennedy BJ, Theologides A. The role of 5-fluorouracil in malignant disease. Ann Intern Med 1961;55:719.

616. Hall BE, Good JW. Treatment of far-advanced cancer with 5-fluorouracil, used alone and in combination with irradiation: incidence and duration of remission and survival-time data in 223 patients. Cancer Chemother Rep 1962;16:369.

617. Eyerly RC. The effects of 5-fluorouracil in patients with incurable cancer. Cancer Chemother Rep 1962;20:89.

618. Hall TC, Cavins JA, Khung CL, et al. Time and vehicle studies of a safe and effective method for administration of 5-fluorouracil. Cancer 1966;19:1008.

619. Vaitkevicius VK, Brennan MJ, Beckett VL. Clinical evaluation of cancer chemotherapy with 5-fluorouracil. Cancer 1961;14:131.

620. Jacobs EM, Luce JK, Wood DA. Treatment of cancer with weekly intravenous 5-fluorouracil. Cancer 1968;22:1233.

621. Silva ARM, Smart CR, Rochlin DB. Chemotherapy of breast cancer. Chemother Breast Cancer 1965;121:494.

622. Moore FD, Woodrow SI, Aliapoulios MA, et al. Carcinoma of the breast: a decade of new results with old concepts. N Engl J Med 1967;277:460.

623. Hortobagyi GN, Blumenschein GR, Tashima CK. Ftorafur, adriamycin, cyclophosphamide and BCG in the treatment of metastatic breast cancer. Cancer 1979;44:398.

624. Marsoni S, Hoth D, Simon R. Clinical drug development: an analysis of phase II trials, 1970–1985. Cancer Treat Rep 1987;71:71.

625. Wilson WL, Schroeder JM, Bisel HF. Phase II study of hexamethylmelamine (NSC-13875). Cancer 1969;23:132.

626. Wilson WL, Bisel HF, Cole D. Prolonged low-dosage administration of hexamethylmelamine (NSC-13875). Cancer 1970;25:568.

627. Wampler GL, Mellette SJ, Kuperminc M, et al. Mexamethylmelamine (NSC-13875) in the treatment of advanced cancer. Cancer Chemother Rep 1972;56:505.

628. Legha SS, Buzdar AU, Hortobagyi GN. Phase II study of hexamethylmelamine alone and in combination with mitomycin C and vincristine in advanced breast carcinoma. Cancer Treat Rep 1979;63:2053.

629. Denefrio JM, Vogel CL. Phase II study of hexamethylmelamine in women with advanced breast cancer refractory to standard cytotoxic therapy. Cancer Treat Rep 1978;62:173.

630. Fabian CJ, Rasmussen S, Stephens R. Phase II evaluation of hexamethylmelamine in advanced breast cancer: a Southwest Oncology Group study. Cancer Treat Rep 1979;63:1359.

631. Martoni A, Pacciarini MA, Pannuti F. Activity of 4-demethoxydaunorubicin by the oral route in advanced breast cancer. Eur J Cancer Clin Oncol 1985;21:803.

632. Pronzato P, Lionetto R, Gulisano M. A phase-II study with oral 4-demethoxydaunorubicin in metastatic breast cancer. Breast Cancer 1985;6:172.

633. Lopez M, Contegiacomo A, Vici P. A prospective randomized trial of doxorubicin versus idarubicin in the treatment of advanced breast cancer. Cancer 1989;64:2431.

634. Chevallier B, Monnier A, Metz R. Phase II study of oral idarubicin (IDR) in elderly patients with advanced breast cancer (Abstract) Proceedings of ECC05, London, 1989.

635. Armand JP, Hurteloup P, Bastit P. Phase II study of oral idarubicin (IDR) in advanced breast cancer. Proc Am Soc Clin Oncol 1986;5:74.

636. De Lena M, Brandi M, Bozzi D. 4-Demethoxydaunorubicin ad-

ministered orally in advanced breast cancer: a Phase II study. Tumori 1988;74:65.

637. Casper ES, Raymond V, Hakes TB. Phase II evaluation of orally administered idarubicin in patients with advanced breast cancer. Cancer Treat Rep 1987;71:1289.

638. Lionetto R, Pronzato P, Conte PF. Idarubicin in advanced breast cancer: a phase II study. Cancer Treat Rep 1986;70:1439.

639. Ahmann DL, Bisel HF, Hahn RG. Phase II clinical trial of isophosphamide (NSC-109724) in patients with advanced breast cancer. Cancer Chemother Rep 1974;58:861.

640. Falkson G, Falkson HC. Further experience with isophosphamide. Cancer Treat Rep 1976;60:955.

641. Band P, Maroun J, Pritchard K. Phase II study of onidamine (LDM) in advanced breast cancer. Proc Am Soc Clin Oncol 1986;5:56.

642. Pronzato P, Amoroso D, Bertelli G. Phase II study of onidamine in metastatic breast cancer. Br J Cancer 1989;59:251.

643. de Graeff A, Mansi JL, Newell DR, et al. A phase II study of lonidamine in advanced breast cancer. Proceedings of ECC05, London, 1989.

644. Buzdar AU, Legha SS, Blumenschein GR. Peptichemio versus melphalan(L-PAM) in advanced breast cancer. Cancer 1982; 49:1767.

645. Sears ME, Haut A, Eckles N. Melphalan (NSC-8806) in advanced breast cancer. Cancer Chemother Rep 1966;50:271.

646. Dodion PF, Piccart MJ, Bartholomeus S. Phase II trial in breast cancer (BRCA) with the new anthracycline antibiotic menogaril (MEN) given orally. (Abstract) Proceedings of ECC05, London, 1989.

647. Long HJ, Schaid DJ, Schutt AJ. Phase II evaluation of menogaril in women with metastatic breast cancer after failure of first-line chemotherapy. Am J Clin Oncol 1988;11:524.

648. Martino S, Piccart MJ, Dodion PF. Phase II study of daily × 3 oral menogaril in advanced breast cancer. Proc Am Soc Clin Oncol 1990;9:52.

649. Moore GE, Bross IDJ, Ausman R. Effects of 6-mercaptopurine (NSC-755) in 290 patients with advanced cancer. Cancer Chemother Rep 1968;52:655.

650. Yap HY, Blumenschein GR, Yap BS. High-dose methotrexate for advanced breast cancer. Cancer Treat Rep 1979;63:757.

651. Sullivan RD, Miller E, Wladyslaw ZZ. Re-evaluation of methotrexate as an anticancer drug. Surg Gynecol Obstet 1967;125:819.

652. Vogler WR, Furtado VP, Huguley CMJR. Methotrexate for advanced cancer of the breast. Cancer 1968;21:26.

653. Andrews NC, Wilson WL. Phase II study of methotrexate (NSC-740) in solid tumors. Cancer Chemother Rep 1967;51:471.

654. Isacoff WH, Eilber F, Tabbarah H. Phase II clinical trial with high-dose methotrexate therapy and citrovorum factor rescue. Cancer Treat Rep 1978;62:1295.

655. Volger WR, Jacobs J, Moffitt S. Methotrexate therapy with or without citrovorum factor in carcinoma of the head and neck, breast and colon. Cancer Clin Trials 1979;2:227.

656. Wilson HE, Louis J. The use of low dosage regimens in the treatments of neoplastic disease. Ann Intern Med 1965;63:918.

657. Schoenbach EB, Colsky J, Greenspan EM. Observations on the effects of the folic acid antagonists, aminopterin and amethopterin, in patients with advanced neoplasms. Cancer 1952;5:1201.

658. Nevinny HB, Hall TC, Haines C, et al. Comparison of methotrexate (NSC-740) and testosterone propionate (NSC-9166) in the treatment of breast cancer. J Clin Pharmacol 1968;8:126.

659. Ahmann D, Bisel H, Hahn R. A phase 2 evaluation of 1-(2-chloroethyl)-3-(4-methyl-cyclohexyl)-1-nitrosourea (NSC-95441) in patients with advanced breast cancer. Cancer Res 1974;34:27.

660. Ingle JN, Brunk SF, Krook JE. Evaluation of mitolactol in women

with advanced breast cancer and prior chemotherapy exposure. Cancer Treat Rep 1983;67:955.

661. Creech RH, Catalano RB, Dierks KM, et al. Phase II study of mitolactol in chemotherapy-refractory metastatic breast cancer. Cancer 1984;68:1499.

662. Tormey DC, Falkson G, Perlin E. Evaluation of an intermittent schedule of dibromodulcitol in breast cancer. Cancer Treat Rep 1976;60:1593.

663. Tormey DC, Simon R, Falkson G. Evaluation of adriamycin and dibromodulcitol in metastatic breast carcinoma. Cancer Res 1977;37:529.

664. Andrews NC, Weiss AJ, Wilson W, et al. Phase II study of dibromodulcitol (NSC-104800). Cancer Chemother Rep 1974;58:653.

665. Crooke ST, Bradner WT. Mitomycin C: a review. Cancer Treat Rev 1976;3:121.

666. van Oosterom AT, Powles TJ, Hamersma E. A phase II study of mitomycin C in refractory advanced breast cancer: a multi-centre pilot study. In: Mouridsen HT, Palshof T, eds. Breast cancer: experimental and clinical aspects. Elmsford, Pergamon, 1980:275.

667. De Lena M, Jirillo A, Branbilla C, et al. Mitomycin C in metastatic breast cancer resistant to hormone therapy and conventional chemotherapy. Tumori 1980;66:481.

668. Creech RH, Catalano RB, Shah MK, et al. An effective low-dose mitomycin regimen for hormonal- and chemotherapy-refractory patients with metastatic breast cancer. Cancer 1983;51:1034.

669. Thompson P, Harvey V. Improved quality of life (QOL) in patients (PTS) with advanced breast cancer responding to treatment with mitoxantrone (MX). Proc Am Soc Clin Oncol 1989;8:34.

670. Mouridsen HT, Cornbleet M, Stuart-Harris R. Mitoxantrone as first-line chemotherapy in advanced breast cancer: results of a collaborative European study. Invest New Drugs 1985;3:139.

671. de Jager R, Cappelaere P, Earl H. Phase II clinical trial of mitoxantrone: 1,4-dihydroxy-5-8-bis(((2-((2-hydroxyethyl)amino)-ethyl)amino)9,10-anthracenedione dihydrochloride in solid tumors and lymphomas. Proc Am Soc Clin Oncol 1982;1:89.

672. Knight WAIII, Von Hoff DD, Tranum B, et al. Phase II trial of dihydroxyanthracenedione (DHAD, mitoxanthrone) in breast cancer: a Southwest Oncology Group (SWOG) study. Proc Am Soc Clin Oncol 1982;1:87.

673. Wilson KS, Paterson AHG. First-line mitoxantrone chemotherapy for advanced breast cancer. Cancer Treat Rep 1986;70:1021.

674. Yap HY, Blumenschein G, Schell F. Dihydroxyanthracenedione: a promising new drug in the treatment of metastatic breast cancer. Ann Intern Med 1981;95:694.

675. Lenzhofer R, Rainer H, Schuster R. Mitoxantrone in the primary treatment of metastasizing breast cancer. Wien Klin Wonchenschr 1984;96:319.

676. Robertson JFR, Williams MR, Todd JH, et al. Mitoxantrone: a useful palliative therapy in advanced breast cancer. Am J Clin Oncol 1989;12:393.

677. Landys K, Borgstrom S, Andersson T, et al. Mitoxantrone as a first-line treatment of advanced breast cancer. Invest New Drugs 1985;3:133.

678. Zubrod CG, Scheiderman M, Frei EIII. Appraisal of methods for the study of chemotherapy of cancer in man: comparative therapeutic trial of nitrogen mustard and triethylene thiophosphoramide. J Chronic Dis 1960;11:7.

679. Mann G, Hortobagyi G, Yap H. A comparative study of PALA, PALA/5-FU, and 5-FU in advanced breast carcinoma. Proc Am Soc Clin Oncol 1982;1:76.

680. Greifenberg B. Pirarubicin: a new drug in the treatment of malignant diseases. In: Berger HG, Buchler M, Reisfeld RA, et al, eds. Cancer therapy: monoclonal antibodies, lymphokines. Berlin, Springer-Verlag, 1989;270.

681. Mathe G, Umezawa K, Oka S. Phase II trials of thp-Adriamycin (pirarubicin), the most efficient and least toxic anthracycline in breast cancer. In: Kuemmerle HP, ed. Advances in experimental and clinical chemotherapy: workshop on pirarubicin. Munich, Ecomed, 1988;51.

682. Scheithauer W, Samonigg H, Depisch D. Activity of 4-O-tetrahydropyranil adriamycin (pirarubicin: THP) in metastatic breast cancer—a phase II study. Proc Am Soc Clin Oncol 1989;8:31.

683. Dorval T, Extra JM, Spielmann M. Thp-Adriamycin (T) (1609 rb) in advanced breast cancer (BC)-compiled data from three phase II studies. Proc Am Soc Clin Oncol 1989;8:54.

684. Lenk H, Wiener N, Tanneberger S. Phase II study of pirarubicin (P) in metastatic breast cancer patients. (Abstract) Book of abstracts: 5th European Conference on Clinical Oncology, 1989.

685. Waldman S, Sridhar KS, Richman S. Phase II trial of pirarubicin (P) in advanced breast CA (BC). Proc Am Soc Clin Oncol 1990;9:50.

686. Mouridsen HT, Kristensen D, Nielsen JH, et al. Phase II trial of prednimustine, 1-1031, (NSC-134087) in advanced breast cancer. Cancer 1980;46:253.

687. Lober J, Mouridsen HT, Christiansen IE. A phase III trial comparing a prednimustine (LEO 1031) to chlorambucil plus prednisolone in advanced breast cancer. Cancer 1983;52:1570.

688. Budman DR, Ginsberg S, Perry M. Phase II trial of spirogermanium in breast adenocarcinoma: a Cancer and Leukemia Group B study. Cancer Treat Rep 1982;66:1667.

689. Falkson G, Falkson HC. Phase II trial of spirogermanium for treatment of advanced breast cancer. Cancer Treat Rep 1983;67:189.

690. Pinnamaneni K, Yap HY, Legha SS. Phase II study of spirogermanium in the treatment of metastatic breast cancer. Cancer Treat Rep 1984;68:1197.

691. Schein PS, O'Connell MJ, Blom J. Clinical antitumor activity and toxicity of streptozotocin. Cancer 1974;34:993.

692. Pandya KJ, Tormey DC, Davis TE. Phase II trial of 6-thioguanine in metastatic breast cancer. Cancer Treat Rep 1980;64:191.

693. Costanza ME, Korzun AH, Rice MA. A phase II study of trimetrexate in previously untreated metastatic breast cancer patients. Proc Am Soc Clin Oncol 1988;7:30.

694. Frei EFI, Carbone PP, Schnider BI. Neoplastic disease. Arch Intern Med 1965;116:846.

695. Armstrong JG, Dyke RW, Fouts PJ, et al. Hodgkin's disease, carcinoma of the breast, and other tumors treated with vinblastine sulfate. Cancer Chemother Rep 1962;18:49.

696. Atkins HL, Gregg HG, Hyman GA. Clinical appraisal of cyclophosphamide in malignant neoplasms. Cancer 1962;15:1076.

697. Wright TL, Hurley J, Korst DR. Vinblastine in neoplastic disease. Cancer Res 1963;23:169.

698. Bleehan NM, Jelliffe AM. Vinblastine sulphate in the treatment of malignant disease. Br J Cancer 1965;19:268.

699. Grinberg R. Vincristine: dosage and response in advanced breast cancer. Cancer Chemother Rep 1965;45:57.

700. Goldenberg IS. Vincristine (NSC-67574) therapy of women with advanced breast cancer. Cancer Chemother Rep 1964;41:7.

701. Gubisch NJ, Norena D, Perlia CP. Experience with vincristine in solid tumors. Cancer Chemother Rep 1963;32:19.

702. Currie VE, Camacho F, Wittes R, et al. Phase II evaluation of vindesine in patients with advanced breast cancer. Cancer Treat Rep 1980;64:693.

703. Smith IE, Powles TJ. Vindesine in the treatment of breast cancer. Cancer Chemother Pharmacol 1979;2:261.

704. Walker BK, Raich PC, Fontana J. Phase II study of vindesine in patients with advanced breast cancer. Cancer Treat Rep 1982;66:1729.

705. Fleishman GB, Yap HY, Bodey GP. Comparability in therapeutic index with continuous 5-day infusion and 5-day bolus vindesine in the treatment of refractory breast cancer. Proc Am Soc Clin Oncol 1982;1:82.

706. Yap HY, Blumenschein GR, Hortobagyi GN. A randomized comparative study of vinblastine (VLB), vindesine (VDS) and vincristine (VCR) in patients (PTS) with refractory metastatic breast cancer. Proc Am Soc Clin Oncol 1981;22:441.

707. Dosik M, Winn R, Koven B. Phase II trial of weekly vindesine in early metastatic breast cancer. Proc Am Soc Clin Oncol 1981;22:445.

708. Morgenfeld EL, Rivaroa EG, Negro A. Vindesine for recurrent metastatic breast cancer. Proc Am Soc Clin Oncol 1988;7:21.

709. Canobbio L, Boccardo F, Pastorino G. A phase II study with a new vinca alkaloid, navelbine (NVB), in the treatment of advanced breast cancer patients. Proc Am Soc Clin Oncol 1989;8:50.

710. Fumoleau P, Delgado FM, Delozier T. Phase II trial with navelbine (NVB) in advanced breast cancer (ABC): preliminary results. Proc Am Soc Clin Oncol 1990;9:21.

711. Marty M, Leandri S, Extra JMD. A phase II study of vinorelbine (NVB) in patients (PTS) with advanced breast cancer (BC). Proc Am Assoc Cancer Res 1989;30:256.

712. Tirelli U, Franchin G, Crivellari D. Phase II study of VM-26 in extensively pretreated breast cancer. Am J Clin Oncol 1984;7:451.

713. Holmes FA, Esparanza L, Yap HY. A comparative study of etoposide and teniposide in refractory metastatic breast cancer (Abstract). Breast Cancer Res Treat 1986;8:93.

714. Vaughn CB, Panettiere F, Thigpen T. Phase II evaluation of VP-16213 in patients with advanced breast cancer: a Southwest Oncology Group study. Cancer Treat Rep 1981;65:443.

715. EORTC. Epipodophyllotoxin VP16213 in treatment of acute leukemias, hematosarcomas, and solid tumors. Br Med J 1973;3:199.

716. Nissen NI, Pajak TF, Leone LA. Clinical trial of VP-16213 (NSC141540) IV twice weekly in advanced neoplastic disease: a study of the Cancer and Leukemia Group B. Cancer 1980;45:232.

717. Fraschini G, Esparza L, Holmes F. High-dose etoposide in metastatic breast cancer. Breast Cancer Res Treat 1989;14:142.

718. Bezwoda WR, Seymour L, Ariad S. High-dose etoposide in treatment of metastatic breast cancer. Oncology 1992;49:104.

719. Palombo H, Estape J, Viholas N. Chronic oral etoposide in advanced breast cancer. (Abstract) Proc Am Soc Clin Oncol 1993;12:216.

720. Cerar D, Cervek J, Cufer T. Salvage chemotherapy with oral etoposide in metastatic breast cancer: preliminary report. (Abstract) Ann Oncol 1992;3(Suppl 5):84.

22.2
High-Dose Chemotherapy for Breast Cancer
WILLIAM P. PETERS

The use of high-dose chemotherapy with autologous cellular support for the treatment of breast cancer remains one of the most contentious therapeutic approaches in medicine. The clinical development and evaluation of this treatment approach has been rapid and has been accompanied by strong positions taken not only by physicians and scientists,[1-4] but also by insurers and public bodies. Arbitrary and capricious denial of insurance coverage for some patients[5] has resulted in litigation, sometimes with enormous punitive awards. The field represents a paradigm that displays both the good and the bad of contemporary medicine and its interface with a rapidly evolving medical care environment. The lessons learned in the development of this field are perhaps useful for other developing fields. Although ongoing prospective randomized clinical trials are being conducted, the outcomes of these studies are unlikely to be available for several more years, creating the awkward situation of dealing with an emotionally charged area on the basis of incomplete data. The purpose of this review is to evaluate the available data and to examine both the strengths and weakness of different analytic techniques. Although definitive conclusions concerning the place of dose-intensified therapy in breast cancer therapy will depend to a large extent on the results of ongoing prospective randomized trials, analysis of the available data is useful to provide insights into the potential value and place for this treatment and to indicate areas where further study will be necessary and potentially fruitful.

History

The development of dose-intensive approaches to breast cancer began in earnest in the early 1980s, with the recognition of and convergence of several therapeutic observations. Breast cancer is a common disease, afflicting more than 183,400 women annually in the United States and resulting in more than 46,000 deaths annually.[6] Despite its frequency, limited curative potential has been demonstrated (some would say none) for any treatment for metastatic breast cancer. Further, identifiable subgroups appear to have a particularly poor prognosis, for example, premenopausal women with hormone-insensitive metastatic breast cancer involving the viscera. The recognition and consensus concerning subgroups of patients with breast cancer who have a particularly poor prognosis provided further reason to explore new therapeutic approaches for these patients, in whom conventional treatment approaches were limited.

Further, evidence was developing in the early 1980s that adjuvant therapy for breast cancer was producing curative results with chemotherapy programs that were not curative in metastatic disease.[7-10] This finding suggested that tumor volume or natural history could prove important for testing of novel treatment approaches; treatments of limited effectiveness in some settings could prove effective if used earlier in the natural history of the disease or in settings of minimal tumor volume.

Previous laboratory and clinical experience was also seminal to the development of high-dose therapy. The experience in Hodgkin's disease and acute leukemia, pioneered by Frei, Holland, DeVita, and others, based on previous laboratory studies, indicated that high-dose and combination chemotherapy were critical to the development of curative treatment approaches. Some of these concepts were most clearly articulated by Frei and Canellos, who highlighted the critical importance of dose intensity. Further, information from experimental model systems, influenced primarily by Schabel and associates,[11-14] demonstrated features of dose-intensive treatment approaches that were previously not appreciated. These investigators at the Southern Research Institute demonstrated, in murine tumor systems, the important concepts of non–cross-resistance and, sometimes, therapeutic synergy among selected alkylating agents. These observations, coupled with the steep dose–response effect of alkylating agents, suggested that if selected alkylating agents were combined at high doses, it might be possible to overcome the effects of intrinsic resistance that appeared to limit the effectiveness of available therapy. Clinical studies using escalated doses of single agents had demonstrated substantial nonmyelosuppressive, nonoverlapping toxicity among selected alkylating agents,[15-18] and this finding offered potential to combine multiple agents at escalated doses. Finally, the experience of the Seattle bone marrow transplantation effort, led by E. Donnall Thomas, indicated that curative results were possible in treatment settings, for example, in patients with relapsed acute myelogenous leukemia, using allogeneic bone marrow transplantation in patients in whom curative results were not possible with any conventional-dose therapy.[19] Taken together, these data suggested that it might be possible to escalate multiple alkylating agents (using autologous bone marrow support) and to increase, in linear–log fashion, the cellular kill of epithelial malignant tumors, such as breast cancer. Coupled with improved supportive care techniques, the basis for early efforts at high-dose combination alkylating agent therapy was established.

The initial phase I trials attempted to combine, in general, multiple alkylating agents using autologous bone marrow support (ABMS).[21] The results demonstrated an unexpectedly high frequency of objective response, including complete responses, even though the patients had frequently received extensive prior chemotherapy. The remissions were of short duration, and morbidity and mortality associated with the transplant were substantial. Further, the toxicities encountered were often novel and differed from those encountered when the escalated drugs were used singly at high doses. Nonetheless, the frequency of response in these highly resistant settings suggested an evaluation of the approach in patients who had received less prior therapy.

A limited number of phase II trials were undertaken in patients with poor-prognosis metastatic breast cancer. These studies demonstrated that, in a small fraction of patients, a single high-dose treatment using ABMS could result in long-term disease-free remission. Figure 22.2-1 shows results from a trial undertaken by the Duke Bone Marrow Transplant Program in which women with hormone-insensitive, measurable, metastatic breast cancer were treated with a single course of high-dose cyclophosphamide, cisplatin, and carmustine (CPB) and ABMS.[20] In this series, the minimum follow-up is now longer than 8 years, with 3 of 22 patients (14%) remaining continuously disease-free at full performance status. These data are particularly compelling in that the outcome cannot be ascribed to any other therapy because the only therapeutic intervention used was high-dose combination alkylating agents with any additional induction with conventional-dose therapy or consolidation with radiation therapy or hormones. These data are at variance with the premise that multiple treatment courses are necessary in breast cancer to result in durable remissions. In these patients, most relapses occurred in pretreatment sites of bulk disease or in areas of prior radiation therapy. These observations suggested that the treatment results might be optimized by using high-dose therapy in a setting of lower tumor volume or earlier in the natural history of the disease.

Two strategies derived from these observations: (1) an attempt to reduce tumor burden rapidly in metastatic disease through the use of intensive but conventional-dose pretransplantation chemotherapy programs, particularly ones not based on alkylating agent therapy; and (2) evalua-

tion of high-dose therapy in the high-risk adjuvant setting in which tumor burden is minimal and natural history of the disease is earlier.

Sequential Induction Therapy Followed by High-Dose Chemotherapy and Autologous Bone Marrow Transplantation

In metastatic disease, the use of high-dose consolidation after conventional-dose induction therapy has been undertaken by a series of groups, with the results summarized in various reviews of the literature. In general, the results are remarkably similar from study to study. Most complete responses occur in patients achieving a complete or partial response to induction chemotherapy. In some centers, and perhaps in most, patients failing to respond to induction chemotherapy are not given high-dose consolidation therapy. The data supporting this selection process are not convincing. With intensive induction chemotherapy programs, most patients are able to achieve an objective response; of the small percentage not responding (15% to 25%), about 10% of these patients are able to achieve durable progression-free remissions. It is not clear from the available data that the discriminatory capability attributed to induction chemotherapy is as strong as has been claimed by some. Other factors, such as bulk or site of disease or prior adjuvant chemotherapy, may prove more robust as predictive factors. Table 22.2-1 lists the clinical characteristics of long-term disease-free remission patients from 2 sequential studies in which all patients entering the study were anticipated to receive high-dose therapy. In the first study, 22 premenopausal women with measurable, hormone-insensitive metastatic breast cancer were treated with a single course of high-dose CPB with ABMS, with no other therapeutic intervention; 3 of 22 (14%) have remained continuously disease-free (Fig. 22.2-1), all patients have been followed-up for longer than 8 years. The pretreatment characteristics of the patients, presented in Table 22.2-1, indicate a predominance of lung and lymph node disease and limited prior adjuvant chemotherapy. A second study used induction chemotherapy with doxorubicin, 5-fluorouracil, and methotrexate (AFM), followed by high-dose consolidation with CPB. Forty-five patients were entered, and 40 were given high-dose therapy; 5 of the 45 (11%) remained continuously disease-free with a minimum follow-up of more than 5 years. Again, the clinical characteristics long-term disease-free survivors are presented in Table 22.2-1 and indicate a predominance of limited-volume disease and minimal prior adjuvant chemotherapy, and they provide some evidence for the value of adjuvant surgery and radiation therapy. Some of these features may not be as relevant today, when a much higher fraction of all patients receive adjuvant chemotherapy, because subsequent studies (albeit with shorter follow-up of all entered patients) have indicated that some patients with liver or other sites of visceral disease can achieve durable

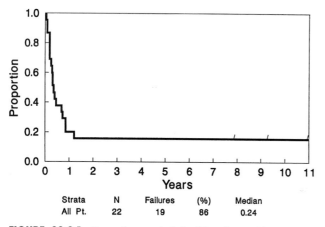

Strata	N	Failures	(%)	Median
All Pt.	22	19	86	0.24

FIGURE 22.2-1 Event-free survival for 22 patients with metastatic breast cancer treated with high-dose cyclophosphamide, cisplatin, and carmustine as first-line therapy for hormone-insensitive disease. Event-free survival includes all relapses and all therapy-related mortality.

TABLE 22.2-1

Pretreatment Characteristics of Patients Achieving Long-Term Disease-Free Survival in Early Studies of High-Dose Therapy for Breast Cancer

Patient	Protocol	Site of Metastases	Comments
1	Upfront*	Pleura, hilum	No adjuvant, no radiation therapy
2	Upfront*	Mediastinum, bone	CMF adjuvant; prior radiation therapy
3	Upfront*	Cervical and supraclavicular lymph nodes	No adjuvant
4	AFM†	Cervical and supraclavicular lymph nodes, breast	No adjuvant, CCR to AFM, surgery then complete response; radiation therapy
5	AFM†	Supraclavicular lymph nodes 2 cm	No adjuvant; complete response to AFM
6	AFM†	Chest wall 4 cm; lymph nodes, lung	No adjuvant; partial response to AFM; complete response post; radiation therapy
7	AFM†	Chest wall 2 cm; internal mammary lymph nodes	No adjuvant; no radiation therapy

CMF, cyclophosphamide, methotrexate, and 5-fluorouracil.

* Protocol using high-dose cyclophosphamide, cisplatin, and carmustine as initial chemotherapy treatment for hormone-insensitive metastatic breast cancer; minimum follow-up was in excess of 8 years for all treated patients.

† Protocol using high-dose cyclophosphamide, cisplatin, and carmustine as consolidation after induction therapy using doxorubicin, 5-fluorouracil, and methotrexate for hormone-insensitive metastatic breast cancer; minimum follow-up was more than 5 years for all treated patients.

remissions. Only time and further study will allow more precise identification of patient populations for which high-dose therapy may be useful.

In an effort to address some of these issues, data concerning autologous bone marrow transplantation (ABMT) for metastatic breast cancer obtained from a survey of North American bone marrow transplantation centers was analyzed. Thirty-three centers supplied information on all the breast cancer autotransplantations performed. The survey requested specific patient information concerning demographics, prior adjuvant chemotherapy, type of induction and transplant therapy used, and dates of diagnosis, treatment, progression, and death. Full details of this survey will be published elsewhere. Data from this survey of North American bone marrow transplantation centers indicate similar findings to the single-institution data. For patients receiving induction therapy followed by ABMT as first-line therapy for metastatic breast cancer, the overall survival at 3 years is 35% (95% confidence interval [CI], 30% to 41%). A comparison of this overall survival with survival in patients derived from three large series of single-institution or cooperative-group patients treated with conventional dose chemotherapy is also presented in Table 22.2-2. The conventional-dose series were selected to include patients under the age of 55 years with hormone-insensitive disease and who had measurable metastatic disease. Although any such comparison of nonrandomized populations is subject to many potential biases, the selection criteria and the availability of actual data for the treatment populations provide information improved from previous comparisons. Nonetheless, the potential for biases affecting this type of analysis is significant and should be recognized by anyone attempting to interpret this information. Subset analysis did not indicate that a disease-free interval from adjuvant therapy of more or less than 1 year

TABLE 22.2-2

Summary Outcome Data at 3 Years for Patients Treated with Autologous Bone Marrow Transplantation and Conventional-Dose Therapy

	Patients	Median Survival (y)	3-Year Overall Survival Rate (95% CI)
PATIENT POPULATIONS			
Stage IV*	1101	2.06	37% (32–42)
Stage IV ER−−PR−†	919	1.88	33% (28–39)
Stage IV induction: partial response‡	254	1.87	34% (27–42)
CONTROL POPULATIONS:			
CALGB ER−§	64	1	5%
SWOG (80% ER−)¶	39	1.2	8%

ER−, estrogen receptor-negative; PR−, progesterone receptor-negative; CALGB, Cancer and Leukemia Group B; SWOG, Southwest Oncology Group.

* Overall survival data for 1101 patients with stage IV breast cancer treated with high-dose chemotherapy as first-line therapy for metastatic disease.

† Stage IV breast cancer patients ER- and PR-negative tumors or patients whose treatment with hormonal therapy fails.

‡ Stage IV breast cancer patients who obtained a partial response to induction therapy prior to proceeding to high-dose consolidation.

§ Metastatic breast cancer treated with conventional-dose chemotherapy as defined in two CALGB trials—protocols 8081 and 8281. Characteristics of patients reported in text[28] attempting to define outcomes for patients similar to patients entering transplant studies.

¶ Outcome summary for metastatic disease patients treated with conventional-dose chemotherapy in SWOG cooperative group trials selected to be similar to patients entering transplant studies as reported.[29]

was an important prognostic factor in this analysis. Patients who had hormone-sensitive tumors not previously treated with hormonal therapy had a better overall survival (61% versus 32% at 3 years) than those with hormone-insensitive tumors, findings consistent with prior experience in the treatment of breast cancer.

These data, taken together, are consistent with the conclusion that, for historically matched control populations, overall survival appears improved with the use of high-dose intensification and autologous cellular support. The potential biases and the limitations of such comparisons must be recognized, and results of prospective, randomized trials are awaited. At least two such trials are being undertaken in patients with metastatic breast cancer. The Duke Bone Marrow Transplant Program initiated in 1988 a prospective, randomized trial of high-dose therapy in patients with measurable, metastatic breast cancer (Fig. 22.2-2). Eligibility requirements include histologically demonstrated, measurable metastatic breast cancer not involving the brain or bone marrow. Prior doxorubicin exposure during adjuvant chemotherapy was required to be less than 300 mg/m², and no prior chemotherapy for metastatic disease was permitted. The patient's tumor was required to be both estrogen receptor– and progesterone receptor–negative or demonstrated to be progressive despite at least one hormonal therapy. Induction chemotherapy was prescribed as AFM, as previously described. Induction therapy with AFM was administered for a maximum of four cycles, a total lifetime doxorubicin exposure of 450 mg/m², or evidence that tumor regression was not continuing. At the end of induction therapy, clinical and radiologic restaging was undertaken. If the patient achieved a complete remission, the patient was randomly assigned to either consolidation with high-dose CPB or to observation. If disease recurrence was demonstrated on the observation arm, patients were then offered high-dose therapy and ABMT. Patients achieving a partial response to the induction therapy were offered high-dose therapy and ABMT without randomization in an effort to convert the response to a complete response; patients

without response or with progressive disease during induction therapy were taken off the study. More than 400 patients have entered into this study, and projected accrual goals are nearing completion; analysis of this trial should be possible within the next year.

A second prospective randomized trial in metastatic disease is being undertaken by the Philadelphia Cooperative Bone Marrow Transplant Group. In this trial, patients with metastatic breast cancer that responds partially or completely to induction therapy are randomly assigned to receive either high-dose consolidation and bone marrow transplantation or continued therapy with conventional-dose therapy.

Autologous Bone Marrow Transplantation for Primary Breast Cancer

The data in metastatic breast cancer indicate that a small fraction of patients achieve durable remissions after a single course of high-dose therapy. The nature of the results prompted comparisons with those seen by the Seattle Transplant Group using allogeneic bone marrow transplantation for relapsed acute leukemia. In this latter circumstance, treatment earlier in the disease, or at a smaller tumor burden while the patient was in the first complete remission, resulted in a substantial improvement in the outcome. Although clearly major differences exist between these diseases and treatments, the demonstration of the value of this strategy suggested that trials in earlier breast cancer could be worthwhile.

Patients with primary breast cancer who are found to have multiple involved lymph nodes at the time of diagnosis remain at high risk for disease recurrence despite the use of surgery, radiation therapy, and conventional-dose chemotherapy. In an analysis of data derived from studies of relapses after surgical treatment of breast cancer, Skipper

FIGURE 22.2-2 Treatment scheme for the AFM randomized trial using CPA/cDDP/BCNU as consolidation after induction therapy with AFM. Patients who achieve a clinical complete remission to the induction therapy are randomly assigned to immediate consolidation with high-dose therapy or to observation with high-dose therapy given at time of progression.

estimated a modal distribution of nearly 10^8 to 10^9 viable clonogenic cancer cells remaining after surgery in patients whose tumors involved four or more axillary lymph nodes to account for the frequency and rate of recurrence. The data suggest that the large number of cells remaining after surgical treatment present formidable barriers to successful treatment with conventional-dose chemotherapy and imply that studies of additional therapy are warranted. In this regard, the initial efforts using high-dose therapy with ABMS have been an approach to this difficult treatment setting. In a study from the Duke Bone Marrow Transplant Program in collaboration with the Cancer and Leukemia Group B (CALGB), 85 patients with primary breast cancer (stage IIA, IIB, or IIIA) involving 10 or more axillary lymph nodes demonstrated an apparent improvement in disease-free survival, compared with selected contemporaneous and historical controls. At present, these difference appear to be as much as 30% to 40% improved over the control series, but such data need to be considered cautiously because the comparisons are based on nonrandomized data. Two large cooperative group prospective randomized trials are underway, and the outcome of these studies will be critical to assessing the role of high-dose therapy in treatment strategy. The designs of these prospective randomized trials are shown in Figure 22.3-3, but at current accrual rates, it is unlikely that analysis of these trials will occur for another 3 to 4 years.

We have completed a survey of the identified North American bone marrow transplant centers requesting primary data on the experience of high-dose treatment in the primary breast cancer setting. Data were secured on 662 patients with a median 13 positive lymph nodes treated with high-dose chemotherapy with bone marrow or peripheral blood support as part of their treatment program. The analysis is shown in Figure 22.2-4 presents the Kaplan-Meier estimated overall and event-free survival for these patients. The data appear to be similar to single-institution data for this patient population. Again, these data were obtained from a survey, and therefore, any comparison of this information with data from other series is potentially fraught with bias. Nonetheless, the consistent experience in the conventional-dose therapy of primary breast cancer has been uniformly poor, suggesting that the strategy used in these high-dose consolidation studies may afford a therapeutic advantage. Again, the results of prospective randomized trials will be of importance in helping to assign the ultimate role of this treatment in the management of breast cancer.

DECLINE OF TREATMENT-RELATED TOXICITY

One of the major concerns raised concerning bone marrow transplantation procedures has been the toxicity associated with high-dose chemotherapy. In contrast to allogeneic bone marrow transplantation, in which graft-versus-host disease contributes substantially to treatment-related morbidity and mortality, bone marrow transplantation for breast cancer has relied on ABMT, in which the graft is rarely associated with toxicity. Further, with the widespread adoption of colony-stimulating factor (CSF)–

primed peripheral blood progenitor cells (PBPCs), morbidity and mortality have decreased and in most major centers are now in the range of 2% to 5%. With the increasing intensity of conventional-dose therapy, the toxicity of bone marrow transplantation is now often less than that associated with multiple courses of intensive conventional-dose therapy.

Several advances in supportive care have enabled bone marrow transplantations for breast cancer to be conducted largely as outpatient procedures at some centers. The use of CSF-primed PBPCs coupled with bone marrow has resulted in a major reduction in the time to neutrophil recovery, the effective elimination of the period of absolute leukopenia, a major reduction in the requirement for platelet transfusions, and a reduced overall morbidity of transplantation.[21] Adoption of a sequential prophylactic oral antibiotic regimen with an empiric once-daily parenteral antibiotic approach has resulted in a major reduction in the frequency of febrile neutropenia, reduced the number of documented bacterial infections, and reduced the requirement for empiric antifungal therapy. Improvements in computerized medical recordkeeping have also resulted in an enhanced capability to permit rapid transitions between outpatient and inpatient care.[22] We have used intensive outpatient clinic support to reduce the number of hospital days associated with high-dose CPB, and ABMT–PBPC support from a median 24.5 days to 5 days, with a consequent reduction in hospital charges of nearly 60%.[23]

Long-Term Effects of High-Dose Therapy

With increasing use of high-dose therapy for primary and metastatic breast cancer and the demonstration of extended remissions, assessment of the long-term effects of high-dose therapy will be important. Only limited information on the long-term effects of high-dose therapy is available. The most important long-term effects of high-dose therapy are, of course, those on disease outcome. The results of randomized and other trials of this therapeutic approach will be of primary importance in this setting. Effects of the treatment approach on long-term toxicity will be critical to assessing the ultimate role of this therapy for patients, however. The potential effects of high-dose therapy on hematopoiesis, immunologic function, pulmonary, hepatic, and renal function, and late malignant disease must be determined. Ultimately, quality of life following high-dose therapy may well be the most important parameter by which to measure the value of high-dose versus conventional-dose therapy. Few data are available on any of these subjects.

We have examined the long-term hematologic reconstitution data for patients treated with high-dose chemotherapy and ABMS. Data indicate that blood counts tend to return toward, but not completely to, normal soon after the completion of high-dose therapy. In my experience, tolerance to conventional-dose chemotherapy after high-

A

C=cyclophosphamide 600 mg/m2 IV d1
A=doxorubicin 60 mg/m2 IV d 1
F=flurouracil 600 mg/m2 IV d 1,8
    repeat cycles q 28 days

B

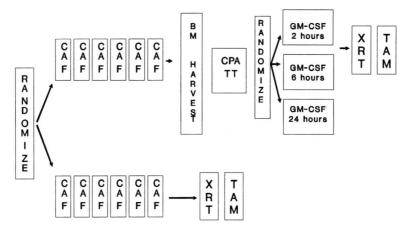

C= cyclophosphamide 100 mg/m2 po qd x 14
A=doxorubicin 30 mg/m2 IV d 1,8
F=flurouracil 500 mg/m2 IV d 1,8
    repeat cycles q 28 days

CPA = cyclophosphamide 6000 mg/m2 IV over 96 hr
TT = ThioTEPA 800 mg/m2 IV over 96 hours

FIGURE 22.2-3 Protocol scheme's for two prospective randomized trials underway using high-dose therapy as consolidation after conventional dose induction therapy. **A.** Intergroup trial (CALGB 9082/SWOG 9114/ NCIC MA-13). **B.** Eastern Cooperative Oncology Group (ECOG 2190) in collaboration with SWOG.

dose chemotherapy improves as the time after the bone marrow transplantation increases. Within the first few months after high-dose therapy, bone marrow tolerance is marginal even for the first cycles of therapy, but by a year or more, posttransplant chemotherapy tolerance is remarkably robust for at least the first few cycles.

Significant reductions in the number of CD4 lymphocytes and an inverted CD4/CD8 ratio persist for extended periods after ABMT.[24] Despite these abnormalities, however, few late infections are encountered in these patients,

except when the patients are treated with corticosteroids or other immunosuppressive agents.[25] When corticosteroids are administered for the treatment of pulmonary drug toxicity or thrombotic microangiopathy, the risk of opportunistic infections such as *Pneumocystis carinii* or other organisms increases dramatically. Antibody production appears mostly unaffected.

Pulmonary toxicity has been encountered after many different high-dose programs, but it has, in general, been manageable. Depending on the treatment setting and

FIGURE 22.2-4 Event-free (**A**) and overall (**B**) survival for eligible patients treated with CAF followed by high-dose CPA/cDDP/BCNU with ABMT/PBPC support and for similar patients selected from two case-controlled data sets from CALGB trials. Vertical bars represent the 95% confidence intervals for each data set determined at the median follow-up of the transplant trial. (Peters WP, Ross M, Vredenburgh JJ, et al. High-dose chemotherapy and autologous bone marrow support as consolidation after standard dose adjuvant therapy for high-risk primary breast cancer. In: Salmon SE, ed. Adjuvant therapy of cancer VII. Philadelphia, JB Lippincott, 1993: 207)

definition, this syndrome can occur in as many as 30% to 40% of treated patients. The syndrome most commonly manifests as cough, fever, dyspnea, and hypoxemia about 6 to 12 weeks after bone marrow transplantation.[26] Radiologic evaluations often demonstrate a peripheral, patchy infiltrate, and one commonly sees a significant decline in the carbon monoxide diffusion in the lungs (DLCO).[27] Treatment with corticosteroids, such as prednisone, usually causes prompt resolution of symptoms, often within 48 hours. Corticosteroid treatment is often required for 6 to 12 weeks before the medication can be completely withdrawn, however. Radiation therapy may exacerbate the syndrome. Long-term residual effects have been uncommon, and most patients return toward normal DLCO 1 year after bone marrow transplantation. Continued follow-up will be required to determine whether this syndrome has any late effects.

An infrequent but serious late complication of high-dose chemotherapy is a syndrome termed thrombotic microangiopathy or hemolytic–uremic syndrome. Occurring an average of 4 months after bone marrow transplantation, the syndrome is characterized by hemolytic

anemia, thrombocytopenia, fever, renal dysfunction, and occasionally altered mental status. An infectious process is often associated. Management is complicated and is frequently unsuccessful. The cause is presumed to be related to the endothelial injury produced by the high-dose chemotherapy with exacerbation from some subsequent event.

Of major concern is the potential for development of secondary malignant diseases or myelodysplastic syndromes (MDSs) in patients treated with high-dose chemotherapy. Only now are sufficient numbers of patients reaching extended periods of follow-up after high-dose therapy. My colleagues and I have analyzed 1054 patients entered into studies of whom 696 received high-dose chemotherapy with CPB; 243 of these patients have been followed-up for more than 2 years after bone marrow transplantation. Five of 1054 enrolled patients (0.5%), 4 of 696 patients treated with high-dose CPB, and 3 of 243 patients more than 2 years after bone marrow transplantation developed either acute leukemia or myelodysplasia. One patient randomized to observation after achieving a complete remission to intensive AFM induction therapy developed acute leukemia after 1 year of observation without ever receiving high-dose therapy, and 1 patient developed acute monocytic leukemia (AML) 6 weeks after bone marrow transplantation. Three other patients developed AML–MDS at 11 to 43 months after high-dose therapy. All the patients had normal cytogenetic features at the time of bone marrow harvest, but 3 had abnormal karyotypes at the time of MDS–AML diagnosis. These cases will be described in detail in a subsequent publication.

High-dose therapy represents an important evolving approach to the treatment of breast cancer. The results of ongoing prospective randomized trials will be of major importance in establishing the role of this therapy in the treatment options for breast cancer. Until these trials have been completed, the best available analyses are the results of single-institution trials and survey data that examine the collected treatment results from multiple institutions. From these uncontrolled data from patients with metastatic disease, high-dose chemotherapy with ABMS or PBPC support appears to offer a modest improved in disease-free and overall survival, compared with conventional-dose regimens in similar patients. At present, the results of high-dose therapy used as consolidation after conventional-dose therapy in high-risk patients with primary breast cancer appear to represent a substantial improvement in disease-free survival compared with results in similar patients who did not receive high-dose consolidation. Only time and continued follow-up will allow greater comfort in interpreting the data concerning high-dose therapy. Major reductions in toxicity associated with the therapy are, however, making the treatment more accessible and less expensive. Some patients can receive nearly their entire bone marrow transplantation as outpatients. The long-term effects of high-dose therapy are only now beginning to become apparent as sufficient numbers of patients are followed-up for long periods after bone marrow transplantation for breast cancer.

References

1. Hryniuk W, Busch H. The importance of dose intensity in chemotherapy of metastatic breast cancer. J Clin Oncol 1984;2:1281.
2. Devita VT. Dose-response is alive and well. J Clin Oncol 1986;4:1157.
3. Hryniuk W, Levine MN. Analysis of dose intensity for adjuvant chemotherapy trials in stage II breast cancer. J Clin Oncol 1986;4:1162.
4. Henderson IC, Hayes DF, Gelman R. Dose-response in the treatment of breast cancer. J Clin Oncol 1988;6:1501.
5. Peters WP, Rogers M. Variation in approval of private health insurance coverage for autologous bone marrow transplantation for breast cancer. N Engl J Med 1994;330:473.
6. Wingo PA, Tong T, Bolden S. Cancer statistics, 1995. CA Cancer J Clin 1995;45:8.
7. Fisher B, Fisher ER, Redmond C. Ten year results from NSABP clinical trials evaluating the use of phenylalanine mustard in the management of primary breast cancer. J Clin Oncol 1986;4:929.
8. Bonadonna G, Valagussa P. Adjuvant systemic chemotherapy for primary breast cancer. J Clin Oncol 1985;3:259.
9. Hortobagyi GN, Frye D, Buzdar AU, et al. Complete Remissions in metastatic breast cancer: a thirteen year follow-up report. Proc ASCO 1988;7:37,143a.
10. Legha SS, Buzdar AU, Smith TL, et al. Complete remission in metastatic breast cancer treated with combination drug therapy. Ann Intern Med 1979;91:847.
11. Schabel FM, Trader MW, Laster WR, et al. Patterns of resistance and therapeutic synergism among alkylating agents. Antibio Chemother 1978;23:200.
12. Schabel FM. Animal models as predictive systems. In: Cancer chemotherapy: fundamental concepts and recent advances. Chicago, Year Book, 1975:323.
13. Steel GG. Growth and survival of tumor stem cells. In: Growth kinetics of tumors Oxford, Clarendon, 1977:244.
14. Schabel FM, Griswold DP Jr, Corbett TH, et al. Testing therapeutic hypothesis in mice and man: observations of the therapeutic activity against advanced solid tumor in mice treated with anticancer drugs that have demonstrated or potential clinical utility for treatment of advanced solid tumors of man. In: Devita VT, Busch H, eds. Methods in cancer research. New York, Academic, 1979:3.
15. Herzig G. In: Brown EB, ed. Progress in hematology. New York, Grune & Stratton, 1981:1.
16. Peters WP, Eder JP, Henner WD, et al. High dose combination alkylating agents with autologous bone marrow support: a phase I trial J Clin Oncol 1986;4:646.
17. Slease RB, Benear JB, Selby GB, et al. High-dose combination alkylating agent therapy with autologous bone marrow rescue for refractory solid tumors. J Clin Oncol 1988;6:1314.
18. Maraninchi D, Piana L, Blaise D, et al. Phase I and II studies of high-dose alkylating agents in poor-risk patients with breast cancer with autologous bone marrow transplantation: proceedings of the Third International Symposium. Houston, University of Texas MD Anderson Hospital, 1987:475.
19. Thomas ED. The use and potential of bone marrow allograft and whole-body irradiation in the treatment of leukemia. Cancer 1982;50:1449.
20. Peters WP, Shpall EJ, Jones RB, et al. High dose combination alkylating agents with bone marrow support as initial treatment for metastatic breast cancer. J Clin Oncol 1988;6:1368.
21. Peters WP, Kurtzberg J, Rosner G, et al. Comparative effects of G-CSF and GM-CSF on priming peripheral blood progenitor cells for use with autologous bone marrow after high-dose chemotherapy. Blood 1993;81:7,1709.
22. Gilbert C, Meisenberg B, Vredenburgh J, et al. Sequential prophylactic ciprofloxacin and rifampin and empiric once daily vancomycin and aminoglycoside for neutropenic fever after high-dose chemotherapy and autologous bone marrow support. J Clin Oncol 1994;12:1005.
23. Peters WP, Ross M, Vredenburgh JJ, et al. The use of intensive clinic support to permit outpatient autologous bone marrow transplantation for breast cancer. Semin Oncol 1994;21:25.
24. Olsen GA, Gockerman JP, Bast RC, et al. Altered immunologic reconstitution after standard-dose chemotherapy or high-dose chemotherapy with autologous bone marrow support. Transplantation 1988;46:57.
25. Peters WP, Ross M, Vredenburgh JJ, et al. High-dose chemotherapy and autologous bone marrow support as consolidation after standard dose adjuvant therapy for high-risk primary breast cancer. J Clin Oncol 1993;11:6,1132.
26. Todd NW, Peters WP, Ost AH, et al. Pulmonary drug toxicity in patients with primary breast cancer treated with high-dose combination chemotherapy and autologous bone marrow transplantation. Am Rev Respir Dis 1993;147:1264.
27. Patz EF, Peters WP, Goodman PC. Pulmonary drug toxicity fol-

lowing high-dose chemotherapy with autologous bone marrow transplantation: CT findings in 20 cases. J Thorac Imaging 1994; 9:129.

28. Mick R, Colin CB, Antman KH, et al. Diverse prognosis in metastatic breast cancer: who should be offered alternative initial therapies. Breast Cancer Res Treat 1989;13:33.

29. Livingston RB. High-dose consolidation for stage IV breast cancer.

In: ASCO educational book. American Society of Clinical Oncology, 1994:74.

30. Peters WP, Ross M, Vredenburgh JJ, et al. High-dose chemotherapy and autologous bone marrow support as consolidation after standard dose adjuvant therapy for high-risk primary breast cancer. In: Salmon SE, ed. Adjuvant therapy of cancer VII. Philadelphia, JB Lippincott, 1993:207.

22.3

Biologic Therapy of Breast Cancer

MARC E. LIPPMAN

The purpose of this chapter is to review the principles of biologic therapy of breast cancer. A variety of strategies that can be used to identify appropriate targets of biologic therapy are presented. A series of approaches in varying stages of preclinical and clinical testing is discussed mechanistically. The therapeutic advantages and potential toxicities of these approaches and their limitations are described insofar as they are currently known.

The principles of biologic therapy of breast cancer are straightforward. Current dogma holds that all breast cancer is due to genetic changes that are either inherited or acquired somatically. Whatever damage to the genome is involved in the evolution of breast cancer, the eventual presentation of invasive breast cancer in women by definition encompasses a series of properties of the tumor that together define the behavior of the tumor. These commonly identified properties, when expressed together, provide a working definition of breast cancer:

- Capacity for unlimited growth
- Invasiveness
- Metastatic potential
- Ability to evoke an angiogenic response
- Acquisition of drug resistance through amplification of genes of target proteins

An essential assumption of biologic therapy is that these phenotypic properties of breast cancer are specifically due to differential protein expression, that is, proteins expressed by the cancer, which are expressed less often or never by other mature tissues in the body, proteins expressed by normal tissue and not made by the cancer, and occasionally, mutated proteins expressed exclusively by the cancer (eg, mutated p53).

The underlying premise of biologic therapies is that sufficient specificity exists among these differentially displayed proteins responsible for the malignant phenotype to be clinically exploitable.

Several specific areas are not considered under biologic therapy in this chapter. First, no consideration is given to a variety of cytokines that can modulate the toxicities of chemotherapy. Promising results with granulocyte colony-stimulating factor and granulocyte–macrophage colony-stimulating unit in ameliorating myelosuppression

due to chemotherapeutic drugs have already been established. Several groups have finally identified a protein with thrombopoietin function, and the gene for this protein has been cloned.[1] Its potential role in the clinical management of breast cancer is obvious, and it will be the subject of intense clinical trials. Second, this discussion does not deal with immunologic approaches to breast cancer because this topic is discussed elsewhere in this book. Rather, I focus on those properties of breast cancer that differentiate it from normal breast epithelium and consider both the identification of further biologic targets and the potential means of altering the concentrations or activities of targeted proteins as a form of therapy.

All these approaches need to be considered in the context of other means by which improved treatment for metastatic breast cancer may be envisioned. Obviously, new agents may become available with worthwhile activity against breast cancer. Paclitaxel (Taxol) and its derivatives represent examples of exciting new agents with potential usefulness in breast cancer. One hopes that we will continue to learn how to use existing therapies more effectively. Aside from alterations in dose intensity with cytokine or stem cell support, a series of innovative scheduling changes can be envisioned as leading to more effective therapy. These include trails based on circadian variations.[2] Finally, one may envision immunologic approaches to tumors either in the form of gene therapy, which increases the immunologic targeting of cancer cells, or in some other form of adoptive immunotherapy. These latter considerations are also discussed elsewhere in this book.

Malignant Phenotype

As mentioned previously, the malignant phenotype of breast cancer is definable as unlimited growth, invasiveness, metastatic potential, the ability to induce an angiogenic response, and the acquisition of drug resistance. Significant potential exists for overlap among the functional roles that proteins contributing to this process may serve. For example, metastases never progress beyond the occult phase without angiogenic capacity; tumor cells without invasive ability probably are unable to metastasize. If each function is absolutely required for the complete malignant phenotype, however, then blocking any of them will strongly inhibit malignant behavior, much as failing to dial one number correctly among several in a combination lock blocks the phenotype of a lock (to lock or unlock) without destroying the lock.

Of paramount significance in the success of biologic therapy is the choice of a target protein. A given breast cancer probably has the potential to exploit several different molecules to achieve the same phenotypic effect. For example, several members of the fibroblast growth factor (FGF) family or the pleiotrophin family may independently be sufficient for an angiogenic response. A cancer is potentially capable of expressing more than one molecule at the same time, or, by a process of selective pressure, clonal evolution of populations of cells exploiting different angiogenic molecules could lead to the failure of a given biologic therapy aimed at only one molecule. If multiple choices for proteins exist for each of the functions that contribute to the malignant phenotype, the overall behavior of the malignant lesion will be highly variable, depending on which particular combination is at work in any particular cancer.

All epithelial malignant tumors, including breast cancer, have the capacity for unlimited growth. Although this growth may not be particularly rapid, normal stromal epithelial boundaries do not limit growth, so-called contact inhibition is not expressed, and, if left untreated, eventually a lethal body burden of tumor will accumulate. Many molecules may contribute to this phenotype. These include growth factors and their cognate receptors, molecules in cell cycle progression or the inactivation of molecules in specific checkpoints, and altered expression of molecules in cell adhesion to basement membrane and other cellular components that may be involved in limiting growth. Failure of apoptotic mechanisms also probably contributes to this phenomenon. Clearly, many signal transduction pathway proteins may also be involved, such as ras, raf, and the various mitogen-activated protein (MAP) kinases. A discussion of their contributions to growth regulation is beyond the scope of this chapter. Alberts and associates[3] provide a useful general introduction and overview. Given the requirement of differential expression of target proteins in breast cancer versus normal cells, however, these may often be less attractive targets because of their lack of specificity.

The definition of breast cancer commonly has the word *invasive* in it. The property of invasion, the ability to extend beyond the lobular units and breast ducts morphologically, can be distinguished readily from expansive growth. Although the larger the primary tumor, the more likely it is to have invasive components, no preordained relationship exists between primary tumor size and the likelihood of invasiveness. Rather, the invasive phenotype depends minimally on the ability of the cancer cells to digest basement membranes, to free themselves from adherence to surrounding cells, and to migrate into new tissue spaces independently of their ability to grow.

The mechanisms by which malignant tumors acquire the ability to metastasize, and the properties that tend to make metastases of given tumors moderately definable by the sites to which they spread, are largely unknown. For example, although breast cancer commonly metastasizes to bone, it rarely involves sites distal to elbow or knee. Nonetheless, clinical observations show that unlimited invasion and growth are separable from metastasis. To some extent, alterations in cell adhesion molecule expression, locomotion, and the ability to disrupt normal tissue planes by mechanisms similar or identical to those involved in invasion are probably essential. Moreover, the ability of microscopic deposits of breast cancer cells to form visible progressive metastases may possibly depend on subsequent genetic events that occur at those sites, including the ability to engender an angiogenic response.

Little question exists that one of the hallmarks of malignant growth is its ability to induce an angiogenic response in normal tissues.[4] Were it not for the ability of breast cancer cells to induce endothelial cell responses, including the specific migration and proliferation of endothelial cells into groups of cancer cells, no tumor would be able to progress beyond a near-microscopic size of a millimeter or two. Finally, most epithelial malignant tumors, including breast cancer, have acquired the genetic ability to amplify individual parts of their genome. When tumors are subjected to stress in the form of some kind of therapy, cells are selected with ever-increasing expression of target proteins, so resistance is seen. This can manifest itself not only as resistance to drugs (as in the amplification overexpression of dihydrofolate reductase, the target enzyme of methotrexate), but as a growth advantage (for example, the overexpression of either the epidermal growth factor (EGF) receptor or erbB-2).

In addition, many breast cancers are aneuploid and clearly have a less tightly regulated ability to replicate DNA in an orderly fashion than do normal cells. This ability leads to an increased frequency of mutations, most of which are actually harmful to the cancer cells. Unfortunately, some have the potential to increase the growth advantages of malignant cells further.

These phenotypic effects that are the hallmarks of invasive breast cancer may be the result of direct genetic alterations in genes responsible for these properties. For example, a point mutation in erbB-2 (HER-2/neu), a cellular growth factor receptor, can lead to its activation in the absence of growth factor.[5] Although this mechanism has not been reported to occur in human breast cancer, it can transform normal mammary epithelium transfected or infected with a point-mutated and thereby activated erbB-2.[6] It is an obvious example by which a genetic event can alter the growth of a breast cell. On the other hand, many other genetic events that eventually lead to breast cancer may have far more complex and indirect mechanisms of action. Inactivation of tumor-suppressor genes such as Rb (which occurs uncommonly in breast cancer),[7] or point mutation of p53 (which occurs up to 50% of the time),[8] may have effects on the transcription of numerous other genes that, although not mutated themselves, are then expressed abnormally, allowing the malignant phenotype to be expressed.

Paradigm of Biologic Therapy

In trying to understand how one may attempt to develop biologic therapies based on the malignant phenotype, a series of assumptions are required. First is that sufficient specificity from normal tissue exists for any given molecule contributing to the malignant phenotype to be biologically exploitable. In the simplest case, the putative gene in breast cancer behavior is uniquely expressed in breast cancer and nowhere else at any time. This situation has not, in fact, been shown to be true for breast cancer, although it has been shown to be true for other malignant diseases. For example, in the activation of the c-abl gene by chromosomal translocation or the numatrin-alk translocation in childhood leukemia, a "new gene" is created by chromosomal rearrangement that does not exist in any normal cell, thus providing a unique target.

Far more commonly, one hopes that proteins in the malignant phenotype, although potentially expressed at other times (developmentally or in other states of injury), exhibit substantial enough differential expression to be targeted with acceptable toxicity.

No matter how rational the approach or how many experiments suggest the uniqueness of the target or the therapy, the only final proof of success must lie in an empiric clinical trial. On the other hand, a host of studies can suggest which targets are more or less likely to be relevant for clinical trials.

Selection of a Biologic Target

A reasonable basis for developing a target for biologic therapy is summarized in Figure 22.3-1.

Through experimentation, a molecule is identified that has some putative role in contributing to the breast cancer phenotype. Two major directions can add validity to this approach. First, one can look for associative data. A molecule that contributes to the malignant process is likely to have either diagnostic or prognostic significance. In this regard, as discussed elsewhere in this book, many growth factors, their receptors, molecules contributing to invasion, metastasis, and angiogenesis have been shown to be useful in dividing breast cancer patients into prognostic subsets with varying outcomes. For example, patients with stage II breast cancer and whose tumors overexpress erbB-2 have substantially worse prognoses than patients whose tumors do not. Similarly, patients whose tumors overexpress urokinase plasminogen activator (uPA), cathepsin D, and other proteolytic enzymes also have a far worse prognosis.

The specificity of molecules in terms of their contribution to the malignant process can partially be ascertained by measurement of these molecules directly in tumor samples or in blood, urine, or nipple fluid aspirates. Molecules that are associated with the presence of the malignant state are clearly of greater interest and may be appropriate targets for biologic therapy. Molecules that correlate well with prognosis and have some diagnostic significance, however, may be of no value as biologic targets unless they contribute to the malignant process, as in the case of CA-15-3 and other shed antigens.

Information on the appropriateness of a target protein can only be derived (short of a clinical trial) from biologic experiments. Thus, in a series of animal models, cell culture systems, and human tumor xenografts, the effects of modulating the expression of a given protein or its activity can be explored as a means of understanding its pathogenetic significance. Most commonly, these experiments take the form of either increasing the level of expression of a given protein (commonly by gene transfer techniques) or inactivating it in one of the many ways described subsequently. If these experiments provide promising data on tumor progression or antitumor effect, and if the toxicities of these therapies appear acceptable, then the molecule can be considered a potential target for evaluation in clinical trials.

Specific Biologic Therapies

A variety of imaginative strategies have been proposed as potential biologic therapies. Some of the most promising are summarized in Figure 22.3-2. The numbers following each approach are keyed to the figure. In every case, these strategies are based on the idea that specific protein products subserve individual aspects of the malignant phenotype. Thus, these strategies attempt to interfere with the synthesis or activities of individually targeted proteins. The usefulness of these strategies rests not only on their ability to block expression or activity of the target protein, but also in the specific and nonspecific toxicities that result from these interventions. For example, were it to be shown that insulin represented an essential autocrine or paracrine growth factor for breast cancer, a strategy that blocked insulin synthesis or activity throughout the organism would obviously engender an unacceptable degree of specific toxicity. Similarly, antibodies directed against a growth factor or a receptor that showed cross-reaction with other species expressed elsewhere in the body would be a source of nonspecific toxicity.

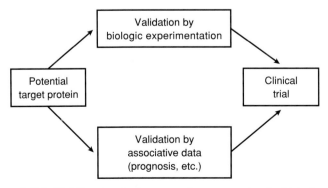

FIGURE 22.3-1 The development of target proteins for biologic therapy.

ANTISENSE STRATEGIES. (See 1 in Figure 22.3-2.) Because proteins are the growth and translational products of messenger RNA (mRNA) molecules, approaches that can interfere with the transcription, transcriptional processing, or translation of specific RNA molecules can potentially have enormous biologic potential. Every amino acid sequence has a unique mRNA that encodes it. Based on the principle of base complementation, one can, in theory, make a nucleotide sequence complementary to only one species of mRNA molecules, a so-called *antisense sequence*. These sequences may have RNA-type or DNA-type sugar phosphate backbones or newer chemically modified sugar phosphate backbones (with altered biochemical properties)

or combinations. General reviews can be found elsewhere.[9,10] Thus, the promise of an antisense strategy has always been its potential for substantial specificity. Current studies are aimed at chemically modifying sugar phosphate backbones for these molecules and enhancing their ability to penetrate cells. Two entirely different mechanisms of antisense technology exist. On the one hand, antisense molecules may be envisioned as drugs that are administered either locally or systemically and then penetrate target cells and interact with their complementary RNA targets. Alternatively, a gene therapy technique exists in which a synthetic gene encoding an antisense sequence is introduced into target cells. These cells then continuously

FIGURE 22.3-2 Biologic therapies for breast cancer.
1a. Antisense molecules targeted to unprocessed mRNA
1b. Antisense molecules targeted to mature mRNA
2. Ribozymes
3. Anti–growth factor receptor antibodies
3a. Immunotoxins; growth factor receptor antibodies linked to toxic moieties
4. Anti–cell surface epitope antibodies
5. Oncotoxins (growth factors linked to toxic moieties)
5a. Growth factor receptor fragments
6. Anti–growth factor antibodies
7. Ligand derived inhibitors of growth factor receptors
8. Inhibitory products of cancer cells
9. Blockade of signal transduction
10. Blockade of cell surface proteolysis with naturally occuring inhibitors
11. Chemical sequestration of growth factor molecules

produce the antisense RNA molecules derived from the transfected gene that then block the eventual expression of the target protein.

Numerous cell culture experiments have demonstrated reasonably high levels of success in blocking expression of specific proteins by either of these approaches. Preliminary clinical trials with antisense molecules have already begun. Two aspects of this approach are illustrated in Figure 22.3-2. In 1A, an antisense sequence against an unprocessed RNA transcript blocks its eventual splicing to a mature mRNA; In 1B, translation is blocked by an antisense sequence that either blocks mRNA interaction with the ribosome or reacts to endonucleose destruction of the mRNA.

RIBOZYME STRATEGIES. (See 2 in Figure 22.3-2.) Some RNA molecules can exhibit enzymatic activity. The seminal work of Cech and colleagues revealed that some naturally occurring RNA structures are capable of specifically cleaving other target RNA molecules.[11] These RNAs, called ribozymes, have two critical elements.[12] First is a recognition sequence, which is the equivalent of an antisense sequence; that is, these elements contain an RNA sequence complementary to the nucleotide on a target messenger RNA. In addition, a configuration of nucleotides near this antisense sequence has the enzymatic ability to hydrolyze the specific target RNA. The antisense nucleotide sequences on the ribozyme that provide recognition for the target RNA are completely interchangeable. Thus, ribozyme molecules can be aimed at any mRNA and can be synthesized at will. Once again, these molecules can be introduced into cells through two potential means: (1) as a drug administered exogenously (no published reports of this situation exist) or (2) by a gene therapy strategy in which a synthetic gene encodes a sequence that is then transcribed into an RNA with the ribozyme sequence. For example, it has been possible to prepare a ribozyme to the angiogenic molecule pleiotrophin.[13] Pleiotrophin is produced by approximately 60% of breast cancers and is a likely candidate as a critical angiogenic molecule. Cells expressing the pleiotrophin ribozyme no longer have detectable intact mRNA for pleiotrophin, and they lose their ability to produce pleiotrophin protein as well as their angiogenic potential. Once again, the attractiveness of the ribozyme strategy lies in its potential for enormous specificity because, in theory, only the oligonucleotide sequence of the target mRNA would be disrupted.

GROWTH FACTOR RECEPTOR ANTIBODIES. (See 3 in Figure 22.3-2.) Investigations have established the critical importance of endocrine, paracrine, and autocrine pathways in cancer progression in general and in breast cancer in particular.[14] All these pathways involve signaling through receptors located on cell surfaces by growth factors that are produced at a distance, by neighboring cells, or by the same cells, respectively. For these growth factors to be able to signal correctly, they must be able to interact with their cognate receptors. For this reason, multiple groups have prepared antibodies to growth factor receptors, in the hope of thereby blocking the ability of ligands (growth factors) to interact with their cognate receptor or potentially blocking other aspects of receptor function required for eventual intracellular signaling such as dimerization. Antibodies to both erbB-2 (Slamon D, personal communication) and the EGF receptor[15] are currently in clinical trial.

One can imagine several variants on this system. For example, such growth factor antibodies either could be conjugated to imaging agents or could be used as a means of targeting a variety of toxic substances or drugs to cancer cells (see 3A in Fig. 22.3–2). Thus, antireceptor antibody toxic conjugates, which are a variant of immunotoxins, as discussed later, might provide a means of substantially increasing their therapeutic index for the delivery of such compounds.

IMMUNOTOXINS. (See 4 in Figure 22.3-2.) Cancer cells display on their surfaces a variety of immunogenic epitopes. Some of these may be specifically involved in cellular signaling, as in growth factor receptors, whereas others may simply represent the expression of proteins displayed at either a higher density or some degree of specificity on cancer cells, such as carcinoembryonic antigen. Antibodies against the former (discussed previously) may have antitumor activity of their own. Those antibodies, or antibodies directed against any cell-surface determinant that is more exclusively expressed on cancer cells, may potentially be conjugated to chemotherapeutic drugs, isotopes, or toxic moieties. These conjugates, known as immunotoxins, have the potential to increase the therapeutic index for drug delivery by selectively targeting the agent to cancer cells. A variety of immunotoxin molecules are currently in clinical trial. For example, a Lewis blood group antibody–doxorubicin conjugate has shown great promise in treating xenografts of human breast cancer in nude mice.[16] This agent is in phase I testing. A variety of biologic and pharmacologic factors will determine the eventual success of these compounds. Because of species differences, the study of human tumors and xenografts may not accurately predict the toxicity of such compounds; however, the potential to achieve even modest increases in therapeutic index may have significant benefit in diseases such as breast cancer in which severalfold alterations in dose intensity have been able to alter response rates substantially.

ONCOTOXINS. (See 5 in Figure 22.3-2.) As mentioned previously, endocrine, paracrine, and autocrine effects all require the interaction of specific growth factors with target receptors. The principle underlying oncotoxins is the coupling of drugs or toxins to growth factors by either chemical or recombinant means. Thus, a chimeric molecule is prepared that has an intact growth factor on one end or the part of the growth factor required for specific receptor binding to the other end of the molecule, which is linked to a toxic moiety or drug.[17] The premise of this therapy is that the growth factor portion of the oncotoxin steers the toxin to its target. Because the interactions of the growth factor with the receptor are often of extremely high affinity, and because the receptor is, one hopes, displayed either uniquely or far more abundantly on the cancer cell, multiple mechanisms exist for increasing the therapeutic index. Several oncotoxins have been explored experimentally, including chimeras of the FGFs, the EGF superfamily, and interleukin-2 (IL-2). In the case of both IL-2[18] and the EGF superfamily,[19] responses in patients have been reported. This is probably one of the most exciting areas for biologic therapy, and many clinical trials can be anticipated over the next several years.

NEUTRALIZING ANTIBODIES. (See 6 in Figure 22.3-2.) One of the earliest mechanisms by which biologic agents were expected to exert antitumor effects was through neutralizing antibodies. The idea of antireceptor antibodies has previously been discussed. One can also imagine neutralizing antibodies to growth factors or other molecules in the malignant process. To some extent, these approaches appear to have received less attention lately, for a variety of reasons. First, the generation of large clinical amounts of monoclonal antibodies is an expensive undertaking. Until recently, technologies to humanize these monoclonal antibodies were not available, so the development of human antimouse antibodies (hama's) was anticipated to be a substantial problem limiting the usefulness of these approaches. Recently, however, recombinant technology has permitted the humanizing of these antibodies. In addition, series of derivative structures such as single-chain antibodies and smaller peptide and nonpeptide binding epitopes have been prepared. This advance has permitted the design of far smaller molecules of interest. The development of the technology of recombinatorial phage-display libraries and similar methods have created the potential of sorting through inconceivably large numbers of potential molecules empirically while enriching for peptides that can, in effect, function as minitopes or neutralizing peptides.[20] None of these have yet entered clinical trial. A variant of neutralizing antibodies against ligands exploits naturally occurring molecules capable of binding growth factors and blocking interaction with functional cell-surface receptors. High-affinity binding proteins for the insulin-like growth factors (IGFs) have been described. Overexpression of these binding proteins or induction of their increased expression by the tumor could block autocrine or paracrine signaling. Alternately, shed extracellular domains of growth factor receptors that retained binding affinity for growth factor but lacked an intracellular signaling mechanism could accomplish the same result. This is schematically shown in 6A.

INHIBITORY LIGANDS AND COMPETITIVE INHIBITORS OF GROWTH FACTOR ACTION. (See 7 in Figure 22.3-2.) One of the most substantial advances in breast cancer therapy has been the development of potent inhibitors of estrogen action. Although the mechanism of action of antiestrogens is complex, their effectiveness is based, at least in part, on antagonism of the interaction of biologically functional estrogens with their cognate receptors. Antiprogestins have also entered the clinical arena. Although one has traditionally referred to these *hormonal therapy* approaches, as compared with *biologic therapy,* this distinction is more

historical than biologically defensible. In the same way, however, one may envision the design of peptide fragments derived or modified from agonistic growth factors that have antagonistic effects. Leutinizing hormone–releasing antagonists and somatostatin analogues are good examples of the antagonism of endocrine growth factor receptors. Success with designing such antagonists for autocrine and paracrine growth factors has been much more difficult to achieve. In part, this has been based on the finding that, for IGFs and the EGF receptor superfamily, complicated loop structures created by disulfide bridges involve multiple parts of the polypeptide chain in receptor interaction. Thus, simple fragments of these peptides are generally biologically inert. Peptides that appear to interact with receptor through a more restrictive linear region of their sequence (eg, the FGFs) have shown themselves more amenable to the design of inhibitory peptides, however. Extraordinary advances in three-dimensional structure analysis of receptors and ligands combined with the ability, usually based on a lead structure and recombinatorial libraries of compounds, have increased the likelihood that these approaches will potentially yield high-affinity antagonists of receptor action. Such drugs would have tremendous application not only in breast cancer, but also in the disruption of other receptor-mediated processes important in many pathogenic states.

INHIBITORY LIGANDS. (See 8 in Figure 22.3-2.) Some ligands are inhibitory in their own right. These include the transforming growth factor β family and tumor necrosis factor and related peptides. Efforts to use these clinically have thus far shown tremendous potential for toxicity, and whether these pleiotrophic regulators of multiple cellular function can ever be developed into specific therapeutic approaches remains to be seen. Targeted delivery systems or gene therapy approaches may possibly prove useful. In addition, in situations in which a growth factor is overexpressed, growth factors or ligands that are stimulatory under normal circumstances can be shown to have profound inhibitory effects. Pharmacologic doses of estrogens can lead to regression of estrogen-receptor–positive breast cancer at a rate equivalent to that induced by tamoxifen. Chronic gonadotropin-releasing hormone stimulation can cause down-regulation of gonadotropin secretion. Human breast cancer cell lines that overexpress EGF, ErbB-2, and FGF receptors have all been reported to be inhibited by treatment with the appropriate growth factors.[21,22] Eventually, this may form the basis of biologic therapy.

INTERFERENCE WITH SIGNAL TRANSDUCTION. (See 9 in Figure 22.3-2.) Once a growth factor or other cell-surface molecule interacts with its cognate receptor, a series of signals must be transmitted intracellularly that alter cellular function, commonly at the transcriptional level. Many cell-surface receptors have enzymatic activity of their own that becomes activated following ligand binding. For example, they are either tyrosine kinases or serine threonine kinases. Multiple efforts have been made toward finding sufficient specificity among the kinase activities to be able to design inhibitors that have specificity for one receptor kinase or another. Although many such experiments have been performed, until recently none of these approaches have thus far shown remarkable specificity. Fry and colleagues have described an inhibitor of the EGF receptor tyrosine kinase that shows up to four orders of magnitude specifity over related cell-surface receptor tyrosine kinases.[23] To be able to block receptor intracellular signaling in addition to blocking interaction of ligand with receptor remains an attractive notion, however.

One of the most exciting approaches to signal transduction inhibition has been developed, based on an improved understanding of the mechanism by which protooncogenes of the ras family are involved in signal transduction. Following the translation of the ras mRNA into protein, a posttranslational modification occurs in the protein that is required for its function. The four terminal amino acids in ras encode a consensus sequence for an enzyme known as farnesyl transferase, which allows the transfer of a farnesyl lipid group onto the ras protein. This allows insertion of the ras protein in the cell membrane. Without this association of ras with the cell membrane, neither normal ras nor oncogenic point-mutated ras is capable of evoking a signal. Several groups of investigators have now isolated inhibitors of farnesyl transferase and have shown that these substances can block malignant behavior of many cells in culture and in human tumor xenografts.[24] These compounds will likely enter clinical trial shortly.

In addition, molecules that can antagonize protein kinase C activity have also been described. Such a molecule is involved in the signaling of many growth factor molecules. A molecule isolated from a bryozoan, named bryostatin, which has potent protein kinase C inhibitory activity, has entered clinical trial.[25]

INHIBITORS OF INVASION AND METASTASIS. (See 10 in Figure 22.3-2.) As stated previously, it is difficult to separate steps involved in invasion and metastasis. A group of steps involving digestion of basement membranes and matrices, motility, and, in the latter case, angiogenesis, may all be involved. A series of molecules that contribute to the invasive process has recently been identified, however. Critical are a series of metalloproteases. They include the collagenases and stromelysins. Associative data have shown that their expression in malignant cells is commonly associated with a worse prognosis. In addition, a group of biologic studies have shown that overexpression of any of several metalloproteases in target cells renders them far more invasive and more likely to induce metastasis. Several inhibitors of these metalloproteases have been isolated. These agents appear to be virtually nontoxic on isolated cells. In vivo, they generally have a broad spectrum of activity against multiple metalloproteases. One of these compounds, Batimastat (BB-94), has been shown to inhibit most metalloproteases and, based on preclinical evaluation, has entered phase I clinical testing.[26]

The most commonly voiced objection to approaches based on invasion and metastasis models is based on a clinical consideration of the disease stage at which therapy is initiated. When most patients with breast cancer present for diagnosis, they presumably either do or do not already have metastatic (albeit occult) disease. That is, once the primary tumor is removed from the patient, no possibility of subsequent metastases from it exists. A treatment that perfectly blocks metastases that is begun at the time of diagnosis would not necessarily have any effect on micrometastases that already exist throughout the body. For this reason, strategies for testing these compounds need to be developed that allow one to examine effects on already existent micrometastases rather than the blockade of metastatic spread at the time of the administration of antimetastatic drug, the usual case in animal experiments.

In the case of breast cancer, at least one genetic element that appears to be involved in the metastatic process has been investigated. The gene, NM23, has been characterized as a so-called antimetastasis gene.[27] The expression of this gene appears to be lost in breast cancers that have become metastatic, as compared with primary tumors. Reexpression of NM23 appears to reduce the metastatic potential of many cells. The lack of expression of NM23 in human breast cancers is associated with a worse prognosis. Based on these prognostic and biologic observations, one could eventually attempt some form of gene therapy in which NM23 expression and function were restored to target cells.

ANTIANGIOGENIC THERAPY. (See 11 in Figure 22.3-2.) As previously mentioned, a critical requirement of all solid tumors is the ability to engender a blood supply. A series of observations in breast cancer generally suggested that the ability of a primary tumor to induce angiogenic responses, as assessed by quantitative capillary counts, correlates with overall survival. In many cases, the individual molecules that are likely candidates for angiogenesis in breast cancer have been identified. These include the vascular endothelial growth factors,[28] the FGFs[29] and the pleiotrophins.[30] These molecules can all be targeted by mechanisms that have previously been described, such as growth factor receptor antibodies, inhibitory peptides, and oncotoxins. In addition, one could specifically target proliferating endothelial cells by other means. For example, a series of heparinoid-like compounds have been described that are capable of tightly binding to the foregoing growth factors, all of which have high-affinity binding to heparin. These heparinoids, such as pentosan polysulfate, can then presumably sequester growth factors outside of cells and can thereby block their availability to their growth factor receptors.[31] In addition, agents that are specifically cytotoxic to endothelial cells could also be used. This approach is shown as 11 in Figure 22.3-2. Pentosan polysulfate has entered early clinical trial. One fungal derivative, fumagillin, is specifically toxic to endothelial cells. A variety of congeners of this derivative have been prepared, and one of them, TMP 470, has entered clinical trial in cancer.[32] These antiendothelial cell strategies are based on the likely observation that endothelial cells within tumors have a far higher rate of turnover in proliferation than do endothelial cells found in normal tissues. The potential for hemorrhagic toxicity, however, is obvious.

The foregoing list is by no means exhaustive. Observations on mechanisms of action of all these pathways have suggested other potential targets for intervention. It is beyond the scope of this chapter to deal with all these other imaginative alternatives, most of which are farther removed from clinical trials at this time.

Biologic Therapy in the Clinical Management of Breast Cancer

To make any firm predictions concerning the activity or role of biologic therapy of breast cancer is premature. Researchers have traditionally imagined that biologic therapies would be most successful against smaller tumor burdens. This viewpoint, although sensible, has no serious credibility and is independent of validation in clinical trials; it will be necessary to await those results before any conclusions can be reached. Multiple observations suggest extraordinary synergism between biologic therapies and chemotherapy and radiotherapy, however.[33] Chemotherapy probably places a far higher proportion of cancer cells at risk for damage than are actually killed. If in conjunction with this damage, the cancer cells were further stressed by some form of biologic therapy, far more substantial anticancer effects might be seen. In fact, clinical trials are already underway testing this premise using anti−erbB-2 receptor antibodies in conjunction with platinum and anti−EGF receptor antibodies in conjunction with doxorubicin.

In addition, many of these biologic therapies can be used together. For example, multiple steps in a given pathway could conceivably be targeted because of the anticipated lack of toxicity of these approaches. Thus, a molecule that targeted a ligand, a molecule that targeted the receptor, and a molecule that targeted signal transduction might all be used simultaneously to increase the effectiveness of the therapy while potentially lessening toxicity.

Although many of these approaches may appear as science fiction to clinicians involved, as they are, on a day-to-day basis with the care of breast cancer patients, the pressure to improve our treatment strategies has encouraged, and will continue to encourage, clinical trials with new approaches. It seems extraordinarily unlikely that therapies based on far more specific knowledge of the biologic behavior of breast cancer will not at some point assume an important role in our approaches to breast cancer.

References

1. Metcalf D. Thrombopoietin—at last. Nature 1994;369:519.
2. Bjarnason GA, Hrushevsky WJM. Circadian cancer chemotherapy: clinical trials. J Infus Chemother 1992;2:79.
3. Alberts B, Bray D, Lewis J, et al. Cell signaling. *In*: Molecular biology of the cell. New York, Garland, 1994;721.
4. Denekamp J. Vascular attack as a therapeutic strategy for cancer. Cancer Metast Rev 1990;9:267.
5. Bargmann CI, Hung MC, Weinberg RA. The neu oncogene encodes an epidermal growth factor receptor-related proteins. Nature 1986;319:226.
6. Muller WJ, Sinn E, Pattengale PK, et al. Single step induction of mammary adenocarcinoma in transgenic mice bearing the activated c-*neu* oncogene. Cell 1988;54:105.
7. Benedict WF, Hong-Ji X, Shi-Xue H, et al. Role of the retinoblastoma gene in the initiation and progression of human cancer. J Clin Invest 1990;85:988.
8. Harris CC, Hollstein M. Clinical implications of the p53 tumor-suppressor gene. N Engl J Med 1993;329:1318.
9. Neckers L, Whitesell L, Rosolen A, et al. Antisense inhibition of oncogene expression. Crit Rev Oncogen 1992;3:175.
10. Denhardt DT. Antisense strategies come of age. N Biol 1992;4:473.
11. Cech T. Self-splicing of group 1 introns. Ann Rev Biochem 1990;59:543.
12. Rossi JJ. Making ribozymes work in cells. Curr Biol 1994;4:469.
13. Czubayko F, Riegel AT, Wellstein A. Ribozyme-targeting elucidates a direct role of pleiotrophin in tumor growth. J Biol Chem 1994;269:21358.
14. Aaronson SA. Growth factors and cancer. Science 1991;254:1146.
15. Mendelsohn J. The epidermal growth factor receptor as a target for therapy with antireceptor monoclonal antibodies. Semin Cancer Biol 1990;1:339.
16. Trail PA, Willner D, Lasch SJ, et al. Cure of xenografted human carcinomas by BR96-doxorubicin immunoconjugates. Science 1993;261:212.
17. Pastan I, FitzGerald D. Recombinant toxins for cancer treatment. Science 1991;254:1173.
18. Hesketh P, Caguioa P, Koh H, et al. Clinical activity of a cytotoxic fusion protein in the treatment of cutaneous T cell lymphoma. J Clin Oncol 1993;11:1682.
19. Goldberg MR, Heimbrook DC, Russo P, et al. Phase I clinical study of the recombinant oncotoxin TP40 in superficial bladder cancer. Clin Cancer Res 1995;1:57.
20. Houghten RA. Combinatorial libraries: finding the needle in the haystack. Curr Biol 1994;4:564.
21. Ennis BW, Lippman ME, Dickson RB. The EGF receptor system as a target for antitumor therapy. Cancer Invest 1991;9:553.
22. Lupu R, Colomer R, Zugmaier G, et al. A candidate ligand of the erbB2 protooncogene interacts directly with both EGF receptor and erbB2. Science 1990;249:1552.
23. Fry DW, Kraker AJ, McMichael A, et al. A specific inhibitor of the epidermal growth factor receptor tyrosine kinase. Science 1994;265:1093.
24. Kohl NE, Mosser SD, deSolms J, et al. Selective inhibition of *ras*-dependent transformation by a farnesyltransferase inhibitor. Science 1993;260:1934.
25. Prendiville J, Crowther D, Thatcher N, et al. A phase I study of intravenous bryostatin 1 in patients with advanced cancer. Br J Cancer 1993;68:418.
26. Wang X, Fu X, Brown PD, et al. Matrix metalloproteinase inhibitor BB-94 (Batimastat) inhibits human colon tumor growth and spread in a patient-like orthotopic model in nude mice. Cancer Res 1994;54:4726.
27. Steeg PS, Cohn KH, Leone A. Tumor metastasis and nm23: current concepts. Cancer Cells 1991;3:257.
28. Neufeld G, Shoshana T, Gitay-Goren H, et al. Vascular endothelial growth factor and its receptors. Prog Growth Factor Res 1994;5:89.
29. Johnson DE, Williams LT. Structural and functional diversity in the FGF receptor multigene family. Adv Cancer Res 1993;60:1.
30. Bohlen P, Kovesdi I. HBNF and MK, members of a novel gene family heparin-binding proteins with potential roles in embryogenesis and brain function. Prog Growth Factor Res 1991;3:143.
31. Zugmaier G, Lippman ME, Wellstein A. Pentosanpolysulfate in-

hibits heparin-binding growth factors released from tumor cells and blocks tumor growth in animals. J Natl Cancer Inst 1992;84:1716.

32. Toi M, Yamamoto Y, Imazawa T, et al. Antitumor effect of the angiogenesis inhibitor AGM-1470 and its combination effect with

tamoxifen in DMBA induced mammary tumors in rats. Int J Oncol 1993;525.

33. Baselga J, Norton L, Masui H, et al. Antitumor effects of doxorubicin in combination with anti-epidermal growth factor receptor monoclonal antibodies. J Natl Cancer Inst 1993;85:1327.

22.4

Cytokinetics and Breast Cancer Chemotherapy

TERESA GILEWSKI • LARRY NORTON

Cancer cells are constantly in a state of flux: in their biochemistry, in their stromal relations, and in their absolute numbers. An increase in cell number, termed *proliferation,* is the product of successful mitoses. *Growth,* the overall increase in tumor size, is largely a consequence of proliferation. Growth also reflects average cell size, vasculature, content of extracellular matrix, edema, hemorrhage, and leukocyte infiltration, however. *Inappropriate growth*—to a size incompatible with the normal function of a host organ—is the key attribute of malignancy. *Cytokinetics,* the study of the dynamics of proliferation and growth, is intimately involved with many other aspects of malignant behavior. For example, the other two key features of malignancy, invasion and metastasis, and the process of carcinogenesis itself, all depend on proliferation.

The design of drug therapy is primarily concerned with proliferation because anticancer drugs are intended to disrupt mitosis as their principal mode of action. This is also their predominant mechanism for producing toxicity. Proliferation is also linked to the development of tumor heterogeneity, including, paradoxically, heterogeneity in sensitivity to anticancer drugs. From a clinical perspective, therefore, the cytokinetics of breast cancer is relevant both to prognostication and to the design of treatment schedules. This chapter focuses on some therapeutic implications of cytokinetic principles, many of which derived originally from studies of cells other than breast cancer cells.

Proliferation, Growth, and Mutation

The proliferation and growth of breast cancer, and any regression in cell numbers or tumor volume that may be induced by drug therapy, are described by a class of mathematic functions called *proliferation curves* or *growth curves.* The two most discussed curves are the *exponential curve* (Fig. 22.4-1) and the *gompertzian curve* (Fig. 22.4-2). Either of these curves could be applied to proliferation or growth, depending on the unit of size measurement: cell number as a function of time for proliferation, or cubic centimeters or milligrams for growth. The two curves are related mathematically, but they have different implications regarding carcinogenesis, clinical course, and re-

sponse to treatment. Although the exponential curve is simpler and therefore easier to work with, evidence is discussed that it is not an accurate reflection of the cytokinetics of human breast cancer.

All proliferation, whether exponential or gompertzian in pattern, is founded in the mitosis of cancer cells. The *mitotic cycle* (also called the *proliferative cycle,* or *cell cycle*) in breast cancer averages about 2 to 4 days, comparable with normal hematopoietic and mucosal progenitors.[1,2] The four phases of the cell cycle—*synthesis* or S-phase, *mitosis* or M-phase, *gap-1* or G_1, and *gap-2* or G_2—were defined originally by autoradiography using radioactively labeled precursors of DNA.[3,4] The percentage of cells in S is termed the *S-phase fraction* (SPF) if it is measured by flow cytometry and the *labeling index* (TLI) if it is measured by the uptake of tritiated thymidine. The adjective *mitotic* is often applied loosely to all cells in late G_1, S, G_2, or M to distinguish these cells from other cells (G_0, S_0, and rarely $G_{2/0}$) without immediate proliferative potential. Like G_1 cells, G_0 cells contain a diploid amount of DNA. S_0 cells are usually less than tetraploid.[5,6] G_0 to G_1 phases lengths in breast cancer cells fit a wide log-normal probability distribution skewed toward longer times. G_0 cells are distinguished operationally from G_1 cells by being smaller, by containing less RNA and protein, by lacking the Ki-67 antigen, and by failing—by several mechanisms—to metabolize the dye rhodamine.[7-12]

A mitotic cell is a member of the *proliferative compartment,* also called the *proliferative fraction,* the *growth fraction,* or the *growth compartment.*[13] A cell in prolonged G_0, S_0, or an arrested G_2 is in the *nonproliferative compartment, nonproliferative fraction, quiescent fraction,* or *quiescent compartment.* The magnitude of the growth fraction is estimated by multiplying the TLI by the duration of the cell cycle divided by the duration of S-phase.[14] The TLI is used because the SPF is contaminated by S_0 cells. For this and probably other reasons, the S-phase fraction is usually larger than the TLI. For most breast cancers the TLI is about 2% to 20%. Because S-phase occupies one quarter to one half the cell cycle, the growth fraction may be estimated at 4% to 80%, with an average of less than 20%. The *cell loss fraction* is the fraction of cells dying by apoptosis or necrosis in any cell cycle phase.[15] Proliferation is the difference between cell production and cell death. Hence, the cell loss fraction is a key determinant of neoplastic

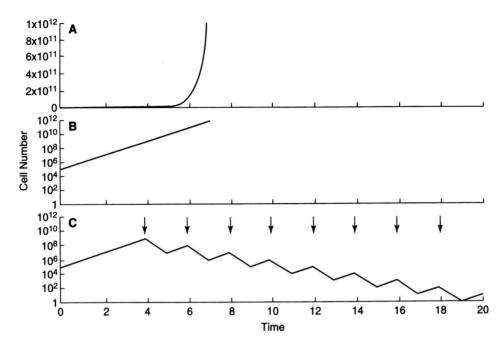

FIGURE 22.4-1 Exponential proliferation. **A.** An exponential curve on an arithmetic scale of cell number, which is the way this curve would appear to the clinician. Note the illusion of little increase in cell number for a long period, followed by an explosive increase in population size. Acute leukemias, germ cell tumors, and some other cancers may follow this pattern, but breast cancers very rarely do. **B.** The same curve on a logarithmic scale of size. Here the constant doubling time is more obvious. **C.** The manner by which an exponential curve may respond to drug therapy. Each dose (signified by an arrow) kills 99% of the cells present. A dose of sufficient efficacy is chosen to reduce the population size to one cell after 8 treatments. Note the slow regrowth after the last cycle: by 20 time units, only about 10 cells remain.

growth: a breast cancer with a large cell loss fraction may appear to be growing slowly in spite of a large growth fraction. This is important because each mitotic cycle carries with it a finite probability of mutation.[16]

Let us say that the probability of an individual cell not mutating during one mitotic cycle is $(1 - x)$. Then the probability $P_{(N-1)}$ of at least one mutation in $(N - 1)$ mitotic cycles,

$$P_{(N-1)} = 1 - (1 - x)^{(N-1)} \qquad (1)$$

approaches unity as the number of mitoses becomes large. Hence, a high cell loss rate that is compensated by a high mitotic rate predisposes toward genetic lability. Concordant with this reasoning is the observation that breast carcinogenesis culminates a long process of preneoplastic proliferation and depends on high rates of cell turnover.[21–24]

Exponential Curves

Most of the pioneering work on tumor growth kinetics was based on the transplantable leukemia L1210 in BDF1 or DBA mice. The growth fraction, cell loss fraction, and cycle duration of this cancer is remarkably stable from a population size of 1 cell to 10^9 cells, which is the lethal cell number, equivalent to about 1 cc of packed cells.[25,26] As a consequence of this stability in proliferative compartments, L1210 grows exponentially, increasing by a constant percentage per constant unit of time regardless of the number of cells present.

The general equation for breast cancer proliferation is

$$N_t = f(t) \cdot N_0^{g(t)} \qquad (2)$$

where:

$$N_t = \text{the number of cancer cells at time } t$$
$$N_0 = \text{the number of cancer cells at time } 0$$
$$f(t) \text{ and } g(t) = \text{functions of } t$$

Time, of course, is a relative value, and any given tumor size may be called N_0 as long as the time of measurement of that tumor size is set to 0. In exponential proliferation, $g(t) = 1$ for all values of t, and $f(t)$ is a simple power function of t:

$$N_t = k^t \cdot N_0 \qquad (3)$$

where:

$$k = \text{a positive constant}$$

Let T_D symbolize a fixed time interval, called the *doubling time.* T_D is the time required for the population of cells to double in number. By equation 3,

$$N_t/N_0 = 2 = k \cdot e^{T_D} \qquad (4)$$

Hence, the doubling time for exponential proliferation is constant at $\log_e(2)/\log_e(k)$ regardless of the magnitude of N_0.

Skipper–Schabel–Wilcox Model

The Skipper–Schabel–Wilcox model, also termed the *log-kill model,* was the first significant proliferation model in modern clinical oncology.[27] It was based on observations of experimental neoplasms like L1210 that are both exponential in proliferative pattern and generally homogeneous in drug sensitivity. When such laboratory tumors are treated with anticancer drugs, the *fraction* of cells killed is

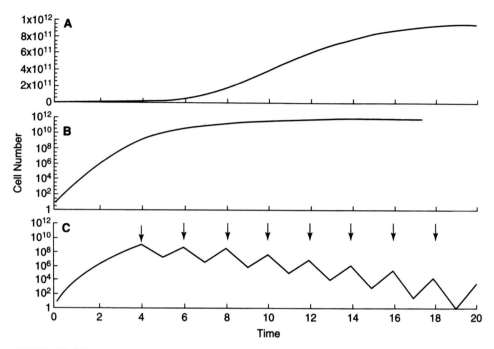

FIGURE 22.4-2 Gompertzian proliferation. This curve differs significantly from the exponential curve in Figure 22.4-1, even though both seem to follow similar patterns around 10^9 cells. **A.** The curve on an arithmetic scale of size. Note that unlike the curve in Figure 22. 4-1*A*, which expands faster and faster, the gompertzian tumor slows down progressively, approaching a plateau size at 10^{12} cells. **B.** The same curve on a logarithmic scale of cell number. Note the constantly increasing doubling time, which eventually approaches infinity. Also note that the number of cells at time zero is much smaller than in Figure 22.4-1*B*: because gompertzian proliferation is rapid at small population sizes, the preclinical period of proliferation is much shorter than for an exponential curve. **C.** Gompertzian regression in response to effective drug therapy. Note that the log-kill is larger when the tumor size at the time (marked by the arrows) of therapy is smaller. However, the rebound after treatment is more rapid for smaller tumor populations as well. Hence, even though only one cell is left after the eighth cycle, by 20 time units almost 10^4 cells are present, 1000 times more cells than in the exponential curve of Figure 22.4-1*C*.

always the same regardless of the number of cells present when the drugs are administered. Let us pick an arbitrary moment and call it time 0. We then measure the number of cancer cells present at time 0 and call that number N_0. If a specified therapy is given at time 0, then N_T, number of cancer cells present at a later time T, is given by

$$N_T = k^{[T-W(T)]} \cdot N_0 \qquad (5)$$

The function $W(T)$ is the total anticancer influence of a therapy by time T. It is actually the definite integral of w(dose,t), which is a function of the dose level of therapy and time after drug administration:

$$W(T) = {}_0\!\!\int^T w(dose,t)dt \qquad (6)$$

For ineffective therapy, w(dose,t) is 0. For therapy effective enough to cause tumor regression, $W(T)$ is greater than T.

As illustrated in Figure 22.4-1*C*, equation 5 means that if a certain dose of a specified drug reduces 10^9 cells to 10^7 (the first cycle of therapy), the same dose of the same drug would reduce 10^6 cells to 10^4 (the fourth cycle), or 10^2 to 1 (the last cycle). These are all examples of a *two-

log kill, equivalent to a 99% decrease in cell number. The function w(dose,t) often rises monotonically with increasing dose, which means that the log-kill often increases with increasing dose.[28,29] In addition, if $w_i(dose_i,t)$ reflects the influence of drug i, the combined effects of drugs i = 1, 2, 3 . . . q is often given by

$$w(dose,t) = \sum_{i=1}^{q} w_i(dose_i,t) \qquad (7)$$

Equation 7 means that if a given dose of drug A or B or C would each kill 90% of the cancer cells, then A plus B would kill 99% and A plus B plus C would kill 99.9% (a three-log kill). A second cycle of A + B + C would kill 99.9% of the cells present at that time. By this model, enough cycles of enough drugs at high enough individual dose levels should be able to kill a high percentage—even all—of the cells. This reasoning was highly influential in the development of the concept of *combination chemotherapy,* which has proved to be one of the most important concepts in modern clinical oncology.[30]

At first analysis, therefore, one would seem to have every reason to believe that aggressive combination chemotherapy should readily cure the micrometastases left after breast cancer surgery.[31,32] If one starts chemotherapy at a time of few cells, then log-kills by the chemotherapy of six or higher should easily eradicate many tumors. Unfortunately, this concept has not proved sound for breast cancer. The adjuvant chemotherapy of primary breast cancer does reduce the probability of patients developing stage IV disease and does result in improved survival. With conventional regimens such as cyclophosphamide, methotrexate, and 5-fluorouracil (CMF), however, the effect is only modest even though each of these three drugs is effective in killing breast cancer cells.[33,34]

Skipper and colleagues have long been aware of the limitations of the log-kill model and have listed many possible reasons for the divergence between theory and experience. They have discussed the possibility that chemotherapy may be adequate to cure, but that it will fail if it is not given for long enough to eradicate all cells. This is clearly not applicable to the adjuvant chemotherapy of primary breast cancer because periods of treatment longer than 4 to 6 months offer no therapeutic advantage.[34] Skipper and coworkers also considered the possibility that most tumors have a fraction of cells that are completely, permanently resistant to all the drugs that we are likely to use. Such cells are rarely found in small aliquots of L1210 and would therefore have to arise spontaneously at some time between the carcinogenic event and the appearance of larger amounts of tumor.[35] By equation 1, the rapidity with which such resistance develops should be associated with the magnitude of proliferative activity. Extending this argument, proliferative activity should relate to other acquired aberrancies, such as aneuploidy and metastatic potential.

Delbruck–Luria Concept

Before we examine the relations among ploidy, metastatic potential, and drug resistance, let us consider the implications of the concept that failure to cure with anticancer drugs is largely due to the existence of cells biochemically resistant to drug action.[36] If resistance is acquired as a function of proliferation, therapy can be successful only if it is initiated while the tumor is too small to have produced such dangerous mutations.[37] Quantitative models have been applied to the problem, how small is small enough? In 1943, Luria and Delbruck studied bacterial cultures that had never been exposed to bacteriophage. These cells spontaneously developed mutations that made them resistant to bacteriophage infection.[38] Exposure to the viruses could then be used to select out the resistant bacteria and thereby to measure the percentage of cells that had randomly acquired resistance. If a mutation had occurred early in the history of a particular culture, there would have been time for this clone to grow to become a significant fraction of all the bacteria present in the culture.

By equation 1, the probability that one individual bacterium will not produce any bacteriophage-resistant mutants after $(N - 1)$ mitoses is $(1 - x)^{(N-1)}$. If each of these $N - 1$ mitoses produces two viable cells, and no cell loss

occurs, N cells will result. Because $\log_e(1 - x) \approx -x$ for small x, the probability of finding not even one resistant bacterium in a culture of N bacteria is

$$1 - P_{(N-1)} = \exp[-x(N - 1)] \qquad (8)$$

Within a decade of the publication of this concept, the same mathematic pattern was successfully applied to the appearance of methotrexate resistance in L1210 cells.[39] This finding confirmed that drug resistance could be acquired spontaneously during cancer cell proliferation; that is, the development of the drug resistance trait does not always require the presence of the drug in question. The application of this concept to clinical practice meant that at the time of first treatment, a cancer could have already developed resistance to a drug to which it had not yet been exposed. Hence, treatment of that cancer with any single drug was likely to fail. Yet, combinations of drugs might work because it was deemed unlikely that any one cell could spontaneously become resistant to many drugs, particularly drugs with different biochemical sites of action.[40] For this reason, only combinations of drugs could possibly eradicate all cancer cells.[40] This line of reasoning became a fundamental principle underlying combination chemotherapy.[41]

Equation 8 is also believed to express a quantitative relation between proliferation and other manifestations of genetic lability. The entry of G_1 cells into S and G_2 cells into M is tightly regulated in normal cells. A prototypic regulatory mechanism may involve a cyclic process in which the $p34^{cdc2}$ protein couples with different cyclin proteins to coordinate a cell's entry into either S or M, but only from the appropriate gap period.[42] Abnormalities in this regulatory process could hinder the normal controls that prohibit rereplication.[43,44] That is, if a G2 cell is sent into S, sections of the genome may be replicated more than once, producing *aneuploidy,* or aberrant levels of DNA per neoplastic cell.[45] Hence, by equation 8, the appearance of aneuploidy should also be a function of the number of mitoses, particularly if some of these mitoses are anomalously rereplicating.

Goldie-Coldman Hypothesis

As described previously, the concept of drug resistance was of great importance in the early history of the development of modern combination chemotherapy. More recently, the quantitative relevance of the Delbruck-Luria model to the treatment of human cancer has been reexamined.[35,46,47] Equation 8 predicts that at a tenable mutation rate of $x = 10^{-6}$, which is an average of 1 mutation per million mitoses, the probability of finding no mutants to any single drug in a total population of 10^5 cells is about 90%.[48] Also by equation 8, however, the probability of the absence of resistant mutants in 10^7 cells is only 0.0045%. If incurability is a consequence of the existence of even one drug-resistant mutant, the Goldie-Coldman hypothesis predicts that the property of incurability should be acquired quickly as a tumor grows from 10^5 to 10^7 cells.

The approximate volume of 10^9 densely packed breast cancer cells is 1 cc. Breast cancers, however, are not composed only of breast cancer cells, but also of benign host tissue such as stromal cells, blood and lymph and their vessels, colloid, collagen, and extracellular fluid. Hence, only a percentage of the tumor mass is actually composed of cancer cells. One cubic centimeter of tumor could contain only 10^7 to 10^8 cells. Therefore, the Goldie-Coldman model would conclude that cancers larger than 0.1 to 1 cc should always be incurable with any single agent. Conversely, smaller cancers should be cured in at least 90% of cases.

The Goldie-Coldman model thereby predicts a major advantage to the perioperative or even preoperative chemotherapy of primary breast cancer. Regarding the design of chemotherapy schedules, the model theorizes that as many effective drugs as possible should be applied as soon as possible, so cells that are already resistant to one drug could be killed before they have a chance to mutate to resistance to other drugs. The best approach, these investigators conclude, would be true combination chemotherapy, giving several drugs simultaneously at full dosages. If the toxicity to normal organs would preclude such a schedule,[49] then the strict alternation of two or more regimens would be the next best approach.[50]

Clinical Critique

The exponential model and the concepts derived therefrom raise many interesting issues of immediate theoretic and practical interest. In human breast cancer, is the growth fraction independent of tumor size? Does high growth fraction imply a high probability of mutations? Does the log-kill model apply? Is equation 8 defensible? What is the evidence in favor of drug resistance as the primary cause of therapeutic failure? Are the predictions of the Goldie-Coldman hypothesis substantiated by clinical experience? What are the shapes of the relations between the doses of anticancer drugs and their efficacies $w_i(dose_i,t)$ in causing cell kill?

The growth fraction seems to be a stable property of an individual breast cancer. TLI measurements of the disease in the breast and in the axilla correlate positively,[51] as do SPF measurements of primary breast cancers and metastatic deposits.[52] Analysis of growth fraction may relate to clinical aggressiveness.[53-55] TLI may be independent of tumor size and of lymph node status,[56] and high values may predict estrogen and progesterone receptor negativity,[57] and low values may predict longer disease-free intervals and longer survival times,[58,59] but this is not a consistent finding.[60] SPF is usually independent of axillary nodal status, tumor size, or menopausal status,[61] but it is frequently high in tumors in younger patients, who tend to have an inferior prognosis,[62-64] and in tumors that are estrogen and progesterone receptor–negative,[61,63,65,66] poorly differentiated,[61] aneuploid,[62,63,67-69] and clinically aggressive.[62,64,70-76] SPF is a less powerful prognostic factor in node-positive patients[68,77] than in node-negative ones,[73]

but although its value is often limited to subgroups,[67,78-85] a consensus review concluded that it is associated with tumor grade as well as the probability of relapse and survival.[86] Similarly, although no clear relation exists between Ki-67 staining and tumor size or histologic grade,[87,88] this antigen is abundant in cancers with poor estrogen receptor content, aneuploidy, high nuclear grade, and rapid relapse after primary surgery.[87] All these data signify that growth fraction, as estimated by TLI and SPF, is positively correlated weakly with some aggressive manifestations, but not others, so factors other than growth fraction alone are important determinants of malignant behavior.

The relation between growth fraction and the probability of response to chemotherapy is difficult to define, because this relation is confounded with the relation between growth fraction and prognosis independent of the influence of the systemic therapy.[51,89] Aneuploid tumors, which tend to have higher growth fractions,[61,90,91] may be more sensitive to chemotherapy or hormone therapy.[92-94] This observation might be artifactual because aneuploid tumors tend to relapse more quickly than diploid ones, so a difference between patients who have or have not received drug treatment will tend to emerge more quickly in aneuploid than in slower-growing diploid cases. This same argument is relevant to more recent observations regarding the value of HER2 expression or SPF in predicting response to higher-dose versus lower-dose chemotherapy in the adjuvant setting.[95] If it is indeed true that aneuploidy predicts for drug sensitivity, however, this would be consistent with equation 5 but contrary to equation 8, because high growth fraction should predispose to the development of drug resistance. One possible explanation is that aneuploid tumors are more sensitive to chemotherapy because they may have lost the capacity to repair DNA damage. Another is that equation 8 is inapplicable to human breast cancer.

Indeed, the clinical application of equation 8 raises many concerns. Aneuploidy is indeed more common among more poorly differentiated tumors.[61,90,91,96,97] Yet, despite promising early reports,[65,77,98] aneuploidy does not predict high degrees of lymph node involvement.[66,99-103] Only 4 of 17 studies demonstrated a statistically significant correlation between axillary nodal status and ploidy.[61] Moreover, most reports find no correlation between ploidy and patient age, menopausal status, tumor size, or tumor hormone receptor content.[61] Some have reported that aneuploidy is more common in estrogen receptor–negative tumors, but this effect is so weak that it is lost in the random variation of other small studies.[65,77,93,99,104] The weakness of equation 8 is also demonstrated by the observation that special histologic types of breast cancer—types that tend to have a better prognosis, such as mucinous, tubular, and papillary—are often diploid.[61] Lobular invasive carcinomas also tend to be diploid, although their prognoses are similar to those of the more common ductal types, which are more likely to be aneuploid. Also contrary to predictions is the observation that medullary carcinomas are usually aneuploid.[105] This is interesting because, when medullary carcinomas are small and do not involve axillary lymph nodes, they exhibit a low probability of distant metastatic dissemination.

Because aneuploidy is associated with poor differentiation and, possibly, low estrogen receptor content, equation 8 would predict that patients with aneuploid tumors should have a worse prognosis. Some analyses have indeed found that patients with diploid tumors have lower relapse rates[77] and longer survival times than those with aneuploid tumors.[74,106–110] Because ploidy correlates with other known prognostic factors,[111] however, many individual studies and multivariate analyses have not found that ploidy is of independent utility.[62,64,68,69,73,75,76,78,112–114] The literature is ambiguous, presenting the opinions of vigorous defenders of ploidy as a prognostic marker[115–119] and of equally fervent opponents.[61,67,84,85,120,121] A consensus conference concluded that ploidy is a weak prognostic factor, but not one of independent value.[86]

It might be argued that even if ploidy is truly unrelated to clinical behavior, equation 8 is still valid concerning the development of metastatic ability. At reasonable packing ratios, 10^7 breast cancer cells would occupy a volume of 0.1 to 1 cc, or a spherical tumor mass 0.58 to 1.24 cm in diameter. Hence, perhaps it is not a coincidence that the mass diameter of 1 cm is critical in human oncology. At about 1 cm in diameter breast cancers frequently become metastatic to the axillary lymph nodes.[122] Also at this size, node-negative breast cancers frequently demonstrate the ability to produce distant metastases.[105,123] Another argument concerning metastatic behavior is based on data from up to the late 19th century, when primary breast cancers were left to grow unimpeded, because no effective therapies were then available. Almost all patients died of metastatic disease (confirmed by autopsy) within 16 years of the presentation of the mass in the breast.[124] Hence, most breast cancers develop metastatic ability if they are allowed to achieve large size, as predicted by equation 8.

Nevertheless, these clinical observations do not constitute firm proofs because alternate explanations of the association between tumor size and malignant behavior exist, as discussed in more detail later. In addition, the changes in the natural history of breast cancer, associated with the introduction of aggressive surgical management of primary tumors in the 1890s, are inconsistent with equation 8. Long-term follow-up of patients treated by radical mastectomy has suggested that at least 30% are cured.[125,126] The mortality rate is about 10% per year in the first year, dropping steadily to about 2% per year by year 25,[127] thereafter approaching the mortality rate of the general population.[128,129] Many of the breast cancers in these series were large and node-positive at the time of surgery. Hence, although all breast cancers have the potential for developing metastases, not all have already done so by the time the mass first appears in the breast. Yet, by equation 8, most breast cancers larger than 1 cm in diameter should have generated mutants with metastatic capacity. That this is not the case raises doubts about the applicability of the model. Consistent with such doubts are data from a major trial that treated patients with primary disease by lumpectomy with or without radiation therapy.[130] The local relapse rate was high in those not receiving radiation, con-

firming the existence of cancer in the remaining, nonirradiated breast. Yet these inadequately treated patients with high local relapse rates did not seem to have a higher metastatic rate than patients treated by lumpectomy and immediate radiotherapy. Even if, on further follow-up, it appears that local recurrence does increase the odds of metastatic spread, this effect is unlikely to be strong. Hence, cancers can grow locally without rapidly developing cells with metastatic capacity.

The mutant cells of greatest importance to all oncologists are those with metastatic potential. The mutant cells of second greatest importance to the chemotherapist are those that demonstrate resistance to anticancer drugs. Do these develop in a manner consistent with equation 8? The clinical pattern for many breast cancer cases is primary treatment of the disease in the breast, then adjuvant chemotherapy, then a disease-free interval, then recurrence that is often retreated with chemotherapy. Responses to such retreatment in the stage IV setting are common, despite previous exposure of the cancers to chemotherapy. In one trial, patients received cyclophosphamide, doxorubicin, and 5-fluorouracil (CAF) with or without tamoxifen as their first treatment for advanced (metastatic) breast cancer.[131] The response rate, response duration, and overall survival were unaffected by prior adjuvant chemotherapy. Ample evidence now indicates that patients with recurrent disease a year or more after adjuvant CMF responded as well to CMF as patients who had been randomly allocated not to receive adjuvant chemotherapy.[132] This must mean that, contrary to the philosophy surrounding equation 8, breast cancer cells that fail to be cured by adjuvant CMF are not universally resistant to CMF.[133]

The interpretation of equation 8 has also led to the hypothesis that chemotherapy cannot be effective unless it is started as soon as possible after diagnosis.[47] Yet a randomized trial in node-positive primary breast cancer found that 7 months of chemotherapy starting within 36 hours of surgery was no more effective than 6 months of chemotherapy starting about a month after surgery.[134] Hence, delay in initiating chemotherapy did not reduce its efficacy. In confirmation, the worldwide overview of all randomized trials found no pattern of improved results with early institution of chemotherapy or even preoperative chemotherapy.[34] Indeed, delayed therapy might convey some advantages. One trial treated node-positive patients with either 8 months of CMF plus vincristine and prednisone (CMFVP) followed by 6 months of vinblastine, doxorubicin, thiotepa, and fluoxymesterone (VATH) or with an equivalent total duration (14 months) of CMFVP alone.[135,136] Patients receiving the VATH experienced better disease-free survival. Hence, total resistance to VATH did not develop rapidly in the cancer cells that failed to be eradicated by the CMFVP.

Doubts about the clinical validity of equation 8 should raise concerns about the use of this equation in the design of chemotherapy schedules. The treatment recommendation most closely associated with the Goldie-Coldman hypothesis is that concerning alternating chemotherapy. According to their hypothesis, if one were to use two treatments, A and B, in the design of a multicycle regimen, then ABABAB will be superior to AAABBB. The reason is that ABABAB will deliver B sooner than AAABBB. If AAABBB were used, cells resistant to A would stand a great chance of mutating to resistance to B during the AAA portion of the regimen. However, clinical experience to date has failed to validate these predictions. In patients with advanced breast cancer, there is no advantage to CMFVP alternating with VATH over CAF or VATH alone.[137] Moreover, in patients with node-positive primary breast cancer, a sequential chemotherapy regimen was found to be superior to an alternating one.[138] The sequential regimen was four 3-week courses of adjuvant doxorubicin (A) followed by eight 3-week courses of intravenous CMF (C), symbolized as

AAAACCCCCCCC

The alternating regimen was two courses of CMF alternating with one course of doxorubicin, repeated four times for a total of 12 courses, symbolized as

CCACCACCACCA

The superiority of the sequential regimen over the alternation regimen casts serious doubt about the therapeutic applicability of equation 8.

If a constructive critique of equation 8 is important to the design of chemotherapy regimens, an understanding of equation 7 is vital, because much drug resistance is relative, rather than absolute. For many drugs w(dose,t) rises with increasing dose, so it may seem that some cells resistant to a given dose level of drug can be killed by a higher dose level.[139,140] In randomized trials in patients with advanced breast cancer,[141] the higher dose regimen proved superior. Retrospective analyses are also supportive.[142] In addition, dose levels of chemotherapy high enough to require maximum hematopoietic rescue, that is, autologous bone marrow transplantation, clearly produce dramatic rates of tumor volume regression and may result in prolonged, unmaintained remissions.[143,144]

The shape of the relation between w(dose,t) and dose is not totally clear for any drug, however. For some agents, some data suggest a strictly proportional relation. A randomized trial using node-positive patients compared three plans of CAF adjuvant treatment.[145] Let Z equal a certain total cumulative dose of chemotherapy: The three regimens gave either $2 \cdot Z$ over 4 months (R_x I), $2 \cdot Z$ over 6 months (R_x II), or Z over 4 months (R_x III). R_x I was superior to R_x III in reducing the rate of recurrence, but no difference has as yet been reported between R_x I and R_x II. Hence, the total anticancer influence of one of these regimens—from equation 6 this is W(T)—seems to be strictly proportional to the total dose administered,

$$W(T) = k \cdot (\text{cumulative dose}) \qquad (9)$$

with T, in this example, equal to 6 months.
The cumulative influence over 6 months of R_x I is $k \cdot 2 \cdot Z$. This cumulative influence is the sum of $k \cdot 2 \cdot Z$ over the first 4 months plus zero for the 2 additional months. R_x II also yields $k \cdot 2 \cdot Z$ over 6 months. R_x III delivers half as much total anticancer influence, that is $k \cdot Z$ over the

first 4 months, then zero for the remaining 2 months, for a total of $k \cdot Z$. Because benefit is related to total cumulative anticancer influence, a proportional dose–response relationship would predict that R_x III should be inferior to both R_x II and R_x III. As is discussed subsequently, if this chemotherapy cures some patients, then R_x I should eventually prove superior to R_x II, because the log-kill accomplished at 4 months from $2 \cdot Z$ given over 4 months should be greater than the log-kill measured at 4 or at 6 months from $2 \cdot Z$ given over 6 months. For some patients given $2 \cdot Z$ over 4 months, the log-kill might be enough to preclude disease regrowth.

A proportional dose–response relation would mean that it would be possible to improve clinical results merely by increasing the dose level of the drugs used.[146,147] This would be a desirable state of affairs, because improvements in hematopoietic technology and other means of ameliorating toxicity now allow us to increase dose level considerably.[148] The problem is that other data suggest that the dose–response relation for some drugs is actually inferior to that predicted by strict proportionality. For example, a recent study of doxorubicin and cyclophosphamide (AC) in the adjuvant setting has yet to find an advantage to a marked escalation of the cyclophosphamide dose (as permitted by the use of granulocyte colony-stimulating factor (G-CSF), with schedule and total duration of treatment held constant.[149] These data would indicate that W(dose,t) is not always proportional to dose level or even strictly rising with increasing dose.

More Clinical Questions

We may now answer tentatively some of the questions raised earlier, but these answers produce new issues. In human breast cancer, the growth fraction seems to be independent of tumor size. What, then, is the biologic determinant of growth? Higher growth fraction does weakly imply a higher probability of mutations. How, then, is proliferation linked to genetic aberrancy? The magnitude of the growth fraction is not a good predictor of therapeutic response. How, then, does chemotherapy work? How are we to optimize the impact of multicycle chemotherapy regimens when the relation between cumulative proliferation and the likelihood of appearance of drug-resistant mutants is more complex than equation 8? How do we optimize treatment when the existence of drug resistance is not the only cause of therapeutic failure, when the predictions of the Goldie-Coldman hypothesis regarding alternating treatments are not substantiated by clinical experience, and when dose–response relations may not always be strictly proportional? To address these issues, we must consider growth curves more relevant to human breast cancer than simple exponential curves.

Gompertzian Curves

The log-kill model and its further developments were based on exponential proliferation, a common pattern in laboratory models such as L1210. Exponential proliferation, equation 3, implies that the doubling time, defined in equation 4, is constant. Many experimental tumors, however, and perhaps all human cancers, do not exhibit a constant doubling time.[150-155] Exponential models may fail to explain clinical observations adequately in breast cancer because the exponential proliferation curve may not be appropriate.

In exponential proliferation, the growth fraction is constant regardless of tumor size. Yet small solid tumors often contain a higher percentage of actively dividing cells than do larger cancers of the same histologic type.[156,157] The gompertzian curve (see Fig. 22.4-2) is the most common proliferation curve used to fit these phenomena. This curve was first proposed in 1825 by Benjamin Gompertz for different applications.[150] In gompertzian proliferation, the functions f(t) and g(t) in equation 2 are not constant, but vary with time t:

$$N_t = N_\infty^{(1 - d^t)} N_0 d^t \qquad (10)$$

A derivation of equation 10 and the theoretic meaning of parameter d are discussed in the next paragraph.

The doubling time in equation 10 is found not by population doubling—which may not in fact ever take place, especially if the tumor is large—but rather by taking the proliferation rate at N_t and calculating what the doubling time would be were proliferation exponential rather than gompertzian. When this procedure is done, the doubling time is discovered not to be constant but rather increasing with increasing N_t. This finding means that were we to assume that a clinical cancer is exponential, we would overestimate the doubling time during the preclinical phase of growth;[158] that is, when the gompertzian model pertains, preclinical cancers proliferate more rapidly than we would predict from observations of clinical cancers. Therefore, it would take less time for the preclinical cancer to reach clinical size than we would estimate for an exponential tumor. For example, it might take one breast cancer cell 2 to 3 years on the average to reach a population size large enough to be palpable in the breast.[152] The exponential model would predict a subclinical growth duration several times longer than this. At the other extreme, as N_t becomes large, the doubling time becomes so long that it approaches infinity. This means that a tumor of large N_t proliferates so slowly that it appears to be at a stable plateau size, N_∞. Whole animals and all normal organs follow gompertzian kinetics: the adult sizes of all parts of the body appear to remain within a narrow range, that is, close to stable plateaus, for the duration of adult life. Some preneoplasias, such as ductal carcinomas in situ of the breast, may grow slowly at plateau sizes for long periods (ie, their values of N_∞ are small, usually no more than one or several cubic centimeters). For malignant cancers, however, the plateau size is so large that it is incompatible with the life of the host.

Speer–Retsky Model

Speer and Retsky and their colleagues questioned the applicability of the exponential model to human breast cancer.[159] Their work was based on a study of survival durations of patients who received no therapy for their breast cancers,[124] on the growth histories of mammographic shadows,[160] and on disease-free durations of patients following mastectomy.[161] These investigators found that simple exponential kinetics could not apply. Furthermore, they derived a computer model in which tumors grow in randomly increasing steps of gompertzian plateaus, with an overall pattern that roughly resembles a bumpy gompertzian curve. This model fits time-to-event data (ie, time to death, time to recurrence), confirming the general applicability of gompertzian-like curves. The long temporary plateaus that they predict have never actually been observed, however.[162] In addition, the model has made a clinical prediction that has not been verified. The prediction was that the postsurgical adjuvant chemotherapy of breast cancer should not be used only immediately after surgery, but that additional chemotherapy should be reapplied at later dates to kill breast cancer cells that are dividing during presumed proliferation spurts. A clinical trial designed to test this hypothesis did not find advantage in the late application of CMF after initial AC adjuvant treatment.[163] The failure of this prediction may be based on the assumption of these investigators that all breast cancers start along the same proliferation path, with heterogeneity developing in random steps over time. If heterogeneity in proliferation is an early property of breast cancer, then the Speer-Retsky model produces curves that for all practical purposes are identical to those of a simple gompertzian model, but with different clinical implications. In fact, the same clinical data that were used to derive the Speer-Retsky model have been fit more parsimoniously, and with greater accuracy, by a family of simple gompertzian curves.[152] The gompertzian model so derived was the simplest proliferation model that could fit the data accurately. As with the Speer-Retsky approach, a family of exponential curves would not work because the predicted time from relapse to death would be too short.

Norton–Simon Model

The foregoing discussion establishes the gompertzian curve as a plausible model of human breast cancer proliferation. Yet if this is the pattern of volume expansion, what is the pattern of volume regression of breast cancer after effective drug therapy? Experimental and clinical data indicate that the pattern of tumor regression mimics the pattern of proliferation that the tumor would have followed had it been left unperturbed at the moment of treatment.[164-166] For exponential tumors, as symbolized by equation 5, the pattern of regression after effective therapy is exponential. Let N_t' stand for the rate of proliferation of an unperturbed tumor (eg, the first derivative of N as a function of t). Using parameter k from equation 3, in exponential proliferation

$$N_t' = \log_e(k) \cdot N_t \qquad (11)$$

Then, by equation 5, the rate of regression $\tilde{N}'_t$ following effective therapy, is given by

$$\tilde{N}'_t = [1 - w(dose,t)] \cdot N'_t \qquad (12)$$

Just as exponential proliferation means a constant fractional gain in population size per unit of time—hence a constant doubling time—exponential regression means a constant proportional cell kill per dose of therapy (see Fig. 22.4-1*C*).

The only distinction between the Skipper-Schabel-Wilcox model and the Norton-Simon model is that the regression of a gompertzian tumor is gompertzian, not exponential. From equations 6, 10, and 12,

$$N'_t = \log_e(d) \cdot \log_e(N_\infty/N_t) \cdot N_t \qquad (13a)$$

$$\tilde{N}'_t = [1 - w(dose,t)] \cdot \log_e(d) \cdot \log_e(N_\infty/N_t) \cdot N_t \qquad (13b)$$

$$N_T = N_\infty \cdot (1 - d^{T-W(T)}) \cdot N_0 \cdot d^{T-W(T)} \qquad (13c)$$

Although it may not be intuitive from inspection of equations 13a through 13c, these equations mean that log-kill are not constant but are greater when the tumor N_0 is small (see Fig. 22.4-2*C*). In interpreting this result, one must remember that, although the log-kill is greater for smaller tumors, the rate of regrowth or recovery from therapy, given by equation 10, is greater as well. Therefore, the overall impact of treatment is modest, unless the tumor cannot regrow. Biochemical methods of achieving permanent G_0 status of the cancer cells would be one way of preventing regrowth, and this is indeed a proper research direction. The most obvious method of preventing tumor regrowth is the eradication of all cancer cells, however.

An aspect of tumor eradication relevant to the design of treatment schedules concerns the observation that breast cancers are heterogeneous in drug sensitivity. For example, let us conceive of the whole breast cancer in an individual patient as a collection of different sublines with different proliferation rates and different sensitivities to treatment. Eradicating some sublines by chemotherapy would leave others to grow. The residual sublines would have a tendency to regrow rapidly by virtue of their gompertzian kinetics. Hence, partially effective therapies, even those killing most of the cells present, could translate in the clinic to only small increases in disease-free survival times.

One subline that may be particularly resistant to chemotherapy is the *stem cell*. These cells are an important class of undifferentiated cells that can form colonies in soft agar,[167] and they are thought to be able to reproduce the whole spectrum of subtypes that make up a mature organ or tumor. Only 0.1% to 1% of the cells in a typical breast cancer have this capacity. Stem cells in G_0 may be recruited into G_1 by the proper environmental signal—death or injury of neighboring cancer cells, drugs, or hormones.[168,169] In the absence of such signals, stem cells may remain in G_0 for long periods and could be a source of therapeutic failure.[170] The pessimistic side of this argument is that more aggressive chemotherapy in the clinic may produce little real survival benefit because of the existence of resistant sublines and their ability to rebound with

gompertzian kinetics from therapy. The optimistic side is that our current adjuvant chemotherapies might actually be bringing us closer to total cellular eradication than we might otherwise be led to suspect by their modest impact on disease-free and overall survival.

The important clinical question, then, is how do we eradicate residual sublines, particularly those that are slowly growing, slowly regressing, and therefore harder to kill.[171] Slower-growing cells should be in the minority by the time of diagnosis because, by then, they should have been overgrown by faster-growing cells. The Norton-Simon model suggests that the best way to cure this heterogeneous population is to eradicate the numerically dominant, faster-growing cells first. Then, the therapy should be directed against the numerically inferior, slower-growing, more resistant cells.[172]

Dose Density

This brings us to the function w(dose,t). If the dose–response relation is rising, increasing dose level is a good way to increase w(dose,t), resulting in a more negative $T - W(T)$ by time T in equation 13c, and a greater chance of eradicating the drug-sensitive subpopulations. How do we increase cell kill if the dose–response relation rises slowly, however, or is even flat at therapeutic dose levels of drug? Increasing dose level, in these cases, results in essentially the same w(dose,t). Here we must recall that the total impact of a therapy between time zero and time T is given by T minus the total anticancer influence W(T). If a fixed W(T) can be given over a shorter T, the impact of therapy will be greater. This is because a shorter T leaves less time for tumor regrowth to occur. Even if w(dose,t) per administration does not increase with increasing dose level, more frequent administrations of treatment will increase cell kill and thereby increase the odds of subline eradication.

Let us imagine giving three cycles of therapy, each at $W(T_1) = Z$, over a total duration of treatment T_1. The total impact of this treatment will be $T_1 - 3 \cdot Z$. If we give the same three cycles at the same dose levels over T_2, which is shorter than T_1, the impact will be $T_2 - 3 \cdot Z$, which is more negative than $T_1 - 3 \cdot Z$ and thereby more cytoreductive. This concept, which might be termed *dose density*, to distinguish it from *dose intensity*, is illustrated in Figure 22.4-3. The concept of dose intensity concerns milligrams of drug per square meter of patient surface area per unit of time (usually a week).[173] It mixes dose level and schedule of administration and assumes that the relation between dose and w(dose,t) is always rising or is even strictly proportional, as described previously. When the dose–response relation is unknown, however, dose density, keeping the dose level constant but decreasing the time between administrations, is a more reliable way of increasing cell kill.

The concept of dose density, plus the conclusion of the Norton-Simon model that faster sublines should be eliminated before slower sublines, may explain the superi-

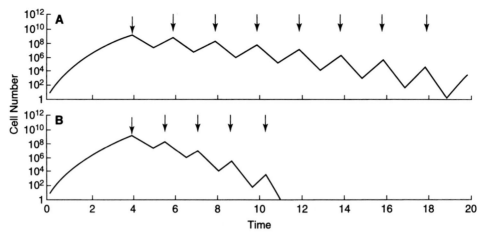

FIGURE 22.4-3 The advantages of dose-dense chemotherapy in a Gompertzian model. **A.** Reproduction of the curve shown in Figure 22.4-2C. Eight cycles of chemotherapy reduces 10^9 cells to one cell that quickly regrows toward recurrence. **B.** A subtle shortening of the cycle length, however, limits regrowth time between administrations, leading to tumor eradication by five cycles. In this simulation, dose level is not increased. If dose level can be increased without sacrificing short intervals between treatments, however, this might be an even more effective plan, because a rising dose-response relationship is found for many chemotherapeutic agents. If the total tumor is composed of several sublines, each with specific sensitivity to a given drug, dose-dense schedules of each drug would be the best way to eradicate each subline.

ority of AAAACCCCCCCC over CCACCACCACCA in the adjuvant setting, as described previously.[138] The first regimen gave eight cycles of CMF over 33 weeks, from the beginning of treatment, and four cycles of doxorubicin over 9 weeks. This means that the dose density of the doxorubicin was high compared with the second regimen, which gave eight cycles of CMF over a similar 30 weeks, but four cycles of doxorubicin over 33 weeks.

In AAAACCCCCCCC, dose density is achieved by *crossover scheduling*, AAAA crossing over to CCCCCCCC. Increasing dose density by crossover scheduling as a means of eradicating subpopulations and improving the results of clinical chemotherapy will require much development in the arena of clinical trials. The concept has laboratory backing: The cure of 10^{11} L1210 cells is best accomplished by using cytosine arabinoside plus 6-thioguanine for 2 or 3 courses, followed by 1 high-dose treatment with cyclophosphamide plus BCNU.[174] Compared to the use of methyl-CCNU alone, the complete remission rate and the median survival time of BDF1 mice bearing the M5076 tumor may be doubled by using 4 doses of methyl-CCNU first, then crossing over to a single dose of L-phenylalanine mustard.[175] L-Phenylalanine mustard by itself has weak activity against this tumor because only a small subpopulation of cells is sensitive just to this drug.

In the clinic, a plan giving multiple cycles of dose-dense doxorubicin followed by multiple cycles of dose-dense cyclophosphamide has been piloted successfully in the adjuvant setting.[176] A prospective determination of comparative efficacy of a similar regimen versus a more traditional combination chemotherapy is in progress by the Southwest Oncology Group. The dose-dense plan exploits the ability of hematopoietic growth factors to ensure frequent administration of adequate dose levels of drug.[177] At present, a pilot study is applying three cycles of dose-dense doxorubicin, followed by three of dose-dense paclitaxel, then three of dose-dense cyclophosphamide, all with G-CSF, in postsurgical patients with node-positive primary breast cancer.[178] The concept is also applicable to patients with stage IV breast cancer responsive to conventional chemotherapy: patients with advanced disease have been treated with dose-dense cyclophosphamide followed by dose-dense thiotepa, and further developments using peripheral blood progenitor cell reinfusions as hematopoietic support are in progress.[179–181] These plans differ from the conventional single-bolus intensification plans that have traditionally been associated with the use of autologous bone marrow reinfusions.[182] Single-bolus plans increase dose level, but dose density depends on multiple cycles.

The rationality of crossover scheduling is supported by models other than that of Norton and Simon. Goldie and Coldman's prediction of the superiority of alternating chemotherapy, CCACCACCACCA, depended on the assumption of symmetry: sublines with equal numbers of cells, equal proliferation rates, and equal mutation rates. Day reconsidered the Goldie-Coldman model, but performed computer simulations of mutation to drug resistance under asymmetric conditions.[183] From this, he formulated a rule similar to that of the Norton-Simon model in that the alternating plan is predicted to be inferior.[184]

Biologic Basis for Gompertzian Proliferation

An intriguing issue, of relevance to the design of therapy and also to an understanding of carcinogenesis, concerns the biologic basis of gompertzian proliferation. An old concept in this regard is that the natural pattern of proliferation is exponential but that a solid tumor outgrows its supply of nutrients (ie, vascularity) and therefore cannot sustain simple exponential proliferation. The default proliferation curve, according to this hypothesis, is gompertzian. This concept is intuitive but contestable in that even small tumors, with rich blood supply, proliferate in a gompertzian manner. In addition, large tumors, with relatively slow proliferation rates, often have more than adequate vascularity. Indeed, the ability to induce neovascularization may be an absolute requirement for a tumor to reach a large size.[185] Other evidence suggests that large tumors may be growing slowly because of decreased cell production rather than increased cell loss.[156,157] Such decreased cell production may be the consequence of longer cell cycle times, because, as we observed, growth fraction is often independent of tumor size.

A starting point in the quest for a tenable biologic model may be the histopathology of breast cancer that is observed microscopically. The geometric relation between invasive ductal breast cancer cells and their stroma is complex. An examination of pathologic specimens reveals that all tumors, of the breast and otherwise, are composed of repeating elements—such as branching tree patterns or multiple nodules—that are self-similar over various scales of size. The most common arrangement in breast cancer is the branching pattern. This is reminiscent of a tissue's vascular supply and is in fact the normal structure of all exocrine glands. The normal breast is composed of lobules and ducts organized into branching tubes. Breast cancers of ductal origin follow similar patterns, but they vary from this normal architecture depending on their degree of differentiation. Well-differentiated tumors follow patterns close to normal, whereas poorly differentiated ones differ so much from this pattern that little resemblance to a branching tree can be discerned, and this pattern is replaced by a solid block of cells.[124] Nevertheless, all these cancers obey the geometric rule that the number of cells (N) in the mass is proportional to its volume (V) raised to a positive power less than or equal to 1[186,187]:

$$N = V^d \qquad (14)$$

A small exponent d means that the number of cancer cells per volume of tumor is relatively small. In general, well-differentiated breast cancers are indeed observed to have a relatively low ratio of cancer cells over total mass volume, because so much of the tumor is composed of normal host cells, fat, or interstital space.[188] Alternatively, poorly differentiated breast cancers are commonly composed of densely packed cancer cells with little intervening stroma.[124] These cancers tend to be more malignant. In geometric terms, their values of d are close to 1. It is mathematically possible for a tumor with high d to have a small plateau size N_∞ and hence be benign, but the histopathologic features of invasive ductal breast cancers do seem to confirm a positive relation between d and malignancy.

How does such a mass, following the rule of equation 14, proliferate and grow? Let us hypothesize that cancer cells define a certain potential proliferation space proportional to the number of cells. This is tenable because the stromal cells in a primary breast cancer are known to make growth factors,[189,190] proteinases,[191] and other biologically active chemicals.[192,193] The production of these chemicals by the stromal cells could be reactive to signals from the cancer cells.[194] A mathematic statement of this phenomenon is that the tumor volume V_1 at one arbitrary time unit after time 0 is proportional to N_0, the number of cells present at time 0:

$$V_1 = a \cdot N_0 \qquad (15)$$

By equation 14,

$$N_1 = V_1^d = a^d N_0^d \qquad (16)$$

Because $V_t = a N_{t-1}$,

$$N_t = a^{\sum_{i=1}^{t} d^i} N_0^{d^t} = N_\infty^{(1-d^t)} N_0^{d^t} \qquad (17)$$

where:

$$N_\infty = a^{[d/(1-d)]} \qquad (18)$$

Equation 17 is equivalent to equation 10. Hence, the fractal geometry of the branching tree pattern generates gompertzian proliferation.

By equation 14, parameters a and d associate the number of cells to the size of the tumor. High values of d (close to one) are associated with a high density of cancer cells and extremely malignant biologic behavior. Lower values of d are associated with lower cell densities and more benign biologic behavior. How does the magnitude of d relate to the pattern of gompertzian proliferation? When d = 1, equation 16 reduces to exponential proliferation, equation 3. Equations 17 and 18 do not apply. It is not unreasonable to associate exponential proliferation with extremely malignant behavior, because exponential proliferation is unbounded from above, growing faster and faster as tumor size increases. When d is less than one, equations 17 and 18 are relevant, and gompertzian proliferation results. In fact, by equation 18, N_∞ is sensitive to d. As shown in Figure 22.4-4, for a fixed value of a, N_∞ changes little for a wide range of values of d, but becomes large quickly as d increases past a threshold (in this case, between 0.75 and 0.85). Does the plateau size N_∞ in gompertzian proliferation relate to the degree of malignancy? A qualified affirmative answer would seem to be intuitive, because a small N_∞ is clearly associated with benign lesions, such as fibroadenomas of the breast. Although benign tumors can sometimes achieve large size while remaining benign, in breast tumors this event is rare. More commonly, extremely malignant cancers tend toward large size, tumor size being one of the most important prognostic variables in primary breast cancer.[105,197] Malignant lesions with great metastatic potential can be found in the breast while they are small, but these lesions would have probably grown to large size were they not excised or irradiated, as suggested by the natural history of stage III breast cancer.

The relation between parameter d and N_∞ may be important in carcinogenesis. Equation 18 means that normal tissues could sustain considerable genetic injury that raises

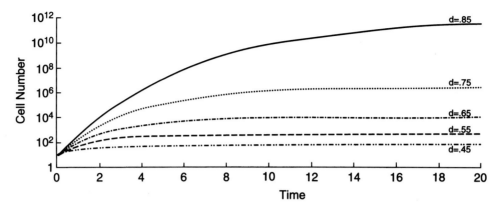

FIGURE 22.4-4 Gompertzian curves for various values of d, where d expresses the relation between the volume of a population and its cellularity (for a fixed value of parameter a, as discussed in the text). Low values of d favor low ratios of premalignant or cancer cells to stroma; large values are more commonly associated with more densely packed cancer cells. In this simulation, low values of d, below 0.75, produce population plateau sizes that are well below the level of clinical appreciation. However, as d changes to between 0.75 and 0.85, the population assumes a characteristic of malignancy: proliferation to a large size. The hypothetic relation between the magnitude of parameter d and the features of invasion and metastasis are discussed in the text. This model is consistent with a prolonged preneoplastic state (with abnormally large but still subthreshold values of d), followed by sudden transformation to malignancy with a small additional increment in parameter d. Alterations in parameter a, which concerns the relation between the preneoplastic or cancer cells and their stroma, could also produce neoplastic conversion, as described in the text.

d, but these tissues could still maintain a benign proliferation pattern with small N_∞. At a critical point of increasing d, however, a threshold is crossed, resulting in high N_∞, consistent with malignancy. This concept is congruous with a long process of evolving preneoplasia. The relevance to invasive breast cancers, evolving from atypical hyperplasias, carcinomas in situ, and perhaps other lesions with small N_∞, is evident.

N_∞ is also affected by parameter a. For example, a gompertzian lesion with d equal to 0.9 achieves a miniscule N_∞ of only 10^6 with parameter a equal to 6. For parameter a equal to 12, the same d yields N_∞ of between 10^9 and 10^{10}. For parameter a equal to 24, however, N_∞ exceeds 10^{12}, clearly a troublesome number for the patient's health. Hence, a small value of parameter a could keep a tumor benign even with densely packed cells. This would be the case were the local environment inhospitable to the growth of the tumor, so the cells could not successfully define a significant potential growth space around them. Even if parameter a is 24, however, N_∞ cannot exceed 10^{10} unless d is greater than about 0.88.

How does high N_∞ relate to invasion and metastasis? Parameters a and d concern the relation between the cancer cells N and their stroma. Large parameter a could be the result of cancer cells that are aggressive in defining a potential growth space, by stromal dissolution, angiogenesis, or any combination of such factors. High d may be caused by any combination of three phenomena[195]:

1. The proliferation of the cancer cells has become so sensitive to stromal factors that they are overstimulated by the stroma.
2. The cancer cells have become autonomous of stromal factors, which could be considered a state of infinite sensitivity.
3. The stroma has lost its capacity to inhibit the proliferation of the cancer cells.

In any event, high a and d imply a loss of normal anatomic constraints, so invasion might well result. In addition, the cells from a tumor with large parameters a and d may be so prone to stimulation by distant tissue (bone, viscera, and so forth),[196] so autonomous of such stimulation, or so uninhibited by distant tissues that they can proliferate and grow in metastatic sites. Thus, proliferation, invasion, and metastasis are linked by geometric considerations. In breast cancer, as in most solid tumors, metastatic potential is a direct function of tumor size.[197] Total autonomy (either because of infinite sensitivity to growth factors, of acrine proliferation, or of inability to be inhibited) would mean that the cancer cells could grow anywhere in the host and might even grow exponentially by virtue of a parameter d equal to 1.

Chemotherapy and Cytokinetics

This analysis may help us to explain one of the most perplexing problems in clinical proliferation curve analysis: how does chemotherapy work? Chemotherapy is hypothesized to be mitotoxic, which means that it is thought to be particularly lethal to mitotic cells. More rapidly proliferating tissues, or tissues in the more rapidly growing phases of their gompertzian curves, are assumed to be more sensitive to chemotherapy because more of their cells are in division and hence at risk.[198] In support of this hypothesis is the evidence that stimulation of MCF-7 cells in vitro with estradiol or epidermal growth factor increases both cell proliferation and cell kill from doxorubicin.[199] Estradiol also enhances the cytotoxicity of melphalan in hormone-responsive cell lines.[200] In the clinic, hormone recruitment of locally advanced breast cancer has resulted in high local response rates to chemotherapy.[201,202]

The advantages of recruitment are slight or nonexistant in the treatment of metastatic breast cancer.[203–205] Moreover, tamoxifen antagonizes the cytotoxicity of melphalan and 5-fluorouracil at dose levels insufficient to cause a G_1–S arrest.[200] Tamoxifen actually enhances the cytotoxicity of doxorubicin and of the alkylating agent 4-hydroxy-cyclophosphamide in this system. When MCF-7 cells are exposed to low levels of doxorubicin, S-phase is not especially damaged.[206] Instead, one sees a slow accumulation of cells in late S, G_2, and M. Hence, some reasons to doubt the mitotoxicity hypothesis exist.

Indeed, from a kinetic viewpoint, mitotoxicity has never been an adequate explanation for the magnitude of the response of clinical breast cancer to chemotherapy. Only about 5% to 6% of the cells in an average breast cancer are in S-phase. Hence, even if our drugs killed all the cells in the growth fraction, less than 20% of the cells in the tumor mass could possibly be killed by a single treatment. Yet volume regressions greater than 90% are frequently seen after single exposures to high-dose chemotherapy.[143] We have also observed that the magnitude of the growth fraction, as estimated by TLI, does not predict chemosensitivity in either locally advanced breast cancer[89] or in the adjuvant setting.[207] Normal tissues such as bone marrow, hair follicles, and alimentary mucosa have higher growth fractions than many breast cancers. Yet these normal tissues can recover quickly from the influence of chemotherapy, whereas the breast cancers may not, giving long periods of disease control off treatment. Many other examples exist of the failure of the mitotoxicity hypothesis to explain experimental and clinical observations.

An alternative concept is that chemotherapy, and even hormonal therapy, may work by resetting the relations between the cancer cells and their stroma as expressed in the foregoing equations. This resetting would result in equation 12. One mechanism for this effect would be the disruption of growth factor loops, which is a primary determinant of cell–stromal interactions. In the laboratory, doxorubicin has been shown to up-regulate epidermal growth factor receptors in HeLa and 3T3 cells.[208] Drug activation of the intracellular signal called *protein kinase C* increases cell kill by cisplatin without increasing drug uptake.[209] Antibodies to growth factor receptors inhibit the growth of human cancer xenografts and synergize in this action with a variety of chemotherapeutic agents.[210] Hence, chemotherapy might work by a growth factor mechanism. In this regard, when hematopoietic cells are deprived of essential growth factors, they die by *apoptosis,* an orderly process of programmed cell death.[211,212] It might not be a coincidence, therefore, that chemotherapy often kills cancer cell by inducing apoptosis.[213]

Current Critical Issues

The gompertzian model allows us to address some of the critical issues in the cytokinetics of breast cancer from a perspective different from the exponential view. The growth fraction may be independent of tumor size because the major biologic determinants of growth are parameters a and d in equations 17 and 18, which express the relation between the cancer cells and their environment, rather than parameter k in equation 3, which concerns the growth fraction only. Proliferation is linked to genetic aberrancy, not merely by the tumor's growth fraction, but also by the tumor's geometry. Profound changes in the geometry of preneoplastic tissues may produce little increase in maximum population size, invasion, and metastatic potential until a critical threshold is crossed, whence malignant behavior suddenly ensues. The magnitude of the growth fraction is not a good predictor of therapeutic response because chemotherapy works by resetting cell–stromal interactions, not just by killing dividing cells. Of most immediate practical relevance, the impact of multicycle chemotherapy regimens may be optimized by schedules that increase dose density, even when dose–response relations are not strictly proportional or even rising with increasing dose.

All these conclusions require much experimental verification, but a framework exists for the interpretation of complex phenomena of proliferation and growth. A major area of interest is the relation between the biochemistry of breast cancer cells and their cytokinetic behavior. What are the influences of growth-promoting and growth-inhibiting hormones on tumor geometry? How does the overexpression of growth factor receptors such as the epidermal growth factor receptor and HER2/*neu* relate to parameters a and d? These questions are now relevant to therapeutics because of the availability of drugs such as tamoxifen and antireceptor monoclonal antibodies.[210,214] Drugs that interfere with signal transduction are soon to be added to the list. Even with conventional chemotherapeutic agents, the best way to achieve dose density and the evaluation of the impact of innovative dose-dense schedules on disease-free and overall survival are topics of current experimentation. Of greatest long-term value may be investigations of preneoplasia and the influences on parameters a and d that convert predisposed normal tissues to high N_∞ cancers. Effective prevention strategies may result from such studies. The discovery of the structure of the breast and ovarian cancer susceptibility gene BRCA1 may provide an important tool for this purpose.[215] Cytokinetics is clearly an important aspect of breast cancer, closely related to fundamental biologic and genetic considerations and deserving of the attention of both laboratory and clinical scientists.

References

1. Hoffman J, Post J. In vivo studies of DNA synthesis in human normal and tumor cells. Cancer Res 1967;27:898.

2. Quastler H, Sherman FG. Cell population kinetics in the intestinal epithelium of the mouse. Exp Cell Res 1959;17:420.

3. Howard A, Pelc SR. Nuclear incorporation of ^{32}p as demonstrated by autoradiographs. Exp Cell Res 1951;2:178.

4. Lajtha LG, Oliver R, Ellis F. Incorporation of ^{32}p and adenine ^{14}C into DNA by human bone marrow cells in vitro. Br J Cancer 1954;8:367.

5. Gelfant S. Cycling–noncycling cell transitions in tissue aging, immunological surveillance, transformation and tumor growth. Int Rev Cytol 1981;70:1.

6. Darzynkiewicz Z. Metabolic and kinetic compartments of the cell cycle distinguished by multiparameter flow cytometry. In: Skehan P, Friedman SJ eds. Growth, cancer and the cell cycle. Clifton, NJ, Humana, 1984:249.

7. Ling MR, Kay JE. Lymphocyte stimulation. New York, Elsevier, 1965.

8. Baserga A. Growth in size and cell DNA replication. Exp Cell Res 1984;151:1.

9. Darzynkiewicz Z, Traganos F, Melamed MR. New cell cycle compartments identified by multiparameter flow cytometry. Cytometry 1980;1:98.

10. Gerdes J, Lemke H, Baisch H, et al. Cell cycle analysis of a cell proliferation-associated human nuclear antigen defined by the monoclonal antibody Ki-67. J Immunol 1984;133:1710.

11. Johnson LV, Walsh ML, Chen LB. Localization of mitochondria in living cells with rhodamine 123. Proc Natl Acad Sci USA 1980;77:990.

12. Chaudhary PM, Roninson IB. Expression and activity of P-glyco-protein, a multidrug efflux pump, in human hematopoietic stem cells. Cell 1991;66:85.

13. Mendelsohn ML. The growth fraction: a new concept applied to neoplasia. Science 1960;132:1496.

14. Killman SA. Acute leukemia: the kinetics of leukemic blast cells in man. Series Hematol 1968;1:38.

15. Steel GG. Cell loss as a factor in the growth rate of human tumors. Eur J Cancer 1967;3:381.

16. Novick A, Szilard L. Experiments with the chemostat on spontaneous mutations of bacteria. Proc Natl Acad Sci USA 1950;36:708.

17. Varmus H. An historical overview of oncogenes. In: Weinberg RA, ed. Oncogenes and the molecular origins of cancer. Cold Spring Harbor, NY, Cold Spring Harbor Laboratory, 1989:3.

18. Vogelstein B, Kinzler KW. The multi-step nature of cancer. Trends Genet 1993;9:138.

19. Weinberg RA. Oncogenes, antioncogenes and the molecular basis of multistep carcinogenesis. Cancer Res 1989;49:3713.

20. Knudson AG. Hereditary cancers: clues to mechanisms of carcinogenesis. Br J Cancer 1989;59:661.

21. Ryser HJ. Chemical carcinogenesis. N Engl J Med 1971;285:721.

22. De Ome KB, Medina D. A new approach to mammary tumorigenesis in rodents. Cancer 1969;24:1255.

23. Davis HH, Simons M, Davis JB. Cystic disease of the breast: relationship to carcinoma. Cancer 1964;17:957.

24. Sandison AT. An autopsy study of the adult human breast: with special reference to the proliferative epithelial changes of importance in the pathology of the breast. Natl Cancer Inst Monogr 1962;8:1.

25. Skipper HE, Schabel FM Jr, Wilcox WS. Experimental evaluation of potential anticancer agents. XIII. On the criteria and kinetics associated with "curability" of experimental leukemia. Cancer Chemother Rep 1964;35:1.

26. Norton L, Simon R. Growth curve of an experimental solid tumor following radiotherapy. J Natl Cancer Inst 1977;58:1735.

27. Skipper HE. Laboratory models: the historical perspective. Cancer Treat Rep 1986;70:3.

28. Goldin A, Venditti JM, Humphreys SR, et al. Influence of the concentration of leukemic innoculum on the effectiveness of treatment. Science 1956;123:840.

29. Roosa R, Weaver CF, DeLamater ED. Importance of transplant size in chemotherapeutic assay with the use of the Gardner lymphosarcoma. Proc Am Assoc Cancer Res 1957;2:243.

30. Holland JF. Clinical studies of unmaintained remissions in acute lymphocytic leukemia. In: The proliferation and spread of neoplastic cells. University of Texas MD Anderson Hospital and Tumor Institute at Houston. 21st Annual Symposium on Fundamental Cancer Research 1967. Baltimore, Williams & Wilkins, 1968:453.

31. Schabel FM. Concepts for the systemic treatment of micrometastases. Cancer 1975;35:15.

32. Shapiro DM, Fugmann RA. A role for chemotherapy as an adjunct to surgery. Cancer Res 1957;17:1098.

33. Early Breast Cancer Trialists' Collaborative Group. Systemic treatment of early breast cancer by hormonal, cytotoxic, or immune therapy. Lancet 1992;339:71.

34. Goldie JH, Coldman AJ. A mathematic model for relating the drug sensitivity of tumors to their spontaneous mutation rate. Cancer Treat Rep 1979;63:1727.

36. Devita VT. Principles of chemotherapy. In: Cancer: principles and practice of oncology, ed 3. Devita VT Jr, Hellman S, Rosenberg SA, eds. Philadelphia, JB Lippincott, 1988:279.

37. Devita VT. The relationship between tumor mass and resistance to treatment of cancer. Cancer 1983;51:1209.

38. Luria SE, Delbruck M. Mutations of bacteria from virus sensitivity to virus resistance. Genetics 1943;28:491.

39. Law LW. Origin of resistance of leukaemic cells to folic acid antagonists. Nature 1952;169:628.

40. Frei E III, Freireich EJ, Gehan E, et al. Studies of sequential and combination antimetabolite therapy in acute leukemia: 6-mercaptopurine and methotrexate. Blood 1961;18:431.

41. Burchenal JH, Cramer MA, Williams BS, et al. Sterilization of leukemic cells in vivo and in vitro. Cancer Res 1951;11:700.

42. Broek D, Bartlett R, Crawford K, et al. Involvement of P34^{cdc2} in establishing the dependency of S phase on mitosis. Nature 1991;349:388.

43. Hartwell LH, Weinert TA. Checkpoints: controls that ensure the order of cell cycle events. Science 1989;246:629.

44. Murray AW, Kirschner MW. Dominoes and clocks: the union of two views of the cell cycle. Science 1989;246:614.

45. Murray AW. Remembrance of things past. Nature 1991;349:367.

46. Goldie JH, Coldman AJ. Application of theoretical models to chemotherapy protocol design. Cancer Treat Rep 1986;70:127.

47. Goldie JH. Scientific basis for adjuvant and primary (neoadjuvant) chemotherapy. Semin Oncol 1987;14:1.

48. Kendal WS, Frost P. Metastatic potential and spontaneous mutation rates: studies with two murine cell lines and their recently induced metastatic variants. Cancer Res 1986;46:6131.

49. DeVita VT, Young RC, Cannellos GP. Combination vs single agent chemotherapy: a review of the basis for selection of drug treatment of cancer. Cancer 1975;35:98.

50. Coldman AJ, Goldie JH. A mathematical model of drug resistance in neoplasms. In: Bruchovsky N, Goldie JH, eds. Drug and hormone resistance in neoplasia. Boca Raton, CRC, 1982:55.

51. Daidone MG, Silvestrini R, Valentinis B, et al. Proliferative activity of primary breast cancer and of synchronous lymph node metastases evaluated by ^{3}H-thymidine-labeling index. Cell Tissue Kinet 1990;23:401.

52. Meyer JS, McDivitt RW. Reliability and stability of the thymidine labeling index of breast carcinoma. Lab Invest 1986;54:160.

53. Meyer JS. Cell kinetics in selection and stratification of patients for adjuvant therapy of breast carcinoma. Natl Cancer Inst Monogr 1986;1:25.

54. Meyer JS, Coplin MD. Thymidine labeling index, flow cytometric

S-phase measurement, and DNA index in human tumors. Am J Clin Pathol 1988;59:586.

55. Tubiana M, Pejovic MH, Koscielny S, et al. Growth rate, kinetics of tumor cell proliferation and long-term outcome in human breast cancer. Int J Cancer 1989;44:17.

56. Silvestrini R, Daidone MG, Mastore M, et al. Cell kinetics of 9200 human breast cancers: consistency of basic and clinical results. Proc Am Assoc Can Res 1992;33:238.

57. Valentinis B, Silvestrini R, Daidone MG, et al. ³H-thymidine-labeling index, hormone receptors, and ploidy in breast cancers from elderly patients. Breast Cancer Res Treat 1991;20:19.

58. Silvestrini R, Daidone MG, Valagussa P, et al. ³H-thymidine-labeling index as a prognostic indicator in node-positive breast cancer. J Clin Oncol 1990;8:1321.

59. Silvestrini R, Daidone MG, Del Bino G, et al. Prognostic significance of proliferative activity and ploidy in node-negative breast cancers. Ann Oncol 1993;4:213.

60. Cooke TG, Stanton PD, Winstanley J, et al. Long-term prognostic significance of thymidine labelling index in primary breast cancer. Eur J Cancer 1992;28:424.

61. Frierson HF. Ploidy analysis and S-phase fraction determination by flow cytometry of invasive adenocarcinomas of the breast. Am J Surg Pathol 1991;15:358.

62. Muss HB, Kute TE, Case LD, et al. The relation of flow cytometry to clinical and biologic characteristics in women with node negative primary breast cancer. Cancer 1989;64:1894.

63. Stal O, Brisfors A, Carstensen J, et al. Interrelations between cellular DNA content, S-phase fraction, hormone receptor status and age in primary breast cancer. Acta Oncol 1992;31:283.

64. Dressler LG. Are DNA flow cytometry measurements providing useful information in the management of the node-negative breast cancer patient? Cancer Invest 1992;10:477.

65. Dressler LG, Seamer LC, Owens MA, et al. DNA flow cytometry and prognostic factors in 1331 frozen breast cancer specimens. Cancer 1988;61:420.

66. McDivitt RW, Stone KR, Craig RB, et al. A proposed classification of breast cancer based on kinetic information. Cancer 1986;57:269.

67. Fisher B, Gunduz N, Costantino J, et al. DNA flow cytometric analysis of primary operable breast cancer. Cancer 1991;68:1465.

68. Witzig TE, Ingle JN, Schaid DJ, et al. DNA ploidy and percent S-phase as prognostic factors in node-positive breast cancer: results from patients enrolled in two prospective randomized trials. J Clin Oncol 1993;11:351.

69. Clark GM, Mathieu M, Owens MA, et al. Prognostic significance of S-phase fraction in good-risk, node-negative breast cancer patients. J Clin Oncol 1992;10:428.

70. Haffty BG, Toth M, Flynn S, et al. Prognostic value of DNA flow cytometry in the locally recurrent, conservatively treated breast cancer patient. J Clin Oncol 1992;10:1839.

71. Winchester DJ, Duda RB, August CZ, et al. The importance of DNA flow cytometry in node-negative breast cancer. Arch Surg 1990;125:886.

72. Arnerlöv C, Emdin SO, Lundgren B, et al. Mammographic growth rate, DNA ploidy and s-phase fraction analysis in breast carcinoma. Cancer 1992;70:1935.

73. O'Reilly SM, Camplejohn RS, Barnes DM, et al. Node-negative breast cancer: prognostic subgroups defined by tumor size and flow cytometry. J Clin Oncol 1990;8:2040.

74. Sigurdsson H, Baldetorp B, Bord A, et al. Indicators of prognosis in node-negative breast cancer. N Engl J Med 1990;322:1045.

75. Dressler LG, Eudey L, Gray R, et al. Prognostic potential of DNA flow cytometry measurements in node-negative breast cancer patients: preliminary analysis of an intergroup study (INT 0076). J Natl Cancer Inst Monogr 1992;11:167.

76. Merkel DE, Winchester DJ, Goldschmidt RA, et al. DNA flow cytometry and pathologic grading as prognostic guides in axillary lymph node–negative breast cancer. Cancer 1993;72:1926.

77. Hedley DW, Rugg CA, Gelber RD. Association of DNA index and S-phase fraction with prognosis of node positive early breast cancer. Cancer Res 1987;47:4729.

78. Ferno M, Baldetorp B, Borg A, et al. Flow cytometric DNA index and S-phase fraction in breast cancer in relation to other prognostic variables and to clinical outcome. Acta Oncol 1992;31:157.

79. Stal O, Carstensen J, Hatschek T, et al. Significance of S-phase fraction and hormone receptor content in the management of young breast cancer patients. Br J Cancer 1992;66:706.

80. Ottestad L, Pettersen EO, Nesland JM, et al. Flow cytometric DNA analysis as prognostic factor in human breast carcinoma. Pathol Res Pract 1993;189:405.

81. Hatschek T, Fagerberg G, Stal O, et al. Cytometric characterization and clinical course of breast cancer diagnosed in a population-based screening program. Cancer 1989;64:1074.

82. Ewers S, Attewell R, Baldetorp B, et al. Prognostic potential of flow cytometric S-phase and ploidy prospectively determined in primary breast carcinomas. Br Cancer Res Treat 1991;20:93.

83. Bosari S, Lee AKC, Tahan SR, et al. DNA flow cytometric analysis and prognosis of axillary lymph node-negative breast carcinoma. Cancer 1992;70:1943.

84. Ewers S, Attewell R, Baldetorp B, et al. Flow cytometry DNA analysis and prediction of loco–regional recurrences after mastectomy in breast cancer. Acta Oncol 1992;31:733.

85. Stanton PD, Cooke TG, Oakes SJ, et al. Lack of prognostic significance of DNA ploidy and S phase fraction in breast cancer. Br J Cancer 1992;66:925.

86. Hedley DW, Clark GM, Cornelisse CJ, et al. Consensus review of the clinical utility of DNA cytometry in carcinoma of the breast. Cytometry 1993;14:482.

87. Brown RW, Allred DC, Clark GM, et al. Prognostic significance and clinical–pathological correlations of cell-cycle kinetics measured by KI-67 immunocytochemistry in axillary node-negative carcinoma of the breast. Br Cancer Res Treat 1990;16:192.

88. Gasparini G, Dal Fior S, Pozza F, et al. Correlation of growth fraction by Ki-67 immunohistochemistry with histologic factors and hormone receptors in operable breast carcinoma. Breast Cancer Res Treat 1989;14:329.

89. Daidone M, Silvestrini R, Valentinis B, et al. Changes in cell kinetics induced by primary chemotherapy in breast cancer. Int J Cancer 1991;47:380.

90. O'Reilly SM, Camplejohn RS, Barnes DM, et al. DNA index, S-phase fraction, histological grade and prognosis in breast cancer. Br J Cancer 1990;61:671.

91. Feichter GE, Mueller A, Kaufmann M, et al. Correlation of DNA flow cytometric results and other prognostic factors in primary breast cancer. Int J Cancer 1988;41:823.

92. Brifford M, Spyratos F, Tubiana-Hulin M, et al. Sequential cytopunctures during preoperative chemotherapy for breast cancer: cytomorphologic changes, initial tumor ploidy and tumor regression. Cancer 1989;63:631.

93. Baildam AD, Zaloudik J, Howell A, et al. DNA analysis by flow cytometry, response to endocrine treatment, and prognosis in advanced carcinoma of the breast. Br J Cancer 1987;55:553.

94. Stuart-Harris R, Hedley DW, Taylor IW, et al. Tumor ploidy, response and survival in patients receiving endocrine therapy for advanced breast cancer. Br J Cancer 1985;51:573.

95. Muss HB, Thor AD, Berry DA, et al. C-erb B-2 expression and response to adjuvant therapy in women with node-positive early breast cancer. N Engl J Med 1994;330:1260.

96. Lawry J, Rogers K, Duncan JL, et al. The identification of informative parameters in the flow cytometric analysis of breast carcinoma. Eur J Cancer 1993;29A:719.

97. Frierson HF. Grade and flow cytometric analysis of ploidy for infiltrating ductal carcinomas. Hum Pathol 1993;24:24.

98. Cornelisse CJ, van de Velde CJH, Caspers RJC, et al. DNA ploidy and survival in breast cancer patients. Cytometry 1987;8:225.

99. Meckenstock G, Bojar H, Wort W. Differentiated DNA analysis in relation to steroid receptor status, grading, and staging in human breast cancer. Anticancer Res 1987;7:749.

100. Owainati AAR, Robins RA, Hinton C, et al. Tumor aneuploidy, prognostic parameters and survival in primary breast cancer. Br J Cancer 1987;55:449.

101. Dowle CS, Owainati A, Robins A, et al. Prognostic significance of the DNA content of human breast cancer. Br J Surg 1987;74:133.

102. Fallenius AG, Franzen SA, Auer GU. Predictive value of nuclear DNA content in breast cancer in relation to clinical and morphologic factors. Cancer 1988;62:521.

103. Remvikos Y, Magdelenat H, Zajdela A. DNA flow cytometry applied to fine needle sampling of human breast cancer. Cancer 1988;61:1629.

104. Horsfall DJ, Tilley WD, Orell SR, et al. Relationship between ploidy and steroid hormone receptors in primary invasive breast cancer. Br J Cancer 1986;53:23.

105. Rosen PP, Groshen S, Kinne DW, et al. Factors influencing prognosis in node-negative breast carcinoma: analysis of 767 T1N0M0/T2N0M0 patients with long-term follow-up. J Clin Oncol 1993;11:2090.

106. Auer GU, Caspersson TO, Wallgren AS. DNA content and survival in mammary carcinoma. Anal Quant Cytol 1980;61.

107. Kallioniemi O-P, Blanco G, Alavaikko M, et al. Tumor DNA ploidy as an independent prognostic factor in breast cancer. Br J Cancer 1987;56:637.

108. Lewis WE. Prognostic significance of flow cytometric DNA analysis in node-negative breast cancer patients. Cancer 1990;65:2315.

109. Clark GM, Dressler LG, Owens MA, et al. Prediction of relapse or survival in patients with node-negative breast cancer by DNA flow cytometry. N Engl J Med 1989;320:627.

110. Balslev I, Christensen J, Bruun Rasmussen B, et al. Flow cytometric DNA ploidy defines patients with poor prognosis in node-negative breast cancer. Int J Cancer 1994;56:16.

111. Batsakis JG, Sneige N, El-Naggar AK. Flow cytometric (DNA content and S-phase fraction) analysis of breast cancer. Cancer 1993;71:2151.

112. Kute TE, Muss HB, Cooper MR, et al. The use of flow cytometry for the prognosis of stage II adjuvant treated breast cancer patients. Cancer 1990;66:1810.

113. Keyhani-Rofagha S, O'Toole RV, Farrar WB, et al. Is DNA ploidy an independent prognostic indicator in infiltrative node-negative breast adenocarcinoma? Cancer 1990;65:1577.

114. Ewers SB, Attewell R, Baldetorp B, et al. Prognostic significance of flow cytometric DNA analysis and estrogen receptor content in breast carcinomas: a 10 year survival study. Breast Cancer Res Treat 1992;24:115.

115. van der Linden JC, Lindeman J, Baak JPA, et al. The multivariate prognostic index and nuclear DNA content are independent prognostic factors in primary breast cancer patients. Cytometry 1989;10:56.

116. Beerman H, Kluin M, Hermans J, et al. Prognostic significance of DNA-ploidy in a series of 690 primary breast cancer patients. Int J Cancer 1990;45:34.

117. Aaltomaa S, Lipponen P, Papinaho S, et al. Nuclear morphometry and DNA flow cytometry as prognostic factors in female breast cancer. Eur J Surg 1992;158:135.

118. Gnant MFX, Blijham G, Reiner A, et al. DNA ploidy and other results of DNA flow cytometry as prognostic factors in operable breast cancer: 10-year results of a randomised study. Eur J Cancer 1992;28:711.

119. Gnant MFX, Blijham GH, Reiner A, et al. Aneuploidy fraction but not DNA index is important for the prognosis of patients with stage I and II breast cancer: 10 year results. Ann Oncol 1993;4:643.

120. Toikkanen S, Joensuu H, Klemi P. Nuclear DNA content as a prognostic factor in $T_{1-2}N_0$ breast cancer. Am J Clin Pathol 1990;93:471.

121. Joensuu H, Toikkanen S, Klemi PJ. DNA index and S-phase fraction and their combination as prognostic factors in operable ductal breast carcinoma. Cancer 1990;66:331.

122. National Cancer Institute (USA). Surveillance, Epidemiology and End Results (SEER) Program: cancer statistics review 1973–1990, Bethesda, National Cancer Institute, 1993.

123. Rosen PP, Groshen S, Kinne DW. Survival and prognostic factors in node-negative breast cancer: results of long-term follow-up studies. J Natl Cancer Inst Monogr 1992;11:159.

124. Bloom H, Richardson M, Harris B. Natural history of untreated breast cancer (1804–1933): comparison of treated and untreated cases according to histological grade of malignancy. Br Med J 1962;2:213.

125. Adair F, Berg J, Joubert L, et al. Long-term follow-up of breast cancer patients: the 30-year report. Cancer 1974;33:1145.

126. Ferguson DJ, Meier P, Karrison T, et al. Staging of breast cancer and survival rates: an assessment based on 50 years experience with radical mastectomy. JAMA 1982;248:1337.

127. Harris J, Hellman S. Observations on survival curve analysis with particular reference to breast cancer. Cancer 1986;57:925.

128. Brinkley D, Haybittle JL. The curability of breast cancer. Lancet 1975;2:95.

129. Rutqvist LE, Wallgren A, Nilsson B. Is breast cancer a curable disease? a study of 14,731 women with breast cancer from the Cancer Registry of Norway. Cancer 1984;53:1793.

130. Fisher B, Redmond C, Poisson R, et al. Eight-year results of a randomized clinical trial comparing total mastectomy and lumpectomy with or without irradiation in the treatment of breast cancer. N Engl J Med 1989;320:822.

131. Kardinal CG, Perry MC, Korzun AH, et al. Responses to chemotherapy or chemohormonal therapy in advanced breast cancer patients treated previously with adjuvant chemotherapy: a subset analysis of CALGB study 8081. Cancer 1988;61:415.

132. Valagussa P, Tancini G, Bonadonna G. Salvage treatment of patients suffering relapse after adjuvant CMF chemotherapy. Cancer 1986;58:1411.

133. Valagussa P, Brambilla C, Zambetti M, et al. Salvage treatment after first relapse of breast cancer: a review. Proceedings of the Third International Conference on Adjuvant Therapy of Primary Breast Cancer, St Gallen, Switzerland, 1988:9.

134. Ludwig Breast Cancer Study Group. Combination adjuvant chemotherapy for node positive breast cancer. N Engl J Med 1988;319:677.

135. Perloff M, Norton L, Korzun A, et al. Advantage of an adriamycin combination plus halotestin after initial CMFVP for adjuvant therapy of node-positive stage II breast cancer. Proc Am Soc Clin Oncol 1986;70:273.

136. Korzun A, Norton L, Perloff M, et al. Clinical equivalence despite dosage differences of two schedules of cyclophosphamide, methotrexate, 5-fluorouracil, vincristine and prednisone (CMFVP) for adjuvant therapy of node-positive stage II breast cancer. Proc Am Soc Clin Oncol 1988;7:12.

137. Aisner J, Korsun A, Perloff M, et al. A randomized comparison of CAF, VATH, and VATH alternating with CMFVP for advanced breast cancer, a CALGB study. Proc Am Soc Clin Oncol 1988;7:27.

138. Buzzoni R, Bonadonna G, Valagussa P, et al. Adjuvant chemotherapy with doxorubicin plus cyclophosphamide, methotrexate, and fluorouracil in the treatment of resectable breast cancer with more than three positive axillary nodes. J Clin Oncol 1991;9:2134.

139. Bruce WR, Meeker BE, Valeriote FA. Comparison of the sensitiv-

ity of normal hematopoietic and transplanted lymphoma colony-forming cells to chemotherapeutic agents administered in vivo. J Natl Cancer Inst 1966;37:233.

140. Griswold OP Jr, Trader MW, Frei E III, et al. Response of drug-sensitive and -resistant L1210 leukemias to high-dose chemotherapy. Cancer Res 1987;47:2323.

141. Tannock IF, Boyd NF, DeBoer G, et al. A randomized trial of two dose levels of cyclophosphamide, methotrexate, and fluorouracil chemotherapy for patients with metastatic breast cancer. J Clin Oncol 1988;6:1377.

142. Crown JPA, Norton L. Issues in chemotherapy: breast cancer. New York, Triclinica, 1993.

143. Peters WP. High-dose chemotherapy and autologous bone marrow support for breast cancer. In: DeVita VT Jr, Hellman S, Rosenberg SA, eds. Important advances in oncology. Philadelphia, JB Lippincott, 1991:135.

144. Peters WP, Ross M, Vredenburgh JJ, et al. High-dose chemotherapy and autologous bone marrow support as consolidation after standard-dose adjuvant therapy for high-risk primary breast cancer. J Clin Oncol 1993;11:1132.

145. Wood WC, Budman DR, Korzun AH, et al. Dose and dose intensity of adjuvant chemotherapy for stage II, node-positive breast carcinoma. N Engl J Med 1994;330:1253.

146. Frei E III, Canellos GP. Dose: a critical factor in cancer chemotherapy. Am J Med 1980;69:585.

147. Devita VT Jr. Dose-response is alive and well. J Clin Oncol 1986;4:1157.

148. Peters WP, Ross M, Vredenburgh J, et al. Role of cytokines in autologous bone marrow transplantation. Hematol Oncol Clin North Am 1993;7:737.

149. Dimitrov N, Anderson S, Fisher B, et al. Dose intensification and increased total dose of adjuvant chemotherapy for breast cancer (BC): findings from NSABP B-22. Proc Am Soc Clin Oncol 1994;13:64.

150. Laird AK. Dynamics of growth in tumors and in normal organisms. Natl Cancer Inst Monogr 1969;30:15.

151. Sullivan PW, Salmon SE. Kinetics of tumor growth and regression in IgG multiple myeloma. J Clin Invest 1972;51:1697.

152. Norton L. A Gompertzian model of human breast cancer growth. Cancer Res 1988;48:7067.

153. Spratt JA, Von Fournier D, Spratt JS, et al. Decelerating growth and human breast cancer. Cancer 1993;71:2013.

154. Spratt JS, Greenberg RA, Hauser LS. Geometry, growth rates and duration of cancer and carcinoma in situ of the breast before detection by screening. Cancer Res 1986;46:970.

155. Demicheli R. Growth of testicular neoplasm lung metastases: tumor-specific relation between two Gompertzian parameters. Eur J Cancer 1980;16:1603.

156. LaLa PK. Age-specific changes in the proliferation of Ehrlich ascites tumor cells grown as solid tumors. Cancer Res 1972;32:628.

157. Watson JV. The cell proliferation kinetics of the EMT6/M/AC mouse tumor at four volumes during unperturbed growth *in vivo*. Cell Tissue Kinet 1976;9:147.

158. Norton L. Mathematical interpretation of tumor growth kinetics. In: Greenspan, EM, ed. Clinical interpretation and practice of cancer chemotherapy. New York, Raven, 1982:53.

159. Speer JF, Petrovsky VE, Retsky MW, et al. A stochastic numerical model of breast cancer that simulates clinical data. Cancer Res 1984;44:4124.

160. Hauser L, Spratt J, Polk H. Growth rates of primary breast cancer. Cancer 1979;43:1888.

161. Fisher B, Slack N, Katrych D, et al. Ten-year follow-up results in patients with carcinoma of the breast in a cooperative clinical trial evaluating surgical adjuvant chemotherapy. Surg Gynecol Obstet 1975;140:528.

162. Norton L. Reply to letter to the editor. Cancer Res 1989;49:6444.

163. Fisher B, Brown AM, Dimitrov NV, et al. Two months of doxorubicin–cyclophosphamide with and without interval reinduction therapy compared with 6 months of cyclophosphamide, methotrexate, and fluorouracil in positive-node breast cancer patients with tamoxifen-nonresponsive tumors: results from the National Surgical Adjuvant Breast and Bowel Project B-15. J Clin Oncol 1990;8:1483.

164. Norton L, Simon R. Growth curve of an experimental solid tumor following radiotherapy. J Natl Cancer Inst 1977;58:1735.

165. Norton L, Simon R. Tumor size, sensitivity to therapy, and the design of treatment schedules. Cancer Treat Rep 1977;61:307.

166. Hill RP, Stanley JA. Pulmonary metastases of the Lewis lung tumor–cell kinetics and response to cyclophosphamide at different sizes. Cancer Treat Rep 1977;61:29.

167. Hamburger A, Salmon SE. Primary bioassay of human myeloma stem cells. J Clin Invest 1977;60:846.

168. Bruce WR, Valeriote FA. Normal and malignant stem cells and chemotherapy. In: The proliferation and spread of neoplastic cells. 21st Annual Symposium on Fundamental Cancer Research 1967. Baltimore, Williams & Wilkins, 1968:409.

169. Till JE, McCullock GA, Phillips RA, et al. Aspects of the regulation of stem cell function. In: The proliferation and spread of neoplastic cells. 21st Ann Symp Fund Cancer Res 1967. Baltimore, Williams & Wilkins, 1968:235.

170. Look AT, Douglass EC, Meyer WII. Clinical importance of near-diploid tumor stem lines in patients with osteosarcoma of an extremity. N Engl J Med 1988;318:1567.

171. Norton L, Simon R. The Norton–Simon hypothesis revisited. Cancer Treat Rep 1986;70:163.

172. Norton L. Implications of kinetic heterogeneity in clinical oncology. Semin Oncol 1985;12:231.

173. Hryniuk WM. Average relative dose intensity and the impact on design of clinical trials. Semin Oncol 1987;14:65.

174. Skipper HE. Analyses of multiarmed trials in which animals bearing different burdens of Ll2lO leukemia cells were treated with two, three, and four drug combinations delivered in different ways with varying dose intensities of each drug and varying average dose intensities. South Res Instit Booklet 7. 1986;42:87.

175. Griswold DP, Schabel FM, Jr, Corbett TH, et al. Concepts for controlling drug-resistant tumor cells. In: Fidler J, White RJ, eds. Design of models for testing cancer therapeutic agents. New York, Van Nostrand Reinhold, 1982:215.

176. Hudis C, Lebwohl D, Crown J, et al. Dose-intensive sequential crossover adjuvant chemotherapy for women with high risk node-positive primary breast cancer. In: Salmon SE, ed. Adjuvant therapy of cancer IV. Philadelphia, JB Lippincott, 1993:214.

177. Gabrilove JL. Colony-stimulating factors: clinical status. In: Devita VT Jr, Hellman S, Rosenberg SA, eds. Important advances in oncology 1991. Philadelphia, JB Lippincott, 1991:215.

178. Hudis C, Seidman A, Baselga J, et al. Sequential high dose adjuvant doxorubicin (A), paclitaxel (T), and cyclophosphamide (C), with G-CSF (G) is feasible for women (pts) with resected breast cancer (BC) and >4 (+) lymph nodes (LN). Proc Am Soc Clin Oncol 1994;13:62.

179. Crown J, Kritz A, Vahdat L, et al. Rapid administration of multiple cycles of high-dose myelosuppressive chemotherapy in patients with metastatic breast cancer. J Clin Oncol 1993;11:1144.

180. Crown J, Raptis G, Vahdat L, et al. Rapid administration of sequential high dose cyclophosphamide, melphalan, thiotepa supported by filgrastim plus peripheral blood progenitors in patients with metastatic breast cancer: a novel and very active treatment strategy. Proc Am Soc Clin Oncol 1994;13:242.

181. Crown J, Vahdat L, Raptis G, et al. Rapidly cycled courses of high-dose chemotherapy supported by filgrastim and peripheral blood progenitors in patients with metastatic breast cancer. Proc Am Soc Clin Oncol 1994;13:243.

182. Ayash LA, Elias A, Wheeler C, et al. Double dose-intensive chemotherapy with autologous marrow and peripheral-blood progenitor-cell support for metastatic breast cancer: a feasibility study. J Clin Oncol 1994;12:37.

183. Day RS. Treatment sequencing, asymmetry, and uncertainty: Protocol strategies for combination chemotherapy. Cancer Res 1986;46:3876.

184. Norton L, Day R. Potential innovations in scheduling in cancer chemotherapy. In: Devita Jr VT, Hellman S, Rosenberg SA, eds. Important advances in oncology 1991. Philadelphia, JB Lippincott, 1991:57.

185. Folkman J, Shing Y. Angiogenesis. J Biol Chem 1992;267:10931.

186. Onoda G, Toner J. Fractal dimensions of model particle packing having multiple generations of agglomerates. J Am Ceram Soc 1986;69:C278.

187. Norton L. Introduction to clinical aspects of preneoplasia: a mathematical relationship between stromal paracrine autonomy and population size. In: Marks PA, Türler H, Weil R, eds. Challenges of modern medicine, vol 1. Precancerous lesions: A multidisciplinary approach. Milan, Ares-Serono Symposia, 1993:269.

188. McDivitt RW, Boyce W, Gersell D. Tubular carcinoma of the breast: clinical and pathological observations concerning 135 cases. Am J Surg Pathol 1982;6:401.

189. Yee D, Paik S, Lebovic G, et al. Analysis of IGF-I gene expression in malignancy-evidence for a paracrine role in human breast cancer. Mol Endocrinol 1989;3:509.

190. Cullen KJ, Smith HS, Hill S, et al. Growth factor messenger RNA expression by human breast fibroblasts from benign and malignant lesions. Cancer Res 1991;51:4978.

191. Basset P, Bellocq JP, Wolf C. A novel metalloproteinase gene specifically expressed in stromal cells of breast carcinomas. Nature 1990;348:699.

192. Garin-Chesa P, Old LJ, Rettig WJ. Cell surface glycoprotein of reactive stromal fibroblasts as a potential antibody target in human epithelial cancers. Proc Natl Acad Sci 1990;87:7235.

193. Smith HS, Stern R, Liu E, et al. Early and late events in the development of human breast cancer. Basic Life Sci 1991;57:329.

194. Shekhar PV, Aslakson CJ, Miller FR. Molecular events in metastatic progression. Semin Cancer Biol 1993;4:193.

195. Frixen U, Behrens J, Sachs M, et al. E-cadherin mediated cell–cell adhesion prevents invasiveness of human carcinoma cell lines. J Cell Biol 1991;117:173.

196. Nicolson GL. Cancer progression and growth: relationship of paracrine and autocrine growth mechanisms to organ preference of metastases. Exp Cell Res 1993;204:171.

197. Koscielny S, Tubiana M, Le MG, et al. Breast cancer: relationship between the size of the primary tumour and the probability of metastatic dissemination. Br J Cancer 1984;49:709.

198. Valeriote F, van Pullen L. Proliferation-dependent cytotoxicity of anticancer agents: A review. Cancer Res 1975;35:2619.

199. Hug V, Johnston D, Finders M, et al. Use of growth-stimulating hormones to improve the *in vitro* therapeutic index of doxorubicin for human breast cancer. Cancer Res 1986;46:147.

200. Osborne CK, Kitten L, Arteaga CL. Antagonism of chemotherapy-induced cytotoxicity for human breast cancer cells by antiestrogens. J Clin Oncol 1989;7:710.

201. Conte PF, Alama A, Beriefli G, et al. Chemotherapy with estrogenic recruitment and surgery in locally advanced breast cancer: clinical and cytokinetic results. Int J Cancer 1987;40:490.

202. Swain SM, Sorace RA, Bagley CS, et al. Neoadjuvant chemotherapy in the combined modality approach of locally advanced nonmetastatic breast cancer. Cancer Res 1987;47:3889.

203. Conte PF, Pronzato P, Rubagotti A, et al. Conventional vs cytokinetic polychemotherapy with estrogenic recruitment in metastatic breast cancer: results of a randomized cooperative trial. J Clin Oncol 1987;5:339.

204. Lippman ME. Hormonal stimulation and chemotherapy for breast cancer. (Editorial) J Clin Oncol 1987;5:331.

205. Lippman ME, Cassidy J, Wesley M, et al. A randomized attempt to increase the efficacy of cytotoxic chemotherapy in metastatic breast cancer by hormonal synchronization. J Clin Oncol 1984;2:28.

206. Bontenbal M, Siewerts AM, Klijn JGM, et al. Effect of hormonal manipulation in doxorubicin administration on cell cycle kinetics of human breast cancer cells. Br J Cancer 1989;60:688.

207. Dressler LG. DNA flow cytometry measurements have significant prognostic impact in the node negative breast cancer patient: an intergroup study (INT 0076). Treatment of early breast cancer: program and abstract. NIH Consensus Development Conference, National Cancer Institute, Office of Medical Applications of Research of the NIH, June 18–21, 1990:99.

208. Zuckiel G, Tritton TR. Adriamycin causes high-regulation of epidermal growth factor receptors in actively growing cells. Exp Cell Res 1983;148:155.

209. Isonishi S, Andrews PA, Howell SB. Increased sensitivity to cis-diamminedichoroplatinum (11) in human ovarian carcinoma cells in response to treatment with 12-O-tetradecanoylphorbol-13-acetate. J Biol Chem 1990;265:3623.

210. Baselga J, Mendelsohn J. The epidermal growth factor receptor as a target for therapy in breast cancerinoma. Br Cancer Res Treat 1994;27:127.

211. Koury MJ, Bondurant MC. Erythropoietin retards DNA breakdown and prevents programmed death in erythroid progenitor cells. Science 1990;248:378.

212. Williams GT, Smith CA, Spooncer E, et al. Haemopoietic colony stimulating factors promote cell survival by suppressing apoptosis. Nature 1990;347:76.

213. Barry MA, Behnke CA, Eastman A. Activation of programmed cell death (apoptosis) by cisplatin, other anticancer drugs, and toxins and hyperthermia. Biochem Pharmacol 1990;40:2353.

214. Lippman ME. The development of biological therapies for breast cancer. Science 1993;259:631.

215. Miki Y, Swensen J, Shattuck-Eidens D, et al. A strong candidate for the breast and ovarian cancer susceptibility gene BRCA1. Science 1994;266:66.

Diseases of the Breast, edited by Jay R. Harris,
Marc E. Lippman, Monica Morrow, and Samuel Hellman.
Lippincott-Raven Publishers, Philadelphia, © 1996.

Specific Sites and Emergencies

23.1
Brain Metastases in Patients With Breast Cancer

J. PETER GLASS ▪ KATHLEEN M. FOLEY

The central nervous system (CNS) manifestations of systemic cancer are becoming increasingly evident, particularly as patients live longer. Intracranial metastases represent the most common metastatic complication of systemic cancer. Brain metastases can rarely be cured, but with early diagnosis and aggressive treatment, palliation is likely.

Incidence and Epidemiology

The overall incidence of brain metastases from breast carcinoma varies from series to series.[1] The incidence ranges from 5.9% in a study of 389 cases conducted by Richards and McKissock to 39% in a series of 218 cases reported by Chu and Hilaris. A clinical study conducted at the University of Tokyo reveals that 16.2% of 616 patients with breast carcinoma had brain metastases. An autopsy study of 1177 cases at Montefiore Hospital and Medical Center in New York demonstrates an incidence of 23.6%.

Brain metastases from breast carcinoma are more likely to occur in women who are premenopausal or in those who are less than 5 years postmenopausal and who have advanced disease.[2] A study by Stewart and coworkers[3] shows that estrogen receptor–negative tumors metastasize to the brain more commonly than do those that are estrogen receptor–positive. Evidence substantiates the premise that the development of brain metastases is delayed in patients who are treated with adjuvant or ablative hormonal therapy for their initial recurrence, but it has not been found to affect overall survival.[2–4]

Presenting Symptoms and Signs

The presenting symptoms and signs of patients with breast carcinoma and brain metastases are similar to those in patients with other solid tumors. The mechanisms by which tumor produces neurologic dysfunction are varied.[5] Localized tumor is, by itself, capable of destroying normal CNS tissue, making possible the identification of the site of metastatic involvement. A brain metastasis may be associated with cerebral edema, which may affect the function of the brain at a site distant to the metastasis. This results in symptoms and signs that are more widespread than those caused by the metastasis itself. Likewise, a brain metastasis and its surrounding edema can cause a shift of cerebral structures, thereby producing various syndromes of herniation. The two most common types of herniation are cingulate and transtentorial (uncal). When the cingulate gyrus herniates under the falx, it compresses the opposite frontal lobe and both anterior cerebral arteries. Such herniation produces bilateral frontal lobe infarctions, causing bilateral lower extremity weakness, changes in mental status, and urinary incontinence. Herniation of the medial portion of the temporal lobe (uncus) into the tentorial notch compresses the ipsilateral oculomotor nerve and the contralateral cerebral peduncle, causing pupillary dilatation and hemiparesis ipsilateral to the side of the lesion. Uncal herniation also can compress the ipsilateral posterior cerebral artery, resulting in occipital lobe infarction. The brain stem may be displaced downward, causing a decrease in the level of consciousness, and there may be obstruction to the flow of cerebrospinal fluid, resulting in hydrocephalus.

The onset of symptoms and signs in patients with brain metastases from breast carcinoma usually is insidious, occurring over a period of days to weeks. Breast carcinoma is typically not hemorrhagic, so a sudden bleed into the tumor that produces a neurologic deficit is highly unlikely, even in the face of thrombocytopenia. Conversely, most metastases occur at the junction of gray and white matter, so that the sudden onset of a focal or generalized seizure disorder is possible. From studies by Posner,[6] if seizures are excluded, acute onset of neurologic signs occurs in less than 10% of patients.

The presenting symptoms and signs in 201 patients with brain metastases are summarized in Table 23.1-1. Of these, headache is discussed in greatest detail because it often is the earliest presenting symptom.

Headache

Headache is the most common presenting complaint in patients with brain metastases, occurring in about half the affected patients. It may be either focal or generalized. In only 40% of patients it is the typical "brain tumor head-

TABLE 23.1-1
Symptoms and Signs in 201 Patients With Brain Metastases

	Cases (%)
SYMPTOM	
Headache	45
Behavioral and mental changes	33
Focal weakness	21
Gait ataxia	22
Seizures (focal 7%, generalized 13%)	20
Speech or language disturbances	14
Limb ataxia	10
Sensory disturbance	10
SIGN	
Impaired cognitive function	12
Hemiparesis (mild to moderate 28%, severe 6%)	34
Aphasia	17
Unilateral sensory loss	16
Papilledema	15
Gait ataxia	14
Visual field loss	13
Limb ataxia	10

(Gamache FW Jr, Galicich JH, Posner JB. Treatment of brain metastases by surgical extirpation. In: Weiss L, Gilbert MA, Posner JB, eds. Brain metastases. Chicago, Year Book, 1980)

ache," which occurs early in the morning, after awakening but before arising, and improves as the day progresses. The headache generally increases in frequency, severity, and duration until it becomes constant and other signs of increased intracranial pressure develop, such as drowsiness, nausea, and vomiting.

The most likely explanation for the pathogenesis of headache that occurs with metastatic disease is that it results from increased intracranial pressure with traction on pain-sensitive structures, including the dura, cranial nerves, and large venous sinuses. Occasionally, particularly in patients with cerebellar metastasis associated with a marked increase in intracranial pressure, the headache may be paroxysmal and may be accompanied by neurologic signs, such as visual obscurations, changes in consciousness, nausea, vomiting, and syncope. Paroxysmal headache is thought to be related to sudden, transient increases in intracranial pressure, referred to as plateau waves. Even though the headache caused by metastatic disease usually is accompanied by increased intracranial pressure, the incidence of associated papilledema is not high, occurring in only 25% to 40% of patients.

Diagnostic Considerations

Computed tomography (CT) of the brain remains the radiographic test most widely available to establish the diagnosis of brain metastasis (Fig. 23.1-1), but magnetic resonance imaging (MRI) is the diagnostic procedure of choice.[7–10] Cerebral arteriography is rarely used to evaluate patients with brain metastases.[10,11]

Although nonspecific, MRI is the most sensitive neuro-radiologic method in establishing the diagnosis of brain metastases, especially when accompanied by the intravenous administration of gadolinium (Fig. 23.1-2). MRI must be performed before surgical treatment because the use of gadolinium may detect other metastatic lesions or show metastatic tumor too small to be visible on CT.[12]

A study by Davis and associates[13] describes comparative imaging results in 23 patients who had postgadolinium MRI to clarify equivocal findings on double-dose delayed CT. Postgadolinium MRI demonstrated more than 67 definite or typical parenchymal metastases whereas double-dose delayed CT revealed only 37. Three patients had 5 or fewer lesions on CT and lesions too numerous to count on MRI. The frequency of equivocal or unconvincing lesions was similar on CT (11) compared with MRI (10). In this series, MRI with enhancement proved superior to double-dose delayed CT for lesion detection, anatomic localization, and differentiation of solitary versus multiple lesions.

Up to 50% of cerebral metastases are single. Although it had been standard practice to assume that the development of a brain lesion seen on CT or MRI in a patient with breast cancer represented metastasis, the prospective series by Patchell and others[14] showed a false-positive rate of 11% when biopsy is performed on a single lesion. Thus, pathologic examination of tissue after biopsy or resection

FIGURE 23.1-1 CT scan before (**A**) and after (**B**) conventional-dose iodinated contrast injection. Nothing is evident before contrast injection, but multiple enhancing metastases are seen afterward.

FIGURE 23.1-2 MRI T1-weighted images before (**A**) and after (**B**) conventional-dose gadolinium infusion. Nothing is seen before the gadolinium infusion, but multiple enhancing metastases are demonstrated afterward.

remains the gold standard for diagnosis of a single brain metastasis.

An innovation in diagnosing brain metastases on MRI is the use of triple-dose gadolinium to bring out metastatic disease and to differentiate single from multiple lesions (Fig. 23.1-3).

Both MRI and cerebral arteriography are superior to CT in differentiating metastatic tumors from meningiomas, which are associated with breast cancer and represent 20% of all tumors affecting the CNS having a female preponderance.[15]

MRI with gadolinium has obvious advantages for patients who are allergic to iodinated contrast agents and is the procedure of choice for this group. Cerebral arteriography is a second-line procedure, following CT or MRI, to clarify tumor blood supply before surgery or to further assess the vascular components of a potentially resectable tumor.

The use of positron emission tomography to differentiate recurrent tumor from radiation necrosis has proven to be valuable but is not infallible. Theoretically, tumor is hypermetabolic and the changes related to radiation are hypometabolic using 18-fluorodeoxyglucose.

Treatment

Several modalities alone or in combination are used to treat brain metastases from breast carcinoma. These include radiation therapy, surgery (by itself or in association with radiation), and systemic or local intraarterial chemotherapy. In this study, the clinician must also consider the efficacy of steroids (glucocorticoids) and anticonvulsants to control symptoms. Only one prospective, randomized study has compared the results of radiation therapy alone with those obtained using both surgery and radiation therapy for single brain metastases from solid tumors.[14] In this study, of 54 patients, 6 patients were excluded because, on biopsy, their lesions were either second primary tumors or benign inflammatory masses. In 48 patients, surgical removal of a brain metastasis followed by radiation therapy prolonged survival, decreased recurrences in the brain, and improved the quality of life compared with patients treated with radiation therapy alone. By 90 weeks, less than 10% of the patients in either group remained alive. Only 3 of the patients in the study had breast cancer, making these data not completely transferable to the decision-making

FIGURE 23.1-3 MRI T1-weighted images after conventional-dose gadolinium infusion (**A**) and triple-dose gadolinium infusion (**B**) The conventional scan appears normal, but the scan after triple-dose gadolinium infusion brings out multiple metastases.

process in the patient with breast cancer. The data, however, favor consideration of surgery followed by radiation therapy as being a useful approach. Each of the therapies is considered in the following sections.

Radiation

The mainstay of the treatment of intracranial metastatic disease has been radiation therapy.[16] It is preferable to surgery when the primary neoplasm is not under control and when widespread metastases occur throughout the body.

The different time-dose fractionation schemes for delivering whole-brain radiation therapy (WBXRT)—that is, 200 cGy in 5 fractions over 1 week, or 4000 cGy in 20 fractions over 4 weeks, or 1500 cGy in 2 fractions within 3 days—has had no influence on overall response rate or duration of response.[17] Median survivals from the time of diagnosis of cerebral metastases until death range from 3 to 6 months. Less than 10% of all patients are alive 1 year after diagnosis.

A pattern has emerged from a review of the overall experience in treating patients with radiation therapy at Memorial Sloan-Kettering Cancer Center.[18-20] About 20% of patients with brain metastases do not complete the prescribed course of radiation therapy because of a rapid deterioration in their general status. Most die of their systemic disease within a short time. About 50% of all patients and 75% of those who receive a full course of radiation therapy benefit from it. The use of rapid, high-dose courses of radiation results in high acute-complication rates.[21] These complications may include headache, nausea, vomiting, fever, and cerebral herniation. Most radiation therapists have abandoned such rapid regimens.

Retreatment

Patients who redevelop neurologic symptoms and signs after an initial course of radiation may be treated again. In a study of Kurup and associates,[22] 56 patients (15 with breast carcinoma) underwent reirradiation. The dosages ranged from 500 cGy delivered in 1 fraction to 4600 cGy delivered in 20 fractions, using 5 fractions per week. Most patients received either 2000 cGy in 5 fractions or 3000 cGy in 10 fractions. The interval between the first and second courses of radiation therapy was 1 to 46 months (median, 5 months).

The second course of radiation produced a response in 42 of the 56 patients. Improvement in neurologic signs occurred within 1 to 12 months (median, 2.5 months). The duration of response was less than 3 months in 26 patients (62%), 3 to 6 months in 12 patients (28.5%), and longer than 6 months in 4 patients (9.5%). The survival data after the second course of radiation treatment were analyzed in 53 patients. Survival ranged from 1 week to 16 months (median, 3.5 months). Only 14 patients (25%)

survived for more than 6 months after the second course of radiation therapy. Seven patients went on to receive a third course of radiation, and 2 patients underwent a fourth treatment course, each time with diminishing responses. No major side effects, such as cerebral radiation necrosis, were reported.

Hazuka and Kinzie[23] reviewed the records of 455 patients undergoing radiation therapy for cerebral metastases at the University of Colorado Health Science Center in Denver. Of these, 44 (9.7%) underwent reirradiation because of suggestive neurologic findings or findings of recurrent disease on imaging studies. Four patients (9%) had breast carcinoma. Patients being treated again received at least two courses of radiation, and one received three. The median interval between the first and second courses was 34 weeks. For the initial course of treatment, all patients were given WBXRT to a dose of 3000 to 3600 cGy (median, 3000 cGy) at 150 to 400 cGy per fraction. Retreatment also consisted of WBXRT in 37 of 42 patients with additional doses of 600 to 3600 cGy (median, 2500 cGy) at 200 to 400 cGy per fraction. The total cumulative doses to brain varied from 3800 to 7500 cGy (median, 6000 cGy).

Survival data were available for 42 of the 44 patients treated again. All patients died with disease. The median survival after the initial course of radiation was 40 weeks, with 10 patients (24%) living more than 1 year. The median survival after retreatment, however, was only 8 weeks, with 1 patient living beyond 1 year. Only 12 patients (27%) demonstrated partial neurologic improvement with reirradiation, and over half (55%) either failed to respond or deteriorated during or soon after their second treatment. Autopsies were performed in 8 patients. Three of these had radiation necrosis. It was concluded that retreatment of brain metastases is seldom worthwhile. Survival usually is short; more importantly, the quality of life frequently is not improved.

Radiation Treatment Results

Cairncross and colleagues[24] have demonstrated that radiation therapy may be curative, not just palliative, in patients with brain metastases. They examined five patients with metastases that had been documented clinically, as well as by radionuclide scan, cerebral arteriography, pneumoencephalography, or CT. All were treated with WBXRT and had no evidence of residual tumor at autopsy. These five patients (one of whom had breast carcinoma) represented about 3% of the patients treated for brain metastases and later examined at autopsy at Memorial Sloan-Kettering Cancer Center. The median survival time of this small group was 9 months, compared with 4 months for patients in whom tumors were found in the brain at autopsy. Two conclusions were reached: namely, that radiation therapy delivered to brain metastases, particularly in patients with radiosensitive tumors, may be more than just palliative; and that all nonterminal patients should be offered such treatment. Moreover, it was thought that if some brain metastases could be sterilized with 2400 to 3900 cGy delivered in conventional fractions (palliative radiation), additional lesions would be more likely to be sterilized by higher, curative doses.

In a study by DeAngeles and coworkers,[25] the role of postoperative radiation therapy after resection of a single brain metastasis was reviewed retrospectively in 98 patients. The researchers concluded that postoperative WBXRT was an important adjunct to complete resection of a single brain metastasis, particularly in patients with limited or no systemic disease who had the potential for long-term survival or even cure, but there was a risk of late neurologic toxicity. They estimated that 5500 to 6000 cGy delivered in 180- to 200-cGy fractions approached the threshold dose for cerebral radionecrosis. Meningeal recurrence was not prevented by WBXRT in this series.

Late Complications

Patients who receive WBXRT or systemic chemotherapy with or without surgery for brain metastases and survive longer than 1 year are at increased risk for developing focal radiation necrosis and treatment-related leukoencephalopathy.[26,27] The latter is a syndrome of progressive and severe memory loss, leading to dementia associated with gait abnormalities (frontal lobe ataxia) and urinary incontinence. Functional survival data in these patients do not exist. In retrospective studies, the incidence rate is about 5%. Debate exists over the offending agent, but radiation therapy in fractions of 300 to 500 cGy a day seems most likely.

To reduce the likelihood of treatment-related leukoencephalopathy, patients who are potential long-term survivors, such as those with breast cancer who present with a brain metastasis before any systemic therapy is given, should receive WBXRT in daily fractions of 180 to 200 cGy to a total of 4000 to 4500 cGy over 4 to 5 weeks. This should have the same efficacy as the higher dose fractions and yet reduce the long-term sequelae. In patients who develop neurologic problems related to brain dysfunction several months to a year after radiation, MRI is essential. New lesions present on these scans should at least undergo biopsy to rule out focal radiation necrosis versus tumor, unless unequivocal evidence of tumor recurrence exists. In the absence of recurrence, patients who demonstrate ventricular enlargement and changes in white matter on CT or MRI should be considered for therapy with corticosteroids and a ventriculoperitoneal shunt. These therapeutic modalities are often temporarily effective in relieving symptoms.[27]

Surgical Therapy

Previously described retrospective analyses comparing the results of surgery for brain metastases with those obtained with radiation therapy showed a modest survival advantage

for surgery or no difference between the two treatment modalities.

Comparing data for radiation therapy alone with surgery followed by radiation therapy might not be strictly possible. It seems that patients undergoing surgery are more likely to be in better physical and neurologic condition than those undergoing radiation. Also, such patients are more likely to have a single brain metastasis and are less likely to have extensive systemic disease. Conversely, patients receiving radiation therapy are more likely to have multiple brain metastases and extensive systemic disease. Thus, the median and long-term survival statistics would be expected to be better for patients treated with surgery than for those undergoing radiation. In the Gamache series,[28] however, about 20% of the patients had significant neurologic deficits when surgery was undertaken, and two thirds of the patients who underwent surgery had metastatic disease outside the CNS. Despite these facts, the results of this study compare favorably with those from the literature on both radiation and surgical treatment.

Other studies of patients receiving surgery for asymptomatic brain metastases followed by radiation therapy[29–31] have shown significantly longer survival because of lower recurrence of these metastases and fewer neurologic-related deaths when compared with studies of patients receiving only radiation therapy and having essentially the same extent of systemic disease.

Surgical removal of a brain metastasis at least guarantees the accuracy of the pretreatment diagnosis, as demonstrated by the Patchell study.[14] Because histologic verification of brain metastases treated with radiation can be obtained only at autopsy, the occasional appearance of a long-term survivor among patients in any radiation therapy series may be the result of diagnostic error. When Posner[32] reviewed a series of patients who received WBXRT for presumptive brain metastases and who were examined at autopsy before 1971, he discovered a 35% error rate. When strict neurologic criteria, including contrast studies such as cerebral arteriography or CT, were followed in establishing the diagnosis of cerebral metastases, the error rate fell to below 2%.[29] Thus, if a patient survives for a long period after radiation, it is possible that the diagnosis was incorrect rather than that radiation therapy was effective.

In a review of single brain metastases from breast cancer, Salvati and associates[33] evaluated 34 patients. Nine underwent surgical removal only, and 25 had surgical removal and WBXRT. A longer survival was seen in patients who underwent surgery and radiation therapy (mean, 28 months). In the 9 patients who did not receive radiation, the mean was 15 months and there was a higher incidence of brain relapse.

Sundaresan and colleagues[34] have written about the reoperation of brain metastases in 21 patients (4 with breast carcinoma) after initial successful resection. Local recurrence was found in 14, with other sites involved in the remaining 7. The time to recurrence ranged from 3 to 30 months. At the time of the second craniotomy, disease was limited to the CNS in 12 (57%) of the patients. The median survival after the second craniotomy was 9 months, giving an actuarial 2-year survival rate of 25%. Neurologic improvement was seen in two thirds of the patients (median duration, 6 months).

Radiosurgery

Stereotactic radiosurgery for treating brain metastases from breast cancer represents an alternate or additive approach to surgery and WBXRT.[36-39] This technique is being evaluated as a front-line approach for patients with a single metastasis but is indicated for use in patients with recurrent, isolated metastases in whom symptoms and signs are attributable to a less than 3-cm lesion in a patient with a Karnofsky status of 70% or more.[35,36] Stereotactic radiosurgery is a technique that delivers a focal, large, single dose of radiation using three-dimensional image processing, stereotactic guidance, and multiple nonconvergent and highly collimated beams. The sharp dose gradient at the treatment field edges markedly reduces the dose of radiation to the surrounding normal structures. Its advantages are that it is minimally invasive, is able to treat surgically inaccessible lesions, and can be done as an outpatient procedure. Although demonstrated to be highly effective in small arteriovenous malformations and small benign tumors, its role in treating breast metastases is under study with several series, suggesting a promising role.[35] From the two large published series of patients treated with radiosurgery for brain metastases, the data for patients with breast metastases show no significant difference of local control of breast metastases compared with other histologic types.[37,38] The median overall survival was 9 to 11 months after radiosurgery, with tumor control rates of 85% at 1 year and 65% to 67% at 2 years. In the study of Flickinger and associates,[37] the 2-year actuarial rates for developing biopsy-proven radiation necrosis or delayed symptomatic edema were 4%±3.8% and 10.8%±5.1%, respectively. The high control rates for radiosurgery in these two series equal those reported for surgical resection, with or without WBXRT. The merits of surgical resection compared with radiosurgery for different patients needs to be defined more thoroughly, however. Ongoing studies to assess survival, local control, and impact on qualify of life should delineate a standardized treatment strategy for this technique.

The surgery and radiosurgery data suggest that aggressive therapy should be restricted to the minority of patients for whom brain metastases represent a life-threatening site of their disease. For patients with few or no symptoms and small lesions, radiosurgery seems to be an alternative to surgery. Whereas radiosurgery is a noninvasive procedure, the same selection criteria should be considered as for those undergoing surgical resection. Surgery or radiosurgery cannot be justified as an adjunct to WBXRT in patients with progressive systemic disease.

Chemotherapy

The use of chemotherapeutic agents in the management of brain metastases has been limited for years because it was assumed that the standard antineoplastic drugs, administered systemically, had restricted accessibility to the brain. However, several investigators have produced evidence that the blood–brain barrier is different within brain tumors than it is in normal tissue.[39] This barrier is broken down in the presence of tumor.

A series of pharmacokinetic studies with different systemic chemotherapeutic agents has demonstrated that lipid solubility is not a requirement for penetration of the blood–brain barrier.[40] Various drugs, such as 5-fluorouracil, cyclophosphamide, bleomycin, and cisplatin, have been found to enter brain tumors in higher concentrations than adjacent, normal brain tissue. This factor suggests that tumor growth circumvents the blood–brain barrier, probably through neovascularization.[41]

Rosner and associates[42] report a series of 100 consecutive patients with symptomatic brain metastases from breast carcinoma, documented by radionuclide scan or CT, treated initially with systemic chemotherapy only. Primary treatment with chemotherapy in these metastases yielded responses in 27 of 52 patients (52%) treated with cyclophosphamide, 5-fluorouracil, and prednisone (CFP); 19 of 35 (54%) who received CFP-methotrexate and vincristine; 3 of 7 (43%) treated with methotrexate, vincristine, and prednisone; and 1 of 6 (17%) who received cyclophosphamide and doxorubicin. In all, 50 of 100 patients demonstrated an objective response to systemic chemotherapy, as documented by radionuclide or CT scans done before and after therapy. There were 10 complete responders, 40 partial responders, 9 patients who remained stable neurologically with no change in the size or number of metastases seen on scan, and 41 patients who failed to respond.

The median duration of remission for the complete responders was 10 months and 7 months for the partial responders. Thirteen of 35 patients who subsequently relapsed in the brain were successfully treated with second-line chemotherapy. The overall median survivals for complete responders and partial responders were 39.5 months and 10.5 months, respectively. This sharply contrasts with patients who were considered nonresponders with a median survival of 1.5 months. Thirty-one percent of all treated patients survived for more than 1 year. These findings indicate that systemic chemotherapeutic agents may play a role in treating brain metastases.

Colomer and colleagues[43] describe a patient having breast cancer with cerebral metastases who responded for more than 2 years to hormonal therapy with tamoxifen. They also reviewed the literature. As can be seen in Table 23.1-2, patients with breast cancer and brain metastases who respond to endocrine treatment tend to have long disease-free intervals or are postmenopausal. Estrogen receptor status was studied in only one case, and it was positive. Patients who responded in the brain also responded at other sites, and overall response was maintained in all reported cases for longer than 1 year (a period ex-

TABLE 23.1-2

Patients With Breast Carcinoma Metastatic to the Brain Responding to Hormonal Therapy

Investigators	Age (menopausal status) at Primary Diagnosis (y)	Time to Brain Metastases (y)	Tumor Sites Other Than the Brain	Cranial Radiation Therapy	Endocrine Therapy	Response Brain	Other Sites	Duration of Response (mo)	Survival (mo)
Carey et al, 1981[44]	43	5	Soft tissue, breast	Prior	TAM	Complete	Partial	14	—
Sparrow & Rubens, 1981[2]			Lung	No	FLU	Partial	Partial	16	—
Girsoli et al, 1981[56]	46	8	No	No	BRC	Complete	—	12★	—
Hansen et al, 1986[57]	38	30	Soft tissue	No	TAM	Partial	Complete	14★	—
Current case	56 (postmenopausal)	0	Bone, breast	No	TAM	Complete	Partial	34	38★

TAM, tamoxifen; FLU, fluoxymesterone; BRC, bromocriptine.

★ Steroids were given initially during > 5 and 7 mo, respectively.

(Colomer R, Cosos D, Del Campo JM, et al. Brain metastases from breast cancer may respond to endocrine therapy. Breast Cancer Res Treat 1988;12:83)

pected in responding patients without brain involvement). It was concluded that hormonal therapy should be considered alone or in conjunction with other forms of therapy in a small subset of breast cancer patients without life-threatening brain involvement who present with clinical or laboratory predictors of response to endocrine drugs.[44]

Twenty-two consecutive patients with brain metastases from breast cancer were treated with a combination of cisplatin and etoposide every 3 weeks by Cocconi and others.[45] Five (23%) achieved a complete response and seven (32%) obtained a partial response, for an overall response rate of 55%. Five patients received radiation therapy after reaching a maximum degree of objective remission with chemotherapy. Median duration of combined complete response plus partial response was 40 weeks. Median duration of survival was 58 weeks. Fifty-five percent of the patients were alive at 1 year. This study demonstrated that this combination treatment is highly effective in managing brain metastases from breast cancer.

In a prospective, nonrandomized study by Boogerd and associates,[46] the response of brain metastases from breast cancer to a standard systemic chemotherapeutic regimen was measured by clinical follow-up and serial CT. Treatment consisted of 4-week courses of cyclophosphamide, methotrexate, and 5-fluorouracil (CMF) in 20 patients, or 3-week courses of cyclophosphamide, doxorubicin, and 5-fluorouracil (CAF) in 2 patients. Seven patients had previously received CMF or CAF as adjuvant treatment for progressive systemic disease. Another seven patients had been previously treated for brain metastases with surgery, radiation therapy, or both. Based on the results of clinical follow-up and CT, a response that lasted at least 6 weeks was seen in 13 patients (59%), including 4 of the 7 patients with recurrent brain metastases. Objective tumor regression occurred after two courses of chemotherapy in

76% of patients and after six courses in 47%. The median duration of neurologic remission in the 13 patients was 30 weeks. The median overall survival was 25 weeks. The response rate of systemic disease paralleled the neurologic response. When compared with a matched group of historic control subjects treated with radiation therapy alone, chemotherapy induced a higher rate of neurologic response and led to a longer survival. These results warrant further studies on the use of chemotherapy in brain metastases from breast cancer.

There have also been reports of complete and partial responses in patients with intraarterial carmustine[47] and intravenous and intraarterial cisplatin.[48,49] Again, the lack of biopsy-proven tumors in these patients should be recognized.

Symptom Control

CORTICOSTEROID THERAPY

The use of corticosteroids before, during, and after surgery or WBXRT invariably produces immediate and sometimes dramatic improvement in neurologic signs.[50–52] These improvements are short lived, however, and surgery or radiation therapy is necessary to control tumor growth. Steroids are used to stabilize or decrease the edema surrounding cerebral metastases. They have no significant oncolytic effect in most metastatic tumors. Standard doses have not been established, but we recommend administering 10 mg of dexamethasone intravenously as a loading dose in stable patients, followed by the administration of 4 mg of the drug intravenously or by mouth every 6 hours with antacid coverage. This treatment regimen should be

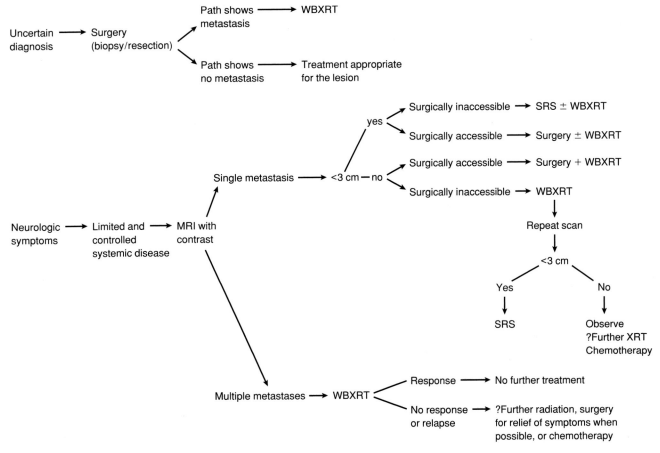

FIGURE 23.1-4 Treatment approach for patients with brain metastases. Chemo, chemotherapy; MRI, magnetic resonance imaging; WBXRT, whole-brain radiation therapy; SRS, stereotactic radiosurgery; XRT radiation therapy.

tapered gradually after surgery or after the full course of radiation therapy to the lowest possible dose that will control symptoms.

ANTICONVULSANT THERAPY

Seizures occur in 20% to 30% of patients with brain metastases. Anticonvulsants should be administered only to patients who have experienced seizures.[53] This practice eliminates the problems of an obligation to a lifetime of medication, compliance, toxicity, and drug–drug interaction. In terms of the use of anticonvulsant medications in patients with brain metastases, phenytoin is the drug of choice. The standard dosage is 300 to 400 mg/day after an initial loading dose of 15 mg/kg. This regimen should achieve therapeutic blood levels of 10 to 20 μg/mL. In patients who have had seizures and are to begin radiation therapy, phenobarbital is the drug of choice because of the risk of erythema multiforme and Stevens-Johnson syndrome in patients receiving cranial radiation and phenytoin.[54] Phenobarbital is given at 30 mg three times a day after a loading dose of 120 mg to establish therapeutic blood levels of 15 to 40 μg/mL.

MANAGEMENT SUMMARY

- The standard treatment approach for patients with brain metastases is outlined in Figure 23.1-4.
- Therapy of brain metastases requires an individualized approach in which the patient's extent of disease, functional status, surgical accessibility, prior treatment for systemic disease, projected survival, potential side effects, and, most importantly, preference have to be seriously weighed.
- The most controversial issue is how to treat the patient with a solitary symptomatic or asymptomatic brain metastasis.[55] In patients with limited systemic disease or disease confined to the CNS, surgical resection is recommended, with radiosurgery providing an alternate therapeutic option. The usefulness of radiation therapy after resection is in question, but the evidence suggests a longer tumor-free interval with such treatment.

References

1. Takakura K, Sano K, Hojo S, et al. Metastatic tumors of the central nervous system. Tokyo, Igaku–Shoin, 1982:113.

2. Sparrow GEA, Rubens RD. Brain metastases from breast cancer: clinical course, prognosis, and influence on treatment. Clin Oncol 1981;7:291.

3. Stewart JF, King RJ, Sexton SA, et al. Oestrogen receptors, sites of metastatic disease, and survival in recurrent breast cancer. Eur J Cancer Clin Oncol 1981;17:449.

4. DiStefano A, Yap HY, Hortobagyi GN, et al. The natural history of breast cancer patients with brain metastases. Cancer 1979;44:1913.

5. Cairncross JG, Posner JB. Neurologic complications of systemic cancer. In: Yarbo JW, Bornstein RS, eds. Oncologic emergencies. New York, Grune & Stratton, 1981:73.

6. Posner JB. Neurologic complications of systemic cancer. Med Clin North Am 1979;63:783.

7. Shi M-L, Wallace S, Libshitz HI, et al. Cranial computed tomography of breast carcinoma. J Comput Assist Tomogr 1982;6:77.

8. Hayman LA, Evans RA, Henck VC. Delayed high iodine dose contrast computed tomography. Radiology 1980;136:677.

9. Shalen PR, Hayman LA, Wallace S, et al. Protocol for delayed contrast enhancement in computed tomography of cerebral neoplasia. Radiology 1981;139:397.

10. Kent DL, Larson FB. Magnetic resonance imaging of the brain and spine. Ann Intern Med 1988;108:402.

11. Sze G, Shin J, Krol G, et al. Intraparenchymal brain metastases: MR imaging vs contrast-enhanced CT. Radiology 1988;168:187.

12. Peretti-Viton P, Margain D, Murayama N, et al. Brain metastases. J Neuroradiol 1991;18:161.

13. Davis PC, Hudgins PA, Peterman SB, et al. Diagnosis of cerebral metastases: double-dose delayed CT vs contrast-enhanced MR imaging. AJNR 1991;12:293.

14. Patchell RA, Tibbs PA, Walsh JW, et al. A randomized trial of surgery in the treatment of single metastasis to the brain. N Engl J Med 1990;322:494.

15. Smith FP, Slavik M, MacDonald JS. Association of breast cancer with meningioma: report of two cases and review of the literature. Cancer 1978;42:1992.

16. Cairncross JG, Kim J-H, Posner JB. Radiation therapy of brain metastases. Ann Neurol 1980;7:529.

17. Borgelt B, Gelber R, Kramer S, et al. The palliation of brain metastases: final results of the first of two studies by the Radiation Therapy Oncology Group. Int J Radiat Oncol Biol Phys 1980;6:1.

18. Chao JH, Phillips R, Nickson JJ. Roentgen-ray therapy of cerebral metastases. Cancer 1954;7:682.

19. Chu FCH, Hilaris BS. Value of radiation therapy in the management of intracranial metastases. Cancer 1961;14:577.

20. Nisce LZ, Hilaris BS, Chu FCH. A review of experience with irradiation of brain metastases. Am J Roentgenol 1971;111:329.

21. Young DF, Posner JB, Chu FCH, et al. Rapid-course radiation therapy of cerebral metastases: results and complications. Cancer 1974;4:1069.

22. Kurup P, Reddy S, Hendrickson FR. Results of re-irradiation for cerebral metastases. Cancer 1980;46:2587.

23. Hazuka MB, Kinzie JJ. Brain metastases: results and effects of re-irradiation. Int J Radiat Oncol Biol Phys 1988;15:433.

24. Cairncross JG, Chernik NL, Kim J-H, et al. Sterilization of cerebral metastases by radiation therapy. Neurology 1979;29:1195.

25. De Angeles LM, Mandell LR, Thaler HT, et al. The role of postoperative radiotherapy after resection of single brain metastasis. Neurosurgery 1989;24:798.

26. Rottenberg DA, Chernik NL, Deck MDF, et al. Cerebral necrosis following radiotherapy of extracranial neoplasms. Ann Neurol 1977;1:339.

27. De Angeles LM, Delattre JY, Posner JB. Radiation induced dementia in patients cured of brain metastases. Neurology 1989;39:789.

28. Gamache FW, Galicich JH, Posner JB. Treatment of brain metastases by surgical extirpation. In: Weiss L, Gilbert HA, Posner JB, eds. Brain metastasis. Boston, GK Hall, 1980:390.

29. Sundaresan N, Galicich JH. Surgical treatment of brain metastases: clinical and computerized tomographic evaluation of the results of treatment. Cancer 1985;55:1382.

30. Patchell RA, Cirrincione MS, Thaler HT, et al. Single brain metastases: surgery plus radiation or radiation alone. Neurology 1986;36:447.

31. Moser RP, Johnson ML. Surgical management of brain metastases: how aggressive should we be? Oncology 1989;3:123.

32. Posner JB. Diagnosis and treatment of metastases to the brain. Clin Bull 1974;4:47.

33. Salvati M, Capoccia G, Orlando ER, et al. Single brain metastases from breast cancer: remarks on clinical pattern and treatment. Tumori 1992;78:115.

34. Sundaresan N, Sachdev VP, DiGiacinto GV, et al. Reoperation for brain metastases. J Clin Oncol 1988;6:1625.

35. Alexander E III, Loeffler JS, Lansford LD, eds. Stereotactic radiosurgery. New York, McGraw–Hill, 1993.

36. Flickinger JC, Loeffler JS, Larson DA. Stereotactic radiosurgery for intracranial malignancies. Oncology 1994;8:81.

37. Flickinger JC, Kondziolka D, Lansford LD, et al. A multi-institutional experience with stereotactic radiosurgery for solitary brain metastases. Int J Radiat Oncol Biol Phys 1994;28:979.

38. Alexander E III, Moriarty TM, Davis RB, et al. Stereotactic radiosurgery for the definitive non-invasive treatment of brain metastases. J Natl Cancer Inst 1994 1995;87:34.

39. Vick NA, Khandekar JD, Bigner DD. Chemotherapy of brain tumors: the "blood–brain barrier" is not a factor. Arch Neurol 1977;34:523.

40. Hasegawa H, Shapiro WR, Posner JB. Chemotherapy of experimental metastatic brain tumors in female Wistar rats. Cancer Res 1979;39:2691.

41. Ushio Y, Posner JB, Shapiro WR. Chemotherapy of experimental meningeal carcinomatosis. Cancer Res 1977;37:1232.

42. Rosner D, Takuma N, Lane W. Chemotherapy induces regression of brain metastases in breast carcinoma. Cancer 1986;58:832.

43. Colomer R, Cosos D, Del Campo JM, et al. Brain metastases from breast cancer may respond to endocrine therapy. Breast Cancer Res Treat 1988;12:83.

44. Carey RW, Davis JM, Zervas NT. Tamoxifen-induced regression of cerebral metastases in breast carcinoma. Cancer Treat Rep 1981;65:793.

45. Cocconi G, Lottici R, Bisagni G, et al. Combination therapy with platinum and etoposide of brain metastases from breast carcinoma. Cancer Invest 1990;8:327.

46. Boogerd W, Dalesio O, Bais EM, et al. Response of brain metastases from breast cancer to systemic chemotherapy. Cancer 1992;69:972.

47. Madajewicz S, West CR, Park MC, et al. Phase II study: intraarterial BCNU therapy for metastatic brain tumors. Cancer 1981;47:653.

48. Kolaric K, Roth A, Jelicic I, et al. Phase II clinical trial of cis-dichlopodiamine platinum (cis-DDP) in metastatic brain tumors. J Cancer Res Clin Oncol 1982;104:287.

49. Lehane DE, Bryan RN, Horowitz B, et al. Intra-arterial cisplatinum chemotherapy for patients with primary and metastatic brain tumors. Cancer Drug Deliv 1983;1:69.

50. Galicich JH, French LA. Use of dexamethasone in the treatment of cerebral edema resulting from brain tumors and brain surgery. Am Pract Dig Treat 1961;12:169.

51. Galicich JH, French LA, Melby J. Use of dexamethasone in treatment of cerebral edema associated with brain tumors. Lancet 1961;1:46.

52. Kofman S, Garvin JS, Nagamani D, et al. Treatment of cerebral metastases from breast carcinoma with prednisone. JAMA 1957;163:1473.

53. Cohen N, Strauss G, Lew R, et al. Should prophylactic anticonvulsants be administered to patients with newly diagnosed cerebral metastases? a retrospective analysis. J Clin Oncol 1988;6:1621.

54. Delattre JY, Safai B, Posner JB. Erythema multiforme and Stevens–

Johnson syndrome in patients receiving cranial irradiation and phenytoin. Neurology 1988;38:194.

55. Posner JB. Surgery for metastases to the brain. (Editorial) N Engl J Med 1990;322:544.

56. Girsoli F, Vincentelli F, Foa J, et al. Effect of bromocriptine on brain metastasis in breast cancer. Lancet 1981;2:745.

57. Hansen SB, Galsgard H, vonEyben FE, et al. Tamoxifen for brain metastases from breast cancer. Ann Neurol 1986;20:544.

23.2

Epidural Metastasis

RONNIE J. FREILICH ▪ KATHLEEN M. FOLEY

Epidural spinal cord compression (ESCC) is one of the true neurologic emergencies that arises in the management of patients with breast cancer. Because the prognosis for good functional outcome is primarily dependent on the degree of impairment at the commencement of treatment, it behooves the clinician caring for patients with breast cancer to have a high degree of suspicion and vigilance about the possible presence of ESCC. Over 91% of patients with ESCC have symptoms for more than 1 week before a diagnosis is made,[1] with a mean duration of pain of 6 weeks.[2] This long period should allow the clinician adequate time to properly investigate when patients have symptoms and signs suggestive of epidural metastasis and to institute appropriate therapy. Compromise of the conus medullaris and cauda equina by epidural metastasis is included in discussion of the presentation, diagnosis, and management of ESCC because the natural history and management of these problems are similar to those for compression of the spinal cord itself.

Pathology

Epidural metastases most commonly arise from metastases to the vertebral column (85%). They arise less commonly from metastases to the paravertebral space (5% to 10%), which either secondarily invade bone and then grow into the epidural space, or invade the epidural space directly through the intervertebral foramen. In rare instances, direct hematogenous spread to the epidural space or to the parenchyma of the spinal cord occurs.[3,4]

The vertebral column is the most frequent site of metastases to bone. Vertebral metastases occur in up to 41% of all patients with cancer[5] and in 60% of patients with breast cancer.[6] The incidence in patients with advanced breast cancer may be as high as 84%.[3] The high incidence of vertebral metastases relates to the fact that cancers of the breast (as well as cancers of the lung and pelvis) are in communication with the Batson vertebral plexus,[7] a low-pressure, valveless venous system that fills when thoracoabdominal pressure is raised (eg, by maneuvers such as coughing, straining, and lifting). The presence of growth factors in bone marrow also may be a contributing factor.[8] Ninety-three percent of patients with breast cancer have known bone metastases at the time of onset of their neurologic deficit, with a median time from the first bone metastasis to ESCC of 11 months (range, 0 to 7.5 years).[1] Breast cancer is commonly associated with multilevel vertebral metastases compared with lung cancer, in which a single level usually is involved.[9] Stark and others[9] demonstrated noncontiguous vertebral involvement in 50% of patients with breast cancer who had abnormal results on plain spine roentgenograms, and epidural tumor was multifocal in 29%. As is anticipated from their origin in the vertebral bodies, most epidural metastases are situated anterior or anterolateral to the spinal cord,[10] which has important implications for therapy; this is discussed later.

Spinal cord damage in ESCC primarily results from direct compression of the spinal cord by tumor, and rarely from compression of radicular arteries that pass through the intervertebral foramen.[3] Axonal swelling and white matter edema occur early in animal models of ESCC, whereas damage to gray matter occurs later.[11] Prolonged cord compression results in necrosis of both gray and white matter. Early spinal cord damage likely results from venous stasis, whereas arteriolar compression by tumor is probably responsible for the late stage of tissue necrosis.[11]

Incidence

The overall incidence of ESCC in patients with cancer is about 5%.[12,13] One study has revealed a similar incidence of 4% in patients with breast cancer.[1] Breast cancer accounts for 7% to 32% of all cases of ESCC in patients with cancer.[9,10,14–19] The median time from the diagnosis of breast cancer to the onset of ESCC is 42 months (range, 0 to 28 years).[1] ESCC may be the initial sign of cancer; this occurs more frequently in a general hospital than in a specialized cancer center.[9,10] In some instances, biopsy of an epidural metastasis is required to establish the diagnosis of cancer.

Clinical Symptoms and Signs

Epidural spinal cord compression resulting from breast cancer occurs most commonly in the thoracic spine,[9,10,20] partly because this is the longest section of the vertebral column, but also because of the pattern of drainage from Batson plexus and the proximity of the primary tumor to the thoracic vertebrae.

The principal symptom of ESCC is pain (Table 23.2-1). It is the initial symptom in 96% of patients and precedes other symptoms by a median of 7 weeks (range, 5 days to 2 years).[10] Pain is of three types: local, radicular, and referred. Local back pain is a constant ache and occurs in almost all patients. Radicular pain results from involvement of nerve roots by the tumor mass and is typically described as a shooting pain. It is more common with cervical and lumbosacral lesions than with thoracic lesions.[10] Radicular pain is typically unilateral with cervical or lumbosacral epidural metastases, and bilateral (bandlike pain or tightness) with thoracic disease. Radicular pain resulting from thoracic epidural metastases may be felt more at the lateral or anterior chest wall than in the back itself. Referred pain occurs at a distant site from the lesion and does not radiate. For example, T12-L1 vertebral lesions may be referred to both iliac crests or both sacroiliac joints, whereas C7-T1 lesions may be referred to the interscapular region or to both shoulders.[21]

The pain of epidural metastasis is worsened by lying supine, possibly because of filling of vertebral veins in this position. Patients typically report that they are unable to sleep lying down and need to sleep sitting up; this information often is not volunteered by patients but must be sought by direct questioning during the taking of the clinical history. The Valsalva maneuver (coughing, sneezing, or straining at stool) exacerbates the pain of epidural metastases as it fills vertebral veins and also raises intracranial pressure, which is then transmitted to the already compromised spinal canal. Pain is also worsened by stretching maneuvers, such as neck flexion in the case of cervical or upper thoracic tumors and straight leg raising with lumbosacral or thoracic lesions. Escalating back pain in patients with cancer is a particularly ominous indicator of

the possibility of ESCC. There may be tenderness over the vertebral column at the site of the lesion, and there may be referred tenderness at the site of referred or radicular pain.

Myelopathy is the other characteristic clinical finding in ESCC. Myelopathic symptoms include limb weakness, numbness and paresthesiae, and sphincter disturbance (urinary retention, urinary urgency and urge incontinence, and constipation). At the time of diagnosis, 76% of patients complain of weakness, 87% are weak on examination, 57% have autonomic dysfunction, 51% have sensory symptoms, and 78% have sensory deficits on examination.[10] In many series, less than 50% of patients are ambulant at diagnosis and up to 25% are paraplegic[1,2,10]; these figures are significant because prognosis is related to clinical deficit at presentation. Signs of a myelopathy include paraparesis or quadriparesis (depending on the spinal level), increased tone, clonus, hyperreflexia, extensor plantar responses, a distended bladder, and a sensory level. There may be a patch of hyperesthesia at the upper aspect of the sensory level. The sensory, motor, and reflex levels are an indication of the level of disease, but the sensory level may be several segments below the site of cord compression. Furthermore, there may be multiple sites of epidural disease. The myelopathy may be incomplete, and a hemicord or Brown-Séquard syndrome may occur, although this is rare.[9,10] Involvement of spinocerebellar tracts in the spinal cord may lead to lower extremity ataxia out of proportion to the degree of weakness.[22] Patients also may present with herpes zoster, presumably because of reactivation of latent virus by compression of the dorsal root ganglion by tumor.[10]

ESCC at the conus medullaris and cauda equina produce different neurologic symptoms and signs, although pain still is a prominent feature, particularly with cauda equina lesions. Conus lesions typically show symptoms of early and marked sphincter disturbance and perineal sensory loss. Anal sphincter tone may be lax, and there may an absent anal wink. Lesions at the cauda equina produce patchy lower motor neuron signs related to the lumbar and sacral nerve roots: hyporeflexia or areflexia, myotomal leg weakness, and dermatomal sensory loss; sphincter disturbance tends to occur late and be less marked than in conus lesions.

TABLE 23.2-1

Symptoms and Signs of Epidural Spinal Cord Compression in 130 Patients From a Large Cancer Hospital

Symptom or Sign	First Symptom (%)	Symptoms at Diagnosis (%)	Signs at Diagnosis (%)
Pain	96	96	—
Weakness	2	76	87
Autonomic dysfunction	0	57	—
Sensory loss	0	51	78
Ataxia	2	3	7
Herpes zoster	0	2	2
Flexor spasms	0	1	1

(After Gilbert RW, Kim J-H, Posner JB. Epidural spinal cord compression from metastatic tumor: diagnosis and treatment. Ann Neurol 1978;3:40)

Investigations

The serious consequences of paraplegia or quadriplegia of untreated ESCC necessitate an orderly and expeditious examination of all patients in whom this diagnosis is suspected. The imaging modalities that have been used in the investigation of ESCC include plain spine roentgenograms, radionuclide bone scans, computed tomography (CT) of the spine, and techniques that definitively image the epidural space: myelography (with or without CT) and magnetic resonance imaging (MRI). Because most patients with ESCC have back pain as the presenting symptom, the investigation of ESCC can be regarded as the examination of patients with breast cancer and back pain. It is not practical or appropriate to perform definitive imaging of the epidural space in every patient with breast cancer who has back pain, and this has led to the development of several algorithms for investigation and treatment.[3,23-26] These algorithms are based on the varied clinical presentations of patients with back pain, as well as the sensitivity and specificity of individual imaging techniques in detecting the presence of epidural metastases. Discussing the available investigational tools is useful in terms of individual clinical presentations (local back pain only with normal neurologic examination, radiculopathy, plexopathy, and myelopathy), after which an algorithm is formulated for investigation and treatment based on these data (Fig. 23.2-1).

NORMAL NEUROLOGIC EXAMINATION FOR LOCAL BACK PAIN

Plain Spine Roentgenograms

Several studies have demonstrated the clinical usefulness of plain roentgenograms in assessing possible epidural disease. Eighty-five percent of patients with epidural metastases

have a vertebral body metastasis seen on plain roentgenogram at the appropriate level.[9,10] This figure varies depending on the type of tumor: epidural disease resulting from breast cancer has been associated with vertebral metastases in 94% to 98% of cases,[9,27] whereas only 32% of patients with lymphoma and ESCC have bony abnormalities on plain roentgenograms.[28] A higher incidence of asymptomatic ESCC (about 10%) exists in patients with multiple vertebral lesions.[29] Plain roentgenograms may be less sensitive in detecting bony disease at certain sites, particularly the C7-T1 vertebrae (which are commonly involved in breast cancer), because overlying bone and mediastinal shadows may obscure the image of these vertebrae. Rodichok and associates[30] found epidural metastases in 25 of 34 (74%) patients with local back pain, no neurologic abnormalities, and an abnormal finding on plain roentgenogram. In contrast, Graus and coworkers[31] found the incidence to be only 12 of 35 (34%). When Graus classified the radiologic abnormalities by the types of changes seen, however, it was found that epidural metastases were present in 7 of 8 (87%) patients with more than

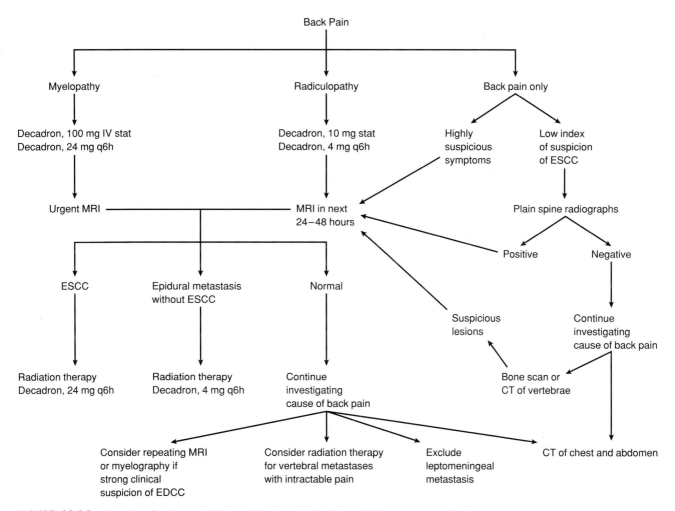

FIGURE 23.2-1 Algorithm for the investigation and treatment of patients with breast cancer and back pain. CT, computed tomography; ESCC, epidural spinal cord compression; IV, intravenously; MRI, magnetic resonance imaging; stat, immediately.

50% vertebral collapse, 4 of 13 (31%) with isolated pedicle destruction, and 1 of 14 (7%) with metastasis restricted to the vertebral body without severe collapse. Both studies demonstrated an incidence of epidural metastasis of 3% or less in patients with normal findings on plain roentgenograms. In another study, epidural metastases were found in 43% of vertebral segments that were asymptomatic but showed abnormal results on plain roentgenograms.[32] Although this study was retrospective and may have been biased toward patients with epidural metastases, it emphasizes the importance of radiographic abnormalities in assessing patients with back pain.

Radionuclide Bone Scans

Bone scintigraphy is a sensitive but less-specific indicator of epidural metastases than plain roentgenograms.[32] In patients with an abnormal finding on bone scan but a normal finding on plain roentgenogram, Portenoy and colleagues[32] found epidural metastases in only 1 of 9 (12%) symptomatic segments (defined as pain or neurologic signs referable to the vertebral segment), and in 0 of 22 (0%) asymptomatic segments. It was concluded that bone scans may, however, play a role in the assessment of back pain: for example, an abnormal result on bone scan may confirm that an epidural metastasis is unlikely in patients with an abnormal finding on roentgenogram. In the study of Rodichok and others,[30] epidural metastases were seen in 15 of 26 (58%) patients with back pain, no neurologic signs, and abnormal findings on bone scan, and in 0 of 7 (0%) patients with normal findings on bone scans. Bone scans were not performed in many cases because the clinical picture and plain roentgenograms led to myelography without the need for a bone scan. The authors determined that bone scans do not contribute significantly more information to the findings from plain roentgenograms.

Computed Tomographic Scanning

Computed tomographic scanning without the instillation of myelographic dye is more sensitive than plain roentgenograms in detecting vertebral and paravertebral metastases, and it has been demonstrated that cortical disruption adjacent to the epidural space is a useful marker of epidural metastasis.[24,33] CT, however, does not adequately visualize the epidural space. Furthermore, CT produces axial images and so only a limited area of the spine can be imaged by this technique. CT scans may be useful in differentiating vertebral collapse due to tumor from that due to osteoporosis.

Summary

In patients with breast cancer and local back pain alone, plain spine roentgenograms are the appropriate first line of investigation. Definitive imaging of the epidural space should be performed if plain films give abnormal results. In patients with a clinical picture that is strongly suggestive of epidural metastasis (eg, back pain that is significantly exacerbated by lying flat and worsened by the Valsalva maneuver), definitive imaging of the epidural space still should be performed, even if a plain roentgenogram gives normal results; in fact, it is reasonable to proceed straight to MRI in this situation. The potential difficulties in interpreting changes at the C7-T1 vertebrae should be considered if this is the site of clinical suspicion. In patients with local back pain with characteristics that are not strongly suggestive of epidural metastasis, definitive imaging of the epidural space is not indicated if a plain roentgenogram gives normal results. Investigations must proceed, however, to determine the cause of the back pain. Bone scan and CT of the vertebrae may be performed because they are more sensitive than plain roentgenograms in detecting bone metastases; if suspicious lesions are seen, particularly on CT, then definitive imaging of the epidural space should be considered. Other investigations that may be performed include CT of the chest or abdomen to exclude lesions such as paravertebral or visceral metastases. The differential diagnosis of back pain also includes leptomeningeal metastases, but usually other clinical clues are present to indicate this diagnosis.

RADICULOPATHY

Radiculopathy is associated with a high incidence of epidural metastases. In the Rodichok series,[30] 27 of 43 (63%) patients with radiculopathy and without signs of spinal cord involvement were found to have epidural metastases, compared with 27 of 61 (44%) with local back pain alone. When plain roentgenograms produced abnormal results, epidural metastases were found in 20 of 22 (91%) patients with radiculopathy. Similarly, in patients with abnormal findings on plain roentgenograms, Graus and coworkers[31] found epidural metastases in 47 of 67 (70%) patients with radiculopathy, compared with 12 of 35 (34%) with local back pain alone. When categorized by roentgenogram abnormality, epidural metastases were found in 6 of 7 (86%) patients with more than 50% vertebral collapse, in 36 of 48 (75%) with isolated pedicle destruction, and in 5 of 12 (42%) with metastasis restricted to the vertebral body without severe collapse. Importantly, in the series of Graus and others[31] and of Rodichok and associates,[30] epidural metastases were found in 9% to 33% of patients with radiculopathy and normal findings on plain roentgenograms.

Given the high incidence of epidural metastases in patients with radiculopathy, even in those with normal findings on plain roentgenograms, it is reasonable to proceed straight to definitive imaging of the epidural space in all patients with breast cancer and radiculopathy. Remember that in lesions of the thorax, which is the most common site of ESCC in breast cancer, radiculopathy presents as bilateral bandlike dermatomal pain, and that in some situations lateral or even anterior chest pain may be more prominent than back pain.

PLEXOPATHY

The possibility of epidural metastasis must be considered in patients with breast cancer and a malignant brachial plexopathy because tumor may infiltrate directly along the plexus to the epidural space. Brachial plexus lesions present with pain (usually in the shoulder girdle and radiating to the elbow, medial side of the forearm, and medial two digits), as well as weakness and sensory symptoms in a segmental distribution. Clinical clues to the presence of epidural metastases in the setting of brachial plexopathy include a panplexopathy (compared with the more usual lower plexopathy with involvement of C-7, C-8, and T-1 nerve roots) and the presence of Horner syndrome (indicating more proximal involvement).[34] The presence of back pain also suggests that the tumor has grown proximally, but back pain may be absent with epidural extension. Patients with brachial plexopathy require imaging of the brachial plexus with CT or MRI, and if vertebral body collapse or erosion is present at the C7-T1 levels, or if a paraspinal mass is seen, then definitive imaging of the epidural space should be performed. Note that epidural tumor is present in about one third of patients with paraspinal lesions and normal results on plain roentgenogram.[31] If MRI is used to image the brachial plexus, the cervical and upper thoracic spine can be imaged at the same time.

MYELOPATHY

Definitive Imaging of the Epidural Space

Definitive imaging of the epidural space is required in patients with myelopathy and in other patients in whom the clinical presentation or investigations strongly suggest the presence of epidural metastases. Myelography had been the traditional mainstay of investigation of ESCC, but MRI is the investigation of choice.

Myelography is performed by the instillation of a contrast agent into the subarachnoid space through a lumbar spinal puncture (Fig. 23.2-2). Water-soluble contrast agents such as Omnipaque are used, rather than the older lipid-soluble agents such as Pantopaque, which produced complications such as arachnoiditis. CT may be performed after myelography to provide axial images through abnormal regions. If a complete spinal block is present on myelography, a cisternal C1-2 puncture must be performed to identify the upper border of the block to allow for adequate treatment planning. CT after myelography may assist in the delineation of this upper border because enough contrast material may get past the block to be seen on CT; however, this occurs in less than half the patients who have complete block.[35] Cerebrospinal fluid should be collected when myelography is performed to exclude leptomeningeal metastasis. Myelography may be contraindicated in patients with a coagulopathy and in patients with raised intracranial pressure from intracerebral metastases. A spinal tap performed in patients with a complete block may worsen the neurologic deficit because of the creation of a pressure differential between the spinal canal above and below the block.[36]

MRI has the following advantages: being noninvasive, producing excellent delineation of soft tissue planes, being sensitive in the detection of vertebral and paravertebral metastases, and providing imaging in three planes (sagittal, coronal, and axial) (Figs. 23.2-3 and 23.2-4). Several studies comparing MRI with myelography in the evaluation

FIGURE 23.2-2 Myelogram showing a complete block to the flow of contrast material. The upper level of the block at T11-12 is delineated by a C1-2 injection (*left*), whereas the lower level of the block at T12-L1 is demonstrated by a lumbar injection (*right*). Right T-12 pedicle erosion is seen on the left side of the diagram.

of patients with suspected ESCC have suggested that MRI is not as sensitive as myelography, particularly in patients with small epidural metastases or metastases that are situated laterally in the spinal canal, and that MRI may underestimate the degree of block seen on myelography.[37-41] The scanning protocols for these studies did not, however, routinely include axial images; sagittal images (with or without coronal images) may easily miss a small or laterally placed metastasis. Other investigators, on the other hand, have shown MRI to be as sensitive as myelography in the detection of epidural metastases, including the detection of small lesions and metastases producing nerve root compression.[42-44] In some instances, MRI has been shown to be superior to myelography: in detecting epidural metastases with more sensitivity, in accurately determining the upper border of a complete block, in imaging multiple sites of spinal block, and in detecting paravertebral and vertebral metastases.[38,40-45] The differences in the findings of these various studies cannot be explained purely on the basis of the strength of the magnet used, because one study that used a 0.5-Tesla magnet found MRI to be as sensitive as myelography.[42] Technical problems such as motion artifact or phase-encoding errors led to the inaccuracy of MRI in some cases.[37,38,42] Although we routinely use MRI as the investigation of choice in ESCC, in some situations MRI scan may give a false-negative result, and repeat MRI or myelography may be indicated if a strong clinical

FIGURE 23.2-3 **A.** Sagittal T1-weighted MRI scans demonstrating epidural spinal cord compression. The vertebral body is completely replaced by tumor and appears hypodense. Tumor extends posteriorly from the vertebral body to compress the spinal cord from its anterior aspect; this is the commonest pathologic feature encountered with epidural metastases. The two scans shown are 4 mm apart; the degree of spinal cord compression appears less severe on the scan on the right, emphasizing the inadequacy of a single midline sagittal image as a screening test for epidural metastasis. The hypodense signal in multiple vertebral bodies indicates diffuse bony metastases in this patient. **B.** In this sagittal T2-weighted MRI sequence, cerebrospinal fluid is white and the spinal cord is gray; disease is better demonstrated on T2-weighted than on T1-weighted images. **C.** This axial T1-weighted image shows the vertebral canal to be almost completely obliterated by tumor extending posteriorly from the vertebral body. Compare this with **D,** in which the spinal cord and epidural space are clearly seen; minor epidural metastases are present anterolateral to the spinal cord.

suspicion of epidural metastases remains. Furthermore, in centers where MRI is not readily available or in situations in which MRI cannot be performed (eg, patients with pacemakers or the occasional patient with severe claustrophobia), myelography should be performed.

An unenhanced MRI scan will establish the diagnosis of ESCC. If results are normal then a contrast-enhanced scan using gadolinium–DTPA should be obtained to look for leptomeningeal metastasis, which may mimic the presentation of ESCC. The entire spine should be imaged, because epidural disease may be present at multiple levels, and, as mentioned earlier, the spinal level indicated by clinical ex-

amination may be several segments below the level of the lesion. We have been able to image the entire spine in two sections. As discussed earlier, axial scans should be obtained in addition to sagittal images. A screening midline sagittal scan is inadequate; multiple sagittal scans using thin slices should be performed to adequately image the spinal canal. We do not routinely obtain coronal images of the spine. Adequate analgesia (including corticosteroids) should be administered before the MRI is performed because the patient must lie motionless for the scan, and lying flat may worsen the back pain. If the patient cannot tolerate the full procedure or if there is not enough time to perform an MRI of

TABLE 23.2-2
Treatment Outcome as Influenced by Pretreatment Ambulatory Status

Investigators	Patients	Tumor Type	Ambulant Before Treatment	Patients Ambulant After Treatment — Nonambulant Before Treatment			Treatment
				Overall	*Paretic*	*Plegic*	
Gilbert et al[10]	235	All	60/80 (75%)	54/155 (35%)	52/116 (45%)	2/39 (5%)	RT = laminectomy + RT
Hill et al[1]	70	Breast	22/23 (96%)	13/29 (45%)			RT = laminectomy
Maranzano et al[68]	105	All	48/50 (96%)	26/55 (47%)	25/45 (56%)	1/10 (10%)	RT
Maranzano et al[69]	56	Breast	29/30 (97%)	18/26 (69%)	17/23 (74%)	1/3 (33%)	RT
Kim et al[2]	59	All	13/13 (100%)	12/46 (26%)	11/31 (35%)	1/15 (7%)	RT ± laminectomy
Sørensen et al[67]	345	All	103/131 (79%)	38/214 (18%)	35/165 (21%)	3/49 (6%)	RT = laminectomy ± RT

RT, radiation therapy.

remain ambulant after treatment: 79% to 100% of patients who are ambulant before treatment remain so, whereas only 18% to 69% of nonambulant patients regain the ability to walk.[1,2,10,67–69] In most series, less than 10% of patients who are paraplegic or quadriplegic before treatment regain the ability to walk.[1,2,10,67–69] As discussed earlier, studies on vertebral body resection have suggested a better prognosis for ambulation for paraplegic patients receiving this treatment.[58,60] In Harrington's study, in which patients received both vertebral body resection and radiation, 6 of 13 patients who were plegic before treatment recovered completely, whereas another 3 of 13 improved.[58] In the Siegal study,[60] 13 of 61 patients were plegic before vertebral body resection, whereas only 1 of 57 was plegic after treatment; it was not stated how many plegic patients became ambulant and how many regained some movement but remained nonambulant.

The median duration of the response to radiation therapy depends on the posttreatment ambulatory status; the pretreatment ambulatory status does not influence the duration of improvement.[69] In the study of Maranzano and others,[69] the median duration of response was 12 months for all patients, 15 months for patients who were ambulant after treatment, and only 2 months for those who were nonambulant after treatment.

The mean survival of patients with breast cancer who develop ESCC is 5 to 14 months, whereas the median survival is 4 to 13 months.[1,19,67,69] One study suggests a longer survival in patients treated with both laminectomy and radiation therapy, compared with those treated by either laminectomy or radiation alone, but these differences may be explained by selection bias.[67] Another study demonstrates no difference in patients treated with surgery or radiation.[1] Posttreatment ambulatory status is the most important factor influencing survival in patients with breast cancer.[1,69] In the study of Maranzano and coworkers,[69] the median survival was 13 months for all patients, 17 months for patients who were ambulant after treatment, and only 2 months for those who were nonambulant after

treatment. The 1-year survival rate for posttreatment ambulant patients in this study was 66% versus 10% for nonambulant patients. The time from diagnosis of breast cancer to the development of ESCC also has been found to be a predictor of survival, with a better survival found among patients who develop ESCC after 3 or more years.[1]

References

1. Hill ME, Richards MA, Gregory WM, et al. Spinal cord compression in breast cancer: a review of 70 cases. Br J Cancer 1993;68:969.
2. Kim RY, Spencer SA, Meredith RF, et al. Extradural spinal cord compression: analysis of factors determining functional prognosis: prospective study. Radiology 1990;176:279.
3. Posner JB. Back pain and epidural spinal cord compression. Med Clin North Am 1987;71:185.
4. Byrne TN. Spinal cord compression from epidural metastases. N Engl J Med 1992;327:614.
5. Byrne TN, Waxman SG. Spinal cord compression: diagnosis and principles of treatment. In: Contemporary neurology series, vol 33. Philadelphia, FA Davis, 1990.
6. Fornasier VL, Horne JG. Metastases to the vertebral column. Cancer 1975;36:590.
7. Batson OV. The vertebral venous system: Caldwell lecture, 1956. In: Weiss L, Gilbert HA, eds. Bone metastasis. Boston, GK Hall, 1981:21.
8. Arguello F, Baggs RB, Duerst RE, et al. Pathogenesis of vertebral metastasis and epidural spinal cord compression. Cancer 1990;65:98.
9. Stark RJ, Henson RA, Evans SWJ. Spinal metastases: a retrospective survey from a general hospital. Brain 1982;105:189.
10. Gilbert RW, Kim J-H, Posner JB. Epidural spinal cord compression from metastatic tumor: diagnosis and treatment. Ann Neurol 1978;3:40.
11. Kato A, Ushio Y, Hayakawa T, et al. Circulatory disturbance of the spinal cord with epidural neoplasm in rats. J Neurosurg 1985;63:260.
12. Barron KD, Hirano A, Araki S, et al. Experiences with metastatic neoplasms involving the spinal cord. Neurology 1959;9:91.
13. Bach F, Larsen BH, Rohde K, et al. Metastatic spinal cord compres-

sion: occurrence, symptoms, clinical presentations and prognosis in 398 patients with spinal cord compression. Acta Neurochir (Wien) 1990;107:37.

14. Torma T. Malignant tumors of the spine and spinal extradural space. Acta Chir Scand Suppl 1957;225:1.

15. White WA, Patterson RH, Bergland RM. Role of surgery in the treatment of spinal cord compression by metastatic neoplasm. Cancer 1971;27:558.

16. Fornasier VL, Horne JG. Metastases to the vertebral column. Cancer 1975;36:590.

17. Greenberg HS, Kim JH, Posner JB. Epidural spinal cord compression from metastatic tumor: results with a new treatment protocol. Ann Neurol 1980;8:361.

18. Dunn RC, Kelly WA, Wohns RNW, et al. Spinal epidural neoplasia: a 15-year review of the results of surgical therapy. J Neurosurg 1980;52:47.

19. Constans JP, de Divitiis E, Donzelli R, et al. Spinal metastases with neurological manifestations: review of 600 cases. J Neurosurg 1983;59:111.

20. Sundaresan N, Digiacinto GV, Hughes JE, et al. Treatment of neoplastic spinal cord compression: results of a prospective study. Neurosurgery 1991;29:645.

21. Foley KM. Pain syndromes in patients with cancer. In: Bonica JJ, Ventafridda V, eds. Advances in pain research and therapy, vol 2. New York, Raven, 1979:59.

22. Hainline B, Tuszynski MH, Posner JB. Ataxia in epidural spinal cord compression. Neurology 1992;42:2193.

23. Lewis DW, Packer RJ, Raney B, et al. Incidence, presentation and outcome of spinal cord disease in children with systemic cancer. Pediatrics 1986;78:438.

24. O'Rourke T, George CB, Redmond J, et al. Spinal computed tomography and computed tomographic metrizamide myelography in the early diagnosis of metastatic disease. J Clin Oncol 1986; 4:576.

25. Portenoy RK, Lipton RB, Foley KM. Back pain in the cancer patient: an algorithm for evaluation and management. Neurology 1987;37:134.

26. Redmond JR, Friedl KE, Cornett P, et al. Clinical usefulness of an algorithm for the early diagnosis of spinal metastatic disease. J Clin Oncol 1988;6:154.

27. Harrison KM, Muss HB, Ball MR, et al. Spinal cord compression in breast cancer. Cancer 1985;55:2839.

28. Haddad P, Thaell JF, Kiely JM, et al. Lymphoma of the spinal extradural space. Cancer 1976;38:1862.

29. Cherny NI, Portenoy RK. Cancer pain: principles of assessment and syndromes. In: Wall PD, Melzack R, eds. Textbook of pain, ed 3. Edinburgh, Churchill Livingstone, 1994:787.

30. Rodichok LD, Ruckdeschel JC, Harper GR, et al. Early detection and treatment of spinal epidural metastases: the role of myelography. Ann Neurol 1986;20:696.

31. Graus F, Krol G, Foley KM. Early diagnosis of spinal epidural metastasis (SEM): correlation with clinical and radiological findings. (Abstract) Proc Am Soc Clin Oncol 1985;4:269.

32. Portenoy RK, Galer BS, Salamon O, et al. Identification of epidural neoplasm: radiography and bone scintigraphy in the symptomatic and asymptomatic spine. Cancer 1989;64:2207.

33. Weissman DE, Gilbert M, Wang H, et al. The use of computed tomography of the spine to identify patients at high risk for epidural metastases. J Clin Oncol 1985;3:1541.

34. Kori SH, Foley KM, Posner JB. Brachial plexus lesions in patients with cancer: 100 cases. Neurology 1981;31:45.

35. Kori SH, Shah CP. Efficacy of metrizamide CT in delineating upper level of epidural metastatic disease. (Abstract) Neurology 1987; 37(Suppl 1):337.

36. Hollis PH, Malis LI, Zappulla RA. Neurological deterioration after lumbar puncture below complete spinal subarachnoid block. J Neurosurg 1986;64:253.

37. Krol G, Heier L, Becker R, et al. MRI and myelography in the evaluation of epidural extension of primary and metastatic tumors. In: Valk J, ed. Neuroradiology 1985/1986. Amsterdam, Elsevier, 1986:91.

38. Heier LA, Krol G, Sundaresan N, et al. MR imaging in evaluation of epidural lesions: comparison with myelography. (Abstract) Radiology 1985;157:150.

39. Krol G, Heier L, Becker R, et al. Value of magnetic resonance imaging in the evaluation of patients with complete and high degree block due to intracranial neoplasm. Acta Radiol 1986; 369(Suppl):741.

40. Hagenau C, Grosh W, Currie M, et al. Comparison of spinal magnetic resonance imaging and myelography in cancer patients. J Clin Oncol 1987;5:1663.

41. Hagen N, Stulman J, Krol G, et al. Epidural disease (ED) in cancer patients: correlation of clinical and imaging findings. (Abstract) Proc Am Soc Clin Oncol 1989;8:88.

42. Smoker WRK, Godersky JC, Knutzon RK, et al. The role of MR imaging in evaluating metastatic spinal disease. AJR 1987; 149:1241.

43. Carmody RF, Yang PJ, Seeley GW, et al. Spinal cord compression due to metastatic disease: diagnosis with MR imaging versus myelography. Radiology 1989;173:225.

44. Williams MP, Cherryman GR, Husband JE. Magnetic resonance imaging in suspected metastatic spinal cord compression. Clin Radiol 1989;40:286.

45. Sarpel S, Sarpel G, Yu E, et al. Early diagnosis of spinal–epidural metastasis by magnetic resonance imaging. Cancer 1987;59:1112.

46. Posner JB, Howieson J, Cvitkovic E. "Disappearing" spinal cord compression: oncolytic effect of glucocorticoids (and other chemotherapeutic agents) on epidural metastases. Ann Neurol 1977; 2:409.

47. Siegal T, Shohami E, Shapira Y, et al. Indomethacin and dexamethasone treatment in experimental neoplastic spinal cord compression. Part 2. Effect on edema and prostaglandin synthesis. Neurosurgery 1988;22:334.

48. Ushio Y, Posner R, Posner JB, et al. Experimental spinal cord compression by epidural neoplasm. Neurology 1977;27:422.

49. Ushio Y, Posner R, Kim JH, et al. Treatment of experimental spinal cord compression caused by extradural neoplasms. J Neurosurg 1977;47:380.

50. Delattre JY, Arbit E, Thaler HT, et al. A dose-response study of dexamethasone in a model of spinal cord compression caused by epidural tumor. J Neurosurg 1989;70:920.

51. Greenberg HS, Kim J-H, Posner JB. Epidural spinal cord compression from metastatic tumor: diagnosis and treatment. Ann Neurol 1980;8:361.

52. Vecht CJ, Haaxma-Reiche H, van Putten WLJ, et al. Initial bolus of conventional versus high-dose dexamethasone in metastatic spinal cord compression. Neurology 1989;39:1255.

53. Sepkowitz KA, Brown AE, Telzak EE, et al. Pneumocystis carinii pneumonia among patients without AIDS at a cancer hospital. JAMA 1992;267:832.

54. Gorter K. Results of laminectomy in spinal cord compression due to tumours. Acta Neurochir (Wien) 1978;42:177.

55. Young RF, Post EM, King GA. Treatment of spinal epidural metastases: randomized prospective comparison of laminectomy and radiotherapy. J Neurosurg 1980;53:741.

56. Findlay GF. Adverse effects of the management of malignant spinal cord compression. J Neurol Neurosurg Psychiatry 1984;47:761.

57. Siegal T, Siegal T, Robin G, et al. Anterior decompression of the spine for metastatic epidural cord compression: a promising avenue of therapy? Ann Neurol 1982;11:28.

58. Harrington KD. Anterior cord decompression and spinal stabilization for patients with metastatic lesions of the spine. J Neurosurg 1984;61:107.

59. Sundaresan N, Galicich JH. Treatment of spinal metastases by vertebral body resection. Cancer Invest 1984;2:383.

60. Siegal T, Siegal T. Surgical decompression of anterior and posterior malignant epidural tumors compressing the spinal cord: a prospective study. Neurosurgery 1985;17:424.

61. Sundaresan N, Galicich JH, Lane JM, et al. Treatment of spinal metastases by vertebral body resection. J Neurosurg 1985;63:676.

62. Fyfe I, Henry A, Mulholland R. Closed vertebral biopsy. J Bone Joint Surg 1983;65:140.

63. Findlay GF, Sandeman DR, Buxton P. The role of needle biopsy in the management of malignant spinal compression. Br J Neurosurg 1988;2:479.

64. Boogerd W, van der Sande JJ, Kröger R, et al. Effective systemic therapy for spinal epidural metastases from breast carcinoma. Eur J Cancer Clin Oncol 1989;25:149.

65. Sanderson IR, Pritchard J, Marsh HT. Chemotherapy as the initial treatment of spinal cord compression due to disseminated neuroblastoma. J Neurosurg 1989;70:688.

66. Cooper K, Bajorin D, Shapiro W, et al. Decompression of epidural metastases from germ cell tumors with chemotherapy. J Neurooncol 1990;8:275.

67. Sørensen PS, Børgesen SE, Rohde K, et al. Metastatic epidural spinal cord compression: results of treatment and survival. Cancer 1990;65:1502.

68. Maranzano E, Latini P, Checcaglini F, et al. Radiation therapy in metastatic spinal cord compression: a prospective analysis of 105 consecutive patients. Cancer 1991;67:1311.

69. Maranzano E, Latini P, Checcaglini F, et al. Radiation therapy of spinal cord compression caused by breast cancer: report of a prospective trial. Int J Radiat Oncol Biol Phys 1992;24:301.

23.3

Leptomeningeal Metastasis

LISA R. ROGERS ▪ KATHLEEN M. FOLEY

Leptomeningeal metastasis occurs when tumor spreads to the leptomeninges that surround the brain and spinal cord. It has emerged as an important diagnostic and therapeutic dilemma in patients with solid tumors. Both prolonged patient survival and enhanced clinical detection contribute to the increased frequency of leptomeningeal metastasis observed in these patients.

The frequency of leptomeningeal metastasis in clinical series of breast cancer patients is estimated at 2% to 5%[1–3]; autopsy series provide a similar estimate of 3% to 6%.[4,5] Leptomeningeal metastasis usually coexists with disseminated systemic disease, but if the systemic disease is stable or responding to therapy, an aggressive approach to diagnosis and treatment is indicated. Determining the diagnosis often is difficult because the presenting neurologic signs can be confused with other central nervous system complications of breast cancer. Neuroimaging and laboratory methods of diagnosis aid in establishing the diagnosis, but are limited by a lack of sensitivity, specificity, or both. Optimal therapy has not been defined; difficulties of drug distribution in the cerebrospinal fluid (CSF) and neurotoxicity are two important factors that impede the success of standard therapies. This chapter reviews the clinical presentation of this disorder, the methods of diagnosis, and the recommended therapeutic approaches.

Clinical Setting

Although the histologic subtype of breast cancer is not described in most series of leptomeningeal metastasis, an unusually high incidence of lobular carcinoma seems to be associated with it. In a clinical series, Harris and associates[6] report that leptomeningeal metastasis occurred in 9 of 56 patients (16%) with lobular carcinoma, but in only 1 of 309 patients (0.3%) with ductal carcinoma, a statistically significant difference. Conversely, parenchymal brain metastasis occurred more commonly in patients with ductal carcinoma, although the difference was not statistically significant. Autopsy studies have confirmed the predilection of lobular carcinoma to spread to the leptomeninges.[5,7] The reason that lobular carcinoma metastasizes to the leptomeninges is not clear, but the pattern of systemic metastasis also differs between these subtypes.[5–7]

A wide interval between the diagnosis of breast cancer and the occurrence of leptomeningeal metastasis is reported; in large series it ranges from a few weeks to more than 15 years.[8,9] In rare instances, leptomeningeal metastasis is the initial manifestation of breast cancer. Many patients with solid tumor have widespread metastatic disease when leptomeningeal metastasis is diagnosed, but in patients with breast cancer the tumor may be inactive or responding to chemotherapy. Of 40 patients reported by Yap and coworkers,[3] the systemic disease was responding or stable in 14 (35%) and there was no evidence of active systemic disease in 12 (30%) when leptomeningeal metastasis was diagnosed. In the remainder, leptomeningeal metastasis occurred during or concurrent with systemic relapse.

Pathophysiology of Leptomeningeal Metastasis

The cerebral and spinal meninges are composed of the dura mater, arachnoid, and pia mater (Fig. 23.3-1). The leptomeninges include the arachnoid and pia mater. The pia is a thin lining, closely adherent to the surface of the brain and spinal cord, separated from the arachnoid by fine trabeculae. It follows the sulci of the cerebral cortex and penetrates the parenchyma of the central nervous sys-

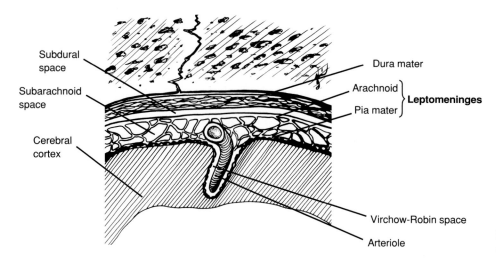

FIGURE 23.3-1 Relation of the cerebral meninges to the brain.

tem in association with arterioles. The associated parenchymal perivascular space is termed the *Virchow-Robin space* (see Fig. 23.3-1). Pathologic evidence suggests several methods by which tumor cells reach the leptomeninges, including hematogenous spread to the vessels of the arachnoid or to the choroid plexus of the ventricles (the latter produces dissemination of malignant cells to the leptomeninges by normal CSF flow) and from direct extension of adjacent metastasis in the cerebral parenchyma or dura, spinal epidural space, or lymphatic paraspinal region.

Autopsy studies demonstrate that when tumor reaches the leptomeninges, it usually grows in a sheetlike fashion along the surface of the brain, spinal cord, and nerve roots.[10] It is usually widely disseminated, but may be limited to portions of the cerebral or spinal leptomeninges. A less common pattern of tumor growth is the formation of multifocal nodules, which typically develop on the nerve roots of the lumbosacral spine and on the ventricular surface of the brain. Leptomeningeal metastasis usually is accompanied by a fibroblastic proliferation of the meninges and rarely is accompanied by an inflammatory response. When tumor enters the subarachnoid space from a parenchymal or dural metastasis, a fibrotic reaction often develops that walls off the tumor and diffuse leptomeningeal dissemination does not occur.[10] Tumor may ensheath meningeal arteries and veins within the subarachnoid space and extend into the Virchow-Robin spaces, resulting in perivascular tumor cuffing and parenchymal invasion. Tumor also may encase or invade the spinal and cranial nerves.

The clinical signs of leptomeningeal metastasis reflect the pathologic process of leptomeningeal infiltration. Cerebral symptoms often result from hydrocephalus, caused by tumor cells proliferating in the basal cisterns and obstructing CSF flow. Cerebral symptoms also can be caused by interference of local cortical function because of direct competition for blood flow and essential metabolites between metabolically active tumor and the underlying cortical tissue or direct parenchymal invasion.[11] Cranial and spinal nerve symptoms result from neoplastic compression or destruction of the nerves.

Clinical Manifestations

A clue to the clinical diagnosis of this disorder is the simultaneous occurrence of multifocal abnormalities at more than one level of the neuraxis (cerebral, cranial nerve, and spinal). A careful neurologic examination often detects signs that are not suggested by the clinical symptoms. In a study of 90 patients with leptomeningeal metastasis from solid tumors (half had breast carcinoma), Wasserstrom and others[9] found that 47 patients complained of symptoms in one area of the neuraxis only, but on examination symptoms and signs were localized to one area of the neuraxis in only 17 patients; 50 had abnormalities in two areas and 23 patients in all three areas. A study of leptomeningeal metastasis in 33 breast cancer patients confirmed these findings; 16 complained of symptoms in only one area, but on examination 27 had involvement of two or three areas.[8]

Spinal symptoms are the most common presentation of leptomeningeal metastasis. The most common complaint is limb weakness, typically involving the lower extremities, that may be accompanied by paresthesias of the extremities and pain in the spine or limbs. Neurologic examination may reveal asymmetric depressed deep-tendon reflexes, limb weakness, and sensory loss. Signs of meningeal irritation are uncommon, such as a positive finding on a straight leg raising test and nuchal rigidity. Cerebral symptoms of leptomeningeal metastasis result, in large part, from the obstruction of CSF flow and include headache, changes in mentation (lethargy, confusion, and memory loss), nausea and vomiting, and imbalance in walking. Seizures and diabetes insipidus are rare. The most common finding of cerebral dysfunction on neurologic examination is a change in mentation. The most common cranial nerve symptom is diplopia. Hearing loss, vision loss, and facial numbness also occur. Paresis of the extraocular muscles is the most common cranial nerve abnormality, followed by facial weakness and diminished hearing.[8,9]

Methods of Diagnosis

The definitive method to diagnose leptomeningeal metastasis is to demonstrate malignant cells in CSF, typically obtained by lumbar puncture. The presence of malignant cells in lumbar CSF indicates that tumor has reached the subarachnoid space (malignant cells should not be identified in the CSF of patients who have isolated parenchymal, dural, or epidural tumor).[12] The initial lumbar CSF cytologic examination gives negative results in up to 46% of patients with leptomeningeal metastasis.[9] The detection of malignant cells depends partly on the amount of CSF available for analysis, and the yield increases with additional spinal taps. In some patients, an alternate site for spinal puncture also increases the yield. Rogers and colleagues[13] found that cytologic examination of cisternal CSF was more sensitive than lumbar CSF in 3 of 12 patients with documented leptomeningeal metastasis. In some instances, the failure to detect malignant cells in CSF reflects adherence of the cells to the leptomeninges, without exfoliation into the CSF. Finally, the failure to detect malignant cells may indicate that the tumor is localized. In an autopsy study of 30 cases of leptomeningeal metastasis, Glass and associates[12] found that 76% of patients with multifocal or disseminated leptomeningeal tumor had positive results on CSF cytologic evaluation, whereas only 58% of patients who had focal disease did. Immunohistochemical staining rarely enhances the detection of carcinoma cells by cytologic evaluation,[14] and flow cytometric study can be a useful adjunct to cytologic examination in some cases of leptomeningeal metastasis,[15] although it has not been well studied in breast cancer patients. If results from CSF cytologic examination are repeatedly negative, definitive diagnosis also can be obtained from a leptomeningeal biopsy.

The lumbar CSF of most patients with leptomeningeal metastasis demonstrates abnormalities of the protein value, the glucose level, or white blood cell count.[9] Elevated protein is the most common abnormality. Up to half of patients also have elevated white blood cells, usually a mononuclear pleocytosis. About one third of patients have depressed CSF glucose. (CSF glucose less than 70% of simultaneous serum glucose is pathologic.) Single or combined CSF tumor markers also can be useful to detect leptomeningeal tumor when the cytologic examination gives negative results, but are limited by a low sensitivity and specificity. CSF β-glucuronidase is elevated in more than half of patients with leptomeningeal metastasis, but it is also elevated in patients with acute and chronic infectious meningitis.[16] CSF carcinoembryonic antigen (CEA) is elevated in some cases of breast carcinoma metastatic to the leptomeninges.[17,18] CSF CEA should be compared with serum CEA, because extremely elevated serum levels can cross the blood–brain barrier. Elevation of the total lactic acid dehydrogenase (LDH) or the percentage of the LDH-5 isoenzyme also can indicate leptomeningeal metastasis.[19,20] However, CSF LDH can also be elevated in infections and other disorders of the central nervous system. The CSF β_2-microglobulin level can be elevated in

leptomeningeal carcinoma,[21] but it is also elevated with central nervous system infection and after intrathecal methotrexate administration. If the CSF value exceeds the serum value, even when normal, this is suggestive of leptomeningeal tumor. A combination of marker assessments can be useful.[22] Elevations of CSF tumor markers must be interpreted cautiously in patients with other sites of central nervous system metastasis in close proximity to the ventricles or leptomeningeal surfaces. Tumor marker values are lower in the ventricular than lumbar CSF, making interpretation from this region difficult. Other CSF markers that have been reported to aid in the diagnosis of leptomeningeal metastasis include HMFG1 antigen,[23] glucosephosphate isomerase,[24] creatine kinase–BB,[25] and tissue polypeptide antigen.[26]

Neuroimaging procedures are indicated in patients who are thought or proven to have leptomeningeal metastasis to exclude parenchymal brain or spinal epidural lesions, which may produce a similar clinical picture, and to determine the extent of disease. They also can supplement the clinical suggestion of leptomeningeal metastasis when results of the CSF cytologic examination are negative. Contrast-enhanced CT scans and gadolinium-enhanced magnetic resonance imaging (MRI) of the brain may reveal hydrocephalus and diffuse abnormal enhancement of the sulci and the leptomeninges of the convexities, tentorium, basal cisterns, and ependyma, with basilar cistern obliteration (Figs. 23.3-2 and 23.3-3).[27–29] Enhanced brain MRI is more sensitive than computed tomographic scanning in detecting leptomeningeal and ependymal enhancement.[28,29] Focal nodular leptomeningeal and cortical enhancement sometimes can be demonstrated by either technique.[27,28] Enhanced MRI lacks sensitivity and specificity, however. In two studies of patients with documented leptomeningeal metastasis, 30% of enhanced brain MRI gave false-negative results.[28,29] Diffuse leptomeningeal enhancement also can be demonstrated in patients who have undergone craniotomy or have adjacent pathologic lesions or leptomeningeal infection.[28] Localized leptomeningeal enhancement can mimic a primary leptomeningeal tumor.[30] Myelography can show varying degrees of subarachnoid block and irregularity of spinal nerve roots. Enhanced MRI is the recommended procedure to demonstrate spinal leptomeningeal tumor[31–33] because it is superior to myelography in detecting diffuse linear enhancement along the spinal cord and nerve roots (Fig. 23.3-4), and in detecting small (2- to 3-mm) tumor nodules.

Often, a high index of suspicion is necessary to make the diagnosis of leptomeningeal metastasis. Signs of cerebral, cranial nerve, or spinal nerve dysfunction, particularly in combination, are suggestive of leptomeningeal metastasis in patients with breast carcinoma. If routine CSF cytologic examination gives negative results, the clinician must rely on other clinical, neuroimaging, and CSF examinations. A presumptive diagnosis can be established, even in the absence of a positive finding on CSF cytologic examination, if the appropriate neuroimaging and CSF findings support this diagnosis, and if infection and other

FIGURE 23.3-2 Axial contrast-enhanced brain CT scan reveals abnormal diffuse enhancement of the leptomeninges, sulci, cisterns, and tentorium. The arrow demonstrates leptomeningeal and sulcal enhancement. The lateral and third ventricles are enlarged, which is consistent with hydrocephalus.

sites of central nervous system metastasis producing the abnormal findings can be excluded.

Treatment

Optimal therapy for leptomeningeal metastasis from breast carcinoma has not been determined. It is difficult to interpret published treatment results because of a nonuniform selection of patients and treatment design. Most studies have used whole-brain or involved-field radiation therapy to bulky disease and symptomatic sites and intra-CSF chemotherapy. Several issues regarding chemotherapy treatment of leptomeningeal metastasis must be considered. Because leptomeningeal metastasis frequently involves the entire neuraxis, treatment must encompass the entire CSF volume. Leptomeningeal tumor develops its own vascular supply, which lacks a blood–brain barrier, but it is difficult to obtain high levels of chemotherapy in the CSF with standard intravenous chemotherapy. For this reason, therapy usually involves administration of chemotherapy directly into

the CSF. An advantage of direct CSF instillation includes permitting a higher concentration of chemotherapy in close proximity to the leptomeninges, because the initial volume of distribution is smaller than the vascular compartment and the clearance half-life is longer in the spinal fluid for some agents.[34] In addition, intra-CSF instillation often reduces or spares systemic dose-limiting toxicity, although the CSF can act as a reservoir for methotrexate, which can slowly leak into the peripheral circulation. A disadvantage to chemotherapy instillation into the CSF is the frequent occurrence of CSF flow abnormalities, which may result in nonuniform distribution of the chemotherapy agent throughout the CSF pathways, reducing efficacy and increasing local toxicity.[35,36]

Chemotherapy can be directly instilled into the lumbar subarachnoid space or the ventricular system via a reservoir device such as an Ommaya system. Intraventricular administration usually is recommended because this assures delivery of drug into the CSF; lumbar punctures may be limited by inadvertent epidural or subdural injection. In addition, a lumbar puncture may be contraindicated if a parenchymal or epidural mass lesion is present. Most importantly, delivery of drug into the ventricular system ensures a more uniform drug distribution. In a study of pharmacokinetics and drug distribution, Shapiro and coworkers[37] found that injection of methotrexate into the ventricular system provided a more uniform distribution of methotrexate in the spine and ventricles than lumbar injection, even when the lumbar injection was successful (Fig. 23.3-5). In addition, the use of a ventricular reservoir allows for repetitive intraventricular administration using novel

FIGURE 23.3-3 Coronal gadolinium-enhanced brain MRI reveals diffuse linear enhancement of the leptomeninges adjacent to the falx, cerebral convexities, and tentorium (*arrow*).

FIGURE 23.3-4 Sagittal gadolinium-enhanced spine MRI reveals thickening and linear enhancement of the leptomeninges adjacent to the distal spinal cord (*dark arrow*) and on the lumbosacral nerve roots (*white arrow*).

therapeutic approaches. If the patient requires a ventriculoperitoneal shunt for hydrocephalus, a subcutaneous reservoir with an on–off device should be included.

Patients who are diagnosed with leptomeningeal metastasis should undergo enhanced MRI of the entire neuraxis to search for bulky disease. Radiation should be administered to symptomatic areas of leptomeningeal metastasis and to bulky disease because intra-CSF chemotherapy penetrates only a short distance into bulky tumor deposits. In addition, bulky tumor deposits limit the flow of CSF, causing an accumulation of excessively high concentration of drugs proximal to the flow obstruction. The use of complete spine radiation is discouraged because radiation to the entire spine may result in severe myelosuppression, particularly in patients who are receiving or have received systemic chemotherapy. Whole-brain radiation can enhance the neurotoxicity of chemotherapy administered into the CSF and should be used only when there are symptoms from the brain or cranial nerves or there is a cranial CSF flow obstruction. Data do not suggest that systemic or intra-CSF administration of corticosteroids is effective in treating leptomeningeal metastasis, but steroids are indicated if there is mass effect within the nervous system.

CSF flow studies should be performed if aggressive therapy with intra-CSF chemotherapy is planned, because these often demonstrate abnormalities of CSF flow in the brain or spine, which result in compartmentalization of CSF pathways.[35,36] Flow abnormalities are present even when enhanced MRI or myelography does not reveal bulky disease.[38] Areas of CSF block prevent homogeneous distribution of chemotherapy and may be an important factor in the failure of intra-CSF chemotherapy to eradicate leptomeningeal tumor and in neurotoxicity. Areas of CSF block identified on flow studies may respond to involved-field radiation therapy, permitting intra-CSF chemotherapy to distribute throughout the CSF. If the blockages do not respond to radiation, these patients probably should receive intraventricular and intralumbar CSF administration to distribute drug more homogeneously, but no data support this.

Response criteria in leptomeningeal metastasis are not standardized. Most reported studies define complete response as the normalization of CSF and improvement of clinical symptoms. Sixty to 80% of patients show response after intra-CSF methotrexate, with or without radiation.[3,8] Response may be durable, even if only a partial response is obtained.[39] Methotrexate seems to provide an improved survival compared with no therapy in most studies, with a median survival ranging from 3 to 6 months[3,8,40–42] and a median survival of 15 months in those who respond.[3,8] Boogerd and coworkers,[41] however, reported similar survivals among patients with similar pretreatment characteristics who were not treated or who were treated with intraventricular methotrexate.

Intra-CSF administration of methotrexate usually is performed two or three times a week initially. The following regimens are used: a dosage based on body surface area (7 mg/m^2); a fixed dose (10 to 20 mg) because the volume of CSF should not vary significantly based on surface area; and a dosage based on monitoring of ventricular methotrexate levels. Monitoring of methotrexate levels is the most appropriate way to assure that cytotoxic concentrations of the drug are obtained[41] but rarely is performed.

Intra-CSF thiotepa has been studied in small numbers of patients with leptomeningeal metastasis from solid tumors, including breast carcinoma. The dosage is usually 10 mg twice weekly. In a comparative randomized study of intraventricular methotrexate versus thiotepa in 52 patients with solid tumors, 25 of whom had breast carcinoma, Grossman and colleagues[42] found a slight survival advantage with methotrexate. Thiotepa has a rapid clearance half-life in the CSF, which may limit its effectiveness. No evidence shows that combination intra-CSF chemotherapy is better than methotrexate alone, and its use is limited by systemic toxicity.[43] Investigational agents available in protocol settings for treating leptomeningeal metastasis from solid tumors include DepoFoam/ara-C,[44] diaziquone,[45] interleukin-2,[46] radioactively tagged monoclonal antibodies,[47] nitrosoureas,[48] and 4-hydroperoxycyclophosphamide.[49]

Neurotoxicity after irradiation of the nervous system

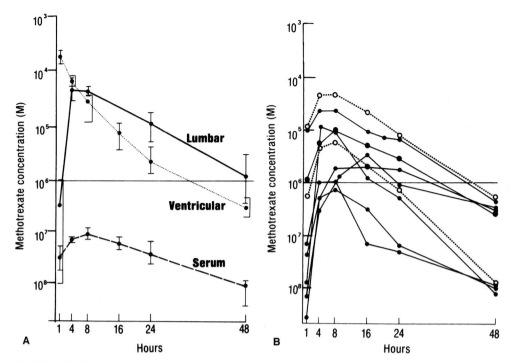

FIGURE 23.3-5 A. Methotrexate distribution (mean ± range) in five studies after administration of 6.25 mg/m² through the Ommaya reservoir. **B.** Intraventricular methotrexate concentration in nine studies after lumbar administration. Solid circles represent seven studies at a methotrexate dose of 6.25 mg/m². Open circles represent two studies at a dose of 12.5 mg/m². (Shapiro WR, Young DF, Mehta BM. Methotrexate: distribution in cerebrospinal fluid after intravenous ventricular and lumbar injections. N Engl J Med 1975;293:163)

and intra-CSF chemotherapy is a significant obstacle to aggressively treating patients with leptomeningeal metastasis. The most common neurologic complication of intra-CSF methotrexate is a transient aseptic meningitis, which develops within hours of injection and produces headache, fever, stiff neck, and confusion. It does not recur on subsequent injections.[9] A subacute encephalomyelitis also can occur. The most significant neurologic complication of intra-CSF methotrexate is a disseminated necrotizing leukoencephalopathy. The risk of leukoencephalopathy is increased with increasing total methotrexate dose, prolonged CSF methotrexate levels, and concurrent cranial radiation.[50] It produces demyelination, predominantly in the cerebral periventricular white matter, with fibrinoid necrosis and thickening and calcification of vascular walls.[51] It may result in apathy, memory loss, gait disturbance, and focal neurologic abnormalities, such as hemiparesis. It is visible on computed tomography or MRI as diffuse tissue density abnormalities in the periventricular white matter. A concentration × time schedule of intraventricular methotrexate produces less neurotoxicity compared with standard-dose schedules in patients with leukemia[52] but has not been studied in breast cancer patients. Focal leukoencephalopathy can result from high local cerebral concentrations of methotrexate around the Ommaya reservoir catheter, particularly if inadvertent separation of the catheter occurs.[53,54] Systemic complications of methotrexate include stomatitis and myelosuppression. Folinic acid should be administered to those at risk for myelosuppression.

Thiotepa can result in myelosuppression, particularly when concurrent systemic chemotherapy is administered. It can also cause a myelopathy after lumbar injection.[55] Clinically significant complications related to the Ommaya reservoir system are rare and include bacterial meningitis and intracerebral hemorrhage.

CSF from the Ommaya reservoir should be sampled at each chemotherapy injection, but because ventricular fluid is not accurate for monitoring tumor markers or cytologic findings, periodic lumbar punctures are necessary for determining CSF response. CSF tumor markers can parallel response to treatments. If neurologic decline occurs, the possibility of treatment-related toxicity or progressive leptomeningeal tumor must be evaluated. If the latter occurs, the chemotherapy agent should be changed, radiation administered to bulky areas, or both. Patients must also be monitored for progression of their systemic disease, although in large series,[3,41] most patients with breast cancer died of progressive leptomeningeal disease or the leptomeningeal disease was an important contributing factor to death.

Prospective studies to evaluate treatment response based on individual clinical variables are necessary to allow the clinician to predict which patients with breast carcinoma will fare best with aggressive treatment of leptomeningeal metastasis. CSF flow studies should be used in planning therapy; some treatment failures in the past may have resulted from compartmentalization of CSF flow, which leads to inadequate drug delivery and excessive toxicity. Ongoing trials of novel chemotherapeutic agents and drugs packaged in novel delivery systems designed for prolonged CSF exposure should improve treatment results in patients with leptomeningeal metastasis of breast carcinoma.

References

1. Sondak V. Leptomeningeal spread of breast cancer: report of case and review of the literature. Cancer 1981;48:395.
2. Hitchins RN, Bell DR, Woods RL, et al. A prospective randomized trial of single-agent versus combination chemotherapy in meningeal carcinomatosis. J Clin Oncol 1987;5:1655.
3. Yap HY, Yap BS, Rasmussen S, et al. Treatment for meningeal carcinomatosis in breast cancer. Cancer 1982;49:219.
4. Tsukada Y, Fouad A, Pickren JW, et al. Central nervous system metastasis from breast carcinoma: autopsy study. Cancer 1983;52:2349.
5. Lamovec J, Zidar A. Association of leptomeningeal carcinomatosis in carcinoma of the breast with infiltrating lobular carcinoma: an autopsy study. Arch Pathol Lab Med 1991;115:507.
6. Harris M, Howell A, Chrissohou M, et al. A comparison of the metastatic pattern of infiltrating lobular carcinoma and infiltrating duct carcinoma of the breast. Br J Cancer 1984;50:23.
7. Smith DB, Howell A, Harris M, et al. Carcinomatous meningitis associated with infiltrating lobular carcinoma of the breast. Eur J Surg Oncol 1985;11:33.
8. Ongerboer de Visser BW, Somers R, Nooyen WH, et al. Intraventricular methotrexate therapy of leptomeningeal metastasis from breast carcinoma. Neurology 1983;33:1565.
9. Wasserstrom WR, Glass JP, Posner JB. Diagnosis and treatment of leptomeningeal metastases from solid tumors: experience with 90 patients. Cancer 1982;49:759.
10. Olson ME, Chernik NL, Posner JB. Infiltration of the leptomeninges by systemic cancer. Arch Neurol 1974;30:122.
11. Siegal T, Mildworf B, Stein D, et al. Leptomeningeal metastasis: reduction in regional cerebral blood flow and cognitive impairment. Ann Neurol 1985;17:100.
12. Glass JP, Melamed M, Chernik NL, et al. Malignant cells in cerebrospinal fluid (CSF): the meaning of a positive CSF cytology. Neurology 1979;29:1369.
13. Rogers LR, Duchesneau PM, Nunez C, et al. Comparison of cisternal and lumbar CSF examination in leptomeningeal metastasis. Neurology 1992;42:1239.
14. Hovestadt A, Henzen-Logmans SC, Vecht CJ. Immunohistochemical analysis of the cerebrospinal fluid for carcinomatous and lymphomatous leptomeningitis. Br J Cancer 1990;62:653.
15. Cibas ES, Malkin MG, Posner JB, et al. Detection of DNA abnormalities by flow cytometry in cells from cerebrospinal fluid. Am J Clin Pathol 1987;88:570.
16. Schold SC, Wasserstrom WR, Fleisher M, et al. Cerebrospinal fluid biochemical markers of central nervous system metastases. Ann Neurol 1980;8:597.
17. Twijnstra A, Nooyen WJ, van Zanten AP, et al. Cerebrospinal fluid carcinoembryonic antigen in patients with metastatic and nonmetastatic neurological diseases. Arch Neurol 1986;43:269.
18. Yap B, Yap H, Fritsche HA, et al. CSF carcinoembryonic antigen in meningeal carcinomatosis from breast cancer. JAMA 1980;244:1601.
19. Fleisher M, Wasserstrom WR, Schold SC, et al. Lactic dehydrogenase isoenzymes in the cerebrospinal fluid of patients with systemic cancer. Cancer 1981;47:2654.
20. Twijnstra A, van Zanten AP, Hart AAM, et al. Serial lumbar and ventricle cerebrospinal fluid lactate dehydrogenase activities in pa-

tients with leptomeningeal metastases from solid and haemotological tumors. J Neurol Neurosurg Psychiatry 1987;50:313.
21. Twijnstra A, vanZanten AP, Nooyen WJ, et al. Cerebrospinal fluid β2-microglobulin: a study in controls and patients with metastatic and non-metastatic neurological diseases. Eur J Cancer Clin Oncol 1986;22:387.
22. Ongerboer de Visser BW, van Zanten AP, Twijnstra A, et al. Sensitivity and specificity of cerebrospinal fluid biochemical markers of central nervous system metastases. Prog Exp Tumor Res 1985;29:105.
23. Moseley RP, Oge K, Shafqat S, et al. HMFG1 antigen: a new marker for carcinomatous meningitis. Int J Cancer 1989;44:440.
24. Newton HB, Fleisher M, Schwartz MK, et al. Glucosephosphate isomerase as a CSF marker for leptomeningeal metastasis. Neurology 1991;41:395.
25. Bach F, Bach FW, Pedersen G, et al. Creatine kinase-BB in the cerebrospinal fluid as a marker of CNS metastases and leptomeningeal carcinomatosis in patients with breast cancer. Eur J Cancer Clin Oncol 1989;25:1703.
26. Bach F, Soletormos G, Dombernowsky P. Tissue polypeptide antigen activity in cerebrospinal fluid: a marker of central nervous system metastases of breast cancer. J Natl Cancer Inst 1991;83:779.
27. Ascherl GF, Hilal SK, Brisman R. Computed tomography of disseminated meningeal and ependymal malignant neoplasms. Neurology 1981;31:567.
28. Sze G, Soletsky S, Bronen R, et al. MR imaging of the cranial meninges with emphasis on contrast enhancement and meningeal carcinomatosis. AJNR 1989;10:965.
29. Chamberlain MC, Sandy AD, Press GA. Leptomeningeal metastasis: a comparison of gadolinium-enhanced MR and contrast-enhanced CT of the brain. Neurology 1990;40:435.
30. Buff BL, Schnick RM, Norregaard T. Meningeal metastasis of leiomyosarcoma mimicking meningioma: CT and MR findings. J Comput Assist Tomogr 1991;15:166.
31. Kramer ED, Rafto S, Packer RJ, et al. Comparison of myelography with CT follow-up versus gadolinium MRI for subarachnoid metastatic disease in children. Neurology 1991;41:46.
32. Phillips ME, Ryals TJ, Kambhu SA, et al. Neoplastic vs inflammatory meningeal enhancement with Gd-DTPA. J Comput Assist Tomogr 1990;14:536.
33. Sze G, Abramson A, Krol G, et al. Gadolinium-DTPA in the evaluation of intradural extramedullary spinal disease. AJNR 1988;9:153.
34. Poplack DG, Bleyer WA, Horowitz ME. Pharmacology of antineoplastic agents in cerebrospinal fluid. In: Wood JH, ed. Neurobiology of cerebrospinal fluid. New York, Plenum, 1980:561.
35. Chamberlain MC, Corey-Bloom J. Leptomeningeal metastasis: 111 indium-DTPA CSF flow studies. Neurology 1991;41:1765.
36. Grossman SA, Trump DL, Chen DCP, et al. Cerebrospinal fluid flow abnormalities in patients with neoplastic meningitis. Am J Med 1982;73:641.
37. Shapiro WR, Young DF, Mehta BM. Methotrexate: distribution in cerebrospinal fluid after intravenous, ventricular and lumbar injections. N Engl J Med 1975;293:161.
38. Chamberlain MC. Comparative spine imaging in leptomeningeal metastases. J Neurooncol 1995;23:233.
39. Siegal T, Lossos A, Pfeffer MR. Leptomeningeal metastasis: analysis of 31 patients with sustained off-therapy response following combined-modality therapy. Neurology 1994;44:1463.
40. Trump DL, Grossman SA, Thompson G, et al. Treatment of neoplastic meningitis with intraventricular thiotepa and methotrexate. Cancer Treat Rep 1982;66:1599.
41. Boogerd W, Hart AAM, van der Sande JJ, et al. Meningeal carcinomatosis in breast cancer: prognostic factors and influence of treatment. Cancer 1991;67:1685.
42. Grossman SA, Finkelstein DM, Ruckdeschel JC, et al. Randomized prospective comparison of intraventricular methotrexate and thiotepa

in patients with previously untreated neoplastic meningitis. J Clin Oncol 1993;11:561.

43. Giannone L, Greco FA, Hainsworth JD. Combination intraventricular chemotherapy for meningeal neoplasia. J Clin Oncol 1986;4:68.

44. Chamberlain MC, Khatibis, Kim JC, et al. A phase I study of Depo-Foam/Ara-C in the treatment of carcinomatous meningitis. Arch Neurol 1993;50:261.

45. Berg SL, Balis FM, Zimm S, et al. Phase I/II trial and pharmacokinetics of intrathecal diaziquone in refractory meningeal malignancies. J Clin Oncol 1992;10:143.

46. Moser RP, Black JB, London WG, et al. Pilot study of intraventricular interleukin-2 for the treatment of leptomeningeal cancer. (Abstract) Proc Annu Meet Am Soc Clin Oncol 1991;10:384.

47. Moseley RP, Benjamin JC, Ashpole RD, et al. Carcinomatous meningitis: antibody-guided therapy with I-131 HMFg1. J Neurol Neurosurg Psychiatry 1991;54:260.

48. Levin VA, Chamberlain M, Silver P, et al. Phase I/II study of intraventricular and intrathecal ACNU for leptomeningeal neoplasia. Cancer Chemother 1983;33:1565.

49. Arndt CAS, Colvin OM, Balis FM, et al. Intrathecal administration of 4-hydroperoxycyclophosphamide in rhesus monkeys. Cancer Res 1987;47:5932.

50. Bleyer WA. Neurological sequelae of methotrexate and ionizing radiation: a new classification. Cancer Treat Rep 1981;65:89.

51. Shapiro WR, Chernik NL, Posner JB. Necrotizing encephalopathy following intraventricular instillation of methotrexate. Arch Neurol 1973;28:96.

52. Bleyer WA, Poplack DG, Simon RM. "Concentration X time" methotrexate via a subcutaneous reservoir: a less toxic regimen for intraventricular chemotherapy of central nervous system neoplasms. Blood 1978;51:835.

53. Lemann W, Wiley RG, Posner JB. Leukoencephalopathy complicating intraventricular catheters: clinical, radiographic and pathologic study of 10 cases. J Neurooncol 1988;6:77.

54. de Waal R, Algra PR, Heimans JJ, et al. Methotrexate induced brain necrosis and severe leukoencephalopathy due to disconnection of an Ommaya device. J Neurooncol 1993;15:269.

55. Hahn AF, Feasby TE, Gilbert JJ. Paraparesis following intrathecal chemotherapy. Neurology 1983;33:1032.

23.4

Brachial Plexopathy in Patients With Breast Cancer

NATHAN I. CHERNY ▪ KATHLEEN M. FOLEY

In patients with cancer, symptoms and signs of brachial plexopathy may be attributable to acute brachial neuritis, trauma to the plexus during surgery or anesthesia, metastatic spread of tumor, transient or permanent radiation injury, or radiation-induced plexus tumors. In patients with breast cancer, the most common causes of such signs are metastatic spread of tumor and radiation injury to the plexus and second primaries. Careful evaluation of the clinical history, symptoms and signs, as well as electrodiagnostic and imaging studies are helpful in diagnosing the cause of a brachial plexopathy.

Tumor Infiltration of the Brachial Plexus (Metastatic Brachial Plexopathy)

Tumor infiltration of the plexus is common because of its proximity to the draining axillary lymph nodes, yet this diagnosis represented only 5% of the neurologic consultations evaluated by one neurology consultation service[1] and 4% of patients referred to a cancer pain service.[2] Early and accurate diagnosis is critical in preventing irreversible nerve damage and chronic neuropathic pain and in determining the prognosis and treatment of tumor.

CLINICAL FEATURES

Pain is the most common symptom, often preceding neurologic signs or symptoms for up to 9 months.[3-7] The pain distribution depends on the site of plexus involvement.

Eighty-five percent of patients with tumor infiltration present with pain that is moderate to severe, typically in the shoulder girdle and radiating to the elbow, medial side to the forearm, and in the fourth and fifth fingers (consistent with involvement of the lower plexus C-7, C-8, and T-1).[3,6,7] Other presentations are occasionally observed including the following: pain localized to the posterior aspect of the arm or to the elbow; a burning or freezing sensation and hypersensitivity of the skin along the ulnar aspect of the arm; or pain referred to either the shoulder girdle or the tip of either the index finger or thumb (consistent with infiltration of the upper plexus C5-6 by tumor rising in the supraclavicular nodes). By the time of diagnosis of a brachial plexus lesion, 98% of patients have pain that is most often reported as severe. In the series by Kori and others,[3] 2 of 78 patients with malignant brachial plexopathy had pain as the only symptom or sign of tumor recurrence and required exploration and biopsy of the plexus to establish the diagnosis.

Paresthesias occur as a presenting symptom in 15% of patients with tumor, in an ulnar distribution from infiltration of the lower plexus, or with a median nerve distribution in lesions of the upper plexus. Lymphedema rarely is a presenting symptom of tumor infiltration of the brachial plexus,[3,7] but it does occur in about 10% of patients, most often in patients who have had previous radiation therapy to the plexus and who subsequently develop recurrent tumor.

Focal weakness, atrophy, and sensory changes in the distribution of the C-7, C-8, and T-1 roots occur in more than 75% of patients. In one series of patients with brachial plexopathy arising from any tumor type, the presenting symptom in 25% of patients was whole-plexus motor weakness (panplexopathy).[3] Patients with a panplexopathy or Horner syndrome have a higher likelihood of epidural extension and should undergo imaging of the epidural space as part of their examination.

In 12 of 78 patients with tumor infiltration of the brachial plexus included in the Kori series,[3] the plexus lesion was the only evidence of tumor and other metastases appeared only after several months. In two patients, the plexus lesion was the only sign of recurrence for 4 years. In one patient, surgical exploration after 2 years of plexopathy signs proved to be normal, but because of progressive worsening of neurologic signs, a second exploration was carried out, confirming tumor recurrence.

ELECTRODIAGNOSTIC STUDIES

Electromyography typically reveals fibrillation potentials and positive waves characteristic of denervation in the distribution of the brachial plexus that is consistent with plexus signs and symptoms.[8-11] A normal finding on electromyography in the cervical paraspinal muscles usually is adequate to exclude the presence of root disease. In the rare instances that myokymia is observed in patients with tumor infiltration of the brachial plexus, it is localized and may be isolated to one muscle group alone[11]; widespread myokymic discharges are strongly suggestive of radiation-induced plexopathy.[10-13] Median somatosensory-evoked potentials have been used in the evaluation of brachial plexopathy, and may be reliable in confirming the presence of an abnormality in the brachial plexus, the C-5, T-1 roots, or the epidural space rostral to the second vertebral body. In a study of 23 patients with tumor infiltration of the brachial plexus, vertebral body disease, and radiation fibrosis,[14] median somatosensory-evoked potentials detected myelopathy in nine patients with epidural disease, but reported myelopathic changes in four patients with normal results on myelograms. In this study, the median somatosensory-evoked potentials did not distinguish tumor infiltration of the brachial plexus from radiation injury. This test may be useful in patients with pain but without evidence of neurologic abnormalities who are at risk for tumor infiltration of the brachial plexus. Exploration of the plexus should be considered for select patients who have suggestive clinical findings and abnormal median somatosensory-evoked potentials.

IMAGING STUDIES

Computed Tomography

Radiographic studies such as computed tomography (CT) and magnetic resonance imaging (MRI) are helpful in determining the cause of brachial plexopathy in patients with breast cancer.[9,15-21] CT provides both soft tissue and bony definition in a two-dimensional anatomic plane. Because thicker slices miss subtle anatomic changes, Cooke and associates[15,16] advocate the use of narrow-section (4-mm) CT with bolus intravenous en-

hancement to examine the root of the neck and axilla. Adequate imaging requires scanning from C-4 to T-6 vertebral bodies using a large gantry aperture to include both axillary fossae[21] so that the symptomatic plexus may be compared with the asymptomatic one. Vascular enhancement allows for identification of vascular structures that relate to the plexus. Because a high concentration of contrast can produce a streaking artifact, some experts recommend that intravenous contrast should be administered contralateral to the suspected lesion.[21] The elements of the brachial plexus are depicted as nodular or linear areas of soft tissue density that can be difficult to identify (Figs. 23.4-1 and 23.4-2).

In 28 of 42 patients with neurologic symptoms affecting the arm or hand evaluated by Cooke and coworkers,[15] changes on CT were seen in 96%. Among 19 postoperative patients with breast cancer and suspected local or regional recurrence, CT correctly identified the recurrence in all 15 biopsy-proven cases. Of interest, in two cases, suspicious areas on the CT scans proved to be residual pectoralis muscle. In the Cascino study[9] of patients with known tumor involving the brachial plexus, CT showed abnormalities in 89% of patients; all but one had a circumscribed mass in the region of the brachial plexus. Paravertebral extension and tumor erosion of bone were frequently demonstrated despite normal findings on plain radiographs and bone scans. In fact, plain radiographs of the spine gave abnormal results in only 4 of 39 patients, whereas CT detected spine abnormalities in 13 of 41 patients. Similarly, bone scans were not helpful and gave false-negative results, especially in patients who had received prior radiation therapy.[22] In this study,[9] computed tomographic studies were reviewed for four abnormalities: soft tissue density changes in the region of the brachial plexus, paravertebral extension of soft tissue masses, bony erosion, and epidural extension. Forty-one of 46 patients with metastatic plexopathy had abnormalities in the region of the symptomatic brachial plexus. Five patients had completely normal results on CT despite proven metastatic plexopathy. All other diagnostic studies (bone scans, myelograms, or cervical spine radiographs) in four of these patients showed normal results as well. One patient had an epidural tumor at C-7, detected on myelography, which was found during surgery to extend out and invade the plexus. In two patients, surgical explorations of the brachial plexus through an anterior approach gave normal results. Postoperative CT demonstrated a mass deep in the brachial plexus. Repeat exploration of the abnormality revealed by CT demonstrated a tumor at biopsy.

Magnetic Resonance Imaging

Although comparative data on the sensitivity and specificity of MRI to CT in evaluating lesions of the brachial plexus is not available, MRI is a clinically useful test that may replace CT and myelography.[23] MRI is a noninvasive procedure that can assess the integrity of the

FIGURE 23.4-1 Diagrams of tomographic anatomy of the normal brachial plexus. **A.** Upper cervical level. Cervical roots (*arrows*) exit through the neural foramina and proceed anterolaterally, behind major blood vessels, to form the plexus. **B.** Lower cervical level. Brachial plexus components (*arrow*) lie behind major blood vessels and between the anterior and medial scalene muscles. **C.** Axillary fossa. The brachial plexus accompanies axillary arteries and veins. The neurovascular bundle (*arrow*), surrounded by fat tissue, lies in a triangle outlined by the chest wall medially, the pectoralis minor anteriorly, and the subscapularis muscle posteriorly. (Adapted from Krol G. Evaluation of neoplastic involvement of brachial and lumbar plexus: imaging aspects. J Back Musculoskel Rehab 1993;3:35)

vertebral bodies and may differentiate tumor from radiation fibrosis as well as fully visualize the adjacent epidural space.[19,20] Clinical experience suggests that full evaluation requires the use of a modified sagittal view (with 15 degrees of angulation) to assess the contents of the cervical foramina and the cervical and upper thoracic spinal cord, axial views to define a paraspinal mass, and coronal views to evaluate the peripheral components of the brachial plexus.[23] T1- and T2-weighted images are useful: a hyperintense appearance on T2-weighted images of a mass in the brachial plexus is characteristic of tumor infiltration and is less frequently seen with radiation fibrosis, and T1-weighted images best define the relation of tumor to the surrounding structures (Fig. 23.4-3).[24] Enhancement after injection of gadolinium has been observed with both tumor infiltration and radiation fibrosis, and the capacity to differentiate between these two diagnoses remains indeterminate.

Because patients with brachial plexus lesions are at high risk for developing epidural cord compression from

FIGURE 23.4-2 Contrast-enhanced CT scan of the brachial plexus in a 57-year-old woman with a history of breast cancer who presented with right arm and hand pain. There is a mass in the right brachial plexus (*arrows*). (Cherny NI, Portenoy RK. Cancer pain: principles of assessment and syndromes. In: Wall PD, Melzack R, ed. Textbook of pain, ed 3. Edinburgh, Churchill Livingstone, 1994:787)

direct tumor infiltration along the plexus into the epidural space, or from hematogenous spread of tumor to the vertebral body,[3,19,22] imaging should include the adjacent epidural space. Imaging of the epidural space is essential if spinal cord compression is suspected and in the evaluation of patients who have any of the clinical findings that are commonly associated with this complication, including panplexopathy, Horner syndrome, vertebral body erosion, or collapse at the C-7 to T-1 levels, or a paraspinal mass detected on CT. Accurate imaging with MRI determines the extent of epidural encroachment (which influences prognosis and may alter the therapeutic approach) and defines the appropriate radiation portals.[25]

For patients who require evaluation of the epidural space but lack access to MRI and those unable to undergo the procedure, myelography remains the investigation of choice. MRI is relatively contraindicated in patients with severe claustrophobia and absolutely contraindicated for all patients with pacemakers. Some metallic implants are MRI safe, and a policy of individual case review with the MRI technicians is encouraged. Patients who would benefit from total spinal imaging, such as those with multifocal pain or multiple spinal metastases (who have a 10% chance of epidural compression remote from the symptomatic site[26]), and those with severe kyphosis or scoliosis, who may not be suitable for MRI scanning because of technical considerations, also may need a different approach. Myelography also may be needed after MRI that produces suboptimal

FIGURE 23.4-3 MRI demonstrating a mass in the axilla involving the brachial plexus and invading the chest wall.

or nondiagnostic results, particularly in the setting of neurologic deterioration.

Ultrasound

Ultrasound examination of the axilla is a useful technique for the identification of metastatic axillary nodes,[27–29] but its role in evaluating malignant brachial plexopathy has not been defined. In evaluating the axilla for nodal disease, ultrasound has been observed to be more sensitive than mammography[28] and digital subtraction angiography,[30] but less sensitive than CT.[30] Hypoechoic masses frequently indicate tumor. Hyperechoic lesions are much less specific and may be either malignant or benign.[30] Color Doppler ultrasonography can detect alterations in blood flow around axillary nodes infiltrated with tumor. In a prospective study involving 51 patients who subsequently underwent axillary dissection,[29] this technique demonstrated a sensitivity of 75%, specificity of 84%, positive predictive value of 94%, and negative predictive value of 84%. These impressive results are substantially better than those observed using other imaging modalities and suggest a potential use of this technique in assessing patients with brachial plexopathy.

TREATMENT

The treatment of tumor infiltration of the brachial plexus depends on the status of the disease, the extent of neurologic involvement, and any prior history of radiation therapy to the brachial plexus. In patients with tumor infiltration of the brachial plexus with evidence of metastatic disease in other sites, systemic chemotherapy is a reasonable approach. In those who have undergone previous radiation therapy to the region, systemic therapies involving either cytotoxic or hormonal therapies may offer the only reasonable antitumor treatment. However, in a patient who has not previously been irradiated if the neurologic signs are rapidly progressive, or if evidence exists of epidural spinal cord compression, radiation therapy is the procedure of choice. MRI or myelography should be used to define the exact radiation ports in these cases.

The dose of radiation therapy employed varies. In several reported series, a dose of 3000 cGy, delivered over a 3-week period or 5000 cGy delivered over 5 weeks represents the most commonly used dose ranges.[3,8,31,32] Clinical evidence suggests that steroids provide pain relief in patients with tumor infiltration of the brachial plexus, and they often are used to provide analgesia during therapy.[33] If the diagnosis of brachial plexus tumor infiltration is made early and effective therapy is instituted, the patient's neurologic symptoms should resolve and a marked reduction in pain should occur. Ampil[32] reviewed the literature, summarizing the results of external irradiation and his own experience, and reported that the total amount of delivered dose, rather than the width of the therapy port, was the most important factor in achieving optimal symptomatic palliation. In his series of 23 patients, significant pain relief was achieved in 4 patients (77%) for a median of 3 months; the observed objective response rate was 46%. In

the series by Nisce and Chu,[34] 12 of 47 patients (25.5%) with metastatic brachial plexopathy and breast cancer had complete pain relief for a mean duration of 15 months, and 23 (49%) had partial pain relief for a mean duration of 6 months. These researchers suggest that higher doses of irradiation (5000 cGy) are more effective than lower doses. In the retrospective review of Kori and others,[3] the treatment of metastatic plexopathy was disappointing. Radiation therapy, in doses of 2000 to 5000 cGy delivered to the plexus, relieved pain in only 46% of cases.[3] Neurologic improvement was minimal, and persistent, chronic pain was the most significant problem. However, if neurologic signs have progressed and the pain has a burning, dysesthetic component, effective tumor therapy may not be associated with a marked improvement in pain. This results, in part, from the fact that nerve injury is not reversible and that a causalgia or neuropathic pain has developed. This type of pain results from injured nerve, and analgesic treatment in these cases can be challenging.[35,36] Among 44 breast cancer patients with definite (31 patients) or probable (13 patients) brachial plexopathy, 9 of the 17 patients (53%) treated with radiation therapy improved.[6] Among patients in whom radiation therapy was no longer a therapeutic option because of prior radiation therapy, the yield from systemic therapies was low: 2 of 7 patients responded to hormonal therapy and only one of six patients responded to chemotherapy.

Radiation Injury to the Brachial Plexus

PATHOPHYSIOLOGY OF RADIATION INJURY

The peripheral nervous system has been thought to be relatively radioresistant, but a series of experimental studies have demonstrated that, under certain conditions, the peripheral nerves are sensitive. Sensitivity to a given dose of radiation depends on several factors: age, the radiation dose, the size of the port, and especially, the premorbid state of the irradiated nerve.[37] In cases of radiation injury to the brachial plexus, the predominant findings are in the upper plexus. When the anatomic relation of the brachial plexus to the surrounding lymph nodes is considered, these findings are not surprising. In 73 of 78 patients with metastatic plexopathy in the Kori series,[3] the initial tumor was located in an area that drains into the lateral group of axillary lymph nodes, which is in close contact with the division of the lower trunk of the plexus, whereas the upper trunk and its divisions are remarkably free of lymph nodes. Thus, when metastatic plexopathy is a result of the spread of tumor through lymphatics, the roots affected are C-8 and T-1. On the other hand, the divisions of the lower trunk run a shorter course through the radiation port, are partially protected by the clavicle, and are less likely to be damaged by irradiation than are the divisions of the upper trunk.

There are three possible types of peripheral nerve damage after radiation therapy.[38] First, a high dose of radiation may cause direct damage to a segment of a nerve trunk or may injure the nerve trunk by causing severe vascular damage. This type of peripheral nerve damage occurs within months to years after irradiation. Second, a peripheral nerve trunk situated within intact tissue that is treated by high-dose radiation can be damaged but only if extensive fibrosis of the adjacent and overlying connective tissues has been present for many years. Finally, a peripheral nerve trunk situated in tissue previously subjected to surgical dissection also can be damaged by a course of irradiation after extensive fibrosis of the adjacent connective tissues has been present for a period of a few months to a few years. The trauma of surgically removing subcutaneous and connective tissues, irradiation, and the subsequent decreased vascularity are all contributing factors in facilitating the development of early and extensive fibrosis of the adjacent connective tissues around the nerve trunk. This fibrosis and decreased vascularity over months to years can destroy peripheral nerves and prevent the regeneration of their proximal normal portions. The degree of connective tissue injury at the time of or preceding radiation therapy may be important in influencing the subsequent development of connective tissue fibrosis.

Three distinct clinical syndromes of brachial plexopathy related to radiation therapy have been reported in patients with breast cancer: (1) reversible or transient brachial plexopathy, (2) radiation fibrosis or radiation injury to the brachial plexus, and (3) acute ischemic brachial plexopathy.[3,4,31,39] All three are uncommon clinical entities, each with a characteristic clinical presentation and course.

TRANSIENT RADIATION INJURY

A transient brachial plexopathy has been described in breast cancer patients immediately after radiation therapy to the chest wall and adjacent nodal areas. In retrospective studies, the incidence of this phenomenon has been variably estimated as 1.4% to 20%[6,31]; clinical experience suggests that lower estimates are more accurate. In a review of 565 patients who were treated with moderate doses (5000 cGy in 5 weeks) of supervoltage radiation therapy, Salner and coworkers[31] identified 8 (1.4%) patients with transient brachial plexopathy, with the onset of symptoms occurring 3 to 14 months after irradiation (median, 4.5 months). The clinical symptoms included paresthesias in the arm and hand, and, less commonly, weakness and pain. Seven of 8 patients received adjuvant chemotherapy; in 6 patients, symptoms began after drug treatment. There was a temporal clustering of these cases, suggesting a neurotropic viral component. The symptoms and signs of paresthesias and weakness did not conform to any anatomic pattern, but most commonly affected the distribution of the lower plexus. Weakness occurred in 5 of 8 patients, and was profound in 2 of them. All patients regained full strength. In 3 patients, residual paresthesias persisted. Fulton[6] retrospectively evaluated 63 patients with breast cancer treated with radiation therapy to the chest wall and adjacent nodal areas, including the brachial plexus, and reported radiation-induced plexopathies in 19, 14 of whom had transient plexopathy and 5 of whom had a permanent plexopathy. He suggested that transient plexo-

pathy did not seem to predispose patients to the development of a radiation-induced permanent plexopathy. In a long-term follow-up of 1624 patients, Pierce and colleagues[40] found that radiation-induced plexopathy was transient in 16 of the 20 cases identified. Mild symptoms, with minimal pain and weakness, were predictive of resolution.

RADIATION FIBROSIS

Radiation fibrosis of the brachial plexus results in progressive and irreversible neurologic dysfunction of the brachial plexus. This entity has been well described in the literature.[3,4,6,37,41–46] The risk of development of chronic brachial plexopathy has been variably estimated as 0.6% to 14%.[3,4,9,10,31,43,47,48]

Symptoms usually develop months to years after radiation therapy,[4,43,49] although in many cases no latency is apparent.[45,50] In the Kori series,[3] the interval from the last dose of radiation to the first symptoms of plexus disorder in patients with radiation fibrosis ranged from 3 months to 26 years (median, 4 years; average, 5.5 years). Kori and coworkers[3] observed that 5 of the 7 patients who received radiation therapy because of local disease developed radiation damage within 1 year, whereas 13 of 15 patients who received radiation therapy to the plexus as prophylaxis developed symptoms after 1 year. No good explanation exists for this finding.

Scheduling factors associated with an increased relative risk of subsequent plexopathy include high total dose[44] and larger fraction size (more than 1900 rad/d).[45,47,51,52] Powell and others[49] compared the incidence of radiation-induced brachial plexopathy in 449 patients who had been randomized to either 4600 rad in 15 fractions or 5400 rad in 27 to 30 fractions. The incidence of radiation plexopathy was only 1% in the high-dose–small-fraction group compared with 5.9% in the low-dose–large-fraction cohort, thus concluding that fractional dose is the major scheduling risk factor.[49] Other factors associated with an increased relative risk include younger age of treatment[45,50] and concurrent cytotoxic therapy.[6,40,45]

Clinical Features

Although pain is a presenting symptom in less than 20% of patients with radiation injury to the brachial plexus, its prevalence increases with time.[3,45,46,50] The pain is commonly described as mild discomfort associated with aching pain in the shoulder or hand. At the time of diagnosis, 65% of patients report discomfort or pain in the arm; in 35% it is severe.[3] Other symptoms include paresthesias in the entire hand in over 50% of affected patients, swelling and heaviness of the arm in 50% of patients, and proximal weakness of the arm in the deltoid distribution in all patients.[3] The paresthesias are commonly reported to occur in the thumb and forefinger but often involve the entire hand. These symptoms often are confused with carpal tunnel syndrome but can be differentiated clinically and by electrodiagnostic studies.

Motor weakness typically involves the muscles innervated by the upper plexus alone or both the upper and lower plexus.[3,4,6,7,10,43,45,50] Weakness in a distribution of the lower plexus is uncommon,[45,50] and Horner syndrome is rarely observed.[7,10,45,50] Lymphedema of the ipsilateral arm was observed in 16 of 22 of patients with radiation fibrosis in the Kori series[3] and in a substantial proportion of those reported by others.[4,7] Olsen and associates[50] found that lymphedema is a common late consequence of radiation therapy that occurs in about 25% of patients, and that it was not predictive of brachial plexus fibrosis. Radiation skin changes were noticed in about one third of the patients with radiation injury, but these changes were not predictive of an underlying plexopathy.[3] Osteoradionecrosis of the ribs and rarely of the humeral head can be observed on plain radiographs.[42]

The natural history of brachial plexus fibrosis is variable. Sensorimotor dysfunction may be incomplete or may progress to a severe paresis.[45,46,50] Even with advanced radiation fibrosis, severe pain is relatively uncommon and its presence should prompt evaluation of the patient for recurrent tumor.[3]

RADIATION-INDUCED ACUTE ISCHEMIC BRACHIAL PLEXOPATHY

Gerard and colleagues[39] have reported a case of subclavian artery occlusion occurring 19 years after a patient with breast cancer was treated with 4000 rad to the breast and axillary area after radical mastectomy. The patient's symptoms occurred acutely after carrying a heavy object and holding her left arm outstretched above the shoulder. A painless weakness developed rapidly in the left arm, with temperature change evolving over the ensuing days. She was evaluated neurologically 2 months later, at which time she had atrophy and fasciculations of the interosseous muscles with distal weakness, grade 3/5, of the entire hand, and the flexor of the wrist and fingers, and 4/5 weakness of the extensors of the wrist and proximal muscles of the arm. Reflexes were absent and she had decreased sensation to pin, light touch, and temperature in the hand and light touch in the entire forearm. Painless induration was present over the left supraclavicular fossa; humeral, radial, and cubital pulses were absent. Electrical studies did not demonstrate any myokymic discharges, and the left paracervical muscles were normal. CT and MRI of the left axillary region and cervical spine gave normal results, as did evaluation of the cerebrospinal fluid. Angiography showed segmental occlusion of the left subclavian artery with collateral revascularization. The lesion seemed to be acute in onset and was nonprogressive and painless, in contrast to the typical progressive nature of radiation fibrosis and the associated pain in up to 35% of patients in that group. At least one other case with this unusual entity has been reported by Mumenthaler and associates.[53]

ELECTRODIAGNOSTIC PROCEDURES

Electrodiagnostic procedures in patients with radiation fibrosis have been demonstrated to show signs of fibrillation and positive waves associated with denervation. Widespread myokymia is strongly suggestive of radiation-induced plexopathy.[10–13,54] Roth and associates[54] electrodiagnostically assessed a patient with radiation fibrosis after radiation therapy for breast cancer who had clinical myokymia, cramps, and pain. They related the myokymia to the existence of a persistent conduction block of several years' duration. Streib and others[55] also reported conduction blocks in two patients treated for breast cancer. Plexus exploration in one of the patients did not reveal constrictive connective tissue or other sources of nerve entrapment. The exact cause of conduction block is not fully understood.

H reflexes of the flexor carpi radialis muscle were studied in 52 controls and 25 cancer patients with radiation-induced brachial plexopathy. In the symptomatic arm, the H-reflex conduction velocity was decreased in 13 patients. Three patients showed H-reflex latency differences in the median nerve.[56]

In a separate study, median sensory-evoked potentials could not distinguish between patients with brachial plexus dysfunction from tumor infiltration and those with radiation fibrosis, but they could detect abnormal nerve function.[14]

RADIOGRAPHIC FINDINGS

The typical appearance of radiation fibrosis of the plexus on CT is a diffuse infiltration and loss of tissue planes without a mass lesion.[9] There is often associated lymphedema in the arm, evident on CT, and occasionally, radiation necrosis of the clavicle or rib or humeral head occurs at the adjacent level.[42] Tumor infiltration of the plexus cannot be differentiated from radiation fibrosis by CT when diffuse infiltration is present. MRI using T1- and T2-weighted images may distinguish radiation changes in bone and soft tissue by their low signal intensity on T2-weighted images. As described earlier, a hyperintense appearance on T2-weighted images of a mass in the brachial plexus is characteristic of tumor infiltration and is less frequently seen with radiation fibrosis.[24] Plain radiographs of the chest and spine may be useful in demonstrating radiation fibrosis of the apex of the lung, clavicle, or both, and rib erosion from radiation necrosis.

TREATMENT

Managing patients with radiation fibrosis begins with the establishment of an accurate diagnosis to rule out metastatic disease. No methods have been proven to reverse neurologic damage. Splinting the arm at the chest wall, preventing subluxation of the shoulder joint, and using intensive physical therapy to manage lymphedema[57,58] are common approaches to managing the musculoskeletal pain syndromes associated with this disorder. Some authors have suggested the use of neurolysis with pedicle omentoplasty to treat radiation fibrosis.[56,59–61] Cumulative anecdotal data suggest that this procedure frequently results in reduced pain and that progression of neurologic deficit can be arrested in some cases.[46,56,59–61] In the largest series, Le Quang[56] reported on 60 patients observed from 2 to

9 years and advocated early surgery as soon as possible after the onset of paresthesias. Surgical exploration of the brachial plexus is difficult, and further injury to the nerve may be associated with a worsening pain syndrome after surgically induced nerve injury.[62] Further studies are necessary to assess the usefulness of this technique to preserve neurologic function and to treat pain.

Other Causes of Brachial Plexopathy and Neuropathic Arm Pain

SECOND PRIMARY TUMORS

Uncommonly, a malignant peripheral nerve tumor or a second primary tumor in a previously irradiated site can account for pain recurring late in the patient's course.[63,64] Primary tumors of the brachial plexus are uncommon,[65,66] and nerve sheath tumors that occur years after radiation therapy are generally thought to be a late effect of the therapy.[63,67]

CARPAL TUNNEL SYNDROME

Among patients with medical histories of breast cancer who were referred for evaluation of arm pain, 4 of 30 were found to have carpal tunnel syndrome.[7] Although electrophysiologic abnormalities that are consistent with carpal tunnel syndrome occur twice as frequently ipsilateral to the resection among women who have undergone mastectomy,[68] it is an infrequent cause of arm pain in this population and the diagnosis requires demonstration of a prolonged sensory latency that is greater than that recorded for the median and ulnar nerves.[69,70]

LYMPHEDEMATOUS BRACHIAL PLEXUS COMPRESSION

Some authors have suggested that lymphedema alone can produce a compression injury of the brachial plexus.[7,68] Ganel and coworkers[68] performed a series of electromyographic studies on women who had undergone mastectomies with or without subsequent radiation therapy. On the basis of an increased prevalence of F-wave latency abnormalities ipsilateral to previous mastectomy in women with lymphedema, he proposed that the lymphedema may indeed cause an entrapment brachial plexopathy. Vecht[7] inferred this diagnosis in one of 28 patients evaluated for arm pain on the basis of normal results on imaging studies and a nonprogressive neurologic deficit in a patient with lymphedema. In the absence of demonstrable reversibility of the neurologic deficit with effective management of the lymphedema, or surgical evaluation of the plexus to exclude recurrent tumor or radiation fibrosis, this diagnosis should be approached with clinical skepticism.

When to Explore the Plexus

The differential diagnosis of tumor infiltration of the brachial plexus, especially as distinguished from radiation injury to the plexus, is generally based on the clinical criteria (Table 23.4-1). However, if these diagnostic approaches fail to define the nature of the neurologic disorder, exploration of the plexus should be considered. Such exploration is rarely undertaken. The following circumstances may lead to the need to explore the plexus:

1. The computed tomographic and MRI results are normal or show no evidence of change from before the onset of symptoms in a patient with progressive pain, neurologic deficit, or both.
2. The site of neurologic involvement is certain (eg, a lesion that can be localized to either the upper or lower plexus). This factor is important in determining the appropriate surgical approach. Upper plexus dysfunction may best be assessed through a supraclavicular approach, whereas involvement of the lower plexus is best assessed through a posterior scapular approach or a high posterior thoracotomy, commonly used to explore apical tumors of the lung.[71]
3. A work-up including tumor markers to establish the full extent of disease has been completed and shows no evidence of diffuse metastatic disease.
4. The onset of symptoms and signs occurs several years after completion of successful antitumor therapy, or treatment for the presumed primary tumor does not appear to be effective.

In a study to assess the role of brachial plexus exploration in defining the cause of the patient's pain and neurologic deficit, Payne and Foley[64] reported a patient with breast cancer who had been previously irradiated to the brachial plexus for extraneural disease who developed pain and weakness in her left upper extremity. Radiographic studies demonstrated evidence of radiation fibrosis in the apex of the lung, but all other studies demonstrated no evidence of breast tumor recurrence. Biopsy of the area of radiation fibrosis revealed adenocarcinoma of the lung as the cause of the patient's progressive plexopathy.

In a second patient with pain and progressive plexopathy and negative radiologic studies, exploration of the plexus revealed no evidence of tumor. About 3 months later the patient developed evidence of a chest wall recurrence and subsequently died of widely metastatic breast cancer. The autopsy showed diffuse infiltration of the brachial plexus as the cause of the patient's symptoms and signs.

In the Kori study,[3] no adverse effects of surgical exploration of the plexus occurred, but the procedure requires an expert surgeon who can carefully distinguish fibrous tissue from nerve tissue using intraoperative neurophysiologic techniques. If the patient is stable neurologically, careful follow-up is the reasonable approach.

TABLE 23.4-1

Causes of Brachial Plexopathy in Patients With Breast Cancer: Distinguishing Clinical Features

Feature	Tumor Infiltration	Radiation Fibrosis	Transient Radiation Injury	Acute Ischemic Injury
Incidence of pain	80%	18%	40%	Painless
Location of pain	Shoulder, upper arm, elbow, 4th and 5th fingers	Shoulder, wrist, hand	Hand, forearm	Hand, forearm
Nature of pain	Dull ache in shoulder, lancinating pains in elbow and ulnar aspect of hand; occasional paresthesias and dysesthesias	Ache in shoulder; prominent paresthesias in C5-6 distribution of hand and arm	Ache in shoulder; prominent paresthesias in C5-6 distribution of hand and arm	Paresthesias in C5-6 distribution of hand and arm
Severity	Moderate to severe (severe in 98%)	Usually mild to moderate (severe in 20%–35%)	Mild	Mild
Course	Progressive neurologic dysfunction: atrophy and weakness in C7-T1 distribution, persistent pain; occasional Horner syndrome	Progressive weakness; panplexus or upper plexus distribution; Horner syndrome uncommon	Transient weakness with complete resolution	Acute nonprogressive weakness and sensory loss
Study findings				
Magnetic resonance imaging	High signal intensity mass on T2-weighted images; may enhance with gadolinium	Low signal intensity lesion on T2-weighted images; generally nonenhancing with gadolinium	No data	Normal
Computed tomography	Mass: circumscribed or diffuse tissue infiltration	Diffuse tissue infiltration	Normal	Angiography demonstrates subclavian artery segmental obstruction
Electromography	Segmental slowing	Diffuse myokymia	Segmental slowing	Segmental slowing

Management of Pain Associated With Brachial Plexopathy

ANALGESIC PHARMACOTHERAPY

An approach to the management of brachial plexus pain is illustrated in Figure 23.4-4. Primary antitumor therapies should be considered for patients with tumor invasion of the brachial plexus. All patients with pain should initially be treated with analgesic pharmacotherapy in accordance with the World Health Organization's Three-Step Analgesic Ladder.[72]

OPIOIDS IN THE MANAGEMENT OF BRACHIAL PLEXUS PAIN

A trial of opioid therapy should be administered to all patients with pain of moderate or greater severity, irrespective of the pathophysiologic mechanism underlying the pain.[73–76] Patients who present with severe pain usually are treated with an opioid customarily used in step 3 of the analgesic ladder. Patients with moderate pain are commonly treated with a combination product containing acetaminophen or aspirin plus a conventional step 2 opioid (codeine, dihydrocodeine, hydrocodone, oxycodone, and propoxyphene).[72,77]

The doses of these combination products can be increased until the maximum dose of the nonopioid coanalgesic is attained (eg, 3000 mg acetaminophen); beyond this dose, the opioid contained in the combination product could be increased as a single agent, or the patient could be switched to an opioid conventionally used in step 3.

Opioids should be administered by the least invasive and most convenient route capable of providing adequate analgesia for the patient. In routine practice, the oral route is usually the most appropriate. Parenteral routes of administration should be considered for patients who have impaired swallowing or gastrointestinal obstruction, those who require the rapid onset of analgesia, and highly tolerant patients who require doses that cannot otherwise be conveniently administered.

Patients with continuous or frequently recurring pain generally benefit from scheduled around-the-clock dosing. All patients who receive an around-the-clock opioid regimen also should be offered a rescue dose, which is a supplemental dose given on an as-needed basis to treat pain that breaks through the regular schedule. The rescue drug is typically identical to that administered on a continuous basis, with the exception of transdermal fentanyl and methadone; the use of an alternative short half-life opioid is recommended for the rescue dose when these drugs are used. Patient-controlled analgesia is a technique of

FIGURE 23.4-4 An approach to the management of pain associated with brachial plexopathy. (Adapted from Cherry NI, Portenoy RK. Cancer pain management: current strategy. Cancer [Suppl] 1993;72:3393)

parenteral drug administration in which the patient controls a pump that delivers bolus doses of an analgesic according to parameters set by the physician.

Patients in severe pain who are opioid-naive generally should begin one of the opioids conventionally used for severe pain at a dose equivalent to 5 to 10 mg intramuscular morphine every 3 to 4 hours. If a switch from one opioid

drug to another is required, the equianalgesic dose table (Table 23.4-2) is used as a guide to the starting dose. The persistence of inadequate pain relief should be addressed through a stepwise escalation of the opioid dose until adequate analgesia is reported or unmanageable side effects supervene. The severity of the pain should determine the rate of dose titration. An understanding of the strategies used to prevent or manage common opioid toxicities is needed to optimize the balance between analgesia and side effects.

ADJUVANT ANALGESICS

Even with optimal management of adverse effects, some patients do not attain an acceptable balance between pain relief and side effects. Several types of noninvasive interventions—including adjuvant analgesics, a switch to another opioid, and the use of psychologic, physiatric, or noninvasive neurostimulatory techniques—should be considered for their potential to improve this balance by reducing the opioid requirement. Adjuvant analgesics are drugs that have a primary indication other than pain but that have analgesic effects in some painful conditions. The use of adjuvant analgesics can contribute substantially to the successful management of pain caused by brachial plexopathy. Numerous drugs are used empirically for this indication, including selected antidepressants, oral local anesthetics, anticonvulsants, and others. For drug selection, it is useful to distinguish between continuous and lancinating neuropathic pain based on the patient's history and physical examination[78] (Table 23.4-3).

ANESTHETIC AND NEUROSURGICAL TECHNIQUES

Invasive anesthetic and neurosurgical techniques should be considered only for patients who are unable to achieve a satisfactory balance between analgesia and side effects from systemic analgesic therapies. Techniques such as intraspinal opioid and local anesthetic administration, intrapleural local anesthetic,[79] or intraventricular opioid administration[80] can potentially achieve this end without compromising neurologic integrity. The use of neurodestructive procedures such as brachial plexus blockade,[81-84] chemical or surgical rhizotomy, or a dorsal root entry zone lesion[85,86] should be based on an evaluation of the likelihood and duration of analgesic benefit, the immediate and long-term risks, the likely duration of survival, and the anticipated length of hospitalization. Patients rarely are treated with a forequarter amputation of the limb for relief of the discomfort of a lymphedematous, functionless arm. Although this approach is not successful in providing significant pain relief, it does improve patient complaints of a heavy, lymphedematous, useless extremity.

MANAGEMENT SUMMARY

- Early diagnosis of tumor infiltration of the brachial plexus is important to prevent the development of chronic neuropathic pain and neurologic dysfunction.
- Evaluation consists of a careful history, a detailed neurologic examination, and MRI or computed to

TABLE 23.4-2
Opioids Conventionally Used in the Management of Severe Pain: Step 3 of the Analgesic Ladder

Drug	Dose (mg) Equianalgesic to 10 mg IM Morphine		Half-Life (h)	Duration of Action (h)	Comments
	IM	PO			
Morphine	10	30 (repeated dose) 60 (single dose)	2–3	3–4	M6G accumulation in renal failure may predispose to additional toxicity; wide range of formulations; on WHO essential drug list
Oxycodone	15	30	2–3	2–4	Formulated as single agent; can be used for severe pain
Hydromorphone	1.5	7.5	2–3	2–4	Wide range of formulations; useful in the elderly
Methadone	10	20	15–190	4–8	Plasma accumulation may lead to delayed toxicity; dosing should be initiated on a PRN basis
Meperidine	75	300	2–3	2–4	*Not recommended for cancer pain;* normeperidine toxicity limits use; contraindicated in patients with renal failure and those receiving MAO inhibitors
Oxymorphone	1	10 (PR)	2–3	3–4	No oral formulation available; less histamine release than other opioids
Levorphanol	2	4	12–15	4–8	Plasma accumulation may lead to delayed toxicity
Fentanyl transdermal system	†	—	—	48–72	Patches available to deliver 25, 50, 75 and 100 μg/h

IM, intramuscularly; MAO, monoamine oxidase; PO, orally; PR, per rectum; WHO, World Health Organization.

† Transdermal fentanyl, 100 μg/h.

(Adapted from Cherny NI, Portenoy RK. Cancer pain management: current strategy. Cancer 1993;72(Suppl):3393)

mographic imaging. Electrodiagnostic studies should be performed if the radiographic studies are normal on examination of soft tissue and bony disease. An evaluation to assess for evidence of metastatic disease should follow and, if results are normal, surgical exploration should be considered to allow for biopsy of adjacent lymph nodes and soft tissue if patients are neurologically progressive.

- In patients who have brachial plexopathy after previous radiation therapy, the history and physical findings and follow-up on CT and MRI may be helpful to distinguish tumor recurrence from radiation fibrosis, but none of these may be definitive. Surgical exploration may be considered if the diagnosis will affect the treatment decision, for example, in a patient with progressive symptoms of brachial plexopathy but without other evidence of distant metastases, in whom documentation of recurrent disease will result in a decision to initiate anti-cancer treatment.

TABLE 23.4-3
Guide to the Selection of Adjuvant Analgesics for Neuropathic Pain Based on Clinical Characteristics

Continuous Pain	Lancinating Pain
Antidepressants	Anticonvulsant drugs
Amitriptyline	Carbamazepine
Doxepin	Phenytoin
Imipramine	Clonazepam
Desipramine	Valproate
Nortriptyline	Baclofen
Trazodone	
Maprotiline	
Paroxetine	
Oral local anesthetics	
Mexiletine	
Clonidine	

(Adapted from Cherny NI, Portenoy RK. Cancer pain management: current strategy. Cancer 1993;72(Suppl):3393)

References

1. Clouston P, De Angelis L, Posner JB. The spectrum of neurologic disease in patients with systemic cancer. Ann Neurol 1992;31:268.
2. Gonzales GR, Elliot KJ, Portenoy RK, et al. The impact of a comprehensive evaluation in the management of cancer pain. Pain 1991;47:141.
3. Kori SH, Foley KM, Posner JB, et al. Brachial plexus lesions in patients with cancer 100 cases. Neurology 1981;31:45.
4. Bagley FH, Walsh JW, Cady B, et al. Carcinomatous versus radiation induced brachial plexus neuropathy in breast cancer. Cancer 1978;41:2154.

5. Tsairis P, Dyck PJ, Mulder D, et al. Natural history of brachial plexus neuropathy. Arch Neurol 1972;27:109.

6. Fulton DS. Brachial plexopathy in patients with breast cancer. Dev Oncol 1987;51:249.

7. Vecht CJ. Arm pain in the patient with breast cancer. J Pain Sympt Manage 1990;5:109.

8. Son Y. Effectiveness of irradiation therapy in peripheral neuropathy caused by malignant disease. Cancer 1967;20:1447.

9. Cascino TL, Kori S, Krol G, et al. CT scan of brachial plexus in patients with cancer. Neurology 1983;33:1553.

10. Lederman RJ, Wilbourn AJ. Brachial plexopathy: recurrent cancer or radiation? Neurology 1984;34:1331.

11. Harper CM, Thomas JE, Cascino TL, et al. Distinction between neoplastic and radiation-induced brachial plexopathy, with emphasis on EMG. Neurology 1989;39:502.

12. Albers JW, Allen AH, Bashow JA, et al. Limb myokymia. Muscle Nerve 1981;4:494.

13. Flaggman PD, Kelly JJ. Brachial plexus neuropathy: an electrophysiological evaluation. Arch Neurol 1980;37:160.

14. Rappaport S, Stacy C, Foley KM. Median nerve somatosensory-evoked potentials are useful in the diagnosis of metastases to the brachial plexus and adjacent spinal roots and epidural space. Ann Neurol 1983;14:143.

15. Cooke J, Powell S, Parsons C. The diagnosis by computerized tomography of brachial plexus lesions following radiotherapy for carcinoma of the breast. Clin Radiol 1988;39:602.

16. Cooke J, Cooke D, Parsons C. The anatomy and pathology of the brachial plexus as demonstrated by computerized tomography. Clin Radiol 1988;39:595.

17. Shea WJ, de-Greer G, Webb WR. Chest wall after mastectomy. Part II. CT appearance of tumor recurrence. Radiology 1987;162:162.

18. Gilbert RW, Kim JH, Posner JB. Epidural spinal cord compression from metastatic tumor: diagnosis and treatment. Ann Neurol 1978;3:40.

19. Hagen N, Stulman J, Krol G, et al. The role of myelography and magnetic resonance imaging in cancer patients with symptomatic and asymptomatic epidural disease. Neurology 1989;39:309.

20. Hagenau C, Grosh W, Currie W, et al. Comparison of spinal magnetic resonance imaging and myelography in cancer patients. J Clin Oncol 1987;5:1663.

21. Krol G. Evaluation of neoplastic involvement of brachial and lumbar plexus: imaging aspects. J Back Musculoskel Rehab 1993;3:35.

22. Kanner R, Martini N, Foley KM. Nature and incidence of postthoracotomy pain. (Abstract) Proc Amer Soc Clin Oncol 1982;1:590.

23. de Verdier HJ, Colletti PM, Terk MR. MRI of the brachial plexus: a review of 51 cases. Comput Med Imag Graph 1993;17:45.

24. Posniak HV, Olson MC, Dudiak CM, et al. MR imaging of the brachial plexus. Am J Roentgenol 1993;161:373.

25. Portenoy RK, Lipton RB, Foley KM. Back pain in the cancer patient: an algorithm for evaluation and management. Neurology 1987;37:134.

26. Stark RJ, Henson RA, Evans SJW. Spinal metastases: a retrospective survey from a general hospital. Brain 1982;105:189.

27. Svensson WE, Mortimer PS, Tohno E, et al. The use of colour Doppler to define venous abnormalities in the swollen arm following therapy for breast carcinoma. Clin Radiol 1991;44:249.

28. Rissanen TJ, Makarainen HP, Mattila SI, et al. Breast cancer recurrence after mastectomy: diagnosis with mammography and US. Radiology 1993;188:463.

29. Walsh J, Dixon JM, Paterson D, et al. Color doppler studies of axillary nodes in patients with breast cancer. Proceedings of the 50th Annual Congress of the British Institute of Radiology, May 18–20, 1992, Birmingham, UK, 1992:142.

30. Tohnosu N, Okuyama K, Koide Y, et al. A comparison between ultrasonography and mammography, computed tomography and digital subtraction angiography for the detection of breast cancers. Surg Today 1993;23:704.

31. Salner AL, Botnick L, Hertzog AG, et al. Reversible transient plexopathy following primary radiation therapy for breast cancer. Cancer Treat Rep 1981;65:797.

32. Ampil FL. Radiotherapy for cacinomatous brachial plexopathy: a clinical study of 23 cases. Cancer 1985;56:2185.

33. Ettinger AB, Portenoy RK. The use of corticosteroids in the treatment of symptoms associated with cancer. J Pain Sympt Manage 1988;3:99.

34. Nisce LZ, Chu FC. Radiation therapy of brachial syndrome from breast cancer. Radiology 1968;91:1022.

35. Portenoy RK. Issues in the management of neuropathic pain. In: Basbaum A, Besson J-M, eds. Towards a new pharmacotherapy of pain. New York, John Wiley & Sons, 1991:393.

36. Hanks GWC, Portenoy RK, MacDonald N, et al. Difficult pain problems. In: Doyle D, Hanks GW, MacDonald N, eds. Oxford textbook of palliative medicine. Oxford, Oxford University, 1993:257.

37. Maruyama Y, Mylrea MM, Logothetis J. Neuropathy following irradiation. Am J Roentgenol 1967;101:216.

38. Cavanagh JB. Effects of x-irradiation on the proliferation of cells in peripheral nerve during wallerian degeneration in the rat. Br J Radiol 1968;41:275.

39. Gerard JM, Franck N, Moussa Z, et al. Acute ischemic brachial plexus neuropathy following radiation therapy. Neurology 1989;39:450.

40. Pierce SM, Recht A, Lingos TI, et al. Long-term radiation complications following conservative surgery (CS) and radiation therapy (RT) in patients with early stage breast cancer. Int J Radiat Oncol Biol Phys 1992;23:915.

41. Stoll BA, Andrews JT. Radiation induced peripheral neuropathy. Br Med J 1966;1:834.

42. Schulte RW, Adamietz IA, Renner K, et al. Humeral head necrosis following irradiation of breast carcinomas: a case report. Radiology 1989;29:252.

43. Thomas JE, Colby MY. Radiation-induced or metastatic brachial plexopathy? JAMA 1972;222:1392.

44. Basso-Ricci S, della Costa C, Viganotti G, et al. Report on 42 cases of post-irradiation lesions of the brachial plexus and their treatment. Tumori 1980;66:117.

45. Olsen NK, Pfeiffer P, Johannsen L, et al. Radiation-induced brachial plexopathy: neurological follow-up in 161 recurrence-free breast cancer patients. Int J Radiat Oncol Biol Phys 1993;26:43.

46. Killer HE, Hess K. Natural history of radiation-induced brachial plexopathy compared to surgically treated patients. J Neurol 1990;237:247.

47. McDermott RS. Cobolt 60 beam therapy: post-radiation effects in breast cancer patients. Can Assoc Radiol J 1971;22:195.

48. Uematsu M, Bornstein BA, Recht A, et al. Long-term results of postoperative radiation therapy following mastectomy with or without chemotherapy in stage I–III breast cancer. Int J Radiat Oncol Biol Phys 1993;25:765.

49. Powell S, Cooke J, Parsons C. Radiation induced brachial plexus injury: follow-up of two different fractionation schedules. Radiother Oncol 1990;18:213.

50. Olsen NK, Pfeiffer P, Mondrup K, et al. Radiation-induced brachial plexus neuropathy in breast cancer patients. Acta Oncol 1990;29:885.

51. Svensson H, Westling P, Larson LG. Radiation-induced lesions of the brachial plexus correlated to dose time fraction schedule. Acta Radiol Ther Phys Biol 1975;14:228.

52. Cohen L, Svenssen H. Cell population kinetics and dose–time relationship for post-radiation injury of the brachial plexus in man. Acta Radiol Oncol 1978;17:161.

53. Mumenthaler M, Narakas A, Billiat RW. Brachial plexus disorders.

In: Dyke JP, Thomas PK, Lambert EH, et al., eds. Peripheral neuropathy, vol 2. Philadelphia, WB Saunders, 1987:1384.

54. Roth G, Magistris MR, Le-Fort D, et al. Postradiation brachial plexopathy: persistent conduction block: myokymic discharges and cramps. Rev Neurol 1988;144:173.

55. Streib E, Sun SF, Leibrock L. Brachial plexopathy in patients with breast cancer: unusual electromyographic findings in two patients. Eur Neurol 1982;21:256.

56. Le Quang C. Postirradiation lesions of the brachial plexus: results of surgical treatment. Hand Clin 1989;5:23.

57. Brennan MJ. Management of lymphedema: review of pathophysiology and treatment. J Pain Symp Manage 1992;7:110.

58. Casley-Smith JR, Casley-Smith JR. Modern treatment of lymphoedema. I. Complex physical therapy: the first 200 Australian limbs. Australas J Dermatol 1992;33:61.

59. Narakas AO. Operative treatment for radiation-induced and metastatic brachial plexopathy in 45 cases, 15 having an omentoplasty. Bull Hosp Joint Dis Orthop Inst 1984;44:354.

60. Uhlschmid G, Clodius L. A new use for the freely transplanted omentum: management of a late radiation injury of the brachial plexus using freely transplanted omentum and neurolysis. Chirurgie 1978;49:714.

61. Brunelli G, Brunelli F. Surgical treatment of actinic brachial plexus lesions: free microvascular transfer of the greater omentum. J Reconstr Microsurg 1985;1:197.

62. Match RM. Radiation-induced brachial plexus paralysis. Arch Surg 1975;110:384.

63. Foley KM, Woodruff JM, Ellis FT. Radiation-induced malignant and atypical peripheral nerve sheath tumors. Arch Neurol 1980;7:311.

64. Payne R, Foley KM. Exploration of the brachial plexus in patients with cancer. Neurology 1986;36(Suppl 1):329.

65. Sharma BS, Banerjee AK, Kak VK. Malignant schwannoma of brachial plexus presenting as spinal cord compression. Neurochirurgia 1989;32:189.

66. Horowitz J, Kline DG, Keller SM. Schwannoma of the brachial plexus mimicking an apical lung tumor. Ann Thorac Surg 1991;52:555.

67. Aho KA, Sainio K. Late irradiation-induced lesions of the lumbosacral plexus. Neurology 1983;33:953.

68. Ganel A, Engel J, Sela M, et al. Nerve entrapments associated with postmastectomy lymphedema. Cancer 1979;44:2254.

69. Dawson DM. Entrapment neuropathies of the upper extremity. N Engl J Med 1993;329:2013.

70. Stevens JC. AAEE minimonograph #26: the electrodiagnosis of carpal tunnel syndrome. Muscle Nerve 1987;10:99.

71. Kline DG, Kott J, Barnes G, et al. Exploration of selected brachial plexus lesions by the posterior subscapular approach. J Neurosurg 1978;48:842.

72. World Health Organization. Cancer pain relief. Geneva, World Health Organization, 1986.

73. McQuay HJ, Jadad AR, Carroll D, et al. Opioid sensitivity of chronic pain: a patient controlled analgesia method. Anaesthesia 1992;47:757.

74. Jadad AR, Carroll D, Glynn CJ, et al. Morphine responsiveness of chronic pain: double blind randomised crossover study with patient controlled analgesia. Lancet 1992;339:1367.

75. Portenoy RK, Foley KM, Inturrisi CE. The nature of opioid responsiveness and its implications for neuropathic pain: new hypotheses derived from studies of opioid infusions. Pain 1990;43:273.

76. Cherny NI, Thaler HT, Friedlander-Klar H, et al. Opioid responsiveness of cancer pain syndromes caused by neuropathic or nociceptive mechanisms: a combined analysis of controlled single dose studies. Neurology 1994;44:857.

77. World Health Organization. Cancer pain relief and palliative care. Geneva, World Health Organization, 1990.

78. Portenoy RK. Adjuvant analgesics in pain management. In: Doyle D, Hanks GW, MacDonald N, eds. Oxford textbook of palliative medicine. Oxford, Oxford University, 1993:187.

79. Myers DP, Lema MJ, de Leon-Casasola OA, et al. Intrapleural analgesia for the treatment of severe cancer pain in terminally ill patients. J Pain Sympt Manage 1993;8:505.

80. Crammond T, Stuart G. Intraventricular morphine for intractable pain of advanced cancer. J Pain Sympt Manage 1993;8:465.

81. Kaplan R, Aurenello Z, Pfisterer W. Phenol brachial plexus block for upper extremity cancer pain. Reg Anesth 1988;13:58.

82. Neill RS. Ablation of the brachial plexus: control of intractable pain due to a pathological fracture of the humerus. Anaesthesia 1979;34:1024.

83. Mullin V. Brachial plexus block with phenol for painful arm associated with Pancoast's syndrome. Anesthesiology 1980;53:431.

84. Swerdlow M. Neurolytic blocks of the neuraxis. In: Patt RB, ed. Cancer pain. Philadelphia, JB Lippincott, 1993:427.

85. Sindou M, Fobe JL. Rhizotomies and dorsal route entry zone lesions in the management of cancer related pain. In: Arbit E, ed. Management of cancer-related pain. Mount Kisko, NY Futura, 1993:341.

86. Zeidman SM, Rossitch EJ, Nashold BSJ. Dorsal root entry zone lesions in the treatment of pain related to radiation-induced brachial plexopathy. J Spinal Disord 1993;6:44.

23.5
Ocular Metastases From Breast Cancer
BERYL McCORMICK

The most common malignant lesion of the human eye is metastatic cancer. In most series of ocular metastases, the primary lesion with the highest incidence of spread to this site is breast carcinoma.[1-7] Through 1976, the question of whether metastatic disease or primary cancer represented the most common ocular malignancy was still a subject of debate.[8] As autopsy studies[2,9] and results of systematic ocular examinations[1] in cancer patients replaced series of case reports in the ophthalmic literature, however, the predominance of metastatic cancer eventually became evident.

Incidence

In an autopsy study confined to examination of the globe in patients dying of cancer, Bloch and Gardner[2] found that 37% of the 52 patients in their series with breast cancer had ocular metastases. In studies reviewing the incidence of breast cancer to both the orbital soft tissues and the globe, a slight but consistent trend is found in favor of more frequent metastases to the choroid or middle layer of the globe than to other areas of the orbit.[1-5,10]

Table 23.5-1 shows the percentage of cases with breast cancer in series of patients with ocular metastases. The first four cited studies list the incidence for both orbital soft tissue disease and intraocular disease, with a ratio of about 4:5. The last three confine themselves to the globe only. With the exception of the Nelson study,[9] the incidence ranges from 40% to 70%. Unlike the others, the Nelson study[9] included patients with leukemia and lymphomas as well as solid tumors.

Stephens and Shields,[7] in a study of 70 patients referred with ophthalmologic symptoms, made special mention of the multiple lesions observed in patients with breast cancer primaries. The observation of bilateral ocular metastatic involvement also is not surprising; this ranges from 22% in the Stephens and Shields[7] series up to 41% in the observations of Mewis and Young[11] and of Rottinger and others.[12]

Simultaneous involvement of the central nervous system and the eye with metastases is common. Because of therapeutic implications, once ocular metastasis has been diagnosed, computed tomography (CT) or magnetic resonance imaging (MRI) should be performed to rule out concomitant CNS involvement. Maor and colleagues[13] documented that 3 of 42 patients with choroidal metastases from breast cancer also had brain metastases; Mewis and Young[11] found that 30 patients (41%) had CNS involvement. In the 30 patients in their series, 15 patients had concurrent involvement, 13 had subsequent involvement, and just 2 had prior involvement.

Breast cancer is also the most likely tumor to metastasize to the eyelids. In a series by Riley[14] combining his results and Mayo Clinic data, 38% of all metastatic lesions in the eyelids were from breast cancer.

The symptoms of choroid metastases that bring the woman to the ophthalmologist include decreased visual acuity and, less frequently, pain, headache, and photophobia.[4–7,15,16] The most important test in establishing the diagnosis is indirect funduscopic examination. According to Reese[17] findings include detachment of the retina, usually posteriorly. The detachment itself is described as having a pinkish white color fading "off into the surrounding normal-appearing retina. Frequently the surface of the tumor had a mottled appearance. Over the involved area there may be an occasional hemorrhage and some pigmentary changes."[17] Reese noticed a grayish or yellowish color to the lesions and, on occasion, multiple foci. For single lesions, this appearance is like that seen with a primary ocular melanoma. Ultrasound is useful in distinguishing the two, with malignant melanomas characteristically showing low reflectivity in the A scan, whereas metastatic tumors lack this pattern. Fluorescein angiograms are useful in evaluating retinal disturbance that may not be clinically evident. Shields[18] also finds value in fluorescein angiography in differentiating choroidal metastases from benign processes, such as hemorrhage, inflammation, and neovascular membranes. Because of the small size of the lesions and nonspecific character of detachments, MRI[20] or CT is not as useful in establishing a differential diagnosis but is helpful in treatment planning.

For patients with metastatic disease to the orbital soft tissues, the most common presenting symptoms are proptosis, ptosis, pain, diplopia, and clinical evidence of a mass.[4–6,16] Rarely a scirrhous carcinoma may cause retraction of the soft tissues and enophthalmos.[20] Imaging of the orbits by contrast-enhanced CT[20] or MRI is essential in work-up of orbital metastases.

Diagnosis

The median time from diagnosis of a primary breast cancer to the development of choroidal metastasis is between 3 and 4 years,[10,15,16] and is the first sign of metastatic spread in about 20% of the patients.[10,15]

Treatment and Prognosis

Appropriate treatment for most ocular metastases is a course of external-beam radiation therapy. This treatment is noninvasive and well tolerated by the patients.

TABLE 23.5-1
Incidence of Ocular Metastases in Patients With Breast Cancer

Investigators	Breast Cancer in Series (%)	Patient Base	Sites
Glassburn et al[5]	49	Radiation referrals	Orbit + globe
Freedman et al[4]	49	Ophthalmic referrals	Orbit + globe
Albert et al[1]	70	Ophthalmic screen	Orbit + globe
Ferry[3]	40	Pathologic ophthalmic registry	Orbit + globe
Stephens & Shields[7]	65	Ophthalmic referrals	Uveal tract
Nelson et al[9]	10	Autopsy	Globe
Bloch and Garner[2]	68	Autopsy	Globe

Treatment planning for patients with choroidal metastases consists of careful review of the ophthalmologist's examination notes and a head CT or MRI. The presence or absence of brain metastases and bilateral disease must be established before the treatment-planning process. Because of the multifocal nature of breast cancer in the eye, the goal of treatment planning is to design a field that encompasses all of the choroid from the equator posteriorly, with a margin. Except in unusual cases of more anteriorly located metastases, radiation to the lens can be avoided by using a lateral field with D-shaped blocks similar to that used in retinoblastoma designed at the time of simulation.[21] Photons with some skin sparing are appropriate for this treatment. In departments in which only high-energy photons are available, the CT or MRI must be evaluated for globe location to ensure that the lateral choroid region is beyond the buildup region of the beam.

Acutely, the patient's vision may deteriorate during or just after the radiation treatments because of shifting subretinal fluid and retinal detachment at this time. Table 23.5-2 shows the results of external-beam radiation therapy in four series of choroid metastases from breast cancer. In the Chu series,[15] doses ranged from 2000 cGy in 2 weeks to 5000 cGy in 5 weeks. In the Mewis and Young series,[11] doses delivered were consistent, ranging from 2500 to 3000 cGy in 10 fractions. The Thatcher series[22] looked at dose–response and documented a threshold dose equivalent of 3250 cGy associated with a complete response. In that series, the median time for improvement was 4 weeks from the start of radiation (range, 4 days to 10 weeks). A fifth series by Maor and others[13] also demonstrated a dose–response curve. In that study, three fraction schemes were used (2500 cGy in 5 fractions, 2500 cGy in 10 fractions, or 3000 cGy in 10 fractions). A response was seen in all patients treated, but those treated at the lower doses later relapsed in the eye.[13]

For patients with orbital soft tissue metastases, a wedged-pair arrangement of photon beams is appropriate in almost all instances. The target volume should include the contents of the bony orbit. Patients with orbital metastases tend to live longer those with choroid metastases.

Freedman and Folk[4] documented a median survival time for breast cancer patients with choroid metastases of 314 days, compared with 794 days for those with orbital metastases, although Ratanatharathorn and coworkers[10] in a small study found the opposite. The anticipated side effects of external-beam radiation include periorbital edema, excessive tearing, and radiation-related inflammation of the conjunctiva. Corneal irritation and dry eye rarely are seen at the doses used in this palliative setting. Radiation-induced cataracts develop late in the lens, because with a wedged-pair field arrangement, this structure cannot be shielded without introducing a lens block that will also shield the target. Because of the increased normal tissue complications and the longer survival time in these patients, a dose of 4000 cGy in 3.5 to 4 weeks is recommended for this group.

Gragoudas[23] recommends using the proton beam for treating selected patients with metastatic disease to the choroid. With limited follow-up, results seem equal, but not superior, to conventional external-beam therapy. Response of choroidal metastases also has been documented in patients receiving endocrine or chemotherapy. Most of these reports are in patients with multiple sites of metastases that require systemic treatment. If a patient can be carefully observed by her ophthalmologist and exhibits no progression of disease, such treatment is appropriate.[24–26] In patients with limited sites of metastases or in whom visual deterioration is noticed, however, external-beam therapy remains the treatment of choice to stabilize and improve these symptoms.

MANAGEMENT SUMMARY

- If metastases are present in the eyes and brain, the limits of the disease must be established.
- Growth of ocular metastases must be assessed in relation to any systemic therapy the patient may have been taking at the time of the diagnosis.
- For cases of progressive visual symptoms, the patient should be referred for palliative external-beam radiation therapy.

TABLE 23.5-2
*Results of External-Beam Radiation Therapy for Choroid Metastases From Breast Cancer**

Investigators	No Response or Stable (%)	PR (%)	CR (%)
Chu et al[15]	37	28	35
Mewis & Young[11]	67	27 (PR + CR)	
Rottinger et al[12]	11	8	62
Thatcher & Thomas[22]	20	51	26

CR, complete response; PR, partial response.

* This structure cannot be shielded without introducing a lens block that will also shield the target.

References

1. Albert DM, Rubenstein RA, Scheie HG. Tumor metastasis to the eye. Part 1. Incidence in 213 adult patients with generalized malignancy. Am J Ophthalmol 1967;63:723.
2. Bloch RS, Garner S. The incidence of ocular metastatic carcinoma. Arch Ophthalmol 1971;85:673.
3. Ferry AP. The biological behavior and pathological features of carcinoma metastatic to the eye and orbit. Trans Am Ophthalmol Soc 1973;71:373.
4. Freedman MI, Folk JC. Metastatic tumors to the eye and orbit. Arch Ophthalmol 1987;105:1215.
5. Glasburn JR, Klionsky M, Brady LW. Radiation therapy for metastatic disease involving the orbit. Am J Clin Oncol 1984;7:145.
6. Reddy S, Saxena VS, Hendrickson F, et al. Malignant metastatic

disease of the eye: management of an uncommon complication. Cancer 1981;47:810.

7. Stephens RF, Shields JA. Diagnosis and management of cancer metastatic to the uvea: a study of 70 cases. Ophthalmology 1979;86:1336.

8. Francois J, Hanssens H, Verbraeken H. Intraocular metastasis as first sign of generalized carcinomatosis. Ann Ophthalmol 1973;8:405.

9. Nelson CC, Hertzberg BS, Klintworth GK. A histopathologic study of 716 unselected eyes in patients with cancer at the time of death. Am J Ophthalmol 1983;95:788.

10. Ratanatharathorn V, Powers WE, Grimm J, et al. Eye metastasis from carcinoma of the breast: diagnosis, radiation treatment and results. Cancer Treat Rev 1991;18:261.

11. Mewis L, Young SE. Breast carcinoma metastatic to the choroid: analysis of 67 patients. Ophthalmology 1982;89:147.

12. Rottinger EM, Heckemann R, Scherer E, et al. Radiation therapy of choroidal metastases from breast cancer. Arch Ophthalmol 1976;200:243.

13. Maor M, Chan RC, Young SE. Radiotherapy of choroidal metastases: breast cancer as a primary site. Cancer 1977;40:2081.

14. Riley FG. Metastatic tumors of the eyelids. Am J Ophthalmol 1970;69:259.

15. Chu FCH, Huh SH, Nisce LZ, et al. Radiation therapy of choroid metastases from breast cancer. Int J Radiat Oncol Biol Phys 1977;2:273.

16. Dobrowsky W. Treatment of choroid metastases. Br J Radiol 1988;61:140.

17. Reese AB: Neoplastic metastasis to the eye and orbit. In: Tumors of the eye, ed 2. New York, Harper & Row, 1963:496.

18. Shields JA. Metastatic tumors of the uvea and retina. In: Shields JA ed. Diagnosis and management of intraocular tumors. St Louis, CV Mosby, 1983:278.

19. Wilms G, Marchal G, Van Fraeyenhoven L, et al. Shortcomings and pitfalls of ocular MRI. Neuroradiology 1991;33:320.

20. Hesselink JR, Davis KR, Weber AL, et al. Radiological evaluation of orbital metastases, with emphasis on computed tomography. Radiology 1980;137:363.

21. McCormick B, Ellsworth RE, Abramson D, et al. Radiation therapy for retinoblastoma: comparison of results with lens sparing versus lateral beam techniques. Int J Radiol Oncol Biol Phys 1988;15:567.

22. Thatcher N, Thomas PRM. Choroidal metastases from breast carcinoma: a survey of 42 patients and the use of radiation therapy. Clin Radiol 1975;26:549.

23. Gragoudas ES. Current treatment of metastatic tumors. Oncology 1989;3:103.

24. MacMichael IM. Management of choroidal metastases from breast cancer. Br J Ophthalmol 1969;53:782.

25. Letson AD, Davidorf FH, Bruce RA. Chemotherapy for treatment of choroidal metastases from breast carcinoma. Am J Ophthalmol 1982;93:102.

26. Brinkley JA. Response of a choroidal metastasis to multiple-drug chemotherapy. Cancer 1980;45:1538.

23.6
Local Treatment of Bone Metastases

ALAN D. AARON ▪ L. CANDICE JENNINGS ▪ DEMPSEY S. SPRINGFIELD

Bone metastasis is a significant problem for a large number of cancer patients. Up to 85% of patients who die of breast, prostate, or lung carcinoma primary tumors have bone involvement at autopsy.[1] Osseous involvement often results in pain, difficulty in ambulation, and a diminishment in a patient's quality of life. Pathologic fractures are debilitating and often result in decreased survival for otherwise stable patients. Patient survival varies widely in patients with metastatic bone disease. Patients with metastatic breast disease survive an average of 34 months once the first metastasis is detected (range, 1 to 90 months).[2] Survival with metastatic prostate cancer averages 24 months, whereas lung cancer patients have a more dismal prognosis of less than 1 year.[1] Most patients with metastatic bone disease are eligible for treatment, whether it be chemotherapy, radiation, or surgical intervention. An understanding of the pathophysiology, clinical presentation, and implications of tumor progression on local bone strength aids the clinician in directing treatment.

Pathophysiology

Metastasis involves a cascade of linked sequential steps that must be traversed before a neoplastic cell successfully establishes a secondary tumor in a distant bony site. Most neoplastic cells at the primary site contain deficient genomes and are unable to initiate distant metastatic spread.[1,3] Two theories of bone metastasis often are cited: the anatomic–mechanical theory proposed by Ewing,[4] and the seed and soil hypothesis of Paget.[5] The mechanistic approach states that metastasis develops in the first organ of tumor cell delivery. This has been graphically demonstrated by Batson[6] using injection studies in primates, which defined a valveless paravertebral venous plexus emanating from the pelvis. Mapping of this plexus was highly predictive for the bony metastatic spread of prostate carcinoma. Increased abdominal pressure or recumbency increases retrograde flow because of the plexus' valveless nature. A similar plexus has been identified in the shoulder girdle and correlated with the bony metastatic spread of breast carcinoma.[6] Although this anatomic approach plays a role in bone metastasis, it is viewed as oversimplified. To accommodate the apparent organ specificity of some metastatic carcinomas, a second theory is under investigation: chemotaxis and osteotropism.

Certain cancers clearly exhibit osteotropism and, predictably, metastasize to bone. Most (80%) such cancers are of the breast, prostate, lung, thyroid, or kidney.[7] The rate of metastasis at autopsy is estimated to be between 37% and 84%, with most emanating from either the breast or prostate.[7] Chemotaxic factors have been isolated and are hypothesized to play a role in directing circulating tumor cells to bone. Animal models of bone metastasis have been developed to study these factors. One such model is the Walker 256 murine carcinoma, a cell line that is predictably metastatic to bone in rats.[8] Bone matrix proteins, such as type I collagen and transforming growth factor β (TGF-β), have been reported to stimulate Walker 256 cell motility and chemotaxis in vitro.[9]

Clinical reports of patients with both Paget disease and metastatic carcinoma describe an increased metastasis rate to pagetoid bones.[10] Modulation of increased bone turnover can affect metastatic rates and has been tested in vivo using the Walker carcinoma rat model. Rice H-500 Leydig cell tumor cells were used to stimulate bone resorption with increased osteoclast number and activity. In Leydig tumor–bearing rats, metastatic deposition of Walker 256 cells adjacent to trabecular bone increased by more than 50%.[8] Conversely, inhibition of bone mineralization, such as with etidronate, reduces the rate of bone metastasis in this model.[11,12] In vitro studies using prostate cancer cell lines have reported increased cellular growth in response to growth factors produced by bone fibroblasts.[13] In this study, lung, normal rat kidney, and NIH 3T3 fibroblastic cell–generated conditioned media were not found to be mitogenic, whereas a bone-derived fibroblast growth factor stimulated prostate cancer cell growth by 180%.[13] Studies also report increased prostate cancer cell proliferation in response to conditioned media from human bone marrow.[14] Although not fully developed, in vivo metastatic models of human breast cancer using nude mice are under study. Intraarterial inoculation into the left ventricle of mice has been shown to reliably result in widespread bony metastasis.[15,16] Quantification and characterization of these systems holds promise for better chemotherapeutic or immunologic modalities to control metastatic dispersal and progression in distant osseous sites. The anatomic–mechanistic and the chemotaxic–osteotropism theories both explain aspects of bone metastasis without being mutually exclusive.

Clinical Presentation and Diagnosis

Patients with bone metastasis frequently come to the clinician with pain. It is characteristically described as dull in character, gradually progressive in intensity, and constant in presentation. Night pain and pain not relieved by rest are especially worrisome. Bone pain often is referred to adjacent joints with delays in diagnosis resulting from inadequate radiographic evaluation. Spinal involvement often presents with localized back pain. Extremity paresthesia from nerve root compression, and especially bladder and bowel impairment or complete paralysis from spinal cord compression, is uncommon. Biochemical tests are not demonstrative of microscopic bony metastatic progression in patients with breast cancer, because the alkaline phosphatase is elevated in only 32% to 53% of patients.[17] When a history of carcinoma exists, plain radiographs of the involved extremity and a bone scan to define the extent of disease are indicated.[18] Although an initial bone scan is performed to adequately stage the disease, radiographic screening of patients with known breast cancer primaries is of little benefit. One study reviewed the results of intensive screening using mammography, chest roentgenography, and bone scanning every 6 months in 1243 consecutive breast cancer patients.[19] Although earlier detection of metastatic disease was demonstrated, this did not affect the overall 5-year survival rate.[19]

Most neoplasms are characterized radiographically by regions of lytic bone destruction, with most of the prostate and about 15% of breast metastases demonstrating sclerotic foci (Fig. 23.6-1). Bone destruction by neoplastic cells results either from direct bone destruction or from secondary bone resorption.[20–22] Studies using the 256 Walker rat model have identified several local factors secreted by neoplastic cells that modulate bone resorption. Osteoclast activity factor, prostaglandins (particularly PGE-2), and epidermoid growth factor have all been implicated in tumor-directed bone resorption from multiple myeloma and metastatic carcinoma[20] (Fig. 23.6-2). Bone sclerosis results mostly from bone formation in response to heightened bone resorption. Stromal bone formation, as evidenced with prostate cancer, can occur to some degree, with ossification of fibrous stromal tissue via intramembranous bone formation.[21,22] In addition, TGF-β, a modulator of fracture repair, has also been implicated in the production of bone in prostatic metastatic deposits.[23]

Radiographs need not be obtained of all additional sites identified on bone scan; however, radiographs should be performed on all painful upper extremity and all lower extremity lesions to evaluate fracture risk. Patients with polyostotic disease and a known primary neoplasm often can be treated without obtaining a biopsy. However, careful observation is needed, with needle biopsy being reserved for patients who do not respond predictably to treatment. This is especially important because a small number of patients may present with multiple metastatic sites and two different primary carcinomas. Needle biopsy is preferred to open procedures because it is minimally invasive and can be performed on an outpatient basis. Lesions that are at risk for fracture can be addressed with surgical stabilization at the time of biopsy, if the results of frozen section confirm carcinoma or metastatic sarcoma. Monostotic lesions, especially in patients younger than 40 years of age, are at increased risk to be a primary sarcoma and need to undergo imaging before biopsy. Computed tomography (CT) or magnetic resonance imaging (MRI)

FIGURE 23.6-1 Lytic breast carcinoma metastasis residing in the proximal femur. Local bone destruction without sclerotic bone production and absence of periosteal reaction are characteristic of osseous metastasis.

is needed to clearly elucidate the full extent of the lesion for proper biopsy planning.[18] A well-planned biopsy is critical in case surgical resection is necessary later and should be performed by a surgeon who will be involved with future definitive surgery. Biopsy incisions generally need to be longitudinal and planned along the lines of a possible larger surgical resection. The biopsy should pass through a single compartment and not violate any neurovascular structures. Drains, when used, are brought out of the incision, and meticulous hemostasis must be obtained before closure, even if a tourniquet is used.

Treatment

Treatment of bone metastasis is aimed at relieving pain, preventing development of pathologic fractures, enhancing mobility and function, and thereby improving survival.[7] Unfortunately, the cause of bone pain subsequent to tumor destruction is poorly understood, with pain resulting from direct tumor progression or biomechanical

weakness from bone loss being the most likely causes. Some reports indicate that this pain is primarily because of perineoplastic soft tissue edema and inflammation. In addition, it has been hypothesized that chemical factors (ie, bradykinin, substance P, and histamines) from damaged bone tissue stimulate the endosteal nerve fibers' pain receptors.[24]

Radiation is effective in alleviating bone pain from tumor progression. Radiation generally is the first treatment employed, especially for solitary metastasis. About 90% of patients experience at least minimal relief of pain, and 54% to 66% obtain complete relief.[7,25] The reason for this response is unknown but has been hypothesized to be because of tumor shrinkage or inhibition of the release of chemical pain mediators from normal bone cells. The speed by which patients respond to radiation therapy varies from days to weeks and does not adhere to a dose–response curve. Early responders (ie, those who respond in less than 2 weeks) probably gain most of their pain relief from a rapid reduction in periosseous inflammation. Late responders may exhibit symptomatic relief because of ossification of weakened regions of bone.[26]

Radiation therapy can be delivered as a single dose or over several days as a fractionated dose. The advantages of single-dose therapy are lower cost and ease of delivery for patients. Comparisons of several retrospective studies demonstrate no appreciable difference in pain relief or relapse rates between these two modalities. A prospective, randomized study by Price and associates[27] confirms these findings by comparing a single treatment of 8 Gy with a fractionated dose of 3 Gy given over 2 weeks (10 treatments).

If single dosing is used, a dose of between 6 and 8 Gy has been recommended by several authors. Hoskin and colleagues[28] report on 270 patients in a prospective randomized trial comparing single-dose delivery of 4 and 8 Gy for bone pain resulting from metastasis. At 4 weeks, the response rates for doses of 4 and 8 Gy were 44% and 69%, respectively. Even though the authors recommend the delivery of 8 Gy when using a single-dose regimen, patients with reduced tolerance could gain adequate control with a single dose of 4 Gy.[28]

Painful relapse because of biomechanical weakness should be treated with operative stabilization. In cases of recurrent tumor growth without compromise of bone strength, retreatment with radiation has been proven to be effective. In a study encompassing 280 sites, 57 sites were retreated once, with 8 being treated a second time.[29] Although a range of dose fractionation schedules was used, 87% of patients achieved measurable pain relief with retreatment.[29]

Multiple lesions require a different approach, which includes medical treatment (hormonal or chemotherapy, radionuclide, or diphosphonate therapy) or radiation therapy (multiple-site or half-body irradiation [HBI]). An extensive review of the use of radionuclides and diphosphonates is given in Chapter 22. Multiple-site and HBI have been reported to be equally effective in controlling the pain related to widespread metastatic disease. Tong and coworkers[26] effectively treated multiple lesions with multi-

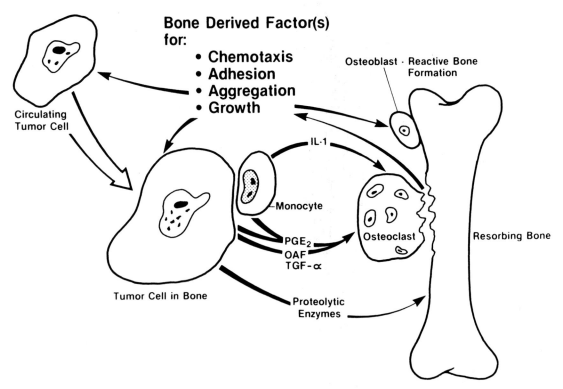

FIGURE 23.6-2 Postulated interrelation between neoplastic cells, host elements, and bone resorption. TGF-α, transforming growth factor α. PGE₂, prostaglandin E₂; OAF, osteoclast-activating factor; IL-1, interleukin-1. (Manishen WJ, Sivananthan K, Orr FW. Resorbing bone stimulates tumor cell growth: a role for the host microenvironment in bone metastasis. Am J Pathol 1986;123:39).

ple separate fields in doses ranging from 15 to 30 Gy. Rapid relief of pain was reported with patients treated with 15 Gy over 1 week, and patients who received 25 to 30 Gy over 2 weeks demonstrated reduced benefit.[26]

HBI usually is applied as a single dose ranging from 6 to 10 Gy, with 60% to 80% of patients gaining pain relief within 2 days of treatment.[30] Acute toxicity, usually manifested as nausea, vomiting, or diarrhea, is commonly seen but is transient and disappears within a few days after treatment. Hematologic toxicity peaks after 2 to 3 weeks, with normal function being restored in most cases after 4 to 6 weeks. Doses greater then 8 Gy increase toxicity considerably, with lower doses being well tolerated. The concomitant administration of chemotherapy can heighten these side effects. Hospitalization is required for upper torso HBI while hydration, antiemetics, and corticosteroids are administered to minimize side effects. Lower torso HBI is more easily tolerated and does not require hospitalization. No studies have compared separate multiple-site treatment with HBI in a prospective, randomized manner.[30]

In lesions responsive to systemic treatment, controlling pain with either hormonal or chemotherapeutic treatment is preferred. One third of unselected women with metastatic breast cancer benefit from hormonal therapy, and at least half of women with hormone receptor–positive tumors respond to hormonal manipulation.[31]

The biomechanical implications of lytic metastasis are profound, even with small cortical defects. Cortical perforations are divided into two categories: stress risers and open-section defects. Stress risers are defined as perforations measuring less than the cross-sectional width of the bone, with open-section defects being considered larger than the local bone diameter. Stress risers decrease torsional rigidity by 60%, with open-section defects further compromising bone strength by almost 90%.[32] A cortical perforation results in a concentration of forces at the edge of the defect because of an asymmetrical redistribution of the stresses experienced during walking (Fig. 23.6-3). Pathologic fractures result if these forces overcome the fatigue strength of the bone cortex.[32]

Structural weakness because of extensive bone destruction is not immediately reversed after medical or radiation treatment, with bone regeneration often being impeded by these modalities. Radiation therapy has been reported to actually increase fracture risk in high doses. In a comparison of two fractionated regimens, a higher fracture rate was reported with doses of 40 Gy (18%) compared with 20 Gy (4%).[26] In such cases, an approach that supports the bone during recovery often is necessary. Upper extremity lesions often can be protected with orthotic devices. Humeral lesions residing in the diaphysis are amenable to lightweight functional bracing. Operative treatment should be reserved for patients with either extensive local

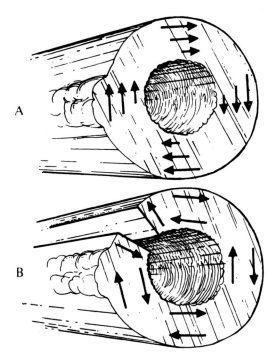

FIGURE 23.6-3 **A.** Under torsional loading, the distribution of shear stress in a cross-section of intact bone is symmetrical and linearly a function of the radius. **B.** An open-section defect causes a redistribution of stresses. Only the stress vectors at the periphery of the cross-section are able to resist the applied torsional load. Thus, an open-section defect severely reduces the ability of the bone to carry the torsional load. (Pugh J, Sherry HS, Futterman B, et al. Biomechanics of pathologic fractures. Clin Orthop 1982;169:109).

bone destruction or lower extremity involvement necessitating the use of an assistive device for ambulation, such as a cane or walker. The lower extremity is less tolerant, largely because of the high degree of stress experienced during ambulation. Impending fractures of the lower extremity generally require surgical stabilization with fracture-fixation devices or prosthetic reconstruction. The use of methylmethacrylate to reconstitute large bone defects permits immediate weight bearing in most cases. Methylmethacrylate maintains excellent rigidity, especially when compressively loaded, and is not adversely affected by radiation.[33]

The indications for prophylactic fixation of impending fractures have not been clearly defined; most of the criteria are generated from retrospective studies of plain radiographs.[7,34,35] Often-quoted radiographic criteria for an impending fracture, which have been cumulated from several studies, follow[7]:

- Cortical bone destruction of 50% or more
- Lesion of 2.5 cm or more in the proximal femur
- Pathologic avulsion fracture of the lesser trochanter.
- Persisting stress pain despite irradiation

These criteria are guidelines, not strict rules. One of the problems with plain radiographs is that bone loss must approach 30% to 50% before it becomes apparent. In addi-

tion, in metastatic lesions characterized by bone production (eg, prostate), clear evidence of bone destruction can be difficult to assess radiographically.

An objective evaluation of these criteria was undertaken in a study by Keene and others,[36] who focused only on breast cancer patients with proximal femoral lesions. In their study, critical dimensions for fracture based on lesion size and percentage of cortical involvement were not identifiable because of similar ranges between patients who experienced fracture and those who did not. The reliability of radiographic evaluation was questioned because lesion size could vary on any two radiographs of the same patient. Bone pain unresponsive to radiation also was evaluated and found not to correlate with fracture risk.[36] To address these inconsistencies, Mirels[37] proposed a scoring system for measuring the risk for pathologic fracture (Table 23.6-1). This system assigns a numerical score to four variables, with a cumulative score of 7 points or less indicating a low risk for fracture (5%). Scores of 9 and above have at least a 33% risk for fracture whereas a score of 8 is suggestive of a 15% fracture risk.[37] This type of scoring system holds the most promise for quantitatively predicting patients at risk for pathologic fractures, with further study being necessary.

Once a pathologic fracture has occurred, aggressive surgical management should be undertaken in most cases. The goals and benefits of rigid fixation of pathologic fractures include pain relief, resumption of ambulation, enhancement of survival, and improved fracture healing. Patients who are unstable medically or who have a life expectancy of less than 4 weeks are not considered surgical candidates. Habermann[34] found that 97% of patients had good to excellent pain relief after internal fixation or prosthetic replacement. Regaining ambulatory status is imperative for patient survival. Harrington[7] reported a success rate of 95% in returning his patients to prefracture ambulatory status with surgical intervention. With current methods, aggressive fracture fixation after pathologic fracture has led to an improved patient survival of 24.6 months, as opposed to survival for historic controls of 11.6 months.[7]

It has been well documented that radiation alone adversely affects fracture healing.[38] On the other hand, successful frac-

TABLE 23.6-1
Quantification of Fracture Risk

	Score		
Variable	1	2	3
Site	Upper limb	Lower limb	Peritrochanter
Pain	Mild	Moderate	Functional
Lesion	Blastic	Mixed	Lytic
Size*	$<1/3$	$1/3-2/3$	$>2/3$

* Expressed as a fraction of bone diameter.

(Mirels H. Metastatic disease in long bones. Clin Orthop 1989;249:256)

FIGURE 23.6-4 A. This patient, who complained of severe pain and inability to ambulate, presented with a large lytic metastasis residing in the left ischium and posterior acetabulum. **B.** CT scan showing a large soft tissue mass and extensive bone involvement with disruption of the acetabular wall. **C.** A cemented total hip arthroplasty with methylmethacrylate and Steinmann pin reconstruction of the acetabulum successfully alleviated the patient's pain and permitted ambulation with a cane.

ture healing is achieved in 90% of patients who survive longer than 6 months, who are surgically stabilized, and who receive a radiation dose of no more than 30 Gy.[39] Delayed fracture healing is a special problem in lesions located in the proximal femur, which is subjected to repeated high stress during weight bearing. One study reported a 44% implant failure rate for femoral lesions compared with an overall failure rate of 33% at 5 years in operatively stabilized pathologic fractures. Improper implant selection was the most frequent problem, with intramedullary fixation or prosthetic replacement augmented with methylmethacrylate being the most successful modality.[40] Periacetabular pelvic lesions are best treated with methylmethacrylate and Steinmann pin–augmented total hip replacement (Fig. 23.6-4). Iliac wing

lesions are best treated with radiation therapy, reserving surgical resection for patients with unrelenting pain resulting from a poor response to radiation therapy or a painful fracture nonunion.

The spine is the most common site for skeletal metastasis. Seventy percent of patients who die from cancer demonstrate vertebral metastasis on postmortem examination.[41] Neurologic signs, such as paraplegia, paraparesis, or sensory level abnormalities, suggest spine involvement but are not reliable. Initial radiographic evaluation generally includes plain radiographs and bone scintigraphy. CT or MRI of the spine is reserved for patients who have vertebral body compression of 50% or greater or neurologic involvement.

FIGURE 23.6-5 **A.** Patient experienced back pain and lower extremity paraparesis; a lateral roentgenogram demonstrates bony collapse with severe compression of the third lumbar vertebral body. **B.** Sagittal MRI revealed nerve root compression resulting from retropulsed tumor and bone fragments. **C.** Anterior vertebral corpectomy was performed, with spinal instrumentation and fusion using an iliac crest bone graft.

Once workup is complete, patients can be divided into five categories, depending on the extent of neurologic involvement or bone destruction[41]:

Category I—no significant neurologic involvement

Category II—bone involvement without collapse or instability

Category III—major neurologic compromise without bone involvement

Category IV—bony collapse without neurologic involvement

Category V—major neurologic impairment combined with vertebral collapse

Most patients fall into category I, II, or III and can be treated nonoperatively with chemotherapy, hormonal manipulation, or radiation. Operative treatment is reserved for patients with either bony collapse and instability (category IV) or with vertebral body collapse that results in retropulsion of bone and disc fragments directly into the cord (category V). The treatment of choice is anterior resection of the diseased vertebral body and reconstruction with bone graft, or methylmethacrylate and spinal instrumentation as needed[42] (Fig. 23.6-5). Advances in spinal instrumentation have resulted in better methods for the stabilization of vertebral body collapse from metastatic disease. Anterior cervical plates, titanium cages, and distraction rods, when used in conjunction with bone graft or cementation, have found wide applicability in cervical and thoracic reconstructions. Posterior instrumentation is occasionally necessary when extreme instability is apparent. The goal of surgery is to prevent neurologic compromise and restore ambulatory ability. At least 62% of initially paraplegic patients regain enough neurologic recovery to walk after surgical decompression. Patients who have rapid, as opposed to chronic, spinal cord compromise and paraplegia exhibit a poor prognosis for recovery of function.[41] Most patients, however, do not have this degree of neurologic compromise and respond well to radiation therapy or chemotherapy without surgery.

Radiation therapy and systemic treatment often provide patients with excellent pain relief and potentially slow the progression of local tumor growth. Surgery and postoperative irradiation should be considered in patients with lesions at risk for fracture. Although further elucidation of these criteria is necessary, various parameters can aid the clinician in selecting the most appropriate course of treatment. The operative management of pathologic fractures often is challenging and is best reserved for orthopedic surgeons familiar with techniques of pathologic fracture fixation. This is particularly true in cases of extensive acetabular and spinal involvement. Continued development of in vivo models of human breast metastasis will improve medical management options for retarding the progression of bone metastasis.

References

1. Nielson OS, Munro AJ, Tannock IF. Bone metastasis: pathophysiology and management policy. J Clin Oncol 1991;9:509.

2. Koenders PG, Beex LVAM, Kloppenborg PWC, et al. Human breast cancer: survival from first metastasis. Breast Cancer Res Treat 1992;21:173.

3. Fidler IJ, Radinsky R. Genetic control of cancer metastasis. J Natl Cancer Inst 1990;82:166.

4. Ewing J. Metastases. In: Neoplastic diseases: a textbook on tumors. Philadelphia, WB Saunders, 1928:77.

5. Paget S. The distribution of secondary growths in cancer of the breast. Lancet 1889;1:571.

6. Batson OV. The role of the vertebral veins in metastatic processes. Ann Intern Med 1942;16:38.

7. Harrington KD. Orthopaedic management of metastatic bone disease. St Louis, CV Mosby, 1988:7.

8. Orr FW, Kostenuik P, Sanchez-Sweatman OH, et al. Mechanisms involved in the metastasis of cancer to bone. Breast Cancer Res Treat 1993;25:151.

9. Magro C, Orr FW, Manishen WJ, et al. Adhesion, chemotaxis, and aggregation of Walker carcinosarcoma cells in response to products of resorbing bone. J Natl Cancer Inst 1985;74:829.

10. Powell N. Metastatic carcinoma in association with Paget's disease of bone. Br J Radiol 1983;56:582.

11. Bassani D, Sabatini M, Scanziani E, et al. Bone invasion by Walker 256 carcinoma, line A in young and adult rats: effects of etidronate. Oncology 1990;47:160.

12. Guaitani A, Sabatini M, Coccioli G, et al. An experimental rat model of local bone cancer invasion and its responsiveness to ethane-1-hydroxy-1,1-bis (phosphonate). Cancer Res 1985;45:2206.

13. Gleave M, Hsieh J, Gao C, et al. Acceleration of human prostate cancer growth in vivo by factors produced by prostate and bone fibroblasts. Cancer Res 1991;51:3753.

14. Chackal-Roy M, Niemeyer C, Moore M, et al. Stimulation of human prostatic carcinoma cell growth by factors present in human bone marrow. J Clin Invest 1989;84:43.

15. Aaron AD, Ergener J, Roach J, et al. Bone metastasis via arterial injection of human breast cancer in nude mice. Orthopedic Research Society, Orlando, February 1995.

16. Vershraegen CF, Kozielski T, Mendoza J. Development of a bone metastasis (M) model from a human breast carcinoma in the nude mouse. Proc Am Assoc Cancer Res 1993;34:70.

17. Coombs RC, Gazet JC, Ford HT, et al. Assessment of biochemical tests to screen for metastasis in patients with breast cancer. Lancet 1980;1:296.

18. Frassica FJ, Gitelis S, Sim FH. Metastatic bone disease: general principles, pathophysiology, evaluation, and biopsy. Instr Course Lect 1992;41:293.

19. Rosselli Del Turco M, Palli D, Cariddi A, et al. Intensive diagnostic follow-up after treatment of primary breast cancer: a randomized trial. National Research Council Project on Breast Cancer Follow-Up. JAMA 1994;271:1593.

20. Manishen WJ, Sivananthan K, Orr FW. Resorbing bone stimulates tumor cell growth: a role for the host microenvironment in bone metastasis. Am J Pathol 1986;123:39.

21. Galasko CSB. Mechanisms of lytic and blastic metastatic disease of bone. Clin Orthop 1982;169:20.

22. Mundy GR. Mechanisms of osteolytic bone destruction. Bone 1991;12(Suppl 1):1.

23. Harris SE, Harris MA, Mahy P, et al. Expression of bone morphogenetic protein messenger RNAs by normal rat and human prostate and prostate cancer cells. Prostate 1994;24:204.

24. Ford HT, Yarmolel JR. Radiation therapy-pain relief and recalcification. In: Stoll BA, Parbhoo S, eds. Bone metastasis: monitoring and treatment. New York, Raven; 1983:34.

25. Schocker JD, Brady LW. Radiation therapy for bone metastasis. Clin Orthop 1982;169:38.

26. Tong D, Gillick L, Hendrickson FR. The palliation of symptomatic

osseous metastases: final results of the Radiation Therapy Oncology Group. Cancer 1982;50:893.

27. Price P, Hoskins PJ, Easton D, et al. Prospective randomised trial of single and multifraction radiotherapy schedules in the treatment of painful bone metastasis. Radiother Oncol 1986;6:247.

28. Hoskins PJ, Price P, Easton D, et al. A prospective randomised trial of 4 Gy or 8 Gy single doses in the treatment of metastatic bone pain. Radiother Oncol 1992;23:74.

29. Mithal NP, Needham PR, Hoskins PJ. Retreatment with radiotherapy for painful bone metastases. Int J Radiat Oncol Biol Phys 1994;29:1011.

30. Salazar OM, Rubin P, Hendrickson FR, et al. Single-dose half-body irradiation for palliation of multiple metastases from solid tumors: final radiation therapy oncology group report. Cancer 1986;58:29.

31. Stoll BA. Natural history, prognosis, and staging of bone metastasis. In: Stoll BA, Parbhoo S, eds. Bone metastasis: monitoring and treatment, New York, Raven, 1983:1.

32. Pugh J, Sherry HS, Futterman B, et al. Biomechanics of pathologic fractures. Clin Orthop 1982;169:109.

33. Murray JA, Bruels MC, Lindberg RD. Irradiation of polymethylmethacrylate. J Bone Joint Surg 1974;56A:311.

34. Habermann ET. The pathology and treatment of metastatic disease of the femur. Clin Orthop 1982;169:70.

35. Parrish FF, Murray JA. Surgical treatment for secondary neoplastic fractures: a retrospective study of ninety-six patients. J Bone Joint Surg 1970;52A:665.

36. Keene JS, Sellinger DS, McBeath AA, et al. Metastatic breast cancer in the femur: a search for the lesion at risk for fracture. Clin Orthop 1986;203:282.

37. Mirels H. Metastatic disease in long bones. Clin Orthop 1989;249:256.

38. Bonarigo BC, Rubin P. Nonunion of pathologic fracture after radiation therapy. Radiology 1967;88:889.

39. Gainor BJ, Buchert P. Fracture healing in metastatic bone disease. Clin Orthop 1983;178:297.

40. Yazawa Y, Frassica FJ, Chao EYS, et al. Metastatic bone disease: a study of the surgical treatment of 166 pathologic humeral and femoral fractures. Clin Orthop 1990;251:213.

41. Harrington KD. Metastatic disease of the spine. J Bone Joint Surg 1986;68A:1110.

42. Clark CR, Keggi KJ, Panjabi MM. Methylmethacrylate stabilization of the cervical spine. J Bone Joint Surg 1984;66A:40.

23.7

Medical Treatment of Bone Metastases

RICHARD L. THERIAULT

Bone is the most common site of breast cancer metastases. Bone disease can be asymptomatic or can result in catastrophic disability. Clinically manifest bone metastasis presents most often as pain, which is either insidious in onset or precipitous, as with pathologic long bone fracture. Patients are often treated for nonspecific musculoskeletal pain for varied lengths of time before metastasis is diagnosed.

Metastases are most prevalent in bone marrow–rich areas of the skeleton, that is, the pelvis, axial vertebral skeleton, and proximal long bones; any skeletal site may be involved, however, including phalanges[1-3] (Table 23.7-1).[1-3] Specific sites of involvement may lead to recognized syndromes, such as base of skull or radicular syndromes, and may provide the impetus for preventive treatment for spinal cord compression, which can lead to paralysis.[4] Bone disease and resulting pain, pathologic fracture, neurologic compromise, and hypercalcemia are formidable clinical problems.[2]

Localization and Diagnosis

The concept that the development of bone metastases is not dependent on vascular circulation flow is supported by estimates of total marrow blood flow to the trabecular bone compartment and the limited vascularity of cortical bone. The vertebral veins are the unifying vascular network with an internal and external, cortical and extracortical, venous system.[5]

Although no good models of bone metastasis from breast cancer exist to track the anatomic development of disease, trabecular bone is involved most often, presumably by hematogenous dissemination of tumor emboli. Paracortical and trabecular tumor growth are believed to be stimulated by factors associated with normal bone remodeling. All histologic breast tumor types metastasize to bone. Bone metastasis can be diagnosed by radionuclide scanning before radiographic detection. Whereas scanning is sensitive, it lacks specificity, and bone radiographs have been reported to be more reliable in assessing response to therapy.[1] Although computed tomography has been suggested as a tool to assess bone disease, its expense and the variability in extent of bone disease do not make it a choice for screening.[6,7] It may show lytic and blastic cortical disease to advantage. Magnetic resonance imaging may be useful in demonstrating trabecular disease and is of value in detecting epidural disease extension, as well as spinal cord compression.[8]

Radiographically, bone metastasis from breast cancer most often appears lytic, followed in frequency by mixed osteolytic–osteoblastic and osteoblastic appearances.[2]

The development of bone metastasis is believed to be a multistep process. A framework for bone metastasis development is shown in Figure 23.7-1.

TABLE 23.7-1
Site of Bone Metastases in Breast Cancer

	Patients (%)		
	Hortobagyi et al[1]	Scheid et al[2]	Tubiana-Hulin[3]
Pelvis	54	79	31
Ribs	54	57	18
Thoracic spine	35	62	37
Lumbar spine	38	72	52
Skull	36	39	12
Cervical spine	24	30	11
Long bones	—	56	23

Bone Remodeling

Bone undergoes constant remodeling in response to mechanical, endocrine, and local environmental factors. Two essential cells participate in the remodeling process and constitute the remodeling unit.[9] The osteoblast is responsible for the production of new collagen matrix, as well as the proteins osteocalcin, osteopontin, and osteonectin. Osteopontin is a bone glycoprotein with an amino acid sequence identical to the fibronectin cell binding sequence. The observation that osteopontin promotes fibroblast and osteoblast attachment and spreading suggests that it serves as a cell attachment factor within bone.[10]

Osteocalcin, also known as bone Gla protein (γ-carboxyglutamic acid), is synthesized by osteoblasts in response to stimulation by 1,25-dihydroxyvitamin D_3.[10-13] It has been suggested to be a useful marker of bone repair in metastatic bone disease, including breast cancer and multiple myeloma.[14-16] Osteocalcin is the most abundant noncollagenous protein found in bone matrix.

Osteonectin also is found in abundance in bone matrix; however, it is not a bone-specific protein.[17,18] Most connective tissues synthesize osteonectin, and it is found in platelets from whence it is secreted into the serum during the clotting process.

The precise functions and cellular interactions of each of these proteins within the bone compartment continue to be actively studied. Specific roles for these in the development of metastasis have not been confirmed.

Osteoblast activation seems to occur sequentially and follows osteoclast activation and local bone dissolution. Osteoblasts are derived from hematopoietic precursors and have receptors for parathyroid hormone (PTH), vitamin D_3, epidermal growth factor, prostaglandins, and a variety of hormones, including estrogen and progesterone. Osteoblasts are necessary for osteoclast activation and functional bone dissolution.[9]

Osteoclasts are derived from the monocyte–macrophage cell line; are mobile within the confines of the skeleton; and respond to a variety of cytokines, both marrow and bone

derived, including macrophage colony-stimulating factor, granulocyte-macrophage colony-stimulating factor, transforming growth factors, and interleukin-6 (IL-6), all of which are produced by activated osteoblasts.[9,19-22] Osteoclasts directly dissolve bone at attachment sites in disparate parts of the skeletal framework. Multiple areas of bone remodeling at multiple skeletal sites is the strongest argument in favor of local factors being the major determinants of bone remodeling. Osteoclasts have receptors for calcitonin, which directly inhibits osteolysis.

The relation between osteoblastic and osteolytic activity is balanced in normal bone remodeling. Osteoblastic–osteolytic activity is said to be coupled. The uncoupling of bone remodeling, as may occur in metabolic bone disease such as osteoporosis, has its counterpart in bone me-

FIGURE 23.7-1 Bone metastasis development.

tastases wherein osteolytic or osteoblastic activity becomes predominant, resulting in defective bone formation.[24]

Tumor-derived products are believed to exert local effects on osteoblast−osteoclast cells, resulting in the radiographic appearance of metastatic breast disease. Lowik and coworkers[25] have demonstrated that PTH and PTH-like protein can stimulate IL-6 production by osteoblasts, which results in osteoclastogenesis. Whereas the predominant clinical picture in breast cancer is lytic disease, dysregulation of the bone remodeling unit may lead to any radiographic appearance.

Factors that activate osteoclasts, such as prostaglandin E and parathyroid hormone−related peptide (PTHrP), may be tumor cell−derived or locally derived factors of the cellular microenvironment, stromal, or endothelial cells; they include colony-stimulating factors, interleukins, and tumor necrosis factor.[26−29] In addition, endocrine effects of vitamin D and estrogens may play a role in the bone remodeling process of neoplastic-affected bone. Trabecular bone is an estrogen sensitive, dependent tissue; however, the target cell for estrogen action, the alteration in cytokine production engendered by estrogen, and the ultimate effect on bone remodeling are unknown.[19]

Tumor Products and Osteoclastic Activity

Breast cancer cells produce a variety of cytokines and growth factors that may influence osteoclast activity. These include PTHrP, transforming growth factor α,[30] prostaglandins (PGE_2), and interleukin-1. PTHrP production has been demonstrated in cultured breast cancer cells and in fresh tumor specimens.[31,32] Immunohistochemical and mRNA expression of PTHrP have been reported to be more common in cells that metastasize to bone.[33−35] Localization of PTHrP has been reported more frequently in bone metastases than other organ sites, suggesting a potential role of PTHrP in the osteotropism of breast cancer metastases.[33,36,37] In addition to direct or indirect effects on osteoclasts, breast cancer cell lines can synthesize factors that can influence osteoblast cells independent of osteoclasts.[29] A variety of other polypeptide bone−derived growth factors have the potential to influence the development of breast cancer metastases.[38] Included among these are fibroblast growth factor, transforming growth factor β, and insulin-like growth factor I.[39,40]

Bone Remodeling and Markers of Osteoclast−Osteoblast Function

The final common pathway for bone destruction is osteoclast activation.[41] Increased osteoclastic activity results in the dissolution of bone matrix. This process is dependent on a proton pump, which maintains an acidic environment at the site of osteoclast bone adherence. Dissolution of bone matrix releases into circulation the breakdown prod-

ucts of bone. Whereas an ideal marker of osteoblast or osteoclast activity has not been determined, the effects of metastatic cells on bone metabolism have been assessed with a number of biochemical and serum protein markers. Acid and alkaline phosphatase have been shown to be abnormally elevated in breast cancer patients with bone metastases.[42,43] Alkaline phosphatase from bone is osteoblast derived and therefore believed to reflect osteoblastic activity. Serum acid phosphatase is an osteoclast- and erythrocyte-derived enzyme. In the absence of red blood cell hemolysis, elevated levels of tartrate-resistant acid phosphatase reflect bone disease and osteolytic activity. Bone alkaline phosphatase may correlate with extent of disease, as determined by radionuclide bone scans and radiographs, as well as response to treatment.[44] However, its levels may be normal in patients with limited bone disease. The combination of alkaline phosphatase and serum osteocalcin has been reported to be an accurate predictor of therapeutic response in bone metastases from breast cancer.[45] CA 15-3, a human breast tumor−associated antigen defined by monoclonal antibodies to breast cancer cells and milk fat globule, has been reported to be a sensitive marker in breast cancer metastases. Its use has been proposed as a method of screening for bone metastases.[46] However, alkaline phosphatase and urinary hydroxyproline excretion may be more sensitive and specific for monitoring disease progress in bone metastases.[47] CA 15-3 has a lower sensitivity for bone metastasis detection than bone scintigraphy and may not reflect the presence of limited bone disease.[48]

Serum osteocalcin, a biologic marker of osteoblastic repair, has been used as an indicator of bone metastasis and as a monitor of disease response to therapy.[49−51]

Collagen type I is the only collagen found in bones and tendons. The carboxy terminal procollagen may be a marker of bone collagen synthesis, bone formation rate and, hence, osteoblastic activity. In a correlative study, Francini and colleagues[52] suggest that alkaline phosphatase, osteocalcin, and procollagen type I may be biologic markers of different stages of osteoblast activity. Procollagen I levels have been shown to correlate with the efficacy of strontium[89] treatment of painful bone metastases.[53]

Products of bone destruction have been measured in the urine and correlated with osteolytic (osteoclast) activity. The most frequently used, hydroxyproline, reflects bone collagen resorption but is not specific, and levels may be influenced by diet and soft tissue destruction by extraskeletal metastases.[54−56]

A urinary product of bone destruction, derived from the measurements of the cross-link proteins pyridinoline and deoxypyridinoline, has been reported to reflect osteolytic activity. These are released into circulation when the collagen matrix degrades during osteoclastic bone resorption.[57−60] Elevated levels of cross-links have been reported for Paget disease, primary hyperparathyroidism, and inflammatory arthritides.[61−64] Preliminary results suggest the use of monitoring metastatic bone disease by measurement of cross-links.[65−67] A serum measurement of pyridinium cross-link levels has been reported, and serum levels ultimately may be an alternative to urinary collection and assay.[65] Table 23.7-2 summarizes available osteolytic-osteoblastic tests, none of which has been sensitive or specific enough to document bone micrometastases.

Bone-Directed Therapy for Metastatic Disease

Osteoporosis, the destruction and loss of trabecular bone, is a direct consequence of estrogen deficiency. The therapeutic strategy of using systemic estrogen replacement therapy for prevention and treatment of bone loss has provided the focus for the development of bone-specific systemic therapies. Whereas many agents have been used (fluorine, estrogens, androgens, calcitonin), the focus has been the use of bisphosphonates. Other antiosteoclast agents, such as gallium nitrate, may be of value in the future.

Bisphosphonates

Bisphosphonates are analogues of pyrophosphate, a natural inhibitor of bone demineralization.[68] The bisphosphonates have a carbon substitution for the oxygen of the pyrophosphate molecule. This substitution makes them resistant to hydrolysis by endogenous phosphatases. Bisphosphonates bind to hydroxyapatite crystals of bone by adsorption, resulting in stabilization of bone mineral. Bone mineral dissolution is thus inhibited. In addition to bisphosphonates inhibiting osteoclast function, they seem to inhibit differentiation and recruitment from the monocyte–macrophage cell line. Bisphosphonates inhibit bone resorption in in vivo experimental systems, including PTH, corticosteroid, and retinoid-induced bone loss. The potency of the bisphosphonates in inhibiting bone resorption varies, as does the inhibition of normal bone mineralization.[69]

TABLE 23.7-2
Bone Metastases Markers of Osteoclast–Osteoblast Activity

	Osteolytic	Osteoblastic
Urinary hydroxyproline	+	
Alkaline phosphatase		+
Bone-specific alkaline phosphatase		+
Tartrate-resistant acid phosphatase	+	
Procollagen type I		+
Pyridinoline	+	
Osteocalcin		+
CA 15-3	−	−
Urinary calcium increased levels	+	

Clinical Use of Bisphosphonates in Metastatic Bone Disease

The inhibition of osteoclastic activity, regardless of the activating factors, formed the basis for trials of bisphosphonates in malignancy-associated hypercalcemia. A number of trials demonstrate the efficacy of etidronate, clodronate, and pamidronate in treating hypercalcemia (Table 23.7-3). These agents have been shown to be superior to others such as calcitonin, corticosteroids, and plicamycin. The safety and lack of toxicity, even in severely ill patients, has been demonstrated.[70]

In addition to the clinical relevance of the hypocalcemic effect of bisphosphonates, a number of studies have shown that bone destruction can be inhibited by treatment with bisphosphonates. However, it is unknown if breast cancer cell tumor growth also is inhibited. In vitro studies in breast cancer have not been done. Inhibition of osteolysis by bisphosphonate use in a Walker 256 carcinosarcoma bone metastasis model seems to be independent of tumor cell growth.[71]

Morton and coworkers[72] reported sclerosis of lytic bone lesions in 25% of pamidronate-treated breast cancer patients, with radiologic stability in an additional 25%.[72] No other systemic chemotherapy or hormonal therapy was administered to patients in this trial. In a similar pamidronate study, Coleman and others[73] demonstrated radiographic evidence of bone healing in 17% of patients and bone disease stabilization in 46% of breast cancer patients treated with pamidronate. A number of prospective studies have shown improvement in skeletal related morbidity with bisphosphonate treatment.[74–80] A double-blind, controlled trial of clodronate demonstrated a reduction in incidence of hypercalcemia, vertebral and nonvertebral fractures, and all skeletal-related morbid events.[81] This trial of 173 patients used an oral clodronate formulation and identical-appearing placebo. In an open, randomized trial of oral pamidronate, reductions in episodes of hypercalcemia, bone pain, fractures, and need for palliative radiation therapy was demonstrated in 173 patients with metastatic bone disease.[82] Neither trial demonstrated a survival advantage for the bisphosphonate-treated group. Improved quality of life, palliation of bone pain, reduction in pathologic fracture frequency, decrease in the need for radiation therapy, and surgical intervention for bone disease have been shown in multiple studies. Biermann and associates[83] have suggested significant reductions in treatment-related costs for metastatic disease if clodronate is used in the treatment of breast cancer.

Bisphosphonate use is hampered by lack of availability of an oral formulation in the United States. A large multicenter study of pamidronate, intravenously administered, is being conducted in women with osteolytic disease being treated with hormonal therapy or chemotherapy. This randomized, placebo-controlled trial may confirm the previous bisphosphonate study observations and provide the basis for an adjuvant trial in breast cancer patients at high risk for metastases.

TABLE 23.7-3
Bisphosphonates in Breast Cancer–Related Skeletal Disease

Investigators	Agent	Bone Pain	New or Progressive Lytic Disease	HCM	Pathologic Fracture	Survival
Elomaa et al[74]	Clodronate	Improved	Reduced	Reduced	Reduced	Improved
vanHolten-Verzantvoort et al[75]	Pamidronate	Improved	NR	Reduced	Reduced	Improved
Thiebaud et al[76]	Pamidronate	Improved	NR	NR	NR	NR
Neri et al[78]	Clodronate	Improved	Stable			
Paterson et al[79]	Clodronate	Improved	Reduced	NR	Reduced (vertebral fracture)	NR
Paterson et al[81]	Clodronate	Improved (indirect assessment)	—	—	Reduced	No benefit
vanHolten-Verzantvoort et al[82]	Pamidronate	Improved	—	—	Reduced	No benefit

HCM, hypercalcemia of malignancy. NR, not reported; PD, progressive disease.

Gallium

Gallium nitrate, the anhydrous salt of gallium and nitric acid, has been shown to inhibit bone resorption by a direct effect on osteoclasts.[84] Bockman and associates[85] have shown an increase in bone calcium and crystallite perfection of hydroxyapatite. Studies have shown that gallium increases calcium and phosphate content of bone at metabolically active sites of bone.[86] Gallium nitrate inhibits accelerated bone turnover in patients with bone metastases, as assessed by reduction in urinary calcium and hydroxyproline excretion.[87] These observations, as well as observations on the treatment of acute hypercalcemia of malignancy,[88–90] suggest that gallium may be a useful agent as a modification of osteoclast activation resulting from the presence of bone metastases. Clinical trials for the treatment and prevention of bone disease have not been initiated.

Bone-Directed Radiation Therapy

Radiation therapy for bone metastases has been used primarily to relieve pain, but it may also prevent pathologic fracture and relieve symptoms resulting from spinal cord or nerve root compression.[91,92] Questions remain unanswered about the use of external-beam radiation therapy for bone metastasis, including dose, schedule, response of disease, duration of response, prevention of fracture, and use of multidisciplinary therapeutic approaches.[93–95]

Systemic therapy for bone metastasis with radioactive bone-seeking agents is an alternative to external-beam radiation therapy. Phosphorus 32–labeled phosphates have considerable hematologic toxicity but do relieve pain.[96,97]

Many agents are being tested in clinical trials; however, only strontium-89 is available for use in clinical practice.[98] Strontium-89 has been in use since Pecher[99] showed excellent pain relief from bone pain from prostate cancer. It is preferentially taken up at sites of active bone mineral turnover, similar to bisphosphonates and gallium, and has a greater uptake in metastatic disease than in normal bone.[100] Strontium mimics calcium uptake into bone and renal excretion. It is a β emitter with a half-life of about 50 days and a tissue penetration of 8 mm.[101]

Most patients treated with strontium-89 have had pain resulting from prostate cancer; nevertheless, response rates for breast cancer, as assessed by pain relief, have been reported as high as 89%. Robinson and associates[101] reported clinical response rates of 80% for bone pain improvement in breast cancer patients, with about 20% of patients becoming pain-free.

Assessment of the role of strontium-89 in palliation of the pain of bone metastases from breast cancer is limited because of the small number of patients, the limited response assessment criteria, and the known variability of clinical presentation and extent of disease.

Strontium-89 toxicity is predominantly hematologic, with about 20% of patients developing thrombocytopenia. The reported studies are inadequate in defining the effect of disease extent, marrow involvement, and prior therapy (chemotherapy and radiation therapy) history on hematologic toxicity for breast cancer patients. The indications for strontium 89 use are not well delineated but include the following: pain refractory to analgesic medication; disease progression after front-line therapy; adequate baseline hematologic parameters; and a life expectancy adequate to derive the anticipated benefit from treatment (generally considered 3 months).[100]

Additional systemic radioisotopes with bone-targeting potential are being studied such as rhenium 186, which is also a β emitter and has shown some promise regarding relief of pain from bone metastasis in about 75% of patients.[97]

Phase I and II studies of samarium-153 have shown pain relief for breast and prostate cancer bone metastases. Dose-limiting toxicity has been hematologic.[102,103] However, too few patients with breast metastases have been treated to confirm the clinical use of these agents for the palliation of pain.

Bone metastases remain a formidable clinical problem. The development of bone-targeted therapeutic interventions to prevent osteoclast activation and to provide palliation of pain, however, may provide benefit in addition to that achieved with the conventional therapy of systemic hormonal and chemotherapeutic agents.

The potential of adjunctive bisphosphonate therapy to prevent or delay development of bone metastasis is an exciting prospect that awaits further laboratory in vitro and in vivo substantiation.

MANAGEMENT SUMMARY

- The diagnosis of bone metastases is typically made on the basis of bone scan and radiographs. In addition, CT (for cortical bone) and magnetic resonance imaging (for trabecular bone) may be useful in defining the extent of the involvement.
- Patients with bone metastases should be continuously examined for potential morbidity, such as pathologic fracture, neurologic compromise, and hypercalcemia.
- Treatment is either local (surgery–external-beam radiation therapy) or systemic (hormonal therapy–chemotherapy), depending on the clinical situation (see Chaps. 22.1 and 23.6).
- In patients with progressive disease after conventional therapies, newer treatment approaches, such as bisphosphonates and systemic radiation therapy using strontium-89, are under investigation. Trials using bisphosphonates with conventional systemic therapy are also underway.

References

1. Hortobagyi GN, Libshitz HI, Seabold JE. Osseous metastases of breast cancer: clinical, biochemical, radiographic, and scintigraphic evaluation of response to therapy. Cancer 1984;53:577.
2. Scheid V, Buzdar AU, Smith TL, et al. Clinical course of breast cancer patients with osseous metastasis treated with combination chemotherapy. Cancer 1986;58:2589.
3. Tubiana-Hulin M. Incidence, prevalence and distribution of bone metastases. Bone 1991;12(Suppl 1):S9.
4. Greenberg JS, Deck MDF, Vikram, et al. Metastases to the base of the skull: clinical findings in 43 patients. Neurology 1981;31:530.
5. Henriques CQ. The veins of the vertebral column and their role in the spread of cancer. Ann R Coll Surg Engl 1962;31:1.
6. Vandemark RM, Shpall EJ, Affronti ML. Bone metastases from breast cancer: value of CT bone windows. J Comput Assist Tomog 1992;16:608.
7. Muindi J, Coombes RC, Golding S, et al. The role of computed tomography and the detection of bone metastases in breast cancer patients. Br J Radiol 1983;56:233.
8. Jones AL, Williams MP, Powles TJ, et al. Magnetic resonance imaging in the detection of skeletal metastases in patients with breast cancer. Br J Cancer 1990;62:296.
9. Huffer WE. Biology of Disease: morphology and biochemistry of bone remodeling: possible control by vitamin D, parathyroid hormone, and other substances. Lab Invest 1988;59:418.
10. Butler WT. The nature and significance of osteopontin. Connect Tissue Res 1989;23:123.
11. Neri B, Cecchettin M, Pacini P, et al. Osteocalcin as a biological marker in the therapeutic management of breast cancer bone metastases. Cancer Invest 1989;7:551.
12. Coleman RE, Mashiter G, Fogelman I, et al. Osteocalcin: a potential marker of metastatic bone disease and response to treatment. Eur J Cancer Clin Oncol 1988;24:1211.
13. Orwoll ES, Deftos LJ. Serum osteocalcin (BGP) levels in normal men: a longitudinal evaluation reveals an age-associated increase. J Bone Min Res 1990;5:259.
14. Pietschmann P, Zielinski C, Woloszcuzuk W. Serum osteocalcin levels in breast cancer patients. J Cancer Res Clin Oncol 1989;115:456.
15. Bataille R, Delmas PD, Chappard D, et al. Abnormal serum bone Gla protein levels in multiple myeloma. Cancer 1990;66:167.
16. Carlson K, Ljunghall S, Simonsson B, et al. Serum osteocalcin concentrations in patients with multiple myeloma: correlation with disease stage and survival. Ann Intern Med 1992;231:133.
17. Malaval L, French M, Delmas PD. Circulating levels of osteonectin in normal subjects and patients with thrombocytopenia. Bone Miner 1990;9:129.
18. Romanowski R, Jundt G, Termine JD, et al. Immunoelectron microscopy of osteonectin and type I collagen in osteoblasts and bone matrix. Calcif Tissue Int 1990;46:353.
19. Horowitz MC. Cytokines and estrogen in bone: anti-osteoporotic effects. Science 1993;260:626.
20. Kahn AJ, Partridge NC. New concepts in bone remodeling: an expanding role for the osteoblast. Am J Otolaryngol 1987;8:258.
21. Wlodarski KH. Basic science and pathology: properties and origin of osteoblasts. Clin Orthop 1988;252:276.
22. Hagel-Bradway S, Dziak R. Regulation of bone cell metabolism. J Oral Pathol Med 1989;18:344.
23. Centrella M, McCarthy TL, Canalis E. Effects of transforming growth factors on bone cells. Connect Tissue Res 1989;20:267.
24. Athanasou NA, Wells CA, Quinn J, et al. The origin and nature of stromal osteoclast-like multinucleated giant cells in breast carcinoma: implications for tumour osteolysis and macrophage biology. Br J Cancer 1989;59:491.
25. Lowik CWGM, van der Pluijm G, Bloys H, et al. Parathyroid hormone and PTH-like protein stimulate interleukin-6 production by osteogenic cells: a possible role of interleukin-6 in osteoclastogenesis. Biochem Biophys Res Commun 1989;162:1546.
26. Hauschka PV, Chen TL, Mavrakos AE. Polypeptide growth factors in bone matrix. Cell Mol Biol 1988;207.
27. Mundy GR, Bonewald LF. Role of TGFβ in bone remodeling. Ann NY Acad Sci 1990;593:91.
28. Krane SM, Goldring MB, Goldring SR. Cytokines 1988;239.
29. Evans CE, Ward C, Braidman IP. Breast carcinomas synthesize factors which influence osteoblast-like cells independently of osteoclasts in vitro. J Endocrinol 1991;128:R5.
30. Grill V, Ho P, Body JJ, et al. Parathyroid hormone-related protein: elevated levels in both humoral hypercalcemia of malignancy and hypercalcemia complicating metastatic breast cancer. J Clin Endocrinol Metab 1991;73:1309.
31. Powell GJ, Southby J, Danks JA, et al. Localization of parathyroid hormone–related protein in breast cancer metastases: increased incidence in bone compared with other sites. Cancer Res 1991;51:3059.

32. Brandt DW, Wachsman W, Deftos LJ. Parathyroid hormone-like protein: alternative messenger RNA splicing pathways in human cancer cell lines. Cancer Res 1994;54:850.

33. Bundred NJ, Walker RA, Ratcliffe WA, et al. Parathyroid hormone related protein and skeletal morbidity in breast cancer. Eur J Cancer 1992;28:690.

34. Kissin MW, Henderson MA, Donks JA, et al. Parathyroid hormone-related protein in breast cancer of widely varying prognosis. Eur J Surg Oncol 1993;99:134.

35. Vargas SJ, Gillespie MT, Powell GJ, et al. Localization of parathyroid hormone-related protein mRNA expression in breast cancer and metastatic lesions by in situ hybridization. J Bone Miner Res 1992;7:971.

36. Bundred NJ, Walker RA, Ratcliffe WA, et al. A humoral role for parathyroid hormone-related peptide in breast cancer. Breast Cancer Res Treat 1991;99:159.

37. Powell GJ, Southby J, Danks JA, et al. Localization of parathyroid hormone-related protein in breast cancer metastases: increased incidence in bone compared with other sites. Cancer Res 1991; 51:3059.

38. Arteaga CL, Carty-Dugger T, Moses HL, et al. Transforming growth factor beta 1 can induce estrogen-independent tumorigenicity of human breast cancer cells in athymic mice. Cell Growth Differ 1993;4:593.

39. Luparello C, Ginty AF, Gallagher JA, et al. Transforming growth factor-beta 1, beta 2, and beta 3, urokinase and parathyroid hormone–related peptide expression in 8701-BC breast cancer cells and clones. Differentiation 1993;55:73.

40. Mundy GR. Mechanisms of osteolytic bone destruction. Bone 1991;12:S1.

41. Coleman RE. Pathophysiology of metastatic bone disease: a rationale for treatment with osteoclast inhibitors. (Abstract) Clin Exp Metas 1992;10:68.

42. Cooper EH, Forbes MA, Hancock AK, et al. Serum bone alkaline phosphatase and CA 549 in breast cancer with bone metastasis. Biomed Pharmacother 1992;46:31.

43. Nguyen M, Bonneterre J, Hecquet B, et al. Plasma acid and alkaline phosphatase in patients with breast cancer. Anticancer Res 1991;11:831.

44. Berruti A, Osella G, Raucci CA, et al. Transient increase in total serum alkaline phosphatase predicts radiological response to systemic therapy in breast cancer patients with osteolytic and mixed bone metastases. Oncology 1993;50:218.

45. Coleman RE, Whitaker KB, Moss DW, et al. Biochemical prediction of response of bone metastases to treatment. Br J Cancer 1988;58:205.

46. O'Brien DP, Horgan PG, Gough DB, et al. CA 15-3: a reliable indicator of metastatic bone disease in breast cancer patients. Ann R Coll Surg 1992;74:9.

47. Francini G, Montagnani M, Petrioli R, et al. Comparison between CEA, TPA, CA 15/3 and hydroxyproline, alkaline phosphatase, whole body retention of ^{99m}Tc MDP in the follow-up of bone metastases in breast cancer. Int J Biol Markers 1990;5:65.

48. Crippa F, Bombardieri E, Seregni E, et al. Single determination of CA 15.3 and bone scintigraphy in the diagnosis of skeletal metastases of breast cancer. J Nucl Biol Med 1992;36:52.

49. Onat H, et al. Osteocalcin: a valuable bone metastasis marker. Eur J Gynecol Oncol 1991;12:399.

50. Neri B, Cecchettin M, Pacini P, et al. Osteocalcin as a biological marker in the therapeutic management of breast cancer bone metastases. Cancer Invest 1989;7:551.

51. Coleman RE, Mashiter G, Fogelman I, et al. Osteocalcin: a potential marker of metastatic bone disease and response to treatment. Eur J Cancer Clin Oncol 1988;24:1211.

52. Francini G, Gonnelli S, Petrioli R, et al. Procollagen type I carboxy-terminal propeptide as a marker of osteoblastic bone metastases. Cancer Epidemiol Biomarkers Prev 1993;2:125.

53. Guerrieri P, Modoni S, Parisi S, et al. Bone formation markers and pain palliation in bone metastases treated with strontium-89. Am J Clin Oncol 1994;17:77.

54. Coombes RC, Dady P, Parsons C, et al. Assessment of response of bone metastases to systemic treatment in patients with breast cancer. Cancer 1983;52:610.

55. Niell HB, Palmieri GM, Neely CL, et al. Postabsorptive urinary hydroxyproline test in patients with metastatic bone disease from breast cancer. Arch Intern Med 1981;141:1471.

56. Gasser AB, DePierre D, Mermiltod B, et al. Free serum hydroxyproline and total urinary hydroxyproline for the detection of skeletal metastases. Br J Cancer 1982;45:477.

57. Coleman RE, Houston S, James I, et al. Preliminary results of the use of urinary excretion of pyridinium crosslinks for monitoring metastatic bone disease. Br J Cancer 1992;65:766.

58. Pyridinium crosslinks as markers of bone resorption. Lancet 1992;340:278.

59. Miyamoto KK, McSherry SA, Robins SP, et al. Collagen cross-link metabolites in urine as markers of bone metastases in prostatic carcinoma. J Urol 1994;151:909.

60. Li F, Pitt PI, Sherwood R, et al. Biochemical markers of bone turnover in women with surgically treated carcinoma of the breast. Eur J Clin Invest 1993;23:566.

61. Uebelhart D, Gineyts E, Chapuy MC, et al. Urinary excretion of pyridinium crosslinks: a new marker of bone resorption in metabolic bone disease. Bone Miner 1990;8:87.

62. Black D, Marabani M, Sturrock RD, et al. Urinary excretion of the hydroxypyridinium cross links of collagen in patients with rheumatoid arthritis. Ann Rheum Dis 1989;48:641.

63. Seibel MJ, Gartenberg F, Silverberg SJ, et al. Urinary hydroxypyridinium cross-links of collagen in primary hyperparathyroidism. J Clin Endocrinol Metab 1992;74:481.

64. Robins SP, Black D, Paterson CR, et al. Evaluation of urinary hydroxypyridinium crosslink measurements as resorption markers in metabolic bone diseases. Eur J Clin Invest 1991;21:310.

65. Demers L, Lipton A, Harvey H, et al. The measurement of pyridinium cross-links in serum of patients with metastatic bone disease. (Abstract) Proc Annu Meet Am Soc Clin Oncol 1993;12:A243.

66. Paterson CR, Robins SP, Horobin JM, et al. Pyridinium crosslinks as markers of bone resorption in patients with breast cancer. Br J Cancer 1991;64:884.

67. Lipton A, Demers L, Daniloff Y, et al. Increased urinary excretion of pyridinium cross-links in cancer patients. Clin Chem 1993;39:614.

68. Fleisch H. Bisphosphonate pharmacology and use in the treatment of tumour-induced hypercalcemia and metastatic bone disease. Drugs 1991;42:919.

69. Averbuch SD. New bisphosphonates in the treatment of bone metastases. Cancer 1993;72:3443.

70. Theriault RL. Hypercalcemia of malignancy: pathophysiology and implications for treatment. Oncology 1993;7:47.

71. Kostenuik PJ, Orr FW, Suyama K, et al. Increased growth rate and tumor burden of spontaneously metastatic Walker 256 cancer cells in the skeleton of bisphosphonate-treated rats. Cancer Res 1993;53:5452.

72. Morton AR, Cantrill JA, Pillai GV, et al. Sclerosis of lytic bone metastases after disodium aminohydroxypropylidene bisphosphonate (APD) in patients with breast carcinoma. BMJ 1988;297:772.

73. Coleman RE, Woll PJ, Miles M, et al. Treatment of bone metastases from breast cancer with (3-amino-1-hydroxypropylidene)-1,1-bisphosphonate (APD). Br J Cancer 1988;58:621.

74. Elomaa I, Blomqvist C, Porkka L, et al. Treatment of skeletal disease in breast cancer: a controlled clodronate trial. Bone 1987;8(Suppl 1):S53.

75. van Holten-Verzantvoort A, Bijvoet OLM, Hermans J, et al. Reduced morbidity from skeletal metastases in breast cancer patients during long-term bisphosphonate treatment. Lancet 1987;983.

76. Thiebaud D, Leyvraz S, von Fliedner V, et al. Treatment of bone metastases from breast cancer and myeloma with pamidronate. Eur J Cancer 1991;27:37.

77. Dodwell DJ, Howell A, Ford J. Reduction in calcium excretion in women with breast cancer and bone metastases using the oral bisphosphonate pamidronate. Br J Cancer 1990;61:123.

78. Neri B, Gemelli MT, Sambataro S, et al. Subjective and metabolic effects of clodronate in patients with advanced breast cancer and symptomatic bone metastases. Anticancer Drugs 1992;3:696.

79. Paterson AHG, Ernst DS, Powles TJ, et al. Treatment of skeletal disease in breast cancer with clodronate. Bone 1991;12:S25.

80. van Holten-Verzantvoort A, Zwinderman A, Aaronson N, et al. The effect of supportive pamidronate treatment on aspects of quality of life of patients with advanced breast cancer. Eur J Cancer 1991;27:544.

81. Paterson AHG, Powles TJ, Kanis JA, et al. Double-blind controlled trial of oral clodronate in patients with bone metastases from breast cancer. J Clin Oncol 1993;11:59.

82. van Holten-Verzantvoort ATM, Kroon HM, Bijvoet OLM, et al. Palliative pamidronate treatment in patients with bone metastases from breast cancer. J Clin Oncol 1993;11:491.

83. Biermann WA, Cantor RI, Fellin FM, et al. An evaluation of the potential cost reductions resulting from the use of clodronate in the treatment of metastatic carcinoma of the breast to bone. Bone 1990;12:S37.

84. Hall TJ, Chambers TJ. Gallium inhibits bone resorption by a direct effect on osteoclasts. Bone Miner 1990;8:211.

85. Bockman RS, Boskey AL, Blumenthal NC, et al. Gallium increases bone calcium and crystallite perfection of hydroxyapatite. Calcif Tissue Int 1986;39:376.

86. Repo MA, Bockman RS, Betts F, et al. Effect of gallium on bone mineral properties. Calcif Tissue Int 1988;43:300.

87. Warrell RP, Alcock NW, Bockman RS. Gallium nitrate accelerated bone turnover in patients with bone metastases. J Clin Oncol 1987;5:292.

88. Warrell RP Jr. Murphy WK, Schulman P, et al. A randomized double-blind study of gallium nitrate compared with etidronate for acute control of cancer-related hypercalcemia. J Clin Oncol 1991;9:1467.

89. Warrell RP, Israel R, Frisone M, et al. Gallium nitrate for acute treatment of cancer-related hypercalcemia. Ann Intern Med 1988;108:669.

90. Warrell RP, Skelos A, Alcock NW, et al. Gallium nitrate for acute treatment of cancer-related hypercalcemia: clinicopharmacological and dose response analysis. Cancer Res 1986;46:4208.

91. Hill ME, Richards MA, Gregory WM, et al. Spinal cord compression in breast cancer: a review of 70 cases. Br J Cancer 1993;68:969.

92. Poulsen HS, Nielsen OS, Klee M, et al. Palliative irradiation of bone metastases. Cancer Treatm Rev 1989;16:41.

93. Bates T. A review of local radiotherapy in the treatment of bone metastases and cord compression. Int J Radiat Oncol Biol Phys 1990;23:217.

94. Okawa T, Kita M, Goto M, et al. Randomized prospective clinical study of small, large and twice-a-day fraction radiotherapy for painful bone metastases. Radiother Oncol 1988;13:99.

95. Bates T, Yarnold JR, Blitzer P, et al. Bone metastasis consensus statement. Int J Radiat Oncol Biol Phys 1991;23:215.

96. Silberstein EB. The treatment of painful osseous metastases with phosphorus-32–labeled phosphates. Semin Oncol 1993;20:10.

97. Friedell HL, Storaasli JP. The use of radioactive phosphorus in the treatment of carcinoma of the breast with wide-spread metastases to the bone. Am J Roentgenol Rad Ther 1950;64:559.

98. Holmes RA. Radiopharmaceuticals in clinical trials. Semin Oncol 1993;20:22.

99. Pecher C. Biological investigations with radioactive strontium and calcium: preliminary report on the use of radioactive strontium in the treatment of bone cancer. Univ Calif Publ Pharmacol 1942;11:117.

100. Porter AT, Davis LP. Systemic radionuclide therapy of bone metastases with strontium-89. Oncology 1994;8:93.

101. Robinson RG, Blake GM, Preston DF, et al. Strontium-89: treatment results and kinetics in patients with painful metastatic prostate and breast cancer in bone. Radiographic 1989;9:271.

102. Turner H, Claringbold PG, Hetherington EL, et al. A phase I study of samarium-153 ethylenediaminetetramethylene phosphonate therapy for disseminated skeletal metastases. J Clin Oncol 1989;7:1926.

103. Turner JH, Claringbold PG. A phase II study of treatment of painful multifocal skeletal metastases with single- and repeated-dose samarium-153 ethylenediaminetetramethylene phosphonate. Eur J Cancer 1991;27:1084.

23.8

Lymphatic Spread of Breast Cancer

CLAUDINE ISAACS

Intrathoracic spread is seen in 57% to 77%[1,2] of patients with metastatic breast carcinoma and may manifest as pulmonary nodules, lymphadenopathy, lymphangitic spread, pleural effusions, or pleural masses. Of the patients with thoracic metastases, 18% to 35% have clinical evidence of lymphangitic disease.[3,4] Autopsy series reveal a higher frequency of lymphatic involvement than is suspected on clinical grounds, with studies showing that only 20% of patients with demonstrated lymphangitic disease were diagnosed before their death.[5]

Lymphangitic carcinomatosis is characterized by widespread neoplastic involvement of the pulmonary lymphatics and has been observed as a terminal event in up to 25% of patients with breast cancer.[5] The diagnosis of this condition often is difficult, given that it tends to present with nonspecific symptoms that may be associated with a wide variety of other disease states.

Clinical Presentation

The clinical syndrome associated with lymphangitic spread to the lungs includes progressive dyspnea, which may be present with minimal exertion, a nonproductive cough, and hypoxemia.[6,7] In addition, associated findings may include fever, weight loss, cyanosis, pleuritic chest pain, tachypnea, tachycardia, and evidence of right-sided heart failure.[7–10] Although these patients often have insidious onset of symptoms, they occasionally suffer a more aggressive clinical picture characterized by a sudden onset of severe dyspnea, high fever, and a rapid development of respiratory compromise more in keeping with an infectious cause.[11]

The severity of symptoms in many patients often is out of proportion to the findings on physical examination. These consist primarily of scattered rales and rhonchi, and occasionally signs of a pleural effusion.[6,7]

Radiologic Findings

The characteristic finding on chest radiograph is a diffuse reticulonodular pattern, frequently more marked in the bases than in the upper lobes.[12–16] Although most commonly bilateral, unilateral or focal disease has been reported.[5] Nonbranching, fine, straight lines pointing toward the hilum (Kerley A lines) and linear densities perpendicular to and abutting the pleura (Kerley B lines) are observed.[12,13,16] The nodular pattern seen on chest radiograph is believed to represent a superimposition of shadows of many tumor-filled lymphatics rather than true nodular metastases.[13] Although a reticulonodular pattern is typical, it is often accompanied by other evidence of pulmonary disease[13,15] (Table 23.8-1). Pleural effusions have been observed in up to 63% of patients[5] (Fig. 23.8-1). Hilar and mediastinal lymphadenopathy also may be observed.[13,17] Up to 40% of patients with characteristic pathologic findings of lymphangitic carcinomatosis have normal results on chest radiograph.[18,19]

Computed tomography, particularly high-resolution scanning with slices obtained every 1.5 to 2 mm, has been touted as a more sensitive radiologic procedure for evaluating lymphangitic spread (Fig. 23.8-2). These scans reveal thickened septal lines, prominent reticular pattern, nodular or beaded thickening of the bronchovascular bundles, and polygonal lines[15,20–22] (Table 23.8-2). Beaded thickening of the bronchovascular bundles is thought to be a finding specific to lymphangitic carcinomatosis. This sign was present on high-resolution computed tomographic scans of inflation-fixed lungs in 19 of 22 patients with pathologically confirmed lymphangitic carcinomatosis, but was not seen in any of 148 control cases with a variety of other lung pathologic processes.[22] The only other condition in which this sign has been described is sarcoidosis.[23]

Other noninvasive tests also have been used for diagnosing lymphangitic carcinomatosis. Ventilation–perfusion scanning demonstrates irregular peripheral perfusion defects with a normal ventilation pattern.[18,24,25] Pulmonary function testing is characterized by a restrictive pattern with decreased vital capacity, total lung capacity, and a reduced D_{LCO},[18,26] and arterial blood gas sampling reveals hypoxemia.[18] The results of these tests tend to be nonspecific and may not be helpful in distinguishing this condition from other disease entities associated with a similar clinical presentation.

TABLE 23.8-1

Findings on Chest Radiograph

Abnormality	Cases (N = 20)
Reticular pattern	12 (60%)
Kerley B lines	11 (55%)
Hilar adenopathy	8 (40%)
Pleural effusion	6 (30%)
3–10 mm nodules	4 (20%)
Nonspecific	5 (25%)
Normal	1 (5%)

(Data from Munk PL, Miller NL, Miller RR, et al. Pulmonary lymphangitic carcinomatosis: CT and pathologic findings. Radiology 1988;166:705)

FIGURE 23.8-1 Chest radiolograph of a 58-year-old woman with a T2, N1, M0 infiltrating ductal carcinoma of the right breast that was diagnosed in 1988. She remained without evidence of disease after a modified radical mastectomy and six cycles of chemotherapy with CMF until February 1994, when she experienced increasing dyspnea on exertion and a nonproductive cough. Transbronchial biopsy confirmed the presence of lymphangitic spread. **A.** Chest radiograph showing bilateral interstitial lung disease more prominent at the bases than in the upper lobes. In addition, a small pleural effusion is seen on the left. **B.** Close-up image of the left base demonstrating interstitial changes compatible with lymphangitic carcinomatosis.

Pathophysiology and Pathologic Diagnosis

The pulmonary lymphatic channels consist of a peripheral network found in the interlobular septa and a deep system found in association with the vessels and bronchi. The deep lymphatics lie in the perivascular and peribronchial spaces located in the pulmonary interstitium.[16,27]

The mechanism by which the tumor cells reach the pulmonary lymphatics has been greatly debated. It had long been thought that lymphangitic carcinomatosis occurred by retrograde spread, with the tumor originally being borne through the lymphatics to the thoracic duct and the hilar lymph nodes, and then to the pulmonary and pleural lymphatic channels.[28-31] Other data suggest that this is probably not the mode of spread, given that the thoracic duct in most patients shows complete absence of disease and that the hilar lymph nodes are infrequently involved. The evidence supports that the cancerous cells reach the intrapulmonary lymphatics by a hematogenous route, with tumor emboli being arrested in the small arterioles.[29,32,33] They are then able to proliferate and eventually gain access to the perivascular lymphatics. From there

they are carried centrally toward the hilar lymph nodes. In addition, an obliterative endarteritis may be seen resulting from thrombosis or intravascular fibrosis. A study of 23 autopsy-confirmed cases of lymphangitic carcinomatosis by Janower and Blennerhassett[16] provides further support that the hematogenous route is the primary mode of spread. Only 11 of the cases showed any involvement of the lymph nodes, whereas 20 of the patients had arterial tumor emboli.

Lymphangitic carcinomatosis frequently is a difficult diagnosis to make on clinical and radiologic grounds alone. In patients with known widespread metastatic disease in whom the diagnosis of lymphangitic spread is suspected, systemic treatment can be initiated without histologic documentation of lung involvement. In patients in whom this is the only potential site of metastatic disease, however, tissue sampling is required for confirmation. However, these patients are frequently ill, and therefore it may be clinically hazardous to attempt invasive procedures to obtain a histologic diagnosis. The procedure of choice, if clinically feasible, is bronchoscopy with either transbronchial biopsy or bronchoalveolar lavage.[34-36] Studies using small groups of patients have suggested that the diagnostic accuracy of bronchoalveolar lavage is at least equivalent to that of transbronchial biopsy.[34,37] If coagulopathy or

FIGURE 23.8-2 Thin-cut CT scan of the chest of the patient in Figure 23.8-1 demonstrating thickened septa peripherally (*arrow*).

other medical contraindications do not exist, then both transbronchial biopsy and bronchoalveolar lavage should be carried out. Bronchial washings and brushings also may yield diagnostic information. In certain instances, these procedures may not provide a diagnosis and an open-lung biopsy should be considered (Fig. 23.8-3).

Other investigators suggest a role for the sampling of pulmonary microvascular blood for cytologic evaluation.[38–40] This is carried out by the withdrawal of blood through a pulmonary artery catheter that is inflated in the wedge position. The cells obtained are stained with the Papanicolaou method and must be examined by an experienced cytopathologist. In a study carried out by Masson and associates,[40] malignant cells were detected in 7 of 8 patients with lymphangitic carcinomatosis. Of the 17 pa-

tients with malignancy but no evidence of pulmonary metastases, 16 had normal results on cytologic evaluation. This method still is experimental; however, in patients who are too ill to undergo a more invasive procedure, this procedure may provide a means of confirming the diagnosis of this disease.

Pathologic examination of material obtained from patients with lymphangitic carcinomatosis demonstrates tumor cells filling the perivascular, peribronchial, and pleural lymphatics.[28,32] Pulmonary arterioles frequently show evidence of occlusion secondary to tumor cells or to a fibrotic process. This intravascular fibrosis is thought to be the result of either a desmoplastic reaction of the intima to the presence of tumor cells or organization of thrombi precipitated by tumor emboli.[28,32,41] This obliterative process leads to the occlusion of both lymphatic and vascular channels. Figures 23.8-4 and 23.8-5 demonstrate characteristic histologic changes seen in patients with this condition.

Given the described pathogenesis of this disease, it is not surprising that the radiographic manifestation is as an interstitial process. The observed thickening of the interstitium likely results from several different factors. The tumor cells themselves cause a distension of the lymphatic channels, both at their site of metastasis and distally. In addition, these malignant cells induce a reactive inflammatory and fibrotic response, leading to further thickening of the interstitium. The final mechanism postulated to play a role is the development of pulmonary edema resulting from lymphatic obstruction by the tumor.[29] Thus, these three processes are believed to be the pathologic correlates of the observed radiologic picture.

TABLE 23.8-2
Findings on Computed Tomography

Abnormality	CT (N = 21)	HRCT (N = 10)
Beaded thickening of bronchovascular bundles	21 (100%)	10 (100%)
Uneven thickened septal lines	18 (86%)	10 (100%)
Diffuse interstitial changes	11 (52%)	
Pleural thickening	10 (48%)	
Polygonal lines	8 (38%)	8★ (80%)
Pleural effusion	6 (29%)	
Discrete nodules	2 (10%)	

CT, computed tomography; HRCT, high-resolution computed tomography.

★ Polygonal lines not seen in seven of these eight patients on conventional 10-mm slice CT.

(Data from Munk PL, Miller NL, Miller RR, et al. Pulmonary lymphangitic carcinomatosis: CT and pathologic findings. Radiology 1988;166:705)

Differential Diagnosis

The vast differential diagnosis of patients with lymphatic spread of breast cancer includes infectious causes, pulmonary edema, drug or radiation toxicity, and throm-

FIGURE 23.8-3 Diagnostic approach to patients with lymphangitic carcinomatosis.

botic or nonthrombotic pulmonary emboli. Differentiating between them may be difficult.

Many chemotherapeutic agents—including cyclophosphamide, methotrexate, melphalan, and mitomycin C—have been associated with the development of pulmonary fibrosis manifesting as progressive dyspnea, dry cough, and at times fever.[42] The radiologic picture often is indistinguishable from that seen with lymphangitic carcinomatosis. The development of pulmonary fibrosis has been reported as early as after the second cycle of mitomycin C and as late as 6 years after the completion of therapy with cyclophosphamide. In certain instances, it can be difficult to distinguish between these two entities and the only means of making a definitive diagnosis is by demonstrating tumor cells within the pulmonary lymphatics.

Radiation pneumonitis progressing on to radiation fibrosis characteristically occurs 1 to 6 months after the completion of therapy and presents with shortness of breath, nonproductive cough, and low-grade fever.[43] The chest radiograph initially demonstrates an indistinct haziness followed by alveolar infiltrates or dense consolidation. Eventually, fibrosis develops with linear markings radiating from the area of pneumonitis toward the hilum or apex. These changes usually are limited to the radiation field; however, in certain instances radiographic changes have been observed in the contralateral lung field.[44] Given the focal nature of the radiologic changes in most cases, the diagnosis of radiation pneumonitis is easily distinguishable from lymphangitic spread.

Perhaps the most difficult condition to differentiate

FIGURE 23.8-4 Notice the presence of lymphatic spaces distended by tumor deposits adjacent to a bronchus (see the ciliated epithelium; *arrow*).

from lymphangitic carcinomatosis is pulmonary tumor emboli.[8,45,46] In a study comparing the clinical and pathologic features of 19 patients with pure arterial tumor emboli with those of 44 women with disease seen only in the lymphatic channels, Soares and coworkers[8] found that the only significant clinical difference between these two groups was a higher incidence of respiratory distress as the main cause of death in those with arterial emboli. Morphologically, right ventricular hypertrophy and dilatation was less common in those with lymphangitic disease. Although these two entities seem to be different pathologically, the distinction between them is of little clinical significance, given that the treatment of both of these conditions is similar.

In addition, pulmonary embolism may present with signs and symptoms similar to those seen with lymphangitic carcinomatosis. Chest radiography, ventilation perfusion scanning, and, on occasion, pulmonary angiography can be used to differentiate these two entities.

Thus, given the nonspecific nature of the clinical and radiologic picture of patients with lymphangitic carcinomatosis, a tissue diagnosis often is necessary to distinguish this condition from other disease states, particularly viral infections, chemotherapy toxicity, and certain cases of radiation pneumonitis.

Prognosis and Treatment

The presence of lymphangitic carcinomatosis is believed to confer a poor prognosis. Autopsy studies have revealed that 18% to 24% of all patients who die of metastatic breast

FIGURE 23.8-5 Lymphatic tumor deposit showing mitotic activity within the lung parenchyma. The presence of lymphoid aggregates (*open arrow*) and interstitial collagen deposition (*closed arrow*) imparts the reticulonodular pattern seen on chest radiograph.

cancer have evidence of lymphangitic involvement.[1,5] In these reports, lymphangitic carcinomatosis was found to account for 50% to 75% of the causes of deaths resulting from respiratory insufficiency. In one of the reports, only 23% of patients were diagnosed with lymphangitic metastases before death.[5] The median survival of this patient population is poor. In a study of patients with intrathoracic metastases from breast cancer, Gawne-Cain and others[3] found that the median survival of patients with lymphangitic carcinomatosis was 5.5 months. Although not a statistically significant difference, a 13.5-month median survival was observed in the patient group as a whole. Similar results have been noticed by others, with some investigators finding that only 25% of women with lymphangitic carcinomatosis were alive at 1 year[5] and others showing an 11% survival rate at 2 years.[4]

Information regarding the effect of treatment in this group of patients is scanty. If lymphangitic carcinomatosis is the sole site of disease in those with metastatic breast cancer, it is recommended that these women be excluded from clinical trials given that they have nonmeasurable disease.[47] Thus, the results on the impact of treatment in these patients, in general, are limited to case reports and small studies. In addition, from the available data, it is often difficult to differentiate between the efficacy of treatment and the patients' underlying poor prognosis.

Results from a Southeastern Cancer Study Group Project Trial[48] in which 362 patients were randomly assigned to treatment with low-dose chemotherapy with cyclophosphamide, methotrexate, 5-fluorouracil, vincristine, and prednisone or to a regimen of cyclophosphamide, doxorubicin, and 5-fluorouracil (CAF) demonstrated that responsiveness to therapy with CAF was related to the site of metastatic disease. Patients with lymphangitic lung disease, pleural effusions, or widespread liver metastases fell into a poor-risk group and had a significantly shorter duration of disease control and survival than did those with nodular lung metastases, soft tissue disease, or bone metastases. The authors concluded that patients with poor-risk disease had a lesser benefit from chemotherapy than did those with a good-risk pattern of metastasis.

A retrospective study published by Lower and Baughman[37] suggests that the percentage of lymphocytes found on bronchoalveolar lavage may be helpful in identifying a subgroup of patients with lymphangitic spread of breast cancer who have an inferior prognosis. In a group of 14 patients treated with steroids and cytotoxic chemotherapy, those who had a normal lymphocyte count on lavage had a median survival of 1.6 months compared with a 15.5-month survival in those with greater than 10% lymphocytes. Although this study was performed on a small cohort of patients, the difference between the results observed in the two patient groups was clinically significant and may be useful in providing prognostic information in this patient population. Larger studies are needed to validate these findings.

Other groups have published survival data in patients with lymphangitic spread. In a small group of patients, Green and colleagues[18] observed a median survival of 1 month in patients who did not show any response to therapy or in those who received supportive care only,

compared with a 7-month median survival in those who responded to treatment with either combination chemotherapy alone or similar therapy with whole-lung irradiation. Anecdotal reports[49] have described survival of up to 4 years in a patient treated with chemotherapy followed by hormonal therapy.

Given the small number of patients in these studies, it is difficult to draw definitive conclusions about the most appropriate therapeutic approach. In general, patients with lymphatic spread tend to have a rapid downhill course if not treated aggressively. Therefore, chemotherapy is recommended if clinically feasible. Hormonal therapy is appropriate, however, in certain groups of patients, including those with relatively asymptomatic minimal disease who are hormone receptor–positive and who have a long disease-free interval from initial diagnosis.

In summary, lymphangitic spread of breast cancer tends to present in an insidious fashion and frequently is difficult to diagnose. It is associated with a poor prognosis, and systemic treatment in the form of chemotherapy generally is recommended.

References

1. Hagemeister FB, Buzdar AU, Luna MA, et al. Causes of death in breast cancer. Cancer 1980;46:162.
2. Lee, YTN. Breast carcinoma: pattern of metastasis at autopsy. J Surg Oncol 1983;23:175.
3. Gawne-Cain ML, Malthouse SR, Reidy JF, et al. Radiographic patterns of intrathoracic disease in breast carcinoma: prognostic implications. Clin Radiol 1993;48:253.
4. Kreisman H, Wolkove N, Schwartz Finkelstein H, et al. Breast cancer and thoracic metastases: review of 119 patients. Thorax 1983;38:175.
5. Goldsmith HS, Bailey HD, Callahan EL, et al. Pulmonary lymphangitic metastases from breast carcinoma. Arch Surg 1967;94:483.
6. Chandler GN, Telling M. Lymphangitis carcinomatosa. BMJ 1952:639.
7. Hauser TE, Steer A. Lymphangitic carcinomatosis of the lungs: six case reports and a review of the literature. Ann Intern Med 1951;34:881.
8. Soares FA, Pinto APFE, Magnani Landell GA, et al. Pulmonary tumor embolism to arterial vessels and carcinomatous lymphangitis. Arch Pathol Lab Med 1993;117:827.
9. Altemus LR, Lee RE. Carcinomatosis of the lung with pulmonary hypertension. Arch Intern Med 1967;119:32.
10. Greenspan, EB. Carcinomatous endarteritis of pulmonary vessels resulting in failure of right ventricle. Arch Intern Med 1934;54:625.
11. Nixon DW, Shlaer SM. Fulminant lung metastases from cancer of the breast. Med Pediatr Oncol 1981;9:381.
12. Mueller HP, Sniffen RC. Roentgenologic appearance and pathology of intrapulmonary lymphatic spread of metastatic cancer. Am J. Roentgenol Rad Ther 1945;53:109.
13. Trapnell DH. Radiological appearances of lymphangitis carcinomatosa of the lung. Thorax 1964;19:251.
14. Chiles C, Ravin CE. Intrathoracic metastasis from an extrathoracic malignancy: a radiographic approach to patient evaluation. Radiol Clin North Am 1985;23:427.
15. Munk PL, Muller NL, Miller RR, et al. Pulmonary lymphangitic carcinomatosis: CT and pathologic findings. Radiology 1988;166:705.
16. Janower ML, Blennerhassett JB. Lymphangitic spread of metastatic cancer to the lung. Radiology 1971;101:267.

17. McLoud TC, Kalisher L, Stark P, et al. Intrathoracic lymph node metastases from extrathoracic neoplasms. Am J Roentgenol 1978;131:403.

18. Green N, Kern W, Levis R, et al. Lymphangitic carcinomatosis of the lung: pathologic, diagnostic and therapeutic considerations. Int J Radiat Oncol Biol Phys 1977;2:149.

19. Alkalay I, Fairfax CW, Bullard JC. Lymphangitic carcinomatosis of the lungs with normal appearing chest x-ray films. Chest 1972;62:229.

20. Davis SD. CT evaluation for pulmonary metastases in patients with extrathoracic malignancy. Radiology 1991;180:1.

21. Hirakata K, Nakata H, Harafake J. Appearance of pulmonary metastases on high resolution CT scan: comparison with histopathologic findings from autopsy specimens. Am J Roentgenol 1993;161:37.

22. Ren H, Hruban RH, Kuhlman JE, et al. Computed tomography of inflation-fixed lungs: the beaded septum sign of pulmonary metastases. J Comput Assist Tomogr 1989;13:411.

23. Bergin CJ, Muller NL. CT of interstitial lung disease: a diagnostic approach. Am J Radiol 1987;148:8.

24. Green N, Swanson L, Kern W, et al. Lymphangitic carcinomatosis: lung scan abnormalities. J Nucl Med 1975;17:258.

25. Pendergrass HP, Hartley SN, Clement PB, et al. Lung perfusion pattern associated with widespread occlusion of the pulmonary vessels and lymphatics. Radiology 1972;105:615.

26. Schwarz MI. Unusual causes of interstitial lung disease. In: Schwarz MI, King TE, eds. Interstitial lung disease. New York, Marcel Dekker, 1988:301.

27. Spencer H. The anatomy of the lung. In: Spencer H, ed. Pathology of the lung vol 1, ed 4. Oxford, Pergamon, 1985:64.

28. Schattenberg MS, Ryan JF. Lymphangitic carcinomatosis of the lungs: case report with autopsy findings. Am J Med 1941;14:1710.

29. Hentzman ER. Lymphangitic metastasis to lung. In: The lung: radiologic–pathologic correlations, ed 2. St Louis, CV Mosby, 1984:413.

30. Yang, S, Lin C. Lymphangitic carcinomatosis of the lungs, the clinical significance of its roentgenologic classification. Chest 1972;62:179.

31. Hendin AS, Deveney CW. Postmortem demonstration of abnormal deep pulmonary lymphatic pathways in lymphangitic carcinomatosis. Cancer 1974;33:1558.

32. Morgan AD. The pathology of subacute cor pulmonale in diffuse carcinomatosis of the lungs. J Pathol Bact 1949;61:75.

33. Spencer H. Secondary tumours in the lung. In: Spencer H, ed. Pathology of the lung, vol 2, ed 4. Oxford, Pergamon, 1985:1085.

34. Levy H, Horak DA, Lewis MI. The value of bronchial washings and bronchoalveolar lavage in the diagnosis of lymphangitic carcinomatosis. Chest 1988;94:1028.

35. Aranda C, Sidhu G, Sasso LA, et al. Transbronchial lung biopsy in the diagnosis of lymphangitic carcinomatosis. Cancer 1978;42:1995.

36. Joyner LR, Scheinhorn DJ. Transbronchial forceps lung biopsy through the fiberoptic bronchoscope. Chest 1975;67:532.

37. Lower EE, Baughman RP. Pulmonary lymphangitic metastasis from breast cancer. Chest 1992;102:1113.

38. Lukl P. Pulmonary microvascular cytology in the dyspneic cancer patient. Arch Pathol Lab Med 1992;116:129.

39. Masson RG, Ruggieri J. Pulmonary microvascular cytology, a new diagnostic application of the pulmonary artery catheter. Chest 1985;88:908.

40. Masson RG, Krikorian J, Lukl P, et al. Pulmonary microvascular cytology in the diagnosis of lymphangitic carcinomatosis. N Engl J Med 1989;321:71.

41. Winterbauer RH, Elfenbein IB, Ball WC. Incidence and clinical significance of tumor embolization to the lungs. Am J Med 1968;45:271.

42. Ginsberg SJ, Comis RL. The pulmonary toxicity of antineoplastic agents. Semin Oncol 1982;9:34.

43. Spain RC, Whittlesay D. Respiratory emergencies in patients with cancer. Semin Oncol 1989;16:471.

44. Smith JC. Radiation pneumonitis: case report of bilateral reaction after unilateral irradiation. Am Rev Resp Dis 1964;89:264.

45. Kane RD, Hawkins HK, Miller JA, et al. Microscopic pulmonary tumor emboli associated with dyspnea. Cancer 1975;36:1473.

46. Case Records of the Massachusetts General Hospital (case 30-1987). N Engl J Med 1987;317:4:225.

47. Hayward JL, Carbone PP, Heuson JC, et al. Assessment of response to therapy in advanced breast cancer. Cancer 1977;39:1289.

48. Smalley RV, Lefante J, Bartolucci A, et al. A comparison of cyclophosphamide, adriamycin, and 5-fluorouracil, vincristine, and prednisone (CMFVP) in patients with advanced breast cancer. Breast Cancer Res Treat 1983;3:209.

49. Hamilton CR, Plowman PN. Prolonged remission of lymphangitis carcinomatosis from breast cancer. Br J Dis Chest 1987;81:400.

23.9
Malignant Effusions

LAWRENCE N. SHULMAN ▪ DAVID J. SUGARBAKER

Malignant effusions from breast cancer occur in the pleural space, pericardial space, and peritoneum. In all three cases, the cause of the effusion is directly related to serosal involvement with metastatic deposits, except in the case of ascites resulting from extensive hepatic metastases. Because patients with breast cancer frequently develop metastatic disease and these locations often are involved with metastases, malignant effusions in these areas are common clinical problems.

Pleural Effusions

NORMAL PHYSIOLOGY

The pleural space exists between the parietal pleura, lining the inside of the chest wall, and the visceral pleura, lining the outside of each lung. This space is normally lubricated to allow smooth and comfortable movement of the lung and chest wall during respiration. In the physiologic state, the pleural space contains 5 to 20 mL of fluid, the content of which reflects the plasma concentrations of glucose and electrolytes, with a similar pH.[1,2] The protein concentration usually is lower than plasma, though, and is generally below 2 g/dL. The fluid is produced by hydrostatic pressure from the parietal pleura and is reabsorbed by the venous and lymphatic channels of the visceral pleura. It is estimated that 5 to 50 L of fluid is produced and reabsorbed by these mechanisms each day.

CHARACTERISTICS OF MALIGNANT PLEURAL EFFUSIONS

Malignant effusions occur when the pleura is involved with metastatic disease, which causes increased capillary leaking, resulting in increased fluid production and blockage of the normal vascular channels responsible for fluid reabsorption. A hallmark of malignant effusion is a high protein level (more than 3 g/dl), classifying it as an exudative fluid. In addition, the glucose level usually is low, possibly reflecting glucose consumption by the malignant cells.[3] The pH of the malignant effusion can be normal or low (below 7.3), and about one third of patients with effusions have effusions with low pH.[4] The effusions with low pH may have low glucose levels and are more likely to have positive cytologic findings on the first fluid evaluation. Breast cancer patients with pleural effusions with low pH also have a mean survival that is shorter than patients with effusions with normal pH (3.5 versus 16.6 months, respectively).[4] This suggests that low pH is an indication of involvement with more aggressive, metabolically active malignant tumor and has been confirmed by others for both breast cancer patients and patients with other tumor types.[5]

CYTOLOGIC EVALUATION

Thoracentesis can provide fluid for cytologic diagnosis, and closed pleural biopsy also can be performed. The cellular component of pleural fluid is concentrated and prepared for cytologic evaluation by either filtration or centrifugation. In either case, cells are stained with Papanicolaou or other appropriate stains for histologic review. Generally, volumes of 100 mL or more are optimal for evaluation. The more fluid that is processed by concentration methods, the more likely malignant cells will be seen, although positive results sometimes can be obtained with only a few milliliters of fluid.

In one series, 81% of breast cancer patients had malignant cells identified on cytologic analysis, and an additional 6% of patients had a malignant diagnosis made with pleural biopsy, for a total diagnostic rate of 87%.[6]

Other techniques of fluid analysis, such as carcinoembryonic antigen determination, have been used to increase diagnostic accuracy of thoracentesis in this patient population, but none have substantially added to the value of standard cytologic analyses and protein determination, and they add to the cost of the procedure.

MALIGNANT PLEURAL EFFUSIONS IN BREAST CANCER PATIENTS

Overall, lung cancer is the most frequent cause of malignant pleural effusion, but breast cancer is second; for women, breast cancer is the most common cause of malignant effusion. In a compilation of studies totalling 811 patients with malignant effusion, 23% of effusions resulted from breast cancer and 35% were from lung cancer.[2] In another series analyzing women separately, 37% of malignant effusions were caused by breast cancer, whereas 20% were the result of genitourinary malignancy (mostly ovarian cancer), and 15% were from lung cancer.[7]

Effusions can be ipsilateral or contralateral to the original breast cancer, and this distinction might give insight into the mechanism of the effusion. Contralateral effusions are likely to be due to hematogenous tumor spread, whereas ipsilateral effusions might be caused by hematoge-

nous spread or direct invasion through the chest wall by tumor resulting from chest wall or nodal recurrence. In one series, 83% of effusions were ipsilateral, 9% contralateral, and 6% bilateral.[8] In another series, 48% were ipsilateral, 42% contralateral, and 10% bilateral.[9] In spite of these discrepant numbers, clearly some patients with breast cancer have chest wall recurrences, and on radiologic evaluation, tumor is seen infiltrating through the chest wall into the pleural space, with resultant malignant effusion. Likewise, gross involvement of the internal mammary nodes occasionally is associated with an ipsilateral effusion.

Malignant pleural effusion rarely occurs as a component of the initial presentation of breast cancer, but more commonly occurs some time after the initial diagnosis of primary breast cancer, at a time when disseminated metastatic disease has developed. Time between initial diagnosis and occurrence of pleural effusions has been reported to be between 20 and 42 months, and in as many as 20% of patients it is the only initial site of metastatic disease.[7,8] The median survival of patients with malignant effusions is the same as for patients with metastatic breast cancer in general, between 1 and 2 years.

TREATMENT

Malignant effusions are troublesome because of the symptoms they cause, most notably shortness of breath, cough, and pain. Shortness of breath occurs primarily because of a ventilation–perfusion mismatch. The affected lung continues to receive deoxygenated blood from the pulmonary arterial vasculature, but because of the presence of the effusion, the lung may not expand with inspiration and ventilate.

Because effusions in these patients result from the presence of pleural metastases, successful systemic treatment of the breast cancer, either with hormonal therapy or chemotherapy, would result in disappearance of the effusion. The ability to accomplish this depends on the effectiveness of the therapy, and even if the therapy is effective, improvement with hormonal therapy or chemotherapy is slow, and the patient must be able to wait for this effect to occur and to understand that a beneficial effect may not be seen. Overall, in patients with newly diagnosed metastatic disease, response to systemic chemotherapy is about 70% and response to chemotherapy in patients with previously treated metastatic disease is variable, but in the range of 10% to 40%. Hormonal therapy can be expected to produce responses in 70% of patients with estrogen receptor–positive tumors and 10% of patients with estrogen receptor–negative tumors. These statistics should be taken into account when evaluating systemic therapy as a component of the treatment of a malignant effusion. The decision to use systemic treatment or local treatment is based on the size of the effusion, the degree of compromise of the patient, and the likelihood that systemic therapy will result in a rapid response.

Local treatment of the effusion consists either of intermittent drainage via percutaneous thoracentesis, chest tube placement and sclerosis, or thoracotomy and sclerosis. Intermittent drainage is effective only if systemic therapy has a simultaneous beneficial impact on the pleural metastases;

otherwise pleural fluid reaccumulates quickly, often at a rate of 1 to 3 L/d.

Chest tube drainage and sclerosis is based on the principle of draining the effusion dry, so that the parietal and visceral pleura are once again in contact with each other, and on instilling a sclerosing agent. Most sclerosing agents are designed to cause fusion of the parietal and visceral pleurae by chemical irritation. If the pleural surfaces become fused, the potential pleural space is obliterated, preventing reaccumulation of fluid. Chemotherapy agents such as thiotepa have been used in the hope that a direct antineoplastic effect would be seen and this effect would prevent reaccumulation of the effusion, but most agents work by chemical irritation of the pleura with resultant pleural fusion.

The success of pleural sclerosis is related to the ability to keep the pleural space dry so that the parietal and visceral pleurae are in contact during the instillation of the sclerosing agent, and with the irritative properties of the sclerosing agent. In practice, a chest tube is placed and attached to suction, and drainage continues until the daily fluid output falls below 100 to 200 mL/d. This often takes several days. In the experience of the authors, modest intravascular depletion with the aid of diuretics occasionally decreases chest tube output to the desired level. Follow-up chest radiographs are performed to evaluate the completeness of the drainage, particularly to determine whether loculated areas of effusion persist, which may require chest tube repositioning or placement of additional chest tubes.

Many drugs have been used as sclerosing agents, including tetracycline, nitrogen mustard, bleomycin, and talc. Reports in the literature of response rates for different agents vary, making it difficult to determine which agent is most effective. These variations are probably the result of differences in techniques, differences in the tumor characteristics of patient populations, and differences in the length of follow-up of the patients, because longer follow-up is associated with an increased failure rate. In some series, patients with various tumors are included, and even when breast cancer patients are examined as a separate group, the patients can be at various stages of their disease, which might effect response rates.

Nitrogen mustard, for instance, has been reported to achieve successful sclerosis in between 25% and 87% of patients.[10–12] In practice, nitrogen mustard is rarely used.

Tetracycline also has been used widely, although it is not available in the necessary formulation in the United States. Reported response rates for tetracycline vary widely. In one report, only 15% of patients receiving tetracycline had a complete response, and an additional 40% achieved partial responses (defined as patients having reaccumulation of some pleural fluid but not requiring repeated drainage).[13] Another study reports a complete response rate of 69%.[14] These authors suggest that the acid pH of the tetracycline solution might be responsible for the beneficial effects of sclerosis, rather than the tetracycline itself; they conducted a randomized trial comparing tetracycline and a placebo solution with a similar pH (2.8). As observed earlier, patients sclerosed with tetracycline had a complete response rate of 69%, whereas patients sclerosed with the acid solution had an 11% response rate.

Because tetracycline is no longer available in the United States in the form necessary for sclerosis, doxycycline has been used in its place. Complete response rates at 1 month after sclerosis of 88% and 78% have been reported for patients treated with chest tube drainage and doxycycline instillation, respectively.[15,16] Clearly this seems to be an acceptable replacement for tetracycline.

Bleomycin also has been used extensively as a sclerosing agent. One series reports a 69% complete response rate and a 12% partial response rate 30 days after bleomycin instillation.[17] At 90 days, 54% of patients were in complete response and 4% were in partial response. When evaluating patients with malignant effusions from breast cancer only, 81% of patients were responders at 30 days and 63% at 90 days. Several other studies report similar results, suggesting this as one of the more effective agents available.[18,19] In a randomized comparison of bleomycin and tetracycline, the reoccurrence of pleural fluid at 90 days after sclerosis was 30% in the group treated with bleomycin and 53% in the group treated with tetracycline, suggesting more prolonged control of the malignant effusion by bleomycin sclerosis when compared with tetracycline sclerosis.[20]

Talc, which causes an intense pleuritis, also has been widely used as a sclerosing agent, and some believe it to be the most effective agent available.[2] Most of the studies involving talc used more extensive surgical procedures, instilling the talc during pleuroscopy or thoracotomy under general or local anesthesia, making it a more cumbersome and risky procedure. A thoracoscopic approach, though, has the advantage of allowing the surgeon to be certain of complete fluid drainage, lysis of adhesions, and even distribution of the talc during insufflation. Using pleuroscopic instillation, Weissburg and coworkers[21] reported a 90% success rate. Other studies suggest control rates of 90% or more, also using either pleuroscopy or open thoracotomy with talc instillation.[22] In one trial randomizing talc versus mustine, the group sclerosed with talc had a 90% response rate compared with 56% for the group treated with mustine.[23] The same group studied talc versus tetracycline, reporting a 92% response rate to talc and a 48% response rate to tetracycline.[24] Another study compared, in a case–control manner, talc instilled through thoracoscopic guidance with chest tube drainage and bleomycin and tetracycline sclerosis.[25] Some centers are using talc instillation through percutaneous chest tube rather than during pleuroscopy or thoracotomy.

Other attempts to use chemotherapy agents instilled within the pleura have had only modest success. One such report by the Lung Cancer Study Group investigated administration of the combination of cisplatin and cytarabine in the management of malignant pleural effusions in patients with various primary tumors.[26] Systemic toxicity was modest, but the complete plus partial response rate was only 49%, and the median duration of response was 9 months for the complete responders and 5 months for the partial responders.

Summary

As shown in Table 23.9-1, several options exist for managing malignant pleural effusions from metastatic breast cancer. A review of the English-language literature evaluating

TABLE 23.9-1
Therapeutic Options for the Management of Malignant Pleural Effusion

PERCUTANEOUS DRAINAGE (THORACENTESIS)

Rapid and transiently effective, but unless the underlying tumor is controlled with systemic therapy, the effusion will rapidly recur.

THORACOSCOPIC INSTILLATION OF TALC

This has the highest success rate of all procedures. It allows direct visualization of the pleural space, assuring complete drainage of the effusion, and lysis of any adhesions. It also ensures relatively even distribution of the talc throughout the pleural space. This can be performed under general anesthesia or local anesthesia with sedation.

CHEST TUBE DRAINAGE AND SCLEROSIS WITH DOXYCYCLINE OR BLEOMYCIN

This procedure is relatively easy but requires chest tube drainage until the pleural fluid output falls below 100–200 mL/d. The success rate is lower than that for talc, but this procedure does not require general anesthesia or operating room time.

reports on 1168 patients suggests that talc insufflation has the highest response rate (93%), but acceptable rates also were found for tetracycline (67%), doxycycline (72%), minocycline (86%), and bleomycin (54%).[27] As a general recommendation, thoracoscopic insufflation with talc or chest tube drainage with sclerosis using doxycycline, minocycline, or bleomycin are reasonable alternatives for the management of malignant pleural effusions.

Pericardial Effusions

Breast cancer patients can develop pericardial effusions because of tumor involvement or radiation pericarditis. Pericardial involvement with tumor can lead to constrictive or effusive pericardial tamponade, either of which can result in cardiovascular collapse and death if not recognized and treated promptly.

HEMODYNAMICS AND PATHOPHYSIOLOGY OF PERICARDIAL TAMPONADE

Increased intrapericardial pressure results in reduced ventricular expansion and diastolic filling.[28] This further results in early closure of the atrioventricular valves. Myocardial muscle fiber length is shortened and stroke volume is reduced. An increase in mean ventricular, left and right atrial, pulmonary venous, and arterial and vena caval pressures occurs. While cardiac output drops, heart rate and peripheral vasoconstriction increase to maintain arterial perfusion and venous return to the heart.

CLINICAL SIGNS OF PERICARDIAL TAMPONADE

Because of the pathophysiology of pericardial tamponade, a number of important signs may be observed in early and later stages of pericardial tamponade, as outlined in Table

23.9-2. One of the most important and early signs is dyspnea on exertion; exertion can unmask deficits in early tamponade because the heart is unable to increase cardiac output in response to the increased oxygen demand of the exercised muscles. As part of this phenomenon, dyspnea on exertion can be severe, although the patient can be reasonably comfortable at rest. In most series, dyspnea is the most common complaint, present in about 75% of patients with tamponade.[29] Arterial blood gases obtained at rest often show normal oxygenation, sometimes causing the clinician to wonder about the cause of the dyspnea on exertion. Because of peripheral vasoconstriction, the patient's extremities may be cool and cyanotic.

A number of physical examination findings have been associated with tamponade, including tachycardia, decreased or absent cardiac impulse, pericardial friction rub, paradoxical movement of the jugular venous pulse, pulsus paradoxicus, atrial fibrillation, and pulsus alternans. Tachycardia can become more pronounced with minimal exertion; this results, as mentioned earlier, from the heart's inability to increase cardiac output with increasing muscle oxygen demand. With significant tamponade, the cardiac impulse is almost always absent. The heart, pumping with reduced stroke volume within a tense pericardial sac, transmits no discernible impulse. Pericardial friction rub sometimes is heard in the early stages of malignant pericardial

TABLE 23.9-2
Symptoms and Signs of Pericardial Tamponade

SYMPTOMS

Dyspnea on exertion

Orthopnea

Tachycardia

Chest pain

CLINICAL SIGNS

Tachycardia

Distant heart sounds

Decreased or absent cardiac impulse

Pericardial friction rub

Hypotension and peripheral vascular constriction

Jugular venous distention

Paradoxical movement of the jugular venous pulse

Pulsus paradoxicus

Pulsus alternans

LABORATORY FINDINGS

Low voltage on electrocardiogram

Electrical alternans

Enlarged globular cardiac silhouette on chest radiograph

Pericardial effusion or thickened pericardium on echocardiography

Diastolic collapse of the right atrium and ventricle on echocardiography

Pericardial effusion or thickened pericardium on computed tomography involvement but may disappear while the effusion becomes larger, and causes complete separation of the pericardium and myocardium. Jugular venous distention may be more pronounced because of increased right atrial pressure, and there may be paradoxical movement of the jugular venous pulse, increasing with inspiration rather than decreasing with inspiration, presumably because of stretching of the heart and pericardium on downward movement of the diaphragms, resulting in increased intrapericardial pressure. Pulsus paradoxicus, defined as a drop of 10 mmHg or more in systolic blood pressure with inspiration, occurs by the same pathophysiologic route as paradoxical movement of the jugular venous pulse. Atrial fibrillation occurs, most likely, because of the direct electrical irritative effects of pericardial metastases. Pulsus alternans and electrical alternans are seen in few cases and represent unclear pathophysiologic processes.[30,31] Low voltage also can be seen on electrocardiogram because of reduced electrical transmission through the fluid-filled pericardial sac.

None of these clinical signs are seen universally in malignant pericardial tamponade, and most, except for tachycardia and absence of cardiac impulse, are seen in only a few patients, so that the clinician must have a high degree of suspicion of pericardial involvement, and proceed, when appropriate, with more definitive testing.[32] In addition, the clinician must distinguish between malignant pericardial tamponade, idiopathic tamponade, and radiation-induced pericarditis. The clinical scenario often is helpful in this differential diagnosis, because, for instance, radiation-induced pericarditis occurs only in patients who received radiation therapy to the pericardium.

DIAGNOSIS

Pericardial tamponade from pericardial effusion or constrictive pericarditis can be suggested by the presence of the clinical signs outlined earlier. Chest radiography sometimes reveals the typical enlarged globular cardiac shadow. In cases of constrictive pericardial tamponade, though, the cardiac shadow may not be enlarged. Pleural effusion is a frequent finding in patients with pericardial tamponade but obviously is not specific.[26]

Echocardiography has been a mainstay in the diagnosis of pericardial effusion and cardiac tamponade. In the case of effusive pericarditis, the fluid-filled pericardial sac can be demonstrated. Fluid often initially collects posteriorly, but with increasing fluid, it usually fills the entire sac. Collapse of the right atrium and right ventricle during diastole is one of the cardinal signs of tamponade physiology, and is important in determining clinical compromise in the patient with a pericardial effusion.[33] While pericardial fluid increases and intrapericardial pressure rises, right atrial collapse occurs first.[34] With increasing intrapericardial pressure, right ventricular collapse during diastole occurs, which has been shown to be highly predictive of tamponade physiology, with a sensitivity of 92% and a specificity of 100% in the series of Singh and others.[34] Once right ventricular collapse occurs, drainage of pericardial fluid is likely to improve cardiac function. During dynamic studies, it has been shown that with removal of pericardial fluid while intrapericardial pressure decreases,

a major improvement in cardiac function occurs at the same time that right ventricular collapse disappears.

Computed tomography is also useful in determining the presence of pericardial effusion and pericardial thickening, which often is seen in malignant pericardial disease.[35] On occasion, it demonstrates pericardial abnormalities not seen on echocardiographic examination. It does not, however, give physiologic information because it is a static study.

PERICARDIAL DISEASE IN BREAST CANCER PATIENTS

Breast cancer is one of the leading causes of malignant pericardial disease, together with lung cancer and non-Hodgkin lymphoma.[32] Pericardial involvement by breast cancer is present in about 25% of patients with metastatic disease by the time of death, but is responsible for death in less than 5% of breast cancer patients.[36] In a large series from the Mayo Clinic, breast cancer patients were divided into three groups; those with effusions discovered incidently on echocardiography, those without any evidence of metastatic breast cancer with symptoms suggestive of pericardial tamponade, and those with known metastatic breast cancer and signs or symptoms of pericardial tamponade.[37] Of the patients discovered incidentally, all had small effusions, and only 1 of 20 patients had clinical signs of pericardial tamponade late in the course of her disease that were believed to result from malignant involvement of the pericardium without histologic confirmation. Of the patients without known metastatic disease but with symptomatic pericardial effusion, 20% required surgical treatment of tamponade but none had definitive evidence of malignant cause of their effusion. All were thought to result from radiation pericarditis. Of 38 patients with known metastatic breast cancer, 15 (39%) had large effusions, 19 (50%) had certain malignant diagnosis, and others may also have had malignant causes of their effusions that were not histologically documented. In this group of patients, surgical therapy was essential for the successful management of the pericardial disease. Pericardiocentesis alone was associated with a high relapse rate, even with concurrent chemotherapy, and treatment with systemic chemotherapy only was associated with a high failure rate and sudden death in several patients. The median survival of patients with known malignant pericardial involvement was 17 months; it was 20 months for patients who had surgical management of their effusions.

TREATMENT

Pericardial tamponade is a medical emergency, is associated with severe symptoms, and can result in sudden death. Most cases seem to result primarily from effusive pericarditis, but some result from constrictive pericarditis, and the treatment approach may be different for the two groups. As noted earlier, patients with symptomatic tamponade should not be treated with systemic therapy alone. The failure rate is high, as is the incidence of sudden cardiac death. Therapeutic options include percutaneous pericardial catheter drainage, surgical placement of a pericardial window, and pericardial stripping.

Tetracycline sclerosis also has been used as a therapy.[38] Pericardial catheters were placed into the pericardial sac and allowed to drain for 12 to 24 hours, after which xylocaine and tetracycline were instilled. One to five instillations were performed, and the authors reported a 68% control rate with no evidence of development of constrictive pericardial compromise. In practice, this is not widely used, in part because patients require continued close monitoring and, often, multiple treatments using sclerosis, whereas pericardotomy usually is successful as a single procedure.

Simple catheter drainage can be life-saving by rapidly relieving critical tamponade because removal of even small amounts of pericardial fluid can result in substantial improvement in cardiac dynamics; however, this procedure has not demonstrated lasting success in most cases because effusions frequently reoccur and sudden death can result.[37]

Most patients are treated with surgical placement of a pericardial window, often using the subxiphoid approach.[39,40] This can be accomplished quickly and safely with a high success rate. More extensive surgical approaches using an anterior thoracotomy approach allowing removal of more of the pericardium also have been used. In one nonrandomized study comparing these two techniques, subxiphoid pericardiotomy was equally effective and had a far lower complication rate than anterior thoracotomy.[41] No difference in survival existed between patients treated with subxiphoid pericardiotomy compared with those treated with anterior thoracotomy, and no patients undergoing subxiphoid pericardiotomy required further treatment of the pericardial effusion. In addition, no patients undergoing subxiphoid pericardiotomy had major complications, whereas half the patients undergoing anterior thoracotomy sustained major complications, including pulmonary embolism, arterial embolism with gangrene, disseminated intravascular coagulation, acute renal failure, pneumonia, sepsis, pleural effusion requiring drainage, and recurrent pericardial effusion. Although this was not a randomized study, pretreatment patient characteristics were similar, suggesting the difference in complication rate was not likely because of patients with more advanced disease being selected for anterior thoracotomy.

Thoracoscopic approaches to pericardiectomy also have been reported using a video-assisted thoracoscopic three-cannula technique. This method allows for a more extensive pericardiectomy than the subxiphoid approach but is a less invasive procedure than thoracotomy. Mack and associates[42] reported on 22 patients, all of whom had successful relief of their pericardial effusion without morbidity or mortality. It seems that the ability to open both the anterior and posterior pericardial cavity makes this superior to the subxiphoid approach, and morbidity and mortality is lower than with thoracotomy.

The presence of pericardial fluid allows for a safer thoracoscopic pericardiectomy. Therefore, we do not advise using catheter drainage in patients in whom a surgical approach is contemplated unless hemodynamic compromise is present. Pericardial fluid protects the myocardium during incision of the pericardium through the thoracoscopic approach. Selection of the right or left side to perform the thoracoscopic pericardiectomy may be dictated by the presence of a pleural effusion, because, if desired, a talc pleurodesis can be performed during the same procedure.

SUMMARY

Options for the management of pericardial effusion are shown in Table 23.9-3. A review of the English-language publications addressing management of malignant pericardial effusions suggests that pericardial drainage by percutaneous catheter is effective at relieving the physiologic features causing tamponade, and in patients with tumors expected to rapidly respond to systemic therapy, this may be all that is needed.[43] When the underlying tumor cannot be expected to respond rapidly to systemic therapy, as might be the case for patients with disseminated breast cancer, placement of a pericardial window by the subxiphoid approach is relatively safe and has a high chance of success. A video-assisted thoracoscopic approach has a high success rate with low morbidity and mortality. For patients in whom this approach is planned, catheter drainage of the pericardial fluid should not be performed unless there is hemodynamic compromise, because the presence of pericardial fluid protects the myocardium and makes the technique safer. Patients with extensive constrictive pericardial involvement may require open thoracotomy and pericardial stripping. These patients represent a minority of patients with breast cancer and pericardial involvement.

TABLE 23.9-3
Management of Malignant Pericardial Tamponade

PERCUTANEOUS CATHETER DRAINAGE

This has the advantage of ease, can be performed rapidly and relatively safely under ultrasound guidance, and can effectively reverse tamponade physiology. Unless the underlying tumor is controlled rapidly with systemic therapy, the effusion is likely to recur.

SUBXIPHOID PERICARDIAL WINDOW

This procedure has low morbidity and mortality and is effective in most patients with malignant pericardial tamponade. The recurrence of effusion and tamponade is uncommon.

VIDEO-ASSISTED THORACOSCOPIC SURGERY (VATS)

This procedure, performed with a three-cannula technique, has a high success rate, low morbidity, and low mortality. It is safer when performed with pericardial effusion present, because the effusion protects the myocardium during the initial incision. Therefore, catheter drainage of the pericardial effusion should not be done unless there is hemodynamic compromise.

THORACOTOMY AND PERICARDIAL STRIPPING

This procedure is associated with a higher complication rate than subxiphoid window placement but is required in a small number of patients with diffuse involvement of the pericardium and resultant constrictive pericarditis.

Ascites

Ascites in patients with breast cancer can occur either from peritoneal serosal implants or from extensive hepatic metastases and resultant portal hypertension. Extensive hepatic metastases with portal hypertension usually occurs as a terminal event, and unless systemic chemotherapy is rapidly effective in reducing the tumor burden, fatal hepatic failure ensues. Ascites in this circumstance is of secondary concern.

Ascites from peritoneal tumor implants is uncommon in breast cancer patients. The abdominal bloating is uncomfortable in itself and often causes early satiety, resulting in decreased oral intake and upward pressure on the diaphragm, which prevents full expansion of the lungs and can cause shortness of breath and dyspnea on exertion. The ascites in itself is not life-threatening because the peritoneal implants are usually only one manifestation of disseminated metastatic disease, with other sites of involvement often being more life-threatening. This is different than the situation in ovarian cancer, where isolated intraabdominal disease is common and often is the major clinical problem for the patient.

In patients with metastatic breast cancer and ascites, the most effective therapy is systemic chemotherapy or hormonal therapy directed at reducing tumor mass, which results in a reduced amount of ascites. If this is not feasible or the ascites is particularly discomforting, then paracenteses can be performed, which transiently improves comfort. Without control of the basic tumor, though, ascitic fluid reaccumulates. The rate of reaccumulation is variable from patient to patient, and some patients have relief of their symptoms for several days and benefit from repeated paracenteses.

Intraabdominal chemotherapy has been widely used in patients with ovarian cancer because the peritoneum frequently is the only site of disease, and in these patients it can clearly have a palliative role. Breast cancer patients usually have other sites of metastatic disease that are frequently more troublesome to them, making intraabdominal chemotherapy an inappropriate option for most breast cancer patients.

Peritoneovenous shunts have been described as therapy for patients with malignant ascites and have been shown to reduce abdominal girth and number of paracenteses in selected groups of patients.[44–46] Complications can be serious, however, with a significant number of patients developing disseminated intravascular coagulation, sepsis, and congestive heart failure. Shunts frequently clot, and there is the theoretic concern that shunts will seed peritoneal tumor cells into the pulmonary circulation, resulting in the development of pulmonary metastases. In practice, peritoneovenous shunts are rarely used to palliate ascites in patients with metastatic breast cancer.

References

1. Leff A, Hopewell PC, Costello J. Pleural effusion from malignancy. Ann Intern Med 1978;88:532.
2. Hausheer FH, Yarbro JW. Diagnosis and treatment of malignant pleural effusion. Semin Oncol 1985;12:54.
3. Silverberg I. Management of effusions. Oncology 1970;24:26.
4. Sahn SA, Good JT. Pleural fluid pH in malignant effusions: diagnostic, prognostic, and therapeutic implications. Ann Intern Med 1988;108:345.
5. Sanchez-Armengol A, Rodriguez-Panadero F. Survival and talc pleurodesis in metastatic pleural carcinoma revisited: report of 125 cases. Chest 1993;104:1482.
6. Prakash UBS, Reiman HM. Comparison of needle biopsy with cytologic analysis for the evaluation of pleural effusion: analysis of 414 cases. Mayo Clin Proc 1985;60:158.
7. Johnston WW. The malignant pleural effusion: a review of cytopathologic diagnoses of 584 specimens from 472 consecutive patients. Cancer 1985;56:905.
8. Raju RN, Kardinal CG. Pleural effusion in breast carcinoma: analysis of 122 cases. Cancer 1981;48:2524.
9. Fentiman IS, Millis R, Sexton S, et al. Pleural effusion in breast cancer: a review of 105 cases. Cancer 1981;47:2087.
10. Weisberger AS, Levine B, Storaasli JP. Use of nitrogen mustard in the treatment of serous effusions of neoplastic origin. JAMA 1955;159:1704.
11. Fracchia AA, Knapper WH, Carey JT, et al. Intrapleural chemotherapy for effusions from metastatic breast carcinoma. Cancer 1970;26:626.
12. Kinsey DL, Carter D, Klassen KP. Simplified management of malignant pleural effusion. Arch Surg 1964;89:389.
13. Gravelyn TR, Michelson MK, Gross BH, et al. Tetracycline pleurodesis for malignant pleural effusions: a 10-year retrospective study. Cancer 1987;59:1973.
14. Zaloznik AJ, Oswald SG, Langin M. Intrapleural tetracycline in malignant pleural effusions: a randomized study. Cancer 1983;51:752.
15. Robinson LA, Fleming WH, Galbraith TA. Intrapleural doxycycline control of malignant pleural effusions. Ann Thorac Surg 1993;55:1115.
16. Heffner JE, Standerfer RJ, Torstveit J, et al. Clinical efficacy of doxycycline for pleurodesis. Chest 1994;105:1743.
17. Ostrowski MJ. An assessment of the long-term results of controlling reaccumulation of malignant effusions using intracavity bleomycin. Cancer 1986;57:721.
18. Bitran JD, Brown C, Desser RK, et al. Intracavitary bleomycin for the control of malignant effusions. J Surg Oncol 1981;16:273.
19. Paladine W, Cunningham TJ, Sponzo R, et al. Intracavitary bleomycin in the management of malignant effusions. Cancer 1976;38:1903.
20. Ruckdeschel JC, Moores D, Lee JY, et al. Intrapleural therapy for malignant pleural effusions: a randomized comparison of bleomycin and tetracycline. Chest 1991;100:1528.
21. Weissburg D, Kaufman M, Zurkowski Z. Pleuroscopy in patients with pleural effusions and pleural masses. Ann Thorac Surg 1980;29:205.
22. Pearson FG, Macgregor DC. Talc poudrage for malignant pleural effusion. J Thorac Cardiovasc Surg 1966;51:732.
23. Fentiman IS, Rubens RD, Hayward JL. Control of pleural effusions in patients with breast cancer: a randomized trial. Cancer 1983;52:737.
24. Fentiman IS, Rubens RD, Hayward JL. A comparison of intracavitary talc and tetracycline for the control of pleural effusions secondary to breast cancer. Eur J Cancer Clin Oncol 1986;22:1079.
25. Hartman DL, Gaither JM, Kesler KA, et al. Comparison of insufflated talc under thoracoscopic guidance with standard tetracycline and bleomycin pleurodesis for control of malignant pleural effusion. J Thorac Cardiovasc Surg 1993;105:743.
26. Rusch VW, Figlin R, Godwin D, et al. Intrapleural cisplatin and cytarabine in the management of malignant pleural effusions: a lung Cancer Study Group trial. J Clin Oncol 1991;9:313.
27. Walker-Renard PB, Vaughan LM, Sahn SA. Chemical pleurodesis for malignant pleural effusions. Ann Intern Med 1994;120:56.

28. Theologides A. Neoplastic cardiac tamponade. Semin Oncol 1978;5:181.

29. Cham WC, Freiman AH, Carstens PHB, et al. Radiation therapy of cardiac and pericardial metastases. Ther Radiol 1975;114:701.

30. Lawrence LT, Cronin JF. Electrical alternans and pericardial tamponade. Arch Intern Med 1963;112:415.

31. Spodick DH. Electrical alternation of the heart: its relation to the kinetics and physiology of the heart during cardiac tamponade. Am J Cardiol 1962;10:155.

32. Posner MR, Cohen GI, Skarin AT. Pericardial disease in patients with cancer: the differentiation of malignant from idiopathic and radiation-induced pericarditis. Am J Med 1981;71:407.

33. Gillam LD, Guyer DE, Gibson TC, et al. Hydrodynamic compression of the right atrium: a new echocardiographic sign of cardiac tamponade. Circulation 1983;68:294.

34. Singh S, Wann S, Schuchard GH, et al. Right ventricular and right atrial collapse in patients with cardiac tamponade: a combined echocardiographic and hemodynamic study. Circulation 1984;70:966.

35. Isner JM, Carter BL, Bankoff MS, et al. Computed tomography in the diagnosis of pericardial heart disease. Ann Intern Med 1982;97:473.

36. Hagemeister FB, Buzdar AU, Luna MA, et al. Causes of death in breast cancer. Cancer 1980;46:162.

37. Buck M, Ingle JN, Giuliani ER, et al. Pericardial effusion in women with breast cancer. Cancer 1987;60:263.

38. Shepherd FA, Ginsberg JS, Evans WK, et al. Tetracycline sclerosis in the management of malignant pericardial effusion. J Clin Oncol 1985;3:1678.

39. Snow N, Lucas A. Subxiphoid pericardiotomy: a safe, accurate, diagnostic and therapeutic approach to pericardial and intrapericardial disease. Am Surg 1983;49:249.

40. Osuch JR, Khandekar JD, Fry WA. Emergency subxiphoid pericardial decompression for malignant pericardial effusion. Am Surg 1985;51:298.

41. Park JS, Rentschler R, Wilbur D. Surgical management of pericardial effusion in patients with malignancies. Cancer 1991;67:76.

42. Mack MJ, Landreneau RJ, Hazelrigg SR, et al. Video thoracoscopic management of benign and malignant pericardial effusions. Chest 1993;103:390S.

43. Vaitkus PT, Herrmann HC, LeWinter MM. Treatment of malignant pericardial effusion. JAMA 1994;272:59.

44. Qazi R, Savlov ED. Peritoneovenous shunt for palliation of malignant ascites. Cancer 1982;49:600.

45. Cheung DK, Raaf JH. Selection of patients with malignant ascites for a peritoneovenous shunt. Cancer 1982;50:1204.

46. Souter RG, Wells C, Tarin D, et al. Surgical and pathologic complications associated with peritoneovenous shunts in management of malignant ascites. Cancer 1985;55:1973.

23.10

Hypercalcemia

RAYMOND P. WARRELL, JR.

Hypercalcemia is the major metabolic complication most commonly experienced by women with breast cancer. Estimates of the incidence of hypercalcemia in breast cancer generally range from 10% to 15%.[1-3] Patients with metastases to both bone and liver may be especially prone to the development of hypercalcemia, with an incidence of up to 31% in one series.[3] Although exceptions exist, hypercalcemia usually is a manifestation of advanced disease.

Etiology

Of all tumor types, breast cancer has been the prototype for hypercalcemia associated with bone metastases. Less than 10% of women with breast cancer develop hypercalcemia in the absence of detectable bone metastases,[3] and for practical purposes, the disorder does not occur with localized disease.

Previously, breast cancer cells were thought to directly resorb bone independent of osteoclasts, possibly by releasing proteolytic enzymes that digested bone matrix.[4] However, these in vitro findings generally have not been confirmed in studies of clinical specimens. Furthermore, as with other types of cancers, no particular relation has existed between the extent of osteolytic disease and the incidence of hypercalcemia.[5,6]

In the mid-1970s, extracts from certain tumors were found to contain factors with osteoclast-activating activity (OAFs). A number of proteins have been shown to stimulate bone-resorptive activity by osteoclasts.[7] For many of these cytokines, such as colony-stimulating factors, interleukin-1, and interleukin-6,[8-10] OAF activity is probably insignificant compared with their mediation of other effects. In most patients, bone resorption is initiated by normal osteoclasts that have been excessively stimulated by locally active factors released or induced by tumor cells. In breast cancer, a number of proteins have been implicated as initiators of osteoclast activation in the development of hypercalcemia; however, the extent of their contribution to the syndrome, mechanisms of action, and interactions with each other are poorly understood. Two of the most important factors are the parathyroid hormone–related protein (PTH-RP) and the transforming growth factors (TGFs).

PARATHYROID HORMONE–RELATED PROTEIN

Of the several factors implicated in the pathogenesis of cancer-related hypercalcemia, the most important is the PTH-RP.[11-14] PTH-RP is a 17,000-kd protein comprised of about 170 amino acids and encoded by a gene mapped to the short arm of chromosome 12.[15] Several bioactive fragments of the peptide have been found in the circulation of hypercalcemic patients,[16-19] a finding that suggests the protein is subject to posttranslational or postsecretory modification. Compared with native human PTH (whose gene is located on chromosome 11), PTH–RP shares only partial amino acid homologic features within the first 13 amino acids (which corresponds to the receptor-binding domain) and thereafter differs entirely. Thus, although the protein seems to be misnamed, it is nonetheless widely distributed, and on immunohistochemical staining, it has been found in a number of normal tissues including heart, parathyroid, thyroid, bladder, uterus, and brain.[19–24] From an evolutionary standpoint, the factor is highly conserved and high levels of PTH–RP have been found in human milk and lactating breast tissue,[25–27] a finding that previously suggested a developmental role. High levels of expression also have been associated with stretch reflexes in smooth muscle, particularly in uterus.[23,24] PTH–RP appears to act only intracellularly to regulate calcium channel fluxes; it has no known extracellular function under normal homeostatic conditions.

Patients with breast cancer were not previously thought to exhibit clinical findings of pseudo- or ectopic hyperparathyroidism (ie, hypophosphatemia, hyperphosphaturia, and hyperchloremia[28]). However, new studies using sensitive assays of biochemical function[29–31] have indicated that many patients have evidence of increased PTH-like activity. Reports show an unexpectedly high incidence—up to 50%—of increased PTH–RP levels in hypercalcemic patients with breast cancer.[16,32–34] Therefore, PTH–RP is considered an important mediator of hypercalcemia in breast cancer, exerting effects both locally at the sites of bone metastases and systemically on the renal tubule.[35] Finally, high levels of PTH–RP expression have been described in breast cancer cells that have metastasized to bone[36,37] and in banked specimens of breast cancers excised at diagnosis from patients who ultimately relapsed in bone.[38] These observations suggest that this protein may partly regulate the osteotropic potential of breast cancers (ie, the propensity of breast cancer to preferentially metastasize to bone). Tests for PTH–RP are commercially available; however, their general use is limited (except, perhaps, as a tumor marker of disease activity). They are primarily useful for distinguishing between unusual causes of hypercalcemia or for occult disease in breast cancer patients previously treated for parathyroid adenomas. Plasma levels of PTH–RP are not influenced by specific antihypercalcemic therapies, such as gallium nitrate or bisphosphonates, irrespective of the drugs' effects on serum calcium.[39–41]

TRANSFORMING GROWTH FACTORS

In vitro, both transforming growth factor α (TGF-α) and transforming growth factor β (TGF-β) have major effects on cell-mediated bone resorption and formation.[42–52] TGF-β is secreted by osteoblasts and may serve as an autocrine regulator of osteoblast growth and differentiation.[46–48] Administration of purified TGF-β to rodents causes a marked increase in osteoid synthesis and bone formation. Conversely, systemic administration of TGF-α stimulates bone resorption and induces hypercalcemia.[42–45,52] Because both TGFs are elaborated by breast cancer cells, an imbalance between resorption and forma-

tion—tightly coupled under normal circumstances—may account for the typically mixed lytic and blastic pattern of skeletal metastases observed in this disease.

Specific identification of the mediators of osteoclast activation in hypercalcemia may become increasingly relevant to clinical practice. As receptors for these proteins and their mechanisms of action are characterized, it becomes possible to design specific pharmacologic inhibitors that reverse their deleterious activities. Antagonists of the PTH–RP,[53] active and passive immunotherapy against PTH–RP,[54,55] and interleukin-1 receptor antagonists[56] all have been developed and are being tested.

Clinical Manifestations and Differential Diagnosis

Symptoms of hypercalcemia are nonspecific and reflect both the severity and the chronicity of the syndrome. Most commonly, patients present insidiously with fatigue, nausea, constipation, polyuria, and dehydration. As the syndrome worsens, mental status deteriorates with increasing confusion and somnolence. Less commonly in breast cancer, hypercalcemic patients present with renal failure, cardiac arrythmias, psychosis, or abdominal complaints resulting from ileus or pancreatitis. A syndrome unique in breast cancer is the occurrence of hypercalcemia and bone pain that occurs shortly after the introduction (and occasionally the withdrawal) of hormonal therapy, the so-called flare phenomenon.[57]

Overwhelmingly, hypercalcemia from breast cancer occurs in women with established disease and bone metastases.[1–3] Diagnostic confusion may arise in patients who develop hypercalcemia while on treatment in the absence of obvious progressive disease. Several reports have noted an increased prevalence of primary hyperparathyroidism in patients with breast cancer.[58,59] However, one evaluation suggests that this incidence is no greater than that in a comparable age-matched population.[60] Classically, patients with hyperparathyroidism exhibit a metabolic alkalosis with hypophosphatemia, hyperchloremia, and hyperphosphaturia because of increased tubular reabsorption of phosphate.[61] Urinary cyclic adenosine monophosphate also is elevated,[62] although this test is unavailable in most clinical laboratories. Furthermore, the use of such nonspecific tests has been greatly diminished by the prevalence of the PTH–RP, which can mimic all of these effects. Because current radioimmunoassays for the intact PTH molecule do not cross-react with PTH–RP or its circulating fragments, the most useful test for distinguishing primary hyperparathyroidism from cancer-related hypercalcemia remains the measurement of serum PTH by a reliable method.[63] As observed earlier, about one half of hypercalcemic women with breast cancer have detectable elevations of plasma PTH–RP levels.[32–35]

Patients with hypercalcemia, localized breast cancer, and a normal serum PTH level pose a more difficult diagnostic problem, and other diagnostic possibilities must be considered. Among the more important causes are excessive ingestion of dietary supplements that include calcium or vitamin D, thiazide usage, granulomatous diseases such as sarcoidosis, hyperthyroidism, or another type of cancer. A careful history and physical examination, combined with directed laboratory studies (eg, chest radiograph, skin testing, and serum vitamin D levels), usually are sufficient to make the diagnosis.[64]

Management

The management of cancer-related hypercalcemia must include a judgment as to severity of the disorder and whether hospitalization is required. A third consideration is whether to specifically treat hypercalcemia in a patient who is terminally ill without other therapeutic options. A general treatment guideline appears in Table 23.10-1. Hospitalization should be recommended for patients with a serum calcium of 12 mg/dL or more (3 mmol/L) or for any patient who has symptoms other than mild fatigue. Aggressively treating patients who are nauseous or mentally impaired is especially important because an inability to maintain oral fluid intake leads to rapid dehydration from polyuria and marked clinical deterioration.

Severity of the illness may not be directly related to the level of serum calcium. Patients with long-standing hypercalcemia tolerate substantially higher levels of serum calcium than patients who experience an abrupt onset. Because malnutrition and hypoproteinemia often accompany hypercalcemia in patients with advanced cancer, simple measurements of total serum calcium may understate the severity of the disorder. It is useful to obtain a determination of ionized serum calcium using an ion-specific elec-

trode. Alternatively, total serum calcium can be adjusted for the level of serum protein using an algorithm such as the following[65]:

$$\text{Corrected [calcium] (mg/dL)}\star$$
$$= \text{measured [calcium] (mg/dL)}$$
$$- \text{[albumin] (g/dL)} + 4.0$$

In this chapter, all references to serum calcium refer to *corrected* values.

HYDRATION AND DIURETICS

Rehydration with intravenous fluids is recommended for all hospitalized patients, and normal saline is the preferred solution except for patients who have gross edema or congestive heart failure. Infusion rates of 200 to 400 mL/h (or higher) can be used in the initial hours of therapy, provided that strict attention is paid to ensuring adequate urinary output and fluid balance. In moderate-to-severe hypercalcemia (total calcium of 12.0 mg/dL or more), saline hydration alone does not generally reduce the serum calcium to normal.[66] Furosemide is commonly administered to increase calciuresis, even though compelling evidence of clinical effectiveness is lacking. If used, furosemide should be given *after* the patient has received adequate fluid replacement to replenish intravascular volume lost from dehydration. Serum potassium and magnesium may be further depleted by furosemide therapy and should be replaced parenterally as needed. With the advent of more effective drugs, the goals of fluid therapy have changed from a mainstay of primary treatment to a rapid restoration of intravascular volume and resumption of urinary output.

CALCITONIN AND CORTICOSTEROIDS

Most forms of hypocalcemic treatment should be delayed until adequate urinary output has been ensured. However, in patients with hypercalcemia that is immediately life-threatening, calcitonin may be extremely useful. Calcitonin has a rapid onset of action (within 2 to 4 hours),[67] causes few serious toxic reactions, and can be used immediately without regard to hydration status or renal function. The drug has some important disadvantages, including nausea, brief duration of action, incomplete effect, rapid loss of activity (the escape phenomenon), and infrequent hypersensitivity reactions. When administered acutely, it is preferable to give large doses (6 to 8 IU/kg) every 6 to 8 hours, generally for a maximum of 2 days. To minimize variability in absorption, intramuscular rather than subcutaneous injections generally should be used. Because calcitonin rarely reduces serum calcium to normal, it should not be relied on as a single agent for hospitalized patients. More potent drugs such as gallium nitrate

TABLE 23.10-1

Determining the Appropriate Level of Care for Patients With Hypercalcemia Related to Breast Cancer

Parameter	Outpatient	Inpatient
Serum calcium level	<12 mg/dL	≥12 mg/dL
Nausea or vomiting	Nothing significant	Yes
Digestion	Able to ingest fluids	Dehydrated
Mental status	Alert	Impaired
Renal function	Normal	Renal insufficiency
Cardiac rhythm	Stable	Arrhythmia
Gastrointestinal status	Mild constipation	Obstipation, ileus
Home status	Companion for supervision	Lives alone
Medical care access	Access to emergency care	Limited access

(Adapted from Warrell RP Jr. Metabolic emergencies. In: DeVita V Jr, Hellman S, Rosenberg SA, eds. Cancer: principles and practice of oncology, ed 4. Philadelphia, JB Lippincott, 1993:2128)

★ Concentrations in milligrams per deciliter can be converted to SI units by multiplying by 0.2495, yielding concentrations expressed in millimoles per liter.

or a bisphosphonate should be added after the patient has been hydrated and urinary output has been established. Despite weak single-agent activity, the combination of calcitonin with a third-generation bisphosphonate or with gallium nitrate may become a standard for acute treatment of life-threatening hypercalcemia.[68]

For most patients with cancer-related hypercalcemia, the addition of corticosteroids does not enhance the effect of calcitonin. Breast cancer may represent an important exception, not because the drugs are synergistic or prevent "escape," but because each agent is independently effective. About 25% of patients with breast cancer experience an objective antitumor effect with the use of corticosteroids alone.[69] Therefore, a partial hypocalcemic effect could be anticipated with or without the use of calcitonin. For acute treatment, larger doses (40 to 100 mg of prednisone or the equivalent per day) are preferred, with tapering of the dose as tolerated to minimize side effects. Disadvantages to acute use in emergencies include a slow onset of action (up to a week) and hyperglycemia, which may further exacerbate dehydration.

PHOSPHATES

The most important action of phosphate is inhibition of calcium resorption from bone.[70] Practically no indications remain for the use of intravenous phosphate in the acute treatment of hypercalcemia. Parenteral phosphates have been associated with a high incidence of acute renal failure, along with less common sequelae such as ectopic calcifications in muscle, heart, lung, and eye.[71,72] However, orally administered phosphate (0.5 to 3 g/d in divided doses) may be especially valuable, particularly for patients who are hypophosphatemic, and this agent represents an important component of hypocalcemic therapy, particularly for outpatients.[73,74] Adverse effects of oral phosphates include nausea and diarrhea. Phosphates should not be used in the presence of significant renal insufficiency or in patients who are already hyperphosphatemic.

MITHRAMYCIN

Mithramycin is directly cytotoxic to osteoclasts,[75] and thus it directly decreases bone resorption by the effector cell. Mithramycin is generally regarded as one of the most potent hypercalcemic agents available, albeit one of the most toxic. Mithramycin is administered at doses ranging from 10 to 50 μg/kg of body weight, with the usual dose being 25 μg/kg, or a total dose of 1.5 to 2 mg. The drug can be administered as a bolus injection or as brief or prolonged infusions. The longer infusions (4 to 6 hours) do not improve the hypercalcemic effect and should probably be avoided because of venous irritation and inconvenience, unless nausea is severe. The onset of action occurs after 24 to 48 hours; therefore, doses should not be repeated more frequently than every 2 to 3 days. Thrombocytopenia, hepatotoxicity, and renal insufficiency are the most important adverse effects of mithramycin, and toxicity may be cumulative.[76]

GALLIUM NITRATE

Gallium nitrate is a potent new drug for treatment of cancer-related hypercalcemia. After localizing in bone tissue,[77] gallium inhibits the proton pump of the osteoclast, thereby impairing its ability to acidify and resorb bone mineral and matrix.[78] This drug also seems to enhance calcium accretion into bone and to promote synthesis of bone collagen.[79-81] These dual actions on formation and resorption may partly account for its potency. Randomized double-blind studies have shown superiority of gallium nitrate relative to both maximally approved doses of calcitonin as well as the bisphosphonate etidronate.[82,83] Randomized studies against pamidronate are near completion.

In unselected individuals with moderate-to-severe hypercalcemia, 80% to 90% of patients can be expected to achieve normocalcemia. The drug does not cause nausea or myelosuppression. The major side effect is renal insufficiency, which can be minimized by ensuring adequate urinary output during acute therapy (about 2000 mL/d). A dose of 200 mg/m^2/d (usually 350 mg) is administered by a continuous intravenous (IV) infusion until the serum calcium has normalized or up to a maximum of 5 days. The use of low-dose subcutaneous injections (40 mg once per day) after acute treatment may extend the duration of normocalcemia in patients for whom effective antitumor therapy is not available. Oral formulations of gallium have been identified, but they are still in early stages of investigation.

BISPHOSPHONATES

Bisphosphonates (formerly called diphosphonates) are synthetic analogues of pyrophosphate that are incorporated into bone and inhibit bone resorption, probably by altering osteoclast activity.[84,85] Clinically important bisphosphonates include etidronate, clodronate, pamidronate, and alendronate.

Etidronate is available as both an IV infusion and as orally administered tablets. Randomized studies indicate that 25% to 40% of hypercalcemic patients treated with etidronate achieve normocalcemia,[83,86,87] a figure that is comparable with calcitonin but weaker than the newer bisphosphonates. Etidronate is most useful for patients with mild-to-moderate hypercalcemia. An IV dosage of 5 to 7.5 mg/kg/d for 3 to 5 days is recommended. The drug should be administered as an infusion over 4 hours to avoid nephrotoxicity.[88] The oral formulation is not recommended for acute treatment. Clodronate (dichloromethylene bisphosphonate) is available in Europe for treatment of hypercalcemia; it is slightly more active than etidronate but significantly less effective than either pamidronate or alendronate.[89]

The most important bisphosphonates are pamidronate (aminohydroxypropylidene bisphosphonate) and alendronate (aminohydroxybutylidene bisphosphonate). Both drugs inhibit bone resorption by similar mechanisms, probably by direct toxicity to osteoclasts. The variety of doses and treatment schedules have made therapeutic comparisons difficult.[90,91] Several studies suggest that the dose of pamidronate can be prescribed according to the severity of hypercalcemia (ie, higher doses for a higher value of serum calcium).[91,92] This concept has not been confirmed by others,[93] possibly because extreme elevations in serum calcium also may reflect the degree of dehydration. However, the response to pamidronate may be somewhat improved with a dose of 90 mg rather than 60 mg[92,94] administered as an intravenous infusion over 2 to 4 hours. (No advantage exists to the previously recommended 24-hour infusion schedule.) The dose can be repeated 3 to 4 days later if the initial response has been inadequate; however, if a patient has not responded to two infusions, treatment should be switched to a different drug such as gallium nitrate or mithramycin. With these doses of pamidronate, about 60% to 70% of unselected patients attain normocalcemia, a proportion somewhat lower than that of gallium nitrate; however, the drug has been shown to be significantly superior when compared with etidronate.[87] Side effects include fever, lymphopenia, and irritation at the infusion site.[95]

Alendronate also has completed clinical trials in the United States and Europe.[96,97] The drug is similar in efficacy and side effects to pamidronate, and a dose of 10 to 15 mg infused over 2 to 4 hours achieves comparable results. An important advantage of alendronate relative to pamidronate is the availability of an oral formulation, although this treatment has not been shown to extend the duration of normocalcemia.

Patients whose hypercalcemia is mediated by the PTH-RP seem to have more resistant hypercalcemia and are less likely to respond to bisphosphonates.[98-102] Because of the high activity and potentially broad activity of these compounds in both cancer and metabolic bone disease, a large number of third-generation bisphosphonate analogues have been synthesized and are being tested.[103]

OUTPATIENT THERAPY

Ambulatory management of the patient with chronic or recurrent hypercalcemia remains a substantial challenge. As with all forms of palliative care, the principal goal is to maintain an optimal quality of life and minimize the need for multiple hospitalizations. Emphasis also must be placed on prevention of recurrence (notwithstanding the obvious benefits of effective antitumor therapy). For such patients, mobility should be maximized by appropriate use of analgesics, physical therapy, site-directed radiation therapy, or orthopedic procedures, if necessary. Low doses of calcitonin administered subcutaneously (4-IU/kg or 100-U total dose daily or three times per week) are occasionally effective; however, many patients experience nausea and potency is low. Chronic therapy with corticosteroids may be useful using low doses of prednisone (5 to 20 mg/d). Long-term side effects include gastrointestinal bleeding, cataract formation, skin thinning, and osteoporosis that may increase the risk of pathologic fractures in patients with established bone metastases. Oral phosphates (see earlier) may also be useful, and the dose can be increased pending tolerance to gastrointestinal side effects. Low doses of mithramycin (eg, 10 μg/kg) administered weekly can be effective; however, nausea, cumulative or-

gan toxicity, and interference with other anti-cancer therapy remain significant problems during chronic treatment.

The availability of bisphosphonates and gallium nitrate has considerably improved the therapy of hypercalcemia in hospitalized patients. The long-term use of both groups of drugs, although still investigational, is being tested for maintenance of normocalcemia after acute control. Oral etidronate has been proposed for the prevention of recurrent hypercalcemia, but available evidence does not suggest that it is beneficial by this route.[104] Pamidronate (60 to 90 mg intravenously every 2 to 3 weeks) and oral alendronate (still investigational) have been proposed for long-term control of patients susceptible to recurrent hypercalcemia. Gallium nitrate (40 mg subcutaneously daily) also has been tested.

Survival after the initial onset of hypercalcemia is extraordinarily difficult to assess because of marked patient heterogeneity. Patients who are treated for a hormonal flare clearly have a better prognosis than patients with extensive hepatic or pulmonary metastases. A series of unselected patients with hypercalcemia from breast cancer reported an overall median survival of 34 weeks; patients who had only mild hypercalcemia and no symptoms or visceral metastases, however, had a median survival in

TABLE 23.10-2
Initiating Appropriate Therapy for Patients With Hypercalcemia Related to Breast Cancer

Outpatient	Inpatient
LEVEL 1	
Increase oral hydration	IV fluids (normal saline 200–400 mL/h)
Eliminate drugs	
Reduce dietary factors (eg, calcium, vitamins)	Furosemide
Cytotoxic chemotherapy	
LEVEL 2	
Oral phosphates	Calcitonin
Corticosteroids	Corticosteroids
	Etidronate (IV)
LEVEL 3	
Calcitonin 100 IU SC QD to TIW	Mithramycin
Mithramycin (10-25 μg/kg IV 1–2x/wk)	
Gallium nitrate (SC)	Gallium nitrate
Pamidronate	Pamidronate
	Alendronate★
LEVEL 4	
Hospitalization	Renal dialysis

★ May be investigational depending on local regulations.

Warrell RP Jr. Metabolic emergencies. In: DeVita V Jr, Hellman S, Rosenberg SA, eds. Cancer: principles and practice of oncology, ed 4. Philadelphia, JB Lippincott, 1993:2128.

excess of 3 years.[1] Such patients obviously should receive aggressive antitumor and hypocalcemic treatments.

MANAGEMENT SUMMARY

- The initial determination in patient management requires assessment of the need for hospitalization. Decision making should evaluate the clinical and psychosocial criteria given in Table 23.10-1.
- Treatment for both hospitalized and ambulatory patients is based on the severity of the disorder and associated symptoms. The levels in Table 23.10-2 correspond to the comparative potency of the treatments.
- Although most hospitalized patients should receive IV fluids, few patients actually achieve normocalcemia with hydration alone. Thus, additional hypocalcemic therapy should be administered after correction of hypovolemia.
- Corticosteroids are most useful for treatment of flare reactions; otherwise, their use is limited.
- For acute emergencies in which a rapid reduction of serum calcium is required, the combination of short-course high-dose calcitonin (8 IU/kg intramuscularly every 6 hours for four doses) plus a potent antiresorptive drug (gallium nitrate, pamidronate, or alendronate) is recommended.

References

1. Brada M, Rowley M, Grant DJ, et al. Hypercalcemia in patients with disseminated breast cancer. Acta Oncol 1990;29:577.
2. Hickey RC, Samaan NA, Jackson GL. Hypercalcemia in patients with breast cancer. Arch Surg 1981;116:545.
3. Coleman RE, Rubens RD. The clinical course of bone metastases from breast cancer. Br J Cancer 1987;55:61.
4. Eilon G, Mundy GR. Direct resorption of bone by human breast cancer cells in vitro. Nature 1978;276:726.
5. Ralston S, Fogelman I, Gardner MD, et al. Hypercalcaemia and metastatic bone disease: is there a causal link? Lancet 1982;2:903.
6. Ralston SH, Fogelman I, Gardner MD, et al. Relative contribution of humoral and metastatic factors to the pathogenesis of hypercalcaemia of malignancy. Br Med J 1984;288:1405.
7. Warrell RP Jr. Metabolic emergencies. In: DeVita V Jr, Hellman S, Rosenberg SA, eds. Cancer: principles and practice of oncology; ed 4. Philadelphia, JB Lippincott, 1993:2128.
8. Lee MY, Leu CC, Lottsfeldt JL, Judkins SA, et al. Production of granulocyte-stimulating and bone cell-modulating activities from a neutrophilia hypercalcemia-inducing murine mammary cancer cell line. Cancer Res 1987;47:4059.
9. Sabatini M, Boyce B, Aufdemorte T, et al. Infusions of recombinant interleukin-1 alpha and beta cause hypercalcemia in normal mice. Proc Natl Acad Sci USA 1988;85:5235.
10. Ishimi Y, Miyaura C, Jin CH, et al. Interleukin-6 is produced by osteoblasts and induces bone resorption. J Immunol 1990;145:3297.
11. Moseley JM, Kubota M, Dieffenbach-Jagger H, et al. Parathyroid hormone−related protein purified from a human lung cancer cell line. Proc Nat Acad Sci USA 1987;84:5048.
12. Suva LJ, Winslow GA, Wettenhall REH, et al. A parathyroid hormone−related protein implicated in malignant hypercalcemia: cloning and expression. Science 1987;237:894.
13. Burtis WJ, Wu T, Bunch C, et al. Identification of a novel 17,000-dalton parathyroid hormone−like adenylate cyclase−stimulating protein from a tumor associated with humoral hypercalcemia of malignancy. J Biol Chem 1987;262:7151.
14. Mangin M, Webb AC, Dreyer B, et al. Identification of a cDNA encoding a parathyroid hormone-like peptide from a human tumor associated with humoral hypercalcemia of malignancy. Proc Natl Acad Sci USA 1988;85:596.
15. Mangin M, Ikeda K, Dreyer BE, et al. Isolation and characterization of the human parathyroid hormone−like peptide gene. Proc Natl Acad Sci USA 1989;86:2408.
16. Burtis WJ, Brady TG, Orloff JJ, et al. Immunochemical characterization of circulating parathyroid-like protein in patients with humoral hypercalcemia of malignancy. N Engl J Med 1990;332:1106.
17. Burtis WJ, Fodero JP, Gaich G, et al. Preliminary characterization of circulating amino- and carboxy-terminal fragments of parathyroid hormone−related peptide in humoral hypercalcemia of malignancy. J Clin Endocrinol Metab 1992;75:1110.
18. Blind E, Raue F, Glotzmann J, et al. Circulating levels of midregional parathyroid hormone−related protein in hypercalcemia of malignancy. Clin Endocrinol 1992;37:290.
19. Pandian MR, Morgan CH, Carlton E, et al. Modified immunoradiometric assay of parathyroid hormone−related protein: clinical application in the differential diagnosis of hypercalcemia. Clin Chem 1992;38:282.
20. Weir EC, Brines ML, Ikeda K, et al. Parathyroid hormone−related peptide gene is expressed in the mammalian central nervous system. Proc Natl Acad Sci USA 1990;87:108.
21. Yamamoto M, Harm SC, Grasser WA, et al. Parathyroid hormone−related protein in the rat urinary bladder: a smooth muscle relaxant produced locally in response to mechanical stretch. Proc Natl Acad Sci USA 1990;87:108.
22. Deftos LJ, Burton DW, Brandt DW. Parathyroid hormone−like protein is a secretory product of atrial myocytes. J Clin Invest 1993;92:727.
23. Thiede MA, Daifotis AG, Weir EC, et al. Intrauterine occupancy controls expression of the parathyroid hormone−related peptide gene in preterm rat myometrium. Proc Natl Acad Sci USA 1990;87:6969.
24. Shew RL, Yee JA, Kliewer DB, et al. Parathyroid hormone-related protein inhibits stimulated uterine contraction in vitro. J Bone Min Res 1991;6:955.
25. Thiede MA, Rodan GA. Expression of a calcium-mobilizing parathyroid hormone−like peptide in lactating mammary tissue. Science 1988;242:278.
26. Budayr AA, Halloran BP, King JC, et al. High levels of a parathyroid hormone−like protein in milk. Proc Natl Acad Sci. USA 1989;86:7183.
27. Stewart AF, Wu TL, Insogna KL, et al. Immunoaffinity purification of parathyroid hormone−related protein from bovine milk and human keratinocyte-conditioned medium. J Bone Min Res 1991;6:305.
28. Galasko CSB, Burn JI. Hypercalcemia in patients with advanced mammary cancer. Br Med J 1971;3:573.
29. Percival RL, Yates AJP, Gray RES, et al. Mechanisms of malignant hypercalcemia in carcinoma of the breast. BMJ 1985;291:776.
30. Isales C, Carcangiu ML, Stewart AF. Hypercalcemia in breast cancer: reassessment of the mechanism. Am J Med 1987;82:1143.
31. Gallacher SJ, Fraser WD, Patel U, et al. Breast cancer−associated hypercalcaemia: a reassessment of renal calcium and phosphate handling. Ann Clin Biochem 1990;27:551.
32. Budayr AA, Nissenson RA, Klein RF, et al. Increased serum levels

of a parathyroid hormone-like protein in malignancy-associated hypercalcemia. Ann Intern Med 1989;111:807.

33. Bundred NJ, Ratcliffe WA, Walker RA, et al. Parathyroid hormone−related protein and hypercalcaemia in breast cancer. BMJ 1991;303:1506.

34. Grill V, Ho P, Body JJ, et al. Parathyroid hormone−related protein: elevated levels in both humoral hypercalcemia of malignancy and hypercalcemia complicating metastatic breast cancer. J Clin Endocrinol Metab 1991;73:1309.

35. Rizzoli R, Caverzasio J, Chapuy MC, et al. Role of bone and kidney in parathyroid hormone−related peptide-induced hypercalcemia in rats. J Bone Mineral Res 1989;4:759.

36. Vargas SJ, Gillespie MT, Powell GJ, et al. Localization of parathyroid hormone−related protein mRNA expression in breast cancer and metastatic lesions by in situ hybridization. J Bone Min Res 1992;7:971.

37. Southby J, Kissin MW, Danks JA, et al. Immunohistochemical localization of parathyroid hormone−related protein in human breast cancer. Cancer Res 1990;50:7710.

38. Bouizar Z, Spyratos F, Deytieux S, et al. Polymerase chain reaction analysis of parathyroid hormone−related protein gene expression in breast cancer patients and occurrence of bone metastases. Cancer Res 1993;53:5076.

39. Gurney H, Grill V, Martin TJ. Parathyroid hormone-related protein and response to pamidronate in tumour-induced hypercalcaemia. Lancet 1993;341:1611.

40. Body JJ, Dumon JC, Thirion M, et al. Circulating PTHrP concentrations in tumor-induced hypercalcemia: influence on the response to bisphosphonate and changes after therapy. J Bone Min Res 1993;8:701.

41. Budayr AA, Zysset E, Jenzer A, et al. Effects of treatment of malignancy-associated hypercalcemia on serum parathyroid hormone−related protein. J Bone Min Res 1994;9:521.

42. Ibbotson KJ, D'Souza SM, Ng KW, et al. Tumor derived growth factor increases bone resorption in a tumor associated with humoral hypercalcemia of malignancy. Science 1983;221:1292.

43. Ibbotson KJ, Twardzik DR, D'Souza SM, et al. Stimulation of bone resorption in vitro by synthetic transforming growth factor-alpha. Science 1985;228:1007.

44. Tashjian AH Jr, Voelkel EF, Lazzaro M, et al. Alpha and beta human transforming growth factors stimulate prostaglandin production and bone resorption in cultured mouse calvariae. Proc Natl Acad Sci USA 1985;82:4535.

45. Stern PH, Krieger NS, Nissenson RA, et al. Human transforming growth factor-α stimulates bone resorption in vitro. J Clin Invest 1985;76:2016.

46. Linkhart TA, Mohan S, Jennings JC, et al. Copurification of osteolytic and transforming growth factor-β activities produced by human lung tumor cells associated with humoral hypercalcemia of malignancy. Cancer Res 1989;49:271.

47. Pfeilschifter J, Seyedin SM, Mundy GR. Transforming growth factor beta inhibits bone resorption in fetal rat long bone cultures. J Clin Invest 1988;82:680.

48. Mundy GR. Hypercalcemic factors other than parathyroid hormone−related protein. Endocrinol Metab Clin North Am 1989;18:795.

49. Canalis E, McCarthy T, Centrella M. Growth factors and the regulation of bone remodeling. J Clin Invest 1988;81:277.

50. Robey PG, Young MF, Flanders KC, et al. Osteoblasts synthesize osteoid and respond to TGF-β in vitro. J Cell Biol 1987;105:457.

51. Insogna KL, Weir EC, Wu TL, et al. Co-purification of transforming growth factor beta-like activity with PTH-like and bone-resorbing activities from a tumor associated with humoral hypercalcemia of malignancy. Endocrinol 1987;120:2183.

52. Guise TA, Yoneda T, Yates AJ, et al. The combined effect of tumor-produced parathyroid hormone-related protein and trans-

forming growth factor-α enhance hypercalcemia in vivo and bone resorption in vitro. J Clin Endocrinol Metab 1993;77:40.

53. Haq M, Kremer R, Goltzman D, et al. A vitamin D analogue (EB1089) inhibits parathyroid hormone−related peptide production and prevents the development of malignancy-associated hypercalcemia in vivo. J Clin Invest 1993;91:2416.

54. Kukreja SC, Shevrin DH, Wimbiscus SA, et al. Antibodies to parathyroid hormone related protein lower serum calcium in athymic mouse models of malignancy-associated hypercalcemia due to human tumors. J Clin Invest 1988;82:1798.

55. Sato K, Yamakawa Y, Shizume K, et al. Passive immunization with anti-parathyroid hormone−related protein monoclonal antibody markedly prolongs survival time of hypercalcemic nude mice bearing transplanted human PTHrP-producing tumors. J Bone Min Res 1993;8:849.

56. Guise TA, Garrett IR, Bonewald LF, et al. Interleukin-1 receptor antagonist inhibits the hypercalcemia mediated by interleukin-1. J Bone Min Res 1993;8:583.

57. Legha SS, Powell K, Buzdar AU, et al. Tamoxifen-induced hypercalcemia in breast cancer. Cancer 1981;47:2803.

58. Vichayanrat A, Avraamides A, Gardner B, et al. Primary hyperparathyroidism and breast cancer. Am J Med 1976;61:136.

59. Farr HW, Fahey TJ Jr, Nash AG, et al. Primary hyperparathyroidism and cancer. Am J Surg 1973;126:539.

60. Axelrod DM, Bockman RS, Wong GY, et al. Distinguishing features of primary hyperparathyroidism in patients with breast cancer. Cancer 1987;60:1620.

61. Boyd JC, Ladenson JH. Value of laboratory tests in the differential diagnosis of hypercalcemia. Am J Med 1984;77:863.

62. Stewart AF, Horst R, Deftos LJ, et al. Biochemical evaluation of patients with cancer-associated hypercalcemia: evidence for humoral and non-humoral groups. N Engl J Med 1980;303:1377.

63. Lufkin EG, Kao PC, Heath H. Parathyroid hormone radioimmunoassays in the differential diagnosis of hypercalcemia due to primary hyperparathyroidism or malignancy. Ann Intern Med 1987;106:559.

64. Strewler GJ, Nissenson RA. Nonparathyroid hypercalcemia. Adv Intern Med 1987;32:235.

65. Payne RB, Carver ME, Morgan DB. Interpretation of serum total calcium: effects of adjustment for albumin concentration on frequency of abnormal values and on detection of change in the individual. J Clin Pathol 1979;32:56.

66. Hosking DJ, Cowley A, Bucknall CA. Rehydration in the treatment of severe hypercalcemia. Q J Med 1981;200:473.

67. Bilezikian JP. Management of acute hypercalcemia. N Engl J Med 1992;326:1196.

68. Ralston SH, Alzaid AA, Gardner MD, et al. Treatment of cancer associated hypercalcaemia with combined aminohydroxypropylidene diphosphonate and calcitonin. Br Med J 1986;292:1549.

69. Kristensen B, Ejlertsen B, Holmegaard SN, et al. Prednisolone in the treatment of severe malignant hypercalcaemia in metastatic breast cancer: a randomized study. J Intern Med 1992;232:237.

70. Herbert LA, Lemann J, Peterson JR, et al. Studies of the mechanism by which phosphate infusion lowers serum calcium concentration. J Clin Invest 1966;45:1886.

71. Shackney S, Hasson J. Precipitous fall in serum calcium, hypotension, and acute renal failure after intravenous phosphate therapy for hypercalcemia: report of two cases. Ann Intern Med 1967;66:906.

72. Carey RW, Schmott GW, Kopald HH, et al. Massive extraskeletal calcification during phosphate treatment of hypercalcemia. Arch Intern Med 1968;122:150.

73. Mundy GR, Wilkinson R, Heath DA. Comparative study of available medical therapy for hypercalcemia of malignancy. Am J Med 1983;74:421.

74. Heath DA. The use of inorganic phosphate in the management of hypercalcemia. Metab Bone Dis Rel Res 1980;2:213.

75. Minkin C. Inhibition of parathyroid hormone stimulated bone resorption *in vitro* by the antibiotic mithramycin. Calcif Tissue Res 1973;13:249.

76. Green L, Donehower RC. Hepatic toxicity of low doses of mithramycin in hypercalcemia. Cancer Treat Rep 1984;68:1379.

77. Bockman RS, Repo MA, Warrell RP Jr, et al. Gallium localization in bone: micron range resolution using synchrotron x-ray microscopy. Proc Natl Acad Sci USA 1990;87:4149.

78. Blair HC, Teitelbaum SL, Tan H-L, et al. Reversible inhibition of osteoclastic activity by bone-bound gallium (III). J Cell Biochem 1992;48:401.

79. Warrell RP Jr, Bockman RS, Coonley CJ, et al. Gallium nitrate inhibits calcium resorption from bone and is effective treatment for cancer-related hypercalcemia. J Clin Invest 1984;73:1487.

80. Repo MA, Bockman RS, Betts F, et al. Effect of gallium on bone mineral properties. Calcif Tissue Int 1988;43:300.

81. Bockman RS, Boskey A, Blumenthal NC, et al. Gallium increases bone calcium and crystallite perfection of hydroxyapatite. Calcif Tissue Int 1986;39:376.

82. Warrell RP Jr, Israel R, Frisone M, et al. Gallium nitrate for acute treatment of cancer-related hypercalcemia: a randomized, double-blind comparison to calcitonin. Ann Intern Med 1988;108:669.

83. Warrell RP Jr, Murphy WK, Schulman P, et al. A randomized double-blind study of gallium nitrate compared to etidronate for acute control of cancer-related hypercalcemia. J Clin Oncol 1991;9:1467.

84. Fleisch H. Bisphosphonates: a new class of drugs in diseases of bone and calcium metabolism. Recent Results Cancer Res 1989;116:1.

85. Carano A, Teitelbaum SL, Konsek JD, et al. Bisphosphonates directly inhibit the bone resorption activity of isolated avian osteoclasts in vitro. J Clin Invest 1990;85:456.

86. Ryzen E, Martodam RR, Troxell M, et al. Intravenous etidronate in the management of malignant hypercalcemia. Arch Intern Med 1985;145:449.

87. Gucalp R, Ritch P, Wiernik PH, et al. Comparative study of pamidronate disodium and etidronate disodium in the treatment of cancer-related hypercalcemia. J Clin Oncol 1992;10:134.

88. Bounameaux HM, Schifferli J, Monatni J-P, et al. Renal failure associated with intravenous diphosphonates (Letter). Lancet 1983;1:471.

89. Ralston SH, Gallacher SJ, Patel U, et al. Comparison of three intravenous bisphosphonates in cancer-associated hypercalcemia. Lancet 1989;2:1180.

90. Body JJ, Borkowski A, Cleeren A, et al. Treatment of malignancy-associated hypercalcemia with intravenous aminohydroxypropylidene diphosphonate. J Clin Oncol 1986;4:1177.

91. Thiebaud D, Jaeger P, Jacquet AF, et al. Dose response in the treatment of hypercalcemia of malignancy by a single infusion of the bisphosphonate AHPrBP. J Clin Oncol 1988;6:762.

92. Nussbaum SR, Younger J, Vandepol CJ, et al. Single-dose intravenous therapy with pamidronate for the treatment of hypercalcemia of malignancy: comparison of 30-, 60-, and 90-mg dosages. Am J Med 1993;95:297.

93. Ralston SH, Boyle IT. Clinical experience with aminohydroxypropylidene bisphosphonate (APD) in the management of cancer-associated hypercalcaemia. In: Burckhardt P, ed. Disodium pamidronate (APD) in the treatment of malignancy-related disorders. Toronto, Hans Huber, 1989:72.

94. Body JJ, Pot M, Borkowski A, et al. Dose-response study of aminohydroxypropylidene bisphosphonate in tumor-associated hypercalcemia. Am J Med 1987;82:957.

95. Gallacher SJ, Ralston SH, Patel U, et al. Side-effects of pamidronate (Letter). Lancet 1989;2:42.

96. Adami S, Bolzicco GP, Rizzo A, et al. The use of dichloromethylene bisphosphonate and aminobutane bisphosphonate in hypercalcemia of malignancy. Bone Min 1987;2:395.

97. Nussbaum SR, Warrell RP Jr, Rude R, et al. Dose-response study of alendronate sodium for the treatment of cancer-associated hypercalcemia. J Clin Oncol 1993;11:1618.

98. Gurney H, Kefford R, Stuart-Harris R. Renal phosphate threshold and response to pamidronate in humoral hypercalcemia of malignancy. Lancet 1989;2:241.

99. Beex L, Hermus A, Smals A. Pamidronate and hypercalcemia of malignancy. (Letter) Lancet 1989;2:617.

100. Ralston SH, Gallagher SJ, Patel U, et al. Pamidronate and hypercalcemia of malignancy. (Letter) Lancet 1989;2:617.

101. Gurney H, Grill V, Martin TJ. Parathyroid hormone–related protein and response to pamidronate in tumour-induced hypercalcaemia. Lancet 1993;341:1611.

102. Body JJ, Dumon JC, Thirion M, et al. Circulating PTHrP concentrations in tumor-induced hypercalcemia: influence on the response to bisphosphonate and changes after therapy. J Bone Min Res 1993;8:701.

103. Shinoda H, Adamek G, Felix R, et al. Structure-activity relationships of various bisphosphonates. Calcif Tissue Int 1983;35:87.

104. Schiller JM, Rasmussen P, Benson AB, et al. Maintenance etidronate in the prevention of malignancy-associated hypercalcemia. Arch Intern Med 1987;147:963.

23.11

Bone Marrow Metastases

STEVEN E. COME ▪ LOWELL E. SCHNIPPER

Bone marrow metastases in breast cancer are associated with a spectrum of clinical and hematologic manifestations. Thirty percent to 60% of patients with metastatic breast cancer have marrow involvement demonstrated by biopsy.[1–4] Two thirds of these patients with marrow metastases have an abnormal complete blood count. Anemia is the most frequent abnormality, with 40% to 60% of patients with bone marrow involvement having a hemoglobin value of less than 12 g/dL, compared with 14% of stage IV patients with no marrow involvement.[1,5] However, the presence of anemia is not diagnostic of marrow metastases because the anemia of chronic disease is a common additional cause of decreased red cell production in this setting. Leukopenia, thrombocytopenia, or both are seen in only 12% to 25% of patients with abnormal bone marrow findings.[1,5,6] One third of patients with metastatic breast cancer and marrow metastases have normal complete blood counts.[1,5,6] Thus, routine hematologic parameters are of limited usefulness in predicting bone marrow involvement. However, in patients with advanced breast cancer, marrow metastases correlate well with the presence of cortical bone involvement. Ingle and coworkers[1] found marrow metastases in 55% of patients with abnormal results on bone films or scans. Moreover, multiple series have demonstrated that only 2% to 8% of patients with stage IV breast cancer and marrow metastases have no evidence of skeletal involvement on combined radiographic and radionuclide studies.[1,2,5,7–9]

A proportion of patients with advanced breast cancer and marrow involvement have more prominent hematologic abnormalities. Myelophthisic anemia has been reported in 12% to 50% of patients with marrow metastases.[5,10–12] This condition, alternatively described as leukoerythroblastic anemia, is a state of diminished bone marrow function associated with infiltration of the marrow cavity by neoplastic cells, fibroblasts, or both and the appearance of red blood cell and granulocytic precursors in the peripheral blood. The pathogenesis of myelophthisic anemia is incompletely understood, but a desmoplastic response to the intramedullary metastases seems to be an important factor. Myelofibrosis is found in 80% of patients with myelophthisic anemia secondary to marrow metastases.[10,11] Tumor, fibrosis, or both replace the marrow space and interfere with hematopoiesis by disrupting the marrow microvasculature. Distortion of the endothelial sinuses permits nondeformable early red cells and granulocytes, normally confined to the marrow, to escape into the circulation.[13] A corresponding increase in the level of colony-forming units in the peripheral blood also has been reported in patients with myelophthisic anemia.[14] Extramedullary hepatosplenic hematopoiesis is a frequent, probably secondary, pathologic finding in these patients.[10,15]

A small number of patients with breast cancer who have myelophthisic anemia develop an associated microangiopathic hemolytic anemia. This syndrome of mechanical intravascular hemolysis occurs when there is a large tumor burden with extensive marrow infiltration and tumor microemboli in the pulmonary and other vascular beds.[16] Another rare occurrence in patients with breast cancer and marrow metastases is the appearance of tumor cells in the peripheral blood. This carcinoma cell leukemia (carcinocythemia) has been observed in patients with underlying myelophthisic anemia and accompanying microangiopathic hemolysis. In some of these patients, prior splenectomy or splenic atrophy has been postulated to diminish the clearance of circulating tumor cells, permitting their accumulation to levels that may reach 25,000/mm^3.[11,13,17,18] In peripheral smears, these cells are larger (25 to 30 μm) than leukemic blasts, often appear in clusters, and have vacuolated basophilic cytoplasm. Intracellu-

lar mucin is present, and the smears stain positive for periodic acid–Schiff.

Clinical Findings and Diagnostic Evaluation of Myelophthisic Anemia

Myelophthisic anemia may occur at any point in the course of breast cancer. Webster and others[19] estimate that the incidence of leukoerythroblastosis in the total breast cancer population is 0.5% per year.[19] In that series, a presenting symptom in three patients was myelophthisic anemia; evaluation revealed the primary breast tumor. Conversely, two patients developed myelophthisic anemia 7 and 12 years, respectively, after the primary diagnosis. Kiely and Silverstein[15] reported on the occurrence of myelophthisic anemia as early as 3 months and as late as 21 years after the initial diagnosis of breast cancer. Patients with myelophthisic anemia may be slightly younger than the overall population of patients with breast cancer.[19]

SIGNS AND SYMPTOMS

The most common symptoms of myelophthisic anemia in patients with breast cancer are those of anemia, including congestive heart failure in the elderly, and bone pain. The latter may reflect the associated cortical bone metastasis or marrow necrosis that is secondary to the myelophthisic process.[13,15] The accompanying physical findings may include tachycardia, signs of increased cardiac output, pulmonary congestion, edema, and focal or diffuse bony tenderness. Although extramedullary hematopoiesis usually is present on pathologic examination, marked splenomegaly is less common, occurring in only 12% to 25% of patients.[15,20] Additional symptoms and signs related to other sites of metastases may be present.

LABORATORY FINDINGS

The most common hematologic abnormality is a normocytic normochromic anemia. Although some patients have a leukoerythroblastic peripheral smear without anemia, the mean hemoglobin levels reported in three series were 7.8 to 8.9 g/dL (range, 6.2 to 11.6 g/dL).[15,19,21] The reticulocyte count usually is slightly increased, but the reticulocyte index is low.[13,15,21] Thrombocytopenia occurs in 70% to 90% of patients; platelet counts are less than 100,000/μL in more than 50% of patients.[15,19,21] Thrombocytosis is seen in less than 10% of cases. The white cell count may be elevated or slightly decreased but usually is normal.

Examination of the peripheral smear in patients with myelophthisic anemia reveals nucleated red blood cells, numbering from 1 to 135 per 100 white blood cells.[15,21] Other morphologic abnormalities may include tear-drop poikilocytosis, anisocytosis, red cell stippling, polychromatophilia, giant platelets, and megakaryocytic fragments.[13] Schistocytes, helmet cells, and burr cells may be present if there is associated microangiopathic hemolysis.[16]

Other frequent laboratory abnormalities appearing in patients with breast cancer who have myelophthisic anemia include elevation of lactate dehydrogenase and alkaline phosphatase levels. Hypercalcemia occasionally is present. Hyperbilirubinemia and evidence of disseminated intravascular coagulation are common in patients with superimposed microangiopathic hemolysis.

BONE MARROW EXAMINATION

In patients with breast cancer, the bone marrow biopsy is more useful than is an aspirate smear or clot section in establishing marrow involvement. In the Ingle series[1] from the National Cancer Institute, biopsy showed abnormalities in 89% of patients with marrow metastases, and biopsy was the only procedure showing abnormalities in 33% of patients. Results of clot sections and aspirate smear were abnormal in 30% to 85% of patients, but tumor was rarely revealed when the biopsy results were normal.[1,5]

The presence of the characteristic peripheral blood findings of myelophthisic anemia in a patient with known metastatic breast carcinoma is essentially diagnostic of marrow involvement.[22] Bone marrow aspiration and biopsy are confirmatory procedures. The bone marrow aspiration in patients with myelophthisic anemia may be a dry tap. The biopsy reveals fibrosis and nests of tumor cells in addition to normal hematopoietic tissue. The relative proportions of tumor and fibrosis are variable.

Differential Diagnosis of Myelophthisic Anemia in Patients With Breast Cancer

The detection of carcinoma cells by bone marrow examination establishes the cause of myelophthisic anemia and eliminates other diagnoses that may be associated with a leukoerythroblastic peripheral smear, including primary hematologic or lymphoreticular malignant disease, tuberculosis, sarcoidosis, histoplasmosis, and lipid storage diseases. However, when the biopsy reveals extensive fibrosis without diagnostic carcinoma cells, differentiation of marrow metastases from agnogenic myeloid metaplasia may be difficult.[15] This differential diagnosis is most important in patients who have previously been treated for primary breast cancer and who were without evidence of metastases before the development of myelophthisic anemia. Because intramedullary metastases are highly correlated with cortical bone involvement, the presence of skeletal pain or evidence of bone metastases on radiographic studies often helps to establish this distinction.[15] Skeletal metastases are frequently sclerotic in patients with extensive marrow fibrosis.[23] In addition, Kiely and Silverstein[15] found that patients with marrow metastases and myelophthisic anemia had less marked splenomegaly than did patients with agnogenic myeloid metaplasia. Leukocytosis, basophilia, tear-drop poikilocytosis, giant platelets, and platelet fragments were more pronounced in agnogenic myeloid metaplasia, whereas normoblastosis was more prominent in patients with marrow metastases.[15] Marked leukocytosis or thrombocytosis is rare in myelophthisic anemia associated with malignant disease.[13,15,19,21]

Determination of the level of urinary hydroxyproline excretion also may be useful in establishing the diagnosis. Elevated levels have been found in patients with breast cancer who have myelophthisic anemia, whereas normal values were reported in patients with breast cancer without marrow metastases and in those with agnogenic myeloid metaplasia.[24]

Myeloproliferative syndromes, which may arise as a consequence of the treatment of breast cancer with alkylating agents or radiation therapy, also must be considered in the differential diagnosis of myelophthisic anemia secondary to marrow metastases. A cumulative risk of about 1.5% has been reported for acute leukemia and myeloproliferative syndromes after adjuvant chemotherapy for breast cancer.[25] Pancytopenia and increased reticulin fibrosis in the marrow are common features of these treatment-induced hematologic neoplasms.[26-28] Dysplastic and cytogenetic changes in hematopoietic cells and an absence of carcinoma cells on marrow examination allow a distinction to be made between this entity and myelofibrosis associated with marrow metastases.

Prognosis of Patients With Advanced Breast Cancer and Bone Marrow Metastases

The prognosis reported for patients with breast cancer who have marrow metastases is variable. In a large series from Sweden, Landys[2] observed a highly significant increased death risk in patients with marrow metastases compared with those without marrow metastases. In contrast, other studies have found that abnormal results on bone marrow biopsy have no correlation to the response rate, duration of response, or survival of patients with advanced breast cancer.[3,4,6,9] In part, this discrepancy likely results from differences in characteristics among patients, considering that several factors influence the prognosis of patients with marrow metastases. The extent of marrow involvement is important as an indicator of the overall tumor burden and hence, the patient's potential resistance to treatment. Furthermore, the degree of marrow compromise may govern the intensity of therapy. In a multivariate analysis of prognostic factors in patients with metastatic breast cancer, a pretreatment hemoglobin value of less than 11 g/dL and a platelet count below $200,000/\mu L$ were found to have a statistically significant negative effect on response to chemotherapy and survival.[29] A decrease in response rate and survival in patients with marrow metastases who require reductions in chemotherapeutic dose also have been reported.[3] The extent of concurrent metastases to other sites is another prognostic factor in patients with marrow metastases, with the combination of visceral, osseous, and soft tissue involvement having a particularly adverse impact.[30] The disease-free interval from the time of the initial diagnosis of breast cancer to the onset of metastases, the timing of the metastases with respect to the menopause, the hormone receptor status of the tumor, and the history of prior treatment are additional prognostic variables in patients with marrow metastases.[5]

Differences in these factors undoubtedly contribute to the wide range of response and survival rates recorded in the subset of patients with breast cancer who have marrow metastases and myelophthisic anemia. West and associates[21] report a median survival of 72 days in 18 patients with breast cancer and myelophthisic anemia at Memorial Hospital. The 7 responding patients had a mean survival of 4.8 months compared with a mean survival of 1.1 months for those who did not respond.[21] In contrast, the observations of Kiely and Silverstein[15] were more optimistic, with 5 of 6 patients surviving for at least 1 year after the onset of myelophthisic anemia; 3 of these patients survived 2 to 4 years. Similarly, Webster and others[19] reported a 2-year survival in 40% of patients with breast cancer and leukoerythroblastosis. In that series, all patients with disease-free intervals of more than 1 year responded to treatment, whereas no responses were observed in patients with disease-free intervals of 1 year or less from the time of the primary diagnosis to the onset of myelophthisic anemia.

Treatment of Patients With Bone Marrow Metastases

The therapeutic approach to patients with breast cancer who have marrow metastases consists of both supportive measures and treatment of the underlying neoplasm. In patients with anemia or thrombocytopenia, transfusions may be necessary before and during therapy. Antibiotics are indicated in patients with fever and neutropenia that occurs as a consequence of either marrow involvement or its treatment. Both hormonal manipulation and chemotherapy may be efficacious in patients with marrow metastases. The choice between these modalities is based on the considerations that apply in general to the management of patients with breast cancer (see Chap. 22).

ENDOCRINE THERAPY

Budd[8] found that 54% of patients with breast cancer who had marrow involvement had estrogen receptor–positive tumors and that an additional 11% had tumors with borderline levels of receptor. Thus, most patients with marrow metastases are potential candidates for endocrine therapy, which may have a particularly high therapeutic ratio when marrow involvement is extensive, such as in those with myelophthisic anemia. Patients with metastases limited to the marrow or with associated osseous or soft tissue involvement who have hormone receptor–positive tumors and disease-free intervals of 0 or in excess of 2 years should receive endocrine therapy. Indeed, endocrine manipulation may be more effective in patients with mye-

lophthisic anemia than in the overall population with advanced breast cancer. Although about 40% of patients with advanced breast cancer respond to endocrine therapy, patients with myelophthisic anemia have reported rates of 50% to 85%.[19]

In premenopausal patients with breast cancer and myelophthisic anemia, ovarian ablation has produced response rates ranging from 25% to 100%, with response durations frequently exceeding 2 years.[19,21] Tamoxifen is a potential alternative to oophorectomy in premenopausal women and is the initial treatment of choice in postmenopausal patients. Other endocrine maneuvers, including adrenalectomy and hypophysectomy, also have produced response in more than half the patients with marrow metastases.[31,32] Androgenic steroids may have a dual role in patients with myelophthisic anemia, providing both an antineoplastic effect and potential stimulation of the residual normal marrow.[13,19]

CHEMOTHERAPY

Chemotherapy is indicated in patients with breast cancer and marrow metastases who have hormone receptor–negative tumors, who have become refractory to hormone maneuvers, or who have clinical features such as a short disease-free interval, rapid progression of disease, or involvement of multiple visceral sites that are unfavorable for the use of endocrine therapy. In particular, patients with pulmonary lymphangitic metastases or microangiopathic hemolytic anemia require prompt initiation of chemotherapy.

Studies from the National Cancer Institute and from the M.D. Anderson Hospital have assessed the impact of chemotherapy on patients with marrow metastases.[3,6] Using a combination of cyclophosphamide, 5-fluorouracil, and either methotrexate or doxorubicin, Ingle and coworkers[6] achieved response rates of 67% in patients with advanced breast cancer and marrow metastases, compared with a response rate of 71% in those without bone marrow involvement. The median duration of response also was comparable for patients with and without marrow involvement. Patients with bone marrow involvement, however, had a greater requirement for hematologic support and a higher incidence of infection. Forty-six percent of patients with marrow metastases required transfusion, compared with only 21% of those without bone marrow involvement. Twenty percent of the group with marrow involvement developed sepsis, which occurred in only 7% of the group without marrow metastases. In this study, chemotherapeutic doses were decreased for patients with leukopenia and thrombocytopenia; half the full dose or less was given when the white blood cell count was below $3000/\mu L$ or the platelet count was below $75,000/\mu L$. Patients with bone marrow involvement had lower white blood cell counts for the first two cycles of therapy and lower platelet counts for the first three cycles of therapy than did those without marrow metastases. Thereafter, for the duration of the 10-cycle treatment plan, the white blood cell and platelet counts were comparable in the two groups.

Rodriguez-Kraul and colleagues[3] treated 48 patients with metastatic breast cancer and marrow metastases with a combination of doxorubicin, cyclophosphamide, methotrexate, 5-fluorouracil, and bacillus Calmette-Guerin vaccine or levamisole. In this series, dose reduction was permitted only for infection or hemorrhage, rather than in cases of myelosuppression. Sixteen of 21 patients (76%) receiving full doses of chemotherapy achieved a response, including 8 (38%) who experienced complete marrow remissions. In contrast, 14 of 27 patients (52%) receiving less than full doses responded, and only 3 (11%) had complete resolution of marrow metastases. Compared with similarly treated patients without marrow metastases, the patients with marrow involvement had more frequent and more severe myelosuppression. Hematologic support was required in 60% of patients with bone marrow involvement, compared with 26% of those without bone marrow metastases. Eleven of 48 patients with marrow metastases were hospitalized at least once for fever and neutropenia. Five episodes of sepsis and three infectious deaths occurred in these patients. The patients with bone marrow involvement had a median duration of response of 16 months, which was equivalent to that in patients without marrow metastases.

Both of these reports demonstrate that chemotherapy with vigorous supportive care may achieve good results in patients with marrow metastases. It is likely, however, that the extent of marrow involvement in these patients was minimal, because marrow metastases were detected by biopsies performed as routine staging procedures rather than as evaluation for cytopenia or abnormal peripheral smears. Only 40% of the patients in the Ingle series[6] were anemic, 27% were leukopenic, and 13% were thrombocytopenic when abnormal results were obtained from marrow biopsy. Only 15 of 48 patients with marrow metastases in the Rodriguez-Kraul study[3] had hematologic abnormalities. Other researchers, however, have demonstrated the feasibility and effectiveness of chemotherapy in patients with more advanced marrow involvement.[33,34] Using a combination of vincristine, doxorubicin, and prednisone, Dady and colleagues[33] obtained four responses, three of which were complete, in patients with bone marrow metastases and profound pretreatment thrombocytopenia. Kiang and others[34] report a complete response in a patient with leukoerythroblastic anemia, thrombocytopenia, myelofibrosis, and splenomegaly. During treatment with cyclophosphamide, methotrexate, 5-fluorouracil, vincristine, prednisone, and halotestin, all abnormalities resolved, including dense reticulin and collagen fibrosis in the marrow.

In patients with severely compromised marrow function, the approach to chemotherapy dosing is controversial. Traditionally, initial doses are reduced, but full-dose therapy may produce improved response rates. The availability of colony-stimulating factors to support granulocyte counts and the potential for platelet support with interleukins or thrombopoietin in the near future may facilitate full-dose treatment. No data that growth factors improve the safety or outcome of therapy are available, however. In these patients, regardless of the chemotherapy dose administered, the necessity of intensive hematologic support must be anticipated. Early in treatment, infection, including sepsis, is common, and neutropenic febrile patients require hospitalization and antibiotics. With response to therapy, however, the hematologic parameters and the safety of ongoing treatment improve.

Detection and Significance of Marrow Micrometastases in Primary Breast Cancer

Using immunocytochemical staining for epithelial antigens, cytologically occult tumor cells can be demonstrated in marrow samples from patients with primary or localized breast cancers. This technique may allow detection of 1 tumor cell in 10^5 to 10^6 marrow cells.[35,36] Coombs and collaborators[37–39] reported a 26% to 28% incidence of marrow micrometastases in patients with localized cancers. Twenty-two percent of patients with T1 or T2 tumors and 39% with T3 or T4 tumors had carcinoma cells present on marrow smears. Furthermore, five of six women with positive axillary nodes, intratumoral vascular invasion, and a negative estrogen receptor finding had marrow micrometastases. Thus, the presence of marrow micrometastases seems to correlate with other poor prognostic factors.

The significance of marrow micrometastases in patients without other evidence of metastases remains to be clarified. In a small series, Cote and associates[40] found that marrow micrometastases detected by monoclonal antibody predicted a significantly higher early recurrence rate in stage I and II breast cancer. Mansi and others[41] reported that the presence of marrow micrometastases correlates with decreased relapse-free survival and recurrence in bone. Mansi and colleagues[39] have also performed serial marrow evaluations in 82 patients with primary breast cancer. Twenty-six percent of patients had micrometastases at diagnosis, but the incidence fell to 2% after removal of the primary tumor, suggesting that a large proportion of micrometastases may be nonviable cells shed into the circulation and subsequently cleared. In this study, the frequency of micrometastases increased to 30% with the appearance of clinically demonstrable nonskeletal metastases and to 100% in those with osseous recurrence. Thus, the micrometastases seemed to be more a marker of disease activity than an independent predictor of the development of overt metastases. Furthermore, the presence or absence or micrometastases did not correlate with the outcome of adjuvant chemotherapy in this group, suggesting that the technique is not sufficiently sensitive to monitor such therapy.

Vaughan and coworkers[42] found cancer cells in cytospins from Dexter-type cell cultures in 57% of histologically negative marrow harvests taken from patients with stage I, II, III, or locally recurrent breast cancer. The persistence of these cells after 4 to 12 weeks in culture may indicate their viability, although not necessarily clonogenicity. In this patient group, 8 of 16 with positive culture results experienced relapse compared with none of 12 with negative culture results during short follow-up. Additional investigations are necessary to determine both the optimal technique for detecting marrow micrometastases and the clinical usefulness of such efforts.

Detection and Significance of Marrow Micrometastases and Tumor Cells in Peripheral Blood Stem Cell Collections in Breast Cancer Patients Receiving High-Dose Chemotherapy

Similar immunocytochemical techniques demonstrate tumor cells in marrow and peripheral blood stem cell (PBSC) harvests from breast cancer patients undergoing intensive chemotherapy and hematopoietic reconstitution. Ross and others[43] found tumor cells in marrow specimens from 67% of such patients, whereas paired PBSC collections from these patients were abnormal in 18%. Twenty-one of 26 immunocytochemically positive specimens were found to be clonogenic. The tumor burden was higher in marrow than in PBSC specimens. Furthermore, Ross and associates[44] observed that the rate of PBSC samples showing abnormalities increased from 5.5% to 19.8% when multiple rather than single collections were analyzed for a given patient. Brugger and others[45] observe that tumor cells are mobilized into the peripheral blood after chemotherapy and treatment with colony-stimulating factors, which are commonly used to increase the yield of hematopoietic progenitor cells during PBSC collection. In this report, the incidence of circulating tumor cells increased from 0% to 21% after such therapy. Furthermore, all breast cancer patients with marrow involvement had detectable tumor cells in PBSC collections harvested after exposure to chemotherapy and colony-stimulating factors. Concern about reinfusion of viable, clonogenic tumor cells after high-dose therapy has led to attempts to purge tumor cells from these collections, using either antibodies, chemotherapy, or positive selection of CD34-positive cells.[46] The significance of tumor cell contamination of marrow and PBSC autografts and the efficacy of techniques to modify this remain under investigation (see Chap. 22.2).

MANAGEMENT SUMMARY

- Bone marrow biopsy is the diagnostic procedure of choice. Hematologic parameters do not predict marrow involvement.
- Both hormonal manipulation and chemotherapy may be effective in patients with marrow involvement. The choice between these modalities is based on considerations that apply in general to the treatment of patients with advanced breast cancer.
- In patients with compromised marrow function, chemotherapy dosing is controversial. Traditionally, initial doses have been reduced, but this strategy may

compromise response rates. The availability of colony-stimulating factors and the introduction of interleukins and thrombopoietin in the near future may facilitate full-dose treatment. No data that growth factors improve safety or outcome of therapy are available, however, and the need for intensive hematologic support may be anticipated in these patients, regardless of the chemotherapy dose administered.
- Immunocytochemical and culture techniques can detect marrow and peripheral blood involvement by tumor not identified on routine cytologic examination. The significance of these micrometastases is under investigation, as are attempts to purge these cells from marrow and stem cell autografts.

References

1. Ingle JN, Tormey DC, Tan HK. The bone marrow examination in breast cancer: diagnostic considerations and clinical usefulness. Cancer 1978;41:670.
2. Landys K. Prognostic value of bone marrow biopsy in breast cancer. Cancer 1982;49:513.
3. Rodriguez-Kraul R, Hortobagyi GN, Buzdar AU, et al. Combination chemotherapy for breast cancer metastatic to bone marrow. Cancer 1981;48:227.
4. Mendoza CB, Moore GE, Crosswhite LH, et al. Prognostic significance of tumor cells in the bone marrow. Surg Gynecol Obstet 1969;129:483.
5. Westberg M, Armitage JD, Corder MP. Bone marrow involvement in breast cancer: unexpected clinical findings. (Abstract) Proc Am Soc Clin Oncol 1982;1:85.
6. Ingle JN, Tormey DC, Bull JM, et al. Bone marrow involvement in breast cancer: effect on response and tolerance to combination chemotherapy. Cancer 1977:39.
7. DiStefano A, Tashima CK, Yap Y, et al. Bone marrow metastases without cortical bone involvement in breast cancer patients. Cancer 1979;44:196.
8. Budd GT. Estrogen receptor profile in patients with breast cancer metastatic to the bone marrow. J Surg Oncol 1983;24:167.
9. Ceci G, Franciosi V, Passalacqua R, et al. The value of bone marrow biopsy in breast cancer at the time of the first relapse. Cancer 1988;61:1041.
10. Delsol G, Guiu-Godfrin B, Guiu M, et al. Leukoerythroblastosis and cancer: frequency, prognosis and physiopathologic significance. Cancer 1979;44:1009.
11. Rubins JM. The role of myelofibrosis in malignant leukoerythroblastosis. Cancer 1983;51:308.
12. Contreras E, Ellis LD, Lee RE. Value of bone marrow biopsy in the diagnosis of metastatic carcinoma. Cancer 1972;29:778.
13. Zucker S. Anemia associated with foreign cells in the marrow (myelophthisis). In: Lichtman MA, ed. Hematology and oncology: the science and practice of clinical medicine. New York, Grune & Stratton, 1989:42.
14. Delforge A, DeCaluwe JP, Ronge-Collard E, et al. Increased levels of myeloid progenitor cells in the blood of patients with metastatic invasion of the marrow. Scand J Haematol 1983;31:275.
15. Kiely JM, Silverstein MN. Metastatic carcinoma simulating agnogenic myeloid metaplasia and myelofibrosis. Cancer 1969;24:1041.

16. Antman KH, Skarin AT, Mayer RJ, et al. Microangiopathic hemolytic anemia and cancer: a review. Medicine 1979;58:377.

17. Carey RW, Taft PD, Bennett JM, et al. Carcinocythemia (carcinoma cell leukemia): an acute leukemia-like picture due to metastatic carcinoma cells. Am J Med 1976;60:273.

18. Myerowitz RL, Edwards PA, Sartiano GP. Carcinocythemia (carcinoma cell leukemia) due to metastatic cancer of the breast. Cancer 1977;40:3107.

19. Webster DJT, Preece PR, Bolton PM, et al. Leukoerythroblastosis in breast cancer. Clin Oncol 1975;1:315.

20. Vaughn MJ. Leukoerythroblastic anemia. J Pathol Bacteriol 1938;42:541.

21. West LD, Ley NB, Pearson DH. Myelophthisic anemia in cancer of the breast. Am J Med 1955;18:923.

22. Weich JK, Hagedorn AB, Linman JW. Leukoerythroblastosis: diagnostic and prognostic significance. Mayo Clin Proc 1974;49:110.

23. Kamby C, Guildhammer B, Vegborg I, et al. The presence of tumor cells in bone marrow at the time of first recurrence of breast cancer. Cancer 1987;60:1306.

24. Wang JC, Aung MK, Tobin MS. Urinary hydroxyproline excretion in myelofibrosis. Blood 1980;55:383.

25. Fisher B, Rockette H, Fisher ER, et al. Leukemia in breast cancer patients following adjuvant chemotherapy or postoperative radiation: the NSABP experience. J Clin Oncol 1985;3:1640.

26. Sultan C, Sigaux F, Imbert M, et al. Acute myelodysplasia and myelofibrosis: a report of eight cases. Br J Haematol 1981;49:11.

27. Feuilhade F, Brun B, Tuhran A, et al. Acute leukemia and breast cancer: apropos of 12 cases observed in the department of oncology at the Henri Mondor Hospital. Bull Cancer (Paris) 1983;70:389.

28. Soffer T, Chan WC, Arynes RK, et al. Myeloproliferative disorder with profound hypereosinophilia associated with chemotherapy for breast cancer. Cancer 1984;54:2356.

29. Hortobagyi GN, Smith TL, Legha SS, et al. Multivariate analysis of prognostic factors in metastatic breast cancer. J Clin Oncol 1983;1:1776.

30. Valagussa P, Brambilla C, Bonadonna G. Advanced breast cancer: are the traditional stratification parameters still of value when patients are treated with chemotherapy? Eur J Cancer 1979;15:565.

31. Frazer ID, Talbot Ch. The response to adrenalectomy of a leucoerythroblastic process due to metastatic carcinoma of the breast. Lancet 1961;1:690.

32. Akinsette FL, Kernohaw IR, Dawson AA. Pituitary ablation for leucoerythroblastosis in carcinoma of the breast. Lancet 1973;2:1050.

33. Dady PJ, Sugarbaker PH, Robertson NH. Combination chemotherapy for thrombocytopenia and bone marrow metastases from breast cancer. BMJ 1977;1:554.

34. Kiang DT, McKenna RW, Kennedy BJ. Reversal of myelofibrosis in advanced breast cancer. Am J Med 1978;64:173.

35. Osborne MP, Wong GY, Asina S, et al. Sensitivity of immunocytochemical detection of breast cancer cells in human bone marrow. Cancer Res 1991;51:2706.

36. Porro G, Menard S, Tagliabue E, et al. Monoclonal antibody detection of carcinoma cells in bone marrow biopsy specimens from breast cancer patients. Cancer 1988;61:2407.

37. Redding WH, Coombs RC, Monaghan P, et al. Detection of micrometastases in patients with primary breast cancer. Lancet 1983;2:1271.

38. Berger U, Bettleheim R, Mansi JL, et al. The relationship between micrometastases in the bone marrow, histopathologic features of the primary tumor in breast cancer and prognosis. Am J Clin Pathol 1988;90:1.

39. Mansi JL, Berger U, McDonnell T, et al. The fate of bone marrow micrometastases in patients with primary breast cancer. J Clin Oncol 1989;7:445.

40. Cote RJ, Rosen PP, Lesser ML, et al. Prediction of early relapse in patients with operable breast cancer by detection of occult bone marrow micrometastases. J Clin Oncol 1991;9:1749.

41. Mansi JL, Berger U, Easton D, et al. Micrometastases in bone marrow in patients with primary breast cancer: an evaluation as an early predictor of bone metastases. BMJ 1987;295:1093.

42. Vaughan WP, Mann SL, Garvey J, et al. Breast cancer detected in cell culture of histologically negative bone marrow predicts systemic relapse in patients with stage I, II, III and locally recurrent disease. (Abstract) Proc ASCO 1990;9:9.

43. Ross AA, Cooper BW, Lazarus HM, et al. Detection and viability of tumor cells in peripheral blood stem cell collections from breast cancer patients using immunocytochemical and clonogenic assay techniques. Blood 1993;82:2605.

44. Ross AA, Cooper BW, Lazarus HM, et al. Different rates of detection of breast cancer cells in peripheral blood stem cell (PBSC) collections in single versus multiple specimens. (Abstract) Proc ASCO 1994;13:64.

45. Brugger W, Bross KJ, Glatt M, et al. Mobilization of tumor cells and hematopoietic progenitor cells into peripheral blood of patients with solid tumors. Blood 1994;83:636.

46. Shpall EJ, Stemmer SM, Bearman SJ, et al. New strategies in marrow purging for breast cancer patients receiving high-dose chemotherapy with autologous bone marrow transplantation. Breast Cancer Res Treat 1993;26:519.

23.12
Management of Discrete Pulmonary Nodules

STEVEN S. MENTZER ▪ DAVID J. SUGARBAKER

Solitary pulmonary nodules are spherical tumors of 4 cm or less in the periphery in the lung. The nodules are asymptomatic and are typically identified by routine radiographic examinations. Solitary pulmonary nodules are not associated with atelectasis or hilar adenopathy. If the nodule is new, based on comparisons with previous chest radiographs, the solitary pulmonary nodule most likely represents either cancer or benign granulomas.[1,2]

In patients with a history of breast cancer, solitary pulmonary nodules may represent recurrent breast cancer. Almost two thirds of patients with recurrent breast cancer develop systemic disease[3,4]; many of these patients have recurrence in the lung. Autopsy series have shown that the distribution of metastases in breast cancer involves the lung in 58% to 77% of cases.[5-7] Clinical series have demonstrated that pulmonary metastases are second only to bone as the first site of recurrent breast cancer. The lung is the first site of recurrence in 15% to 25% of patients with metastatic breast cancer.[3,8,9] In more than half of these patients with a lung recurrence, a solitary pulmonary nodule is the presenting symptom.[10] Other common sites of metastatic disease include the pleura and intrathoracic lymph nodes.[3,9]

Alternatively, the solitary pulmonary nodule may represent a primary lung cancer. Lung cancer is the most common fatal malignancy in both sexes. The incidence of lung cancer is 13% of all cancers in women; however, lung cancer represents 23% of all cancer deaths in women.[11] In patients who develop lung cancer, 10% to 15% have a solitary pulmonary nodule.[2] About 20% of these patients are nonsmokers. The solitary pulmonary nodule represents a primary lung cancer in more than 50% of patients with breast cancer[1,10,12] (Table 23.12-1).

The most common benign pathologic diagnosis of a solitary pulmonary nodule is a granuloma. Granulomas can occur in response to inhaled particulate matter or a variety of infectious pathogens. The histopathologic evaluation of granulomatous lesions typically involves special histochemical studies to exclude acid-fast bacilli, fungal forms, or common inhaled particulates. Although granulomatous lesions can be routinely cultured, most granulomas are sterile and do not require further therapy.

Diagnosis

Pulmonary nodules are commonly evaluated by chest computed tomography (CT). CT further characterizes the nodular lesion and identifies additional intrathoracic disease. The chest CT of a potential malignancy routinely includes examination of the liver and adrenal glands because these organs frequently are associated with intrathoracic disease. A complete chest CT is useful because it provides important anatomic information about other common metastatic sites for breast cancer: specifically, the lung, liver, intrathoracic lymph nodes, and pleura.[8,9,3,13]

TABLE 23.12-1
*Histopathologic Findings After Resection of Pulmonary Nodules**

		Histopathologic Diagnosis (%)		
Study	N	Lung Cancer	Breast Cancer	Benign
Cahan et al† [44]	78	63	30	5
Casey et al[10]	42	52	43	5
Mentzer et al‡ [12]	59	47	34	8

* The patients in these series had histories of breast cancer and pulmonary nodules (typically solitary) on chest radiograph.

† Reported series of solitary pulmonary nodules. This report follows previous report from Cahan and colleagues.[44]

‡ Four patients in this series had metastatic lesions identified from nonbreast occult primary tumors.

Common metastatic sites for lung cancer are intrathoracic lymph nodes, pleura, liver, and adrenal glands.

CT clearly is more sensitive than chest radiography in detecting pulmonary metastases.[14,15] Chest computed tomographic scans can detect peripheral nodules as small as 2 to 3 mm. In patients with a discrete nodule on chest radiography and a history of extrathoracic malignancy, CT may detect additional nodular lesions.[13,16] A limitation of chest CT is that many of these nodules are benign.[14-16] Despite the limited specificity of chest CT, the use of CT can be enhanced with attention to other clinical factors, and CT can be used for surgical planning.[15]

Magnetic resonance imaging (MRI) has been used to evaluate lung nodules. This preliminary work suggests that conventional MRI does not have sufficient spatial resolution to provide any additional information to that provided by CT. The additional time and expense of chest MRI has precluded its routine use.

The primary limitation of chest CT of the discrete pulmonary nodule is that the images cannot distinguish between primary and metastatic cancer. Metastases are typically spherical without any associated adenopathy. Primary lung cancers are typically spiculated, but lung cancers can also be spherical. The CT scan is particularly useful in identifying benign characteristics. Granulomas can be totally calcified or have central or laminar calcification. These observations virtually exclude the diagnosis of malignant diseases.[1]

Cytologic study to confirm a malignant diagnosis has a limited role in evaluating the solitary pulmonary nodule. Cytologic specimens are typically obtained from sputum, bronchoscopic washing, and transthoracic needle biopsy. Specimens for sputum cytologic study should be obtained from early morning sputum on 3 consecutive days. Specimens should be appropriately collected to prevent oral contamination and carefully preserved to facilitate interpretation.[17] Sputum cytologic study can yield a malignant diagnosis in 80% of patients with a large central tumor.[18] The yield of sputum cytologic study decreases to less than 25% with more peripheral lesions and diminishing size of the malignancy.[18] In patients undergoing bronchoscopic examination, endoscopic brushings and airway lavage of a peripheral lesion improve the cytologic yield to more than 70%.[19] Both sputum and bronchial cytologic study are limited by sample size. In addition, inflammatory exudates, excessive blood, or poor preservation decrease the tumor detection rate. Cytologically atypical cells in the lung often are associated with inflammatory disorders, further complicating the cytologic diagnosis of malignancy.

Transthoracic needle biopsy performed by fluoroscopic or CT guidance provides the cytologic specimen directly from the peripheral lung nodule. It provides the positive diagnosis of malignancy in 80% to 90% of patients with a malignant nodule.[20-22] The procedure is performed on an outpatient basis with a small risk of pneumothorax (about 10%).[21,23] The major problem with transthoracic needle biopsy is the appreciable false-negative rate. For example, Charing and others[20] have shown that in 38 patients with no malignant cells identified by the technique, 25 were subsequently confirmed to have a lung malignancy. Another problem is that cytologic study rarely positively establishes a benign diagnosis. Even when bacterial or fungal forms are identified in a cytologic specimen, it is difficult to exclude the possibility of a coexistent malignant disease. Bronchoscopy also has a limited role in evaluating the solitary pulmonary nodule. Bronchoscopy can facilitate cytologic diagnosis by airway washing, cytologic brushings, or bronchoalveolar lavage. These diagnostic approaches may be useful in establishing a diagnosis of infection caused by pulmonary pathogens such as *Mycobacterium tuberculosis.* Although infections with *M tuberculosis* commonly result in nodular lesions, the patient must be carefully monitored to exclude coexistent carcinoma. An additional bronchoscopic approach is fluoroscopically directed transbronchial biopsy. Transbronchial biopsies are useful in documenting diffuse parenchymal disease, such as lymphangitic carcinoma of the lung. The diagnostic yield of transbronchial biopsy in peripheral lung nodules falls to about 20% to 50%, depending on the size and location of the lesion.[1,24] Other limitations of transbronchial biopsy in solitary pulmonary nodules are the small sample size (about 300 alveoli), the small risk of pneumothorax, and the potential delay in establishing a definitive diagnosis.

The most reliable approach to establishing a diagnosis in a patient with a solitary pulmonary nodule is surgery. Surgery provides an adequate tissue for cytomorphologic, immunohistochemical, and special protein studies. In contrast to other diagnostic approaches, surgery avoids the sampling and interpretative errors that might delay definitive therapy. In the past, the major limitation with surgery was the morbidity associated with a standard thoracotomy. This limitation has resolved with the development of videothoracoscopic surgery.

Thoracoscopy

The thoracoscope provides an opportunity to diagnose and treat diseases of the chest with minimal morbidity.[25] Thoracoscopic surgery involves a videothoracoscope and generally two working ports to facilitate manipulation of the lung and other intrathoracic structures[26] (Fig. 23.12-1). Working through these three access ports, a variety of surgical procedures can be performed. The advantages of thoracoscopic video optics and miniaturized instrumentation have led to their incorporation in a variety of thoracic surgical procedures. Because these procedures are performed with variable incision lengths, this spectrum of surgical procedures has led to the more inclusive term of video-assisted thoracic surgery (VATS).[27]

Videothoracoscopy is a surgical approach that requires general anesthesia and a fully equipped operating room. To facilitate visualization of the lung and hemithorax, single-lung ventilation is required. Differential lung ventilation can be established with a double-lumen endotracheal tube or an inflatable bronchial blocker. Both techniques facilitate the deflation of the ipsilateral lung. Bronchoscopy is routinely performed at the beginning of the procedure to confirm placement of the double-lumen endotracheal tube or the bronchial blocker. Bronchoscopy also provides an opportunity to identify any potential oc-

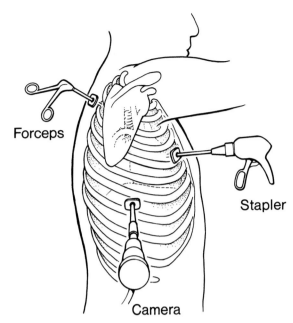

FIGURE 23.12-1 Videothoracoscopy is performed in the lateral thoracotomy position. Thoracoscopy access ports are positioned to triangulate the area of interest and to facilitate the manipulation of intrathoracic structures. With single-lung ventilation, deflation of the ipsilateral lung provides an opportunity to examine the contents of the hemithorax. The solitary pulmonary nodule can be identified and resected to facilitate the histopathologic diagnosis. If the preliminary frozen section diagnosis is consistent with a primary lung metastasis, the thoracoscope can be used to surgically stage the ipsilateral hemithorax.

cult endobronchial lesions.[28] The contraindications to thoracoscopy are obliterative pleural scarring or an inability to tolerate single lung ventilation. In most cases, patients with minimal pleural thickening and symmetric lung disease seen on plain chest radiography are candidates for thoracoscopic procedures.

The morbidity of thoracoscopy is minimized by the small incisions used in this procedure. When pulmonary resections are performed, a chest tube drain is used to evacuate residual air and facilitate lung expansion. Depending on the extent of the resection, the tube may be indwelling for less than an hour or for more than a few days.

Patients do experience some discomfort at the site of the access ports. This bruising pain can persist for several weeks. In addition, patients may complain of some numbness of the anterior chest wall. Both of these symptoms presumably are secondary to intraoperative compression of the intercostal nerve. Localized discomfort is minimized with use of intercostal nerve blocks with local anesthetics at the conclusion of the procedure. More invasive analgesic techniques, such as epidural analgesics, rarely are necessary after videothoracoscopic procedures. The typical thoracoscopic resection requires only an overnight hospitalization.

The primary benefits of thoracoscopy is the enhanced flexibility it provides in illuminating difficult diagnostic problems. Videothoracoscopy provides a panoramic view of the ipsilateral hemithorax. This view includes the visceral and parietal pleural surfaces, the internal chest wall, and the internal mammary, hilar, and paratracheal lymph nodes.

In the patient with a history of breast cancer, videothoracoscopy provides an opportunity to examine the pleural surfaces for any evidence of malignancy. Small amounts of pleural fluid can be sent for cytologic examination, and biopsy can be performed directly on pleural nodules. Internal mammary, hilar, and paratracheal lymph nodes can be inspected and potentially can undergo biopsy. In most cases, the solitary pulmonary nodule can be identified by digital palpation. The objective of surgery is the resection of the nodule with grossly negative tumor margins. Adequate margins are obtained to ensure local control of the metastatic nodule and adequate sampling of a benign nodule.

Intraoperative frozen-section histologic study of the lung nodule is routinely performed. If the nodule has special cytomorphologic features characteristic of the primary breast cancer, then no further staging is necessary. The benign appearance of the granulomatous lesions suggests that culturing of the nodule for mycobacterial and fungal pathogens may be appropriate. Alternatively, the frozen-section histopathologic study may suggest the possibility of a primary lung cancer. For example, squamous cell differentiation, a small cell carcinoma appearance, or bronchoalveolar morphologic features would indicate a primary lung cancer. With these histopathologic findings, a careful staging of hilar (N1) and ipsilateral peritracheal (N2) paratracheal lymph nodes should be performed.

The clinical context and patient risk factors dictate the usefulness of a completion lobectomy at the time of videothoracoscopy. In the case of a primary lung cancer, growing evidence demonstrates that a limited resection of a primary lung nodule is associated with an increased risk of local recurrence.[29] Although definitive evidence is lacking, there seems to be a trend toward an impact on survival as well.[29] The cumulative evidence at this time suggests that lobectomy is the standard cancer operation for patients with primary T1, N0, M0 or T2, N0, M0 lung cancers.

In the patient with staged disease and a definitive diagnosis of lung cancer, VATS anatomic resections often can be performed during the same anesthetic. The anatomic resection of a segment of lobe can be performed with significantly less morbidity than is associated with a standard thoracotomy. The development of improved thoracoscopic instruments should make VATS anatomic resections commonplace in the future. If an accurate histopathologic diagnosis cannot be established at the time of the thoracoscopic procedure, any further resection should be delayed. An advantage of videothoracoscopy is that it is minimally invasive. After the final pathologic specimen has been obtained, patients will be physically capable of undergoing subsequent thoracotomy or VATS lobectomy.

The aggressive natural history of primary lung cancer underscores the importance of establishing a definitive histopathologic diagnosis of lung carcinoma. A definitive diagnosis, however, may be difficult to establish with peripheral adenocarcinomas. Peripheral adenocarcinomas can be ambiguous lesions, presenting a challenge to the pathologist and clinician in discriminating breast metastases from primary lung cancer.

In patients with a solitary breast metastasis, resecting the nodule may have some therapeutic value. Staren and others[30] report a mean survival of 58 months after resection of a solitary pulmonary nodule. Lanza and colleagues[24] reviewed 37 cases of surgical resection of a solitary nodule and found a 49.5% actuarial 5-year survival rate.[31] The authors[31] also found a correlation between a longer disease-free interval and improved survival after metastasectomy. This relation is consistent with studies of metastases of other histologic types.[32-34] Although these retrospective studies are preliminary, the results suggest that the surgical resection of solitary pulmonary nodules may result in long-term survival for selected patients.

The potential benefit of multiple metastasectomies has been proposed for sarcoma, germ cell tumors, and other selected tumors.[32-34] These tumors, however, are unique in their tropism for the lung. In contrast to these diseases, breast cancer does not demonstrate a selective pattern of pulmonary metastasis. A potential therapeutic value of the resection of multiple metastases in breast cancer is unlikely.

Pathology

About 80% of primary tumors of the lung have a pathologic diagnosis of adenocarcinoma. Similarly, 80% of the metastatic lesions in the lung are adenocarcinoma.[5] Because of their histologic similarity, the distinction between primary lung adenocarcinoma and metastatic breast cancer can be difficult. The association of a peripheral location, pleural retraction, anthracotic pigment, and central scarring were previously thought to be characteristic of lung primaries. These features, however, can be mimicked by metastatic adenocarcinoma of the breast.[35]

Occasionally, the morphologic features of the lung lesion may be identical to the breast primary. Characteristic features, such as comedo differentiation or characteristic ductal pattern, may permit a definitive diagnosis of metastatic breast cancer. More commonly, cytomorphologic dissimilarity exists between the primary and the metastatic lesion. This potential discrepancy is one of the primary limitations of diagnostic approaches based on cytologic study alone.

The characteristic morphologic features of lung primary adenocarcinoma can be used to establish a diagnosis of primary lung cancer. Lung adenocarcinomas are commonly heterogeneous and can demonstrate areas of bronchoalveolar differentiation. Another characteristic of a lung primary is the presence of composite histologic features. An example of a composite histologic type is adenosquamous differentiation or adenocarcinoma with a small cell carcinoma element. These composite tumors are uncommon and only observed in about 10% of non-small cell cancers.

Special studies occasionally can be helpful in distinguishing primary lung carcinoma from metastatic breast cancer. A problem with immunohistochemical or receptor protein studies is that breast cancer metastases can lose the expression of these distinguishing features. In addition, recurrent breast cancers in the lung are estrogen receptor–positive in only 25% of cases.[36] Confounding this observation is the finding that primary lung cancers can express a variety of unexpected proteins. For example, estrogen receptors are expressed in about 30% of primary lung adenocarcinomas.[37] Similarly, progesterone receptors have described in about 15% of primary lung cancers.[37]

In addition to diagnostic cytomorphologic features, the most discriminating pathologic feature of breast metastases to the lung is immunohistochemical staining for gross cystic disease fluid protein,[38] which is associated with apocrine differentiation. It has not been reported in primary lung carcinomas and can effectively exclude the diagnosis of a lung primary.[39] The limitation of staining for gross cystic disease fluid protein is that the antigen is present in only 30% to 50% of breast cancer patients.[38,40] Furthermore, primary breast cancers that express this protein may lose antigen expression when they recur systemically. Despite the low frequency of lung nodules expressing the protein, it is the only marker that seems to distinguish lung primaries from breast metastases.

Several new approaches are likely to help distinguish primary and metastatic cancers in the future. The development of new monoclonal antibodies suggests that immunohistochemical study may contribute to the definitive diagnosis of lung cancer.[41–43] The cytogenetic features of the tumor also may be helpful. Lung cancers, such as small cell carcinoma, seem to express characteristic chromosomal deletions. Small cell carcinoma, for example, typically demonstrates a deletion of the short arm of chromosome 3 (3P). This deletion is rarely seen in patients with breast cancer. Although uniform cytogenetic abnormalities have not been identified for adenocarcinoma of the lung or breast, this is an area that has the potential to contribute to the discrimination of primary lung carcinoma and metastatic breast cancer.

MANAGEMENT SUMMARY

- Patients with a history of breast cancer and discrete pulmonary nodules need a tissue diagnosis to exclude benign disease or primary lung cancer.
- Lung cancer is the most common cause of death in women with cancer. The diagnosis of a lung primary must be considered in a patient with pulmonary adenocarcinoma.
- A cytologic diagnosis of malignancy rarely is sufficient to exclude a primary lung cancer, and a benign cytologic diagnosis is at risk for sampling error. Thoracoscopy provides a minimally invasive approach to obtain definitive tissue for histopathologic study and staging information regarding the pleura, ipsilateral paratracheal, and internal mammary lymph nodes.

ACKNOWLEDGMENT
Supported in part by NIH Grant HL47078.

References

1. Swensen SJ, Jett JR, Payne WS, et al. An integrated approach to evaluation of the solitary pulmonary nodule. Mayo Clin Proc 1990;65:173.

2. Anderson RW, Arentzen CE. Carcinoma of the lung. Surg Clin North Am 1980;60:793.

3. Nikkanen TA. Recurrence of breast cancer: a retrospective study of 569 cases in clinical stages I–III. Acta Chir Scand 1981;147:239.

4. Valagussa P, Bonadonna G, Veronesi U. Patterns of relapse and survival following radical mastectomy: analysis of 716 consecutive patients. Cancer 1978;41:1170.

5. Abrams HL, Spiro R, Goldstein N. Metastases in carcinoma: analysis of 1000 autopsied cases. Cancer 1950;3:74.

6. Saphir O, Parker ML. Metastasis of primary carcinoma of the breast with special reference to spleen, adrenal glands and ovaries. Arch Surg 1941;42:1003.

7. Warren S, Witham EM. Studies on tumor metastasis. 2. The distribution of metastases in cancer of the breast. Surg Gynecol Obstet 1933;57:81.

8. Kamby C, Rose C, Ejlertsen B, et al. Stage and pattern of metastases in patients with breast cancer. Eur J Cancer Clin Oncol 1987;23:1925.

9. Kamby C, Vejborg I, Kristensen B, et al. Metastatic pattern in recurrent breast cancer: special reference to intrathoracic recurrences. Cancer 1988;62:2226.

10. Casey JJ, Stempel BG, Scanlon EF, et al. The solitary pulmonary nodule in the patient with breast cancer. Surgery 1984;96:801.

11. Boring CC, Squires TS, Tong T. Cancer statistics, 1994. CA Cancer J Clin. 1994;44:7.

12. Mentzer SJ, DeCamp MM, Harpole DH, et al. Thoracoscopic evaluation of intrathoracic malignancy in patients with breast cancer 1994 (Submitted).

13. Scott WW, Jr, Fishman EK. Detection of internal mammary lymph node enlargement: comparison of CT scans and conventional roentgenograms. Clin Imaging 1991;15:268.

14. Chalmers N, Best JJ. The significance of pulmonary nodules detected by CT but not by chest radiography in tumour staging. Clin Radiol 1991;44:410.

15. Davis SD. CT evaluation for pulmonary metastases in patients with extrathoracic malignancy. Radiology 1991;180:1.

16. Fernandez EB, Colon E, McLeod DG, et al. Efficacy of radiographic chest imaging in patients with testicular cancer. Urology 1994;44:243,248.

17. Walts AE. Cytologic techniques for the diagnosis of pulmonary neoplasms. In: Marchevsky AM, ed. Lung biology in health and disease: surgical pathology of lung neoplasms. New York, Marcel Dekker, 1990:29.

18. Ng AB, Horak GC. Factors significant in the diagnostic accuracy of lung cytology in bronchial washing and sputum samples. II. Sputum samples. Acta Cytol 1983;27:397.

19. Ng AB, Horak GC. Factors significant in the diagnostic accuracy of lung cytology in bronchial washing and sputum samples. I. Bronchial washings. Acta Cytol 1983;27:391.

20. Charig MJ, Stutley JE, Padley SP, et al. The value of negative needle biopsy in suspected operable lung cancer. Clin Radiol 1991;44:147.

21. Cristallini EG, Ascani S, Farabi R, et al. Fine needle aspiration biopsy in the diagnosis of intrathoracic masses. Acta Cytol 1992;36:416.

22. Zakowski MF, Gatscha RM, Zaman MB. Negative predictive value of pulmonary fine needle aspiration cytology. Acta Cytol 1992;36:283.

23. Collins CD, Breatnach E, Nath PH. Percutaneous needle biopsy of lung nodules following failed bronchoscopic biopsy. Eur J Radiol 1992;15:49.

24. Wang KP, Haponik EF, Britt EJ, et al. Transbronchial needle aspiration of peripheral pulmonary nodules. Chest 1984;86:819.

25. Mentzer SJ, Sugarbaker DJ. Thoracoscopy and video-assisted thoracic surgery. In: Brooks DC, ed. Current techniques in laparoscopy. Philadelphia, Current Medicine, 1994:20.

26. Landreneau RJ, Mack MJ, Hazelrigg SR, et al. Video-assisted thoracic surgery: basic technical concepts and intercostal approach strategies. Ann Thorac Surg 1992;54:800.

27. McKneally MF, Lewis RJ, Anderson RJ, et al. Statement of the AATS/STS Joint Committee on Thoracoscopy and Video Assisted Thoracic Surgery. J Thorac Cardiovasc Surg 1992;104:1.

28. King DS, Castleman B. Bronchial involvement in metastatic pulmonary malignancy. J Thorac Surg 1943;12:305.

29. Ginsberg RJ, Rubinstein L, and the Lung Cancer Study Group. Patients with T1N0 non-SCLC lung cancer. Lung Cancer 1991;7(Suppl):83.

30. Staren ED, Salerno C, Rongione A, et al. Pulmonary resection for metastatic breast cancer. Arch Surg 1992;127:1282.

31. Lanza LA, Natarajan G, Roth JA, et al. Long-term survival after resection of pulmonary metastases from carcinoma of the breast. Ann Thorac Surg 1992;54:244,248.

32. Brandt B, Ehrenhaft JL. Surgical management of pulmonary metastasis. Curr Probl Cancer 1980;4:1.

33. Kaiser D, Ennker IC, Hartz C. Video-assisted thoracoscopic surgery: indications, results, complications, and contraindications. Thorac Cardiovasc Surg 1993;41:330.

34. Mentzer SJ, Antman KH, Attinger C, et al. Selected benefits of thoracotomy and chemotherapy for sarcoma metastatic to the lung. J Surg Oncol 1993;53:54.

35. Marchevsky AM. Metastatic tumors of the lung. In: Marchevsky AM, ed. Lung biology in health and disease: surgical pathology of lung neoplasms. New York, Marcel Dekker, 1990:231.

36. Johnson FE, Rosen PP, Menendez-Botet C, et al. Estrogen receptor protein in visceral metastases from breast carcinoma. Am J Surg 1981;142:252.

37. Beattie CW, Hansen NW, Thomas PA. Steroid receptors in human lung cancer. Cancer Res 1985;45:4206.

38. Wick MR, Lillemoe TJ, Copland GT, et al. Gross cystic disease fluid protein-15 as a marker for breast cancer: immunohistochemical analysis of 690 human neoplasms and comparison with alpha-lactalbumin. Hum Pathol 1989;20:281.

39. Chaubert P, Hurlimann J. Mammary origin of metastases: immunohistochemical determination. Arch Pathol Lab Med 1992;116:1181.

40. Monteagudo C, Merino MJ, LaPorte N, et al. Value of gross cystic disease fluid protein-15 in distinguishing metastatic breast carcinomas among poorly differentiated neoplasms involving the ovary. Hum Pathol 1991;22:368.

41. Ioachim HL, Pambuccian S, Giancotti F, et al. Reactivity of lung tumors with lung-derived and non-lung-derived monoclonal antibodies. Int J Cancer Suppl 1994;8:132-133.

42. Kawai T, Torikata C, Suzuki M. Immunohistochemical study of pulmonary adenocarcinoma. Am J Clin Pathol 1988;89:455.

43. Souhami RL, Beverley PC, Bobrow LG, et al. Antigens of lung cancer: results of the second international workshop on lung cancer antigens. J Natl Cancer Inst 1991;83:609.

44. Cahan WG, Castro EB, Huvos AG. Primary breast and lung carcinoma in the same patient. J Thorac Cardiovasc Surg 1974;68:546.

Diseases of the Breast, edited by Jay R. Harris,
Marc E. Lippman, Monica Morrow, and Samuel Hellman.
Lippincott-Raven Publishers, Philadelphia, © 1996.

24

Special Therapeutic Problems

24.1
Male Breast Cancer

MICHAEL P. MOORE

Carcinoma of the male breast is an uncommon phenomenon, accounting for less than 1% of all breast cancers. It is estimated that 1000 new cases will be diagnosed in the United States in 1996 and will account for 300 deaths.[1]

Breast cancer in men has been traditionally thought to be substantially different from that in women. As more becomes known of this relatively rare entity, the similarities of the disease between genders become more striking than the differences. Cause, predisposition based on family history, prognosis, and response to treatment are remarkably similar between the sexes.

Family history of breast cancer is present in about 30% of males with breast cancer.[2-4] Multiple cases of male breast cancer within a family are unusual but have been reported to occur among siblings[2] and between uncle and nephew.[3] A review of familial breast cancer in males has described 10 families with sufficient evidence to suggest a familial distribution. The most common scenario in this group was female breast cancer, but rare male involvement was noted.[5] This finding suggests that a familial form of breast cancer exists in which both males and females show an increased risk for developing breast cancer. Inclusion of male breast cancer has not routinely been considered as a component of such familial syndromes as the Li-Fraumeni syndrome.[6] As BRCA1 and other breast cancer genes become more widely applicable, the genetic relations of male breast may be better understood.

The risk for breast cancer increases with age in males but lacks the early premenopausal peak seen in females.[7] For this reason, the greatest incidence occurs 5 to 10 years later in males with the peak at 60 years of age. The annual incidence increases steadily from 35 years of age, with 0.1 case per 100,000 men to 11.1 cases at age 85 years or greater.

Various factors specific to males have been implicated as possibly contributing to the development of male breast cancer.[8-13] These include undescended testes, orchiectomy, orchitis, late puberty, infertility, obesity, hypercholesterolemia, estrogen use, and environmental exposure.[10,11] Some evidence suggests that male breast cancer may develop in persons with relative androgen deficiency.[10]

The global distribution of male breast cancer is similar to that of female breast cancer, with areas virtually devoid of both male and female disease and an increased reported incidence among males in those areas with higher rates for females. Certain exceptions exist. For example, in Egypt, male breast cancer is quite common and is related to schistosomiasis.

Radiation exposure may be related to an increased risk for the disease, with cancer developing 12 to 36 years after exposure.[13-16] The risk in men seems similar to the risk in women; exposure to radiation doses greater than 50 to 100 cGy increases the risk for cancer, and the risk increases if the exposure occurs at a young age.[13,17] Occupational or environmental exposure may exert an effect on the development of male breast cancer. A review of the occupation of males with breast cancer has shown a disproportionate frequency of chronic work exposure to heat, suggesting that increased environmental temperatures may

859

potentiate the development of breast cancer in men.[18] Potential etiologies may involve testicular dysfunction secondary to heat exposure and are consistent with the theory that male breast cancer may develop in response to relative androgen deficiency.[10]

Because of the unusual nature of male breast cancer and the potential of an endocrinologic basis, several studies have evaluated estrogen metabolism. The studies have used small sample sizes and lack an agreement or trend in their results.[19-23] Ballerini and colleagues[19] reported no difference in testosterone, estradiol, prolactin, follicle-stimulating hormone (FSH) and luteinizing hormone (LH) between 10 men with breast cancer and matched controls. Excretion of estrogen metabolites was no different in 19 patients with cancer compared with controls.[20] Olsson and coworkers[23] reported increased prolactin and decreased FSH levels with no difference in LH, estradiol, or testosterone levels in 15 men with breast cancer compared with controls. Several additional studies, again involving small sample sizes, reported elevated estriol production, lower levels of estrone, and estrogen breakdown products in men with breast cancer.[21,22]

Exogenous hormone therapy clearly promotes breast cancer in several susceptible species of experimental animals, but similar data in human males are lacking. Breast cancer is rarely reported in men undergoing estrogen therapy for prostate cancer, and a breast mass in such a patient is more often metastatic than primary.[24] Anecdotal reports have described breast cancer in male-to-female transsexuals taking estrogen to promote secondary sexual characteristics.[25,26]

Excess circulating estrogen secondary to compromised hepatic metabolism may explain the increased incidence of male breast cancer seen in several parts of the world. In parts of Africa, hepatic dysfunction is common, secondary to bilharziasis, cirrhosis, and chronic malnutrition, and is associated with an increased incidence of male breast cancer. Schistosomiasis (and related hepatic dysfunction) is associated with an increased rate of male breast cancer in Egypt.

Patients with Klinefelter syndrome have a risk for breast cancer that approaches that of females.[27] The breasts of these men are hypertrophic, secondary not only to gynecomastia but also to the development of acini and lobules. Although Klinefelter syndrome is associated with an increased risk for breast cancer, it is rare and therefore accounts for less than 1% of male breast cancer.

Pathology

The distribution of the histopathologic findings of breast cancer differs between males and females primarily because lobules are routinely not developed in the male breast. An early series from Memorial Hospital documented the absence of infiltrating lobular carcinoma in males.[28] Nance and Reddick[29] described infiltrating carcinoma of the male breast, and Heller and colleagues[30] reported an updated series from Memorial and similar to females infiltrating ductal carcinoma accounted for over 80% of all lesions. Intraductal carcinoma was more common in females (5% versus 3.8%), and this difference increases as screening mammography detects more ductal carcinoma in situ (DCIS) in the screened female population.[30] Infiltrating lobular carcinoma in males is quite unusual and has been only reported in rare instances.[29] Lobular carcinoma in situ has not been reported. All other types of breast cancer—including medullary, papillary, colloid, and Paget disease—have been reported in men.

Hormone Receptors

Estrogen receptor protein is present in male breast cancer in a higher percentage of patients than in women with breast cancer.[31-36] Rosen and colleagues[32] described positive estrogen receptor protein results in 75% of 8 male cancers, and Mercer and coworkers[34] found 94% of the lesions to be positive for estrogen receptor protein and 93% to be positive for progesterone receptor protein. Other series have confirmed these findings, and no correlation seems to exist between patient age, histologic grade of the lesion, stage, or nodal status. In a collected series of 47 patients, 80% were estrogen receptor protein–positive, and over 30% with metastatic disease responded to hormonal manipulation.[31]

Diagnosis and Natural History

The most common presentation of male breast cancer is a painless, unilateral breast mass. It is most often eccentric, slightly irregular, and quite firm. Mammographically detected lesions in asymptomatic men or in those presenting with a normal breast examination and ipsilateral axillary node are quite rare.[37,38] Nipple discharge is an unusual presentation of the disease and, if present, is often bloody or serosanguineous. Treves and colleagues[39] reported that such discharge was associated with cancer 80% of the time and accounted for nearly 14% of the male breast cancers.

Differential diagnosis of a breast mass in a male routinely must distinguish between gynecomastia and cancer. Gynecomastia remains the most common cause of either unilateral or bilateral breast mass. Although more commonly bilateral and symmetric with well-defined discoid margins, histopathologic confirmation is the only sure differential between benign and malignant disease. Fine-needle aspiration cytology depends highly on the experience of both the clinician and the cytopathologist. Although this technique may become more useful as experience increases, fine-needle aspiration cytology is not widely used in the differentiation of a male breast lesion. Mammography may be useful in differential diagnosis, but the gold standard remains biopsy.[37] Although gynecomastia remains the most common differential of a breast mass, it is not thought to be related to an increased risk for breast cancer.

Treatment

The historical treatment of choice for male breast cancer had been radical mastectomy. This approach had been advocated because of the theoretical or realized proximity of the lesion to the pectoralis major muscle. In addition, the stage at presentation may be more advanced in men than women and thus may necessitate a radical mastectomy. The current trend is toward modified radical mastectomy. Kinne and colleagues[40] described 36 consecutive cases at Memorial Hospital, 27 of whom were treated by modified radical mastectomy. Similar findings were reported by Hodson and also showed similar survival and local control between radical and modified radical mastectomy.[41] A review of 104 patients treated at several institutions since 1975 showed that 67% were treated with modified mastectomy.[33] Breast conservation has not been an issue in male breast cancer.

Prognosis and Survival

Carcinoma of the male breast is staged similarly to female breast cancer, using the American Joint Committee Clinical Staging System. As in women, axillary nodal status is the strongest predictor of outcome. A multivariate analysis of prognostic factors in 166 male breast cancers showed that age at diagnosis, tumor size, and nodal status were significant prognosticators, with nodal status proving strongest.[42] Prognosis in 335 cases was reported by Guinee and coworkers[43] and showed that both clinical axillary nodal status and clinical tumor size were predictive of outcome. A patient with palpable axillary nodes had double the risk for disease-related death, and an increase in tumor diameter of 3 cm carried a similarly increased risk for treatment failure. Although fixation to the skin or chest wall, as well as ulceration of tumor are more commonly reported in males than females, neither finding was predictive of outcome in multivariate analysis.[42]

Overall survival is often stated to be worse for men than for women with breast cancer.[44] When corrected for disease stage, survival seems to be similar, although men more commonly have advanced disease. A recent analysis of male breast cancer showed that 30% of men had advanced disease at presentation. A collection of men with breast cancer described 335 cases with an 84% 10-year survival rate in node-negative patients and a 44% survival rate for node-positive patients. They concluded that the prognosis of breast cancer is the same in male and female patients when compared stage for stage.[43] A similar analysis of compiled cases reported 5-year survival rates at 100% for node-negative disease and 60% for node-positive disease.[33]

Again it was concluded that the survival rates were quite similar to those of female breast cancer (Table 24.1-1).

Adjuvant Therapy

Adjuvant radiotherapy has been used in the treatment of male breast cancer. Although local control may be slightly improved, no improvement exists in overall survival. Improvement in local control may reflect advanced disease stage in men, rather than a biological difference in the disease between genders.

Hormonal ablation in the treatment of metastatic disease dates to the report of Farrow and colleagues[50] from Memorial Hospital in New York. They observed response from orchiectomy to symptomatic metastatic disease. Since the time of their report, orchiectomy has become the standard of care for metastatic disease. Recently, tamoxifen has been used as first-line treatment in receptor-positive disease and has shown response rates from 50% to 80%.[35,42,49,51,52]

Multiple reports have described the utility of adjuvant chemotherapy, but the disease is too uncommon to allow randomized clinical trials of systemic therapy.[53] General recommendations regarding patient selection for treatment resemble those for female patients. All patients with positive nodes and those selected node-negative patients who are at high risk for recurrence are treated with systemic therapy.

Several small series have described the efficacy of hormonal manipulation or chemotherapy in the treatment of male breast cancer. A review of hormone manipulation reported an overall response rate of 51%, but a rate of 71% was noted if the patient was positive for estrogen

TABLE 24.1-1
Survival in Male Breast Cancer

Investigators	5-Year Survival	
	Node-Negative Disease	Node-Positive Disease
	n	
Crichlow, 1972[44]	79	28
Heller et al, 1978[30]	90	NA
Yap et al, 1979[45]	77	38
Ramantanis et al, 1980[46]	57	31
Appleqvist & Salmo, 1982[47]	67	57
Erlichman et al, 1984[48]	77	37
Borgen et al, 1992[33]	100	60
Guinee et al, 1990[49]	90	74

NA, not available.

receptor protein. Patients who respond to first-line hormonal manipulation are more likely (70%) to respond to a second attempt.[40]

The efficacy of adjuvant chemotherapy in male breast cancer has also been reported. Because of the relative rarity of the disease, benefit is usually determined in comparison with historic controls and is fraught with the usual inaccuracies of such studies. A study from the M.D. Anderson Cancer Center reported such results in seven patients with stage II and four with stage III cancers and concluded that adjuvant therapy reduced the risk for recurrence and favorably influenced survival.[51,53] Similar results were reported from the National Cancer Institute, where 24 node-positive patients were treated with cyclophosphamide, methotrexate, and 5-fluorouracil. The 5-year survival rate of 80% exceeded that of historic controls, and the investigators concluded that adjuvant chemotherapy was beneficial in the treatment of node-positive disease.[54]

References

1. Boreng C, Squires T, Tong T, et al. Cancer statistics 1994. CA Cancer J. Clin 1994;44:18.
2. LaRaja R, Pagnozzi J, Rothenberg R. Cancer of the breast in three siblings. Cancer 85;55:2709.
3. Rosenblatt K, Thomas D, McTiernan A, et al. Breast cancer in men: aspects of familial aggregation. J Natl Cancer Inst 1991;83:849.
4. Kozak FK, Hall JG, Baird PA. Familial breast cancer in males: a case report and review of the literature. Cancer 1986;58:2736.
5. Kozak F, Hall J, Band P. Familial breast cancer in males: a case report and review of the literature. Cancer 1986;58:2736.
6. Malkin D. The Li-Fraumeni syndrome. Princ Pract Oncol Updates 1993;7:1.
7. Young J, Percy C, Asire A. Surveillance, epidemiology and end results: incidence and mortality data. (NIH Pub 81-2330). Natl Cancer Inst Monogr 1981;57:74.
8. Lenfant-Pejovic MH, Mlika-Cabanne N, Bouchardy C, et al. Risk factors for male breast cancer: a Franco-Swiss case-control study. Int J Cancer 1990;45:661.
9. Mabuchi K, Bross DS, Kessler I. Risk factors for male breast cancer. J Natl Cancer Inst 1985;74:371.
10. Thomas DB, Jiminez LM, McTiernan A, et al. Breast cancer in men: risk factors with hormonal implications. Am J Epidemiol 1992; 135:734.
11. Casagrande J, Hanische R, Pike M. A case-control study of male breast cancer. Cancer Res 1988;48:1326.
12. Mani S, Ahmad YH, Papac RJ. Male breast cancer: risk factors and clinical features. Proc Annu Meet Am Soc Clin Oncol 1992; 11:A157.
13. Eldar S, Nash E, Abrahamson J. Radiation carcinogenesis in the male breast. Eur J Surg Oncol 1989;15:274.
14. Greene M, Goedert J, Bech-Hansen N. Radiogenic male breast cancer with in vitro sensitivity to ionizing radiation and bleomycin. Cancer Invest 1983;1:379.
15. Hauser A, Lerner I, King R. Familial male breast cancer. Am J Med Genet 1992;44:839.
16. Jauchum J. Occupational exposure to electromagnetic fields and breast cancer in men. Am J Epidemiol 1992;135:1423.
17. Yahalom J, Petrek JA, Biddinger PW, et al. Breast cancer in patients irradiated for Hodgkin's disease: a clinical and pathologic analysis of 45 Events in 37 patients. J Clin Oncol 1992;10:1674.
18. Mabuchi A, Bross D, Kessler I. Risk factors in male breast cancer. J Natl Cancer Inst 1985;74:371.
19. Ballerini P, Recchione C, Cavalleri A, et al. Hormones in male breast cancer. Tumori 1990;76:26.
20. Scheike O, Svenstrup B, Frandson B. Metabolism of estradiol 17-β in men with breast cancer. J Steroid Biochem 1973;4:489.
21. Zumoff B, Fishman J, Cassouto J, et al. Estradiol transformation in men with breast cancer. J Clin Endocrinol Metab 1966;26:960.
22. Dao T, Morreal C, Nemoto T. Urinary estrogen excretion in men with breast cancer. N Engl J Med 1973;289:138.
23. Olsson H, Alm P, Aspegren K, et al. Increased plasma prolactin levels in a group of men with breast cancer: a preliminary study. Anticancer Res 1990;10:59.
24. Schlappack OK, Braun O, Maier U. Report of two cases of male breast cancer after prolonged estrogen treatment for prostatic carcinoma. Cancer Detect Prev 1986;9:319.
25. Pritchard T, Pankowsky D, Crowe J, et al. Breast cancer in a male to female transsexual. JAMA 1988;259:2278.
26. Symmers W. Carcinoma of the breast in trans-sexual individuals after surgery and hormonal interference with primary and secondary sex characteristics. Br Med J 1968;2:83.
27. Evans D, Crichlow R. Carcinoma of the male breast and Klinefelter's syndrome: is there an association? CA Cancer J Clin 1987;37:246.
28. Holleb A, Freeman H, Farrow J. Cancer of the male breast. NY State Med J 1968;68:836.
29. Nance KV, Reddick RL. In situ and infiltrating lobular carcinoma of the male breast. Hum Pathol 1989;20:1220.
30. Heller K, Rosen P, Schottenfeld D. Male breast cancer: a clinicopathologic study of 97 cases. Ann Surg 1978;188:60.
31. Friedman M, Hoffman P, Dandolos E. Estrogen receptors in male breast cancer. Cancer 1981;47:134.
32. Rosen P, Botet C, Nisselbaum J. Estrogen receptor protein in lesions of the male breast. Cancer 1976;37:1866.
33. Borgen P, Wong G, Vlamis V, et al. Current management of male breast cancer: a review of 104 cases. Annals Surg 1992;215:451.
34. Mercer RJ, Bryan RM, Bennett RC. Hormone receptors in male breast cancer. Aust NZ Surg 1984;54:215.
35. Ribeiro G, Swindell R. Adjuvant tamoxifen for male breast cancer. Br J Cancer 1992;65:252.
36. Pacheco MM, Oshima CF, Lopes MP. Steroid hormone receptors in male breast diseases. Anticancer Res 1986;6:1013.
37. Dershaw DD, Borgen PI, Deutch BM, et al. Mammographic findings in men with breast cancer. Am J Roentgenol 1993;160:267.
38. Balich SM, Khandekhar JD, Sener SF. Cancer of the male breast presenting as an axillary mass. J Surg Oncol 1993;53:68.
39. Treves N, Robbins G, Amoroso W. Serous and serosanguineous discharge from the male nipple. Arch Surg 1956;73:319.
40. Kinne D, Hakes T. Male breast cancer. In: Harris J, Hellman S, Henderson IC, et al, eds. Breast diseases. Philadelphia, JB Lippincott, 1991:782.
41. Hodson GR, Urdaneta LF, Al-Jurf AS, et al. Male breast carcinoma. Am Surgeon 1985;51:47.
42. Hulthorn R, Friberg S, Hulthorn KA. Male breast carcinoma. II. A study of the total material reported to the Swedish Cancer Registry 1958-1967 with respect to treatment, prognostic factors and survival. Acta Oncol 1987;26:327.
43. Guinee VF, Olsson H, Moller T, et al. The prognosis of breast cancer in males. Cancer 1993;71:154.
44. Crichlow R. Carcinoma of the male breast. Surg Gynecol Obstet 1972;134:1011.
45. Yap H, Tashima C, Blumenschein G, et al. Male breast cancer: a natural history study. Cancer 1979;44:748.

46. Ramantanis G, Besbeas S, Garas J. Breast cancer in the male: a report of 138 cases. World J Surg 1980;4:621.

47. Appleqvist P, Salmo M. Prognosis in carcinoma of the male breast. Acta Chir Scand 1982;148:499.

48. Erlichman C, Murphy K, Elhakim T. Male breast cancer: a 13-year review of 89 patients. J Clin Oncol 1984;2:903.

49. Guinee VF, Moller T, Olsson H, et al. Clinical prognostic factors in male breast cancer: eleven-center study, international cancer patient data exchange system. Proc Annu Meet Am Soc Clin Oncol 1990;9:A138.

50. Farrow J, Adair F. Effects of orchiectomy on skeltal metastases from cancer of the male breast. Science 1942;95:654.

51. Jaiyesimi I, Buzdar A, Sahin A, et al. Carcinoma of the male breast. Ann Intern Med 1992;117:771.

52. Chi JC, Juler GL, Rosen AO. Treatment modalities and survival in male breast carcinoma. Proc Annu Meet Am Soc Clin Oncol 1988;7:A94.

53. Patel HZ, Buzdar AU, Hortobagi GN. Role of adjuvant chemotherapy in male breast cancer. Cancer 1989;64:1583.

54. Bagley C, Wesley M, Young R, et al. Adjuvant chemotherapy in males with cancer of the breast. Am J Clin Oncol 1987;10:55.

24.2
Phyllodes Tumors

JEANNE A. PETREK

Phyllodes tumor (formerly called cystosarcoma phyllodes) is a rare distinctive fibroepithelial tumor that occurs only in the breast. The entity produces a spectrum of diseases ranging from the benign (with significant risk for local recurrence) to the malignant (sometimes with rapidly growing metastases). During the past 150 years, since being described by Johannes Muller in 1838,[1] who called it cystosarcoma phyllodes, it has had at least 62 synonymous designations.[2] Believing that the tumor was entirely benign, Muller stressed its difference from breast cancer and apparently chose the term *sarcoma,* not to indicate the rare malignant subgroup but to describe the fleshy appearance.

It was only in 1931 at Memorial Hospital in New York that the first case of metastatic phyllodes tumor was described.[3] Nevertheless, the name cystosarcoma phyllodes overstates the malignant potential of most such tumors; thus, it is unduly alarming to patients and physicians alike. The term *sarcoma* is not objectionable when it refers to the malignant and borderline varieties, both of which are infrequent. *Cysto* implies that the lesion contains macroscopic cysts, although this is not always the case.

As for other terms, *fibroadenoma phyllodes* would be appropriate, especially if applied only to those tumors that are deemed, after careful pathologic study, to be almost certainly benign. It has the merit of alerting surgeons that they are addressing an unusual tumor that shares some characteristics with fibroadenoma (but not with sarcoma). If this term were used for benign phyllodes tumors that can have a local recurrence rate of 20%, the term would be acceptable. The malignant category could be called *cystosarcoma phyllodes.* The name for the borderline category of this tumor would still be problematic.

Thus, most agree that the best name is *phyllodes tumor* with the extra qualification according to the pathologist's assessment of its microscopic appearance and therefore its likely behavior—benign, malignant, or borderline. All these tumors would remain classified under a single term. The nomenclature is not entirely new and merely reminds one of the original term (*cystosarcoma phyllodes*).

Macroscopic Appearance

The size of phyllodes tumors varies from 1 cm[4] to larger than 40 cm.[5] In modern series, it is common to diagnose most such tumors in the smaller sizes.[6] Most phyllodes tumors, benign or malignant, appear well circumscribed grossly, although they lack a true capsule. This may occur because, being so hypercellular, they present a hard barrier that compresses and pushes upon the softer surrounding breast tissue.

Muller[1] described the lesion as grayish white and resembling a head of cauliflower. The barely visible surface projections make complete surgical excision with narrow margins difficult, and inadvertent amputation predisposes to tumor recurrence. The cut surface is slimy or mucoid and tends to bulge outward. Firm, fibrous areas alternate with soft fleshy areas and, occasionally, with cysts filled with clear or semisolid bloody fluid. Yellow fatty areas as well as areas of hemorrhage and necrosis can occur. Leaflike ("phyllodes")—papillary protrusions of stromal connective tissue lined with epithelium—often extend into the cystic areas.

Microscopic Appearance

Histologically, phyllodes tumor, like fibroadenoma, is composed of epithelial elements and a connective tissue stroma. Cuboidal epithelium, resembling ductal epithelium of the surrounding breast tissue, lines the canaliculi, which appear as ductal spaces. These epithelial areas can become irregularly flattened in rapidly growing lesions, presumably by the pressure of the enlarging stroma. The epithelium may be hyperplastic and may have varying degrees of atypia in benign or malignant states. Apocrine and squamous metaplasia of the epithelial elements, although rare, has also occurred.[4] Rare case reports have described cases in which the epithelium had changes indicative of carcinoma.[7]

Characteristics of the stroma alone, however, determine whether a phyllodes tumor should be classified as benign or malignant, just as the appearance of the connective tissue distinguishes benign phyllodes tumor from fibroadenoma (Table 24.2-1 and Fig. 24.2-1). In general, stroma from malignant phyllodes tumor contains marked cellularity with pleomorphism and nuclear atypia, increased mitotic activity, and overgrowth of the stromal element[8,9] (Fig. 24.2-2). Often the malignant areas are focal and can be overlooked if multiple areas are not sampled.[10,11]

Two common stromal patterns exist. In the first, cells are spindle shaped, resembling a fibrosarcoma. In the second, the cells are looser and myxoid in appearance, resembling a myxoliposarcoma.[4,12] Both patterns are usually found intermixed in the same tumor. The stroma can also show multidirectional differentiation into mesenchymal elements, which are (in order of frequency) fibrosarcoma, liposarcoma, chondrosarcoma, osteosarcoma, and leiomyosarcoma.[4,9]

Histologic Classification and the Clinical Course

The association of histologic appearance with the clinical course has been studied in various retrospective surveys, including several recent reviews (Table 24.2-1). In the 1950s, the large series of Lester and Stout[11] (58 patients) and that of Treves and Sunderland[8] (77 patients) tried to relate the clinical behavior of phyllodes tumors to two characteristics of the stroma—cellular atypia and increased mitotic activity. Both groups found this classification unreliable, because some patients with characteristics of malignancy had a benign course, and patients with metastases had tumors with only benign or borderline characteristics.

In 1967, Norris and Taylor[13] used the same two characteristics—cellular atypia and mitotic activity—and added a third, tumor margin (pushing versus infiltrating), as determinants of malignant potential. These three criteria, when considered together, are more reliable.

Pietruszka and Barnes,[14] refining the criteria of Norris and Taylor, attempted to correlate clinical behavior with classification as benign (0 to 4 mitoses in 10 high-power fields [HPFs]), borderline (5 to 9 mitoses in 10 HPFs, pushing or infiltrating margins, minimal stromal cellular atypia), or malignant (10 or more mitoses in 10 HPFs, infiltrating margins, moderate to marked stromal cellular atypia). Although mitotic rate was the most important determinant, the authors found increased predictability with the combination criteria. Metastases occurred only in the malignant tumors. Nevertheless, only 23.5% of patients diagnosed with a malignant phyllodes tumor developed metastatic disease.

Studies from the Northwestern University Hospitals[15,16] in Chicago have used a grading system (based on cellularity, pleomorphism, differentiation, mitoses, and vascularity) to be an indicator of aggressive behavior. Their studies with flow cytometric analysis of DNA ploidy and proliferative index also correlated with the grading system.[16]

Although the role of flow cytometric analysis continues to be evaluated, several reports have not shown this tool to be particularly useful. Five series[17-21] published in the early 1990s using small sample sizes (range, 8 to 30 patients) have evaluated the correlation of flow cytometry with standard pathologic variables and clinical behavior. Three studies showed poor correlation[17,18,20]; one showed that DNA content is a significant predictor on multivariate analysis[21]; and one concluded that S-phase may "complement the traditional histologic analysis."[20] Electron microscopy has not contributed to the differentiation of benign from malignant tumors.[22]

Stromal overgrowth (at expense of epithelial elements) has been found to be a reliable, and perhaps most important, single predictor of aggressive behavior in many recent studies.[12,15,16,23-27] The only large series (77 patients) in which this factor was not predictive is from the Swedish Cancer Registry.[23] Stromal overgrowth has been most commonly defined as disproportionate proliferation of the stromal components so that at least one 40-power field (other than in the large papillary regions) contains no ductal epithelium.[27]

Probably because of the diverse criteria, the percentage of all phyllodes tumors classified as malignant ranges between 23%[10] and 50%.[28] One review[29] concluded that the accepted incidence of histologically malignant tumors is about 25%. Metastases occur in 6.2%[30] to 22%[31] of all cases.

Precise classification by individual pathologists of this uncommon tumor into benign, borderline, and malignant categories is partially responsible for this wide range. Referral patterns favor malignancy in series from specialized institutions, such as Memorial Sloan-Kettering Cancer Center[4,10] or the Armed Forces Institute of Pathology.[13]

TABLE 24.2-1

Histologic Considerations in the Classification of Phyllodes Tumors as Benign, Borderline, and Malignant

ACCEPTED AND STANDARD CHARACTERISTICS

Cellular atypia[8,11,13-16]

Miotic activity[8,11,13-16]

Tumor margins[13,14]

Stromal overgrowth[12,15,16,23-27]

NONSTANDARD OR UNPROVEN CHARACTERISTICS

Vascularity[15,16]

Flow cytometric analyses[15-21]

Pleomorphism[15-16]

Electron microscopic characteristics[22]

FIGURE 24.2-1. Benign cystosarcoma phyllodes. **A.** Low-power view showing characteristic epithelium-lined clefts, which outline islands of stroma composed of spindle cells and collagen. **B.** High-magnification view showing thin layers of benign epithelial cells and benign stroma. Mitoses and nuclear pleomorphism are absent from the stroma.

Haagensen[30] believes that a realistic figure of metastatic disease from all phyllodes tumors is that from his series (6.2%), originating in a general surgical center.

Histogenesis

The origin of phyllodes tumors has been difficult to investigate, presumably because of its relative rarity and because incipient tumors and microscopic disease are rarely encountered. One author[32] believes that most phyllodes tumors arise in preexisting fibroadenomas. Occasionally patients have been aware of small lumps in their breasts for as long as 45 years before growth of the nodule, biopsy, and diagnosis of phyllodes tumors.[33] In some tumors, the more dense fibrous parts appear localized into a distinctly ovoid outline, an appearance that has been interpreted as the residual benign fibroadenoma that gave rise to phyllodes tumors.[30] Most authors do not comment on the tumor's origin or state that the lesion probably arises de novo from breast parenchyma.[8]

FIGURE 24.2-2. Malignant cystosarcoma phyllodes. **A.** Low-magnification view showing highly cellular stroma and relatively inconspicuous epithelium. **B.** At higher magnification, the cellular stroma reveals considerable nuclear pleomorphism and several mitotic figures.

Steroid Receptors

Estrogen and progesterone receptor analyses have recently been performed on tumor tissue from patients with phyllodes tumors. Variability of results has been noted[34-36] and may reflect, in part, the relative amounts of epithelium (which contains the receptors) compared with stroma in the tumors. Hormonal treatment has no known value because only the stromal component metastasizes.

Clinical and Radiologic Features

In almost all cases, a phyllodes tumor (whether benign or malignant) is discovered as a painless breast mass that is smooth, rounded, and multinodular. Most patients have continuous growth, although some patients have had rapid growth in a previously stable, long-standing nodule. When the tumor enlarges, it often does so rapidly, but this occurrence does not necessarily indicate malignancy. The shiny, stretched, and attenuated skin with varicose veins can overlie a phyllodes tumor. In these circumstances, skin ulceration is due to ischemia, secondary to stretching and pressure. With ulceration due to carcinoma, the ulcerated skin also has dimpling, or peau d'orange. The nipple may be effaced but is not invaded or retracted.

A notable feature of phyllodes tumor is the usual absence of suspicious axillary lymph nodes, despite a large mass, a situation infrequent with breast cancer. Axillary lymph node enlargement can occur (in as many as 20% of cases in one series).[13] This finding is virtually never the result of metastatic disease but is usually due to necrotic, and sometimes infected, tumor.

The mammographic appearance of phyllodes tumors is very much like that of fibroadenoma, with smooth, polylobulated margins, although some margins may be irregular, suggesting local invasion.[37-39] Similarly, these tumors cannot be differentiated ultrasonographically from fibroadenomas and well-circumscribed malignant tumors.[37,38] On ultrasonography, fluid-filled elongated clefts may be found within an otherwise solid mass with no significant posterior shadowing. A diagnosis of phyllodes tumor should therefore be considered if cysts with a solid, circumscribed lesion are noted.

Patient Characteristics

Phyllodes tumors are rare, reported to be about 2%[8,11,30] to 4.4%[40] as numerous as fibroadenomas diagnosed in the same institution. A recent population-based study from California noted a higher risk in Latino women compared with white or Asian women. The risk for malignant phyllodes tumors in their study overall was 2.1 per million women.[41]

The mean age of tumor onset in patients evaluated in large series occurs in the fourth decade,[4,10,14,30] which is 10 to 20 years older than the mean age for fibroadenoma. A wide range is recorded in most series, and phyllodes tumor has been recorded in prepubertal and adolescent ages.[42,43] The mean age of patients with benign phyllodes is younger than that of patients with malignant phyllodes.[4,32] Bilaterality is rare with either benign[13,30] or malignant tumors. A 30% incidence of bilaterality was found only in one report[44] and is a notable exception.

Phyllodes tumor is rarely, if ever, found in men. The largest recent series is from the Armed Forces Institute of Pathology.[45] All reported cases in men seem to occur in the presence of gynecomastia and lobular development.[45]

Histologically malignant epithelium is rare, as witnessed by the few cases reported. Intraductal cancer,[7,13,30,46] infiltrating duct cancer,[46,47] lobular carcinoma in situ (lobular neoplasia), and squamous carcinoma,[7,8,30,48] all have been described. A recent study from Denmark[49] has reached similar conclusions about the rarity of this tumor's occurrence. Nevertheless, as any associated carcinoma is quite rare, principles of management for phyllodes tumors should not generally address this possibility.

Natural History

LOCAL–REGIONAL RECURRENCE

Numerous investigators have concluded that, overall, phyllodes tumors recur locally in perhaps 20% of the cases.[9,30,32,50] The recurrence may be as easily excised or, as shown by the rare case report, may be quite aggressive, invading the chest wall and thoracic cavity.[10,51]

In general, little difference exists in the tendency for benign versus malignant tumors to recur locally. A series of malignant phyllodes tumors (not necessarily metastatic)[52] at Memorial Hospital found a low (8%) local recurrence rate. This probably occurred because more extensive margins were obtained, compared with benign phyllodes tumors which have a higher local recurrence rate. In another series,[29] half of patients had a local recurrence in the course of their metastatic disease.

Most locally recurrent tumors are histologically similar to the original lesion. In the Memorial Hospital series, only 2 of the 28 locally recurrent benign lesions had histologic "malignant transformation" at reexcision.[52] Other authors reported malignant transformation of the recurrence less commonly than in the Memorial Hospital series.[30,53,54]

The Memorial Hospital series[52] reported earlier recurrences when the original lesion was classified as malignant (6 to 24 months), rather than benign (18 to 24 months). In a recent large series of 216 consecutive patients, the Milan authors[55] noted similar findings. They found an average interval to local recurrence of 32 months for benign, 22 months for malignant, and 18 months for borderline phyllodes tumors.

Regional lymph node metastases rarely develop from

malignant phyllodes tumors. Clinical enlargement of the lymph nodes is present in about 20%,[13,56] although that finding is probably due to necrotic tumor or other factors, given that the incidence of lymph node metastases in various series of malignant phyllodes tumor is less than 5%.[56,57] It appears that only one patient with axillary lymph node metastases has been reported as cured.[58]

SYSTEMIC RECURRENCE

All reported metastatic lesions except one[59] have resembled sarcomas, being devoid of all the epithelial elements. Less than 5% of all phyllodes tumors (benign, borderline, or malignant) metastasize. About one fourth of those classified as histologically malignant metastasize, depending, as always, on the histologic criteria used for classification.

Metastatic lesions have been reported as early as the initial diagnosis of the primary tumor and as late as 12 years after diagnosis.[29] In a review of all reported cases of metastatic phyllodes tumors (67 cases), Kessinger and colleagues[29] found that the average survival time after diagnosis of metastasis was 30 months. The longest survival after diagnosis with metastatic disease was 14.5 years. The most common site of the initially diagnosed distant metastasis was the lungs. After lungs, the bones, liver, heart, and distant lymph nodes were metastatic sites in a roughly descending order of frequency.[29,56]

Management Considerations

INITIAL DIAGNOSIS OF PHYLLODES TUMOR

Because of its similarity to fibroadenoma on physical examination, mammography and during operation, phyllodes tumors are often enucleated—excised with no margin—which is the standard procedure for fibroadenoma. About 20% of phyllodes tumors recur locally if excised with no margin or with a margin of only a few millimeters. The proportion may be somewhat higher with borderline or malignant varieties and lower with benign tumors. Local recurrence rates as high as 20%,[52] 28%,[30] and 33%[13] have been reported.

Even when agreeing with the general number of 20% local recurrence, authors differ as to whether immediate reexcision should be done to obtain the recommended margin of 2 cm when an unsuspected phyllodes is diagnosed on permanent section. At Memorial Hospital—where patients are informed of these statistics and of the alternatives, risks, and benefits—most patients undergo reexcision about 4 weeks later.

In review of 106 patients with benign phyllodes tumors done in Singapore, Chua and colleagues[60] concluded that, because only 16% of patients undergoing presumptive surgery for fibroadenoma develop a local recurrence, a policy of close follow-up is usually acceptable. If, however, microscopic assessment shows definite transection of the tumor, Chua recommends immediate reoperation. A pitfall

in the "watch-and-wait" policy is shown by the fact that 7 of 106 patients on long-term follow-up had pseudorecurrences, with only scar tissue and benign fibrocystic changes found during a second operation.[61]

The largest series reported thus far described 216 consecutive patients and also addressed the question of phyllodes tumor found unexpectedly on permanent section analysis.[55] With various breast resection procedures, 7.9% of the benign phyllodes tumors recurred. The investigators found no difference in local recurrence rates with narrow versus no margins. Five of 55 patients were treated with enucleation, and 5 of 52 with narrow (otherwise undefined) resections. In the small group of malignant phyllodes 23.3% recurred, and, in the borderline group, 19.6% recurred. This finding is logical, given that the borderline and malignant varieties recur earlier, probably because of faster growth, although benign phyllodes eventually have a similar local recurrence.

Methods that have been evaluated but that do not have an important place in the management of phyllodes tumors include preoperative fine-needle aspiration of all apparent fibroadenomas or intraoperative frozen section. Theoretically, this approach could lead to identification of phyllodes tumor and would lead the surgeon to perform a wide (rather than a close) excision as the initial surgical procedure.

To diagnose a phyllodes tumor on fine-needle aspiration, the smear must yield a dimorphic pattern of stromal elements (tissue fragments or single spindle cells) and benign epithelial tissue. Fine-needle aspiration failed in 22%[62] and 86%[28] of cases in two recent reports, respectively; in another recent report containing four benign phyllodes tumors,[63] 2 were mistakenly diagnosed as carcinoma, 1 was suspicious for carcinoma and 1 was summarized descriptively as "benign duct epithelium."

Performing an intraoperative frozen section on all apparent fibroadenomas is not judicious. Apart from the great expense and intraoperative time involved for the rare occurrence, the differentiation of benign phyllodes from cellular fibroadenoma can be difficult using a frozen section. Further, the sarcomatous element in phyllodes tumors can be mistakenly diagnosed as an undifferentiated carcinoma, thereby leading to unnecessary radical procedures.

SPECIAL CONSIDERATIONS OF MALIGNANT PHYLLODES TUMORS

Most authors agree on the initial wide excision for benign phyllodes tumors; however, for histologically malignant phyllodes tumors, some authors,[13,29,32,33,49,54,59] particularly in the past, have recommended total mastectomy as routine initial treatment.

Haagensen[30] was one of the first to advocate a wide excision if the tumor-to-breast size would permit, instead of a mastectomy, given that the object is local control. With multicentricity not an issue as it is in breast cancer, breast preservation has been accomplished without local recurrence after diagnosis of malignant phyllodes tumors in more recent series.[56,57]

Because regional lymph node metastases rarely occur with phyllodes tumors, it is virtually never necessary to do a formal axillary dissection.[13,56,57] If clinically enlarged and suspicious lymph nodes exist, excisional biopsy of the lymph nodes invariably proves these lymph nodes to be hyperplastic.

LOCAL RECURRENCE

For the local recurrence of a benign phyllodes tumor, reexcision with at least a 2- to 3-cm margin is advised. As noted, almost all recurrences retain the histologic pattern of the primary tumor, and more aggressive treatment to address the small possibility of malignant transformation is not advised. Rarely, with a large tumor relative to a small breast size, the recommended margin necessitates a mastectomy. Sometimes, the wide excision or mastectomy includes a portion of the pectoralis fascia or even a portion of full-thickness pectoralis muscle (if necessary) for 2 to 3 cm of posterior margin.

With local recurrence after a malignant phyllodes has been initially treated with wide margins of 2 to 3 cm, a total mastectomy is most often recommended. Although acknowledging that no patient with a malignant phyllodes treated by simple mastectomy in his practice had a recurrence, Haagensen[30] pointed out that, with local recurrence after local excision, mastectomy was successful at that time. Even in patients with metastatic disease, he believes that aggressive initial treatment would not have mattered, because blood-borne metastases to the lungs appeared within a few months.

SYSTEMIC DISEASE

Thus far, therapy for metastatic disease has been discouraging, with no sustained remissions from radiation,[10,11,59,64,65] additive hormones,[10] castration,[32,66] or chemotherapy.[29,59,64] A recent report attempted to evaluate the role of radiation in this disease. It concluded that little has been published, probably because of early experience, which found no effect of radiation, and the early results which deterred further attempts.[67] No reported cases exist to support response to hormonal manipulation,[10,13,29,64,65] even if hormone receptors were present. Ifosfamide and, secondly, doxorubicin may be the most active on metastatic disease.[64,68,69]

At the opposite end of the spectrum are the rare cases that prove fatal by direct extension without distant metastases.[14,70] As is the case with sarcomas in general, distant pulmonary metastases may be resectable for possible cure.[9,58]

MANAGEMENT SUMMARY

- Because of the similarity to fibroadenoma on physical examination and mammography and during operation, phyllodes tumors are often enucleated or excised with narrow margins, which is standard treatment for fibroadenoma. In this situation, a local recurrence rate of 20% may be expected.
- If permanent histology shows phyllodes tumor at the margin, reoperation to obtain a 2-cm negative margin is recommended. For smaller negative margins, reoperation for wider excision and close follow-up have both been recommended.
- The use of systemic therapy for metastatic disease of phyllodes tumor is based on the guidelines for treating sarcomas, not breast cancer.

References

1. Muller J. Uber den feineran Bau und die Forman der krankhaften Geschwilste. Berlin, G Reimer, 1838.
2. Fiks A. Cystosarcoma phyllodes of the mammary gland: Muller's tumor. Virchows Arch 1981;392:1.
3. Lee B, Pack G. Giant intracanalicular fibroadenomyxoma of the breast. Am J Cancer 1931;15:2583.
4. McDivitt RW, Stewart FW, Berg JW. Tumors of the breast. In: Atlas of tumor pathology, series 2, fascicle 2. Washington, DC, Armed Forces Institute of Pathology, 1968.
5. Lee B, Pack G. Giant intracanalicular fibroadenomyxoma: the so-called cystosarcoma phyllodes mammae of Johannes Muller. Ann Surg 1931;93:250.
6. Bartoli C, Zurrida S, Veronesi P, et al. Small sized phyllodes tumor of the breast. Eur J Surg Oncol 1990;16:215.
7. Rosen PP, Urban JA. Coexistent mammary carcinoma and cystosarcoma phyllodes. Breast 1975;1:9.
8. Treves N, Sunderland D. Cystosarcoma phyllodes of the breast: a malignant and a benign tumor. Cancer 1951;4:1286.
9. Hart WR, Bauer RC, Oberman HA. A clinicopathogic study of twenty-six hypercellular periductal stromal tumors of the breast. Am J Clin Pathol 1978;70:211.
10. Treves N. A study of cystosarcoma phyllodes. Ann NY Acad Sci 1964;114:922.
11. Lester J, Stout A. Cystosarcoma phyllodes. Cancer 1954;7:335.
12. Azzopardi JG. Sarcomas of the breast. In: Bennington JL, ed. Problems in breast pathology, vol 2. Major problems in pathology. Philadelphia, WB Saunders, 1979.
13. Norris HJ, Taylor HB. Relationship of histologic features to behavior of cystosarcoma phyllodes: analysis of ninety-four cases. Cancer 1967;20:2090.
14. Pietruszka M, Barnes I. Cystosarcoma phyllodes: a clinicopathologic analysis of 42 cases. Cancer 1978;41:1974.
15. Hines JR, Murad TM, Beal JM. Prognostic indicators in cystosarcoma phyllodes. Am J Surg 1987;153:276.
16. Murad TM, Hines JR, Beal J, et al. Histological and clinical correlations of cystosarcoma phyllodes. Arch Pathol Lab Med 1988;112:752.
17. Rowell MD, Perry RR, Hsiu JG, et al. Phyllodes tumors. Am J Surg 1993;165:376.
18. Keelan PA, Myers JL, Wold LE, et al. Phyllodes tumor: clinicopathologic review of 60 patients and flow cytometric analysis in 30 patients. Hum Pathol 1992;23:1048.
19. Grimes MM. Cystosarcoma phyllodes of the breast: histologic features, flow cytometric analysis, and clinical correlations. Mod Pathol 1992;5:232.
20. Palko MJ, Wang SE, Shackney SE, et al. Flow cytometric S fraction as a predictor of clinical outcome in cystosarcoma phyllodes. Arch Pathol Lab Med 1990;114:949.

21. El-Naggar AK, Ro JY, McLemore D, et al. DNA content and proliferative activity of cystosarcoma phyllodes of the breast. Am J Clin Pathol 1990;93:480.

22. Kesterson GHD, Georgiade N, Seigler HF, et al. Cystosarcoma phyllodes: a steroid receptor and ultrastructure analysis. Ann Surg 1988;190:640.

23. Cohn-Cedermark G, Rutqvist LE, Rosendahl I, et al. Prognostic factors in cystosarcoma phyllodes: a clinicopathologic study of 77 patients. Cancer 1991;68:2017.

24. Kario K, Maeda S, Mizuno Y, et al. Phyllodes tumor of the breast: a clinicopathologic study of 34 cases. J Surg Oncol 1990;45:46.

25. Hawkins RE, Schofield JB, Fisher C, et al. The clinical and histologic criteria that predict metastases from cystosarcoma phyllodes. Cancer 1992;69:141.

26. Inoshita SI. Phyllodes tumor (cystosarcoma phyllodes) of the breast. Acta Pathol Jpn 1988;28:21.

27. Ward RM, Evans HL. Cystosarcoma phyllodes: a clinicopathology study of 26 cases. Cancer 1986;58:2282.

28. Salvadori B, Cusumano F, Del Bo R, et al. Surgical treatment of phyllodes tumors of the breast. Cancer 1989;63:2532.

29. Kessinger A, Foley JF, Lemon HM, et al. Metastatic cystosarcoma phyllodes: a case report and review of the literature. J Surg Oncol 1972;4:131.

30. Haagensen CD. Diseases of the breast, ed 2. Philadelphia, WB Saunders, 1975:227.

31. Oberman HA. Cystosarcoma phyllodes: a clinicopathologic study of hypercellular periductal stromal neoplasms of the breast. Cancer 1965;18:697.

32. McDivitt RW, Urban JA, Farrow JH. Cystosarcoma phyllodes. Johns Hopkins Med J 1966;120:33.

33. Maier WP, Rosemond GP, Wittenberg R, et al. Cystosarcoma phyllodes mammae. Oncology 1968;22:145.

34. Pashof T. Estradiol binding protein in cystosarcoma phyllodes of the breast. Eur J Cancer Clin Oncol 1980;16:591.

35. Porton WM, Poortman J. Estrogen receptors in cystosarcoma phyllodes of the breast. Eur J Cancer Clin Oncol 1981;17:1147.

36. Brentani MM, Nagai MA, Oshimi CTF, et al. Steroid receptors in cystosarcoma phyllodes. Cancer Detect Prev 1982;5:211.

37. Buchberger W, Strasser K, Heim K, et al. Phyllodes tumor: findings on mammography, sonograph, and aspiration cytology in 10 cases. Am J Roentgenol 1991;157:715.

38. Dorsi CJ, Feldhaus L, Sonnenfeld M. Unusual lesions of the breast. Radiol Clin North Am 1983;21:67.

39. Cosmacini P, Zurrida S, Veronesi P, et al. Phyllodes tumor of the breast: mammographic experience in 99 cases. Eur J Radiol 1992;15:11.

40. Dyer NH, Bridger JE, Taylor RS. Cystosarcoma phyllodes. Br J Surg 1966:450.

41. Bernstein L, Deapen D, Ross RK. The descriptive epidemiology of malignant cystosarcoma phyllodes tumors of the breast. Cancer 1993;71:3020.

42. Amerson JR. Cystosarcoma phyllodes in adolescent females: a report of seven patients. Ann Surg 1971;71:849.

43. Gibbs BR Jr, Roe RD, Thomas DF. Malignant cystosarcoma phyllodes in a pre-pubertal female. Ann Surg 1968;167:229.

44. McDonald JR, Harrington SW. Giant fibro-adenoma of the breast: cystosarcomas phylloides. Ann Surg 1950;131:243.

45. Ansah-Boateng Y, Tavassoli F. Fibroadenoma and cystosarcoma phyllodes of the male breast. Mod Pathol 1992;5:114.

46. Klausner JM, Lelcuk S, Ilia B, et al. Breast carcinoma originating in cystosarcoma phyllodes. Clin Oncol 1983;9:71.

47. Philip PJ. Carcinosarcoma of the breast. J R Coll Surg Edinb 1976;21:229.

48. Cornog JL, Mobini SE, Enterline HT. Squamous carcinoma of the breast. Am J Clin Pathol 1971;55:410.

49. Christensen L, Nielsen M, Madsen PM. Cystosarcoma phyllodes: a review of 19 cases with emphasis on the occurrence of associated breast carcinoma. Acta Pathol Microbiol Immunol Scand 1986;94:35.

50. Contarini O, Urdaneta LF, Hagan W, et al. Cystosarcoma phyllodes of the breast: a new therapeutic proposal. Am Surg 1982;48:157.

51. Ross DE. Malignancy occurring in cystosarcoma phyllodes. Am J Surg 1954;88:243.

52. Hajdu S, Espinosa MH, Robbins GF. Recurrent cystosarcoma phyllodes: a clinicopathologic study of 32 cases. Cancer 1975;38:1402.

53. Al-Jurf A, Hawks WA, Crile G Jr. Cystosarcoma phyllodes. Surg Gynecol Obstet 1978;146:358.

54. Rix DB, Tredwell SJ, Forward AD. Cystosarcoma phyllodes (cellular intracanalicular fibroadenoma): clinicopathologic relationships. Can J Surg 1971;14:31.

55. Zurrida S, Bartoli C, Galimberti V, et al. Which therapy for unexpected phyllode tumour of the breast? Eur J Cancer 1992;28:654.

56. Reinfuss M, Mitus J, Smolak K, et al. Malignant phyllodes tumours of the breast: a clinical and pathological analysis of 55 cases. Eur J Cancer 1993;29A:1252.

57. Palmer ML, De Risi, DC, Pelikan A, et al. Treatment options and recurrence potential for cystosarcoma phyllodes. Surg Gynecol Obstet 1990;170:193.

58. Fernandez BB, Hernandez FJ, Spindler W. Metastatic cystosarcoma phyllodes: a light and electron microscopic study. Cancer 1976;37:1737.

59. West L, Weiland LH, Clagett OT. Cystosarcoma phyllodes. Ann Surg 1971;173:520.

60. Chua CL, Thomas A, Ng BK. Cystosarcoma phyllodes: a review of surgical options. Surgery 1989;105:141.

61. Chua CL, Thomas A. Cystosarcoma phyllodes tumors. Surg Gynecol Obstet 1988;166:302.

62. Stanley MW, Tani EM, Rutqvist LE, et al. Cystosarcoma phyllodes of the breast: a cytologic and clinicopathologic study of 23 cases. Diagn Cytopathol 1989;5:29.

63. Dusenbery D, Frable WJ. Fine needle aspiration cytology of phyllodes tumor: potential diagnostic pitfalls. Acta Cytologica 1992;36:215.

64. Burton GV, Hart LL, Leight GS Jr, et al. Cystosarcoma phyllodes: effective therapy with cisplatin and etoposide chemotherapy. Cancer 1989;63:2088.

65. Vorherr H, Vorherr VF, Kutvirt DM, et al. Cystosarcoma phyllodes: epidemiology, pathohistology, pathobiology, diagnosis, therapy, and survival. Arch Gynecol 1985;236:173.

66. Geist D. Cystosarcoma phyllodes of the female breast. Am Surg 1964;30:105.

67. Hopkins ML, McGowan TS, Rawlings G, et al. Phylloides tumor of the breast: a report of 14 cases. J Surg Oncol 1994;56:108.

68. Hawkins RE, Schofield JB, Wiltshaw E, et al. Ifosfamide is an active drug for chemotherapy of metastatic cystosarcoma phyllodes. Cancer 1992;69:2271.

69. Turalba CIC, El-Mahdi AM, Ladaga L. Fatal metastatic cystosarcoma phyllodes in an adolescent female: case report and review of treatment approaches. J Surg Oncol 1986;33:176.

70. Aronson W. Malignant cystosarcoma phyllodes with liposarcoma. Wis Med J 1966;65:184.

24.3

Paget Disease

ROSEMARY B. DUDA

In 1874, Sir James Paget described a rare form of breast cancer characterized by eczematous changes of the nipple that precede the clinical detection of breast cancer.[1] Because cancer of the breast generally developed 1 year after the presenting nipple or areolar lesion, Paget suggested that the nipple lesion was benign but possibly responsible for inducing the underlying malignancy. This association of nipple eczematous changes and breast cancer was based on the clinical observation of 15 patients.

The incidence of Paget disease has been reported to range from 0.7% to 4% of all breast cancers.[2–9] The age of onset of Paget disease is similar to that of other breast cancers, with no predisposing factors identified.[10] Paget disease has been described as a unilateral nipple and areolar change that includes various findings, ranging from a recurrent areolar vesicle to a chronic, moist, erythematous and eczematoid lesion, to a dry and psoriatic lesion, to a red and granular erosion. The lesion appears first on the nipple then progresses to the areola but rarely involves the surrounding skin of the breast. About 62% of patients present with crusty, scaly erosions or discharge.[11] Serous or serosanguineous discharge may be presenting symptoms and are frequently prominent in the later stages of the disease. Pruritus, burning, and hypersensitivity are frequently reported as early and prominent symptoms.[11] The differential diagnosis includes contact dermatitis, eczema, amelanotic melanoma, subareolar duct papillomatosis, basal cell carcinoma, intraductal papilloma, and duct ectasia.[12] Delays in diagnosis of 1 year or longer are frequently reported.[3,8]

Paget disease is almost always accompanied by an underlying malignancy, either an invasive ductal carcinoma or intraductal carcinoma.[3,5,6,9,11,13] Ashikari and colleagues[5] evaluated 96 patients with clinical signs of Paget disease confined to the nipple and areola. Sixty-three of these patients had an intraductal carcinoma, and 33 patients had an infiltrating ductal carcinoma found in the mastectomy specimen. Only 3.5% had axillary nodal metastasis. Lobular, medullary, and papillary carcinoma have also been reported in association with Paget disease. Paone and Baker[9] identified 19 patients with Paget disease clinically confined to the nipple and 31 patients with a palpable mass, most of which were immediately adjacent to the nipple in the subareolar location. All had an intraductal or invasive ductal carcinoma identified in the mastectomy specimen; however, 6 cases failed to show any connection between the Paget disease in the nipple and the underlying carcinoma.

Palpable masses are present in about 60% of all patients presenting with Paget disease.[5,14,15] In many of the patients without palpable masses, mammographic findings of microcalcifications, a mass, areolar thickening, subareolar densities or architectural distortion are detected.[9,14,16] Among 34 patients who had clinical findings suggestive of Paget disease, the mammograms of 17 patients (50%) were normal, those of 10 patients (29%) showed nipple, areolar, or subareolar abnormalities, and 7 mammograms (21%) showed evidence of suspicious masses or calcifications. Of the mammograms of 24 patients with no clinical evidence of Paget disease but with Paget cells found in the nipple at histopathologic examination, 19 (79%) showed a suspicious mass or microcalcifications, four (17%) showed abnormalities of the nipple or areola, and only one was normal.[17]

A small number of patients present with Paget disease without clinical or radiographic evidence of an underlying malignancy.[5,18–21] Ashikari and colleagues[5] identified 6 cases from a total of 214 specimens (2.8%) that had no evidence of an invasive or noninvasive cancer after a resection. Lagios and coworkers[21] described 2 of 6 patients with Paget disease confined to the nipple epidermis, and El-Sharkawi and Waters[15] identified 1 of 4 patients with Paget disease confined to the nipple after surgical resection. Paget cells have also been described microscopically in the histologic evaluation of the nipple and areola without any clinical or radiographic signs of the disease.[5,11,22]

Paget did not delineate the histologic findings of this disease, but they were subsequently described microscopically by others.[23–27] The Paget cells (Fig. 24.3-1) are characterized as large rounded or ovoid intraepidermoid cells with abundant pale cytoplasm and enlarged polymorphic and hyperchromatic nuclei and large nucleoli. The cells often contain diastase-resistant periodic acid-Schiff–positive granules with frequent mitoses. Paget cells may lie singly, primarily among the basal epidermal cells, tending to flatten at the surface, or may form small nests, sometimes as ductal or glandular structures. The number of cells in the specimen varies greatly, from a few isolated cells to complete replacement of portions of the epidermis. Ulceration is found in advanced cases. Paget cells do not invade the corium, which otherwise shows signs of chronic inflammation. The surrounding epidermis is often hyperplastic with hyperkeratosis.[3]

Origin of the Paget Cell

Controversy exists about the origin of the Paget cell. The epidermotropic theory postulates that the malignant cell originates in the breast parenchyma and migrates upward along the duct to the nipple epithelium. Toker[28] presented evidence of epidermotropic migration of Paget cells based on a thorough histologic examination of a mastectomy specimen that contained an invasive carcinoma 3 cm from the nipple. Paget cells were meticulously traced within the epithelium of a single duct from the mass to the nipple.

FIGURE 24.3-1 Histologic section of a mastectomy specimen of a 73-year-old white woman showing Paget disease of the nipple. **A.** Nests of malignant cells are visible within the squamous epithelium of the nipple at 25× magnification. **B.** The same findings are shown at a 40× magnification. The specimen was found to contain an underlying intraductal comedo-type carcinoma.

The other main theory hypothesizes that the Paget cell originates in the intraepidermis and is to be considered an independent in situ carcinoma, possibly as a multicentric breast cancer.[3] Several immunohistochemical profiles have been performed on the Paget cells and the underlying carcinomas and support the epidermotropic theory, whereas ultrastructural studies support the theory of in situ transformation. Cohen and colleagues,[29] described an identical profile for seven or more antigens for Paget cells and the underlying carcinoma in 18 of 20 patients (90%). Concordant immunostaining between Paget cells and associated carcinomas has been reported for low-molecular-weight cytokeratin,[30] epithelial membrane antigen,[31] carcinoembryonic antigen,[32,33] κ-casein,[34] α-lactalbumin,[35] carcinoma-associated antigens,[36] and c-*erb*B-2 oncoprotein.[37–39] These studies suggest that the Paget cells and the underlying carcinoma cells originate from the same neoplastic population. The discordant results in a few cases suggest, however, that, in a minority of instances, Paget

cells may arise in the epidermis from multipotent cells in the basal layer.[29] The in situ theory is supported by a demonstrated lack of continuity of malignant cells in some cases between the nipple epithelium and the breast carcinoma,[5,7] the absence of underlying carcinoma in some cases or the occurrence of Paget disease in ectopic nipples,[5,9,18,21] and ultrastructure studies that show plasma membrane specializations such as desmosomes between Paget cells and adjacent cells that mitigate against the migratory nature of Paget cells.[9,40,41] Alterations of epidermal cells adjacent to Paget cells suggest an in situ transformation of normal epidermal cells into Paget cells.[40]

Treatment and Prognosis

The treatment of Paget disease of the breast has evolved as our understanding of the biologic nature of breast cancer evolves. Initially, all breast cancers were treated using radical surgery, either alone or with radiation and chemotherapeutic treatments. The trend is now toward more conservative, breast-preserving therapy.[42–44] This is also the case with Paget disease. More recent approaches to Paget disease divide it into two categories, those with clinical disease only and those with Paget disease and a palpable mass. Those who present with limited disease are now frequently selected for conservative treatment. The prognosis depends on the presence of an invasive breast cancer associated with Paget disease, particularly the presence of axillary lymph nodes positive for metastatic disease. No evidence of Paget cells in axillary nodes has been documented. Earlier accounts by several authors[5,9,11,13,22] have described the use of a radical and total mastectomy, with or without radiation, as the treatment of choice for Paget disease. In the series reported by Maier and colleagues,[11] 99 of 137 patients were treated by a radical mastectomy and 31 by a total mastectomy. One patient was treated with radiation and an oophorectomy alone. This patient survived 6 years after the diagnosis. Because of widespread disease at the time of diagnosis, the others had biopsy alone and no further treatment. The overall 5-year survival rate for this series was 52.3% for those who had a radical mastectomy and ranged from 37.6% to 67% for those treated with a total mastectomy. The survival rate was poorer in those patients with a palpable mass if they also had positive axillary nodes. If the nodes were negative, then the two groups had equivalent survival rates. Rissanen and Holsti[13] treated patients with Paget disease without a mass using local excision (including the nipple and areola plus a wedge of underlying breast tissue) and radiation treatments, local excision alone, total mastectomy and radiation therapy, and a biopsy alone with radiation therapy. Patients who presented with Paget disease and a palpable mass were treated using radical mastectomy and radiation therapy. In this series, an 83% (10 of 12 patients) 5-year survival rate was noted in the group with Paget-disease with no palpable mass compared with a 0% (none of 9 patients) rate for those with Paget disease and a palpable mass, when all treatments were combined. The poor survival in the group with a palpable breast mass probably reflects the presence of metastatic disease in the axillary nodes.

Paone and Baker[9] described 50 patients diagnosed with Paget disease. Twenty-five patients were treated with a radical mastectomy, 12 with a modified radical mastectomy, 8 with a total mastectomy, and 5 with an excision of the nipple, areola, and underlying breast parenchyma. A trend toward more conservative surgical procedures was noted in the later years of the series. An underlying intraductal carcinoma or infiltrating ductal carcinoma was identified in all patients. For the 19 patients with Paget disease and no palpable mass, no axillary metastases or deaths occurred. For those 31 patients who presented with a palpable mass, the 10-year overall survival rate was 43.5% for node–negative patients and 9.9% for node-positive patients. No significant difference existed for those who had radical compared with modified radical mastectomy. All 5 patients treated with a nipple and wedge resection survived without disease recurrence. The overall length of survival of those treated with conservative therapy was not reported.

Several studies have evaluated the role of breast-conserving therapy—surgery alone, radiation alone, or a combination of the two.[7,15,21,45,46] To date, no completed randomized trial has evaluated breast conservation treatment in comparison with mastectomy. The European Organization for Research and Treatment of Cancer (EORTC) is, however, conducting a nonrandomized clinical trial to evaluate the adequacy of breast-conserving therapy for patients with Paget disease and intraductal carcinoma without invasion in the retroareolar ducts. These patients must have a complete resection of the nipple, areola, and underlying carcinoma followed by 50 Gy of radiation treatments to the entire breast. This clinical trial is accruing eligible patients, and therefore results are not yet available.[47] With an increased clinical awareness of breast cancer, a larger number of patients with Paget disease may be diagnosed with disease confined to the nipple, areola, and subareolar area and may respond well to breast-conserving therapy.

Lagios and colleagues[21] described 6 patients with Paget disease with no palpable breast or axillary masses and normal mammograms. One patient had been diagnosed with intraductal carcinoma 12 months before the diagnosis of Paget disease. One patient had been treated with a modified radical mastectomy and 5 had undergone excision of the underlying breast tissue and the affected nipple–areola complex. Normal-appearing areolar tissue was not resected. One patient treated with conservative surgery also had an axillary nodal dissection, and 3 had random four-quadrant biopsies. Two of the five patients treated conservatively had disease confined to the epidermis of the nipple with no underlying intraductal or infiltrating ductal carcinoma. Three had intraductal carcinoma involving a single lactiferous duct to depths of 4, 6, and 8 mm without other evidence of any carcinoma within the resected nipple complex. The patient who had been treated with a modified radical mastectomy had Paget disease of the nipple and involvement of a single lactiferous duct to a depth of 15 mm with no other evidence of any invasive or noninvasive disease. Of the 5 patients treated with breast conserving therapy, one experienced recurrence of Paget disease at 12 months in the remaining nipple–areola complex. This tumor was resected and the patient was free of any other recurrence at 43 months. The last reported follow-up for these patients is 50 months (range, 30 to 69 months), with no further recurrences. Fourquet and colleagues[45] described 20 selected patients with Paget disease confined to the nipple and areola. Seventeen were treated with radiation alone, and 3 were treated with either a nipple excision or an excision of the nipple and areola and subsequently treated with radiation. The breast tissue received a dose of cobalt-60 irradiation ranging from 50 to 65 Gy, and the tumor dose ranged from 55 to 83 Gy, including therapy delivered as electrons. The axillary, supraclavicular, and internal mammary lymph nodes were included in the radiation field. The median follow-up period was 7.5

years. Three recurrences were noted, all in the nipple or areola and all representing Paget disease without any evidence of intraductal or infiltrating ductal carcinoma. No axillary node recurrences or deaths secondary to breast cancer occurred. The 3 patients who had recurring disease were treated by either total mastectomy or modified radical mastectomy and were free of any further recurrence at 28, 77, and 98 months of observation. The actuarial 7-year probability of living 7 years disease-free with breast conserving therapy is 81% in this study.

Bulens and colleagues[7] described 13 patients with Paget disease confined to the nipple or areola and no clinical or radiographic evidence of any breast parenchymal or axillary abnormality who were treated with breast irradiation alone. Five patients also had an axillary node dissection. These patients received 30 to 65 Gy of cobalt-60 photons and an electron boost to a total of 60 to 70 Gy. After a mean follow up of 58.6 months (range, 15 to 118 months) and a median follow-up of 52 months, no local or distant recurrence was noted in any patient. Stockdale and colleagues[46] described 30 patients (19 of whom had no palpable masses or mammographic abnormalities, 3 of whom had palpable masses) and concluded that conservative treatment with radiation only is appropriate for those with Paget disease and no palpable masses but not for those with palpable cancers. All three patients with palpable cancers had recurrent disease after radiation treatment alone, compared with no recurrences in 16 of 19 patients with Paget disease and no palpable or radiographic underlying carcinomas. El-Sharkawi and Waters[15] described four patients with limited Paget disease and no clinical or radiographic evidence of underlying carcinoma. Three were treated with local radiation to the nipple and periareolar region after biopsy. No evidence of recurrence was seen in this highly select population of elderly patients. The one patient treated with a modified radical mastectomy had no underlying carcinoma in the specimen. This report suggests that local radiation to the nipple and areola (and not to the entire breast) may provide for adequate local therapy in selected patients.

Special Presentations

Male breast cancer is uncommon, comprising less than 1% of all breast cancers.[48] Therefore, Paget disease of the male breast is especially rare. Several authors have described Paget disease in men and caution about the importance of a correct differential diagnosis.[49-55] No difference in histologic features or presenting symptoms[54] exists between men and women; however, the 5-year survival rate is reported to be consistently poorer (20% to 30%) for men.[56,57] The treatment of choice has been either a radical mastectomy or modified radical mastectomy, with no reported cases of conservative management. The poorer prognosis in men may be related more to advanced disease stage at the time of diagnosis rather than to an aggressive biology. If Paget disease can be detected at an early stage

prior to a palpable mass, conservative therapy may be an appropriate option.

Paget disease has also been reported in several unusual situations. Two reports have described four patients who developed Paget disease in the nipple after subcutaneous mastectomy as treatment for breast cancer.[58,59] Three of 584 patients (0.5%) described by Shearman and Watts[58] were found to have Paget disease of the nipple at 18 months after surgery for two patients and at 4 years for the third patient. Two patients were treated with radiation therapy but subsequently had resection of the nipple. One specimen contained no residual carcinoma, the other contained intraductal carcinoma in one lactiferous duct. The third patient was treated primarily with an excision of the nipple and underlying breast tissue in which an infiltrating ductal carcinoma was identified.

Few reports have described Paget disease occurring after a conservative excision for invasive and noninvasive breast cancer treated without radiation therapy[21,60] and after breast-conserving therapy with a wide resection and radiation therapy.[61-64] Peterse and colleagues[62] described 1 of 25 recurrences as Paget disease, Schnitt and associates[63] describe 2 of 15 patients who had recurrences after breast-conserving therapy for Paget disease. Menzies and co-workers[61] reported a series of 356 patients, 338 of whom were treated with breast-conserving therapy and 38 who developed a local recurrence. Three of these 38 recurrences were confirmed to be Paget disease after an average of 19 months' delay in diagnosis. The nipple changes were believed to be consistent with postradiation changes and were not suspicious. Two of these three patients had an underlying intraductal carcinoma, and one had an infiltrating ductal carcinoma. These findings warrant an early biopsy in the presence of what may otherwise be considered benign or innocuous postradiation nipple changes.

Molecular Studies

Protooncogenes and oncogenes are hypothesized to be involved in the regulation of normal cellular growth and differentiation. Several investigators have evaluated the expression of c-erbB-2 expression in Paget disease and the underlying carcinoma when present.[37-39] Wolber and associates[37] evaluated c-erbB-2 expression using polyclonal antiserum directed against the 14 amino acid segment of the oncoprotein and found that 15 of 19 specimens (79%) of Paget disease expressed positive membrane staining. Fourteen specimens had underlying carcinoma, 7 of which had an infiltrative component. Concordant membrane staining was done in 12 of 14 specimens; 2 cases of Paget disease stained positive, whereas the underlying carcinoma was negative for c-erbB-2 expression.

Lammie and colleagues[38] evaluated c-erbB-2 expression in the paraffin-embedded tissues of 45 patients with Paget disease using the antibody 21N, which was raised against a peptide from the C terminus of the oncoprotein. Positive immunostaining was seen in 41 of the Paget cells (92%), and in 80% of the cases most of the tumor cells stained. Membrane positivity was always associated with cytoplasmic granular staining. Underlying carcinoma was identified in 42 cases, pure intraductal carcinoma in 15, infiltrating carcinoma and intraductal carcinoma in 26 cases, and pure infiltrating ductal carcinoma in one case. The intraductal carcinomas were of the comedo, solid, and (occasionally) cribriform type. Concordant immunostaining was noted in 40 of 42 cases, 37 showing positive staining. Of these 37 cases, 14 were intraductal carcinoma of the comedo type, 22 were infiltrating ductal carcinoma with an intraductal component, and 1 was pure invasive cancer, with staining similar in the invasive and noninvasive components and the proportion of cells staining similar for the Paget cells and the underlying carcinoma. Meissner and coworkers[39] evaluated 23 cases of Paget disease for c-*erb*B-2 expression with the monoclonal antibody 3B5, which was directed at the intracellular domain of the oncoprotein. All 23 of the paraffin-embedded tumor cells but none of the normal epidermal cells exhibited distinct membrane staining. An underlying carcinoma was identified in 18 patients, and all invasive and noninvasive carcinomas showed unequivocal membrane staining. Mori and associates[65] examined the expression of the ras oncoprotein p21 expression in four cases of Paget disease. All four cases exhibited positive immunostaining, 3 had an underlying carcinoma, and all showed positive membrane staining. The intensity of staining was similar in the Paget cells and underlying carcinoma. No staining was noted among normal keratinocytes. Estrogen receptor content was evaluated in 6 patients with Paget disease by immunocytochemical analysis.[66] Four of the 6 cases showed positive staining for estrogen receptors. Analysis of the estrogen receptor status by the radioligand assay and immunocytochemistry in three invasive carcinomas showed a receptor content similar to that seen in the Paget cells. These studies suggest a common genetic alteration in the Paget cells and the underlying carcinoma, and they support the epidermotropic theory of origin of the Paget cell.

Summary

Paget disease of the breast is rare and is typically but not always associated with an underlying invasive or noninvasive carcinoma. For those who present with Paget disease and a palpable mass, the treatment and prognosis are governed by the histologic features of the palpable mass and the status of the axillary nodes. For those who present with early signs of Paget disease and no palpable mass, the prognosis appears to be excellent, and conservative management of the patient could be considered. The final results of the EORTC clinical trial should provide important information about the results of conservative therapy for carefully selected patients. No definitive recommendations should be made until the results of a randomized trial are available. Many proponents of conservative therapy for patients with Paget disease, however, recommend the use of wide local excision alone, wide local excision plus radiation therapy, and radiation therapy alone. Based on the current information available, it appears reasonable to treat a patient with Paget disease limited to the nipple or areola with a wide local excision of the nipple, areola, and underlying breast tissue alone. A wide excision alone may also be considered for those with a small, noncomedo carcinoma in the underlying ductal tissue associated with Paget disease. For those patients with an associated underlying invasive carcinoma or comedotype intraductal carcinoma who prefer a conservative approach, a wide local excision with radiation appears appropriate. Because mammograms may not detect an underlying microscopic carcinoma, resection of the underlying ductal tissue is critical for appropriate therapeutic management.

MANAGEMENT SUMMARY

- Detailed mammographic evaluation of the ipsilateral breast is important to identify other areas of involvement.
- For patients with Paget disease and a separate lesion in the breast parenchyma, modified radical mastectomy is usually required; the use of systemic therapy follows the same guidelines as those for other patients with breast cancer (see Chap. 17.2).
- For patients with Paget disease limited to the nipple–areolar complex, breast-conserving treatment, along with mastectomy, should be considered following the guidelines for treatment of DCIS discussed in Chapter 11; in patients electing breast-conserving treatment, resection should include underlying ductal tissue.

References

1. Paget J. On disease of the mammary areola preceding cancer of the mammary gland. St Bartholomew's Hosp Rep 1874;10:87.
2. Dockerty MB, Harrington SW. Preclinical Paget's disease of the nipple. Surg Gynecol Obstet 1951;93:317.
3. Ordonez NG, Awalt H, Mackay B. Mammary and extramammary Paget's disease: an immunocytochemical and ultrastructural study. Cancer 1987;59:1173.
4. Ascensao AC, Marques MSJ, Capitao-Mor M. Paget's disease of the nipple: clinical and pathological review of 109 female patients. Dermatologica 1985;170:170.
5. Ashikari R, Park K, Huvos AG, et al. Paget's disease of the breast. Cancer 1970;26:680.
6. Chaudary MA, Millis RR, Lane B, et al. Paget's disease of the nipple: a ten-year review including clinical, pathological, and immunohistochemical findings. Breast Cancer Res Treat 1986;8:139.
7. Bulens P, Vanuytsel L, Rijnders A, et al. Breast conserving treatment of Paget's disease. Radiother Oncol 1990;17:305.
8. Nance FC, DeLoach DH, Welsh RA, et al. Paget's disease of the breast. Ann Surg 1970;171:864.

9. Paone JF, Baker PR. Pathogenesis and treatment of Paget's disease of the breast. Cancer 1981;48:825.
10. Osteen RT. Special therapeutic problems: Paget's disease of the nipple. In: Harris JR, Hellman S, Henderson IC, eds. Breast diseases. Philadelphia, JB Lippincott, 1987:589.
11. Maier WP, Rosemond GP, Harasym EL, et al. Paget's disease of the female breast. Surg Gynecol Obstet 1969;128:1253.
12. Sanchez JA, Feller WF. Paget's disease of the breast. Am Fam Physician 1987:145.
13. Rissanen PM, Holsti P. Paget's disease of the breast. The influence of the presence or absence of an underlying palpable tumor on the prognosis and of the choice of treatment. Oncology 1969;23:209.
14. Baker RR. Breast cancer: strategies for the 1990s. Surg Clin North Am 1990;70:963.
15. El-Sharkawi A, Waters JS. The place for conservative treatment in the management of Paget's disease of the nipple. Eur J Surg Oncol 1992;18:301.
16. Hoeffken W, Lanyi M. Mammography: technique, diagnosis, differential diagnosis, results. Philadelphia, WB Saunders, 1977:178.
17. Ikeda DM, Helvie MA, Frank TS, et al. Paget disease of the nipple: radiologic–pathologic correlation. Radiology 1993;189:89.
18. Kister SJ, Haagensen CD. Paget's disease of the breast. Am J Surg 1970;119:606.
19. Silverberg SG, Chitale PR. Assessment of significance of proportions of intraductal and infiltrating tumor growth in ductal carcinoma of the breast. Cancer 1973;32:830.
20. Cheatle GL, Cutler M. Paget's disease of the nipple: review of the literature. Clinical and microscopical studies of seventeen breasts by means of whole serial sections. Arch Pathol 1931;12:435.
21. Lagios MD, Westdahl PR, Rose MR, et al. Paget's disease of the nipple: alternative management in cases without or with minimal extent of underlying breast carcinoma. Cancer 1984;54:545.
22. Freund H, Maydovnik M, Laufer N, et al. Paget's disease of the nipple. J Surg Oncol 1977;9:93.
23. Darier J. La maladie de Paget du mamelon. CR Soc Biol Paris 1889;1:225.
24. Jacobaeus HC. Paget's Disease und sein Verhaltnis zum Milchdrunsenkarzinom. Virchows Arch Pathol 1904;178:124.
25. Inglis K. Paget's disease of the nipple with special reference to the changes in the ducts. Am J Pathol 1946;22:1.
26. Muir R. The pathogenesis of Paget's disease of the nipple and associated lesions. Br J Surg 1935;22:728.
27. Muir R. Further observations on Paget's disease of the nipple. J Pathol Bacteriol 1939;49:299.
28. Toker C. Some observations on Paget's disease of the nipple. Cancer 1961;14:653.
29. Cohen C, Guarner J, DeRose PB. Mammary Paget's disease and associated carcinoma: an immunohistochemical study. Arch Pathol Lab Med 1993;117:291.
30. Ordonez NG, Awalt H, Mackay B. Mammary and extramammary Paget's disease: an immunocytochemical and ultrastructural study. Cancer 1987;59:1173.
31. Kirkham N, Berry N, Jones DB, et al. Paget's disease of the nipple: immunohistochemical localization of milk fat globule membrane antigens. Cancer 1985;55:1510.
32. Kariniemi AL, Forsman L, Wahlstrom T, et al. Expression of differentiation antigens in mammary and extramammary Paget's disease. Br J Dermatol 1984;110:203.
33. Nadji M, Morales AR, Girtanner RE, et al. Paget's disease of the skin: a unifying concept of histogenesis. Cancer 1982;50:2203.
34. Bussolati G, Pich A, Alfani V. Immunofluorescence detection of casein in human mammary dysplastic and neoplastic tissues. Virchows Arch A Pathol Anat Histopathol 1975;365:15.
35. Lee AK, DeLellis RA, Rosen PP, et al. Alpha-lactalbumin as an immunohistochemical marker for metastatic breast carcinomas. Am J Surg Pathol 1984;8:93.
36. Mariani-Costantini R, Andreola S, Rilke F. Tumour-associated antigens in mammary and extramammary Paget's disease. Virchows Arch A Pathol Anat Histopathol 1985;405:333.
37. Wolber RA, DuPuis BA, Wick MR. Expression of c-erbB-2 oncoprotein in mammary and extramammary Paget's disease. Am J Clin Pathol 1991;96:243.
38. Lammie GA, Barnes DM, Millis RR, et al. An immunohistochemical study of the presence of c-erbB-2 protein in Paget's disease of the nipple. Histopathology 1989;15:505.
39. Meissner K, Riviere A, Haupt G, et al. Study of neu-protein expression in mammary Paget's disease with and without underlying breast carcinoma and in extramammary Paget's disease. Am J Pathol 1990;137:1305.
40. Sagebiel RW. Ultrastructural observations on epidermal cells in Paget's disease of the breast. Am J Pathol 1969;57:49.
41. Sagami S. Electron microscopic studies in Paget's disease. Med J Osaka Univ 1963;14:173.
42. Fisher B, Bauer M, Margolese R, et al. Five-year results of a randomized clinical trial comparing total mastectomy and segmental mastectomy with or without radiation in the treatment of breast cancer. N Engl J Med 1985;312:666.
43. Veronesi U, Saccozzi R, DelVecchio M, et al. Comparing radical mastectomy with quadrantectomy, axillary dissection and radiotherapy in patients with small cancers of the breast. N Engl J Med 1981;305:6.
44. Harris JR, Lippman ME, Veronesi U, et al. Breast cancer. N Engl J Med 1992;327:390.
45. Fourquet A, Campana F, Vielh P, et al. Paget's disease of the nipple without detachable breast tumor: conservative management with radiation therapy. Int J Radiat Biol Phys 1987;13:1463.
46. Stockdale AD, Brierley JD, White WF, et al. Radiotherapy for Paget's disease of the nipple conservative alternative. Lancet 1989; Sept:664.
47. EORTC 10873 Phase II Study. Breast conserving therapy in Paget's disease of the nipple.
48. Treves N, Holleb AI. Cancer of the male breast: a report of 146 cases. Cancer 1955;8:1239.
49. Crichlow RW, Czernobilsky B. Paget's disease of male breast. Cancer 1969;24:1033.
50. Nehme AE. Paget's disease of the male breast: a collective review and case report. Am Surg 1976;42:289.
51. Gupta S, Khanna NN, Khanna S, et al. Paget's disease of the male breast: a clinicopathologic study and a collective review. J Surg Oncol 1983;22:151.
52. Satiani B, Powell RW, Mathews WH. Paget's disease of the male breast. Arch Surg 1977;112:587.
53. Ho TCN, St Jacques M, Schopflocher P. Pigmented Paget's disease of the male breast. J Am Acad Dermatol 1990;23:338.
54. Serour F, Birkenfeld S, Amsterdam E, et al. Paget's disease of the male breast. Cancer 1988;62:601.
55. Sano Y, Inoue T, Aso M, et al. Paget's disease of the male breast: report of a case and histopathologic study. J Dermatol 1989;16:237.
56. Lancer HA, Moschella SL. Paget's disease of the male breast. J Am Acad Dermatol 1982;7:393.
57. Haagensen CD. Diseases of the breast. Philadelphia, WB Saunders, 1971;783.
58. Shearman CP, Watts GT. Paget's disease of the nipple after subcutaneous mastectomy for cancer with primary reconstruction. Ann R Coll Surg 1968;68:17.
59. Mendez-Fernandez MA, Henly WS, Geis RC, et al. Paget's disease of the breast after subcutaneous mastectomy and reconstruction with a silicone prosthesis. Plast Reconstr Surg 1980;65:683.

60. Plowman PN, Gilmore OJA, Curling M, et al. Paget's disease of the nipple occurring after conservative management of early infiltrating breast cancer. Br J Surg 1986;73:45.

61. Menzies D, Barr L, Ellis H. Paget's disease of the nipple occurring after wide local excision and radiotherapy for carcinoma of the breast. Eur J Surg Onc 1989;15:271.

62. Peterse JL, vanDongen JA, Bartelink H. Recurrence of breast carcinoma after breast conserving treatment. Eur J Surg Onc 1988;14:123.

63. Schnitt SJ, Connolly JL, Recht A, et al. Breast relapse following primary radiation therapy for early breast cancer. II. Detection,

64. Markopoulous CH, Gazet JC. Paget's disease of the nipple occurring after conservative management of early breast cancer. Eur J Surg Oncol 1988;14:77.

65. Mori O, Hachisuka H, Nakano S, et al. Expression of ras p21 in mammary and extramammary Paget's disease. Arch Pathol Lab Med 1990;114:858.

66. Tani EM, Skoog L. Immunocytochemical detection of estrogen receptors in mammary paget cells. Acta Cytol 1988;32:825.

pathologic features, and prognostic significance. Int J Radiat Oncol Biol Phys 1985;11:1277.

24.4
Other Cancers in the Breast
LORI JARDINES

Other cancers that occur in the breast include lymphomas, sarcomas and melanoma. These malignancies behave in a fashion similar to smaller tumors elsewhere in the body.

Primary Breast Lymphoma

Primary breast lymphomas are thought to arise from the periductal and perilobular lymphoid tissue[1] or from intrammammary lymph nodes. The major presenting sign and symptom of a primary breast lymphoma is a breast mass that may or may not be painful.[2-5] Primary lymphoma of the breast is an uncommon lesion, accounting for 0.04% to 0.5% of all breast malignancies[2,6-8] and less than 3% of extranodal non-Hodgkin lymphomas.[7,9,10] Therefore, the diagnosis of this disease is usually made only after biopsy. The clinical and histologic criteria for diagnosis of a primary breast lymphoma are (1) close association between the breast tissue and infiltrating lymphoma (Fig. 24.4-1), (2) no evidence of widespread lymphoma and no history of previous extramammary lymphoma, and (3) documentation of the breast as the principal organ involved and thus the primary site.[2,11] Because no uniform histologic staging and classification systems exist for primary breast lymphoma, it is difficult to compare and contrast the results of published trials.

PATHOLOGY

Most cases of primary breast lymphoma are diffuse, intermediate grade, B-cell lymphomas.[5,6] T-cell lymphomas have rarely been reported.[7] In pregnant or postpartum women, this disease tends to have the histologic appearance of a high-grade Burkitt lymphoma.[12] Estrogen receptors have been identified in primary breast lymphomas;[7,12] it is doubtful, however, that antiestrogens would be beneficial in treating estrogen receptor–positive breast lymphoma because estrogen stimulation of lymphoid cells does not lead to cellular proliferation.[13] Fine-needle aspiration cytology of a breast mass may be helpful in diagnosing lymphoma.[14,15] As with lymphomas at other sites, the diagnosis and cell typing are established by excisional biopsy. Primary breast lymphoma may be confused with poorly differentiated carcinoma on frozen section, and the diagnosis is most often made based on the permanent sections.[11] In addition to routine histopathology, immunohistochemistry has been used to classify primary breast lymphomas.[12,16] The polymerase chain reaction test has been used to analyze for certain genetic alterations in breast lymphomas.[12]

CLINICAL PRESENTATION AND RADIOGRAPHIC FEATURES

The most common presenting complaint is that of a painless breast mass.[2-5,8] Most tumors are larger than 5 cm (range 1 to 12 cm) at diagnosis.[2,6-8,11,12,17] Less commonly, the patient complains of breast swelling without a dominant mass.[7,17] Occasionally, associated ipsilateral axillary adenopathy may be present at the time of presentation. B symptoms are uncommon with a localized breast lymphoma.[4,15] Primary breast lymphoma is most frequently seen in women[6,14,18] and rarely in men.[5] Bilateral synchronous or metachronous breast involvement may occur in as many as 25% of patients.[2,5] Mean age at diagnosis is 60 years (range, 13 to 86 years).[2,6-8,11,12,17] The disease appears to have a bimodal age distribution with a peak in incidence at 38 years and again at 58 years.[7] Younger patients are more likely to have bilateral, diffuse disease associated with pregnancy or the postpartum period.[7]

No mammographic abnormality is specific for primary breast lymphoma, with findings varying from a discrete well-circumscribed nodule with benign features to a lesion with spiculated borders.[19] In one study of 26 patients with primary breast lymphoma who underwent mammography,[15] 2 patients had examinations suggestive of lymphoma, 16 had examinations suggestive of carcinoma, and 8 had examinations consistent with benign breast disease.

FIGURE 24.4-1 A primary non-Hodgkin lymphoma of the breast is visible on the left. It is contained within normal breast tissue, which is on the right.

TREATMENT AND PROGNOSIS

After the diagnosis of primary breast lymphoma is established, the patient must be carefully evaluated, because therapy is based on the stage of disease. The initial staging evaluation begins with a detailed history and physical examination, laboratory studies, chest roentgenogram, computed tomography of the abdomen and pelvis, bilateral lower extremity lymphangiogram and bilateral bone marrow biopsies. No consistent approach has been taken to pretreatment staging of primary breast lymphoma; however, thorough evaluation identifies occult disease, leading to a change in stage in 50% of patients.[4]

Surgical treatment of primary breast lymphoma has ranged from biopsy to radical mastectomy.[2,4,6-8,12,14,15,17] Radical surgery is not indicated in treating primary breast lymphoma, given that local disease can be controlled with radiation therapy. Five-year overall survival for patients with stage I and IIE disease has ranged from 72% to 85% at 5 years in recent studies.[14,18] Disease-free survival at 5 years has been reported as 39%.[18] Brustein and colleagues[17] recently analyzed the disease-free and overall survivals for patients with stage IE and IIE cancers separately at both 5 and 10 years. At 5 years, the disease-free and overall survivals were significantly better in the stage IE patients, but by 10 years, they were about equal in both groups. Certain groups have attempted to identify prognostic factors for primary breast lymphoma, and an association appears to exist between disease stage,[4] tumor size,[17] histologic characteristics[4,7,11] and outcome.

Chemotherapy and radiotherapy are used to treat primary breast lymphomas and their use varies according to the disease stage and histologic subtype.

Primary Breast Sarcomas

The term *stromal sarcoma* had been coined by Berg and colleagues[20]; however, others have felt that sarcomas in the breast should be classified on the basis of the cell of origin.[21,22] Therefore, the diagnosis of stromal sarcoma should be reserved for those rare sarcomas that arise from the specialized periductal or perilobular stroma.[22] Primary breast sarcomas, with the exception of angiosarcomas, behave like sarcomas that arise elsewhere in the body. Cystosarcoma phyllodes is not a true sarcoma, because its diagnosis is based on the presence of epithelial elements within a cellular stroma. Due to differences in therapy offered for tumors of epithelial origin, carcinosarcoma and sarcomatoid carcinoma must be differentiated from true sarcomas.

INCIDENCE AND HISTOLOGY

The breast is an uncommon site for soft tissue sarcomas and these tumors account for less than 1% of all breast malignancies.[21-23] As in other parts of the body, soft tissue sarcomas are a heterogeneous group of tumors. The most common histologic types of soft tissue sarcomas of the breast, excluding angiosarcomas, are malignant fibrous histiocytoma, liposarcoma, and fibrosarcoma.[22-37] In most series true stromal sarcomas are extremely unusual[22,35,38]; however, in a recent report, stromal sarcomas accounted for 37% of primary breast sarcomas after angiosarcomas were excluded.[39] One large series in the literature evaluated patients with primary breast sarcomas.[39] Most studies of breast sarcoma are either single case reports or are reports of 10 to 20 patients treated in various ways. Hormone receptors have been identified in some primary breast sarcomas, but their clinical significance, if any, is not known.[31]

CLINICAL AND RADIOGRAPHIC FINDINGS

Primary breast sarcomas are more common in women, with the exception of leiomyosarcomas, where men are affected to almost the same extent as women.[28-30] The most common presenting complaint is that of a painless, mobile, breast mass.[21,22,36,38,39] The patient may also note a recent, rapid increase in the size of a long-standing breast mass.[36,37] Skin retraction or ulceration, nipple discharge or nipple retraction may be seen but are not common physical findings.[21,31] The average tumor size is 4 to 6 cm (range, 0.5 to 40 cm).[21,22,31,36,39,40] No predilection exists for either the right or left breast, and bilaterality is extremely uncommon. The median age at diagnosis is in the sixth decade of life (range, second to ninth decade)[21,22,35,36,38] Axillary lymph nodes may be palpable at the time of the initial examination, but they are rarely involved with tumor.[21,39]

The only mammographic finding diagnostic of a breast sarcoma is the presence of osseous trabeculae within a mass, indicating an osteogenic sarcoma.[34] On mammograms, sarcomas may have smooth borders, they may be lobulated like fibroadenomas, or they may be indistinct[41] (Fig. 24.4-2B). Sarcomas imaged mammographically are usually masslike and dense when compared with the surrounding breast tissue.[41] The size of the lesion seen on mammograms correlates with the clinical examination. The diagnosis may be made using a core needle biopsy or fine-needle aspiration cytology, which may allow for treatment planning before a surgical procedure. If this sampling does not supply an adequate amount of tissue, either an excisional or incisional biopsy should be done, depending on the size of the lesion.

PROGNOSIS AND TREATMENT

Surgery is the treatment of choice for primary breast sarcomas. The extent of surgery has ranged from excision to radical mastectomy.[21,22,36,38] Callery and colleagues[22] found a 53% incidence of local failure when local excision was used. Additionally, after the recurrence was identified only one third of patients were salvageable with further treatment.[22] With mastectomy, the local failure rate was only 8%.[22] Pollard and colleagues[36] found that the local recurrence rate for wide excision and total mastectomy were virtually identical and higher than that observed for radical mastectomy. Until recently, most authors agreed that mastectomy was the treatment of choice and that the extent of surgery was based on the need for wide surgical margins. Gutman and colleagues[39] have suggested that the extent of surgery should be guided by the size of the tumor and that no survival advantage is associated with mastectomy, provided that negative surgical margins can be attained. Routine axillary lymph node dissection is not indicated due to the rarity of nodal metastases in this disease. Lymph node dissection should be performed only to allow complete resection of the primary tumor or if nodes are clinically positive.[20,22,35]

Prognostic factors affecting outcome with primary breast sarcomas are difficult to assess due to the small numbers of patients with the disease and differences in classification of histologic types among the reports in the literature. The relation between size of the primary tumor and outcome is not clear, with two studies identifying this as a prognostic factor.[39,40] The microscopic characteristics of the tumor borders seem to influence outcome, with an infiltrating pattern associated with diminished survival.[21,36,40] The degree of cellular differentiation and histologic grade also appear to be important in predicting outcome.[21,22,37,40] The effect of mitotic activity as a sole predictor of prognosis is not clear,[21,36,37,40] but, when combined with other factors, mitotic activity may be important in assessing risk of failure.[37]

Survival varies according to the series. Callery and colleagues[22] described 25 patients with primary breast sarcoma with an actuarial 5-year survival rate of 91%; however, the length of follow-up was short.[22] Johnstone and colleagues[38] found 68% and 66% actuarial disease-free and overall survival rates, respectively. In this series, there were no local failures and patients died secondary to metastatic disease. Norris and Taylor[40] studied 32 patients with primary sarcomas of the breast and found a 73% 5-year survival rate. In this series, 18 patents were without evidence of disease and 4 were alive with disease. Common sites of distant metastases were lung, bone, liver, and brain.[36,37]

Angiosarcoma of the Breast

Angiosarcoma was first described in 1887 and is seen to a greater proportion in the breast than at other sites.[42] Since that time, some 200 cases have been reported in the literature.[43–47] There are relatively few long-term survivors because of the aggressive nature of this disease and the development of distant metastases. A recent study challenges this and reported a 10-year overall survival rate of 51% for patients with this malignancy.[39] Some angiosarcomas of the breast have been seen after radiation therapy, are viewed as a complication of that treatment, and are reviewed in detail in the chapter on complications of radiation therapy.

INCIDENCE AND PATHOLOGY

It is estimated that angiosarcoma accounts for as many as 9% of all breast sarcomas.[48] It has been suggested, however, that the true incidence of angiosarcoma is not known, because a tendency exists to classify many well-differentiated angiosarcomas as benign hemangiomas.[43,45,47] In one study, half the lesions were initially diagnosed as benign vascular neoplasms.[47] The diagnosis is made by identifying specific microscopic findings that include hyperchromatic nuclei, interanastomosing vascular channels, and the presence of these vessels within the breast parenchyma.[42,45] On the basis of other histologic features, breast angiosarcomas have been divided into groups[42] or defined as well, moderately, or poorly differentiated.[45] These classifications have been used to identify microscopic features associated with outcome.

CLINICAL AND RADIOGRAPHIC FEATURES

Women are most often affected and usually present with a painless mass that is often rapidly growing.[42–45,49] Skin retraction or peau d'orange has been seen but is relatively

FIGURE 24.4-2 Bilateral mammography of a patient with a primary breast sarcoma located in the upper outer quadrant of the left breast.

uncommon.[47] The average tumor size is approximately 5 cm (range, 1 to 14 cm).[42–45,49] The average age at presentation ranges from 34 to 46 years, with the youngest patients diagnosed in their teens. The right and left breasts are affected almost equally. Bilateral disease is not uncommon and is usually associated with pregnancy. Contralateral breast involvement may be due to either development of a second primary tumor or metastatic spread.[43] Common sites of metastasis are bone, skin, lung, ovary, and liver.[43–45] Vascular tumor of the breast should be completely excised and thoroughly examined to distinguish other vascular lesions such as atypical angiomatous lesions, cavernous hemangiomas, or benign perilobular hemangiomas from angiosarcomas.[42] The atypical microscopic angiomas should be completely excised because they may represent an early-stage angiosarcoma.[42]

TREATMENT AND PROGNOSIS

Histologic features may represent the most important prognostic factor.[44] Outcome may be predicted on the basis of certain histologic features where lesions were graded as well, moderately, or poorly differentiated.[45] Merino and colleagues[45] found that patients with moderately and poorly differentiated tumors had similar outcomes where 6 of 10 patients with these histologic grades died of disease and 1 of 10 was alive with disease. Four out of five patients with well-differentiated tumors were alive and disease-free at 2 to 24 years after diagnosis.[45] Donnell and colleagues[42] and Rosen and associates[44] used another system based on histologic features and divided tumors into types I, II, or III low grade, intermediate grade, and high grade, respectively. Using this classification system, type I and type II patients behave similarly. Disease-free survival for patients with type I histology is 76%; with type II, 70%; and with type III, 15%. Overall survival at 10 years was 81%, 68%, and 14% for types I, II, and III, respectively.[44]

Angiosarcoma of the breast is an aggressive malignancy, and, in most series, most patients die of their disease.[43–45,50] The recommended primary treatment for angiosarcoma of the breast is total mastectomy; however, more extensive local surgery may be indicated to attain wide negative margins.[42–45] Because of the rarity of regional nodal metastases, axillary lymph node dissection is indicated only if necessary to excise the primary lesion.[44] Rarely, a patient with a small lesion can be treated with quadrantectomy.[44] Some patients who have local recurrence only have been treated with reexcision to achieve long-term survival.[46]

Metastases to the Breast

INCIDENCE AND CHARACTERISTICS

Hematogenous metastases from nonbreast primary cancers are uncommon with only some 340 cases reported in the literature.[51–69] The incidence may be underestimated because some may only be detected at postmortem examination.[70] The most common source of metastatic disease to the breast is a contralateral breast primary tumor. Hematogenous metastases from nonbreast primary cancers are most frequently secondary to lymphomas or leukemias, melanoma, and lung cancer, particularly small cell carcinoma.[51,52,68,71,72] Less commonly, ovarian adenocarcinomas, soft tissue sarcomas, gastrointestinal adenocarcinomas, and genitourinary tumors may metastasize to the breast.[51,54–68,71,72]

Metastasis to the breast from nonbreast primary cancers is more commonly seen in women, and the average age at diagnosis is in the late thirties to forties.[52,71] In Arora and Robinson's series[52] 14 of the 15 women with metastatic melanoma to the breast were premenopausal. This finding may be associated with hormonal influences in the trafficking of melanoma cells to the breast, given that estrogen receptors have been identified in some melanoma cells.[52] The disease usually presents as a circumscribed solitary mass, which, if superficial, may be fixed to the skin.[71,72] Most often, only one breast is involved with metastatic disease; in one series, however, about one third of the patients with metastatic melanoma were found to have bilateral breast involvement.[52] In one study, the breast was the initial site of clinically evident metastatic disease in 31% of patients.[71]

Mammography in patients with disease metastatic to the breast generally shows findings that include most commonly single or multiple masses with distinct or semidiscrete borders and, less commonly, skin thickening or axillary adenopathy.[51,72] Patients with metastatic disease to the breast from lymphoma or leukemia may also show a diffuse increase in stromal density on mammography.[51] Calcifications were observed in one patient with metastatic ovarian cancer in whom the calcifications were secondary to psammoma bodies.[51]

Fine-needle aspiration cytology is useful in distinguishing metastatic disease to the breast from a primary carcinoma if the lesion has cytologic features that are not usually seen in primary breast cancer.[67–69,72] The diagnostic accuracy of aspiration cytology can be enhanced by comparing the histologic features of the material aspirated from the breast with the cytologic features of the primary neoplasm. Electron microscopy and immunocytochemistry of the aspirated material can also be helpful in determining the cell of origin.[72] When cytology is not helpful, open biopsy may be necessary to distinguish a breast primary from metastatic disease. On biopsy, metastatic disease should be suspected when a periductal or perilobular distribution of the malignant tumor cells exists without ductal or lobular carcinoma in situ.[71]

Patients may present with either synchronous or metachronous bilateral adenocarcinoma of the breast. In both instances, it is important to determine whether the disease is related to two primary lesions or whether the patient has a single breast primary tumor with metastatic disease to the contralateral breast. Metastasis from one breast to the other generally occurs through the lymphatics across the midline.[51] Several criteria have been suggested to aid in making this distinction and fall into clinical, pathologic, and mammographic categories. Clinical factors that favor the presence of a contralateral metastatic breast cancer include a medial location of the primary as well as the secondary lesion,[73–75] a short disease-free interval,[76,77] multiple lesions within the breast,[73–78] and the presence of metastatic disease at other sites. New primary lesions are located within the breast parenchyma, whereas metastases tend to be located in fatty or subcutaneous tissues.[73–78] Presence of in situ disease suggests a second and new primary lesion. In such cases, a different histology is identified and the degree of histologic differentiation is greater than that of the original lesion.[79] Mammographic features associated with a contralateral breast primary include a solitary nodule, the presence of microcalcifications, and the absence of skin thickening.[80] Radiographic findings associated with metastatic disease in the contralateral breast are similar to those observed with metastases from other sites.[51]

PROGNOSIS AND TREATMENT

Prognosis is generally poor after disease metastatic to the breast is identified, with most patients dying within 1 year of diagnosis.[71,72] Long-term survivors have been reported after the treatment of malignancies metastatic to the breast, most of whom had either melanoma or lymphoma.[71,72] Treatment should be focused on the primary lesion; in some instances, however, surgery, radiation therapy, or chemotherapy can be useful to provide palliation.

When a patient develops disease metastatic to the contralateral breast, it is treated in the same manner as metastatic disease to any other soft tissue site. When it is uncertain as to whether the lesion is a new breast primary lesion or is metastatic from the contralateral breast, most recommend treating the patient as if it is a new breast primary tumor and treating the patient for cure.

Cutaneous Melanomas of the Breast

Primary melanomas arising from the skin of the breast are uncommon, occurring more frequently in men.[81-84] The diagnosis and surgical treatment for melanoma arising in this region are the same as those for melanoma arising elsewhere.

INCIDENCE AND PATHOLOGY

Malignant melanoma arising in the skin of the breast accounts for 0.3% to 3.8% of all cutaneous melanomas.[82-84] The average age at diagnosis is 40 years, with women being diagnosed at a younger age than the men.[81,82,84] Most lesions are superficial spreading melanomas of Clark level II or III.[83,84] Criteria for high-risk melanomas of the breast are the same as those for melanomas located elsewhere on the body and include vertical growth phase, ulceration, Clark level III or higher, and thickness greater than 1.5 mm.[84,85]

PROGNOSIS AND TREATMENT

In early reports in the literature, radical mastectomy and extended radical mastectomy were frequently used as the surgical treatment for melanoma involving the skin of the breast.[81,83] Other authors have reported success with wide excision of the primary lesion.[82,84] The extent of resection should be based primarily on the thickness of the lesion where 1-cm margins are adequate for melanomas less than 1 cm and for lesions thicker than 1 cm, 2- to 3-cm margins are adequate.[86] Closure of the wound can be accomplished in various ways that include primary closure or use of split thickness skin graft. In one report, a latissimus dorsi flap was used to improve cosmetic outcome in female patients.[84] The role of elective lymph node dissection remains controversial; if a patient has palpable axillary adenopathy, however, a therapeutic lymph node dissection should be done.

The prognosis for melanoma involving the skin of the breast is good; Greenberg and colleagues[84] reported a 72% survival rate with an average follow-up of 58 months. With an average follow-up of 57 months, Roses and associates[82] reported no deaths in 21 patients; follow-up was short in this series, however.

References

1. Adair FE, Hermann JB. Primary lymphosarcoma of the breast. Surgery 1944;16:836.
2. Wiseman C, Liao KT. Primary lymphoma of the breast. Cancer 1972;29:1705.
3. Liu FF, Clark RM. Primary lymphoma of the breast. Clinic Radiol 1986;37:567.
4. Schouten JT, Weese JL, Carbone PP. Lymphoma of the breast. Ann Surg 1981;194:749.
5. Arber DA, Simpson JF, Weiss LM, et al. Non-Hodgkin's lymphoma involving the breast. Am J Surg Pathol 1994;18:288.
6. DeBlasio D, McCormick B, Straus D, et al. Definitive irradiation for localized non-Hodgkin's lymphoma of breast. Int J Radiat Oncol Biol Phys 1989;17:843.
7. Hugh JC, Jackson FI, Hanson J, et al. Primary breast lymphoma: an immunohistologic study of 20 new cases. Cancer 1990;66:2602.
8. Lamovec J, Jancar J. Primary malignant lymphoma of the breast: lymphoma of the mucosa-associated lymphoid tissue. Cancer 1987;60:3033.
9. Smith MR, Brustein S, Straus D. Localized non-Hodgkin's lymphoma of the breast. Cancer 1987;59:351.
10. Freeman C, Berg JW, Cutler SJ. Occurrence and prognosis of extranodal lymphomas. Cancer 1972;29:252.
11. Dixon JM, Lumsden AB, Krajewski A, et al. Primary lymphoma of the breast. Br J Surg 1987;74:214.
12. Bobrow LG, Richards MA, Happerfield LC, et al. Breast lymphomas: a clinicopathologic review. Hum Pathol 1993;24:274.
13. Danel L, Vincent C, Rousse F, et al. Estrogen and progesterone receptors in some human myeloma cell lines and murine hybridomas. J Steroid Biochem 1988;30:363.
14. Dixon JM, Anderson TJ, Lamb J, et al. Fine needle aspiration cytology, in relationship to clinical examination and mammography in the diagnosis of a solid breast mass. Br J Surg 1984;71:593.
15. Giardini R, Piccolo C, Rilke F. Primary non-Hodgkin's lymphomas of the female breast. Cancer 1992;69:725.
16. Cohen PL, Brooks JJ. Lymphomas of the breast: a clinicopathologic and immunohistochemical study of primary and secondary cases. Cancer 1991;67:1359.
17. Brustein S, Kimmel M, Lieberman PH, et al. Malignant lymphoma of the breast. Ann Surg 1987;205:144.
18. Smith MR, Brustein S, Straus DJ. Localized non-Hodgkin's lymphoma of the breast. Cancer 1987;59:351.
19. Meyer JE, Kopans DB, Long JC. Mammographic appearance of malignant lymphoma of the breast. Radiology 1980;135:623.
20. Berg JW, DeCrosse JJ, Fracchia AA, et al. Stromal sarcomas of the breast. Cancer 1962;15:418.
21. Barnes L, Pietruszka M. Sarcomas of the breast. Cancer 1977;40:1577.
22. Callery CD, Rosen PP, Kinne DW. Sarcoma of the breast. Ann Surg 1985;201:527.
23. Khanna S, Gupta S, Khanna NN. Sarcomas of the breast: homogeneous or heterogenous. J Surg Oncol 1981;18:119.
24. Smola MG, Ratschek M, Samonigg H, et al. The impact of resection margins in the treatment of primary sarcomas of the breast: a clinico-pathological study of 8 cases with review of literature. Eur J Surg Oncol 1993;19:61.
25. DeDycker RP, Schumacher T, Neumann RLA. High-dose interferon-beta in treatment of spindle-cell sarcoma of breast. Eur J Cancer 1990;26:925.
26. Langham MR Jr, Mills AS, DeMay RM, et al. Malignant fibrous histiocytoma of the breast. Cancer 1984;54:558.
27. Austin RM, Dupree WB. Liposarcoma of the breast: a clinicopathologic study of 20 cases. Hum Pathol 1986;17.
29. Chen KTK, Kuo TT, Hoffmann KD. Leiomyosarcoma of the breast. Cancer 1981;47:1883.
30. Pardo-Mindan J, Garcia-Julian G, Altuna ME. Leiomyosarcoma of the breast. Am J Clin Pathol 1974;62:477.
31. Pitts WC, Rojas VA, Gaffey MJ, et al. Carcinomas with metaplasia and sarcomas of the breast. Am J Clin Oncol 1991;95:623.
32. Roditi G, Prasad S. Case report: radiology of stromal sarcoma of the breast with ossifying pleural metastases. Br J Radiol 1994;67:212.
33. Jernstrom P, Lindberg AL, Meland ON. Osteogenic sarcoma of the mammary gland. Am J Clin Pathol 1963;40:521.
34. Elson BC, Ikeda DM, Andersson I, et al. Fibrosarcoma of the breast: mammographic findings in five cases. AJR 1992;158:993.

35. McGregor GI, Knowling MA, Este FA. Sarcoma and cystosarcoma phyllodes tumors of the breast: a retrospective review of 58 cases. Am J Surg 1994;167:477.

36. Pollard SG, Marks PV, Temple LN, et al. Breast sarcoma: a clinicopathologic review of 25 cases. Cancer 1990;66:941.

37. Terrier PH, Terrier-Lacombe MJ, Mouriesse H, et al. Primary breast sarcoma: a review of 33 cases with immunohistochemistry and prognostic factors. Breast Cancer Res Treat 1989;13:39.

38. Johnstone PAS, Pierce LJ, Merino MJ, et al. Primary soft tissue sarcomas of the breast: local–regional control with post-operative radiotherapy. Int J Radiat Oncol Biol Phys 1993;27:671.

39. Gutman H, Pollock RE, Ross MI, et al. Sarcoma of the breast: implications for extent of therapy. Surgery 1994;116:505.

40. Norris HJ, Taylor HB. Sarcomas and related mesenchymal tumors of the breast. Cancer 1968;22:22.

41. D'Orsi CJ, Feldhaus L, Sonnenfeld M. Unusual lesions of the breast. Radiol Clin North Am 1983;21:67.

42. Donnell RM, Rosen PP, Lieberman PH, et al. Angiosarcoma and other vascular tumors of the breast. Am J Surg Pathol 1981;5:629.

43. Chen KTK, Kirkegaard DD, Bocian JJ. Angiosarcoma of the breast. Cancer 1980;46:368.

44. Rosen PP, Kimel M, Ernsberger D. Mammary angiosarcoma. Cancer 1988;62:2145.

45. Merino MJ, Berman M, Carter D. Angiosarcoma of the breast. Am J Surg Pathol 1983;7:53.

46. Savage R. The treatment of angiosarcoma of the breast. J Surg Oncol 1981;18:129.

47. Rainwater LM, Martin JK Jr, Gaffey TA, et al. Angiosarcoma of the breast. Arch Surg 1986;121:669.

48. Myerowitz RL, Pietruska M, Barnes EC. Primary angiosarcoma of the breast. JAMA 1978;239:403.

49. Rosner D. Angiosarcoma of the breast: long-term survival following adjuvant chemotherapy. J Surg Oncol 1988;39:90.

50. Hunter TB, Martin PC, Dietzen CD, et al. Angiosarcoma of the breast. Cancer 1985;56:2099.

51. Paulus DD, Libshitz HI. Metastasis to the breast. Radiol Clin North Am 1982;20:561.

52. Arora R, Robinson WA. Breast metastases from malignant melanoma. J Surg Oncol 1992;50:27.

53. Hunter GJ, Choi NC, McLoud TC, et al. Lung tumor metastasis to breast detected by fluorine-18 fluorodeoxyglucose PET. J Nucl Med 1993;34:1571.

54. Ooijen BV, Slot A, Henzen-Logmans C, et al. Cervical cancer metastasising to the breast: report of two cases. Eur J Surg 1993;159:125.

55. Moir GC, Carpenter R, Bass P, et al. Metastatic carcinoid for the breast: an unusual screen-detected breast cancer. Eur J Surg Oncol 1993;19:92.

56. Hamby LS, McGrath PC, Cibull ML, et al. Gastric carcinoma metastatic to the breast. J Surg Oncol 1991;48:117.

57. Alvarez RD, Gleason BP, Gore H, et al. Coexisting intraductal breast carcinoma and metastatic choriocarcinoma presenting as a breast mass. Gynecol Oncol 1991;43:295.

58. Allen FJ, Van Velden JJ. Prostate carcinoma metastatic to the male breast. Br J Urol 1991;67:434.

59. Lesho EP. Metastatic renal cell carcinoma presenting as a breast mass. Post Graduate Med 1992;91:145.

60. Younathan CM, Steinbach BG, DeBose CD. Case report metastatic cervical carcinoma to the breast. Gynecol Oncol 1992;45:211.

61. Ron IG, Inbar M, Halpern M, et al. Endometrioid carcinoma of the ovary presenting as primary carcinoma of the breast: a case report and review of the literature. Acta Obstet Gynecol Scand 1992;71:80.

62. Sham JST, Choy D. Breast metastasis from nasopharyngeal carcinoma. Eur J Surg Oncol 1991;17:91.

63. Kattan J, Droz JP, Charpentier P, et al. Ovarian dysgerminoma metastatic to the breast. Gynecol Oncol 1992;46:104.

64. Loredo DS, Powell JL, Reed WP, et al. Ovarian carcinoma metastatic to breast: a case report and review of the literature. Gynecol Oncol 1990;37:432.

65. Duda RB, August CZ, Schink JC. Ovarian carcinoma metastatic to the breast and axillary node. Surgery 1991;110:552.

66. Yamasaki H, Saw D, Zdanowitz J, et al. Ovarian carcinoma metastasis to the breast case report and review of the literature. Am J Surg Pathol 1993;17:193.

67. Kumar PV, Esfahani FN, Salimi A. Choriocarcinoma metastatic to the breast diagnosed by fine needle aspiration. Acta Cytol 1991;35.

68. Gorczyca W, Osszewski W, Tuziak T, et al. Fine needle aspiration cytology of rare malignant tumors of the breast. Acta Cytol 1992;36:918.

69. Silverman JF, Feldman PS, Covell JL, et al: Fine needle aspiration cytology of neoplasm metastatic to the breast. Acta Cytol 1987;31:291.

70. Di Bonito L, Luchi M, Giarelli L, et al. Metastatic tumors to the female breast: an autopsy study of 12 cases. Path Res Pract 1991;187:432.

71. Hajdu SI, Urban JA. Cancers metastatic to the breast. Cancer 1972;29:1691.

72. Sneige N, Zachariah S, Fanning TV, et al. Fine-needle aspiration cytology of metastatic neoplasms in the breast. Am J Clin Pathol 1989;92:27.

73. Finney GG, Finney GG, Montague ACW, et al. Bilateral breast cancer, clinical and pathological review. Ann Surg 1972;175:635.

74. Fisher ER, Fisher B, Sass R, et al. Pathologic findings from the National Surgical Adjuvant Breast and Bowel Project (Protocol No. 4). XI. Bilateral breast cancer. Cancer 1984;54:3002.

75. Harvey EB, Britton LA. Second cancer following cancer of the breast in Connecticut, 1935–82. Natl Cancer Inst Monogr 1985;68:99.

76. Leis HP. Managing the remaining breast. Cancer 1980;46:1026.

77. Lewision EF. The follow-up examination of the contralateral breast: from the viewpoint of the surgeon. Cancer 1969;23:809.

78. Lewison EF, Neto AS. Bilateral breast cancer at the Johns Hopkins Hospital: a discussion of the dilemma of the contralateral breast. Cancer 1971;28:1297.

79. Chaudary MA, Millis RR, Hoskins EOL, et al. Bilateral primary breast cancer: a prospective study of disease incidence. Br J Surg 1984;71:711.

80. Egan RI. Bilateral breast carcinomas: role of mammography. Cancer 1976;38:931.

81. Papachristou DN, Kinne DW, Rosen PP, et al. Cutaneous melanoma of the breast. Surgery 1979;85:322.

82. Roses DF, Harris MN, Stern JS, et al. Cutaneous melanoma of the breast. Ann Surg 1978;189:112.

83. Ariel IM, Caron AS. Diagnosis and treatment of malignant melanoma arising from the skin of the female breast. Am J Surg 1972;124:384.

84. Greenberg BM, Hamilton R, Rothkopf DM, et al. Management of cutaneous melanomas of the female breast. Plast Reconstr Surg 1987;80:409.

85. Balch CM, Cascinelli N, Drzewiecki, KT, et al. A comparison of prognostic factors worldwide: epidemiologic features of melanoma prognostic factors. In: Balch CM, Houghton AN, Milton GW, et al, eds. Cutaneous melanoma ed 2. Philadelphia, JB Lippincott, 1992:188.

86. Singletary SE, Balch CM, Urist MM, et al. Surgical treatment of primary melanoma: epidemiologic features of melanoma prognostic factors. In: Balch CM, Houghton AN, Milton GW, et al, eds. Cutaneous melanoma, ed 2. Philadelphia, JB Lippincott, 1992:269.

24.5
Breast Cancer and Pregnancy
JEANNE A. PETREK

Pregnancy–Associated Breast Cancer

The traditional definition of pregnancy-associated breast cancer holds that the diagnosis of breast cancer is made during pregnancy or within 1 year afterward. With that definition, one review[1] noted an incidence between 0.2% and 3.8% in 32 series from the past several decades.

Diagnosed breast cancers occur in 1 in 3000 to 10,000 pregnancies,[2,3] making the malignancy almost as common as cancer of the uterine cervix.[4] The incidence of pregnancy-associated breast cancer among patients less than 40 years old using the traditional definition is about 15%.[1] As more women bear children in their 30s and even 40s, ages when breast cancer is more common, the incidence of pregnancy-associated breast cancer will undoubtedly rise.

Determining the effect of the hormonal milieu of pregnancy on a breast cancer is a problem. Although pregnancy and breast cancer are only rarely concurrent, a great number of patients have had an unknown subclinical breast cancer while pregnant, given that the occult preclinical tumor growth phase is several years.[5] This issue has only recently been addressed.

A 1994 study of young breast cancer patients at nine American and European cancer centers demonstrated that the recency of pregnancy (up to 4 years) was associated with a worse prognosis.[6] For each additional year in the time between pregnancy and breast cancer diagnosis, the risk of dying decreased by 15%. The effect of recent pregnancy could substantially contribute to the observation of the poorer prognosis in the young,[7,8] considering that the reproductive rate is high in the young and that the documented effect lingers for 4 years.[6]

Prognosis of Breast Cancer Diagnosed During Pregnancy and Lactation

The earliest reports, from more than a century ago, noted a dismal prognosis. Kilgore and Bloodgood[9] reported no survivors, and White's collective series[11] reported a 17% 5-year survival rate. Haagensen and Stout[10] reported only an 8.6% overall 5-year survival rate.

Harrington[12] is credited with reviving optimism at the Mayo Clinic in 1937 by finding a 61% 5-year survival rate among patients with negative lymph nodes. Unfortunately, presentation with lymph node metastases was then, and remains, common in pregnant women. Nine papers published during the 1960s,[13–21] reporting patient numbers from 29 to 117, found a rate of positive lymph nodes ranging from 53% to 74% (median, 65%). Four similar papers[3,22–24] published during the 1970s found a rate of positive lymph nodes of 56% to 81%. Few studies have attempted to put these percentages into the context of age, decade of diagnosis, and similar demographics by designating a nonpregnant comparison group.

At Memorial Hospital in New York, I compared 56 patients with pregnancy-associated breast cancer (American Joint Committee on Cancer stage I, II, or III) diagnosed between 1960 and 1980 with nonpregnant control patients from a consecutive mastectomy series of the same age who were diagnosed and treated at the same hospital during the same period by the same physicians.[25] Sixty-two percent of the pregnancy-associated patients had positive lymph nodes compared with 39% of their nonpregnant counterparts. Only 31% of the pregnant patients had pathologic tumors less than 2 cm compared with 50% of the control group. The findings are similar to other studies that also include comparison groups.[17,26–28] Only 4 Memorial Hospital patients were lost before 5-year follow-up (and 1 patient before a 10-year follow-up). These 5 were known to have metastatic disease at the time they were lost to follow-up.

The patients with pregnancy-associated breast cancer with negative lymph nodes had a 82% 5-year survival rate compared with an 82% rate for their nonpregnant counterparts. The pregnant patients with positive lymph nodes had a 47% 5-year survival rate compared with a 59% rate in the control patients. Among pregnant patients who were eligible, there was a 77% 10-year survival rate for those with negative lymph nodes and a 25% rate for those with positive lymph nodes. In comparison, the 10-year survival rate was 75% for nonpregnant patients with negative nodes and 41% for nonpregnant patients with positive nodes. The differences in 5- and 10-year survival times in patients grouped by stage were not statistically significant.

Table 24.5-1 presents the results of similar recent studies of patients presenting with operable breast cancer. The similarity between the 5-year survival rates among these studies from three different countries is striking. The only modern series with nonpregnant controls (matched for age, stage and calendar year at diagnosis) that shows a significantly worse survival rate is a small series from Norway in which only 6 of 20 patients had negative lymph nodes.[29] The survival times cannot be compared with those of other series, since the patients with metastatic disease were not separated. There is no obvious explanation for such a poor prognosis.

TABLE 24.5-1

Proportion of Operable Patients Presenting With Negative Lymph Nodes and Proportion Surviving 5 Years According to Lymph Node Status

| | Patients With Negative Lymph Nodes (%) | 5-Year Survival Rate (%) | |
		Negative Lymph Nodes	Positive Lymph Nodes
Investigators			
Deemarsky & Neishtadt, 1980[28]	32	73	43
King et al, 1985[26]	38	82	36
Ribiero et al, 1986[27]	28	79	45
Petrek et al, 1991[25]	39	82	47

The largest study thus far concerns 118 women with pregnancy-associated breast cancer treated in Toronto from 1958 to 1987. They found no statistically significant difference in survival between pregnant and nonpregnant patients when matched by age, stage, and year of diagnosis.[30] The pregnant women had a 2.5-fold higher risk of diagnosis with metastatic breast cancer and a significantly decreased chance of a stage I diagnosis. A 1992 study published in a Japanese cancer journal also with a large number of patients showed similar findings.[31]

In summary, almost all reports note a worse overall survival rate for patients with pregnancy-associated breast cancer. When the pregnancy-associated breast cancer patients are evaluated with nonpregnant controls, however, the pregnancy-associated group has an equivalent survival rate at least in the early stages. Overall, pregnancy-associated breast cancer bears a worse prognosis, since it is regularly associated with more advanced disease at presentation. It is unknown whether this is due to a more aggressive growth pattern secondary to the biologic effects of pregnancy, delayed diagnosis secondary to the breast changes of pregnancy, or a combination of the two.

Considerations of the Developing Fetus in Staging and Treatment

In cancer diagnosis and treatment, dangers to the fetus include those of development, such as the teratogenicity possibly caused by radiation therapy, chemotherapy, and general anesthesia. In addition to congenital abnormalities, various other risks, such as intrauterine growth retardation or prematurity and possible postnatal neoplasia, must also be considered. The overall effects on the fetus of chemotherapy and radiation therapy without consideration of specific diseases have been reviewed elsewhere.[32]

RADIATION RISK TO THE FETUS

In both rodents and humans, the principal effect of radiation during the preimplantation period (from conception to days 10 to 14) is embryo death. The second period,

organogenesis (lasting from days 10 to 14 through week 8), is undoubtedly the most sensitive to ionizing radiation. There is a 20% incidence of severe malformations (often involving the central nervous system) in mice with exposures as low as 18 cGy and a 100% incidence with 200 cGy.[33] In the pregnant women of Hiroshima and Nagasaki, an air dose of 1 to 9 cGy during weeks 6 through 11 of pregnancy resulted in an 11% incidence of microcephaly and mental retardation in children, compared with 4% in a nonirradiated Japanese control population.[34]

Radiation exposure beyond 8 weeks is much less likely to produce congenital abnormalities than during the organogenesis period. In humans, microcephaly has been observed after radiation exposure during the early fetal period, but, dose-for-dose, the incidence is four to five times less than after exposure during the earlier organogenesis period.[34] After about 30 weeks of gestation, radiation-induced congenital defects are extremely rare.[35]

The atomic bomb experience and animal experimentation data led to the conclusion that 5 cGy is the dose level for early pregnancy at which radiation-induced anomalies become meaningful. The American Academy of Pediatrics and other organizations support the conclusion of the American College of Radiology that interruption of pregnancy is not routinely recommended if the fetus was exposed to less than 5 cGy.[1] (In this discussion, it is not considered that even low doses could have genetic effects that are manifested only in subsequent generations derived from this offspring.)

Another theoretic risk of radiation is carcinogenesis in the offspring. Although some retrospective studies indicate an association between prenatal x-ray exposure (usually through maternal pelvimetry) and future childhood cancers, this is not universally accepted. Even so, the reported risk of leukemia at 10 years after a 2-cGy exposure is only 1 in 2000 versus 1 in 3000 in unexposed controls.[36] Blood-borne carcinogenesis (transplacental) has been reviewed elsewhere.[37]

FETAL RISK FROM STAGING PROCEDURES DURING PREGNANCY

Accurate staging and appropriate treatment depend on comprehensive evaluation for metastatic disease, and most tests use ionizing radiation. Published estimates of the approximate fetal and maternal exposures are available.[38] The radiation dose to the embryo, fetus, or even a particular fetal organ can also be specifically calculated by a medical physicist when the relevant parameters are known (for x-ray examinations—beam quality, kilovoltage, exposure time, distance, film size, view; for nuclear medicine procedures—type of agent, total activity, target organ, effective half-life).[39]

Some guidelines can be made for recommended staging tests. There is no contraindication to chest radiography, which is sometimes performed with abdominal and pelvic shielding. Late in pregnancy, with the gravid uterus directly under the diaphragm, fetal shielding would obscure the lower lung parenchyma. Nevertheless, exposing the third-trimester fetus to chest radiography presents no great concern.

In regard to evaluation for bone metastases, serum alkaline phosphatase is elevated because of pregnancy itself. Conventional radiography, excluding the pelvis and abdomen, can be performed (eg, skull, long bones). There is no adequate substitute for a bone scan. A recent article noted modification of the bone-scanning technique for pregnant patients.[40] If the bone scan result will not change the immediate treatment, it should be delayed until after delivery. Therefore, in a patient with clinical stage I or II disease, bone scan can usually be avoided, since the incidence of diagnosable bone metastases is so low.[41] In clinical stage III pregnant patients, however, who have an increased rate of bone metastases found on bone scan, it is possible that this test changes treatment.

Magnetic resonance imaging is highly accurate and seems safe for the fetus. Recent reports on its use for fetal imaging in prenatal diagnosis contain limited follow-up of the infants with no adverse effects reported.[42,43] It is particularly useful for the diagnosis or confirmation of bone metastases, liver metastases, or even brain metastases (although a head computed tomographic scan with abdominal shielding should yield only small amounts of fetal exposure).

BREAST PRESERVATION IN THE PREGNANT WOMEN

The fetal dose can be estimated by thermoluminescent dosimeters placed in an anatomic phantom shielding. However, the standard breast radiation therapy course of about 5000 cGy exposes the fetus to from 10 cGy early in pregnancy to 200 cGy or more late in pregnancy and so should be rejected as a treatment option.

The developing fetus receives up to several percent of the total breast dose. The radiation leakage from the radiation unit should not exceed 0.1% of the direct beam exposure rate, as measured from a meter from the radiation source.[44] A larger amount of radiation, however, reaches the fetus from internal scatter by the mother's tissues (which cannot be reduced by external shielding). The quantity of such radiation depends on the distance of the fetus from the field center, the field size, and the energy source of the radiation. A 6-meV linear accelerator pro-

duces less fetal dose by internal scatter than a 1.25-meV cobalt-60 unit.

For example, when the fetus is of less than 12 weeks' gestation (ie, is still in the true pelvis and perhaps 40 cm from field center), the dose from a field that is 10×10 cm and is produced by a 4-meV unit would be in the range of 0.2% to 0.3% of the tumor dose. This could result in an exposure of 10 to 15 cGy early in pregnancy for a breast treatment course of 5000 cGy. Toward the end of pregnancy, if a fetal part is 10 cm distant, it would receive 200 cGy for the same treatment course.

Much of the information about radiation (and also chemotherapy) must be obtained in reports on lymphoma and leukemia. A recent report from M.D. Anderson Cancer Center[45] evaluated 14 patients with Hodgkin disease who had various fields of radiation of 3500 to 4000 cGy while in the second or third trimester. This is about three fourths of the dose necessary for breast cancer. With specialized techniques, they were able to decrease the total estimated *mid*-fetus dose to 1.4 to 13.6 cGy. The dose to the closest fetal part was not estimated.

Likewise, radiation after mastectomy involves similar doses to the chest wall and poses the same hazard to the fetus. Because, even with medial breast cancers, postmastectomy irradiation is of arguable benefit in routine patients, it should be postponed in similarly staged pregnant women. Postmastectomy irradiation in late stage is often indicated because of the high risk of local recurrence. Nevertheless, it is probably wisest to delay the radiation therapy until the patient is no longer pregnant. If local recurrence occurs before delivery, it can be excised to the extent possible to enable further postponement of irradiation at least until late in pregnancy, when fetal risk is greatly lessened.

BREAST PRESERVATION DURING PREGNANCY WITH DELAYED RADIATION

To accomplish breast preservation in the pregnant woman, lumpectomy during pregnancy followed by radiation therapy after delivery has been suggested. To advocate this approach one must extrapolate from the data obtained in nonpregnant women. A pregnant woman's breast, however, with the large interanastomosing network of ducts and sizable lymph and blood vessels, is not anatomically and physiologically similar to the less active breast of a premenopausal woman. The duct structure itself might predispose to lengthy intraductal spread. It is not certain that the same results after lumpectomy and irradiation will occur with lumpectomy during pregnancy and delayed postpartum radiation.

A situation due to endogenous hormones changing the breast anatomic structure and resulting in increased local recurrence rates (with quadrantectomy and no radiation) is hypothesized in a recent Milan study.[46] The researchers found a 3.8% local recurrence rate in women over 55 years of age, a 8.7% rate in women aged 46 to 55 years, and a 17.5% rate in women aged 45 years or less. The investigators surmised that treatment response differed by age because of the duct structure. After menopause, the complex structure of the breast disappears, and the breast becomes "a fatty organ with scattered islands of fibroepithelial tissue without connection between them."[46] The anatomic difference between the pregnant breast and the nonpregnant breast of the same individual seems greater than that between premenopausal and postmenopausal breasts. The local recurrence rate after breast conservation in pregnant women is unknown, since there are no published series.

Chemotherapy During Pregnancy

Chemotherapeutic agents are minimally selective and usually affect rapidly proliferating cells, which makes the developing fetus a prime target for teratogenesis. The fetal effect is related to drug dosage, to gestational age, to synergism when combined with other drugs or radiation, and to the individual drug, working, as they do, through different mechanisms and at different molecular sites. As Garber[47] stated in her 1989 review, which included limited follow-up of infants, "The teratogenic effects of the approximately 20 cytotoxic agents in general use must be extracted from more than 300 anecdotal reports and interviews." Most reports involve leukemia and lymphoma.[48–54]

The placenta may create a biologic barrier for some antineoplastic agents, although most apparently readily traverse the placenta[51,55]; doxorubicin has been particularly studied in this regard.[56–58] There are several excellent reviews of fetal effects.[47,52,54,59,60]

For chemotherapy administered during the first trimester, Schapira and Chudley[61] reviewed eight reports with 71 patients and found an aggregate fetal malformation rate of 12.7%. In Sweet and Kinzie's series[52] and Nicholson's series,[60] which was as large, about 40% of infants exposed to chemotherapy in utero were of low birthweight, and the concern is one of future growth and development.

A 1992 report[62] noted statistically significant lower birthweights than matched controls due to both significantly lower gestational age (prematurity) and substantial intrauterine growth retardation. Even the infants born markedly underweight or premature have been called "normal," although this term lacks definition. Garber[47] noted that anecdotal reports routinely state childhood normalcy without providing details, even with infants born markedly underweight or premature.

Also of great concern is the unknown effects that can appear in childhood after chemotherapy exposure during fetal development. Only recently are the long-term effects of chemotherapy given to children being reported, such as with doxorubicin, a common drug for breast cancer. Doxorubicin therapy, in the absence of radiation, has been associated with late echocardiographic abnormalities in 65% of childhood leukemia survivors.[63] These abnormalities are progressive and may result in congestive heart failure, among other disorders.[64] The long-term effects of

individuals exposed to chemotherapy in utero, rather than at childhood, have not been studied.

Adjuvant chemotherapy is the standard of care for premenopausal patients with systemic breast cancer and axillary nodal metastases, and there is general agreement that patients with tumors larger than 1 cm who have no axillary node metastases also benefit. Even if effects on the fetus could be ruled out, any course of chemotherapy during pregnancy is serious for many reasons, including the possible complications of sepsis and hemorrhage during unplanned labor and delivery. For all of these reasons, one might consider a delay of several weeks to allow a pregnant woman to deliver before the initiation of chemotherapy. Such delays are found in nonpregnant women with postsurgical complications and with the use of radiation therapy sequentially before chemotherapy.[65] The greatest permissible time lapse before effective adjuvant chemotherapy is unknown. Adjuvant chemotherapy in women who are pregnant must be resolved on a patient-by-patient basis.

Metastatic Disease in the Fetus and Placenta

Only melanoma and lymphosarcoma have been reported to cause actual fetal metastases.[66] Placental metastases have been reported in 30 patients with solid tumors, including several breast cancers.[67] Microscopic examination of the placenta, especially of the intervillous space, is important, since only half the patients had visible metastases.[68]

Anesthetic Considerations

General anesthesia is necessary for a mastectomy or axillary dissection and rarely for an adequate wide excision. General anesthesia during pregnancy is difficult because of increased blood volume, increased heart rate and cardiac output, increased platelet count and fibrinogen level, supine positional hypotension, decreased pulmonary functional residual capacity, elevated diaphragms, prolonged gastric emptying, hypervascularity of the respiratory tract mucosa, and so on. As compared with the risks of teratogenesis from radiation therapy and chemotherapy, those associated with the general anesthetic drugs are almost nonexistent.

Despite the fact that nitrous oxide and halothane interfere in vitro with nucleic acid synthesis, no deleterious effects can be detected in humans.[69] These potent inhalational agents have the theoretic advantage of relaxing uterine musculature and forestalling premature labor. In fact, premature labor seems to depend more on the surgical site (it is more common with lower abdominal or pelvic operations) than on anesthetic technique and is not likely with breast operations. In any event, obstetricians have several drugs for reversal of premature labor. Fetal monitoring should be used whenever possible, so that patterns of fetal distress may be followed immediately by fine adjustments of anesthetic technique.

A large population-based study from Sweden studied 5405 nonobstetric operations during pregnancy and compared them with 720,000 pregnancies without general anesthesia.[70] The major problems found were increased incidence of low birthweight, due both to prematurity and to intrauterine growth retardation, and an increased incidence of infants born alive who died within 7 days. On the positive side, the incidence of congenital anomalies was not increased in women who had first-trimester operations, and general anesthesia with nitrous oxide was not associated with an increased incidence of adverse outcomes. These adverse effects are not necessarily attributable to the surgical operation, since the illness that necessitated the surgery must have had a significant role.[70]

The Question of Therapeutic Abortion

The traditional view of concurrent breast cancer and pregnancy as an especially dreaded situation may have contributed to zealous enthusiasm for abortion in the past, usually combined with oophorectomy. For example, Haagensen and Stout[10] recommended refusing mastectomy to any breast cancer patient diagnosed during pregnancy or lactation as categorically incurable (although they later changed this opinion[71]). In 1953, Adair,[72] at Memorial Hospital in New York, noticed longer crude survival rates after therapeutic abortion, especially for patients with positive axillary lymph nodes (these differences were not statistically significant).

Thereafter, the opinion on the uniformly lethal nature of concurrent breast cancer and pregnancy as well as the unquestioned value of therapeutic abortion gradually began to change. Holleb and Farrow,[21] also at Memorial Hospital, reported in 1962 on 24 patients treated with radical mastectomy, and abortion was not associated with a better survival. The most recent reports are from the mid-1980s[26,73] and also show no survival advantage after therapeutic abortion.

In a 1989 article reporting on 154 pregnant patients between 1931 and 1985, Clark and Chua[74] stated that therapeutic abortion is associated with decreased survival. There was a 5-year survival rate of 20% with therapeutic abortion, a 28% rate with live birth, and a 50% rate for those who were fortunate enough to have a spontaneous abortion. Overall, the whole group had advanced disease, with only 19% documented with negative lymph nodes and 10% with primary tumors less than 2 cm. However, the characteristics of the patients in the three groups is unknown. Similar findings in 100 cases of gestational breast cancer seen between 1926 and 1972 were published by the Petrov Research Institute of Oncology in Leningrad.[28]

In all these data, reported numbers are small and data were collected over long intervals. Cases were not precisely staged. Most importantly, any beneficial effect of abortion would be disguised by the selection factor, since it appears that the more advanced cases were more likely to undergo therapeutic abortion.

For example, in a series of 63 pregnant patients at the Mayo Clinic,[26] a 5-year survival rate of 43% was reported in the group with interrupted pregnancies compared with 59% in group that were delivered of full-term infants. Of the 20 stage I patients, however, 17 were delivered of infants and only 3 had their pregnancies interrupted. There was an excellent 5-year survival rate of 86% on the 17 patients who were allowed to give birth. Only 1 of 3 patients with interrupted pregnancies survived, for a 5-year survival rate of 33%. Stage I is a broad group, however, and most clinicians are able to predict the patients who have poor prognoses (such as those in stage I with extensive lymphatic invasion or anaplastic tumors). The inclination is to recommend abortion to them but not to the other patients in stage I.

Therapeutic abortion is strongly recommended if the issue is fetal damage from the proposed chemotherapy or radiation treatments. Treatment is always simplified with therapeutic abortion early in pregnancy. In the end, it is the mother who must make as informed a decision as possible about the pregnancy.

When combined with standard therapy, any additional benefit of routine therapeutic abortion cannot be demonstrated in the published reports. Nevertheless, because survival rates are generally equivalent between those continuing pregnancy and those whose pregnancies are aborted, and the patients with more advanced disease underwent abortions preferentially, abortion may be beneficial but that fact is disguised by patient selection.

Steroid Hormone Receptors

Little is known about the accuracy and ultimate value of steroid hormone receptor status during pregnancy. Pregnancy may result in false-negatives in two ways. Increasing estrogen and progesterone concentrations are known to down-regulate estrogen receptor levels in some cell lines,[75] and thus actual estrogen receptor levels could be suppressed below a threshold detectable by the ligand-binding assay. Furthermore, routine ligand-binding assays (without exchange techniques) depend on the availability of unbound receptor; in pregnancy, all binding sites may already be occupied by endogenous hormone. In the nonpregnant state, only up to 35% of cytosol receptor was occupied by endogenous steroid, so that most was available for assay.[76]

When the receptor assay is performed during pregnancy, unbound estrogen should first be removed by treatment of cytosol with dextran-charcoal.[77] Exchange assays should then be performed to detect occupied estrogen receptor.[78,79] Because most laboratories are not experienced in these techniques, the frozen tissue should be shipped to a laboratory where the procedures are routinely performed.

Immunohistochemical staining assays are arguably more accurate in pregnant women since the occupied receptor should still stain. One report compared the receptor status by immunohistochemistry to ligand-binding assay of pregnant versus nonpregnant women.[80] No retrospective data on pregnant patients with accurate hormone receptor status exist for formulating recommendations on therapeutic abortions, hormonal manipulation, or subsequent pregnancies.

Pregnancy Safety After Breast Cancer

TIMELINESS OF THE ISSUE

Many women with breast cancer have sought medical advice about the safety of pregnancy after successful breast cancer treatment and even more are expected in the future as a result of two trends of the 1980s that are continuing into the 1990s. Breast cancer incidence continues to rise in all age groups. The numbers are enormous, since 10% to 20% of the 182,000 cases in the United States in 1994 occurred in women of childbearing age.[81]

Furthermore, women who have postponed their first childbirth for personal, educational, or professional reasons can have more breast cancer risk factors, since they are often white, college educated, and socioeconomically privileged. Whatever the associations, the National Center for Health Statistics[82] reported that the numbers of first births among women aged 30 to 34 increased by 140% and among women aged 35 to 39 by 124% in the 16-year period from 1970 to 1986, and subsequent births are also more common in older women.

The importance of the hormonal milieu as a determinant of breast cancer growth and patient survival has been recognized for almost a century. Beatson's[86] original 1896 description of the efficacy of bilateral oophorectomy as a treatment for premenopausal women with breast cancer stimulated a large body of research examining endocrine manipulation.

One would expect that the influence of such a profound hormonal event as pregnancy (with total estrogen levels 1000 times that of a menstruating woman) would have been carefully studied. Despite the singular value of subsequent pregnancy as an issue to the modern young breast cancer survivor, a 1991 review[84] could find only 563 total patients reported on in 12 articles since 1946.

Virtually all hormonal events (age at first full-term pregnancy, age at menarche and menopause, usage of postmenopausal hormone replacement) have been proven to have an effect on breast cancer development. After successful breast cancer treatment, the issue is not only a new primary breast cancer but, more importantly, the stimulation of dormant systemic micrometastases by gestational hormones.

Unfortunately, the hormones of pregnancy are complex as well as intense and include steroids beyond estrogen and progesterone, as well as peptide hormones. How each of these substances relates to carcinogenesis and cancer promotion is unknown. Because physicians have stressed the complete rehabilitation of cancer patients, including reconstruction and psychosocial aspects, it follows that patients, on completion of therapy, wish to reassume and continue their life roles, including becoming mothers of their children. It behooves physicians to give the best advice possible to women with breast cancer.

PROGNOSIS

The earlier literature stated that at least 7% of women who did not have oophorectomies underwent one or more pregnancies and 70% of these pregnancies were to be expected in the first 5 years after breast cancer treatment.[85] From the meager amount of older literature on the topic, it has been generally observed that women with breast cancer who subsequently become pregnant have good survival, often the same or better than patients with no subsequent pregnancies.[1]

Eight of White's[11] patients who became pregnant (67%) lived at least 5 years and 58% lived 10 years. A similar finding was recorded by Rissanen,[86] whose 53 patients had 5- and 10-year survival rates of 77% and 69%, respectively. Fifty percent of patients in Cheek's series[87] survived 5 years. Holleb and Farrow[21] reported on 52 patients with an overall 5-year survival rate of 52%, whereas a 75% 5-year survival rate was reported by Cooper and Butterfield[88] in 32 patients.

The case-matching studies attempt to eliminate the obvious factor of pregnancy occurring only in those with a good prognosis. Ninety-six patients with subsequent pregnancies were matched by Peters and Meakin[17] with respect to age and clinical stage. The patients with subsequent pregnancies not only had longer survival times than those without subsequent pregnancies but also had longer disease-free intervals when cases of recurrence were compared. Furthermore, when the factor of selection through early death was minimized by considering only those who became pregnant within 6 months after mastectomy, 54% were found to survive 5 years.

In a more recent analysis, Cooper and Butterfield[88] matched each of 40 patients who subsequently became pregnant with two controls as determined by the clinical stage, age, status of lymph node involvement, and equal survival at least to the time of pregnancy. The patients with subsequent pregnancies still had a survival time superior to that of the controls.

There were three reports from the 1980s. Memorial Sloan-Kettering Cancer Center[89] published their results of 41 patients collected over 30 years. No detrimental effect of subsequent pregnancy was noted, even among patients with positive axillary lymph nodes or among those whose pregnancies occur less than 2 years after mastectomy.

In a 1986 nationwide French study, the 10-year survival rate of 68 patients who had subsequent pregnancies was 71%. The survival of the negative-node patients was 90% at 10 years, and there was no difference between cases and controls.[90]

Ariel and Kempner[91] noted in 1989 that subsequent pregnancies did not affect overall prognosis. They found no demonstrable detrimental effect of subsequent pregnancies on patients after breast cancer, even in those who had positive nodes. The 10-year survival rate was 56% for the 16 patients with positive lymph nodes who become pregnant and 55% for some 300 similar patients in their practice who did not become pregnant.

Table 24.5-2 presents studies from four countries published within the past several years that demonstrate similar survival after subsequent pregnancies. The good survival rates are particularly striking, since the numbers include unselected patients of any stage.

INTERVAL BETWEEN BREAST CANCER DIAGNOSIS AND PREGNANCY

In the simplest analysis, the interval between breast cancer diagnosis and pregnancy affects prognosis, since women who defer a pregnancy for many years are also those who have remained disease-free for longer periods. Four groups of investigators have examined the question of the timing of the subsequent pregnancy on breast cancer prognosis.

Clark and Chua[74] found that 72% of their patients became pregnant within 2 years of treatment. Those who became pregnant within 6 months had a comparatively poor prognosis—a 5-year survival rate of 53.8% compared with a 78% 5-year survival rate among those who waited 6 months to 2 years to become pregnant after diagnosis. Those who waited 5 years or more to become pregnant had 100% 5-year survival from that point. They concluded that a wait of at least 6 months from completion of treatment was to be recommended.

The recent French series[90] and the Memorial Hospital series[89] did not find a statistically significant difference between outcome of patients who conceived based on the interval between breast cancer treatment and conception.

In a report 30 years ago, Peters and Meakin found that the 5-year survival rate was 50% when the pregnancy occurred within 1 year of treatment, 83% when the pregnancy occurred 1 to 2 years after treatment, and 100% when the conception occurred more than 2 years after treatment.[17] Recurrence rates for breast cancer are highest just after treatment, which can provide the important reason for deferral for a time.

MORE THAN ONE SUBSEQUENT PREGNANCY

Among women who became pregnant after breast cancer, 18%[27] to 35.3%[88] have had more than one pregnancy. Clark and Reid[24] found that 25% of those who became pregnant did so more than once and that those who had multiple pregnancies appeared to have improved survival.

The fact of multiple pregnancies by itself affects prognosis for the same reason that interval affects prognosis: women who have more than one pregnancy are also those who have remained disease-free for greater periods in order to achieve the multiple pregnancies. Rissanen[86] found that 34% of patients in his series had two or more posttreatment pregnancies and did as well as those with one pregnancy.

PROBLEMS OF RELIABLE DATA COLLECTION

How much reliance can be placed on these reports? Because pregnancy is not coded as a disease or coded in any other way by the record room or tumor registry, cases from the previous decades are all found by memory, as is the situation with the Memorial Hospital series.[89] Even if a chart or tumor registry review of all premenopausal women had been undertaken, the occurrence of subsequent pregnancy may not be noted.

The methods sections of these papers ignore the question of the denominator, the total number of subsequently pregnant patients. The most recent and largest series states simply, "We have reviewed a total of 413 patients whose case histories are currently available."[74] Because cases over the decades have been obtained in these reports from the many clinicians' memories, and since it is human nature to remember those who have been seen more recently, the design of these studies is predisposed to find and report on the patients who are alive.

For all of these reasons, each report probably contains a small fraction of such patients from that institution. For example, consider a typical series, that from Memorial Sloan-Kettering Cancer Center: during 30 years, 41 stage

TABLE 24.5-2
Survival of Patients With Breast Cancer of Any Stage and With Subsequent Pregnancies

Investigator	Country	Total Patients	Overall 5-Year Survival Rate (%)
Harvey et al, 1981[89]	United States	41	80
Mignot et al, 1986[90]	France	68	71
Ribiero et al, 1986[27]	England	53	69
Clark & Reid, 1989[24]	Canada	136	78

I and II patients were found who became pregnant after breast cancer treatment, and they had an outstanding 80% 5-year survival rate.[89]

Based on the numbers and ages of women seen in those 30 years (as I was able to obtain from the Memorial Hospital tumor registry), however, and assuming only 7% of women with breast cancer who are less than 40 years old became pregnant, this study should have reported on at least 450 women. Therefore, the patients reported from Memorial Hospital represent a highly selected subset, possibly 10% or so of the total who became pregnant after breast cancer treatment.

This phenomenon seems to be acknowledged in a recent French language report.[90] A questionnaire survey of the French Gynecology Society of French obstetricians found only 68 women in all of France who had subsequent pregnancies after breast cancer treatment. They had a good survival, similar to the control group, but one must wonder about the several hundred women who went unreported and who had subsequent pregnancies after being treated for breast cancer.

In their 1989 article, the most recent report on this topic, Clark and Chua[74] updated the Toronto patients reported by Peters and Meakin in 1965.[17] The question about the denominator of the total number of women with subsequent pregnancies after breast cancer treatment is applicable here. Clark and Chua[74] commented in their introduction that "1500 new patients with breast cancer annually" were seen at their institution, and one third that number was seen in 1958. Although tabulation cannot be performed from these numbers, the reported 136 breast cancer patients with subsequent pregnancies over 50 years probably represents a small proportion.

In summary, the effect of subsequent pregnancy on breast cancer prognosis is uncertain, since the reported patients probably represent a small and selectively obtained group of patients from any institution.

MANAGEMENT SUMMARY

- Modified radical mastectomy is the preferred local management of breast cancer during pregnancy. There is much experience about pregnancy and general anesthesia as a result of the more than 50,000 various surgical procedures performed annually on pregnant women.
- Radiation therapy should be avoided during any trimester because of the dose (mainly due to internal scatter) that is absorbed by the fetus. Limited breast resection during pregnancy with radiation therapy delayed until after delivery has been recently suggested. There are not yet any reports on the local recurrence rates or survival rates with such a breast-conservation schedule.
- Therapeutic abortion cannot be proved beneficial in patient series. The existing reports are inadequate, however, since they are based on small numbers and employ patient selection in which women with more advanced disease appear more likely to undergo abortion. The value of therapeutic abortion is uncertain, with the exception that breast cancer treatment is greatly simplified with no concern of fetal effects from the treatment modalities.
- Chemotherapy during pregnancy must be considered on a case-by-case basis because of the risk of fetal damage, particularly early in pregnancy. If the patient is in the third trimester, it is often best to postpone chemotherapy until after full-term delivery, early delivery by induction of labor, or cesarean section. There is no absolute contraindication to most chemotherapeutic agents during the latter half of the pregnancy, however. Some patients choose this approach after being fully informed of the potential advantages and disadvantages.

References

1. Wallack MK, Wolf JA Jr, Bedwinek J, et al. Gestational carcinoma of the female breast. Curr Probl Cancer 1983;7:1.
2. Saunders CM, Baum M. Breast cancer and pregnancy: a review. J R Soc Med 1993;86:162.
3. Anderson JM. Mammary cancers and pregnancy. BMJ 1979;1:1124.
4. Allen HH, Nisker JA. Cancer in pregnancy: therapeutic guidelines. In: Allen HH, Nisker JA, eds. Cancer in pregnancy: an overview. New York, Futura, 1988:3.
5. Moolgavkarsh, Day NE, Stevens RG. Two-stage model for carcinogenesis: epidemiology of breast cancer in females. J Natl Cancer Inst 1980;65:559.
6. Guinee VF, Olsson H, Moller T, et al. Effects of pregnancy on prognosis for young women with breast cancer. Lancet 1994;343:1587.
7. de la Rochefordiere A, Asselain B, Campana F, et al. Age as prognostic factor in premenopausal breast carcinoma. Lancet 1993;341:1039.
8. Adami HO, Malker B, Holmberg L, et al. The relationship between survival and age at diagnosis in breast cancer. N Engl J Med 1986;315:559.
9. Kilgore AR, Bloodgood JC. Tumors and tumor-like lesions of the breast in association with pregnancy. Arch Surg 1029;18:2079.
10. Haagensen CD, Stout AP. Carcinoma of the breast: criteria of operability. Ann Surg 1943;118:859, 1032.
11. White TT. Carcinoma of the breast and pregnancy. Ann Surg 1954;139:9.
12. Harrington SW. Carcinoma of the breast: results of surgical treatment when the carcinoma occurred in course of pregnancy or lacation and when pregnancy occurred subsequent to operation, 1910–1933. Ann Surg 1937;106:690.
13. Byrd BF, Bayer DS, Robertson JC, et al. Treatment of breast tumors associated with pregnancy and lactation. Ann Surg 1962;155:940.
14. Bunker ML, Peters MV. Breast cancer associated with pregnancy or lactation. Am J Obstet Gynecol 1963;85:312.
15. Montgomery TL. Detection and disposal of breast cancer in pregnancy. Am J Obstet Gynecol 1961;81:926.
16. Miller HK. Cancer of the breast during pregnancy and lactation. Am J Obstet Gynecol 1962;83:607.
17. Peters VM, Meakin JW. The influence of pregnancy in carcinoma of the breast. Prog Clin Cancer 1965;1:471.
18. Mickal A, Torres JE, Mule JG. Carcinoma of breast in pregnancy and lactation. Am Surg 1963;29:509.

19. Rosemond GP. Carcinoma of the breast during pregnancy. Clin Obstet Gynecol 1963;6:994.

20. DeVitt JE, Beattie WG, Stoddart TG. Carcinoma of the breast and pregnancy. Can J Surg 1964;7:124.

21. Holleb AI, Farrow JH. The relation of carcinoma of the breast and pregnancy in 283 patients. Surg Gynecol Obstet 1962;115:65.

22. Applewhite RR, Smith LR, DeVicenti F. Carcinoma of the breast associated with pregnancy and lactation. Am Surg 1973;39:101.

23. Crosby CH, Barclay THC. Carcinoma of the breast: surgical management of patients with special conditions. Cancer 1971;28:1628.

24. Clark RM, Reid J. Carcinoma of the breast in pregnancy and lactation. Int J Radiat Oncol Biol Phys 1978;4:693.

25. Petrek JA, Dukoff R, Rogatko A. Prognosis of pregnancy-associated breast cancer. Cancer 1991;67:869.

26. King RM, Welch JS, Martin JL, et al. Carcinoma of the breast associated with pregnancy. Surg Gynecol Obstet 1985;160:228.

27. Ribiero GG, Jones DA, Jones M. Carcinoma of the breast associated with pregnancy. Br J Surg 1986;73:607.

28. Deemarsky LJ, Neishtadt EL. Breast cancer and pregnancy. Breast 1980;7:17.

29. Tretli S, Kvalheim G, Thoresen S, et al. Survival of breast cancer patients diagnosed during pregnancy or lactation. Br J Cancer 1988;58:382.

30. Zemlickis D, Lishner M, Degendorfer P, et al. Maternal and fetal outcome after breast cancer in pregnancy. Am J Obstet Gynecol 1992;166:781.

31. Ishida T, Yokoe T, Kasumi F, et al. Clinicopathologic characteristics and prognosis of breast cancer patients associated with pregnancy and lactation: analysis of case-control study in Japan. Jpn J Cancer Res 1992;83:1143.

32. Boice JD Jr. Fetal risk to radiotherapy and chemotherapy exposure in utero. Cancer Bull 1986;38:293.

33. Hall EJ. Effects of radiation on the developing embryo. In: Hall EJ, ed. Radiobiology for the radiologist. New York, Harper & Row, 1973:231.

34. Miller R, Mulvihill S. Small head size after atomic radiation. Teratology 1976;14:355.

35. Orr JW, Shingleton HM. Cancer in pregnancy. Curr Probl Cancer 1983;8:1.

36. Miller RW. Epidemiological conclusions from radiation toxicity studies. In: Late effects of radiation. London, Taylor & Francis, 1970.

37. Miller RW. Transplacental carcinogenesis. Cancer Bull 1986;38:300.

38. Brent RL. The effects of ionizing radiation, microwaves, and ultrasound on the developing embryo: clinical interpretations and applications of the data. Curr Probl Pediatr 1984;14:61.

39. Mossman KL, Hill LT. Radiation risks in pregnancy. Obstet Gynecol 1982;60:237.

40. Baker J, Ali A, Groch MW, et al. Bone scanning in pregnant patients with breast carcinoma. Clin Nucl Med 1987;12:519.

41. Harbert JC. Efficacy of bone and liver scanning in malignant disease: facts and options. In: Nuclear medicine annual. New York, Raven, 1982.

42. Adzick NS, Harrison MR. The unborn surgical patient. Curr Probl Surg 1994;31:1.

43. Mattison DR, Angtuaco T. Magnetic resonance imaging in prenatal diagnosis. Clin Obstet Gynecol 1988;31:353.

44. National Council on Radiation Protection and Measurements. Report #39: basic radiation protection criteria. Washington, DC, NCRP, 1971.

45. Woo SY, Fuller LM, Cundiff JH, et al. Radiotherapy during pregnancy for clinical stages IA–IIA Hodgkin's disease. Int J Radiat Oncol Biol Phys 1992;23:407.

46. Veronesi U, Luini A, Del Vecchio M, et al. Radiotherapy after breast-preserving surgery in women with localized cancer of the breast. N Engl J Med 1993;328:1587.

47. Garber JE. Long-term follow-up of children exposed in utero to antineoplastic agents. Semin Oncol 1989;16:437.

48. O'Dell RF. Leukemia and lymphoma complicating pregnancy. Clin Obstet Gynecol 1979;22:859.

49. Pizzuto J, Aviles A, Noreiga L, et al. Treatment of acute leukemia during pregnancy: presentation of nine cases. Cancer Treat Rep 1980;64:679.

50. Sanz MA, Rafecas FJ. Successful pregnancy during chemotherapy for acute promyelocytic leukemia. N Engl J Med 1982;306:939.

51. Williamson RA, Karp LE. Azathioprene teratogenicity: review of the literature and case report. Obstet Gynecol 1981;58:247.

52. Sweet DL, Kinzie J. Consequences of radiotherapy and antineoplastic therapy for the fetus. J Reprod Med 1976;17:241.

53. Caligiuri MA, Mayer RJ. Pregnancy and leukemia. Semin Oncol 1989;16:388.

54. Reynoso EE, Shepherd FA, Messner HA, et al. Acute leukemia during pregnancy: the Toronto leukemia study group experience with long-term follow-up of children exposed in utero to chemotherapeutic agents. J Clin Oncol 1987;5:1098.

55. Willemse PHB, van der Sude, Sleufer DT. Combination chemotherapy and radiation for stage IV breast cancer during pregnancy. Gynecol Oncol 1990;36:281.

56. Turchi JJ, Villasis C. Anthracyclines in the treatment of malignancy in pregnancy. Cancer 1988;61:435.

57. Karp GI, von Oeyen P, Valone F, et al. Doxorubicin in pregnancy: possible transplacental passage. Cancer Treat Rep 1983;67:773.

58. d'Incalci M, Broggini M, Buscaglia M, et al. Transplacental passage of doxorubicin. Lancet 1983;1:75.

59. Doll DC, Ringenberg S, Yarbro JW. Antineoplastic agents and pregnancy. Semin Oncol 1989;16:337.

60. Nicholson HO. Cytotoxic drugs in pregnancy. J Obstet Gynecol Br Emp 1988;75:307.

61. Schapira DV, Chudley AE. Successful pregnancy following continuous treatment with combination chemotherapy before conception and throughout pregnancy. Cancer 1984;54:800.

62. Zemlickis D, Lishner M, Degendorfer P, et al. Fetal outcome after in utero exposure to cancer chemotherapy. Arch Intern Med 1992;152:573.

63. Lipschultz SE, Colan SD, Gelber RD, et al. Late cardiac effects of doxorubicin therapy for acute lymphoblastic leukemia in childhood. N Engl J Med 1991;324:808.

64. Lipschultz SE, Colan SD. The use of echocardiography and holter monitoring in the assessment of anthracycline-treated patients. In: Green DM, D'Angio GJ, eds. Cardiac toxicity after treatment for childhood cancer. New York, Wiley-Liss, 1993;54.

65. Recht A, Come SE, Gelman RS, et al. Integration of conservation surgery, radiotherapy, and chemotherapy for the treatment of early-stage, node-positive breast cancer: sequencing, timing and outcome. J Clin Oncol 1991;9:1662.

66. Potter JF, Schoeneman M. Metastases of maternal cancer to the placenta and fetus. Cancer 1970;25:380.

67. Smythe AR, Underwood PB, Kreutner A. Metastatic placental tumors: report of three cases. Am J Obstet Gynecol 1973;125:1149.

68. Fox H. Non-trophoblastic tumors of the placenta. In: Fox H, ed. Pathology of the placenta. Philadelphia, WB Saunders, 1978:357.

69. Pedersen H, Finster M. Anesthetic risks in the pregnant surgical patient. Anesthesiology 1979;51:439.

70. Mazze RI, Kallen B. Reproductive outcome after anesthesia and operation during pregnancy: a registry study of 5405 cases. Am J Obstet Gynecol 1989;161:1178.

71. Haagensen CD. The treatment and results in cancer of the breast at

the Presbyterian Hospital, New York. Am J Roentgenol 1949; 62:328.

72. Adair FE. Cancer of the breast. Surg Clin North Am 1953;33:313.

73. Nugent P, O'Connell TX. Breast cancer and pregnancy. Arch Surg 1985;120:1221.

74. Clark RM, Chua T. Breast cancer and pregnancy: the ultimate challenge. Clin Oncol 1989;1:11.

75. Read LD, Greene GL, Katzenellenbogen BS. Regulation of estrogen receptor messenger ribonucleic acid and protein levels in human breast cancer cell lines by sex steroid hormones, their antagonists, and growth factors. Mol Endocrinol 1989;3:295.

76. Sakai F, Saez S. Existence of receptors bound to endogenous estradiol in breast cancers in premenopausal and postmenopausal women. Steroids 1976;27:99.

77. Sarrif WM, Durant JR. Evidence that estrogen-receptor-negative progesterone-receptor–positive breast and ovarian carcinoma contain estrogen receptor. Cancer 1981;48:1215.

78. Katzenellenbogen JA, Johnson HJ Jr, Carlson KE, et al. Studies on the uterine, cytoplasmic estrogen binding protein: thermal stability and ligand dissociation rate. An assay of empty and filled sites by exchange. Biochemistry 1973;12:4092.

79. Garola RE, McGuire WL. An improved assay for nuclear estrogen receptor in experimental and human breast cancer. Cancer Res 1977;37:3333.

80. Elledge RM, Ciocca DR, Langone G, et al. Estrogen receptor, and her-2/neu protein in breast cancers from pregnant patients. Cancer 1993;71:2499.

81. Boring CC, Squires TS, Tong T. Cancer statistics, 1993. CA Cancer J Clin 1993;43:7.

82. Ventura SJ. First births to older mothers 1970–1986. Am J Public Health 1989;79:1675.

83. Beatson GT. On the treatment of inoperable cases of carcinoma of the mamma: suggestions for a new method of treatment. Lancet 1896;2:162.

84. Danforth DN. How subsequent pregnancy affects outcome in women with a prior breast cancer. Oncology 1991;5:23.

85. Donegan WL. Pregnancy and breast cancer. Obstet Gynecol 1977;50:244.

86. Rissanen PM. Pregnancy following treatment of mammary carcinoma. Acta Radiol Ther Phy Biol 1969;8:415.

87. Cheek JH. Cancer of the breast in pregnancy and lactation. Am J Surg 1973;126:729.

88. Cooper DR, Butterfield J. Pregnancy subsequent to mastectomy for cancer of the breast. Ann Surg 1970;171:429.

89. Harvey JC, Rosen PP, Ashikari H, et al. The effect of pregnancy on the prognosis of carcinoma of the breast following radical mastectomy. Surg Gynecol Obstet 1981;153:723.

90. Mignot L, Morvan F, Berdah J, et al. Pregnancy after breast cancer: results of a case-control study. Presse Med 1986;15:1961.

91. Ariel I, Kempner R. The prognosis of patients who become pregnant after mastectomy for breast cancer. Int Surg 1989;74:185.

24.6

Occult Primary Cancer With Axillary Metastases

ALAIN FOURQUET ▪ ANNE DE LA ROCHEFORDIÈRE ▪ FRANÇOIS CAMPANA

Breast cancer can sometimes present as an isolated axillary adenopathy without any radiologically detectable breast tumor. These occult primary cancers are staged as T0, N1 (stage II in the UICC/AJC classification). This staging requires that proper clinical *and* mammographic investigations be done to rule out the presence of a small breast tumor. If this is accomplished, axillary metastases of occult breast primary cancer represent a rare clinical entity first described by Halsted in 1907.[1]

Frequency

The incidence of an occult primary tumor with axillary metastases is low. Incidence rates ranged from 0.3% to 0.8% of operable breast cancers in the largest reported series.[2–5] Some 300 cases have been reported in the published literature during the past 50 years. Because these series are limited and management policies have varied widely over this period, it is difficult to compare characteristics of the patients, management, and results of treatment. Interpretation of these comparisons should only be done with caution.

Of some 13,000 patients with nonmetastatic primary breast cancer registered in the Institut Curie data base be-

tween 1981 and 1993, 26 (0.2%) had tumors that presented as an isolated axillary adenopathy, a figure that seems slightly lower than those of other series. Many of these were in patients with suspicious mammograms.[2,6,7,8] Presumably, the recent use of higher-quality mammograms has decreased the rate of occult breast carcinoma and therefore the incidence of occult primary with axillary metastases.

The characteristics of the patients with T0, N1 breast cancer are similar to those of patients with typical stage II disease. The series from the Institut Curie included 49 patients treated between 1960 and 1993. This series represents an update from a previously published study.[9] The median patient age was 58 years (range, 36 to 79 years). Thirty patients (61%) were postmenopausal. Thirteen patients (26%) had family histories of breast cancer. Twenty-three patients (47%) had left axillary nodes and 26 (53%) had right axillary nodes. This predominant right laterality was also reported by Rosen and Kimmel[10] and Kemeny and colleagues.[11]

Diagnosis

AXILLARY ADENOPATHY

Isolated axillary adenopathy is a benign condition in most patients. Lymphomas are the most frequent malignant tumors.[12]

Adenocarcinoma in areas other than the breast include thyroid, lung, gastric, pancreatic, and colorectal cancer.[13] These tumors, however, probably do not have isolated axillary metastases as the only presentation of disease, and an extensive search for primary adenocarcinoma other than breast cancer is not recommended.[3,8,11] A thorough clinical examination and chest radiography may prove sufficient. Tumor markers may help in the diagnosis of metastatic colon or pancreatic cancers.

Axillary adenopathy usually consists of one or two involved nodes, sometimes with large diameters. The median axillary node size at presentation in the patients treated at the Institut Curie was 30 mm (range, 10 to 70 mm). The initial diagnosis of malignancy was achieved by node excision in 22 of 49 patients, by fine-needle aspiration in 19 patients, and by core needle biopsy (drill biopsy) in 8 patients.

A primary breast cancer located in the axillary tail of the breast may be confounded with an axillary node. The presence of normal lymph node structure on the pathologic sample usually leads to the diagnosis of metastasis to a lymph node. The recognition of a metastatic lymph node can, however, be difficult because of massive involvement with extension of the tumor into the axillary fat and disappearance of the lymphoid patterns.

BREAST CANCER

Bilateral mammography should always be performed in the presence of metastatic adenocarcinoma in an axillary lymph node. Baron and colleagues[2] reported an overall 44% accuracy in the diagnosis of occult breast cancer in a series of 34 patients in which only 9 were considered suspicious. Nonetheless, any suspicious mammographic image should be removed for pathologic analysis. Studies suggest that magnetic resonance imaging (MRI) of the breast may improve the accuracy of conventional mammography in detecting breast cancer. Promising results describing the use of MRI in characterizing nonpalpable but radiologically detectable breast lesions have been published.[14,15] The role of MRI in screening a clinically and mammographically normal breast has not been evaluated, however, and remains under investigation. Therefore, the systematic use of MRI in searching for a breast tumor in occult primary cancers with axillary adenopathy should not be recommended, except in the setting of controlled prospective evaluations.

In patients who have nonpalpable breast masses and normal mammograms, the mammary origin of a metastatic adenocarcinoma to an axillary lymph node cannot be established with certainty. Therefore, the diagnosis of occult breast cancer can only be highly presumed based on a bundle of elements including sex, age, isolated adenopathy, and histologic diagnosis of adenocarcinoma.

High estrogen or progesterone receptor levels found in the metastatic axillary nodes can help to confirm a primary breast tumor[16]; however, one series[2] reported that half of occult breast cancer cases were found to be negative for estrogen receptors. Because surgical excision of the palpable node was often the first diagnostic procedure, rarely was an attempt made to analyze the receptors by biochemical methods. In the Institut Curie series, receptor analysis was done in only 10 of the 49 tumors (20%) and was positive in 5 of 10. Immunohistochemical detection of hormone receptors can now be done in paraffin-embedded tissue.[17]

Natural History

After removal of an axillary adenopathy, a breast cancer eventually developed in the untreated breast in 20 of 53 patients (38%) described in the literature, with recurrence intervals ranging from 5 months to 64 months (Table 24.6-1). Patient samples were limited in these series, however, and follow-up periods varied widely.

The number of pathologically involved lymph nodes seen after axillary dissection is high. Rosen and Kimmel[10] reported a median of three involved nodes (range, 1 to 65 nodes) in 48 patients. Nineteen patients in the Institut Curie series had an axillary dissection as initial treatment. The median number of involved nodes was 4 (range, 1 to 15). Eleven of the 49 patients in the series had distant metastases: 3 (27%) in the brain, 5 (45%) in the liver, 1 as a cervical node, and 2 in multiple sites. None had isolated bone metastases. Seven patients had contralateral disease, which occurred in the contralateral breast alone in four patients. Of note, three patients had isolated contralateral axillary node metastases.

Treatment and Results

Mastectomy and axillary node dissection has been the most commonly used treatment in this group of patients. The combined analysis of 11 published series has shown that

TABLE 24.6-1
Occurrence of Breast Cancer in Nontreated Breasts

Investigators	Breast Failures/ Nontreated Breasts	Delay (mo)
Atkins & Wolff[18]	5/9	9 to 17
Ellerbroek et al[19]	5/9	NA
Feigenberg et al[7]	0/4	
Feuerman et al[20]	0/1	
Haagensen[4]	2/3	12, 24
Halsted[1]	2/3	12, 24
Kemeny et al[11]	0/7	
Klopp[21]	1/1	48
Van Ooijen[22]	3/14	16 to 56
Institut Curie	2/2	9 to 67

NA, not available.

breast cancer was found in the mastectomy specimens of 128 of 185 patients (69%; Table 24.6-2). Invasive tumors were found in 117 of 185 patients (63%). One study[19] reported that no tumor was found in any of 10 mastectomy samples. These data, along with the fact that nearly 40% of the patients who received no form of breast treatment will eventually have disease recurrence in the breast, support the recommendation to treat the breast when no tumor can be detected clinically or mammographically.

Two recent studies reported the results of breast-conserving treatment of T0, N1 cancer. The group from M.D. Anderson Cancer Center[19] treated 25 of 35 patients with breast preservation; the breast was irradiated in 16, and no breast treatment was given to 9. Breast recurrences occurred in 12% of the irradiated breast group and in 56% of the nonirradiated breast group. Survival did not differ between those who underwent mastectomy and those who did not. In the Memorial Sloan-Kettering series,[2] 7 of 35 patients had a breast-conserving treatment, with radiotherapy in 6. Five-year survival rates were similar between this group and patients who had a mastectomy. Of the 49 patients treated between 1960 and 1993 at the Institut Curie, 3 had mastectomies. Two patients underwent neither mastectomy nor breast irradiation. Both eventually had breast cancer at 9 months and 67 months, respectively. Forty-four patients received whole-breast irradiation (median dose, 60 Gy; range, 52 to 70 Gy). Breast recurrence occurred in 9 of 44 patients; the 8-year risk for ipsilateral breast recurrence was 9%. All patients who had disease recurrence were treated by mastectomy. The 8-year breast-preservation rate was 91%. The results of these studies therefore support the use of irradiation as an alternative to mastectomy.

After axillary node dissection, should irradiation be delivered to the remaining lymph nodes? Few data are available in the literature to support any treatment options. A substantial risk for nodal involvement of the upper axilla can be suspected, however, based on the fact that three or four involved nodes are expected to be found in half of the patients. In patients with axillary node involvement associated with an invasive breast cancer, irradiation of the upper axilla is typically delivered when four or more nodes are involved.[24] Therefore, by analogy with other stage II tumors, irradiation of the upper axilla can be recommended in these instances. Forty-eight of 49 patients treated at the Institut Curie received nodal irradiation. In most instances, only the upper axilla and supraclavicular nodes were treated after complete axillary nodal dissection, whereas the whole axilla was treated when a simple adenectomy had been performed. There were three axillary node recurrences. One was isolated, but two of three were associated with a breast recurrence. The indications for internal mammary node irradiation are currently debated for patients with a breast mass and central or medial tumor or axillary involvement. Recommendations about treatment of the internal mammary nodes in patients with occult primary tumors and axillary adenopathy are difficult to formulate, because the evaluation of internal mammary node irradiation in this rare form of breast cancer is impossible on the basis of limited retrospective series. Because the location of the primary tumor is unknown, the Institut Curie policy supports irradiation of the internal mammary nodes in all patients.

The reported 5-year actuarial survival rates after treatment of occult breast cancer with axillary metastases range from 36% to 79% (Table 24.6-3). The 5-year survival rate estimate in the 49 patients treated at the Institut Curie was 80% with a median follow-up of 109 months (range, 9 to 383 months). The survival rate was 77% at 8 years. These figures seem higher than those observed after treatment of patients with stage II disease and detectable breast tumor. This has been emphasized by several authors.[3,5,11,20]

TABLE 24.6-2
Pathologic Report After Mastectomy

Investigators	Years	Patients With Mastectomy	In Situ Carcinoma	Invasive Carcinoma	Carcinoma (%)
Ashikari et al[6]	1946–75	34	3	20	67
Bhatia et al[16]	1977–85	11	2	9	100
Baron et al[2]	1975–78	28	4	16	71
Ellerbroek et al[19]	1956–87	10	0	0	0
Feigenberg et al[7]	1971–74	4	0	3	80
Feuerman et al[20]	1949–61	2	0	1	50
Fitts et al[3]	1948–63	11	0	7	70
Haagensen[4]	1916–66	13	0	12	92
Kemeny et al[11]	1973–85	11	2	3	45
Owen et al[5]	1907–50	27	0	25	92
Patel et al[8]	1952–79	29	0	16	60
Weigenberg & Stetten[23]	1937–48	5	0	5	100

TABLE 24.6-3
*Five-Year Survival Rates for Patients
With Occult Breast Carcinoma*

Investigators	Patients	Follow-Up (mo)	Actuarial Survival Rate (%)
Ashikari et al[6]	42	NA	79
Baron et al[2]	35	58 (mean)	75
Ellerbroek et al[19]	35	121 (mean)	68
Feuerman et al[20]	47	NA	36★
Kemeny et al[11]	18	NA	57
Institut Curie	49	109 (median)	80

NA, not available.

★ Crude survival rate.

However, these survival rate estimates are derived from small series of patients with various durations of follow-up and heterogeneous treatment modalities. Rosen and Kimmel[10] attempted to evaluate the results more precisely by matching a series of 48 patients with occult breast primary and axillary node metastases with a series of patients with stage II breast cancer who presented with palpable breast tumors (T1, N1 and T2, N1). Although the difference was not statistically significant, higher overall survival and size- or node status–adjusted survival rates were observed in the group of patients with occult primary tumors.

Reliable prognostic analyses are difficult to perform because of the multiple selection biases in the retrospective series and the small sample size. Rosen and Kimmel[10] showed that survival was determined by the number of axillary nodes involved, with patients with less than four involved nodes doing better than those with more than four nodes involved. Baron and colleagues[2] showed that estrogen receptor–positive patients fared better than estrogen receptor–negative patients. None of the factors analyzed in the series from the Institut Curie showed any influence on overall survival. Several prognostic factors appeared when the endpoint was the occurrence of distant metastases, however. Our findings corroborated those indicating that metastasis-free interval was shorter in patients with more than four involved axillary nodes: the 8-year metastasis-free intervals were 88% and 48%, respectively ($P = .02$). Postmenopausal patients had a higher metastasis-free interval than did premenopausal patients (86% versus 65%; $P < .05$).

Is there a role for adjuvant systemic treatment in patients with occult primary breast cancer? As mentioned previously, because of the rarity of this disease and the multiple selection biases, the efficacy of systemic therapy in patients with T0, N1 breast cancer is impossible to ascertain. By analogy with stage II, node-positive breast cancer, the general tendency is to use the same criteria

(ie, axillary node involvement) to prescribe systemic chemotherapy or hormone therapy. However, no data in the literature support this attitude, which may be disputable if one admits that occult primary tumors of the breast with axillary metastases have a better prognosis than other stage II cancers. Eighteen of the 49 patients treated at Institut Curie received adjuvant chemotherapy, with a regimen of cyclophosphamide, doxorubicin, and 5-fluorouracil. Patients who received chemotherapy were slightly younger and had more involved nodes than those who did not, but these differences were not statistically significant. The 5-year metastasis-free interval was 71%±24% in the 18 patients who received chemotherapy and 89%±12% in the 31 patients who did not ($P = .04$). This apparently detrimental effect of chemotherapy may be explained by the fact that, in this group of patients, chemotherapy did not reverse the adverse prognostic influence of massive nodal involvement. Little is known about the effect of hormone therapy in these patients. Of 10 patients who received tamoxifen for at least 2 years in the Institut Curie series, only 1 developed distant metastases 7 years after diagnosis. The numbers are too small to make significant statistical comparisons, but these results suggest that hormone treatment may be effective and support its use, at least in patients who have high hormone receptor levels.

The common policy in most institutions is to give adjuvant systemic therapy to patients with involved axillary nodes. Although the outcome of patients with occult primary and axillary metastases seems slightly better than that of patients with stage II node-positive breast cancer, this finding needs to be confirmed by larger series. Therefore, adjuvant systemic treatment should be given to such patients.

MANAGEMENT SUMMARY

Occult primary breast cancer presenting as an axillary lymph node is rare and represents a clinical entity with an outcome better than that of patients with stage II breast cancer and palpable mass and axillary involvement. The heterogeneity of treatment, as well as the limited number of patients studied in the published literature, makes it difficult to standardize treatment options.

However, several guidelines can be used:

- After the diagnosis of adenocarcinoma has been established by surgical removal of an isolated axillary mass, extensive work-up evaluation is not necessary. A thorough clinical examination, chest radiographs, bilateral mammograms, and tumor markers are sufficient to establish a high presumption of axillary metastases of mammary origin.
- An axillary dissection should be done to provide prognostic indicators (number of involved nodes) as well as sufficient material for hormone receptor dose.
- The breast should be treated. Breast-conserving treat-

ment by whole-breast irradiation to a dose of 50 to 55 Gy limits the risk for disease recurrence and is an alternative to mastectomy.

- Irradiation of the upper axilla and supraclavicular area, to a maximum dose of 45 Gy, is recommended in patients with more than three involved axillary nodes.
- By analogy to the indications for patients with stage II node-positive breast cancer (who always receive some type of adjuvant systemic treatment), adjuvant chemotherapy or hormone therapy should be given to patients with occult primary tumors with axillary metastases, even though their outcomes appear to be slightly better.

References

1. Halsted W. The results of radical operations for the cure of carcinoma of the breast. Ann Surg 1907;46:1.
2. Baron PL, Moore MP, Kinne DW, et al. Occult breast cancer presenting with axillary metastases: updated management. Arch Surg 1990;125:210.
3. Fitts WT, Steiner GC, Enterline HT. Prognosis of occult carcinoma of the breast. Am J Surg 1963;106:460.
4. Haagensen CD. The diagnosis of breast carcinoma. In: Haagensen CD. Diseases of the breast. Philadelphia, WB Saunders, 1971:486.
5. Owen HW, Dockerty MB, Gray HK. Occult carcinoma of the breast. Surg Gynecol Obstet 1954;98:302.
6. Ashikari R, Rosen PP, Urban JA, et al. Breast cancer presenting as an axillary mass. Ann Surg 1976;183:415.
7. Feigenberg Z, Zer M, Dinstman M. Axillary metastases from an unknown primary source: a diagnostic and therapeutic approach. Isr J Med Sci 1976;12:1153.
8. Patel J, Nemoto T, Rosner D, et al. Axillary lymph node metastasis from an occult breast cancer. Cancer 1981;47:2923.
9. Campana F, Fourquet A, Ashby MA, et al. Presentation of axillary lymphadenopathy without detectable breast primary (T0N1b breast cancer): experience at Institut Curie. Radiother Oncol 1989;15:321.
10. Rosen PP, Kimmel M. Occult breast carcinoma presenting with axillary lymph node metastases: a follow-up study of 48 patients. Hum Pathol 1990;21:518.
11. Kemeny MM, Rivera DE, Teri JJ, et al. Occult primary adenocarcinoma with axillary metastases. Am J Surg 1986;152:43.
12. Pierce EH, Gray HK, Dockerty MB. Surgical significance of isolated axillary adenopathy. Ann Surg 1957;145:104.
13. Copeland EM, McBride CM. Axillary metastases from unknown primary sites. Ann Surg 1973;178:25.
14. Boetes C, Mus RD, Barentsz JO, et al. Characterization of suspect breast lesions by using a gadolinium-enhanced dynamic TurboFlash substraction technique. (Abstract) Radiology 1993;189:405.
15. Gilles R, Lucidarme O, Meunier M, et al. Intraductal carcinomas: diagnosis by dynamic contrast-enhanced substraction MRI. (Abstract) Eur J Cancer 1994;30A(Supp 2):32.
16. Bhatia SK, Saclarides TJ, Witt TR, et al. Hormone receptor studies in axillary metastases from occult metastases. Cancer 1987;59:1170.
17. Pertschuk LP, Kim DS, Nayer K, et al. Immunocytochemical estrogen and progestin receptor assays in breast cancer with monoclonal antibodies: histopathologic, demographic and biochemical correlations and relationship to endocrine response and survival. Cancer 1990;66:1663.
18. Atkins H, Wolff B. The malignant gland in the hospital. Guys Hospital Rep 1960;1:109.
19. Ellerbroek N, Holmes F, Singletary E. Treatment of isolated axillary metastases in patients with an occult primary consistent with breast. (Abstract) Int J Radiat Oncol Biol Phys 1989;17(Suppl 1):178.
20. Feuerman L, Attie JN, Rosenberg B. Carcinoma in axillary lymph nodes as an indicator of breast cancer. Surg Gynecol Obstet 1962;114:5.
21. Klopp CT. Metastatic cancer of axillary lymph node without a demonstrable primary lesion. Ann Surg 1950;131:437.
22. Van Ooijen B. Axillary nodal metastases from an occult primary consistent with breast origin. (Abstract) Eur J Cancer 1993;29A(Suppl 6):S67.
23. Weigenberg HA, Stetten D. Extensive secondary axillary lymph node carcinoma without clinical evidence of primary breast lesion. Surgery 1951;29:217.
24. Harris JR, Recht A. Conservative surgery and radiotherapy. In: Harris JR, Hellman S, Henderson CI, et al, eds. Breast diseases, ed 2. Philadelphia, JB Lippincott, 1991:413.

24.7

Lymphedema

JEANNE A. PETREK ▪ ROBERT LERNER

Lymphedema is a common and troublesome problem: the cosmetic deformity cannot be disguised with normal clothing, physical discomfort and upper extremity disability are associated with the enlargement, and recurrent episodes of cellulitis and lymphangitis can be expected. Added to the physical symptoms is the distress caused unintentionally by clinicians interested in cancer recurrence, who trivialize the nonlethal nature of lymphedema. The appearance of arm swelling is more distressing than that of a mastectomy since the latter can be easily hidden, but the disfigured arm and hand are constant reminders of the disease to the woman herself and are a subject of curiosity to others.

About 15% to 20% of women experience lymphedema after breast cancer treatment. It is estimated that at least 1 to 2 million breast cancer survivors are alive today after lymphadenectomy and that 400,000 of them cope daily with the disfigurement, discomfort, and disability of arm and hand swelling.

Anatomy and Physiopathologic Factors

Large molecules that reach the interstitial space by filtration or cellular metabolism and secretion are not effectively removed except by the lymphatic system. If they accumulate, as in the case with obstructed transport due to axillary treatment, effective osmotic pressure develops and causes excessive fluid in the interstitial space, or lymphedema.[1] It has been estimated that almost half of the total circulating plasma protein is returned daily to the venous system through the lymphatic system by way of the thoracic duct.[2] Lymphatic vessels differ from blood vessels in that the basement membrane is virtually absent,[3] which probably allows for intercellular diffusion of plasma proteins and lipids that are too large for reabsorption through the venous system.[4] Normally, lymphatic pressure is zero or negative; it becomes positive with lymphedema.

The most superficial lymphatics, sometimes called *primary lymphatics,* are valveless and constitute a complex dermal network of capillary-like structures.[5] These drain into secondary lymphatics, larger subdermal channels with valves, that run roughly parallel with the superficial veins. The secondary lymphatics drain into a third deeper layer in the subcutaneous fat just above the fascia. The deeper subcutaneous lymphatics have valves and a muscular layer in the wall for active, unidirectional transport. Intramuscularly, a less elaborate system of lymphatics parallels the deep arteries and drains the muscle compartment. It is believed that the superficial and deep systems effectively function independently except in abnormal states.[5]

Presentation and Progression

Lymphedema is the result of a functional overload of the lymphatic system in which lymph volume exceeds transport capabilities. The build-up of interstitial macromolecules leads to an increase in oncotic pressure in the tissues, producing more edema. Persistent swelling and stagnant protein eventually lead to fibrosis and provide an excellent culture medium for repeated bouts of cellulitis and lymphangitis. With dilatation of the lymphatics, the valves become incompetent, causing further stasis. The muscle compartments below the deep fascia appear to be spared of the disease process.

Lymphedema can begin insidiously at variable periods after axillary treatment. It can range from a mild, barely noticeable swelling in the early stages to a seriously disabling enlargement later. The skin appears brawny because of the fibrosclerosis of the protein-rich fluid. With repeated episodes of cellulitis and lymphangitis, the skin becomes indurated, leathery, and hyperkeratotic.

In the presence of extensive axillary tumor involvement, a combination of venous and lymphatic obstruction can occur. Noninvasive studies, such as color flow Doppler to evaluate the axillary vein patency and computed tomography (CT) or magnetic resonance imaging (MRI) to evaluate bulky tumor involvement, may be useful. Invasive studies have almost no role: venography and lymphangiography results are unlikely to influence management, and they have high complication rates. Clodius[6] reported that the increase in swelling following lymphangiography was permanent in many patients. Rarely, the use of lymphoscintigraphy can be helpful if the diagnosis of lymphedema is in question.[7]

Assessment

Various methods have been used to measure the lymphedematous arm. The traditional method is a tape-measured arm circumference 10 cm below or 10 cm above either the olecranon or the lateral epicondyle. Such measurements vary according to the degree the soft tissues are constricted with the tape. Furthermore, it is wise to measure at least one location of the lower arm and two locations of the upper arm (instead of relying on a single value), since the shape of the arm can differ before and after swelling. Measurement of the arm volume by water displacement is more accurate and results in a single value, but the technique is unwieldy and infrequently used. Other more sophisticated methods (of little clinical use) include dichromatic differential absorptiometry[8] and CT scanning.[9]

No standard degree of enlargement constitutes lymphedema. Although a 2-cm difference between arms is the most common definition, such swelling could be severe in a thin arm and unnoticeable in others. Even natural variation sometimes allows up to a 2-cm greater circumference in the dominant and overused extremity.[10] Thus, it is important to measure both arms and to do so preoperatively if accurate lymphedema assessment is sought.

Nevertheless, about half of patients with documented minimal enlargement (1 to 2 cm) suffer symptoms of arm heaviness.[11] A simple mail questionnaire found that half of the patients who suffered arm swelling had never reported this problem to any physician.[12]

Incidence

The reported incidence of lymphedema varies greatly and depends in part on the methods used to define lymphedema, the completeness of the patient population follow-up, and the interval between axillary treatment and measurement. For example, in the early era, when the halstedian radical mastectomy and modified radical mastectomy were the only treatments for breast cancer, the incidence of lymphedema in a review by American investigators Britton and Nelson[13] ranged between 6.7% and 62.5% among nine reports; a similar review by British researchers Hughes and Patel[14] found a range of 41% to 70% among several reports.

In patients treated from 1988 to 1990 at Johns Hopkins University in Baltimore on cooperative group protocols,[15] the incidence of lymphedema was 16% (defined as a difference in circumference between arms of 2 cm or more) at more than 1 year after breast cancer treatment. With only 43% of patients evaluated, the lymphedema incidence may be higher, since patients may not return to the physician associated with the complication.

At Memorial Hospital in New York, 282 patients were measured for lymphedema at routine follow-up visit.[16] The median interval between treatment and measurement was 39 months (range, 7 to 109 months). The 5-year actuarial rate of lymphedema (defined as a circumference 2.5 cm larger on the treated side) was 16%.

With careful volumetric measurements, a report from the Royal Marsden[10] noted that 25.5% of the breast cancer patients who returned for follow-up over the course of 6 months had a more than 200-mL volume increase in the ipsilateral arm after axillary treatment. The interval between primary therapy and data collection was less than 5 years in 50%, 5 to 10 years in 30% and more than 10 years in 20%.

A report from Denmark on 57 consecutive patients who underwent modified radical mastectomy procedures reported a lymphedema incidence of 17% at a median follow-up of 42 months.[17] In the small number of patients available for analysis, the investigators concluded that chest wall radiation therapy increased the lymphedema incidence and that systemic chemotherapy did not.

The fact that the incidence of lymphedema continues with the newer techniques of breast conservation is suggested by the similar incidence of lymphedema when the more common treatment changed from radical mastectomy to modified radical mastectomy.[13–14] Furthermore, in three reports cited earlier,[10,15,16] most patients underwent breast conservation. In 1992, Ivens and colleagues[18] reported that 18% of 126 consecutive patients treated solely with breast conservation had measurable arm swelling after 4 years.

The incidence of lymphedema remains the same or may be higher with the use of breast conservation, since scatter radiation from the breast field can be absorbed at the level of the dissected axillary lymphatic tissue, and axillary radiation is known to be synergistic with axillary dissection in producing lymphedema.

In summary, the objective lymphedema incidence in six reports published within the past 10 years, as noted in Table 24.7-1, was about 20%.[10,15–19] The range was 16% to 25.5% of the study populations measured at various intervals after axillary dissection with arm circumferences or volumetric equipment. It is striking that the reported proportion of patients with lymphedema is similar, since these patients underwent different procedures for breast cancer treatment in three different countries.

Etiology

Almost all studies in previous decades and within the past 10 years find that the incidence and the degree of lymphedema are correlated to the general extent of surgical dissection.[10,18–23] In fact, the linear relation of lymphedema and the extent of dissection can be shown best when the extent of dissection is none, sampling (usually retrieving three to eight lymph nodes), or standard dissection.[20] Two large studies could not demonstrate a relation between extent of dissection and lymphedema.[16,24] This may have occurred because rather small differences in extent were assessed (eg, when the highest three to six lymph nodes were added to a standard dissection).[16]

Axillary radiation therapy to the dissected area was a strong predictor of lymphedema in all studies that evaluated the issue.[10,20,22,24] Beyond these two factors, a wide range of possible etiologic factors has not been evaluated systematically. Little agreement exists about the several variables that have been studied.

Older age at diagnosis was reported to be a significant factor in one study,[21] was unrelated to lymphedema incidence in another,[10] and curiously was not mentioned in others. In one report, there was a tendency to greater lymphedema when the dominant hand was on the operated side,[18] but another report could not confirm this.[10] Patient weight (height was not recorded) was a significant factor in two studies,[16,23] but obesity was not evaluated in other studies.

One study, which evaluated surgical technique, found a higher incidence of lymphedema when the pectoralis

TABLE 24.7-1
Incidence of Objective Lymphedema in Reports From 1986 to 1993

Investigator	Country	Total Patients	Patients With Lymphedema (%)	Follow-Up Median	Methods and Definitions of Lymphedema
Kissin et al[10]	England	200	25.5	5 y (1–10+ y)	Volumetric, >200 mL
Lin et al[15]	United States	122	16	1.5 y	Circumference, >2 cm
Werner et al[16]	United States	282	16	39 mo (7–109 mo)	Circumference, >2.5 cm
Ryttov et al[17]	Denmark	57	17	42 mo (32–48 mo)	Circumference, >2.5 cm
Ivens et al[18]	England	106	10	2 y	Volumetric, >200 mL
Pezner et al[19]	United States	74	14	14 mo (5–41 mo)	Circumference, >2 cm

muscle was split.[19] In a retrospective report that evaluated only postoperative fluid formation in 49 consecutive patients,[25] the authors found a correlation with lymphedema incidence, but other factors such as age, obesity, and extent of axillary surgery were not evaluated. Similar findings were reported in relation to seroma formation in an older retrospective study.[26]

Reasons for the scanty evaluation of lymphedema include (1) the prolonged course for development, (2) lack of contact with the original surgeon or the radiotherapist, and, most importantly, (3) as for other issues concerning the quality of life, lymphedema has been viewed as less important than the eradication of cancer and detection of recurrence. The last factor may be changing, since we now have a government award to systematically evaluate the incidence, time course, and etiologic factors in some 500 long-term survivors of a consecutively treated cohort.

Prevention

CONSIDERATIONS OF THE EXTENT OF AXILLARY TREATMENT

Because it is accepted that the magnitude of surgical dissection and the addition of axillary radiation are important factors in lymphedema development (and there is no agreement on other factors), it is crucial to individualize and optimize the extent of axillary treatment for each patient.

Axillary dissection is indicated for staging and local control, and for the potential influence (estimated to be small, probably about 5%) of unexcised positive nodes on overall survival rate. Several modern series with no dissection and radiation only of nonsuspicious axillae found low axillary failure rates of 2% to 5%.[27–29] One third of axillae that are clinically nonsuggestive, however, contain pathologically proven lymph node metastases.[30,31] Therefore, axillary dissection is a requisite for precise lymph node status, such as is required for systemic adjuvant therapy individualized by the number of positive nodes.

If a patient with nonsuggestive lymph nodes undergoes lumpectomy and is judged not to be a candidate for systemic therapy (perhaps because of advanced age or severe medical illnesses), either observation only with delayed nodal dissection if necessary or axillary radiation along with the breast is a reasonable option. If a patient undergoes general anesthesia and mastectomy, lymph node dissection of an appropriate extent should be included.

If a patient with breast cancer has clinically suspicious (or sometimes difficult-to-examine lymph nodes), the recommendation is different. The radiation dose required to control clinically suspicious lymph nodes is greater than that required to control subclinical (small) involvement and is associated with a greater incidence of complications and axillary recurrence. Axillary lymphadenectomy is indicated for local control (even when not necessary for staging) for clinically suspicious nodes.

In the United States, for the purposes of staging, no axillary dissection is currently recommended for patients with small areas of intraductal carcinoma (in which the incidence of positive lymph nodes is 1%) and a low axillary dissection for intraductal carcinoma, which is large, palpable, or possessing microinvasion of 1 to 2 mm (in which the positive node incidence may reach 5%). "Low" axillary dissection means level I, or somewhat less, perhaps preserving 1 cm of fatty tissue along the inferior vein to avoid the general area of the lymphatic trunks.

A level I or II dissection for staging is undertaken for typical invasive cancers. Even then, the scope of the dissection can be scaled to the disease. For a 1-cm invasive cancer, a level "I and ½," with preservation of 0.5 to 1 cm of tissue under the vein and the second intercostobrachial nerve can be appropriate. All three levels are suitable for a cancer with obviously positive lymph nodes. Although hardly foolproof, obtaining a frozen section on the largest or most suspicious lymph node can help confirm the clinical decision about the extent of axillary lymphadenectomy and can help tailor the operation to the disease.

For precise radiation technique, it is helpful to indicate the medial (highest) extent of the axillary dissection of every case with a radiopaque clip so that the surgical boundary is marked. The radiation therapist can then accurately avoid the dissected area, when, for example, the supraclavicular area is included for inner quadrant breast cancers.

PREVENTION AFTER AXILLARY TREATMENT

Because controlling lymphedema requires daily attention and since "curing" lymphedema has not been accomplished, emphasis must be placed on prevention. All patients are instructed in the same arm and hand care precautions, which may, however, be too severe for those at low risk and not aggressive enough for those at the highest risk. The scanty studies available have not defined the cause of lymphedema and its risk categories.

Because lymphedema development may occur even several decades after the axillary treatment,[32] all patients are admonished to follow these demanding precautions for the remainder of their lives. The precautions are related to two principles—not increasing lymph production (which is directly proportional to blood flow) and not further impeding the lymph transport through lymphatic channels. Heat such as that in a sauna or that caused by significant infections or vigorous arm exercise increases blood flow and thereby lymph production. Obstruction of lymph flow can result from tight arm garments, from repeated infections with ensuing fibrosis and stenosis of lymphatic vessels, and from an inactive arm held in a dependent position.

To avoid arm swelling and infection, the patient is instructed as follows:

1. Avoid vaccinations, injections, blood pressure monitoring, blood drawing, and intravenous administration in that arm.
2. Avoid puncturing or injuring the skin in any way. Use

meticulous skin, nail, and cuticle care. Pay immediate attention and use standard first-aid care on all small or large injuries. Use antibiotics liberally.

3. Avoid constricting sleeves or jewelry, and wear a padded bra strap to avoid constriction.
4. Avoid heat, including sunburns, tanning, baths, and saunas.
5. Avoid violent exercises and strenuous exertion. Participate in vigorous aerobic arm exercise only when the arm is supported by a antilymphedema compression garment or bandage.

Treatment

The treatment of established lymphedema varies from none at all to (particularly in the past) a host of aggressive surgical procedures. Between the extremes are various combined conservative treatments, the most important of which are compression garments, centripetal massage and exercises, pneumatic compression, and a program of complete (or complex) decongestive physiotherapy (CDP).

Therapeutic nihilism—that is, no treatment at all—is deplorable but common. Too often a woman is told that she "should be thankful to be alive" and that she "must learn to live with it." Once lymphedema is established, it is permanent and almost always progressive.[33] The sooner the treatment is started, the less treatment is required to prevent further progression.

CONSERVATIVE TREATMENT

Garments

Elevation is helpful in reducing swelling from lymphedema through use of gravity. It is impractical during the day, however, and the patient is unlikely to maintain the elevated position for long periods overnight.

A patient with lymphedema should be fitted with an elastic sleeve from wrist to axilla, especially after swelling reduction. If the hand is swollen, a glove with or without fingertips is necessary. The physician that prescribes the support garment should be aware of the different products available and order the proper compression class for each patient. These classes are as follows:

I   20 to 30 mmHg   III 40 to 50 mmHg
II 30 to 40 mmHg   IV   50 to 60 mmHg

For upper extremity lymphedema, a class II or III support is generally required.

The person measuring the lymphedematous arm and hand should be trained in fitting such garments and in instructing the patient in proper application. Too often, this task is left to a clerk in a surgical supply store who has no specific training and experience. A separate gauntlet or handpiece allows the patient to remove the glove to wash the hands without removing the entire sleeve.

Medications

Diuretics, widely prescribed in the United States for lymphedema, are both useless and detrimental.[33] Although they may be beneficial for high-body-sodium, low-protein edema, they are not effective in high-protein edemas such as lymphedema, since the high proteins in the interstitial space cause fluid retention. Although the diuretics can temporarily mobilize water, the osmotic pressure from the increased protein in the interstitial space causes rapid reaccumulation of edema.

Benzopyrones belong to a group of drugs that include the bioflavonoids and the coumarins. The former occur widely in nature, especially in fruits and vegetables. Benzopyrones improve chronic lymphedema[34] by stimulating macrophage activity for increased proteolysis and thereby removal of stagnant, excess protein in the tissue spaces, which results in less oncotic pressure and edema fluid.

A randomized, double-blind, placebo-controlled, crossover trial of 5,6-benzo-α-pyrone in 31 patients with lymphedema after axillary treatment has demonstrated its efficacy.[35] The patients received 400 mg of the active drug or placebo, each for 6 months. Although the effect was mild, it was statistically significant. In the drug group, the circumference of the arm was reduced from 17% above normal to 13% above normal ($P < .01$), and the volume was reduced from 46% above normal to 26% above normal ($P < .001$). There was no improvement, and sometimes worsening, in the placebo group.

There are several benzopyrones used clinically. None has been approved by the US Food and Drug Administration. Some of these are 5,6-benzo-α-pyrone, also known as Coumarin, 56-BaP, or 1,2-benzopyrone, ortho-β-hydroxyethyl-rutoside, marketed as HR, paroven, or troxerutin; venalot, a mixture of troxerutin and 56-BaP; and rutin. Although *coumarin* is the correct common chemical name of 5,6-benzo-α-pyrone, this agent is not an anticoagulant like its derivatives, the bis-4-hydroxycoumarins.

Several European and Australian researchers[34-37] have concluded that 5,6-benzo-α-pyrone produces a slow reduction of lymphedema and that the drugs should be included in physical rehabilitation programs. The benzopyrones are relatively nontoxic and have no effect on blood coagulation. Two to 5% of patients complain of gastrointestinal disturbances, which can be minimized by taking the medication with meals.

The modern pneumatic compression devices are pumps that provide gradient pressures and sequential rhythmic pumping from distal to proximal to milk the fluid out of the extremity. The various devices have been shown to be effective in many studies.[38-40] Although theoretically attractive to use machinery for the pumping action on the arm lymphatics, lymphedema actually involves the whole quarter of the ipsilateral trunk, the area in addition to the arm that the obstructed axillary channels would normally drain. Forcing protein-rich edema fluid toward the shoulder, an area already congested, may be the reason for failure of long-term improvement of some patients. In particular, pneumatic compression therapy appears less useful in advanced lymphedema, possibly because of the greater skin thickening and fibrosis of deeper tissues.

Complete (or Complex) Decongestive Physiotherapy

Widely available in Europe for many years, CDP takes into account the fact that lymphedema exists in an entire body quadrant, although it is most noticeable and distressing in the arm and hand. Professor Foeldi and others are credited with explaining the pathophysiology of lymphostasis and demonstrating the superiority of CDP[41-43] to the medical community.

CDP must be done by skilled, specially trained therapists. During phase I (treatment phase), the patient is given one or two daily 75-minute treatments over 1 to 4 weeks. Lymphedema should be treated as early as possible to prevent further progression and to avoid infections and other complications. The earlier the treatments are begun, the fewer are needed and the easier it is to achieve an excellent result.

In phase II, the maintenance phase, the patient maintains and optimizes the results by applying some of the techniques learned in the treatment phase: wearing an elastic sleeve during the day, bandaging the affected limb overnight, and doing a series of exercises for 10 minutes twice a day while wearing the bandages. Phase II is continued indefinitely or until the limb is no longer enlarged. Patients are reevaluated every 6 months to assess progress and to measure for a new elastic sleeve.

Each CDP treatment (phase I) consists of four steps:

1. Meticulous skin and nail care, including the eradication of any infection.
2. Manual lymph drainage, a delicate massage technique that stimulates lymph vessels to contract more frequently and that channels lymph and edema fluid toward adjacent, functioning lymph basins. Manual lymph drainage begins with stimulation of the lymph vessels and nodes in adjacent basins (neck, contralateral axilla, ipsilateral groin), which is followed by manual decongestion, in segmental order, of the involved trunk, shoulder, arm, forearm, wrist, and hand. Edema fluid and obstructed lymphatics are made to drain toward the venous angle, toward functioning lymph basins across the midline of the body, down toward the groin, over the top of the shoulder, around the back, and so forth.
3. Compression bandaging is done immediately after manual lymph drainage. Bandages are applied from the fingertips to the axilla with maximal pressure distally and minimal pressure proximally. This is done by using many layers of minimally elastic cotton bandages beneath which layers of foam rubber are inserted to ensure uniform pressure distribution or to increase pressure in areas that are particularly fibrotic. The bandage does not constrict blood flow but increases diminished skin and interstitial pressures. This prevents any reaccumulation of evacuated edema fluid and also prevents the ultrafiltration of additional fluid into the interstitial space.
4. The bandaged patient is next guided through a series of remedial exercises with the muscles and joints functioning within a closed space. The exercises increase lymph flow in all available lymph channels and in collateral pathways that are used to make the passage to the venous angle.

CDP has been used in thousands of patients in specialty clinics in New York City and Princeton for the past 5 years. Since then, other CDP clinics have opened in Cleveland, San Antonio, Fort Worth, Miami, and many other cities. Physical therapists are being trained to master the CDP techniques at the Princeton center and by various schools in Europe and Australia.

CDP is safe, noninvasive, and effective. It is also cost-effective, since it ultimately transfers the burden of care from clinic to patient. It does not cure the lymphedema but restores the limb to normal or near-normal. CDP also trains patient and family to continue the maintenance at home, to prevent any progression of the lymphedema, and to further improve lymphatic circulation.

SURGICAL PROCEDURES

Many operations have been used in the past century to improve the status of a lymphedematous upper limb. Philosophically, these can be loosely grouped as re-creation or imitation of lymphatic channels, bridging of the lymphedematous area to normal lymphatic areas, and resection or debulking of lymphedematous tissue.

The most biologically based concept, re-creation of lymph channels, is composed of older procedures, such as Handley's 1908 operation[44] involving implantation of threads in the attempt to form new lymph channels, to the newest microsurgical techniques of lymphovenous anastomosis,[33,45-48] lymph vessel transplantation,[49] and the interposition of small caliber veins to replace scarred or absent lymph vessels.[50]

Numerous bridging operations have been designed. Kondoleon[51] advised excision of the deep fascia to improve drainage between a patent deep lymphatic system and an obstructed superficial system. Thompson[52] surgically implanted deepithelialized dermis into the deep muscle compartment so that obstructed lymph channels might drain freely into normal deep lymphatics, the so-called buried dermal flap. Goldsmith[53,54] used transposed greater omentum for lymph transport from obstructed basins.

Resections involving debulking of the greatly expanded subcutaneous tissue (with or without the skin) down to the level of the muscle fascia have been attempted, often worsening the lymphedema. These include the Charles, Homans, and Sistrunk operations.[12,55] In this decade, there has been a renewal of interest in resections, with the trial of liposuction[56] for lymphedema. Although no follow-up studies have been offered, it is unlikely that liposuction will be any more successful than the previous resective procedures. The ultimate resective procedure, which has been used only as a last resort, is amputation.[57]

Summary

Because managing the disabling symptoms of lymphedema requires daily attention, and since curing of lymphedema has not been accomplished, emphasis must be placed on prevention. Measures to control lymphedema include centripetal massage, elevation, a custom-made compression garment, intermittent pneumatic compression equipment, the program of CDT popularized in Europe, and oral benzopyrones, which are mildly effective but which have not yet been released in the United States. The list of the diverse multiple operations attempted for this incapacitating condition in the past decades suggests one fact: none is successful.

There are no specific guidelines regarding the sequenced use of various modalities discussed in this chapter for lymphedema treatment. The use of the modalities depends on their availability, their effectiveness in a particular situation and the interest of the patient in following through with that technique. It is of great benefit, however, to begin treatment and thereby to control early lymphedema. Otherwise, there is progression to moderate and severe lymphedema, at which time treatment is more difficult and less effective.

Choices with mild lymphedema include the CDT program and elevation and a sleeve. The options for severe lymphedema are CDT and a combination of modalities in whatever fashion appears most effective by the supervising rehabilitation specialist.

References

1. Cragg PA. Cardiovascular system. In: Bray JJ, Cragg PP, Macknight ADC, et al. eds. Lecture notes human physiology, ed 2. Boston, Blackwell Scientific, 1989:371.
2. Witte MH, Honto D, Witte CL. Clinical and experimental techniques to study the lymphatic system. Vasc Surg 1977;11:20.
3. Mayerson HS. On lymph and lymphatics. Circulation 1963;28:839.
4. Patterson RM, Ballard CL, Wasserman K, et al. Lymphatic permeability to albumen. Am J Physiol 1958;194:120.
5. Crockett DJ. Lymphatic anatomy and lymphedema. Br J Plast Surg 1965;18:12.
6. Cloduis L. In: lymphedema. Stuttgart, Georg Thieme, 1977:155.
7. Golueke PJ, Montgomery RA, Petronis JD, et al. Lymphoscintigraphy to confirm the clinical diagnosis of lymphedema. J Vasc Surg 1989;10:306.
8. Bolin FP, Preuss LE, Beninson J. Di-chromatic differential absorptiometry for assessment of lymphedema. Int J Nucl Med Biol 1980;7:449.
9. Stewart G, Hurst PAE, Thomas ML, et al. CAT scanning in the management of the lymphedematous limb. Immun Haematol Res 1988;2:241.
10. Kissen MW, della Rovere QG, Easton D, et al. Risk of lymphedema following the treatment of breast cancer. Br J Surg 1986;7:580.
11. Brennan MJ. Lymphedema following the surgical treatment of breast cancer: a review of pathophysiology and treatment. J Pain Sympt Manage 1992;7:110.
12. McCaffrey JF. Lymphedema: its treatment. In: Paterson AHG, Lees AW, eds. Fundamental problems in breast cancer. Boston, Martinus Nijhoff, 1987,259.
13. Britton RC, Nelson PA. Causes and treatment of post-mastectomy lymphedema of the arm: report of 114 cases. JAMA 1962;180:95.
14. Hughes JH, Patel AR. Swelling of the arm following radical mastectomy. Br J Surg 1966;53:4.
15. Lin PP, Allison DC, Wainstock J, et al. Impact of axillary lymph node dissection on the therapy of breast cancer patients. J Clin Oncol 1993;11:1536.
16. Werner RS, McCormick B, Petrek JA, et al. Arm edema in conservatively managed breast cancer: obesity is a major predictive factor. Radiology 1991;180:177.
17. Ryttov N, Holm NV, Qvist N, et al. Influence of adjuvant irradiation on the development of late arm lymphedema and impaired shoulder mobility after mastectomy for carcinoma of the breast. Acta Oncol 1988;27:667.
18. Ivens D, Hoe AL, Podd CR, et al. Assessment of morbidity from complete axillary dissection. Br J Cancer 1992;66:136.
19. Pezner RD, Patterson MP, Hill LR, et al. Arm lymphedema in patients treated conservatively for breast cancer: relationship to patient age and axillary node dissection technique. Int J Radiat Oncol Biol Phys 1986;12:2079.
20. Yeoh EK, Denham JW, Davies SA, et al. Primary breast cancer. Acta Radiol Oncol 1986;25:105.
21. Delouche G, Bachelot F, Premont M, et al. Conservation treatment of early breast cancer: long-term results and complications. Int J Radiat Oncol Biol Phys 1987;13:29.
22. Aitken RJ, Gaze MN, Rodger A, et al. Arm morbidity within a trial of mastectomy and either nodal sample with selective radiotherapy or axillary clearance. Br J Surg 1989;76:568.
23. Larson D, Weinstein M, Goldberg I, et al. Edema of the arm as a function of the extent of axillary surgery in patients with stage I–II carcinoma of the breast treated with primary radiotherapy. Int J Radiat Oncol Biol Phys 1986;12:1575.
24. Dewar JA, Sarrazin D, Benhamou E, et al. Management of the axilla in conservatively treated breast cancer: 592 patients treated at Institut Gustave-Roussy. Int J Radiat Oncol Biol Phys 1987;13:475.
25. Tadych K, Donegan WL. Postmastectomy seromas and wound drainage. Surg Gynecol Obstet 1987;165:483.
26. West JP, Ellison JB. A study of the causes and prevention of edema of the arm following radical mastectomy. Surg Gynecol Obstet 1959;109:359.
27. Recht A, Pierce SM, Abner L, et al. Regional nodal failure after conservative surgery and radiotherapy for early-stage breast carcinoma. J Clin Oncol 1991;9:988.
28. Halverson KJ, Taylor ME, Perez CA, et al. Regional nodal management and patterns of failure following conservative surgery and radiation therapy for stage I and II breast cancer. Int J Radiat Oncol Biol Phys 1993;26:593.
29. Sarrazin D, Le M, Arriagada R, et al. Ten year results of a randomized trial comparing a conservative treatment to mastectomy in early breast cancer. Radiother Oncol 1989;14:177.
30. Kinne DW. Primary treatment of breast cancer: surgery. In: Harris JR, Hellman S, Henderson IC, eds. Breast diseases, ed 2. Philadelphia, JB Lippincott, 1991:347.
31. Haagensen CD: Diseases of the breast, ed 3. Philadelphia, WB Saunders, 1986:658.
32. Brennan MJ, Weitz J. Lymphedema 30 years after radical mastectomy. Am J Phys Med Rehabil 1992;71:12.
33. Lerner R, Requena R. Upper extremity lymphedema secondary to mammary cancer treatment. Am J Clin Oncol 1986;9:481.
34. Casley-Smith JR, Gaffney RM. Excess plasma proteins as a cause of chronic inflammation and lymphedema. J Pathol 1981;133:243.
35. Casley-Smith JR, Morgan RG, Piller NB. Treatment of lymphedema of the arms and legs with 5,6-benzo-[alpha]-pyrone. N Engl J Med 1993;16:329.

36. Piller NB, Clodius L. The role of the mononuclear phagocytic system in lymphedema, etc. Lymphologic 1980;4:35.

37. Cluzan R, Miserey G, Alliot F. Principles and results of physiotherapeutic therapy in mechanical lymphatic insufficiency of secondary or primary nature. Phlebologie 1988;41:401.

38. Zelikovski A, Deutsch A, Reiss R. The sequential pneumatic compression device in surgery for lymphedema of the limbs. J Cardiovasc Surg 1983;24.

39. Richmand DM, O'Donnell TF, Zelikovski A. Sequential pneumatic compression for lymphedema. Arch Surg 1985;120:1116.

40. Bastien MR, Goldstein BG, Lesher JL Jr, et al. Treatment of lymphedema with a multicompartmental pneumatic compression device. J Am Acad Dermatol 1989;20:853.

41. Foeldi E, Foeldi M, Clodius L. The lymphedema chaos. Lancet Ann Pl Surg 1989;22:6.

42. Foeldi M. Treatment of lymphedema. (Editorial) Lymphology 1994;27:1.

43. Foeldi E, Foeldi M, Weissleder H. Conservative treatment of lymphedema of the limbs. Angiol J Vasc Diseases 1985;36:171.

44. Handley WS. Lymphangioplasty. Lancet 1908;1:783.

45. Degni M. New microsurgical technique of lymphaticovenous anastomosis for treatment of lymphedema. Lymphology 1981;14:G1.

46. Laine HB, Howard JM. Experimental lymphaticovenous anastomosis. Surg Forum 1963;14:111.

47. Nielubowicz J, Olszewski W. Surgical lymphaticovenous shunts in patients with secondary lymphedema. Br J Surg 1968;55:440.

48. O'Brien BM, Mellow CG, Khazanchi RK, et al. Long-term results after microlymphatico-venous anastomoses for the treatment of obstructive lymphedema. Plast Reconstr Surg 1990;85:562.

49. Baumeister RG, Siuda S. Treatment of lymphedemas by microsurgical lymphatic grafting: what is proved? Plast Reconstr Surg 1988;85:64.

50. Campisi C. The autologous vein grafts in reconstructive microsurgery for lymph stasis. In: Olszewski WL, ed. Lymph stasis: pathophysiology, diagnosis and treatment. Boca Raton, CRC, 1991.

51. Kondoleon E. Die chirurgische Behandlung der elefantiastischen Oedema durch eine neue Methode der Lymphableiatung. Muench Med Wochyschr 1912;59:2726.

52. Thompson N. The surgical treatment of advanced postmastectomy lymphedema of the upper limb. Scand J Plast Reconstr Surg 1969;3:56.

53. Goldsmith HS. Long-term evaluation of omental transposition for chronic lymphedema. Ann Surg 1974;180:847.

54. Goldsmith HS, Los Santos R. Omental transposition in primary lymphedema. Surg Gynecol Obstet 1967;125:607.

55. Stone EJ, Hugo NE. Lymphedema. Surg Gynecol Obstet 1972;135:626.

56. O'Brien B, Khazanchi RK, Kumar PAV, et al. Liposuction in the treatment of lymphoedema: a preliminary report. Br J Plast Surg 1989;42:530.

57. Aitken DR, Minton JP. Complications associated with mastectomy. Surg Clin North Am 1983;63:1331.

24.8
Managing Menopausal Symptoms

RENA VASSILOPOULOU-SELLIN

Epidemiologic Considerations of Menopause After Breast Cancer

The rising incidence of breast cancer is due primarily to the increasing recognition of early-stage disease, including lesions in situ. The consequent expectation that therapy for patients with limited disease will result in improved disease-free and overall survival rates means that, among the growing population of aging women, an increasing number will have histories of breast cancer. The adverse health consequences of prolonged estrogen deficiency in older women and the need to develop appropriate therapeutic strategies to manage the symptoms of menopause are relatively recent medical concerns. Because many women now survive well into their eighth decade, their reproductive (estrogen-sufficient) lifespan represents a smaller percentage of their overall life expectancy. Many women now live for several decades without the benefit of ovarian estrogen. For most aging women who are long-term survivors of breast cancer and who are likely to remain in good health, the history of breast cancer recedes in importance over time. When other medical conditions arise, however, the prior diagnosis of breast cancer often creates special dilemmas in the choice of safe and effective treatments, particularly compared with the option of estrogen replacement therapy (ERT) in patients without cancer.

Health Consequences of Estrogen Deficiency

At the conclusion of the reproductive lifespan, ovarian estrogen production gradually decreases, usually after 50 years of age. During the subsequent decades, complex multisystem changes, attributable to estrogen deficiency, characterize the menopausal years[1] (Table 24.8-1). Hot flashes and vasomotor instability are the most frequent and distressing subjective developments, usually motivating women to seek treatment.[2,3] Genitourinary atrophy often leads to dyspareunia and may predispose patients to bladder infections.[4,5] The most serious health hazard for aging women, however, is the progressive increase in cardiovascular disease, which remains the leading cause of death among older women, with mortality exceeding that from all other causes including breast cancer.[6-9]

Accelerated bone loss also occurs in most aging wo-

TABLE 24.8-1
Physiologic Consequences of Estrogen Deprivation and Nonhormonal Treatment Alternatives

Estrogen Deficiency	Treatment Alternatives
Vasomotor instability	Bellergal, clonidine, progesterone, herbal remedies
Genitourinary atrophy	Topical estrogen creams
Dyspareunia	Vaginal lubricants
Osteoporosis prevention	Calcium, bisphosphonates, calcitonin, (?) fluoride
Cardiovascular disease dyslipidemia-related	Bile acid–binding resins, fibric acid derivatives, HMG-CoA reductase inhibitors, nicotinic acid, antioxidants

(Vassilopoulou-Sellin R. Estrogen replacement therapy in women at increased risk for breast cancer. Breast Cancer Res Treat. 1993;28:167)

men, and clinically significant osteoporosis develops in many;[10-13] this bone loss represents the most common metabolic bone disease in postmenopausal women and is responsible for the development of over 1 million fractures annually. Extended or permanent nursing care in rehabilitation facilities is needed for 25% of patients after experiencing a hip fracture, a factor that contributes to substantial health care costs in addition to significant suffering and more than 50,000 associated deaths per year. Although family history, body habitus, and lifestyle choices contribute to an individual's risk for developing osteoporosis, estrogen deficiency is the single most significant causative factor.[14-18]

The medical community has therefore focused appropriately on the long-term health hazards of estrogen deficiency, and a concerted effort has been made to develop sensible and effective health maintenance strategies for aging women. Among postmenopausal women, however, concerns about prevention of even the most serious hazard—future heart disease—are of less concern than immediate climacteric symptoms.[19-21] The severity of these symptoms and the fear of osteoporosis motivate most women to seek medical care and appear central to their interest in, or avoidance of, postmenopausal estrogen use.

Management of Menopause in Women With Histories of Breast Cancer: the Dilemma of Estrogen Replacement

Women previously diagnosed and treated for breast cancer are, as a group, exposed to estrogen deficiency more often and for longer periods than are women in the general population. Both preoperative and adjuvant cytotoxic chemotherapy are increasingly incorporated into treatment protocols for localized breast cancer. This approach

improves survival but generally precipitates premature ovarian failure in these patients. Thus, more of these women with prolonged life expectancy develop early menopause after treatment for early breast cancer. In addition, for women in whom menopause has been surgically induced, ERT is almost always discontinued when breast cancer is diagnosed. In both groups, it is frequently necessary to delineate nonhormonal alternatives for the management of health issues linked to estrogen deficiency because these patients are, as a matter of conventional practice, excluded from estrogen replacement programs. This approach stems from long-held concerns that estrogen may adversely affect the course of breast cancer. (The role of estrogen in the pathophysiology of breast cancer is reviewed in Chapter 3.3 and is not reiterated here.) In general terms, most existing clinical studies focus on the discussion of risks and benefits for women who do not have breast cancer. No direct evidence exists to provide guidelines for estrogen administration after treatment for breast cancer. As the number of women who have been successfully treated for localized breast disease increases, it will become important to determine whether their exclusion from ERT is appropriate. Nevertheless, until appropriate clinical trials help to resolve this problem, nonhormonal alternatives constitute the standard of care and are the focus of this review.

The Role of Estrogen in the Management of Menopause in Women With No History of Breast Cancer

The efficacy of ERT in preventing or correcting the complex sequelae of estrogen deficiency and in reducing mortality has been well established by multiple studies beyond the scope of this discussion. ERT reduces cardiovascular mortality in postmenopausal women,[22-25] in part because of its favorable impact on the patient's lipid profile. Estrogens promote the decrease of low-density lipoprotein (LDL) and total cholesterol and the increase of high-density lipoprotein (HDL) cholesterol, but direct effects on the heart and vasculature have also been observed.[26-32] Vasomotor and genitourinary symptoms in menopausal women are readily treatable with ERT. In addition, ERT can reduce or prevent the development of osteoporosis and its related morbidity and mortality;[33-35] ERT is effective in maintaining bone mass, in slowing loss of bone, and (more important) in reducing the risk for vertebral and hip fractures.[36,37]

Nonhormonal Therapies for the Management of Menopause

CARDIOVASCULAR HEALTH

The fact that cardiovascular disease constitutes the major threat to the health of aging women has been amply emphasized in recent years.[30] Constitutional factors include a family history of coronary disease at a young age, hypertension, a history of claudication or stroke, diabetes mellitus, and hyperlipidemia.[38] Lifestyle considerations such as obesity, physical inactivity, and smoking are also important. Clearly, smoking cessation, weight regulation, and physical fitness are important goals for the preservation of cardiovascular health and for the maintenance of a sensible, healthful life-style in general. Meticulous control of hypertension and diabetes is critically important for the prevention of vascular complications in all affected patients, regardless of their age and gender. The panoply of available medications and therapeutic algorithms are outlined in standard medical textbooks.[39]

Regarding hyperlipidemia, most studies of medical interventions have established therapeutic principles[29] primarily by studying populations of men; it is has been assumed that the benefits of similar nonhormonal treatments should also apply to women, although direct data remain sparse. Bile acid sequestrants such as colestipol and cholestyramine resin are used to lower LDL cholesterol levels; elevation of tryglyceride levels may be exacerbated with these agents, and appropriate monitoring is needed. Nicotinic acid effectively reduces triglyceride and LDL cholesterol levels and is often obtained as an over-the-counter preparation; however, intolerance is relatively common because of its complex pattern of primarily gastrointestinal side effects. More recently, HMG coenzyme-A reductase inhibitors have been developed as potent cholesterol-lowering agents. Liver dysfunction and myopathy are potential side effects of these compounds, and appropriate monitoring is required. Fibric acids are used to lower triglyceride levels, and probucol is available to reduce LDL cholesterol levels. These agents may be used individually or in combination to achieve the desired lipid-lowering effect.[29]

OSTEOPOROSIS

Progressive osteopenia occurs with advancing age; in women, the rate of bone loss is accelerated after the development of estrogen deficiency.[40–43] Nevertheless, clinically significant osteoporosis with disabling vertebral or hip fractures is not an inevitable sequela of old age. The description of a "thin framed, sedentary, white smoker" outlines several important risk factors for osteoporosis. Although all correlations of estrogen deficiency continue to show its strong association with osteoporosis, hereditary and racial influences on bone mass are becoming increasingly appreciated.[16,44,45] Nonhormonal treatments for established osteoporosis include exercise and supplementation of calcium, calcitonin, vitamin D, and fluoride.[46,47]

The prevention of calcium and vitamin D deficiency are important measures for the maintenance of skeletal integrity; calcium supplementation significantly slows bone loss in healthy postmenopausal women[48–50] and is generally included in treatment regimens. Whether pharmacologic administration of vitamin D can have a significant impact on the development of vertebral or hip fracture remains controversial,[51] but its effect is supported by evidence from two recent studies showing that low-dose

vitamin D[53] and calcitriol[54] were associated with decreased rates of hip and vertebral fractures, respectively.

Calcitonin is an approved treatment modality for osteoporosis;[55] it prevents bone loss and has important analgesic properties, although no solid evidence suggests that it reduces the incidence of hip fracture. Associated side effects of nausea and flushing can, however, be frequent and especially disturbing in women with a history of cancer and prior exposure to chemotherapy.

Fluoride has been an attractive agent for the treatment of osteoporosis because it appears to increase bone formation; although several studies have shown that fluoride administration increases bone mineral density, whether it may paradoxically increase the risk for fractures remains controversial.[56,57] Most recently, low-dose[58] and slow-release[59] sodium fluoride therapy, in combination with calcium, has been shown to be beneficial in terms of vertebral fractures; if confirmed, this relatively safe drug may provide another promising therapeutic alternative.

In the past few years, bisphosphonates have emerged as an effective and well-tolerated group of compounds that support, and even enhance, bone mineral density for several years;[60–63] the potential impact of these compounds on the long-term morbidity and mortality associated with skeletal fractures remains under investigation, but results of initial studies appear promising.

The benefit of exercise in the prevention of osteoporosis is an intuitive concept that has been difficult to document.[64,65] Although immobilization and weightlessness result in significant bone loss, neither endurance nor weight-bearing exercise programs have been easily shown to prevent or reverse menopause-induced osteopenia.

Perhaps the single most important measure that can reduce the cost and suffering associated with osteoporosis is the prevention of accidental falls, which represent the most frequent immediate cause of hip fractures.

CLIMACTERIC HOT FLUSHES

This most prominent perimenopausal and postmenopausal symptom affects over 70% of women and may persist for several years, although it usually abates spontaneously after 2 years.[66] Sensations of heat, sweating, flushing, and anxiety may be accompanied by irritability and a sense of panic.[67–69] The pathophysiology of hot flushes remains unclear, but they are considered to be a consequence of dysfunctional thermoregulation,[70] which may be mediated by alterations of central catecholamine secretion.[71] This presumed etiology has guided the design of nonhormonal therapies.

Bellergal (a combination of phenobarbital, ergotamine, and belladona) has been used to treat hot flushes for many years and has shown modest efficacy in some women. Blurred vision, dry mouth, and gastrointestinal symptoms are frequent side effects, and these lead most women to abandon bellergal treatment after several months.

Clonidine is a centrally active α-agonist that was initially developed as an antihypertensive medication. Several studies show that it can alleviate both the frequency and severity of hot flushes associated either with estrogen deficiency[72] or with tamoxifen administration.[73] Drowsiness and dry mouth are frequent side effects but are usually not severe enough to warrant interrupting therapy. Orthostatic symptoms, however, may become limiting and should be monitored closely, especially at the beginning of treatment. Other α-agonists and antidopaminergic agents have also been used with moderate success.

Progestational agents are often considered in the management of hot flushes;[74] because progesterone is an ovarian hormone with significant potential impact on breast tissue proliferation, it should not be used until carefully designed studies have determined its safety.

OTHER CLIMACTERIC SYMPTOMS

Genitourinary atrophy, bladder dysfunction with stress incontinence and infections, dyspareunia, and decreased libido frequently occur at the time of menopause and are attributed to estrogen deficiency. Emotional symptoms such as irritability, nervousness, depression, insomnia, and inability to concentrate are also described by many women,[19,75] but their causal relation to estrogen deficiency remains a matter of debate. The efficacy of nonhormonal interventions for these problems remains disappointing. Several herbal remedies are advocated in the lay literature and by the health food industry; information about their efficacy remains anecdotal, although they are widely used. It is important to remember that estrogenic compounds are widely distributed in natural foodstuffs;[76] because the potential influence of environmental estrogens on breast cancer remains a concern,[77] caution should be exercised in the use of herbal remedies for the treatment of menopausal symptoms.

ROLE OF TAMOXIFEN

Tamoxifen is an effective antineoplastic agent that is used widely and for prolonged periods in postmenopausal women with breast cancer. Early concerns that this antiestrogen may have deleterious effects on the cardiovascular and skeletal systems have, fortunately, proved unwarranted. On the contrary, this compound has significant estrogenic activity in various tissues.

Tamoxifen administration is associated with a decrease in total and LDL cholesterol levels; modest elevation of triglyceride levels has also been noted.[78-82] The effects on HDL cholesterol levels are less consistent. These beneficial effects persist for at least 2 years of continuous therapy. The expectation that these favorable lipid changes will result in a reduction in cardiovascular morbidity and mortality remains to be substantiated but is supported by a recent observation that fewer tamoxifen-treated patients (5 versus 16 patients among 747 participants) suffered fatal heart attacks.[83] A retrospective analysis of women receiving adjuvant therapy with tamoxifen for a median of 6 years showed that this therapy significantly reduced the incidence of hospital admissions for cardiac disease; no decrease in such hospitalizations was noted for thromboembolic disease.[84]

Equally promising is evidence that tamoxifen may exert a weak estrogenic effect on the skeleton and thus prevent postmenopausal bone loss, as measured both by bone mineral density surveillace[85-88] and by transiliac crest bone biopsy results.[89] Long-term benefit in terms of vertebral and hip fracture reductions, however, has yet to be shown. In addition, tamoxifen tends to exacerbate climacteric vasomotor symptoms[90] and depression,[91] and may have additional toxicities. The potential for combined estrogen and tamoxifen programs in the long-term management of menopause for women who have completed treatment for breast cancer thus remains undefined.

Estrogen Replacement in Women With Histories of Breast Cancer

The omission of estrogen from health maintenance programs designed for women who have previously been treated for breast cancer has been the rule for many years. This proscription is based on indirect but well-established experimental and clinical evidence that ovarian hormone manipulation has important effects on breast physiology and tumor growth. The concern that ERT may stimulate the growth of occult micromatastases or activate new primary lesions has contributed to the current standard practice, and caution is urged.[92-94]

The emerging skepticism about our current practice in this group of patients with prior breast cancer is reflected in many recent editorials and commentaries.[92-101] The importance of developing appropriate guidelines specifically for women with breast cancer is now being discussed,[102,103] and the need for specifically designed clinical trials is being emphasized by many investigators.[92,93,95,100] A prospective, randomized clinical study is under way to assess the safety of ERT in women with histories of localized (stage I or II), estrogen receptor–negative breast cancer;[104] additional studies are needed to extend such observations for additional subgroups of women with breast cancer and to evaluate different hormone replacement regimens so that objective guidelines can be developed.

Increasingly, patients express concern about the lack of information about ERT for their particular condition and about personal health risks linked to estrogen deficiency.[105] Equally important, many of these women obtain estrogen preparations in an unsupervised manner and outside the environment of oncologic surveillance. The need to obtain direct pertinent information cannot be overemphasized.

Whether the use of supplemental, low-dose estrogen has any effect on disease recurrence or longevity in postmenopausal women who have had breast cancer is unknown, but several lines of evidence cast doubt on the assumption that endogenous estrogens have any adverse effect. Available studies suggest that women who develop breast cancer while receiving estrogen replacement may have improved outcomes compared with women with breast cancer who are not receiving estrogen, perhaps because the estrogen users tend to have smaller lesions and earlier-stage disease at the time of diagnosis.[106-109] Whether this finding represents some effect of estrogen on the biology of breast cancer or a favorable detection bias resulting from improved surveillance and early diagnosis remains to be defined. Women who become pregnant after the diagnosis and treatment of breast cancer do not have an increased risk for disease recurrence or death from breast cancer.[110–112] Finally, in two recent small, uncontrolled studies, no adverse effects were reported in women who elected to receive ERT after being diagnosed with breast cancer.[113,114]

In older women, most breast cancers develop several years after the onset of estrogen deficiency, but these tumors tend to be estrogen-receptor–positive lesions and to respond to hormonal manipulation. In contrast, development of breast cancer is infrequent in younger women with higher ambient estrogen levels, but the tumors in these women tend to be estrogen receptor–negative and relatively resistant to hormonal manipulation. Thus, both the incidence and hormonal dependence of breast cancer do not correlate with the estrogenic millieu in most women.

Summary

During the course of normal aging, women develop gradual but irreversible estrogen deficiency toward the end of their fifth decade. Although menopause marks the conclusion of reproductive capability, it does not necessarily create the need for medical intervention. Many women experience mild and self-limited climacteric symptoms and are not at risk for heart or bone disease by virtue of their individual health profiles. For such women, no management strategies are required. Others have an increased risk for heart disease but not osteoporosis (or vice versa), whereas for some women the climacteric symptoms are overwhelming and overshadow all other considerations. The appropriate approach to these various potential menopausal scenaria clearly differs for each person, and therapeutic decisions must be individualized.

In general, adopting a healthful life-style (characterized by nutritional discretion, weight control, and physical fitness) does much to prevent or alleviate the potential chronic complications of estrogen deficiency. Careful control of coexisting diabetes, hypertension, or hyperlipidemia is necessary and often sufficient to reduce cardiovascular morbidity and mortality. Adequate calcium supplementation and prevention of accidental falls (through appropriate use of footware or cane support) are safe and effective, although underemphasized, measures for the prevention of osteoporosis-related morbidity and cost. Nonhormonal lubricants may sufficiently alleviate dyspareunia, but topical estrogen application is often needed to palliate genitourinary symptoms. Moreover, nonhormonal remedies rarely offer a satisfactory solution to climacteric vasomotor and mood changes. Because estrogen deficiency is central to the pathophysiology of the many postmenopausal changes outlined in this review, it is intuitively apparent that the reversal of estrogen deficiency should provide a unified approach to therapy when medical intervention is needed, especially for women with multisystem complaints and other health concerns. Accordingly, ERT is considered the standard of care in most circumstances for women without breast cancer; the exact regimen or the duration of estrogen administration is tailored to the individual needs of each person.

Women with histories of breast cancer present with the same range of menopausal symptoms and health concerns as do women without that history, but the severity and duration are often exaggerated because of chemotherapy-induced premature menopause. Although the available therapies for menopausal symptoms are the same for all postmenopausal women, the chosen treatment for patients with histories of breast cancer often differs because ERT is excluded. The guidelines for nonhormonal therapies for these hormonal symptoms do not differ from the principles of care that apply to women without breast cancer. Whether and for which women the potential risks of estrogen administration outweigh the known advantages of this approach is becoming a subject of thoughtful and critical discussions that are expected to provide objective guidelines. It is appropriate to suggest that nonhormonal measures should be carefully and vigorously explored as a first approach; when vaginal estrogen administration is needed, we suggest that the dose be gradually increased as needed for control of genitourinary symptoms. Serial measurement of serum estrogen and gonadotropin levels can be used to monitor against the unwanted potential systemic absorption of topical estrogen. In patients with resistant symptoms or health risks, carefully supervised systemic estrogen administration may be required.

References

1. Bungary GT, Vessey MP, Mc Pherson CK. Study of symptoms in middle life with special reference to the menopause. Br Med J 1980;2:181.
2. McKinley SM, Brambilla PJ, Posner JG. The normal menopause transition. Maturitas 1992;14:103.
3. Wiklund I, Karlberg J, Lindgren R, et al. A Swedish version of the Women's Health Questionnaire: a measure of postmenopausal complaints. Acta Obstet Gynecol Scand 1993;72:648.
4. Scotti RJ, Ostergard DR. The urethral syndrome. Clin Obstet Gynecol 1984;27:525.
5. Notelovitz M. Gynecologic problems of menopausal women: changes in genital tissues. Geriatrics 1978;33:24.
6. Wenger NK, Speroff L, Packard B. Cardiovascular health in women. N Engl J Med 1993;329:247.
7. Rosenberg L, Hennekens CHE, Rosner B, et al. Early menopause and the risk of myocardial infarction. Am J Obstet Gynecol 1981;139:47.
8. Mathews KA, Meihlahn E, Kuller LH, et al. Menopause and risk factors for coronary heart disease. N Engl J Med 1989;321:641.
9. Heart and strokes facts. Dallas, Am Heart Association, 1992.
10. Richelson LS, Wahner HW, Melton LJ III, et al. Relative contributions of aging and estrogen deficiency to postmenopausal bone loss. N Engl J Med 1984;1273.
11. Wasserman SHS, Barzel VS. Involution osteoporosis. N Engl J Med 1986;314:1676.

12. Riggs BL, Melton LJ III. Osteoporosis, the state-of-art. Semin Nucl Med 1987;17:283.

13. A special conference: osteoporosis. National Conference on Women's Health Series, Bethesda, October 30, 1987.

14. Richelson LS, Wahner HW, Melton LJ, et al. Relative contributions of aging and estrogen deficiency to postmenopausal bone loss. N Engl J Med 1984;311:1273.

15. Nordin BEC, Need AG, Bridges A, et al. Relative contributions of years since menopause, age and weight to vertebral density in postmenopausal women. J Clin Endocrinol Metab 1992;74:20.

16. Slemenda CW, Christian JC, Williams CJ, et al. Genetic determinants of bone mass in adult women: a reevaluation of the twin model and the potential importance of gene interaction on heritability estimates. J Bone Miner Res 1991;6:561.

17. Mitlak BH, Nussbaun SR. Diagnosis and treatment of osteoporosis. Annu Rev Med 1993;44:265.

18. Gambacciani M, Spinetti A, De Simone L, et al. The relative contributions of menopause and aging to postmenopausal vertebral osteopenia. J Clin Endocrinol Metab 1993;77:1148.

19. Utian WH, Schiff I. NAMS-Gallup survey on women's knowledge, information sources, and attitudes to menopause and hormone replacement therapy. Menopause 1994;1:39.

20. Leather AT, Holland EFN, Studd JWW. The clinical problems of women referred to a specialist menopause clinic. J Soc Med 1993;86:385.

21. Morse CA, Smith A, Dennerstein L, et al. The treatment-seeking woman at menopause. Maturitas 1994;18:161.

22. Henderson BE, Paganini-Hill A, Ross RK. Estrogen replacement therapy and protection from acute myocardial infarction. Am J Obst Gynecol 1988;159:312.

23. Stamper MJ, Colditz GA, Willett WC, et al. Postmenopausal estrogen therapy and cardiovascular disease: ten-Year follow-up from the Nurse's Health Study. N Engl J Med 1991;325:745.

24. Nachtigall LE, Nachtigall RH, Nachtigall RD, et al. Estrogen replacement therapy. II: A prospective study in the relationship to carcinoma and cardiovascular and metabolic problems. Obstet Gynecol 1979;54:74.

25. Nabulsi AA, Folsom AR, White A, et al. Association of hormone-replacement therapy with various cardiovascular risk factors in postmenopausal women. N Engl J Med 1993;328:1069.

26. Williams JK, Adams MR, Klopfenstein HS. Estrogen modulates responses of atherosclerotic coronary arteries. Circulation 1990;81:1680.

27. Pines A, Fishman EZ, Levo Y, et al. Menopause-induced changes in left ventricular wall thickness. Am J Cardiol 1993;72:240.

28. Pines A, Fishman EZ, Levo Y, et al. The effects of hormone replacement therapy on normal postmenopausal women: measurements of Doppler-derived parameters of aortic flow. Am J Obstet Gynecol 1991;164:806.

29. Denke MA, Grundy SM. Hypercholesterolemia in elderly persons: resolving the treatment dilemma. Ann Intern Med 1990;112:780.

30. Wenger NK, Speroff L, Packard B. Cardiovascular health and disease in women. N Engl J Med 1993;329:247.

31. Penotti M, Nencioni T, Gabrielli L, et al. Blood flow variations in internal carotid and middle cerebral arteries induced by postmenopausal hormone replacement therapy. Am J Obstet Gynecol 1993;169:1226.

32. Orimo A, Inoue S, Ikegami A, et al. Vascular smooth muscle cells as target for estrogen. Biochem Biophys Res Commun 1993;195:730.

33. Ettinger B, Genant HK, Cann CE. Postmenopausal bone loss is prevented by treatment with low dosage estrogen with calcium. Ann Intern Med 1987;106:40.

34. Lindsay R, Hart DM, Forrest C, et al. Prevention of spinal osteoporosis in oophorectomized women. Lancet 1989;2:1151.

35. Riggs BL, Melton LJ. The prevention and treatment of osteoporosis. N Engl J Med 1992;327:620.

36. Weiss NS, Ure CL, Ballard JH, et al. Decreased risk of fractures of the hip and lower forearm with postmenopausal use of estrogens. N Engl J Med 1980;303:1195.

37. Naessen T, Persson I, Adami HO, et al. Hormone replacement therapy and the risk for first hip fracture: a prospective, population-based cohort study. Ann Intern Med 1990;113:95.

38. Ettinger B. Hormone replacement therapy and coronary heart disease. Obstet Gynecol Clin North Am 1990;17:741.

39. Disorders of the cardiovascular system. Isselbacher KJ, Braunwald E, Wilson JD, et al, eds. In: Harrison's principles of internal medicine. New York, McGraw-Hill, 1994:939.

40. Riggs BL, Melton LJ. The prevention and treatment of osteoporosis. N Engl J Med 1992;327:620.

41. Notelovitz M. Osteoporosis: screening, prevention and management. Fert Steril 1993;59:707.

42. Recker RR. Clinical review 41: current therapy for osteoporosis. J Clin Endocrinol Metab 1993;76:14.

43. Mitlak BH, Nussbaum SR. Diagnosis and treatment of osteoporosis. Annu Rev Med 1993;44:265.

44. Luckey MM, Meier DE, Mandeli JP, et al. Radial and vertebral bone density in white and black women: evidence for radial differences in premenopausal bone homeostasis. J Clin Endocrinol Metab 1989;69:762.

45. Liel Y, Edwards J, Shary J, et al. The effects of race and body habitus on bone mineral density of the radius, hip and spine in premenopausal women. J Clin Endocrinol Metab 1988;66:1247.

46. Peck WA, Riggs BL, Bell NH, et al. Research directions in osteoporosis. Am J Med 1988;84:275.

47. Harward MP. Nutritive therapies for osteoporosis: the role of calcium. Med Clin North Am 1993;77:889.

48. Nilas L. Calcium intake and osteoporosis. World Rev Nutr Diet 1993;73:1.

49. Dawson-Hughes B, Dallal GE, Krall EA, et al. A controlled trial of the effect of calcium supplementation on bone density in postmenopausal women. N Engl J Med 1990;323:878.

50. Reid IR, Ames RW, Evans MC, et al. Effect of calcium supplementation on bone loss in postmenopausal women. N Engl J Med 1993;328:460.

51. Ott SM, Chestnut CH. Calcitriol is not effective in postmenopausal osteoporosis. Ann Intern Med 1989;110:267.

53. Chapuy MC, Arlot ME, Duboeuf F, et al. Vitamin D3 and calcium to prevent hip fractures in elderly women. N Engl J Med 1992;327:1637.

54. Tilyard MW, Spears GFS, Thomson J, et al. Treatment of postmenopausal osteoporosis with calcitriol or calcium. N Engl J Med 1992;326:357.

55. Fatourechi V, Heath H. Salmon calcitonin in the treatment of postmenopausal osteoporosis. Ann Intern Med 1987;107:923.

56. Heaney RP, Baylink DJ, Johnston CC, et al. Fluoride therapy for the vertebral crush fracture syndrome. Ann Intern Med 1989;111:678.

57. Riggs BL, Hodgson SF, O'Fallon EYS, et al. Effect of fluoride treatment on the fracture rate in postmenopausal women with osteoporosis. N Engl J of Med 1990;322:802.

58. Riggs BL, O'Fallon, Hodgson SF, et al. Clinical trial of fluoride therapy in postmenopausal osteoporotic women: extended observations and additional analysis J Bone Min Res 1994;9:265.

59. Pack CYK, Sakhall K, Piziak V, et al. Slow-release sodium fluoride in the management of postmenopausal osteoporosis: a randomized controlled trial. Ann Intern Med 1994;120:625.

60. Watts NB, Harris ST, Genant HK, et al. Intermittent cyclical etidronate treatment of postmenopausal osteoporosis. N Engl J Med 1990;323:73.

61. Harris ST, Watts NB, Jackson RD, et al. Four-year study of intermittent cyclic etidronate treatment of postmenopausal osteoporosis:

three years of blinded therapy followed by one year of open therapy. Am J Med 1993;95:557.

62. Storm T, Thamsborg G, Steiniche T, et al. Effect of intermittent cyclical etidronate therapy on bone mass and fracture rate in women with postmenopausal osteoporosis. N Engl J Med 1990;322:1265.

63. Etidronate for postmenopausal osteoporosis. Med Lett 1990; 32:111.

64. Forwood MR, Burr DB. Physical activity and bone mass: exercises in futility. Bone Miner 1993;21:89.

65. Jaglal SB, Kreiger N, Darlington G. Past and recent physical activity and risk of hip fracture. Am J Epidemiol 1993;138:107.

66. Greendale GA, Judd HL. The menopause: health implications and clinical management. J Am Geriatr Soc 1993;41:426.

67. Oldenhave A, Netelenbos C. Pathogenesis of climacteric complaints: ready for a change? Lancet 1994;343:649.

68. Kronnenberg F. Hot flushes: epidemiology and physiology. Ann NY Acad Sci 1990;592:52.

69. Tulandi T, Samarthji L. Menopausal hot flush. Obstet Gynecol Surv 1985;40:553.

70. Casper RF, Yen SSC. Neuroendocrinology of menopausal flushes: an hypothesis of flush mechanism. Clin Endocrinol 1985;22:293.

71. Rosenberg J, Larsen SH. Hypothesis: pathogenesis of postmenopausal hot flush. Med Hypotheses 1991;35:349.

72. Clayden JR, Bell JW, Pollard P. Menopausal flushing: double-blind trial of a non-hormonal medication. BMJ 1974;1:409.

73. Goldberg RM, Loprinzi CL, O'Fallon JR, et al. Transdermal clonidine for ameliorating tamoxifen-induced hot flushes. J Clin Oncol 1994;12:155.

74. Loprinzi CL, Michalak JG, Onella SK, et al. Megestrol acetate for the prevention of hot flashes. N Engl J Med 1994;331:347.

75. Studd JWW, Smith RNJ. Estrogen and depression in women. Menopause 1994;1:33.

76. Miksicek RJ. Commonly occuring plant flavonoids have estrogenic activity. Mol Pharmacol 1993;44:37.

77. Cotton P. Environmental estrogenic agents area of concern: medical news and perspectives. JAMA 1994;271.

78. Dnistrian AM, Schwartz MK, Greenberg EJ, et al. Effect of tamoxifen on serum cholesterol and lipoproteins during chemohormonal therapy. Clin Chim Acta 1993;223:43.

79. Bagdade JD, Wolter J, Subbaiah PV, et al. Effects of tamoxifen treatment of plasma lipids and lipoprotein lipid composition. J Clin Endocrinol Metab 1990;70:1132.

80. Love RR, Wiebe DA, Newcomb PA, et al. Effects of tamoxifen on cardiovascular risk factors in postmenopausal women. Ann Intern Med 1991;115:860.

81. Schapira DV, Kumar NB, Lyman GH. Serum cholesterol reduction with tamoxifen. Breast Cancer Res Treat 1990;17:3.

82. Thangaraju M, Kumar K, Gandhirajan R, et al. Effect of tamoxifen on plasma lipids and lipoproteins in postmenopausal women with breast cancer. Cancer 1994;73:659.

83. Stewart HJ, for the Scottish Cancer Trials. Breast group: the Scottish Trial of Adjuvant Tamoxifen in Node-Negative Breast Cancer. J Natl Cancer Inst Monogr 1992;11:117.

84. Rutqvist LE, Mattsson A, for the Stockholm Breast Cancer Study Group. Cardiac and thromboembolic morbidity among postmenopausal women with early-stage breast cancer in a randomized trial of adjuvant tamoxifen. J Natl Cancer Inst 1993;85:1398.

85. Fornander T, Rutqvist LE, Sjoberg HE, et al. Long-term adjuvant tamoxifen in early breast cancer: effect on bone mineral density in postmenopausal women. J Clin Oncol 1990;8:1019.

86. Love RR, Mazess RB, Barden HS, et al. Effects of tamoxifen on bone mineral density in postmenopausal women with breast cancer. N Engl J Med 1992;326:852.

87. Neal AJ, Evans K, Hoskin PJ. Does long-term administration of

88. Wright CDP, Garrahan NJ, Stanton M, et al. Effect of long-term tamoxifen therapy on cancellous bone remodeling and structure in women with breast cancer. J Bone Mineral Res 1994;9:153.

89. Wright CDP, Garrahan NJ, Stanton M, et al. Effect of long-term tamoxifen on cancellous bone remodeling and structure in women with breast cancer. J Bone Mineral Res 1994;9:153.

90. Love RR, Cameron L, Connell BL, et al. Symptoms associated with tamoxifen treatment in postmenopausal women. Arch Intern Med 1991;151:1842.

91. Cathcart CK, Jones SE, Pumroy CS, et al. Clinical recognition and management of depression in node negative breast cancer patients treated with tamoxifen. Breast Cancer Res Treat 1993;27:277.

92. Lobo RA. Hormone replacement therapy: oestrogen replacement after treatment for breast cancer? Lancet 1993;341:1313.

93. Marchant DJ. Estrogen-replacement therapy after breast cancer: risk versus benefits. Cancer 1993;71:2169.

94. Spicer DV, Pike MC. Hormone replacement after breast cancer. Lancet 1993;342:183.

95. Stoll BA, Parbhoo S. Treatment of menopausal symptoms in breast cancer patients. Lancet 1988;1278.

96. Bluming, AZ. Hormone replacement therapy: benefits and risks for the general postmenopausal female population and for women with a history of previously treated breast cancer. Semin Oncol 1993;20:662.

97. Creasman WT. Estrogen replacement therapy: is previously treated cancer a contraindication? Obstet Gynecol 1991;77:309.

98. Theriault RL, Vassilopoulou-Sellin R. A clinical dilemma: estrogen replacement therapy in postmenopausal women with a background of primary breast cancer. Ann Oncol 1991;2:709.

99. Powles TJ, Hickish T, Casey S, et al. Hormone replacement after breast cancer. Lancet 1993;342:60.

100. Cobleigh MA, Berris RF, Bush T, et al. Estrogen replacement therapy in breast cancer survivors, a time for change. 1994;272:540.

101. Vassilopoulou-Sellin R. Estrogen replacement therapy in women at increased risk for breast cancer. Breast Cancer Res Treat 1993;28:167.

102. National Cancer Institute-Sponsored Conference of Breast Cancer in Younger Women. Monogr Natl Cancer Inst 1994;16:1.

103. National Cancer Institute, Division of Cancer Prevention and Control Working Group. Clinical trials of hormone replacement therapy in patients with a history of breast cancer. NIH Workshop, November 1993.

104. Vassilopoulou-Sellin R, Theriault RL. Randomized prospective trial of estrogen replacement therapy in women with a history of breast cancer. J Natl Cancer Inst Monogr 1994;16:153.

105. Vassilopoulou-Sellin R, Zolinski C. Estrogen replacement therapy in women with breast cancer: a survey of patient attitudes. Am J Med Sci 1992;304:145.

106. Byrd BF, Burch JC, Vaughn WK. The impact of long-term estrogen support after hysterectomy: a report of 1016 cases. Ann Surg 1977;185:574.

107. Hunt K, Vessey M, McPherson K. Mortality in a cohort of long-term users of hormone replacement therapy: our updated analysis. Br J Obstet Gynaecol 1990;97:1080.

108. Bergkvist L, Adami H, Persson I, et al. Prognosis after breast cancer diagnosis in women exposed to estrogen and estrogen–progestorone replacement therapy. Am J Epidemiol 1989;130:221.

109. Jones G, Ingram D, Mattes E, et al. The effect of hormone replacement therapy and prognostic indices in women with breast cancer. Med J Austr 1994;161:106.

110. Sutton R, Buzdar AU, Hortobagyi GN. Pregnancy and offspring after adjuvant chemotherapy in breast cancer patients. Cancer 1990;65:847.

tamoxifen affect bone mineral density? Eur J Cancer 1993; 29A:1971.

111. Danforth DN. How subsequent pregnancy affects outcome in women with a prior breast cancer. Oncology 1991;5:23.

112. Sankila R, Heinävaara S, Hakulinen T. Survival of breast cancer patients after subsequent term pregnancy: "healthy mother effect." Am J Obstet Gynecol 1994;170:818.

113. Stoll BA. Hormone replacement therapy in women treated for breast cancer. J Cancer Clin Oncol 1989;25:1909.

114. Wile AG, Opfell RW, Margileth DA. Hormone replacement therapy in previously treated breast cancer patients. Am J Surg 1993;165:372.

24.9

Breast Cancer in Underserved Minorities

JON F. KERNER

In 1986, the US National Cancer Institute (NCI) published its cancer control objectives for the United States for the years 1990 and 2000.[1] Included were three objectives related to breast cancer:

1. Dietary objectives to reduce the total fat consumption of the US population from 38% of total calories from fat in 1980 to less than 35% by 1990 and to 25% by the year 2000.
2. Screening prevalence objectives to increase the use of clinical breast examinations (CBEs) from 43% in 1980 to 70% in 1990 and 80% by the year 2000 and to increase the use of mammography (among women 50 to 70 years of age) from 14% in 1980 to 45% in 1990 and 80% by 2000.
3. Treatment objectives to increase the application of state-of-the-art treatment for selected cancer sites, including breast cancer.

The projected reductions in breast cancer mortality, which would be achieved if these objectives were met, were estimated to be 25% from reducing fat, 16.0% from expanding use of breast cancer screening services, and 14.3% from expanding access to the best available breast cancer treatment.

During the decade in which these objectives were formulated and published, the US population became significantly more ethnically diverse. For example, the US black female resident population grew from over 14 million in 1980 to over 16 million in 1990 (an increase of 14.4%). The US Hispanic female resident population grew from almost 7.4 million in 1980 to just under 11 million in 1990 (+49.6%), and the US Asian or Pacific Islander female resident population increased by 111%. Simultaneously, the US white female resident population increased by only 6.7%.[2] This increasing diversity was accompanied by endemic poverty, experienced disproportionately by black and Hispanic minorities. Table 24.9–1 displays data for white, black, and Hispanic individuals, children under 18, and families with female heads of household and children under 18. The proportion of these populations who live below the poverty level remained approximately the same or increased slightly in the 1980s for one or more segments of all ethnic groups.

What are the implications of endemic poverty and increasing cultural diversity with respect to the achievement of these national breast cancer control objectives? With respect to our understanding of the epidemiology of breast cancer in the United States, national cancer incidence and mortality data do not capture information on ethnic or socioeconomic diversity within our at-risk populations. Data on this disease are largely limited to black–white racial comparisons that, although informative, probably mask large variations among ethnic and socioeconomic status (SES) groups that are important to our understanding of the public health problem represented by breast cancer. Regional and local cancer data provide some in-

TABLE 24.9-1

Percentage of Persons and Families With Female Heads of Household Below the Poverty Level for US Whites, Blacks, and Hispanics in 1980 and 1990

Individuals and Families by Race or Ethnicity*	Percentage in 1980	Percentage in 1990
ALL PERSONS		
Black	32.5	31.9
Hispanic	25.7	28.1
White	10.2	10.7
CHILDREN <18†		
Black	42.1	44.2
Hispanic	33.0	37.7
White	13.4	15.1
FAMILIES‡		
Black	56.0	56.1
Hispanic	57.3	58.2
White	35.9	37.9

* The race groups black and white include both Hispanics and non–Hispanics. The ethnic group Hispanic includes people of any race.

† Related children under 18 years of age in families.

‡ Families with female householder, no husband present, and children under 18 years of age.

(United States Department of Health and Human Services. Health United States 1992 and Healthy People 2000 review. DHHS publ no. [PHS] 1993:1232) sights into ethnic group variation. Socioeconomic data are lacking at all levels, however, and investigators must estimate the impact of SES using ecologic analyses of census tract information.[3,4]

Behavioral data do exist for certain breast cancer risk factors (eg, height, weight, reproductive history, and diet). Some surveys have even oversampled black and Hispanic populations to explore risk factors in more depth among these historically underrepresented populations. National and state budgetary limitations, however, often reduce needed sample sizes, limit efforts to provide bilingual interviewers, and preclude properly translated interview instruments. These limitations, in turn, fail to ensure full participation by minorities, particularly non–English-speaking ones, who may be at high risk.[5] With respect to case-control and cohort studies, which attempt to identify risk factors that could lead to new prevention initiatives, those dealing with underserved minorities are rare.[6–8]

Turning to early detection of breast cancer, the literature is replete with behavioral studies documenting that older, lower-income, less-educated, and ethnic minority populations make less use of available mammography and CBE services than their younger, better-educated, white, middle-class counterparts. Why these differences persist is rarely explained, however. Several intervention studies have been designed and implemented to promote the use of mammography and CBEs, with some early success shown. The key health care system factors that deter medically underserved women from seeking breast cancer screening have not been eliminated, however, nor have they been overcome.

Much less studied are consequences of the need for the medically underserved to seek diagnostic resolution of an abnormal mammogram or abnormal CBE in a health care system with insufficient resources to address their needs. These women are more likely to be without insurance, or to receive Medicaid, or otherwise to be financially compromised by the process. In addition, few studies have examined the variation in access to the best available treatment services for underserved minority breast cancer patients in the United States. In this chapter, what is known about minority and medically underserved women at risk for developing breast cancer is reviewed in relation to the opportunities for these women to benefit from the best available breast cancer prevention, early detection, diagnosis, and treatment services.

Epidemiology and Prevention

Breast cancer incidence rates among medically underserved populations vary by population and source of data. Nationally, breast cancer rates among black and white women show that, although the gap between age-adjusted incidence rates is narrowing, white women (all ages combined) continue to have higher rates of the disease than black women.[9] Black women under the age of 40 years have a higher incidence of breast cancer than white

women. Limited data on breast cancer incidence among other underserved minorities are collected on a state or local basis and are irregularly published.[10–12] Native Hawaiians have the highest age-adjusted breast cancer incidence rates. Mexican Americans from New Mexico, residents of Puerto Rico, and Native Americans have the lowest rates.[13] A significant problem in tracking cancer incidence among certain minority groups, such as Hispanics, is that of ethnic group identification in both numerator (ie, cancer incidence registry) and denominator (ie, census) data. Thus, ethnic group variation among Hispanics is virtually impossible to assess, because the quality of the ethnicity and country-of-origin identification in the cancer incidence registries and the census varies widely from one region of the United States to another.[14]

Black–white differences in the relative risk of dying from breast cancer, and also from other causes, are displayed in Table 24.9–2. Although age-adjusted breast cancer mortality among white women increased by only 0.4% from 1980 to 1990, breast cancer mortality among black women increased by 18% and exceeded mortality rates for white women throughout the decade.[10] Similar patterns of either larger increases in all-neoplastic mortality or smaller decreases in all-cause mortality were experienced between black and white women.

Older women in general, and older black women in particular, also experienced larger increases in breast cancer mortality from 1973 through 1990.[10] During this period, black women 65 years old and older had a 30.3% increase in breast cancer mortality, black women 50 years old and older had a 22.4% increase in breast cancer mortality, followed by white women 65 years old and older, who experienced a 14.3% increase in breast cancer mortality. During the same period, white women under the age of 50 years experienced a 12.5% reduction in breast cancer mortality, despite a 5.9% increase in incidence. White women under the age of 65 years had a 7.2% decline in mortality despite

TABLE 24.9-2

Age-Adjusted Death Rates* for US Black and White Females in 1980 and 1990 From All Causes Combined, All Neoplasms Combined, and Breast Cancer

Population	Year	All Causes	All Neoplasms	Breast Cancer
Black	1980	631.1	129.7	23.3
	1990	581.6	137.2	27.5
Percentage of Change		−7.8%	+5.8%	+18%
White	1980	411.1	107.7	22.8
	1990	369.9	111.2	22.9
Percentage of Change		−10.0%	+3.2%	+0.4%

* Rates are per 100,000 population.

(United States Department of Health and Human Services. USDHHS: Health United States 1992 and Healthy People 2000 review. DHHS publ no. (PHS) 1993:1232.)

a 14.6% increase in incidence; and black women under the age of 50 years had only a 2.5% increase in mortality despite a 16.2% increase in incidence. Clearly, being older and black puts one in double jeopardy of dying from breast cancer.

Well-established breast cancer risk factors include older age, a family history of breast cancer, early menarche, late age at first childbirth, late age at menopause, history of benign breast disease, and exposure to ionizing radiation.[15] These established risk factors share two things in common: (1) the increased relative risk (RR) of developing breast cancer associated with them is modest (RR, 1.5 to 2); and (2) none lends itself to simple preventive interventions.[17] Although diet,[16] alcohol,[17,18] and, most recently, cigarette smoking[19] have all been reported as potential risk factors for breast cancer and lend themselves to breast cancer prevention interventions, analytic epidemiologic data suggest weak associations, no association, or contradictory associations.[20]

Few studies have examined variation in cancer risk factors among medically underserved populations,[9] although some investigators have speculated on the way in which differential exposure to risk factors may explain racial and ethnic group variation in cancer incidence.[13,21] For breast cancer, black women and white women have been shown to share four risk factors at a comparable magnitude: age at first full-term birth, parity, surgical menopause, and history of benign breast disease.[9] On the other hand, family history appears to manifest itself differently among black and white women. The odds of a black woman's developing breast cancer with a first-degree relative with breast cancer (odds ratio [OR], 1.61) are comparable to those of a black woman with a second-degree relative with breast cancer (OR, 1.71); the odds are lower than those of a white woman with a first-degree relative with breast cancer (OR, 2.16), and they are higher than those of a white woman with a second-degree relative (OR, 1.44) with breast cancer. In addition, the impact of early age at menarche was not significant for black women, compared with a small but significant increase in risk for white women who reached menarche at age 12 years or under (OR, 1.26). Thus, this study contradicted earlier suggestions that early age at menarche might explain higher breast cancer incidence rates among young black women.[22] Despite more than a decade of awareness, the higher rates of breast cancer among black women under 40 years of age compared with white women under 40 years of age remain largely unexplained.

Although older women in general have higher incidence and higher mortality rates of breast cancer than younger women, older women are also more likely to develop and die of competing disease causes. Thus, the absolute risk of dying of breast cancer declines with increasing age because of competing mortality risks. Mor and coworkers[23] pointed out that, in 1987, 2.9% of all deaths among women aged 65 to 74 years were from breast cancer, whereas for women aged 75 to 84 years, the figure is 1.7%. Should the incidence and mortality rates of competing diseases (eg, cardiovascular disease) continue to decline through the year 2000, however, then the percentage of disease and death attributed to breast cancer will rise.

Turning to primary prevention, current intervention studies focus on tamoxifen, retinoids, and a low-fat diet.

Also proposed as preventive measures, but not yet in trial, are an increase in physical activity before menarche, to delay its onset, and the use of leutinizing hormone–releasing hormone agonists to reduce the number of ovulatory menstrual cycles among premenopausal women.[24] Given the multifactorial cause of breast cancer, the likelihood that any one of these approaches will have marked impact on overall breast cancer incidence seems limited.

Of importance to medically underserved minority populations is that epidemiologic research on which these interventions are based usually fails to include the medically underserved. Moreover, researchers testing prevention interventions have had enormous difficulty in recruiting these populations to participate. Thus, poor women, less-educated women, nonwhite women, women who cannot speak English, and older women are often severely underrepresented, if they are represented at all, in these studies. This is particularly a concern for molecular and genetic epidemiologic studies, in which failure to involve underserved minorities may limit the biologic variability observed and may seriously compromise the external validity of study conclusions. Prevention trials based on these new markers of breast cancer risk may be similarly compromised.

Part of the difficulty in involving medically underserved minorities is that many of these studies focus on convenience samples recruited through the academic medical centers where the investigator's research is supported. Reaching out to involve underserved minority communities can pose significant practical as well as methodologic difficulties (eg, difficulty in completing follow-up in cohort studies). Moreover, many underserved minority communities are reluctant to participate in these observational studies, given a history of decades of study with little or no evidence that individual participation contributes to the health or well-being of their communities and some particularly notorious evidence that participation is synonymous with exploitation.[25] The net effect is that the underserved are understudied, and the potential benefits of epidemiologic research leading to primary prevention are not experienced by those who may need them most.

To involve medically underserved minorities in descriptive epidemiologic studies may require linking these types of research to interventional research that is evaluating health services (eg, cancer screening) that are desired and appreciated by the underserved population of interest. Thus, collecting molecular markers from medically underserved patients recruited for a cancer screening trial,[26] with full informed consent, can provide an excellent opportunity to study biologic variation in a high-risk population that would be unlikely to consent to a strictly observational study design alone. Moreover, remuneration for time involved in study participation may be critical in low-income communities.

Early Detection of Breast Cancer

The incidence of TNM stage II, III, and IV breast cancer declined for black and white women between 1983 and 1990, and the incidence of in situ and stage I disease increased during the same period.[10] Data from the Surveillance, Epidemiology and End Results (SEER) program and from regional studies have documented, however, that minority breast cancer patients remain more likely to be diagnosed with late-stage disease than most white breast cancer patients. For example, in 1990, just over 11% of both black and white breast cancer patients in SEER were diagnosed with in situ disease, whereas 29.8% of black women were diagnosed with TNM stage I disease compared with 42.5% of white women.[10] Black women had higher percentages of patients diagnosed with TNM stage II, III, or IV disease, compared with white women. Hispanics are also less likely than whites to be diagnosed with early-stage breast cancer.[27]

Later stage of breast cancer at diagnosis among medically underserved female populations can be explained by two principal factors. First, limited access to and less use of baseline (prevalence screening) and routine (incidence screening) CBE and mammography. Second, even when breast cancer screening use increases, or perhaps because it increases, more delay in diagnostic resolution and higher rates of incomplete clinical follow-up of abnormal breast cancer screening test findings may be observed. Both lower rates of screening use and inadequate or delayed clinical follow-up among the medically underserved can, in turn, be explained by patient behavior, clinician behavior, and health care system barriers and inequities.

With respect to the use of breast cancer screening services, the rate of baseline and routine mammography use is generally lower than that of routine CBE and virtually all adult women have had at least one CBE in their lifetime.[28] Although current guidelines for annual CBEs are relatively clear and are agreed on by providers, elderly women,[29] low-income patients, and ethnic and racial minorities have lower prevalence of use rates,[30] with the rate-limiting barrier among many of the medically underserved being the absence of a regular source of primary care.[31] Among providers, some efforts have focused on improving the quality of the CBE, and some investigators have even suggested that a high-quality CBE is as effective as, and perhaps more cost-effective than, a screening mammogram in detecting breast cancer at an early enough stage to improve prognosis and to reduce mortality.[32] In the absence of a regular primary care provider, public education campaigns are particularly important and have focused on making women aware of the importance of routine screening, knowledgeable about sources of screening, active initiators of the screening process, and adherent to recommended screening guidelines.[30]

The rates of mammography use are far less clear. In general, national prevalence estimates of breast cancer screening may report "ever screened" or "screened within the past year." The first estimate is usually higher than the second, indicating that some women in any screening program are screened for the first time (ie, the prevalence screen). Reports tend to group these women with those who have been previously screened when trying to determine who uses screening and who does not.[33] Factors that predict individual mammographic screening include age, education, income, the interaction of these factors, and

urban or rural residence. Reasons reported for not being screened continue to show failure of the physician to recommend mammography as the most prevalent (30.7%), followed by not thinking it was needed (22.3%), or not having a problem (14.3%).[35] In addition to income, both inconvenience and the price of mammography have been barriers to use.[34] The frequency with which cost was mentioned as a reason for not having had a mammogram increased from 2.5% in 1987 to 7.2% in 1990.[35]

Although baseline and routine mammography use rates have increased over time,[35] elderly, low-income, and racial and ethnic minority populations are at particularly high risk for mammography underuse,[36] particularly with respect to regular incidence screening.[37] Whereas, for CBE, having a regular source of care increased the likelihood that a medically underserved woman would be screened, this is not necessarily the case for mammography. Gemson and associates[38] reported that medical practices in which 50% or more of the patients were black were less likely to follow mammography guidelines than medical practices in which 50% or more of the patients were white. Black and Hispanic women are most likely to have undergone mammography when their regular source of care was a hospital emergency department or an outpatient clinic, compared with white, non–Hispanic women, who were most likely to have had mammography if they were part of a prepaid health plan.[39]

In a study of women at higher risk because they had a first-degree relative with breast cancer, Lerman and colleagues[40] showed that psychologic distress about breast cancer had a significant impact on reducing annual mammography adherence among the women in the study who had less than a high school education. Adherence among the women in the study who had more than a high school education appeared unaffected by the level of anxiety about breast cancer. Thus, the response to perceiving oneself at risk for breast cancer appears to vary based on one's educational background, and medically underserved populations with less than a high school education may avoid seeking breast cancer screening services when they perceive themselves to be at risk.

Women may come in for early cancer detection with a symptom or without. Although cancer screening is differentiated from case finding, in part, on the basis of this distinction,[41] many women may go to a breast cancer screening program because of a perceived problem. This is particularly true in low-income and ethnically diverse communities, where specialized programs for the early detection of cancer may be more user-friendly than the usual public hospital clinic programs. In addition, before increased health insurance coverage of screening mammography, recording a symptom to justify billing a diagnostic procedure was a common practice.

Love[42] notes that a decision to seek care requires an understanding of the medical implications of symptoms and a belief in the benefits of diagnosis and treatment. Among some populations, particularly low-income and minority populations, fatalism about cancer and negativism about cancer therapy are widespread.[43] Although knowledge of cancer symptoms and belief in the possibility of early detection and cure may lead to prompter action, the experience among medically underserved populations of reduced cancer survival in general, and reduced breast cancer survival in particular,[10] may lead them to be more pessimistic about the efficacy of early detection and treatment and may lead to delay in seeking care.

What are the implications of the combination of health care system barriers and differential risk perception among low-income and medically underserved populations? Before having screening, low-income women may be anxious about their risk of developing the disease, they may be fatalistic about breast cancer outcomes, and they may face considerable financial and health care system barriers. Thus, low-income women are less likely to seek breast cancer screening. If, on obtaining a first breast-screening examination, a medically underserved woman's findings are negative for cancer, and her perception of risk goes down,[44] then this woman may be less likely to return for a routine annual or biannual screening follow-up examination than a woman who maintains a certain level of concern and views routine breast cancer screening as part of her overall health priorities. For a disadvantaged woman with a finding that is suspicious for cancer or one that requires short-term follow-up, barriers to obtaining a definitive diagnosis combined with fatalism about outcomes may lead to delayed or discontinued follow-up of abnormal findings.

Clinical Follow-Up, Diagnosis, and Treatment

Relatively limited attention has been paid to a problem that occurs in the interval between screening for and treatment of breast cancer: delays or incomplete clinical follow-up of abnormal mammographic and clinical breast findings. As previously noted, in 1986, the NCI set 45% as its target for annual mammogram prevalence and 70% for CBEs among women 50 years of age and older.[1] By 2000, these targets were to be 80% prevalence for both procedures. Assuming that 20% of these women would have some abnormality that required clinical follow-up, then almost 3.5 million women in 1990 would have required clinical follow-up, if the 45% mammography goal alone had been achieved. To date, official public health attention to this matter has been limited to recommendations for the development of breast (and cervical) cancer clinical follow-up practice guidelines for physicians and the development of office-based clinical follow-up systems.[45]

The several steps from the discovery of an abnormal breast screening finding through the diagnostic resolution and treatment for cancer include the following:

- What happens in the interval between the screening encounter and the notification of an abnormal finding
- What transpires between patient notification and patient action
- What the patient brings to the diagnostic encounter

- What happens during the diagnostic encounter
- What transpires from diagnosis through treatment

Although, on average, two procedures are performed to evaluate each abnormal breast-screening examination,[46] the appropriate time span from notification of abnormal results to diagnostic resolution has not been established, and the endpoint of this period is variously defined in the literature as time to first diagnostic test, time to biopsy, time to completion of workup, or time to diagnostic resolution.[47]

In a survey of a 10% random sample of US mammography facilities,[48] only 27.1% of the facilities reported having complete clinical follow-up information on all patients, and an additional 46.5% of the facilities reported having such information on 50% or more of their patients. In a study of procedures to improve follow-up for referrals of patients at risk for cancer,[49] standardized communication from a nurse after examination, combined with one written and one telephone reminder and a patient form to be returned after compliance, improved complete follow-up from 68.2% in the control group to 89% in the experimental group. Half the patients who were eligible for the intervention were not included in the study, however, because of direct physician referral, because of a missed opportunity by the nurses to see the patient, or because the nurses were too busy.

Perhaps as important as *when* feedback about abnormal findings is provided to patients is *how* it is provided. Little is known about how women differ in their reactions to abnormal cancer screening test results.[50] Ideally, no screening program should be initiated without a specific plan for effectively communicating abnormal results and procedures for follow-up.[50] Research on cancer prevention and control intervention has tested some mechanisms for improving patient willingness to complete follow-up. In a large randomized trial involving more than 2000 women with an abnormal Papanicolaou (Pap) smear,[51] three clinic-based interventions were tested, in a factorial design, to increase return rates for screening follow-up: a slide–tape program on Pap smears (before the index smear), a personalized follow-up letter and pamphlet (after the index smear), and transportation incentives (bus passes and parking permits).

The study reported high overall rates of loss to follow-up (29%), with rates ranging among participating clinics from 13% to 42%. Transportation incentives, particularly for medically underserved participants, emerged as the single most effective intervention. For more advantaged patients, the combination of personalized follow-up and the slide–tape presentation was the only intervention that improved clinical follow-up.

Based on follow-up interviews, and because only a third of the patients who received bus passes reported using them, it was suggested that the positive effects of transportation incentives may in part be explained by their psychologic impact on the patients.[51] Patients who received bus passes reported having had a sense of urgency conveyed to them about the importance of clinical follow-up. Moreover, the receipt of the pass conveyed to the patients the concern of the clinic staff for their health and well-being.

The perception of the health care system by patients with abnormal cancer screening findings can be affected both by prior experience with the system and by their experience in trying to set up a diagnostic follow-up appointment. For medically underserved patients, the time and effort entailed in negotiating public health systems may be prohibitive. Similarly, the psychologic consequences of waiting for weeks or even months for an initial appointment can be profound. System barriers may promote delay or denial because of a perception that the "cure" may be seen as worse than the disease[46] and because any slowness in the system to respond to the patient's need for clinical follow-up may communicate a lack of urgency.

Results of large-scale surveys that focus on black–white differences in cancer knowledge and behaviors,[52] and in access to care,[53] point to a need for further research to address the unique experiences of black patients that give rise to negative perceptions and attitudes regarding health care delivery. Underlying this concern is the question whether these attitudes are associated with lower SES or whether they constitute a pattern common to most blacks regardless of their SES. Although a review conducted by the American Cancer Society concluded that income rather than race was responsible for black–white differences in knowledge and behaviors,[54] income alone may not account for the differences.

Findings that blacks continue to face repeated incidents of racial discrimination[55] suggest that attitudes of minority groups toward health care may be shaped by such experiences, and an understanding of these attitudes may be essential to addressing the reluctance or inability of some women to pursue diagnostic resolution after having abnormal CBE or mammographic results. Support for this assertion can be found in the results of a national survey that revealed significant race differences in the use of health care even after controlling for the effects of income, health status, age, and sex.[56]

Thus, experiences that transcend lines of social class among blacks emerge as potentially significant in explaining reduced access to care and differences in perceptions of the quality of care received. For example, Hunter and associates[56] found that factors associated with stage of disease at diagnosis were expressed differently among black and white breast cancer patients. Among black patients, indicators of access to health care, lack of mammography use, and increased body mass index contributed significantly to stage differences, whereas income was marginally associated with stage among whites. In addition, having a CBE by a physician, a history of patient delay, and nuclear grade of the tumor explained up to 50% of the excess risk of stage III or IV tumors versus stage I or II (N0) among black women compared with white women.

The context of the diagnostic encounter may play an important role in determining subsequent patient behavior.[57] Whether screened by a primary care physician or through an inreach or outreach cancer-screening program, the patient whose breast cancer screening shows the need for clinical follow-up will have a limited, if any, prior relationship with the clinical follow-up service providers to whom she is referred. In the absence of such a personal relationship, and without the advocacy role of a personal physician, previous experience with the health care system will help to determine the response of the patient to the diagnostic encounter as well as any follow-up recommendations made.

When low-income and ethnically diverse patients receive care, what does the health care system convey to them? "When I went into the system (with an abnormality) I knew I was poor, but then the system made me feel poor." This statement was often made by cancer patients and their families in a series of national hearings held by the American Cancer Society in 1989.[54] Scheduling clinical follow-up for weeks or months after a sign or symptom of cancer is detected, onerous financial and medical clearances for diagnostic and subsequent treatment procedures, and the inability to communicate with the provider are all significant barriers. These barriers to quality of care are common in the underresourced health care systems serving many low-income and culturally diverse populations.

When black women with breast cancer are compared with white women with breast cancer, many differences emerge that could contribute to poorer survival (overall and within stage of disease at diagnosis).[58] Black breast cancer patients are less likely to be married, they often have a lower SES and less formal education, and they are more likely to list a publicly funded facility as a usual source of care than white breast cancer patients. Black breast cancer patients have more comorbid illnesses, are more likely to be overweight, and are more likely to be current smokers. With respect to their prognosis and treatment, black women with breast cancer are diagnosed with more advanced disease, are more likely to have poorly differentiated and estrogen receptor–negative tumors, and are less likely to have undergone therapeutic surgery or to have received radiation therapy than white women with breast cancer.

Many of these factors are interrelated, and based on the finding that 40% of black–white differences in overall survival rates was explained by more advanced disease at diagnosis and another 15% was explained by histologic or pathologic differences, Hunter and coworkers concluded[56] that public health resources should focus primarily on promoting the early detection of breast cancer. Although treatment differences explained no new additional survival variance after controlling for stage and tumor characteristics, treatment was measured crudely (as present or absent) and stage-specific black–white survival differences were not examined because of reduced sample sizes. Thus, variation in the quality of multidisciplinary breast cancer patient management in relation to stage-specific survival differences among blacks and whites has not yet been examined.

Although various guidelines for the optimal treatment of breast cancer have been published[59] and promoted, variation in access to and patterns of therapeutic surgical therapy, radiation therapy, and systemic therapy persist.[60] Patterns-of-care studies of regional and hospital variation in treatment of breast cancer have documented that substantial variation exists, and this variation is related in part to geographic locale (urban versus rural), type of hospital (teaching versus nonteaching), physician characteristics (years in practice, solo practice), and patient characteristics (age, health insurance).[61-64] Assuming that medically underserved populations are more likely to be seen in resource-limited health care institutions, where access to the most advanced care may be more limited, then physician and patient alike may be handicapped in providing and receiving the best that multidisciplinary breast cancer management has to offer.

Beyond geographic and institutional variation in available breast cancer treatment resources, better understanding of patient and physician interactions in treatment decision making is important,[63,64] particularly as it relates to the medically underserved. From the provider's perspective, family practice residents believe that poor patients are more likely to miss appointments than others, are more likely to be late for appointments, and are less knowledgeable about their illnesses.[65] One in four residents believed that poor patients did not appreciate the work of their physicians and nurses, and 43% claimed that the poor are more difficult patients. Finally, many of these residents indicated that the poor are unlikely to practice preventive health behaviors (72%), they are unlikely to be compliant with their medical regimens (60%), and they cared less than others about their health (41%).

Poor and ethnically diverse patients tend to view the health care system as cold, unfriendly, and insensitive to their particular needs. Providers regard these patients as noncompliant and unappreciative. Given these views, the prospects of ensuring clinical follow-up and access to the most advanced care for many of these patients appear dim. Distrust of the health care system is linked with noncompliance.[66] Thus, building a community's confidence in their medical providers may be as important for breast cancer control as improving access to primary care and ensuring adequate early-detection facilities. Similarly, educating providers about the unique problems that poor people face in adhering to providers' advice is important. Improving the image of community health care can be achieved by directing new and expanded resources toward community-based and culturally appropriate disease detection and clinical follow-up programs that also ensure a promise of early detection leading to cure for all patients.[67]

Discussion

With respect to breast cancer, as well as many other cancers, the medically underserved are understudied, they are not well understood by many in the medical and academic research community, and they are attended by health care institutions that are underfunded and often do not have the resources necessary to ensure access to the best possible cancer screening, clinical follow-up, diagnosis, and treatment. At the same time, medically underserved women are more likely to be diagnosed with late-stage breast cancer, and some groups (eg, black women) bear the greatest

breast cancer mortality burden in the United States. Although the short-term emphasis on increasing use of existing breast cancer screening resources may contribute to downstaging breast cancer in these high-risk women, both the inaccessibility of screening services for many women and the barriers to prompt and effective clinical follow-up, diagnosis, and treatment suggest that the long-term burden of breast cancer will continue to grow for the medically underserved.

When resources are limited, triaging service resources to those patients and communities with the greatest breast cancer burden would appear to be a logical first step. In the absence of any serious progress toward health care reform, however, those who need the most care will undoubtedly continue to receive the least. Efforts to involve these high-risk populations in cancer research could conceivably also play a role in improving access to the most advanced prevention, early detection, and treatment trials for breast cancer. If this is to be accomplished, however, serious efforts to involve leaders of the medically underserved community in the design and implementation of this research will be necessary to ensure that the research will be accepted by the community and that the interventions tested have a reasonable chance of proving themselves cost-effective and maintaining themselves beyond the initial research grant funding.

If solutions to the inclusion problems in breast cancer prevention and treatment trials exist, they will not likely be facilitated by the National Institutes of Health–imposed requirement for proportional representation in publicly funded research. On the contrary, where class, racial, ethnic, or age differences are of potential scientific importance, then overrepresentation of medically underserved minorities will be required to ensure sufficient statistical power to explore and test group differences. Conversely, when being a member of an underserved minority is unlikely to contribute to variation in the risk markers of interest, then proportional representation becomes an arbitrary evaluation standard with no internal or external validity. This requires a scientific judgment call, in which the evidence is often limited and is usually insufficient. Nevertheless, the effort made to consider the alternatives, and specifically to address the mechanisms for obtaining minority oversampling where necessary, will be superior to the current system of rubber-stamping all research in which underserved minorities are proportionately represented in the proposed design but are rarely accrued in the actual study.

For all breast cancer intervention research, involving, from the very beginning of the study design, community, medical, and scientific leaders that reflect the cultural background of the study populations of interest will help to ensure acceptance when field accrual begins. Formative research (eg, focus groups) to explore community attitudes toward the intervention can also help to identify potential trouble spots before the trials begins. Of equal importance is the need to develop mechanisms by which the community studied is provided feedback in an educationally and culturally appropriate manner as to the final results of the study. Such community debriefings are extremely rare, given the pressure to publish study findings in the professional literature. In the long run, however, efforts to provide the study subjects with the findings of the study in a user-friendly format greatly contribute to the trust necessary for individuals to volunteer and to participate fully.

Whether focused on service delivery or inclusion in research, academic health centers must take the lead in forging partnerships with the medically underserved communities in their regional service area.[68] Of the 126 academic health centers in the United States, 75% have medically underserved minority populations in their local area.[69] Essential characteristics of these partnerships include community-based leadership and ownership of specific programs, training and use of community health workers, joint planning for research, and services targeted to meet community health problems.[69] In the absence of such joint efforts, initiatives to reduce breast cancer mortality among the medically underserved are unlikely to be effective.

References

1. Greenwald P, Sondik E, eds. Cancer control objectives for the nation: 1985–2000. Natl Cancer Inst Monogr 1986;2:105.
2. National Center for Health Statistics. Health, United States, 1992. Hyattsville, MD, Public Health Service, 1993.
3. Baquet CR, Horm JW, Gibbs T, et al. Socioeconomic factors and cancer incidence among blacks and whites. J Natl Cancer Inst 1991;83:551.
4. Krieger N. Social class and the black/white crossover in the age-specific incidence in breast cancer: a study linking census-derived data to population-based registry records. Am J Epidemiol 1990;131:804.
5. Kerner JF, Breen N, Tefft M, et al. Tobacco use among multi-ethnic latino populations. Am J Public Health (in press).
6. Nomura AMY, Lee J, Kolonel LN, et al. Breast cancer in two populations with different risk for the disease. Am J Epidemiol 1984;119:496.
7. Schatzkin A, Palmer JR, Rosenberg L, et al. Risk for breast cancer in black women. J Natl Cancer Inst 1987;78:213.
8. Mayberry RM, Stoddard-Wright C. Breast cancer risk factors among black women and white women: similarities and differences. Am J Epidemiol 1992;136:1445.
9. Miller BA, Gloeckler Ries LA, Hankey BF, et al, eds. SEER Cancer Statistics Review 1973–1990. Bethesda, National Cancer Institute, NIH publ no. 93-2789, 1993.
10. Trapido EJ, Chen F, Davis K, et al. Cancer in south Florida Hispanic women: a 9-year assessment. Arch Intern Med 1994;154:1083.
11. Polednak AP. Cancer incidence in the Puerto Rican–born population of Connecticut. Cancer 1992;70:1172.
12. Wolfgang PE, Semeiks PA, Burnett WS. Cancer incidence in New York City Hispanics, 1982–85. Ethnic Dis 1991;1:263.
13. Baquet CR, Ringen K, Pollack ES, et al. Cancer among blacks and other minorities: statistical profiles. Bethesda, National Cancer Institute, NIH publ. no. 86-2785, 1986.
14. Trapido EJ, Obeso JL, Stein NS, et al. Unidos po la salud para vivir bien cancer data report: National Hispanic Leadership Initiative on Cancer of the National Coalition of Hispanic Health and Human Service Organizations. Washington, DC, 1995.
15. Harris JR, Lippman ME, Veronesi U, et al. Breast cancer. N Engl J Med 1992;327:319.
16. Wynder EL, Cohen LA, Rose DP, et al. Dietary fat and breast cancer: where do we stand on the evidence? J Clin Epidemiol 1994;47:217.
17. Gapstur SM, Potter JD, Sellers TA, et al. Increased risk of breast cancer with alcohol consumption in postmenopausal women. Am J Epidemiol 1992;136:1221.
18. Friedenreich CM, Howe GR, Miller AB, et al. A cohort study of alcohol consumption and risk of breast cancer. Am J Epidemiol 1993;137:512.
19. Calle EE, Miracle-McMahill HL, Thun M, et al. Cigarette smoking and risk of fatal breast cancer. *Am J Epidemiol* 1994;139:1001.
20. Willett W. Response to Wynder et al's paper on dietary fat and breast cancer. J Clin Epidemiol 1994;47:223.
21. Cancer incidence among NYC Hispanics. NY State J Med 1990:44.
22. Gray GE, Henderson BE, Pike MC. Changing ratio of breast cancer incidence rates with age of black females compared with white females in the United States. J Natl Cancer Inst 1980;64:461.
23. Mor V, Pacala JT, Rakowski W. Mammography for older women: who uses, who benefits? J Gerontol 1992;47:43.
24. Bernstein L, Ross RK, Henderson BE. Prospects for the primary prevention of breast cancer. Am J Epidemiol 1992;136:42.
25. Thomas SB, Quinn SC. Public health then and now: the Tuskegee syphilis study, 1932 to 1972. Am J Public Health 1991;81:1498.
26. Mandelblatt J, Traxler M, Lakin P, et al. Breast and cervical cancer screening of poor, elderly, black women: clinical results and implications. Am J Prev Med 1993;3:133.
27. Chen F, Trapido EJ, Davis K. Differences in stage at presentation of breast and gynecologic cancers among whites, blacks, and hispanics. Cancer 1994;73:2838.
28. Breen N, Kessler L. Current trends in cancer screening. MMWR (in press).
29. King EU, Resch N, Rimer B, et al. Breast cancer screening practices among retirement community women. Prev Med 1993;22:1.
30. The national strategic plan for the early detection and control of breast and cervical cancer. Bethesda, Centers for Disease Control and Prevention, Food and Drug Administration, National Cancer Institute, 1994.
31. Mandelblatt J. Screening elderly, poor, black women for breast and cervical cancer. Cancer prev 1993:1.
32. Miller AB. Screening for breast cancer: is too much being attempted? Breast Cancer Res Treat (in press).
33. Breen N, Kessler L. Changes in use of screening mammography: evidence from the 1987 and 1990 national health interview surveys. Am J Public Health 1994;84:62.
34. Urban N, Anderson GL, Peakcock S. Mammography screening: how important is cost as a barrier to use. Am J Public Health 1994;84:50.
35. Mammography and breast examination: results from the behavioral risk factor surveillance system, 1992. Oncology 1993;7:48.
36. Whitman S, Ansell D, Lacey L, et al. Patterns of breast and cervical cancer screening at three public health centers in an inner city urban area. Am J Public Health 1991;81:1651.
37. Mandelblatt J, Traxler M, Lakin P, et al. Mammography and Papanicolau smear use by elderly poor black women. J Am Geriatr Soc 1992;40:1001.
38. Gemson DH, Elinson J, Messeri P. Differences in physician prevention practice patterns for white and minority patients. J Commun Health 1988;13:53.
39. Fox SA, Stein JA. The effect of physician–patient communication on mammography utilization by different ethnic groups. Med Care 1991;29:1065.
40. Lerman C, Daly M, Sands C, et al. Mammography adherence and psychological distress among women at risk for breast cancer. J Natl Cancer Inst 1993;85:1074.
41. Winawer SJ, Kerner JF. Sigmoidoscopy: case finding versus screening. (Editorial) Gastroenterology 1988;95:527.
42. Love N. Why patients delay seeking care for cancer symptoms: what you can do about it. Cancer Eval 1991;89:151.
43. American Cancer Society. Cancer and the poor: a report to the

nation: findings of regional hearings conducted by the American Cancer Society. Atlanta, American Cancer Society, 1989.

44. Lerman C, Trock B, Rimer BK, et al. Psychological and behavioral implications of abnormal mammograms. Ann Intern Med 1991;114:657.

45. The national strategic plan for the early detection and control of breast and cervical cancers. Bethesda, Centers for Disease Control and Prevention, Food and Drug Administration, 1994:30.

46. Kerlikowski K, Grady D, Barclay J, et al. Positive predictive value of screening mammography by age and family history of breast cancer. JAMA 1993;270:2444.

47. Kerlikowski K. Follow-up after abnormal screening mammography. Breast Cancer Res Treat (in press).

48. Houn F, Brown ML. Current practice of screening mammography in the United States: data from the National Survey of Mammography Facilities. Radiology 1994;190:209.

49. Manfredi C, Lacey L, Warnecke R. Results of an intervention to improve compliance with referrals for evaluation of suspected malignancies at neighborhood public health centers. Am J Public Health 1990;80:85.

50. Lerman CE, Rimer BK. Psychosocial impact of cancer screening. Oncology 1993;7:67.

51. Marcus AC, Crane LA, Kaplan CP, et al. Improving adherence to screening follow-up among women with abnormal pap smears. Med Care 1992;30:216.

52. Jepson C, Kessler LG, Portnoy B, et al. Black–white differences in cancer prevention knowledge and behavior. Am J Public Health 1991;81:501.

53. Blendon RJ, Aiken LH, Freeman HE, et al. Access to medical care for black and white Americans: a matter of continuing concern. JAMA 1989;261:278.

54. American Cancer Society. Cancer and the poor: a report to the nation: findings of regional hearings conducted by the ACS, 1989.

55. Feagin JR. The continuing significance of race: anti-black discrimination in public places. Am Soc Rev 1991;56:101.

56. Hunter C, Redmond CK, Chen VW, et al. Breast cancer associated with stage at diagnosis in black and white women. J Natl Cancer Inst 1993;85:1129.

57. Celantano D. The Lerman/Rimer article reviewed. Oncology 1993;7:72.

58. Eley JW, Hill HA, Chen VW, et al. Racial differences in survival from breast cancer. JAMA 1994;272:947.

59. NIH Consensus Conference. Treatment of early-stage breast cancer. JAMA 1991;265:391.

60. Ayanian JZ, Guadagnoli E. Variations in breast cancer treatment by patient and provider characteristics. Breast Cancer Res Treat (in press).

61. Samet JM, Hunt WC, Farrow DC. Determinants of receiving breast conserving surgery. Cancer 1994;73:2344.

62. Ayanian JZ, Kohler BA, Abe T, et al. The relation between health insurance coverage and clinical outcomes among women with breast cancer. N Engl J Med 1993;329:326.

63. Iscoe NA, Goel V, Wu K, et al. Variation in breast cancer surgery in Ontario. Can Med Assoc J 1994;150:345.

64. Whelan T, Marcellus D, Clark R, et al. Adjuvant radiotherapy for early breast cancer: patterns of practice in Ontario. Can Med Assoc J 1993;149:1273.

65. Price JH, Desmond SM, Snyder FF, et al. Perceptions of family practice residents regarding health care and poor patients. J Fam Pract 1988;27:615.

66. Greenwald HP, Becker SW, Nevitt MC. Delay and noncompliance in cancer detection: a behavioral perspective for health planners. Milbank Memorial Fund Quarterly/Health and Society 1978:56.

67. Kerner JF, Dusenbury L, Mandelblatt JS. Poverty and cultural diversity: challenges for health promotion among medically underserved populations. Annu Rev Publ Health 1993;14:355.

68. Levine DM, Becker DM, Bone LR, et al. Community–academic health center partnerships for underserved minority populations. JAMA 1994;272:309.

69. Health professions education for the future: schools in service to the nation. Report of the Pew Health Professions Commission. Durham, Pew Health Professions Commission, 1993.

Diseases of the Breast, edited by Jay R. Harris,
Marc E. Lippman, Monica Morrow, and Samuel Hellman.
Lippincott-Raven Publishers, Philadelphia, © 1996.

Patient Rehabilitation and Support

25.1
Psychologic Reactions to Breast Cancer Diagnosis, Treatment, and Survival

JULIA H. ROWLAND ▪ MARY JANE MASSIE

Breast cancer, the most common form of cancer among American women, will be diagnosed in more than 183,400 women in 1995, and an estimated 46,240 women will die of the disease.[1] Whereas an exact understanding of the causes and control of breast cancer continues to elude researchers, rapid advances in detection and treatment have led to increases in the disease-free survival among women diagnosed with breast cancer.[1-3] Most women diagnosed today can expect to be cured of or live for long periods with their disease. Unlike treatment for other chronic diseases such as diabetes and heart disease, however, the treatments for cancer are more toxic and intensive. The result is increasing demands on patients' physical reserves and on their psychologic and social resources to survive and manage the illness.

Specific developments in breast cancer care have drawn attention to the key role of psychosocial factors in prevention, detection, treatment, and outcome.[4] Improvements in and broader use of screening mammography has led to an increase in numbers of women whose cancers are diagnosed at earlier stages and to questions of who gets screened. The greater availability of options for surgical management (eg, lumpectomy plus radiation versus mastectomy with or without breast reconstruction with implants or autologous tissue) has expanded women's role in the decision-making process. More extensive use of aggressive multimodal treatment regimens has increased sensitivity to issues of patient–doctor and family communication and patient adherence. Finally, identification of genetic markers of breast cancer risk and the evaluation of chemopreventive agents has raised awareness of the psychologic toll on unaffected women who are at increased risk for this disease, sometimes referred to as the "worried well."[5]

All of these changes have occurred in the context of greater demand by patients for involvement in their own care, consumer activism, attention to ethical and informed consent issues, use of quality-of-life assessment in treatment outcomes, and emphasis on cost efficacy in care. The consequence of these changes is a growing demand for medical professionals to recognize and address the psychosocial impact of breast cancer across the course of care.

Although breast cancer is a major stress for any woman, there is great variability in women's psychologic responses. This chapter outlines the normal and abnormal responses to cancer and those factors that may increase a woman's risk for poor adaptation. In addition, because of their growing importance, the role of family in women's adaptation and the special concerns related to sexual functioning are addressed.

Factors Affecting Psychologic Impact

Three sets of factors contribute to psychologic response: the sociocultural context in which treatment options are offered, the psychologic and psychosocial factors that the woman and her environment bring to the situation, and the medical factors or physical facts the woman must confront in terms of disease stage, treatment, response, and clinical course (Table 25.1-1). To provide comprehensive care to every woman, each of these areas must be assessed, and problems must be addressed across the illness trajectory.

SOCIOCULTURAL CONTEXT

To understand and interpret the data on women's responses to breast cancer, it is critical to appreciate the context within which diagnosis and treatment occur, both medically and socially. The broader changes in public attitudes toward cancer over the last century are reviewed elsewhere.[6] Several specific changes that have taken place in the scientific understanding of and medical approach to breast cancer in the last decade have had a significant impact on how this disease is viewed by the public. Primary among these changes have been growing attention to the patient's role in decision making across the course of cancer care, increased demand for and greater public

TABLE 25.1-1

Factors Contributing to the Psychologic Responses of Women to Breast Cancer

---

CURRENT SOCIOCULTURAL CONTEXT, TREATMENT OPTIONS, AND DECISION MAKING

Changes in surgical management from a uniform approach

   Breast-conserving management; more acknowledged uncertainty

Social attitudes

   Public figures disclose having had breast cancer

   Autobiographic accounts of and "how to" guides for treatment of breast cancer in popular press

Ethnical imperative for patient participation in treatment issues; legal imperative for knowledge of treatment options

Variations in care by ethnicity, location, age

Public awareness of treatment and research controversies; advocacy for more funding and lay oversight

PSYCHOLOGIC AND PSYCHOSOCIAL FACTORS

Type and degree of disruption in life cycle tasks caused by breast cancer (eg, marital, childbearing)

Psychologic stability and ability to cope with stress

Prior psychiatric history

Availability of psychologic and social support (partner, family, friends)

MEDICAL FACTORS

Stage of cancer at diagnosis

Treatment received: mastectomy/lumpectomy and radiation, adjuvant chemotherapy, hormonal therapy, bone marrow transplant

Availability of rehabilitation

   Psychologic (partner, support groups)

   Physical (reconstruction)

Psychologic support provided by physicians and staff

---

involvement in the assessment of research into the prevention and treatment of breast cancer in particular, and more federal support for research on the psychosocial and behavioral aspects of cancer.

Decision Making

The importance of patient involvement in treatment choices is the result of the following: a broader range of options offered at time of diagnosis; greater intensity of treatments recommended for most women, even those with early-stage disease; and increased public demand for informed consent. Today, women with a diagnosis of breast cancer are aware of the plurality of views about primary breast cancer treatment. Most recognize that no best treatment exists, that they have options, and that their preference can be considered in the decision. Women often are provided with survival statistics associated with each mode of treatment, although physicians may vary in the emphasis placed on them. The increased dialogue between physician and patient about treatment reduces some of the stresses formerly faced by women in an earlier period when there was little discussion about management of the disease. However, the new psychologic burden of responsibility for making the right choice can increase anxiety when it is already great.

Over the course of initial care, women face three major decision points. The first of these is at the time of initial discovery of the lump. Most women consult their gynecologist or trusted and accessible physician when they find a lump (64% to 70% of which are found by women themselves).[7] How quickly a woman decides to seek evaluation of her lump or to follow-up on a recommended course of action depends on a number of variables, including sociodemographic status, knowledge, attitudes and beliefs about cancer, personality and coping styles, and nature of the existing doctor–patient relationship.[8] It is well established that the earlier her tumor is detected, the more likely a woman's breast cancer is to be curable. However, presence of advanced disease does not always imply delay.[9] Furthermore, responsibility for delay may rest with the physician, the woman, or both. One study suggested that survival rates are higher in women who themselves delayed diagnosis than in women whose physicians were responsible for the delay.[10] Concerns that delay in seeking care may account for the poorer survival in African American women have not been supported. Epidemiologic data have shown that biologic risk factors may play a more important role in survival than access to treatment.[11] Greater public awareness of the importance of screening mammography, emphasis on the importance of early detection, private and public programs and funding for access to care, and efforts to decrease physician delay in referral for further evaluation all decrease the delay of treatment.[12]

At the time of consultation with a surgeon, the woman is faced with her second set of decisions: whether to accept a one- or two-step procedure; if given a choice, whether to undergo mastectomy or lumpectomy plus irradiation; and whether to seek a second opinion or care elsewhere. In 18 states, the law and clinical practice dictate that the surgeon must inform the woman that she has the option of a two-stage surgical procedure, which separates the diagnostic biopsy from the primary treatment procedure. In these states, the two treatment options of mastectomy or lumpectomy with irradiation must be presented as well, although how this is done varies widely by state.[13] Some insurance carriers mandate a second opinion before the performance of any elective procedure. Research has shown that these laws make a difference; in those states that mandate informed decision making, more women receive lumpectomy.[14,15] At the same time, whereas these policies provide a valuable impetus for women to obtain thorough medical evaluation and information, they also introduce other sets of opinions. The woman whose second or third opinion differs dramatically from the first has the difficult task of deciding which physician she trusts and which treatment plan to accept. Meanwhile, considerable time can be lost.

In the past few years, a number of cancer centers across the country have developed multidisciplinary breast clinics to address the need for women to seek opinions from diverse specialists. In these centers, women usually are seen after their initial biopsy and meet with a surgeon, medical oncologist, radiation oncologist, and in some centers, other breast specialists including a pathologist, radiologist, plastic surgeon, mental health professional, and clinical research nurse. The concept behind this one-stop visit is to provide the woman with information about all of her treatment options in a comprehensive setting and to outline for her treatment that can be tailored to her specific cancer and to her personal needs. Clinical experience suggests that such programs are helpful in reducing the stress experienced by women around decision making and facilitating information gathering. However, studies are needed to demonstrate the benefits of this approach compared with the more common practice of multiple consultations.

During the diagnostic workup period, the woman must cope simultaneously with the need to keep her distressing emotions of anxiety and fear within tolerable limits while making the difficult decision about treatment for a potentially fatal disease. To accomplish this, she must assimilate new medical information that, in itself, produces anxiety. One study has shown that before and after breast biopsy, anxiety and information overload compromise some women's decision-making ability, making informed decisions difficult, even at best.[16] Valanis and Rumpler[17] observed that a woman's previous experiences, her personal and demographic characteristics, her social support network (family and friends), and her physician influence her treatment selection.

The current legal climate, which dictates that full and complete disclosure of information be given by the doctor in a uniform manner to all women, fails to take into account the wide variation in women's reactions to the information and the range of ways of dealing with the decisions about treatment. Ideally, the method of giving information should be individualized for each patient. Emphasis on informed decision making places a heavy responsibility on the physician to be cognizant of the individual patient's physical and psychologic needs and to tailor the

discussion and recommendations with that in mind. At times, it may mean tempering a woman's demands for unrealistic treatment, acquiescing to another woman's desire to defer a final decision to her physician or significant other, or in some cases, reassuring a woman that she need not reach a decision instantly but has a few days to research her options and come to an appropriate choice. (A broader review of women's response styles and physician–patient communication issues is provided elsewhere.[18–20])

When faced with breast cancer, some women find themselves emotionally paralyzed by the decision-making process. They may be overwhelmed by the knowledge that they have breast cancer and by its potential threat to their lives. For these women, even the options are too painful to consider. They often benefit from referral for psychiatric consultation. It is helpful for them to have the pressure temporarily removed by postponing surgery and to be able to review the events and possible treatments in a setting in which they can express concerns and fears and identify the reasons for their response. A useful procedure is for the mental health consultant or specially trained nurse clinician to take them, step by step, through each treatment option, asking at each juncture, "How would you respond to that?" By this method, with reduced anxiety, it usually becomes clear that certain aspects of one or the other treatment are more acceptable to the patient. These women can then return to their surgeon ready to proceed with treatment.

Although many women report the decision-making process as highly stressful, research indicates that women who are given a choice about treatment do better than those who are not.[21–24] In their work, Ashcroft and co-workers[21] found that when women were given a choice of treatment, in this case between mastectomy or limited resection plus radiation therapy, they adapted well to both types of treatment. Levels of anxiety and depression for both groups were similar to those in other surgical patients, and no evidence of profound anxiety and depression was present at 1 year. In their study, Morris and Royle[22] found that both women who were *not* offered a choice in treatment and their husbands had high levels of anxiety and depression preoperatively and up to 2 months after surgery. By contrast, women and their husbands who were offered a choice showed similar mood levels to patients with benign disease or those undergoing noncancer surgery. Other studies show that the quality of physician communication during this phase is a critical determinant of subsequent psychologic well-being in breast cancer patients.[25] Although most women when confronted with breast cancer want to have information, clinicians need to be aware that not all women wish to make the final decision about treatment.[26] A woman's need for information must be assessed separately from her desire to participate in or delegate treatment choice.

Public Attitudes

A sense of public distrust has grown toward the medical community in general and cancer research in particular. Some of this arises from confusion about the state of progress in the war on cancer.[27] In addition, the public and some researchers remain uncertain about the attributable risk of a variety of epidemiologic factors (eg, use of exogenous hormones such as oral contraceptives and hormone replacement, exposure to environmental carcinogens such as pesticides, and dietary risks).[28] Finally, several specific events have fueled public concern. These include questions raised at the US Food and Drug Administration (FDA) hearings about the safety of silicone and saline implants, publication of early reports that tamoxifen may have more serious long-term effects than anticipated,[29] and media reports challenging the results of clinical trials whose outcomes have influenced the course of breast cancer care.

While at times creating fear, rage, and confusion for women who believed that their treatment or lives were affected, disclosure of this information has empowered a sector of the population to become more vocal advocates for better research on breast cancer prevention and treatment. The Breast Cancer Coalition, represented largely by breast cancer survivors and the healthcare professionals caring for them, was successful in lobbying substantial funds from the Department of Defense earmarked for breast cancer research. Lay advocates also have been specifically included in clinical trials' oversight committees.

The net effect of this movement is growing attention to the need for more research on prevention and for more methods to increase survival. Included in this is emphasis on the role of complementary approaches to care, often involving efforts to change people's life-style to reduce risk or improve coping responses to promote adaptation. Importantly, it has also resulted in greater opportunity for physician–patient dialogue and teamwork in facing the challenges of breast cancer care.

PSYCHOLOGIC VARIABLES

In her classic review, Meyerowitz[30] delineated the psychosocial impact of breast cancer in three broad areas: psychologic discomfort (anxiety, depression, and anger); changes in life patterns (consequent to physical discomfort, marital or sexual disruption, and altered activity level); and fears and concerns (mastectomy or loss of breast, recurrence, and death). Although women may have many more treatment options, the psychologic concerns remain the same. In addition to these variables, the life stage at which the cancer occurs, previous emotional stability (personality and coping style), and the presence of interpersonal support should be included.

Age, or the point in the life cycle at which breast cancer occurs, and what social tasks are threatened or interrupted, are of prime importance. The threat to a sense of femininity and self-esteem occurs in all women, but it may be more difficult for a young woman whose attractiveness and fertility are paramount, especially for those who are single and without a partner. In their review, Mor and colleagues[31] highlight several factors that may put younger women at greater risk for problems in adapting. These include the following: the "off-timedness" of a diagnosis in the younger patient; disruption of primary role as caregiver and, increasingly, as breadwinner; and women's perception of having more to loose (including careers and chance to see offspring grow up). An estimated 14% of breast cancers occur in women younger than 45 years of age, with most of these (78%) in women between the ages of 35 and 44 years.[28] Whereas premenopausal women thus constitute a small proportion of those diagnosed with breast cancer, the special issues related to their cancer risk, survival, and care were the focus of a conference sponsored by the National Cancer Institute.[32] At the other end of the spectrum, breast cancer diagnosed in a woman older than 65 years may be experienced in the presence of other major losses, particularly of a spouse, which means that she must adjust to concurrent life stresses. Fotopoulos and Cook,[33] reporting from a multicenter psychologic study of breast cancer, noticed a high level of distress in older women. Such reports, coupled with findings that indicate older women are significantly less likely to receive appropriate surgical care or rehabilitation,[34] suggest that women at both ends of the developmental continuum are at particular risk for problems in adapting to breast cancer.

The second variable contributing to adaptation relates to the patient herself, that is, her personality and coping patterns. Each woman has her own style of adaptation to stress, which is a remarkably abiding quality. Studies of breast cancer patients suggest that women who use an active, problem-solving approach to the stresses of illness exhibit a less distressed mood and better adaptation.[35–37] In addition, because adaptation to illness is necessarily a dynamic process, those who exhibit flexibility in their efforts cope better. For example, Glanz and Lerman[4] observe that although information-seeking and problem-solving skills may be critical during treatment planning, use of denial and avoidant coping strategies during active chemotherapy or radiation may be more helpful in reducing or minimizing treatment side effects. The relative efficacy of each style thus may be situation specific.[38] Finally, women who are able to draw on and use available social resources and support adapt better as well.[39] By contrast, women at risk for poor coping are those who exhibit a passive, helpless, hopeless, or pessimistic stance in the face of illness, are rigid in their use of coping strategies, and tend to be socially isolated or to reject help when offered. Further studies suggest that women who exhibit a pattern of active, fighting spirit to their disease have a better quality of life and also may survive longer than women who seem to give up.[40]

In the context of any discussion of coping responses, the relation between attitudes and cancer survival, as well as risk, has become a growing area of public interest and psychooncologic research. Because breast cancer is a prevalent neoplasm and one with great psychologic impact, possible role of psychologic variables in risk and survival has been explored extensively. The question of a potential role for emotions in vulnerability to breast cancer and its progression has received much attention in the public press. Many women express concern that they brought it on themselves or that their attitude is bad and that they or their lifestyle may be making the cancer worse. In a study of what women attributed to having caused their breast cancer, Taylor and colleagues[36] found that 41% of women from their well-educated sample believed that they were responsible for the development of the disease and that stress was a major contributor to its development. In an ongoing study that we are conducting at Georgetown among women 4 to 12 months after treatment for node-negative breast cancer, 35 of 131 women interviewed (27%) indicated that they believed that stress, emotions, or both contributed to their illness; 18% believed that such factors played a major role in disease onset.

The belief that they may be responsible for their own illness and its outcome has become an added psychologic burden for many women with breast cancer. Indeed, it is a hazard for those who, based on these beliefs, seek questionable and unproved therapies as primary treatment for their breast cancer, either never starting or discontinuing conventional treatments. Publication in the public media of early and controversial findings about emotions in breast cancer is a growing concern. For these reasons, oncologists must be familiar with the status of psychologic research in breast cancer risk and survival to answer their patients' questions on the subject and provide clarification and reassurance. For an extensive review of the research on psychologic factors in cancer risk and survival, the reader is referred to reports by Holland[41] and Bovbjerg,[42] as well as reviews by Levenson and Bemis,[43] and Spiegel.[44]

Prior personal association with breast cancer can also influence adjustment. The memory of a mother's, sister's, or grandmother's death from breast cancer, or that of a close friend, makes the diagnosis seem far more ominous and may result in greater levels of psychologic distress during and after treatment. Some women with a high investment in their bodies cannot tolerate even the idea of loss or damage to a breast. Such women are at risk for delay in seeking consultation when a symptom occurs; they may also be at risk for problems in adaptation after treatment, particularly if hoped-for attempts to preserve cosmetic appearance are less than expected or must be abandoned because of the extent of disease.

Finally, adjustment depends on the response from other significant people: first from spouse or partner and also from family and friends. Because of the importance of social support to women's adaptation, this is addressed at greater length under the section on family adaptation.

Prolonged anxiety or depression is not an expected reaction to a cancer diagnosis. Of the 50 studies of the prevalence of depression in individuals with cancer conducted over the last 27 years, 17 included women with breast cancer.[45] Reported rates of depression in these 17 studies range from 1.5% to 50%. Most of this variance can be attributed to the lack of standardization of methodology and diagnostic criteria. The common stress reactions around the time of diagnosis and during early treatment can be quickly evaluated and managed by the patient's physician, nurse, or specially designated cancer counselor. However, some women have greater problems and benefit from psychologic management by psychiatrists and psychologists, who often are collaborating members of the treatment team (see Table 25.1-2).

Consultation usually is requested for women with the following characteristics: are at high genetic risk for breast

TABLE 25.1-2
Women With Breast Cancer Who Should Be Considered for Psychiatric Evaluation

Those who present with current symptoms or a history of:
   Depression or anxiety
   Suicidal thinking (attempt)
   Substance or alcohol abuse
   Confusional state (delirium or encephalopathy)
   Akathisia from neuroleptic antiemetics
   Mood swings, insomnia, or irritability from steroids
Those who:
   Have a family history of breast cancer
   Are very young, old, pregnant, nursing, single, or alone
   Are adjusting to multiple losses and managing multiple life stresses
   Seem paralyzed with cancer treatment decisions
   Fear death during surgery or are terrified by loss of control under anesthesia
   Request euthanasia
   Seem unable to provide informed consent

cancer and request prophylactic mastectomy; are cancerphobic and considering prophylactic mastectomy; are unable to make a decision about treatment; and have a psychiatric history of an anxiety or depressive disorder, substance abuse, or other mental illness. The patient who is a management problem for the physician and staff, or who is unable to comply with hospital rules, also needs psychiatric consultation. Rarely are patients so depressed that they are frankly suicidal during evaluation and treatment. However, if suicidal thinking is expressed, a formal psychiatric evaluation should be requested. Patients who have questionable ability to consent to treatment or who refuse treatment (secondary to mental retardation or severe psychiatric symptoms) require careful evaluation.

Many patients during workup or during the perioperative period have anxiety or insomnia that interferes with their usual functioning; to help patients sleep, physicians prescribe low-dose anxiolytics (ie, 0.25 to 1 mg of alprazolam or lorazepam orally three or four times daily) or hypnotics (ie, 0.125 to 0.25 mg of triazolam at bedtime as needed).[46] When anxiety and insomnia cannot be controlled with these medications or when surgical or medical staff observe a significant degree of depression manifesting as frequent crying episodes, irritability, inability to concentrate, or remarks indicating hopelessness or helplessness or suicidal thoughts, psychiatric consultation is indicated. Psychiatric consultants use the crisis intervention model of support that combines support of the patient and evaluation and support of her significant others. Anxiolytic, hypnotic, or antidepressant medication, along with emotional support, usually restores a woman to her prior level of function. The newer antidepressant medications (ie, fluoxetine, paroxetine, and sertraline) are effective and have fewer uncomfortable side effects than tricyclic medications.

MEDICAL VARIABLES

The stage of breast cancer at diagnosis, the treatment required, the prognosis, and the rehabilitative opportunities available constitute the medical variables that influence psychologic adjustment. Central, however, is the relationship to the supportive surgeon, radiotherapist, or oncologist, who, ideally, is sensitive to the concerns of the patient, communicates clearly, and monitors emotional as well as physical well-being. Both the expanded length and intensity of treatments and the recognition that women treated for breast cancer must be followed for the remainder of their lives, have placed an added burden on healthcare providers who are expected provide support across the course of care, often involving years of follow-up. The office or clinic nurse and treatment staff become the patient's "second family." Receptionists and radiation therapy technicians additionally contribute actively to the social environment that the patient experiences. Whereas some clinicians and staff welcome this added demand, others are uncomfortable with the expected intimacy and care, particularly around psychosocial issues. One model to address this demand involves training nurse clinicians to provide continuity of care and serve as patient advocates. Other models include screening patients for psychosocial needs and then triaging them to care, and assigning specific support or assessment tasks on the basis of staff interest and expertise.[47,48] Depending on the types of medical interventions experienced, the problems faced by women may vary.

Mastectomy

Because it was for so long the standard treatment for breast cancer, and still continues to be recommended for large numbers of women, there is considerable research on the impact of loss of one or both breasts on women's physical, social, and emotional functioning. Among the effects documented are feelings of mutilation and altered body image, diminished self-worth, loss of a sense of femininity, decrease in sexual attractiveness and function, anxiety, depression, hopelessness, guilt, shame, and fear of recurrence, abandonment and death.[30,49] Whereas mourning for the loss of a cherished body part and the threat to life are universal, the extent to which other sequelae are experienced seems variable. Research indicates that from 10% to 56% of women studied 1 to 2 years after mastectomy experience some degree of social or emotional impairment.[50,51] Although most women report improvement in emotional and physical well-being over time, for a significant minority (20% to 25%) of these problems may persist beyond 2 years after treatment.[52]

However, few studies of mastectomy were controlled. A large prospective study by Bloom and collaborators[53] compared levels of psychosocial functioning in four groups of women, none of whom had a history of prior significant psychiatric disturbance or medical illness. The groups consisted of women who had a mastectomy for stage I or II breast cancer (145 patients), women who had a cholecystectomy (their surgical control group, 90 patients), women who had a biopsy for benign breast disease (87 disease-free at-risk women) and a group who had no surgery in the prior year (90 healthy controls). Although women with breast cancer showed greater psychologic distress than surgical or healthy controls, related to social and interpersonal relationships, these emotionally healthy women did not experience serious psychiatric sequelae such as suicidal ideation. Only women with stage II disease who had undergone chemotherapy had significantly higher distress at 1 year. The others had returned to near-normal levels of function. Thus, women who are well adjusted before they have a mastectomy, and whose disease is in an early stage, can expect at 1 year to have a quality of life equal to unaffected peers, a finding since replicated in other controlled studies.[54] In addition to more advanced disease, other predictors of poorer adaptation in this study were additional concurrent illness or stress, expectation of poor support from others, and a tendency to perceive events in life as less under one's own control.

There has been a dramatic shift away from more radical surgical approaches to breast cancer based on scientific evidence that systemic versus more extensive local management therapy was more critical to survival.[55] This also has been advanced by the hope that, by sparing breast tissue, much of the psychosocial morbidity associated with the disease could be reduced.

Lumpectomy and Irradiation

Since 1980, more than two dozen studies have examined the differences on social and emotional as well as sexual functioning among women undergoing mastectomy or lumpectomy with irradiation[56-66] (Table 25.1-3). Despite the variability in methods employed, the early pattern of results was consistent: women who received breast-sparing surgery were less self-conscious, had a better body image, reported greater satisfaction with sexual activity, and manifested a somewhat better overall adjustment. In particular, women in the conservation group believed that they were less sexually inhibited, had sex more frequently, and reported that their husbands were more sexual and affectionate than did women undergoing mastectomy.

Although the overall data suggest that women receiving lumpectomy and irradiation have, as a group, adapted well,[67,68] three important criticisms have been leveled at this research. First, most of these studies evaluated women within the first year and often the first few months of their treatment. Thus, it was not known whether these early differences would persist over time. Indeed, some evidence suggests that women in the conservation group fare no differently from,[69,70] or may do worse than their mastectomy peers in the long term.[71]

The concern also exists that the populations of women undergoing each option were self-selected and perhaps differed before surgery. Of the studies reviewed, all were conducted after surgery was completed, and in most cases women or their physicians had chosen between one or the other option. The four exceptions to this were the studies by Schain and colleagues,[57] de Haes and Welvaart,[60] Fallowfield and coworkers,[62] and Lasry and others.[64] In

TABLE 25.1-3
Controlled Studies of Psychologic Response to Mastectomy (M) Versus Limited Resection and Radiation (LRR)

Study	Subjects LRR	Subjects M	Satisfaction With Body Image	Marital Adjustment	Satisfaction With Sexual Function	Psychologic Adjustment	Fear of Recurrence
Sanger and Reznikoff[56]	20	20 modified	LRR: more positive feelings	Equal	—	Equal	—
Schain et al[57]	18	20 modified	LRR: less negative feelings	Equal	Equal	Equal	Equal (M=80%; LRR=83%)
Steinberg et al[58]	21	46 modified	LRR: more positive feelings	Equal	LRR: report husbands more sexual	Equal depression, anxiety; LRR better in general	Equal
Bartelink et al[59]	114	58 modified	LRR: less self-conscious	—	LRR: less sexually inhibited	—	M greater
Taylor et al[36]	26	31 simple/modified 9 radical	LRR: less concern about disfigurement	Equal	LRR: report more frequent sex, more affectionate husbands	LRR: best overall adjustment	—
de Haes and Welvaart[60]	21	18 radical	LRR: less negative feelings	Equal	Equal	Equal	Equal (older patients less fearful)
Baider et al[61]	32	32 modified	—	M: slightly less conflict than LRR	Equal	Equal	—
Fallowfield et al[62]	48	53 modified	—	—	Equal	M: slightly fewer problems (32% vs 38% for LRR)	LRR more?
Ganz et al[63]	19	31 modified	LRR: less uncomfortable with changes	Equal	Equal	Equal, but more M (42%) than LRR (18%) report decrease in overall quality of life	Equal
Lasry et al[64]	36 LRR, 44 L only	43 total	LRR and L: less negative feelings	—	—	Equal (LRR slightly lower than L or M)	Equal
Wellisch et al[65]	11 LRR, 14 L only	27 total	LRR: more positive feelings	Equal	Equal; however, within M significant decrease in libido	Equal	M more worried
Margolis et al[66]	32	20 modified, 2 modified + reconstruction	LRR: more positive feelings (especially in nude)	—	LRR: report higher quality of relationship	M: higher report of transient suicidal thoughts	—

L, limited resection; LRR, limited resection and radiation; M, mastectomy.

each of these studies the women were randomized to receive either mastectomy or limited resection and irradiation. The data of Schain's group[57] and that of de Haes and Welvaart[60] demonstrate more positive feelings about body image among the lumpectomy and irradiation group but little difference with respect to the other parameters measured. In contrast, Fallowfield and colleagues[62] found no significant differences between the groups; if anything, the lumpectomy group seemed to do somewhat worse. The data of Lasry and others[64] fell in between: lumpectomy patients had a better body image than mastectomy patients, but women receiving irradiation exhibited higher levels of depression. A further confound to interpretation of the results of the studies is that younger women, already at increased risk for psychosocial problems in adaptation to breast cancer by virtue of age and developmental stage disruption, tend to select breast conservation.

Given the expected dramatic emotional benefit that saving the breast was expected to provide, the differences seen are less than might have been predicted.[72,73] In some cases, although statistically significant, the differences observed do not seem to be clinically significant. Breast conservation is not a psychosocial panacea,[71] rather, it serves to provide a woman with options in her care that may facilitate her particular adaptation.

Two critical factors that continue to influence the surgical decision-making process are attitudes about cancer and irradiation. The thought of leaving tumor cells in the breast is intolerable for some women who feel more secure with mastectomy. Other women fear irradiation or are unable to devote 6 weeks to daily radiation therapy treatments because of family or work demands or distance from a treatment center. Personality characteristics also influence a woman's decision. Women selecting lumpectomy plus irradiation over mastectomy have been found to be more concerned about insult to body image, more dependent on their breasts for self-esteem, and believed they would have had difficulty adjusting to loss of the breast to mastectomy.[21,74,75] In contrast, patients choosing mastectomy perceived the breast containing cancer as an offending part that should be removed, and they were more fearful of the side effects of irradiation. Whereas it has been suggested that older women may be more likely to select mastectomy,[75] there is some concern that this may reflect as much a bias in the provision of treatment options as personal preference.[76]

The percentage of stage I patients on whom a partial mastectomy or lumpectomy is performed increased from 23.3% in 1983 to 36.5% in 1987; for patients younger than 50 years, this figure increased from 29.9% in 1983 to 41.9% in 1987.[77] Although it is not clear what percentage of women nationally are *offered* a choice, in one prospective study of women who were, almost half (49%) chose conservation.[78] These figures are comparable with patterns of care in other large cancer centers as well as those reported abroad. In their survey of consultant surgeons in Great Britain, Morris and colleagues[79] found that only 39.1% would perform mastectomy whereas 64.4% would perform conservative surgery. Most surgeons in this study also said they would offer a choice of treatments.

Remember that it is only in the last decade that American women have routinely been given a choice between lumpectomy or mastectomy; even today this is mandated by fewer than half the states. Little is understood about *how* women make their decisions. It is likely that a significant proportion of decisions are made on the nature of the care that is available.[14,15,34] For women diagnosed in communities that are removed from major medical centers, mastectomy may simply be a more practical and safe treatment choice. Another deciding factor may be the availability of high-quality radiation therapy. Restricted access to implants and to plastic surgeons having extensive experience with transverse rectus abdominis muscle (TRAM) flap reconstruction has already limited the availability of reconstructive options. Cultural and ethnic values also may direct or even dictate choice, although the role of these is poorly understood. Research and clinical experience suggest that physician recommendation continues to exert the most significant influence on treatment choice for most women.[21,74]

Clinical experience indicates that many women who are treated by breast conservation may not feel the emotional effect of the experience until they begin the daily routine of radiation therapy. Spared the loss of their breast, these women often feel they should be grateful and not complain. Evidence indicates that they elicit, or at least perceive themselves as receiving less emotional support from others than women undergoing mastectomy.[71] It is often only when the irradiation starts, with daily visits to the clinic, exposure to others with cancer, cumulative fatigue, and realization of what they have gone through that patients react with distress. Physicians and staff should be aware of these delayed reactions because they, too, may perceive these women as having less severe psychologic trauma. It has become clear that women undergoing radiation are at higher risk of psychologic disturbance than has been assumed, in particular, depressive symptoms.[64,80] Although these may result from the side effects of irradiation, which vary widely in the degree of discomfort and fatigue produced, mood states need to be monitored.

Women undergoing irradiation therapy experience initial anxiety, which is usually allayed after a few treatments. It often returns, however, when end of treatment is approaching because of fear of regrowth of tumor without treatment, as well as in anticipation of the loss of close observation and frequent visits with the doctor and staff. To ease the transition, patients should be made aware of when treatment will end and the common paradoxic increase in distress. Reassurance should be provided about staff availability by telephone contact and by systematic scheduling of follow-up appointments. Fears of disease recurrence remain high in many women and reach distressing levels before follow-up visits and scans and while waiting for test results. Anxiety returns to usual levels with news of normal findings.

Reconstruction

The FDA hearings, opened in November 1991, on the safety of silicone gel–filled breast implants brought to the attention of the public and the medical community several important questions: How many women seek implants? What are the benefits of their use? What are the medical risks associated with these devices? These questions were no more keenly felt than among the estimated half million breast cancer survivors with implants.

It is uncertain among those women choosing or undergoing mastectomy, what percentage do so with the intention of seeking reconstruction. Before the implant hearings, national figures suggested that as many as 30% of eligible patients might pursue breast reconstruction.[77] The American Society of Plastic and Reconstructive Surgeons reported that a total of 42,888 breast reconstructions were performed by their 3000 members in 1990; this represented a 25% increase over figures gathered in 1988 and a 114% increase from 1981.[81] Fears associated with implants and more restricted access to implants likely has reduced these figures, even allowing for increased use of autologous tissue reconstructions. Nevertheless, far from being abandoned, postmastectomy breast reconstruction continues to be an important cosmetic and rehabilitative option pursued by a subset of women undergoing mastectomy.

Despite the fact that breast reconstruction for cancer has been available much longer than breast conservation, few studies have systematically examined the psychosocial impact of mastectomy alone compared with mastectomy plus reconstruction. Only two studies to date compare women selecting each of the three different surgical options[66,68] (lumpectomy versus mastectomy alone versus mastectomy with reconstruction); all of this research involved implant populations, and women undergoing reconstruction were not evaluated separately from those receiving mastectomy.

Three empirical studies compare women receiving conservation versus those undergoing mastectomy with reconstruction. The first of these included a small sample (9 patients) and found no differences between groups in quality of life, mood, marital satisfaction, or sexual satisfaction 1 year after surgery.[82] A Japanese study compared 42 women with breast conservation with 48 women undergoing immediate reconstruction with myocutaneous flaps.[83] No differences in sexual satisfaction or fear of recurrence were found between groups an average of 3 years after surgery. Conservation group members were less self-conscious about their appearance and stated they would be more likely to choose the same treatment again than women in the reconstruction group. In a retrospective study, 72 women who had partial mastectomy were compared with 146 women who had undergone immediate reconstruction, predominantly with implants, an average of 4 years after surgery.[84] No differences were observed between groups in overall psychosocial adjustment to illness, body image, or satisfaction with relationships or sexual life. However, women who had breast reconstruction reported less frequent breast caressing and more loss of pleasure with this activity. They also tended to be less likely to achieve orgasm with noncoital sexual stimulation. Factors predictive of greater psychosocial distress included a conflicted marriage, feeling unattractive, sexual dissatisfaction, less education, and treatment with chemotherapy.

The largest prospective study to date examined the psychologic variables characteristic of who seeks reconstruction and women's response to reconstruction. One hundred fifty women who sought consultation for reconstruction after mastectomy were evaluated along surgical and psychologic parameters; 83 of the 117 women undergoing reconstruction were reassessed postoperatively.[85] In addition, a matched comparison sample of 50 women who had not sought reconstruction was studied.[86]

On interview and self-report, women seeking consultation for reconstruction were psychologically well adjusted and functioning at a high level. Although they harbored some emotional pain related to cancer and the mastectomy, they were generally well informed about the nature of the surgery and approached reconstruction with realistic expectations of potential benefits to them both psychologically and physically. The reasons most frequently cited for seeking surgery were to be rid of the prosthesis, to feel whole again, to reestablish symmetry, and to diminish self-consciousness about appearance. These motives have been echoed in other study samples.[87,88]

The study's results underscored the positive effects of breast reconstruction. With few exceptions, the net effect of the surgery was to increase both observed and stated satisfaction with levels of psychologic, social, and sexual function. Most of the women (83%) stated they were happy or absolutely delighted with the overall results, and most found that the surgical results met or surpassed their expectations. Response to reconstruction was found to be independent of a woman's age, her social class, or her plastic surgeon's estimate of the success of the procedure. However, women who pursued reconstruction primarily to please their significant other or with the expectation of improving sexual and social relations were at risk of disappointment. Time since cancer surgery also modified response such that the farther the woman was since mastectomy, the greater her satisfaction with the overall results. Finally, satisfaction was found to be related to having thorough preoperative information, especially for additional procedures on the remaining breast (eg, symmetry), and to have the opportunity to express concerns and fears about results after the procedure.

When women seeking reconstruction were compared with those who had not, the two groups resembled each other in many aspects.[86] No differences were seen between the groups in general satisfaction, the ability to resume daily activities after the mastectomy, levels of self-esteem, feelings of attractiveness, sexual functioning, or self-reported psychologic symptoms. Women who did not undergo reconstruction reported greater comfort with use of external prostheses, had less knowledge about reconstruction, and, importantly, attached greater importance to their breasts. There was also a suggestion that women in the reconstruction group believed that their husband or sexual partner more frequently avoided touching or looking at the mastectomy site than did husbands or partners of the nonreconstruction group. Further comparisons between women who consulted and went on to have reconstruction and those who sought consultation, but opted not to pursue additional surgery, suggest that women who are at increased risk for subsequent emotional or surgical disappointment after reconstructive procedures may select themselves out at the time of consultation.

Concerns that women seeking reconstruction may do so because of inappropriate, neurotic reasons were not supported by our own or other investigators' research.[87-90] Most women sought surgery for themselves; 60% of women stated that their husband or significant other was neutral (recognized that she needed to make the decision herself) or even opposed to their desire for reconstruction (claiming it was not important to their relationship). The importance of personal versus public body image was a consistent theme also echoed by patients in Daniel's study.[91] After reconstruction, many women found themselves less preoccupied with their health and the fact that they had cancer; they no longer had the constant reminder of the physical defect. Increased sexual activity and increases in sexual responsiveness have been reported as well.[92,93] For some older women, the request for breast reconstruction may serve as a catalyst for better adjustment to the midlife crises that are complicated by diagnosis of cancer.[94] The fact that women of all ages (range, 28 to 68 years) sought out and shared similar hopes for breast reconstruction lends support to the contention that attractiveness is not primarily a concern of younger women; older women may react as strongly as younger women to breast loss.

Because most of the research among women undergoing reconstruction was conducted at a time when mastectomy was still the primary treatment of choice, it is not clear how many of these women might have selected breast conservation if it had been available to them. At the same time, many women today may select mastectomy precisely because they believe reconstruction will provide an acceptable cosmetic outcome while avoiding the more limited surgery and irradiation. Clearly, these studies need to be replicated in the context of the changes in treatment. They also need to be expanded to address cultural and ethnic issues, because it is clear that cultural beliefs and practices influence both women's choice of options and outcomes.[95-97]

Furthermore, little research has been done evaluating the psychosocial outcomes for women undergoing reconstruction using abdominal flaps (TRAM surgery). Use of autologous tissue for reconstruction has the advantage of eliminating many of the medical (eg, rejection, encapsulation, and altered mammographic imaging) and device-related (eg, rupture, deflation, and leakage) problems associated with implants. The cosmetic outcomes can be as good as or better than implant as well. On the negative side, these procedures require lengthy exposure to anesthesia and major abdominal surgery, and, although reportedly low, a risk for failure exists. (See Chapter 19 for a discussion of these issues.) Because long-term follow-up data on the cosmetic or physical sequelae associated with such reconstruction are unavailable, it is difficult to provide women with information on which to make their decision.

Key concerns of women about reconstruction include the cost of the surgery, the length of time under anesthesia, number of procedures required, the safety of the techniques used in both the potential for complications and, in the case of implants, the risk of masking recurrent cancer or promoting recurrent or autoimmune disease, and cosmetic results achievable.[98] Surgeons differ in their approach to this latter concern. Some prefer to use written materials only, others show pictures of reconstructed breasts, whereas many use some combinations of these approaches and, at times, may refer a woman to a previously reconstructed patient for more details. In our own research and that of others, several additional issues appeared of importance in counseling women considering or undergoing these procedures.[99,100] These include the need for discussion of all facets of the surgical steps (including number and length of hospitalizations), a thorough review of the surgical procedures planned to achieve symmetry of the breasts and to create a nipple, and consideration of timing of the procedure. The psychologic impact of the timing of reconstruction has been the focus of additional studies.

IMMEDIATE VERSUS DELAYED RECONSTRUCTION. Physician support for immediate reconstruction (versus delayed: that performed more than a week after mastectomy) is based on the perception of the absence of medical contraindications to immediate reconstruction and anticipation of significant benefits to the woman in sparing her the pain of disfigurement and loss that accompany mastectomy.[101] The American Society of Plastic and Reconstructive surgeons reported that of reconstructions performed in 1990 by member surgeons, 38% were immediate and 62% delayed.[81]

Research with women undergoing immediate reconstruction has shown high levels of patient satisfaction with surgical results and significantly less psychosocial morbidity than in those who undergo mastectomy alone.[101-105] Patients undergoing immediate reconstruction were less depressed and experienced less impairment of their sense of femininity, self-esteem, and sexual attractiveness than their peers who delayed or did not seek reconstruction. As with findings on lumpectomy versus mastectomy, however, researchers have noticed that initial differences in adjustment may be minimal and disappear over time.[104] In addition, although Schain and others[104] suggest that immediate reconstruction does not interfere with the necessary mourning process associated with threat to life and breast loss, clinicians have reported this as a problem in long-term follow-up of these patients. It is an issue that needs further study.

Adjuvant Chemotherapy

The news that adjuvant chemotherapy is needed demands psychologic adjustment to another treatment modality. This involves a lengthened treatment period and awareness of the threat to life implicit in the need for systemic therapy. Some women in this group describe their early weeks of treatment as having been characterized by one piece of bad news after another. The third decision point in the course of cancer encompasses deciding whether to undergo adjuvant treatment and, if more than one treatment is proposed, which drugs or protocol to choose.

Anticipation of chemotherapy can be difficult. Women's fears of the side effects arise from common knowledge of the distressing sequelae of chemotherapy in general. Because many women with early breast cancer receive some form of adjuvant therapy, the association of these treatments with more serious disease has diminished. Women anticipating and undergoing adjuvant therapy are told the specific drugs they will receive, their side effects, and the transient nature of most of these. Despite having fears, few women refuse treatment and most comply with their regimen.[106] Reactive anxiety and depression should be treated to assist in the woman's adjustment.

Meyerowitz and colleagues[107] studied women with breast cancer during chemotherapy and 2 years after completing it. Among those disease-free at 2 years, 23% reported difficulty with personal and family relationships during treatment and 44% had continuing physical problems 2 years later. Despite this, 89% stated they would recommend adjuvant chemotherapy to friends in a similar situation. Many reported that they had coped with treatment by staying busy, getting information about the treatment, and keeping a positive, hopeful outlook. In this study, 41% of women reported that the treatment had been easier than they expected. Clinical experience suggests that some women cope with the short-term adverse psychologic effects by focusing on delayed benefits (eg, reassurance that they have done everything possible to eradicate their disease).

Many of the common side effects of adjuvant chemotherapy, once feared and dreaded by patients, are now well controlled with pharmacologic and behavioral interventions. Nausea and vomiting is generally well controlled with the use of antiemetic drugs.[108] The introduction of ondansetron (Zofran) has dramatically reduced the incidence of nausea and vomiting in the adjuvant setting. The use of simple behavioral interventions (hypnosis, distraction, and relaxation exercises) provides a means of regaining a sense of self-control over symptoms while also reducing anxiety.[109,110] Anticipatory nausea and vomiting are particularly susceptible to control by this means.[111] The negative impact on patients' quality of life of this conditioned response was stressed by Hughson and colleagues.[112] Their work emphasized the importance of early intervention for patients experiencing severe nausea and vomiting. Their study also revealed significantly more depression among patients receiving adjuvant chemotherapy compared with those who underwent adjuvant radiation therapy alone, underscoring the value of providing early counseling for these women.

Three additional troublesome side effects of adjuvant therapy that have psychologic consequences are hair loss, weight gain, and problems with concentration. Although anticipated, the impact of alopecia for women undergoing chemotherapy often is devastating. Some women report this as more distressing than the breast surgery itself, in part because it is a visible indicator of disease, but also because it is overtly disfiguring. In our own research, women rated hair loss to be as distressing as learning of their diagnosis. Early discussion of the expected changes, information about wigs, and referral to the American Cancer Society–sponsored Look Good . . . Feel Better program all help to reduce distress caused by hair loss.[113]

The cause of weight gain remains unclear.[114] A study by Huntington[115] revealed that half the patients gained more than 4.5 kg (10 lb). No difference was found by treatment regimen (cyclophosphamide, methotrexate, and 5-fluorouracil [CMF] versus CMF plus vincristine and prednisone), estrogen receptor status, age, or menopausal status, although a decrease in activity level was found in those who experienced weight gain. At least one study has shown that weight may be negatively associated with mortality.[116] The added insult to self-esteem posed by significant weight gain suggests that more attention should be paid to this problem. The introduction of exercise programs during chemotherapy is increasingly being considered, along with nutritional guidance.

Difficulty with concentration and memory also are reported by many women undergoing chemotherapy. Not well researched or clearly documented, these symptoms may be associated with the stress of illness, antiemetic drugs, the chemotherapy itself, and possibly with hormonal changes secondary to chemotherapy-induced menopause.

A final, troublesome effect of chemotherapy in younger women is premature menopause.[117] Both the threatened or actual loss of fertility and acute onset of menopause anticipated with adjuvant treatment may cause distress in the woman who is premenopausal at diagnosis. Unlike the symptoms associated with natural menopause, the hot flashes, nightsweats, vaginal dryness, and atrophy caused by chemotherapy-induced menopause produce more severe discomfort. The latter symptoms may lead to dyspareunia. Although instruction in the use of vaginal lubricants is helpful, thinning of the vaginal mucosa still may result in irritation on intercourse. A further effect of chemotherapy is the loss of libido likely associated with a reduction in circulating androgens.[118] For many women, loss of desire is the most difficult sequelae to treat. In these cases, use of androgen supplements may be considered (see Chap. 24.8).[118,119]

Although longitudinal data are lacking, it can be expected that early loss of ovarian function also increases the risk in these young patients of later morbidity associated with osteoporosis and cardiovascular disease.[120,121] In a randomly selected survey of 224 breast cancer survivors, differences were found in women's concerns about these health issues according to menopausal status.[122] Premenopausal women were more concerned about osteoporosis (82% versus 66% for postmenopausal) and heart disease (92% versus 73%), and that estrogen replacement therapy might precipitate cancer recurrence (98% versus 73%). At the same time, they were more willing to consider estrogen replacement therapy under medical supervision (59% versus 40%). Discussion of these issues early in the course of care and referral for evaluation for risk and intervention is appropriate. Although estrogen replacement in these women remains controversial, it is being investigated.[123]

Psychologic preparation for chemotherapy is essential and should incorporate patient educational materials, nursing input, and an outline by the physician of the disease and treatment-related expectations. It is equally important to anticipate and plan for emotional reactions to ending treatment when, as with radiation therapy, fears of recurrence peak. Our clinical experience suggests that women experience more severe reactive anxiety and depression during this part of the treatment than at an earlier period, perhaps because of their greater awareness of prognosis. One symptom in particular that may continue to distress patients long after treatment has ended is fatigue. Noted clinically, the prevalence and cause of posttreatment fatigue is not well studied. In one sample of 60 women, 87.5% reported fatigue as a serious and unexpected side effect of chemotherapy.[124] Whereas careful work-up to rule out underlying depression or any medical cause of persistent fatigue is warranted, many women benefit from reassurance that it may take months, not weeks, before they feel their energy level is back to preillness levels.

Adjuvant Hormonal Therapy

Increasing use of tamoxifen in the adjuvant setting has drawn attention to the psychologic and sexual impact of hormonal therapies. Although used more commonly for postmenopausal patients, tamoxifen is sometimes given to premenopausal women as part of their adjuvant therapy. Although an antiestrogen, research has shown that tamoxifen may have weak estrogenic effects on the vaginal mucosa. Some older women find that the associated increase in hot flashes with use of this drug are a side-limiting factor. By contrast, we have had some younger patients report that tamoxifen provides relief from the vaginal dryness and loss of libido that accompany chemotherapy-induced premature menopause. Reports of a small but unexpected number of deaths from tamoxifen-related uterine cancer and concern over ocular toxicities with prolonged use have made many patients and physicians anxious about continued or long-term use of this drug.[29,125] The outcome that has been the recommendation of many is careful gynecologic monitoring. Whether this includes endometrial biopsy, transvaginal ultrasound, or both and at what intervals remains unclear, however.[126] A variety of hormonal manipulations are given for recurrent disease, including tamoxifen, megestrol acetate, progestins, aminoglutethimide, luteinizing hormone–releasing hormone analogues and estrogens. Aminoglutethimide has been associated with severe vaginal atrophy.[127] Megace increases appetite and results in significant weight gain for many women. As noted earlier, alterations in appearance resulting from hormonal therapy may result in embarrassment and loss of self-esteem. Counseling about expected changes is important.

Bone Marrow Transplant

The last decade has seen increasing use of bone marrow transplantation (BMT) as a treatment for cancer. This modality has been applied in the area of solid tumors such as ovarian and breast cancer. Although much has been written about the psychologic stages in, and patients' adaptation to BMT, investigators have focused largely on samples of patients treated for hematologic cancers, predominately with allogeneic transplants.[128–130] Long-term follow-up of patients undergoing BMT suggests that although most patients do well, 15% to 20% may continue to experience distress and might benefit from psychologic or psychiatric intervention. At least one study reports that despite the additional strain and longer hospitalization associated with BMT, no difference could be seen in psychologic or social functioning between BMT survivors and those treated with conventional chemotherapy alone.[132] As observed earlier, however, it is not known to what extent this is true for women diagnosed with breast cancer undergoing these procedures.

Breast cancer patients undergoing BMT represent the vanguard of survivors. Less is known about their experience and how it may be the same as or different from those treated with allogeneic transplant, or in an earlier period without benefit of growth factor support, effective antiemetics and shorter hospitalization. As a consequence, anticipatory anxiety may be high. What is clear is that as with other intensive therapies, the toll on quality of life often is significant. As a consequence, the equation must be balanced by hope for the results and the desire to live. For this reason, ensuring that optimal support is provided across the course of transplant and follow-up is critical. Whereas psychiatric problems may or may not alter survival, they can dramatically impact quality of survival and should be rapidly diagnosed and treated.[133]

Advanced Disease

Supportive care for patients with advanced breast cancer is aimed at comfort and control of symptoms. Different metastatic sites, especially bone, lung, and brain, present special supportive problems. Bone pain often is difficult to control, and confusional states must be monitored and treated. As discussed in Chapter 25.3, the use of support groups may influence both quantity and quality of survival significantly in this group of women.

Advanced care is best provided at home with support from the family and, if needed, a home health aide. However, a hospice setting with home care components also serves the needs of many patients well. Central to the success of a supportive program is a sense of continuity of care with physicians and staff and continued support of family and friends. Psychiatric consultation should be considered when distress is not responsive to the usual supportive measures. It is extremely helpful to have a psychiatric consultant who is knowledgeable about the problems faced by women with breast cancer, ideally as a member of a multidisciplinary team.[134]

Among the psychiatric symptoms of most concern, anxiety and depression are the most frequent and the most disabling. Depression may reach significant proportions. Although suicide is unusual, suicidal ideation is common. A management approach that combines psychologic support with psychopharmacologic use of antidepressants often is helpful. Amitriptyline is beneficial for its antidepressant, analgesic, and sedative properties when given at bedtime in doses of 50 to 75 mg. Anxiety may be high and distressing, especially in the presence of hypoxia or prolonged pain. Anxiolytic drugs, particularly diazapam and alprazolam, also are helpful for control of symptoms. It is best to give these drugs at regular intervals initially to achieve control, thereafter tapering the dose or prescribing the drug on an as-needed basis. In general, if given control of their own dose initially, women will take too little to be effective. Agitated behavior associated with metabolic encephalopathy, resulting often from hypercalcemia or from narcotic side effects, may require control by administration of a neuroleptic in small doses.

Because it is such a prevalent concern in more advanced stages of disease, attention to pain is important.[135,136] Cancer patients who experience pain are more likely to exhibit higher levels of mood disturbance and functional disability than those who have little or no pain.[137] Spiegel and Bloom[138] found that for women with metastatic breast cancer, beliefs about the meaning of the pain in relation to the illness predicted level of pain better than site of metastasis. In their research, Glajchen and colleagues[139] found that 64% of patients surveyed cited communication barriers as an impediment to pain relief. Attitudinal barriers to compliance with medical treatment were cited by over half the respondents, including stoicism and fear of narcotic addiction. Thus, addressing the meaning and response to pain from the perspective of the patient is as important as an explanation of proposed control techniques.

Interventions

The use and variety of psychosocial interventions applied in the cancer setting in general, and in breast cancer care in particular, have grown in the last decade.[140-142] Although varying greatly by the type (eg, individual versus group), orientation (eg, behavioral versus cognitive versus supportive), duration (time-limited versus open-ended), and timing (eg, before, during or after treatment), as well as target populations served (early versus advanced, younger than 40 years versus older, partnered versus single, or mixed), the fundamental purpose of interventions developed has been the same: to provide each woman with the skills or resources necessary to cope with her illness and improve the quality of her life. The various types of educational and supportive interventions in use in the breast cancer setting are reviewed in Chapter 25.3. However, three points need to be made regarding their use in the overall care of patients and families.

First, taken as a whole, researchers have found that those who received an intervention designed to improve knowledge or coping or to reduce distress did better than those who did not (the control group often being standard care). Specifically, patients provided with or randomly assigned to some form of individual or group intervention experienced less anxiety and depression,[143,144] had an increased sense of control,[145] had improved body image,[146] reported greater satisfaction with care[147] and better sexual function,[148,149] and exhibited improved medication adherence.[150] Importantly, no studies show women who received additional help to do worse than their standard-care peers.

Second, use of psychosocial interventions is increasing. Surveys show that most cancer treatment centers in the United States provide counseling services to their patients and families.[151,152] This reflects the patient demand for supportive care and the growing recognition that addressing psychosocial issues may improve outcomes for patients. In their seminal study, Spiegel and colleagues[153] found that women with metastatic cancer who participated in a year of weekly supportive group therapy with self-hypnosis for pain (50 patients), survived an average of 18 months longer from time of randomization, compared with a control group (36 patients). To explain their surprising findings, Speigel and colleagues[153] emphasize the multiple support functions such groups serve.

Third, whereas it might be argued that an individually tailored intervention should result in the best outcome for any given patient, this may not be suitable or even desirable in all cases. Indeed, most cancer patients resist being singled out for individual therapy and feel burdened by any label that might suggest that they are mentally ill and not simply medically ill. In addition, increasing evidence shows that participation in group activity offers a uniquely supportive and normalizing experience for many cancer patients struggling to deal with the realities of their new or continued status as cancer survivors. In studies that have specifically compared use of individual with group interventions, groups were as effective as individual counseling or support in reducing patient distress.[146,147] Krupnick and coworkers[154] have developed a model that uses groups to educate and support patients across the course of care that can be tailored to the needs of the oncology community being served.

Special Issues

Three changes in how breast cancer is diagnosed and treated have important ramifications for clinicians in their management of patients. These include increased awareness of the familial nature of breast cancer, greater involvement of family in patient care, and growing attention to the impact of breast cancer treatment on women's sexual functioning. Psychologic issues related to being at genetic risk for breast cancer are covered in Chapter 9. In the remaining two sections, the special issues related to the care of other family members and the role of sexual quality of life in rehabilitation are reviewed.

ROLE AND CARE OF THE FAMILY

Research into the impact of social support and health has blossomed in the last decade.[155-157] One consistent finding is that a positive relationship exists between social support and health or illness outcome.[158] This has been no more dramatically illustrated than in the context of cancer where adequate social support has been found to be integral to positive adjustment[159] and to length of survival.[153,160] For most patients, primary support comes from the family. At the same time, however, new stresses have taxed this resource. Greater demands on family decision making, the lengthened course of treatment with more aggressive therapies, and shift of care into the outpatient setting all have renewed the focus on the family in the management of care.

When people are ill, they tend to feel less in control, less powerful, and more inferior, especially when they must rely on others. At the same time, serious illness of any kind increases the ill person's need for closeness to others to counteract feelings of insecurity and vulnerability. The need for love and support often heightens in patients over time, both as a reaction to the effects of disease and treatment and the fear that others will no longer love or care for them. Fears of abandonment and rejection, experienced by other critically ill patients, often are keenly felt by the cancer patient. Absence of social support, or loss of a significant person who withdraws during the patient's illness, becomes an additional stressor that may be more painful emotionally than the illness itself.[161]

Active involvement of the family clearly serves a range of patient needs, from the most basic, namely, provision of emotional support (the psychic fuel that keeps a patient going) to the practical (eg, transportation to therapy sessions and financial resources to support these services), to the more abstract (eg, providing meaningful roles and hence functional goals toward which the patient can strive). For their part, the oncology team may count on the family member to be an advocate, a careprovider, and a one-person cheering section on behalf of the patient.

Despite their recognized importance, the role of partners and family in patient care have been the focus of few studies. Work by Wellisch and colleagues[162] indicates that involvement of the husband in the decision-making process, hospital visitation, early viewing of scars, and early resumption of sexual activity were important for optimal functioning of couples. Open dialogue appears critical to this process. Sabo and colleagues[163] found that the tendency for some men to assume a protective guardian stance was sometimes a deterrent to effective and open communication. Maguire[164] found that husbands of mastectomy patients reported more distress than a control group of husbands whose wives had benign breast disease up to a year after surgery. Similarly, Baider and Kaplan-DeNour[165] reported that both patients and partners reported moderate degrees of emotional distress related to mastectomy. Further, they found that patients' and husbands' levels of adjustment were significantly related; if one partner was experiencing difficulties adjusting, the other was also likely to be having problems. Northouse[166] reported that when asked what helped them cope with illness during hospitalization and 1 month later, both patients and husbands identified emotional support, information, attitude, and religion as important factors. In her research, patients and partners who reported higher levels of social support reported fewer adjustment difficulties at both 3 days and 30

days after surgery. However, younger couples may be at particular risk for problems.[167]

The vital nature and complexity of the relationship of spouse or partner and family to patient well-being is especially obvious when this system goes awry. When such situations occur, it is critical to remember that support is a two-way street: the source of the problem may arise in the provider of support (family member) as well as in the recipient, and commonly involves both. The impact of cancer can be as devastating to a family member as to the patient. Spouses may feel angry, ashamed, and vulnerable to illness themselves. Clinicians working with families of cancer patients suggest that they may at times need to be viewed as second-order patients. Seeing that partners have a support network and chance to air conflicting emotions can be critical to ensuring that they will be available to patients when needed. Toward this end, it is helpful for staff to acknowledge the difficult task faced by family members, to provide opportunities for them to talk about questions and reactions, both with the patient and alone, and to ensure that backup supports are available and provision made to give family members relief, especially if care is going to be complex or long term. Family members must also be permitted to limit care to those areas in which they are most comfortable and effective.

For their part, patients may not always welcome or correctly interpret care extended by family.[168] They may resist help because of concern about what others will think, cultural taboos associated with asking for help, or the sense of dependency and helplessness that such support engenders. The overly solicitous and jollying efforts of well-meaning spouses can make patients feel angry and isolated. When family members are expected to play an active role in specific rehabilitative or support tasks, it is necessary to explain to them how to go about doing so and to negotiate with the patients as to what is comfortable. Because patients' status and needs change over time, periodic review of the type and level of support provided is essential. In working with patients who feel guilty about asking for or accepting assistance, it is helpful to emphasize that requests for aid make the spouse or family member feel useful in a time of crisis. Shifting perspective on help requests decreases patient concerns about being a burden and also serves to strengthen patients' sense that they can actively direct, not merely passively receive, aid.

The traumatic effect on children, both sons and daughters, is great when the mother develops breast cancer. Behavioral disorders, conflicts with parents, and regressive and acting-out behaviors in children have been seen to increase during a parental illness.[169–171] Lichtman and colleagues[171] observed deterioration of the mother–child relationship in 12% of women with breast cancer whom they studied. Problems were more likely to arise in situations in which the mother had a poor prognosis, extensive surgery, poor psychologic adjustment, or, to a smaller extent, difficulty adjusting to chemotherapy or radiation therapy. A prior history of parent–child conflicts also places the relationship at risk during the mother's illness. Mother's relationships with their daughters were significantly more stressed than those with their sons. Daughters were more likely to show signs of fearfulness, withdrawal, and hostility, perhaps emanating from their greater fears of developing the disease and the greater demands placed on daughters. These findings parallel those reported by Litman[170] and Wellisch,[172] who noticed that mothers rely more often on daughters than sons during illness and that adolescent daughters may be particularly vulnerable to disruption in their lives.

The monitoring of all children, especially when the mother's breast cancer is advanced, is important. The opportunity for parents to discuss how and what to tell their children about the mother's illness early in the course of care also is important and should include advice on tailoring these conversations to meet appropriate developmental needs of their offspring. Two books by Fine[173] and Leshan,[174] as well as a publication put out by the National Cancer Institute, *When Someone in Your Family Has Cancer*, may be useful in this process.

Attention has become focused on the overall psychologic adjustment and quality of life of adult first-degree relatives of patients. In one study, 27% of women at increased family risk exhibited clinically elevated levels of psychologic distress that warranted intensive counseling.[175] In a population based study of first-degree relatives of breast cancer patients, 53% of women surveyed reported intrusive thoughts about breast cancer, 33% reported impairments in daily functioning because of breast cancer worries, and 20% reported sleep disturbance.[176] The frequency and severity of the symptoms observed were consistent with those found in populations exposed to a traumatic stressor. In another study, daughters of breast cancer patients reported significant decrements in the frequency of sexual activity and sexual satisfaction compared with age-matched controls.[177,178] These patterns of response in female family members warrant special attention because excessive psychologic distress potentially can interfere with family function and adherence to subsequent breast cancer screenings,[175,176] an issue addressed in greater detail in Chapter 8.

A number of books are available that may be helpful to both women and their families dealing with the challenges imposed by breast cancer. These include Kathy LaTour's *Breast Cancer Companion*, Wendy Harpham's *After Cancer*, and Andy Murcia and Bob Stewart's book, *Man to Man*. Each is thoughtfully written, highlights the problems families can expect, and provides resources for dealing with these. In addition, the National Coalition for Cancer Survivorship, based in Silver Spring, Maryland, has produced a useful volume with Consumer Reports entitled, *Charting the Journey*, which, as its title implies, discusses the practical problems that arise from diagnosis through survivorship, and solutions to each.

QUALITY OF LIFE AND SEXUAL FUNCTIONING

Although there has been extensive research on the psychosocial consequences of breast cancer, little of this work addressed the impact of disease and treatment on sexual functioning. Early studies focused on loss of breast and its impact on sexual relationships. These older, longitudinal studies, conducted among women treated with radical or modified radical mastectomy, reported significant sexual problems in 30% to 40% of samples assessed.[50,51] However, studies have since shown that the sexual disruption that occurs is independent of type of surgical treatment.[67,71,76] In her review of breast cancer on sexuality, body image, and intimate relationships, Schover[179] notes the lack of detail and specificity of available data on sexuality after breast cancer treatment, with most studies limiting the assessment to overall satisfaction or information on the frequency of intercourse. She observes that the premature and severe menopausal impact of systemic therapy may be the most common culprit in causing sexual dysfunction. As observed earlier, with increasing numbers of women receiving chemotherapy or hormonal therapy, this less-explored area of sexual morbidity needs attention.

In their review of sexuality and cancer in women, Schultz and associates[180] describe the range of psychologic reactions to cancer that threaten sexual function, including threats to the following:

- Sexual identity and self-esteem, such as disturbances of mood, gender, and sexual identity and body image.
- Personal control over body functions, such as disease-related symptoms (eg, pain, fatigue, nausea) that interfere with or inhibit sexual functioning.
- Intimacy, such as loss of social contacts that have potential for intimate physical expression, or the disintegration of established patterns of achieving physical pleasure and intimacy, or myths related to contagion.
- Reproductive function, such as the direct impairment of fertility or the fear of recurrence with pregnancy

In addition to these psychologic reactions, some women experience less joy and vigor, as well as an underlying uncertainty about their health and the vulnerability of their bodies to further assault.[181] All of these factors affect the sexual response in the breast cancer survivor.

In research conducted by Ganz and colleagues,[182,183] 227 early-stage breast cancer patients were assessed at four points in time during the first year after surgery; some of these women were reassessed at 2 years (69 patients) or 3 years (70 patients) after surgery. Their data suggest that a subset of women may be at risk for psychosexual distress after treatment. Specifically, 1-year problems and frequencies for the at-risk group included not feeling sexually attractive (54%), not being interested in having sex (44%), decreased frequency of sexual intercourse (58%), difficulty becoming sexually aroused (42%), difficulty with lubrication (50%), and difficulty achieving orgasm (41% low risk and 56% at risk). Of the 70 women assessed at 3 years, 43% continued to be uncomfortable with body changes, 47% reported disinterest in sex, and many continued to experience specific sexual dysfunction, including difficulty with arousal (48%), lubrication (64%), and orgasm (52%). Important in their research was the finding that survivors seem to attain maximum recovery from the physical and emotional trauma by 1 year after surgery. Further, in spite of relatively good physical and emotional recovery achieved, a number of problems persist beyond 1 year, in particular, those associated with sexual rehabilitation.

The emotional distress, pain, fatigue, and insult to the patient's body image and self-esteem caused by the diagnosis and treatment of breast cancer can damage sexual functioning, even among individuals who had a strong and satisfying sexual relationship before illness. When illness occurs in the context of preexisting problems or before relationships are fully established, the outcome may be devastating. Despite heightened sensitivity to sexual issues, in practice, provision of effective sexual interventions remains highly variable, in part because of staff avoidance.

Auchincloss[184] found that staff resistance or reluctance to address patient's sexual concerns clusters around four broad themes. First, many professionals whose focus is on treatment and management of illness believe that the sexual consequences or treatment are not their concern. Auchincloss argues strongly that, as with any other side effect of treatment, the responsibility for monitoring sexual sequelae rests with the oncology team. Second, many staff members are reluctant to raise the topic of sex because they believe that little information is available to remedy problems. This attitude is being slowly replaced while the field of sex therapy has grown. Education about effective therapies for problems such as vaginal dryness, painful intercourse, and lack of desire is acknowledged and available. Third, belief that the patient is principally (or solely) concerned with her cancer prevents other staff from raising sexual issues. Work by Vincent and colleagues[185] challenges the accuracy of this perception. In their study, 80% of patients interviewed desired more information about sexual issues, although 75% expressed reluctance to broach the subject themselves. Finally, some staff personnel may simply be too embarrassed to discuss sex.

Auchincloss[184] stresses that with time, education, patience, and practice, most health professionals can come to believe that they have something to offer patients who are anxious, distressed over new problems, and unsure of how to go about asking for help. Caregivers should be reassured that patients often feel an enormous sense of relief to have a problem acknowledged, to know that it is not uncommon, and that help is available through suitable referral. In short, it is the staff's obligation to raise the issue of potential or actual impact of illness and treatment on this area of function and to discuss sexual rehabilitation options with every patient from the adolescent to the elderly.

Sexual rehabilitation starts ideally before treatment with a good social and sexual history. With regard to patients for whom specific impairment of sexual function might be anticipated (eg, premature menopause in young chemotherapy patient), discussion of these effects is essential. Raising the topic of sexual function early, by letting the patient know it is an appropriate focus of concern and that the health care provider is willing to discuss it, opens the door for future dialogue in this area and helps to ensure that problems with sexual function will be addressed. Auchincloss[184] cautions, however, against initiating sexual discussions during periods of acute stress (eg, treatment setbacks, recurrences, family or work crises), and places a high premium on finding a private space for conducting such interviews. Some teams may wish to designate one staff member to initiate conversations or to follow-up on those introduced by the primary physician. The primary nurse often is best suited for this position. Establishing this role is important, because it is as undesirable to have everyone asking about sexual function as to have no one address this area. When specific questions arise, the nurse needs to know what the patient has been told and by whom so as to focus questions for patients, direct their inquiries to the appropriate staff member, clarify or reinforce information provided, and serve as an advocate for the patient. Above all, it is necessary for team members to know about efforts in this area and to coordinate their input with that of others.

It is beyond the scope of this chapter to go into the particular types of problems that may occur or their treatment. There are, nevertheless, a number of excellent resources in the growing field of sexual rehabilitation of cancer patients.[186,187] An excellent manual for patients, *Sexuality and the Woman Who Has Cancer and Her Partner*, is available through the American Cancer Society. In addition, there are a small number of programs around the country that train sex counselors and therapists. For women with more difficult sexual problems, or longstanding issues further compounded by treatment, referral to a qualified sex therapist should be considered. Names of trained professionals for referral or workshop purposes can be obtained from the American Association of Sex Educators, Counselors and Therapists, based in Washington, DC.

Summary

Breast cancer remains the most common tumor in women; it has a unique and, at times, complex psychologic impact, but one to which psychologically healthy women respond well without developing serious psychologic symptoms. Increased use in primary treatment of breast-conserving procedures is reducing the negative effect on self-image and body image. However, ethical and legal constraints relating to treatment options have added substantially to decision-making dilemmas and to fears of recurrence, which, by virtue of the detailed information given about survival statistics, may persist for an indefinite period. Greater emphasis is needed on providing support to women during the decision-making period. In addition, as newer therapies such as intensive chemotherapy and BMT are introduced, research on their immediate and delayed psychosocial impact are needed. Broader dissemination of information from the psychologic studies of adaptation to the available treatment options will help in efforts to determine the best treatment to meet patients' physical and emotional needs.

Special attention must be directed to the psychologic well-being of the immediate relatives of women with breast cancer, especially their partners and offspring. In addition, greater attention is needed to the quality of life of women themselves, especially with respect to sexual functioning, across the course of illness and recovery. Data indicate that addressing the psychosocial needs of breast cancer patients improves quality of survival and may even enhance length of survival.

References

1. Wingo PA, Tong T, Bolder S. Cancer Statistics, 1995. CA Cancer J Clin 1995;45:8.
2. Hankey BF, Miller B, Curtis R, et al. Trends in breast cancer in younger women in contrast to older women. Natl Cancer Inst Monogr 1994;16:7.
3. Early Breast Cancer Trialists' Collaborative Group. Treatment of early breast cancer, vol 1. Worldwide evidence 1985–1990. Oxford, Oxford University, 1990.
4. Glanz K, Lerman C. Psychosocial impact of breast cancer: a critical review. Ann Behav Med 1992;14:204.
5. Lerman C, Rimer BK, Engstrom PF. Cancer risk notification: psychosocial and ethical implications. J Clin Oncol 1991;9:1275.
6. Holland JC. Historical overview. In: Holland JC, Rowland JH, eds. Handbook of psychooncology: psychological care of the patient with cancer. New York, Oxford University, 1989:3.
7. Rosato FE, Rosenberg AL. Examination techniques: role of the physician and patient in evaluating breast diseases. In: Bland KI, Copeland EM III, eds. The breast: comprehensive management of benign and malignant diseases. Philadelphia, WB Saunders, 1991:409.
8. Holland JC. Fears and abnormal reactions to cancer in physically healthy individuals. In: Holland JC, Rowland JH, eds. Handbook of psychooncology: psychological care of the patient with cancer. New York, Oxford University, 1989:18.
9. Robinson E, Mohilever J, Zidan J, et al. Delay in diagnosis of cancer: possible effects on the stage of disease and survival. Cancer 1984;54:1454.
10. Vernon SW, Tilley BC, Neale AV, et al. Ethnicity, survival and delay in seeking treatment for symptoms of breast cancer. Cancer 1985;55:1563.
11. Ragland KE, Selvin S, Merrill DW. Black–white differences in stage-specific cancer survival: analysis of seven selected sites. Am J Epidemiol 1991;133:672.
12. Rimer BK. Understanding the acceptance of mammography by women. Ann Behav Med 1992;14:197.
13. Nayfield SG, Bongiovanni CG, Alciati MH, et al. Statutory requirements for disclosure of breast cancer treatment alternatives. J Natl Cancer Inst 1994;86:1202.
14. Nattinger AB, Gottlieb MS, Veum J, et al. Geographic variation in the use of breast-conserving treatment for breast cancer. N Engl J Med 1992;326:1102.
15. Farrow DC, Hunt WC, Samet JM. Geographic variation in the treatment of localized breast cancer. N Engl J Med 1992;326:1097.
16. Scott DW. Anxiety, critical thinking and information processing during and after breast biopsy. Nurs Res 1983;32:24.
17. Valanis BG, Rumpler CH. Helping women to choose breast cancer treatment alternatives. Cancer Nurs 1985;8:167.
18. Rowland JH, Holland JC. Psychological reactions to breast cancer and its treatment. In: Harris JR, Hellman S, Henderson IC, et al, eds. Breast diseases, ed 2. Philadelphia, JB Lippincott, 1991:849.
19. Emanuel EJ, Emanuel LL. Four models of the physician–patient relationship. JAMA 1992;267:2221.
20. Siminoff LA. Cancer patient and physician communication: progress and continuing problems. Ann Behav Med 1989;11:108.
21. Ashcroft JJ, Leinster SJ, Slade PA. Breast cancer-patient choice of treatment: preliminary communication. J R Soc Med 1985;78:43.
22. Morris J, Royle GT. Offering patients a choice of surgery for early breast cancer: a reduction in anxiety and depression in patients and their husbands. Soc Sci Med 1988;26:583.
23. Glynn Owens R, Ashcroft JJ, Leinster SJ, et al. Informal decision analysis with breast cancer patients: an aid to psychological preparation for surgery. J Psychosoc Oncol 1987;5:23.
24. Fallowfield LJ, Hall A, Maguire GP, et al. Psychological outcomes of different treatment policies in women with early breast cancer outside a clinical trial. Br Med J 1990;301:575.
25. Lerman C, Daly M, Walsh WP, et al. Communication between patients with breast cancer and health care providers: determinants and implications. Cancer 1993;72:2612.
26. Cassileth BR, Zupkis RV, Sutton-Smith K. Information and participation preferences among cancer patients. Ann Intern Med 1980;92:832.
27. Weiss R. How goes the war on cancer? are cases going up? are death rates going down? Washington Post Health, February 14, 1995:12.
28. Velentgas P, Daling JR. Risk factors for breast cancer in younger women. Monogr Natl Cancer Inst 1994;16:15.
29. van Leeuwen FE, Benraadt J, Coebergh JW, et al. Risk of endometrial cancer after tamoxifen treatment of breast cancer. Lancet 1994;343:448.
30. Meyerowitz BE. Psychosocial correlates of breast cancer and its treatment. Psychol Bull 1980;87:108.
31. Mor V, Malin M, Allen S. Age differences in the psychosocial problems encountered by breast cancer patients. Monogr Natl Cancer Inst 1994;16:191.
32. Breast cancer in younger women. Proceedings of a conference held at the National Institutes of Health, Bethesda, January 28, 1993. Monogr Natl Cancer Inst 1994;16.
33. Fotopoulos S, Cook MR. Psychological aspects of breast cancer: age. Am Psycholog Assoc Meet, Montreal, Quebec, September, 1980.
34. Hynes DM. The quality of breast cancer care in local communities: implications for health care reform. Med Care 1994;32:328.
35. Penman DT. Coping strategies in adaptation to mastectomy (doctoral dissertation). New York, Yeshiva University, 1979.
36. Taylor SE, Lichtman RR, Wood JV, et al. Illness-related and treatment-related factors in psychological adjustment to breast cancer. Cancer 1985;55:2506.
37. Hilton BA. The relationship of uncertainty, control, commitment, and threat of recurrence to coping strategies used by women diagnosed with breast cancer. J Behav Med 1989;12:39.
38. Suls J, Fletcher B. The relative efficacy of avoidant and non-avoidant coping strategies: a meta-analysis. Health Psychol 1985;4:249.
39. Rowland JH. Interpersonal resources: social support. In: Holland JC, Rowland JH, eds. Handbook of psychooncology: psychological care of the patient with cancer. New York, Oxford University, 1989:58.
40. Pettingale KW, Morris T, Greer S, et al. Mental attitudes to cancer: an additional prognostic factor. Lancet 1985;1:750.
41. Holland JC. Behavioral and psychosocial risk factors in cancer: human studies. In: Holland JC, Rowland JH, eds. Handbook of psychooncology: psychological care of the patient with cancer. New York, Oxford University, 1989:705.
42. Bovbjerg D. Psychoimmunology and cancer. In: Holland JC, Rowland JH, eds. Handbook of psychooncology: psychological care of the patient with cancer. New York, Oxford University, 1989:727.
43. Levenson JL, Bemis C. The role of psychological factors in cancer onset and progression. Psychosomatics 1991;32:124.
44. Spiegel D. Psychosocial aspects of cancer. Curr Opin Psychiatry 1991;4:889.
45. DeFlorio M, Massie MJ. A review of depression in cancer: gender differences. Depression (in press).
46. Jacobsen PJ, Massie MJ, Kinne DW, et al. Hypnotic efficacy and

safety of triazolam administered during the post-operative period. Gen Hosp Psychiatry 1994; 16:419.

47. Wieder S, Schwartzfeld J, Fromewick J, et al. Psychosocial support program for patients with breast cancer at Montefiore Hospital: team effort. Q Rev Bull 1978; 4:10.

48. Weisman AD, Worden JW. The existential plight of cancer: significance of the first 100 days. Int J Psychiatry Med 1976–77; 7:1.

49. Lewis FM, Bloom JR. Psychosocial adjustment to breast cancer: a review of selected literature. Int J Psychiatry Med 1978–79; 9:1.

50. Maguire GP, Lee EG, Bevington DJ, et al. Psychiatric problems in the first year after mastectomy. BMY 1978; 279:963.

51. Morris T, Greer HS, White P. Psychological and social adjustment to mastectomy: a two-year follow-up study. Cancer 1977; 77:2381.

52. Irvine D, Brown B, Crooks D, et al. Psychosocial adjustment in women with breast cancer. Cancer 1991; 67:1097.

53. Psychological Aspects of Breast Cancer Study Group. Psychological response to mastectomy: a prospective comparison study. Cancer 1987; 59:189.

54. Hughson AV, Cooper AF, McArdle CS, et al. Psychosocial consequences of mastectomy: levels of morbidity and associated factors. J Psychosom Med 1988; 32:383.

55. General Accounting Office. Breast conservation versus mastectomy: patient survival in day-to-day medical practice and in randomized studies. Washington, DC, November 15, 1994.

56. Sanger CK, Reznikoff M. A comparison of the psychological effects of breast-saving procedures with the modified mastectomy. Cancer 1981; 48:2341.

57. Schain W, Edwards BK, Gorrell EV, et al. Psychosocial and physical outcomes of primary breast cancer therapy: mastectomy vs excisional biopsy and irradiation. Breast Cancer Res Treat 1983; 3:377.

58. Steinberg MD, Juliano MA, Wise L. Psychological outcome of lumpectomy versus mastectomy in the treatment of breast cancer. Am J Psychiatry 1985; 142:34.

59. Bartelink H, van Dam F, van Dongen J. Psychological effects of breast conserving therapy in comparison with radical mastectomy. Int J Radiat Oncol Biol Phys 1985; 11:381.

60. de Haes JCJM, Welvaart K. Quality of life after breast cancer surgery. J Surg Oncol 1985; 28:123.

61. Baider L, Rizel S, Kaplan-DeNour A. Comparison of couples adjustment to lumpectomy and mastectomy. Gen Hosp Psychiatry 1986; 8:251.

62. Fallowfield LJ, Baum M, Maguire GP. Effects of breast conservation on psychological morbidity associated with diagnosis and treatment of early breast cancer. BMJ 1986; 293:1331.

63. Ganz PA, Schag CC, Polinsky ML, et al. Rehabilitation needs and breast cancer: the first month after primary therapy. Breast Cancer Res Treat 1987; 10:243.

64. Lasry J-CM, Margolese RG, Poisson R, et al. Depression and body image following mastectomy and lumpectomy. J Chron Dis 1987; 40:529.

65. Wellisch DK, DiMatteo R, Silverstein M, et al. Psychosocial outcomes of breast cancer therapies: lumpectomy versus mastectomy. Psychosomatics 1989; 30:365.

66. Margolis G, Goodman RL, Rubin A. Psychological effects of breast-conserving cancer treatment and mastectomy. Psychosomatics 1990; 31:33.

67. Keibert GM, de Haes JCJM, van de Velde CJH. The impact of breast-conserving treatment and mastectomy on the quality-of-life of early-stage breast cancer patients: a review. J Clin Oncol 1991; 9:1059.

68. Fallowfield LJ. Psychosocial adjustment after treatment for early breast cancer. Oncology 1990; 4:89.

69. Maunsell E, Brisson J, Deschenes L. Psychological distress after initial treatment for breast cancer: a comparison of partial and total mastectomy. J Clin Epidemiol 1989; 42:765.

70. Omne-Ponten M, Holmberg L, Sjoden P-O. Psychosocial adjustment among women with breast cancer stages I and II: six-year follow-up of consecutive patients. J Clin Oncol 1994; 12:1778.

71. Levy SM, Haynes LT, Herberman RB, et al. Mastectomy versus breast conservation surgery: mental health effects at long-term follow-up. Health Psychol 1992; 11:349.

72. Zevon MA, Rounds JB, Karr J. Psychological outcomes associated with breast conserving surgery: a meta-analysis. Paper presented at the 8th Annual Meeting of the Society of Behavioral Medicine, Washington, DC, March 1987.

73. Fallowfield LJ, Hall A. Psychosocial and sexual impact of diagnosis and treatment of breast cancer. Br Med Bull 1991; 47:388.

74. Margolis GJ, Goodman RL, Rubin A, et al. Psychological factors in the choice of treatment for breast cancer. Psychosomatics 1989; 30:192.

75. Wolberg WH, Tanner MA, Romsaas EP, et al. Factors influencing options in primary breast cancer treatment. J Clin Oncol 1987; 5:68.

76. Ganz PA. Treatment options for breast cancer: beyond survival. N Engl J Med 1992; 326:1147.

77. Miller BA, Ries LAG, Hankey BF, et al, eds. Cancer statistics review: 1973–1989. Bethesda, National Cancer Institute, NIH publ no. 92-2789; 1992.

78. Wolberg WH. Surgical options in 424 patients with primary breast cancer without systemic metastases. Arch Surg 1991; 126:817.

79. Morris J, Royle GT, Taylor I. Changes in the surgical management of early breast cancer in England. J R Soc Med 1989; 82:12.

80. Monroe AJ, Biruls R, Griffin AV, et al. Distress associated with radiotherapy for malignant disease: a quantitative analysis based on patients' perceptions. Br J Cancer 1989; 60:370.

81. American Society of Plastic and Reconstructive Surgeons 1990 Statistics. Arlington Hts, IL, ASPRS, 1991.

82. Pozo C, Carver CS, Noriega V, et al. Effects of mastectomy versus lumpectomy on emotional adjustment to breast cancer: a prospective study of the first year postsurgery. J Clin Oncol 1992; 10:1292.

83. Noguchi M, Kitagawa H, Kinoshita K, et al. Psychologic and cosmetic self-assessments of breast-conserving therapy compared with mastectomy and immediate breast reconstruction. J Surg Oncol 1993; 54:260.

84. Schover LR, Yetman RJ, Tuason LJ, et al. Partial mastectomy and breast reconstruction: a comparison of their effects on psychosocial adjustment, body image, and sexuality. Cancer 1995; 75:54.

85. Rowland JH, Holland JC, Chaglassian T, et al. Psychological response to breast reconstruction: expectations for and impact on postmastectomy functioning. Psychosomatics 1993; 34:241.

86. Rowland JH, Dioso J, Holland JC, et al. Breast reconstruction after mastectomy: who seeks it, who refuses. Plast Reconstr Surg 1995; 95:812.

87. Goin JM, Goin MK. Breast reconstruction after mastectomy. In: Goin JM, Goin MK. Changing the body: psychological effects of plastic surgery. Baltimore, Williams & Wilkins, 1981:163.

88. Clifford E. The reconstruction experience: the search for restitution. In: Georgiade NG, ed. Breast reconstruction following mastectomy. St. Louis, CV Mosby, 1979:22.

89. Houpt P, Dijkstra R, Storm van Leeuwen JB. The result of breast reconstruction after mastectomy for breast cancer in 109 patients. Ann Plast Surg 1988; 21:517.

90. Gilboa D, Borenstein A, Floro S, et al. Emotional and psychosocial adjustment of women to breast reconstruction and detection of subgroups at risk for psychological morbidity. Ann Plast Surg, 1990; 25:397.

91. Daniel E. Breast reconstruction post-mastectomy: a psychosocial study. Dissert Abstr Int 1984; 46:1741B.

92. Teimourian B, Adham M. Survey of patients' response to breast reconstruction. Ann Plast Surg 1982; 9:321.

93. Gerard D: Sexual functioning after mastectomy: life vs lab. J Sex Marital Ther 1982; 8:305.

94. Goin MK, Goi JM. Midlife reactions to mastectomy and subsequent breast reconstruction. Arch Gen Psychiatry 1981;38:225.

95. Filiberti A, Tamburini M, Murru L, et al. Psychologic effects and esthetic results of breast reconstruction after mastectomy. Tumori 1986;72:585.

96. Mueller SC, Cioroiu M, LaRaja RD, et al. Postmastectomy breast reconstruction: a survey of general and plastic surgeons. Plast Reconstr Surg 1988;82:555.

97. van Dam FSAM, Bergman RB. Psychosocial and surgical aspects of breast reconstruction. Eur J Surg Oncol 1988;14:141.

98. Schain WS, Jacobs E, Wellisch DK. Psychosocial issues in breast reconstruction: intrapsychic, interpersonal, and practical concerns. Clin Plast Surg 1984;11:237.

99. Winder AE, Winder BD: Patient counseling: clarifying a woman's choice for breast reconstruction. Patient Educ Counsel 1985;7:65.

100. Matheson G, Drever JM. Psychological preparation of the patient for breast reconstruction. Ann Plast Surg 1990;24:238.

101. Noone RB, Frazier TG, Hayward CZ, et al. Patient acceptance of immediate reconstruction following mastectomy. Plast Reconstr Surg 1982;69:632.

102. Dean C, Chetty U, Forrest APM. Effects of immediate breast reconstruction on psychosocial morbidity after mastectomy. Lancet 1983;1:459.

103. Stevens LA, McGrath MH, Druss RG, et al. The psychological impact of immediate breast reconstruction for women with early breast cancer. Plast Reconstr Surg 1984;73:619.

104. Schain WS, Wellisch DK, Pasnau RO, et al. The sooner the better: a study of psychological factors in women undergoing immediate versus delayed breast reconstruction. Am J Psychiatry 1985;142:40.

105. Wellisch DK, Schain WS, Noone BR, et al. Psychosocial correlates of immediate versus delayed reconstruction of the breast. Plastic Reconstr Surg 1985;76:713.

106. Taylor SE, Lichtman RR, Wood JV. Compliance with chemotherapy among breast cancer patients. Health Psychol 1984;3:553.

107. Meyerowitz BE, Watkins IK, Sparks FC. Psychosocial implications of adjuvant chemotherapy: a two-year follow-up. Cancer 1983;52:1541.

108. Grunberg SM, Hesketh PJ. Control of chemotherapy-induced emesis. N Engl J Med 1993;329:1790.

109. Redd WH. Behavioral approaches to treatment-related distress. CA Cancer J Clin 1988;38:138.

110. Carey MP, Burish TG. Etiology and treatment of the psychological side effects associated with cancer chemotherapy: a critical review and discussion. Psychol Bull 1988;104:307.

111. Andrykowski MA. The role of anxiety in the development of anticipatory nausea in cancer chemotherapy: a review and synthesis. Psychosom Med 1990;52:458.

112. Hughson AVM, Cooper AF, McArdle CS, et al: Psychological impact of adjuvant chemotherapy in the first two years after mastectomy. BMJ 1986;293:1268.

113. Manne SL, Girasek D, Ambrosino J. An evaluation of the impact of a cosmetics class on breast cancer patients. J Psychosoc Oncol 1994;12:83.

114. Denmark-Wahnefried W, Winer EP, Rimer BK. Why women gain weight with adjuvant chemotherapy for breast cancer. J Clin Oncol 1993;11:1418.

115. Huntington M. Weight gain in patients receiving adjuvant chemotherapy for carcinoma of the breast. Cancer 1985;65:572.

116. Senie RT, Rosen PP, Rhodes P, et al. Obesity at diagnosis of breast carcinoma influences duration of disease-free survival. Ann Intern Med 1992;116:26.

117. Schover LR. Sexuality and body image in younger women with breast cancer. Monogr Natl Cancer Inst 1994;16:177.

118. Kaplan JS. A neglected issue: the sexual side effects of current treatments for breast cancer. J Sex Marital Ther 1992;18:3.

119. Sherwin BB. A comparative analysis of the role of androgen in human male and female sexual behavior: behavioral specificity, critical thresholds, and sensitivity. Psychobiology 1988;16:416.

120. Henderson BE, Paganini-Hill A, Ross RK. Decreased mortality in users of estrogen replacement therapy. Arch Intern Med 1991;151:75.

121. Dupont WD, Page DL. Menopausal estrogen replacement therapy and breast cancer. Arch Intern Med 1991;151:67.

122. Vassilopoulou-Sellin R, Zolinski C. Estrogen replacement therapy in women with breast cancer: a survey of patient attitudes. Am J Med Sci 1992;304:145.

123. Vassilopoulou-Sellin R, Theriault RL. Randomized prospective trial of estrogen-replacement therapy in women with a history of breast cancer. Monogr Natl Cancer Inst 1994;16:153.

124. Tierney A, Leonard R, Taylor J, et al. Side effects expected and experienced by women receiving chemotherapy for breast cancer. Br Med J 1991;302:272, 1991.

125. Pavlidis NA, Petris C, Briassoulis E, et al. Clear evidence that long-term, low-dose tamoxifen treatment can induce ocular toxicity. Cancer 1992;69:2961.

126. Uziely B, Lewin A, Brufman G, et al. The effect of tamoxifen on the endometrium. Breast Cancer Res Treat 1993;26:101.

127. Physician's desk reference, ed 49. Oradell, NJ, Medical Economics, 1995:878.

128. Lesko LM. Bone marrow transplantation. In: Holland JC, Rowland JH, eds. Handbook of psychooncology: psychological care of the patient with cancer. New York, Oxford University, 1989:163.

129. Winer EP, Sutton LM. Quality of life in patients after bone marrow transplantation. Oncology 1994;8:19.

130. Wolcott DL, Fawzy FI, Wellisch DK. Psychiatric aspects of bone marrow transplantation: a review and current issues. Psychiatr Med 1987;4:299.

131. Wolcott DL, Wellisch DK, Fawzy FI, et al. Adaptation of adult bone marrow transplant recipient long-term survivors. Transplantation 1986;41:478.

132. Lesko LM, Ostroff JS, Mumma GH, et al. Long-term psychological adjustment of acute leukemia survivors: impact of bone marrow transplantation versus conventional chemotherapy. Psychosom Med 1992;54:30.

133. Jenkins PL, Lester H, Alexander J, et al. A prospective study of psychosocial morbidity in adult bone marrow transplant recipients. Psychosomatics 1994;35:361.

134. Hoffman RS. The psycho-oncologist in a multidisciplinary breast treatment center. In: Cooper CL, ed. Stress and breast cancer. New York, John Wiley & Sons, 1988:171.

135. Portenoy RK, Foley KM. Management of cancer pain. In: Holland JC, Rowland JH, eds. Handbook of psychooncology: psychological care of the patient with cancer. New York, Oxford University, 1989:369.

136. Breitbart W. Psychotropic adjuvant analgesics for cancer pain. Psychooncol 1992;1:133.

137. Massie MJ, Holland JC. The cancer patient with pain: psychiatric complications and their management. J Pain Symptom Manage 1992;7:99.

138. Spiegel D, Bloom JR. Group therapy and hypnosis reduce metastatic breast carcinoma pain. Psychosom Med 1983;4:333.

139. Glajchen M, Fitzmartin RD, Blum D, et al. Psychosocial barriers to cancer pain relief. Cancer Pract 1995;3:76.

140. Massie MJ, Holland JC, Straker N. Psychotherapeutic interventions. In: Holland JC, Rowland JH, eds. Handbook of psychooncology: psychological care of the patient with cancer. New York, Oxford University, 1989:455.

141. Andersen BL. Psychological interventions for cancer patients to enhance the quality of life. J Consult Clin Psychol 1992;60:552.

142. Fawzy FI, Fawzy NW, Arndt LA, et al. Critical review of psychosocial interventions in cancer care. Arch Gen Psychiatry 1995;52:100.

143. Maguire P, Tait A, Brooke M, et al. The effects of counseling

on the psychiatric morbidity associated with mastectomy. BMJ 1980;281:1454.

144. Spiegel D, Bloom JR, Yalom I. Group support for patients with metastatic cancer. Arch Gen Psychiatry 1981;38:527.

145. Bloom JR, Ross RD, Burnell G. The effect of social support on patient adjustment after breast surgery. Patient Counsel Health Educ 1978;1:50.

146. Farash JL. Effects of counseling on resolution of loss and body image disturbance following mastectomy. Dissert Abstr Int 1979;39:4027.

147. Cain EN, Kohorn EI, Quinlan DM, et al. Psychosocial benefits of a cancer support group. Cancer 1986;57:183.

148. Capone MA, Good RS, Westie KS, et al. Psychosocial rehabilitation of gynecologic oncology patients. Arch Phys Med Rehabil 1980;61:128.

149. Telch CF, Telch MJ. Group coping skills instruction and supportive group therapy for cancer patients: a comparison of strategies. J Consult Clin Psychol 1986;54:802.

150. Richardson JL, Shelton DR, Krailo M. The effect of compliance with treatment on survival among patients with hematologic malignancies. J Clin Oncol 1990;8:356.

151. Pressberg BA, Levenson JL. A survey of cancer support groups provided by National Cancer Institute clinical and comprehensive centers. Psychooncol 1993;2:215.

152. Coluzzi PH, Grant M, Doroshow JH, et al. Survey of the provision of supportive care services at National Cancer Institute–designated cancer centers. J Clin Oncol 1995;13:756.

153. Spiegel DS, Bloom JR, Kraemer HC, et al. Effect of psychosocial treatment on survival of patients with metastatic breast cancer. Lancet 1989;2:888.

154. Krupnick JL, Rowland JH, Goldberg RL, et al. Professionally led support groups for cancer patients: an intervention in search of a model. Intl J Psychiatry Med 1993;23:275.

155. Wortman CB. Social support and the cancer patient: conceptual and methodologic issues. Cancer 1984;53:2339.

156. House J, Landis NR, Umberson D. Social relationships and health. Science 1988;241:540.

157. Cohen S, Syme SL, eds. Social support and health. New York, Academic, 1985.

158. Wallston BS, Alagna SW, DeVellis BM, et al. Social support and physical health. Health Psychol 1983;2:367.

159. Nelles WB, McCaffrey RJ, Blanchard CG, et al. Social supports and breast cancer: a review. J Psychosoc Oncol 1991;9:21.

160. Funch DP, Marshall J. The role of stress, social support and age in survival from breast cancer. J Psychosom Res 1983;27:77.

161. Dunkel-Schetter C, Wortman C. The interpersonal dynamics of cancer: problems in social relationships and their impact on the patients. In: Friedman JS, DiMatteo RM, eds. Interpersonal issues in health care. New York, Academic, 1982:69.

162. Wellisch DK, Jamison KR, Pasnau RO. Psychosocial aspects of mastectomy. II. The man's perspective. Am J Psychiatry 1978;135:543.

163. Sabo D, Brown J, Smith C. The male role and mastectomy: support groups and men's adjustment. J Psychosoc Oncol 1986;4:19.

164. Maguire P. The repercussions of mastectomy on the family. Int J Family Psychiatry 1981;1:485.

165. Baider L, Kaplan-DeNour A. Couples' reactions and adjustment to mastectomy: a preliminary report. Int J Psychiatry Med 1984;14:265.

166. Northouse LL. The impact of breast cancer on patients and husbands. Cancer Nurs 1989;12:276.

167. Northouse LL. Breast cancer in younger women: effects on interpersonal and family relations. Monogr Natl Cancer Inst 1994;16:183.

168. Fisher JD, Nadler A, Whitcher-Alagna S. Recipient reactions to aid. Psychol Bull 1982;91:27.

169. Wellisch DK. Family relationships of the mastectomy patient: interactions with the spouse and children. Isr J Med Sci 1981;17:993.

170. Litman TJ. The family as a basic unit in health and medical care: a social behavioral overview. Soc Sci Med 1974;8:495.

171. Lewis FM. The impact of cancer on the family: a critical analysis of the research literature. Patient Educ Counsel 1986;11:269.

171. Lichtman RR, Taylor SE, Wood JV. Relations with children after breast cancer: the mother–daughter relationship at risk. J Psychosoc Oncol 1985;2:1.

172. Wellisch DK. Adolescent acting out when a parent has cancer. Int J Fam Ther 1979;1:238.

173. Fine J. Afraid to ask: a book for families to share about cancer. New York, Lothrop, Lee & Shepard, 1984.

174. Leshan E. When a parent is very sick. Boston, Little, Brown, 1986.

175. Kash KM, Holland JC, Halper MS, et al. Psychological distress and surveillance behaviors of women with a family history of breast cancer. J Natl Cancer Inst 1992;84:1074.

176. Lerman C, Daly M, Sands C, et al. Mammography adherence and psychological distress among women at risk for breast cancer. J Natl Cancer Inst 1993;85:1074.

177. Wellisch DK, Gritz ER, Schain W, et al. Psychological functioning of daughters of breast cancer patients. Part I: Daughters and comparison subjects. Psychosomatics 1991;32:324.

178. Wellisch DK, Gritz ER, Schain W, et al. Psychological functioning of daughters of breast cancer patients. Part II: Characterizing the distressed daughter of the breast cancer patient. Psychosomatics 1992;33:171.

179. Schover LR. The impact of breast cancer on sexuality, body image, and intimate relationships. CA Cancer J Clin 1991;41:112.

180. Schultz WCMW, Van de Wiel HBM, Hahn DEE, et al. Sexuality and cancer in women. Annu Rev Sexual Res 1992;3:151.

181. Quigley KM. The adult cancer survivor: psychosocial consequences of cure. Semin Oncol Nursing 1989;5:63.

182. Schag CA, Ganz PA, Polinsky ML, et al. Characteristics of women at risk for psychosocial distress in the year after breast cancer. J Clin Oncol 1993;11:783.

183. Ganz PA, Coscarelli A, Fred C, et al. Breast cancer survivors: psychosocial concerns and quality of life. Breast Cancer Res Treat (in press).

184. Auchincloss SS. Sexual dysfunction in cancer patients: issues in evaluation and treatment. In: Holland JC, Rowland JH, eds. Handbook of psychooncology: psychological care of the patient with cancer. New York, Oxford University, 1989:383.

185. Vincent CE, Vincent B, Greiss FC, et al. Some marital–sexual concomitants of carcinoma of the cervix. South Med J 1975;68:552.

186. Schover LR, Jensen SB. Sexuality and chronic illness: a comprehensive approach. New York, Guilford, 1988.

187. Vaeth, JM, ed. Body image, self-esteem, and sexuality in cancer patients, ed 2. Basel, Karger, 1986.

25.2

Rehabilitation Management for Women With Breast Cancer: Maximizing Functional Outcomes

LYNN H. GERBER

Breast cancer and its treatments present substantial challenges to women in terms of return to optimal functional status and good quality of life. The impact of this diagnosis on physical, psychological, and socioeconomic well-being must be evaluated and treated if good outcomes are to be realized. Rehabilitation specialists—including physiatrists and physical, occupational, and recreation therapists—are able to evaluate and treat problems that interfere with function as a result of disease sequelae or treatments. These health care professionals can provide comprehensive restorative or preventive measures to help patients resume normal or nearly normal activity. Such approaches have included ameliorating pain; reducing, controlling or preventing edema; restoring shoulder range of motion (ROM) and strength; and guiding patients through stage-appropriate activities and daily routines for the duration of their disease. Treatment of lymphedema is addressed in Chapter 24.7.

Rehabilitation is a process that engages the patient in a therapeutic alliance with rehabilitation specialists to help the patient reach her desired functional goals, when possible. This alliance is critical for progress to be made and is invaluable in educating and preparing the patient for what may lie ahead. Figure 25.2-1 provides an example of patient assessment for rehabilitation. The educational process often forms the infrastructure on which the therapeutic alliance is based and aids in adjustment to illness. Figure 25.2-2 is a checklist for providing patient education to those undergoing breast surgery.

This chapter addresses the rehabilitation, evaluation, and treatment of problems faced by women with breast cancer.

Rehabilitation Problems

Four major problems presented to the rehabilitation team by patients with breast cancer population include: lymphedema (discussed elsewhere), decreased shoulder mobility, pain and fatigue, and need for psychosocial support to foster good functional outcome and independence.

Breast cancer may present in several ways. The patient may be asymptomatic but have a positive mammogram. Conversely, she may experience bone pain, discomfort in the axilla, or arm swelling. The treatment plan for primary management of breast cancer clearly is based on the best treatments shown to control or eradicate disease, and also on the wishes of the patient. Nonetheless, the choices are varied and are often driven by medical as well as functional, psychological, and cosmetic considerations. Determinations of these components are frequently done by rehabilitation specialists, whose evaluations consist of mea-

surements of upper extremity ROM and mobility; strength; change in limb girth; severity of pain in the shoulder girdle, cervical spine, and chest wall; and magnitude of fatigue. Also included in the assessment are questions aimed at determining the patient's ability to do needed daily routines for maintaining personal hygiene, home and work environment activities, and hobbies. Level of pain and fatigue associated with activity is assessed. An in-depth interview is conducted to determine the patient's life goals, her view of her personal roles and their importance, and her coping style and problem-solving ability. Based on the information gathered, we are able to develop a comprehensive treatment plan for each patient.

Specifically, women with breast cancer report problems resulting from disease or its treatment that include arm and forearm swelling, limitation in ROM, weakness in grip strength or shoulder girdle strength, shoulder stiffness, chest wall tenderness, pain in the arm, and numbness along the inner aspect of the arm. Psychologic distress, a decrease in feelings of femininity, and decreased sexual interest have also been described. Physical and psychologic problems should not be viewed as entirely separate entities. Some evidence suggests that physical problems often produce psychologic distress, and women report psychologic distress more often when associated physical problems involve the upper extremity.[1]

Most of the signs and symptoms associated with breast cancer and its primary treatments are treatable. One exception is the medial arm pain and paresthesias associated with axillary dissection. Although the intensity of the symptoms subsides, the overall condition persists. It has been my clinical observation that education about this condition often relieves patient anxiety and renders the problem of little clinical significance.

Mobility and Strength

Shoulder mobility is in good measure influenced by the nature and extent of surgery, the radiation port and dosing schedule, and the timing and type of physical therapeutic interventions.[2-7] Shoulder motion is usually affected by the extent of axillary dissection. Flexion, external rotation, and abduction (the true articular shoulder movements) are the most likely to be affected and are often the most difficult to restore if lost. Shoulder pain is a significant clinical problem that requires treatment to improve comfort and function. Additionally, pain control is essential if ROM exercises are to be successful, because increases in

MEDICAL RECORD	**BREAST SURGERY PHYSICAL THERAPY EVALUATION**

History

Referring Physician:	Surgery Date:	Type of Surgery: ○ MRM ○ Lumpectomy & Axillary Dissection ○ Other

Stage of Cancer:	Involved Side: ○ Right ○ Left	Handedness: ○ Right ○ Left

Past Medical History:
 	
○ Preexisting Shoulder Dysfunction:
 	
○ Previous Cancer Treatment: ○ Chemotherapy
                                                    ○ Radiation
                                                    ○ Other
	Previous Level of Function:
	Activity Level:
	
	Vocation:
	
	Recreational Activities:

Social History:	Family History of Breast Cancer:

PREOPERATIVE

SUBJECTIVE/OBJECTIVE EVALUATION

Subjective

Patient's Main Concerns/Goals: _____

_____

Objective

Observation: Appearance/Symmetry (scapula, skin, swelling): _____

_____

            Posture: _____

Pain Levels (0–10)/(areas of discomfort): _____

Cervical Spine Screening (note limitations): _____

Upper Extremity	R		L		Strength	R	L
Range of Motion	A*	P*	A*	P*			
Shoulder					Shoulder		
Flexion					Flexion		
Abduction					Abduction		
Internal rotation					Internal rotation		
External rotation					External rotation		
Elbow					Pectoralis major		
Flexion					Serratus anterior		
Extension					Elbow		
Supination					Flexion		
Pronation					Extension		
Wrist					Supination		
Flexion					Pronation		
Extension					Wrist		

Girth Measurements	R	L	Flexion		
MCP			Extension		
Palm			Grip		
US			Volumetric Measurement (mL)		
10 cm			*Active/Passive		
20 cm			Sensation:		
30 cm					
40 cm			Functional Status:		
50 cm					

Patient Identification	Breast Surgery Physical Therapy Evaluation NIH-2730 (4-93) P.A. 09-25-0099 File in Section Page 1

FIGURE 25.2-1 Example of patient assessment for rehabilitation.

TREATMENT/EDUCATION

o Discussed Rehabilitation Course

(Refer to Treatment/Education Checklist on Last Page)

o Prosthesis/Bra Shown, If Appropriate

ASSESSMENT

PLAN

POSTOPERATIVE	Postop Day Number:	Number of Drains:

SUBJECTIVE/OBJECTIVE EVALUATION

Subjective

Patient's Main Concerns/Goals: _____

_____

Objective

Observation: Appearance/Symmetry (scapula, skin, swelling, dressings): _____

_____

Posture/Upper Exremity Positioning (scapular winging): _____

Sensory Changes (hypersensitivity, numbness): _____

Pain Levels (0–10)/(areas of discomfort): _____

Cervical Spine Screening (note limitations): _____

Willingness to Move Involved Upper Extremity: _____

Quality of Movement (free moving, with caution, tense, guarding. . .): _____

Girth Measurements	R	L	Functional Status/ADL Difficulties:
MCP			
Palm			
US			
10 cm			
20 cm			**TREATMENT/EDUCATION:**
30 cm			(Refer to Treatment/Education Checklist on Page 4)
40 cm			Functional Status:
50 cm			
Volumetric Measurement (mL)			

ASSESSMENT

Goal: o Completion of checklist elements by discharge.

PLAN

DISCHARGE	Discharge Postop Day Number: _____

SUBJECTIVE/OBJECTIVE EVALUATION

Subjective: _____

Objective

Observation: Appearance/Symmetry (scapula, skin, swelling, dressings): _____

_____

Posture/Upper Exremity Positioning (scapular winging): _____

Sensory Changes (hypersensitivity, numbness): _____

Pain Levels (0-10)/(areas of discomfort): _____

Cervical Spine Screening (note limitations): _____

Page 2

Upper Extremity	R		L				R	L
Range of Motion	A*	P*	A*	P*	Strength			
Shoulder					Shoulder			
Flexion					Flexion			
Abduction					Abduction			
Internal rotation					Internal rotation			
External rotation					External rotation			
Elbow					Pectoralis major			
Flexion					Serratus anterior			
Extension					Elbow			
Supination					Flexion			
Pronation					Extension			
Wrist					Supination			
Flexion					Pronation			
Extension					Wrist			
Girth Measurements			R	L	Flexion			
MCP					Extension			
Palm					Grip			
US					Volumetric Measurement (mL)			
10 cm					*Active/Passive			
20 cm					Functional Status/ADL Difficulties:			
30 cm								
40 cm								
50 cm								

TREATMENT/EDUCATION

(Refer to Treatment/Education Checklist on Page 4)

ASSESSMENT

PLAN

o Schedule patient for follow-up (first clinic appoinment following discharge).

o Provide prescription for breast prothesis/bra.

_____   _____
Signature of Therapist   Date

Page 3

TREATMENT/EDUCATION CHECKLIST FOR BREAST SURGERY PHYSICAL THERAPY

EDUCATED/DISCUSSED WITH PATIENT:

o Sensation changes expected
o Lymphedema precautions
o Prosthesis information
o Posture realignment
o Shoulder movement guidelines:

The active range of motion progression for the involved upper extremity is as follows:			
Postoperative Day	Shoulder Flexion	Shoulder Abduction	Shoulder Int/Ext Rotation
1–3*	45	45	to tolerance
4–6*	45–90	45	to tolerance
7+ or when drains removed	to tolerance	to tolerance	to tolerance
*Gentle accessory mobilization of the glenohumeral joint may also be included.			

o Lifting precautions: (<5 pounds for 2 weeks)
     (<10 pounds for 6 weeks)
o General conditioning recommendations
o Exercise guidelines if receiving radiation treatment
o Breast self-examination and its importance
o Self-monitoring of edema
o Relaxation techniques

PATIENT TAUGHT AND PERFORMED:

o Elevation/positioning of involved upper extremity
o Pumping exercises
o Deep breathing exercises (emphasizing upper chest and rib cage expansion)
o Cervical range-of-motion exercises
o Shoulder shrugs/retractions
o Elbow flexion/extension/supination/pronation
o Active shoulder range-of-motion exercises (avoid incisional stretch pain)
o Home exercise program
o Other: _____

Page 4

FIGURE 25.2-2 Checklist for providing patient education.

ROM are difficult to achieve in the presence of substantial pain. Published data suggest that ROM can be restored and preserved with postoperative physical therapy. Timing of therapy is important. Immediate shoulder mobilization may increase axillary drainage and may delay wound healing.[8,9] Yet, delaying therapy until a clinical problem is present may have a substantial negative effect on eventual functional outcome.[6] It is critical to be clear about which shoulder movements should be performed and when. For example, restricting abduction while permitting internal and external rotation preserves joint integrity without stressing the suture line and hence can be well tolerated. Patients undergoing modified radical mastectomy are more likely to have complications than are those with

less extensive surgical procedures and therefore should be referred earlier in their postoperative course to prevent shoulder dysfunction or to treat problems while they remain relatively minor, when possible.[10]

Pain and Fatigue

Pain is a frequent complaint in breast cancer patients and can be of several types. These pain syndromes are summarized in Table 25.2-1. The natural history of the symptom, how soon after surgery it occurs, its distribution, and intensity often indicate its origin. For example, medial arm

TABLE 25.2-1
Common Sequelae of Mastectomy or Axillary Dissection, or Both

Sequelae	Patients Affected %
PAIN OR DISCOMFORT	
Incisional	90–100
Paresthesia of the arm	90–100
Hypesthesia of the arm	90–100
Cords	40–50
Pectoralis spasm	20–30
Chest wall	25–35
Trigger point	<10
EDEMA	
One arm, transient	≤50
Arm requiring Jobst sleeve (increase >2 cm)	18
Breast	90–100
NEURAPRAXIA	
Serratus anterior	15
Others	15
Limitation in range of motion	Initially, 100 After 9 mo, 2

dysesthesia occurs immediately postoperatively and is a result of cutting the medial brachial cutaneous nerve; hand dysesthesiae are probably referred from the cervical spine or possibly a carpal tunnel syndrome frequently secondary to arm edema and subsequent to axillary dissection. Occasionally, patients complain of phantom breast pain, a sensation that reminds them of their operated breast. Patients undergoing mastectomy occasionally indicate that the breast feels intact. Radiation treatments have been shown to cause chest wall pain that persists for several years beyond completion of radiation therapy.[11] The cause of this pain remains unclear; however, periostitis may contribute to the problem.

Shoulder stiffness is a frequently reported symptom. The causes are multiple but are probably related to local edema, bleeding, postoperative immobilization due to pain, and subsequent postoperative scarring of tissue. This symptom is frequently associated with the inability to put the arm through ROM. One particular syndrome is the development of pain and a sense of tightness in the axilla (and sometimes the elbow) associated with the presence of ropy, cordlike material. These cords are thought to be sclerosed lymphatics, characteristically developing 6 to 8 weeks after surgery. Patients experience some modest loss of ROM, which is temporary and is restored after spontaneous rupture of these cordlike structures.

Fatigue has not been documented to be a significant or common complaint of patients with breast cancer. Clinical wisdom has suggested, however, that patients undergoing breast cancer surgery and radiation therapy do experience fatigue. This may be a result of the physiological effects of anesthesia, surgery, or radiation. Disruption of normal sleep cycles may also occur as a result of pain and anxiety. Many clinicians have commented that they do not encourage their patients to return to vigorous physical activity or aerobic or fitness training programs, in part because they are often ignorant about the patients' presurgical level of exercise or are not aware that these patients might benefit from a fitness program. The benefits of regular exercise apply to this population of patients as well as those without breast cancer.[12] Exercise has been shown to positively affect mood, to restore a more normal sleep cycle, to assist in weight reduction, to retard osteoporosis, and to improve stamina. Exercise may be especially important because estrogen replacement may not be an option for these women. Also, the benefits of exercise groups with respect to socialization and support in the postoperative period are often highly valued by these patients. Return to normal activity, including vocational and avocational activity that requires full ROM and arm positioning over the head for good functional outcome, is not contraindicated for this population after drains are removed from the axilla and healing has occurred.

The resumption of activity that had been typical for the patient before the diagnosis and treatment of breast cancer is a reasonable goal and helps in the control of pain, reduction of fatigue, and promotion of a sense of well-being.

Functional Outcomes

Ultimately, the outcomes of breast cancer treatment and management should be viewed in terms of patient functioning in most domains of her life. Is the patient functioning well, doing what she needs and wishes to do, and perceiving herself as doing well. Function is a blend of physical, psychologic, social, and vocational parameters. It must be seen and measured in the context of the individual patient and her environment. Patients working outside the home and those who have had less extensive surgery tend to return to their life activities sooner than their counterparts who worked inside the home.[13] Patients who underwent breast-sparing procedures reported less psychologic distress than those who had mastectomies.[14] Outcome measures used to determine how well a patient is doing functionally often show different findings between patient self-report and health care professional reports.[15] Some investigators are examining the relation between psychologic distress and survivorship. The hypothesis is that those who have a more supportive environment are able to reduce stress and to function better. These factors may positively influence survivorship. The functional outcomes measured in such studies include physical activity, stamina, indices of mood, and return to prior activity.

Treatment

Published observations about the efficacy of rehabilitation for patients with breast cancer usually describe interventions related to the major rehabilitation problems facing patients with breast cancer. These include lymphedema, mobility, management of pain and fatigue, and functional outcomes. Most of what is reported reflects a cumulative experience of a center or group of practitioners. Occasionally, controlled trials designed to evaluate treatment efficacy are done.

Work done at the National Institutes of Health (NIH) and at other institutions that treat patients with cancer has suggested that structured rehabilitation programs offered routinely to all patients promotes good physical and psychological well-being and function. These programs traditionally include ROM exercises, light aerobic conditioning, evaluation and treatment, and education about lymphedema, management of pain using nonpharmacologic intervention, and strategies to help promote function and quality of life. Recently, efforts to reduce stress and anxiety have been added.

Many medical centers have recognized the value of a comprehensive program for patients with breast cancer. Memorial Sloan-Kettering Hospital in New York was one of the pioneers in this area and developed a program that addressed the physical, psychosocial, and general support needs of their patients. Their program begins on postoperative day 1 with hand squeezing and advances to shoulder exercises on day 2. A nurse is available to provide guidance and answer questions about do's and don'ts.[16] In addition, they use volunteers from the Reach to Recovery program, which introduces newly diagnosed or treated women to those who have had their disease for a longer period. Treatment outcomes from this approach indicate a high level of patient satisfaction and a relatively high rate of return to work.[13]

The program developed at NIH is comprehensive also and was developed after many years of clinical experience with patients with breast cancer. All patients who undergo axillary dissection are referred to rehabilitation and are provided standard treatment aimed at promoting arm mobility (Table 25.2-2), controlling shoulder girdle and chest wall pain and upper extremity edema, and promoting full functional recovery, when possible.[8] Several groups have indicated that immediate shoulder mobilization may complicate wound healing and produce an increased incidence of infection.[17–20] We tend to use early (rather than immediate) shoulder mobilization strategies.[11]

To support mobilization, an overhead pulley, topical heat and cold to the shoulder and possibly the axilla, and (occasionally) transcutaneous nerve stimulation for pain relief can be used. Often, shoulder exercises are done with the patient recumbent to support the scapula and should be performed in that position if serratus anterior palsy is present. To maintain sustained progress, heat and cold may need to be used throughout the mobilization program to preserve a pain-free or nearly pain-free status. These modalities should not be used in an irradiated field during the time of radiation. Active and active-assisted movement is the preferred form of exercise. That is, the patient should put the arm through ROM; with assistance if necessary, rather than have the arm passively moved. We usually provide the patient with written instructions and diagrams showing shoulder flexion, rotation, and abduction ROM.

TABLE 25.2-2
Recommended Postoperative Shoulder Mobilization Schedule

Postoperative Day	Flexion (Degrees)	Abduction (Degrees)	Internal and External Rotation
1–2*	40	40	To tolerance
3*	45	45	To tolerance
4–6*	45–90	45	To tolerance
7	To tolerance	To tolerance	To tolerance
Drains out†	To tolerance	To tolerance	To tolerance

* Gentle accessory mobilization of glenohumeral joint may also be included.

† Active assistive range-of-motion exercises are added or an overhead pulley is used at this time when needed.

If pain interferes with range, we add heat to the stretch program.

Fatigue may have its origin in the psyche, the peripheral muscle, or the cardiovascular system. The treatment of fatigue should include introduction of relaxation strategies. The use of guided imagery to improve energy and natural sleep cycles has been suggested as beneficial in various settings. Relaxation strategies have helped with anticipatory nausea before chemotherapy.

Muscle weakness in the shoulder girdle muscles may contribute to fatigue and certainly contributes to decreased function. Isometric exercise for the rotator cuff, often using a resistive band (Theraband) and gradually advancing to isotonic exercise, is recommended on a daily basis.

The benefits of aerobic exercise have been described in terms of ameliorating sleep disturbance, improving mood, lowering cholesterol levels, and improving feelings of well-being and self-efficacy. We recommend light aerobic conditioning to start. Bicycle ergometry, walking, and aqua therapy are the initial recommendations. Resumption of usual activity is encouraged after the suture line is well healed. Precautions are always taken to prevent sunburn or injury to the affected side.

Some women, when presented with a diagnosis of breast cancer, wish to have their treatment options described for them. This helps to reduce stress and anxiety and helps them plan for the future. Making informed choices at each step becomes a goal for these women and should stimulate health care professionals to be fully informed and support the patient's needs. Decision making reflects a composite of issues that include prognosis, length and toxicity of medication, impact of surgical and radiation therapy on the body, and its ramifications on psychosexual well-being. The multidisciplinary approach to management usually enhances the likelihood that the patient will obtain the support that she needs but does not always receive as part of her primary treatment planning. Several programs are routinely offering such comprehensive programs.[11,16,21,22]

TABLE 25.2-3
Schema for Clinical Management of Rehabilitation Needs of Breast Cancer Patients

Problem	Preoperative Evaluation	Postoperative Evaluation				
		0–2 Weeks	2–12 Weeks	3–6 Months	6–12 Months	>1 Year
Edema	Obtain baseline measurements; If edema present, determine cause	Instruct in preventive arm care; If edema present: <2 cm without erythema Rx: elastic stockinette, elevation, hand pumping 2–4 cm without erythema Rx: Jobst sleeve >4 cm without erythema Rx: compression pump Any, with erythema Rx: antibodies	Same as 0–2 wk; Also maintain antigravity position as much as possible	>2 cm—compression sleeve, overhead hand pumping, arm elevation >4 cm—compression sleeve, compression pump >6 cm—compression pump; with erythema Rx: antibiotics	Same as 3–6 mo With pain rule out metastasis	Same as 3–6 mo With pain rule out metastasis
Shoulder motion	Obtain baseline measurements: If <145 degrees of flexion or abduction <60 degrees of ER/IR Rx: Heat and ROM exercise Precautions must be taken for proper arm position intraoperatively		Begin use of pulley: If <145 degrees of flexion or abduction <60 degrees of ER/IR Use of heat, ice (except when patient is being actively irradiated). Active and passive stretch. If no progress by week 8, add NSAIDS to regimen and check monthly	Determine ROM: If <160 degrees of flexion, 145 degrees of abduction, 60 degrees of ER/IR Rx: ROM exercises with assistance from physical therapist	Determine ROM: If <160 degrees of flexion, 145 degrees of abduction, or 60 degrees of ER/IR and if ROM exercises not effective Rx: Scan, NSAIDS, intraarticular steroids	Sams as 6–12 mo
Muscle strength	Obtain baseline measurement of shoulder complex strength, particularly stabilizers of scapula	Evaluate strength: If weakness, especially serratus anterior, support scapula during ROM exercises	Evaluate strength of shoulder girdle muscle Strength should be returning by end of this period Maintain ROM If weakness continue to support scapula during exercises	Evaluate strength of shoulder girdle muscles If abnormal strength, determine cause. Postoperative weakness should be resolved by 6 mos	Same as 3–6 mo	Same as 3–6 mo
Prosthesis	NA	Fluff, or when would heals, permanent prosthesis	Same as 0–2 wk	Consider reconstruction	Same as 3–6 mo	Same as 3–6 mo
Psychologic support	Orientation to surgery, radiation, and common postoperative problems	Support group and relaxation techniques, if appropriate	Same as 0–2 wk	Same as 0–2 wk	Same as 3–6 mo	Same as 3–6 mo

ER, external rotation; IR, internal rotation; ROM, range of motion.

Immediate reconstruction of the breast, although not commonly done, obviates the need for a breast prosthesis. Women not undergoing breast reconstruction should be counseled about the availability of fluff, which can be pinned to a shirt or camisole or placed in a bra. This may be used until a definitive prosthesis can be provided. Usually, 3 to 6 weeks are needed to permit healing, longer if chest wall edema or wound complications are present.

A summary of the interventions that are often needed in the management of patients with breast cancer is listed in Table 25.2-3. Monitoring the parameters of shoulder mobility, strength, upper extremity swelling, and pain should be maintained throughout the life of the patient. Educating the patient will ensure adequate monitoring, but treatment for the myriad problems that may arise is often best left to rehabilitation professionals who can combine various interventions in a coordinated fashion to promote optimal function.

References

1. Maunsell E, Brisson J, Deschenes L. Arm problems and psychological distress after surgery for breast cancer. Can J Surg 1993;36:315.
2. Aitken RJ, Gaze MN, Rodger A, et al. Arm morbidity within a trial of mastectomy and either nodal sample with selective radiotherapy or axillary clearance. Br J Surg 1989;76:568.
3. Sarin R, Dinshaw KA, Shrivastava SK, et al. Therapeutic factors influencing the cosmetic outcome and late complications in the conservative management of early breast cancer. Int J Radiat Oncol Biol Phys 1993;27:285.
4. Norby PA, Apte-Kakade S. Rehabilitation after conservative breast cancer surgery: management of lymphedema and limited range of motion. Oncol Nurs Forum 1990;17(2 Suppl):209.
5. Pollard K, Callum KG, Altman DG, et al. Shoulder movement following mastectomy. Clin Oncol 2:343, 1976.
6. Atkins H, Hayward JL, Klugman DJ, et al. Treatment of early breast cancer: a report after 10 years of a clinical trial. BMJ 1972;2:423.
7. Eisenberg HS, Goldenberg IS. Measurement of quality of survival of breast cancer patients. In: Hayward JL, Bulbrook RD, eds. Clinical evaluation in breast cancer. New York, Academic, 1966:93.
8. Lotze MT, Duncan MA, Gerber LH, et al. Early vs delayed shoulder motion following axillary dissection. Ann Surg 1981;193:288.
9. Flew TJ. Wound drainage following radical mastectomy: the effect of restriction of shoulder movement. Br J Surg 1966;66:302.
10. Gutman H, Kersz T, Barzilai T, et al. Achievements of physical therapy in patients after modified radiacal mastectomy compared with quadrantectomy, axillary dissection and radiation for carcinoma of the breast. Arch Surg 1990;125:389.
11. Gerber L, Lampert M, Wood C, et al. Comparison of pain, motion and edema after modified radical mastectomy vs. local excision with axillary dissection and radiation. Breast Cancer Res Treat 1992; 21:139.
12. Winningham ML, MacVicar MG, Bondoc M, et al. Effect of aerobic exercise on body weight and composition in patients with breast cancer on adjuvant chemotherapy. Oncol Nurs Forum 1989;16: 683–9.
13. Winick L, Robbins GF. Physical and psychological readjustment after mastectomy. Cancer 1977;39:478.
14. Schain W, Edwards B, Gorrell R, et al. Psychosocial and physical outcomes of primary breast cancer therapy: mastectomy vs excisional biopsy and irradiation. Breast Cancer Res Treat 1983;3:377.
15. Sneeuw KC, Aaronson NK, Yarnold JR, et al. Cosmetic and functional outcomes of breast conserving treatment for early stage breast cancer. Radiother Oncol 1992;25:153–9.
16. Winick L, Robbins GF. The postmastectomy rehabilitation group program: structure, procedure and population demography. Am J Surg 1976;132:599.
17. Hladiuk M, Huchcroft S, Temple W, et al. Arm function after axillary dissection for breast cancer: a pilot study to provide parameter estimates. J Surg Oncol 1992;50:47.
18. Jansen RF, van Geel AN, de Groot HG, et al. Immediate versus delayed shoulder exercises after axillary lymph node dissection. Am J Surg 1990;160:481.
19. Van der Horst Ch MAM, Kenter JAL, DeJong MT, et al. Shoulder function following early mobilization of the shoulder after mastectomy and axillary dissection. Neth J Surg 1985;37:105.
20. Dawson I, Stan K, Heslinga JM, et al. Effect of shoulder immobilization on wound seroma and shoulder dysfunction following modified radical mastectomy: a randomized prospective clinical trial. Br J Surg 1989;76:311.
21. Sachs S, Davis JM, Reynolds SA, et al. Comparative results of postmastectomy rehabilitation in a specialized and a community hospital. Cancer 1981;48:1251.
22. Gaskin TA, LoBuglio A, Kelly P, et al. STRETCH: a rehabilitative program for patients with breast cancer. South Med J Suppl 1987;467.

25.3

Support Programs

JANET WOLTER

In 1992, a minisymposium presented to the National Cancer Advisory Board addressed some of the issues of living with cancer. One part was devoted to psychosocial interventions and began by decrying both the "mindless mutualism" that deemphasizes the importance of psychosocial support for patients with cancer and the obverse extreme viewpoint that suggests without any empirical research that "mind over matter" has failed if patients develop or experience progression of cancer.[1] "The complex interrelationship of mind and body and its influence on vulnerability to disease and disease progression"[1] is undergoing scientific exploration. A fascinating analysis of Alameda County, California, vital statistics showed that people who lacked social and community ties were more likely to die of all causes than were those with such ties (relative risk, 2.3 for men and 2.8 for women) independent of socioeconomic status, health practices, or state of health at the beginning of the study.[2] It is not surprising, then, that psychosocial support influences adjustment to cancer, and clinical observations in various settings suggest that factors ranging from pain control to mortality can be altered by such support.[1,5] The study of psychosocial parameters has been hindered by methodologic difficulties. Not only does no single instrument exist to measure stress, pain, coping, and so forth, but no battery of instruments has been used universally. The Profile of Mood States (POMS) and Time Without Symptoms and Toxicity (TWIST) are mentioned most frequently, but several studies used questionnaires or interview questions developed for the specific project and often without external validation. Nevertheless, with few exceptions, studies have led to the overall impression that support enhances both mental and physical health.[3]

In addition to measurement problems, heterogeneity of subjects in terms of disease stage, treatment of primary cancer, and treatment of advanced disease often confound interpretation of psychosocial data.[4] Rowland[5] stresses that the relative importance of various kinds of support not only differs between individuals but also may change over time. Silberfarb and colleagues[6] interviewed newly diagnosed patients, those at first recurrence, and those with advanced disease and found the first recurrence to be more stressful than either of the other states. Taylor and coworkers[7] found that, regardless of whether the prognosis was good or poor, high levels of social support led to better adjustment.

One review tabulated 11 studies from 1982 to 1989.[4] Although this report evaluated various cohorts using supports differing in both content and duration, individual studies have shown beneficial effects on mood[8] (Fig. 25.3-1), pain[9] (Fig. 25.3-2), coping,[10] adjustment[11] (patients with gynecologic cancers were studied but were

believed by the authors to be generalizable), and survival.[12] A study using the Global Adjustment to Illness Scale (GAIS) found that patients with higher levels of anxiety and hostility and those who were able to externalize their conflicts (the "feisty" ones) appeared to live longer than those who were less hostile and more passive.[13] One recent retrospective review[14] failed to show a survival advantage, but prospective trials now in progress should yield more definitive data.

Definitions

The term *support groups* includes several different entities that have specific connotations to professionals in the behavioral sciences but that are sometimes used interchangeably by medical practitioners. All function on the basis of mutual aid.[15] *Mutual aid* is a general term that refers to any gathering of people who depend on each other to accomplish a common goal (Cella and Yellen[16]) or to face a common stress (Vugia[17]). Examples of mutual aid groups include medieval guilds, fraternal organizations, labor unions, Alcoholics Anonymous (among others), all with either a unified goal or a shared stress (and often both).

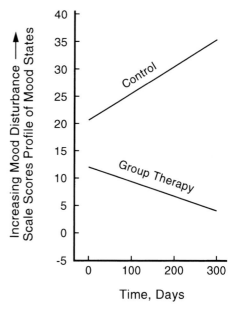

FIGURE 25.3-1 Mood changes. (Spiegel D. Psychosocial intervention in cancer. J Natl Cancer Inst 1993;85:1198)

FIGURE 25.3-2 Pain control. (Spiegel D. Psychosocial intervention in cancer. J Natl Cancer Inst 1993;85:1198)

Although the need must have existed forever, the first support group for patients with cancer was described in 1973.[16] Some basic terms are defined below:

- Self-help group—usually a group of patients with similar problems who meet without a professional facilitator; may be led by a patient
- Support group—a professional facilitator (MD, RN, MSW, and so forth) meets with the group and helps to direct it.
- Group coping skills instruction—a group with a facilitator who teaches problem solving, stress management, and so on.[15]
- Traditional psychotherapy group
- Conglomerate groups that include sources of information, advocacy, referrals to small support groups, and workshops

Who Joins

One of the problems inherent in evaluating support groups is that participants are self-selected. Women in the free-standing groups actively seek help. In institution-based groups, where participation may be presented to a captive audience, refusal to participate is always an option. Although it is popularly believed that people seek support groups when other sources of support are perceived to be inadequate, one interesting report found that people attending groups were more likely to have shared their concerns with their families and friends than were members of a control group,[7] suggesting perhaps that familiarity

with communication of concerns might make group interactions more acceptable.

The demographic characteristics of persons who join support groups have been documented in several geographic areas and were found to be similar. Although this chapter addresses a disease affecting women, women outnumber men four to one in cancer support groups. Participants tend to be more affluent and better educated. The elderly are underrepresented, as are people of color.[7,16,18]

People who seek support groups do so because they expect to feel better and usually are satisfied with what transpires. Although general satisfaction is achieved[8,10,16,18,19] a small but important group of women who expect only optimism are frightened by the intensity of some of the discussions or by the death of another member and leave the group.[16] All sources agree that the benefits outweigh the potential difficulties.

Goals of Support Groups

The goals of support groups depend somewhat on the cohort of patients for whom they are organized. The needs of recently diagnosed patients differ from those of patients with stage IV disease, and each group needs to state its purpose, identifying the major stresses of the target members.[17] The duration of the group, number of participants, (six or seven is often mentioned as ideal), inclusions of family members, and the inclusion or exclusion of drop-ins all must be addressed. Attention must also be paid to meeting hour and duration (usually 60 to 90 minutes) babysitting, and availability of transportation. The essential shared goals of all groups are as follows[16]:

- To provide emotional support
- To maintain the social identity of participants
- To provide education
- To provide tangible environmental support
- To provide a social affiliation

Additional goals, more appropriate in groups with advanced disease include the following[8]:

- To detoxify dying
- To focus and clarify problems and to define personally appropriate solutions
- To address the importance of using remaining time in the most satisfying way

One interesting report defined the goals from the patients' viewpoint rather than the groups' viewpoint and, after an extensive survey, found these five needs to be paramount[20]:

The need for hope
The need for honesty
The need for information
The need for emotional expression
The need to discuss issues related to death and dying

When the goals are met, groups often achieve a high degree of cohesion, with members visiting one another outside of meeting times and exhibiting less tension, depression, fatigue, confusion, and maladjusted coping mechanisms.[8]

How Support Groups Work

The traditional psychotherapy group uses self-exploration in a group setting. Here, a change in the person is the goal, and support is a by-product. The other models, with or without a facilitator, do not try to change the individual but rather to find a sense of belonging (which sometimes brings about change). The teaching of coping skills may be the prime objective in groups dedicated to that end, but the learning of coping skills occurs, to some extent, in all groups.[15]

Common themes of discussion in cancer support groups include internal concerns such as fear of dying, loss, denial, and spiritual questions. Interpersonal themes concern spousal and marital problems, dependency, and problems of communication about therapy and prognosis with friends and family. Social themes include the stigma of cancer, work role changes and life-style concerns. Cancer-related concerns include coping with the side effects of therapy, communication with health care providers, the role of unproven remedies, and financial burdens.[16,17] "The objectives of the group are to provide encouragement and reinforcement to members, to communicate mutual respect for member individuality, to share information that can help other members cope, and to discuss advantages of various coping strategies offered by participants or the facilitator."[16] Not only do support groups provide a safe place where members who share the common concern of cancer diagnosis and therapy can discuss their concerns and share information, they also provide a forum for shared catharsis.[16]

What Is Available

Given the upsurge of interest in support groups seen during the past 20 years, it is estimated that several million people have participated in support programs. The American Cancer Society led the way with Reach to Recovery. This program, begun when the only surgical option available was mastectomy, trained women who had had the operation and who had survived at least 2 years to visit women who had recently undergone the surgery to provide support, as well as a soft temporary prosthesis and information booklets.

Other early support groups such as I Can Cope included women with breast cancer but were applicable to all tumor sites and stages.

Currently, hospitals and oncology practices in each community are either the sponsors of or are aware of the location of support groups of all kinds and thus represent local sources of referral.

The growth of an organization called Y-Me is an example of the current intense interest that has been generated by the area of psychosocial support. Y-Me is a multipurpose type of breast cancer support organization founded in Chicago in 1978 by two women with breast cancer. They were MSWs acquainted with the possibilities of mutual aid and were appalled by the lack of help and information available to them. The organization has grown steadily through the years and now has 19 chapters throughout the United States. In addition to a national hotline, answered only by trained volunteers, it supports conversation groups and hundreds of workshops and educational sessions, drawing on health professionals of all kinds to educate participants. The hotline of the central office (each chapter also has its own hotline) received 17,000 calls in 1993, and 9000 women attended conversation and workshop sessions. Referrals are given to appropriate support groups. Advocacy for breast cancer research and funding has been a natural corollary.

Many different groups offer support for patients with breast cancer and provide advice about such diverse subjects as risk factors and screening, swimming pool exercises for arm mobility, and where to buy a wig if alopecia occurs because of chemotherapy. A most comprehensive booklet is published biannually by the National Alliance of Breast Cancer Organizations (NABCO). Its 51 pages include information about treatment choices, reconstruction, how to find a breast cancer support group, educational print and video materials for both patients and health professionals, resources available in Spanish, and lists of national and regional breast cancer support groups. Copies are available for $3 from NABCO, 1180 Avenue of the Americas, New York, NY 10036, telephone, (212) 719-0154. The Cancer Information Service of the NCI (800-4-CANCER) and the Komen Alliance (800-I'M AWARE) can also provide information.

Summary

Public acknowledgment of the "increasing evidence that providing psychotherapeutic support services for cancer patients and their families is a low-cost, highly effective addition to other medical treatment"[21] is manifested by the Senate Appropriations Committee. Its recommendations for fiscal year 1995 include a statement that the NCI should require supportive psychotherapeutic services for cancer patients and their families in programs funded by the government.

Rowland[5] stated that "a consistent finding in research among patients is that illness is frequently associated with considerable difficulty in interpersonal relationships. A second finding, which can be viewed perhaps as a corollary to the first, is that one of the most important "buffers" against harmful effects of the stress of illness is the presence or availability of persons in the patient's environment with whom the experience can be shared. This role is usually filled by a member (or members) of the nuclear family (spouse, child, or parent), but may be an extended family member or friend(s). Research indicates that the presence of positive social support not only diminishes the psychic distress of cancer, but may be also important in modulating survival as well. Conversely, absence of social support, or loss of a significant person who withdraws during the patient's illness, becomes an additional stressor that may be more painful than the illness itself.

Many ongoing clinical trials include assessments of quality of life, interventions are being examined both as part of treatment trials and independently, and instruments of measurement are being refined. If these trials mature and are positive, modification of the social support systems of patients with cancer and interventions with few negative consequences can be included in future treatment plans.

References

1. Spiegel D. Psychosocial intervention in cancer. J Natl Cancer Inst 1993;85:1198.
2. Berkman LF, Syme SL. Social networks, host resistance and mortality: a nine-year follow-up study of Alameda County residents. Am J Epidemiol 1979;109:186.
3. Levy SM, Heiden LA. Personality and social factors in cancer outcome. In: Personality and disease. New York, John Wiley & Sons, 1990.
4. Nelles WB, McCaffrey RF, Blanchard CG, et al. Social supports and breast cancer: a review. J Psychosoc Oncol 1991;9:21.
5. Rowland JH. Interpersonal resources: social support. In: Holland JC, Rowland JH, eds. Handbook of psychooncology. New York, Oxford University, 1989.
6. Silberfarb PM, Maurer LH, Crouthamel CS. Psychosocial aspects of neoplastic disease. I. Functional status of breast cancer patients during different treatment regimens. Am J Psychiatry 1980;137:450.
7. Taylor SE, Falke RL, Shoptaw SJ, et al. Social support, groups, and the cancer patient. J Consult Clin Psychol 1880;54:608.
8. Spiegel D, Bloom JR, Yalom I. Group support for patients with metastatic cancer. Arch Gen Psychiatry 1981;38:527.
9. Spiegel D, Bloom JR. Group therapy and hypnosis reduce metastatic breast carcinoma pain. Psychosoc Med 1983;45:333.
10. Ferlic M, Goldman A, Kennedy BJ. Group counseling in adult patients with advanced cancer. Cancer 1979;43:760.
11. Cain EN, Kahane EL, Quinlan DM, et al. Psychosocial benefits of a cancer support group. Cancer 1986;57:185.
12. Spiegel D, Bloom JR, Kraemer HC, et al. Effect of psychosocial treatment on survival of patients with metastatic breast cancer. Lancet 1989;2:888.
13. Derogatis L, Abeloff M, Melisaratos N. Psychological coping mechanisms and survival time in metastatic breast cancer. JAMA 1979;242:1504.
14. Gellert GA, Maxwell RM, Siegel BS. Survival of breast cancer patients receiving adjunctive psychosocial support therapy. J Clin Oncol 1993;11:66.
15. Telch CF, Telch MJ. Group coping skills instruction and supportive group therapy for cancer patients: a comparison of strategies. J Consult Clin Psychol 1986;54:802.
16. Cella DF, Yellen SB. Cancer support groups: the state of the art. Cancer Pract 1993;1:56.
17. Vugia HD. Support groups in oncology: building hope through the human bond. J Psychosoc Oncol 1991;9:89.
18. Deans G, Bennett-Emslie GB, Weir J, et al. Cancer support groups: who joins and why. Br J Cancer 1988;58:670.
19. Berger K, Bostwick J. A woman's decision: breast care, treatment, and reconstruction, ed 2. St Louis, Quality Medical, 1994;324.
20. Young-Brockopp D. Cancer patient's perceptions of five psychosocial needs. Oncol Nurs Forum 1982;931.
21. Cancer Lett 1994;30:3.

25.4
Nursing Care in Patient Management and Quality of Life
KAREN HASSEY DOW ▪ MADELINE M. BARNICLE

Quality-of-life issues are integral to the management of women with breast cancer. The term *quality of life* includes an assessment of functional, psychologic, social (home and work), and existential well-being. Maintaining and improving quality of life has been a major focus of nursing care. This chapter focuses on quality-of-life care issues during and after treatment and includes management of physical effects during treatment and the psychologic and social implications to consider after treatment is completed. In addition, the effects of breast cancer on specific minority groups are addressed.

Helping Women to Decide on Initial Treatment

The complexity of breast cancer treatment and the alternatives facing women can be overwhelming and confusing.[1,2] Decisions about primary treatment, adjuvant therapy, and hormonal therapy must be made when women face a potentially life-threatening diagnosis. Studies suggest that concerns about radiation therapy versus surgery as well as about body image, preference for type of information (written or visual), desire for participation in decision making, and prior knowledge about breast cancer treatment are important factors to consider in helping women decide about primary treatment.[3-5] Ward and colleagues[2] found that concerns about radiation therapy and body integrity were the most important factors considered. Women rated active participation in decision making as highly important and preferred people as sources for information over written or visual materials. Hughes[4] found that neither the amount of information during the consultation visit nor the manner of presentation influenced patient preference for treatment.

Pierce[3] outlined several useful steps to help women in the decision making process: perceive the salience of information about treatment alternatives; work through decision-making conflict; seek additional information; understand the risks and benefits of each treatment; and deliberate about treatment choice. One study described an innovative, useful, and cost-effective method to help women decide about treatment.[5] This intervention strategy uses a simple technique of "preference cards" to delineate the specific roles that the treatment team and patient play in the decision-making process. The oncology nurse facilitates questions from the patient and uses preference cards to help determine the degree of the patient's desired involvement in decision making. The intervention emphasizes the patient's concerns, assesses the extent of desired participation, and helps to identify additional questions. This technique was successfully incorporated into a busy outpatient department and can be adapted to other settings.

Physical Effects of Breast-Conserving Surgery and Radiation Therapy

After decisions about primary treatment are made, women and their families have specific questions about treatment side effects. Fortunately, many of the unnecessary fears and concerns associated with the early history of radiation therapy (eg, major skin effects, rib fractures, and unappealing cosmetic results) have abated. Women receiving breast-conserving surgery and radiation therapy are often surprised by the relative lack of acute side effects. It is important to convey to women that the few physical side effects associated with radiation are transitory and usually subside within a few weeks after treatment ends. Major physical side effects of breast-conserving surgery and radiation therapy include fatigue, skin changes, and breast soreness.[6-9] Another consideration is that radiation treatments require daily visits over a 4- to 5-week period, which may require adjustments in work, social, and recreation patterns.

FATIGUE

Fatigue is a common side effect of radiation therapy and occurs commonly among cancer patients in general.[10-12] Blesch and colleagues[10] evaluated the occurrence of fatigue

among a sample of patients with breast (44 patients) and lung cancer (77 patients). Almost all patients (99%) experienced fatigue. The level of pain correlated significantly with fatigue. Although fatigue does not subside entirely, several interventions can decrease its occurrence. One can conserve energy; simplify techniques for bathing, grooming, dressing, food shopping, and child care; engage in health and fitness programs based on level of endurance; do rhythmic walking exercises; and use flexibility, strengthening, and relaxation techniques.[10,12] In addition, Dimensions of Caring is an available support program specifically designed for patients with cancer that provides instructions about fatigue, its causes, and ways to cope with it. The program includes videotape instructions, newsletters, and written materials.

SKIN EFFECTS

Enhancing skin comfort during radiation therapy is a major part of nursing care.[6,9] Radiation-induced skin effects range from slight peeling, dryness, tanning, and itchiness to moist desquamation. Teaching women to manage their skin during radiation therapy ideally begins before or at the start of treatment. Patients are evaluated weekly and as needed as therapy progresses. Women at risk for reactions include those receiving adjuvant chemotherapy, older women, and large-breasted women. Particularly susceptible areas include the inframammary fold and supraclavicular areas. Teaching guidelines for skin care during radiation therapy include the following:

1. Use lukewarm water in shower and bath.
2. Lubricate skin with water-based moisturizer containing no perfumes.
3. Do not use deodorant on the underarm of the treated breast.
4. Wear loose-fitting cotton garments and avoid wool and other scratchy fabrics against skin.
5. Do not wear an underwire bra.
6. Protect irradiated skin from sun, wind, and temperature extremes.
7. Apply cool wet packs to skin if itchy; add oatmeal soap for soothing relief.
8. Use an antihistamine for generalized itching, or apply a thin layer of 0.5% corticosteroid cream to affected area.

Patients may also experience heaviness in the treated breast and soreness or fullness in the breast and affected arm during radiation. They should be instructed to wear a firm support bra without underwire. Athletic support bras may also be used.

Managing Side Effects of Chemotherapy

A person's ability to cope with the demands of chemotherapy can vary; for example, younger women may experience more intense anxiety than older women.[13] Patients are willing to endure debilitating side effects when the goal is cure. Patients receiving therapy for metastatic disease may be more vulnerable and less willing to cope with effects of chemotherapy. Women often experience intense fear and uncertainty on the initial day of chemotherapy. These feelings can be diffused by having the patient meet with the oncology nurse before treatment and by providing the opportunity to ask questions and tour the treatment facility. Patients also benefit from frequent contact with the oncology nurse, either in person or by telephone. The nurse can also assess the patient to identify any psychosocial factors that may predispose to noncompliance with treatment or severe toxicity to chemotherapy.

Most patients choose to keep their lives as normal as possible during chemotherapy; they may continue to work and request a treatment schedule that permits recovery from side effects on days off from work. Others may request treatment on weekends or evenings. Patient and family awareness of toxicities and methods to maximize coping help to maintain quality of life during therapy. Symptom distress is a major concern for women receiving adjuvant chemotherapy.[14-18] The most common physical symptoms are nausea and vomiting, hair loss, weight gain, and fatigue. Other side effects include mucositis, infection, hemorrhagic cystitis, and neurotoxicity.

NAUSEA AND VOMITING

Chemotherapy-induced nausea and vomiting can be divided into three categories: acute, delayed (occurring more than 24 hours after therapy), and anticipatory, a classic conditioned response from inadequate antiemetic therapy. Reports of nausea and vomiting range from 70% to 100% in patients receiving cyclophosphamide-containing regimens.[19,20] Nausea and vomiting occur less frequently in patients over 65 years of age[21] or in those receiving sequential methotrexate and 5-fluorouracil with leucovorin rescue.[22] The emetogenic potentials of various breast cancer protocols are predictable; however, a woman's personal risk characteristics must also be assessed. Women who are anxious or young or who have histories of motion sickness or previous exposure to chemotherapy are at increased risk for nausea and vomiting.[23] Antiemetic regimens must be individualized for each patient. Inadequate control of nausea and vomiting can lead to persistent psychologic and physical complications, such as anticipatory nausea and vomiting and dehydration. These complications can be avoided through follow-up communication with the patient at home.

Substantial improvements in the control of nausea and vomiting have occurred during the past decade. The discovery that higher doses of metoclopramide exhibited 5-HT3 antagonist activity gave rise to a new class of agents, the 5-HT3 antagonists or serotonin antagonists. The available information detailing the central and peripheral neurologic pathways of chemotherapy-induced emesis provides rationale for effective antiemetic combinations. The most effective antiemetic regimen for emetogenic protocols includes a neurotransmittor blocking agent, a corticosteroid, and a benzodiazepine or antihistamine.[23] A serotonin antagonist combined with a corticosteroid offers the same benefit with less sedation.[24-26] Not all regimens, however, require the addition of a serotonin antagonist. One must consider cost because patients may not have insurance coverage for oral medications.

Patients considered to be at low risk should be reassured that nausea and vomiting are unlikely to occur and should be given a prescription for metoclopramide or prochlorperazine to be used as needed. Patients at high risk or those receiving chemotherapy of predictable emetogenic potential require scheduled combinations of antiemetics. Tables 25.4-1 and 25.4-2 review common chemotherapeutic agents, their risk potential, and antiemetic options.

In chemotherapy regimens with high emetogenic potential (eg, doxorubicin and cyclophosphamide), the use of serotonin antagonists has significantly improved control of acute nausea and vomiting. Previously, 70% to 80% of patients experienced nausea and vomiting.[19] Women even endured continuous sedation to achieve relief. Most women can now continue with their daily activities if they are using combined antiemetic therapy. Several studies have evaluated the effectiveness of ondansetron in highly emetogenic chemotherapy.[24-28] Results indicate that ondansetron was effective in controlling chemotherapy-induced nausea and vomiting. No doubt, the serotonin antagonists have improved the quality of life for patients by alleviating the distressful intensity of side effects. Ondansetron has shown efficacy, but comparison studies with newer serotonin antagonists are needed. Ondansetron has not consistently shown efficacy in delayed nausea; however, metochloramide and dexamethasone or dexamethasone alone has shown favorable results. In addition, cost factors need to be taken into account when using ondansetron in differing protocols of antiemetic intensity.

Anticipatory nausea and vomiting are less likely to occur in women receiving short-term adjuvant chemotherapy;[29,30] however, they are not uncommon in patients receiving longer regimens (cyclophosphamide, methotrexate, 5-fluorouracil) or in patients with metastatic disease who require ongoing therapy. Symptoms of anticipatory nausea and vomiting are difficult to manage, so emphasis is placed on tailoring antiemetic regimens to individual patient requirements. Benzodiazepines and psychoonocology have shown efficacy in controlling symptoms.

One of the more challenging sensations to treat is the unrelenting nausea described by patients taking oral cyclophosphamide. Patients report feelings similar to morning sickness, burning, gnawing, and hunger that may be relieved by eating. Strategies to minimize this unpleasant sensation include taking a long-acting antiemetic such as prochlorperazine, eating small amounts of low-calorie foods more frequently, and taking the total daily cyclophosphamide dose at one time, preferably in the morning. Some patients report relief with antacids.

ALOPECIA

Alopecia includes body hair loss (eyelashes, eyebrows, and pubic hair). Patients report that hair loss is one of the most distressing side effects of chemotherapy.[31] Although

TABLE 25.4-1
Common Antiemetic Regimens

Classification	Drug	Dose/Schedule	Schedule	Side Effects	Comments
BENZODIAZEPINES					
Central nervous system depressants—interfere with afferent nerves from cerebral cortex Sedatives Anxiolytics	Lorazepam (Ativan)	Tablets: 0.5, 1, 2 mg Parenteral: 2–4 mg/mL	q3–4h prn	Sedation Amnesia Confusion	Effective for anticipatory nausea and vomiting Use with caution in patients with hepatic or renal dysfunction
PHENOTHIAZINES					
Dopamine antagonists	Prochlorperazine (Compazine)	Tablets: 5, 10, 25 mg SRTs: 10, 15 mg Rectal suppositories: 25 mg IV: 20–40 mg	q4–6h q10–12h q4–6h q3–4h	Sedation (less common with SRTs) Orthostatic hypotension	Extrapyramidal side effects more common before age 30 y Side effects can be cumulative in elderly patients Extrapyramidal symptoms
Inhibit vomiting center by blocking afferent impulses through vagus nerve	Thiethylperazine (Torecan)	Tablets: 10 mg Suppl: 20 mg	q4–6h q6h	Dizziness Drowsiness	Diphenhydramine combats extrapyramidal symptoms or dystonic reactions
SUBSTITUTED BENZAMIDES					
Accelerates gastric emptying 5-HT$_3$ antagonists	Metoclopramide (Reglan)	Tablets: 5–10 mg IV: 1–3 mg/kg	q2–3h	Sedation Diarrhea Anxiety Fatigue	Extrapyramidal symptoms common Use with caution in patients with renal dysfunction
STEROIDS					
Antiprostaglandin synthesis (exact mechanism unknown)	Dexamethasone (Decadron)	PO: 10–40 mg IV: 4–20 mg		Insomnia Euphoria Anxiety Hypertension Edema Mild epigastric burning	Rapid infusion causes perineal itching Compatible with ondansetron and granisetron
ANTIHISTAMINES					
Histamine H$_1$ receptor antagonists	Diphenhydramine (Benadryl)	PO: 25–50 mg IV: 12.5–50 mg	q6h q4–6h	Sedation Hypotension	Prevent extrapyramidal side effects Use cautiously in elderly
SEROTONIN ANTAGONISTS					
	Ondansetron (Zofran)	PO: 4–8 mg IV: 32 mg IV: 0.15 mg/kg	bid q24h 3 doses	Headache Hypotension Constipation Sedation	Most effective in acute phase of nausea
	Granisetron (Kytril)	IV: 10 μg/kg	q24h		

SRTs, sustained-release tablets.

TABLE 25.4-2
Combination of Antiemetic Options*

Chemotherapy Combinations	Antiemetic Combinations
LOW EMETOGENIC POTENTIAL—PATIENT AT LOW RISK	
Taxol	Prochlorperazine, 15 mg q12h, *or*
Novantrone and thiotepa	Thiethylperazine 10 mg q6h, *or*
Methotrexate and 5-fluorouracil with leucovorin rescue	Metoclopramide, 10 mg tid, *and/or*
	Lorazepam, 1 mg q3–4h†
MODERATE EMETOGENIC POTENTIAL—PATIENT AT RISK	
Cyclophosphamide, methotrexate, and 5-fluorouracil	Prochlorperazine, 15–30 mg SRT q12h, *plus* lorazepam, 1 mg
	Ondansetron, 0.15 mg/kg, *plus* dexamethasone 20 mg IV at bedtime
Cyclophosphamide, doxorubicin; and 5-fluorouracil (low dose)	Lorazepam, 1 mg, *plus* diphenhydramine, 50 mg, *plus* prochlorperazine, 15 mg
	Take home:
	Prochlorperazine SRT, 15 mg q12h prn, *plus* lorazepam, 1 mg q4h prn
	Granisetron, 0.1 μg/kg; *plus* dexamethasone, 20 mg
MODERATE EMETOGENIC POTENTIAL	
	Prochlorperazine, 15–20 mg IV over 30 min, *plus* dexamethasone, 10 mg IV, *plus* diphenhydramine, 25 mg IV
	At bedtime:
	Lorazepam, 1 mg, *plus* diphenhydramine, 25 mg, *plus* prochlorperazine 15 mg
	For delayed nausea:
	Prochlorperazine, 15–30 mg PO q12h, *or* Zofran, 8 mg bid, *or* Dexamethasone, 8 mg PO bid for 2 d followed by 4 mg bid for 2 d
	Metoclopramide, 1–2 mg/kg 30 min *plus* diphenhydramine, 25–50 mg IV, *plus* dexamethasone, 10–20 mg IV
	At bedtime:
	Lorazepam, 1 mg, *plus* diphenhydramine, 25 mg, *plus* prochlorperazine, 15–30 mg
HIGH EMETOGENIC PROTOCOL	
Doxorubicin	Ondansetron, 0.15 mg/kg or one 32-mg dose a day, *or*
Cyclophosphamide	Granisetron, 0.1 μg/kg, *plus* dexamethasane, 20 mg
Cyclophosphamide, doxorubicin, and 5-fluorouracil (high dose)	Dexamethasone, 20 mg IV
	At bedtime:
	Lorazepam, 1–2 mg PO, *plus* diphenhydramine, 50 mg PO, *plus* prochlorperazine, 15–30 mg PO
	For delayed nausea:
	Prochlorperazine SRT, 15–30 mg PO q12h for 2 d, *plus* lorazepam, 1 mg q4h prn
	Ondansetron, 8 mg bid for 2 d, *plus* lorazepam, 1 mg PO q4h prn, *plus* prochlorperazine SRT, 15–30 mg q12h for 2d
	Dexamethasone, 8 mg bid for 2 d followed by 4 mg bid for 2 d
	For anticipatory nausea:
	Lorazepam, 1 mg PO 30 min before treatment
	Lorazepam, 0.5–2 mg IV before treatment (avoid before vesicant chemotherapy)
	Consider behavioral therapy options

SRT, sustained-release tablet

* Combinations are based on out patient treatment; establishment of level of risk is emphasized.

† Lorazepam is best used in combination with above.

mastectomy scars are devastating, hair loss can be publicly stigmatizing. Patients are able to adapt when they are prepared for the change and when they understand that it is temporary. Chemotherapeutic drugs cause partial or complete atrophy of the hair root bulb and constriction of the hair shaft, which can break easily with any tension. Drug combinations with minimal or low risk for hair loss include methotrexate and 5-fluorouracil with leucovorin rescue, mitoxantrone, thiotepa, and vinblastine. Oral cyclophosphamide causes generalized hair thinning, especially at the crown. With standard 6-month chemotherapeutic regimens, women with thicker hair may not require a wig. Women with fine, sparse hair usually need a wig after the fourth cycle. Certain measures can minimize or delay hair loss; a shorter hair style decreases weight on the hair shaft and makes cyclophosphamide-induced hair loss less noticeable. Useful interventions for hair loss include the following:

1. Cut hair in a manageable and easy to maintain style before chemotherapy.
2. Use a mild, protein-based shampoo and conditioner.
3. Use electric hair dryer on lowest setting.
4. Avoid electric curlers and curling irons, hair spray, and hair dye, which can increase the fragility of hair.
5. Avoid excessive brushing and hair combing.
6. Purchase a wig to fit normal hair color and style.
7. Consider Look Good . . . Feel Better program.

Complete hair loss can be expected with higher doses of doxorubicin and cyclophosphamide. Some practical suggestions are to purchase a wig ("cranial prosthesis") before hair loss. Wigs can be thinned and shaped to the woman's natural hair style. Some insurance companies will pay part of the cost of the wig if they receive a letter and prescription from the physician. Programs addressing appearance changes such as Look Good . . . Feel Better are very helpful in helping women deal with hair loss.

The use of hair-preservation techniques are controversial and ineffective with higher doses of doxorubicin and cyclophosphamide. Opponents believe it creates a drug sanctuary, rendering the scalp vulnerable to metastasis. This risk needs to be considered when treating patients with curative intent. When oral cyclophosphamide is given, hair-preservation techniques are not practical, because the drug is taken orally. Hypothermia applied 15 to 20 minutes before and 20 to 30 minutes after treatment can be effective for women receiving less than 30 mg/m^2 doxorubicin and may contribute to the patient's quality of life.

WEIGHT GAIN

Weight gain occurs in 50% to 90% of women receiving adjuvant therapy.[32-35] Weight gain of up to 20 pounds is a particular problem among premenopausal women.[32] The underlying mechanisms of energy imbalance among women are unknown, but decreased physical activity, increased dietary intake, hormonal changes, and depression have been postulated.[32-25] Decreased fat intake[36] and a

regular exercise program result in decreased weight gain. Women who exercised routinely reported a significantly higher quality of life.[37] Chlebowski and colleagues[34] evaluated the feasibility of integrating a program based on dietary fat reduction into adjuvant treatment protocol. Nearly 300 postmenopausal women receiving adjuvant therapy were randomly assigned into either a dietary intervention group, receiving a program of individualized instruction for reducing total fat, or a dietary control group with minimal dietary counseling. Significantly reduced ($P < .001$) fat intake was observed in the intervention group at 3 months and was maintained throughout 24 months of follow-up. A 50% reduction in daily fat-gram intake and a lower body weight were noted. Findings showed that substantial and sustained dietary fat reduction within the multimodal treatment management of women undergoing treatment can be achieved at relatively low cost.

EXERCISE MANAGEMENT

Aerobic exercise has shown both physical and psychologic benefit among women receiving radiation therapy or chemotherapy for breast cancer.[38-42] MacVicar and colleagues[39] evaluated the effect of 10-week aerobic interval training on functional capacity among 45 women receiving chemotherapy for stage II breast cancer. Patients were stratified by baseline functional capacity and were randomly assigned into one of three groups. Experimental subjects completed a 10-week, thrice-weekly exercise training program. Patients receiving placebo participated in 10 weeks of nonaerobic stretching and flexibility exercises. The control group maintained normal exercise activities. Results showed that exercise was effective in improving the functional capacity in the experimental group.

Gaskin and associates[40] described an 8-week muscle-strengthening and flexibility and exercise rehabilitation program, Strength Through Recreation Exercise Togetherness Care Help (STRETCH). Results indicated improved range of motion, posture, and psychosocial support benefits for the participants.

Mock and colleagues[41] evaluated the effects of a regular walking program for 14 women receiving adjuvant chemotherapy. Nine women assigned to the experimental arm participated in a rehabilitation walking program and support group, and 5 women in the control group received usual care without structured exercise or support group. Exercise consisted of a self-paced walking program four or five times a week for 20 to 45 minutes. Results indicated that physical performance increased in the experimental walking group and that physical activity decreased in the usual care group. Findings also showed a significantly lower symptom intensity for the exercise group.

Mock and Dow[42] evaluated the effect of the walking exercise program for women receiving adjuvant therapy and for women receiving radiation therapy. Preliminary study results indicates improved physical performance, decreased symptom intensity, and improved quality of life and adaptation to breast cancer. Results of the few studies on exercise and breast cancer indicate improved perceptions of decreased symptom intensity and improved physical capacity, suggesting an important potential cost-effective contribution to the rehabilitation of women with breast cancer.

MUCOSITIS

The incidence of chemotherapy-induced mucositis is less than 20%.[43,44] It occurs most frequently in patients receiving antimetabolites, antitumor antibiotics, and plant alkaloids. The risk for stomatitis is not the same for all patients nor does it occur equally with similar drug regimens. Lack of a universal grading system has led to wide variations in oral care regimens.[43] Generally, consistency in using an oral care regimen offers the best protection against mucositis. Pretreatment strategies to prevent and decrease the incidence of oral complication include a baseline oral assessment, treatment of preexisting dental disease and patient education.[44] Table 25.4-3 outlines oral care protocols for mucositis.

Patients who develop mucositis with the first cycle of chemotherapy are likely to experience oral problems with continued treatment. McCarthy and Skillings[45] investigated the orofacial complications of 34 women receiving combination chemotherapy. The incidence of mucositis was 21% and was greatest in women with oral lesions at baseline, women older than 50 years of age, and women with poor oral hygiene, decreased performance status, anemia, or dentures. Other factors reported to increase risk are tobacco, alcohol, and compromised organ function, which allows the drug to remain in circulation for longer periods. Patients with compromised renal function receiving sequential methotrexate and 5-fluorouracil with leucovorin rescue may have delayed elimination of methotrexate, thus increasing risk for mucositis.

Effective oral care protocols include a cleansing method, lubricants, measures to relieve pain and inflammation, and measures to prevent or treat infection.[46] Normal saline or sodium bicarbonate solution are commonly suggested to enhance removal of debris. The effectiveness of hydrogen peroxide rinses is inconsistent; they break down granulating tissue and have a displeasing taste. Chlorhexidine mouthwash has been used prophylactically with significant reductions in mucositis in patients undergoing bone marrow transplantation and who are at high risk for oral infections.[47] The value of prophylactic antifungal agents is controversial. These agents may not prevent mucositis, but they can assist in maintaining integrity of mucosa.

INFECTION

Immunosuppression increases a patient's vulnerability to oral bacterial, fungal, and viral infections, particularly among those receiving dose-intensive therapy. Identifying an infectious process early through culture allows for appropriate antimicrobial therapy. Presenting with a classic raised cottage cheese—like plaque, *Candida albicans* is the most common fungal infection. Treatment is topical, with

TABLE 25.4-3
Interventions for Stomatitis

POTENTIAL STOMATITIS

Assess oral cavity daily.

Use routine oral hygiene:
  Use oral care in the morning and at bedtime
  Use soft toothbrush and nonastringent fluoride toothpaste; floss with unwaxed dental floss.
  Avoid alcohol-containing mouthwashes.
  Apply lip lubricant.

Use oxidizing agent as needed for mucolytic areas:
  Rinse mouth with sodium bicarbonate solution (1 tsp in 8 oz of water).
  Rinse mouth with warm water and saline.

Use prophylactic chlorhexidine mouth rinse (for high-risk patients)

MILD OR MODERATE STOMATITIS

Assess oral cavity twice daily.

Continue oral care as above:
  Increase frequency.
  Alternate oxidizing agent with warm saline if crusts are present.
  Omit flossing if gums bleed or are painful.
  Remove and clean dentures; replace only for meals.

Assess for evidence of infections: Any suspicious lesions should undergo culture assay.

Apply topical anesthetics before meals and as needed:
  Lidocaine HCL viscous 2% or 5%:
    Apply directly to lesion.
    Dilute in 1 tbsp saline; swish and spit.
  Benzocaine (Cetacaine or Hurricane) spray: Use one or two sprays as needed.
  Stomatitis cocktail (equal parts lidocaine viscous, diphenhydramine elixir, and Maalox, well shaken):
    Swish and spit 15–30 mL every 4 hours as needed.
    Swish and swallow if throat is sore.
  Zilactin (tannic acid 7%, hydroxypropyl cellulose) (available without a prescription): Apply directly to lesion.
  Benzocaine (Oratect) gel: Apply topically directly to lesion.
  Dyclonine (Dyclone) 0.5%–1% solution: Swish and spit 15 mL. (Also available as extrastrength Sucrets lozenges or spray.)

Use oral analgesics for systemic pain control.

Adapt diet to ensure adequate nutrition and hydration:
  Eat soft, bland, nonirritating foods.
  Take high-protein nutritional supplements.
  Maintain adequate fluid intake.

Patients at home with moderate to severe mucositis require frequent communication by phone and office visits as needed.

SEVERE STOMATITIS

Assess oral cavity every 8 hours.

Assess for evidence of infection: Any suspicious lesions should undergo culture assay.

Clean the mouth every 2 hours:
  Alternate warm saline mouthwash with antifungal or antibacterial oral suspension.
  Rinse with oxidizing agent for mucolytic areas.

Avoid trauma to the gums, use toothettes if bleeding occurs.

Maintain integrity of the lips with a lubricant.

Avoid wearing dental prostheses.

Continue with local and systemic measures to ensure comfort, nutrition, and hydration.

nystatin rinses, clotrimazole troches, ketoconizole, or fluconazole. Herpes simplex is the most common viral infection and initially causes a tingling and itching sensation followed by eruption of a small vesicle. Immunosuppressed patients are at risk for reactivation of infections. Acyclovir can be used to prevent reactivation in patients who are at high risk and who are seropositive.[48] Bacterial infections such as *Pseudomonas* and *Streptococcus* require broad-spectrum antibiotics in addition to vigorous oral hygiene. Cryotherapy has been shown to decrease the incidence and severity of stomatitis. This intervention has improved outcomes for patients receiving leucovorin and 5-fluorouracil and has been reported to be effective for patients experiencing doxorubicin-induced mucositis.[49–51]

HEMORRHAGIC CYSTITIS

Hemorrhagic cystitis can range from microscopic hematuria to frank bleeding and develops in 2% to 40% of patients receiving cyclophosphamide.[52] This figure can be expected to rise with increased use of dose intensification. Emphasis is placed on prevention through hydration and patient education. Patients at low risk who are receiving oral therapy are instructed to take the medication early in the day and to drink at least 80 oz of fluid daily. High-risk patients require urine dipstick testing, hyperhydration, frequent voiding, and diuresis. Patients are instructed to report dysuria, irritation, or suprapubic pain. Complaints are evaluated by urine culture. Therapy is reinstated cautiously, because the patient is at risk of recurrent problems. For patients receiving potentially curable therapy, effective control is required to avoid discontinuation of cancer treatment.

NEUROTOXICITY

Patients receiving vincristine, vinblastine, cisplatin, 5-fluorouracil, and taxol are at risk for neurotoxic complications. With vinca alkaloids, peripheral, cranial nerve, and autonomic neuropathies can be dose limiting.[53] Peripheral neuropathies present with loss of sensation beginning at the fingertips and spreading to the wrists and from the toes to the ankles; an objective early sign is loss of the Achilles tendon reflex. With additional therapy, progressive muscle pain, weakness, motor changes, and hypersensitivity to heat and intolerance to cold can occur.[54]

Acute cerebellar dysfunction can occur in high-risk individuals such as the elderly and in association with 5-fluorouracil, particularly with bolus administration. Effects are dose limiting and are reversible after withdrawal of medication. Vinca alkaloids can affect specific cranial nerves, causing ptosis, diplopia, facial nerve palsies, and jaw pain. Peripheral neuropathies have been reported in up to 96% of patients treated with taxol beginning 2 to 4 days after the infusion and lasting 24 to 72 hours. Patients report myalgias and arthralgias, primarily in the lower extremities.[55] The autonomic neuropathies of vinca alkaloids range from mild constipation to paralytic ileus. For high-risk individuals such as the elderly and analgesic users,

preventive measures include use of stool softeners, diet modification, and increased fluids. Patients are instructed to report changes in bowel habits early so appropriate measures can be instituted. Alterations in dosing are considered appropriate when patients are unable to perform fine, coordinated movements such as buttoning clothes or writing, or if they experience muscle pain. Therapy may be reinstituted at 50% of the normal dose when symptoms abate.[53] Symptoms may not completely disappear, however.

SUMMARY

The management of physical symptoms related to primary and adjuvant therapy requires that the oncology team maintain consistency in teaching, support, collaboration, coordination of care, and communication with patients and family members.[56–58] Information and professional support are critical factors in a woman's adjustment to breast cancer. Table 25.4-4 lists useful organizations that provide information on breast cancer side effects, management, and support.

Quality-of-Life Changes After Cancer Treatment

The end of treatment is associated with a decrease in physical side effects and a return to a certain sense of normalcy and routine. Many women, however, experience numerous psychologic and social adjustments that can be expected after treatment ends. These include concerns about managing relationships with children, spouse, and other family members and addressing fears of cancer recurrence. Older women may express concerns about loss of physical function and about becoming a burden. Age differences have also been noted between older and younger women receiving breast cancer treatment. Younger women experienced significantly more deterioration in their mental health and well-being than did older women.[59] Young women may express concerns about fertility and sexuality.[60–65] Women need to have reassurance that their concerns are usual and that assistance is available.

SEXUALITY AND FERTILITY CONCERNS

Attention to sexuality issues affecting women of age is an important part of the recovery process.[65] The impact of treatment on sexuality is subtle and may relate more to a woman's feelings of desirability, lovemaking practices, and enjoyment of sex.[65] Young women are also increasingly concerned about the effects of treatment on fertility. Because many young women have postponed having children until later in life, increasing numbers desire pregnancy after treatment for breast cancer.[66,67] Issues such as effects of treatment on fertility, potential risks associated with treatment, appropriate waiting period before pregnancy,

TABLE 25.4-4
Useful Publications and References

AMERICAN CANCER SOCIETY

1599 Clifton Road, NE
Atlanta, GA 30329

This organization makes available a variety of breast cancer education and support materials at no charge.

DIMENSIONS OF CARING

c/o Healthmark
40 West 23rd Street
New York, NY 10010-5201
1-800-ENABLE

This is a support program for patients with fatigue. It provides information on fatigue, its causes, and ways to cope. Print and videotape materials are available.

LOOK GOOD . . . FEEL BETTER

800-395-LOOK

This public service program, sponsored by the Cosmetic, Toiletry and Fragrance Association Foundation and the American Cancer Society, helps women to change and improve their appearance after cancer treatment. Print and videotape materials are available to patients and professionals.

NATIONAL ALLIANCE OF BREAST CANCER ORGANIZATIONS (NABCO)

1180 Avenue of the Americas
2nd Floor
New York, NY 10036
212-719-0154

This is a not-for-profit resource for information about breast cancer, which acts as an advocate for breast cancer patients. NABCO has an extensive and excellent reference, *Breast Cancer Resource List*, which provides information and referrals, on all aspects of breast cancer.

NATIONAL CANCER INSTITUTE (NCI)

Cancer Information Service
800-4-CANCER

The NCI provides general information on cancer and makes available booklets and pamphlets about breast cancer at no charge.

NATIONAL COALITION FOR CANCER SURVIVORSHIP (NCCS)

1010 Wayne Avenue
Silver Spring, MD 20910
301-650-8868

This is a national network composed of individuals with cancer, their families, health care professionals, and organizations dedicated to supporting people with a history of cancer. NCCS is also a clearinghouse for information and advocacy activities, and has an excellent publication, *Network Directory of National Cancer Support Services*.

NATIONAL LYMPHEDEMA NETWORK

2211 Post Street
Suite 404
San Francisco, CA 94111
800-541-3259

This is a not-for-profit organization that provides counseling, support, and information about the prevention and treatment of lymphedema.

KOMEN ALLIANCE

Susan G. Komen Foundation
Occidental Towers
5005 LBJ Freeway, Suite 37-0
Dallas, TX 75244
214-450-1777

This is a comprehensive program that focuses on sponsoring research, education, and support for patients with breast cancer.

Y-ME

18220 Harwood Avenue
Homewood, IL 60430
708-799-8228
800-221-2141

Y-Me provides support and counseling through a national toll free hotline.

YWCA ENCORE PROGRAM

Program National Headquarters
726 Broadway
New York, NY 10003
212-614-2700

This organization provides support and rehabilitative exercise for women with breast cancer at various YWCA locations across the United States.

---

management during pregnancy, and spousal and family concerns are important to consider.

EFFECTS OF BREAST CANCER ON CHILDREN

Breast cancer is a disease that affects the entire family.[68–72] Issel and colleagues[70] interviewed 81 children aged 6 to 20 years whose mothers had breast cancer and asked how they coped and what type of supports they used. Research-

ers found that children used four distinct coping strategies (1) some anticipated their mother's needs by acting as though they were in her shoes; (2) some tried to maintain a sense of normalcy; (3) some spent more time doing things with the family; and (4) some talked openly about their feelings with other family members. The major supports provided for the children were parents, family members, peer support, and adult family friends. Few professional supports were used.

Mothers with breast cancer report a variety of concerns about their children, ranging from daily disruptions (becoming sick during chemotherapy) to existential questions about dying and leaving the children.[69-71] Day-to-day concerns include ways to talk to their children about having breast cancer without unnecessarily frightening them. Hoke[71] reported that strengths and vulnerabilities, cognitive capacities, developmental level age, and gender are the major influences on children's response to maternal breast cancer. Hoke suggests several intervention strategies in working with children (1) maintain clear and open communication with children about cancer; (2) share information and feelings about the disease; and (3) correct children's beliefs about cancer and allay unnecessary fears. Despite the growing body of information, teaching aids, and books available to parents, many are still reluctant to talk about cancer because they believe that their children's distress will increase. Children are acutely aware of a parent's cancer, however, even when it is not openly discussed.[71] Innovative support groups have been specifically designed for children.[73-75] In a few instances, early identification of major adjustment requires professional consultation.

EFFECTS OF BREAST CANCER ON THE SPOUSE AND SIGNIFICANT OTHER

Breast cancer has a significant effect on the spouse and significant other.[76-79] Northouse[76-78] conducted several studies on spousal adjustment to breast cancer. Her research indicates that (1) both patients and husbands reported levels of distress higher than those in the normal population; (2) women reported more role adjustment problems than their spouse; and (3) individuals with higher levels of social support had fewer adjustment difficulties.

Spouses rarely have the opportunity to take advantage of available social supports.[80,81] An innovative intervention using partners as support for women, however, has helped to facilitate the adjustment of women and their partners to breast cancer.[80]

ADJUSTMENT TO WORK

Work issues can be major hurdles in adjustment after breast cancer.[82,83] Women are often diagnosed during their peak earning and professional lives and may need to continue working. They are plagued by worries about insurance and health benefits. Some cancer survivors stay in a position of "job lock," in which they are reluctant to leave a job because they fear that health benefits will be taken away. In the day-to-day workplace, it can be difficult for women to disclose a breast cancer diagnosis for fear that they will be stigmatized. Although the public's attitudes about breast cancer are changing and because of breast cancer's major prevalence in the lay press and literature, women with breast cancer need to be instructed on the disclosure of their cancer history, the desire to maintain productivity, and the assessment of their physical capabilities.

Effects of Breast Cancer in Minority Groups

Culture and ethnicity play a major part in decisions for treatment and adjustment after therapy.[84-87] Kagawa-Singer[84] found that the significance of the breast in sexuality and body image has traditionally had less sexual meaning among Asian cultures than in the Western culture. This deemphasis on the breast as a sexual organ may be a factor in Asian women's underuse of breast-conserving surgery. Other aspects, such as interpersonal interaction, social support, and quality of life, differ among Asian American women and thus have different meanings for support after treatment.

American Indian women are a second cultural group for which few breast cancer services are available.[85-87] Access to services is difficult because women must travel long distances to receive care. In addition, poverty and lower education among American Indian groups further hamper access to care. Brant[87] found that American Indian women do not prefer invasive procedures such as mastectomy, commonly misunderstand that chemotherapy is different from radiation therapy, do not comprehend how a cancer treatment that has so many side effects can be beneficial, and often prefer to rely on traditional medicine for healing. Researchers involved with American Indian women stress that interventions are more effective when members of their own tribes provide the health teaching about screening and treatment.

Managing Recurrent Disease

Quality-of-life issues in the management of recurrent and disseminated disease are also important.[88-90] Mahon[88] found that an assessment of the patient's perception of recurrence is important, as are its impact on the family, social activities, and roles. Dow[89] found that young women believed that recurrence was the same as death. Women need to have information about the next course of treatment for recurrence and a realistic evaluation of recovery and longevity. Managing recurrence after breast-conserving surgery and radiation therapy should include teaching about mastectomy and emotional support. Women often believe that they have somehow "failed" and need a great deal of emotional support through the mastectomy and follow-up adjuvant therapy.

Summary

Nursing care activities in patient care management are focused on improving physical, psychologic, social, and spiritual well-being. Activities include acute side effect management, exercise intervention, and psychosocial support and education. In addition, needs of ethnic minorities must be considered when planning comprehensive care.

References

1. Cawley M, Kostic J, Cappello C. Informational and psychosocial needs of women choosing conservative surgery/primary radiation for early stage breast cancer. Cancer Nurs 1990;13:90.
2. Ward S, Heidrich S, Wolberg W. Factors women take into account when deciding upon type of surgery for breast cancer. Cancer Nurs 1989;12:344.
3. Pierce PF. Deciding on breast cancer treatment: a description of decision behavior. Nurs Res 1993;42:22.
4. Hughes KK. Decision making by patients with breast cancer: the role of information in treatment selection. Oncol Nurs Forum 1993;20:623.
5. Neufeld KR, Degner LF, Dick JA. A nursing intervention strategy to foster patient involvement in treatment decisions. Oncol Nurs Forum 1993;20:631.
6. Hassey K. Radiation therapy for breast cancer: a historic review. Semin Oncol Nurs 1985;1:181.
7. Hagopian G, Rubenstein J. Effects of telephone call interventions on patients' well-being in a radiation therapy department. Cancer Nurs 1990;13:339.
8. Wilson CA, Strohl RA. Radiation therapy as primary treatment for breast cancer. Oncol Nurs Forum 1982;9:12.
9. Witt ME, McDonald-Lynch A, Lydon J. Enhancing skin comfort during radiation therapy. Oncol Nurs Forum, 1990;17:276.
10. Blesch KS, Paice JA, Wickham R, et al. Correlates of fatigue in people with breast or lung cancer. Oncol Nurs Forum 1991;18:81.
11. Nail L, King K. Fatigue. Semin Oncol Nurs 1987;3:257.
12. Winningham ML, Glass EC, MacVicar MG. Rhythmic walking: exercise for people living with cancer. Columbus, OH, James Cancer Hospital and Research Institute, Ohio State University, 1990.
13. Jacobsen PB, Bovbjerg GH, Redd WH. Anticipatory anxiety in women receiving chemotherapy for breast cancer. Health Psychol 1993;12:469.
14. Ehlke G. Symptom distress in breast cancer patients receiving chemotherapy in the outpatient setting. Oncol Nurs Forum 1988;15:857.
15. Knobf M. Physical and psychological distress associated with adjuvant chemotherapy in women with breast cancer. J Clin Oncol 1986;4:678.
16. Doig B. Adjuvant chemotherapy in breast cancer: a review of the literature. Cancer Nurs 1988;11:91.
17. Greene D, Nail L, Fieler V, et al. A comparison of patient reported side effects during three chemotherapy regimens for breast cancer. Cancer Pract 1994;2:57.
18. Goodman M. Adjuvant systemic therapy of stage I and II breast cancer. Semin Oncol Nurs 1991;7:175.
19. Hortobagyi GN, Body GP, Buzdac AU, et al. Evaluation of high dose versus standard FAC chemotherapy for advanced breast cancer in protected environment units: a prospective study. J Clin Oncol 1987;5:354.
20. Smalley RV, Carpenter J, Bartolucci A, et al. A comparison of cyclophosphamide, adriamycin, 5-fluorouracil (CAF) and cyclophosphamide, methotrexate, 5-fluorouracil, vincristine, prednisone (CMFVP) in patients with metastatic breast cancer. Cancer 1977;40:625.
21. Gelman RS, Taylor SG IV. Cyclophosphamide, methotrexate and 5-fluorouracil chemotherapy in woman more than 65 years old with advanced breast cancer: the elimination of age trends in toxicity by doses based on creatinine clearance: J Clin Oncol 1984;2:2:1404.
22. Fischer B, Redmond C, Dimitrov NV et al. A randomized clinical trial evaluating sequential methotrexate and fluorouracil in the treatment of patients with node-negative breast cancer who have estrogen receptor–negative tumors. N Engl J Med 1989;320:473.
23. Pisters KMW, Kris MG. Management of nausea and vomiting caused by anticancer drugs: state of the art. Oncology 1992;6:99.
24. Bonneterre J, Chevallier B, Metz R, et al. A randomized double blind comparison of ondansetron and metochlopromide in the prophylaxis of emesis induced by cyclophosphamide, fluorouracil and doxorubicin. J Clin Oncol 1990;8:6:1063.
25. Levitt M, Warr D, Yelle L, et al. Ondansetron compared with dexamethasone and metochlopramide as antiemetics in the chemotherapy of breast cancer with cyclophosphamide, methotrexate, and fluorouracil. N Engl J Med 1993;328:1081.
26. Jones AL, Hill AS, Soukop M, et al. Comparison of dexamethasone and ondansetron in the prophylaxis of emesis induced by moderately emetogenic chemotherapy. Lancet 1991;338:483.
27. Cubeddu LX, Hoffman IS, Fuenmayor NT, et al. Antagonism of serotonin S3 receptors with ondansetron prevents nausea and emesis induced by cyclophosphamide-containing chemotherapy regimens. J Clin Oncol 1990;8:1721.
28. Fraschini G, Ciociola A, Esparza L, et al. Evaluation of three oral dosages of ondansetron in the prevention of nausea and emesis associated with cyclophosphamide–doxorubicin chemotherapy. J Clin Oncol 1991;9:1268.
29. Razavi D, Delvaux N, Farvacques C, et al. Prevention of adjustment disorders and anticipatory nausea secondary to adjuvant chemotherapy: a double-blind, placebo-controlled study assessing the usefulness of aprazolam. J Clin Oncol 1993;11:1384.
30. Friedlander M, Kearsley JH, Tattersall MHN. Oral lorazepam to improve tolerance of cytotoxic therapy. Lancet 1981;1:1316.
31. Cline BW. Prevention of chemotherapy induced alopecia: a review of the literature. Cancer Nurs 1984;6:221.
32. Demark-Wahnefried W, Winer EP, Rimer BK. Why women gain weight with adjuvant chemotherapy for breast cancer. J Clin Oncol, 1993;11:1418.
33. Camoriono JK, Loprinzi CL, Ingle JN, et al. Weight change in women treated with adjuvant therapy or observed following mastectomy for node-positive breast cancer. J Clin Oncol 1990;8:1327.
34. Chlebowski RT, Blackburn GL, Buzzard IM, et al. Adherence to a dietary fat intake reduction program in postmenopausal women receiving therapy for early breast cancer: the Women's Intervention Nutrition Study. J Clin Oncol 1993;11:2072.
35. Foltz AT. Weight gain among stage II breast cancer patients: a study of five factors. Oncol Nurs Forum 1985;12:21.
36. Rose DP, Connolly JM, Chlebowski RT, et al. The effects of a low fat dietary intervention and tamoxifen adjuvant therapy on the serum estrogen and sex hormone binding globulin concentrations of post menopausal breast cancer patients. Breast Cancer Res Treat 1993;27:253.
37. Winningham ML, MacVicar MG, Bondoc M, et al. Effect of aerobic exercise on body weight and composition in patients with breast cancer. Oncol Nurs Forum 1989;16:683.
38. Young-McCaughan S, Sexton DL. A retrospective investigation of the relationship between aerobic exercise and quality of life in women with breast cancer. Oncol Nurs Forum, 1991;18:751.
39. MacVicar MG, Winningham ML, Nickel JL. Effects of aerobic interval training on cancer patients' functional capacity. Nurs Res 1989;38:348.
40. Gaskin TA, LoBuglio A, Kelly P, et al. STRETCH: a rehabilitation program for patients with breast cancer. South Med J 1989;82:467.
41. Mock V, Burke MB, Sheehan P, et al. A nursing rehabilitation program for women with breast cancer receiving adjuvant chemotherapy. Oncol Nurs Forum 1994;21:899.
42. Mock V, Dow KH. An exercise rehabilitation program for women

in treatment for breast cancer. Presented at the First Massachusetts Breast Cancer Research Symposium, Boston, May, 1994.

43. Miaskowski C. Management of mucositis during therapy. Natl Cancer Inst 1990;9:95.

44. NIH Consensus Development Conference Statement. Oral Complications of cancer chemotherapies. Natl Cancer Inst Monogr 1990;9:3.

45. McCarthy GM, Skillings JR. Orofacial complications of chemotherapy for breast cancer. Oral Surg Oral Med Oral Pathol 1992;74:172.

46. Daeffler R. Oral hygiene measures for patients with cancer, Part I. Cancer Nurs 1990;3:347.

47. Ferretti GA, Raybould TP, Brown AT, et al. Chorhexidine prophylaxis for chemotherapy and radiotherapy induced stomatitis: a randomized double blind trial. Oral Surg Oral Med Oral Pathol 1990;69:331.

48. Saral R. Management of acute viral infection. Natl Cancer Inst Monogr 1990;9:107.

49. Mahood DJ, Dose AM, Loprinzi CL, et al. Inhibition of fluorouracil-induced stomatitis by oral cryotherapy. J Clin Oncol 1991;9:449.

50. Twelves CJ, Seymour AM. Mouth cooling to prevent doxorubicin-induced stomatitis. Ann Oncol 1991;2:695.

51. Gabrilove JL, Jakubowski A, Sher H, et al. Effect of granulocyte colony stimulating factor on neutropenia and associated morbidity due to chemotherapy for transitional cell carcinoma of the urothelium. N Engl J Med 1988;318:1414.

52. Levine LA, Richie JP. Urological complications of cyclophosphamide. J Urol 1989;141:1063.

53. Goodman M. Managing the side effects of chemotherapy. Semin Oncol Nurs 1989;5:2:29.

54. Weiss HD, Walker MD, Wiernick PH. Neurotoxicity of commonly used antineoplastic agents. N Engl J Med 1974;291:75.

55. Martoni A, Zamagn C, Gheka A, et al. Antihistamines in the treatment of taxol induced paroxystic pain. Natl Cancer Inst 1993;85:676.

56. Oakes J, Teasdale K. Emotional support can precipitate recovery: Setting up a counselling service for breast cancer patients. Prof Nurse, 1992;7:778.

57. Carey RL, Jevne R. Development of an information package for post-mastectomy patients on adjuvant therapy. Oncol Nurs Forum 1986;13:78.

58. Suominen T. Breast cancer patients' opportunities to participate in their care. Cancer Nurs 1992;15:68.

59. Vinokur A, Threatt B, Vinokur-Kaplan D, et al. The process of recovery from breast cancer for younger and older patients. Cancer 1990;65:1242.

60. Carter B. Long-term survivors of breast cancer: a qualitative descriptive study. Cancer Nurs 1993;16:354.

61. Dow KH. The enduring seasons in survival. Oncol Nurs Forum, 1990;17:511.

62. Woods NF, Earp JA. Women with cured breast cancer a study of mastectomy patients in North Carolina. Nurs Res 1978;27:279.

63. Feather BL, Wainstock JM. Perceptions of postmastectomy patients. Part II. Social support and attitudes towards mastectomy. Cancer Nurs 1989;12:301.

64. Feather BL, Wainstock JM. Perceptions of postmastectomy patients. Part I. The relationships between social support and network providers. Cancer Nurs 1989;12:293.

65. Schover LR. The impact of breast cancer on sexuality, body image, and intimate relationships. CA Cancer J Clin 1991;41:112.

66. Hassey K. Pregnancy and parenthood after treatment for breast cancer. Oncol Nurs Forum 1988;15:439.

67. Dow KH, Harris JR, Roy C. Pregnancy after breast conserving surgery and radiation therapy. Natl Cancer Inst Monogr 1994;16:131.

68. Hilton BA. Issues, problems, and challenges for families coping with breast cancer. Semin Oncol Nurs 1993;9:88.

69. Hymovich DP. Child-rearing concerns of parents with cancer. Oncol Nurs Forum 1993;20:1355.

70. Issel LM, Ersek M, Lewis FM. How children cope with mother's breast cancer. Oncol Nurs Forum 1990;17:5.

71. Hoke L. When a mother has breast cancer: parenting concerns and psychosocial adjustment in young children and adolescents. In: Dow KH, ed. Contemporary issues in breast cancer. Boston, Jones & Bartlett (in press).

72. Lewis F. Strengthening family supports. Cancer 1990;65:752.

73. Call D. School-based groups: a valuable support for children of cancer patients. J Psychosoc Oncol 1990;8:97.

74. Taylor-Brown J, Acheson A, Farber J. Kids can cope: a group intervention for children whose parents have cancer. J Psychosoc Oncol 1993;11:41.

75. Greening K. The "bear essentials" program: helping young children and their families cope when a parent has cancer. J Psychosoc Oncol 1992;10:47.

76. Northouse L, Swain A. Adjustment of patients and husbands to the initial impact of breast cancer. Nurs Res 1987;36:221.

77. Northouse L. Social support in patients' and husbands' adjustment to breast cancer. Nurs Res 1988;37:91.

78. Northouse L. The impact of breast cancer on patients and husbands. Cancer Nurs 1989;12:276.

79. Zahlis EH, Shands ME. The impact of breast cancer on the partner 18 months after diagnosis. Semin Oncol Nurs 1993;9:83.

80. Samarel N, Fawcett J, Tulman L. The effects of coaching in breast cancer support groups: a pilot study. Oncol Nurs Forum 1993;20:795.

81. Cella D, Yellen S. Cancer support groups: the state of the art. Cancer Pract 1993;1:56.

82. Berry DL. Return-to-work experience of people with cancer. Oncol Nurs Forum 1993;20:905.

83. Carter B. Surviving breast cancer: a problematic work re-entry. Cancer Pract 1994;2:135.

84. Kagawa-Singer M. Issues affecting Asian American and Pacific American women with breast cancer. In: Dow KH, ed. Contemporary issues in breast cancer. Boston, Jones & Bartlett (in press).

85. Burhansstipanov L, Barry K. Cancer education resources for American Indians and Alaska Natives. Bethesda, National Cancer Institute, NIH publ no. 94-3706, 1993.

86. Burhansstipanov L, Dress C. Native american monograph no. 1: documentation of the research needs of American Indians and Alaska Natives, Bethesda, National Cancer Institute, NIH publ no. 93-3603, 1993.

87. Brant J. Breast cancer challenges in American Indian women. In: Dow KH, ed Contemporary issues in breast cancer. Boston, Jones & Bartlett, (in press).

88. Mahon SM. Managing the psychosocial consequences of cancer recurrence: implications for nurses. Oncol Nurs Forum 1991;18:577.

89. Dow K. On the nature and meaning of locally recurrent breast cancer. In: Quality of life: a nursing challenge. Philadelphia, Meniscus. 1992;1:27.

90. McEvoy MD, McCorkle R. Quality of life issues in patients with disseminated breast cancer. Cancer 1990;66:1416.

26

Diseases of the Breast, edited by Jay R. Harris,
Marc E. Lippman, Monica Morrow, and Samuel Hellman.
Lippincott-Raven Publishers, Philadelphia, © 1996.

Organizing a Comprehensive Breast Center

CATHY COLEMAN · GAIL S. LEBOVIC

Breast health care has become an international priority. The complexity of the diagnosis and treatment of breast diseases, and in particular breast cancer, makes breast health care a rapidly growing subspecialty area of medicine. A multidisciplinary model has become the standard of care and works best when all services and health care professionals work together to minimize duplication and maximize patient satisfaction.

As early as 1931, Dr. Cushman D. Haagensen recognized the need for a workable model to provide comprehensive patient care. He developed a clinical subspecialty in breast disease and stressed the absolute necessity for coordinated breast health care. Haagensen emphasized six essential elements required to achieve optimal breast care[1]:

- A spirit of cooperation between physician subspecialists based on guidance by the pathologist
- Compassionate patient care
- Devoted employees and medical staff
- Modern medical facilities specializing in cancer care
- Meticulous data collection and patient follow-up
- Support and encouragement for clinical and laboratory research

These basic principles are still applicable today and remain the foundation on which to build a multidisciplinary breast program or center.

The development of a model for delivery of comprehensive breast health care has been influenced by political, clinical, and economic factors. Many such models have been presented previously and have proved successful.[2–12] Decreasing health care dollars and increasing health care costs have created the need for a more cohesive approach, however. This need has spawned the evolution of a *conceptual framework* for the development of comprehensive breast centers (Fig. 26-1). Key components of patient care are shown not only as they integrate and complement each other, but also as they remain focused on the central core—the patient and family. Each of these important elements must be united programmatically and operationally, within and between appropriate clinical settings.

This conceptual framework is intended to assist in the creation of an organizational structure, clinical program, business plan, and facility that provides synergy and excellence for all breast care services.

The first step in implementing the conceptual framework requires an outline of clearly defined goals. These goals include the following:

- To contribute to a reduction in morbidity and mortality from breast disease
- To develop a continuum of patient-centered and research-based clinical services
- To define measurable determinants of quality assurance for each program or service
- To support participation in local, regional, or national research trials
- To translate new research findings into clinical practice in a timely manner
- To provide innovative educational programs for patients, providers, and the public
- To promote integrated and efficient systems of patient care delivery
- To achieve and maintain a high degree of patient, employee, and clinical staff satisfaction
- To manage clinical and fiscal operations in a prudent fashion

Achieving these goals necessitates a much different infrastructure from that commonly used in more limited programs that may focus on only one particular area of patient care. When planning a comprehensive breast program, existing individual and institutional preferences influence the initial and sequential expansion of services. These preferences must then be carefully integrated into existing programs within the institution and local medical community. This instills a sense of unity among programs, departments, and staff. Regardless of size, scope, or setting, any breast program should be considered successful if it contributes to the specific goals of the sponsoring organization and the health needs of the community.

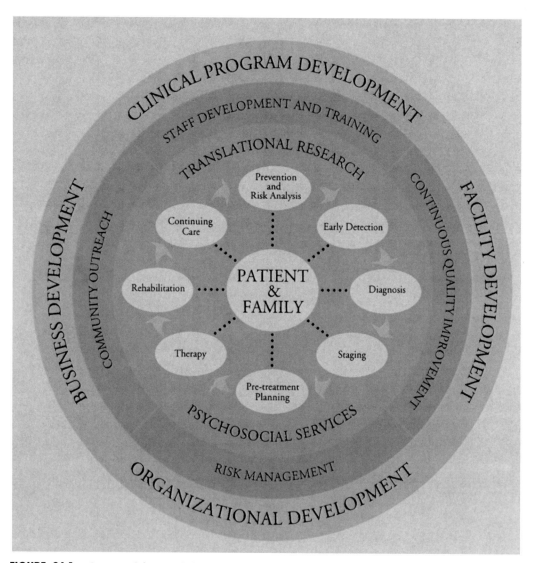

FIGURE 26-1. Conceptual framework for a comprehensive breast program.

Organizational Development

To succeed, a comprehensive program must be carefully planned from its inception. The organizational structure of a breast center requires a combination of effective leadership, a responsive human resources department, and a focused management team. From the outset, programs organized with leadership in oncology create a sense of continuity of patient care and commitment to ongoing research. Furthermore, this facilitates future accreditation by the American College of Surgeons or designation by the National Cancer Institute.[13–19]

A well written mission statement provides continuing focus. An example follows: "This breast center has been established to provide comprehensive, compassionate and cost-effective breast health and breast cancer care to women in our community. Our team of medical and allied health experts in breast health and breast cancer works together with health care consumers to provide women and their families a coordinated range of services in a supportive and comfortable environment" (Alta Bates Comprehensive Breast Center, Berkeley, 1993). Participation in the drafting of a mission statement by the medical staff and employees of the center creates a sense of partnership and teamwork.

The human resources department is responsible for recruitment and retention of highly skilled and dedicated staff. Unfortunately, this department is often an underused resource. Trained staff within the human resources department can often help to facilitate change and to assist with conflict resolution as the breast center or program develops and expands its services.

The management team should strive to create an atmosphere that encourages diverse employee groups, physicians, and research scientists to work harmoniously together. An effective management team can help to transform conflict into constructive, collaborative exchange. These efforts can then be used to change or improve delivery of patient care services.

Achieving collaboration is not always easy. Durant[6] has suggested that the "inertia of the old system" in which a single physician controls patient management is a substantial obstacle in developing multidisciplinary breast clinics.[6] Breast center leaders should anticipate other potential barriers to collaboration that can interfere with healthy teamwork and organizational development. These include a history of antagonism, competition for patients, community politics, and poor communication. Management strategies to overcome such problems include effective listening skills, continuous clarification of goals and objectives, honest and direct communication, recruitment of team members with good human relations skills, and encouragement of equal participation and involvement of all group members.[20-23] The process of developing collaboration also requires time. Rabinowitz[24] believes that the art of engendering physician involvement results in "creative synergy" when program planners allow time for spirited discussions and debate and convey patience during the temporary impasses that are a natural part of group dynamics and the development process.

Collaboration can also be promoted by establishing clearly defined roles and responsibilities. This is an essential component of the initial phase of development. The organizational structure needs to include roles with authority and those that are advisory. The medical director serves as a salaried staff or a volunteer leader for the medical staff and is appointed or elected. This physician oversees all clinical activities, strategic planning, and program development at the breast center. The medical director is also directly responsible for all patient care–related issues and monitors quality assurance. This physician leader delegates responsibilities to the other team members as appropriate, for example, the coordination of tumor board meetings, community outreach programs, and continuing education programs for medical and ancillary staff members.

Physicians' duties are further divided within different specialties of the medical staff. Each section has a division chief who manages the clinical and research activities within the department and reports to the medical director. The division chief is responsible for administrative duties, patient satisfaction, and quality of care. The division chiefs also serve on a professional advisory or planning committee, which is accountable for the critical decisions made during all phases of development. This oversight committee, cochaired by the medical director and administrative director, may function as a subgroup of the cancer committee or as an independent medical staff task force reporting directly to the executive board of the institution.

The administrative director works with the medical director to formulate a strategic plan and to direct the center's daily operations, quality of care, fiscal management, and staff recruitment. This individual must coordinate the nursing, technical, and clerical staffs within each department and must serve as the intermediary among patients, staff, physicians, and other department managers. In addition, the administrative director serves on the advisory committee along with other ancillary staff.

Patient and consumer involvement is also desirable and necessitates a role in the organizational structure of a comprehensive breast center. This can be accomplished by creating a community or patient advisory board, which has the following functions:

- To identify unmet needs in clinical or service delivery
- To promote awareness of the facility
- To raise funds for the organization
- To create a liaison for breast cancer support and advocacy groups
- To provide volunteer peer counseling and other services

These groups generate enthusiasm, energy, and support for many facets of the program and serve, once again, as a constant reminder of the center's focus on the patient, family, and community needs.[15-16,25-26] Both patients and health care providers are served best by a clearly defined organizational structure.

Clinical Program Development

Clinical program development is guided by combining and applying basic principles common to nursing and medicine—assessment, planning, implementation, and evaluation. In health care today, none of these essential

TABLE 26-1
Strategies for Conducting Effective Pretreatment Planning Conferences

Designate conference leaders who are active and directive rather than passive (an active leader provides guidance, voices opinions, participates actively and encourages interaction).

Conduct case presentation in a progressive disclosure format where information is provided in stages with discussion at the end of each stage, rather than an entire case presentation followed by discussion.

Provide educational and managerial leadership training opportunities for practicing physicians if they function as conference chairpersons.

Encourage prospective rather than retrospective case presentations.

Promote inclusion of a broad range of specialists and caregivers to address early diagnosis, quality of life, ethics, legal issues, or other relevant topics.

Use principles of adult learning (develop educational objectives, reference lists, handouts, provide session summaries).

Operate within the financial and time constraints of practicing physicians, conference chairpersons, hospital cancer committees, and tumor registrars.

Invite noncancer specialists such as primary care physicans, health educators, basic scientists, and epidemiologists.

Invite opinion leaders or representatives from local professional groups to assist in the application of new data or new treatments into clinical practice (eg, department chair of pathology if new prognostic test is desired by clinicians).

Describe stage-specific investigational treatment options.
Offer continuing education units.

(Data from references 27–30)

TABLE 26-2
Business Development: Key Objectives

PREPARATION OF FINANCIAL ANALYSIS & BUDGET[52-55]

Establish center's goals and objectives.

   Relative to organizational mission and strategic plan.

Define services:

   Clinical

   Community outreach (educational, free screening, etc.)

   Research

Forecast patient volume projections:

   By department

   Consider cross-training

Analyze and project patient payor mix:

   Self-pay

   Commercial

   Managed care

   Medicaid

   Medicare

   Other

Project operating expenses:

   Equipment needs

   Medical supplies

   Marketing costs

   Equipment maintenance

   Training expenses

   Educational materials

Prepare budget:

   Project expected income from clinical operations, grants and charitable contributions

   Categorize variable and fixed expenses

   Assess direct (cash flow) and indirect benefits (public relations, etc.) of program

Obtain administrative approval.

Conduct ongoing operational and budget analysis.

Monitor trends in profit or loss.

CREATION OF A RESULTS ORIENTED MARKETING PLAN[25,26,42,43,51,55-63]

Assess image in community relative to other providers.

Develop satisfaction surveys (patient, staff, physician, other).

Conduct SWOT analysis (strengths, weaknesses, opportunities, threats).

---

tasks should stand alone, nor should the responsibility of clinical program development depend on any one department to achieve success. Rather, the sum of the parts ultimately provides for success of the whole. A multidisciplinary, comprehensive breast center is meant to provide the services needed to educate, screen, and treat patients with regard to all aspects of breast health care. The continuum of care in breast health and disease includes eight program areas ranging from prevention to continuing care (see Fig. 26-1).

   The center should focus on providing a balanced approach to breast health care, with all departments contributing equally to clinical program development. Each component of patient care is developed both independently and in concert with other program services after an assess-

ment of relevant clinical research trials and psychosocial interventions is completed. This results in the provision of patient-centered and research-driven care, a concept intrinsic to this comprehensive model.

   Realistically, many centers are unable to offer all services. The pretreatment planning process is an essential part of any breast care program and must be included, however. Crucial decisions related to survival and quality of life are made during the initial phase of treatment planning after review and evaluation of the diagnostic and prognostic information available for each patient. The most effective means of achieving this for both patients and caregivers is through regularly scheduled pretreatment planning meetings. Research indicates that the educational process of these case-management conferences can be im-

TABLE 26-2
Business Development: Key Objectives (*Continued*)

CREATION OF A RESULTS ORIENTED MARKETING PLAN[25,26,42,51,55-63] (*Continued*)

S: How your center is different in scope or quality (eg, people, programs, facilities, research, accreditation)

W: Perceived weakness (eg, situated in competitive market, lack of leadership, poor staff morale, perceived as too low quality or high-priced for market, under or overstaffed department)

O: How to improve your position (eg, recruit medical director, provide education and training, create advertising campaign, consider a joint business venture)

T: Anticipate internal or external factors (eg, staff turnover, outdated technology or equipment, decreasing reimbursement)

Review existing referral sources and identify changing patterns, trends related to demographics, etc.

    Target internal customer groups:

        Hospital employees

        Medical staff leadership

        Breast center staff

        Hospital auxiliary and volunteer groups

        Students

        Foundation board

    Target external customer groups:

        Referring physicians and their office staff

        Business and industry organizations

        Community organizations

        Managed care providers

        Patients

        Families

        General public

COORDINATION OF MANAGED CARE CONTRACTS[51,54-56,64-68]

Assess number of existing contracts (quality and quantity).

Prioritize plans or companies that share similar values or philosophy.

Develop patient care guidelines based on objective quality indicators.

Build effective working relationships with medical directors of plans to assess educational, clinical, financial needs and limitations.

Create packages and products that are based on realistic operations and reasonable return on investment.

Implement data systems to track and forecast operational efficiency, patient care audits, continuous quality improvement, tumor registry data, and financial status.

proved.[27-30] Recommendations for conducting effective conferences are outlined in Table 26-1. Final treatment options can then be made to the referring physician, patient, and family after complete review and discussion.

As illustrated in Figure 26-1, the comprehensive model strives to provide clinical research options and psychosocial support within each area of clinical care. When physicians and basic scientists work side by side, exciting opportunities for integrating new research findings into clinical practice become more feasible.[31-39] This process of *translational research* is being encouraged and supported by the National Cancer Institute, as evidenced by three "disease-specific" specialized programs of research excellence (SPORE) grants (for research in breast, lung, and prostate cancer).[40] Biotechnology and pharmaceutical companies are also exploring new frontiers, and many centers choose to collaborate directly with them in bringing new investigational therapies, products, or services to their communities.

Psychosocial services, including clinical trials, should be encouraged for patients, families, and health care profes-sionals throughout the continuum of care. Compelling new findings and interventions related to quality of life, patient–physician communication styles, sexual concerns, pain-management techniques, alternative or complementary therapies, and rehabilitation functions need to be evaluated and offered within the centers.[34,41-50] Thus, planning efforts related to clinical program development must start with a complete review of the literature, with special emphasis on two often underfunded and underappreciated disciplines—clinical research and psychosocial oncology.

Business Development

Breast cancer can be a devastating disease emotionally, physically, and financially. It is an extraordinarily expensive disease to treat, and the economic consequences borne by US private industry are enormous. Estimated costs in 1990 included $937 million for treatment costs, $567 million in disability costs, and $2.71 billion in lost earnings due to premature death.[51] A significant difference is seen in cost of treatment for early versus advanced stages of breast cancer. Early stages can be treated effectively for approximately $10,000 to $40,000, whereas the cost of a bone marrow transplant for advanced breast cancer has been estimated to range from $90,000 to $200,000. Provision of a complete range of breast care services will allow closer monitoring of operational expenses while improving stage-specific treatment costs.

Creating a realistic business plan is complicated and multifaceted. Successful development requires the consultation of financial experts and professionals in marketing and strategic planning. Key objectives in structuring an effective business plan are summarized in Table 26-2. Ongoing analysis and review of the plan should involve close collaboration among financial, operational, and clinical staff members. This process may not be easy, however, so regularly scheduled discussions among these parties should be a priority to ensure financial viability.

A well-managed center offers the opportunity to respond with greater efficiency to patients' needs. Ultimately, this productivity should result in an overall cost benefit as well. Although data supporting the cost-effectiveness of such centers is sparse, such a center incorporates many principles intrinsic to managed health care systems that have proved beneficial. Emphasis is placed on developing coordinated, cost-effective care, but not withholding appropriate care. The role of case managers becomes critically important in effecting the integration of clinical and research goals within financial constraints, particularly when considering the treatment of high-cost patients, such as those with advanced breast cancer. Although whether comprehensive breast centers result in a net decrease in cost remains to be proved, they provide greater convenience and satisfaction to both patients and providers.

Facility Development

When considering the feasibility of a comprehensive breast center, many institutions find their existing services to be scattered and inconvenient. By centralizing the majority of services, accessibility to the patient is greatly improved, thereby decreasing frustration and strengthening the patient's ability to focus on treatment and recovery. Seamless integration of services allows information to be processed quickly and results in a coordinated treatment plan.

Ideally, this works best when most of the services provided by the center are physically contained within one facility or at a designated area within a larger building. Many comprehensive programs are housed within large institutions and a separate building is not required for a successful clinical program. Table 26-3 addresses both potential advantages and disadvantages when contemplating construction of a freestanding breast center. Often, financial constraints limit physical restructuring to match the ideal plan.

The planning and oversight of facility design require a significant amount of cooperation among internal and external groups. An architectural and engineering firm with extensive experience in health care should be retained for the project, so they can assess and construct the building to accommodate patient flow patterns. Early establishment of program requirements dictates the amount of square footage needed, the allocation of appropriate space,

TABLE 26-3
Planning a Comprehensive Breast Center Facility: Advantages and Disadvantages

Advantages	Disadvantages
PHYSICAL PLANT (SEPARATE FACILITY)	
Identifies center of excellence	May be expensive to rebuild or remodel
Increases sense of commitment to goals	May duplicate existing facilities
Attracts physician specialists	May limit expansion of future programs
Creates user friendly environment for patient and family	May be geographically inconvenient for medical staff
Creates nonhospital environment	
Has designated parking area	
PATIENT CARE ISSUES	
Centralizes patient services and medical records	May duplicate existing services
Enhances treatment planning process	Volume of patients may not justify cost
Decreases fragmentation of patient care	Limits patients' choice to center's medical staff
Encourages communication and collaboration	
RESEARCH	
Streamlines data collection from specific patient subgroups	Separate or satellite facility may be duplicative
Has direct access to medical records	Need separate animal care facility for basic research
Readily integrates research into clinical practice	Quality control monitoring may be more of a problem
ADMINISTRATION	
Facilitates efficiency and productivity monitoring	May duplicate departmental job tasks
Facilitates packaging of services for managed care contracts	No clear data prove cost-effectiveness
Implements changes more easily under one roof	Creates new cost center for institution
Improves management oversight	Spin-off revenue may be difficult to track
PERSONNEL	
Is conducive to cross-training	May be labor intensive during start-up
Enhances communication	May duplicate staffing ratios
Fosters team building	May encounter resistance to change
Promotes specialization	

and planning for special instrumentation (eg, computerization, surgical facilities). Bringing the staff into the process of designing workstations, educational libraries, conference rooms, and employee lounges helps to enhance team building and a sense of personal ownership of both the space and the program. Weekly construction team meetings, including technical consultants and subcontractors, are initiated during the planning phase and continue through completion of the center. Discussions among medical space planners, clinical providers, and patients will result in a facility that is functionally compatible with efficient operations, economic limitations, and environmental concerns. Behavioral psychologists and interior designers can minimize anxiety induced by a high-tech environment with the creative use of lighting and decor. For example, aquariums, artwork, sculptures, attractive wall murals, colorful mobiles, and fresh flowers and plants contribute to a more relaxed, life-affirming, and healing atmosphere.

Summary

The emergence of comprehensive breast centers has contributed to the development of patient-centered and research-based clinical services. When these centers or programs are organized to deliver care in a convenient, user-friendly facility, staffed with a highly skilled, specialized team of caring professionals, patient and provider satisfaction should improve. The multidisciplinary approach to breast care requires the expertise of physician specialists functioning as team leaders or coleaders. These physicians, trained as both clinicians and scientists, are practicing "the high art of combining honesty about what they know as scientists with humility and hopefulness about what they do not know as clinicians."[44] Balancing this scientific uncertainty with realistic hope may be the most important challenge facing us as we await the translation of new breakthroughs from molecular medicine, genetics, and oncology into clinical practice.

References

1. Haagensen CD. Diseases of the breast, ed 2. Philadelphia, WB Saunders, 1971:V.
2. Silverstein MJ, et al. The Breast Center: a multidisciplinary model. In: Fundamental problems in breast cancer. Boston, Martinus Nijhoff, 1987:47.
3. August DA, Carpenter LC. Benefits of a multidisciplinary approach to breast care. J Surg Oncol 1993;53:161.
4. Brady AM, Foster J. The development of site specific centers: the breast clinic. Oncol Issues 1992;7:12.
5. Coleman C. The role of the comprehensive breast center. Nurse Pract Forum 1993;4:110.
6. Durant JR. How to organize a multidisciplinary clinic for the management of breast cancer. Surg Clin North Am 1990;70:977.
7. Eklund GW, Cardenosa G. Team approach benefits breast cancer patients. Diagn Imag 1992;14:67.
8. American Hospital Association, Section for Maternal and Child Health. Why care about breast care? 1992:1.
9. Harness JK, Oberman HA, et al, eds. Breast cancer: collaborative management. Chelsea; MI, Lewis, 1988:3.
10. Lee CZ, Coleman C, Link J. Developing comprehensive breast centers. Part 1. Introduction and overview. J Oncol Manage 1992;1:1.
11. Lee CZ, Coleman C, Link J. Developing comprehensive breast centers, Part 2. Critical success factors. J Oncol Manage 1992;1:6.
12. Propst S. Developments in breast cancer care: same-day diagnosis through multidisciplinary tumor evaluation. Health Care Advisory Board. Oncology Issue Tracking, November 5, 1993.
13. Harness JK, Organ CH. Surgeons as leaders of multidisciplinary cancer care. Work in progress, Department of Surgery, University of California, Davis, August 1994.
14. Coleman C. The breast cancer team: roles, conflicts and interfaces. Innov Oncol Nurs 1992;8:1.
15. Scott ML. Establishing a partnership: community involvement and the cancer program. Semin Oncol Nurs 1993;9:44.
16. Lamkin L. Assessment, development, and evaluation of cancer programs. Semin Oncol Nurs 1993;9:17.
17. Henke-Yarboro C, Yarbro JW. Historical development of cancer programs. Semin Oncol Nurs 1993;9:3.
18. Joint Commission on Accreditation of Healthcare Organizations. Accreditation manual for hospitals, vol 1. Standards. 1993:29.
19. Bennis W. On becoming a leader. Reading, MA, Addison-Wesley, 1989:106.
20. California Department of Health Services. Requests for applications for regional demonstration partnerships; June 1994.
21. Krumm S. Collaboration between oncology clinical nurse specialists and nursing administrators. Oncol Nurs Forum 1992;19(Suppl):21.
22. Suters ET. The unnatural act of management. New York, Harper Business, 1992:40.
23. MacDonald SA. Organizational approaches to cancer program development. Semin Oncol Nurs 1993;9:8.
24. Rabinowitz B. Comprehensive breast centers: engendering physician involvement. J Oncol Manage 1994;3:52.
25. National Breast Cancer Coalition. Call to action. Newsletter 1994;1:2.
26. Cancer Letter. Breast cancer action plan calls for more Federal coordination, patient participation. 1994;10:1.
27. McGuire R. Tumor board meetings: too little, too late. Oncology Times, April 1990:7.
28. Nyquist JG, Gates JG, Radecki SE, et al. Investigation into the educational process of cancer case conferences. Acad Med 1990;65(Suppl):35.
29. Nyquist JG, Gates JD, Radecki SE, et al. Improving the educational process of cancer case conferences. Acad Med 1992;67(Suppl):1.
30. Greco J. Changing physicians' practices. N Engl J Med 1993;329:1271.
31. Kripke: translational research is greatest opportunity today. Cancer Lett 1994;20:3.
32. Lippman ME. Oncogenes and breast cancer. N Engl J Med 1988;319:1281.
33. Thompson WD. Genetic epidemiology of breast cancer. Cancer (Suppl) 1994;74:279.
34. Winer EP. Quality-of-life research in patients with breast cancer. Cancer (Suppl) 1994;74:410.
35. Pittsburgh institutions form data network in breast cancer. Cancer Economics, February 1994:3.
36. Antman K, Schnipper LE, Frei E. The crisis in clinical cancer research. N Engl J Med 1988;319:46.
37. Taylor-Papadimitriou J, Fentiman IS. Breast cancer. In: Sidebottom E, ed. Cancer surveys, vol 18. Cold Spring Harbor, NY, Cold Springs Harbor Laboratory, 1993.
38. Henderson MM. Ethical issues: Changing attitudes and practices. Cancer Detect Prev 1994;18:323.

39. Hall DC, Adams CK, et al. Improved detection of human breast lesions following experimental training. Cancer 1980;46:408.

40. Cancer Letter NCI to fund more spores in FY'95 recompetition 1994;20:4.

41. Hilakivi-Clarke L, Rowland J, Clarke R, et al. Psychosocial factors in the development and progression of breast cancer. Breast Cancer Res Treat 1994;29:141.

42. Schain WS. Physician–patient communication about breast cancer: A challenge for the 1990s. Surg Clin North Am 1990;70:917.

43. Davis Spingarn N. Health care reform: an absolute necessity. NCCS Networker 1994;8(2):3.

44. Lerner M. Choices in healing. Cambridge, MA, MIT, 1994:7.

45. Tannock IF. Treating the patient, not just the cancer. N Engl J Med 1987;317:1535.

46. Contavespi V. Faith healing. Forbes, July 4, 1994:134.

47. Dackman L. Up front: sex and the post mastectomy woman. New York, Viking/Penguin, 1991.

48. Lee-Feldstein A, Anton-Culver H, Feldstein PJ. Treatment differences and other prognostic factors related to breast cancer survival. JAMA 1994;271:1163.

49. Kelly, PT. Cancer risk counseling for individuals and families at increased cancer risk. Cancer Bull 1994;46:275.

50. Kaye R. Spinning straw into gold. New York, Simon & Schuster, 1991.

51. National Cancer Institute. Breast cancer screening programs make good business sense. Natl Cancer Inst Fact Sheet, February 1994.

52. Lewis GW, Taylor RB, Mealor RS. What cancer program managers must know: the fiscal and regulatory challenge. Semin Oncol Nurs 1993;9:59.

53. Slochberger WT. The administrator's role in strategic management. Administrat Radiol 1988;7:50.

54. Tan S. Indispensable partners, providers and managed care contractors. Administrat Radiol 1992;11:67.

55. Faltermayer E. A health plan that can work. Fortune, June 14, 1993:88.

56. Straub W, Dey AA. So you want to get into the breast imaging business. Administrat Radiol, July 1989:14.

57. Armtec Medical Marketing, The Armtec report on breast cancer: the disease, the market, and the opportunity. Elm National Oncology Database, 1993.

58. Gilden KM. The challenge of cancer care marketing. Semin Oncol Nurs 1993;9:51.

59. Herzlinger RE. Healthy competition. Atlantic Monthly, August 1991:69.

60. Mathison BJ. Designing a results-oriented marketing plan for breast cancer services. J Oncol Management, 1993;2:34.

61. US Dept Health and Human Services. The national strategic plan for the early detection and control of breast and cervical cancers. Atlanta, US Government Printing Office, 1993:8.

62. Peters T. Thriving on chaos. New York, Harper Collins, 1991:37.

63. Yamamoto JK. Author helping women cope with breast cancer. Hokubei Mainichi Newspaper, San Francisco, August 19, 1994:A1.

64. Kneece J. Stopping the drain of dollars spent on breast cancer. Administrat Radiol 1994;13:27.

65. Kneece J. Breast care: what about tomorrow? Mammogr Today, July/August, 1994:22.

66. McDermott KC. Healthcare reform: past and future. Oncol Nurs Forum 1994;21:827.

67. Ogorzalek LL. Quality management issues. Semin Oncol Nurs 1993;9:32.

68. Swanson GM. May we agree to disagree, or how do we develop guidelines for breast cancer screening in women? J Natl Cancer Inst 1994;86:903.

27

Basic Tools for Advancing Knowledge in Breast Cancer

Diseases of the Breast, edited by Jay R. Harris,
Marc E. Lippman, Monica Morrow, and Samuel Hellman.
Lippincott-Raven Publishers, Philadelphia, © 1996.

27.1

Techniques in Molecular Biology

DAVID MALKIN

In the four decades since the initial identification and characterization of the double helix structure of DNA, an explosion of knowledge has occurred in the field of molecular biology—the study of living organisms in terms of the properties of their constituent molecules. Of course, the concept that such molecules existed was critical to the establishment of Mendel's basic laws of genetics established more than a century earlier. Mendel defined the *gene* as the most basic unit of genetic information. It was not until 1945, however, that Emil Schrödinger promoted the view that the laws of physics, until then thought to be accountable for many natural phenomena, might be inadequate to explain the fundamental properties of genetic material. In particular, the ability to maintain absolute stability from generation to generation appeared to defy established physical principles. "We shall assume the structure of the gene to be that of a huge molecule, capable only of discontinuous change, which consists in a rearrangement of the atoms and leads to an isomeric molecule. The rearrangement [mutation] may affect only a small region of the gene, and a vast number of different rearrangements may be possible."[1] Thus, physical theory attracted many physicists to study biology and molecular biology when these fields were yet in their infancy.

A gene does not function autonomously but relies heavily on its abilities to interact with other cellular components. Although the "average" gene is in fact a huge molecule, it nevertheless represents only part of a vast length of genetic material known as the *genome,* which contains many genes. Of the 50,000 to 100,000 genes thought to compose the human genome, only a small fraction have been isolated, and fewer still have a known function. Each gene is a nucleic acid sequence of the DNA molecule that carries the information defining a particular polypeptide (protein). The search for and characterization of each gene and its encoded protein have constituted a fairly tedious process carried out in innumerable laboratories that has relied on various labor-intensive but highly effective molecular biologic techniques. In the past 5 years, a concerted international effort has led to initiation of the Human Genome Project, the ultimate goal of which is to define the human genome and to use this information, as well as the application of molecular techniques, to solve fundamental problems of biology and human disease.

This chapter outlines some of these molecular biologic techniques as they might apply to diseases of the breast. Obviously, none of the methods is particularly unique to this group of disorders, and virtually all have been used in many biologic systems, ranging from the most primitive unicellular organisms to complex vertebrates, including humans. The chapter also describes the use of these techniques to increase our understanding of the flow of genetic information, in both normal and pathologic cellular pathways, and of the interactive nature of these biologic processes. A more detailed description of many of these techniques and their molecular foundation may be found in various textbooks, including *Genes V* by Lewin;[1] *Recombinant DNA—A Short Course* by Watson and colleagues;[2] *Molecular Biology of the Cell,* 2nd edition, by Alberts and colleagues;[3] and *Molecular Cloning—A Laboratory Manual,* 2nd edition, by Sambrook and associates.[4]

The reader is initially introduced to some general concepts of the basic elements of molecular analysis—the gene, DNA, RNA, and protein. This discussion is followed by an outline of the most commonly used and well-established fundamental molecular techniques and an evaluation of novel techniques of detection for molecular genetic aberrations at each of these genetic targets. Finally, some of the methods used for genetic manipulation are discussed, and their applications to the understanding of biologic functions are evaluated.

The application of molecular biologic theory and techniques will probably lead medical sciences into the next century. It will be incumbent on all clinicians to have at least a fundamental understanding of molecular biology so that they can interact with molecular biologists and develop preventive and therapeutic applications to their full potential in the alleviation or elimination of many human diseases.

General Concepts

DNA

The genetic code that defines the uniqueness of all organisms is carried in the ordered sequence of nucleotides that makes up the general structure of DNA. In the nucleus, DNA is condensed into chromatin along a chromosome. In humans, if each DNA molecule were unwound and laid end to end, the DNA from one cell would be a meter long. An important feature of the structure of the DNA molecule is that it is independent of the particular sequence of its component nucleotides. Although the particular sequence may in fact affect the gross molecular structure and conformation of the molecule, the sequential code of nucleotides ultimately dictates the sequence of amino acids that forms the corresponding polypeptide, or protein. The relation between the DNA sequence and the corresponding sequence of protein is called the *genetic code*. The primary sequence of its constitutive amino acids dictates the structure or enzymatic activities of each unique protein. Characteristic segments within the nucleotide sequences are often similar, or even identical, between genes encoding proteins with similar biologic functions. In addition, certain sequences are conserved phylogenetically through the animal or plant kingdoms. Such conservation is thought to indicate that these regions are important in the function of the protein. Other regions of the DNA molecule contain nucleotide sequences that are recognized as binding sites for molecules that regulate functions of DNA sequences upstream or downstream of that particular region.

Each nucleic acid consists of a chemically linked sequence of four subunits, each of which is composed of a nitrogenous base, a pentose sugar, and a phosphate group. The *pyrimidines* and *purines* represent the two types of nitrogenous bases. Adenine and guanine are the two purines, and are found in both RNA and DNA; cytosine and thymine are the two pyrimidines found in DNA, whereas cytosine and uracil are the pyrimidines found in RNA. The bases are usually referred to by their first letters—A, G, C, T, and U. Two types of pentose are found in nucleic acids. In DNA, it is 2-deoxyribose, whereas in RNA, ribose is the sugar. The base-sugar-phosphate linked group is called a *nucleotide,* and these nucleotides represent the building blocks from which the nucleic acids are constructed. Thus, the nucleotides are linked together to form a polynucleotide chain, referred to as the backbone of the molecule.

As originally demonstrated by Watson and Crick[5] in 1953, DNA is a double-stranded helix in which only two types of nucleotide base pairings can occur: adenine with thymine and guanine with cytosine. The model requires the two polynucleotide chains to run in opposite directions, one strand running in the 5′→3′ direction and the other in the 3′→5′ direction.

The complementarity of base pairing explains three important characteristics of DNA structure and function. First, as outlined previously, it is the basis on which the linear arrangement of nucleotides on the one DNA strand specifies with absolute fidelity the structure and sequence on the opposite strand.

Second, the complementarity of the double helix provides DNA with the ability to encode its own replication. Each of the parental strands may act as a template for the synthesis of a complementary daughter strand. In a zipper-like fashion, the two parental strands separate, so that each becomes a template. Each daughter duplex is identical to the original parent. In this manner, the original nucleotide sequence may be replicated again and again. It is this principle that was the basis for development of the polymerase chain reaction (PCR) technique that has revolutionized molecular biology. The complex interaction of enzymes that unwind strands, remove nucleotides, add nucleotides, and "correct" errors of pairing are described in detail in most genetics and biochemistry textbooks and are beyond the scope of this chapter.

Third, the complementary DNA sequence indirectly mediates the synthesis of proteins. In any given region of the genome, only one of the two strands of DNA encode a protein. For this reason, the genetic code is written as a sequence of bases rather than as base pairs. The code is read in groups of three consecutive nucleotides, each group representing one amino acid. Each trinucleotide sequence is termed a *codon*. The triplet code is outlined in Table 27.1-1. The starting point at which the codons are read (in a 5′→3′ direction) represents the way in which the nucleotide sequence is ultimately translated into a protein. The so-called reading frame for the entire subsequent sequence can be altered by the insertion or deletion of a single base. The resulting *frameshift* leads to the generation of a completely different reading frame that would alter the entire amino acid sequence and function of the protein.

Mutations of the DNA sequence may lead to altered

TABLE 27.1-1
The Genetic Code

RNA Codons	Amino Acid	Abbreviations	
GCA, GCC, GCG, GCU	Alanine	ala	A
AGA, AGG, CGA, CGC, CGG, CGU	Arginine	arg	R
GAC, GAU	Asparatic acid	asp	D
AAC, AAU	Asparagine	asn	N
UGC, UGU	Cysteine	cys	C
GAA, GAG	Glutamic acid	glu	E
CAA, CAG	Glutamine	gln	Q
GGA, GGC, GGG, GGU	Glycine	gly	G
CAC, CAU	Histidine	his	H
AUA, AUC, AUU	Isoleucine	ile	I
UUA, UUG, CUA, CUC, CUG, CUU	Leucine	leu	L
AAA, AAG	Lysine	lys	K
AUG	Methionine	met	M
UUC, UUU	Phenylalanine	phe	F
CCA, CCC, CCG, CCU	Proline	pro	P
AGC, AGU, UCA, UCC, UCG, UCU	Serine	ser	S
ACA, ACC, ACG, ACU	Threonine	thr	T
UGG	Tryptophan	trp	W
UAC, UAU	Tyrosine	tyr	Y
GUA, GUC, GUG, GUU	Valine	val	V
UAA, UAG, UGA	Stop		

protein structure, which may lead to altered or abrogated protein function. In this manner, many protein functions have been elucidated from the position of the mutations within their encoding DNA sequence. Spontaneous mutations, resulting from normal cellular mechanisms or random interactions with environmental factors (mutagens), occur at characteristic background rates in all organisms. Such mutations are necessarily rare events, and particularly damaging ones are selected against during evolution. Treatment of cells and tissues with mutagens, either in vitro or in vivo, can induce mutations.

Any base pair of the DNA molecule can be mutated. Two principle mechanisms exist that lead to the occurrence of a point mutation, which changes a single base pair. Either a chemical modification of the DNA directly changes one base to a different base, or an error of DNA replication leads to the incorrect base insertion into the polynucleotide chain during DNA synthesis. Two terms are used to describe the types of base changes. *Transitions* represent the substitution of one pyrimidine for another, or of one purine for another. *Transversions,* which are generally less common, represent the substitution of a purine for a pyrimidine or vice versa. Rarely, mutagens are analogues of the usual bases, such as bromouracil (BrdU), which is an analogue of thymine. Base analogues may be inappropriately incorporated into the DNA strand in place of one of the regular bases. The ambiguous pairing properties of these analogues permit the base to change its structure and thus to pair with a selection of potential bases. In each replicating cycle of the duplex, the mistaken incorporation can occur as long as the analogue is present. For the most part, point mutations do not induce a frameshift as do insertions or deletions. If the point mutation leads to the substitution of a particular amino acid with a termination codon, however, the encoded protein may be prematurely truncated and its function altered, or completely destroyed.

Chemical modification of one of the four bases can also lead to functional alteration of the DNA molecule. The most commonly modified base is 5-methylcytosine, which is generated by the enzymatic addition of a methyl group to a small proportion of the cytosine residues of DNA. These sites then become hot spots for spontaneous point mutations, which are exclusively G-C to A-T transitions. DNA replication itself will not maintain the presence of methylcytosine. Rather, the methyl group needs to be added at each successive generation. As with point mutations, insertions, or deletions, base pair methylation can be reversed. In this manner, modification of the DNA sequence can occur after it has been synthesized. After a mutation has passed through one generation of replication, however, it inevitably becomes a permanent part of the genetic information.

Mutations in DNA are not completely random events. Some sites are more frequently mutated than expected from a random distribution, whereas other codons or nucleotides are rarely altered. The hot spots for mutations vary and depend on the inducing mutagen. Not all hot spots are sites for all types of mutation. Furthermore, not all DNA mutations actually result in a detectable change in phenotype. Such mutations are referred to as *silent mutations*. They may involve base changes that do not alter the amino acid coded for in the corresponding protein. Other silent mutations do change the amino acid, but the switch does not affect the protein's activity. Rarely, although one mutation may in itself significantly alter protein function, the occurrence of a second mutation elsewhere in the DNA sequence might compensate for this effect and restore the protein's activity.

The complementary nature of the double helix, the ordered sequence of nucleotides and the naturally occurring means by which DNA is altered provide the biochemical bases for the principal techniques of recombinant DNA technology.

RNA

Several complex steps are required for genetic information contained within the DNA nucleotide sequence to be converted successfully to a functionally intact protein. It is the *transcription* of the genome into RNA that reflects much of the complexity of this system.

RNA is synthesized from the DNA template (Fig. 27.1-1). Although they are almost always single stranded, RNA molecules do have complex structures. They frequently have short double-helical regions, which form when two sections of an RNA nucleotide chain lie in a hairpin fold in the correct "antiparallel" orientation to form base pairs. The tertiary structures of certain RNA species, particularly transfer RNA (tRNA, described later), are important to their ultimate function. The four bases in the RNA polynucleotide chain are A, G, C, and U. Although, like DNA, base pairings are usually A-T and G-C; occasionally, weaker G-U pairings can be identified.

RNA polymerase II is the enzyme principally involved in the transcription of genes from DNA sequence into RNA. The RNA copy of the DNA that is to become protein is termed *messenger RNA* (mRNA). This RNA sequence is complementary to the template strand and identical to the coding strand of DNA. The startpoint of transcription occurs at the *promoter* region of the gene (see Fig. 27.1-1). The promoter sequence actually surrounds the first base pair that is to be transcribed into RNA. The promoter's function is to be recognized by proteins that control the rate and degree of transcription. In this way, promoters and adjacent transcription control sites differ from other nucleotide sequences, the primary roles of which are exerted through transcription or translation. The information for promoter function is provided directly by DNA sequence, and its structure represents the actual signal. Conservation of bases over only very short consensus sequences is typical of these regulatory sites. Most promoters have a *TATA box,* usually located about 25 base pairs upstream of the starting point. This A-T base pair element tends to be surrounded by G-C–rich sequences. The fixed position of the TATA box is critical to the positioning of the RNA polymerase. Another important sequence about 70 bases upstream of the start point is the *CAAT box*. This region plays an important role in determining the efficiency of the promoter but does not appear to play a role in promoter specificity. Other upstream elements have been characterized and are known to modify the rate of transcription from specific promoters in either a positive or negative way. They act, therefore, to regulate gene expression during both embryologic development and cellular differentiation. From the promoter region, the RNA polymerase enzyme travels along the template, synthesizing RNA, until it reaches a *terminator* sequence (see Table 27.1-1). It might seem that RNA polymerase transcribes genes in an indiscriminate fashion, but other proteins, known as *transcription regulators,* ensure when particular genes are ready for transcription. For a short stretch, as the RNA polymerase moves along the unwinding DNA molecule, the DNA is in a single-stranded conformation. Within a few bases (as soon as the enzyme has passed by), the DNA duplex reforms. In this fashion, the integrity of the DNA molecule is maintained during transcription.

The nucleic acid sequence of the gene includes not only the *coding region* found in the mRNA, which corresponds to the amino acid sequence of the protein, but also additional intervening sequences that lie within the coding

FIGURE 27.1-1 DNA is transcribed to RNA and translated to protein. Regulatory elements and the CCAAT and TATA boxes are involved in the positive and negative signaling of the initiation of transcription from the start codon ATG. Introns are spliced out from precursor mRNA recognized by specific sequences at the splice-donor and splice-acceptor sites. A stop codon and poly(A) tail at the end of the gene delineate the termination of the template DNA. mRNA is translated into protein in a process mediated by ribosomes moving along the mRNA in a 5′→3′ direction.

region, thus interrupting the sequence that represents the protein. Thus, the *exons* are the regions of the gene represented in the mRNA, whereas *introns* are regions that are absent from the mRNA. The process in which introns are removed from the RNA to yield an mRNA that consists only of exons is known as *RNA splicing*. This processing of the gene and RNA occurs in the nucleus. In addition to splicing out of the introns, a series of some 200 adenine residues is added to the terminal end of the mRNA molecule, which is then said to be polyadenylated. Subsequently, the mRNA is transported to the cytoplasm and translated into protein.

Translation of mRNA to protein occurs on the ribosomes within the cell. Each ribosome consists of two subunits, which contain several proteins in association with a long RNA molecule known as ribosomal RNA (rRNA). The generation of the protein's polypeptide change is mediated by yet another small RNA species termed *transfer RNA* (tRNA). A tRNA is able to recognize only the one amino acid to which it is covalently linked. The tRNA contains a trinucleotide sequence, the anticodon, which is complementary to the codon that represents its amino acid. The anticodon allows the tRNA to recognize the codon through complementary base pairing. The ribosome moves along the mRNA, permitting sequential amino acids to be assembled into proteins.

As noted earlier, the relation of triplet codons to their respective amino acids is referred to as the genetic code. Because any of the four possible nucleotides can occupy any of the three positions of the codon, there are 4^3, or 64, possible trinucleotide sequence combinations. There are therefore more codons than the 20 amino acids from which proteins are synthesized. This apparent discrepancy is resolved by the observation of *degeneracy;* that is, almost every amino acid is represented by several codons. Only methionine and tryptophan carry unique trinucleotide sequences. Similar amino acids are represented by related codons, presumably in an attempt to minimize the effects of mutations. Three codons (UAA, UAG, and UGA) are used specifically to terminate protein synthesis, and one of these *stop (termination) codons* marks the end of every gene. Ultimately, the order of the amino acids in a protein confers its three-dimensional conformation as well as its biologic and biochemical activities. Alteration of the amino acid sequence almost inevitably alters these characteristics.

RESTRICTION FRAGMENTS

On isolation of a segment of DNA, a critical step in obtaining its sequence is to generate a nucleotide map. The identification of *restriction enzymes* that recognize specific short DNA sequences and cleave the DNA strands at those particular sites was a critical development for this technique. These restriction enzymes are produced by bacteria as part of a restriction–modification system that protects the organism from invasion by foreign DNA. Several hundred restriction enzymes that recognize more than 150 specific nucleotide sequences have been identified. Each restriction enzyme recognizes a specific target in double-stranded DNA, usually a sequence of four to six base pairs, and the enzyme cuts the DNA at each and every point at which its target sequence occurs. Different enzymes recognize different target sequences, although some enzymes recognize the same sites (Table 27.1-2). When a panel of enzymes are used to cut DNA, the resulting identification of points of breakage represents a *restriction map*. The distances between breaks varies depending on the sequence of the DNA. In a DNA molecule of random nucleotide sequences, a six-base recognition sequence for a restriction enzyme would be expected to occur once in every 4096 bases (ie, 1 in 4^6 bases). Thus, in human DNA, which is approximately 3×10^9 base pairs long, this enzyme would cut the DNA into several million fragments. These fragments can be separated by size by *gel electrophoresis*. In this technique, the cut DNA is placed at the top of a gel made of either agarose or polyacrylamide. As an electric current is passed through the gel, each fragment moves down the gel at a rate that is inversely proportional to the log of its molecular weight. Because DNA is negatively charged, it will tend to migrate to the positive electrode. The DNA fragments can be visualized with ultraviolet light after the gel is stained with ethidium bromide. This compound intercalates between DNA base pairs and fluoresces when exposed to ultraviolet light. The series of bands that is generated is calibrated against a standard restriction digest of known molecular size. Each band corresponds to a fragment of particular size. The data from this restriction digest can be used to construct a (relatively primitive) map of the original fragment of DNA that one started with. By introducing other enzymes in a sequential fashion, one can generate more complex and accurate maps.

RESTRICTION FRAGMENT-LENGTH POLYMORPHISMS

The coexistence of more than one genetic variation in the population constitutes a *genetic polymorphism*. Any site at which multiple alleles exist as stable components in the population is, by definition, polymorphic. Because the DNA sequence at these sites varies, the restriction maps of the DNA sequences are also distinguishable from each other. Restriction maps of different individuals are therefore useful to detect genomic polymorphisms, which are identified as a change in the pattern of fragments produced by cleavage with a restriction enzyme. When a restriction site is present in one individual and absent in another, the extra cleavage in the first generates two fragments, whose additive size corresponds to the single fragment in the second genome. It is thought that most restriction-site polymorphisms in the genome do not actually affect the phenotype. The genetic mutation, usually a point mutation, does not alter the amino acid sequence of the encoded protein. In addition, restriction site polymorphisms frequently occur in intronic sequences that are not known to be associated with any biologic function.

The difference in restriction maps between two individuals is known as a *restriction fragment-length polymorphism* (RFLP). It can be used as a genotypic genetic marker in the same way as phenotypic markers. Often, recombination

TABLE 27.1-2
Characteristics of Some Restriction Sites

Recognition Sequence and Cleavage Points	Restriction Endonuclease	Characteristics
... ↓ ... GG CC ...CC↑GG...	*Hae*III	4 bases, flush ends
... ↓ ... GTT AAC ...CAA↑TTG...	*Hpa*I	6 bases, flush ends
... ↓ ... TCG A ...A GC↑T...	*Taq*I	4 bases, cohesive ends
...↓ ... GAATTC ... CTTAAG↑...	*Eco*RI	6 bases, cohesive ends
... ↓ ... CTPy PuAC ...GAPu↑PyGT...	*Hind*II	6 bases, ambiguity, cohesive ends
... ↓ ... G ANT C ...C TNA↑G...	*Hinf*I	5 bases, ambiguity, cohesive ends

Py, pyrimidine (C,T); Pu, purine (A,G); N, any nucleotide.

frequency can be measured between a restriction marker and a visible phenotypic marker, and thus provide the basis for linking genetic loci at the molecular level to a particular phenotype. Thus, if a restriction marker is associated with a phenotypic characteristic, the restriction site must be located near or at the gene responsible for the phenotype. Several such disease-associated genes might be in this region, so that, although genetic mapping cannot prove that any particular gene is responsible for the disease, it can exclude target or candidate genes. The high frequency of genetic polymorphisms in the human genome means that each individual has a unique constellation of restriction sites. The *haplotype* of that individual refers to the particular combination of sites found in a specific region.

The mapping of RFLPs has led to the construction of a linkage map for the entire human genome. This map is being used to localize a wide variety of genes associated with human disease. One example has been the localization of a breast cancer susceptibility locus (BRCA1) to a region of approximately 5 centimorgans on chromosome 17q21,[6–8] and BRCA2 on chromosome 13q24. The use of RFLP mapping assisted in narrowing the region to a manageable length whereby classic cloning techniques may be used to isolate the actual genes.

Fundamental Techniques

POLYMERASE CHAIN REACTION

Most genes of interest are present as a single copy, or, at most, as a few copies, in the human genome. If 10 µg of DNA were used as a template for Southern blot analysis,

as little as 10^{-5} µg of the specific gene might be detected. Thus, even when radioactive phosphorus or biotin is used to label probes, up to a week's exposure would be required to visualize specific bands. PCR, described in 1985,[9] is a powerful procedure that allows selected regions of the genome to be amplified by a factor of 10^6 or more in an in vitro reaction. Although PCR is a conceptually simple procedure that has now been almost completely automated in its execution, it depends on knowledge of the exact DNA sequence of at least part of the region to be amplified. The procedure is graphically represented in Figure 27.1-2. It is essentially a series of three-step cycles, with the cycles repeated 20 to 40 times to give an exponential increase of the product. At 100% efficiency in each cycle, a double-stranded DNA segment would be predicted to yield 2^{20} (more than 10^6) copies after 20 cycles. In practice, however, efficiencies are less than 100%. Nevertheless, it is relatively easy to produce 10^6 to 10^8 copies of a DNA template in a few hours.

The essential requirement for PCR is a pair of oligonucleotides, or primers, complementary to nucleotide sequences at the ends of the double-stranded DNA fragment that is to be amplified. These primers can be as short as 12 or as long as 60 base pairs. They are synthesized on machines that chemically bond successive nucleotides to produce the desired nucleic acid. One artificially generated primer is made to be complementary to a selected end of the sense strand and the other complementary to a selected end of the antisense strand. The amplified region therefore lies between these two selected ends. It is possible to amplify several kilobases of DNA using this technique.

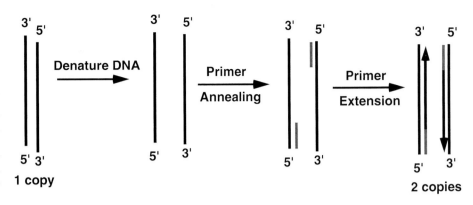

FIGURE 27.1-2 The principle of the polymerase chain reaction (PCR). Three steps in each cycle are denaturation of the double-stranded DNA, usually through heating, annealing of sequence specific primers to opposite ends of the target region, and extension of the primers with a temperature-stable DNA polymerase. Repetition of the sequence generates copies of the DNA between the primers in an exponential manner: repeat for n cycles yields approximately 2^n copies.

The PCR reaction mixture includes, in addition to the primers and DNA template, a thermostable bacterial polymerase that is derived from *Thermus aquaticus* (*Taq* polymerase), free deoxynucleotides, and cofactors or buffer for the enzymatic reaction. The mixture of all the reagents is transferred into a small Eppendorf tube that is placed in a programmable heating block that varies the temperature conditions for the sequential steps in the amplification reaction. Initially, the DNA is heat-denatured at 91° to 94°C for a few minutes. Rapid cooling of the mixture allows the primers to anneal to the appropriate selected ends of the fragment. By varying this temperature, one can increase or decrease the specificity of primer annealing. The temperature is then raised to 72° to 80°C—the optimal temperature range for polymerase activity—to synthesize the target sequence. The cycle is repeated, and after completion of the desired number of cycles, the amplified fragment can be visualized by gel electrophoresis.

It is possible to analyze RNA by PCR; however, it is necessary to first convert the RNA to DNA using the retroviral enzyme reverse transcriptase. The DNA is then amplified in the manner described. The major difficulty with analysis of an RNA sample is the requirement that the sample be fresh. The ubiquitous presence of RNA-degrading enzymes (RNases) often disrupts the molecule sufficiently that a viable template is not available.

PCR has revolutionized both molecular diagnosis and recombinant DNA technology. It has been applied to genetic screening for mutation detection, detection of residual disease in patients after cancer therapy, diagnosis based on specific genetic markers, and the generation of probes for various other molecular biologic techniques including many of those described here. In recognition of this significant advance, Dr. Kary Mullis, who originated and developed the concept and many of its practical applications, received the 1993 Nobel Prize in Medicine and Physiology.

GENE MUTATION ANALYSIS

DNA Sequencing

DNA sequencing is one of the most fundamental tools in the biologic sciences. The ultimate definition of a gene mutation, often initially detected through a deletion or by screening, is in the determination of the exact alteration in the nucleotide sequence. The power of DNA sequence analysis is in the ability of polyacrylamide gels to resolve nucleic acid fragments that differ in length by only a single base. In 1977, Maxam and Gilbert[10] designed a method of sequencing that uses chemical reagents to effect base-specific cleavage. Single-stranded DNA is subjected to four different reactions that cleave randomly at one of four sites: C, T and C, A and G, or G. The resulting strands are separated by size, and comparison of the band patterns from the four reactions permits analysis of the sequence of the parental DNA template. Although this method is still widely used, the technique of Sanger and colleagues[11] first reported in the same year and termed *chain-termination DNA sequencing* is now more commonly used. This technique involves the synthesis of a DNA strand by a DNA polymerase in vitro using a single-stranded DNA template. The reaction is done simultaneously in four tubes, each of which contains a mixture of nucleotides. Synthesis is initiated only at the site at which an oligonucleotide primer anneals to the DNA template. The DNA polymerase catalyses the sequential addition of the appropriate nucleotide to the growing chain. Synthesis is terminated by the incorporation of a nucleotide analog that cannot support continued elongation of the DNA molecule; hence the name chain termination. The chain-termination nucleotide analogues are the 2′,3′-dideoxynucleoside 5′-triphosphates (ddNTPs) that lack the 3′-OH group necessary for DNA chain elongation. Four separate reactions (A, C, G, and T) are performed, each with a different ddNTP, to give complete sequence information. The DNA fragments that act as sequence templates are typically radiolabeled by either tagging the nucleotides or primers with ^{35}S. The reaction products are then separated by size in adjacent lanes of a high-resolution denaturing polyacrylamide gel and detected using autoradiography. The sequence is interpreted from the pattern of alternating bands in the lanes corresponding to the terminal base of the fragment (Fig. 27.1-3). The accuracy of DNA sequencing is high and can be improved by independently sequencing both strands of a DNA molecule. Any sites at which complementarity is lost are identified as possible sequencing errors, and these can be confirmed on resequencing.

Commonly, the DNA template for sequencing is

FIGURE 27.1-3 A DNA single-strand sequence is shown. Each band represents the next in the sequence of bases that make up the nucleotide sequence. Each lane is dedicated to one of the four nucleotides. The three-base sequence CGG (*left*) represents arginine (Arg), which becomes glutanine (Gln) with one base change (*right*). WT, wild-type; MT; mutant; A, adenine; G, guanine; C, cytosine; T, thymidine.

formed when the product of PCR amplification of the fragment of interest is cloned into a plasmid vector. This technique is facilitated by the addition of restriction sites within the primers. Multiple clones must be sequenced, however, to compensate for the possible errors introduced by the *Taq* polymerase used in the PCR. To overcome this problem, direct sequencing of PCR products is preferred, and many methods have been described. Most of these techniques require time-consuming procedures to purify the PCR product or synthesis of a separate primer that anneals within the PCR fragment to be used specifically for sequencing.

A more recent advance in DNA sequencing technology has been the development of automated sequencing instruments based on laser-induced fluorescence. These instruments replace the radioactive labels and autoradiography used in chain-termination sequencing with fluorescent labels and automated detection and interpretation. A particularly important strategy takes advantage of the spectral discrimination possible with fluorescence to permit all four sequencing reactions to be separated by electrophoresis in a single lane. Four different flurophores (dyes) are attached to the oligonucleotide primer, which then becomes attached to the polynucleotide product of the extension reaction. Each reaction (A, G, C, and T) is represented by a distinct dye. The products of each reaction are combined and then separated by electrophoresis in a single lane similar to that in conventional DNA sequencing. During the electrophoresis, a laser scans a

fixed position near the bottom of the gel, exciting fluorescence in the dye primers. A high-sensitivity detector measures the fluorescence as the tagged DNA bands migrate past this point in the gel. The DNA sequence is determined by the temporal order of the colored bands as they pass through the detector. These data are stored, analyzed, and converted to conventional DNA sequence by a computer.

After DNA sequences are generated, they are entered into one or more of several internationally accessible computer data bases, including GenBank and the European Molecular Biology Laboratory (EMBL). These data bases permit other investigators to perform homologic comparisons among proteins and nucleic acids that have already been entered, provide others with access to the data, and permit interesting regions of the genes to be screened for functionally important domains.

Single-Strand Conformational Polymorphism Analysis

To determine the frequency and characteristics of gene mutations, it is often necessary to analyze large numbers of samples concurrently. Studies of this magnitude have recently been made practical by the introduction of screening techniques that allow rapid and efficient detection of DNA sequence alterations without the need to sequence the entire gene of interest.

One such method for localizing single base pair differences in a DNA segment is Single-strand conformational polymorphism (SSCP) analysis[12,13] (Fig. 27.1-4). This technique relies on the property that folding of single-stranded nucleic acid sequences is determined by weak stabilizing forces such as base stacking and intrastrand base pairing, which depend on single nucleotide interactions. Changes in environmental conditions (including temperature and the presence of a denaturant) are likely to result in a conformational change, which is detected in SSCP analysis on a polyacrylamide gel as an alteration in mobility of the polynucleotide strand. Small fragments (usually less than 300 bases in length) of the DNA are amplified using PCR, the double strand is heat denatured into its two complementary single strands, and the sample is then run side by side on a nondenaturing gel. The gene being studied can be arbitrarily divided into short segments, each run on a different gel, or, in some cases, two or more fragments can be run together in what is known as multiplex SSCP. Each fragment can be qualitatively compared with similar fragments on the same gel. It has been shown that the pattern of band separation is reproducible for specific mutations, although occasional variations in band intensity and mobility occur as a result of slight variations in the electrophoretic conditions. Certain mutations are more readily identifiable under more or less stringent electrophoretic conditions. The technique is most effective in regions of the DNA fragment that are not excessively rich in guanine–cytosine (GC) content. Several studies have shown that SSCP can identify over 85% of known mutations and has a low false-negative rate. The sensitivity of the method decreases with increased size of the PCR product. This factor can, in some cases, be overcome by

FIGURE 27.1-4 Single-strand conformational analysis of a 235–base pair fragment encompassing exon 7 of the p53 tumor-suppressor gene in genomic DNA extracted from 18 brain tumors. Extra bands or band shifts in lanes 2, 10, 14, and 15 indicate probable gene sequence alterations that can then be confirmed by DNA sequencing. The technique is qualitative and does not itself identify the precise nature of the base pair alterations.

restriction digestion of a larger amplification fragment before electrophoresis. Although the amplification products are usually performed with the addition to ^{32}P or ^{35}S to the reaction, nonradioactive detection by fluorescence labeling, silver staining, and ethidium bromide staining has also been used successfully.[14–16] For both SSCP analysis and denaturant gradient gel electrophoresis (described later), the assay determines the existence of a sequence difference within the fragment. The precise nature of this alteration must be determined by sequencing.

Denaturant Gel Electrophoresis

An alternative screening technique to SSCP is denaturant gradient gel electrophoresis (DGGE).[17] This method and a recent modification, constant denaturant gel electrophoresis (CDGE),[18,19] both rely on strand dissociation of DNA fragments in discrete sequence-dependent melting domains. Under the correct denaturing conditions, the local biochemical pertubation induced by a single base pair change leaves the strand unfolded to a particularly minor or significant degree. This dissociation causes an abrupt decrease in mobility, which is visible on an acrylamide gel containing a gradient of denaturant. A long GC-rich region (GC clamp) attached to one end of the fragment holds that end together and increases resolution. The addition of the GC clamp increases the number of detectable mutations from 40% of all single-base changes to close to 100%.[17,19] By selecting a specific denaturant concentration based on computer-generated melting curves, maximum separation between wild-type and mutant fragments can be achieved. The modification incorporated by CDGE is to run gels with a constant denaturant that avoids the use of a gradient by selection of a specific denaturant concentration at which maximum separation between the wild-type and mutant fragments occurs. CDGE enables the fragments to migrate with a consistently different rate through the whole gel and allows separation of several centimeters between mutant and wild-type fragments.[19] When both normal and mutant fragments are present in the sample, heteroduplex formation between these noncomplementary species is often observed as multiple bands.

One of the greatest advantages of CDGE or DGGE over traditional SSCP analysis is lack of the need for radioisotope-labeled probes to detect fragments. Instead, ethidium bromide staining is used to visualize the bands.

GENE PRODUCTS

Southern Blot Analysis

As DNA sequencing and PCR revolutionized the ability to accurately detect the minutest base pair alterations and to manipulate nucleic acid fragments, respectively, the Southern blot provided a powerful tool with which to yield a physical position to a DNA fragment of interest. It is a procedure of such wide applicability that it came to bear the name of its inventor, Ed Southern. The Southern blot[20] is one of the most reliable methods by which to detect genes and rapidly screen for alterations. It is frequently a good preliminary step in mutation analysis. Detailed knowledge of the gene structure and sequence is not required, so it is possible to do a preliminary screen with a probe of interest immediately after it has been isolated. The Southern blotting procedure is outlined in Figure 27.1-5.

A sample of genomic DNA, usually 5 to 10 μg, is initially digested by one or more restriction enzymes and resolved in one dimension by agarose gel electrophoresis. Low-molecular-weight DNA, representing smaller fragments, tends to run farther into the gel than high-molecular-weight fragments. After electrophoresis, the gel is incubated in an alkaline solution, which denatures the DNA strands embedded within. Because DNA fragments cannot be handled directly on an agarose gel, the DNA is transferred (blotted) to a solid matrix on which hybridization reactions can occur. Nitrocellulose membranes confer a particular ability to trap single-stranded size-sorted DNA fragments. The DNA is immobilized on the membrane by being baked in an oven. This filter, or blot, can now be placed in a hybridization solution with a radioactively labeled probe that has been rendered single stranded by rapid boiling and quenching. Only fragments that are complementary to a particular probe hybridize with it.

FIGURE 27.1-5   Southern analysis of a series of breast cancer tumors for presence of estrogen receptors reveals a normal pattern in lane 1 (HT415) and loss of alleles in three samples (28T, 29T, and possibly 51T) as represented by deletion of specific bands. A probe labeling a ubiquitous DNA species of 2.1 kb demonstrates the consistency of DNA concentration from sample to sample. (Courtesy of Dr. Irene Andrulis, Samuel Lunenfeld Research Institute, Toronto)

After excess and nonspecifically bound probe is washed off, the hybridization can be visualized through autoradiography. Each complementary sequence gives rise to a band at a position on the gel that is determined by the size of the DNA fragment. The size of the DNA fragments can be estimated by correlating the observed band positions with marker DNA fragments of known molecular weight. The amount of DNA in the sample can be estimated by the intensity of the autoradiographic signal.

Southern blotting permits a particular sequence of DNA to be detected by hybridization in the midst of an innumerable number of DNA fragments. The technique detects large deletions and insertions as represented by the presence of junction fragments or changes in band intensities in blots. It should be noted that, as long as some of the sequence of the probe is complementary to the target, it will hybridize. Further, the probe also satisfactorily hybridizes to fragments of DNA that it only partly covers, yielding several different fragments after Southern blotting. If they alter the restriction sites that were originally used to digest the genomic DNA, point mutations

in the DNA fragment can also be detected. Two restriction endonucleases, MspI and TaqI, have four-base recognition sites in the DNA sequence (CCGG and TCGA, respectively). Because these contain the mutation-prone dinucleotide sequence CpG, they are particularly useful restriction enzymes to scan for mutations by Southern blot.[21] Southern blot analysis has also been used to identify related genes, such as oncogenes, within cells of different species. For example, when DNA fragments from several species are digested with a restriction enzyme, run on an agarose gel, blotted, and hybridized with a mouse probe, the probe recognizes homologous sequences not only of mouse DNA but also of the DNA in the other species. Similarities in these gene sequences are shown by the presence of bands on the autoradiograph in lanes from each DNA sample. The implication of such a "zoo blot" is that the fragments of DNA have been conserved through evolution and presumably represent functionally important regions of the genome.

Pulse-Field Gel Electrophoresis

Although Southern blot analysis has proved to be a powerful tool in molecular biology, it has certain shortcomings. In particular, fragments larger than 20 kilobases are poorly resolved on conventional agarose gels. To overcome this problem, several related methods have been developed that use alterations in the electrical field applied to the DNA and that increase the resolution of the larger fragments. Basically, pulses of current rather than a constant field are used. This pulse-field gel electrophoresis (PFGE) causes the DNA molecules to align in a linear fashion within the field. The size range in which fragments resolve depends on the position of electrode placement and the duration of the pulses. By using some of the variations of PFGE, it is possible to separate fragments as large as 7×10^6 base pairs. The use of restriction endonucleases that recognize larger sequences (8′ base pair sequences) yields a manageable number of fragments that can then be probed with the DNA sequence of interest. The ability of PFGE to resolve large fragments has permitted construction of physical maps of genomes from primitive organisms as well as of small chromosomes. The genome of *Escherichia coli*, which is approximately 10×10^6 base pairs long, has been mapped in this fashion,[22] as have the maps of other bacterial, yeast, and mammalian chromosomes, including human.[23]

Northern Blot Analysis

Northern blotting or transfer is a variation of the Southern technique, differing in that mRNA is the target material for hybridization. The sequence of manipulations is similar to that used for Southern blotting, but there are some important differences. First, fragmentation of RNA is usually not necessary, because mRNA species are already in the size range that is appropriate for electrophoresis and transfer. Second, denaturation of the molecule is required before transfer to disrupt the secondary structure of the unique mRNA species. Without this step, the structure would probably interfere with electrophoretic separation. The electrophoresis itself is also done under denaturing conditions to maintain the looser structure. Third, special precautions must be used in extracting and manipulating the RNA to avoid ubiquitous RNases from destroying the molecule and rendering the Northern analysis uninterpretable. The initial agarose gel electrophoresis usually indicates whether the RNA quality is adequate for analysis.

The size of the RNA sample that is probed can be estimated by correlating the band positions on the gel with marker RNA fragments of known molecular weight in a manner similar to that used for DNA fragments on a Southern blot. An estimate of the amount of RNA in the sample is estimated from the intensity of the autoradiographic signal. Thus, Northern analysis can show both quantitative and qualitative information on steady-state mRNA transcripts and can identify the presence of amplified gene expression. This has been applied to N-*MYC* expression in different clinical stages of neuroblastoma, or hybrid transcripts in rearranged genomic loci, such as the novel eight-kilobase *BCR-ABL* transcript that is expressed in chronic myelogenous leukemia and represents the molecular alteration of the t(9;22) chromosomal translocation.[24,25]

RNase Protection Analysis

Northern analysis provides data on the approximate size of an mRNA transcript but does not indicate the 5′ or 3′ ends with any precision or give information on the exon–intron structure of the DNA template from which the mRNA is derived. The nuclease S_1 protection assay, or RNase protection assay, is one method to accomplish this and can also be used to better quantitate particularly minute amounts of RNA. The basic method involves the protection of double-stranded hybrids from the degrading action of nucleases. A hybrid is formed between mRNA and a complementary DNA probe. The addition of nucleases specifically degrades single-stranded DNA or RNA and leaves double-stranded structures intact. These complexes are then analysed by polyacrylamide gel electrophoresis (Fig. 27.1-6). The extent to which the RNA protects the radiolabeled DNA probe from degradation indicates the structure of the RNA. Because conditions for annealing RNA–DNA are highly selective, S_1 nuclease protection analysis is very sensitive. If sufficient amounts of RNA are available, one mRNA molecule in 100 cells can be detected.

Western Blot Analysis

To follow convention, the electrophoretic blotting technique used to detect and analyze proteins has been designed Western analysis. Protein isolated from tissues, blood, or cells is subjected to electrophoresis on polyacrylamide gels that often contains a detergent—sodium dode-

FIGURE 27.1-6 Schematic representation of RNase protection analysis to determine full-length message versus abnormal patterns. See text for details. (Courtesy of Dr. Carolyn Felix, Children's Hospital of Philadelphia)

cylsulfate—to separate the molecules by their molecular weight. The separated protein is then transferred to a filter using high-voltage electrophoresis. This process is distinguished from RNA or DNA transfer, which is based on capillary action and compressive forces. Enzyme-linked or isotopically labeled antibodies that are species specific are applied to the filter. After recognizing their specific protein, the antibodies bind, and the protein antibody bands can then be visualized by either autoradiographic or calorimetric methods.[4,26,27]

In Situ Hybridization

The technique of in situ hybridization is based on the principle that a labeled nucleic acid probe, when rendered single stranded by heat denaturation, binds specifically to complementary sequences in fixed tissue or on a spread of denatured metaphase chromosomes. After binding has occurred and excess labeled probe has been removed, the location of the probe can be visualized by either radiographic or fluorescein-based methods, depending on what tag was used on the probe. Traditionally, probes were labeled with tritium. After hybridization and washing, the slides were dipped in a photographic emulsion and stored for various periods. Disintegration of the radioactive tritium produced silver grains in the emulsion, which could be scored against specific regions of tissue or chromosome. The disadvantages of this method include the high background of silver grains, the long incubation times required to obtain sufficient numbers of silver grains, and the lack of precise localization of the signal due to scatter of the silver grains around the region of hybridization. For these reasons, nonisotopic methods of labeling of probes with fluorochromes have been developed. This modification is known as fluorescent in situ hybridization (FISH). After hybridization, the signal can be visualized directly by either

fluorescent microscopy or laser-scanning confocal microscopy. This technique is more rapid, less labor intensive, and less prone to scatter than isotope-based in situ hybridization. Further, using different fluorochromes for different probes, it is possible to perform two-color or multicolor fluorescence. In this manner, the relative positions of probes can be deduced. This tool becomes particularly valuable when mapping the relative chromosomal positions of different, closely spaced genes (Fig. 27.1-7).

As has been alluded to, in situ hybridization can be used to locate DNA sequences on chromosomes or to detect the presence of RNA or viral DNA. The method is facilitated by the current ability to generate specific probes by the cloning of DNA sequences or the synthesis of oligonucleotides. For in situ hybridization to succeed, it is critical that the target nucleic acid be retained intact in situ, that it not be degraded by nucleases, and that it be accessible for hybridization to the probe. Unlike the hybridization of nucleic acids in solution for Southern, Northern, and Western analyses, the target in situ nucleic acid is much less accessible to the probe. Therefore, its stability is often markedly decreased under these conditions. The theoretic foundation for this form of hybridization is poorly understood, and aspects of the procedures of in situ hybridization are frequently done on a largely empiric basis. Careful interpretation of results must therefore consider the sensitivity, specificity, and resolution of the particular method used.

Several factors affect the sensitivity of in situ hybridization. They include the accessibility of the target, the method of probe labeling and detection, the length of the probe, whether the probe is RNA or DNA, and whether it is single or double stranded. Maximal sensitivity is frequently required and can be significantly limited by the level of nonspecific background staining, particularly where silver staining is used. The specificity of the binding

FIGURE 27.1-7 FISH analysis of tumors. Neuroblastoma with 70 copies of N-*myc* present as a homogeneously staining region (HSR) on chromosome 4. In the interphase nuclei of the tumor, the yellow-green domain of amplified DNA can easily be seen (*white areas*). The N-*myc* probe is labeled with biotin and detected with avidin conjugated to a yellow fluorochrome. The preparation is counterstained with propidium iodide, giving the red fluorescence of DNA (*gray areas*). (Courtesy of Dr. Jeremy Squire, The Hospital for Sick Children, Toronto).

of the probe and target binding is influenced by the stringency with which the probe is washed after hybridization occurs as well as by the extent of similarity between the probe and sequences related to but distinct from the target sequence. Nonspecific signals can occur from several sources and may resemble background "noise." Resolution of the signal of probe–target binding can vary from subcellular localization, or even subnuclear localization, to greater than the cell diameter. The specific technique is frequently modified to optimize the degree of the signal for the particular target to be identified.

Cloning Genes

Molecular cloning may be defined as the isolation and amplification of specifically defined DNA fragments. It is a process that involves the manipulation of DNA with various enzymes followed by isolation of the desired nucleic acid sequence by screening of the DNA with specific probes. In addition to the previously described restriction endonucleases that are important in cutting the DNA into several fragments, a group of enzymes known as *ligases* are of critical importance in cloning experiments. DNA ligase reseals the cohesive ends of two DNA fragments. A third ingredient in cloning procedures are constructs called *vectors,* which are primarily plasmids and bacteriophage DNA. Vectors have been designed that allow expression of mRNA and protein products encoded by the cloned fragment. Figure 27.1-8 outlines the procedure of genomic cloning of small fragments of DNA into a vector. Essentially, genomic DNA is cut into fragments by the addition of restriction enzymes. These fragments can then be specifically ligated into a vector containing a site that has also been cut with restriction enzymes and that is able to accept the foreign DNA. After being transferred into a bacterium such as *E coli,* small plasmids, which are circular DNA molecules, use the enzymes of the organism to replicate separately (autonomously) from the bacterial chromosome. Plasmids often contain drug-resistance genes, which render the bacterium that harbors the plasmid resistant to antibiotics such as ampicillin or kanamycin. If the foreign DNA that has been ligated into the plasmid positionally disrupts the drug resistance gene, recombinants (ie, bacterial plasmids with foreign DNA inserts) can be isolated. This is because only plasmids with disrupted drug-resistance genes are sensitive to the antibiotic. Commercially available plasmids also use the *LACZ* gene as a marker for the presence of inserts. Typically, the bacteria are grown on X-gal, an artificial substrate for the *LACZ*-encoded enzyme, and, in the presence of a *LACZ* gene promoter, bacteria with intact plasmids produce blue colonies on agar. Where the plasmids have incorporated foreign DNA, the colonies are white. A combination of drug resistance and color selection can be used to select for bacteria that carry a DNA insert of interest.[4]

Unfortunately, plasmids do not accommodate large vectors; for these, the development of bacteriophage vectors has been significant. They are capable of accepting DNA fragments of up to 20 kilobases. To handle even larger amounts of DNA, fragments are incorporated into specialized vectors such as cosmids or yeast artificial chromosomes. The former have the part of the plasmid genome that allows autonomous replication and the phage sequences required for packaging into the phage virion.[28] The average insert size for a yeast artificial chromosome is 350 kilobases, which represents a huge increase on the maximal insert of a plasmid vector.

A key step in the cloning of novel genes is the initial preparation of *libraries,* or banks of recombinant vectors, in which all the original inserted DNA sequences corresponding to the complete genome are represented at least once. In practice, such an all-inclusive library is difficult to achieve, and several different libraries may be required to augment the chances of total representation. Two types of library are commonly used. The first is prepared from genomic DNA, which is first digested with a rare cutter-restriction enzyme. After being mixed with a similarly precut vector, the DNA fragments are allowed to be ligated into the vector and the plasmids are plated with susceptible bacteria on agar. Bacteria infected with the vector are lysed, and clear areas known as *plaques* form on the agar surface. The surface can then be screened with a probe to detect the desired recombinant DNA clone. This screening process is similar to the Southern blotting technique. The colonies, or plaques, are transferred to membranes, which are then treated to denature the DNA and hybridized with the single-stranded probe. Positive spots are detected by autoradiography and, when the filter is overlaid on the agar plate, the corresponding colony

Mendelian disorder—clear mode of inheritance

↓

Find DNA markers consegregating with disease gene locus

↓

Establish firm genetic linkage to a marker

↓

Localize to specific chromosomal region

↓

Search for more closely linked markers

↓

Chromosome walk and jump to disease gene locus

↓

Clone gene and determine nucleotide sequence

↓

Compare DNA sequences of normal and affected individuals

↓

Infer amino acid sequence of protein product

↓

Isolate protein product of normal and disease genes

FIGURE 27.1-8 Reverse genetics, or positional cloning, is represented here in a flow diagram in which the clinical observation of a mendelian disorder, such as hereditary early-onset breast cancer, ultimately yields cloning of a responsible gene and protein. Isolation of the protein is a critical step in understanding the pathogenesis of the disease.

containing the DNA insert can be identified. This technique can identify one recombinant molecule among millions of host genomic fragments. The colony with the relevant DNA insert can be grown to microgram or gram quantities for further analysis, which usually includes DNA sequencing to confirm the presence of the potentially novel gene. As one might expect, these DNA libraries can be reused indefinitely, employing different probes that recognize different DNA sequences to isolate other DNA segments and genes.

The second, and particularly powerful, method of cloning is to develop a cDNA library.[4] For this method, mRNA that has been isolated from specific cells or tissue is reverse transcribed to single-stranded DNA copies. DNA polymerase is used to generate double-stranded DNA fragments, which are then cloned into vectors. A particular advantage to cDNA libraries is that they are limited to only the transcribed portion of genes. They are therefore much less complex than genomic libraries. They provide amplified copies of specific sequences representative of the particular tissue or cell from which they have been derived.

Cloning genes whose protein products are unknown and whose existence is often inferred solely through a disease phenotype is more difficult than when at least part of the sequence is known. In these cases, reverse genetics or positional cloning is required. This tedious process is initiated by the establishment of genetic linkage to DNA markers, followed by mapping of the whole set of markers to a specific region of the chromosome. More closely linked markers are then sought, markers that ideally bracket and close in on the disease gene locus. These close markers can then provide starting points for sophisticated manipulations, including chromosome walking and jumping, in which successive sequences between markers are examined for functional genes. After a candidate gene is identified, it can be cloned and sequenced and its function deduced from structural homologies with other known proteins. This approach and variations on it were used to clone a gene localized to the long arm of chromosome 17 called *BRCA1* that has been implicated in the predisposition to early-onset hereditary breast and breast–ovarian cancer.[6–8]

The ultimate step in the confirmation that an isolated gene is important in the development of disease in an individual is the demonstration that the gene has a specific sequence difference, which may be as minimal as a single nucleotide change, between affected and unaffected individuals. The identification of point mutations in the coding region of the p53 tumor-suppressor gene in affected members of families with the Li-Fraumeni syndrome who are at particularly high risk for the development various cancers, including breast cancer, exemplifies the candidate gene approach to characterization of a disease gene.[29,30]

The eventual cloning of the entire human genome represents a major undertaking of the Human Genome Project. It is expected that the identification and characterization of these genes will lead to an explosion of research into the functional properties of the proteins that they encode. It is hoped that eventually, with the advent of genetic therapeutic technology, this work will directly lead to intervention strategies and the prevention or successful treatment of various human diseases.

Genetic Manipulation

TRANSGENIC ANIMALS

Organisms that carry genetic material that has been artificially introduced into the germline are said to be *transgenic*. The inserted transgene may be a segment of genomic DNA from either a homologous or heterologous species, or even from lower organisms, including prokaryotes and viruses. Cotransfer of regulatory sequences with the gene permits directed expression of the transgene in specific cells or tissue types; sometimes, when less specific expression is desired, ubiquitous regulatory sequences are used.

Three basic mechanisms have been developed for the introduction of foreign genes into the germline:

1. DNA can be directly injected into the pronucleus of a mouse embryo using a microscope that permits manipulation of the embryo.
2. Retroviral vectors can carry the foreign gene and transfer it into the embryo on "controlled" infection.
3. Embryonic stem cells can be manipulated to act as carriers of the transgene into the recipient blastocyst cells (see later).

After any of these forms of microinjection is completed, the embryos carrying the transgene are transplanted into pseudopregnant foster mothers. At birth, DNA is extracted from the offspring and assayed for the presence of the introduced foreign DNA. Assuming that the transgene does not alter the fertility of the offspring, they can then be bred, so that a certain fraction of the positive animals ultimately carries the transgene in the germline, the newly acquired trait frequently being transmitted through a classic mendelian mode of inheritance.[31–33]

The transgene is usually subject to normal gene regulation, and the introduction of the foreign DNA can often lead to the development of novel phenotypes. Ectopic or increased expression of certain oncogenes and aberrant expression of tumor-suppressor genes often generate phenotypes that become models for understanding the function of the gene and its encoded protein. Stable lineages of transgenic mice have been developed that express oncogenes and present reproducible preneoplastic or neoplastic phenotypes. When driven by a promoter of mouse mammary tumor viruses, c-*MYC* transgenic mice develop mammary adenocarcinomas, whereas under the regulation of an immunoglobulin promoter, the same transgene yields pre-B and B-cell lymphomas. Similarly, cyclin D transgenic mice develop, with a somewhat lower yield, mammary adenocarcinomas.[34] This observation shows the direct association of the expression of these genes with the development of their respective tumors. It is also possible that the abnormal expression of the gene in certain tissues or cell types is not associated with an altered phenotype, indicating the absent role of the gene in the malignant transformation of that tissue.

EMBRYONIC STEM CELL TRANSFER

A powerful technique for the introduction of foreign genes into the germline and generation of transgenic mice takes advantage of cultured embryonic stem cells. These are pluripotent cells derived from the mouse blastocyst (the early stage of embryonic development that precedes implantation of the fertilized egg in the uterus). The embryonic stem cells can be altered in vitro and then reunited with the blastocyst cells to form chimeric animals. Genes are transfected into the embryonic stem cells by electroporation, chemical methods, or microinjection. When the donor carries an additional genomic sequence, such as a drug resistance marker or a particular enzyme, the cells that have incorporated the desired gene can be selected. PCR can also be used to assay the transfected embryonic stem cells for successful integration of the donor DNA. After the embryonic stem cells have reunited with the recipient blastocyst, some tissues derived from the chimera are of blastocyst origin, whereas others are derived from the injected embryonic stem cells. To determine whether the embryonic stem cells contributed to the germline lineage, the chimeric mouse is crossed with a mouse that lacks the donor trait. Any progeny that carry the trait must be derived from germ cells descended from the injected embryonic stem cells. In other words, the entire mouse has been generated from an original embryonic stem cell. Among the most sophisticated applications of this application is the introduction of a gene that undergoes homologous recombination with a target gene. In this manner, the normal function of a gene can be disrupted and animal models of the consequences of such disruption can be developed. An example of this process is the generation of mice homozygous or heterozygous for disrupted p53 function. These mice have an increased and more rapid tendency to develop various tumors, including adenocarcinoma of the breast.[35] Other mouse models of breast carcinogenesis are being developed as genes involved in this disease are isolated and characterized.

GENE THERAPY

Transgenic mice have become an important tool in both the development of gene therapy protocols and the eventual correction of genetic defects or reversion of malignant transformation. Because the goal of gene therapy is to introduce a gene into a patient's body to replace or to repair defective gene function, many of the methodologic principles developed in the study of transgenic animals may find their application in humans. The augmentation of healthy recipient genes is the most studied and practical approach. It is being used in clinical trials of the addition of a functional adenosine deaminase gene to patients with severe combined immunodeficiency syndrome.[36,37]

Perhaps the most critical problems that have impeded the translation of preclinical and animal studies of gene therapy into effective clinical protocols have been the significant technical limitations of most procedures.[36] For example, although retroviral vectors carrying transgenes are able to transduce nearly all target cells, their entry into cells depends on the presence of an appropriate receptor on the target cell, most of which are not known. Furthermore, it may be necessary to induce cell mitosis to assist viral integration into the DNA of the target cell. Finally, it is often difficult to maintain more than transient integration of viral DNA, since the retroviruses are themselves unstable in the milieu of the host cell. Much effort has been dedicated to the development of gene therapy protocols based on hematopoietic disease in which the transgene is introduced into bone marrow stem cells of the host, which are then a continual source of genetically modified hematopietic cells during the patient's lifetime. By increasing the number of transducible stem cells, and by optimizing the transfer of the transgene into them, it may be possible to correct many genetic defects that affect the hematopoietic system. The correction of the malignant phenotype of solid tumors remains the more significant challenge.

Perhaps the most difficult challenge of all is that few human disorders, including both malignant and nonmalignant diseases of the breast, result from single-gene defects. Until effective methods of multigene therapy are developed, it is unlikely that this mode of treatment will find universal use. It is nevertheless important to recognize that only 40 years have passed since the discovery of the double helix. There is every reason to maintain unbridled optimism that the technical and theoretic developments in molecular biology will ultimately lead to the better prevention, screening, treatment, and cure of human disease.

ACKNOWLEDGMENTS

This investigation was supported by Grant no. 3128, awarded by the National Cancer Institute of Canada and Grant no. MT-11616, awarded by the Medical Research Council of Canada.

References

1. Lewin B, Genes V. ed 5. New York, Oxford University, 1994
2. Watson JD, Hopkins NH, Roberts JW, et al. Molecular biology of the gene, ed 4. Menlo Park, CA Benjamin Cummings, 1987.
3. Alberts B, Bray D, Lewis J, et al. Molecular biology of the cell, ed 2. New York, Garland, 1989.
4. Sambrook J, Fritsch EF, Maniatis T. Molecular cloning: a laboratory manual, ed 2. Cold Spring Harbor, NY, Cold Spring Harbor Laboratory, 1989.
5. Watson JD, Crick FH. Molecular structure of nucleic acids: a structure for deoxyribonucleic acid. Nature 1953;171:964.
6. Hall JM, Lee MK, Newman B, et al. Linkage of early-onset familial breast cancer to chromosome 17q21. Science 1990;250:1684.
7. Easton DF, Bishop DT, Ford D, et al. Genetic linkage analysis in familial breast and ovarian cancer: results from 214 families. Am J Hum Genet 1993;52:678.
8. Albertsen HM, Plaetke R, Ballard L, et al. Genetic mapping of the

BRCA1 region on chromosome 17q21. Am J Hum Genet 1994; 54:516.

9. Mullis KB, Faloona FA. Specific synthesis of DNA in vitro via a polymerase-catalysed chain reaction. Methods Enzymol 1987; 155:335.

10. Maxam AM, Gilbert W. A new method for sequencing DNA. Proc Natl Acad Sci USA 1977;74:560.

11. Sanger F, Nicklen S, Coulson AR. DNA sequencing with chain-terminating inhibitors. Proc Natl Acad Sci USA 1977;74:5463.

12. Orita M, Iwahana H, Kanazawa H, et al. Detection of polymorphisms of human DNA by gel electrophoresis as single-strand conformation polymorphisms. Proc Natl Acad Sci USA 1989;86:2766.

13. Iwahana H, Yoshimoto K, Itakara M. Detection of point mutations by SSCP of PCR-amplified DNA after endonuclease digestion. Biotechniques 1992;12:64.

14. Yap EP, McGee JO. Nonisotopic SSCP detection in PCR products by ethidium bromide staining. Trends Genet 1992;8:49.

15. Makino R. F-SSCP: fluorescence-based SSCP analysis. PCR Methods Applic 1992;2:10.

16. Ainsworth PJ, Surh LC, Coulter MMB. Diagnostic single strand conformational polymorphism (SSCP); a simplified non-radioisotopic method as applied to Tay-Sachs B1 variant. Nucleic Acids Res 1991;19:405.

17. Myers RM, Maniatis T, Lerman LS. Detection and localization of single base changes by denaturing gradient gel electrophoresis. Meth Enzymol 1987;155:501.

18. Sheffield VC, Cox DR, Lerman LS, et al. Attachment of a 40-base pair G+C-rich sequence (GC-clamp) to genomic DNA fragments by the polymerase chain reaction results in improved detection of single-base changes. Proc Natl Acad Sci USA 1989;86:232.

19. Hovig E, Smith-Sorensen B, Brogger A, et al. Constant denaturant gel electrophoresis, a modification of denaturing gradient gel electrophoresis, in mutation detection. Mutat Res 1991;262:63.

20. Southern EM. Detection of specific sequences among DNA fragments separated by gel electrophoresis. J Mol Biol 1975;98:503.

21. Cooper DN, Youssoufian H. The CpG dinucleotide and human genetic disease. Hum Genet 1988;78:151.

22. Smith CL, Econome JG, Schutt A, et al. A physical map of the *Escherichia coli* K12 genome. Science 1987;236:1448.

23. O'Brien SJ. Genetic maps 1987: a compilation of linkage and restriction maps of genetically studied organisms, vol. 4. Cold Spring Harbor, NY, Cold Spring Harbor Laboratory, 1987.

24. Shtivelman E, Lifshitz B, Gale RP, et al. Fused transcript of *ABL* and *BCR* genes in chronic myelogenous leukemia. Nature 1986;315:550.

25. Grosveld G, Verwoerd T, Van Agthoven T, et al. The chronic myelocytic cell line K562 contains a breakpoint in *BCR* and produces a chimeric *BCR/c-ABL* transcript. Mol Cell Biol 1986;6:607.

26. Towbin H, Staehelin T, Gordon J. Electrophoretic transfer of proteins from polyacrylamide gels to nitrocellulose sheets: procedure and some applications. Proc Natl Acad Sci USA 1979;76:4350.

27. Burnette WN. "Western blotting." electrophoretic transfer of proteins from sodium dodecylsulfate polyacrylamide gels to unmodified nitrocellulose and radiographic detection with antibody and radioiodinated protein A. Ann Biochem 1981;112:195.

28. Saito I, Stark GR. Charomids: cosmid vectors for efficient cloning and mapping of large or small restriction fragments. Proc Natl Acad Sci USA 1986;83:8664.

28a. Miki Y, Swensen J, Shattuck-Eidens D, et al. A strong candidate for the breast and ovarian cancer susceptibility gene BRCA1. Science 1994;266:66.

28b. Futreal PA, Liu Q, Shattuck-Eidens D, et al. BRCA1 mutations in primary breast and ovarian carcinomas. Science 1994;266:120.

29. Malkin D, Li FP, Strong LC, et al. Germ line *p53* mutations in a familial syndrome of breast cancer, sarcomas, and other neoplasms. Science 1990;250:1233.

30. Srivastava S, Zou ZQ, Pirollo K, et al. Germ line transmission of a mutated p53 gene in a cancer-prone family with Li-Fraumeni syndrome. Nature 1990;348:747.

31. Palmiter RD, Brinster RL. Germ-line transformation of mice. Annu Rev Genet 1986;20:465.

32. De Tolla I. Transgenic animal models. Comp Pathol Bull 1990;22:1.

33. Hogan B, Constantini F, Lacy E. Manipulating the mouse embryo. Cold Spring Harbor, NY, Cold Spring Harbor Laboratory, 1986.

34. Wang TC, Cardiff RD, Zukerberg L, et al. Mammary hyperplasia and carcinoma in MMTV-cyclin D1 transgenic mice. Nature 1994;369:669.

35. Donehower LA, Harvey M, Slagle BL, et al. Mice deficient for p53 are developmentally normal but susceptible to spontaneous tumors. Nature 1992;356:215.

36. Mulligan RC. The basic science of gene therapy. Science 1993;260:926.

37. Salmons B, Gunzberg WH. Targeting of retroviral vectors for gene therapy. Hum Gene Ther 1993;4:129.

27.2
Techniques in the Interpretation of Clinical Trials

REBECCA GELMAN

The statistical techniques relevant for design and analysis of clinical trials are usually taught in 10 to 20 graduate-level courses, and the subjects of data base and forms design, protocol writing, and data monitoring could easily extend over a similar number of courses (although education in these subjects is far more likely to take place in on-the-job training and at workshops). New statistical methods are appearing in the medical literature more rapidly after publication in the statistical literature than they were 20 years ago, making it impossible to squeeze even a superficial survey of relevant techniques into a single course or book. As stated in a recent article in the *Journal of the American Medical Association,* "Already the standard methods taught in an introductory [statistics] course would leave a reader unable to judge a high percentage of articles published in the *New England Journal of Medicine,* and that proportion is likely to increase with time."[1]

This chapter will also leave a reader unable to judge the quality of a high percentage of literature reports on breast cancer trials. A single book on clinical trials[2–8] can be compared with a beginning course in cooking. A successful cooking course teaches a student to prepare one particular (and simple) dinner for friends; a successful clinical trials book can teach a student to design and analyze one particular (and simple) clinical trial. In this analogy, a chapter about clinical trials should be considered an antacid. It does not teach anyone how to cook or how to appreciate good cooking. It merely ameliorates some of the symptoms caused by bad cooking or overconsumption. Unfortunately, the indigestion caused by clinical trials is more varied than the indigestion caused by food, and not all types can be treated by a single brand of antacid. The indication for this chapter is indigestion caused by controversies in statistical power and confidence intervals, survival analysis, trial monitoring, subgroup analyses, and metaanalysis.

Quantification of Treatment Differences: Power and Confidence Intervals

POWER

Here is a common cause of indigestion. A journal article on one randomized trial states that treatment C is associated with significantly longer survival than treatment D, but another journal article on a similar trial states that treatment C and D do not differ in survival. How do we explain these inconsistent results? A clinician might look first at the authors of the two articles and decide which are more experienced or reliable. Or the clinician might look first at specifics of eligibility and at the patient mix on the two trials. A statistician will most likely look first for statements about the power of the two trials. People who read the medical literature should be interested in the statistical power of clinical trials because there are two major explanations for a comparison that fails to be statistically significant:

1. The null hypothesis is true. (In breast cancer, the most common null hypothesis amounts to a statement that two treatments have the same effect on some specified outcome measure.)
2. The alternative hypothesis is true, but the trial did not have enough power to detect this.

So if readers do not know the power of the trial, they cannot choose the most likely explanation for a nonsignificant comparison. People who plan clinical trials should be interested in power because no one wants to do all the work involved in conducting a trial if it was planned in such a way that it is highly likely to have an ambiguous result. What is power?

One can think of a statistical test as a type of diagnostic test. In both cases, we are trying to find out about "the true state of the world"—for example, does patient P really have disease S, or is treatment C really associated with longer survival than treatment D? (For this example, assume that the null hypothesis of the study is that treatments C and D have the same survival, and the alternative hypothesis is that C has longer survival.) We try to predict the true state of the world from test results (eg, a blood glucose level 2 hours after eating or the value of a log-

rank test of survival). Usually, these results are compared to a single cut-off value, such as 130 mg/dL for the blood glucose level or 3.84 for the log-rank test. (In these examples, high numbers are predictive for the patient having diabetes or for the treatments having different survival.) Either test could have a false-positive result: a nondiabetic patient could have a high glucose level, or two similar treatments could have a large log-rank value. For the statistical test, the probability of a false-positive result is called the *significance* level or *P value*. (For the diagnostic test, 1 minus the probability of a false-positive result is called the *specificity*.) Either test could have a false-negative result: a diabetic patient could have a low glucose level, or two treatments could have a log-rank value near 0 even if treatment C truly is associated with longer survival than treatment D. In both cases, 1 minus the probability of a false-negative result is called the *sensitivity* of the test. For the statistical test, this value is more commonly called the *power* of the clinical trial.

Not all diagnostic tests have the same sensitivity, and not all clinical trials have the same power. It is desirable to have a large power, and most clinical trialists would consider a power less than 80% to be inadequate (since it would correctly decide in favor of the alternative hypothesis less than four times out of five when the alternative is true). Larger powers than this (eg, 90% or 95%) are appropriate for clinical trials the results of which would affect large numbers of future patients, because in such a case an error in deciding which treatment is better would affect more people.

The calculation of power is based on three quantities—the size of the relevant treatment effect, the largest tolerable probability of a false-positive result (the significance level), and the effective sample size. The relevant treatment effect is either the smallest treatment difference it is clinically important to detect (for a trial with the alternative hypothesis that treatments are different) or the largest difference that is clinically unimportant (for a trial with the alternative hypothesis that treatments are equivalent). How the difference is expressed depends on the endpoint chosen, the difference measure used, and the statistical test to be used; "difference" here need not be subtraction but could be a ratio or a more complicated expression. It is important that the difference specified be both clinically relevant (would this much of an improvement be important to the patient?) and scientifically realistic (based on past studies of these and other treatments, is it reasonable to expect these treatments to differ this much in effect?). For instance, a 40% increase in response percent (eg, from 50% to 90%) in a trial of two combination chemotherapies for metastatic breast cancer would be highly unusual, so such a large difference would probably not be realistic. Similarly, a doubling of median survival time in a trial of adjuvant therapy among a group of patients with primary breast cancer would also be unrealistic. In addition, if not all patients are expected to complete the treatment, the relevant treatment effect refers to the effect in the "average" patient, *not* the effect in a patient who completes all therapy as specified in the protocol.

The most common significance level in the medical

literature is .05, but there is nothing magic about this particular number (although a few journal editors have mistakenly made it sacred by demanding that each published article contain at least one *P* value of .05 or less). In trials whose results affect large numbers of future patients, a smaller significance level (eg, .01 or even .001) might be appropriate. In *equivalence* trials, a larger significance level (eg, a false-positive probability of .10 or .20) is frequently considered tolerable in order to obtain a larger than usual power (eg, a false-negative probability of .05); it is really a question of which error is considered more disastrous and whether a 1 in 20 chance of a disastrous outcome is considered small enough. If the nonequivalence of treatments A and B is possible only if B is better than A, a *one-sided* significance level is used (eg, when A is placebo and B is a treatment without any possible detrimental effect). Otherwise, a *two-sided* significance level is used. Generally, a two-sided calculation should be done unless a significant result in one direction (eg, A better than B) would be ignored and would not be reported as an important difference.

The effective sample size is determined by which endpoint is being studied. For example, in a study of response percentages, the effective sample size is the number of patients included in the analysis; in a study of time to event (eg, death), the effective sample size is the number of observed *events* (eg, deaths). (The number of patients who have died is always smaller than the number of patients entered on the trial multiplied by the death rate as read from an actuarial curve, unless all patients still alive have follow-up longer than the last death time.) In planning a clinical trial based on time to event, one must estimate the number of events that will have occurred at the time of analysis. In reporting a trial, one knows the actual number of events that have occurred. The difference between these two numbers (expected and actual number of events) can make a slight difference between planned power and power calculated at time of analysis. Power calculation methods are detailed elsewhere.[9–22]

Table 27.2-1 shows how the power of a particular clinical trial depends on the relevant endpoint and difference measure. (This example is based on results from a Ludwig Breast Cancer Study Group Trial.[23]) All the power calculations assume the same number of randomized patients (2000), the same duration of accrual (2 years), the same median follow-up (5 years), the same two-sided significance level (.05), the same statistical test (log-rank), and the same statistical distribution for time to event (negative exponential). The size of the treatment effect is measured in three ways common in breast cancer literature: the difference between treatments in the percentage of patients who have the event within the first 5 years of follow-up, the ratio of the average hazard rates over the first 5 years, and the odds ratio at 5 years. (*Hazard rate* is the instantaneous risk of the event, which is mathematically equivalent to the derivative of the log of cumulative percentage survival. The *odds ratio* is the ratio of failure percentages divided by the ratio of nonfailure percentage. To many people, the hazard ratio and odds ratio numbers in Table 27.2-1 seem to represent a bigger treatment difference than the numbers for difference in failure percentages. However, the three numbers in each row of Table 27.2-1 are merely different ways to quantitate the identical difference between treatments. In any trial in which a small percentage of patients have had the event of interest, the difference in failure percentages looks small compared with the equivalent hazard ratio or odds ratio.) From Table 27.2-1, one might conclude that the trial has adequate power for reasonable treatment differences in some endpoints (eg, disease-free interval) but not others (eg, systemic disease-free survival and overall survival).

There have been several surveys of the medical literature that show that most trials do not have enough patients to have a good chance of detecting even large differences in treatment outcome, let alone reasonable differences. Freiman and colleagues[24] reviewed 71 "negative" trials (not restricted to cancer studies) in major medical journals and found that 50 of the trials had at least a 10% risk of missing a 50% "therapeutic improvement." Zelen and coworkers[25] surveyed articles

TABLE 27.2-1
Power for Various Endpoints Based on Ludwig III*

Endpoint	5-Year Failure-Free Percent		Difference in 5-Year Failure Free Percent	Hazard Ratio	Odds Ratio	Power
	Observation	*CMFpT*				
Disease-free interval	31	66	35	2.8	4.3	.88
Disease-free survival	30	57	27	2.1	3.1	.74
Systemic disease-free survival	37	58	21	1.8	2.4	.46
Survival						
Breast cancer deaths only	61	76	15	1.8	2.0	.16
All deaths	59	70	11	1.5	1.6	.11

* Assuming 2000 patients, 2 years of accrual, 5-year median follow-up.

on randomized trials appearing in *Cancer* between 1977 and 1979 and found the median trial size to be 50 per treatment (range, 10 to 400; 70% had fewer than 100 patients per treatment). Mosteller and colleagues[26] reviewed cancer trials referenced in the 1978 book *Randomized Trials in Cancer: A Critical Review by Sites*.[27] They found 108 randomized breast cancer trials with a distribution of sample sizes was similar to that found by Zelen—median size, 45 per treatment; range, 5 to 750. In the small survey my colleagues and I conducted in 1984,[28] the median accrual for randomized trials in metastatic breast cancer was 57 per treatment (range, 21 to 110); the median accrual for randomized adjuvant trials was 190 per treatment (range, 36 to 614). These surveys probably overestimate the median size of clinical trials because small "negative" trials do not always get published. To put these surveys in perspective, Table 27.2-2 uses the methods given in references 11 and 16 to calculate what differences would have an 80% chance of being detected as significant in trials with 25, 50, 100, 200, 500, 1000, and 2000 patients per treatment. For example, it would take 100 patients per treatment to have a power of 80% to detect a difference in true response percentages of 20% (50% on one arm and 70% on the other), yet many published trials accrue only half this many patients. The survival example assumes an exponential survival curve (which may not be appropriate for adjuvant breast cancer[29] but which is a common simplifying assumption in sample size calculations) and that the worse treatment is associated with a median survival of 10 years and that accrual takes 2 years. It also assumed that there are either 3 or 8 years of additional follow-up after accrual ends (for a 5- or 10-year study, respectively). Not until the sample size reaches 500 does the detectable difference become at all reason-

able. There are many who would argue that even 2000 patients per treatment is not enough, since a 1-year improvement in median survival time would be of great clinical importance in a disease that kills some 50,000 women a year in the United States.

Unfortunately, there is no standard place in a medical journal article where one can find power statements. The power of a trial can be given in the materials and methods section, the results section, or the discussion. It is often completely absent, especially in trials that have significant results (in which case the probability of a false-negative result is not directly relevant). For purposes of comparing different trials in the literature, however, and for gauging how well a trial was planned, it would be useful to include statements about power in all articles on clinical trials.

CONFIDENCE INTERVALS

An X% *confidence interval* (CI) for a parameter is an interval that has the property that, if the trial is replicated identically many times, X% of such CIs will include the true parameter value. Of course, in actual practice, no trial is replicated exactly, so the more common interpretation is that the X% CI from a particular trial has an X% chance of containing the true parameter. The ends of the CI are called *confidence limits*. The true parameter is never observed; it is estimated from the data. A common parameter for use with CIs is the mean. For example, one may read that "the average [an estimate of mean] number of bone scans a patient has during the first 5 years of follow-up is 6, with a 95% CI [for the true mean] of 3 to 7." Another common parameter for use with CIs is the true percentage. For example, one may read that "there was 70% response [the observed percentage, an estimate of true percentage] on this therapy, with 95% confidence limits [for the true percentage] of 46% and 88%. (The phrases about "observed" and "true" parameters are often omitted because they are assumed to be "understood".) There is a common misperception that CIs are always symmetric about the observed parameter (eg, average ± twice the standard deviation [SD]). In fact, CIs are symmetric only when the true distribution of the parameter is symmetric, and this is often not the case with biologic measurements. CIs for percentages are often approximated by gaussian (ie, normal) distributions, but these approximations are inaccurate if the number of patients they are based on is less than 30, or for any number of patients if the percentage being estimated is not between 20% and 80%. The confidence interval for a mean is gaussian if the sample size is large enough, but means are not often used in breast cancer clinical trials (and are inappropriate for time-to-event data because of censoring).

CIs are easiest to calculate if the underlying distribution is gaussian, in which case the interval is symmetric, and this has resulted in the vast overuse of gaussian confidence limits (and hence the high prevalence of symmetric CIs) in the medical literature. However, some investigators have noted that "the experimental

TABLE 27.2-2

Differences That Could Be Detected With Significance Level .05 and Power 0.80

Patients per Treatment	Larger Response Percent if Lower One is:		Longer Median Survival if Shorter One is 10 Years, Accrual Takes 2 Years, and Additional Follow-Up is:	
	50%	70%	3 Years	8 Years
25	89	99.8	180	44
50	79	93	44	26
100	71	87	26	19
200	65	83	19	16
500	59	78	15	13
1000	56	76	13	12
2000	55	74	12	11.5

fact is that for most physiologic variables the distribution is smooth, unimodal, and skewed, and that mean ± 2 standard deviations does not cut off the desired 95%.''[30]

One can also make CIs for treatment differences (or ratios or more complicated functions) of a parameter; for example, "the observed treatment difference in percentage response was 8%, with 95% CI [for the true difference] of 1% to 12%." If one did a test of how far this difference in percentage is from 0, a trial that had a 95% CI that does not include 0 would also find the difference to be significant [ly different from 0] with a two-sided *P* value <.05. (However, the usual test of a difference in response percentage is the Fisher exact test,[31] which is not a test of how far the difference is from 0 and does not correspond to a CI for this difference.) At any rate since 1 − CI percentage corresponds to a significance level, it is clear that there is nothing sacred about a 95% CI, just as there is nothing sacred about a 5% significance level. There are times when a 99% CI or a 90% CI is more relevant; however, the most common CI in the medical literature is 95%.

Some authors and journal editors[32,33] have stated that CIs are a better way to summarize results of a clinical trial than hypothesis tests (and significance levels and power). There are two main reasons given for this attitude. First, a CI reminds the reader that parameter estimates from a study are only estimates (not true values), and have variability associated with them. If the study were exactly replicated, one would not expect to get exactly the same parameter estimates because of the play of chance. Second, a CI gives the reader an idea of the likely magnitude of a parameter, whereas a hypothesis test tells the reader only that one particular value (often 0) is or is not likely. In one of the above examples, the difference in response percentage was significantly greater than 0, with *P*<.05. Even the estimated difference (8%) does not help a reader who would not choose the better treatment unless it was likely to increase response rate by at least 5% (perhaps because the better treatment has more toxicity or is more inconvenient). If provided with the 95% CI of 1% to 12%, this reader would know he or she should not yet make the treatment with the higher response percentage the standard. On the other hand, if the 95% CI were 8% to 40%, the reader would be justified in switching to the better treatment.

There are three main disadvantages of CIs in clinical trials. The first is that CIs are made for *parameters,* and they usually correspond to *parametric tests,* that is, tests based on the known mathematical distribution of a particular parameter. Most tests used in clinical trials, however, are *nonparametric,* because no one knows the true mathematical distribution of most of the parameters of interest (eg, median survival, or the difference in 5-year survival rates from a Kaplan-Meier curve, or the percentage of patients who have a longer disease-free interval on treatment A than treatment B). Making an incorrect assumption about the mathematical distribution can often have a big effect on the calculated significance level and hence also on the accuracy of a CI. It is unlikely that a clinical trial will be large enough to adequately test a particular distribution

assumption, precisely because the interesting significance levels correspond to values in the tails (ends) of a distribution (eg, the most extreme 5%) and distributions that are similar in the middle may easily be different in the tails. It is true that most power calculations for nonparametric tests make distribution assumptions, but at least the significance level of the test does not depend on such assumptions. It is also true that most nonparametric tests could be turned into CIs by using computer-intensive methods (eg, the bootstrap[34]), but these CIs are for parameters that may not have intuitive appeal (eg, the truncated integral of the product of the cumulative survival on treatment A multiplied by the derivative of the cumulative survival on treatment B).

A second disadvantage of a CI is that it applies to a single parameter. Most distributions that seem to fit real data can differ in several parameters. For example, even gaussian distributions can differ in terms of standard deviation as well as mean. Even if there is a single obvious parameter for describing the effect of one treatment, the difference between treatments may not be so simply described. One can do multiple simultaneous CIs for several parameters, or one can calculate confidence regions for two (or three) parameters. One can even calculate confidence curves for censored survival curves, although there is no straightforward generalization for the *difference* between censored survival curves. Although these extensions of CIs maintain the first advantage of CIs (reminding a reader that estimates have variability), it is not clear that they always maintain the second advantage (giving the reader the idea of likely magnitude of a parameter).

The third disadvantage is that CIs for treatment differences are often difficult to compute and do not have simple formulas. The difference between two gaussian distributions is another gaussian distribution, which greatly simplifies the calculation of the CI. The gaussian distribution is almost unique in this respect, however. The difference between two binomial distributions is not binomial; the difference between two negative exponential distributions is not negative exponential; and so on. Computers can be used to calculate such CIs, but the programs are not widely available. One can make the same complaint about most power calculations. If the null hypothesis is one of "no difference," however, the significance level is usually easier to calculate.

These disadvantages do not mean that CIs should be abandoned in clinical trials. If only to emphasize that estimates have statistical variability, it would be best for each estimate reported (eg, response percents, survival curves, toxicity percents, nadir white blood cell counts, and estimated treatment differences in these parameters) to have some sort of CI reported with it. This is because humans have a tendency to underestimate statistical (and biologic) variation. Most people who are told that a 20-patient trial had a 20% response rate assume the true response percentage is somewhere between 15% and 25%; in fact, this is close to a 28% CI (and would not cover the true response rate 72% of the time by chance alone, even if one did not have to worry about patient selection). The 95% CI is 6% to 44%. Because the CIs corresponding to the most common statistical tests used in clinical trials are difficult to calculate and interpret for the reasons given earlier, however, it does not seem necessary for every test to be accompanied by a CI.

Analysis of Survival Data

ESTIMATION

In a clinical trial, the outcome variable may be the time between two events. Examples are survival (time from randomization or diagnosis to death), disease-free survival (time from primary treatment to first metastases or recurrence), and duration of response (time from first documentation of partial response to first documentation of relapse). In all of these measures, the date of the first event is known for all patients; the date of the second event may be unknown for some patients, either because no information is available or because the event has not yet occurred for these patients. Such patients are said to be *censored* for survival; the time from diagnosis to the date last known alive is called the *censored survival time*.

To estimate the survival curve of a group of patients, one typically uses either the *life table* (also called the actuarial method)[2,35,36,37] or the modification of that method proposed by Kaplan and Meier.[38–41] These methods assume that the censored patients are just like the uncensored patients in their true survival experience, and that the mechanism causing patients to have censored survival times is statistically independent of their true survival times. When the mechanism causing censoring is related to the patients' true survival times, the actuarial method is inappropriate or misleading. Two examples are patients who are lost to follow-up (and therefore censored) for reasons related to therapy or disease status and patients who are censored for death from the cause of primary interest because they die of competing causes. One cannot say a priori how patients lost to follow-up affect the analysis. It may sometimes be advisable to count patients who are lost because they are too sick to continue on study as relapses or recurrences rather than censored observations. One can also accommodate this type of censoring by making mathematical assumptions about the nature of the relation between survival and censoring. Figure 27.2-1 presents data from a lung cancer clinical trial[42] with 61 patients of whom 33 had died and 28 were either still alive at the time of analysis or were lost to follow-up because of metastases. The uppermost curve is the usual Kaplan-Meier actuarial estimate. The two straight-line curves are estimates that reflect different assumptions about the relation between survival and censoring. The fourth curve is the estimate obtained when all 61 survival times were available. Clearly, the Kaplan-Meier curve did not provide a good estimate of the survival experience in this group.

The setting in which competing causes result in censoring a patient for the event of interest can arise when deaths not attributable to cancer are counted as censored. It also can occur when the endpoint is local recurrence and the

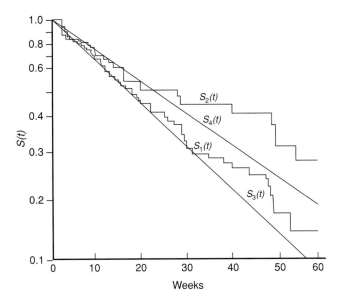

FIGURE 27.2-1 Semilog graphs of four estimates calculated from data: $S_1(t)$, empirical estimate calculated from complete data; $S_2(t)$, constant-sum (Kaplan-Meier) estimate calculated from censored data; $S_3(T)$, cone-model estimate calculated from censored data; $S_4(t)$, constant-sum exponential estimate calculated from censored data. (After Lagakos SW, Williams JS. Models for censored survival analysis: a cone class of variable sum models. Biometrika 1978;65:181).

occurrence of distant recurrence or death leads to censoring. One approach[43] to this problem is to reorient the analysis to first analyze time to first unfavorable event—time to death from any cause, time to first recurrence (counting death as a recurrence), or time to failure in any site. If there is no difference in this time, type of first unfavorable event (eg, local failure versus distant failure versus death) can be analyzed. When such compound endpoints are unacceptable, specific mathematical assumptions about the relation between types of failure may allow actuarial-type estimates to be computed.[44]

COMPARING THE SURVIVAL TIMES OF TWO GROUPS OF PATIENTS

Deciding whether one of two treatments is associated with better survival time would not necessarily be easy even if the two true survival curves were exactly known. Although it is possible to obtain consensus about which of two integers is larger, it may be difficult or impossible for a group of people to agree on which of two curves is better. For example, treatment A could be associated with a higher early mortality rate but a lower late mortality rate than treatment B. Or treatment C could be associated with a higher proportion of patients surviving at each follow-up time than treatment D even though, if we restrict our attention to patients surviving 5 years or more, treatment D is associated with a higher proportion surviving at each follow-up time (this situation is sometimes referred to as *crossing hazard rates*). In either setting, it is difficult to designate a better treatment. The problem of comparing two curves becomes even more difficult when the curves are estimated from data, because of the sampling variability that must be considered. In addition, the estimate of the late part of the curve is always less reliable than the estimate of the earlier part. A data set with many censored values exacerbates this problem.

Sometimes survival curves appear to differ early in the follow-up period and then to come together (Fig. 27.2-2*A*). Sometimes the opposite happens—the curves are similar at first and differ only later in the follow-up period (see Fig. 27.2-2*B*). Not all statistical tests are equally effective in these two situations. This means that a test that is likely to produce a significant result in comparing the curves in Figure 27.2-2*A* might be unlikely to produce a significant result in comparing the curves in Figure 27.2-2*B*. Before a trial begins, one must decide which type of survival difference (early or late) would be of most interest and choose the test statistic accordingly. It would be misleading and inappropriate to try several tests and to report the most significant or to choose the test after viewing the data.

Two of the most commonly used tests of differences in survival curves are the *log-rank test* (variations are known as the proportional hazards test, the Mantel-Haenszel test, the generalized Savage test, or the exponential order scores test[39,44-47]), and the *generalized Wilcoxon test* (variations are known as the Gehan modification of the Wilcoxon test, the Gilbert modification of the Wilcoxon test, and the Breslow test[48-51]). The distributions of these test statistics follow approximate chi-square (χ^2) distributions. The generalized Wilcoxon test is more sensitive to differences in survival distributions that occur earlier in time, and the

log-rank test is more sensitive to differences that occur later in time. As Fleming and colleagues[52] and Lagakos[53] point out, both statistics can be expressed as the weighted sum of statistics from a series of 2×2 contingency tables, with each table corresponding to the number of deaths and number of patients at risk at each observed death time.

As an example, in Figure 27.2-2*A*, the Wilcoxon *P* value of .002 suggests a survival advantage for treatment 2, whereas the log-rank *P* value of .12 suggests that neither treatment offers a survival advantage. In contrast, the Wilcoxon *P* value for the curves in Figure 27.2-2*B* is .16, suggesting no survival difference in the treatments, whereas the log-rank *P* value of .02 suggests that there is a survival advantage to treatment 2.

If the mechanism that causes censoring is related to the true survival time, both the generalized Wilcoxon and the log-rank tests give incorrect significance levels. In a randomized trial, a necessary (but not sufficient) condition for independent censoring is identical follow-up and data collection schedules for both regimens. Planning such identical data collection is not always enough. In a multiinstitutional study of a 6-month induction regimen versus a 16-month induction regimen for metastatic breast cancer,[95] the outcome variable of interest was time to failure. Although follow-up data were supposed to be submitted every 6 months, institutions would often wait until the end of the induction period to submit data unless the patient failed earlier. This resulted in dependent censoring, with far more patients on the 16-month regimen censored when the first analysis was performed at the end of the accrual period. The log-rank test result calculated at that time was nonsignificant; median survival was estimated as

FIGURE 27.2-2   Illustration of different results from log-rank and modified Wilcoxon tests. **A.** Early difference in survival curves. **B.** Late difference in survival curves.

4 months for patients on the shorter regimen and 4.7 months for those on the longer regimen. Analysis of the data available a year after accrual ended showed median survival to be 5.7 months on the shorter regimen and 10.2 months on the longer regimen, a significant difference. Had censoring been independent of survival, the log-rank test performed when accrual ended would have detected the significant difference in survival.

Monitoring

BIAS AND VALIDITY

It has been said that "power tends to corrupt, and absolute power corrupts absolutely."[54] Having just spent several pages arguing that large statistical power is desirable, how can I apply this statement to clinical trials? A large, and hence powerful, trial that controls most bias is good. A large, and hence powerful, trial that does not control bias is bad, because it will be more readily believed than a small trial, even though the results are mostly due to bias rather than "the true state of the world." The term *bias* refers to any factor other than treatment and chance that might influence outcome. Various categorizations of bias have been made.[55,56]

- Selection bias (eg, patients at higher risk choosing a less toxic treatment or physicians putting poorly compliant patients on a less toxic treatment)
- Eligibility bias (eg, patients unable to start adjuvant chemotherapy within a month of mastectomy being excluded from analysis of that regimen, but "control" patients having no such reason for exclusion)
- Diagnostic bias (as diagnostic and staging tests get better, survival appears to improve within each stage, even if overall survival remains the same)
- Bias due to changes in definitions (especially of endpoints) or follow-up or ancillary therapy or supportive care
- Bias due to regression to the mean (eg, metastatic patients starting a new treatment when they have new or worsening symptoms, some of whom appear to respond simply because their bad symptoms were a transient phenomenon)

Bias affects both internal and external validity of a trial. *Internal validity* refers to the quality of comparisons done within the trial's population (most importantly, comparisons of outcome variables in various treatment groups, but it can also involve prognostic factor models or the relations of some outcomes to the risk of other outcomes or the comparison of results in various clinics). Without a large amount of internal validity, the trial cannot teach us anything. *External validity* determines how generalizable the trial results are, since it refers to how similar the study patients, treatments, follow-up, and other procedures are to usual care in some well-specified subset of patients with breast cancer. Even a trial with little external validity, but decent internal validity, provides useful information on treatment comparisons, although it may require a verification study or a "translational" study before a new treatment is adopted as standard.

There are several design features that can help control bias: clear definitions of eligibility and endpoint variables (including toxicity), institutional logs to document what types of patient are not entering the trial, randomization, blinding of the patient to which treatment she is receiving, blinding of the person collecting endpoint data to which treatment the patient is receiving, and specifying the same follow-up schedule for all patients. Unfortunately, designing a trial well is not enough; there need to be some monitoring to ensure that the design is working as planned.

Monitoring is also important for preserving the power of a trial. For example, a trial may be planned to have 80% power to detect a difference between treatments A and B, assuming that 90% of the patients actually receive the treatment to which they are randomly assigned. If only half of the patients actually receive their randomized treatment (and half receive the other treatment on the trial), the trial will have zero power (because the treatment mix in the two groups is identical); the power is larger than zero but less than 80% for "noncompliance" between 50% and 90%. If there is a group of patients for which it is known a priori that neither treatment "works," these patients do not contribute to power and the effective sample size does not include them, so power will be lower than that calculated from the total number of patients. If endpoints are vaguely defined, random noise in coding them also decreases power. To prevent any of these three situations from eroding the power of a trial, it is necessary to monitor these features over the course of a trial, with adjustment of sample size or procedures as needed to maintain power.

Monitoring of clinical trials has been in the news recently[57] because of some fraudulent data involving eligibility of some patients from an institution in the National Surgical Adjuvant Breast and Bowel Project (NSABP). The problem was widely covered in the public press, accrual to all NSABP clinical trials was temporarily halted, and Congress held hearings on clinical trial monitoring. In reaction, the National Cancer Institute (NCI) established a Clinical Trials Monitoring Branch, which has been working on new guidelines for monitoring federally sponsored clinical trials in cancer. The establishment of such guidelines should be federal, since the cost of monitoring is usually by far the most expensive aspect of a trial, and funds for this purpose will have to come from the federal government and drug companies that would be required to follow US Food and Drug Administration (FDA) monitoring guidelines. (This does not imply that all trials should be monitored to the same extent. Different guidelines could be established for different trials, depending on such things as their phase, the subjectiveness of their primary endpoints, the relative difficulty of diagnoses and so forth.) Of course, federal guidelines will not help in judging trials not done in the United States and may not help in judging the numerous "unfunded" cancer trials that examine topics in nondrug (eg, surgical or radiation) therapy or questions such as scheduling or combining treatments already approved by the FDA. The most a reader of the clinical literature can hope for is that such federal guidelines are widely accepted even by trials not required to follow them, and that statements to the effect that "federal guidelines for monitoring clinical trials were followed with the following exceptions" become common in medical journals.

TYPES OF MONITORING

Recently, attention has focussed on the auditing policies of groups conducting clinical trials[57]; that is, how often and for what percentage of patients and data items are the data on forms or in a computer data base compared to the patient's medical record. (Paradoxically, the NSABP problem that precipitated the interest in auditing was *not* discovered on an audit but through a simple comparison of dates on different forms.) The NCI currently requires that each institution participating in a clinical oncology group have an on-site audit at least once every 3 years, although the number of patients and trials audited varies. Auditing, however, is not the only form of monitoring. Monitoring can also include the following[21,22,58–60]:

- Periodic examination of whether a physician, institution, clinic, or laboratory qualifies to participate in a trial (eg, has a properly constituted IRB, passes quality-control tests, is licensed or certified by the relevant group)
- Asking questions during the randomization phone call to establish whether a patient is eligible
- Review of clinic logs or the conduct of surveys to determine what types of eligible patients are not being asked to participate in a study
- Computer or visual checks of data provided for completeness and reasonableness and for consistency over time (sometimes called *logical checks*)
- Periodic production of tables of accrual and toxicity and balance of prognostic factors
- Workshops or surveys to discuss common data abstraction problems and evaluate whether there are major misunderstandings about eligibility requirements, informed consent, randomization procedures, endpoint definitions, toxicity definitions, or reporting procedures
- Double-keying or other methods of preventing computer data entry errors
- Checks that treatment is not begun before patient consent and randomization
- Pill counts or analysis of blood samples to see how much drug a patient is taking (or whether they are taking drugs from treatment arms to which they were not assigned)
- Medical reviews of the judgment calls of primary physicians (eg, eligibility, whether toxicity is related to treatment, tumor response)
- Requirement that two (or more) local physicians examine the patient and agree on eligibility or endpoints
- Centralized review of pathology or scans or other patient materials
- Statistical evaluation of whether variation is larger than expected (eg, institutional differences in patient mix or endpoints) or smaller than expected (eg, a too-perfect linear relation within patient between time and some laboratory value)
- Statistical review of the assumptions on which sample size was based as well as formal sequential analysis of results.

Clearly, for clinical oncology groups, the cost of monitoring includes not only the costs of auditing but also most of the costs associated with data management and statistical offices. Indeed, some have argued that clinical trials are burdened by too much monitoring, not only because of costs but also because monitoring may harm the external validity of a trial, since physicians in practice who use the results of clinical trials and patients treated in accordance with such results are seldom subject to any (let alone so much) checking of eligibility, treatment compliance, and treatment outcome.[57,61] Others seem to believe that fraud, error, and sloppiness is widespread in clinical trials and that results should not be believed unless all possible steps are taken to weed them out.[8] (Surveys of monitoring results in clinical oncology groups have shown that fraud is the rarest problem, affecting less than 0.5% of patients and less than 0.1% of endpoint evaluations, and that sloppiness is the most common problem.[57,62] It is possible that fraud is more of a problem in other cancer trials.) I think that an attitude between these two extremes is justifiable. Clinical trial results affect more patients than the results of individual physician practice, and treatments used on clinical trials are often new and hence less familiar than standard treatment, so clinical trials should be subject to more monitoring than general practice. On the other hand, the amount of effort expended in monitoring any aspect of a trial should be proportional to how much errors in that aspect would affect the internal validity of the trial. Consideration of a few aspects is given in the following sections.

MONITORING OF ELIGIBILITY

Some investigators[63] believe that all patients entered on a randomized study, whether eligible or not, should be included in the analysis. If this is done, there is little reason to spend much time verifying eligibility. The arguments in favor of general inclusion are as follows:

1. On average, randomization should distribute these ineligible patients equally to all treatments.
2. Statistical tests (especially permutation tests) would not be exactly correct without including all patients.
3. The number of "mistakes" made in entering an ineligible patient on the trial is likely to underestimate the number of "mistakes" made in treating unsuitable patients when the therapy becomes standard.
4. One can never be sure that ineligibility was determined in an unbiased way.
5. The enrollment of ineligible patients can help determine that eligibility criteria were too strict.

Other investigators[65] believe that ineligible patients should not be included in the analysis, arguing:

1. There is no clearly defined group to whom the results of the therapies in ineligible patients can be extrapolated.
2. Knowing randomization balances "on average" is small comfort when your trial winds up with an imbalance of ineligible patients on different treatments.
3. The efficacy of breast cancer therapy on a patient who does not have breast cancer simply is not relevant to decisions about the treatment's efficacy in breast cancer (although toxicity may be relevant).
4. The effects of breast cancer therapy on a breast cancer patient whose concomitant diseases are contraindications for the therapy may be important from the point of view of reconfirming the validity of contraindications but not for deciding on the benefit of the therapy in patients without contraindications.

Different institutions at the National Institute of Health take different attitudes, with inclusion of all patients randomized being the rule in National Institute of Allergy and Infectious Diseases–sponsored trials and exclusion of ineligible patients being much more common on NCI-sponsored trials. Both sides of the argument have merit. For this reason, the most helpful reports are those that analyze the trial both ways—with and without the ineligible patients. Second in terms of helpfulness are reports that omit only patients with the most extreme types of ineligibility (eg, those in whom the major endpoint could not be defined or in whom one of the treatments would be on the border of malpractice because of the high probability of serious toxicity).

In any case, if any patients are omitted from analysis because of ineligibility, it is the responsibility of the authors of the article to convince the reader that the determination of eligibility was unbiased, since biased eligibility determination decreases the internal validity of a trial. To be unbiased, the eligibility determination must *not* depend in *any* way on the treatment assignment or the outcome. An example of an eligibility determination that depends on treatment is a trial that randomizes at the time of mastectomy to adjuvant chemotherapy or control and then requires the chemotherapy (but not the control) patients to be recovered enough to start therapy within 3 weeks of the operation. An example of an eligibility criterion that depends on outcome is one that standardly appears in phase II drug protocols but is not often specifically mentioned in reports: a patient must receive 2 months of therapy to be eligible (or "evaluable") for response analysis.

Eligibility does affect the external validity of a trial. In the recent past, there has been some attempt to lessen eligibility requirements in breast cancer clinical trials, precisely to make such trials more generalizable. Some common eligibility requirements of the past were always too restrictive (eg, requiring all trial participants to be free of any history of mild hypertension or hyperglycemia). Some eligibility requirements of the past have become outdated because of recent changes in general practice (eg, the less frequent use of bone and liver scans to rule out metastases in node-negative patients, or the longer time between diagnosis and completion of primary therapy). Indeed, the part of the NSABP controversy involving nonfraudulent

randomization of patients more than a month after primary diagnosis seems moot, since that group and most others have extended the permissible time period in more recent trials. To the extent that the fewer eligibility requirements remaining in more recent protocols are more likely to represent proven and serious medical contraindications for the trial therapies, it may be more important now than in the past to monitor eligibility because of ethical considerations.

One minor note on eligibility monitoring is that it is difficult for a reader to interpret the phase *eligibility could not be verified*. This phrase can mean that eligibility documentation has not yet been sent to a central office. Or it can mean that radiographs and scans were not available for review at the randomizing institution on the day of a surprise audit (which is not an unusual problem in the current system in which a patient's diagnosis, primary treatment, and laboratory tests may be done at different hospitals). Or it can be a euphemism for "this patient was entered fraudulently."

MONITORING OF RANDOMIZATION

To evaluate the importance of monitoring randomization, one must first understand the goals and methods of randomization. Randomization is the main way to eliminate conscious and unconscious bias in treatment comparisons. It also balances, on average, the treatments in a trial with respect to both known and unknown prognostic factors. (The phrase *on average* means that there will be balance among treatments for all factors if there is an infinitely large number of trials studying the same issue). Randomization is a process by which treatments are assigned to patients by a chance mechanism such that each patient has a particular prespecified probability of being assigned to each treatment in the trial. (Usually, these prespecified probabilities are equal, because for a fixed total accrual, equal numbers of patients on each treatment produce the most power. It is possible, however, to have unequal probabilities.) One important feature of randomization is that neither the physician nor the patient knows which treatment the patient will receive before he or she is entered on the trial. Any other arrangement would not eliminate the possibility that the choice of entering the trial was influenced by the treatment assignment. Even prerandomization methods,[66] which sometimes have the patient randomly assigned to a treatment before she knows she has been entered on the trial, do not violate this provision because they consider all randomized patients to be "entered," even if they do not agree to receive the randomized treatment.

Randomizing by patient birth date, patient hospital number, order of appearance at a clinic, or sealed envelopes is suspect. Most modern trials are randomized by a phone call to a central office or by a computer program in which the patient identification must be entered before a treatment is assigned. In such cases, monitoring of randomization is relatively easy. It involves verifying that there has been no attempt to obtain a randomization assignment outside the usual procedures, checking that no patient undergo randomization twice, establishing that no patient received trial treatment before randomization, and carefully documenting the reasons a randomly assigned patient did not receive the treatment assigned by randomization. (In general all patients should be analyzed as randomized rather than by the treatment actually received.) The results of most clinical trials are probably not suspect if one or two cases had randomization irregularities; more randomization irregularities than this call for extensive discussion and make the trial suspect.

It has been argued that few patients are willing to undergo randomization if the process is completely explained to them, and so randomization itself decreases the external validity of a trial.[67] In a disease as heterogeneous as breast cancer, however, nonrandomized trials are subject to so much bias and imbalance in unknown prognostic factors that they lack internal validity, making external validity a moot point. For example, even the best historically controlled study can be misleading. Pocock[68] examined 19 instances in which a clinical trials group used the same treatment in two consecutive trials. "If historical comparisons of this type are without bias, one would not expect any notable difference in survival for two groups receiving the same treatment. In fact, the 19 changes in death rate ranged from −46% to +24%, and in four instances the difference was statistically significant (each $P<.02$)." Similar examples exist in the breast cancer literature. Changing one of the treatments in an Eastern Cooperative Oncology Group (ECOG) randomized trial of metastatic breast cancer resulted in significant changes in the response rate, response duration, time to failure, and survival time of patients given the treatment that *remained* the same; these changes were significant even when adjusted (in statistical models) for the possible effect of institution and 35 prognostic factors.[69] Similar unexplainable differences exist in the survival experience of adjuvant chemotherapy breast cancer patients treated with L-phenylalanine mustard (L-PAM) on two successive NSABP protocols.[70,71] The reliability of historical controls is challenged even more directly when the results of historically controlled trials show significant differences[72] that are not verified by the results of randomized trials.[73] It would certainly be counterproductive to require so much monitoring of randomized trials that nonrandomized trials become the norm in deciding oncology questions.

MONITORING TREATMENT COMPLIANCE

Treatment compliance can be easy to monitor (eg, documenting that the patient was injected once with the trial vaccine) or complicated to monitor (eg, deciding if the dose modifications in a yearlong seven-drug chemotherapy were justified by patient toxicity). As mentioned earlier, for some trials, treatment compliance can affect both power and generalizability. To estimate the effect of compliance on these topics, however, it is not necessary for all patients to be monitored, but only that a large enough sample be monitored to estimate degree and percentage of compliance. To preserve internal validity of a trial, noncompliers should never be omitted from analysis. This is because it is impossible to prove that the decision to depart from protocol guidelines was unaffected by the patient's treatment assignment or outcome. Fortunately, the practice of omitting these patients has decreased in breast cancer reports, so there are not many recent bad examples.

As an example, several cancer studies have shown it is more difficult to give complex treatment precisely as planned than to give simple treatment precisely as planned. So a trial comparing radiation therapy plus chemotherapy to either modality alone is likely to find more protocol violations in the combined-therapy regimen. As another example, many studies involving placebos, including the NSABP B-05 adjuvant trial of L-PAM versus placebo,[74] have shown that patients who take full-dose placebos have better outcomes than patients who are less compliant on their placebo regimen. So it would obviously be a mistake to omit less compliant patients from chemotherapy arms but not observation arms.

With the exception of bone marrow transplant regimens, most breast cancer chemotherapy is given to outpatients rather than to inpatients, and surgery also involves much less inpatient time than in the past. This, combined with a recent trend to more complicated treatments, has made monitoring treatments increasingly difficult. Many protocols now state that treatment modification algorithms are "guidelines" rather than "rules." There is still a role for close monitoring of treatment in phase I and early phase II trials, but it is hard to justify on phase III trials unless the primary scientific question involves dose or schedule.

USE OF MONITORING RESULTS

Some types of monitoring are educational or corrective in and of themselves (eg, the keeping of clinic logs to see what types of patients are not approached to participate in trials, workshops to discuss common data abstraction problems, double-keying to prevent data entry errors). Other types of monitoring require plans on how to use the results (eg, amending the protocol to clarify definitions and procedures, scheduling extra workshops, penalizing noncompliant physicians or institutions, reporting suspected fraud to relevant bodies, modifying the sample size). Fraud is of more concern than mistakes or sloppiness, because it is more difficult to detect, and one worries that an investigator who is found to have committed fraud on one study or for one reason (eg, to make more patients eligible) may have committed undetected fraud on other studies or for other reasons (eg, to make one treatment look better than another). Luckily, fraud appears to be relatively rare.[57]

Most mistakes and sloppiness that have been detected by monitoring and that affect internal validity have tended to make the treatments on a randomized trial look more similar with respect to endpoints than they really are; that is, they lower power. Such mistakes usually do not make treatments look more different than they really are. This is because, even though some errors may occur more on one treatment than another, there are so many different types of errors that they will tend to be distributed on both treatments, just by chance. So how a trial was monitored is more of an issue in trials reporting treatment equivalence than in trials reporting treatment difference.

Subgroups

Another recently controversial issue is subgroup analysis.[75] Analysis of treatment effects for multiple subgroups of patients within a trial seems to be more common in reports on breast cancer studies than in reports on other primary cancers. For example, one study of postmenopausal positive-node patients under the age of 65 years[76] did statistical tests to compare the three treatments not only in the entire study, but also in 10 subgroups: age 55 years or under, age over 55 years, one to three positive nodes and estrogen receptor (ER)–negative, one to three positive nodes and ER–positive, more than three positive nodes and ER–negative, more than three positive nodes and ER–positive, ER–negative, ER–positive, one to three positive nodes, and more than three positive nodes. Had the trial included premenopausal or node-negative women, there probably would have been even more subgroup analysis. There are many reasons for this proliferation of subgroup analyses. Breast cancer trials usually involve a large number of patients monitored for a long time, so they are often expensive, and there is a great temptation to "put the money to good use" by answering several questions at once. Historically, some patient subgroups have been treated differently (eg, node-positive versus node-negative, premenopausal versus postmenopausal, hormone receptor–positive versus hormone receptor–negative, patients with visceral metastases versus patients with only bone metastases), so that investigators reporting on a trial combining several of these groups feel obliged to publish separate estimates and statistical tests to enable the reader to compare the new study with previously published studies. In addition, enough treatments are known to have some benefit in breast cancer that there is a desire to provide guidance on which treatments work best for which patients. In particular, there is a strong incentive to identify patient subgroups that do *not* need systemic, or more toxic, therapy at primary diagnosis or at diagnosis of relatively asymptomatic metastases. Also, breast cancer investigators share with other cancer investigators the need to use differences in treatment effects in subgroups to formulate biologic hypotheses about mechanisms of action of their treatments.

COMMONLY USED SUBGROUPS

Corresponding to this plethora of reasons for subgroup analyses are a large number of factors commonly used alone and in combination to form subgroups in analysis of breast cancer trials. Readers of breast cancer literature will have no difficulty listing the most common of these factors. Table 27.2-3 is based on surveys of factors used of trials in primary and adjuvant therapy in subgroup analyses as well as in eligibility criteria, randomization stratification, and stratified tests or statistical models.[77–79] (The

overall analysis of treatment in a trial that requires eligible patients to be postmenopausal is from one point of view equivalent to a subgroup analysis by menopause in another trial. Stratified tests and statistical models are appropriate methods of combining subgroup analyses.) From this table, it is clear that the most common subgroups before 1985 were based on nodal status, menopausal status (or age), and ER status. In addition, many of these older trials excluded patients with lumpectomies, who were over age 65 to 70 years, or who had TNM stage III (using the older UICC definition), and so some of the investigators must consider type of surgery, older age, and tumor size to be important subgroups. Since 1985, there has been a great increase in the number of factors considered to be of importance in early breast cancer trials, particularly in node-negative studies. The NCI consensus conference on treatment of node-negative patients[80] mentioned tumor size (up to 1 cm versus more than 1 cm), ER and progesterone receptor status, nuclear grade, histologic type, and proliferative rate (ploidy and S-phase fraction) as factors that should be studied further to identify node-negative patients who might obtain more (or less) benefit from systemic treatment. More recent analyses have involved various genetic markers (eg, Her-2/neu, rb, and p24).

Trials on metastatic breast cancer are far less likely than trials of adjuvant therapy to report subgroup analyses and far more likely to report the results of stratified tests and statistical models. Perhaps this is because metastatic trials tend to have smaller accrual (although a larger percentage of patients have died by the time of analysis) and because there are even more "accepted" prognostic factors.

The goals of subgroup analyses are laudable. Unfortunately, there are a number of problems with the naive interpretation of tests done on multiple subgroups: data-derived categories, multiple comparisons, and quantitative versus qualitative interactions.

DATA-DERIVED CATEGORIES

If one wants to compare treatments within subgroups, one has to be able to categorize patients into subgroups. If the characteristic used for this categorization is *continuous* (having many possible values; eg, age or S-phase fraction) and there is no single, widely accepted cutoff for this characteristic, many cutoffs are possible. Some investigators[81] have examined all possible (or many of the possible) cutoffs to choose the cutoff that produces the biggest difference in outcome between categories, and there are recursive partitioning computer programs that automate this search.[82] If the cutoff is chosen to minimize the P value of the subgroup comparison, however, that significance level can no longer be interpreted as the probability that the observed difference is due to chance. In fact, the P value calculated from such data-derived grouping is far smaller than the true P value. This is because, even in the case of a characteristic that truly makes no difference, if enough different cutoffs are examined, the chances are high that at least one will be significant just by chance. Table 27.2-4 shows the true P value[83,84] for χ^2 tests based on choosing the best cutoff when all cutoffs in the central

TABLE 27.2-3
Common Subgroups for Early Breast Cancer Trials in the Period 1975–1985

	Pocock & Lagakos[70] Stratification Survey	Gelman & Zelen[71] Stratification, Eligibility, Analysis Survey	Oxford[72] Metaanalysis
NODAL STATUS			
Positive vs negative	XX	XX	X
1–3 vs >3	XX	XX	X
Clearance vs sampling★			X
MENOPAUSAL STATUS			
Pre and peri vs post	XX	XX	X
AGE			
<50 vs ≥50 y		X	XX
≤65 or 70 y (upper limit)		X	
			X
ESTROGEN RECEPTOR STATUS			
Positive vs negative	X	X	X
Moderately positive vs very positive		X	X
TUMOR SIZE			
<2 vs >2 cm	X	X	
<3 vs >3 cm	X		
<5 vs >5 cm (often ineligible)	X	X	
PRIMARY TREATMENT			
Total vs radical	X		
Radiation vs no radiation	X		
Lumpectomy (ineligibility)		X	

X, commonly used factors; XX, almost universally used factors.

★ Used in connection with number of positive nodes: patients with less than four positive nodes after axillary sampling were categorized with patients with unknown number of positive nodes.

C% of the data are tried. (For example, if 5% of the patients are under 37 years old and 5% are over 69 years old, the central 90% are between 37 and 69.) This table is based on a predefined outcome variable that is binary (eg, response versus no response, or surviving at least 5 years versus dead before 5 years), and the calculations assume that 50% of the patients have each of the two possible outcomes (since this case has the most statistical power). So even if only the middle third of the data is searched for the best cutoff, a calculated P value of .01 corresponds to a true P value of .06 to .07 and a calculated P value of .05 corresponds to a true P value of .21 to .24.

MULTIPLE COMPARISONS

If one does a statistical test of the difference between treatment A and treatment B in k nonoverlapping subgroups, each test having a 5% false-positive error rate (ie, a 5% chance of being declared significant even if treatments A and B have identical effects), one has a probability of $1 - .95^k$ of finding at least one test to be statistically significant at $P < .05$ just *by chance*. In a study in which treatment is compared within premenopausal, ER-negative patients with three or more positive nodes, the reader should assume a similar comparison was made within all eight subgroups defined by nodal status (one to three versus more than three), menopausal status (premenopausal versus postmenopausal), and ER status (positive versus negative). The reader should not interpret $P < .05$ as referring to an event that would happen by chance only 1 time in 20; such an event actually would happen by chance 1 time in 3.

There are several ways around this problem of multiple comparisons. If all k subgroups are independent (ie, nonoverlapping), it is easy to adjust the significance levels. The Bonferroni method[85] is to do each of the k tests with a cutoff corresponding to

TABLE 27.2-4
True Significance Level (P value) for χ^2 Test When Best Cutoff in Central C% of Data Is Used

Central C%	Calculated P=.05					Calculated P=.01				
	33	50	80	90	100	33	50	80	90	100
TOTAL SAMPLE SIZE										
100	.21	.26	.43	.46	.54	.06	.08	.13	.15	.15
200	.21	.28	.44	.53	.62	.06	.08	.14	.17	.19
∞	.24	.31	.49	—	1.00	.07	.09	.16	.21	1.00

$$\alpha' = 1 - \sqrt[k]{1 - \alpha}$$

where:
α = desired overall false-positive error rate

$$\sqrt[k]{1 - \alpha} = \text{the } k^{\text{th}} \text{ root of } 1 - \alpha$$

For example, with $\alpha = 0.05$ and $k = 8$, only tests with $P < .0064$ would be declared significant. Equivalently, one could multiply all significance levels by 7.8 (=.05/.0064) and use a cutoff of .05. (Since $1 - \sqrt[k]{1 - \alpha}$ is approximately equal to α/k, the Bonferroni method is sometimes approximated by multiplying all significance levels by k.)

Holm's method[86] is to obtain a significance level for each of the k comparisons and then to order these significance levels from smallest to largest (say, $P_1, P_2, \ldots, P_k$). One then compares P_1 to α/k, as in the approximate Bonferroni method. If $P_1 < \alpha/k$, one declares the relevant test to be significant at the α level and then goes on to compare P_2 to $(\alpha/k-1)$. If $P_2 < \alpha/(k-1)$, one declares the relevant test to be significant at the α level and then goes on to compare P_3 to $\alpha/(k-2)$, and so on. When some significance level P_m is not smaller than the relevant cutoff $\alpha/(k-m+1)$, the corresponding test *and* tests corresponding to all larger significance levels are declared nonsignificant. Holm's method has the same overall false-positive error probability (α) as the Bonferroni method and has greater power. Both methods have very low power however, when compared with the test of A versus B in the entire study group.

Also, both methods were designed for independent tests and so are not highly accurate when subgroups are overlapping. For example, a trial that tests the difference between treatments A and B in the whole study group, separately in ER-positive and ER-negative patients, separately in premenopausal and postmenopausal women, and separately in patients with one to three or more than three positive nodes has seven overlapping subgroups. Methods for adjusting P values for multiple overlapping subgroups are available but generally require computer simulations to obtain cutoff values. Gray[87] described such a method for adjusting log-rank significance levels and gave an example of a postmenopausal adjuvant breast cancer trial of three treatments in which all three pairwise comparisons

were done in each of 11 overlapping subgroups. The most significant comparison was of CMFP versus control for the ER-negative subgroup, with a P value of .006, uncorrected for multiple comparisons. Computer simulations resulted in a corrected P value of .06, 10 times as large as the uncorrected one.

QUANTITATIVE VERSUS QUALITATIVE INTERACTIONS

Even if significance levels have been appropriately adjusted for multiple comparisons, a trial in which two treatments differ significantly in premenopausal women but not in postmenopausal women does not necessarily correspond to a case in which the biologic effects of the treatments differ in the two groups. Statistical significance is a function of sample size and variability as well as the true difference in treatment effects. Perhaps the two treatments behave the same in the two groups but the postmenopausal group had fewer patients (or, in the case of survival analysis, fewer deaths) than the premenopausal group, or perhaps the postmenopausal group had a greater variety of prognoses. It is also possible that competing causes of death are obscuring a treatment difference in the older, postmenopausal group. At any rate, the question of whether the P values for treatment difference differ in premenopausal and postmenopausal women is not really relevant. Treatment A could be significantly better than treatment B in premenopausal women and nonsignificantly different in postmenopausal women while the true difference between treatments A and B could be identical in the two subgroups. We really want to know whether the estimate of benefit of A over B is significantly larger in premenopausal women than in postmenopausal women. A test of the interaction between treatment and menopausal status answers this question.

The most common of such interaction tests are quantitative.[88-90] In a quantitative interaction,[91] switching from one subgroup to another changes the true *magnitude* of the difference between treatment effects on outcome. It is possible that the direction of the difference is also changed (ie, that one treatment is truly better than the other in one subgroup but truly worse than the other in another subgroup), but this is not required for a quantitative interaction. A quantitative interaction also occurs when treatment A is better than treatment B in both subgroups but the benefit in using A is bigger for one subgroup than another. Quantitative interaction tests are more relevant in clinical trials than multiple-treatment comparisons in subgroups, but they have a disadvantage: they depend on the mathematical properties of the model being used to relate outcome to treatment. If the wrong type of model is chosen, one can find a spurious interaction or fail to find a real one. For example, if the true relation between response percent and treatment and menopausal status is log-linear[92] and there truly is no interaction on the log-linear scale but the investigator fits a logistic model[93] to the data set, there will appear to be a significant interaction between treatment and menopausal status. Similarly, if the true relation is logistic and there truly is no interaction on the logistic scale, an investigator who fits a log-liner model to a data set finds a significant interaction. The same problem arises with additive and multiplicative models. Suppose that treatment B is associated with 10% response in young patients and 30% response in old patients and treatment A is associated with 20% response in young patients. If the relation of treatment to response is additive, one would expect treatment A to be associated with 40% response in old patients (ie, 20% + 20%). If the relation of treatment to toxicity is multiplicative, one would expect treatment A to be associated with 60% response in old patients (ie, 20% × 3). If the wrong model (additive or multiplicative) is chosen, a spurious interaction is introduced. Because the correct mathematical form of the relation between outcome and treatment is seldom known, it is not surprising that significant interactions are often reported.

Such quantitative interactions (whether spurious or real) are often clinically unimportant, however. In the earlier example of an induced interaction, treatment A has more response than treatment B in both subgroups. As long as the benefit of A over B is large enough to be worth the extra cost or toxicity of A in each subgroup, the choice of treatment to use would be unaffected by the presence of a significant quantitative interaction.

In a qualitative (or crossover) interaction,[94] switching from one subgroup to another changes the *direction* of the difference in treatment groups. Tests for qualitative interactions[91] have two benefits over tests for quantitative interactions: they are far less affected by the mathematical model used to relate outcome to treatment and they are always clinically important (since they imply that different subgroups should get different treatments).

Metaanalysis: Statistical Methods for Combining Data From Different Studies

It is not unusual for a clinical question in breast cancer to be associated with several separate but similar randomized trials. The results of the separate trials are often not identical and can be contradictory. Hence, medical journals include many breast cancer literature reviews that attempt to draw overall conclusions from the wealth of published reports. In recent years, the case has been made that, in a common disease such as breast cancer, treatments of only small to moderate benefit could prolong many lives.[79] Very large numbers of patients are required to detect small to moderate treatment differences (see Table 27.2-2), and one way of obtaining large numbers is to combine the data from many moderate-sized trials.

COMBINED GROUP ANALYSIS AND STRATIFIED TESTS

Some of the literature reviews[95–97] use statistical methodology to combine data. In 1976, Glass[98] coined the term *metaanalysis* to describe the use of such statistical methodology. The terms *overview, pooled analysis,* and *combined analy-*

sis were used earlier and continue to be popular.[79,99] The statistical methods used differ primarily in how much homogeneity of studies is assumed. Conceptually, the simplest way of combining data from several randomized trials using the same two treatments (call them A and B) and the same definition for some outcome variable would be to combine all data on patients treated with A, to combine all data on patients treated with B, and then to compare these two large groups using one of the statistical tests described earlier. Let us call this combined group analysis. This method assumes complete homogeneity between trials. It could easily happen, however, that some trials show treatment A better than treatment B and some show B better than A, whereas the combined group analysis shows no difference at all between treatments A and B. In this case, the combined group analysis could be misleading, and an analysis of why the trials differ in results would be much more informative. The power of the analysis could be improved by treating the individual trials as strata and using a stratified test. Stjernsward[95] used a stratified χ^2 test on 5-year survival percents to evaluate the benefit of adjuvant radiation therapy for breast cancer. More recently, the Oxford overview[97] used a stratified log-rank test to evaluate (separately) adjuvant chemotherapy and adjuvant hormonal therapy in breast cancer.

COMBINING *P* VALUES

A simpler and cruder way of combining studies involves combining results rather than patient data. L.H.C. Tippet, R.A. Fisher, and K. Pearson independently proposed methods of combining *P* values in 1931 to 1933.[100–102] The simplest of these methods is the sign test. Suppose there are five trials comparing treatments A and B and that in all five a survival analysis shows A better than B (although not necessarily significantly better). Under the null hypothesis that A and B are associated with the same survival, the probability that all five of five trials would favor A is $.5^5$, or .03125. So this is evidence that A is associated with longer survival than B. In general, if there are a total of *N* trials and A appears to be better in *k* of them, the *P* value associated with this distribution of trials results is the probability that one observes *k* successes in *N* trials of a binomial random variable with probability of success of .5. This probability can be read directly from a table of binomial probabilities.[103] This method has been used by Stjernsward and Day[96] in combining evidence from trials of adjuvant radiation therapy. Its advantages are that it is simple to calculate and the data needed for its calculation are always available in published reports of clinical trials. Its disadvantages are that all trials are equally weighted (eg, a trial of 5 patients monitored for 2 years counts the same as a trial of 5000 patients monitored for 10 years) and that no estimate of the size of the treatment effect is obtained. In both a stratified test and a combined group analysis, the result of each trial is weighted proportionally to the number of events (eg, death or response) in the trial. Hence, the stratified tests and the combined group tests are more sensitive to small differences than the sign test. In addition, both stratified tests and combined group tests produce estimates and CIs for the treatment effect.

RANDOM EFFECTS MODELS

Stratified tests and the sign test assume that some appropriate measure of treatment difference is approximately the same for all trials. Although homogeneity of differences is a more reasonable assumption than homogeneity of outcomes within treatment groups, it has often been criticized.[104–107] There is a group of models, called *random-effects models*,[108] that allow one to test whether the treatment differences are more heterogeneous than could be expected from the sizes of the trials and, if so, to account for this extra variation in a stratified test. Himmel and colleagues[109] used such a model in analyzing published reports of adjuvant chemotherapy in breast cancer. One would expect that random-effects models, by using larger variance estimates for some trials, would result in less significant *P* values, on average, than the stratified test described earlier (sometimes called *fixed-effects models*). Berlin and colleagues[110] compared the results of 22 metaanalyses analyzed by the stratified log-rank test of Peto[97] and the random effects model of DerSimonian and Laird.[108] In the 14 metaanalyses that both methods agreed in classifying as nonheterogeneous, the two methods chose the same 5 to be significant and resulted in similar *P* values for all 14. Of the remaining 8 heterogeneous metaanalyses, 2 were found to be nonsignificant by both methods. However, 3 of the 6 metaanalyses found to be significant by the Peto method were found to be nonsignificant by the DerSimonian and Laird method. Hence, one advantage of the random-effects models is that they are less likely to declare treatment A significantly better than treatment B if the trials in the metaanalysis are too heterogeneous to justify this. One disadvantage of random-effects models is that they assume that the trials being analyzed represent a random sample of all such trials that could be done. This is clearly not the case; both the design and the results of earlier trials affect the design of later trials.

TIME HETEROGENEITY

There is one other type of heterogeneity to worry about in combining data from many studies when the outcome variable used is the time until an event—for example, survival time. Even if one is willing to assume homogeneity of differences over trials, one may not be willing to assume homogeneity of differences over time. That is, the difference between treatments A and B may not be constant over time. For example, in the first year after randomization, A may be twice as good as B as measured by the odds ratio of death; in the second year, A may be only 80% better; in the third year, 40% better; and in the fourth year, the two treatments may be associated with the same risk of death. There is some evidence that differences in survival time and time to recurrence in patients who undergo adjuvant chemotherapy (or hormonal therapy) and control patients are not constant over time.[111] In addition,

many established prognostic factors[112] do not have a constant effect on the hazard of recurrence or death, so the "average" benefit of treatments that are truly of benefit to only some patient subgroups would also be expected to change over time. If either of these assertions are true, combining data from trials with different lengths of follow-up could be misleading. Also, it may be that the trials followed longest are not typical of the studies being combined. If so, the results of the combined analysis might change drastically when more follow-up is obtained on recently started trials.

PUBLICATION BIAS

The widespread discussion of metaanalysis that followed the presentation of breast cancer adjuvant chemotherapy and hormonal therapy overviews has had some useful ancillary results in the areas of publication bias, quality of clinical trials, the arithmetic construct, and comparisons of metaanalyses. The dangers of reviewing only published studies have been clearly stated,[113] and in one case[114] (ovarian cancer), the conclusions from reviewing only published studies have been shown to differ from the conclusions drawn when all available studies are reviewed. The problem is that trials with no significant treatment differences, especially trials too small to have adequate power, are less likely to be published than trials with a significant treatment difference.[115] In addition, there is a natural tendency for investigators to publish reports at a point in follow-up when differences are large rather than at earlier or later follow-up times when differences are not as impressive. Increased discussion of such publication bias may lead to more complete registries of clinical trials,[114] the organization of public record journals to ensure publication of at least minimal data on all randomized trials, and the development of better methods for estimating the effect of unavailable data on the conclusions of literature reviews.[113]

ARITHMETIC CONSTRUCTS

The phrase *arithmetic construct* has been used[116] to refer to the fallacy of assuming that a trial that randomizes the treatment consisting of A plus B against treatment with only A is estimating the same treatment B "effect" as a trial that randomizes B against observation (or placebo). As two counterexamples, consider that breast cancer patients treated with radiation-induced castration plus prednisone may have better outcomes than patients treated with radiation-induced castration alone,[117] and patients treated with CMF plus prednisone may have better outcomes than patients treated with only CMF,[118] and yet prednisone alone may have no antineoplastic effect in breast cancer. After the original presentation of the breast cancer adjuvant treatment overview, it was pointed out that estimates of the magnitude of tamoxifen benefit came from combining trials of tamoxifen versus no systemic adjuvant therapy with trials of chemotherapy plus tamoxifen versus chemotherapy alone. The subsequent publication[79] summarized the effects of tamoxifen separately for these two types of trials. The arithmetic construct is a potential problem in interpreting the conclusions of many clinical trials, not just in interpreting a metaanalysis. The examples of fallacious conclusions using the arithmetic construct that were published in the wake of the adjuvant therapy overview may help physicians recognize this type of logical fallacy wherever it occurs.

COMPARISON OF METAANALYSES: HYPOTHESIS FORMATION

Some investigators believe that the main benefit of overviews is that the evaluation of the arithmetic construct and other trial differences can lead to the formation of important hypotheses deserving of further study. For example, if a metaanalysis of treatment Y in premenopausal patients showed Y not to be of benefit and a metaanalysis of treatment Y in postmenopausal patients showed Y to be of benefit, reasonable investigators would try to hypothesize why the difference occurs. Some would argue that the large number of subsets of interest in breast cancer make metaanalyses mandatory, since no trial has a large enough accrual to evaluate treatment differences in each of these subsets. The problem is that inconsistent definitions, different percentages of misclassification, and incomplete availability of all prognostic variables can make the results of such subset analyses dubious.[119] It is *very* important to realize that studies that compare metaanalyses are subject to all the biases that occur when comparing *nonrandomized* treatments. Selection bias undoubtedly exists.[120] Even if all trials have the same eligibility criteria, the patients who enter a trial of X versus control differ from the patients who enter a trial of A plus X versus A.[121] The patients who enter the first trial of X versus Y differ from the patients who enter subsequent trials of X versus Y, particularly if some results of the first trial are known when the subsequent trials start. These differences may be subtle or difficult to document if they do not involve major prognostic factors, but they may still have a profound effect on the outcome. There are also sources of bias that are likely to be bigger in comparisons of metaanalyses than in comparisons of two nonrandomized treatments:

- Quality bias (one type of trial may by chance be associated with a higher loss to follow-up or more misclassification errors)
- Geographic bias (the types of patients, the treatments available to them, and the factors influencing their agreement to randomization may differ by location, whereas many historical control studies of treatments are restricted to one hospital)
- Competing risk bias (the effects of breast cancer treatment may differ in populations at different risks of noncancer death, whether effects are evaluated by comparing treatments using deaths from all causes or only breast cancer–related deaths)

Given these biases, comparisons of metaanalyses are useful to the extent they encourage the formation of testable hypotheses, the keeping of patient logs and other methods of assessing how patients are selected for trials,

and the standardization of collection of data items and follow-up. Comparisons of metaanalyses are detrimental to the extent they are treated as hypothesis *tests*.

COMPARISON OF METAANALYSES AND SINGLE CLINICAL TRIALS

Metaanalyses are by their nature retrospective, since at least some results of some of the included clinical trials are known at the time the metaanalysis is done. Most well-known proponents of metaanalysis agree that the gold standard of clinical research is the large-scale clinical trial, not the metaanalysis (eg, Sacks and associates,[99] Chalmers and colleseagues,[115] Wittes,[122] Hennekens and coworkers,[123] Demets[124]). Many argue that metaanalyses should be used in hypothesis formation rather than hypothesis testing, so that a successful metaanalysis is one that is followed by a large randomized trial.[125,126] A large randomized trial has often been the result of cardiac metaanalyses. For example, in the mid-1980s, an overview of 6000 patients on 33 trials of fibronolytic drugs given within 24 hours of the start of myocardial infarction symptoms indicated a statistically significant survival benefit,[127] which led to the design and activation of two large trials that verified this benefit (GISSI-2 with 37,000 randomized patients and ISIS-2 with 17,000 patients randomized to four treatments). As another example,[128] eight trials of a 24-hour infusion of magnesium in a total of 3000 patients with myocardial infarctions showed a statistically significant benefit in 1-month mortality, which was not substantiated by a later randomized trial (ISIS-4 with 58,000 patients and a slightly detrimental effect of the drug on 1-month mortality).

Up to now, breast cancer metaanalyses not only have not resulted in new randomized trials, they have also resulted in early termination of ongoing trials.[129] Even Peto and Collins, who once stated that metaanalyses are the only practical way to evaluate treatments with "moderately sized benefits," urge "future trials . . . should plan to obtain sufficient number of events to contribute substantially to such overviews. In many cases, this implies the need for randomized trials that are much larger than is currently standard."[130]

Simon[131] has pointed out that "research reviews have always been regarded as subjective; the determination of what evidence is relevant . . . is not straightforward" and that this same critique applies to metaanalyses. The problem according to Demets[124] is that "procedures for deciding what to combine are not yet adequately developed." Deciding whether the studies included in a metaanalysis are all apples, apples and oranges, or apples and oranges and carrots and airplanes requires a careful evaluation of the treatments involved, the patient populations represented, the quality of the trials, and the medical context during which the trials were performed.[132] There are no general rules for what is "similar enough."

It can be argued that any multicenter (or even multidoctor) clinical trial is also a matter of mixing apples and oranges. A single clinical trial probably has a log order[133] less heterogeneity than a metaanalysis does, however, and this should keep the carrots and airplanes out of the fruit salad. For this reason, I agree with those who believe that metaanalyses are useful for hypothesis generation. For deciding on the relative effectiveness of two treatments, however, there is no substitute for large, well-designed clinical trials. The Oxford overview of adjuvant breast cancer therapy has been invaluable in encouraging international cooperation, obtaining data on almost all known relevant trials and thus eliminating publication bias, and forming important hypotheses with regard to length of tamoxifen treatment or the relative benefits of hormonal therapy and chemotherapy in various patient subgroups. It is now time to "spend our creative energies designing simpler, larger multicentre or multi-country studies with common protocols [and] standardized therapy."[124]

References

1. Altman DG, Goodman SN. Transfer of technology from statistical journals to the biomedical literature: past trends and future predictions. JAMA 1994;272:129.
2. Pocock SJ. Clinical trials: a practical approach, New York, John Wiley & Sons, 1983.
3. Buyse ME, Staquet MJ, Sylvester RJ, eds. Cancer clinical trials: methods and practice, Oxford, UK, Oxford University, 1984.
4. Miké V, Stanley KE, eds. Statistics in medical research. New York, John Wiley & Sons, 1982.
5. Friedman LM, Furberg CD, DeMets DL. Fundamentals of clinical trials, ed 2. Littleton, MA, PSG, 1985.
6. Dawson-Saunders B, Trapp RG. Basic and clinical biostatistics. Norwalk, CT, Appleton & Lange, 1989.
7. Shapiro SH, Louis TA. Clinical trials. New York, Marcel Dekker, 1983.
8. Spilker B. Guide to clinical trials. New York, Raven, 1991.
9. Fleiss JL. Statistical methods for rates and proportions. New York, John Wiley & Sons, 1981;38:260.
10. Feigl P. A graphical aid for determining sample size when comparing two independent proportions. Biometrics 1978;34:111.
11. Casagrande JT, Pike MC, Smith PG. The power function of the exact test for comparing two binomial distributions. Appl Stat 1978;27:176.
12. George SL, Desu MM. Planning the size and duration of a clinical trial studying time to some critical event. J Chron Dis 1974;27:15.
13. Peto R, Pike MC, Armitage P, et al. Design and analysis of clinical trials requiring prolonged observation of each patient. Br J Cancer 1976;34:585, 1977;35:1.
14. Lesser ML, Cento SJ. Tables of power for the F-test for comparing two exponential survival distributions. J Chron Dis 1981;34:533.
15. Schoenfeld DA, Richter JR. Nomograms for calculating the number of patients needed for a clinical trial with survival as an end-point. Biometrics 1982;38:163.
16. Bernstein D, Lagakos SW. Sample size and power determination for stratified clinical trials. J Stat Comput Simul 1978;8:65.
17. Lehmann EL. Nonparametrics: statistical methods based on ranks. San Francisco, Holden-Day, 1975;69.
18. Freedman LS. Tables of the number of patients required in clinical trials using the logrank test. Stat Med 1982;1:121.
19. Wald A. Sequential analysis. New York, John Wiley, 1947.
20. Bross I. Sequential medical plans. Biometrics 1952;8:188.
21. Pocock SJ. Interim analyses for randomized clinical trials: the group sequential approach. Biometrics 1982;38:153.
22. O'Brien PC, Fleming TR. A multiple testing procedure for clinical trials. Biometrics 1979;35:549.
23. Gelber RD, Geldhirsch A. Methodology of clinical trials: investigating endocrine mechanisms in breast cancer. In: Cavalli F, ed. Endocrine therapy of breast cancer, New York, Springer-Verlag, 1986:51.
24. Freiman JA, Chalmers TC, Smith H, et al. The importance of beta, the type II error, and sample size in the design and interpretation of the randomized controlled trial. N Engl J Med 1978;290:690.
25. Zelen M, Gehan E, Glidewell O. Biostatistics. In: Hoogstraten B, ed. Cancer research: the impact of the cooperative groups. New York, Masson 1980:291.
26. Mosteller F, Gelbert JP, McPeek B. Reporting standards and research strategies for controlled trials. Control Clin Trials 1980;1:37.
27. Staquet MJ, ed. Randomized trials in cancer: a critical review by sites. New York, Raven, 1978.
28. Gelman R, Zelen M. Interpreting clinical data. In: Harris JR, Hellman S, Henderson IC, Kinne DW, eds. Breast diseases. Philadelphia, JB Lippincott 1987:708.
29. Gore SM. Assessing methods: transforming the data. BMJ 1981;283:548.
30. Elveback LR, Guillier CL, Keating FR Jr. Health, normality, and the ghost of Gauss. JAMA 1970;211:69.
31. Fisher RA. Statistical methods for research workers, ed 12. Edinburgh, Oliver & Boyd, 1954.
32. Dawson-Saunders B, Trapp RG. Basic and clinical biostatistics. Norwalk, CT, Appleton & Lange, 1990:96.
33. Gardner MJ, Altman DG. Confidence intervals rather than P values: estimation rather than hypothesis testing. BMJ 1986;292:746.
34. Hall P. The bootstrap and edgeworth expansion. New York, Springer-Verlag, 1992:96.
36. Berkson J, Gage RP. Calculation of survival rates for cancer. Proc Mayo Clin, 1950;25:270.
37. Cutler SJ, Ederer F. Maximum utilization of the life table method in analyzing survival. J Chron Dis 1958;8:699.
38. Kaplan EL, Meier P. Nonparametric estimation from incomplete observations, J Am Stat Assoc 1958;53:457.
39. Gelber RD, Zelen M. Planning and reporting of clinical trials. In: Calabresi P, Schein PS, Rosenberg SA, eds. Medical oncology: basic principles and clinical management of cancer. New York, Macmillan, 1985:418.
40. Lee ET. Statistical methods for survival analysis, Belmont, CA, Wadsworth, 1980.
41. Gross AJ, Clark VA. Survival distributions. In: Reliability applications in the biomedical sciences. New York, John Wiley & Sons, 1975:23.
42. Lagakos SW, Williams JS. Models for censored survival analysis: a cone class of variable sum models. Biometrika 1978;65:181.
43. Gelman R, Gelber R, Henderson IC, et al. Improved methodology for analyzing local and distant recurrence. J Clin Oncol 1990;8:548.
44. Prentice RL, Kalbfleisch JD, Peterson AV, et al. The analysis of failure times in the presence of competing risks. Biometrics 1978;34:541.
45. Peto R, Peto J. Asymptotically efficient rank test procedures. J R Stat Soc A 1972;135:185.
46. Savage IR. Contributions to the theory of rank order statistics. Ann Math Stat, 1956;27:590.
47. Mantel N. Evaluation of survival data and two new rank order statistics arising in its consideration. Cancer Chemother Rep 1966;50:163.
48. Gehan EA. A generalized Wilcoxon test for comparing arbitrarily singly-censored data. Biometrika 1965;52:203.
49. Elandt-Johnson RC, Johnson NL. Survival models and data analysis. New York, John Wiley & Sons, 1980:225.
50. Breslow N. A generalized Kruskal-Wallis test for comparing K

samples subject to unequal patterns of censorship. Biometrika 1970;57:579.

51. Tarone RE. On the distribution of the maximum of the logrank statistic and modified Wilcoxon statistic. Biometrics, 1981;37:79.

52. Fleming TR, Green SJ, Harrington DP. Performing serial testing of treatment effects. In: Baum M, Kay R, Scheurlen H, eds. Clinical trials in early breast cancer: second heidelberg symposium. Boston, Birkhauser Verlag, 1982:469.

53. Lagakos SW. Inference in survival analysis: nonparametric tests to compare survival distribution. In: Mike V, Stanley KE, eds. Statistics in medical research: methods and issues with applications in cancer research. New York, John Wiley & Sons, 1982:340.

54. Dalberg JEE (Lord Acton). Letter to Bishop Modell Creighton, 1887.

55. Sackett DL. Bias in analytic research. J Chron Dis 1978;32:51.

56. Feinstein AR. Clinical epidemiology: the architecture of research. Philadelphia, WB Saunders, 1985.

57. Cohen J. Clinical trial monitoring: hit or miss. Science 1994;264:1534.

58. Rosner GL, Tsiatis AA. The impact that group sequential tests would have made on ECOG clinical trials. Stat Med 1989;8:505.

59. Pocock SJ. Interim analysis for randomized clinical trials: the group sequential approach. Biometrics 1982;38:153.

60. O'Brien PC, Fleming TR. A multiple testing procedure for clinical trials. Biometrics 1979;35:549.

61. Peto R, Collins R, Gray R. Large-scale randomized evidence: large, simple trials and overviews of trials. Ann NY Acad Sci 1994;703:314.

62. Weiss RB, Vogelzang NJ, Peterson BA, et al. A successful system of scientific data audits for clinical trials: a report from CALGB. JAMA 1993;270:459.

63. Armitage P. Exclusions, losses to follow-up, and withdrawals in clinical trials. In: Shapiro SA, Louis TA, eds. Clinical trials: issues and approaches. New York, Marcel Dekker, 1983.

64. Falkson G, Gelman R, Falkson CI, et al. Factors predicting for response, time to treatment failure, and survival in women with metastatic breast cancer treated with DAVTH: a prospective ECOG study. J Clin Oncol 1991;9:2153.

65. Sacket DL. On some prerequisites for a successful clinical trial. In: Shapiro SH, Louis TA, eds. Clinical trials: issues and approaches. New York, Marcel Dekker, 1983.

66. Zelen M. A new design for randomized clinical trials. N Engl J Med 1979;300:1242.

67. Hellman S, Hellman DS. Of mice but not men: problems of the randomized clinical trial. N Engl J Med 1991;324:1585.

68. Pocock SJ. Randomized clinical trials. (Letter) BMJ 1977;1:1661.

69. Tormey D, Gelman R, Falkson G. Prospective evaluation of rotating chemotherapy in advanced breast cancer. Am J Clin Oncol 1983;6:1.

70. Fisher B, Redmond C. Studies of the NSABP. In: Salmon SE, Jones SE, eds. Adjuvant therapy of cancer. New York, Elsevier-Dutton Holland, 1977:67.

71. Fisher B, Redmond C, Fisher ER. A summary of findings from NSABP trials of adjuvant therapy. In: Salmon SE, Jones SE, eds. Adjuvant therapy of cancer IV. New York, Grune & Stratten, 1984:185.

72. Gutterman JU, Cardenas JO, Blumenschein GR, et al. Chemoimmunotherapy of disseminated breast cancer: prolongation of remission and survival. BMJ 1976;2:1222.

73. Muss HB, Richards F, Cooper MR, et al. Chemotherapy vs. chemoimmunotherapy with methanol extraction residue of bacillus Calmette-Guerin in advanced breast cancer: a randomized trial by the Piedmont Oncology Association. Cancer 1981;47:2295.

74. Redmond C, Fisher B, Wieand HS. The methodologic dilemma in retrospectively correlating the amount of chemotherapy received

in adjuvant therapy protocols with disease-free survival. Cancer Treat Rep 1983;67:519.

75. Nowak R. Problems in clinical trials go far beyond misconduct. Science 1994;264:1538.

76. Taylor SG IV, Kalish LA, Olson JE, et al. Adjuvant CMFP versus CMFP plus tamoxifen versus observation alone in postmenopausal, node positive breast cancer patients: three year results of an Eastern Cooperative Oncology Group study. J Clin Oncol 1985;3:144.

77. Pocock SJ, Lagakos SW. Practical experience of randomization in cancer trials: an international survey. Br J Cancer 1982;46:368.

78. Gelman R, Zelen M. Interpreting clinical data. In: Harris JR, Hellman S, Henderson IC, et al., eds. Breast disease. Philadelphia, JB Lippincott, 1987:702.

79. Early Breast Cancer Trialists' Collaborative Group (EBCTCG). Treatment of early breast cancer, vol 1. Oxford, Oxford University, 1990.

80. NIH Consensus Development Conference. Treatment of early stage breast cancer. In: NIH Consensus Development Conference consensus statement. 1990;8: June 18–21.

81. Clark GM, Dressler LG, Owens MA et al. Prediction of relapse or survival in patients with node-negative breast cancer by DNA flow cytometry. N Engl J Med 1989;320:627.

82. Breiman L, Friedman JH, Olshen RA, Stone CJ. Classification and regression trees. New York, Wadsworth International, 1983.

83. Miller R, Siegmund D. Maximally selected chi square statistics. Biometrics 1982;38:1011.

84. Halpern J. Maximally selected chi square statistics for small samples. Biometrics 1982;38:1017.

85. Ingelfinger JA, Mosteller F, Thibodeau LA, et al. Biostatistics in clinical medicine. New York, Macmillan, 1983:169.

86. Hochberg Y, Tamhane AC. Multiple comparison procedures. New York, Wiley & Sons, 1987:55.

87. Gray RJ. A simultaneous inference procedure for clinical trials. Commun Statist Theory Meth 1987;16:499.

88. Simon R. Patient subsets and variation in therapeutic efficacy. Br J Clin Pharm 1982;14:473.

89. Shuster J, Van Eys J. Interaction between prognostic factors and treatment, Control Clin Trials 1983;4:209.

90. Thall PF, Lachin JM. Assessment of stratum-covariate interactions in Cox's proportional hazards regression model. Stat Med 1986;5:73.

91. Gail M, Simon R. Testing for qualitative interactions between treatment effects and patient subsets. Biometrics 1985;41:361.

92. Bishop YM, Fienberg SE, Holland PW. Discrete multivariate analysis: theory and practice. Cambridge, MA, MIT, 1975.

93. Hosmer DW, Lemeshov S. Applied logistic regression. New York, Wiley & Sons, 1989.

94. Peto R. Statistical aspects of clinical trials. In: Halnan KE, ed. Treatment of cancer. 1982:867.

95. Stjernsward J. Decreased survival related to irradiation postoperatively in early operable breast cancer. Lancet 1974;1:1285.

96. Stjernsward J, Day N. Rebuttal of two articles by Dr. Levitt et al. Cancer 1977;40:381.

97. Early Breast Cancer Trialist's Collaborative Group. Effect of adjuvant tamoxifen and of cytotoxic therapy on mortality in early breast cancer: an overview of 61 randomized trials among 28,896 women. N Engl J Med 1988;319:1681.

98. Glass GV. Primary secondary and meta-analysis of research. Educ Res 1976;5:3.

99. Sacks HS, Barrier J, Reitman D, et al. Metaanalyses of randomized controlled trials, N Engl J Med 1987;316:450.

100. Tippett LHC. The method of statistics. London, Williams & Norgate, 1931.

101. Fisher RA. Statistical methods for research workers, ed 4. London, Oliver & Boyd, 1932.

102. Pearson K. On a method of determining whether a sample of given

size n supposed to have been drawn from a parent population having a known probability integral has probably been drawn at random. Biometrika 1933;25:379.

103. Beyer WH, ed. CRC handbook of tables for probability and statistics, ed 2. Boca Raton, CRC, 1983:194.

104. Levitt SH, McHugh RB. Early breast cancer and post-operative irradiation. (Letter) Lancet 1975;1:1258.

105. Levitt SH, McHugh RB, Song CW. Radiotherapy in the post-operative treatment of operable cancer of the breast II. Cancer 1976;39:933.

106. Levitt SH, McHugh RB. Reply to rebuttal letter by Drs. Stjernward and Day. Cancer 1977;40:382.

107. Goodman SW. Have you ever seen a meta-analysis you didn't like? Ann Intern Med 1991;114:244.

108. DerSimonian R, Laird N. Meta-analysis in clinical trials. Control Clin Trials 1986;7:177.

109. Himmel HN, Liberati A, Gelber RD, et al. Adjuvant chemotherapy for breast cancer: a pooled estimate based on results from published randomized control trials. JAMA 1986;256:1148.

110. Berlin JA, Laird NM, Sacks HE, et al. A comparison of statistical methods for combining event rates from clinical trials. Stat Med 1989;8:141.

111. Zelen M, Gelman R. The assessment of adjuvant trials in breast cancer. Natl Cancer Inst Monogr 1986;1:36.

112. Gray RJ. Flexible methods for analyzing survival data using splines, with applications to breast cancer prognosis. J Am Stat Assoc 1992;87:942.

113. Begg CB. A measure to aid in the interpretation of publicised clinical trials. Stat Med 1985;4:1.

114. Simes RJ. Publication bias: the case for an international registry of clinical trials. J Clin Oncol 1986;4:1529.

115. Chalmers TC, Leven H, Sacks HS, et al. Meta-analysis of clinical trials as a scientific discipline I: control of bias and comparison with large co-operative trials. Stat Med 1987;6:315.

116. Gelber RD, Goldhirsch A. The concept of an overview of cancer clinical trials with special emphasis on early breast cancer. J Clin Oncol 1986;4:1696.

117. Meakin JW, Alt WEC, Beale FA, et al. Ovarian irradiation and prednisone following surgery and radiotherapy for carcinoma of the breast. Br Cancer Res Treat 3 1983;(Suppl):45.

118. Tormey DC, Gelman R, Band PR, et al. Comparison of induction chemotherapies for metastatic breast cancer. Cancer 1982;50:1235.

119. Gelber RD, Goldhirsch A. Interpretation of results from subset analyses within overviews of randomized clinical trials. Stat Med 1987;6:371.

120. Norton L. Commentary. Stat Med 1987;6:333.

121. Gelber RD. Discussion. Stat Med 1987;6:379.

122. Wittes RE. Discussion. Stat Med 1987;6:277.

123. Hennekens CH, Buring JE, Hebert PR. Implications of overviews of randomized trials. Stat Med 1987;6:397.

124. Demets DL. Methods for combining randomized clinical trials: strengths and limitations. Stat Med 1987;6:341.

125. Furberg CD, Morgan TM. Lessons from overviews of cardiovascular trials. Stat Med 1987;6:295.

126. Collins R. Discussion. Stat Med 1987;6:338.

127. Fibrinolytic Therapy Trialists' Collaborative Group. Indications for fibrinolytic therapy in suspected acute myocardial infarction. Lancet 1994;343:311.

128. Teo KK, Yusuf S, Collins R, et al. Effects of intravenous magnesium in suspected acute myocardial infarction: overview of randomized trials. BMJ 1991;303:1499.

129. Norton L. Discussion. Stat Med 1987;6:289.

130. Collins R, Gray R, Godwin J, Peto R. Avoidance of large biases and large random errors in assessment of moderate treatment effects: the need for systemic overviews. Stat Med 1987;6:245.

131. Simon R. The role of overviews in cancer therapeutics. Stat Med 1987;6:389.

132. Wittes RE. Problems in the medical interpretation of overviews. Stat Med 1987;6:269.

133. Wittes RE. Discussion. Stat Med 1987;6:278.

INDEX

Page numbers followed by *f* indicate illustrations; *t* following a page number indicates tabular material.

A

Abandonment, legal considerations, 129–130
Abdominal metastases, of infiltrating lobular carcinoma, 423
Abortion, therapeutic, with breast cancer in pregnancy, 887
Abscess, breast
  after breast cancer treatment, 659
  after breast-conserving treatment, 527
  diagnosis, 52
  fine-needle aspiration biopsy, 154
  management, 124
  nonpuerperal, 50–51
    clinical features, 51
    etiology, 50–51
    pathogenesis, 50–51
    treatment, 51
  puerperal, 51–52
  subareolar, 50
    clinical features, 51
    recurrence, 51
    treatment, 51
  treatment, 52
AC. *See* Doxorubicin and cyclophosphamide
Accessory nipple(s), 2
A cells, superficial (luminal), 9
Acines, 9
AC → CMF. *See* Doxorubicin and cyclophosphamide → cyclophosphamide, methotrexate, and fluorouracil
Actinomycin D, response to, in metastatic breast cancer, 692*t*
Actinomycosis, of breast, 52
Acute nonlymphatic leukemia, radiation-induced, 536

Acute-phase reactants, breast cancer metastases and, 639
Adenoid cystic carcinoma, 394, 414–416
  axillary metastases, 416
  clinical presentation, 414
  and cribriform carcinoma, differentiation, 415
  electron microscopic studies, 415
  gross pathology, 414–415
  histologic grades, 415
  in males, 414
  microscopic pathology, 415*f*, 415–416
  mucin histochemistry, 415
  prognosis for, 416
  recurrence, 416
Adenolipoma, pathology, 37
Adenoma(s)
  ductal, 37
  lactating, pathology, 33
  of nipple
    papillary, 34
    pathology, 34
  pathology, 33
  pleomorphic, 33
  syringomatous, 33
  tubular, pathology, 33
Adenomyoepitheliomas, 37
Adenosis
  apocrine, 29
  microglandular
    and cancer, 34
    epidemiology, 34
    microscopic pathology, 403
    pathology, 34, 36*f*
  sclerosing, 29, 30*f*
    microscopic pathology, 403
Adenovirus-induced tumors, in rats, 237

Adjuvant systemic therapy. *See* Chemotherapy, adjuvant; Treatment of breast cancer
Adolescent, male, gynecomastia in. *See* Gynecomastia
Aerobic exercise, for breast cancer patient
  benefits, 944, 945
  management, 956–957
African Americans. *See* Blacks
Age
  argyrophilia in breast cancer and, 424
  bone loss and, 903–904, 905
  breast cancer and, 110–111
  breast cancer incidence and, in whites, 190, 192*f*
  breast cancer risk and, 160–161, 163*f*
  at carcinogen exposure, and incidence of tumors, in animal models of breast cancer, 335, 336*f*
  at diagnosis of breast cancer
    cancer susceptibility genes and, 326
    correlation with S-phase fraction, 468, 468*t*
    infiltrating lobular carcinoma and, 420
    invasive breast cancer local recurrence and, 497–499, 498*t*
    medullary carcinoma and, 404
    metaplastic breast cancer and, 411
    prognostic significance, 464–465
    tubular (well-differentiated) breast cancer and, 402
  at first full-term pregnancy
    and breast cancer risk, 162–163, 188–189, 189*t*
    breast cancer risk and, 188–189, 189*t*

Age (*continued*)
  gynecomastia and, 54
  infiltrating lobular carcinoma and, 420
  male breast cancer and, 859
  of malpractice lawsuit claimants,
      comparative average indemnity
      by, 130, 131t
  at menarche, breast cancer risk and,
      163–164, 186–187
  at menopause, breast cancer risk and,
      164, 187–188, 188t
  metaplastic breast cancer and, 411
  palpable breast masses and, 110
  phyllodes tumors and, 866
  and psychological impact of breast
      cancer diagnosis, 922
  and relative risk of dying from breast
      cancer, in minority groups,
      911–912
  specific risk associated with, and
      BRCA1 gene in breast cancer,
      326–327
  squamous carcinoma and, 416
AGM-1470, 278
  antiangiogenic effects, 296. See also
      TNP-470
  in combination therapy, 296
Agnogenic myeloid metaplasia,
      differential diagnosis, in breast
      cancer patient, 849
AJCC. See American Joint Committee
      on Cancer
Alcohol
  cardioprotective effects, 209
  intake
      breast cancer and, 208f, 208–209
      breast cancer prevention and, 346
Alendronate, for hypercalcemia,
      843–844
Alkaline phosphatase
  as indicator of recurrent breast cancer
      in bone, 639
      in liver, 634t, 639, 639t
  as marker of osteoblastic activity,
      821–822
Allelic deletion. See Loss of
      heterozygosity
Alopecia, with chemotherapy,
      management, 929, 953–956
Alprazolam, for breast cancer patient,
      923
  with advanced breast cancer, 931
Alveolar buds, 9
Alveolus, 9
Amastia, 2, 3
Amazia, 2, 3
American Cancer Society, 959t
American College of Radiology
      Reporting and Data System
      (BIRADS), 76–77
American Indians, effects of breast
      cancer in, 960
American Joint Committee on Cancer,
      staging system, 457–459, 459t
9-Amino-camptothecin, 703
Aminoglutethimide
  adjuvant therapy with, for

postmenopausal breast cancer,
    566
  adverse effects, 930
  for breast cancer metastases, 684
      dose-intensity considerations,
          684–685
      enzyme reactions blocked by, 684,
          685f
      with hydrocortisone, 684, 685
      sites of action, 684, 684f
      toxicity, 684, 685t
      tumor flare with, 688–689, 689t
Amitriptyline, for patient with advanced
      breast cancer, 930
Amonafide, 595
  response to, in metastatic breast
      cancer, 692t
Amphiregulin, 221, 225, 272
  in breast development, 18
  steroid hormone regulation of, 276,
      276t
Amsacrine, response to, in metastatic
      breast cancer, 692t
Anaerobes, in nonpuerperal breast
      abscesses, 51
Analgesics
  for brachial plexopathy, 804, 805f
      adjuvant, 805, 806t
  for breast pain, 103
Androgen(s)
  for breast cancer metastases, 687
  tumor flare with, 688–689, 689t
Anemia
  with bone marrow metastases,
      847–848
  myelophthisic. See Myelophthisic
      anemia
Anesthesia
  for biopsy, 133
      in pregnancy and lactation, 123
  for excisional breast biopsy, 136
Aneusomy
  in breast cancer, 447
  in proliferative breast disease, FISH
      investigations, 447
Angiogenesis, 284
  in breast cancer, 286–287
      control, 293–298
      growth factors and, 277–278
      prognostic significance, 399–400,
          477–478
  in breast cancer metastases, 286
  contrast-enhanced imaging and, 84
  factors regulating, 293–294, 294f
  growth factors and, 293–294
  inhibitors, 286
      possible therapeutic applications,
          290
  modulators
      negative, 293
      positive, 293
  process, 286
  prognostic significance, 293
  proteases in, 294
  therapy directed against, 290, 478. See
      also Antiangiogenic agents

combination therapies, 296
    conventional, 294–295
    novel, 295–296
    outlook for, 296
Angiogenic factors, 399–400
Angiogenin, in angiogenesis, 286
Angiomatoses, 37
Angiosarcoma of breast, 878–880
  clinical features, 878–879
  incidence, 878
  pathology, 878
  prognosis for, 879–880
  radiographic features, 878–879
  treatment, 879–880
Animal models, of breast cancer,
      235–244
  chemically induced rodent mammary
      tumors, 235–236
  dietary fat and, 201
  endocrine effects on immune function
      and, 239–240
  future directions in, 241
  human tumor xenografts, 237–240,
      238t
  immunodeficient mouse models, 239
  prevention strategies for, 335–336,
      337f
  principles and rationale for, 235
  transgenic mouse models, 240–241
  virally induced rodent mammary
      tumors, 236–237
ANN. See Artificial neural network
Anovulation, physical activity and, 187,
      187f
Anthracyclines
  antiangiogenic effects, 295
  for metastatic breast cancer, 693–697
Anthrapyrazoles, 595
  for metastatic breast cancer, 696
Antiangiogenic agents, 478
  mechanism of action, 278
Antibiotic(s), for puerperal mastitis, 124
Antibody(ies). See also Monoclonal
      antibodies
  B-72.3, in breast cancer, prognostic
      significance, 402t
  in biologic therapy of breast cancer,
      302
  epithelial membrane antigen, in
      immunohistochemical
      detection of micrometastases,
      432–433
Anticipatory nausea and vomiting, with
      chemotherapy, 953
Antidepressants, for breast cancer patient,
      923
  with advanced breast cancer, 930
Antiemetic regimens, 953, 954t
Antiemetics, 929, 953
Antiestrogen(s). See also Tamoxifen
  effects on breast cancer, growth factors
      and, 274
  for gynecomastia, 59
  for metastatic breast cancer, 680–681
Antigen(s). See also Carcinoembryonic
      antigen

blood group-related, in breast cancer, 299
breast cancer, 298–300
breast mucin, as indicator of recurrent breast cancer, 640
carcinofetal, in breast cancer, 298–299
epithelial membrane, polyclonal antibody, in immunohistochemical detection of micrometastases, 432–433
human leukocyte, up-regulators, in immunotherapy, 304
mammary cancer, as indicator of recurrent breast cancer, 640
mammary serum, as indicator of recurrent breast cancer, 640
melanoma-associated. *See* MAGE-1
proliferating cell nuclear, prognostic significance in breast cancer, 469
Thomsen-Friedenreich, 299
tumor-associated
    as indicator of recurrent breast cancer, 639–642, 641*t*
    as indicators of clinical course, in treatment of metastatic breast cancer, 641*f*, 641–642, 642*f*
Antihistamines, antiemetic regimen, 954*t*
Antihormones, antiangiogenic activity, 295
Antioxidants, breast cancer risk and, 205–208, 346
Antiprogestational agents, effects on breast cancer, growth factors and, 274
Antiprogestins, for breast cancer metastases, 683–684
Anxiety
    with advanced breast cancer, 930–931
    breast cancer diagnosis and, 923
    with mammographic screening, 343–344
    with risk assessment, 349–350
Anxiolytics, for breast cancer patient, 923
    with advanced breast cancer, 931
Apocrine adenosis, 29
Apocrine carcinoma, 413–414
    clinical features, 413–414
    in male, 414
    pathology, 413–414
    prognosis for, 414
Apocrine metaplasia, 413
    with phyllodes tumors, 863–864
Apoptosis
    epithelial, postlactation, 18
    growth factors and, 277
    during mammary involution, 2
A → CMF. *See* Doxorubicin, cyclophosphamide, methotrexate, and fluorouracil
Areola, 5
    reconstruction, 613–615, 616*f*, 617*f*
Argentaffin granules, 424
Argovac cutting needle, 155, 156*f*

Argyrophilia
    in breast cancer, 424
        age distribution, 424
        in males, 424
        microscopic pathology, 424–425
        in mucinous carcinoma, 408, 424–425
Argyrophil reaction, 424
Arithmetic constructs, 1001–1002
Arm. *See also* Shoulder
    edema. *See also* Lymphedema
        with radiation therapy, 532–533
    function, after axillary dissection, 510–511
Aromatase inhibitors, for breast cancer metastases, 684–686
Artificial neural network, in mammography, 91
Ascites, in breast cancer patients, 839
Ascorbic acid. *See* Vitamin C
Asian Americans, effects of breast cancer in, 960
Aspiration. *See* Fine-needle aspiration biopsy; Needle aspiration
Asymmetric density, on mammography
    incidence of malignancy with, 119*t*
    as indication for biopsy, 119*t*
Atamestane, 686
Ataxia-telangiectasia, 175, 178
    gene, chromosomal location, 178
Attributable proportion, 215–216
Atypical lobular hyperplasia, 370
Audit, breast imaging, 74
Autocrine factors, 15, 16, 293, 294*f*
    in breast cancer, 273, 274*f*
    in breast cancer onset, 273–276
    in breast cancer progression, 272, 273*t*, 273–276
Autoimmunity, and mammary duct ectasia and periductal mastitis, 49
Autonomic neuropathy, with vinca alkaloids, 958
Autoradiography
    technical considerations, 466*t*
    tumor proliferation measurement, 466
Autosomal dominant inheritance, 171–172, 172*f*
    of breast cancer, 171–172
AVCF. *See* Doxorubicin, vincristine, cyclophosphamide, and 5-fluorouracil
Axillary adenopathy, 892–893
Axillary artery and vein, 4*f*, 6*f*, 8
Axillary dissection
    arm function after, 510–511
    with breast-conserving treatment, technique, 525–526
    complications, 510
    contraindications to, 512
    effects on survival, 509
    extent
        lymphedema and, 899
        and radiation therapy, 531
        and reported incidence of axillary

involvement in breast cancer, 380–381
    indications for, 512
    local control in axilla and, 510, 510*t*
    lymphedema after
        extent of surgery and, 899
        prevention, 899–900
    for occult primary with axillary metastases, 893–894
    prognostic information provided by, 511–512
    rehabilitation problems with, 939
    role in breast cancer treatment, 511–512
    sentinel node removal in, 511–512
    sequelae, 944*t*
    seroma formation with, 510
    therapeutic utility, 462, 508–509
Axillary lymph nodes
    anatomy, 5–8, 6*f*, 7*f*
    apical, 5
    classification, 382
    dissection. *See* Axillary dissection
    ductal carcinoma in situ in, 359–360
    enlargement
        with medullary carcinoma, 405
        with papillary carcinoma, 410
    involvement in breast cancer, 379–384, 380*t*
        classification, 381–382
        detection, 383
            physical examination in, 381
        extent of treatment, lymphedema and, 899
        histology, prognostic significance, 381, 382*t*
        immunohistochemical detection, 383–384
        level, prognostic significance, 381–382, 508–509
        number of nodes involved, and prognosis, 381–382, 382*t*, 383*t*, 508–509, 511
        with occult primary, 892–896
        prognostic significance, 379, 380*t*, 381, 382*t*, 382–383, 383*t*, 462–463, 463*f*, 508–509
        recurrence risk, after nodal sampling, 510, 510*t*
        survival and, 381–383, 382*t*, 383*t*
        tumor location and, 379, 380, 380*t*, 381*t*
        tumor size and, 379, 380, 380*t*, 381*t*, 382–383, 383*t*
    levels, 5, 508, 508*f*
    medullary carcinoma in, 405
    pathologic examination, 431–432
    physical examination, and detection of involvement in breast cancer, 381, 381*t*
    skip metastases to, 509, 509*t*
    subclavicular, 5
    surgery. *See also* Axillary dissection
        complications, 510–512
        indications for, 507–512
        techniques, 507–512

Axillary sampling, 509–510
Axillary sheath, 4f
Axillary tail of Spence, 3
Axillopectoral muscle, abnormalities, 8
Azacytidine, response to, in metastatic
    breast cancer, 692t
3′-Azido-2′,3′-dideoxythymidine, 698

B
Back pain, in breast cancer patient
    with bone metastases, 812
    computed tomography in, 782
    with epidural metastases, 780
    investigations, 780–785, 781f
    local, neurologic examination for,
        781–782
    neurologic examination for, 781–782
    radionuclide bone scans in, 782
    spinal roentgenograms in, 781–782
Bacteriophage vectors, 983
B-72.3 antibody, in breast cancer,
    prognostic significance, 402t
56-BaP, for lymphedema, 900
Basement membrane
    in breast development, 18–19
    constituents, 19
    production, 21
    remodeling, 19
Base pairing, complementarity, 972
Base pair methylation, 973
Bases, 972
Basilic vein, 6f
B cells (chief cells), basal, 9
BCNU, response to, in metastatic breast
    cancer, 692t
Becquerel, Henri, 489
Behavioral modification, and natural
        killer (NK) cell activity,
        301–302
Bellergal, for hot flushes, 905
Benign disorders, 27–65
    blood flow with, 75
    cancer risk with, 27, 31–32, 32t, 164
    fine-needle aspiration biopsy,
        ultrasound-guided, 154
    follow-up studies, 27
    histology, breast cancer risk and,
        31–32, 32t, 164
    pathology, 27–41
Benign lesions, in pregnancy, 123
Benzodiazepines, antiemetic regimen,
        954t
Benzo(a)pyrene
    cells immortalized by treatment with,
        251
    for lymphedema, 900
Benzopyrones, for lymphedema, 900
Bias, 993–994
    in comparisons of metaanalyses, 993
    competing risk, in comparisons of
        metaanalyses, 1002
    diagnostic, 993
    due to changes in definitions, 993
    due to regression to the mean, 993

eligibility, 993
    geographic, in comparisons of
        metaanalyses, 1002
    lead-time, 308
    length, 308
    publication, and metaanalysis, 1001
    quality, in comparisons of
        metaanalyses, 1002
    selection, 993
Biceps brachii muscle
    long head, 6f
    short head, 6f
Biochemical metaplasia, 424
Biologic therapy, future of, 596
Biomarkers
    attributable proportion and, 215–216
    in epidemiologic studies, 214
    exposure effect, and cancer, 216, 216f
    expression, 214
    prevention and, 214
Biopsy
    anesthesia for, 133
        in pregnancy and lactation, 123
    of breast mass
        breastfeeding and, 123
        indications for, 115, 118, 119t, 120
    of chest wall recurrence, 138
    core-cutting needle. *See* Core-cutting
        needle biopsy
    dedicated prone stereotactic core
        biopsy table for, 145, 145f
    excisional, 136–137, 139
        of clinically occult
            mammographically detected
            lesions, 139
        preoperative needle localization,
            139
        specimen management after, 137,
            137f
        technique, 136f, 136–137
    fine-needle aspiration. *See* Fine-needle
        aspiration biopsy
    incisional, 137
        specimen management after, 137,
            137f
    indications for, 72–74
        mammographic, 118, 119t
            incidence of malignancy by, 118,
                119t
    large-core needle. *See* Large-core
        needle biopsy, ultrasound-
        guided
    for mammographic abnormalities
        indications for, 118, 119t, 120
        results, 118–120, 119t
    mammographically initiated, positive
        predictive value, 73–74,
        144–145
    needle. *See also* Fine-needle aspiration
        biopsy; Large-core needle
        biopsy
        ultrasound-guided, factors affecting,
            152
    during pregnancy and lactation
        delay in, 123
        special considerations, 123

punch, of skin lesions, 137–138, 138f
    of recurrent cancer, 659–660
    of regional adenopathy, 138
    skin. *See* Skin biopsy
    stereotactic core, 144–152
    surgical
        disadvantages, 144
        stereotactic core biopsy and,
            comparison, 147–148, 148t
    techniques, 133–158
Bioptycut device, 135
Biopty gun, 155
Birth characteristics, and breast cancer
        risk, 165
Bisantrene, 696
    response to, in metastatic breast
        cancer, 692t
Bisphosphonates
    for bone metastases, 822–823, 823t
    for hypercalcemia, 843–844
    mechanism of action, 822
    for osteoporosis, 905
    pharmacology, 822
Blacks. *See also* Underserved minorities
    with breast cancer
        prognosis for, 465
        survival, 672, 673f
            factors affecting, 915
    endemic poverty in, 910, 910t
    relative risk of dying from breast
        cancer, 911, 911t
Black/White Cancer Survival Study, 672
Bladder cancer, metastases to breast, 426
Blastomycosis, of breast, 52
Bleomycin
    response to, in metastatic breast
        cancer, 692t
    as sclerosing agent, 835
Blindness, and breast cancer risk, 166
Blood group-related antigens, in breast
        cancer, 299
Body mass index, breast cancer risk and,
        204–205
Bone, breast cancer metastases to. *See*
        Metastases of breast cancer, to
        bone
Bone loss
    age-related, 903–904, 905
    prevention
        estrogens and, 349
        tamoxifen therapy and, 348
Bone marrow
    examination, in breast cancer patients,
        849
    micrometastases to. *See also*
        Micrometastases
        detection, 304
Bone marrow metastases. *See* Metastases
        of breast cancer, bone marrow
Bone marrow transplantation
    with dose-intensive adjuvant
        chemotherapy, 560–561
    for metastatic breast cancer, 708–709
    psychologic considerations, 930
    in vitro and in vivo education

combined with, for breast cancer, 304

Bone metastases. *See* Metastases of breast cancer, to bone

Bone pain, with bone metastases, 812
treatment, 813

Bone remodeling, 820–821
and markers of osteoclast–osteoblast function, 821–822, 822t

Boyden chamber chemoinvasion assay, 252

Brachial artery, 6f

Brachial plexopathy, in breast cancer patient, 796–808
acute ischemic, radiation-induced, 802, 804t
adjuvant analgesics for, 805, 806t
analgesic pharmacotherapy for, 804, 805f
anesthetic techniques for, 805, 806t
computed tomography, 797, 798f, 799f
differential diagnosis, 804t
electrodiagnostic studies, 797
with epidural metastases, 782–783
imaging studies, 797–800
magnetic resonance imaging, 797–800, 799f
management summary, 806–807
metastatic, 796–800
clinical features, 796–797, 804t
neurosurgical techniques for, 805
opioids for, 804–805, 806t
pain management in, 804–806, 806t
radiation-induced, 533, 533t
with second primary, 803
treatment, 800, 804–806
ultrasound, 800

Brachial plexus, 6f
exploration, indications for, 803–804
lymphedematous compression, 803
radiation fibrosis, 801–802
clinical features, 801–802, 804t
electrodiagnostic procedures, 802
radiographic findings in, 802
treatment, 802–803
radiation injury to, 800–803
pathophysiology, 800–801
transient, 801, 804t
tomographic anatomy, 797, 798f
tumor infiltration of, 796–800
clinical features, 796–797, 804t

Brain
breast cancer metastases to. *See* Metastases of breast cancer, central nervous system; Metastases of breast cancer, to brain
herniation, with cerebral metastases, 769–770

BRCA1 gene, 170, 172, 173f, 227
in breast cancer, 174, 221
age-specific risk associated with, 326–327
breast cancer risk estimation and, 180–181

in breast–ovarian cancer syndrome, 175–177, 185
and cancer progression, 288
chromosomal location, 174–175, 976
cloning, 984
genomic structure, 175, 175f
male breast cancer and, 180
mutations, 172, 173f, 175f, 175–177
and breast–ovarian cancer syndrome, 175–177
testing for, 327–328

BRCA2 gene, 172, 176, 180
in breast cancer, 174, 221
breast cancer risk estimation and, 181
chromosomal location, 976
mutation carriers, linkage analysis, 172–173

BrdU. *See* Bromodeoxyuridine

Breast(s)
abnormalities
acquired, 3
congenital, 2–3
muscular, 8
adult, morphology, 3–5, 4f
anatomy, 1–14
microscopic, 9, 10f
muscular, 6f, 8
neural, 8
architectural distortions, 116
asymmetry, 68, 69f, 116
blood supply, 5
developing, traumatic injury, 3
development, 1–14
abnormalities, 2–3
biochemical control, 15–25
hormone action in, 15–16
microanatomy, 9, 9t
modulators, hierarchy of, 15–16, 16f
molecular biology, 1–2
normal, during puberty, 3
edema, 69
embryology, 1
fullness, premenstrual, 10
lobes, 579
lymphatic drainage, 5–8, 7f
microanatomy, 4
morphology, 3–9
microscopic, in menstrual cycle, 9–10, 11t
normal, nodular irregular texture, 70
phases, 3, 3t
physiology, 9–12
tissue aging, 189, 191f
trauma
fat necrosis and, 62
gynecomastia associated with, 56
mechanism of injury, 61

Breast cancer
adenoid cystic. *See* Adenoid cystic carcinoma
adenosquamous, low-grade, 412–413
advanced, psychologic considerations, 930–931
age at diagnosis
cancer susceptibility genes and, 326

correlation with S-phase fraction, 468, 468t
prognostic significance, 464–465
age distribution, 110–111
angiogenesis in. *See* Angiogenesis
animal models. *See* Animal models; Transgenic mice
antigens, 298–300
apocrine, 413–414
autocrine factors in, 273, 274f
axillary node involvement in. *See* Axillary lymph nodes
biochemical metaplasia, 424
biologic therapy, 302–304
in blacks, prognosis for, 465
blood flow to, 75
blood vessel invasion, 399, 399f
calcifications in, 78–79, 79f, 115–117
cell adhesion in, 284–285
cell lines
antiestrogen resistant (ER+ cells), 249–250
BT 20 (mutant ER), 247
BT474 (ER––PR+), 247
characterization, 254–255
culture conditions, 255
establishment, 254–255
estrogen receptor (ER) content, 245
estrogen receptor negative (ER–), 245
DNA studies, 264
invasiveness assays, 252–253, 277
estrogen receptor positive (ER+), 245, 252–253, 277
hormone-independent but responsive
selected against 4-hydroxytamoxifen, 250
selection against 4-hydroxytamoxifen, 250
LY-2, 249
MCF-7, 245–246, 254
growth factor and receptor gene transfection studies in, 276–277
selected against benzothiophene in vitro, 249
selected against tamoxifen in vivo, 249–250
MCF-7/III, invasiveness and metastasis assays, 252
MCF-7 K3, 247
MCF-7/LCC1, 246–247
invasiveness and metastasis assays, 252
MCF-7/MIII, 246–247
MCF-7 MKS, 247
MDA-MB-134 (ER+), 248
MDA-MB-175 (ER+), 248
MDA-MB-231, 248
MDA-MB-361, 248
MDA-MB-435, 248
hematogenesis metastasis model in nude mouse, 278
metastasis assays, 252–253
MDA-MB-436, 248

Breast cancer, cell lines (*continued*)
    MDA-MB-453, 248
    MDA-MB-468, 275
    MDA-MB designated, 248
    new
        characterization, 255
        tumorigenicity, determination,
          255
    selected against benzothiophene in
      vitro, 249
    selected for drug resistance
      to doxorubicin, 250–251
      to steroidal antiestrogens, 250
    selected for hormone independence
      in vitro, 247
      in vivo, 246–247
    SkBr3, 249
    sources, 245
    steroid-dependent (ER+–PR+),
      245–246
    steroid-independent (ER±–PR±),
      246–248
    steroid-responsive, 246–248
    steroid-unresponsive (ER−–PR−),
      247–248, 248–249
    T47D, 246, 254
    T47D$_{CO}$ (ER−–PR+), 247–248
    transduced with MRD1 gene, 251
    transfected with FGF-4, 247
    ZR-75-1, 246, 254
        growth factor and receptor gene
          transfection studies in,
          276–277
  cells
    colonization of metastasis site, 287
    motility, 286
  clinical presentation, 67, 110
  computer-aided diagnosis, 90–93, 92*f*,
    93*f*
  cosmetic outcome, after conservative
    surgery and radiation therapy,
    494–496, 495*t*, 496*t*
  curability, 376*f*, 376–377, 377*f*
  cure, 375, 376
    clinical, 377
    personal, 377
    statistical, 376–377
  cystic hypersecretory, 419*f*, 419–420
  cytologic diagnosis, 154
    false-negative, 154–155
    false-positive, 155
  demographics, 159–168
  diagnosis, delay in
    due to physician, reasons for, 131,
      131*t*
    medicolegal aspects, 125–126
  dietary factors and, 201–212
  digital mammography, 89–90, 90*f*
  disregulated proliferation in, 21
  early detection, clinical significance,
    629–633
  effects
    in minority groups, 960
    on patient's children, 932–933,
      959–960
    on patient's spouse and significant
      other, 932, 960

  with endocrine features, 424–425
    clinical presentation, 424
    gross pathology, 424
    microscopic pathology, 424–425
    prognosis for, 425
    treatment, 425
  endocrine metaplasia, 424
  environmental factors in, 159–168
  epidemiology, 159–220
  epithelial growth in, defective
    regulation, 20–21
  estrogen and progesterone receptor-
    negative, 21
  estrogen receptors and. *See* Estrogen
    receptor(s)
  etiology, biological factors in,
    221–306. *See also* Growth
    factor(s); Oncogene(s); Tumor-
    suppressor gene(s)
  evaluation, medicolegal aspects,
    125–132
  evolution, 267–268, 268*f*
  extramammary recurrences, early
    detection, benefits, 629
  familial. *See* Familial breast cancer
  family history. *See* Family history of
    breast cancer
  within fibroadenoma, 46
  fine-needle aspiration biopsy. *See*
    Fine-needle aspiration biopsy
  gene(s), 162, 169, 299–300
  genetic alterations in, 221, 222*t*, 445
    models, 445
  genetic instability, 445
  genetic linkage analysis, 172–173,
    173*f*
  genetics, 168–169, 170
    in nonwhites, 170
  genetic susceptibility to
    counseling about, 327–328
    testing for, 327–328
  grade, prognosis and, 396
  grading, 395
    Fisher system. *See* Breast cancer,
      grading, nuclear
    histologic, 395–396
    nuclear, 395–396, 396*f*, 464
    Scarff-Bloom-Richardson (SBR)
      system, 464
  growth rate, 377–378
  heterogeneity, 394
  high-risk patients. *See* High-risk
    patients
  in Hispanics, prognosis for, 465
  histology, prognostic significance, 462
  histopathology, prognostic
    significance, 462–464
  hormonal receptor status,
    determination, in fine-needle
    aspirates, 154
  hormone responsivity, 20–21
  imaging, new methods for, 84–98
  immune response to, 300–302
  immunohistochemical markers, as
    prognostic indicators, 401, 402*t*
  immunohistochemical scoring systems,

    advantages and disadvantages,
      466, 466*t*
  immunology, 298–306
  immunotherapy, 298–306
  impact in United States, 159
  incidence, 159–161
    age-specific rates, in whites, 190,
      192*f*
    geographic variation
      among whites in United States,
        160, 162*f*
      international, 159–160, 160*f*
    migrant studies, 160, 160*t*
    race/ethnicity and, in United States,
      160, 161*t*
    time trends, 161, 164*t*
  infiltrating
    ductal. *See* Ductal carcinoma,
      infiltrating
    lobular. *See* Lobular carcinoma,
      infiltrating
    prognostic factors for, 462
    size at diagnosis, and prognosis, 80
  inflammatory, 425–426, 426*f*
    clinical features/presentation,
      425–426, 590
    combined modality treatment, 591*t*,
      591–592
    cutaneous findings in, 425–426
    dermal lymphatic invasion, 591
    dermal tumor emboli, 426
    diagnosis, 586
    dose-intensive therapy for, 595
    HER-2/neu oncogene in, 426
    local–regional therapy for,
      591–592
    lymphocytic reaction in, 425–426,
      426*f*
    management strategy, 596, 596*f*
    microscopic findings in, 425
    occult, 426
    pathology, 425–426
    in pregnancy, infection versus, 124
    prevalence, 590
    prognostic factors, 595
    staging, 586
    treatment, 585–599, 590–592, 591*t*
  inherited. *See also* Familial breast
    cancer
    clinical characteristics, 169
    frequency, 170–171
    genetics, 171–175
  in situ. *See* Carcinoma in situ
  in vitro models, 245–261
    acquired antiestrogen resistance in
      (ER+ cells), 249–250
    cautions with, 254
    epithelial-mesenchymal transition
      and, 19, 21, 253
    normal breast epithelial cells and
      their derivatives, 251–252, 274
    oncogene expression and in vitro
      metastatic potential, 253–254
    for studying invasion and metastasis,
      252–264

for studying multidrug (MDR1/ gp170) resistance, 250–251
interval (arising between screening examinations), 315
intraductal, apocrine carcinoma, 413–414
  prognosis for, 414
invasion
  coordinate regulation with metastasis, 287–288
  genes regulating, 285*t*
  genetic events associated with, 288
  process, 284
  proteinase inhibitors and, 285–286
  proteinases in, 285–286
  redundant mechanisms for, 284
invasive. *See* Invasive breast cancer
invasive potential
  in vitro assays for, 252–253
  measures, prognostic utility in breast cancer, 476–477
juvenile. *See* Breast cancer, secretory
lipid-rich, 419
locally advanced
  combined modality approach to, 587–589, 588*t,* 589*t*
    clinical trials, 588, 588*t*
    combinations and sequences of modalities, 589, 589*t*
    local control rate after, 588–589, 589*t*
  definition, 585
  diagnosis, 586
  dose-intensive therapy for, 595
  induction chemotherapy for, 586–587, 587*t,* 588*t*
  local therapy, 587–589, 588*t,* 589*t*
  management strategy, 596, 596*f*
  prognostic factors, 595
  staging, 586
  treatment, 585–599
    breast preservation after induction chemotherapy, 589–590
    historical perspective on, 585–586
local recurrence
  after conservative surgery, 657–661
    adjuvant chemotherapy for, 661
    breast-conserving surgery for, 660–661
    mammographic appearance, 658, 658*f*
    management, 661
    mastectomy for, 660
    presenting signs and symptoms, 657–658
    pretreatment evaluation, 659–660
    prognosis for, 658–659, 659*f*
    radiologic findings, 658, 658*f*
    reirradiation, 661
    treatment results, 660–661
  after conservative surgery and radiation therapy, 492–494, 493*t,* 494*t*
    margin involvement in, 501–502, 502*t*

patient risk factors, 498*t,* 498–499
  risk factors for, 496–504
  treatment factors in, 502–504
  tumor risk factors, 499–501, 500*f*
after mastectomy
  distant metastases with, 657
  hyperthermia therapy, 655
  intraarterial regional chemotherapy, 655–656
  intralesional therapy, 656
  management, 657
  photodynamic therapy, 655
  presenting signs and symptoms, 649
  pretreatment evaluation, 652
  prognosis for, 650–652, 651*f*
  radiation therapy, 652*t,* 652–654, 653*t*
  reirradiation, 654
  sites of further recurrence, 652, 652*t*
  subsequent morbidity and spread, 649–650
  surgical treatment, 654–655
  systemic therapy, 656–657
  topical treatment, 656
  treatment results, 652–657
  definition, 649
  with distant metastases, 649
  sites, 488–489, 489*f*
local treatment. *See* Local treatment of breast cancer
loss of differentiation in, 21
lymphatic spread, 827–833. *See also* Metastases of breast cancer, lymphatic
  chest radiography, 827, 827*t,* 828*f*
  clinical presentation, 827
  computed tomography, 827, 829*f,* 829*t*
  differential diagnosis, 829–831
  pathologic diagnosis, 828–829, 830*f,* 831*f*
  pathophysiology, 828–829
  prognosis for, 831–832
  radiologic findings, 827, 827*t,* 828*f,* 829*f,* 829*t*
  treatment, 831–832
lymphatic tumor emboli, 397–398, 398*f*
  extratumoral, 397–398
  prognostic significance, 398–399
lymphoplasmacytic infiltration, prognostic significance, 396–397
magnetic resonance imaging, 84–89, 85*f,* 86*f,* 87*f,* 88*f*
male. *See* Male breast cancer
mammographic appearance, 72, 72*f,* 77–82, 115
  margins, 80–81, 115
medullary. *See* Medullary carcinoma
menopausal status at diagnosis, prognostic significance, 465
metachronous, 880

metaplasia, 411. *See also* Metaplasia
  heterologous, 411
  homologous, 411
metaplastic, 411–413
  age at diagnosis, 411
  age distribution, 411
  clinical presentation, 412
  diagnostic criteria, 411
  frequency, 411–412
  gross pathology, 412
  heterologous, 411
  homologous, 411
  microscopic pathology, 412*f,* 412–413
  with osteoclast-like giant cells, 417
  prognosis for, 412–413
  pseudosarcomatous, 411
  squamous, 411
metastagenicity, 376
metastases. *See* Metastases of breast cancer
microinvasive
  axillary metastases, 521
  breast-conserving treatment with, 521–522
  definition, 521
  management, 521–522
  survival with, 521
microvessel density in. *See also* Angiogenesis
  prognostic significance, 400, 478
minimal, 521
molecular epidemiology. *See* Molecular epidemiology
molecular pathology, 445–456
mortality, 159–161, 669, 670*f*
  international geographic variation, 159–160, 160*f*
  in screening trials, 312–314, 313*f,* 314*f*
  by site of involvement, 669, 670*f*
  time trends, 161, 163*f,* 164*t*
mucinous. *See* Mucinous carcinoma
multifocal versus multicentric, 79
National Cancer Institute cancer control objectives for, 910
natural history, 375–391
negative immunoregulation exerted by, 301
nipple discharge with. *See* Nipple discharge
node-negative. *See also* Axillary lymph node(s)
  adjuvant therapy for, 463, 464*t*
  frequency, 463–464, 464*t*
  Ki67 in, prognostic significance, 469, 469*t*
  survival, by tumor size, 463*t,* 463–464
node-positive. *See also* Axillary lymph node(s)
  prognosis for, 463
    correlation with S-phase fraction, 468, 468*t*
noninvasive, prognostic factors for, 462

Breast cancer, noninvasive (*continued*)
  autosomal dominant inheritance, 171–172, 172f, 173f
  epidemiology, 169–171, 170t
  explanations for, 168–169
  frequency, 170–171
  genetic linkage analysis, 172–173, 173f
  genetics, 171–175
  historical perspective on, 168
  inheritance patterns, 170
  in males, 179–180
  in nonwhite populations, 170
  occult primary, with axillary metastases, 892–896
    adjuvant therapy for, 895
    and breast cancer occurrence in untreated breast, 893, 893t
    breast-conserving treatment for, 894
    diagnosis, 892–893
    frequency, 892
    mammography in, 893
    management summary, 895
    mastectomy for, 893–894
    natural history, 893
    pathology, 893–894, 894t
    survival, 894–895, 895t
    treatment, 893–895
  onset, autocrine and paracrine factors in, 273–276
  operable versus inoperable, 585
  orderly. *See* Breast cancer, tubular (well-differentiated)
  with osteoclast-like giant cells, 417f, 417–418, 418f. *See also* Osteoclast-like giant cells, carcinoma containing
  papillary. *See* Papillary carcinoma
  paracrine interactions in, 273, 274f
  pathogenesis
    biologic factors in, 221–306. *See also* Growth factor(s); Oncogene(s); Tumor-suppressor gene(s)
    endogenous hormones in, 190–193
    model, 189–190, 191f, 192f
  patient characteristics, prognostic significance, 464–465
  perineural invasion, 400, 400f
  positron emission tomography, 93–95, 94f, 95f
  predictive factors in, 461–485
    definition, 461
  pregnancy and. *See* Pregnancy, breast cancer and
  premenopausal, 110–111
  prevention, 335–354, 912
    agents, target problems, 336, 337f, 338f
    alcohol intake and, 346
    antiestrogens for, 338–339
    biologic considerations, 335–341
    clinical considerations, 341–354, 342t
    contraception and, 337–338
    diet in, 345–346
    endocrine strategies, 336, 338f

estrogen replacement therapy and, 348–349
    ethical implications, 350–351
    exercise and, 346–347
    future considerations, 339
    life-style factors in, 345–347
    and medically underserved minorities, 912
    medical strategies, 347–348
    pseudopregnancy and, 336–337
    psychologic considerations, 349–350
    synthetic retinoids for, 338
    windows of opportunity for, 336, 338f
  primary
    distribution of residual carcinoma in relation to, 488–489, 489f
    location, and prognosis, 379, 380t
    multiple, risk factors for, 165
    natural history, 378–379, 380f, 380t
    site
      distribution by quadrant, 379
      nomenclature for, 379
      and prognosis, 379, 380t
    size, and prognosis, 379, 380t
  primary therapy, evaluation of patients after, 629–647
  progesterone receptors and. *See* Progesterone receptor(s)
  prognosis for, factors affecting, 394–395
  prognostic factor models, 478–479
  prognostic factors, 461–485
    definition, 461
    examples, 461, 462
    histopathologic features, 462–464
    historical perspective on, 461–462
  progression, autocrine and paracrine factors in, 272, 273t, 273–276
  proliferation, measures, 465, 465t
    prognostic significance in breast cancer, 465–469
    technical considerations, 466, 466t
  protective factors, 185t
  pseudosarcomatous metaplasia, 411–412
    microscopic pathology, 412, 413f
    prognosis for, 413
  psychologic evaluation of patient with, indicators for, 923, 923t
  psychologic impact
    decision making and, 920–921, 945–947
    factors affecting, 919–931, 920t
    medical variables in, 920t, 924–931
    psychologic variables in, 920t, 922–923
    public attitudes and, 921–922
    sociocultural context and, 920t, 920–922
  radiation-induced
    after contralateral radiation therapy, 535–536
    after radiation therapy, 535–536
  radiographic attenuation, 81–82

radiotherapy, pathologic changes associated with, 38f, 39
  recurrence
    after conservative surgery, 657–661
      local, 657–661
    cure versus prolongation of survival, 630–631, 631f, 632f
    detection, 635–643
    factors affecting, 463
    first site of relapse, predictive factors, 635
    histologic documentation, 673–674
    isolated (solitary), definition, 649
    local. *See* Breast cancer, local recurrence
    local–regional, after mastectomy or breast-conserving therapy, 649–667
    natural history, 669–672
    nursing management, 960
    physical palliation for, 632
    prevalence, 669
    regional, definition, 649
    in regional lymph nodes, 379–385, 661–662
      management, 662
      pretreatment evaluation, 662
      prognosis for, 662
      radiation therapy for, 662
      signs and symptoms, 661–662
      subsequent morbidity and spread, 662
      surgery for, 662
      systemic therapy for, 662
      treatment results, 662
    screening for
      cost, 633
      effective treatment and, 630–632
      emotional support and, 632–633
      routine, 630–633
      serologic assays in, 634t, 639, 639t
    sites, 669
    skin involvement in, 426
  reference tumor, distribution of residual carcinoma in relation to, 488–489, 489f
  risk. *See also* High-risk patients
    absolute, 323, 324t
    age and, 160–161, 163f
    age at menarche and, 186–187
    discussion of, with patient, 328
    environmental exposures and, 166, 166t
    estimating, in clinical setting, 180–182
    estimation, 180–182
    with fibroadenoma, 46
    hair dyes and, 165
    by histologic category of benign disease, 31–32, 32t
    lifetime
      analytic, with family history of breast cancer, 181t, 181–182
      empiric, with family history of breast cancer, 181t, 181–182

medical history and, 164–165
occupational exposures and, 166
physical activity and, 165
prenatal exposures and, 165
quantification, 341–342
radiation and, 165–166
relative, 323
smoking and, 165
with solitary intraductal papilloma, 42, 43t
risk factors, 20, 162–166, 186–190
demographic, 162
environmental, 166, 166t
familial, 162
hormonal, 185t, 185–200
interaction with inherited breast cancer risk, 180
in medically underserved minorities, 912
menstrual, 163–164
in racial/ethnic groups, 911, 912
reproductive, 162–163
screening. *See* Screening
secretory, 418f, 418–419
single-photon emission computed tomography, 96
solid circumscribed. *See* Medullary carcinoma
spontaneous hemorrhage into, 62
spread. *See also* Metastases of breast cancer
along mammary ducts, 378
by direct infiltration, 378
Halsted model, 386, 387t
lymphatic, 378–379
mechanisms, 378–379
Spectrum paradigm, 386–387, 387t
Systemic view, 386, 387t
squamous. *See* Squamous carcinoma
squamous metaplasia, 411–412
in medullary carcinoma, 405
microscopic pathology, 412, 412f
with phyllodes tumors, 863–864
prognosis for, 413
stage I, treatment, induction chemotherapy in, 590
stage II, treatment, induction chemotherapy in, 590
stage III
local therapy, 587–589
management, historical perspective on, 585
treatment
breast preservation after induction chemotherapy, 589–590
combined modality treatment, survival effects, 592t, 593f, 593–595, 594f
stage IV, no evidence of disease, treatment, 716–717
staging, 457–459
applications, 457
chest wall, 458
clinical (TNM or cTNM), 457
Columbia Clinical Classification, 457, 458t

cT size, 457
definition, 457
dimpling of skin or nipple retraction, 457
inflammatory carcinoma, 458
multiple simultaneous ipsilateral (infiltrating, grossly measurable) cancers, 457
Paget disease of nipple, 457
pathologic (pTNM), 457
inevaluable nodes for (pNX), 457
inevaluable tumor for (pTX), 457
pT size, 457
simultaneous bilateral cancers, 457
TNM system, 457–459
steroid receptor-positive, 20–21
steroid receptor status, correlation with S-phase fraction, 468, 468t
survival, 161, 164t
adjuvant therapy and, 572–573, 573t
after recurrence, 630–631, 631f, 632f
diet and, 209
disease-free, 549, 631, 631f, 632f
local treatment and, 385–388
overall, 549, 631, 631f, 632f
race and, 672
by tumor size, for node-negative patients, 463t, 463–464
synchronous, 880
tissue compartmentalization in, defective regulation, 21–22
T0, N1, 892
treated, survival in, plotting, 375–376, 376f
treatment. *See* Treatment of breast cancer
tubular (well-differentiated), 401–404
age distribution at diagnosis, 402
clinical presentation, 402
differential diagnosis, 403
gross pathology, 402–403
invasive, 393–394
microscopic pathology, 403, 403f, 404f
with osteoclast-like giant cells, 417
pathologic definition, 401–402
prognosis for, 403–404
recurrence after mastectomy, 404
treatment, 404
tubulolobular, 421
tumor grade, prognostic significance, 464
tumor location
axillary node involvement and, 379–380, 381t
prognostic significance, 379, 380t
tumor size
axillary node involvement and, 379–380, 380t, 381t
prognostic significance, 382–383, 383t
correlation with S-phase fraction, 468, 468t

at diagnosis, and prognosis, 79–80
and metastases, 379, 380f
prognostic significance, 379, 380f, 380t, 463t, 463–464, 464t
tumor-suppressor genes and, 173–175
in underserved minorities, 910–918
clinical follow-up, 914–916
diagnosis, 914–916
early detection, 912–914
epidemiology, 911t, 911–912
health care and service needs, 916–917
prevention, 911–912
research needs, 916–917
treatment, 914–916
untreated, survival in, plotting, 375–376, 376f
virulence, 376
well-differentiated, 401
in whites, prognosis for, 465
work issues after, 960
Breast Cancer Chemotherapy Questionnaire, 551
Breast Cancer Detection Demonstration Project (BCDDP)
breast cancer risk in, with atypical hyperplasia, 31–32
data, risk estimation from, 324–325
nonrandomized clinical trial of breast cancer screening, 312
Breast Cancer Linkage Consortium, 176
Breast Cancer Prevention Trial, participation, risk estimation for, 325, 325f
Breast cancer susceptibility gene(s), 185–186, 186f
BRCA1. *See* BRCA1 gene
BRCA2. *See* BRCA2 gene
p53. *See* p53 gene
risk attributable to, 170–171
Breast care, optimal. *See also* Comprehensive breast program
principles, 963
Breast-conserving treatment
after induction chemotherapy, 589–590, 590t
axillary dissection with, technique, 525–526
breast abscess after, 527
combined with radiation therapy, clinical trials, 490–492, 491f, 492t, 493f, 493t
complications, 525–527, 527
contraindications to, 506, 506t
cosmetic outcome, 494–496
adjuvant chemotherapy and, 496
and extent of resection, 495, 495t, 496t
factors affecting, 495t, 495–496, 496t
scoring system for, 494
with ductal carcinoma in situ, 361–364, 362t, 363f, 364f, 365
guidelines for, 505–507
guidelines for patient selection, 505–507

Breast-conserving treatment (*continued*)
  historical perspective on, 488–489, 579
  ideal procedure for, search for, 580t, 581f, 581–583, 582f, 582t
  indications for reexcision, 526t, 526–527
  local disease recurrence after, 657–661
    breast-conserving surgery for, 660–661
    management, 661
    mastectomy for, 660
    pretreatment evaluation, 659–660
    prognosis for, 658–659, 659f
    reirradiation, 661
    signs and symptoms, 657–658, 658f
    systemic therapy, 661
    treatment results, 660–661
  for local disease recurrence after previous breast-conserving surgery, 660–661
  with microinvasive cancer, 521–522
  for occult primary with axillary metastases, 894
  Paget disease after, 873
  patient selection for, guidelines for, 505–507
  physical effects, 952
  principles and rationale for, 488–489
  psychologic outcome, 505
  radiation therapy after, technique, 529–532
  for recurrent cancer, 660–661
  role of biopsy in, 150–151
  safety, Milan Trial I and, 579–581, 580f, 580t
  sequence of chemotherapy and radiation therapy in, 519–521
  technique, 525–527
  trials
    from Danish Breast Cancer Group, 491, 492t, 493t
    from EORTC, 491, 492t, 493t
    from Institut Gustave-Roussy, 490–491, 492t, 493t
    from Milan National Cancer Institute, 490–491, 492t, 493t, 579–584
    from National Cancer Institute Early Breast Cancer Trial, 491, 492t, 493t
    from NSABP, 491, 492t, 493f, 493t
Breastfeeding
  and breast mass biopsy, 123
  protective effects against breast cancer, 163
Breast implant(s)
  for breast reconstruction, 603–604
  FDA evaluation and classification, 604, 620
  foreign-body granulomatous inflammation with, 38–39
  and risk of breast cancer, 165
  rupture, traumatic, 61
Breast lesion(s)
  nonpalpable

fine-needle aspiration biopsy, 153–155
  high suspicion, management, 149f, 149–150
  low-intermediate suspicion, management, 149f, 149–150
  management, 118, 149–150
  needle-localized biopsy
    accuracy, factors affecting, 141–142
    anesthesia for, 141
    incision for, 142, 143f
    needle placement for, 139–141
    specimen handling and examination, 142–143
    surgical principles, 142
  preoperative imaging-guided needle localization, 139–141
    guides for, 139–140
    mammographically guided, 140–141
    needle positioning, 141
    stereotactic needle placement, 141
  surgical approach to, 141–143
    accurate localization for accurate excision, 141–142
    anesthetic techniques, 141
    excised specimen, handling, 142–143
    principles, 142, 143f
  ultrasound-guided percutaneous needle biopsy, 152–158
palpable
  age distribution, 110
  biopsy techniques, 133–138
  diagnosis, 133–135
  fine-needle aspiration biopsy, 133–135
  mammography, 74–75
  management, 110
  treatment, two-step procedure, 133
  ultrasound, 75–76, 76f
solid
  fine-needle aspiration biopsy, 112, 154
  work-up, 112
spiculated, 72, 72f, 73, 73f, 81, 81f
triple diagnosis, 113, 113f, 134
Breast mass(es)
  aspiration cytodiagnosis, in pregnancy and lactation, 123
  automated detection, on mammography, 91, 93f
  benign, mammographic appearance, 115
  biopsy
    breastfeeding and, 123
    indications for, 115, 118, 119t, 120
  with breast lymphoma, 876
  with breast sarcoma, 877–878
  cystic versus solid, differentiation, 111
  diagnostic workup, 110–111, 111f
  differential diagnosis, in males, 860–861
  examination, 70

indeterminate, management, 115
  initial diagnostic work-up, 110–111, 111f
  malignant
    mammographic appearance, 115
    probability of, correlation with mammographic appearance, 72, 72f, 73f
  with mammary duct ectasia and periductal mastitis, 49–50
  mammographic appearance, 115
  on mammography, 115–116, 116f
    adjunctive assessment, 82
    analyzing, 79–82
    incidence of malignancy with, 119t
    as indication for biopsy, 119t
    location, 81, 82f
    size, 79–80
    x-ray attenuation, 81–82
  management, summary, 114
  needle aspiration, 111
  and nipple discharge, cancer risk with, 107
  nonpalpable. *See* Breast lesion(s), nonpalpable
Breast milk
  ejection, mechanisms, 12
  proteins, genes encoding, regulation, 19–20
  secretion, 12
  synthesis, 12
Breast mucin antigen, as indicator of recurrent breast cancer, 640
Breast–ovarian cancer syndrome, 175f, 175–177
Breast pain, 99–106
  and breast cancer, 130–131
  classification, 99–100
  clinical assessment, 99
  with costochondritis, 100
  cyclic, 100
    versus noncyclic, 99
  diet and, 100
  etiology, 100–101
  evaluation, 99–100
  histologic correlates, 100
  hormones and, 100–101
  with mammary duct ectasia and periductal mastitis, 49–50
  noncyclic, 99–100
  nonmammary causes, 100
  prevalence, 99
  spontaneous resolution, 101
  treatment, 101–104
    algorithm for, 104, 104f
    analgesics for, 103
    hormonal, 102–103
    nonhormonal, 103
    nutritional, 101–102
    psychiatric, 103–104
    summary, 104
    surgical, 104
Breast preservation, in pregnant woman, 885
  with delayed radiation, 885–886
Breast reconstruction, 601–628

autogenous tissue for, 604
with available tissue and saline
    implants, 604*f*, 605, 605*f*, 615*t*
breast management team and,
    601–602
delayed, 602–603
endoscopically assisted, 611–612,
    613*f*, 614*f*
flap procedures, 606–609, 615*t*
    gluteus maximus flap, microvascular
        tissue transfer technique, 611,
        612*f*, 613*f*
    latissimus dorsi extended flap, 607,
        615*t*
    latissimus dorsi musculocutaneous
        flap, 607, 608*f*, 609*f*, 615*t*
    TRAM flap, 607–609, 608*f*, 610*f*,
        615*t*
        microvascular tissue transfer
            technique, 610–611, 611*f*,
            615*t*
immediate, 602, 602*f*
    versus delayed, psychologic
        considerations, 928
    oncologic considerations in,
        528–529
management of opposite breast in,
    615, 618*f*
microvascular tissue transfer technique,
    610–611, 611*f*, 612*f*, 613*f*,
    615*t*
nipple–areolar reconstruction,
    613–615, 616*f*, 617*f*
with prophylactic mastectomy, 617
psychologic considerations, 601,
    926–928
with saline implant, 604*f*, 605, 615*t*
surgery for, 601–619
techniques, 603*f*, 603–611
    comparison, 615*t*
timing, 602–603
tissue expansion for, 605–606, 606*f*,
    615*t*
Breast self-examination, 307
    in breast cancer screening, 318–319
Breast surgery. *See* Treatment of breast
    cancer, surgical
Breslow test, 992
Bromocriptine
    for breast cancer metastases, 687
    for breast pain, 103
Bromodeoxyuridine (bromouracil;
    BrdU), 973
    in tumor proliferation measurement,
        466, 466*t*
Brush-1 gene, 228
    regulation, and breast cancer
        metastasis, 288
Bryostatin-1, anti-PKC activity, 22
BSE. *See* Breast self-examination
BT 20 (mutant ER) cells, 247
BT474 (ER−, PR+) cells, 247

C
CA15–3, as indicator of recurrent breast
    cancer, 640–641, 641*f*, 641*t*,
    642, 642*f*

CA549, as indicator of recurrent breast
    cancer, 640, 641*t*
CAAT box, 974
CAD. *See* Computer-aided diagnosis
Cadherins, 284, 285. *See also* E-cadherin
CAF. *See* Cyclophosphamide,
    doxorubicin, and fluorouracil
Caffeine
    consumption, and breast pain, 100,
        101
    intake, breast cancer and, 209
CAF therapy. *See* Cyclophosphamide,
    doxorubicin, and fluorouracil
Calcification(s), 28
    in benign lesions, 115–116
    of duct ectasia, 115
    eggshell, 78, 115
    of fat necrosis, 79*f*
    with lucent centers, 78, 115
    magnification mammography, 78, 82
    in malignancy, 115–117
    on mammography
        adjunctive assessment, 82
        analyzing, 77–79
        in breast cancer, 78–79, 79*f*
        casting, 79
        clustered, 79
        of comedocarcinoma, 79, 80*f*
        crescent-shaped, 78, 78*f*
        diffusely scattered, 79
        distribution, 79
        eggshell, 78, 115
        heterogeneous, 78–79, 79*f*
        location, 77
        lucent-centered, 78, 115
        morphology, 77–78, 77–79, 78*f*,
            79*f*
        number, 77
        regional, 79
        rod-shaped, 78, 78*f*
        sedimented, in cysts, 78, 78*f*
        segmental, 79
        size, 77, 78–79
        skin, 77, 78
        spherical, 78, 79*f*
        vascular, 78
    microfocal spot magnification, 116,
        117*f*, 118*f*
    pleomorphic, with mass, 82
    risk categories, 115–116
    size, diagnostic significance, 82
Calcitonin
    for hypercalcemia, 842–843
    in mammary carcinoma, 424
    for osteoporosis, 905
Calcitriol, in prevention of osteoporosis,
    905
Calcium, serum. *See also* Hypercalcemia
    measurement, 842
CALGB. *See* Cancer and Leukemia
    Group B
Calle, Robert, 490
Calusterone, for breast cancer metastases,
    687
Camptothecins, for metastatic breast
    cancer, 703

Canada, randomized clinical trial of
    breast cancer screening
    Canada NBSS1, 311*t*, 312, 314, 316*t*
    Canada NBSS2, 311*t*, 312, 313, 313*f*,
        316*t*, 318
    concerns raised about, responses to,
        315, 317*t*
Cancer and Leukemia Group B, study of
    dose-intensive adjuvant
    chemotherapy, 559, 560*t*
Cancer and Steroid Hormone Study,
    171
Cancer Research Campaign, of
    postoperative radiation therapy,
    513*t*, 514–515, 515*f*, 516*f*
Cancer susceptibility gene(s), 326
    testing for, 327–328
Candidal intertrigo, of inframammary
    fold, 52
Candidate gene(s), 984
Candidiasis, in breast cancer patient,
    957–958
Cap cells, 18
Capsular synovial hyperplasia, 39
Carboplatin
    for metastatic breast cancer, 704, 704*t*
    response to, in metastatic breast
        cancer, 692*t*
    with VP-16, for metastatic breast
        cancer, 704, 704*t*
Carcinoembryonic antigen
    in breast cancer, 298–299, 423
        as indicator of recurrence, 639–
            641, 640*t*, 641*f*, 641*t*, 642*f*
        prognostic significance, 401, 402*t*,
            642
    cerebrospinal fluid, 638
    with leptomeningeal metastases, 791
Carcinofetal antigens, in breast cancer,
    298–299
Carcinogenesis
    continuum of, events in, 213, 213*f*,
        336, 337*f*
    estrogen receptor expression in,
        267–268, 268*f*
    genetic alterations in, 445
    time course
        in animal models, 335, 336*f*
        in women, 335
    two-hit hypothesis, 174
Carcinoid tumor
    of breast, primary, 425
    metastases to breast, 425, 426
Carcinoma en cuirasse, 649, 650*f*
Carcinoma in situ, 355–373
    ductal, 355–368
        axillary lymph node involvement in,
            359–360
        classification, 355–359, 359*t*
        clinging carcinoma, 357
        comedo-type, 355–356, 356*f*,
            357–358
        cribriform
            with anaplasia, 358–359
            with necrosis, 358–359
        cribriform-type, 356, 356*f*, 358*f*

Carcinoma in situ, ductal (*continued*)
  differential diagnosis, 30–31,
    360–361
  distribution in breast, 359–360
  EORTC classification, 359, 359t
  histology, prognostic significance,
    364–365
  incidence, 355–359
  intermediately differentiated, 358,
    358f
  and lobular carcinoma in situ
    coexisting, 360–361
    comparison, 360
  management, summary, 366
  microinvasion, 360
  microinvasive carcinoma and,
    comparison, 521
  micropapillary–cribriform,
    358–359
  micropapillary-type, 356–357, 357f
  multicentricity, 359–360
  multifocality, 359
  natural history, 361
  with necrosis, 359
  nipple involvement in, 360
  noncomedo-type, 357–358
  nonpure comedo type, 359
  nuclear grade classification system,
    358–359
  occult invasion in, 360
  papillary-type, 356–357
  pathology, prognostic significance,
    364–365
  presentation, 355–359
  progression to invasive cancer, 361
  pure comedo type, 359
  recurrence
    after breast-conserving treatment,
      361–364, 363f, 364f
    predictive factors for, 364–365
  solid-type, 357
  stereotactic core biopsy, 150
  treatment
    breast-conserving, outcomes,
      361–364, 363f, 364f
    options, 361–366, 362t, 363f,
      363t, 364f
    outcomes, 363f, 363–364, 364f
    predictive factors for, 364–365
    selection, 365–366
  variants, 357
  without necrosis, 359
lobular, 355, 369–373
  breast cancer development with,
    370–372, 371t
  breast cancer risk with, 371–372
  calcifications and, 369
  differential diagnosis, 370
  distribution in breast, 369
  in fibroadenoma, 46
  follow-up studies, 370–371, 371t
  histology, 371, 371t
  incidence, 369
  laterality, 371, 371t
  malignant potential, 370–371, 371t
  mammographic findings in, 369
  management summary, 372

  natural history, 370–372, 371t
  pathology, 369–370, 370f
  treatment, 369
Carcinosarcoma, 411–412, 877
Cardiomyopathy, doxorubicin-induced,
    570
  radiation therapy and, 537
Carmustine, response to, in metastatic
    breast cancer, 692t
Carotenoids, 205
Carpal tunnel syndrome, in breast cancer
    patient, 803
Carryover contamination, 451
Cartilage-derived inhibitor, as
    angiogenesis inhibitors,
    286–287
Case-control trials, of screening, 312
CASH Study, 171
Casting, 79
Cathepsin(s), 286
  cathepsin B, in breast cancer, 22
  cathepsin D
    in breast cancer, 22
      prognostic significance, 402t
    overexpression, in breast cancer,
      286
    prognostic utility in breast cancer,
      476
  cathepsin L, in breast cancer, 22
CBE. *See* Clinical breast examination
CCNU, response to, in metastatic breast
    cancer, 692t
CD44, 284–285
CDGE. *See* Constant denaturant gel
    electrophoresis
CDK4, in metastasis, 22
CDK inhibitors, 20
cDNA library, 984
Cell adhesion molecules, 284–285
Cell-cell adhesion, in mammary
    epithelium, 21
Cell cycle, cell proliferation in,
    regulation, 466
Cell-cycle kinases, 19
Cells, genetically engineered, as
    immunogens, in
    immunotherapy of breast
    cancer, 303
Cell-substrate interactions, 21
Cell-substratum adhesion
  and differentiation, 22
  and metastasis, 22
Cellular therapy, for breast cancer,
    303–304
β-Cellulin, 221, 272
Cellulitis
  after breast cancer treatment, 659
  management, 124
Censored survival time, 991
Central lung distance, 530
Central nervous system, breast cancer
    metastases to. *See* Metastases of
    breast cancer, central nervous
    system; Metastases of breast
    cancer, to brain

Cephalic vein, 4f, 6f
c-erbB-2, 226, 229, 272. *See also*
    HER-2/neu
  in breast cancer, 217–218
  in breast cancer progression, 277
  monoclonal antibodies, possible
    therapeutic applications, 290
  in Paget disease, 873–874
  receptor, 223
  transfection studies, of breast cancer
    invasion and metastasis, 288
  transgenic mice, mammary tumors
    and, 240–241
c-erbB-3, 223, 226, 272
  ligands, 472t
  receptor, ligands, 472t
c-erbB-4, 272
  ligands, 472t
Cerebellar dysfunction, with adjuvant
    therapy, 958
Cerebral edema, with cerebral
    metastases, 769
Cerebrospinal fluid
  carcinoembryonic antigen in, 638
    with leptomeningeal metastases, 791
  chemotherapy in, for leptomeningeal
    metastases, 792–793, 793f
Cervical cancer, metastases to breast, 426
CGH. *See* Comparative genomic
    hybridization
CGS 20267, 686
Chain-termination DNA sequencing,
    977
Chemoendocrine therapy, adjuvant
  benefits, 566–569
  clinical trials, 566
  in postmenopausal patients, 568t,
    568–569
  in premenopausal patients, 566–569
Chemohormonal therapy, for metastatic
    breast cancer, 713–714, 714t
Chemoimmunotherapy, for metastatic
    breast cancer, 715
Chemoprevention, 347–348
  for high-risk patients, 331
Chemotherapy
  adjuvant
    alternating regimen, 556, 557t
    benefits, 552–561
    cardiac complications, 570
    clinical trials, 548
      absolute benefit in, 550
      disease-free survival in, 549f,
        549–551
      endpoints, 549–551
      hazard ratio in, 549–550
      metaanalysis, 551
      multiple subset analysis in, 551
      overall survival in, 549f, 549–551
      positive results, interpretation,
        551
      proportional benefit in, 550
      results interpretation, 548–552
    dose-intensive, 559–561, 560t
      and bone marrow transplantation,
        560–561

doxorubicin-based regimens, 556–557, 557t
historical perspective on, 548
longer-duration versus shorter-duration, 555–556
long-term adverse effects, 570–571
for male breast cancer, 861–862
new agents for, 561
optimal regimen, 554–561
and ovarian ablation, in premenopausal patients, 567
perioperative, 557–558
in postmenopausal patients, 552t, 553
postoperative
  in node-negative patients, 553–554, 554t, 555t
  in node-positive patients, 552–553
postoperative radiation therapy with, 515–518, 517t
premature menopause with, 570
in premenopausal patients, 552t, 552–553
preoperative, 558–559
primary, 558–559
of primary cancer, 548–578
psychologic considerations, 928–930
quality of life estimates with, 551–552
randomized clinical trials
  historical perspective on, 548
  results interpretation, 549–551
rationale for, 548
for recurrent cancer, 661
regimens, 562t
single-agent versus combination regimen, 554–555
summary, 561, 562t
and tamoxifen
  in postmenopausal patients, 568t, 568–569
  in premenopausal patients, 567t, 567–568
toxicity, 551–552, 569–571
  acute, 569t, 569–570
concentration difficulties with, management, 929
for epidural spinal cord compression, 786
fatigue with, 930
future of, 595–596
hair loss with, 953–956
  management, 929
induction (neoadjuvant), 558–559
  for locally advanced cancer, 586–587, 587t, 588t
  breast preservation after, 589–590, 590t
intraarterial regional, for local recurrence after mastectomy, 655–656
intra-cerebrospinal fluid, for leptomeningeal metastases, 792–794, 793f

leukemia risk with, 570–571
for locally advanced breast cancer, 586, 586t
for local recurrence after mastectomy, 656–657
memory difficulties with, management, 929
for metastatic breast cancer, 693–713
  agents, 692t–693t, 693–705
    anthracyclines, 693–697
    anthrapyrazoles, 696
    camptothecins, 703
    cyclophosphamide-based combinations, 697
    5-fluorouracil, 697–698
    ifosfamide, 704–705
    methotrexate, 698
    mitomycin, 705
    plant alkaloids, 698–703
    platinum compounds, 703–704
    taxanes, 699–703
    vinca alkaloids, 698–699
  dose intensity, 707–708
  drug resistance in, 705–706
  duration of therapy, 709–711
  in elderly, 712–713
  and hormonal therapy, comparison, 713
  non–cross-resistant regimens, 706–707, 707t
  number of drugs, 706
  principles, 705–709
  response to, predictive factors, 711–712
nausea and vomiting with, management, 929, 953, 954t, 955t
neoadjuvant, 558–559
  for locally advanced cancer, 586–587, 587t, 588t
  breast preservation after, 589–590, 590t
oral care during, 957
in pregnancy, 886
premature menopause with, 929
prospects for, 595–596
psychologic preparation for, 929–930
quality of life and, 709–711
side effects, management, 952–958
weight gain with, management, 929
Chest tube drainage, for malignant effusions, 835
Chest wall
  breast cancer recurrence in, biopsy, 138
  muscles, 6f
  reconstruction, after radiation therapy, 612–613, 614f, 615t
  vascular anatomy, 6f
Child(ren), of breast cancer patient
  cancer's effects on, 959–960
  psychological considerations in, 932–933
Chlorambucil, response to, in metastatic breast cancer, 692t

Cholesterol, serum, tamoxifen's effects on, 347–348
Chondrolipoma, 37
Chondromatous lesions, 37
Chorionic gonadotropin, and breast changes during pregnancy, 10
Choristoma, 37
Chromosome 17
  in molecular genetic studies of breast cancer, 447
  studies, in breast cancer, 174–175
Chronic cystic mastitis, 27
Cingulate herniation, with cerebral metastases, 769–770
Circumscribed scleroderma, 659
CIs. *See* Confidence intervals
Cisplatin
  for metastatic breast cancer, 703–704
  neurotoxicity, 958
  response to, in metastatic breast cancer, 692t
  with VP-16, for metastatic breast cancer, 703–704, 704t
Cisplatin, doxirubicin, and cyclophosphamide, for metastatic breast cancer, 704, 704t
Cisplatin and cytarabine, for malignant effusions, 835
Clear cell hidradenoma, 33
Clinging carcinoma, 357
Clinical breast examination, 110–114, 307
  abnormalities on, 110–114
  in breast cancer screening, 318
  interpretation, 111, 113
  and mammography, complementary nature, 128. *See also* Triple diagnosis
  medicolegal aspects, 125–126
  nonrandomized clinical trials, 312
  in pregnancy, 122
  in premenopausal women, interpretation, 111
  schedule, by risk status, 329t
  in triple diagnosis, 113
  underuse, in minority groups, 911
Clinical data, interpretation techniques, 986–1005
Clinical evaluation, 67–98
Clinical trial(s)
  eligibility for, monitoring, 994–995
  fraudulent, 993, 996
  interpretation, 986–987
  monitoring, 993–994
  outcome variables, 991
  randomization, monitoring, 995–996
  statistical power in, 987–988, 988t
  subgroup analysis, 997–1000
    commonly used subgroups, 997, 998t
    data-derived categories, 997–998, 999t
    multiple comparisons, 998–999
    quantitative versus qualitative interactions, 999–1000

Clinical trial(s) (*continued*)
  treatment compliance in, monitoring, 996
Clodronate. *See also* Bisphosphonates
  for hypercalcemia, 843
  for metastatic bone disease, 823*t*
Clomiphene citrate, for gynecomastia, 59
Clonal-dominance hypothesis, of metastatically competent cells, 287
Clonidine, for hot flushes, 905–906
Cloning, genes, 983*f*, 983–984
  positional, 983*f*, 984
CMFP. *See* Cyclophosphamide, methotrexate, fluorouracil, and prednisone
CMFPT. *See* Cyclophosphamide, methotrexate, fluorouracil, prednisone, and tamoxifen
CMF therapy. *See* Cyclophosphamide, methotrexate, and fluorouracil
CMFVP. *See* Cyclophosphamide, methotrexate, fluorouracil, vincristine, and prednisone
c-*neu*, protein
  ELISA, 642
  prognostic significance, 642
CNS, breast cancer metastases to. *See* Metastases of breast cancer, central nervous system; Metastases of breast cancer, to brain
COC. *See* Oral contraceptives, combination
Coding region, in mRNA, 974
Codon, 972
Cohort study, of screening, 312
Collagenase(s), 294
Collagenous spherulosis, 37, 415–416
Collecting ducts, 4
Colon cancer
  diet and, 202
  incidence, in patients with previous history of breast cancer, 629
  inherited, 178
Colony-stimulating factor, 16*f*
  action on mammary epithelium, 17
Colony-stimulating factor 1, in mammary development, 18
Colorectal cancer, metastases to breast, 426–427
Colostral milk, secretion, in neonate, 1
Colostrum
  formation, in pregnancy, 11–12
  lactoglobulin in, 12
  regulatory molecules in, 17
  secretion, 12
Columbia Clinical Classification, 457, 458*t*
  of breast cancer, 457, 458*t*
Comedomastitis. *See* Mammary duct ectasia, and periductal mastitis
Comedonecrosis, 79
Comparative genomic hybridization, 445, 447–448, 449*f*
  advantages, 448

Compensatory damages, 130
Competing risk bias, in comparisons of metaanalyses, 1002
Complex sclerosing lesions, 34
Comprehensive breast program
  business development, 966*t*–967*t*, 967–968
  clinical program development, 965–967
  collaborative approach, 964–965
  community advisory board, 965
  conceptual framework for, 963, 964*f*
  facility development, 968–969
  freestanding center, advantages and disadvantages, 968, 968*t*
  goals, 963
  management team, 964–965
  mission statement, 964
  organizational development, 964–965
  patient advisory board, 965
  personnel recruitment and retention, 964
  translational research in, 967
Computed tomography
  of brain metastases, 770–772, 771*f*
  of leptomeningeal metastases, 791, 792*f*
  of orbital metastases, 809, 810
  with pericardial effusions, 837
  of solitary pulmonary nodule, 853
Computer-aided diagnosis
  of breast cancer, 90–93, 92*f*, 93*f*
  in mammography, view stations for, 92–93
Concentration difficulties, with chemotherapy, management, 929
Confidence intervals, 989–991
  disadvantages, 990
Confidence limits, 989
Constant denaturant gel electrophoresis, 979
Constipation, with adjuvant therapy, 958
Constitutional 11q;22q chromosomal translocations, 178–179
Contraceptives, injectable, breast cancer risk and, 194–195
Cooper, Astley, 99
Cooper ligaments, 5, 69
Cooper regimens, for metastatic breast cancer, 697
Coping strategies, and psychologic impact of breast cancer diagnosis, 922–923
Coracobrachialis muscle, 6*f*
Core-cutting needle biopsy, 135
  seeding of needle track in, 135
  technique, 135, 135*f*
Corticosteroids, for hypercalcemia, 842–843
Costochondritis, breast pain with, 100
Costocoracoid ligament, 8
Coumarin, for lymphedema, 900
Cowden syndrome, 175, 177–178
CPT-11, 595

Cranial neuropathy, with adjuvant therapy, 958
Cripto, in breast cancer invasion and metastasis, 288
Cripto-1, 221, 272
Curie, Pierre and Marie, 489
C–V flap, for nipple–areolar reconstruction, 614, 616*f*
Cyclic adenosine monophosphate, 16, 16*f*
Cyclin(s), 225
  breast cancer and, 228–229
  cyclin D$_1$, 228
  cyclin E, 228
  in mammary epithelial cell cycle, 20
  as measure of proliferation, 465*t*
Cyclin-dependent kinases, 20
  breast cancer and, 228–229
  inhibitors, breast cancer and, 228–229
β-Cyclodextrin tetradecasulfate, 290
Cyclophosphamide
  nausea and vomiting with, 953
  response to, in metastatic breast cancer, 692*t*
Cyclophosphamide, doxorubicin, and fluorouracil
  adjuvant chemotherapy regimens based on, 556–557, 557*t*, 562*t*
  cycle interval, 562*t*
  cycles, 562*t*
  dose and schedule, 562*t*
  efficacy
    correlation with S-phase fraction, 467
    and HER-2/neu status, 474
  intravenous
    cycle interval, 562*t*
    cycles, 562*t*
    dose and schedule, 562*t*
Cyclophosphamide, methotrexate, and fluorouracil
  adjuvant therapy
    intravenous, in node-negative patients, 562*t*
    regimens based on, 556–557, 557*t*
    standard regimen, 562*t*
    toxicity, acute, 569*t*, 569–570
  cycle interval, 562*t*
  cycles, 562*t*
  dose and schedule, 562*t*
  efficacy
    correlation with pretreatment thymidine labeling index, 467
    correlation with S-phase fraction, 467
    and HER-2/neu status, 473, 474
  intravenous
    cycle interval, 562*t*
    cycles, 562*t*
    dose and schedule, 562*t*
  for metastatic breast cancer, 697
    dose intensity, 708, 709*t*
  perioperative, 558
  postoperative radiation therapy with, 515–518, 517*t*
  super-CMF regimen, 708, 709*t*

Cyclophosphamide, methotrexate, fluorouracil, and prednisone, postoperative radiation therapy with, 516

Cyclophosphamide, methotrexate, fluorouracil, prednisone, and tamoxifen, postoperative radiation therapy with, 516

Cyclophosphamide, methotrexate, fluorouracil, vincristine, and prednisone

  adjuvant therapy, 556, 557*t*, 562*t*

  cycle interval, 562*t*

  cycles, 562*t*

  dose and schedule, 562*t*

Cylindroma, 414

Cyst(s), 27–28

  aspiration, 111–112, 133

    indications for, 75

    ultrasound-guided, 154

  blue dome, 28*f*

  breast cancer risk and, 28–29

  excisional biopsy, after aspiration, 111–112

  fine-needle aspiration biopsy

    technique, 134

    ultrasound-guided, 154

  fluid

    analysis, indications for, 154

    bloody, 111, 134

    cytopathologic analysis, 111–112, 134

    with malignancy, characteristics, 111, 134

  gross, 28, 28*f*

  mammographic appearance, 73*f*, 81, 81*f*

  management, 111–112, 112*f*

  spontaneous hemorrhage into, 62

  ultrasound, 75, 76*f*

Cystic hypersecretory carcinoma, 419*f*, 419–420

Cystosarcoma phyllodes, 877. *See also* Phyllodes tumors

Cytogenetics, 466

  of breast cancer, 446

  comparative genomic hybridization in, 447–448, 449*f*

  fluorescence in situ hybridization in, 446–447, 447*f*

  molecular, 446. *See also* Comparative genomic hybridization; Fluorescence in situ hybridization; Primed in situ labeling

  primed in situ labeling in, 447, 448*f*

  traditional, 446

Cytokine(s), 19. *See also specific cytokine*

  genes, insertion into tumor cells, for immunotherapy of breast cancer, 303

  in immune response to breast cancer, 302

  monoclonal antibodies against, in biologic therapy of breast cancer, 302

receptors, on breast cancer, and immune response to cancer, 302

  therapy, for breast cancer, 303–304

Cytosine arabinoside, response to, in metastatic breast cancer, 692*t*

Cytotoxic agents, antiangiogenic effects, 295

  in combination therapy, 296

D

Dacarbazine, response to, in metastatic breast cancer, 692*t*

Daidzein, 345–346

Danazol

  for breast cancer metastases, 687

  for breast pain, 102

  for gynecomastia, 59

  mechanism of action, 102

  pharmacology, 102

Daughter(s), of breast cancer patient, psychologic considerations in, 932–933

DCIS. *See* Carcinoma in situ, ductal

DDT exposure, and breast cancer risk, 166

Degeneracy, in genetic code, 975

Denaturant gradient gel electrophoresis, 452, 979

Depression

  with advanced breast cancer, 930–931

  breast cancer diagnosis and, 923

  with tamoxifen therapy, 571

Detection, definition, 71

Dexamethasone (Decadron), antiemetic regimens, 954*t*, 955*t*

DF3, as indicator of recurrent breast cancer, 641*t*

DGGE. *See* Denaturant gradient gel electrophoresis

Diabetic mastopathy, pathology, 39

Diagnosis, definition, 71–72

Diagnostic bias, 993

Diagnostic test(s)

  sensitivity, 987

  specificity, 987

Diazepam, for patient with advanced breast cancer, 931

Diet

  breast cancer and, 201–212

  breast cancer prevention and, 335, 345–346

  breast cancer survival and, 209

  breast pain and, 100

  colon cancer risk and, 202

Diethylstilbestrol, adjuvant therapy with, 566

Dihydrotestosterone, for gynecomastia, 59

Dimensions of Caring, 959*t*

7,12-Dimethybenz(*a*)anthracene, rodent mammary tumors induced by, 236

Diphenhydramine (Benadryl), antiemetic regimens, 954*t*, 955*t*

Discrete pulmonary nodules. *See* Solitary pulmonary nodule(s)

Disease-free survival, 549

Diuretics

  for breast pain, 103

  contraindications to, in lymphedema, 900

DMPA. *See* Medroxyprogesterone acetate, depot

DNA, 972–974

  double helix, 972

  fluorescence in situ hybridization, 446–447, 447*f*, 982, 982*f*

  microinjection, 984

  oxidative damage, 215

  replication, 972

  sequencing, 977–978, 978*f*

    chain-termination, 977

DNA libraries, 983–984

DNA polymerase, as measure of proliferation, 465*t*

Docetaxel (Taxotere), 595

  for metastatic breast cancer, 702–703, 703*t*

    response to, 692*t*

  toxicity, 702

Documentation, medicolegal aspects, 126

Donné corpuscles, 12

Doppler imaging, of breast lesions, 75

Doxorubicin (Adriamycin)

  adjuvant therapy, 556–557, 557*t*

    regimens based on, 556–557, 557*t*

  antiangiogenic effects, 295

  cardiac toxicity, prevention, 592

  cardiomyopathy caused by, 570

    radiation therapy and, 537

  for metastatic breast cancer, 693–695, 694*f*

    comparison with other agents, 696–697

    response to, 692*t*

Doxorubicin, cyclophosphamide, methotrexate, and fluorouracil

  adjuvant therapy with, 562*t*

  cycle interval, 562*t*

  cycles, 562*t*

  dose and schedule, 562*t*

Doxorubicin, vincristine, cyclophosphamide, and 5-fluorouracil, adjuvant chemotherapy, 556, 557*t*

Doxorubicin and cyclophosphamide

  adjuvant therapy, 556, 557*t*, 562*t*

    toxicity, acute, 569*t*, 569–570

  cycle interval, 562*t*

  cycles, 562*t*

  dose and schedule, 562*t*

Doxorubicin and cyclophosphamide → cyclophosphamide, methotrexate, and fluorouracil, adjuvant chemotherapy, 556, 557*t*

Doxycycline, as sclerosing agent, 835

Droloxifene, 680–681

Ductal adenomas, 37

Ductal carcinoma
  cystic hypersecretory, 357
  infiltrating
    argyrophilia, 424–425
    cytologic diagnosis, 154
    with endocrine features, 425
    in fibroadenoma, 46
    lipid-rich, 419
    prognostic factors for, 462
  intraductal component
    cytologic features, 393
    growth pattern, 393
    prognostic significance, 401, 401f
  invasive, 393–401
    angiogenesis, as prognostic factor,
        399–400
    blood vessel invasion, 399, 399f
    classification, 393
    clinical presentation, 395
    elastosis, 400–401
    grading, 395–396, 396f, 397f
    gross pathology, 395
    with heterogeneous histology, 393,
        394f
    histologic patterns, 393–395, 394f
    histologic types, 393
    intraductal carcinoma pattern and
        distribution in, as prognostic
        factor, 401, 401f
    with invasive lobular carcinoma,
        393
    lymphatic tumor emboli in,
        397–399, 398f
    lymphoplasmacytic infiltration,
        396–397
    microinvasion, 401, 401f
    microscopic pathology, 395–401,
        396f
    not otherwise specified, 393
    with osteoclast-like giant cells, 417
    perineural invasion, 400, 400f
    prognostic factors for, 396–401,
        462
    sarcomatous metaplasia, 412, 413f
    stroma in, 400–401
  with lymphocytic reaction, 396–397
  medullary, 396–397
  microinvasive, 401, 401f
  nonmedullary, 396–397
  with productive fibrosis, 393
Ductal carcinoma in situ. *See* Carcinoma
    in situ, ductal
Duct excision, 108f, 109
Duty, medicolegal concept of, 127
Dye injection, as guide for preoperative
    localization of clinically occult
    lesions, 140

E
E-cadherin
  expression in tumor, 253
  in mammary epithelium, 21
Eccrine spiradenoma, 33
Echocardiography, with pericardial

effusions and cardiac
    tamponade, 837
Edema. *See also* Lymphedema
  postoperative, 944t
    management, 946t
    preoperative evaluation and, 946t
Edinburgh Trial
  of postoperative radiation therapy,
      513t, 514–515, 515f, 516f
  randomized clinical trial of breast
      cancer screening, 310, 311t,
      312–314, 313f, 316t
Effective sample size, 988
Effusions
  malignant. *See* Malignant effusions
  pleural. *See* Pleural effusions
EIC. *See* Extensive intraductal
    component
Elastosis, in invasive duct carcinoma,
    400–401
Elderly
  chemotherapy in, 712–713
  hyperlipidemia treatment in, 905
  tamoxifen for
    as adjuvant therapy, 564–565
    as primary therapy, 524–525
Electrocautery, intraoperative damage to
    biopsy specimen by, 429–430,
    430f
Electromagnetic radiation, breast cancer
    risk and, 165–166
Eligibility bias, 993
Elliptinium
  derivatives, 595
  response to, in metastatic breast
      cancer, 692t
EMBL. *See* European Molecular Biology
    Laboratory
Embryonic stem cell transfer, 985
Endocrine-growth factor regulation,
    hierarchy, 15, 16f
Endocrine metaplasia, 424
Endocrine therapy for breast cancer. *See
    also* Tamoxifen
  adjuvant, benefits, 561
  for metastases. *See also* Hormonal
      therapy
    combination regimens, 689–691,
        690t
    response to
      factors affecting, 691–693
      predictive markers for, 691–693
  response to, predicting
    with discordant receptor phenotype,
        262
    by estrogen receptor status, 262
    by progesterone receptor status, 263
Endometrial cancer, tamoxifen use and,
    571–572, 629, 678, 930
Endothelial cell proliferation
  drugs targeted against, antiangiogenic
      effects, 296
  inhibitors based on, 296
  neoangiogenesis and, 293, 295
  therapy directed against, 295–296

Energy intake, childhood or adolescent,
    breast cancer risk and, 204
Epidermal growth factor, 16f, 272
  action, on mammary epithelium, 17
  in angiogenesis, 286
  in breast development, 2
  family, 272
  steroid hormone regulation of, 276,
      276t
Epidermal growth factor family, in
    biochemical control of breast
    development, 17–18
Epidermal growth factor receptor(s), 272
  in breast cancer, as target for therapy,
      302
  family
    in breast cancer, 221–226, 472
    overexpression, clinical significance,
        225–226
  ligands, 472t
  ligand systems, overexpression, clinical
      significance, 225–226
  monoclonal antibodies against,
      therapeutic applications, 290,
      473
  pathway, 224–225
  as predictive factor, 472–473
  prognostic significance in breast
      cancer, 472–473
  –protooncogene, 222–223
  signal transduction cascade from, 224f,
      224–225
  status, as prognostic factor, 223
  as therapeutic target, 473
Epidophyllotoxin, for metastatic breast
    cancer, 699, 700t
Epidural metastases. *See* Metastases of
    breast cancer, epidural
Epidural space, definitive imaging, 783f,
    783–785, 784f, 785f
Epidural spinal cord compression,
    779–789
  incidence, 779
  investigations, 780–785
  myelography in, 783f, 783–785
  pathology, 779
  prognosis for, 787, 787t
  signs and symptoms, 779–780, 780t
  treatment, 785–786
Epiglycanin, 299, 301
Epinephrine, in mammary carcinoma,
    424
Epirubicin, for metastatic breast cancer,
    695–696
  response to, 692t
Epithelial cells
  heterotypic adhesion to myoepithelial
      cells, 21
  homotypic adhesion of, 21
  normal, 251–252
    benzo(a)pyrene-immortalized 184
        and B5 lineages, 251
    derivatives, 251–252
    immortalized, 274
    MCF-10A, 252

transformation with oncogenes, 252, 274
Epithelial membrane antigen, polyclonal antibody, in immunohistochemical detection of micrometastases, 432–433
Epithelial-mesenchymal transition, 19, 21, 253
Epithelial-related calcifications, 28
Epithelial system, of breast
  cell cycle, 20
  growth, defective regulation, in cancer, 20–21
  nomenclature, 4–5, 5*t*
Epitheliosis. *See* Papillomatosis
EPO. *See* Evening primrose oil
EREs. *See* Estrogen-responsive elements
ERK-1 kinase, 225
ERK-2 kinase, 225
Erythema, 69
  of inflammatory carcinoma, 69
E-selectin, in metastasis, 22
Esorubicin, 696
  response to, in metastatic breast cancer, 692*t*
Estradiol
  exposure, breast cancer risk and, 185–186, 186*f*
  metabolism
    breast cancer risk and, 192, 215
    in breast epithelial cells, 185–186, 186*f*
  transport, in breast epithelial cells, 185–186, 186*f*
Estradiol mustard, response to, in metastatic breast cancer, 692*t*
Estramustine, response to, in metastatic breast cancer, 692*t*
Estrogen(s), 19
  breast cancer and, 20–21, 261
  in breast development, 3, 17
  breast pain and, 100–101
  cellular effects, 261–262
  cumulative exposure to, and breast cancer risk, 186–187
  deficiency, health consequences, 903–904, 904*t*
  effects
    on breast cancer, growth factors and, 274
    on tumor initiation and growth, in rat models of carcinogenesis, 336
  endogenous, in breast cancer pathogenesis, 190–192, 192*t*
  exposure, breast cancer risk and, 185, 185*t*
  in lobuloalveolar growth, 17
  metabolism, male breast cancer and, 860
  stromal inductive effect, 17
  therapy, for prostatic carcinoma, and breast cancer, 427
  tumor flare with, 688–689, 689*t*

Estrogen/androgen ratio, gynecomastia and, 54–55
Estrogen receptor(s), 262
  alternative splicing, 268
  breast cancer and, 261–271
    background, 261–262
    DNA studies, 264
    ER−, PR− tumors, proliferative rate, 262*t*
    ER−, PR+ tumors, 266–267, 267*f*
      proliferative rate, 262*t*
    ER+, PR− tumors, 265*f*, 266
      proliferative rate, 262*t*
    ER+, PR+ tumors, proliferative rate, 262*t*
    prognostic significance, 223, 262, 469–471, 470*f*
    and proliferative rate, 262, 262*t*
    protein studies, 263–264
  B-variant allele, 264–265, 265*f*
  clones C.4, C.5, and C.26, 265, 265*f*
  expression, in breast cancer evolution, 267–268, 268*f*
  in fibroadenomas, 46
  functional domains, 262–263
  in immune system cells, 239
  in male breast cancer, 860
  monoclonal antibodies to, 263–264
  PvuII RFLP, 264
  and response to endocrine therapy for breast cancer metastases, 691
  from tamoxifen-resistant patients, 265–266
  variants, 19
    from breast tumors with discordant receptor phenotype, 266*f*, 266–267
    from ER+, PR− tumors, 265*f*, 266
    from ER−, PR+ tumors, 266–267
    exon 5 deletion, 266–267, 267*f*
    isolated from clinical samples, 264–266, 265*f*
Estrogen recruitment, in treatment of metastatic breast cancer, 714–715, 715*t*
Estrogen replacement therapy
  in breast cancer prevention, 348–349
  breast cancer risk and, 195–198, 197*t*, 348–349
  in management of menopause
    in women with history of breast cancer, 904, 906–907
    in women with no history of breast cancer, 904
  postmenopausal, in high-risk women, 330–331
Estrogen-responsive elements, 262
Ethnicity, prognostic significance in breast cancer, 465
Etidronate, for hypercalcemia, 843
Etoposide, response to, in metastatic breast cancer, 692*t*
European Molecular Biology Laboratory, 978
Evening primrose oil, for mastalgia, 101–102

Exemustane, 686
Exercise
  for breast cancer patient
    benefits, 944, 945
    management, 956–957
  in breast cancer prevention, 346
  in prevention of osteoporosis, 905
Exon(s), 975
Expert witnesses, 129
Exponential order scores test, 992
Exposure(s)
  measurement, 214–215
  and molecular biomarkers, and cancer, 216, 216*f*
Extensive intraductal component, invasive breast cancer with
  mammography, 500
  pathophysiology, 500–501
  recognition, 500
  and risk of local recurrence, 499–500, 500*f*, 582–583
External abdominal oblique muscle, 4*f*, 6*f*
External intercostal muscle, 6*f*
Eye, metastases to. *See* Metastases of breast cancer, ocular

F
FACM. *See* 5-Fluorouracil, doxorubicin, cyclophosphamide, and methotrexate
Fadrazole, 686
FAK (focal adhesion kinase), in breast cancer, 22
Familial breast cancer, 168–185, 227, 326. *See also* Breast cancer, inherited; Hereditary breast cancer syndromes
Family, of breast cancer patient
  books and publications for, 933
  care of, 931–933
  role in treatment, 931–933
Family history of breast cancer
  breast cancer risk and, 31–32, 32*t*, 169–170, 170*t*, 326
    historical perspective on, 169
    population-based studies, 169
  in first-degree relative
    breast cancer risk and, 31–32, 32*t*, 169–170, 170*t*, 326
    breast cancer risk estimation and, 169–170, 326
    Claus model, 326–327, 327*t*
  male breast cancer and, 859
  as predictor of screening, 319–320
Fat, dietary
  breast cancer and, 201–204
    animal studies, 201
    case-control studies, 202–203
    cohort studies, 202*t*, 203*f*, 203–204
    international correlation (ecologic) studies, 201
    intervention studies, 204
    secular trends in, 201–202

Fat, breast cancer and (*continued*)
    in special populations, 202
  and breast pain, 100
  intake, during adjuvant therapy, 956
  reduction, effects on breast pain, 101
Fatigue, in breast cancer patient
  with chemotherapy, 930
  with radiation therapy, 952
  rehabilitation and, 943–944
  treatment, 945
Fat necrosis, 62–63, 63*f*, 64*f*
  calcifications of, 79*f*
  causes, 62
  clinical features, 62–63
  diagnosis, 63
  oil cyst form, 81
Fatty acids
  and breast pain, 100
  dietary, carcinogenesis and, 345
FDG. *See* Fluorodeoxyglucose
FEC. *See* 5-Fluorouracil, epirubicin, and
    cyclophosphamide
Fenretinide, 207
  response to, in metastatic breast
    cancer, 692*t*
Fentanyl
  for brachial plexopathy, 806*t*
  transdermal system, pharmacology,
    806*t*
Ferguson reflex, 12
Fertility, after cancer treatment,
    958–959
Fetus
  breast cancer staging and, 884–886
  breast cancer treatment and, 884–886
  metastatic disease in, 886
  radiation risk to, 884
Fiber, dietary, breast cancer and, 204
Fibroadenolipomas. *See* Hamartoma(s)
Fibroadenoma(s), 45–47
  ancient, 33
  aspiration cytology, 47
  breast cancer risk with, 46
  calcified, 115
  cancer within, 46
  cell of origin, 45
  clinical features, 45, 46–47
  clonal analysis, 46
  complex, breast cancer risk with, 46
  core biopsy, histology, 147*f*
  core needle biopsy, 47
  cytogenetics, 45–46
  cytologic diagnosis, 154
  differential diagnosis, 47
  epidemiology, 45
  estrogen receptors in, 46
  etiology, 45–46
  excision, 137
  excisional biopsy, 47
  giant, 33, 47
  histology, 33
  hormonal influence on, 46
  infarction, 33
  juvenile, 33, 47
  mammographic appearance, 45, 75*f*
  management, 46–47
  multiple, 47

natural history, 47
pathology, 32–33, 33*f*
postmenopausal, 46
progesterone receptors in, 46
variants, 33, 47
Fibroblast growth factor(s), 16*f*
  action, on mammary epithelium, 17
  in angiogenesis, 286
    inhibition, 295
  angiogenesis and, 293–294
  in angiogenesis and metastasis, 277,
    278
  basic, 400
  in breast cancer, 273
  in breast development, 2
  in normal and malignant breast, 275
  tumor cell motility and, 286
Fibroblast growth factor 4, cells
    transfected with, as in vitro
    model of breast cancer, 247
Fibrocystic disease, 27
Fibromatosis of the breast
  with familial multicentric fibromatosis,
    37
  with Gardner syndrome, 37
  pathology, 36–37
  treatment, 36–37
Fibronectin
  in breast cancer, 423
  gene, regulation, and breast cancer
    metastasis, 288
Fine-needle aspiration biopsy, 133–135,
    152
  advantages, 133–134
  of breast abscess, 154
  of breast cancer, ultrasound-guided,
    154
  of cysts, technique, 134
  cytologic, 586
    with metastatic disease to breast,
      880
  cytopathological analysis, 134
  in diagnosis of malignancy, 112
  diagnostic accuracy, 134
  hematoma secondary to, 61
  historical perspective on, 133
  interpretation, 134
  of malignant tumors, ultrasound-
    guided, 154
  of palpable breast mass, 133–135
  of solid mass, 112, 154
  of surgical scar lesions, 134
  technique, 134–135
  in triple diagnosis, 113, 134
  triple-negative diagnostic test and, 134
  ultrasound-guided
    of benign lesions, 154
    of cysts, 154
    failures, 154–155
    of fluid collections, 154
    limitations, 154–155
    of lymph node metastases, 154
    of malignant tumors, 154
    of nonpalpable breast lesions,
      153–155
      instrumentation, 153

needle insertion technique, 153,
    153*f*
patient preparation, 153
sampling technique, 153–154
technical considerations, 153–154
of solid masses, 154
and ultrasound-guided large-core
    needle biopsy, comparison,
    155–157
FISH. *See* Fluorescence in situ
    hybridization
Fisher, Bernard, 490
Fish oil consumption, carcinogenesis
    and, 345
Fistula(s)
  mammary, 50
    nonpuerperal, 50–51
  milk, and biopsy of breast mass, in
    lactating woman, 123
Fletcher, Gilbert, 490
Florid intraductal hyperplasia, 29*f*
Florid papillomatosis, 44
  of the nipple ducts, 34
Flow cytometry
  S-phase fraction by, 467–469
    technical considerations, 466*t*
  technical considerations, 466*t*
  tumor proliferation measurement, 466
Floxuridine, response to, in metastatic
    breast cancer, 692*t*
Fludarabine, response to, in metastatic
    breast cancer, 692*t*
Fluid collections
  aspiration, ultrasound-guided, 154
  fine-needle aspiration biopsy,
    ultrasound-guided, 154
Fluorescence in situ hybridization,
    446–447, 447*f*, 982, 982*f*
  advantages and disadvantages, 446
Fluoride, for osteoporosis, 905
Fluorodeoxyglucose, in breast cancer
    imaging with PET, 94*f*,
    94–95, 95*f*
5-Fluorouracil
  for metastatic breast cancer, 697–698
    response to, 692*t*
  neurotoxicity, 958
5-Fluorouracil, doxorubicin,
    cyclophosphamide, and
    methotrexate
  adjuvant chemotherapy, 556, 557*t*
  for metastatic breast cancer, dose
    intensity, 708, 709*t*
5-Fluorouracil, epirubicin, and
    cyclophosphamide, adjuvant
    chemotherapy regimen, 556,
    557*t*
Fluoxymesterone, for breast cancer
    metastases, 687
Follicle-stimulating hormone
  and breast morphology, during
    menstrual cycle, 10
  in normal breast development during
    puberty, 3
Foreign material, reactions to, 38–39
Foreseeability, legal concept of, 127

Formestane, for breast cancer metastases, 685–686
  side effects, 686
Fracture(s), pathologic
  with bone metastases, 815
  management, 816–818
  risk for, quantification, 815*t*, 816
Frameshift, 972
Fraud, legal considerations, 129
Ftorafur, response to, in metastatic breast cancer, 692*t*
Fumagillin, 296. *See also* Pentosan polysulfate
Functional outcomes, of breast cancer treatment, 944
Funduscopy, with ocular metastases, 809

G
Gadolinium diethylenetriaminepentaacetic acid, 84–87
Gail model of risk estimation, 324–325, 325*f*, 342, 343
Galactic band, 1
Galactocele, high fat content, 81
Galactography
  in evaluation of nipple discharge, 108
  with mammary duct ectasia and periductal mastitis, 50
Galactorrhea, causes, 107
Gallium nitrate
  for bone metastases, 823
  for hypercalcemia, 843
  response to, in metastatic breast cancer, 692*t*
Gastric cancer, metastases to breast, 426
GCDP. *See* Gross cystic disease protein
Gd-DTPA. *See* Gadolinium diethylenetriaminepentaacetic acid
Gelatinase(s), 294
  in breast cancer, 22
  in invasive breast cancer, 277–278
Gel electrophoresis, 975
  denaturant, 979
  pulse-field, 980
Gemcitabine, 595
GenBank, 978
Gene(s)
  in breast cancer, 299–300
  candidate, 984
  definition, 971
Generalized Savage test, 992
Generalized Wilcoxon test, 992
Gene therapy, 985
Genetic code, 972, 973*t*, 975
Genetic linkage analysis, 172–173
Genetic manipulations, 984–985
Genetic polymorphism, 975
Genetic testing, 327–328
Genistein, 345–346
Genome, 971
Geographic bias, in comparisons of metaanalyses, 1002

Gestodene, 337–338
Gestrinone
  for breast pain, 102
  pharmacology, 102
Glucocorticoids, in lobuloalveolar growth, 17
Glutathione peroxidase, breast cancer risk and, 207–208
Gluteus maximus muscle flap, for breast reconstruction, microvascular tissue transfer technique, 611, 612*f*, 613*f*
Glycogen, in breast cancer, 401
Goserelin, for breast cancer metastases, 686–687
Göteborg Study, randomized clinical trial of breast cancer screening, 310, 311*t*
Gothenburg, randomized clinical trial of breast cancer screening, 310, 312–314, 313*f*
Granisetron (Kytril), antiemetic regimen, 954*t*
Granular cell tumors
  neurogenic origin, 36
  pathology, 35–36
  treatment, 36
Granulocyte-macrophage–colony-stimulating factor
  in immune response to breast cancer, 301
  immunosuppressive effects, 301
Granulomatous mastitis, 39
Gray (unit), 490
GRB2. *See* Growth factor receptor–binding protein 2
Gross cystic disease fluid protein-15, in breast cancer, 423
  prognostic significance, 402*t*
Gross cystic disease protein, as indicator of recurrent breast cancer, 641*t*
Group coping skills instruction, definition, 949
Growth factor(s)
  angiogenesis and, 277–278, 293–294, 294*f*
  apoptosis and, 277
  in breast cancer, 20–21
    metastases and, 277–278
    steroid hormone regulation, 276*t*, 276–277
    in tumor onset, 273–276
    in tumor progression, 273–276, 276–277
    in tumor proliferation, 276–277
  classes, 272–273
  endocrine function, 17
  families, 272–273, 274*f*
  heparin-binding
    in angiogenesis, 293
    angiogenesis and, 293
    inhibitors, antiangiogenic activity, 295–296
  inhibitors, antiangiogenic activity, 295
  juxtacrine, 15
  in malignancy, 19

  in normal and neoplastic breast, 272–283
  prognostic significance in breast cancer, 472*t*, 472–474
  receptors, 15
    prognostic significance in breast cancer, 472*t*, 472–474
    sex steroid-regulated, in breast cancer, 276*t*, 276–277
    type I, 472
      ligands, 472, 472*t*
  secretion, 15
  secretory routing, 15
  synthesis, 15
  in tumorigenesis, 218–219
Growth factor receptor–binding protein 2, 224
  biochemical function, 19
Growth hormone, 19
  in breast development, 17
  in lobuloalveolar growth, 17
Gynecomastia, 54–60
  age and, 54
  associated conditions, 55–56, 56*t*, 57*t*
  differential diagnosis, 56–57, 860–861
  drug-related, 57, 57*t*, 58–59
  estrogen/androgen ratio and, 54–55
  evaluation, 56–58, 57*t*, 58*f*
  florid stage, 54, 59
  histology, 54, 59
  idiopathic, 56, 58
  inactive stage, 59
  medical therapy, 59–60
  neonatal, 54
  pathogenesis, 54–55, 56*t*
  pathophysiology, 54–55, 56*t*
  prevalence, 54, 55*f*
  prevention, 58–59
  pubertal, 54, 55, 59
    transient or persistent, 57–58
  surgical therapy, 59
  treatment, 59–60

H
Haagensen, Cushman D., 963
Hair dyes, breast cancer risk and, 165
Hair loss, with chemotherapy, 953–956
  management, 929, 953–956
Hair preservation techniques, 956
Halsted, William, 487, 579
Halsted ligament, 6*f*, 7*f*, 8
Hamartoma(s), 47, 81
  clinical features, 47
  incidence, 47
  mammographic findings with, 47
Hand, Learned, 127
Haplotype, 976
Hazard ratio, 549–550
Headache
  with brain metastases, 770
  brain tumor, characteristics, 770
Health insurance, and genetic test results, 328

Health Insurance Plan of New York, randomized clinical trial of breast cancer screening, 310, 311*t,* 312–314, 313*f,* 316*t*

Heart, radiation-related injury, 536–537

Heat shock proteins, 19, 471–472

Heidelberg trials, of postoperative radiation therapy, 513*t,* 515, 515*f,* 516*f*

Height, breast cancer risk and, 204–205, 205*f*

Hemangiomas
    of mammary subcutaneous tissue, 37
    perilobular, 37
    venous, 37

Hematoma
    breast, 61*f,* 61–62
    clinical management, 62
    postoperative
        after excisional breast biopsy, 61–62
        aspiration, ultrasound-guided, 154
        secondary to fine-needle aspiration, 61

Hemorrhagic cystitis, management, 958

Heparin-binding epidermal growth factor, 221, 272, 275

Hepatocyte growth factor
    angiogenesis and, 293
    in breast cancer, 273
    tumor cell motility and, 286

Hepatoma, tamoxifen use and, 571

HER-3. *See* c-erbB-3

HER-4. *See* c-erbB-4

Hereditary breast cancer syndromes, 175–179

Heregulin(s), 221, 272
    heregulin-1, 223, 224, 225
    heregulin α, 272

HER-2/neu. *See also* c-erbB-2
    CAF therapy efficacy and, 474
    CD8 lymphocytes against, 300
    detection, 473
    gene
        amplification, prognostic significance, 473
        in breast cancer, 299–300, 450
        chromosomal location, 175, 473
        immunotherapy and, 300
        in inflammatory carcinoma, 426
        prognostic significance, 299–300, 402*t,* 473–474, 474*t*
    in inflammatory breast cancer, 426
    monoclonal antibodies against, 302
        therapeutic applications, 302
    as predictive factor, 473–474
    protein, 299–300
        CD8 cytotoxic T lymphocytes against, 300
        vaccine, 303
    receptor, ligands, 472*t*
    status, CMF therapy efficacy and, 473, 474
    and tamoxifen resistance, 474
    treatment resistance and, 473–474
    vaccine, in biologic therapy of breast cancer, 303

Hexamethylmelamine, response to, in metastatic breast cancer, 692*t*

Hidradenoma, clear cell, 33

High-density lipoprotein(s), tamoxifen's effects on, 347–348

High-risk patients
    breast cancer prevention trials in, tamoxifen in, 338–339
    management, 323–334
        by chemoprevention, 331
        by close surveillance, 328–329
        options for, 328–332
        by prophylactic mastectomy, 329–331
    oral contraceptives for, 331
    postmenopausal hormone replacement therapy in, 331–332
    screening, 319

Hispanics. *See also* Underserved minorities
    breast cancer in, prognosis for, 465
    endemic poverty in, 910, 910*t*

Histones, as measure of proliferation, 465*t*

History-taking, medicolegal aspects, 125–126

Hookwire system(s), as guide for preoperative localization of clinically occult lesions, 139–140, 140*f*

Hormonal manipulation, for male breast cancer, 861–862

Hormonal therapy
    adjuvant, psychologic considerations, 930
    adverse effects, 930
    for breast cancer metastases, 674–693
        agents, 675–687
            androgens, 687
            antiestrogens, 680–681
            antiprogestins, 683–684
            aromatase inhibitors, 684–686
            LHRH agonists, 686–687
            optimal sequencing, 687–688, 688*t*
            progestins, 681–683
            tamoxifen, 675–680
        historical perspective on, 674–675
        response rate with, 674, 674*t*
            and steroid receptor status, 674–675, 675*t*
    for locally advanced breast cancer, 586, 586*t*
    for local recurrence after mastectomy, 656–657

Hormone(s)
    antiangiogenic activity, 295
    autocrine (or intacrine), 15, 16
    in breast cancer etiology, 185–200
    breast pain and, 100–101
    endogenous, in breast cancer pathogenesis, 190–193, 192*t*
    exogenous, in breast cancer pathogenesis, 193–198, 194*t*
    in normal breast development during puberty, 3
    paracrine, 15

Hormone-induced tumor flare, 688–689, 689*t*

Hormone replacement therapy
    breast cancer risk and, 195–198, 197*t*
    in high-risk patients, 331–332

Hospice care, 930

Hot flushes
    climacteric, 905–906
    with tamoxifen, 677

4HPR. *See* N-4-Hydroxyphenyl retinimide

HR, for lymphedema, 900

hsps. *See* Heat shock proteins

Human chorionic gonadotropin, in breast cancer, 424
    prognostic significance, 402*t*

Human Genome Project, 971, 984

Human leukocyte antigen(s), up-regulators, in immunotherapy, 304

Husband, of breast cancer patient, 932, 960

Hydromorphone
    for brachial plexopathy, 806*t*
    pharmacology, 806*t*

Hydroxyl radicals, 215

N-4-Hydroxyphenyl retinimide, in breast cancer prevention, 338

Hydroxyproline, urinary, as marker of bone destruction, 822

17-Hydroxysteroid dehydrogenase, 185–186, 186*f*

Hydroxytamoxifen, estrogen receptor binding, 263

Hydroxyurea, response to, in metastatic breast cancer, 692*t*

Hypercalcemia, 840–847
    bisphosphonates for, 843–844
    calcitonin for, 842–843
    clinical features, 841–842
    corticosteroids for, 842–843
    differential diagnosis, 841–842
    diuretic therapy for, 842
    etiology, 840
    gallium nitrate for, 843
    hydration therapy for, 842
    management, 842*t,* 842–844
        summary, 842*t,* 844*t,* 845
    mithramycin for, 843
    outpatient treatment, 844
    phosphates for, 843

Hyperlipidemia, treatment, in elderly, 905

Hyperplasia(s), of breast, 2
    atypical
        breast cancer risk and, 29–30
            hormonal milieu and, 31–32
        differential diagnosis, 30
        ductal, 29, 31*f*
        lobular, 29, 31*f*
        pathology, 29–37, 31*f,* 32*t*
        nodular lactational. *See* Adenoma(s), lactating

Hypnotics, for breast cancer patient, 923

Hypodermic needle, as guide for preoperative localization of

clinically occult lesions, 139, 140f
Hypoplasia, of breast, 2
Hysterectomy, breast cancer risk and, 164, 187

I
I-CAM-1, in metastasis, 22
I Can Cope, 950
ICI 182,780, 680–681
Idarubicin, 696
  response to, in metastatic breast cancer, 692t
Ifosfamide, for metastatic breast cancer, 704–705
  response to, 692t
Imaging
  breast cancer, new methods for, 84–98
  of breast lesions, 71–84
    audit, 74
    monitoring results, 74
    double reading, 71
Immunofluorescence, detection of micrometastases, 432–433
Immunoglobulin superfamily, in cell–cell adhesion, 285
Immunohistochemical markers, as prognostic indicators in breast cancer, 401, 402t
Immunohistochemistry
  frozen, technical considerations, 466t
  of micrometastases, 432–433
  p53, and clinical outcome, 475
  permanent, technical considerations, 466t
  scoring systems, advantages and disadvantages, 466, 466t
  tumor proliferation measurement, 466
Immunophilin, 273
Immunoregulation, negative, exerted by tumor, 301
Immunotherapy
  adjuvant, 569
  of breast cancer, 298–306
Implant(s). See Breast implant(s)
Incision(s)
  biopsy, in needle-localized biopsy of nonpalpable mass, 142, 143f
  circumareolar, 108f, 109, 142, 143f
  for excisional breast biopsy, 136, 136f
Indurative mastopathy, 34
Infection(s)
  and biopsy of breast mass, in lactating woman, 123
  breast. See also Mastitis
    in lactation, 124
    in pregnancy, inflammatory cancer versus, 124
    uncommon, 52–53
  in immunosuppressed patient, management, 957–958
  and mammary duct ectasia and periductal mastitis, 49

Inflammation, noninfectious, of breast, 51–52
Inflammatory carcinoma, 425–426, 426f
Inflammatory disorders, 37–39
Inflection point, of survival curves, 376
In situ hybridization, 982f, 982–983
  fluorescent, 446–447, 447f, 982, 982f
Inking, of margins of excisional biopsy, 428, 429f, 430f
Insulin, in lobuloalveolar growth, 17
Insulin-like growth factor(s), 16f
  action on mammary epithelium, 17
  in breast cancer, 273
  in breast development, 18
  IGF-1
    in breast development, 17
    in lobuloalveolar growth, 17
  IGF-2, steroid hormone regulation of, 276, 276t
  tumor cell motility and, 286
Insulin-like growth factor binding protein-3, steroid hormone regulation of, 276, 276t
Insulin-like growth factor binding protein-4, steroid hormone regulation of, 276, 276t
Integrin(s), 284
  in cell-substrate adhesion, 21
  in metastasis, 22
Intercostal arteries and veins, 4f, 5
Intercostobrachial nerve, 6f
Interferon(s)
  in immunotherapy, for breast cancer, 304
  INF-α, as angiogenesis inhibitor, 286–287
  INF-β, as angiogenesis inhibitor, 286
  INF-γ, gene, insertion into mouse adenocarcinoma, 303
  up-regulation of HLA antigens, 304
Intergroup Trial, of postoperative adjuvant chemotherapy in node-negative patients, 554, 554t
Interleukin(s)
  IL-1
    angiogenesis and, 293
    up-regulation of HLA antigens, 304
  IL-2
    effects on breast cancer, 302
    gene, insertion into mouse adenocarcinoma, 303
    therapy, for breast cancer, 303–304
  IL-4
    angiogenesis and, 293–294
    gene, insertion into mouse adenocarcinoma, 303
    receptors, in breast cancer, 302
  IL-6, effects
    on breast cancer, 302
    on ER+ and ER− breast cancer cells, 287
  IL-8, angiogenesis and, 293–294
  IL-10, immunosuppressive effects, 301
Internal intercostal muscle, 6f

Internal mammary artery and vein, 4f, 5, 6f, 7f
Internal mammary lymph nodes. See Lymph node(s), internal mammary
International Breast Cancer Study Group, adjuvant therapy trials, 670
Intertrigo, candidal, of inframammary fold, 52
Interval cancers, 315
Intracranial pressure, increased, with cerebral metastases, 770
Intraductal carcinoma
  in fibroadenoma, 46
  in invasive breast cancer
    mammography, 500
    pathophysiology, 500–501
    recognition, 500
    and risk of local recurrence, 499–500, 500f, 582–583
Intron(s), 975
Invasive breast cancer, 393–444
  atypical medullary, 396
  axillary dissection in, role of, 511–512
  axillary node involvement, and risk of local recurrence, 499
  cribriform, 360, 393–394
  duct. See Ductal carcinoma, invasive
  with extensive intraductal component
    mammography, 500
    pathophysiology, 500–501
    recognition, 500
    and risk of local recurrence, 499–500, 500f, 582–583
  growth factors in, 277
  histology, and risk of local recurrence, 499–500
  local management, 487–547. See also Breast-conserving treatment
    guidelines for, 505–507
    historical perspective on, 487–489
  local recurrence
    after radiation therapy with conservative surgery, 492–494, 494t
    risk factors for, 496–497
      adjuvant chemotherapy as, 503–504
      age at diagnosis as, 497–499, 498t
      extent of resection as, 502–503
      margin involvement as, 501–502, 502t
      patient risk factors, 497–499, 498t
      radiation treatment factors, 502–503
      treatment factors, 502–504
      tumor risk factors, 499–501, 500f
    with lymphatic vessel invasion, and risk of local recurrence, 501
    margin involvement, and risk of local recurrence, 501–502, 502t
    prognostic factors for, 462
    radiation therapy, postoperative

Invasive breast cancer, radiation therapy (*continued*)
    indications for, 512–519
      with systemic therapy, 515–519
      without systemic therapy, trials, 513t, 513–515
    radiation therapy for
      with conservative surgery
        clinical trials, 490–492, 491f, 492t, 493f, 493t
        cosmetic outcome, 494–496
        local recurrence after, 492–494, 494t
        retrospective studies, 492–505
      historical perspective on, 489–490
      reexcision, indications for, 526t, 526–527
      tamoxifen therapy, as primary therapy for elderly patients, 524–525
    tubular, 393–394
    tumor size, and risk of local recurrence, 499
Iodine, for mastalgia, 100, 102
4-Iodotamoxifen, 681
Ionizing radiation, breast cancer risk and, 165–166
IP-10, 303
Irinotecan, 703
IRS-1, biochemical function, 19
Isoflavonoids, breast cancer risk and, 209

J
JAK kinases, 19, 225
Japan
    breast cancer incidence in, 189–190
    cohort study of breast cancer screening, 312
JCRT. *See* Joint Centers for Radiation Therapy
JNK kinase, 225
Joint Centers for Radiation Therapy
    Adjuvant Chemotherapy Trial, 518
    locoregional recurrence series, 650–652, 651f
    radiation therapy technique, 529–532
    on sequencing of radiation therapy and chemotherapy, 519–520
    trial of conservative surgery, 522–523
    trial of postoperative radiation therapy with adjuvant therapy, 517t
Juvenile fibroadenomas, 33, 47
Juvenile papillomatosis, 34, 44
    characteristics, 43t
    recurrent, 44
    in women with positive family histories, 44
Juxtacrine action, 222
Juxtacrine factors, 15

K
Kaplan-Meier estimate, 991, 991f
Keratins, ductal luminal, in breast cancer, 21
Kerley A lines, 827

Kerley B lines, 827
Ketononestrol aziridine, estrogen receptor binding, 263
17-Ketosteroid reductase, 55
Keynes, Geoffrey, 490
Ki67
    measurement, technical considerations, 466t
    prognostic significance in breast cancer, 469, 469t
      correlation with thymidine labeling index, 469
Klinefelter syndrome, 57
    male breast cancer and, 860
Komen Alliance, 950, 959t

L
Labor, premature, 886–887
α-Lactalbumin, 273
    in breast cancer, 423
      and argyrophilia, 425
      prognostic significance, 402t
Lactation, 12
    breast abnormalities in, 122–125
      diagnosis, 122–124
      management summary, 124
      needle aspiration for cytologic analysis, 123
      pathologic diagnosis, 123–124
    breast cancer risk and, 189, 190f
    breast examination in, 122
    diagnostic biopsy in
      delay in, 123
      special considerations, 123
    hormones of, 17
    mammography in, 122–123
    nipple discharge in, blood in, 124
    ultrasound in, 122–123
Lactiferous sinuses, 4
Lactoferrin, 273
    in lactation, 17
LACZ gene, 983
Laminin receptor, prognostic utility in breast cancer, 477
Langer lines, 136, 136f
Large-core needle biopsy, 152
    ultrasound-guided, 155
      factors affecting, 152
      instrumentation, 155
      needle insertion technique, 155, 156f
      patient preparation, 155
      results, 156f
      technique, 156f
      ultrasound-guided fine-needle aspiration biopsy and, comparison, 155–157
Lateral cutaneous nerve, 6f
Lateral pectoral nerve, 6f, 7f, 8
Lateral thoracic artery and vein, 4f, 5, 6f, 7f
Latissimus dorsi muscle, 4f, 8
    extended flap, for breast reconstruction, 607, 615t

musculocutaneous flap
    for breast reconstruction, 607, 608f, 609f, 615t
      skin paddle for, 609f, 615t
    for chest wall reconstruction, after radiation therapy, 613, 615t
L-CAM, in mammary epithelium, 21
LCIS. *See* Carcinoma in situ, lobular
Lead-time bias, 308
Leiomyomas, 37
Length bias, 308
Leptomeningeal metastases. *See* Metastases of breast cancer, leptomeningeal
Leukemia
    acute nonlymphatic, radiation-induced, 536
    chemotherapy-related, 570–571
    metastases to breast, 880
Leukocyte count, of breast milk
    with milk stasis, 52
    with noninfectious breast inflammation, 52
    with puerperal mastitis, 52
Leukoencephalopathy, treatment-related, 774
Leuprolide
    for breast cancer metastases, 687
    for medical oophorectomy, 338
Levorphanol
    for brachial plexopathy, 806t
    pharmacology, 806t
Life-style factors, in breast cancer prevention, 345–347
Li-Fraumeni syndrome, 175, 177, 227
    genetics, 984
Ligase(s), 983
Light exposure, and breast cancer risk, 166
Linear accelerator, 489
Linkage analysis, 172–173, 327
    of familial breast cancer, 172–173, 173f
γ-Linolenic acid
    and breast pain, 100, 101–102
    for mastalgia, 101–102
Lipid-rich carcinoma, 419
Lipoma(s), 81
    pathology, 37
Liver, breast cancer metastases to, evaluation, 634t, 637–638
Liver cancer, tamoxifen and, 678
Liver function tests, breast cancer metastases and, 634t, 639, 639t
Lobectomy, 579
Lobular carcinoma, infiltrating, 420–424
    age at diagnosis, 420
    age distribution, 420
    alveolar, 421, 422f
    argyrophilia, 424–425
    bilateral, 420
    calcifications in, 420
    classic, 421
    clinical presentation, 420–421
    cytology, 421, 422f
    distribution in breast, 420

estrogen receptor status, 420–421
in fibroadenoma, 46
fibronectin and, 423
frequency, 420
gross pathology, 421
histopathology, 420
historical perspective on, 420
metastases
abdominal, 423
central nervous system, 423
ovarian, 423
uterine, 423
microscopic pathology, 420, 421–423,
422f
mixed, 421
neurosecretory granules in, 421–423
with osteoclast-like giant cells, 417
prognosis for, 423–424
prognostic factors for, 462
recurrence, 423–424
solid, 421
survival, 423–424
trabecular, 421, 422f
variants, 421, 422f
prognosis for, 423
Lobular carcinoma in situ. *See*
Carcinoma in situ, lobular
Lobule(s), breast
characteristics, 9, 9t
types, 9, 9t
Lobuloalveolar differentiation, 17
Local anesthetics, for excisional breast
biopsy, 136
Local treatment of breast cancer
effects on survival, 385–388
for invasive cancer, 487–547
for locally advanced cancer, 587–589,
588t, 589t
Log-rank test, 992, 992f
LOH. *See* Loss of heterozygosity
Lomustine, response to, in metastatic
breast cancer, 692t
Long thoracic nerve of Bell, 8
Lonidamine, response to, in metastatic
breast cancer, 692t
Look Good...Feel Better, 956, 959t
Lorazepam (Ativan)
antiemetic regimens, 954t, 955t
for breast cancer patient, 923
Losoxantrone, response to, in metastatic
breast cancer, 692t
Loss of heterozygosity, 174f, 174–175,
221, 288
identification, Southern blot
technique, 449–450
Low-density lipoprotein(s), tamoxifen's
effects on, 347
Ludwig Breast Cancer Study Group
Trial, statistical power in, 988,
988t
Lumpectomy
breast reconstruction after, 611–612,
613f, 614f
complications, 527
and irradiation, psychologic impact,
924–926, 925t

reexcision for involved margins, 150
technique, 525
Lung(s), breast cancer metastases to,
evaluation, 634t, 638
Lung cancer
metastases to breast, 426, 880
radiation-induced, 536
Luteinizing hormone
and breast morphology, during
menstrual cycle, 10
in normal breast development during
puberty, 3
Luteinizing hormone-releasing hormone
agonists
for breast cancer metastases, 686–687
mechanism of action, 686
for breast pain, 103
LY-2 cells, 249
Lymphangitic carcinomatosis, 827–833.
See also Breast cancer,
lymphatic spread; Metastases of
breast cancer, lymphangitic
spread
Lymphatics. *See also* Lymph node(s)
primary, 897
secondary, 897
Lymphedema, 896–903
anatomy, 897
assessment, 897
clinical presentation, 897
etiology, 898–899
incidence, 897–898, 898t
pathophysiology, 897
prevalence, 896
prevention, 899–900
after axillary treatment, 899–900
progression, 897
treatment, 900–901
complete (or complex) decongestive
physiotherapy for, 901
conservative approach, 900–901
management summary, 902
medications for, 900–901
support garments for, 900
surgical procedures, 901
Lymph node(s)
apical, 7f
axillary. *See* Axillary lymph nodes
axillary vein, 5, 7f
central, 5, 7f
examination, 69–70
external mammary, 5, 7f
internal mammary
anatomy, 5–8, 7f
involvement in breast cancer,
384–385, 385f, 385t
relation to axillary node
involvement, 384
interpectoral (Rotter), 5, 7f
intramammary
mammographic appearance, 81, 82f
radiation therapy, 531–532
level I, 7f
level II, 7f
level III, 7f
metastases to, 661–662

immunologic detection, 304
ultrasound-guided fine-needle
aspiration, 154
palpation, 69–70
paramammary, 5
regional
in breast cancer, 379–385
breast cancer recurrence in,
661–662
management, 662
presenting signs and symptoms,
661–662
pretreatment evaluation, 662
prognosis for, 662
subsequent morbidity and spread,
662
surgery and radiation therapy for,
662
systemic therapy for, 662
treatment results, 662
scapular, 5, 7f
supraclavicular
involvement in breast cancer, 385
radiation therapy, 531–532
Lymphocele, postoperative, aspiration,
ultrasound-guided, 154
Lymphocyte(s)
CD4
cytotoxic, in immune response to
breast cancer, 300
in immune response to breast
cancer, 300–301
possible suppressive effects, 301
CD8
against HER-2/neu, 300
in immune response to breast
cancer, 300–301
Lymphoma(s)
metastases to breast, 427, 880
primary breast, 426–427, 876–877
clinical presentation, 876
histology, 877f
mammographic appearance, 876
pathology, 876
prognosis for, 877
radiographic features, 876
treatment, 877
Lymph vessels, of breast, 5

M
Macrophage(s), in immune response to
breast cancer, 301
MAD, 686
MAGE-1
in breast cancer, 300
immunotherapy and, 300
in melanoma, 300
Magnetic resonance imaging
of brain metastases, 770–772, 771f,
772f
of breast, 84–89, 85f, 86f, 87f, 88f
contrast enhancement, 84–85, 85f,
86f, 86–87
to decrease biopsies of false-positive
mammograms, 85–86

Magnetic resonance imaging (*continued*)
   with epidural metastases, 783–785,
      784*f*–785*f*
   in epidural spinal cord compression,
      783–785, 784*f*–785*f*
   for high-risk patients, 329
   indications for, 88–89
   of leptomeningeal metastases, 791,
      793*f*
   of orbital metastases, 809, 810
   of recurrent cancer, 659–660
   of residual or recurrent tumor, 87*f*,
      87–88, 88*f*
   signal intensity of benign versus
      malignant lesions, 86–87
   of silicone implant rupture, 625, 626*f*
   three-dimensional, 84–85
Magnification mammography, 80, 82,
      115
   of calcifications, 78
   of microcalcifications, 116, 117*f*, 118*f*
Male breast cancer, 859–863
   adenoid cystic, 414
   adjuvant therapy, 861–862
   apocrine carcinoma, 414
   argyrophilia in, 424
   diagnosis, 860
   and electromagnetic fields, 166
   epidemiology, 859
   estrogen metabolism and, 860
   familial, 179–180
   family history of breast cancer and,
      859
   geographic distribution, 859
   versus gynecomastia, 57
   hormone receptors in, 860
   incidence, 859
      age-related, 859
   Klinefelter syndrome and, 860
   mortality, 859
   natural history, 860–861
   nodal involvement in, and outcome,
      861
   occupational exposures and, 859–860
   pathology, 860
   prognosis for, 861
   prostatic carcinoma and, 427
   radiation-related, 859
   risk, age and, 859
   risk factors for, 859–860
   staging, 861
   survival, 861, 861*t*
   treatment, 861
Malignant effusions, 833–840. *See also*
      Ascites; Pericardial effusions;
      Pleural effusions
Malmö Trial, randomized clinical trial of
      breast cancer screening, 310,
      311*t*, 312–314, 313*f*, 316*t*
Malpractice, 125
Malpractice insurance, 130
Malpractice lawsuit(s)
   claimants
      age, comparative average indemnity
         by, 130, 131*t*
      distribution by menopausal status,
         130, 131*t*

discovery process, 128–129
   outcomes review, 130*t*, 130–131,
      131*t*
   patient motivations for, 128
   settlements, 130, 130*t*, 130–131, 131*t*
   summons, receiving, 128–129
   summons and complaint in, 128–129
   trial, 128–129
Mammalian son of sevenless (mSOS),
      224
Mammary cancer antigen, as indicator of
      recurrent breast cancer, 640,
      641*t*
Mammary-derived growth factor 1, in
      breast cancer, 273
Mammary-derived growth inhibitor, 273
Mammary duct ectasia, 37–38, 38*f*,
      49–50
   clinical features, 49–50
   definition, 49
   etiology, 49
   nipple discharge with, 49–50, 109
   pathogenesis, 37–38, 49
   and periductal mastitis, 49–50
      carcinoma with, 50
      histopathology, 49
      incidence, 49
      periaolar inflammation with, 49
   treatment, 50
Mammary dysplasia, 27
Mammary epithelial cell cycle, 20
Mammary fistula(s), 50
   treatment, 50
Mammary gland(s)
   accessory, 2
   development
      hormonal control, 16–18, 17*f*
      molecular biology, 1–2
   differentiated cell types, 16
   differentiation, hormonal control,
      16–18
   growth, hormonal control, 16–18
   proliferative processes in, 18
Mammary ridge, 1
Mammary serum antigen, as indicator of
      recurrent breast cancer, 640,
      641*t*
Mammary tissues, accessory, 1
Mammillary fistula, 50
Mammography, 74–75, 75*f*
   abnormalities on, 114–122
      interpretation, 117–120
      management recommendations,
         120, 121*f*
      results, 117–120
      types, 115–117
   adherence, and psychologic distress in
      women at risk for breast
      cancer, 913
   adjunctive assessment, 82
   artificial neural network in, 91
   asymmetric density on
      incidence of malignancy with, 119*t*
      as indication for biopsy, 119*t*
   benefits
      in older women, 315, 318, 344

or lack of benefits, in younger
      women, 111, 313–314,
      315–318, 317*t*
   breast appearance on, and risk of
      breast cancer, 164–165
   of breast cancer, 77–82
   breast masses on, analyzing, 79–82
   of breast sarcoma, 878, 879*f*
   calcifications seen on, analyzing,
      77–79
   carcinogenic potential, 309
   computer-aided diagnosis in, 91–93
   cost, 71
   diagnostic, 111, 115
      definition, 115
      medicolegal considerations,
         127–128
   digital, 89–90, 90*f*, 146, 147*f*
      advantages, 89
      contrast sensitivity, 89–90
      detectability of lesions on, 89–90
      detectors for, 89
      display system, 90
      in interventional procedures, 90
      spatial resolution, 89–90
   in evaluation of nipple discharge, 108
   indications for biopsy on, 118, 119*t*
   in lactation, 122–123
   lesions detected by, analyzing, 76–77
   magnification, 82
   in males, 860–861
   masses on, 115–116, 116*f*
   with metastatic disease to breast, 880
   microcalcifications on, 115–116, 117*f*,
      118*f*
   with occult primary with axillary
      metastases, 893
   in Paget disease, 870
   of palpable mass, 74–75
   periodic follow-up, 144–145
   positive predictive value, 72
   in pregnancy, 122–123
   of primary breast lymphoma, 876
   recommended schedule for, in
      younger women, 317–318
   risk–benefit analysis, 165–166, 343
      for younger age groups, 111,
         313–314, 315–318, 317*t*, 344
   schedule, by risk status, 329*t*
   screening, 144
      anxiety related to, 343–344
      barriers to, 319–320
      batch interpretation, 71
      benefit for older women, 315, 318,
         344
      breast cancer mortality and, 114,
         144, 312–314, 313*f*, 314*f*
      controversies about, 309–310
      controversy about, 315–318, 317*t*
      definition, 115
      detection thresholds, 72–73
      versus diagnosis, 71–72, 72*f*, 73*f*
      effectiveness, evidence for, 312–314
      efficacy, 71
      evaluation, 309
      lack of benefit in younger women,

potential reasons for, 315–317, 317t
limitations, 343–344
medicolegal considerations, 127–128
nonrandomized clinical trials, 312
prescription, in risk management, 342–344, 343f
prescriptions, 342–344, 343f
randomized clinical trial, 309–310
at reduced cost, 71
risk-benefit analysis, 343
in older women, 315, 318, 344
in younger women, 111, 313–314, 315–318, 317t, 344
trends in, 114
trials, overview, 309–310, 311t
with silicone implant, 624f, 625
spot compression views, 82, 115
teleradiology-transmitted, detectability of lesions on, 90, 90f
in triple diagnosis, 113, 134
underuse, in minority groups, 911
Mammography Quality Standards Act, 74, 125
Mammostatin, 273
Manchester Regional I trial, of postoperative radiation therapy, 513t, 514–515, 515f, 516f
Mantel-Haenszel test, 992
MAP kinases, 19, 224f, 224–225
Maspin, 285
gene, regulation, and breast cancer metastasis, 288
Mastalgia. *See* Breast pain
Mastectomy
and breast-conserving surgery, comparison, 490–491, 491f, 492t
complications, 527–529
for ductal carcinoma in situ, 361, 362t, 365
historical perspective on, 386, 487–489, 548
and immediate reconstruction, oncologic considerations in, 528–529
local disease recurrence after, 649–657
hyperthermia for, 655
local therapy, 655–656
management, 657
photodynamic therapy, 655–656
pretreatment evaluation, 652
prognosis for, 650–652, 651f
radiation therapy, 652–654
in-field tumor recurrence and, 653, 653t
reirradiation, 654
signs and symptoms, 649, 650f
sites, 652, 652t
subsequent morbidity and spread of, 649–650
surgery, 654–655
systemic therapy, 656–657
treatment results, 652–657

for local disease recurrence after breast-conserving surgery, 660
for male breast cancer, 861
modified radical, 527
definition, 488
historical perspective on, 488
incision for, 527
indications for, 488
with reconstruction, 603f
skin-sparing procedure, 527
technique, 527
modified radical (Patey), 8
operative mortality, 528
phantom breast syndrome after, 528
prophylactic, 329–331, 344–345, 345f, 615–617
breast cancer occurring after, 330, 344
candidates for, 344–345, 345f
decision-making for, 330, 344–345
efficacy, analysis, 330
indications for, 330, 344
for lobular carcinoma in situ, 372
residual breast tissue remaining after, 330, 344
timing for, 330
psychologic impact, 924, 925t, 932
psychologic outcome, 505
radical, 588
historical perspective on, 487–488, 585
indications for, 488
for recurrent cancer, 660
safety, 528
sequelae, 944t
seroma formation after, 528
skin flap necrosis after, 528
skin-preserving, with reconstruction, 603f
specimen, pathologic examination, 430–431
subcutaneous, for breast pain, 104
survival after, and survival after breast-conserving surgery, comparison, 490–491, 491f, 492t
technique, 527–529
total, technique, 527–528
wound infection with, 528
Mastitis
periductal, 37–38, 38f, 49–50. *See also* Mammary duct ectasia, and periductal mastitis
clinical features, 49–50
etiology, 49
pathogenesis, 49
treatment, 50
plasma cell. *See* Mammary duct ectasia, and periductal mastitis
puerperal, 51–52, 124
differential diagnosis, 51–52
epidemic, 51
sporadic, 51
suppurative, 124
in neonates and infants, 53
tuberculous, 52

Mastitis obliterans. *See* Mammary duct ectasia, and periductal mastitis
Matrigel, 252, 277
MCF-10A cells, 252
MCF-7 cells, 245–246
selected against benzothiophene (LY117018) in vitro, 249
selected against tamoxifen in vivo, 249–250
MCF-7 K3 cell line, 247
MCF-7/LCC1 cell line, 246–247
MCF-7/MIII cell line, 246–247
MCF-7 MKS cell line, 247
MDA-MB-231 cells, 248
MDA-MB-435 cells, 248
MDR1/gp170 expression, models for studying, 250–251
Medial cutaneous nerve of forearm, 6f
Medial pectoral nerve, 7f, 8
Median nerve, 6f, 7f
Medical Device Amendment Act (1976), 620
Medical history, of breast problem, 67, 67t
Medically underserved populations. *See* Underserved minorities
Medical record, medicolegal aspects, 126
Medications, abstention from, for breast pain, 103
Medicolegal considerations, in breast cancer evaluation and treatment, 125–132
Medroxyprogesterone acetate
adjuvant therapy with, 566
for breast cancer metastases, 681–683
adverse effects, 681t, 681–682
dosage and administration, 681
depot, breast cancer risk and, 194–195
Medullary carcinoma, 404–405
age at diagnosis, 404
axillary metastases, 405
bilateral, 404
clinical presentation, 404
cytologic diagnosis, 154
distribution in breast, 404
gross pathology, 404–405
histopathology, 405
immunohistochemistry, 405
microscopic pathology, 405, 406f
prognosis for, 405, 407f
squamous metaplasia in, 405
ultrastructure, 405
Medulloblastoma, metastases to breast, 427
Megace, adverse effects, 930
Megestrol acetate, for breast cancer metastases, 681–683
adverse effects, 681t
dosage and administration, 682
dosage form, 682
dose intensity considerations, 682t, 682–683
mechanism of action, 682
pharmacology, 682
side effects, 682

MEK kinase, 225
Melanoma
  cutaneous, of breast, 881
    incidence, 881
    pathology, 881
    prognosis for, 881
    treatment, 881
  metastases to breast, 426, 880
Melanoma-associated antigen. *See*
      MAGE-1
Melphalan, response to, in metastatic
      breast cancer, 692*t*
Memory difficulties, with chemotherapy,
      management, 929
Men
  breast cancer in. *See* Male breast
        cancer
  Paget disease in, 873
  phyllodes tumors in, 866
Menarche, age at
  breast cancer risk and, 163–164,
        186–187
  trends in, 187
Mendelian inheritance, 171
Meninges, cerebral, relation to brain,
        790, 790*f*
Meningioma(s), and metastatic disease,
        differentiation, 638–639, 772
Meningitis, carcinomatous, 423
Menogaril, 696
  response to, in metastatic breast
        cancer, 692*t*
Menopausal status. *See also*
        Postmenopausal patients;
        Premenopausal patients
  at diagnosis of breast cancer,
        prognostic significance, 465
  and psychological impact of breast
        cancer diagnosis, 922
Menopause
  after breast cancer, epidemiologic
        considerations, 903
  age at, breast cancer risk and, 164,
        187–188, 188*t*
  breast changes with, 12
  cardiovascular health and, 904–905
  climacteric symptoms with, 905–906
  estrogen replacement therapy and
    after breast cancer, 904
    in women with no history of breast
          cancer, 904
  hot flushes and, 905–906
  management, nonhormonal therapies
        for, 904–906
  osteoporosis and, 905
  premature
    with adjuvant chemotherapy, 570
    with chemotherapy, 929
Menstrual cycle
  breast changes in, 18
  microscopic breast morphology in,
        9–10, 11*t*
  and timing if breast surgery, 507, 508*t*
Meperidine, for brachial plexopathy,
        806*t*

6-Mercaptopurine, response to, in
      metastatic breast cancer, 692*t*
Mercapturic acid pathway (MAP) kinase
      kinase, 19
Messenger RNA, 974
  translation, 974*f,* 975
Metaanalysis/metaanalyses, 1000–1003
  arithmetic constructs and, 1001–1002
  combined group analysis, 1000
  combining *P* values, 1000–1001
  comparisons
    bias in, 1002
    hypothesis formation, 1002
    and selection bias, 1002
    with single clinical trials,
          1002–1003
  definition, 1000
  fixed-effects models, 1001
  hypothesis formation in, 1002
  methods for, 1000–1003
  publication bias and, 1001
  random effects models, 1001
  stratified tests, 1000
  time heterogeneity and, 1001
Metabolic encephalopathy, in patient
        with advanced breast cancer,
        931
Metalloprotease(s), 294
Metalloproteinases, 285–286
Metaplasia, 411. *See also* Squamous
        metaplasia
  agnogenic myeloid, differential
        diagnosis, in breast cancer
        patient, 849
  apocrine, 413
    with phyllodes tumors, 863–864
  biochemical, 424
  definition, 411
  endocrine, 424
  heterologous, 411
  homologous, 411
  pseudosarcomatous, 411–412
    microscopic pathology, 412, 413*f*
    prognosis for, 413
  sarcomatous, in invasive ductal
        carcinoma, 412, 413*f*
  synovial, 39
Metaplastic carcinoma. *See* Breast cancer,
        metaplastic
Metastagenicity, definition, 376
Metastases of breast cancer. *See also*
        Breast cancer, recurrence;
        Micrometastases
  antimetastatic therapy for,
        development, 289–290
  axillary. *See also* Axillary lymph nodes,
        involvement in breast cancer
    with occult primary, 892–896
  to bone
    bisphosphonates for, 822–823, 823*t*
    bone-directed therapy for, 822
    clinical presentation, 812–813, 813*f*
    development, 820, 820*f*
    diagnosis, 812–813, 813*f,* 819–820
    differential diagnosis, 847
    evaluation, 634*t,* 636–637, 637*t*

fracture risk with, 815*t,* 815–816
    gallium nitrate for, 823
    hormonal therapy, 815
    localization, 819–820
    local treatment, 811–819
    lytic, biomechanical considerations,
          815, 815*f*
    management summary, 824
    markers of osteoclast–osteoblast
          function in, 821–822, 822*t*
    medical treatment, 819–826
    pathologic fractures with, 815
      management, 816–818
      risk for, quantification, 815*t,* 816
    pathophysiology, 811–813, 814*f*
    radiation therapy, 813–814
    radiation therapy for, bone-directed,
          823–824
    sites, 819, 820*t*
    treatment, 813–818, 816*f,* 817*f*
  bone marrow, 847–853. *See also*
        Myelophthisic anemia
    chemotherapy for, 850–851
    clinical features, 848–849
    detection, 432–433
    endocrine therapy for, 850
    frequency, 847
    hematologic findings with, 847
    prognosis for, 849–850
    treatment, 850–851
  bone marrow transplantation for,
        708–709
  to brain
    chemotherapy, 775–776, 776*t*
    diagnostic considerations, 770–772,
          771*f*
    epidemiology, 769
    headache with, 770
    hormonal therapy, 775–776, 776*t*
    incidence, 769
    management summary, 777, 777*f*
    radiation therapy, 773
      late complications, 774
      results, 773–774
    radiosurgery, 775
    retreatment, 773
    signs and symptoms, 769–770, 770*t*
    surgical therapy, 774–775
    symptom control, 776–777
      anticonvulsant therapy for,
            776–777
      corticosteroid therapy for, 776
    systemic therapy, late complications,
          774
    treatment, 772–773
  central nervous system, evaluation,
        634*t,* 638–639
  chemohormonal therapy, 713–714,
        714*t*
  chemoimmunotherapy, 715
  chemotherapy for, 693–713
    agents, 692*t*–693*t,* 693–705
      anthracyclines, 693–697
      anthrapyrazoles, 696
      camptothecins, 703

cyclophosphamide-based
combinations, 697
5-fluorouracil, 697–698
ifosfamide, 704–705
methotrexate, 698
mitomycin, 705
plant alkaloids, 698–703
platinum compounds, 703–704
taxanes, 699–703
vinca alkaloids, 698–699
dose intensity, 707–708
drug resistance in, 705–706
duration of therapy, 709–711
in elderly, 712–713
and hormonal therapy, comparison,
713
non–cross-resistant regimens,
706–707, 707t
number of drugs, 706
principles, 705–709
response to, predictive factors,
711–712
choroidal, 808–810
clandestine, prognostic significance,
384
colonization, 287
to contralateral breast, 880
coordinate regulation with invasion,
287–288
detection, as investigational endpoint,
633
distant, 388t, 388–389, 389f
at diagnosis, frequency, 284, 289
time course to appearance of,
388–389, 389f
distribution at first recurrence, 634t,
634–635
early, detection, 635–643
endocrine therapy. *See also* Hormonal
therapy
combination regimens, 689–691,
690t
response to
factors affecting, 691–693
predictive markers for, 691–693
epidural, 779–789
chemotherapy for, 786
incidence, 779
investigations, 780–785
myelopathy with, 783–785
pathology, 779
plexopathy with, 782–783
prognosis for, 787, 787t
radiation therapy for, 786
radiculopathy with, 782
signs and symptoms, 779–780, 780t
surgery for, 786
treatment, 785–786
corticosteroids for, 785–786
extraskeletal, survival and, 671, 672f
first recurrence
organ distribution, 634t, 634–635
site, predictive factors, 635
symptoms, 635–636, 636t
Fisher model, 386, 387t
genes regulating, 284, 285t

genetic events associated with, 288
growth factors and, 277–278
Halsted model, 386, 387t
hormonal therapy, 674–693
agents, 675–687
androgens, 687
antiestrogens, 680–681
antiprogestins, 683–684
aromatase inhibitors, 684–686
LHRH agonists, 686–687
optimal sequencing, 687–688,
688t
progestins, 681–683
tamoxifen, 675–680
historical perspective on, 674–675
response rate with, 674, 674t
and steroid receptor status,
674–675, 675t
incidence, 633–635
intramedullary, differential diagnosis,
847
leptomeningeal, 789–796
clinical features, 789
computed tomography, 791, 792f
diagnosis, methods, 791–792, 792f
frequency, 789
histologic subtype and, 789
magnetic resonance imaging, 791,
793f
pathophysiology, 789–790, 790f
signs and symptoms, 790–791
time frame for, 789
treatment, 792–795
to liver
evaluation, 634t, 637–638
serologic assays for, 634t, 639, 639t
lymphangitic spread
clinical features, 827
computed tomography, 827, 829f
differential diagnosis, 829–831
pathologic diagnosis, 828–829
pathophysiology, 828–829
prognosis for, 831–832
radiologic findings, 827, 827t, 828f,
829f, 829t
treatment, 831–832
lymphatic, 827–833
mechanisms, 378–379, 383
natural history, 669–672
newly diagnosed, patient evaluation,
672–673
nodal, 8
ocular, 808–811
with concomitant CNS metastases,
810
diagnosis, 809
incidence, 808–809, 809t
management summary, 810
prognosis for, 809–810
treatment, 809–810, 810t
organ involvement in, 669
organ screening for, 634t, 634–635
organ-specific, 287
palliation, 674
patterns, adjuvant therapy and,
670–671

placental, 886
prevalence, 669
process, 284
pulmonary, 853–858. *See also* Solitary
pulmonary nodule(s)
evaluation, 634t, 638
lymphangitic spread, 827
redundant mechanisms for, 284, 285
regulation, 284, 285t
research techniques, 289
risk factors for, 633–634
screening for
after primary therapy
current practices, 642–643
management summary, 643
candidates for, 633–634
routine, 630–632
cost, 633
effective treatment and, 630–632
as emotional support, 632–633
serologic assays in, 634t, 639, 639t
time frame for, 634
sites, 633–635, 634t, 669
evaluation, 636–639
by histologic type, 670, 671t
survival and, 671–672, 672f
skeletal, 818
survival and, 671, 672f
Spectrum model, 386–387, 387t
spinal, 818
stage IV, no evidence of disease,
treatment, 716–717
symptoms associated with, 635–636,
636t
Systemic model, 386, 387t
and therapy, 284
thoracic, 827
timing, 633–635
treatment, 669–734
for cure versus prolongation of
survival, 630–631, 631f, 632f
goals, 674
hormonal recruitment strategies,
714–715, 715t
for palliation, 632
recommendations for, 716f, 717
special considerations for, 717, 717f
tumor-associated antigens as
indicators of clinical course,
641f, 641–642, 642f
tumor size and, 379, 380f
vertebral, 779, 818
Metastases to breast, 426–427, 427f, 880
characteristics, 880
distribution in breast, 427
incidence, 880
in males, 427
and primary tumor of breast,
differentiation, 427
prognosis for, 880
treatment, 880
Metastasis, 19, 811–812
clonal-dominance hypothesis, 287
Metastasis-suppressor gene nm32,
chromosomal location, 175

Methadone
  for brachial plexopathy, 806t
  pharmacology, 806t
Methotrexate
  antiangiogenic effects, 295
  intra-CSF administration, for
    leptomeningeal metastases,
    792–794, 793f
  for metastatic breast cancer, 698
  response to, 692t
Methylaminopurine, 16f
Methylaminopurine kinase pathway,
    224f, 224–225
Methyl-6-CCNU, response to, in
    metastatic breast cancer, 692t
6-Methylene-amdrostadienedione, 686
Methylxanthines
  and breast pain, 100
  dietary exclusion, 101
Metoclopramide (Reglan), antiemetic
    regimens, 954t, 955t
Mgf, 20
MiB1
  measurement, technical considerations,
    466t
  as measure of proliferation, 465t
Mice. See also Transgenic mice
  breast cancer models, 235, 236–237,
    335–336
  immunodeficient, mammary tumors
    and, 239
  nude, human tumor xenografts in,
    237–240
Microcalcifications
  automated detection
    difference image approach, 91, 92f
    on mammograms, 91–93, 92f
  in breast cancer, 115
  digital mammography, 147f
  on digital mammography, 89–90
  magnification mammography, 115,
    116, 117f, 118f
  mammographic appearance, 115
  on mammography, 115–116, 117f,
    118f
    incidence of malignancy with, 119t
    as indication for biopsy, 119t
  and mass
    incidence of malignancy with,
      119t
    as indication for biopsy, 119t
Microglandular adenosis
  and cancer, 34
  epidemiology, 34
  microscopic pathology, 403
  pathology, 34, 36f
Microinvasive carcinoma. See Breast
    cancer, microinvasive
Micrometastases
  bone marrow
    detection, 432–433
      in peripheral blood stem cell
        collections, in high-dose
        chemotherapy patients, 852
      in primary breast cancer,
        851–852
    management summary, 852

significance
    in peripheral blood stem cell
      collections, in high-dose
      chemotherapy patients, 852
    in primary breast cancer,
      851–852
  detection, 432–433
    immunofluorescent method,
      432–433
    immunohistochemical method,
      432–433
    molecular method, 433
    in peripheral blood, 433
    reverse transcriptase polymerase
      chain reaction method, 433
  prognostic significance, 384
Micronutrients, breast cancer risk and,
    205–208
Microvessel density
  in breast cancer, prognostic
    significance, 400, 478
  and tumor angiogenesis, 293
Mifepristone. See RU 486
Milan National Cancer Institute, breast
    conservation trials, 490–492,
    492t, 493t, 579–584
  of adjuvant chemotherapy regimens,
    556, 557t
  Milan I, 579–581, 580f, 580t, 583f
Milan National Cancer Institute, breast
    conservation trials, Milan II
    (quadrantectomy–radiotherapy
    treatment), 500, 580t, 581,
    581f
Milan National Cancer Institute, breast
    conservation trials
  Milan II
    (quadrantectomy–radiotherapy
    treatment), 582, 583f
  Milan III (conservative surgery with/
    without radiotherapy), 522,
    522t, 582t, 582–583, 583f
  of postoperative adjuvant therapy in
    node-negative cancer, 554,
    554t
  of preoperative adjuvant
    chemotherapy, 558
  recent results, 583f, 583–584
Mild hyperplasia of the usual type, 28
Milk
  components, 19–20
  regulatory molecules in, 17
  secretion, 17, 19
Milk box, 20
Milk fistula, and biopsy of breast mass,
    in lactating woman, 123
Milk of calcium, 78, 78f, 115
Milk stasis, 51–52
Milk streak, 1
Miltefosine, 595
Minorities. See Blacks; Hispanics;
    Underserved minorities
Mithramycin
  for hypercalcemia, 843
  response to, in metastatic breast
    cancer, 692t

Mitogen-activated kinase pathway,
    224–225
Mitogenic cascade, 225
Mitolactol, response to, in metastatic
    breast cancer, 692t
Mitomycin, for metastatic breast cancer,
    705
  response to, 692t
Mitosin, as measure of proliferation, 465t
Mitotic index, 465t, 465–466
  prognostic significance in breast
    cancer, 466–467
Mitoxantrone, for metastatic breast
    cancer, 695
  response to, 693t
Mixed tumor of the breast, 411–412
MMP-1, in invasive breast cancer,
    277–278
MMP-2, 19
  in invasive breast cancer, 277–278
MMP-3, in invasive breast cancer,
    277–278
MMP-9, in invasive breast cancer, 278
MMPs, in breast cancer, 22
Moderate or florid hyperplasias of the
    usual type, 29
Molecular biology
  techniques, 971–986
  textbooks on, 971–972
Molecular cytogenetics, 446. See also
    Comparative genomic
    hybridization; Fluorescence in
    situ hybridization; Primed in
    situ labeling
Molecular epidemiology, 213–220
  attributable proportion in, 215–216
  methodologic issues, 213–214
  odds ratio in, 214
  study design, 214
Molecular genetics, 446
Molecular pathology
  of breast cancer, 445–456
    limitations, 445–446
  clinical applications, 452–454
  future applications, 452–454
Molecular screening, 327–328
Mondor disease, 62, 63f, 69, 69f
Monitoring, 993–997
  of eligibility, 994–995
  of randomization, 995–996
  results, use of, 996–997
  of treatment compliance, 996
  types, 994
Monoclonal antibodies
  against c-erbB-2, possible therapeutic
    applications, 290
  against cytokines
    in biologic therapy of breast cancer,
      302
    in immunotherapy, 302
  against epidermal growth factor
    receptor, therapeutic
    applications, 290, 473
  against estrogen receptor, 263–264
  against HER-2/neu protein

in biologic therapy of breast cancer, 302
in immunotherapy, 302
in immunofluorescent detection of micrometastases, 432–433
against *p53* gene protein, 475
against progesterone receptor, 263–264
Montague, Eleanor, 490
Montgomery glands, 5
development of, 1
Morgagni tubercles, 5
Morphea, postirradiation, 659
Morphine
for brachial plexopathy, 806*t*
pharmacology, 806*t*
MPA. *See* Medroxyprogesterone acetate
mRNA. *See* Messenger RNA
msh2 gene, 229
mSOS. *See* Mammalian son of sevenless (mSOS)
mta-1 gene, regulation, and breast cancer metastasis, 288
mts-1 gene, regulation, and breast cancer metastasis, 288
MUB-1 peptide
antibodies, 299
structure, 299
MUC-1, immunotherapy, 303
Mucin(s)
in breast cancer, 299, 401, 423. *See also* Mucinous carcinoma
embolism, with mucinous carcinoma, 409
as indicators of recurrent breast cancer, 640, 641*t*
Mucin-based treatments, in breast cancer, 302–303
Mucinous carcinoma, 405–409
clinical presentation, 407
cytologic diagnosis, 154
differential diagnosis, 408–409
gross pathology, 407
microscopic pathology, 407–409, 408*f*
with osteoclast-like giant cells, 417
prognosis for, 409
recurrence after mastectomy, 409
Mucocele-like lesions, 37
Mucopolysaccharides, in breast cancer, 401
Mucositis, chemotherapy-induced, management, 957
Muir syndrome, 175, 178
Mullis, Kary, 977
Murine mammary tumor virus, 235
superantigens and, 301
tumors induced by, 236–237
Muscle strength
postoperative, management, 946*t*
preoperative evaluation, 946*t*
Mutagens, 973
Mutation(s), 972–974
analysis, 977–979
effects on protein structure and function, 972–973
silent, 974

Mutation screening methods, 452
Mutual aid, definition, 948
Myelofibrosis, with bone marrow metastases, 848
Myelography
with epidural metastases, 783, 783*f*
in epidural spinal cord compression, 783*f*, 783–785
Myelopathy
of epidural metastases, 780
with epidural metastases, 783–785
Myelophthisic anemia
bone marrow examination in, 849
with bone marrow metastases, 848
clinical features, 848–849
differential diagnosis, in breast cancer patients, 849
laboratory findings in, 848–849
signs and symptoms, 848
Myeloproliferative syndromes, differential diagnosis, in breast cancer patient, 849
Myoepithelial cells, 9

N
NABCO. *See* National Alliance of Breast Cancer Organizations
NAF (*neu* activating factor), 223, 224, 272
Nafarelin, for breast pain, 102
National Alliance of Breast Cancer Organizations, 950, 959*t*
National Cancer Institute, 959*t*
cancer control objectives, for breast cancer, 910
Cancer Information Service, 950
National Coalition for Cancer Survivorship, 959*t*
National Health and Nutrition Examination Survey (NHANES) I, breast cancer risk and attained height in, 204–205
National Institutes of Health (NIH), rehabilitation program for breast cancer patient, 945
National Lymphedema Network, 959*t*
National Surgical Adjuvant Breast and Bowel Project. *See* NSABP
Natural killer (NK) cells, in immune response to breast cancer, 301–302
Nausea and vomiting, with chemotherapy
anticipatory, 953
management, 929, 953, 954*t*, 955*t*
Navelbine, 561
NDF (*neu* differentiating factor), 223, 224, 272
Necrosis
breast, warfarin-induced, 63–64
cribriform ductal carcinoma in situ with, 358–359
fat. *See* Fat necrosis

radiation-induced. *See* Radiation necrosis
skin flap, after mastectomy, 528
NED. *See* Breast cancer, stage IV, no evidence of disease
Needle(s)
anchored, as guide for preoperative localization of clinically occult lesions, 140
core biopsy, 145
Needle aspiration. *See also* Fine-needle aspiration biopsy
for cytologic analysis, during pregnancy and lactation, 123
Needle biopsy, transthoracic, of solitary pulmonary nodule, 853
Needle localization
preoperative, mammographically guided, 140–141
general considerations, 141
guides introduced parallel to chest wall, 141
locating occult lesion by, 140
patient preparation, 140–141
stereotactic needle placement, 141
for surgical excision, 139–140
dye injection, 140
guides for
anchored needles, 140
hookwire systems, 139–140, 140*f*
hypodermic needles, 139, 140*f*
selection, 139–140
preoperative, 139–140
Needle track seeding, in core biopsy, 135, 149
Negligence, 125
Negligent referral, legal considerations, 129
Neoangiogenesis, 278, 293, 295
and metastasis, 278
neu activating factor, 223, 224, 272
neu-differentiating factor, 223, 224, 272
Neurapraxia, postoperative, 944*t*
neu-related protein, circulating, as prognostic indicator in breast cancer, 642
Neurilemomas, 37
Neurofibromas, 37
Neuropathic pain, adjuvant analgesics for, 805, 806*t*
Neurotoxicity
management, 958
of treatment for leptomeningeal metastases, 794
Night pain, with bone metastases, 812
Nijmegen trial, nonrandomized clinical trial of breast cancer screening, 312
Nipple(s), 5
accessory, 2
adenoma, pathology, 34
ectopic, 2
examination, 69
papillary lesions, 44
reconstruction, 613–615, 616*f*, 617*f*

Nipple(s) (*continued*)
  retraction, with mammary duct ectasia
    and periductal mastitis, 49–50
Nipple discharge, 106–110
  blood in, in pregnancy and lactation,
    124
  cancer and, 107–109
  characterization, 107
  cytologic analysis, 124
  diagnostic evaluation, 107f, 107–108
  with duct ectasia, 109
  frequency, 106
  with intraductal papillomas, 42
  in male breast cancer, 860
  with mammary duct ectasia and
    periductal mastitis, 49–50, 109
  mammary fistulas and, 50
  with Paget disease, 870
  with papillary carcinoma, 409
  pathology, 109, 109f
  surgical treatment, 108f, 109
Nipple inversion
  breast abscesses and, 50
  with mammary duct ectasia and
    periductal mastitis, 49–50
  mammary fistulas and, 50
9-Nitro-camptothecin, 703
Nitrogen mustard
  response to, in metastatic breast
    cancer, 693t
  as sclerosing agent, 835
N-Nitrosomethylurea, rodent mammary
    tumors induced by, 236
NMU. *See N*-Nitrosomethylurea
Nodular lactational hyperplasia. *See*
    Adenoma(s), lactating
Nonencapsulated sclerosing lesion, 34
Non-Hodgkin lymphoma, of breast,
    876, 877f
Nonparametric tests, 990
Nonproliferative lesions
  breast cancer risk and, 29
  pathology, 27–29, 28f
Nonrandomized clinical trials, of
    screening, 312
Nonsense mutations, 452
Northern blot analysis, 450, 980–981
NSABP Trial(s)
  B-04, 387–388, 509, 510, 513t,
    514–515, 515f
  B-05, 515
  B-06, 387–388, 491, 492t, 493f, 493t,
    522, 522t
  B-11, 556, 557t
  B-12, 556, 557t
  B-13, 504
  B-14, 504, 521, 572, 677
  B-15, 556, 557t, 569
  of breast-conserving treatment, 491,
    492t, 493f, 493t
  of dose-intensive adjuvant
    chemotherapy, 559–560, 560t
  fraudulent data in, 993
  of local-regional treatment, 387
  participation in, data considered for,
    325, 325f

of perioperative adjuvant
    chemotherapy, 557–558
of postoperative adjuvant
    chemotherapy in node-negative
    patients, 554, 554t
of preoperative adjuvant
    chemotherapy, 558–559
Nucleic acid(s), 972
Nucleoside diphosphate kinase A, 475
Nucleotide(s), 972
Nulliparity, breast cancer risk and,
    162–163, 188–189
Nurses' Health Study, breast cancer risk
    in, with atypical hyperplasia,
    31–32
Nursing care, 951–962

O
Oat cell carcinoma, pulmonary,
    metastases to breast, 426
Occult lesion. *See also* Breast cancer,
    occult primary; Breast lesion(s),
    nonpalpable
  mammographically guided
    preoperative needle
    localization, 140
Occupational exposures, breast cancer
    risk and, 166
Octreotide, for breast cancer metastases,
    687
Ocular metastases. *See* Metastases of
    breast cancer, ocular
Odds ratio, 214
Oligodeoxynucleotides, antisense,
    therapeutic possibilities, 295
Onapristone, for breast cancer
    metastases, 684
Oncofrance trial, 556, 557t
Oncogene(s), 216–218
  activation
    in breast cancer, 221
    in cancer, 173
  as biomarkers for molecular screening,
    218
  in breast cancer, 221–235, 222t,
    299–300
  c-erbB-2. See c-erbB-2
  c-erbB-3. See c-erbB-3
  c-erbB-4, 223, 226
    receptor, ligands, 472t
  c-ets, 225
  c-fos, 226–227
  c-jun, 225, 226–227
  c-junB, 226
  c-myb, 226
  c-myc, 225, 226–227
    in breast cancer, 218
  c-raf-1, 224
  c-ras, 225, 229
  erbB, 223
  erbB-2, 221–222, 222
    amplification, in breast cancer, 447
    gene copy number, cell–cell
      heterogeneity for, 447

overexpression
    in breast cancer, 447
    prognostic significance, 447
    product, as prognostic factor, 223
  erbB-4, 221–222
  expression, in epithelial cells, and in
    vitro metastatic potential,
    253–254
  HER-2, 223
  HRAS, in breast cancer, 218
  hst/int, in breast cancer, 449
  INT2, in breast cancer, 218
  myc, 229
    in breast cancer, 450
    mutation, in breast cancer, 449
  neu, 223
    transfection studies, of breast cancer
      invasion and metastasis, 288
  nuclear, signal
    transduction–associated,
    226–227
  p53. *See p53* gene
  p21ras
    in breast cancer, 300
    mutations, immunotherapy and, 300
  products, as biomarkers for molecular
    screening, 218
  ras
    in metastases, 289
    transfection studies, of breast cancer
      invasion and metastasis,
      287–288
  transformation of human mammary
    epithelial cells, 252
  transformation of immortalized human
    mammary epithelial cells, 252
  Wnt-1, 2
Ondansetron (Zofran), 929, 953
  antiemetic regimens, 954t, 955t
Ontario trial, of conservative surgery
    with and without radiation
    therapy, 522, 522t
Oophorectomy
  breast cancer risk and, 187
  effects on tumor initiation and
    growth, in rodent models of
    carcinogenesis, 336
  medical, in breast cancer prevention,
    338
  and tamoxifen therapy, comparison,
    679–680
Opioids
  for brachial plexopathy, 804–805,
    806t
  pharmacology, 806t
Oral care, during chemotherapy, 957
Oral contraceptives
  breast cancer prevention and,
    337–338
  breast cancer risk and, 20, 193–194,
    194t, 195t, 196t, 349
  combination, breast cancer and,
    193–194, 194t, 195t
  in high-risk patients, 331
Orchiectomy, for male breast cancer,
    861

Organochlorine exposure, breast cancer
    risk and, 166, 192, 215
Ortho-β-hydroxyethyl-rutoside, for
    lymphedema, 900
Oslo trials, of postoperative radiation
    therapy, 513*t*, 515, 515*f*, 516*f*
Osteoblast(s), in bone remodeling, 821
Osteocalcin
    in bone remodeling, 820
    serum, as marker of osteoblastic
        activity, 821–822
Osteoclast(s)
    activity, tumor products and, 821
    in bone remodeling, 821
    factors affecting, 821
Osteoclast-like giant cells, carcinoma
        containing
    in intralymphatic tumor emboli,
        417–418, 418*f*
    mammary, 417*f*, 417–418, 418*f*
        age distribution, 417
        axillary metastases, 418
        distribution in breast, 417
        gross pathology, 417
        histopathology, 417
        microscopic pathology, 417, 417*f*
        progesterone receptor status, 418
        recurrence, 418
        systemic metastases, 418
    organ distribution, 417
Osteonectin, in bone remodeling,
    820–821
Osteopontin, in bone remodeling, 820
Osteoporosis
    postmenopausal, 904, 905
    treatment, 349
Osteotropism, of cancer, 812
Ovarian ablation
    adjuvant, 565*t*, 565–566
    chemotherapy and, in premenopausal
        patients, 567
    premature
        with adjuvant chemotherapy, 570
        with chemotherapy, 929
    second cancers caused by, 570–571
    and tamoxifen therapy, comparison,
        679–680
Ovarian cancer
    incidence, in patients with previous
        history of breast cancer, 629
    metastases to breast, 426
Overall survival, 549
Oxidative metabolism, markers,
    214–216
Oxycodone
    for brachial plexopathy, 806*t*
    pharmacology, 806*t*
Oxymorphone
    for brachial plexopathy, 806*t*
    pharmacology, 806*t*
Oxytocin
    actions, 12
    in breast development, 17
    in lactation, 17
    synthesis, 12

P
Paclitaxel (Taxol), 561, 595
    dosage and administration, 701–702,
        702*t*
    infusion duration, 702, 702*t*
    maximum tolerated dose, 701
    for metastatic breast cancer, 699–701
        response to, 693*t*
    neurotoxicity, 958
    side effects, 701
    structure, 699, 701*f*
PAF. *See* Phenylalanine mustard, plus
        doxorubicin and 5-fluorouracil
PAFT. *See* Phenylalanine mustard, plus
        doxorubicin, 5-fluorouracil,
        and tamoxifen
Paget cell(s), 870, 871*f*
    origin, 870–871
Paget disease of bone, and bone
        metastases, 812
Paget disease of breast, 69, 870–876
    after breast-conserving treatment, 873
    associated malignancy, 870
    clinical features, 870
    differential diagnosis, 870
    estrogen receptor status in, 874
    histology, 870, 871*f*
    incidence, 870
    mammographic findings in, 870
    management summary, 874
    in men, 873
    molecular studies, 873–874
    nipple discharge with, 870
    oncogene and protooncogene
        expression in, 873
    postmastectomy, 873
    prognosis for, 871–873
    special presentations, 873
    treatment, 871–873
PAI-1, in breast cancer, 22
Pain
    back. *See* Back pain
    with bone metastases, 812–813
    breast. *See* Breast pain
    in breast cancer patients, rehabilitation
        and, 943–944
    control
        in brachial plexopathy, 804–806,
            806*t*
        in patient with advanced breast
            cancer, 931
    of epidural metastases, 779–780, 780*t*
    night, with bone metastases, 812
    postoperative, 943–944, 944*t*
    shoulder. *See also* Brachial plexopathy
        postoperative, 939–943
        rehabilitation and, 939–943
PALA, response to, in metastatic breast
        cancer, 693*t*
Palpable masses. *See* Breast mass
Pamidronate. *See also* Bisphosphonates
    for hypercalcemia, 843–844
    for metastatic bone disease, 822–823,
        823*t*
Papillary adenoma of the nipple, 34
Papillary apocrine change, 28

Papillary carcinoma, 409–411
    age at diagnosis, 409
    axillary involvement in, 410
    clinical presentation, 409–410
    cystic, 409
    differential diagnosis, 410
    epidemiology, 409
    gross pathology, 410
    invasive versus noninvasive, 409
    microscopic pathology, 410, 411*f*
    nipple discharge with, 409
    with osteoclast-like giant cells, 417
    prognosis for, 410–411
    solid, 409
    terminology, 409
    WHO Histological Classification, 409
Papillary lesions, 42–45
    of nipple, 44
        breast cancer risk with, 44
        clinical features, 44
        concurrent carcinoma with, 44
        differential diagnosis, 44
        epidemiology, 44
        morphologic growth pattern, 44
        treatment, 44
    subtypes, 42
Papilloma(s)
    intraductal, 29
        histology, 109, 109*f*
        nipple discharge with, 42
        pathology, 34, 35*f*
    multiple peripheral, 42–43, 43*t*
        breast cancer risk with, 43
        characteristics, 42–43, 43*t*
        local recurrence, 43
        mammographic findings with, 42
    and papillary carcinoma,
        differentiation, 410
    solitary intraductal, 42, 43*t*
        breast cancer risk with, 42, 43*t*
        characteristics, 42, 43*t*
        clinical presentation, 42
        epidemiology, 42
        local recurrence, 42
        mammographic findings with, 42
        natural history, 42
        nipple discharge with, 109
        surgical biopsy, 42
        treatment, 42
Papillomatosis, 34
    breast cancer risk with, 44
    differential diagnosis, 43
    florid, 44
    juvenile, 34, 44
        characteristics, 43*t*
        recurrent, 44
        in women with positive family
            histories, 44
    pathology, 43–44
    treatment, 44
Paracrine factors, 15, 16, 293, 294*f*
    in breast cancer onset, 273–276
    in breast cancer progression, 272,
        273*t*, 273–276
Paraffin, foreign-body granulomatous
    inflammation with, 38–39

Paralytic ileus, with adjuvant therapy, 958

Parametric tests, 990

Paraplegia, with epidural spinal cord compression, 780

Parathyroid hormone–related protein, 840–841

Paravertebral venous plexus, 811–812

Parenchyma, 4

Parity, breast cancer risk and, 162–163, 188t, 188–189

Paroven, for lymphedema, 900

Pathologic examination
of breast specimens, 427–432
of excisional biopsy specimen, 428–430
of excision margins, 429, 429f, 430f

Patient education, for breast surgery, 939, 943f

Patient evaluation, clinical standards, medicolegal aspects, 125–127

Peau d'orange, 69, 590

Pectoralis major muscle, 6f, 7f, 8
abnormalities, 8
anatomy, 4f

Pectoralis minor muscle, 6f, 7f, 8
abnormalities, 8

Pectoral muscle, abnormalities, 3

PEM. *See* Polymorphic epithelial mucin

Pentosan polysulfate, 290
HBGF-inhibiting actions, 296

Peptide hormones, in breast development, 19

Percutaneous needle biopsy, ultrasound-guided. *See also* Fine-needle aspiration biopsy, ultrasound-guided; Large-core needle biopsy, ultrasound-guided
of nonpalpable breast lesions, 152–158
recommendations for, 157
stereotaxic guidance and, comparison, 157, 157t

Pericardial disease, in breast cancer patients, 837
management, 838t, 838–839
treatment, 837–838

Pericardial effusions, 836–839
malignant, management, 838t, 838–839

Pericardial tamponade
diagnosis, 837
hemodynamics, 836
management, 838t, 838–839
pathophysiology, 836
signs and symptoms, 836t, 836–837
treatment, 837–838

Pericardial window, 838

Periductal mastitis, 37–38, 38f, 49–50. *See also* Mammary duct ectasia, and periductal mastitis
clinical features, 49–50
definition, 49
etiology, 49
pathogenesis, 49
treatment, 50

Perilobular hemangiomas, 37

Peripheral neuropathy, with adjuvant therapy, 958

Personality, and psychological impact of breast cancer diagnosis, 922

Pesticide exposure, and breast cancer risk, 166

Peters, Vera, 490

PF. *See* Phenylalanine mustard, plus 5-fluorouracil

PFGE. *See* Pulse-field gel electrophoresis

PFT. *See* Phenylalanine mustard, plus 5-fluorouracil and tamoxifen

p53 gene, 170, 172, 227–228
age-specific risk associated with, 326–327
in breast cancer, 174, 216, 221, 299, 450
angiogenesis and, 293
and cancer progression, 288
chromosomal location, 175, 474
functions, 452
in Li-Fraumeni syndrome, 177
mutations, 216–217
in breast cancer, 449
correlation with carcinogen exposure, 217
detection, 474
spectra, 217
strand bias and, 217
nonsense mutations, 452
normal cellular role, 452
PCR analysis, 451–452
prognostic significance, 402t, 466, 474–475, 475t
protein
antibodies, 299
prognostic significance, 299
as tumor marker, 216–217
immunohistochemistry, and clinical outcome, 475
monoclonal antibodies, 475

Phantom breast syndrome, 528

Phenothiazines, antiemetic regimen, 954t

Phenylalanine mustard
plus doxorubicin, 5-fluorouracil, and tamoxifen, adjuvant therapy, 556, 557t
plus doxorubicin and 5-fluorouracil, adjuvant chemotherapy, 556, 557t
plus 5-fluorouracil, adjuvant chemotherapy, 556, 557t
plus 5-fluorouracil and tamoxifen, adjuvant chemotherapy regimen, 556, 557t

Phosphates, for hypercalcemia, 843

Phospholipase C γ, 16f

Phospholipase D, 16f

N-Phosphonacetyl-HL-aspartic acid, 698

Phosphorylase B kinase, 16f

Phyllodes tumors, 863–869
age distribution, 866
associated carcinomas, 866
benign, 864, 865f
clinical course, 864–865
clinical features, 866

grading, 864
histogenesis, 865
histologic classification, 864t, 864–865
histopathology, 863–864
initial diagnosis, 867
macroscopic appearance, 863
malignant, 864, 865f
special considerations with, 867–868
mammographic appearance, 866
management, 867–868
summary, 868
in men, 866
microscopic appearance, 863–864
natural history, 866–867
patient characteristics, 866
radiologic features, 866
recurrence
local–regional, 866–867
management, 868
systemic, 867
size, 863
skin findings with, 866
steroid receptors, 866
stromal patterns, 864
systemic disease, management, 868
ultrasound, 866

Physical activity, breast cancer risk and, 165, 187, 187f

Physical examination, of breasts, 67–70. *See also* Breast self-examination; Clinical breast examination
abnormalities on, 110–114
in pregnancy and lactation, 122
technique, 67–70, 68f, 69f, 70f

Physicians Insurers Association of America
Breast Cancer Study of 1990, 130–131
Breast Cancer Study of 1995, 130

Phytochemicals, anticarcinogenic, breast cancer and, 209

Phytoestrogens
carcinogenesis and, 345–346
dietary, breast cancer risk and, 192

PIAA. *See* Physicians Insurers Association of America

Pierquin, Bernard, 490

Pirarubicin, 696
response to, in metastatic breast cancer, 693t

Placebo(s), in clinical trials, 996

Placenta, metastatic disease in, 886

Placental lactogen
in breast cancer, prognostic significance, 402t
and breast changes during pregnancy, 10

Plaque(s), bacterial, 983

Plasma cell mastitis. *See* Mammary duct ectasia, and periductal mastitis

Plasmids, 983

Plasmin, in breast cancer, 22

Plasmin activator inhibitor, 294

Plasminogen activator(s)
activity, 285

prognostic utility in breast cancer, 476–477, 477*t*
urinary-type, 16*f*
urokinase-type. *See* Urokinase plasminogen activator
Plasminogen activator inhibitor(s)
in breast cancer, 285
prognostic utility in breast cancer, 476–477, 477*t*
Platelet-derived endothelial growth factor, in angiogenesis, 286
Platelet-derived growth factor(s)
in breast cancer, 273
tumor cell motility and, 286
Platelet factor 4, as angiogenesis inhibitor, 286–287
Platinum compounds, for metastatic breast cancer, 703–704
Pleiotrophin
angiogenesis and, 277, 278, 293
in breast cancer, 273
metastasis and, 277, 278
in tumor growth, 295
Pleura, normal physiology, 833
Pleural effusions, 833–836
malignant
in breast cancer patients, 834
characteristics, 833–834
cytologic evaluation, 834
treatment, 834–836
Pleural sclerosis, for malignant effusions, 835–836
Plexopathy, with epidural metastases, 782–783
Pneumatic compression therapy, for lymphedema, 900–901
Pneumocystis carinii, prophylaxis, with steroid therapy, 786
Pneumocystography, 154
Point mutation, 973
Poland syndrome, 2–3
Polychlorinated biphenyls, exposure to, and breast cancer risk, 166
Polymastia, 2
Polymerase chain reaction, 445, 450*t*, 450–451, 453, 976–977, 977*f*
carryover contamination, 451
gene-level analysis using, 451–452
in situ, 451
limitations, 451
mutation screening, 452, 453
principles, 972
products, DNA sequencing analysis, 452
quality control, 451
Polymorphic epithelial mucin, 299
gene, transfection into B cells, 303
Polyoma-induced tumors, in mice, 237
Polythelia, 2
Positional cloning, 983*f*, 984
Positive predictive value
of mammographically initiated biopsy, 73–74, 144–145
of mammography, 72
of screening tests, 308
Positron emission tomography

of breast, 93–95, 94*f*, 95*f*
of breast cancer, staging applications, 94–95
in chemohormonal therapy, 95
computed tomography and, comparison, 93
disadvantages, 95–96
limitations, 95
magnetic resonance imaging and, comparison, 93
of recurrent tumor versus radiation necrosis, 772
tracers, standardized uptake value, 95
whole-body, 95, 95*f*
Posterior humeral circumflex artery and vein, 6*f*
Postirradiation morphea, 659
Postlactational breast, involution, 2
Postmenopausal patients
adjuvant aminoglutethimide for, 566
adjuvant chemoendocrine therapy in, 568*t*, 568–569
adjuvant chemotherapy in, 552*t*, 553
and tamoxifen, 568*t*, 568–569
adjuvant tamoxifen therapy in, 561–563, 906
chemotherapy and tamoxifen in, 568*t*, 568–569
estrogen replacement therapy for, in high-risk women, 330–331
fibroadenomas in, 46
osteoporosis in, 904, 905
Poverty
endemic, by race/ethnic group, 910, 910*t*
race/ethnicity and, 910, 910*t*
Power, statistical, 987–989, 988*t*, 989*t*
PPS. *See* Pentosan polysulfate
Predisposition testing, for breast cancer genes, 327–328
Prednimustine, response to, in metastatic breast cancer, 693*t*
Pregnancy
age at first full-term
and breast cancer risk, 162–163
breast cancer risk and, 188–189, 189*t*
anesthetic considerations in, 886–887
breast abnormalities in, 122–125
diagnosis, 122–124
management summary, 124
needle aspiration for cytologic analysis, 123
pathologic diagnosis, 123–124
breast cancer and, 883
radiologic findings with, 122–123
breast cancer diagnosed during, prognosis for, 883–884, 884*t*
breast cancer in, 883–892
staging, fetal considerations, 884–886
steroid hormone receptors in, 887–888
therapeutic abortion with, 887
treatment, fetal considerations, 884–886

breast changes in, 10*f*, 10–12
breast examination in, 122
chemotherapy during, 886
diagnostic biopsy in
delay in, 123
special considerations, 123
effects on tumor initiation and growth, in rodent models of carcinogenesis, 336
mammography in, 122–123
nipple discharge in, blood in, 124
protective effects against breast cancer, 162–163, 165
safety, after breast cancer, 888–890
data collection about, problems with, 889–890
and interval between cancer diagnosis and pregnancy, 889
management summary, 890
and more than one subsequent pregnancy, 889
prognosis for, 888–889, 889*t*
timeliness of issue of, 888
ultrasound in, 122–123
Pregnancy-specific β_1-glycoprotein, in breast cancer, prognostic significance, 402*t*
Premature labor, 886–887
Premenopausal patients
adjuvant chemoendocrine therapy in, 566–569
and ovarian ablation, 567
adjuvant chemotherapy in, 552*t*, 552–553
and tamoxifen, 567*t*, 567–568
adjuvant tamoxifen therapy in, 561–563
breast cancer in, 110–111
chemotherapy and ovarian ablation in, 567
chemotherapy and tamoxifen in, 567*t*, 567–568
clinical breast examination in, interpretation, 111
tamoxifen's role in, 679
Pretreatment planning conference, effective, strategies for conducting, 965*t*, 966–967
Primary carcinoid tumor of breast, 425
Primary care provider, definition, 125–126
Primed in situ labeling, 447, 448*f*
Primer(s), for polymerase chain reaction, 976–977, 977*f*
PRINS. *See* Primed in situ labeling
Procarbazine, response to, in metastatic breast cancer, 693*t*
Prochlorperazine (Compazine), antiemetic regimens, 954*t*, 955*t*
Profile of Mood States, 948
Progestational agents
for breast cancer metastases, 681–683
for hot flushes, 906
Progesterone(s), 19
and breast pain, 100
for breast pain, 103

Progesterone(s) (*continued*)
  effects on tumor initiation and growth, in rat models of carcinogenesis, 336
  endogenous, in breast cancer pathogenesis, 192–193
  exposure, breast cancer risk and, 185, 185t
  in lobuloalveolar growth, 17
Progesterone receptor(s), 19, 262
  breast cancer and, 261–271
    background, 261–262
    DNA studies, 264
    prognostic significance, 262, 469–471, 470f
    proliferative rate and, 262, 262t
    protein studies, 263–264
  in fibroadenomas, 46
  functional domains, 262–263
  in male breast cancer, 860
  monoclonal antibodies to, 263–264
  variants, 19
Progestin(s)
  in breast cancer, 20–21
  for breast cancer metastases, 681–683
  cellular effects, 261–262
  effects on breast cancer, growth factors and, 274
  orally active, site-specificity, 337
Progestogens, and breast morphology, during menstrual cycle, 10
Prolactin, 19
  and breast changes during pregnancy, 10
  and breast pain, 100–101
  in lactation, 12, 17
  in lobuloalveolar growth, 17
Prolactin-inhibiting factor, and breast changes during pregnancy, 10
Proliferating cell nuclear antigen, prognostic significance in breast cancer, 469
Proliferation, measures, prognostic significance in breast cancer, comparison, 469
Proliferative breast disease
  diagnosis, 30–31
  inheritance, 179
  without atypia
    breast cancer risk and, 29
    pathology, 29, 29f, 30f
Promoter region, 974
Proportional hazards test, 992
Prostatic carcinoma, metastases to breast, 426–427
Prostheses, management, 946t, 947
Protease(s)
  in angiogenesis, 294
  angiogenesis and, 293, 294f
  inhibitors, angiogenesis and, 293, 296
  in invasive breast cancer, 277–278
Protein(s), synthesis, 972–973, 974, 974f
Protein C deficiency, with warfarin-induced necrosis, 64
14–3–3-Protein family, 224
Protein kinase C, 16f
  in breast cancer, 21–22

Proto-oncogene(s)
  c-*erbB*-2. *See* c-*erbB*-2
  met, in breast cancer, 273
Pseudoangiomatous hyperplasia of mammary stroma, 37
Pseudoepithelialization, 39
Pseudogynecomastia, 56–57
pS2 gene, prognostic significance in breast cancer, 471
Psychiatric treatment, for breast pain, 103–104
Psychologic considerations
  in adjuvant chemotherapy, 928–930
  in adjuvant hormonal therapy, 930
  in breast cancer patient, 919–938
    factors affecting, 919–931, 920t
  in breast cancer prevention, 349–350
  in breast reconstruction, 601, 926–928
  in surgical treatment of breast cancer, 505
  in women at risk for breast cancer, mammography adherence and, 913
Psychologic evaluation, of patient with breast cancer, indicators for, 923, 923t
Psychologic impact
  of breast cancer
    decision making and, 920–921, 945–947
    factors affecting, 919–931, 920t
    medical variables in, 920t, 924–931
    psychologic variables in, 920t, 922–923
    public attitudes and, 921–922
    sociocultural context and, 920t, 920–922
  of lumpectomy and irradiation, 924–926, 925t
  of mastectomy, 924, 925t
  on couple, 932
Psychologic outcome, of breast cancer treatment, 505, 944
  and survivorship, 944
Psychologic support, of breast cancer patient
  postoperative, 946t
  preoperative, 946t
  programs for, 948–951. *See also* Support groups
Psychosocial data, interpretation, 948
Psychosocial intervention(s), for breast cancer patient, 931, 948
Psychosocial support, effects on cancer patient, 948
Publication bias, and metaanalysis, 1001
Pulse-field gel electrophoresis, 980
Punch biopsy, 137–138, 138f
Purines, 972
P value(s), 462, 987
  combining, in metaanalysis, 1000–1001
Pyrimidines, 972
Pyrrolidino-4-iodotamoxifen, 681

Q
Q-TWiST, 551–552
Quadrantectomy, 525, 579
Quadriplegia, with epidural spinal cord compression, 780
Quality bias, in comparisons of metaanalyses, 1002
Quality of life, 308
  of breast cancer patient, 933–934
  changes, after cancer treatment, 958–960
  chemotherapy and, 709–711
  definition, 951
  effects of follow-up care, 633

R
Race
  breast cancer survival and, 672, 673f
  prognostic significance in breast cancer, 465
Radial scar(s)
  core biopsy, 151
  histologic diagnosis, 151
  mammographic appearance, 73f, 81
  pathology, 34–35
Radiation
  absorbed dose, units, 490
  breast cancer risk and, 165–166
Radiation necrosis
  cerebral, 774
  soft tissue, 534
Radiation pneumonitis, 534–535, 535t
Radiation therapy
  after breast-conserving treatment, technique, 529–532
  antiangiogenic activity, 295
  arm edema with, 532–533
  for bone metastases, 813–814
  bone sarcoma caused by, 536
  brachial plexus injury with, 533
  with breast-conserving treatment
    clinical trials, 490–492, 491f, 492t, 493f, 493t
    cosmetic outcome, 494–496, 495t, 496t
    historical perspective on, 490
    local recurrence, 492–494, 493t, 494t
      margin involvement in, 501–502, 502t
      patient risk factors, 498t, 498–499
      risk factors for, 496–504
      treatment factors in, 502–504
      tumor risk factors, 499–501, 500f
    retrospective studies, 492–505
    survival, and survival after mastectomy, comparison, 490–491, 491f, 492t
  carcinogenesis induced by, 535–536
  cardiac complications, 536–537
  chest wall reconstruction after, 612–613, 614f, 615t
  complications, 532–537, 1002

decreased arm mobility with, 533
dose distribution, 530
for epidural spinal cord compression, 786
and excision, for ductal carcinoma in situ, 362–363, 363*t*, 365
fatigue with, 952
half-body, for bone metastases, 814
historical perspective on, 489–490
immobilization for, 529–530
of lymph nodes, 531
nodal, 531
for occult primary with axillary metastases, 894
physical effects, 952
postoperative
    complications, 533
    definition, 512
    indications for, 512–519
    Stockholm trial, 513–514, 514*t*
    with systemic therapy, 515–519, 517*t*
    technique, 518–519
    without systemic therapy, trials of, 513*t*, 513–515, 514*t*, 515*f*, 516*f*
in prepubertal females, 3
pulmonary complications, 534–535
rib fractures with, 533–534, 534*t*
skin effects, 659, 952
soft-tissue sarcoma caused by, 536
supplemental dose to primary site (boost), 530–531
tamoxifen and, 521
technique, 529–532
tumor vasculature and, 295
whole-brain, for brain metastases, 773
    late complications, 774
    results, 773–774
Radiculopathy, with epidural metastases, 782
Radiotherapy, pathologic changes associated with, 38*f*, 39
Radium, 489
Raf-1 kinase, 19
Randomized clinical trial(s)
    of adjuvant chemotherapy
        historical perspective on, 548
        results interpretation, 549–551
    monitoring, 995–996
    of screening, 308, 310–312, 311*t*
        Canada NBSS1, 311*t*, 312, 314, 316*t*
        Canada NBSS2, 311*t*, 312, 313, 313*f*, 316*t*, 318
        concerns raised about, responses to, 315, 317*t*
        Edinburgh Trial, 310, 311*t*, 312–314, 313*f*, 316*t*
        Göteborg Study, 310, 311*t*, 312–314, 313*f*
        Health Insurance Plan of New York, 310, 311*t*, 312–314, 313*f*, 316*t*
        international, 310–312

Malmö Trial, 310, 311*t*, 312–314, 313*f*, 316*t*
Stockholm Study, 310, 311*t*, 312–314, 313*f*, 316*t*
Swedish, 310
Swedish Two-County Study, 310, 311*t*, 312–314, 313*f*, 314–315, 316*t*
of screening mammography, 309–310
Range of motion
    assessment, preoperative, 939
    rehabilitation, 939–943
Ras, biochemical function, 19
Rat(s), breast cancer models, 235–236, 237, 335
Reactive disorders, 37–39
Rectus abdominis muscle, 6*f*
Rectus sheath, 6*f*
5α-Reductase, 55
Referral, negligent, legal considerations, 129
Regional adenopathy, biopsy, 138
Rehabilitation
    clinical management, 945–947, 946*t*
    fatigue and, 943–944
    interventions (treatments) in, 945–947, 946*t*
    management, for breast cancer patient, 939–947
    pain and, 943–944
    patient assessment for, 939, 940*f*–942*f*
    problems, for breast cancer patient, 939
    for shoulder mobility, 939–943
    shoulder pain and, 939–943
Relative risk (RR), 215–216, 323
Renal cancer, metastases to breast, 426
Restriction enzymes, 975
Restriction fragment length polymorphism, 975–976
Restriction fragments, 975
Restriction map, 975
Retinoblastoma gene, 227–228, 229
    in breast cancer, 450
Retinol, 205
Reverse genetics, 983, 983*f*, 984
Reverse transcriptase, 977
Rhabdomyosarcoma, metastases to breast, 427
Rhenium-186, in treatment of bone metastases, 824
Rib fracture, post–radiation therapy, 533–534, 534*t*
Ribosomal RNA, 975
Ribozyme targeting, 295
Risk, 323–324. *See also* Breast cancer, risk factors; High-risk patients
    absolute, 323, 324*t*
    analytic, estimation, 181–182
    empiric, 180–181
    estimation
        Gail model, 324–325, 325*f*, 342, 343
        from multivariate models, 341–342
    perception, in medically underserved populations, effects on

treatment-seeking behavior, 913–914
    quantification, 341–342
    relative, 215–216, 323
    status, knowledge of, negative consequences, 328, 341, 350
RISK (computer program), 325
Risk assessment
    anxiety with, 349–350
    communicating results from, 328, 342
    ethical implications, 350–351
    program, development of, 332
    psychologic considerations, 349–350
Risk counseling, 327–328
    ethical implications, 350–351
    program, development of, 332
    psychologic considerations, 349–350
Risk history, 323–324
Risk management
    mammographic screening prescription in, 342–344, 343*f*
    medicolegal aspects, 125–127
RNA, 972, 974–975
    splicing, 975
    structure, 974
    synthesis, 974, 974*f*
RNA polymerase II, 974
RNAse mismatch analysis, 452
RNase protection analysis, 981, 981*f*
Rodent(s)
    breast cancer models, 235
    mammary tumors in
        chemically induced, 235–236
            with 7,12-dimethybenz*(a)*anthracene, 236, 330
            with *N*-nitrosomethylurea, 236
        virally induced, 236–237
            with adenovirus, 237
            with murine mammary tumor virus, 236–237
            with polyoma virus, 237
Roentgen, Wilhelm, 489
RR. *See* Relative risk
RU 486 (Mifepristone)
    for breast cancer metastases, 683–684
        dosage and administration, 683
        side effects, 683
    mechanism of action, 19
Ruffini-like bodies, 5

S
Saline implant(s), 604
Samarium-153, in treatment of bone metastases, 824
Sappey subareolar plexus, 5
Sarcoidosis, pathology, 39
Sarcoma(s)
    after breast cancer treatment, 659
    primary breast, 877–878
        clinical features, 877–878
        histology, 877
        incidence, 877
        mammographic findings with, 878, 879*f*

Sarcoma(s), primary breast (*continued*)
  prognosis for, 878
    radiographic findings, 877–878
    skin findings with, 877–878
    treatment, 878
  radiation-induced, 536
  stromal, 877
Sarcomatoid carcinoma, 877
SBLA syndrome, 175
Scapular circumflex artery and vein, 6*f*
Scatter factor, 277
  angiogenesis and, 293
  in breast cancer, 273
Schrödinger, Emil, 971
Schwannomas, 37
Scleroderma, circumscribed, 659
Sclerosing adenosis, 29, 30*f*
  microscopic pathology, 403
Sclerosing papillary proliferation, 34
Screening, 307–332
  adherence to, 319–320
  breast cancer mortality and, 307, 308
  breast self-examination in, 318–319
  case-control trials, 312
  case fatality rate and, 308
  case finding, 308
  clinical breast examination in, 318
  cohort study, 312
  definition, 307
  effectiveness
    intermediate measures, 314–315,
      316*t*
    measures, 308
  evaluation, principles for, 309
  for extramammary recurrences,
    advantages and disadvantages,
    630
  false-negatives, consequences, 309,
    343
  false-positives
    negative consequences, 309
    physiologic consequences, 309
  for high-risk patients, 319, 328–329
  labeling and, 309
  mammographic
    algorithm, for women <40,
      342–344, 343*f*
    barriers to, 319–320
    breast cancer mortality and, 114,
      144, 307, 312–314, 313*f*, 314*f*
    controversies about, 309–310
    evaluation, 309
    prescription, in risk management,
      342–344, 343*f*
  molecular, 327–328
  negative consequences, 309
  for new primary cancers, after primary
    therapy of breast cancer, 629
  nonrandomized clinical trials, 312
  outcomes, 308
  overdiagnosis and, 309
  patient risk categories and, 328–329,
    329*t*
  patients' decisions to seek, factors
    affecting, 913–914
  randomized clinical trials, 308,
    310–312, 311*t*

  international, 310–312
  rationale for, 307
  research needs, 320
  for second primary breast cancer, 629
  survival and, 308
  tests
    evaluation, 307–308
    positive predictive value, 308
    sensitivity, 308
    specificity, 308
  trials, 310–312
    metaanalyses of, 314, 315*t*
  unanswered questions about, 320
Seat belt injury, subcutaneous rupture of
    breast due to, 61, 61*f*
Secretory carcinoma, 418*f*, 418–419
Secretory component, in breast cancer,
    prognostic significance, 402*t*
Secretory disease of the breast. *See*
    Mammary duct ectasia, and
    periductal mastitis
SEER. *See* Surveillance, Epidemiology
    and End Results Program
Segregation analysis, 326
Seizure(s), with cerebral metastases, 770
  treatment for, 776–777
Selectins, 284
  E-selectin, in metastasis, 22
Selection bias, 993
Selenium, breast cancer and, 207–208
Self-help groups, definition, 949
Semustine, response to, in metastatic
    breast cancer, 692*t*
Sensitivity
  definition, 308
  of diagnostic test(s), 987
Serotonin antagonists
  antiemetic effects, 953
  antiemetic regimen, 954*t*
Serratus anterior muscle, 4*f*, 8
Serum glutamic oxaloacetic transaminase,
    breast cancer metastases and,
    639
Seventh-Day Adventists
  breast cancer in, 202, 209
  colon cancer in, 202
Sex hormone-binding globulin, 55
Sex steroids, and breast changes during
    pregnancy, 10
Sexual functioning, of breast cancer
    patient, 933–934
Sexuality, after cancer treatment,
    958–959
*Sexuality and the Woman Who Has Cancer
    and Her Partner,* 934
Sexual rehabilitation, of breast cancer
    patient, 934
SHBG. *See* Sex hormone-binding
    globulin
SH-2 domains, 19
Shoulder
  mobility, rehabilitation for, 939–943
  motion
    postoperative, 939
      management, 946*t*
    preoperative evaluation, 946*t*

  postoperative mobilization, 945, 945*t*
  postoperative stiffness, 944
Shoulder pain. *See also* Brachial
    plexopathy
  postoperative, 939–943
  rehabilitation and, 939–943
Sialyl-Tn, in treatment of breast cancer,
    302–303
Sialyl-Tn-crotyl, immunization, in breast
    cancer, 302–303
Signal transduction, in mammary
    epithelial cells, 19
Signet ring cell(s), tumor markers and,
    423
Signet-ring cell carcinoma, intraductal,
    357
Significance, statistical, 987
Silicone
  biologic effects, 621–622, 622*f*
  chemical properties, 620–621
  exposure to, 621
    clinical implications, 622–623
  foreign-body granulomatous
    inflammation with, 38–39
  gels, 621
  oils, 621
  rubbers, 621
Silicone autoimmune disease, 620–628
  clinical assessment, 623–626, 624*f*
  clinical features, 622, 623, 623*t*
  clinical implications, 622–623
  clinical staging, 623, 623*t*
  clinical treatment options, 626*f*,
    626–627, 627*f*
  epidemiologic studies, 622
  historical background, 620
  signs and symptoms, 623*t*, 623–624
  surgical management, 626*f*, 626–627,
    627*f*
Silicone implant(s)
  benefits, 622
  breast cancer detection and, 624–625
  capsular contracture, 625, 625*f*, 626,
    626*f*
  chemical properties, 621
  explantation, 626*f*, 626–627, 627*f*
  FDA classification, 620
  FDA evaluation, 604
  gel bleed, 621
  immunogenic response to, 621–622
  leakage, 621
  lumpectomy and radiation therapy in
    patient with, 602*f*
  magnetic resonance imaging, 625,
    626*f*
  mammography with, 624*f*, 625
  physical examination of breasts with,
    625
  and risk of breast cancer, 165
  rupture
    assessment for, 625, 625*f*
    imaging, 625
  sensitivity to, genetic predisposition
    to, 622
  serologic findings with, 625–626
  silicone gel exposure and, 621

ultrasound, 625, 625*f*
Single photon emission computed tomography
of breast cancer, 95–96
for cardiac imaging, 96
Single-strand conformation polymorphism analysis, 452, 453*f*, 474, 978–979, 979*f*
Skate flap, for nipple–areolar reconstruction, 614, 616*f*
Skin
of breast, 4–5
retraction, 68–69
in breast cancer, 457
in breast cancer recurrence, 426
calcifications, on mammography, 77, 78
radiation therapy's effects on, 659, 952
Skin biopsy, 137–138, 138*f*
Skin findings
with breast sarcoma, 877–878
with phyllodes tumors, 866
Small-cell lung cancer, metastases to breast, 880
Smoking, breast cancer risk and, 165
Socioeconomic status, race/ethnicity and, 910*t*, 910–911
Solar radiation, breast cancer risk and, 165–166
Solid circumscribed carcinoma. *See* Medullary carcinoma
Solitary pulmonary nodule(s)
diagnosis, 854–855
histopathology, 854, 854*t*
management, 853–858
summary, 857
pathology, 856–857
with recurrent breast cancer, prevalence, 853
thoracoscopy, 855*f*, 855–856
Somatostatin, for breast cancer metastases, 687
SOS, biochemical function, 19
Southern blot, 449–450, 979–980, 980*f*
disadvantages, 449–450
Soybeans, consumption, carcinogenesis and, 345–346
Specificity, definition, 308
Specimen(s)
axillary lymph nodes, pathologic examination, 431–432
biopsy
intraoperative thermal (electrocautery) damage to, 429–430, 430*f*
pathologic examination, 428–430
from excisional biopsy
frozen section control, 428
gross examination, 428–429
inking, 428, 429*f*, 430*f*
intraoperative thermal (electrocautery) damage to, 429–430, 430*f*
management, 137, 137*f*
pathologic examination, 428–430
receptor control, 428

from incisional biopsy
management, 137, 137*f*
pathologic examination, 428
mastectomy, pathologic examination, 430–431
from nonpalpable lesions, management, 142–143
pathologic examination, 427–432
small, pathologic examination, 428
from stereotactic core biopsy, radiography, 147–150, 148*f*
SPECT. *See* Single photon emission computed tomography
S-phase fraction, 465*t*
by flow cytometry, prognostic significance in breast cancer, 467–469, 468*t*
measurement, technical considerations, 466*t*
Spinal cord compression, epidural, by breast cancer metastases, 779
computed tomography, 782
corticosteroids for, 785–786
incidence, 779
investigations, 780–785
pathology, 779
plain spine roentgenograms, 781–782
prognosis for, 787, 787*t*
radiation therapy, 786
radiculopathy with, 782
radionuclide bone scans, 782
signs and symptoms, 779–780, 780*t*
surgery for, 786
treatment, 785–786
Spindle cell carcinoma, 417
Spiradenoma, eccrine, 33
Spirogermanium, response to, in metastatic breast cancer, 693*t*
Spironolactone, gynecomastia associated with, 56
Spitalier, J. M., 490
Sporotrichosis, of breast, 52
Spouse, of breast cancer patient, 932, 960
S-100 protein, in breast cancer, prognostic significance, 402*t*
Squamous carcinoma, 416–417
age distribution, 416
clinical presentation, 416
distribution in breast, 416
gross pathology, 416
histogenesis, 416
metastatic to breast, microscopic pathology, 416–417
microscopic pathology, 416–417
prognosis for, 417
Squamous metaplasia, 411–412
associated conditions, 416
benign, 416
of lactiferous ducts, 50
in medullary carcinoma, 405
microscopic pathology, 412, 412*f*
with phyllodes tumors, 863–864
prognosis for, 413
SSCP. *See* Single-strand conformation polymorphism analysis

Standards of care, legal aspects, 127, 129
Staphylococci, in nonpuerperal breast abscesses, 51
Staphylococcus aureus
in mastitis, 124
in puerperal mastitis, 51
STAT family of transcription factors, 19, 20
Statistics, 986
Stat proteins, 225
Statute of limitations, 128, 129
Stereotactic core biopsy, 144–152
accuracy, 147–148, 148*t*
advantages and disadvantages, 150–151
automated biopsy gun, 145–146
complications, 148*t*, 148–149
core biopsy needle, 145–146
cost, 151
of ductal carcinoma in situ, 150
equipment, 145, 145*f*
follow-up of benign lesions, 150
future trends in, 151
indications for, 150–151
malignancy diagnosed by, surgical treatment, 150–151, 151*t*
management, 149*f*, 149–150
of microcalcifications, 147–150, 148*f*
problems with, 150–151
procedure, 145–146, 146*f*, 147*f*
specimen radiography, 147–150, 148*f*
surgical biopsy and, comparison, 147–148, 148*t*
Stereotactic needle placement
for mammographically guided preoperative needle localization, 141
for percutaneous needle biopsy, and ultrasound-guided needle placement, comparison, 157, 157*t*
Steroid(s)
antiemetic regimen, 954*t*
in breast development, 19
Steroid–growth factor interaction, in malignant epithelium, 274
Steroid receptor(s)
function, 19
prognostic significance in breast cancer, 469–472
and response to endocrine therapy for metastatic breast cancer, 674–675, 675*t*
Stockholm Study, randomized clinical trial of breast cancer screening, 310, 311*t*, 312–314, 313*f*, 316*t*
Stockholm Trial, of postoperative radiation therapy, 513*t*, 513–514, 514*t*
Stomatitis, chemotherapy-induced, management, 957, 957*t*
Stop (termination) codon, 975
Streptococci, α-hemolytic, in nonpuerperal breast abscesses, 51

Streptozocin, response to, in metastatic breast cancer, 693*t*
Stroma, 4
Stromal fibrosis, radiation-induced, 39
Stromal sarcoma, 877
Stromelysin, 294
  in breast cancer invasion and metastasis, 288
  stromelysin-3, 286
    in invasive breast cancer, 277
Strontium-89
  toxicity, 824
  in treatment of bone metastases, 823–824
Subareolar duct of papillomatosis, 34
Subclavius muscle, 6*f*, 7*f*
  origin, 8
Subgroup analysis, 997–1000
  data-derived categories for, 997–998, 999*t*
  multiple comparisons, 998–999
  of quantitative versus qualitative interactions, 999–1000
  subgroup formation, factors used in, 997, 998*t*
Subscapular artery and vein, 5, 6*f*
Subscapular vein, 7*f*
Substituted benzamides, antiemetic regimen, 954*t*
Superantigens, murine mammary tumor virus and, 301
Supervoltage, 489
Support. *See* Psychologic support
Support groups
  definition, 948, 949
  discussion themes, 950
  goals, 949–950
  members, 949
  objectives, 950
  types available, 950
Supraclavicular lymph nodes. *See* Lymph node(s), supraclavicular
Suramin, 290
Surveillance
  close, for high-risk patients, 328–329
  management, medicolegal aspects, 126–127
Surveillance, Epidemiology and End Results Program
  data on breast cancer detection in minority women, 913
  tumor grading data, 464
Survival data, analysis, 991–993
  comparing survival times of two groups of patients, 991–993, 992*f*
Survivor guilt, 349–350
Sweat gland carcinoma of breast, 414
Swedish trial, of conservative surgery with and without radiation therapy, 522, 522*t*
Swedish Two-County Study, randomized clinical trial of breast cancer screening, 310, 311*t*, 312–314, 313*f*, 314–315, 316*t*

Swiss cheese disease, 34
Synovial metaplasia, 39
Syphilis, of breast, 52

T
Talc, as sclerosing agent, 835
Tamoxifen
  adjuvant therapy, 561–565
    benefits
      ancillary, 347, 571–572
      in patients with ER-poor tumors, 563–564, 564*t*
    in elderly patients, 564–565
    in node-negative and node-positive patients, 563
    optimal duration, 563, 564*t*
    in postmenopausal patients, 561–563
    in premenopausal patients, 561–563
    psychological considerations, 930
    summary, 565
    toxicity, 571–572
    trials, 561–563, 563*t*
  antiangiogenic effects, 295
  antiestrogen effects, 347
  bone resorption blocked by, 348, 571, 906
  in breast cancer prevention, 338–339, 347
  for breast pain, 102–103
  carcinogenic potential, 338–339, 571–572
  cardiovascular disease and, 347–348, 571
  chemotherapy and
    in postmenopausal patients, 568*t*, 568–569
    in premenopausal patients, 567*t*, 567–568
  depression with, 571, 906
  dose intensity considerations, 678*t*, 678–679
  effects
    on lipids, 906
    on tumor initiation and growth
      in mouse models of carcinogenesis, 336
      progesterone and, 336
      in rat models of carcinogenesis, 336
  estrogenic effects, 906, 930
  for gynecomastia, 59
  hot flashes with, 677
  liver cancer and, 678
  for male breast cancer, 861
  mechanism of action, 19, 347
    non-receptor-mediated, 675–676
  menopausal symptoms with, 571, 906, 930
  metabolism, 675, 676*f*
  ocular toxicity, 571, 678, 930
  and oophorectomy, comparison, 679–680
  pharmacology, 102, 675

  plus aminoglutethimide, for breast cancer metastases, 690, 690*t*
  plus aminoglutethimide, danazol, and medroxyprogesterone acetate, plus medroxyprogesterone acetate, 689–690, 690*t*
  plus aminoglutethimide and danazol, for breast cancer metastases, 689, 690*t*
  plus danazol, for breast cancer metastases, 689, 690*t*
  plus fluoxymesterone
    for breast cancer metastases, 689, 690*t*
    tumor flare with, 688–689, 689*t*
  plus medroxyprogesterone acetate, for breast cancer metastases, 690, 690*t*
  for postmenopausal patients, 906
  as primary therapy, for elderly patients, 524–525
  and radiation therapy, 521
  reduced incidence of contralateral breast cancer with, 571
  resistance
    HER-2/neu and, 474
    mechanisms of, 676–677
  role in premenopausal women, 679
  thromboembolic events and, 678
  toxicity, 348, 677*t*, 677–678, 906
  tumor flare with, 688–689, 689*t*
  uterine cancer and, 571–572, 629, 678, 930
  vaginal secretions and, 677
Tamoxifen aziridine, estrogen receptor binding, 263
Taq polymerase, 977, 978
TATA box, 974
Taxanes, 595
  for metastatic breast cancer, 699–703
Taxol. *See* Paclitaxel
Taxotere, 561
T cell(s)
  CD4
    cytotoxic, in immune response to breast cancer, 300
    immunosuppressive effects, 301
  CD8, cytotoxic, against HER-2/neu, 300
  cytotoxic, recognition of tumor-associated antigen, 299
  γ-δ, in immune response to breast cancer, 300
  in vitro and in vivo education, combined with bone marrow transplantation, for breast cancer, 304
T47D cell line, 246
T47D$_{CO}$ (ER−, PR+) cells, 247–248
Technetium-99m, 96
Technetium-99m sestamibi, 96
Telomerase, 229
Teniposide, response to, in metastatic breast cancer, 693*t*
Terminal duct–lobular unit

epithelial cell atypicality in, radiation-related, 39
proliferative activity, 9, 9t
Terminator sequence, 974
Testolactone
for breast cancer metastases, 687
for gynecomastia, 59–60
Testololactone, 686
Testosterone, for breast cancer metastases, 687
Tetracycline, as sclerosing agent, 835
TF antigen. *See* Thomsen-Friedenreich antigen
Thalidomide, antiangiogenic activity, 296
Thallium-201, 96
Thermal injury, intraoperative damage to biopsy specimen by, 429–430, 430f
Thiethylperazine (Torecan), antiemetic regimens, 954t, 955t
Thioguanine, response to, in metastatic breast cancer, 693t
Thiotepa
intra-CSF administration, for leptomeningeal metastases, 794
response to, in metastatic breast cancer, 693t
Thomsen-Friedenreich antigen, 299
Thoracoacromial artery and vein, 4f, 5, 6f, 7f
Thoracodorsal artery and vein, 5, 7f
Thoracodorsal nerve, 8
Thoracoepigastric vein, thrombophlebitis, 69, 69f. *See also* Mondor disease
Thoracoscopy, 855f, 855–856
Thrombospondin
angiogenesis and, 286–287, 293
possible therapeutic applications, 290
Thymidine labeling index, 465t, 466
as predictive factor, 467
prognostic significance in breast cancer, 467, 467t
technical considerations, 466t
Thyroid hormone(s), for breast pain, 103
Thyrotropin-releasing hormone, prolactin responsiveness to, and breast pain, 101
Time Without Symptoms and Toxicity, 948
TIMP. *See* Tissue inhibitors of metalloproteinases
Tissue compartmentalization, in breast biochemical regulation, 21
defective regulation, in cancer, 21–22
Tissue expansion, for breast reconstruction, 605–606, 606f, 615t
Tissue inhibitors of metalloproteinases, 284, 286
angiogenesis and, 293
as angiogenesis inhibitors, 286–287
possible therapeutic applications, 290
Tissue plasminogen activator, 16f

as indicator of recurrent breast cancer, 641t
TNM staging, 457–459, 459t
TNP-470, 278, 290
antiangiogenic effects, 296
Topoisomerase II, as measure of proliferation, 465t
Topotecan, 703
Toremifene, for breast cancer metastases, 680
TRAM flap
for breast reconstruction, 607–609, 608f, 610f, 615t
microvascular tissue transfer technique, 610–611, 611f, 615t
for chest wall reconstruction, after radiation therapy, 613, 614f
fat necrosis in, 62
Transcription, 974, 974f
Transcription factors, 19
Transcription regulators, 974
Transfection studies, of breast cancer invasion and metastasis, 284, 285t, 287–288, 289
Transfer RNA, 975
Transforming growth factor(s), 272
action, on mammary epithelium, 17
TGF-α, 221, 223, 225, 272
angiogenesis and, 286, 293–294
in breast development, 2, 17–18
effects on bone resorption and formation, 841
modulation of cellular transformation, 275
in normal and malignant breast, 274–275
overexpression, and murine mammary cancer, 275
steroid hormone regulation of, 276, 276t
TGF-β, 16f, 272
in angiogenesis, 286
in breast development, 2
effects on bone resorption and formation, 841
effects on breast cancer, 273
family, 19, 272–273
in biochemical control of breast development, 17–18
immunosuppressive effects, 301
in normal and malignant breast, 275–276
steroid hormone regulation of, 276, 276t
tumor cell motility and, 286
Transgenic animals, 984–985
Transgenic mice
c-erbB-2, mammary tumors and, 240–241
c-myc, mammary tumors and, 241, 984
cyclin D, 984
gene therapy in, 985
mammary tumors and, 240–241

MMTV-myc, mammary tumors and, 241, 984
TGF-α, mammary tumors and, 240
TGF-α−myc, 227
v-Ha-ras, mammary tumors and, 241
Transition, in mutation, 973
Translation, of mRNA, 975
Translational research, 967
Transtentorial herniation, with cerebral metastases, 769–770
Transverse thoracic muscle, 6f
Transversion, in mutation, 973
Trauma, breast, 61f, 61–62
Treatment of breast cancer. *See also* Chemotherapy
absolute benefit, versus proportional benefit, 550
adjuvant systemic therapy, 585
follow-up, 634
adjuvant systemic therapy of primary cancer, 548–578. *See also* Chemotherapy; Endocrine therapy for breast cancer, adjuvant; Immunotherapy, adjuvant; Tamoxifen, adjuvant therapy
benefits, 552–561
clinical trials
endpoints, 549f, 549–551, 550t
metaanalysis, 551
overview, 551
randomized, 549–551
results interpretation, 548–552
cost-effectiveness, 572
historical perspective on, 548
quality of life estimates and, 551–552
rationale for, 548
recommendations for, 573–574, 574t
survival and, 572–573, 573t
treatment decision-making, 572–574
treatment toxicity, 551–552
breast-conserving surgery. *See* Breast-conserving treatment
combined-modality approach, 585–586
advantages and disadvantages, 586, 586t
characteristics, 586, 586t
development, 586, 586t
future of, 596
future porspects, 595–596
for locally advanced cancer, 587–589, 588t, 589t
sequence and combinations for, 596
survival effects, 592t, 593f, 593–595, 594f, 594t
tolerance, 592–593
toxicity, 592–593
decision making in
nursing's role in, 951–952
and psychologic impact on patient, 920–921, 945–947
for early-stage cancer, 487–584

Treatment of breast cancer (*continued*)
  endocrine. *See* Endocrine therapy for
    breast cancer
  family's role in, 931–933
  functional outcomes, 944
  historical perspective on, 585–586
  for inflammatory cancer, 590–592,
    591*t*
  leukemia risk with, 570–571
  local. *See* Local treatment of breast
    cancer
  for locally advanced cancer, 585–599
  local–regional, NSABP trials, 387
  medicolegal aspects, 125–132
  NSABP trials
    B-11, 556, 557*t*
    B-12, 556, 557*t*
    B-15, 556, 557*t*, 569
    breast-conserving surgery
      combined with radiation therapy,
        retrospective studies, 492–505
      without radiation therapy, 522*t*,
        522–524
    B-04 trial, 387–388, 509, 510,
      513*t*, 514–515, 515*f*
    B-05 trial, 515
    B-06 trial, 387–388, 491, 492*t*,
      493*f*, 493*t*, 522, 522*t*
    B-13 trial, 504
    B-14 trial, 504, 521, 572, 677
    local–regional therapy, 387
    surgical
      historical perspective on,
        487–489, 489*f*
      psychologic outcome, 505
      timing of surgery, 507, 508*t*
  primary therapy
    evaluation of patients after,
      629–647
    screening for new primary cancers
      after, 629
      current practices, 642–643
      management summary, 643
  prognostic significance, 394–395
  psychologic outcome, 505
  social support and, 931–933
  surgical
    breast-conserving. *See* Breast-
      conserving treatment
    historical perspective on, 548
    in menstrual cycle, 507, 508*t*
    timing for, 507, 508*t*
Triazolam, for breast cancer patient, 923
Trigger point, 42
Trigger spots, 104
Trimetrexate, response to, in metastatic
    breast cancer, 693*t*
Triple diagnosis, of masses, 113, 113*f*,
    134
Troxerutin, for lymphedema, 900
Tru-Cut needle, 135, 135*f*, 155
TSP. *See* Thrombospondin
Tuberculosis, of breast, 52
Tubular (well-differentiated) carcinoma.
    See Breast cancer, tubular
    (well-differentiated)
Tubulolobular carcinoma, 421

Tumor-associated antigen(s)
  clinical course in treatment of
    metastatic breast cancer and,
    641*f*, 641–642, 642*f*
  recurrent breast cancer and, 639–642,
    641*t*
Tumor cell–derived collagenase-
    stimulatory factor, 277–278
Tumor flare, hormone-induced,
    688–689, 689*t*
Tumorigenesis, estrogen receptor
    expression in, 267–268, 268*f*
Tumor markers, immunologic detection,
    304
Tumor necrosis factor
  in immune response to breast cancer,
    301
  TNF-α
    in angiogenesis, 286
    up-regulation of HLA antigens, 304
  in treatment of breast cancer, 304
  up-regulation of HLA antigens, 304
Tumor progression, 213, 213*f*
  integration of genetic changes during,
    229
Tumor suppressor–cell cycle controls,
    228, 228*f*
Tumor-suppressor gene(s)
  BRCA1. *See* *BRCA1* gene
  BRCA2. *See* *BRCA2* gene
  in breast cancer, 173–174, 185,
    216–218, 221, 222*t*, 227–228
  functions, 173–174
  germ-line mutations in, malignancy
    and, 174, 185, 186*f*
  identification, through loss of
    heterozygosity, 174*f*, 174–175
  inactivation
    in breast cancer, 221
    malignancy and, 173–174, 185,
      186*f*
  NF1, chromosomal location, 175
  nm23, 228
    prognostic significance in breast
      cancer, 475
    regulation, and breast cancer
      metastasis, 288
    transfection studies, of breast cancer
      invasion and metastasis, 288
  p53. *See* *p53* gene
  prognostic significance in breast
    cancer, 474–475
Two-hit hypothesis, of carcinogenesis,
    174
Tyrophostins, 225
Tyrosine kinases, signal transduction
    from, 224*f*, 224–225

U
Ulcer(s), skin, with phyllodes tumors,
    866
Ultrasound, 75–76. *See also* Fine-needle
    aspiration biopsy, ultrasound-
    guided; Large-core needle
    biopsy, ultrasound-guided

  adjunctive assessment with, 82
  of breast lesions, 82
  in lactation, 122–123
  palpable masses and, 75–76, 76*f*
  in pregnancy, 122–123
  of recurrent cancer, 659
  of silicone implant rupture, 625, 625*f*
Uncal herniation, with cerebral
    metastases, 769–770
Underserved minorities, breast cancer in,
    910–918
  clinical follow-up, 914–916
  diagnosis, 914–916
  early detection, 912–914
  epidemiology, 911*t*, 911–912
  health care and service needs,
    916–917
  prevention, 911–912
  research needs, 916–917
  treatment, 914–916
uPA. *See* Urokinase plasminogen
    activator
Urokinase plasminogen activator, 294
  in breast cancer, 22, 285
    prognostic significance, 476–477,
      477*t*
Uterine cancer
  metastases to breast, 426
  metastatic breast cancer as, 423
  in patients with previous history of
    breast cancer, 629
  tamoxifen and, 571–572, 629, 678,
    930
Utrecht Study, nonrandomized clinical
    trial of breast cancer screening,
    312

V
Vaccine(s)
  in biologic therapy of breast cancer,
    302–303
    HER-2/neu, 303
  with genetically engineered cells as
    immunogens, 303
Vaccinia growth factor, 272
Validity, 993–994
  external, 993
  internal, 993
Varicocele tumor. *See* Mammary duct
    ectasia, and periductal mastitis
Vascular endothelial growth factor, 400
  in angiogenesis, 286
    inhibition, 295
  angiogenesis and, 293–294
  in angiogenesis and metastasis, 277,
    278
  in breast cancer, 273
Vascular endothelium, in mammary
    development, 18
Vascular lesions, benign, 37
V-CAM-1, in metastasis, 22
Vectors, 983
VEGF. *See* Vascular endothelial growth
    factor

Venous hemangiomas, 37
Vimentin
 in breast cancer, 21
  prognostic significance, 402t
 expression in tumor, 253
Vinblastine
 for metastatic breast cancer, 698–699
  response to, 693t
 neurotoxicity, 958
Vinca alkaloids, for metastatic breast cancer, 698–699
Vincristine
 for metastatic breast cancer, 698–699
  response to, 693t
 neurotoxicity, 958
Vindesine, for metastatic breast cancer, 698–699
 response to, 693t
Vinorelbine, 595
 for metastatic breast cancer, 698–699, 699t
 response to, 693t
Virchow-Robin space, 790, 790f
Virulence, definition, 376
Vitamin A
 breast cancer and, 205–207, 206t
 breast cancer risk and, 346
Vitamin B₁, for breast pain, 102
Vitamin B₆, for breast pain, 102
Vitamin C
 breast cancer and, 207
 breast cancer risk and, 346
Vitamin D
 and breast cancer risk, 166

supplementation, in prevention of osteoporosis, 905
Vitamin E
 breast cancer and, 207
 breast cancer risk and, 346
 for breast pain, 102
Vitamins, for mastalgia, 102
VM-26, response to, in metastatic breast cancer, 693t

W
Walker 256 murine carcinoma, 812
Warfarin, breast necrosis induced by, 63–64
WBXRT. *See* Radiation therapy, whole-brain; Whole-brain radiation therapy
WDNM1 gene, regulation, and breast cancer metastasis, 288
WDNM2 gene, regulation, and breast cancer metastasis, 288
Weight, breast cancer risk and, 189, 190t
Weight gain
 with adjuvant therapy, management, 956
 with chemotherapy, management, 929
Western blot analysis, 981–982
Whites
 breast cancer in, prognosis for, 465
 breast cancer survival in, 672, 673f
 endemic poverty in, 910, 910t
 relative risk of dying from breast cancer, 911, 911t
Whole-brain radiation therapy, for of recurrent tumor, 773–774
 corticosteroid therapy with, 776
Wigs, 956

Wilcoxon test, generalized, 992, 992f
Witch's milk, 1
Wnt gene family, in breast development, 2
Wnt genes
 growth factor-like function, 18
 as oncogenes, 18
Womorulin, in mammary epithelium, 21
Work issues, after breast cancer, 960
Worried well, 919
Wound infection, with mastectomy, 528

X
Xenografts, human tumor, 237–240, 238t
 in animal models of breast cancer, 235, 237–240
 endocrine-responsive, 238–239
 endocrine-unresponsive, 239
 immunodeficient mouse models, 239
X-rays, discovery, 489

Y
Y-Me, 950, 959t
YWCA Encore Program, 959t

Z
ZK119010, 680
ZR-75-1 cell line, 246
Zuska disease, 50